The Cervical Spine

The Cervical Spine

FOURTH EDITION

The Cervical Spine Research Society Editorial Committee

Charles R. Clark, M.D.

Chairman
Dr. Michael Bonfiglio Professor of Orthopaedic Surgery

Edward C. Benzel, M.D.
Bradford L. Currier, M.D.
John P. Dormans, M.D.
Jiří Dvořák, M.D.
Frank Eismont, M.D.
Steven R. Garfin, M.D.
Harry N. Herkowitz, M.D.
Christopher G. Ullrich, M.D. F.A.C.R.
Alexander R. Vaccaro, M.D.

LIPPINCOTT WILLIAMS & WILKINS
A **Wolters Kluwer** Company
Philadelphia • Baltimore • New York • London
Buenos Aires • Hong Kong • Sydney • Tokyo

Acquisitions Editor: Robert Hurley
Developmental Editor: Julia Seto
Project Manager: Bridgett Dougherty
Manufacturing Manager: Benjamin Rivera
Marketing Manager: Sharon Zinner
Production Services: Print Matters, Inc.
Compositor: Compset, Inc.
Printer: Maple Press

© 2005 by LIPPINCOTT WILLIAMS & WILKINS
530 Walnut Street
Philadelphia, PA 19106 USA
LWW.com

Library of Congress Cataloging-in-Publication Data

The cervical spine / the Cervical Spine Research Society, Editorial Committee,
    Charles R. Clark, chairman ; Thomas B. Ducker . . . [et al.].—4th ed.
        p. ; cm.
    Includes bibliographical references and index.
    ISBN 0-7817-3576-9
        1. Cervical vertebrae—Diseases.   2. Cervical vertebrae—Abnormalities.
    3. Cervical vertebrae—Wounds and injuries.   I. Clark, Charles R. (Charles
    Richard), 1950–   II. Ducker, Thomas B., 1937–   III. Cervical Spine
    Research Society. Editorial Committee.
        [DNLM: 1. Cervical Vertebrae. 2. Spinal Diseases. WE 725 C4194 2004]
    RD531.C47 2004
    616.7′3—dc22
                                                                    2004057604

10 9 8 7 6 5 4 3 2 1

Preface

This, the fourth edition of *The Cervical Spine*, embodies the basic principles for which the Cervical Spine Research Society was originally founded in 1973. I believe one of the most important purposes of our Society is to expand our understanding of the cervical spine and consequently improve the care of our patients. This text incorporates information derived in large extent from the study of the cervical spine by members of our Society. The continued growth of our knowledge of the cervical spine and the conditions that afflict it has been significant and a text such as ours needs to be periodically updated. This new edition reflects the latest advances in our knowledge regarding conditions that affect the cervical spine and the exciting new developments in treatment. Truly, our founding members, as well as our entire Society, should be extremely proud of this text.

A work of this scope is not possible without the efforts of many individuals. The entire membership of the Cervical Spine Research Society must be acknowledged for the exchange of ideas as well as contributions they have provided throughout the years, largely at our annual meetings. Such ideas have been the stimulus for this text, although it is impossible to thank the countless individuals involved with this work here, it is important to recognize those individuals who played an integral part in the development of this edition. First and foremost are the members of the Editorial Committee: Jiří Dvořák, M.D., Edward C. Benzel, M.D., Christopher Ullrich, M.D., Harry Herkowitz, M.D., Alexander Vaccaro, M.D., John Dormans, M.D., Steven Garfin, M.D., Frank Eismont, M.D., and Bradford Currier, M.D. In addition, I wish to thank all of the individuals at Lippincott Williams & Wilkins, and in particular Robert Hurley, who have been a major driving force throughout. Lastly, yet most importantly, I wish to thank Peggy Stover for her tremendous secretarial skills, and my wife Barbara and daughters Kathy and Heather for their patience, understanding, and encouragement, during the many hours of editing this text.

It has been a pleasure working with the members of the Editorial Committee as well as all the members of our Society in the development and implementation of this 4th Edition of *The Cervical Spine*.

Charles R. Clark, M.D.
Chairman, Editorial Committee

Dedication

This book is dedicated to my family and in particular, my grandchildren Christopher and Lily, as well as to all of the dedicated families whose loved ones contributed to this book.

C.R.C.

The Cervical Spine Research Society
Editorial Committee

Contributors

Jean-Jacques Abitbol, M.D.
University of California at San Diego
San Diego, CA

Todd J. Albert, M.D.
Associate Professor and Vice Chairman
Department of Orthopaedics
Thomas Jefferson University Medical College
Attending Surgeon
Rothman Institute
Department of Orthopaedics
Thomas Jefferson University Hospital
Philadelphia, PA

Mohammed J. Al-Sayyad, M.D., F.R.C.S.C.
Division of Pediatric Orthopaedic Surgery,
Cincinnati Children's Hospital Medical Center
University of Cincinnati College of Medicine
Cincinnati, OH

Howard S. An, M.D.
Morton International Professor
Department of Orthopaedic Surgery
Rush Medical College
Director of Spine Fellowship
Rush Presbyterian St. Lukes Medical Center
Chicago, IL

Paul A. Anderson, M.D.
Associate Clinical Professor
Department of Orthopedic Surgery and
*   Rehabilitation*
University of Washington Medical School
Seattle, WA

D. Greg Anderson, M.D.
Assistant Professor
Department of Orthopaedic Surgery
University of Virginia
Spinal Surgeon
Department of Orthopaedic Surgery
University of Virginia Medical Center
Charlottesville, VA

M. Darryl Antonacci, M.D.
Attending Spine Surgeon
Lenox Hill Hospital
New York, NY
Consultant Spine Surgeon
Shriners Hospital for Children
Philadelphia, PA

Ronald I. Apfelbaum, M.D.
Professor
Department of Neurosurgery
University of Utah/University Hospital
Salt Lake City, UT

Stefano Bandiera, M.D.
Attending Surgeon
Department of Orthopedics, Traumatology, and
*   Spine Surgery*
Ospedale Maggiore
Bologna, Italy

Daxes M. Banit, M.D.
Spine Fellow
Charlotte Orthopedic Specialists, P.A.
Charlotte, NC

Paolo Beck-Peccoz, M.D.
Full Professor
Institute of Endocrine Sciences
University of Milan
Chief
Department of Endocrinology
Ospedale Maggiore
Milan, Italy

Edward C. Benzel, M.D.
Director, Spinal Disorder
Cleveland Clinic Foundation
Department of Neurosurgery
Cleveland, OH

Mark Bernhardt, M.D.
Clinical Professor
Department of Orthopaedic Surgery
University of Missouri–Kansas City School of
*   Medicine*
Kansas City, MO
Spine Surgeon
Dickson-Diveley Midwest Orthopaedic Clinic
Kansas City Orthopaedic Institute
Leawood, KS

Randal R. Betz, M.D.
Shriners Hospital for Children
Philadelphia, PA

Scott D. Boden, M.D.
Professor
Department of Orthopaedic Surgery
Emory University School of Medicine
Director
The Emory Spine Center
Emory Healthcare
Atlanta, GA

Nikolai Bogduk, M.D., Ph.D., D.Sc.
Professor
Department of Pain Medicine
University of Newcastle
Head
Department of Clinical Research
Royal Newcastle Hospital
Callaghan, NSW, Australia

Christopher M. Bono, M.D.
Orthopaedic Surgeon
University of California at San Diego
San Diego, CA

Stefano Boriani, M.D.
Head
Department of Orthopedics, Traumatology, and
*   Spine Surgery*
Ospedale Maggiore
Bologna, Italy

Craig D. Brigham, M.D.
Chief
Department of Spine Surgery
Carolinas Medical Center
Quality Assurance Chairman
Miller Orthopaedic Clinic
Charlotte, NC

Andrew R. Brodbelt, M.D.
Prince of Wales Medical Research Institute
University of New South Wales
Department of Neurosurgery
Prince of Wales Hospital
Randwick, NSW, Australia

Richard S. Brower, M.D.
Clinical Associate Professor
Northeastern Ohio Universities College of
*   Medicine*
Rootstown, OH
Chief, Spine Service
Department of Orthopaedics
Summa Health System
Akron, OH

Lee Buono, M.D.
Chief Resident
Department of Neurosurgery
Thomas Jefferson University
Philadelphia, PA

James P. Burke, M.D., Ph.D.
Director of Spine Services
Department of Specialized Surgery
Altoona Hospital
Altoona, PA

Andrew L. Carney, M.D.
Clinical Associate Professor
Departments of Orthopaedics and of
*   Neurosurgery and Radiology*
University of Illinois
Chicago, IL

Charles W. Cha, M.D.
Clinical Instructor
Department of Orthopedic Surgery
Emory University
Emory Spine Center
Atlanta, GA

Jens R. Chapman, M.D.
Professor
Department of Orthopaedics
University of Washington
Seattle, WA

Gordon K. T. Chu, M.D., M.Sc., FRCS(C)
Clinical and Research Fellow
Department of Neurosurgery
University Health Network–Toronto Western
*   Hospital*
Toronto, Ontario, Canada

Charles R. Clark, M.D.
Professor
Department of Orthopaedics
University of Iowa Hospitals and Clinics
Iowa City, IA

David H. Clements, M.D.
Department of Orthopaedic Surgery
Temple University Hospital
Philadelphia, PA

Jeffrey D. Coe, M.D.
Medical Director
Center for Spinal Deformity and Injury
Community Hospital of Los Gatos
Los Gatos, CA

Paul R. Cooper, M.D.
Professor
Department of Neurosugery
New York University Medical Center
New York, NY

Lawson A. B. Copley, M.D.
Assistant Professor of Orthopedics
Department of Orthopedic Surgery
University of Texas Southwestern Medical
*   Center*
Division of Children's Orthopedics and Sports
*   Medicine*
Children's Medical Center of Dallas
Dallas, TX

Jerome M. Cotler, M.D.
Everett J. and Marian Gordon Professor
Department of Orthopaedic Surgery
Jefferson Medical Collge of Thomas Jefferson
*   University*
Philadelphia, PA

Alvin H. Crawford, M.D.
Department of Orthopaedic Surgery
Children's Hospital of Cincinnati
Cincinnati, OH

H. Alan Crockard, M.D., D.Sc. FRCS(Ed)
Department of Neurosurgery
National Hospital for Neurology and
*   Neurosurgery*
London, United Kingdom

Bradford L. Currier, M.D.
The Mayo Clinic
Rochester, MN

Lukasz Curylo, M.D.
Assistant Professor
Department of Orthopedic Surgery
University of Rochester Medical Center
Rochester, NY

Alan Dacre, M.D.
Orthopedic Surgeons P.S.C.
Billings, MT

Bruce V. Darden II, M.D.
Fellowship Director
Charlotte Spine Center
Charlotte Orthopaedic Specialists
Charlotte, NC

Károly M. Dávid, M.D., FRCS(SN)
Consultant Neurosurgeon
Department of Neurosurgery
Oldchurch Hospital
Romford, Essex, United Kingdom

Curtis A. Dickman, M.D.
Director of Spine Research
Associate Chief of Spine Surgery
Department of Neurological Surgery
Barrow Neurological Institute
Phoenix, AZ

John F. Ditunno, Jr., M.D.
Professor
Department of Rehabilitation Medicine
Jefferson Medical College
Thomas Jefferson University
Philadelphia, PA

John P. Dormans, M.D.
Chief
Department of Orthopaedic Surgery
Children's Hospital of Philadelphia
Philadelphia, PA

Denis S. Drummond, M.D.
Emeritus Chief of Orthopaedic Surgery
Professor
Department of Orthopaedic Surgery
University of Pennsylvania Health System
Philadelphia, PA

Thomas B. Ducker, M.D.
Professor
Johns Hopkins University
Baltimore, MD
Neurosurgeon
Annapolis Neurosurgery
Annapolis, MD

Edward J. Dunn, M.D.
Professor
Department of Orthopaedic Surgery
University of Massachusetts Medical School
Worcester, MA

Jiří Dvořák, M.D.
Chefarzi Neurologie
Zurich, Switzerland

Frank J. Eismont, M.D.
University of Miami
Coral Gables, FL

Richard Ellenbogen, M.D.
Chief
Division of Neurosurgery
Associate Professor
Department of Surgery
Uniformed Services University of the Health
* Sciences*
Walter Reed Army Medical Center
Washington, DC

Sanford E. Emery, M.D.
Associate Professor
Department of Orthopaedics
University Hospitals of Cleveland Spine
* Institute*
Case Western Reserve University
Cleveland, OH

Joseph A. Epstein, M.D., F.A.C.S.
Clinical Professor
Department of Neurological Surgery
Albert Einstein College of Medicine
Bronx, NY
Chairman Emeritus
Department of Surgery
Division of Neurosurgery
Long Island Jewish Medical Center
New Hyde Park, NY

Nancy E. Epstein, M.D.
Clinical Professor
Department of Neurological Surgery
Albert Einstein College of Medicine
Bronx, NY
Department of Surgery
Division of Neurosurgery
Winthrop University Hospital
Mineola, NY

Thomas J. Errico, M.D.
Chief of the Spine Service
New York University
Hospital for Joint Diseases
New York, NY

Todd A. Fairchild, M.D.
Department of Orthopaedics and
* Rehabilitation*
Yale University School of Medicine
New Haven, CT

Michael G. Fehlings, M.D., Ph.D., FRCS(C)
Professor and Krembil Chair in Neural Repair
* and Regeneration*
Division of Neurosurgery
University of Toronto
Neurosurgeon
Division of Neurosurgery
University Health Network
Toronto, Ontario, Canada

Jeffrey S. Fischgrund, M.D.
Spine Surgeon
Department of Orthopaedics
William Beaumont Hospital
Royal Oak, MI

John M. Flynn, M.D.
Associate Professor
Department of Orthopaedic Surgery
University of Pennsylvania
Attending Surgeon
Division of Orthopaedic Surgery
Children's Hospital of Philadelphia
Philadelphia, PA

Nestor Galvez-Jimenez, M.D., M.Sc.
Consultant in Neurology
Department of Neurology
Cleveland Clinic Florida
Naples, FL
Consultant in Neurology
Department of Neurology
Cleveland Clinic Hospital
Cleveland, OH

Steven R. Garfin, M.D.
Professor, Chair
Department of Orthopaedics
University of California at San Diego
UCSD Medical Center
San Diego, CA

Timothy A. Garvey, M.D.
Assistant Professor
Department of Orthopaedics
University of Minnesota
Orthopaedic Surgeon
Abbott Northwestern Hospital
Minneapolis, MN

Kenneth F. Gavin, C.O.
Director of Orthotics and Prosthetics
Division of Orthotics and Prosthetics
Colorado Springs Orthopaedic Group
Colorado Springs, CO

Peter C. Gerszten, M.D., M.P.H.
Assistant Professor
Department of Neurological Surgery
University of Pittsburgh
Pittsburgh, PA

Alexander J. Ghanayem, M.D.
Chief
Division of Spine Surgery
Department of Orthopaedic Surgery
Loyola University Medical Center
Maywood, IL

Sanjitpal S. Gill, M.D.
Fellow
Emory Spine Center
Department of Orthopaedic Surgery
Emory University School of Medicine
Atlanta, GA

John A. Glaser, M.D.
CIO
Partners HealthCare System
Boston, MA

Vijay Goel, Ph.D.
Professor
Department of Bioengineering
University of Toledo
Co-Director
Spine Research Centre
Toledo, OH

Barth A. Green, M.D., F.A.C.S.
Professor and Chairman
Department of Neurological Surgery
Professor
Department of Orthopedics and Rehabilitation
University of Miami School of Medicine
Coral Gables, FL
Chief of Neurosurgical Services
Jackson Memorial Hospital and Miami Veterans
  Affairs Medical Centers
Miami, FL

Dieter Grob, M.D., Ph.D.
Medical Director
Head of Spine Surgery/Orthopaedics
Schulthess Clinic
Zurich, Switzerland

Zbigniew Gugala, M.D., Ph.D.
Department of Orthopaedic Surgery
Baylor College of Medicine
Houston, TX

Maurice R. Hanson, M.D.
Department of Neurology
Cleveland Clinic Florida
Naples, FL

Yoshihisa Hasegawa, M.D.
Chief
Department of Nuclear Medicine
Osaka Medical Center for Cancer and
  Cardiovascular Diseases
Osaka, Japan

Amir Hasharoni, M.D., Ph.D.
Clinical and Research Fellow in Spine Surgery
Department of Orthopedic Surgery
New York University
Hospital for Joint Diseases
New York, NY

John G. Heller, M.D.
Emory Clinic Spine Center
Decatur, GA

Harry N. Herkowitz, M.D.
Chairman
Department of Orthopaedic Surgery
William Beaumont Hospital
Royal Oak, MI

Jerome M. Hershman, M.D.
Distinguished Professor
Department of Medicine
University of California, Los Angeles School of
*   Medicine*
Associate Chief
Endocrinology and Diabetes Division
VA Greater Los Angeles Healthcare System
Los Angeles, CA

B. David Horn, M.D.
Assistant Professor
Department of Orthopaedic Surgery
Hospital of the University of Pennsylvania
Attending Orthopaedic Surgeon
Children's Hospital of Philadelphia
Philadelphia, PA

Harish S. Hosalkar, M.D.
Department of Orthopaedics
Great Ormond Street Hospital for Children
London, United Kingdom

John K. Houten, M.D.
Assistant Professor
Department of Neurosurgery
Albert Einstein College of Medicine
Director of Spinal Neurosurgery
Department of Neurosurgery
Montefiore Medical Center
Bronx, NY

Louis G. Jenis, M.D.
Clinical Assistant Professor
Department of Orthopaedic Surgery
Tufts University School of Medicine
Orthopaedic Spine Surgeon
Department of Orthopaedic Surgery
New England Baptist Hospital
Boston, MA

Nigel R. Jones, M.D.
Professor of Neurosurgery
Department of Surgery
University of Adelaide
Adelaide, Australia

Christopher D. Kager, M.D.
Neurosurgeon
Department of Neurosurgery
Lancaster Neuroscience and Spine
*   Associates*
Lancaster, PA

Iain H. Kalfas, M.D.
Chairman
Department of Neurosurgery
Cleveland Clinic Foundation
Cleveland, OH

James D. Kang, M.D.
Associate Professor
Department of Orthopaedic Surgery
University of Pittsburgh Medical Center
Pittsburgh, PA

Christopher P. Kauffman, M.D.
Assistant Clinical Professor
Department of Orthopaedic Surgery
University of California at San Diego
La Jolla, CA
UCSD Medical Center–Hillcrest
San Diego, CA

Choll W. Kim, M.D.
Orthopedic Surgeon
UCSD OrthoMed
La Jolla, CA 92037

Scott H. Kitchel, M.D.
Assistant Clinical Professor
Department of Orthopedic Surgery
Oregon Health and Sciences University
Portland, OR

Paul Klimo, Jr.
Department of Neurosurgery
University of Utah School of Medicine
Salt Lake City, UT

Samir Lapsiwala, M.D.
Resident
Department of Neurosurgery
University of Wisconsin
Madison, WI

Christian Lattermann, M.D.
Visiting Clinical Instructor
Department of Orthopaedic Surgery
University of Pittsburgh Medical Center
Pittsburgh, PA

Lawrence Lenke, M.D.
Orthopaedic Surgeon
Washington University
St. Louis, MO

Steven P. Leon, M.D.
Neurosurgeon
Long Island Neuroscience Specialists
East Patchogue, NY

Alan M. Levine, M.D.
Director
Alvin and Lois Lapidus Cancer Institute
Sinai Hospital of Baltimore
Baltimore, MD

**Isador H. Lieberman, M.D., FRCS(C), BSc,
  MBA**
Professor of Surgery
Department of Orthopaedics
Cleveland Clinic
*Lerner College of Medicine at Case Western
  University*
Director
Minimally Invasive Surgery Center
Director
Center of Advanced Skills Training
Department of Orthopaedics & Spinal Surgeon
The Cleveland Clinic Foundation
Cleveland, OH

Ronald W. Lindsey, M.D.
Professor
Department of Orthopaedic Surgery
Baylor College of Medicine
Attending Physician
The Methodist Hospital
Houston, TX

Adam C. Lipson, M.D.
Neurosurgeon
University of Washington
Seattle, WA

Stephen J. Lipson, M.D.
Clinical Professor
Harvard Medical School
Orthopaedic Surgeon-in-Chief
Beth Israel Deaconess Medical Center
Boston, MA

Steven C. Ludwig, M.D.
Assistant Professor
Co-Director of Spine Surgery
Department of Orthopaedic Surgery
University of Maryland School of Medicine
Baltimore, MD

William G. Mackenzie, M.D.
Assistant Professor
Department of Orthopaedics,
Jefferson Medical College
Alfred I. duPont Hospital for Children
Wilmington, DE

Shunji Matsunaga, M.D.
Associate Professor
Department of Orthopaedics
Kagoshima University
Kagoshima, Japan

William McCormick, M.D.
Neurosurgeon
West Islip, NY

Robert A. McGuire, Jr., M.D.
Professor and Chairman
Department of Orthopedics
University of Mississippi Medical Center
Jackson, MS

Anis O. Mekhail, M.D.
Assistant Clinical Professor
University of Illinois at Chicago
Chicago, IL

Sohail K. Mirza, M.D.
Associate Professor
*Departments of Orthopedics and Neurological
  Surgery*
University of Washington
Seattle, WA

William Mitchell, M.D.
Assistant Professor
Department of Neurosurgery
New Jersey Neuroscience Institute
Seton Hall University
Edison, NJ

M. J. Mulcahey, M.S., O.T.R./L.
*Director of Rehabilitation Services and Clinical
  Research*
Philadelphia Shriners Hospital
Associate Professor
College of Allied Health Sciences
Temple University
Philadelphia, PA

Marion Murray, Ph.D.
Professor
Department of Neurobiology and Anatomy
MCP Hahnemann University School of Medicine
Philadelphia, PA

Hironobu Nakamura, M.D., D.Med., Sc.
Professor
Department of Radiology
Osaka University Medical School
Osaka, Japan

Katsuyuki Nakanishi, M.D.
Department of Radiology
Osaka University Medical School
Osaka, Japan

Shun-ichi Nakano, M.D.
Director
Department of Nuclear Medicine
The Center for Adult Diseases
Osaka, Japan

Arthur P. Nestler, R.N.
Clinical Nurse
Department of Neurological Surgery
University of Pittsburgh Medical Center
Presbyterian Universtiy Hospital
Pittsburgh, PA

Bruce E. Northrup, M.D.
Clinical Associate Professor
Department of Neurosurgery
Thomas Jefferson University Hospital
Philadelphia, PA

Kozo Okada, M.D.
Director
Okada Orthopaedic Clinic
Matsuyama, Japan

Keiro Ono, M.D.
Emeritus Professor
Department of Orthopaedic Surgery
Osaka University Medical School
Emeritus Director
Department of Orthpaedic Surgery
Osaka Koseinenkin Hospital
Osaka, Japan

Manohar M. Panjabi, Ph.D., D.Tech.
Professor
Departments of Orthopaedics and Rehabilitation
 and Mechanical Engineering
Orthopaedic Biomechanics Laboratory
Yale University School of Medicine
New Haven, CT

Shahram Partovi, M.D., C.M.
Department of Neuroradiology
Barrow Neurological Institute
Phoenix, AZ

Chetan K. Patel, M.D.
Coffee Regional Medical Center
Douglas, GA

Odysseas Paxinos, M.D.
Visiting Research Associate
Department of Orthopaedic Surgery and
 Rehabilitation
Loyola University
Chicago, IL

Frank X. Pedlow, Jr., M.D.
Emory Clinic Spine Center
Decatur, GA

Lourens Penning, M.D.
Emeritus Professor
Department of Medical Sciences
University of Groningen
Consultant Professor
Department of Radiology
University Hospital
Groningen, The Netherlands

Luca Persani, M.D., Ph.D.
Associate Professor
Institute of Endocrine Sciences
University of Milan
Milan, Italy
Head
Laboratory of Experimental Endocrinology
IRCCS Istituto Auxologico Italiano
Cusano Milanino, Italy

Peter D. Pizzutillo, M.D.
Professor
Department of Orthopaedic Surgery and
 Pediatrics
MCP Hahnemann School of Medicine
Chief
Section of Orthopaedic Surgery
St. Christopher's Hospital for Children
Philadelphia, PA

Mark A. Prévost, M.D.
Clinical Instructor
Department of Orthopaedics
University of Mississippi Medical Center
Jackson, MI

Bogdan P. Radanov, M.D.
Associate Professor of Psychiatry
Psychiatrischen Universitätspoliklinik
Bern, Switzerland

Glenn R. Rechtine II, M.D.
Professor
Department of Neurological Surgery
College of Medicine
Shands Hospital
University of Florida
Gainesville, FL

Takashi Sakou, M.D.
Department of Orthopedic Surgery
Kagoshima University
Kagoshima, Japan

Rick C. Sasso, M.D.
Assistant Professor
Department of Orthopaedic Surgery
Indiana University School of Medicine
Vice-Chairman
Department of Orthopaedic Surgery
St. Vincent Hospital
Indiana Spine Group
Indianapolis, IN

Kazuhiko Satomi, M.D., Ph.D.
Professor and Subchief
Department of Orthopaedic Surgery
Kyorin University
Mitaka-shi, Tokyo

Daniel M. Schwartz, M.D.
Professor
Department of Ophthalmology
University of California at San Francisco
San Francisco, CA

Suken A. Shah, M.D.
Department of Orthopaedics
Alfred I. DuPont Hospital for Children
Wilmington, DE

Henry H. Sherk, M.D.
Professor
Department of Orthopaedic Surgery
Drexel University College of Medicine
Attending Physician
Department of Orthopaedic Surgery
Hahnemann University Hospital
Philadelphia, PA

Jeff S. Silber, M.D.
Assistant Professor
Department of Orthopaedic Surgery
Long Island Jewish Medical Center
New Hyde Park, NY

Andrew V. Slucky, M.D.
Chief
Spinal Surgery Service (Orthopaedics)
Summit–Alta Bates Medical Center
Oakland, CA

Paul D. Sponseller, M.D.
Department of Orthopaedics
John Hopkins Hospital
Baltimore, MD

Michael P. Steinmetz, M.D.
Chief Resident
Department of Neurosurgery
The Cleveland Clinic Foundation
Cleveland, OH

Marcus A. Stoodley, M.D.
Prince of Wales Medical Research Institute
University of New South Wales
Department of Neurosurgery
Prince of Wales Hospital
Randwick, NSW, Australia

Narayan Sundaresan, M.D.
Central Park Neurosurgery
New York, NY

Martin Sutter, M.D.
Department of Neurology
Schulthess Klinik
Zurich, Switzerland

Masakazu Takemitsu, M.D.
Department of Orthopaedic Surgery
Asahikawa Medical College
Asahikawa, Hokkaido, Japan

Charles H. Tator, M.D., Ph.D.
Professor and Campeau Family Chair
Department of Surgery
Division of Neurosurgery
University of Toronto
Staff Neurosurgeon
Professor
Department of Surgery
Division of Neurosurgery
Toronto Western Hospital
Toronto, Ontario, Canada

Gregory Trost, M.D.
Associate Professor and Director of Spinal
  Surgery
Department of Neurosurgery
University of Wisconsin
Madison, WI

Eeric Truumees, M.D.
Orthopaedic Director
Gehring Biomechanics Laboratory
Bioengineering Center
Wayne State University
Detroit, MI
Attending Spine Surgeon
Department of Orthopaedic Surgery
William Beaumont Hospital
Royal Oak, MI

Christopher G. Ullrich, M.D., F.A.C.R.
Neuroradiology Section
Charlotte Radiology PA
Charlotte, NC;
Chief
Department of Radiology
Carolinas Medical Center
Charlotte, NC

Alexander R. Vaccaro, M.D.
The Rothman Institute
Philadelphia, PA

Michael J. Vives, M.D.
Assistant Professor
Department of Orthopaedics
University of Medicine & Dentistry of New Jersey
Newark, NJ

Stan Vohanka, M.D.
Department of Neurology
Schulthess Klinik
Zurich, Switzerland

Eiji Wada, M.D., D.M.Sc.
Chief
Spinal Section
Department of Orthopaedic Surgery
Hoshigaoka Koseinenkin Hospital
Osaka, Japan

Michael Y. Wang, M.D.
Assistant Professor
Department of Neurological Surgery
LAC+USC Medical Center
Department of Neurosurgery
USC University Hospital
Los Angeles, CA

William C. Warner, Jr., M.D.
Associate Professor
Department of Orthopaedic Surgery
University of Tennessee-Campbell Clinic
Chief of Surgery
Department of Orthopaedics
LeBonhem Children's Hospital
Memphis, TN

Robert G. Watkins, M.D.
Center for Orthopedic and Spinal Surgery
Los Angeles, CA

Robert G. Watkins IV, M.D.
Los Angeles Spine Surgery Institute
Los Angeles, CA

Steven E. Weber, D.O.
Orlando Orthopaedic Center
Orlando, FL

James N. Weinstein, D.O., M.S.
Professor
Department of Orthopaedic Surgery
Dartmouth Medical School
Hanover, NH
Chairman
Department of Orthopaedic Surgery
Dartmouth Hitchcock Medical Center
Lebanon, NH

William C. Welch, M.D.
Professor
University of Pittsburgh
Chief
Department of Neurological Surgery
Presbyterian Universtiy Hospital
Pittsburgh, PA

Augustus A. White III, M.D., Ph.D.
Master
Oliver Wendell Holmes Society
Orthopaedic Surgeon-in-Chief Emeritus
Department of Orthopaedic Surgery
Beth Israel Deaconess Medical Center
Boston, MA

Lytton Williams, M.D.
Associate Clinical Professor
USC School of Medicine
Los Angeles, CA

Beth A. Winkelstein, Ph.D.
Assistant Professor
Department of Bioengineering and
  Neurosurgery
University of Pennsylvania
Philadelphia, PA

Willard B. Wong, M.D.
Spine Surgeon
Department of Precision Orthopaedics
Salinas Valley Memorial Hospital
Salinas, CA

Kazuo Yamashita, M.D.
Co-Director
Department of Orthopaedic Surgery
Osaka National Hospital
Osaka, Japan

Isakichi Yamaura, M.D.
Clinical Professor
Department of Orthopaedic Surgery
Tokyo Medical & Dental University
Director
Department if Orthopaedic Surgery
Kudanzaka Hospital
Tokyo, Japan

Kazuo Yonenobu, M.D., D.M.Sc.
Clinical Professor
Department of Orthopaedic Surgery
Osaka University Medical School
Vice Director
National Osaka-Minami Hospital
Osaka, Japan

James J. Yue, M.D.
Orthopaedic Surgeon
Yale Orthopaedic Associates
New Haven, CT

Thomas A. Zdeblick, M.D.
Professor and Chairman
Department of Orthopedics and Rehabilitation
University of Wisconsin
Madison, WI

Seth M. Zeidman, M.D.
Assistant Professor
Departments of Neurosurgery and Critical Care
  Medicine
Uniformed Services University of the Health
  Sciences
Department of Neurosurgery
Johns Hopkins University School of Medicine
Baltimore, MD

Jack E. Zigler, M.D.
Clinical Associate Professor
Department of Orthopaedic Surgery
University of Texas–Southwestern School of
  Medicine
Dallas, TX
Co-Director
Fellowship Training Program
Texas Back Institute
Plano, TX

Geoffrey P. Zubay, M.D.
Neurosurgical Medical Clinic, Inc.
San Diego, CA

Contents

Section V: Trauma: Fractures and Dislocations

Section VI: Spinal Cord Injury

Section VII: Tumors and Spinal Infection

Section VIII: Inflammatory Conditions

Section IX: Degenerative Diseases

Section X: Complications

The Cervical Spine

SECTION I

Anatomy, Physiology, and Biomechanics

CHAPTER 1

Anatomy of the Cervical Spine

John G. Heller, Frank X. Pedlow Jr., and Sanjitpal S. Gill

The neck comprises the region between the thoracic inlet and the base of the head. The musculature of the neck controls the motion of the head and neck as well as the organs (respiratory and digestive) of the neck. The musculofascial arrangement of the neck allows for the protected passage of the blood supply to the head as well as to the upper respiratory and digestive tracts while also allowing complex motion of the head and neck and between the neck's internal structures. The cervical spinal column serves to support the head on top of the trunk while allowing its motion about three axes. It also serves as a protective conduit for the spinal cord and nerve roots, its various articulations, and its complex musculature, allowing again for a high degree of motion.

A thorough knowledge of the anatomy of the neck and cervical spine is essential to an understanding of function and pathological anatomy as well as the rationale for and performance of surgical procedures. This chapter discusses the normal anatomy of the cervical spine and related structures of the neck. Recent qualitative and quantitative studies using cadaveric dissection, computed tomography, and magnetic resonance imaging (MRI) have continued to add to our knowledge of the dimension of and the clinically relevant relations between cervical spine structures. An improved knowledge of anatomy has led to a better understanding of normal and pathological states, advanced our ability to diagnose and treat conditions, and helped reduce the risks associated with surgical procedures.

OSSEOUS ELEMENTS

The cervical spine consists of three atypical and four typical cervical vertebrae. The typical cervical vertebrae, C3 to C6, comprise a vertebral body, a vertebral arch, and several processes for muscular attachment and articulations (Fig. 1.1). The vertebral body supplies the strength and support for two-thirds of the vertebral load. The depth of the vertebral body at the inferior end plate is consistently larger than the depth of the superior end plate except at C7 (1). The upper surface is typically concave from side to side and convex in an anterior-to-posterior direction. On its lower surface, it is convex from side to side and concave in the anterior-to-posterior direction, with the anterior lip of the concavity at times overlapping the vertebral body below. The upper projection on the lateral superior surface of the caudal vertebrae is called the *uncus* (or *hook*) and is related intimately with the convex lateral inferior surface of the cephalad vertebrae called the *enchancure* (*anvil*). These "articulations" also have been called the *uncovertebral joints* or *joints of Luschka* (Fig. 1.2). The vertebral body is composed of cancellous bone covered by a thin layer of cortical bone, the posterior aspect of which is perforated by multiple vascular foramina for the basivertebral veins. The upper and lower end-plate width and depth increase from C2 to C7, with width ranging from 17 to 23.4 mm and depth ranging from 15.6 to 18.1 mm. Thus, the vertebral body width is usually greater than the corresponding depth. The vertebral body height on the posterior wall on the midsagittal plane remains relatively constant from C3 through C7, ranging from 10.9 to 12.8 mm (2).

From the posterolateral aspect of the vertebral bodies project pedicles that together with the laminae form the vertebral arch. The vertebral arch encloses the vertebral foramen, which combines with foramina at other levels to form the spinal canal. From C3 to C7, the average pedicle height is 7 mm and the width 5 to 6 mm (2). From C3 to C7, the angle made by the pedicle with the sagittal plane decreases from 40 degrees to 29 degrees (2). Laminae project posteromedially from the pedicles and join in the midline. In the cervical region, the laminae are shorter and thinner but generally wider than those in the thoracic and lumbar spine. The laminar height (rostral-to-caudal distance) decreases from C2 to C4 and then progressively increases to C7. The minimum height is at C4 (10.4 ± 1.1 mm). Laminar width (medial-to-lateral distance) progressively decreases from

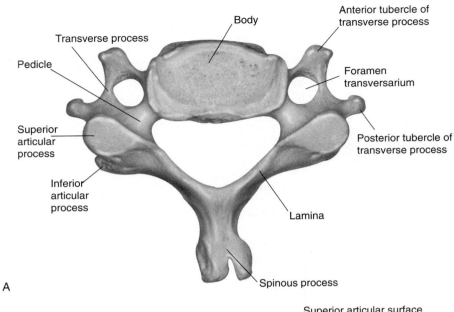

A

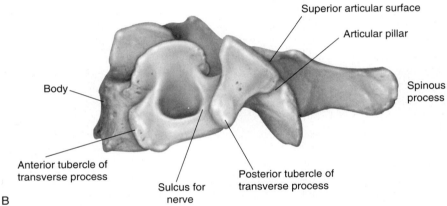

B

FIG. 1.1. Typical cervical vertebra.
A: Cranial view. **B:** Lateral view.

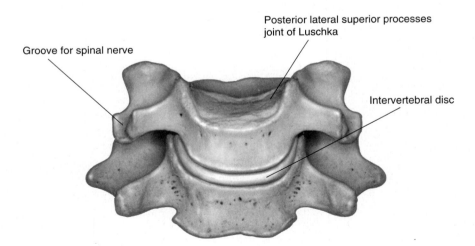

FIG. 1.2. Lower cervical vertebra, showing joints of Luschka and their relation to disc, intervertebral foramen, and facets.

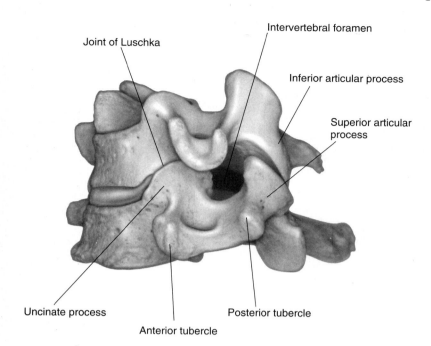

Joint of Luschka

Intervertebral foramen

Inferior articular process

Superior articular process

Uncinate process

Posterior tubercle

Anterior tubercle

FIG. 1.3. Borders of the intervertebral foramen.

C3 to C7. The laminar thickness (anterior-to-posterior distance) is the least at C5 (1.9 ± 0.6 mm). The slope angle, measured as the tilt of each lamina in relation to the horizontal plane of the vertebral body, is 111.7 ± 9.3 degrees at C2 and then sharply decreases to 101.2 ± 5.5 degrees at C3. From C3 to C7, the slope angle slowly increases (3).

The spinous process projects posteriorly from the junction of the laminae. The lateral mass forms at the junction of the lamina and pedicle and gives rise to the superior and inferior articular processes or facets. The superior facet at each level faces upward and posteriorly; the inferior facet faces downward and anteriorly. A superior facet articulates with the corresponding inferior facet of the vertebral body cephalad to form the osseous elements of the zygapophyseal joints. A vertebral notch is located on the superior and inferior aspect of each pedicle, deeper on the lower aspect, such that adjacent notches contribute to the intervertebral foramen, through which the spinal nerve exits the spinal canal. A transverse process projects laterally from the junction of each pedicle and lamina and is composed of two contributing elements. The posterior root, developmentally a true transverse process, arises from the junction of the pedicle and the lamina. The anterior root of the transverse process, developmentally a rib or costal process, arises from the side of the vertebral body. The two roots of the transverse process are connected laterally by the costotransverse bar or lamella, which combines with the anterior and posterior roots and the pedicle to surround the foramen transversarium. In addition, each element of the transverse process ends laterally in a projection, the anterior and posterior scalene tubercles, respectively. The anterior tubercle of C6 is large and called the *carotid tubercle* or

Chassaignac's tubercle. The costotransverse bar has a groove for the existing spinal nerve on its upper surface, representing the most lateral aspect of the intervertebral foramen, which is bound superiorly and inferiorly by the pedicle, posteriorly by the facets, and anteriorly by the intervertebral discs, uncovertebral joints, and vertebral bodies (Fig. 1.3). The vertical diameter of the foramen is approximately 9 mm, the horizontal diameter is 4 mm, and the length ranges from 4 to 6 mm (4). Foramina exit at an angle of 45 degrees from the midsagittal plane. The costotransverse bar of the lower cervical vertebrae often has a middle scalene tubercle for attachment of a portion of the scalenus medius.

The first, second, and seventh cervical vertebrae are considered atypical. C1, or the axis, lacks a body and a spinous process. It is a ringlike structure consisting of two lateral masses connected by a short anterior arch and a longer posterior arch. It is the widest cervical vertebra, with its anterior arch approximately half as long as its posterior arch (Fig. 1.4) Located in the midline on the anterior arch is the anterior tubercle for the attachment of the anterior longitudinal ligament and the longus colli muscles. The posterior arch corresponds to the lamina of the other vertebrae. On its upper surface is a wide groove for the vertebral artery and the first cervical nerve. In 1% to 15% of the population, a bony arch may form, thereby converting this groove into the arcuate foramen, through which passes the same structures (5). On the posterior arch is a posterior tubercle for attachment of the ligamentum nuchae. The lower surface is notched, which contributes to the formation of the C2 intervertebral foramen.

The lateral masses of C1 give rise to a superior and inferior articular facet. The superior articular facet is elongated

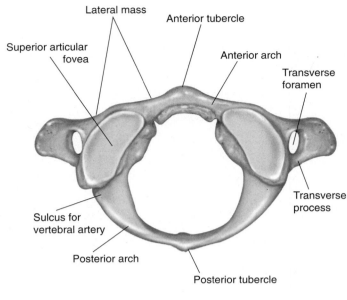

A

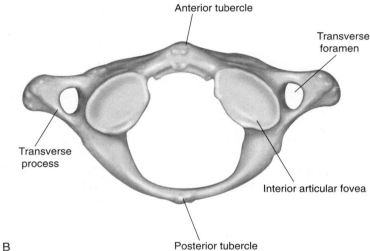

B

FIG. 1.4. The atlas. **A:** Cranial view. **B:** Caudal view.

and kidney-shaped, facing inward and upward to support the occipital condyles, with which it articulates on each side. The inferior articular facets are flatter and more circular, facing downward and inward to articulate with the articular surfaces of the second cervical vertebra. The transverse process is larger than that of other cervical vertebrae and is composed solely of a posterior tubercle that, with the costotransverse bar that attaches to the lateral mass, contains the foramen transversarium. The vertebral artery passes through the foramen transversarium of C1 before turning sharply medially and posteriorly to course behind the superior articular process.

The axis or second cervical vertebra is also known as the *epitrophysis*. It is characterized by a dens or odontoid process that projects upward from the body of C2 to articulate with the posterior aspect of the anterior arch of C1 (Fig. 1.5). The dimensions of the dens are highly variable: Its mean height

is 37.8 mm, its external transverse diameter 9.3 mm, internal transverse diameter 4.5 mm, mean anteroposterior (AP) external diameter 10.5 mm, and internal diameter 6.2 mm (6). Lateral to the dens, the body has a facet for the lower surface of the lateral mass of C1, which is large, slightly convex, and faces upward and outward. It is not a true superior articular process because the articular surface arises directly from the body and pedicle lateral to the dens. The zone between the lamina and the lateral mass is not well defined and comprises a large pedicle that is 10 mm long and 8 mm wide (7). It projects superiorly and medially in an anterior direction. The lower surface of the lateral mass has a forward-facing facet that articulates with the superior articular process of C3. The laminae of C2 are thick, and the spinous process is large and bifid. The transverse process ends in a single tubercle and contains a foramen transversarium. The C2 spinal nerve exits posterior to the superior

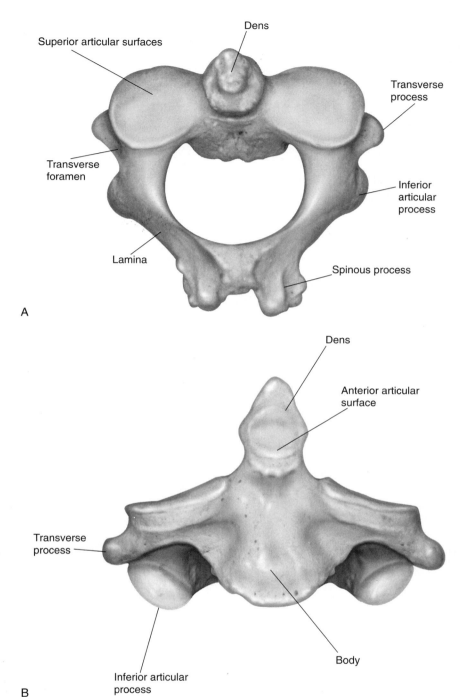

FIG. 1.5. The atlas. **A:** Cranial view. **B:** Anterior view.

articular surface of C2 rather than anterior to the articular complex, as spinal nerves do at other levels.

Large pedicles and a deeper spinal canal are two factors that allow increased mobility at C2 without cord encroachment. The density of the trabecular bone of C2 varies: It is very dense near the center of the tip of the dens and lateral masses beneath the superior articular surface, and hypodense in the area of the trabecular bone immediately beneath the dens. An area of cortical thickening on the

anterior surface of C2, known as the *promontory* of the axis, underlies the insertion of the anterior longitudinal access (8).

The seventh cervical vertebra is characterized by a long spinous process and has thus been given the name *vertebrae prominens*. This spinous process does not bifurcate, and the junction between it and the lamina is not well defined. It ends in a thick tubercle that attaches to the ligamentum nuchae. There is rarely a foramen transversarium at C7, and when present it usually does not contain the vertebral artery. The transverse process is large, and although the costal component of the transverse process is usually small, it may develop secondarily to form a cervical rib.

The occipital condyles have also been thoroughly characterized (9). The occipital condyles are the paired lateral prominences of the occipital bone that form the foramen magnum together with the basioccipital segment anteriorly and the supraoccipital (or squamosal) segment posteriorly. The occipital condyles are commonly oval or bean-shaped and slope inferiorly from lateral to medial in the coronal plane. The condyles make an angle of 25 to 28 degrees with the midsagittal plane. The occipitoatlantal articulations are cup-shaped paired joints between the concave occipital condyles and the concave superior atlantal facets. Within the base of each occipital condyle, the hypoglossal nerve (cranial nerve XII), a meningeal branch of the ascending pharyngeal artery, and an emissary vein pass through the hypoglossal (anterior condyloid) canal. Anterior to the condyles, the condylar foramen carries anastomotic venous channels from the sigmoid sinus to the suboccipital venous plexus; posteriorly, an indentation known as the *condyloid fossa* exists on the skull base. Cranial nerves (CN) IX to XI, the inferior petrosal sinus, the internal jugular vein, and the posterior meningeal artery travel lateral to the occipital condyles in the jugular foramen.

The cervicothoracic junction is a transitional region, like C2, exemplified by certain differences in the seventh cervical vertebra from other cervical vertebrae. At this level, the spinal canal decreases in size to the dimensions of the thoracic spine. The inferior articular process of C7 articulates with T1 to form a facet joint that is more thoracic in nature in that it is more perpendicular in the transverse plain. The seventh cervical vertebra also has a thinner lateral mass than other cervical vertebrae. The length, height, and width of the pedicles increase from C7 to T1 as the angle between the perpendicular of the posterior aspect of the vertebral body and the axis of the pedicle decreases. An and colleagues (7) described the morphologic characteristics of the pedicles of C7, T1, and T2. The C7 pedicle has an average inner diameter of 5.2 mm in a mediolateral plane and an angulation medially in a posterior anterior direction of 34 degrees. Xu and associates (10) found the thickness of the lateral mass of C7 to average 6.8 mm, with pedicular widths of 6.2 mm and height of 7 mm. They measured the angle between the pedicle axis and the posterior aspect of the lateral mass to be 170 degrees in the transverse plane and 76.2 degrees in the sagittal plane (10). Jones and coworkers (11) found that cervical pedicle screws demonstrated a significantly higher resistance to pull-out forces than did lateral mass screws. However, the variability in pedicle morphometry and orientation influences the capability of placing pedicle screws in the cervical spine.

The spinal canal is formed by sequential vertebral foramina and is triangular with rounded edges. It has a greater lateral than AP width and is more spacious in the upper cervical spine, with sagittal diameters averaging 23 mm at C1 and 20 mm at C2. In comparison, the average diameter from C3 through C6 ranges between 17 and 18 mm and decreases to 15 mm at C7 (2). Thus, the cross-sectional area of the cervical spinal canal is greatest at C2 and smallest at C7.

ARTICULATIONS, LIGAMENTS, AND INTERVERTEBRAL DISCS

The osseous elements of the cervical spine and skull are connected to one another by various joints and ligamentous structures. These structures combine to form distinct articular complexes at the atlantooccipital and the atlantoaxial levels. Intervertebral discs are located between the vertebral bodies of all cervical vertebrae except C1 and C2 (Fig. 1.6).

The atlantooccipital complex is composed of two membranous attachments between C1 and the occiput and the two synovial atlantooccipital joints laterally. The atlantooccipital joints are formed between the superior articular facet of the atlas and the occipital condyle. These joints contain a synovial membrane and are surrounded by a capsular ligament. Also contributing to the complex are the anterior and posterior atlantooccipital membranes connecting the anterior and posterior arch of C1 with the corresponding margin of the foramen magnum. The anterior atlantooccipital membrane blends on its lateral edges with the capsular ligaments of the synovial joints and inferiorly with the anterior longitudinal ligament. The posterior atlantooccipital membrane blends laterally with the capsular ligaments of the synovial joints and is pierced on each side just above the posterior arch of C1 by the vertebral artery in the first cervical nerve (Fig. 1.7).

The atlantoaxial complex is composed of three synovial joints, one median and two lateral (Fig. 1.7). The lateral atlantoaxial joints consist of an encapsulated synovial joint between the inferior articular facet of C1 and the superior articular surface of C2. The capsule is reinforced posteriorly by an accessory ligament that extends from the posterior aspect of C2 superiorly and laterally to the lateral mass of C1. The median atlantoaxial joint forms between the anterior arch and transverse ligament of C1 and the dens. It is a pivot joint with synovial membrane and capsular ligaments anteriorly and posteriorly to the dens. The cruciate (cruciform ligament) is composed of the transverse ligament of the atlas and the superior and inferior ligamentous extensions that connect it to the anterior edges of the foramen magnum and posterior aspects of the C2 body, respectively. The transverse ligament attaches laterally to tubercles located on the posterior aspect of the anterior arch of C1, where it blends with the lateral mass (Fig. 1.8). The length of the transverse ligament averages 21.9 mm.

The axis has three other connections to the occipital bone. The apical ligament extends from the tip of the dens to the anterior edge of the foramen magnum and has an

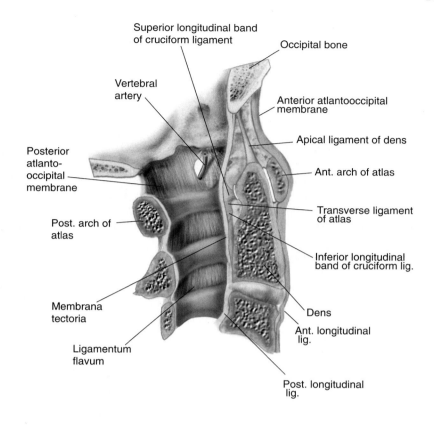

FIG. 1.6. Median section at craniocervical junction, revealing atlantooccipital and atlantoaxial ligaments and membranes.

average length of 23.5 mm and a 20-degree anterior tilt (12). The alar ligaments extend from the tip of the dens to the medial aspects of each occipital condyle, with a small insertion also on the lateral mass of the atlas (13). They average 10.3 mm long. Sometimes there is a ligamentous connection between the base of the dens and the anterior arch of the atlas, called the *anterior atlantodental ligament* (13). The tectorial membranes extend from the posterior body of C2 and the posterior longitudinal ligament to the upper surface of the basilar portion of the occipital bone and the anterior aspect of the foramen magnum. This membrane covers all other occipitoaxial ligaments as well as the dens. Thus, anterior to the spinal canal at the level of the craniocervical junction, the ligaments are arranged with the anterior atlantooccipital membrane most anteriorly followed (in an anterior-to-posterior direction) by the apical alar, the cruciate, and, most posteriorly, the tectorial.

The bodies of the cervical vertebrae are connected by two longitudinal ligaments and the intervertebral discs. The anterior longitudinal ligament is a broad, thick ligament that runs longitudinally anterior to the vertebral body and disc (Fig. 1.9). It is joined loosely to the periosteum of the anterior vertebral bodies and closely to the annulus fibrosis of the anterior vertebral disc and attaches superiorly to the anterior tubercle of the atlas. The posterior longitudinal ligament (PLL) lies within the vertebral

canal on the posterior aspect of the vertebral bodies and intervertebral discs. Superiorly, it is continuous with the tectorial membrane and thus attaches to the occipital bone and anterior aspect of the foramen magnum. As it descends, it narrows behind each vertebral body but spreads out at the disc level, where it is adherent to the annulus fibrosis. Hayashi and associates (14) described two layers: a superficial and deep layer. The deep layer surrounds the vertebral body and laterally is continuous with the lateral extension of the anterior longitudinal ligament in the intervertebral foramen. A more superficial layer is closely related to the dura mater and laterally separates from the deep layer, enveloping the dura mater, nerve roots, and vertebral artery. The venous plexus is located between the layers of the PLL—not in the epidural space, as previously thought (15).

The intervertebral discs are fibrocartilaginous joints that create shock-absorbing pads or cushions between the borders of adjacent cervical vertebrae, with the most cephalad disc at the C2-C3 level. Each disc consists of an inner nucleus pulposus surrounded by a circumferential annulus fibrosis; the border between the two becomes more difficult to distinguish with increasing age and degeneration. These two components are separated from the vertebral bone above and below by a thin cartilage end plate. The nucleus pulposus is a semigelatinous central portion that contains

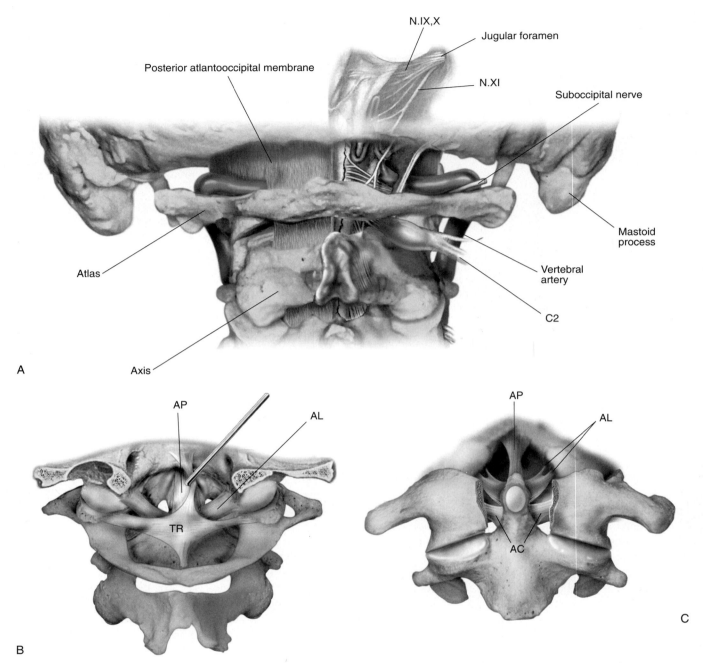

FIG. 1.7. Posterior view of the ligaments of the atlas and axis. **A:** Vertebral artery as it pierces posterior atlantooccipital membrane. **B:** Posterior membrane, posterior arch of atlas and axis, and posterior rim of foramen magnum removed. **C:** Anterior view with anterior arch of atlas removed. AP, apical ligament; TR, transverse ligament; AL, alar ligaments; AC, accessory ligaments.

collagen fibers, connective tissue cells, and cartilage cells with large amounts of amorphous extracellular material. It is held in shape by the cartilage end plates, the annulus fibrosis, and the uncovertebral joints laterally. The annulus fibrosis consists of spirally arranged and layered laminar collagenous fiber bundles with each ring of fiber arranged at right angles to the previous. The fibers are connected circumferentially to the vertebral end plate and to the ante-

rior and posterior longitudinal ligaments. Posterolaterally, the cervical discs are bound by the uncovertebral process, and inferiorly and superiorly the annulus fibrosis is firmly attached to adjacent vertebral end plates. End plates consist of a thin layer of hyaline cartilage resting on the subchondral bone of the vertebral body, which distributes stress over the body. The cartilage plays a role in the growth of the vertebral body and nutrition for the disc.

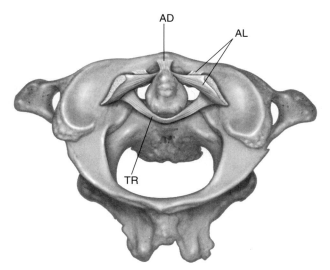

FIG. 1.8. Axial view of cervicocranium from above, demonstrating the relations among the transverse (TR), alar (AR), and atlantodental (AD) ligaments.

Tanaka and coworkers (16) characterized the relation of the disc to the nerve root at the intervertebral foramen in the middle to lower cervical spine. At the entrance zone of the intervertebral foramen, the C4-5 disc was most likely proximal to the C5 nerve root (33%) or just anterior to the C5 nerve root (67%). For the C5-6 disc and the C6-7

disc, the relation between the disc and the nerve root was most likely an axillary type (72% and 89%, respectively). With the C8 nerve root, 78% of nerve roots did not contact the C7-T1 disc at the entrance zone of the foramen but contacted the disc at the lateral exit zone of the foramen.

The vertebral arches are connected by the synovial joints between articular processes of adjacent vertebrae and by the accessory ligaments between the laminae, the transverse processes, and the spinous processes (Fig. 1.10). The facet joints, or zygapophyseal joints, are diarthrodial joints with articular cartilage and menisci and are formed between the adjacent articular processes of sequential vertebral levels. Each zygapophyseal joint is surrounded by a fibrous capsule and is lined by a synovial membrane. Different types of menisci have been described in the cervical facet joints based on age, location, and degree of degeneration (17). Mechanical, receptive, and nociceptive nerve endings have been located in the facet capsules of cervical zygapophyseal joints (18).

The facet joints of the cervical region are oriented more horizontally than those in other regions of the spine. The upper facet joints begin with an angle approximately 45 degrees superiorly in the transverse plane and gradually assume a more vertical position as they descend to the thoracic region. The superior articular facet faces from a generally more medial toward a lateral projection

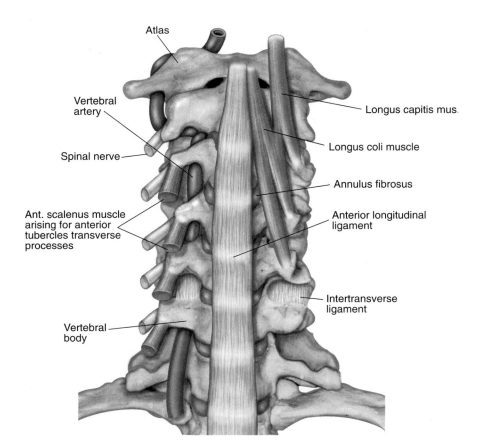

FIG. 1.9. Anterior cervical spine and associated ligaments and muscles.

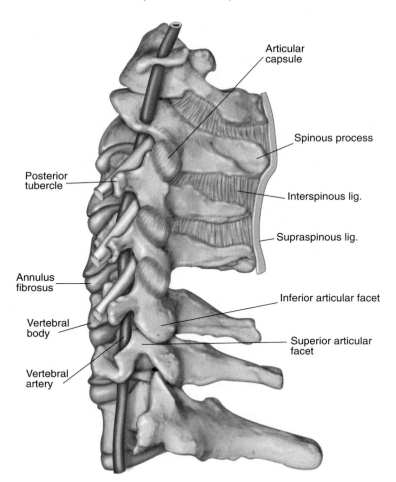

FIG. 1.10. Lateral view of cervical spine, demonstrating facets and capsular and interspinous ligaments.

as the cervical spine is descended. Facet widths increase from C3 to T1, with facet depth greatest in the upper three vertebrae and then decreasing from C5 to T1 (19). The interfacet distance varies between 9 and 16 mm (average, 13 mm) (2). The capsular ligament of each facet is oriented posteriorly at a 45-degree angle to the transverse plane (20).

The supraspinous ligament of the thoracic region continues into the cervical region as the ligamentum nuchae. This is a triangular membrane that forms a median fibroseptum between the muscles of the two sides of the posterior cervical region. It extends approximately from the external occipital protuberance to the spine of the seventh cervical vertebra. There are deep attachments to the external occipital crest, the posterior tubercle of the atlas, and the spinous processes of C2 through C7. The interspinous ligament is poorly developed in the cervical region and is found between the spinous processes from the ligamentum flavum to the tip of the process. It often has a thin, filmy appearance. The intertransverse ligaments between the transverse processes of the cervical spine are also weak and replaced by the intertransversalis muscles (21). The ligamentum flavum consists mainly of elastic fibers and connects the inferior and superior aspects of adjacent laminae, extending laterally

to blend into the capsule of the facet joints (Fig. 1.11). The ligaments arise from the undersurface of the lamina above and insert on the superior edge of the lamina below. The ligamenta flava are discontinuous in the midline; the small fissure allows the exit of veins.

From a biomechanical standpoint, the anterior ligamentous complex (anterior and posterior longitudinal ligaments) has a higher failure stress and Young's modulus than the posterior complex (interspinous ligament, joint capsules, and ligamentum flavum). However, the posterior ligamentous complex has a higher failure strain ($\Delta L/L_0$) than the anterior complex (22).

NEURAL ELEMENTS

Spinal Cord

The spinal cord extends from the foramen magnum above, where it is continuous with the medulla oblongata. With its surrounding meninges, it lies within the vertebral or spinal canal, which is formed by sequential vertebral foramina. The anterior wall of the spinal canal is formed by the posterior border of the intervertebral discs and cervical vertebral bodies. The lateral wall consists of the

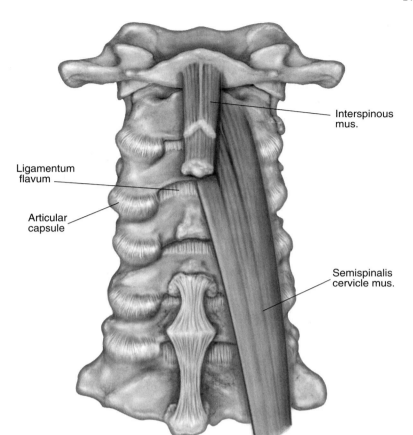

Interspinous mus.

Ligamentum flavum

Articular capsule

Semispinalis cervicle mus.

FIG. 1.11. Posterior view of cervical spine, revealing ligamentum flavum as it blends into articular capsule of the facet joints.

pedicles and successive intervertebral foramina, through which the spinal nerves exit. Posteriorly, the articular processes laterally and the ligamentum flavum and the lamina medially and posteriorly form the final borders of the spinal canal.

The spinal cord exhibits considerable individual variation in size. Its morphology also changes at different levels (23). It is cylindrical and slightly flattened in the AP direction, and thus usually has a larger transverse than AP diameter. The spinal cord enlarges from C3 to C6, where it usually attains a maximal transverse diameter of 13 to 14 mm (24). Okada and associates (25), using MRI analysis, found that the spinal cord reached a maximal transverse area of 85.8 ± 7.2 mm^2 at the C4 to C5 level, whereas a cadaveric study by Kameyama and colleagues (26) found a maximal transverse area of 58.3 ± 6.7 mm^2 at C6, which corresponds to the large number of nerve roots innervating the upper extremities.

On the posterior surface of the cord is a posterior median sulcus and two posterior lateral sulci (Fig. 1.12). The region along the posterior lateral sulcus where the posterior rootlets enter the spinal cord is termed the *dorsal* or *posterior root entry zone*. The range of distance from the midline to the posterior root entry zone is 2.5 to 4.5 mm. The longitudinal length of the posterior root entry zone ranges from 8 to 14 mm, depending on the cervical level. The pos-

terior root entry zone decreases in length and moves closer to the midline in the lower cervical and upper thoracic spinal cord (15). The number of posterior rootlets ranges from 5 to 16 at each level. Also present on the posterior cord are small arteries, veins, and the posterior spinal medullary vessels.

On the anterior surface of the spinal cord is the anterior median fissure, which contains the anterior spinal artery and small veins. Ventral root filaments exit the anterior lateral aspect of the cord at regular intervals at the ventral lateral sulcus at regions termed the *anterior root exit zones* (AREZ). Anterior root exit zones range from 1 to 3 mm from the midline, and the average distance tends to decrease in the lower cervical spinal cord. The transverse and longitudinal lengths of the AREZ range from 1.5 to 3 mm and 10 to 18 mm, respectively. The AREZ tends to decrease in longitudinal and transverse length in the lower cervical spinal cord. About 20 nerve rootlets leave the AREZ at each level; the number decreases in the lower cervical spine (15).

When cut, transverse sections of the spinal cord consist of an inner butterfly-shaped gray substance composed of nerve-cell bodies of efferent and interneural neurons and the surrounding white substance composed of nerve fibers and glia of either ascending or descending tracts (Fig. 1.13). The gray matter consists of cell columns that extend the

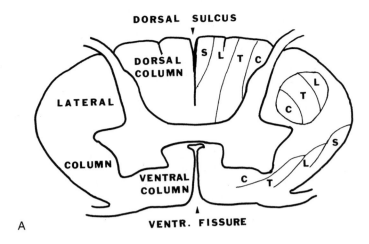

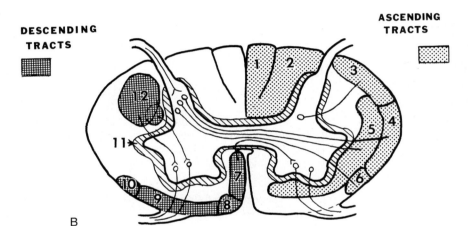

FIG. 1.12. Cross-sectional anatomy of the ascending and descending columns of the cervical spinal cord. **A:** Segmental arrangement of the tracts of the ventral, lateral, and posterior columns: sacral (*S*), lumbar (*L*), thoracic (*T*), cervical (*C*). **B:** Tracts of the spinal cord: (*1*) fasciculus gracilis, (*2*) fasciculus cuneatus, (*3*) dorsal spinocerebellar, (*4*) ventral spinocerebellar, (*5*) lateral spinothalamic, (*6*) spinoolivary, (*7*) anterior corticospinal, (*8*) tectospinal, (*9*) vestibulospinal, (*10*) olivospinal, (*11*) intersegmental or propriospinal, (*12*) lateral corticospinal. (From: Parke WW, Sherk HH. Normal adult anatomy. In: Sherk HH, Dunn EJ, Eismont FJ, et al., eds. The cervical spine, 2nd ed. Philadelphia: JB Lippincott, 1988: 11–32, with permission.)

length of the spinal cord. Although the configuration varies at different levels, in general each half of the spinal cord has a posterior gray column or horn that extends in a posterior lateral direction almost to the surface of the cord and an anterior gray column or horn that extends anteriorly but does not reach the surface. A gray commissure connects the gray substance from the two sides and encircles the central canal. The posterior horn of the gray matter contains somatosensory neurons, whereas the anterior horn contains somatomotor neurons. Throughout the white matter are ascending and descending fibers that are organized into distinct tracts. The white matter is organized into three columns: posterior, lateral, and anterior.

The posterior column lies between the posterior horns of the gray matter, divided by the posterior median septum in the midline. On each side, it is composed of the fasciculus cuneatus laterally and the fasciculus gracilis medially, which are divided by the posterior intermediate septum. The posterior column is an ascending column of proprioception and vibratory and tactile sensation. Tracts from the lower portion of the body are placed more medially in the

posterior column, whereas fibers from tracts entering higher in the body are placed more laterally.

The lateral column is located between the anterior and posterior root entry zones. This region contains the lateral corticospinal tract and the lateral spinothalamic tract. The lateral corticospinal tract is a descending pathway concerned with voluntary discrete and skillful motor function. This tract, the small anterior corticospinal tract, and the very small anterior lateral corticospinal tract make up the cortical spinal system. At the pyramidal decussation of the medulla, 75% to 90% of axons of the corticospinal system decussate, forming the crossed lateral corticospinal tract and the uncrossed anterior corticospinal tract. Corticospinal tract fibers are arranged so that the more cephalad fibers are arranged medially in the descending tract. The lateral spinothalamic tract transmits ascending impulses, allowing discernment of pain and thermal sense from the contralateral side. The posterior spinocerebellar tract is an uncrossed tract that ascends along the posterior lateral periphery of the spinal cord and is most likely involved in fine coordination of individual limb movement and posture.

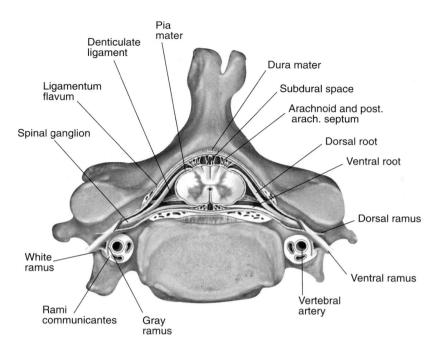

Pia mater
Denticulate ligament
Dura mater
Subdural space
Arachnoid and post. arach. septum
Ligamentum flavum
Dorsal root
Ventral root
Spinal ganglion
Dorsal ramus
White ramus
Ventral ramus
Rami communicantes
Vertebral artery
Gray ramus

FIG. 1.13. Cross section of the spinal cord with its meningeal coverings.

The anterior column lies between the anterior median fissure and the anterior root entry zone. Important tracts in this region are the anterior corticospinal tract and the anterior spinothalamic tract. The ascending fibers of the anterior spinothalamic tract convey impulses associated with light touch. As mentioned, the anterior corticospinal tract is a descending uncrossed tract concerned with fine motor skills.

A *segment* of the cord is a portion of the cord to which are attached the corresponding pair of ventral and dorsal roots. The anatomy of the anterior and posterior root entry zones already has been mentioned. In the lower cervical spine, the anterior and posterior root entry zones are located approximately one disc level higher than the corresponding intervertebral foramen through which will pass the nerve root formed from its rootlets (15,27). The rootlets pass obliquely laterally and caudally within the canal, entering the root sleeve where the sensory and motor roots are separated by the interradicular septum, a lateral extension of the dura mater. Each dorsal root presents an oval enlargement, the spinal ganglion, as it approaches or enters the intervertebral foramen. Just distal to this ganglion, the dorsal and ventral roots combine to form a spinal nerve. Just before the formation of the cervical nerve, the anterior root is at an anterior inferior position within the intervertebral foramen just posterior to the uncovertebral junction, whereas the posterior root is related to the superior articular process.

The cervical nerve root occupies usually one-third of the foraminal space in a normal spine, usually the inferior aspect, with the superior aspect being filled with fat and associated veins. The ventral (motor) roots emerge from the dura mater more caudally than the dorsal (sensory) roots,

and the ventral roots course along the caudal border of the dorsal roots within the intervertebral foramina. Thus, compression of the ventral roots, dorsal roots, or both depends on the anatomic structures around the nerve roots, such as a prolapsed disc (ventral root compression) or osteophytes from the facet joint (dorsal root compression). The most likely site of compression of the radicular nerve is at the entrance zone of the intervertebral foramen because the medial entrance zone of the foramen is smaller in diameter than the lateral exit zone, whereas the nerve roots are widest at their takeoff from the central thecal sac and become more narrow laterally (16).

The first cervical spinal nerve exits between the occiput and C1; nerves C2 to C7 exit above the correspondingly numbered vertebrae. The eighth cervical nerve root exits the intervertebral foramen formed between the seventh cervical vertebra and the first thoracic vertebra. The dorsal root ganglion is usually located between the vertebral artery and the superior articular process. In the sagittal plane, cervical nerve roots C3 through C8 in the intervertebral foramina lie midway between the posterior midpoints of the lateral masses situated an average of 5.5 mm above or below each lateral mass point (28). Thus, cervical nerve roots enter their intervertebral foramina and leave the spinal canal at the level of the disc and above the pedicle of the same numbered level, except for C8, which exits above the T1 pedicle. Each nerve root goes on to supply a specific dermatome or myotome, with considerable overlap (especially with the high incidence of intradural connections between the dorsal rootlets of C5, C6, and C7) and variations existing in sensory and motor patterns between individuals because of the complex anastomoses of epispinal axons and nerve rootlets as well as gross anatomic variations of the brachial plexus (6,16,29–31).

Meninges

The spinal cord is surrounded by three meninges, the outermost being the spinal dura mater, a dense, tough, fibrous tube extending from the foramen magnum, where it continues with the dura mater of the brain. It is slightly adherent to the foramen magnum and the C2 and C3 vertebral bodies. Between the dura mater and the posterior vertebral wall lie epidural fat and loose connective tissue, with an internal vertebral venous plexus located between the superficial and deep layers of the posterior longitudinal ligament. Spinal roots enter a tubular prolongation of the dura mater called a *dural sheath* as they approach the intervertebral foramina. At approximately the level of the spinal ganglion, the sheaths of the two roots blend to form a sheath that continues into the epineurium of the spinal nerve. The lower cervical roots descend intradurally and may angulate as they turn toward the intervertebral foramina. The subdural space is a potential space between the arachnoid and the dura mater that contains a thin film of fluid and communicates with lymphatic vessels and nerves.

The arachnoid is a delicate translucent membrane that is continuous with the cerebral arachnoid through the foramen magnum. Laterally, it continues with the dural sheath for a short distance. The subarachnoid space contains cerebrospinal fluid as well as blood vessels and nerve rootlets and is the interval between the arachnoid and the pia mater. It is partly subdivided by the denticulate ligaments and a variable fibrous condensation, the subarachnoid septum, which extends backward from the cord in the midsagittal plane.

The pia mater, the outer lining of the cord, consists of both reticular tissue and collagenous fibers. The reticular tissue invests the spinal cord, passing posteriorly into the anterior median fissure, and invests the rootlets, becoming continuous with similar elements of the arachnoid. It forms the posterior median septum. The collagenous fibers extend to the reticulum layer and contain vessels on the cord surface. Anteriorly in the midsagittal plane, it forms the linea splendens, which ensheathes the anterior spinal artery. Laterally, the pia mater extension forms a longitudinal septum, the denticulate ligament, which fuses with the arachnoid and dura mater via small noncontinuous processes that help to anchor the spinal cord. These processes begin at the foramen magnum and are located on each side of the cord in the interval between two adjacent spinal nerves. The denticulate ligament attaches to the spinal cord roughly halfway between the dorsal and ventral root entry zones.

Spinal Nerves

Just beyond the dorsal root ganglion and usually just outside the intervertebral foramina, the cervical spinal nerves divide into dorsal and ventral primary rami. The first cervical nerve exits the vertebral canal through an orifice in the posterior atlantooccipital membrane just above the posterior arch of the atlas and posteromedial to the lateral mass of the atlas. Its ventral primary ramus unites with the second cervical ventral primary ramus and contributes fibers to the hypoglossal nerve; this is also known as the superior root of the ansa cervicalis, the inferior root that consists of fibers from the ventral primary rami of cervical nerves C2 and C3. The cervical plexus is formed by the ventral rami of the upper four cervical nerves and is located on the surface of the levator scapulae and scalenus medius and beneath the internal jugular vein and sternocleidomastoid. The dorsal primary ramus of C1 enters the suboccipital triangle, and its terminal branches supply the muscles of this region (Fig. 1.14). There is usually no cutaneous branch of the dorsal primary ramus of C1, also known as the *suboccipital nerve.*

The second cervical nerve emerges between the posterior arch of the atlas and the lamina of the axis just posterior to its lateral mass. Its dorsal rami are much larger than its ventral rami and are the largest of all the cervical dorsal rami. The medial branch of the dorsal rami, or greater occipital nerve, runs transversely in the soft tissue dorsal to the C2 lamina, turning upward in the submuscular position and eventually entering the scalp with the occipital artery through an opening above the aponeurotic sling between the trapezius and the sternocleidomastoid (32).

Cervical nerves C3 to C8 exit the vertebral canal through the intervertebral foramina, the borders of which have already been described. The principal branch of the third cervical dorsal rami is the third occipital nerve, which curves dorsally and medially around the superior articular process of C3 and crosses behind the C2-C3 zygapophyseal joint, supplying it. It runs medially toward the midline, where it turns dorsally and superiorly, supplying the posterior cervical musculature and terminating in cutaneous branches for the occipital and mastoid regions. The dorsal rami for cervical nerves C4 to C8 arise from the spinal nerve just outside the intervertebral foramina and divide into medial and lateral branches. The lateral branches of C4 to C7 supply the longissimus cervicis and splenis cervicis, with the lateral branches of C8 supplying the iliocostal cervicis. The medial branches of these nerves have an overlapping cutaneous innervation supplying the multifidus and interspinales muscles and sending branches to the facet joints rostral and caudal to it (32).

As stated, the anterior rami of cervical nerves C1 to C4 form the cervical plexus, and those from C5 to T1 form the brachial plexus. The cervical plexus is arranged in a series of loops from which peripheral branches arise. This arrangement results in overlap of the cutaneous sensory distribution. A loop formed between branches of the first through third cervical nerves gives branches that form the ansa cervicalis. The superior root of the ansa cervicalis is formed between the first and second cervical nerves and

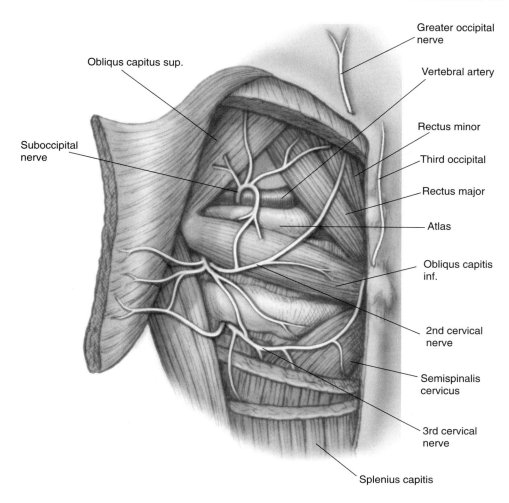

Greater occipital nerve

Vertebral artery

Rectus minor

Third occipital

Rectus major

Atlas

Obliqus capitis inf.

2nd cervical nerve

Semispinalis cervicus

3rd cervical nerve

Splenius capitis

Obliqus capitus sup.

Suboccipital nerve

FIG. 1.14. Dorsal primary divisions of the first through third cervical nerves.

gives off a branch to the hypoglossal nerve. The inferior root, or nervus descendens cervicalis, consists of fibers of cervical nerves C2 and C3. The ansa cervicalis lies superficial to the carotid sheath and supplies all the strap or infrahyoid muscles except for the thyrohyoid. The cervical plexus also gives rise to superficial cutaneous branches, including the lesser occipital, greater auricular, and transverse cervical nerves (Fig. 1.15).

The phrenic nerve originates chiefly from cervical root 4. It forms at the lateral border of the scalenus anterior and runs vertically across the front of the scalenus under cover of the internal jugular vein and sternomastoid. It is located behind the prevertebral fascia and is crossed by the transverse cervical artery. The cervical plexus also communicates with cranial nerves X, XI, and XII, and via rami communicantes with the sympathetic chain. The ventral rami, forming the brachial plexus, exit the intervertebral foramina between the anterior and middle scalene muscles and lie in the posterior triangle under cover of the platysma and deep fascia.

Innervation of Specific Regions

The osseous and ligamentous structures of the cervical spine are surrounded by a continuous network of interlacing nerve fibers (Fig. 1.16). The ventral plexus of the anterior longitudinal ligament and the dorsal plexus of the PLL are connected at the level of the intervertebral foramen by branches of rami communicantes. These nerves receive contributions from the sympathetic trunk rami communicantes and the perivascular nerve plexus of the segmental arteries. Anteriorly, branches from the perivascular nerve plexus may reach the anterior longitudinal ligament nerve plexus by coursing both superiorly and deep to the longus colli muscle.

The nerve plexus of the PLL receives innervation from the sinuvertebral nerve (Fig. 1.16), which has been well described in the literature. It has both somatic and autonomic origins and originates from the ventral ramus of the spinal nerves, the rami communicantes of the sympathetic trunk, and the perivascular vertebral arterial nerve plexus (33). Autonomic fibers also may come from the vertebral nerve, which is formed by gray rami communicantes in the mid-cervical region, or from the stellate ganglion in the lower cervical region. After its origin from the ventral ramus, the sinuvertebral nerve runs back through the intervertebral foramen anterior to the spinal nerve, posterior to the vertebral artery, and arrives at the posterior aspect of the disc and the posterior vertebral body. It then branches rostrally and

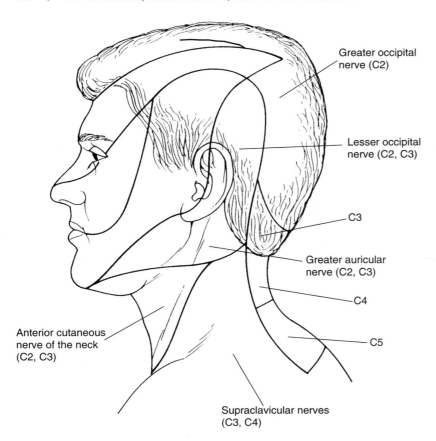

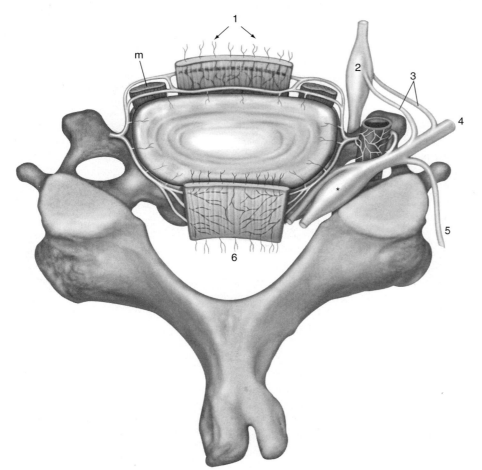

FIG. 1.15. Cutaneous sensory distribution of branches of cervical spinal nerves on the back of the head and neck. (From: Parent A, ed. *Carpenter's human neuroanatomy*, 9th ed. Baltimore: Williams & Wilkins, 1996, with permission.)

FIG. 1.16. Schematic diagram of the nerve plexus of the anterior longitudinal ligament (*1*) and the posterior longitudinal ligament. (*2*) Sympathetic trunk, (*3*) rami communicantes, (*4*) ventral ramus of spinal nerve, (*5*) dorsal ramus of spinal nerve, (*m*) longus coli muscle, and (*asterisk*) spinal ganglion.

caudally, running along the lateral edge of the PLL, parallel to the ventral spinal branches of the segmental arteries, and branching to the periosteum, intraspinal veins, and the outer annulus fibrosus of the disc above and below the level of nerve origin. The sinuvertebral nerve of cervical nerve C3 ascends rostrally in a similar manner, crossing the dorsal surface of the tectorial membrane and entering the cranial fossa, supplying the dura of the clivus. It joins the sinuvertebral nerves of C1 and C2 to innervate the ligaments of the atlantoaxial joint.

The ventral spinal dura is innervated by a dense longitudinally oriented nerve plexus receiving contributions from the sinuvertebral nerve, the nerve plexus of the PLL, and the perivascular nerve plexus of segmental artery branches. The dorsal dura is supplied by dorsal nerves that originate from the ventral plexus at the level of the intersleeval parts of the dura but do not reach the midline portion of the dorsal dura. Ventral nerves may extend up to eight segments. Thus, a large amount of overlap exists between adjacent nerves (34).

The cervical zygapophyseal joints from C3-C4 through C8-T1 are supplied by medial branches of the cervical dorsi rami. Each joint is supplied by a branch above and below its location. The C2-C3 joint is supplied by the third occipital nerve as it crosses the posterior aspect of this articulation. The upper cervical synovial joints (the atlantooccipital and the lateral atlantoaxial joints) are not innervated by the cervical dorsal rami but receive branches from the C1-C2 ventral rami (35). The intervertebral disc is innervated at its posterior aspect by branches of the sinuvertebral nerve and at its lateral aspect by branches of the vertebral nerve (35,36).

VASCULAR STRUCTURES OF THE CERVICAL SPINE

Vertebral Artery and Other Major Arteries

The major source of blood for the osseous and neural elements of the cervical spine is the vertebral arteries, which arise from the first part of the subclavian artery medial to the scalenus anterior and ascend behind the common carotid artery between the longus colli and the scalenus anterior (Fig. 1.17). They are crossed by the inferior thyroid artery and on the left by the thoracic duct. In the lower cervical region, they lie anterior to the ventral rami of the seventh and

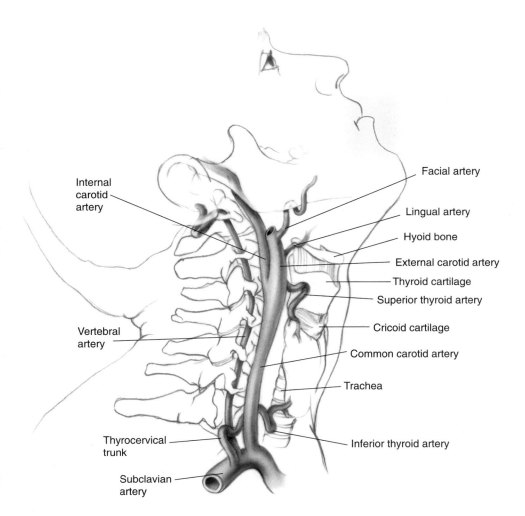

Internal carotid artery

Facial artery

Lingual artery

Hyoid bone

External carotid artery

Thyroid cartilage

Superior thyroid artery

Cricoid cartilage

Vertebral artery

Common carotid artery

Trachea

Thyrocervical trunk

Inferior thyroid artery

Subclavian artery

FIG. 1.17. Arteries of the neck.

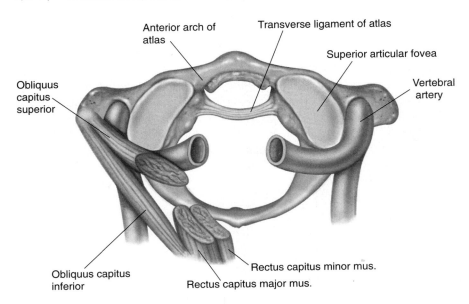

FIG. 1.18. Cranial view of the course of the vertebral artery in the upper cervical spine.

eighth cervical nerves and to the transverse process of the seventh cervical vertebra.

The vertebral artery enters the transverse foramen of C6 and ascends through the cephalad transverse foramen to the level of the atlas. In this region, it lies anterior to the ventral rami of cervical nerves C6 to C2 and is surrounded by a venous plexus and sympathetic nerve fibers. The vertebral artery migrates posteriorly to anteriorly from C3 to C6 and travels posteriorly at C7. The distance between the medial margins of the foramen transversaria ranges from 25.0 to 31.2 mm from C3 to C7 (1). The transverse interforaminal distance, and thus the transverse distance between vertebral arteries at the same cervical level, increases slightly from C3 to C6, as does the distance of the vertebral artery from the anterior border of the spinal canal. This relates the vertebral artery more closely to the anterior border of the spinal canal, and thus the origin of the neural foramina, at more cephalad levels (37,38).

Throughout its course between transverse foramina as it ascends the cervical spine, the vertebral artery is encased in a fibrous osteomuscular tunnel, fixing it to adjacent structures via a trabeculated collagen network (39). At the level of the atlas, the vertebral artery turns posteromedially, coursing transversely behind the lateral mass and over the posterior arch of C1 (Fig. 1.18). The artery then passes through the posterior atlantooccipital membrane, turning anteriorly and cephalad through the foramen magnum. The vertebral arteries then join to form the basilar artery. Just before forming the basilar artery, the vertebral arteries give off branches anteriorly that join to form the single anterior spinal artery. Anomalies of the vertebral artery in the region of C1-C2 include fenestration or intraspinal coursing and have been found to have a prevalence of 0.3% to 2% (40).

The ascending cervical artery originates from either the thyrocervical trunk or from the inferior thyroid artery, and it accompanies the phrenic nerve, rising on the transverse process along the medial border of the scalene, anterior to the cervical vertebrae. It gives off muscular branches and branches to the vertebral arteries and the neural elements. The deep cervical artery, which arises either alone from the subclavian artery or from the costocervical trunk, rises between the transverse process of C7 and the neck of the first rib, ascending between the semispinalis capitis and cervicis toward the spinous process of C2. It also gives off branches to the vertebral canal at the lower regions of the cervical spine. The occipital artery usually originates from the posterior surface of the external carotid artery in the upper cervical spine. It may give off branches to the nuchal musculature, which communicate with branches of the vertebral artery and thus also can contribute to the blood supply of the spinal cord.

Blood Supply to the Spinal Cord

The blood supply to the spinal cord arises from a pattern of arterial supply contained within three longitudinal channels on the surface of the spinal cord (Fig. 1.19). One channel is anteromedial in position, and the other two are posterolateral. The three channels are reinforced at irregular intervals by medullary feeders from segmental arteries. Before they join to form the basilar artery, each vertebral artery gives off a single branch, which then joins to form the anterior spinal artery. The anterior spinal artery courses in a caudal direction in the anterior median fissure on the anterior surface of the spinal cord. In this position, it is reinforced by medullary arteries and supplies most of the spinal cord, except for the posterior funiculus and the major portion of the posterior gray columns (41).

The two posterior spinal arteries arise from either the vertebral artery or the posterior inferior cerebellar arteries. They course in the posterior lateral sulcus of the spinal cord

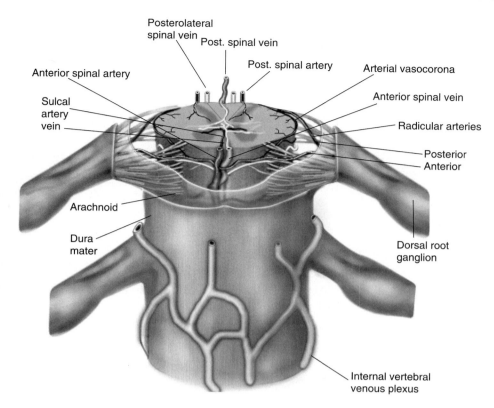

Posterolateral spinal vein
Post. spinal vein
Post. spinal artery
Arterial vasocorona
Anterior spinal artery
Anterior spinal vein
Sulcal artery vein
Radicular arteries
Posterior
Anterior
Arachnoid
Dura mater
Dorsal root ganglion
Internal vertebral venous plexus

FIG. 1.19. Arterial supply and venous drainage of spinal cord.

and give rise to plexiform channels on the surface of the cord on each side. These channels also are reinforced by medullary arteries. This reinforcing segmental supply of the spinal cord is provided by medullary arteries derived primarily from the spinal branches of the ascending cervical, deep cervical, and vertebral arteries (41,42). The ventral and dorsal nerve roots are supplied by radicular branches of the spinal arteries.

Blood Supply to the Vertebral Body

The blood supply of the vertebral body originates from segmental vessels off the vertebral arteries. At each level, these branches exit, passing anteriorly beneath the longus colli supplying the anterior vertebral body and the anterior longitudinal ligament. Another branch enters the intervertebral foramina and passes anteriorly and superiorly, supplying the posterior vertebral body and the posterior longitudinal ligament. Other branches pass laterally from within the spinal canal, supplying the laminae and radicular branches to the spinal cord. The outer surface of the laminae is supplied by other branches of the vertebral artery that pass dorsally before entering the intervertebral foramina (42).

The vascular supply to the dens is unique and worth mentioning. It is supplied by paired ascending anterior and posterior arteries, all of which arise from the vertebral arteries. These arteries rise along the borders of the dens to form an apical arcade, which anastomoses with the carotid system via anterior and posterior horizontal arteries

(43–45). The alar and accessory ligaments also make vascular contributions, as does an intraosseous supply from the body of the axis.

Venous Drainage of the Cervical Spine

Venous drainage of the spinal cord occurs via an anterior and posterior channel system, each consisting of three veins running longitudinally (Fig. 1.19). Anteriorly, the veins run parallel to the anterior spinal artery in the median fissure. Posteriorly, one vein lies centrally in the posterior median sulcus, and the other two are closely related to the dorsal longitudinal arteries more laterally. These medullary veins empty into radicular veins, which in turn drain into the intervertebral veins.

The venous drainage of the spinal cord and vertebral bodies also consists of an anterior and posterior internal vertebral venous plexus and the basivertebral veins, which drain the vertebral bodies (Fig. 1.20). The anterior internal vertebral plexus consists of a series of valveless sinuses that are most prominent in the canal in the midportion of the vertebral body just medial to the pedicles and least appreciable at the level of the intervertebral disc and centrally (15). There is free communication across the midline with veins of the opposite side as well as with the basivertebral veins. Although originally believed to lie in the epidural space, the anterior internal vertebral plexus has been found to be localized between the two layers of the PLL (15). The posterior internal vertebral plexus is located in the epidural

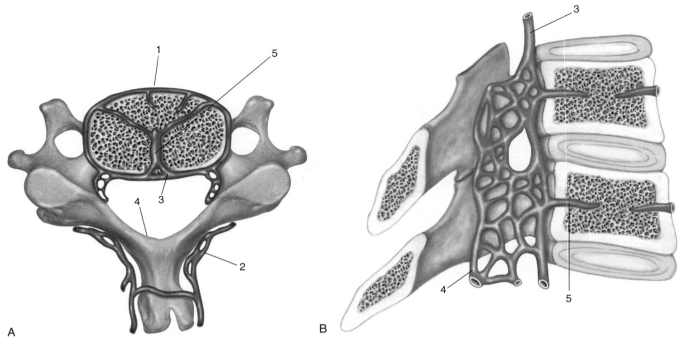

FIG. 1.20. A and **B:** Vertebral column venous plexus in sagittal and transverse sections. (*1*) Anterior external venous plexus, (*2*) posterior external venous plexus, (*3*) anterior internal plexus, (*4*) posterior internal plexus, (*5*) major drainage of body.

space, has connections with the anterior plexus, and receives the venous drainage from the dura. The intervertebral veins, through the intervertebral foramina, connect the internal venous drainage of the spinal cord and vertebral bodies with the vertebral veins, the deep cervical veins, the suboccipital venous plexus, and the external anterior and posterior vertebral venous plexus (24). The posterior external vertebral plexus consists of valveless veins located on the posterior surface of the vertebral arches. It drains into the deep cervical vein.

FASCIA AND MUSCULATURE OF THE CERVICAL SPINE

Cervical Fascia

Beneath the skin in the cervical spine is located the superficial fascia, which is continuous over the clavicle with the superficial fascia of the pectoral and deltoid regions. This layer is continuous around the entire neck and contains both the platysma and the external jugular vein. All fascia deep to the superficial fascia are considered deep cervical fascia (Fig. 1.21).

Deep to the superficial fascia, structures are anatomically compartmentalized by an organized deep fascia and potential interfascial spaces. This allows the complex motion and functions of the neck and its structures and allows dissection between fascial planes with an awareness of the structures that cross compartments. Descriptions and nomenclature vary in descriptions of the arrangement of

fascial layers in the cervical spine (21,24,29,42,46). In general, there are three principle deep layers: a superficial, middle, and deep layer, with some descriptions separating the middle layer into muscular and visceral compartments. Added to this group is the carotid sheath, the only paired compartment in the neck.

The investing layer, or superficial layer of the deep cervical fascia, surrounds all other fascial compartments in the neck. Superiorly, it is attached to the external occipital protuberance, the superior nuchal line, the ligamentum nuchae, and the spinous processes of the cervical vertebrae. Anteriorly and medially, it is attached to the mastoid process and the lower border of the mandible as well as the zygomatic arch, the styloid process, and hyoid bone. Its inferior attachments are to the clavicle, the sternum, the acromion, and the spine of the scapula. In its circumferential pattern, it divides to surround both the trapezius and the sternocleidomastoid and forms the roof of the posterior and anterior triangles of the neck. About the sternum, it divides into a superior and deep layer, which attaches to the front and back of the manubrium. The interval between these two fascial layers is termed the *suprasternal space.*

The middle cervical fascia, or the middle layer of deep fascia, encases the infrahyoid or strap muscles of the cervical spine. It is the most anterior fascial compartment inside the outer investing layer of fascia and is just anterior to the visceral compartment of fascia. It joins the visceral fascia at musculature insertions.

The carotid sheath encases the carotid artery, the internal jugular vein, and the vagus nerve. It is located lateral to the

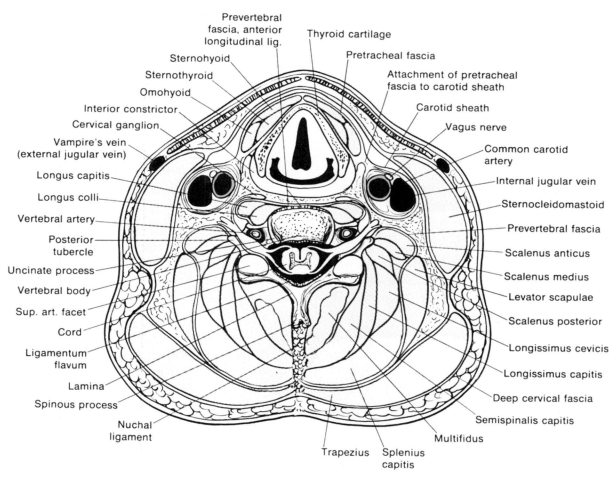

FIG. 1.21. Representation of fascial layers of the cervical spine at levels of C5 in cross section. (From: Hoppenfeld S, deBoer P. *Surgical exposures in orthopaedics: the anatomic approach,* 2nd ed. Philadelphia: JB Lippincott, 1994, with permission.)

visceral compartment and anterior to the prevertebral fascial compartment. The carotid sheath is fused with the investing fascia anterolaterally, and anteromedially it is fused with the pretracheal fascia. Posteriorly, it has a loose attachment with the prevertebral fascia. Branches of the external carotid artery leave the carotid sheath starting at the level of the upper border of the thyroid cartilage. The superior laryngeal branch of the vagus nerve travels behind both carotid arteries before leaving the carotid sheath and traveling to the visceral fascia and eventually dividing into its terminal branches. The hypoglossal nerve passes superficial to both carotid arteries, whereas the glossopharyngeal nerve passes between the carotid arteries, penetrating the carotid sheath. The cervical sympathetic chain is located on the longus colli and is related to the posterior surface of the carotid sheath; it is imbedded in the prevertebral fascia.

The pretracheal or visceral fascia (visceral middle layer of deep cervical fascia) surrounds the thyroid gland and forms its sheath. It surrounds the trachea and esophagus as well as the larynx and pharynx. At approximately the level of C6, the larynx meets the trachea and the pharynx meets

the esophagus. The retropharyngeal space is the space located between the prevertebral and visceral fascia at the pharyngeal level.

The prevertebral or deep layer of the deep cervical fascia encases the cervical spine and all musculature anteriorly and posteriorly associated with its movements. Posteriorly, it is attached to the ligamentum nuchae in the midline. Anteriorly, it is attached to the anterior longitudinal ligament of the anterior cervical spine and covers the longus capitis and colli muscles. Some authors refer to an additional fascial layer, the alar fascia, located anterior to the vertebral bodies between the prevertebral and pretracheal fascia. Laterally, the prevertebral fascia encases the scalenus muscles and attaches to the transverse processes of the cervical vertebrae and also forms the floor of the posterior triangle. As the brachial plexus and the subclavian artery course toward the axilla, they are encased within a prolongation of the prevertebral fascial layer, which forms the axillary neurovascular sheath (46). Superiorly, the prevertebral fascia attaches to the external occipital protuberance, the superior nuchal line, the mastoid process, and the base of the skull.

Inferiorly, it attaches to the outer aspects of the first and second rib in the thorax and the pleural dome.

Musculature

The musculature of the neck and cervical spine may be divided into the anterolateral and posterior muscle groups. These two groups then may be further subdivided.

Anterolateral Muscles

The anterolateral muscles may be divided into the superficial cervical, lateral cervical, suprahyoid, infrahyoid, anterior vertebral, and lateral vertebral muscles (29,46). The superficial cervical muscles of the cervical spine include the platysma anterolaterally and the trapezius posteriorly (Fig. 1.22). The platysma is a broad muscle originating from the superior fascia of the pectoral and deltoid region. It rises over the clavicle obliquely and travels superomedially across the neck, inserting on the mandible and the subcutaneous tissue and skin in the lower fascial region. The composition and thickness of the muscular fibers may vary. It acts to move the lip and corner of the mouth laterally and inferiorly and is innervated by the facial nerve.

The sternocleidomastoid originates from the sternal and clavicular heads to rise superiorly and laterally across the anterior lateral neck and insert into the lateral surface of the mastoid process. It acts to bend the head laterally to the same side and to rotate the head to the opposite side. The anterior fibers of both sides work together to flex the head, and the posterior fibers work to extend the head. The nerve supply is from the accessory spinal nerve (CN XI) and the second and third cervical nerves.

The suprahyoid muscles as a group raise the hyoid bone during swallowing and help in opening the mouth when the hyoid bone is stabilized by the infrahyoid muscles. The digastric muscle consists of an anterior and posterior belly; these bellies originate from the lower border of the mandible and the mastoid notch of the temporal bone, respectively. The two bellies end in a tendon that inserts on the body in the greater horn of the hyoid bone. The anterior belly is supplied by the trigeminal nerve (CN V), and the posterior belly is supplied by the facial nerve (CN VII). The stylohyoid muscle is located anteriorly and superiorly to the posterior belly of the digastric, arising from the styloid process and inserting on the body of the hyoid. It is supplied by the facial nerve (CN VII). The mylohyoid muscle is located just superior to the anterior belly of the digastric and is a flat, broad muscle that forms the floor of the oral cavity. It arises from the mylohyoid line of the mandible and inserts into a median raphe, where fibers from each side join, and into the body of the hyoid. This muscle is supplied by the trigeminal nerve (CN V). The geniohyoid lies medial to the mylohyoid, originating from the inferior mental spine of the symphysis menti, and inserts into the hyoid bone. It is supplied by the first cervical nerve via the ansa cervicalis.

The infrahyoid muscles act as a group to depress the larynx and hyoid after these structures have been raised with the pharynx during swallowing. The omohyoids act as an accessory respiratory muscle. The sternohyoid is a thin straplike muscle that arises from the medial aspect of

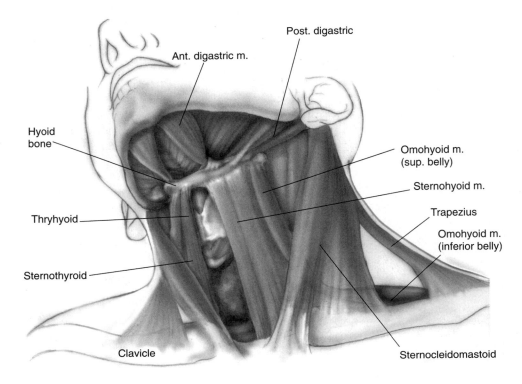

FIG. 1.22. Superficial muscles of the anterior neck.

Labels: Ant. digastric m. · Post. digastric · Hyoid bone · Thryhyoid · Sternothyroid · Clavicle · Omohyoid m. (sup. belly) · Sternohyoid m. · Trapezius · Omohyoid m. (inferior belly) · Sternocleidomastoid

the clavicle and the posterior manubrium and inserts into the body of the hyoid. The sternothyroid is located just posterior to the sternohyoid, arising from the posterior manubrium and the first rib and inserting into the oblique line in the lamina of the thyroid cartilage. The thyrohyoid arises almost as a continuation of the sternothyroid from the oblique line of the lamina of the thyroid cartilage. It inserts on the great horn of the hyoid bone. The omohyoid consists of an inferior and superior belly. The inferior belly arises from the scapula and superior transverse ligament of the scapular notch. It travels anteriorly, transversely, and slightly superiorly to a position behind the sternocleidomastoid, at which point it turns sharply and rises superiorly just lateral to the sternothyroid, inserting on the lower aspect of the hyoid bone. The infrahyoid muscles are all supplied by the first, second, and third cervical nerves via the ansa cervicalis, except for the thyrohyoid, which is supplied by the first cervical nerve.

The longus colli is located on the anterior aspect of the cervical spine (Fig. 1.23) and consists of three portions: The superior oblique portion originates from the anterior tubercle of the transverse processes of the third through

fifth cervical vertebrae and inserts on the tubercle of the anterior arch of the atlas; the inferior oblique portion arises from the anterior surface of the vertebral bodies T1 to T3 and inserts on the anterior tubercles of the transverse processes C5 to C6; and the vertical portion arises from the anterior bodies of C7 to T3 and inserts on the anterior bodies of C2 to C4. This muscle acts to flex the neck and allows some rotation of the cervical spine. It is supplied by the ventral rami of the second through sixth cervical spinal nerves.

The longus capitis originates from tendinous slips from the anterior tubercles of the transverse processes of the third through sixth cervical vertebrae, rising to insert on the basilar portion of the occipital bone. It is a flexor of the upper cervical spine and head and is supplied by the first through the third cervical spinal nerves.

The rectus capitis anterior, located just deep to the superior aspect of the longus capitis, originates from the anterior surface of the lateral mass and the root of the transverse process of C1. It inserts on the foramen magnum anteriorly and on the basilar portion of the occipital bone. This muscle flexes the head and stabilizes the atlantooccipital joint and

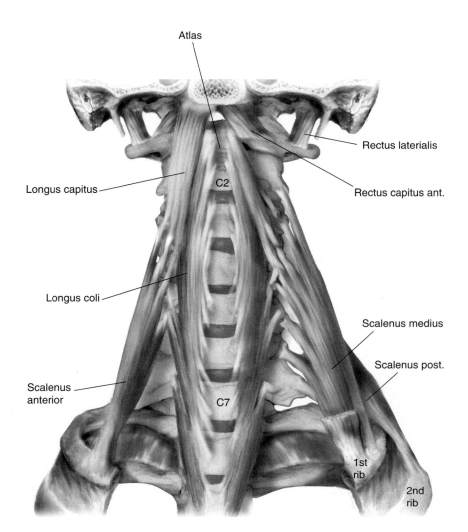

FIG. 1.23. Anterior and lateral vertebral muscles.

Atlas

Rectus laterialis

Longus capitus

C2

Rectus capitus ant.

Longus coli

Scalenus medius

Scalenus post.

Scalenus anterior

C7

1st rib

2nd rib

is supplied by the first and second cervical nerves. The rectus capitis lateralis originates from the superior surface of the transverse process of C1 and inserts on the inferior surface of the jugular process of the occipital bone. This muscle causes ipsilateral lateral bending of the head and stabilizes the atlantooccipital joint. It is supplied by the first and second cervical nerves.

The scalenus anterior lies deep to the sternocleidomastoid arising from the anterior tubercle of the transverse process of C3 to C6 and inserts on the scalene tubercle on the inner ridge of the upper aspect of the first rib (Fig. 1.23). It is supplied by the ventral rami of C5 and C6. The scalenus medius originates from the posterior tubercle of the transverse process of C2 through C7 and inserts on the upper first rib behind the subclavian groove. It is supplied by the ventral rami of C3 through C8. The scalenus posterior arises from the posterior tubercle of the transverse process at C4 through C6 and inserts on the outer surface of the second rib just deep to the attachment of the scalene anterior. It is supplied by C7 and C8. The subclavian vein crosses the first rib just anterior to the insertion of the scalenus anterior, and the subclavian artery crosses the first rib behind the scalenus anterior in the subclavian groove. These muscles

as a group act to flex and rotate the neck while raising the rib on which they insert.

Posterior Muscles

The posterior musculature of the cervical spine and neck can be divided into superficial and deep groups. The deep group then can be subdivided into a superficial and deep layer. To this is added the muscles of the suboccipital region. The most superficial muscle on the posterior aspect of the neck is the trapezius (Fig. 1.24), which arises from the external occipital protuberance and the medial aspect of the superior nuchal line of the occipital bone, the spinous processes of C7-T1 through T12, the supraspinal ligament, and the ligamentum nuchae. It has a complex insertion on the clavicle, the acromion, the spine, and the tubercle of the scapula. Its actions relative to the neck are that it draws the head to the same side and turns the face to the opposite side. The trapezius also draws the head backward into extension when both sides act together. Where the two muscles from each side join in the midline, they are attached to the spinous processes of the cervical and thoracic region by a long triangular aponeurosis. The muscle is supplied by the

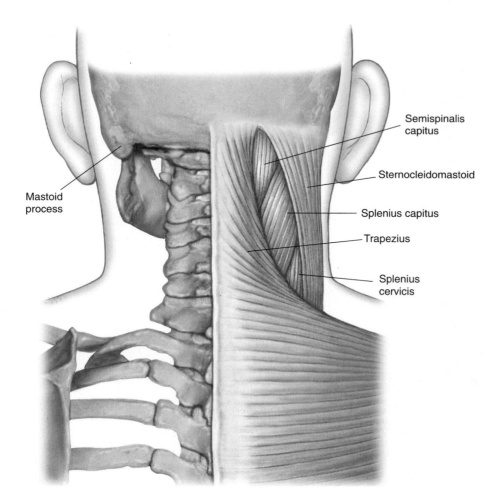

Mastoid process

Semispinalis capitus

Sternocleidomastoid

Splenius capitus

Trapezius

Splenius cervicis

FIG. 1.24. Superficial muscles of the posterior neck.

spinal accessory nerve (CN XI) and the third and fourth cervical nerves.

The superficial layer of the deep cervical musculature can be called the *transversocostal group* of muscles (Figs. 1.25 and 1.26). All muscles are supplied by the dorsal rami of the cervical nerves. The splenius capitis arises from the ligamentum nuchae and spinous processes of C7 and T1 through T3 and inserts on the lateral portion of the occipital bone, the superior nuchal line, and the mastoid process of the temporal bone. This muscle rotates the head to the same side and also extends the head. The splenius cervicis arises from the spinous processes of T3 through T6, rising to insert on the transverse processes of C1 through C3. This muscle rotates the cervical spine to the same side and may extend the neck. The erector spinae of the cervical region are divided into lateral, internal, and medial divisions. The iliocostalis cervicis of the lateral division arises from the angles of the third, fourth, fifth, and sixth ribs, rising to insert on the posterior tubercles of the transverse processes of C4 through C6. This muscle acts to extend, laterally flex, and rotate the spine in the cervicothoracic region. Like all muscles in the erector spinae group, this muscle is supplied by dorsal primary divisions of the spinal nerves. The longissimus cervicis of the intermediate division arises from tendinous slips off the tips of the transverse processes of T1 through T5 and inserts onto the posterior tubercles of the transverse processes of C2 through C6. It acts to extend and laterally bend the vertebral column. The medial division of the erector spinae includes the splenius cervicis and the splenius capitis, which arises from the spinous processes of C7 and at times T1 and T2 and inserts into the spinous process of C2 and at C3 and C4. It is just medial to and sometimes indistinguishable from the semispinalis capitis

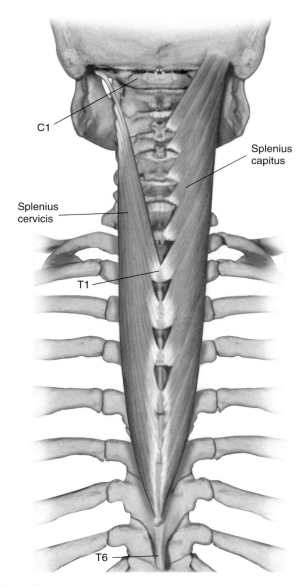

FIG. 1.25. Superficial layer of the deep cervical musculature of the posterior neck.

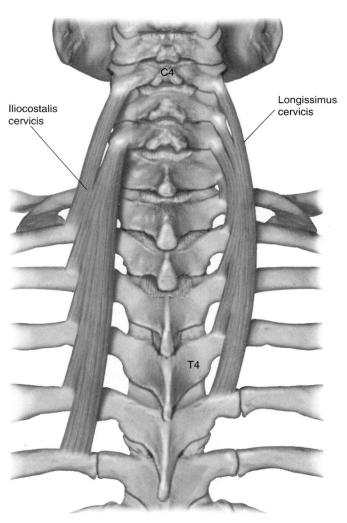

FIG. 1.26. Superficial layer of the deep cervical musculature of the posterior neck.

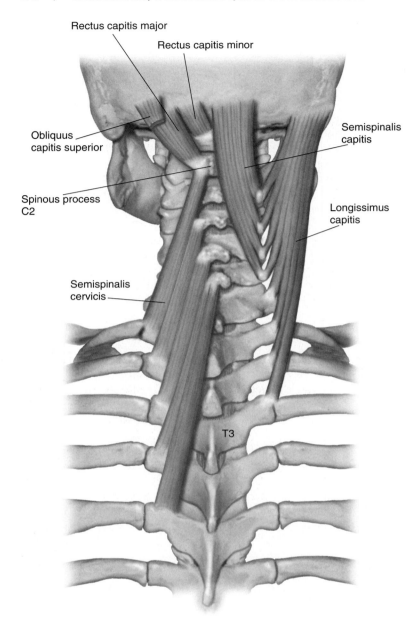

FIG. 1.27. Deep layer of deep posterior cervical musculature.

and originates and inserts with it. These two muscles extend the vertebral column.

The deep layer of the deep cervical musculature is termed the *transversospinal group* (Fig. 1.27). The semispinalis cervicis arises from the transverse processes of T1 through T5 and inserts into the spinous processes of C2 through C5. The semispinalis capitis, which overlies the semispinalis cervicis, lies deep to the splenius and just medial to the longissimus muscles. It arises from the transverse processes of C7 through T6 and from the articular processes of C4 through C6 and inserts between the superior and inferior nuchal lines of the occipital bone. The semispinalis cervicis extends and rotates the vertebral column to the opposite side, whereas the semispinalis capitis extends and rotates the head to the opposite side. Both are supplied by dorsal primary divisions of cervical nerves.

The multifidus muscles lie deep to the semispinalis cervicis in the cervical spine and arise from the articular processes of the lower four cervical vertebrae. The muscles ascend obliquely, ascending two to five vertebral levels, and insert on the spinous process at the higher level. The multifidus muscles laterally flex, extend, and rotate the vertebral column to the opposite side. They are supplied by the dorsal primary divisions of the cervical spinal nerves. The rotatores are just deep to the multifidus; they arise from the transverse processes of one vertebra and ascend to insert either on the spinous process of the next vertebra above (breves) or the spinous process of two above (longi). They rotate the vertebral column to the opposite side and are supplied by dorsal primary divisions of the spinal nerves.

The interspinale-intertransverse group are muscles that pass from one vertebral segment to the next (Fig. 1.28). The interspinale cervicis consists of six pairs of muscles that

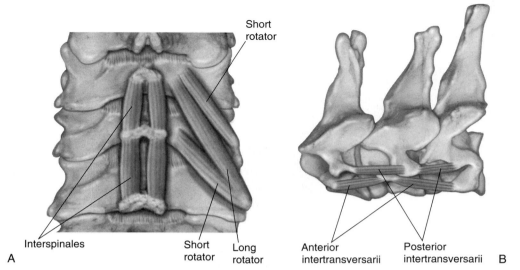

FIG. 1.28. A and **B:** The interspinale-intertransverse group of short muscles on the posterior cervical spine.

segmentally connect the spinous processes of adjoining vertebrae from C2 through T2. These muscles act to extend the cervical spine. The intertransverse cervicis consists of paired anterior and posterior muscles connecting the anterior and posterior tubercles of contiguous transverse processes, respectively. These muscles allow lateral bending and extension of the vertebral column and are supplied by both ventral and dorsal primary rami spinal nerves.

The suboccipital muscles consists of four paired muscles lying deep to the semispinalis cervicis in the most cephalad portion of the dorsal cervical region (Fig. 1.29). The rectus capitis posterior major originates from the spinous process of C2, ascending to insert on the lateral part of the inferior nuchal line of the occipital bone and the bone just below

this line. This muscle extends the head and rotates it to the same side. The rectus capitis posterior minor lies just medial to the major and passes from the tubercle on the posterior arch of the atlas to the inferior nuchal line and the portion of the occipital bone just medial to it. This muscle acts to extend the head. The obliquus capitis inferior arises from the apex of the spinous process of the axis and inserts into the inferior and dorsal aspect of the transverse process of the atlas. This muscle rotates the head to the same side via its effect on the atlas. The obliquus capitis superior arises from the superior surface of the transverse process of the atlas, blending with the insertion of the obliquus capitis inferior. It rises to insert on the occipital bone between the superior and inferior nuchal lines and extends the head and

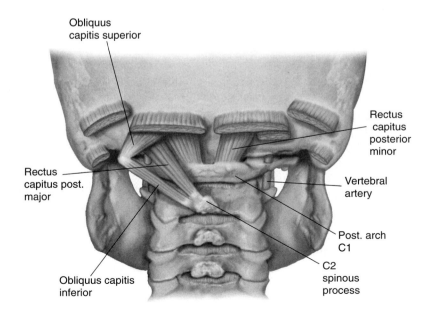

FIG. 1.29. Suboccipital muscles.

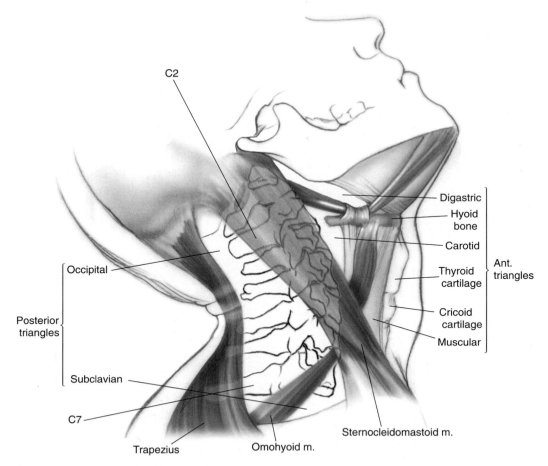

FIG. 1.30. Triangles and surface anatomy of the neck.

bends it to the same side. All the muscles in the suboccipital region are supplied by a branch of the dorsal primary rami of the suboccipital nerve.

The region between the obliqui and the rectus capitis posterior major is termed the *suboccipital triangle*. It is situated deep to the semispinalis capitis, and its floor is formed by the posterior atlantooccipital membrane and the posterior arch of the atlas. Its contents include the vertebral artery and the suboccipital nerve (the dorsal rami of the first cervical nerve).

Triangles of the Neck

The sternocleidomastoid divides the cervical region into two anatomic compartments called the *anterior* and *posterior triangles* (Fig. 1.30). The anterior triangle is bound by the midline anteriorly, the anterior border of the sternocleidomastoid posteriorly, and the inferior border of the mandible superiorly. It is subdivided into the submandibular (or digastric), carotid, and muscular triangles.

The submandibular triangle is bound by the two bellies of the digastric muscle and the inferior border of the mandible. It contains a submandibular gland, facial artery and vein, mylohyoid artery and nerve, and, in the posterior region, a portion of the parotid gland and the external

carotid artery. The internal carotid artery, jugular vein, and glossopharyngeal and vagus nerves are deeper in the triangle. The remaining anterior triangle is divided by the superior belly of the omohyoid muscle into the carotid and muscular triangles.

The contents of the carotid triangle (located above the omohyoid) include the common carotid artery and its bifurcation and the internal jugular vein, all of which are overlapped by the anterior border of the sternocleidomastoid. The superior thyroid, lingual, and facial branches of the external carotid artery; portions of cranial nerves X, XI, and XII; the larynx; pharynx; and the superior laryngeal nerve with its terminal branches, as well as the ansa cervicalis, are all found in this region. Sometimes included as a subdivision of the anterior triangle is the submental triangle, which forms directly above the hyoid bone between the right and left anterior bellies of the digastric muscles.

The posterior triangle of the cervical region is bound anteriorly by the posterior border of the sternocleidomastoid, inferiorly by the middle third of the clavicle, and posteriorly by the anterior border of the trapezius muscle. The inferior belly of the omohyoid divides the posterior triangle into the occipital and omoclavicular or subclavian triangles. The contents of the posterior triangle include the accessory nerve, the brachial plexus, the third part of the subclavian artery, the dorsal scapular nerve, the long thoracic nerve, the nerve to the subclavius, the suprascapular nerve, and the transverse cervical artery. A line drawn from the posterior margin of the sternocleidomastoid at the level of the cricoid cartilage to the midpoint of the clavicle usually indicates the location of the brachial plexus and the posterior triangle of the neck (42). The brachial plexus lies deep to both the investing and prevertebral layer of fascia. The accessory nerve lies on the levator scapula on the floor of the posterior triangle. This roof is pierced by the lesser occipital, greater auricular, and supraclavicular nerves, all of which emerge just behind the posterior border of the sternocleidomastoid muscle. The subclavian artery lies inferior to the inferior belly of the omohyoid in the omoclavicular triangle as it courses from its origin at the medial border of the anterior scalene, behind the anterior scalene, and laterally toward the border of the first rib. Just posterior and anterior to this is located the brachial plexus, which traverses the inferior portion of the occipital triangle, crossing between the anterior and middle scalene muscles, behind the inferior belly of the omohyoid, over the first rib, and inferior to the clavicle.

SUPERFICIAL ANATOMY AND RELATED STRUCTURES OF THE CERVICAL SPINE

Anteriorly in the cervical spine, palpation of certain landmarks correlates well with cervical vertebral level. The carotid tubercle, an enlargement of the anterior tubercle of the transverse process of C6, can be palpated at times. In addition, the cricoid cartilage, which is easily palpable just beneath the thyroid cartilage, is located at the level of the C6 vertebral body. Usually, the hyoid bone is located at the level of the C2-3 intervertebral disc, and the superior aspect of the thyroid cartilage is located at the level of the C4-5 intervertebral disc (Fig. 1.30).

Structures in the neck other than those already discussed deserve to be mentioned because of their importance in the understanding of the pathoanatomy of certain clinical conditions or in the surgical treatment of disorders of the cervical spine (Fig. 1.31). The thyroid gland is situated in the neck opposite cervical vertebrae 5 through 7. It is enclosed in a fibrous capsule and has a sheath that is derived from the pretracheal layer of the deep cervical fascia. It consists of two lobes connected by an isthmus in the midline, with the isthmus lying anterior to the trachea at

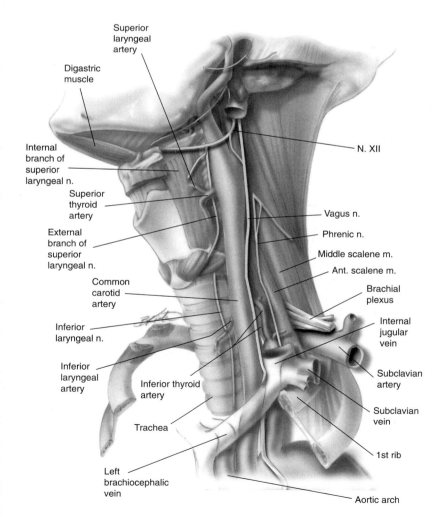

FIG. 1.31. Relations between important nerves and vascular structures of the lateral neck.

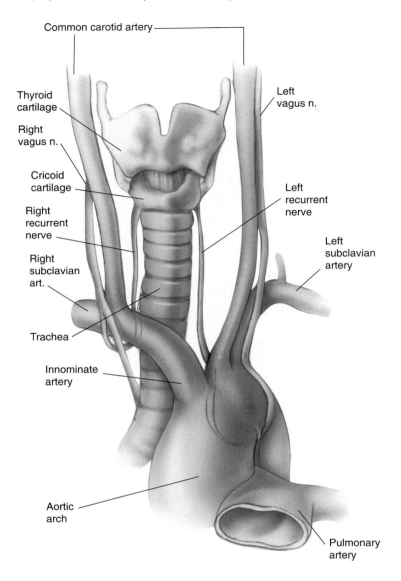

Common carotid artery

Thyroid cartilage

Right vagus n.

Cricoid cartilage

Right recurrent nerve

Right subclavian art.

Trachea

Innominate artery

Aortic arch

Left vagus n.

Left recurrent nerve

Left subclavian artery

Pulmonary artery

FIG. 1.32. Course of the recurrent laryngeal nerves.

approximately the level of the second, third, and fourth tracheal rings. The level of the inferior thyroid artery's entrance into the right thyroid lobe usually coincides with the right recurrent laryngeal nerve's entrance into the tracheoesophageal groove. Both the trachea and the esophagus continue from their respective laryngeal and pharyngeal origins at the level of C6. The trachea is related anteriorly to the esophagus, which in turn is related anteriorly to the longus colli and cervical vertebral bodies.

The common carotid artery arises from the brachiocephalic trunk on the right and on the left directly from the arch of the aorta. The common carotid usually does not give off any branches in the neck and divides at the level of C4 beneath the sternocleidomastoid. Before its division, it is crossed by the omohyoid at the level of the cricoid cartilage (C6), above which it lies under the anterior border of the sternocleidomastoid. The external carotid artery begins in the carotid triangle, where it is partly covered by the sternocleidomastoid and crossed by the hypoglossal nerve.

Its most relevant branch in the neck is the superior thyroid artery, which originates below the level of the tip of the greater horn of the hyoid bone and under the cover of the sternocleidomastoid. It runs forward in the carotid triangle deep to the omohyoid, sternohyoid, and sternothyroid and is related to the external laryngeal nerve. It enters the thyroid gland at its apex and divides into multiple branches.

The glossopharyngeal nerve (CN IX) is found in the submandibular region at the angle of the mandible, where it passes from behind the internal jugular vein, crosses between the internal and external carotid artery, passes deep to the styloid process and styloid muscles, curves forward around the stylopharyngeus deep to the hyoglossus, and enters the constrictors of the pharynx. The vagus nerve descends in the neck within the carotid sheath between the internal jugular vein and the carotid artery. The superior laryngeal branches of the vagus pass deep to both the internal and external carotid artery and leave the carotid sheath traveling with the superior thyroid artery and then dividing into internal and external branches prior to entering the visceral fascia. The internal branch of the superior laryngeal nerve is sensory and supplies the mucosa of the larynx above the vocal folds. It is important in initiating the cough reflex. The external branch supplies the motor function to the cricothyroid muscle.

The recurrent laryngeal nerves innervate all laryngeal muscles except the cricothyroid and supply the mucous membrane of the larynx below the vocal folds (Fig. 1.32). These nerves arise from different levels on each side of the body secondary to the different embryologic development of the aortic arches. The right recurrent laryngeal nerve leaves the carotid sheath more proximally than the left, winds around the first part of the subclavian artery, and enters the tracheoesophageal groove in the visceral fascia at approximately the level of the inferior thyroid arteries' entrance to the thyroid gland. Although the right recurrent laryngeal nerve usually runs in front of and lateral to the inferior thyroid artery, this relationship is variable. The left recurrent laryngeal nerve leaves the vagus at the level of the aortic arch, loops beneath the ligamentum arteriosum, and then arises in the tracheoesophageal groove to reach the larynx. In 0.5% to 1% of the population, the right recurrent laryngeal nerve may leave the vagus at the level of C6 and go directly to the larynx (47). In this situation, it is termed a *nonrecurrent* or *inferior laryngeal nerve*. This is sometimes, although not always, associated with an anomaly of the right subclavian artery.

The hypoglossal nerve supplies the motor function of the tongue. In the upper cervical spine, it crosses anterior to both the internal and external carotid artery and beneath the occipital artery. It then travels superficial to the hyoglossal and passes deep to the digastric and myoglossal muscles. It enters the tongue between the hyoglossal and myoglossal.

The cupula pleura is the pleura covering the apex of the lung as it projects into the neck through the thoracic inlet. It is a continuation of the costal and mediastinal pleura and begins at the internal border of the first rib, rising to a level from 2.5 to 5.0 cm above the sternal end of the first rib (46). Thus, its superior limit in the neck is at the level of the spinous process of C7, or approximately 3 cm above the medial third of the clavicle (42,46). The cupula pleura is covered by a superior extension of the endothoracic fascia termed the *suprapleural membrane (Sibson fascia)*. Muscular fibers extending from the transverse process of C7 to the fascia supporting the cupula pleura and the inner border of the first rib are termed the *scalenus pleuralis* or *scalenus minimus muscle* (46).

The cervical portion of the sympathetic trunk consists of three or four ganglia connected by an intervening cord or cords in a complex and variable arrangement (Fig. 1.33). The superior cervical ganglion extends from the level of the first to the second or third cervical vertebra lying behind the internal carotid artery on the surface of the longus capitis muscle. The middle cervical ganglion is usually located at

the level of C6, with the vertebral ganglion commonly found at the level of C7. The cervicothoracic or stellate ganglion is usually found at the level of C7 or T1, anterior to the spinal nerves exiting at these levels. It lies anterior to the seventh cervical transverse process and posterior to the vertebral artery. Because the longus colli muscles diverge laterally in the lower cervical spine whereas the sympathetic trunk converges medially at C6, the sympathetic trunk is more vulnerable to injury during anterior lower cervical spine procedures: The sympathetic trunk is closer to the medial border of the longus colli at C6 than at C3 (48).

Preganglionic autonomic fibers in the cervical sympathetic trunk originate from the gray matter of the upper thoracic spinal cord, reaching the thoracic part of the sympathetic trunk via rami communicantes from thoracic ventral roots and then ascending to the cervical portion of the sympathetic

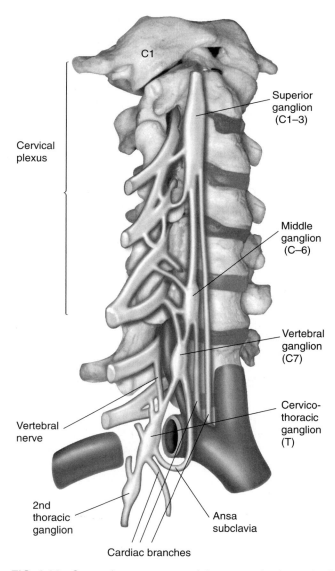

FIG. 1.33. General arrangement of the sympathetic trunk of the right lateral aspect of the cervical spine.

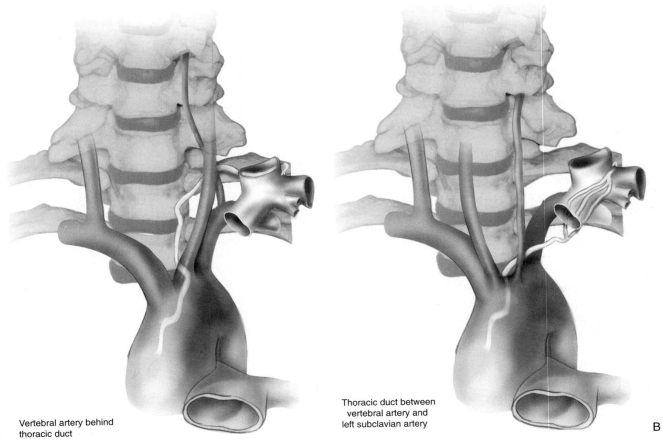

Vertebral artery behind
thoracic duct

A

Thoracic duct between
vertebral artery and
left subclavian artery

B

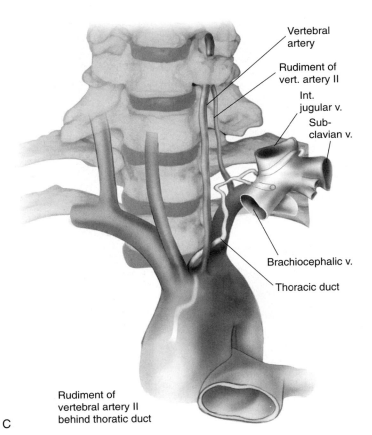

Vertebral
artery

Rudiment of
vert. artery II

Int.
jugular v.

Sub-
clavian v.

Brachiocephalic v.

Thoracic duct

Rudiment of
vertebral artery II
behind thoratic duct

C

FIG. 1.34. A, B, and **C:** Variations in the relation of the thoracic duct to the great vessels and its entrance into the venous system. (From: Lang J. *Clinical anatomy of the cervical spine.* New York: Thieme Medical Publishers, 1993, with permission.)

trunk. Postganglionic fibers communicate with the cervical spinal nerves at the level of the primary rami via rami communicantes. The sympathetic fibers from the vertebral and cervicothoracic ganglia to the vertebral artery form a vertebral plexus that accompanies the artery as it ascends the cervical spine. Some fibers also form the vertebral nerve, a separate nerve located posterior to the vertebral artery that ascends to the level of C1 or C2.

The thoracic duct passes through the thoracic inlet and arches laterally at the level of C7 (Fig. 1.34). It passes in front of the sympathetic trunk, the vertebral artery, the phrenic nerve, and the scalenus anterior, separated from these structures by the prevertebral layer of fascia. The duct is located posterior to the common carotid artery, the vagus nerve, and the internal jugular vein. It ends by opening into either the junction of the left internal jugular and subclavian vein or one of these structures individually. The thoracic duct receives lymph from the left side of the head and neck and most of the body.

The ansa cervicalis, located on the surface of the carotid sheath anteromedially, possesses a superior root that connects it with the hypoglossal nerve and an inferior root that connects it with branches of the second and third cervical nerves. The phrenic nerve arises chiefly from the fourth cervical spinal nerve but may receive an accessory root from the fifth cervical nerve and fibers from the third cervical spinal nerve. It is formed at the lateral border of the scalenus anterior and runs vertically and inferiorly across the front of the scalenus anterior beneath the anterior jugular vein and the sternocleidomastoid. It is located behind the prevertebral fascia and is crossed by both the transverse cervical and suprascapular arteries. The ascending cervical artery may be located medially, and the phrenic nerve passes between the subclavian artery and vein and continues on its course into the thorax.

REFERENCES

1. Oh S-H, Perin NI, Cooper PR. Qualitative three-dimensional anatomy of the subaxial cervical spine: implication for anterior spinal surgery. *Neurosurgery* 1996;38:1139–1144.
2. Panjabi M, Duranceau J, Goel V, et al. Cervical human vertebrae. Quantitative three-dimensional anatomy of the middle and lower regions. *Spine* 1993;16:861–874.
3. Xu R, Burgar A, Ebraheim NA, et al. The quantitative anatomy of the laminas of the spine. *Spine* 1999;24:107–113.
4. Czervionke LF, Daniels DL, Ho PSP, et al. Cervical neural foramina: correlative anatomic and MR imaging study. *Neuroradiology* 1988; 169:753–759.
5. Stubbs D. The arcuate foramen: variability in distribution related to race and sex. *Spine* 1992;17:1502–1504.
6. Heller JG, Alson MD, Schaffler MB, et al. Quantitative internal dens morphology. *Spine* 1992;17:861–966.
7. An HS, Gordin R, Renner K. Anatomic considerations for plate-screw fixation of the cervical spine. *Spine* 1991;16(Suppl): S548–S551.
8. Heggeness M, Doherty B. The trabecular anatomy of the axis. *Spine* 1993;18:1945–1949.
9. Leone A, Cerase A, Cesare C, et al. Occipital condylar fractures: a review. *Radiology* 2000;216:635–644.
10. Xu R, Ebraheim N, Yeasting R. Anatomy of C7 lateral mass and projection of pedicle axis on its posterior aspect. *J Spinal Disord* 1995;8:116–120.
11. Jones EL, Heller JG, Silcox DH, et al. Cervical pedicle screws versus lateral mass screws: anatomic feasibility and biomechanical comparison. *Spine* 1997;22:977–982.
12. Panjabi M, Oxland T, Parks E. Quantitative anatomy of the cervical spine ligaments. Part I: upper cervical spine. *J Spinal Disord* 1991;4:2 70–276.
13. Dvorak J, Panjabi M. Functional anatomy of the alar ligaments. *Spine* 1987;12:183–189.
14. Hayashi K, Yabuki T, Kurokawa T, et al. The anterior and the posterior longitudinal ligaments of the lower cervical spine. *J Anat* 1977;124: 633–636.
15. Kubo Y, Waga S, Kojima T. Microsurgical anatomy of the lower cervical spine and cord. *Neurosurgery* 1994;34:895–902.
16. Tanaka N, Fujimoto Y, An HS, et al. The anatomic relation among the nerve roots, intervertebral foramina, and intervertebral discs of the cervical spine. *Spine* 2000;25:286–291.
17. Yu S, Sether L, Haughton VM. Facet joint menisci of the cervical spine: correlative MR imaging and cryomicrotomy study. *Radiology* 1987;164:79–82.
18. McLain R. Mechanoreceptor endings in human cervical facet joints. *Spine* 1994;19:495–502.
19. Milne N. The role of zygapophyseal joint orientation and uncinate processes in controlling motion in the cervical spine. *J Anat* 1991; 178:189–201.
20. Panjabi M, Oxland T, Parks E. Quantitative anatomy of the cervical spine ligaments. Part II: middle and lower cervical spine. *J Spinal Disord* 1991;4:277–285.
21. Yeager VL, Cooper MH. Surgical anatomy of the cervical spine surrounding structures. In: Young PH, ed. *Microsurgery of the cervical spine*. New York: Raven Press, 1991.
22. Yoganandan N, Kumaresan S, Pintar FA. Geometric and mechanical properties of the human cervical spine ligaments. *J Biomech Eng* 2000;122:623–629.
23. Elliott HC. Cross-sectional diameters and areas of the human spinal cord. *Anat Rec* 1945;93:287–293.
24. Lang J. *Clinical anatomy of the cervical spine*. New York: Thieme Medical Publishers, 1993.
25. Okada Y, Ikata T, Katoh S, et al. Morphologic analysis of the cervical spinal cord, dural tube and spinal canal by magnetic resonance imaging in normal adults and patients with cervical spondylotic myelopathy. *Spine* 1994;19:2331–2335.
26. Kameyama T, Hashizume Y, Ando T, et al. Morphometry of the normal cadaveric cervical spinal cord. *Spine* 1994;19:2077–2081.
27. Payne E, Spillane P. The cervical spine: an anatomical-pathological study of 70 specimens (using a special technique) with particular reference to the problem of cervical spondylosis. *Brain* 1957;80:571–596.
28. Xu R, Ebraheim NA, Nadaud MC, et al. The location of the cervical nerve roots on the posterior aspect of the cervical spine. *Spine* 1995;20:2267–2271.
29. Hollingshead WH. *Anatomy for surgeons*, vol. 3, 3rd ed. Philadelphia: Harper and Row, 1982.
30. Parke WW, Watanabe R. Lumbosacral intersegmental epispinal axons and ectopic ventral nerve rootlets. *J Neurol* 1987;67:269–277.
31. Schwartz HG. Anastomoses between cervical nerve roots. *J Neurosurg* 1956;13:190–194.
32. Bogduk N. The clinical anatomy of the cervical dorsal rami. *Spine* 1982;7:319–320.
33. Groen G, Baljet B, Drukker J. Nerves and nerve plexuses of the human vertebral column. *Am J Anat* 1980;188:282–296.
34. Groen G, Baljet B, Drukker J. The innervation of the spinal dura mater: anatomy and clinical implications. *Acta Neurochir* 1988;92:39–46.
35. Bogduk N, Marsland A. The cervical zygapophyseal joints as a source of neck pain. *Spine* 1988;13:610–617.
36. Ferlic DC. The nerve supply of the cervical intervertebral disc in man. *Bull Johns Hopkins Hosp* 1963;113:247–251.
37. Ebraheim N, Lu J, Brown J. Vulnerability of vertebral artery in anterolateral decompression for cervical spondylosis. *Clin Orthop* 1996;322:146–151.
38. Vaccaro R, Ring D, Scuderi G. Vertebral artery location in relation to the vertebral body as determined by two-dimensional computed tomography evaluation. *Spine* 1994;19:2637–2641.
39. Chop P, de Miranda Neto NH, Lucas GA, et al. The vertebral artery: its relationship with adjoining tissues in its course intra and intertransverse processes in man. *Rev Paul Med* 1992;110: 245–250.

40. Sato K, Watanabe T, et al. Magnetic resonance imaging of C2 segmental type of vertebral artery. *Surg Neurol* 1994;41:45–51.

41. Dommisse GF. The blood supply of the spinal cord. *J Bone Joint Surg Br* 1974;56:225.

42. Gardner E, Gray D, O'Rahilly R. *Human anatomy*. Philadelphia: WB Saunders, 1975.

43. Althoff B, Goldie IF. The arterial supply of the odontoid process of the axis. *Acta Orthop Scand* 1977;48:622–629.

44. Schatzker J, Rorabeck CH, Waddell JP. Fractures of the dens (odontoid process): an analysis of thirty-seven cases. *J Bone Joint Surg Br* 1971;53:392–405.

45. Schiff DCM, Parke WW. The arterial supply to the odontoid process. *J Bone Joint Surg Am* 1973;55:1450–1456.

46. Clemente C, ed. *Gray's anatomy*, 30th American ed. Philadelphia: Lea and Febiger, 1985.

47. Sanders G, Uyeda RY, Karlan MS. Nonrecurrent inferior laryngeal nerves and their association with a recurrent branch. *Am J Surg* 1983;146:501–503.

48. Ebraheim NA, Lu J, Yang H, et al. Vulnerability of the sympathetic trunk during the anterior approach to the lower cervical spine. *Spine* 2000;25:1603–1606.

CHAPTER 2

Developmental Anatomy
of the Normal Cervical Spine

Henry H. Sherk

The normal processes that occur during the *in utero* development of the spine are governed by a single family of genes. These have been conserved with remarkable consistency since the Cambrian era 600 million years ago. They were first discovered in study of the chromosomes of fruit flies, which had developed mutations manifested by two sets of wings. These genes, known as the *homeobox* or *Hox genes,* regulate the sequential development of the midline axial structures of the individual, controlling differentiation and segmentation from the cranial to the caudal ends. Each homeotic gene product controls a domain of 60 amino acids, known as the *homeodomain,* and the coding sequence is known as the *homeobox.* In the fruit fly, normal sequential expression of the homeobox genes results in the development of the head and proboscis, then the antennae, and then the thorax and attached wings, followed by the development of the abdomen. The genes that control this orderly development are activated in sequence, and the timing of the expression of each gene allows for the normal development of the head, thorax, abdomen, and their related structures.

Mammals possess gene clusters similar to those of the fruit fly. These clusters, known as the Hoxa, Hoxb, Hoxc, and Hoxd genes, are found on chromosomes 7, 17, 12, and 2, respectively, in mice. As in the fruit fly, these genes are activated sequentially and are expressed maximally in neighboring segments of the developing individual. In mammals, however, the expression of the genes overlaps to a degree, so that a single genetic defect may not result in observable deformity of the spine or appendicular skeleton. In the fruit fly, the genetic control appears to be more structure specific.

The homeobox genes continue to be the focus of research on normal and flawed development of mammals and other species, and new knowledge continuously becomes available. The processes of development, however, have been studied and well understood. The remainder of this chapter focuses on the developmental anatomy of the spine, particularly the cervical spine, during embryonic, fetal, and postnatal life.

The spinal column develops largely through the process of enchondral ossification, which is the culmination of a chain of events beginning in the third week of gestation when mesenchyme differentiates out of the mesoderm into segmented somites. These structures develop on either side of the notochord; they distend the thin overlying ectoderm and are clearly visible as uniform blocks of tissues on either side of the developing individual (Fig. 2.1). During the fourth week of embryonic life, the somites differentiate into the sclerotome and myodermatomes. The former structure gives rise to the spinal column. The mesenchymal cells of the sclerotome migrate dorsally to give rise to the vertebral arches that eventually surround the spinal cord as the pedicles and laminae. Sclerotomal cells also migrate ventrally to form the vertebral bodies, discs, and costal processes (Fig. 2.2). At about 6 weeks of embryonic life, the sclerotomes undergo a metamorphosis, which heretofore has been termed the process of *resegmentation.* This event involves vertebration of the notochord and formation of discs to maintain flexibility and motion as well as to transmit the stresses of weight bearing (Fig. 2.3).

In resegmentation, the caudal half of one sclerotome is said to fuse with the cranial half of the adjacent sclerotome (Fig. 2.4), occurring at the same time that the mesenchyme of the sclerotomes migrates ventrally to surround the notochord. The combination of events results in formation of a vertebral body with intervertebral discs. This hypothesis focuses on the vertebral body as the major developmental spinal structure and implies that the intervertebral disc is a secondary element that arises from a splitting apart of the sclerotomes to permit motion of the spinal column. Resegmentation as a theory of development made it possible to

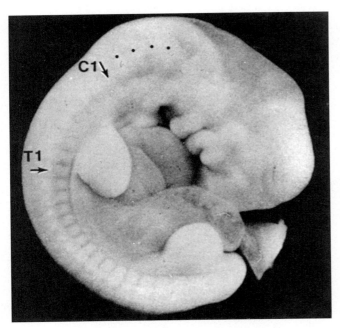

FIG. 2.1. A 5.5-mm human embryo showing the external manifestations of the somites. The relations of the cervical somites to the limb bud presage that the nerves will be involved in the brachial plexus. The black dots rostral to the cervical somites indicate the position of the precervical somites that will form the basiocciput.

explain the spanning of the discs by muscles of the myoder-matome to provide for voluntary motion. The muscles at each myodermatome, according to this theory, are related developmentally to the caudal half of the upper vertebra and the cranial half of the lower vertebra, crossing the intervertebral disc between the two halves.

The reality of spinal development is probably more complex. The intervertebral disc is probably the essential feature phylogenetically as well as ontologically, and the central portion of each sclerotome gives rise to the disc, which permits motion between vertebral segments. The vertebral body originates from a continuous mass of cells that surrounds the notochord to form a recognizable centrum. The caudal half of the more distal somite gives rise to a portion of the neural arch and the transverse process at each level, and the caudal half gives rise to the costal process. In the thoracic spine, this structure becomes a rib, but in the cervical and lumbar spine it forms part of the transverse process. The costal process component of the sclerotome also gives rise to the hypochordal bow. In the neck, this structure becomes the anterior arch of the atlas, but more distally it forms the thick portion of the anterior longitudinal ligament at each level. The costal process and the hypochordal bow are the vestiges of the hemal or ventral arch in other vertebrate species such as birds and reptiles. Voluntary motion activated by contraction of muscles

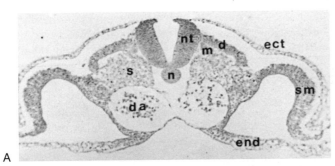

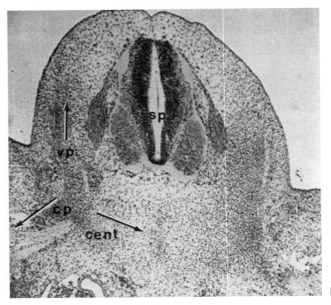

FIG. 2.2. A: Thoracic somite cross section from a 20-somite chick embryo. The neural tube (*nt*) lies dorsal to the nonsegmental notochord, and the somite shows its differentiation into the dermatome (*d*), myotome (*m*), and sclerotome (*s*). The endoderm (*end*) and ectoderm (*ect*) enclose the somatic meso-derm (*sm*) in the lateral region. **B:** Further development of the sclerotome into vertebral anlagen is indicated in the cross section of the mesenchymal (membranous) vertebra in a 9-mm pig embryo. This sclerotomal cell migration to preform the vertebra is indicated by a dorsal mass to form the vertebral process (*vp*), a ventral mass to form the centrum (*cent*), and a lateral mass to form the costal process (*cp*).

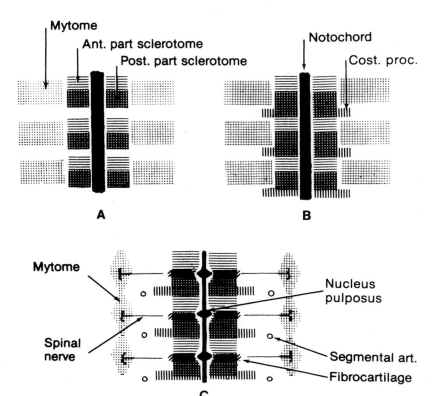

FIG. 2.3. Schema of the resegmentation of the vertebral primordia and their eventual relation with other segmented structures.

is made possible by the spanning of the segments by muscles that link the transverse processes of the proximal vertebra with the transverse processes of the subjacent one (Fig. 2.5).

Once the embryo has metamorphosed, the structure of the spinal column is established. The vertebral components are initially mesenchyme, but they rapidly begin the process of chondrification and then ossification. The former begins in the upper-level somites of the occiput and proceeds distally. Mesenchymal vertebral anlagen chondrifies in dual centers on either side of the notochord and in the base of the laminae. The process of ossification begins at the cervicothoracic junction and proceeds caudally and cranially. Ossification *in utero* takes place in five centers, replacing the cartilage of the chondrified vertebral anlagen. These five centers are the centrum of the vertebral body, the two neural arches, and the two costal processes. At birth in the cervical spine, the centrum, neural arches, and the costal processes at each level have ossified, but these structures have not fused (Figs. 2.6 and 2.7).

The formation of the upper cervical spine results in the development of the occipitoatlantoaxial complex, which although uniquely different from subaxial vertebrae reflects only a variation of the developmental process described earlier. The basiocciput arises from the fusion of the proximal occipital sclerotomes. These structures are perforated by the foramina of the roots to the twelfth (hypoglossal)

cranial nerve. The apex of the dens and its ligaments arise from the fusion of the "cervical 0" (C0) sclerotome and the C1 sclerotome. The central portion of the dens reflects the fusion of the C0 and the C1 sclerotomes. The anterior arch of the atlas is the enlarged hypochordal bow of the C0 sclerotome; with the anterior part of the lateral mass of the atlas, it is the first contribution of the costal process to the structure of the mature atlas. The dorsal arch of the atlas arises from the C0 and C1 sclerotomes. The atlas vertebra at birth is ossified only in the lateral masses, but ossification proceeds rapidly in the anterior and posterior arches on each side. These ossification centers usually fuse both dorsally and ventrally to complete the mature structure of the atlantal ring by late childhood (about 10 years); occasionally, however, a secondary ossification center develops in the anterior arch at age 6 years.

The apex of the dens with the associated apical and alar ligaments is the vertebral body formed by the contribution of the C4 through C0 somites. This structure does not ossify until midchildhood, and the relatively late ossification may cause some confusion in interpretation of anteroposterior and lateral roentgenograms in children.

The central portion of the odontoid process is formed by a continuous mass of cells about the notochord between the C0 and C1 sclerotomes. The apex of the dens and the dens proper form as a single structure. The main portion of the dens ossifies from paired ossific nuclei; just before birth,

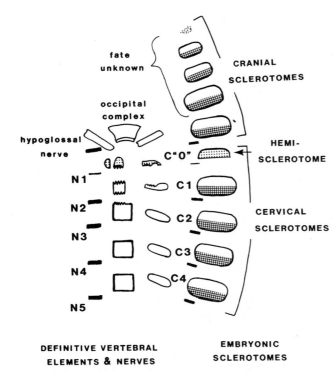

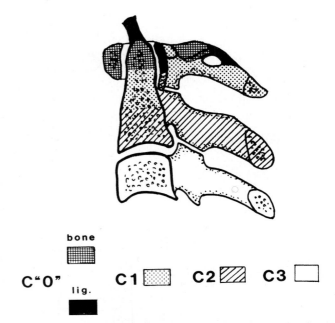

FIG. 2.4. Diagram of arrangement of the craniocervical sclerotomes and their segmentally related definitive vertebral elements and nerves. The cranial and cervical sclerotomes were most likely committed to the cervical region, but expansion of the brain case in amniotes incorporated them into the skull, along with their related nerves. (Preamniotes have only ten cranial nerves.) In mammals, the contributions of the cranial sclerotomes to the skull above the occiput have been lost or obscured, but the occipital complex, with its segmental hypoglossal nerve, is known to be of vertebral origin. With the simultaneous expansion of the skull and the requirements of increased craniocervical mobility, an "orphan" sclerotome, which is cranial in most reptiles and cervical in mammals, became the precursor to proatlas components; it is here designated the "cervical zero" (C0) sclerotome. Its derivatives, arising from only the cranial half of a sclerotome, would be primarily centrum and arch elements without disc primordia.

FIG. 2.5. The definitive contributions of the first three sclerotome segments to the atlantoaxial complex and its ligaments. The hemisclerotome C0 provides the upper part of the odontoid process, the hypochordal anterior arch, and the dorsal part of the superior atlas facet, as well as the alar, transverse (upper part), and retroarticular ligaments (shown in black). The conventionally designated C1 sclerotome then provides the remainder of the posterior arch and the inferior part of the odontoid process.

these nuclei fuse across the midline. At birth, therefore, the dens has a truncated oval appearance radiographically because the apical segment has not yet ossified and the dens has not fused into the vertebral body of the axis. The latter event does not occur until at least 4 years of age. The mesenchyme that forms the axis vertebral body arises in the second and third cervical segments. The expected intervertebral disc of the C1 sclerotome lying between the dens and axis does not develop. It is the analogue of the synchondrosis between the dens and axis. This structure disappears when the dens fuses to the axis vertebral body after age 4 years. The complexity of the upper cervical spine from the standpoint of this development may be a factor in the frequency of congenital malformations in this region (Fig. 2.8).

The primary ossific nuclei of the cervical spine have all developed and manifested themselves by the time the fetus reaches the end of fetal life. The nuclei rapidly enlarge and replace the chondrified portions of the spine until the secondary ossification centers appear. The first of these centers is the apical nucleus of the dens.

Additional ossification centers appear at the tips of the transverse processes and spinous processes. They usually manifest themselves by age 10 in girls and age 12 in boys. They enlarge to fill the cartilaginous anlage of the transverse or spinous processes and then fuse with the subjacent primary ossific nucleus at age 13 in girls and at age 17 in boys.

The vertebral ring epiphyses make their appearance at about the same time the transverse and spinous process secondary centers appear. These epiphyses give rise to the dense cortical bone rimming each of the vertebral bodies from the caudal surface of C2 distally to the cranial surface of S1. In the cervical spine, lateral roentgenograms clearly show their development first as a density anteriorly on the caudal surface of each vertebra and shortly thereafter on the cranial surface. At birth and in young children, the intervertebral disc appears deceptively large on roentgenograms,

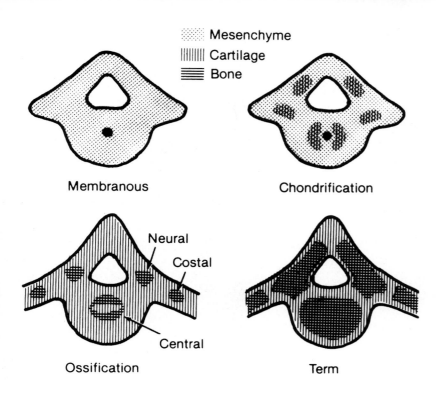

Mesenchyme
Cartilage
Bone

Membranous

Chondrification

Neural
Costal
Central

Ossification

Term

FIG. 2.6. Schematic of the sequential changes in the development of a vertebral element. The basic form of a vertebra preexists in two distinct types of tissue (membranous mesenchyme and cartilage) before the definitive ossification from the indicated centers occurs.

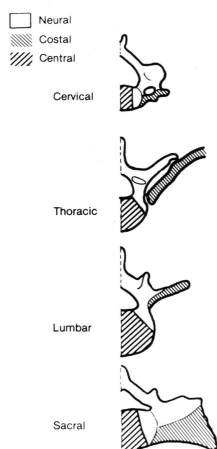

Neural
Costal
Central

Cervical

Thoracic

Lumbar

Sacral

FIG. 2.7. Regionally comparative schematic of the relative contributions of the three primary ossific centers to the typical vertebra of each of the four major spinal areas. The neurocentral synchondrosis lies well within the definitive body in all regions, but the neural ossific centers provide the greatest contribution to the body in the cervical region.

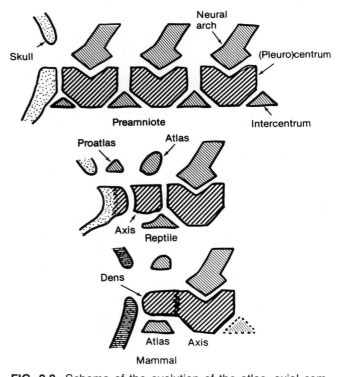

Skull

Neural arch

(Pleuro)centrum

Preamniote

Intercentrum

Proatlas   Atlas

Axis   Reptile

Dens

Atlas   Axis

Mammal

FIG. 2.8. Schema of the evolution of the atlas–axial complex. The progressive reduction in the number of elements illustrated indicates that several segments eventually became incorporated in the skull, whereas the most cranial of the definitive cervical elements formed the craniocervical articulations. The intercentrum (hypochordal bar) is considered the antecedent of the anterior arch of the atlas, and the proatlas may become represented by the apical secondary center of ossification for the dens.

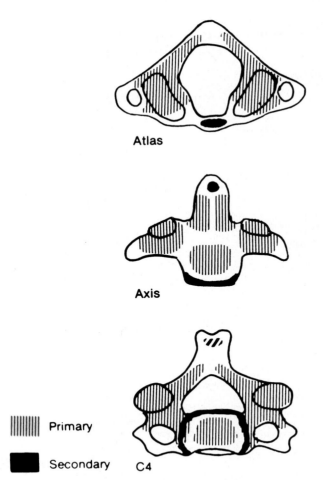

Atlas

Axis

Primary

Secondary   C4

FIG. 2.9. Schematic of the ossification centers in the cervical vertebrae. The first two cervical vertebrae have atypical numbers of ossific centers. The atlas has but two primaries that correspond to the neural arch centers of the conventional elements. The secondary center that forms in the anterior arch is considered the phyletic remnant of the hypochordal bar (intercentrum) of lower vertebrates. The axis has five primary and two secondary centers. The dens ossifies from bilobed centers representing the original central center of C1. The apical secondary center may be a developmental representation of the original proatlas. The inferior secondary center of the axis forms the ring apophysis, as in other vertebrae. The typical cervical vertebra, as represented here by C4, arises from the conventional three primary and two secondary centers for the ring apophysis. A secondary center of the tip of the spinous process (*cross-hatched*), although constant in more inferior elements, appears only sporadically in cervical vertebrae, being more frequent in the lower (C6, C7) elements.

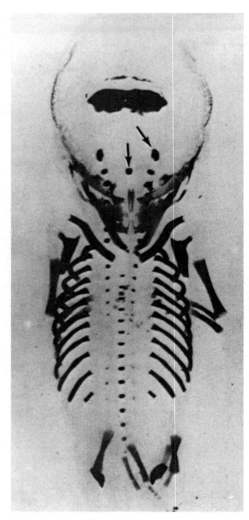

FIG. 2.10. A cleared alizarin-stained fetus of 54-mm crown–rump length (CRL). Differential commencement of ossification in various spinal regions is apparent. The center for the centrum is first to appear in the lower thoracic and lumbar regions, whereas the two neural arch centers appear first in the cervical region. Ossification centers for the occipital bone are indicated by arrows. The lateral two centers form the exoccipital contributions, and the central one gives rise to the basioccipital center.

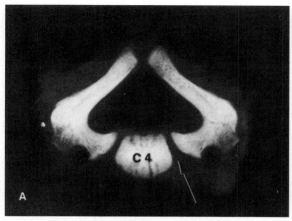

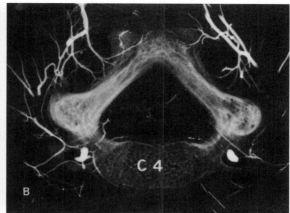

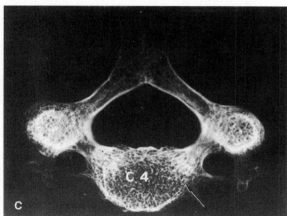

FIG. 2.11. Progressive ossification of cervical vertebrae, as typified by C4. **A:** The extent of ossification in a fetus of 34 weeks. The costal contribution shows no evidence of ossification. The neurocentral synchondrosis is more medially situated in cervical vertebrae (*arrow*), allowing a greater contribution to the centrum from the neural arch than that in more inferior segments. **B:** A roentgenogram of C4 from a 6-year-old cadaver that had been arterially injected with barium sulfate. The neurocentral synchondroses are still radiologically demonstrable (*arrow*), and the ossification of the costal contribution has completed the anterior part of the vertebral foramen. **C:** A vertical radiograph of C4 from an adult. The original position of the neurocentral synchondrosis is no longer radiologically discernible (*arrow*). The definitive tuberosities of the spine have formed, and the anterior and posterior tuberosities of the transverse processes are fully ossified. Although these tuberosities may be from secondary centers in the thoracolumbar region, only an occasional secondary center appears in the tuberosity of the spine in the cervical vertebrae.

and indeed the disc has been suggested to be wider in this age group than in adults. This appearance, however, results from a relatively small volume of visibly ossified material in the primary ossific nucleus. As that structure enlarges and fills more of the cartilaginous anlage and as the secondary ring of apophyses appears, the intervertebral disc takes on the normal adult size and proportion. A fusion of the secondary ring apophyses to the primary ossific nucleus of the vertebral bodies occurs at about age 13 in girls and age 17 in boys. This event marks the cessation of growth of this portion of the spine. Injuries and various disease states can cause premature closure or result in a delay of closure of the secondary physes and alter these normal patterns of maturation (Figs. 2.9 to 2.12).

The physeal anatomy of the cervical spine provides for the growth and enlargement of this portion of the spinal column. In this regard, it is of some interest that despite the considerable elongation and filling out of the neck from infancy to adult life, the cervical cord changes relatively little in diameter and length. The central nervous system—that is, the brain and spinal cord—have reached an advanced state of development at birth and therefore have less potential for growth than other body structures.

A late-developing anatomic feature of the subaxial spine is the appearance of the joints of Luschka. Histologic examination of the lateral and posterior margins of the intervertebral discs, even in very young subjects, shows that loose fibrous and vascular tissue occupies the space between the uncus projecting upward from the superior surface of the caudal vertebra and the echancrure of the inferior surface of the more rostral vertebra. In children, this area begins to show fissuring; as a person matures into adult life, the fissuring occupies a greater proportion of the intervertebral space. The cleft that develops in adults in this location, the joint of Luschka, has some of the characteristics of a synovial joint (a joint space containing synovial fluid between two bony surfaces and a fibrous and vascular matrix surrounding the joint space). At one time, a controversy arose concerning the nature of the joint of Luschka and whether it was a true joint or reflected only adaptive changes. It now appears that the cleft in the lateral margin of the cervical intervertebral discs develops normally in the process of maturation. The clefting proceeds with continued alteration in the chemistry of the proteoglycans of the disc; as a result, most normal people have extensive fissuring in the disc spaces. With continued aging, these changes grow more

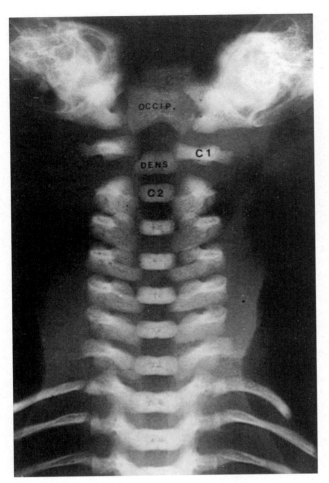

FIG. 2.12. Anteroposterior roentgenogram of a 30-week fetal cervical spine. The bilobed centers of ossification positioned about the central ossification of C2 constitute the dens. The intervening cartilage is the homologue of the first intervertebral disc, and its ossific replacement is frequently deficient in adults. Because no secondary centers are yet apparent, the apex of the dens and the arches of the atlas are represented only in cartilage.

evident and, accelerated by injury or disease, may produce structural changes (Fig. 2.13).

SELECTED READING

Angelvine JB. Clinically relevant embryology of the vertebral column and spinal cord. *Clin Neurosurg* 1973;20:95–113.

Bagnali KM, Harris PF, Jones PRM. A radiographic study of the human fetal spine. 2. The sequence of development of ossification centers in the vertebral column. *J Anat* 1977;124:791–802.

Bailey DK. The normal cervical spine in infants and children. *Radiology* 1952;59:712–719.

Barson AJ. The vertebral level of termination of the spinal cord during normal and abnormal development. *J Anat* 1970;106:489.

Dalgleish AE. A study of the development of thoracic vertebrae in the mouse, assisted by autoradiography. *Acta Anat* 1985;122:91–95.

Ehrenhaft JL. Development of the vertebral column as related to certain congenital and pathological changes. *Surg Gynecol Obstet* 1943;76:282.

Fesmire FM, Listen RC. The pediatric cervical spine: developmental anatomy and clinical aspects. *J Emerg Med* 1982;7:131–142.

Galis F. Why do almost all animals have seven cervical vertebrae? Developmental constraints, Hox genes, and causes. *J Exp Zool* 1999;285:19–26.

Hensinger RN. Osseous anomalies of the craniovertebral junction. *Spine* 1986;11:322.

Keynes RJ, Stern CD. Mechanisms of vertebrate segmentation. *Development* 1988;103:413–429.

MacAlister A. Notes on the developments and variations of the atlas. *J Anat Physiol* 1983;27:519.

McGinnis W, Krumlauf R. Homeobox genes and axial patterning. *Cell* 1992;68:283–302.

Moore KL. *The developing human*, 4th ed. Philadelphia: WB Saunders, 1988.

Noback CR, Robertson GG. Sequences of appearance of ossification centers in the human skeleton during the first five prenatal months. *Am J Anat* 1951;89:1.

Odgen JA. Postnatal development of the cervical spine. *Orthop Trans* 1982;6:89.

Pattern BM. Embryological states in the establishment of myeloschisis with spina bifida. *Am J Anat* 1953;93:365.

Rosier RN, Reynolds PR, O'Keefe RJ. Molecular and cell biology in orthopedics. In: Buckwalter JA, Einhorn TA, Simon SR, eds. *Orthopaedic basic science*, 2nd ed. Chicago: American Academy of Orthopedic Surgeons, 1999:19–76.

Sensenig EC. The early development of the human vertebral column. *Carnegie Contrib Embryol* 1949;33:21.

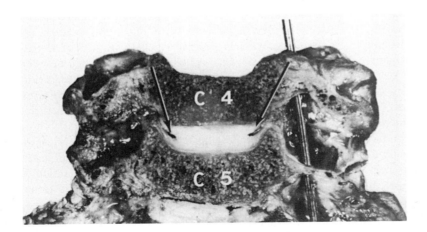

FIG. 2.13. Frontal section of a C4 disc, with arrows indicating the uncovertebral "joints." These do not appear until the latter part of the first decade and are not uniform with regard to the level or side of their occurrence.

Sensenig EC. The development of the occipital and cervical segments and their associated structure in human embryos. *Carnegie Contrib Embryol* 1957;36:143–151.

Sherk HH, Parke WW. Developmental anatomy of the cervical spine. In: Sherk HH, Dunn EJ, Eismont FJ, et al., eds. *The cervical spine*, 2nd ed. Philadelphia: JB Lippincott, 1989:1–33.

Subramanian V, Meyer BI, Grusc P. Disruption of the murine homeobox gene Cd x1 affects axial skeletal identities by altering the mesodemial expression domains of Hox genes. *Cell* 1995;83:641–653.

Synder RG, Schneider LW, Owings CL, et al. *Anthropometry of infants, children, and youths to age 18 for product safety design SP-450.* Warrendale, PA: Pennsylvania Society of Automotive Engineers, 1977.

Taylor JR. Growth of human intervertebral discs and vertebral bodies. *J Anat* 1975;120:49–68.

Vontorklus D, Gehle W. *The upper cervical spine.* New York: Grune & Stratton, 1972.

Weus LH. Congenital deficiency of the vertebral pedicle. *Anat Rec* 1963; 145:193.

CHAPTER 3

Functional Anatomy of Joints, Ligaments, and Discs

Alexander J. Ghanayem and Odysseas Paxinos

The human cervical spine has a unique anatomy adapted to accommodate the needs of the highly mobile head–torso transitory zone. Normal cervical motion in every plane, both simple and complex, is checked by anatomic restraints that protect the spinal cord and accompanying neurovascular structures. Most of the information on the protection provided by these restraints is derived from postmortem analysis of fatal cervical spine injuries and biomechanical studies of cadaveric specimens (1–4). Clinical and radiographic studies have also aided in defining the normal function of cervical joints and soft tissues (5–11). Disturbance of the anatomy or the physical and mechanical properties of the elements of the cervical spine may lead to clinical symptoms. The upper cervical spine segment (C0-C1-C2) and the lower cervical spine (C3 through C7) have distinct anatomic and functional features and are described separately.

UPPER CERVICAL SPINE

The upper cervical spine includes the occipitoatlantal (C0-C1) and the atlantoaxial (C1-C2) joint complexes (Figs. 3.1 to 3.3). Anatomic characteristics include the absence of intervertebral discs, the absence of ligamenta flava, and the distinct shape of C1 and C2. Motion is coupled between the two joints, which share a common embryonic origin. Instead of an intervertebral disc in the occipitoatlas level, the developmental process results in the formation of the apical and alar ligaments as well as the cranial portion of the dens. In the atlantoaxial level, the caudal part of the C1 somite and the cranial part of the C2 somite fuse to form the odontoid process. The odontoid process begins to fuse with the body of C2 at 4 years of age; this fusion is complete by age 7. Almost one-third of adults will have a remnant of cartilaginous tissue between the odontoid and the body of C2 (12).

Bony morphology and the attachments of ligaments that can span over two articulations define the kinematics of the C0-C1-C2 complex. The complex is responsible for 40% of total cervical flexion-extension and 60% of total cervical rotation. Although in this chapter functional anatomy is described separately for the C0-C1 and C1-C2 segments, one should remember that these two motion segments are intimately linked and the motion is coupled.

Occipitoatlantal Junction

Motion in the sagittal plane is the primary function at the occipitoatlantal junction and is reported on average as being between 13 degrees (13) and 25 degrees (10). The C0-C1 joints have a cup-shaped configuration that is deeper in the frontal plane. Flexion of C0-C1 is limited by the tip of the dens impinging on the anterior margin of the foramen magnum, on what Werne (13) has described as the bursa apicis dentis. The tectorial membrane inserts at the body of C2 and the anterior rim of the foramen magnum and limits extension. Flexion at C0-C1 rolls the upper part of the membrane taut, which limits further flexion at the C1-C2 level. Translation at this junction is minimal under normal conditions. Flexion and extension should result in no more than 1 mm of translation between the basion and tip of the dens (14).

Axial rotation and lateral bending in C0-C1 is limited to about 5 degrees on each side and is controlled by the capsules and the alar ligaments (Fig. 3.4). The alar ligaments are symmetrical on both sides and about 10 to 13 mm long, with one portion connecting the dens to the occiput and the remaining ligament connecting the dens to the atlas (15,16). During left lateral bending, the right upper component (connected to the occiput) and the left lower component (connected to the ring of C1) become taut. When the head

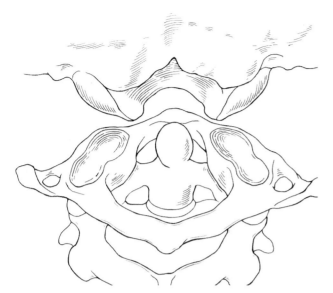

FIG. 3.1. Posterior view of the occipitoatlantal articulation. The occipitoatlantal articulation has been rotated forward to allow visualization of the articulation between the base of the skull and the saddle-type surface of the axis.

rotates to the left, both components of the right ligament become taut. The instantaneous axis of rotation (IAR) for the C0-C1 articulation has not been defined, although the x-axis is considered to pass through the mastoids and the z-axis is considered to be 2 to 3 mm above the tip of the dens.

Compressive sagittal plane translation (z-axis) is minimum under normal conditions because of the cup-shaped articular anatomy. Distraction of the joint complex is restricted mainly by the tectorial membrane, with minor contribution from the alar ligaments. The apical ligament and anterior and posterior atlantooccipital membranes have not been found to contribute against distraction (13,15,17–19).

Atlantoaxial Junction

The atlantoaxial (C1-C2) complex is composed of two facet joints and the unique atlantodental articulation. Stability at this highly mobile junction is primarily dependent on ligamentous structures. Sagittal plane motion (flexion-extension) in C1-C2 has been reported by several authors to be on average 11 degrees and may be facilitated by a rounded tip of the dens (8,13,20). Rotation in the upper cervical spine represents 60% of the entire cervical spine rotation and has been reported to be between 39 degrees (21) and 47 degrees (13) on each side. Lateral bending is negligible (13,21).

The IAR for sagittal plane motion is located in the region of the middle third of the dens, and for axial rotation it is located in the central axis of the dens (13). Posterior translation is prevented by mechanical abutment of the anterior portion of C1 on the dens. Anterior translation is prevented primarily by the transverse ligament (Fig. 3.4). The paired alar ligaments, through their anterior atlantodental component, provide secondary restraint (5,15). The accessory atlantoaxial ligaments and capsular ligaments are tertiary stabilizers. Up to 3 mm of anterior translation of C1 on C2, as measured at the anterior atlantodental interval (AADI), is normal (Fig. 3.2). Fielding and others noted that for this interval to increase, the transverse ligament must be attenuated (22). As the AADI increases to 5 mm or greater, the transverse ligament and accessory stabilizing ligaments have been ruptured. The transverse ligament also protects the atlantoaxial joint from a rotary dislocation. With the transverse ligament intact, a complete bilateral dislocation

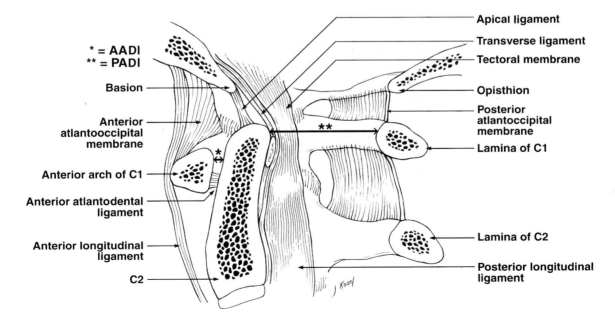

* = AADI
** = PADI

Apical ligament
Transverse ligament
Tectoral membrane
Basion
Opisthion
Posterior atlantooccipital membrane
Anterior atlantooccipital membrane
Lamina of C1
Anterior arch of C1
Anterior atlantodental ligament
Anterior longitudinal ligament
Lamina of C2
C2
Posterior longitudinal ligament

FIG. 3.2. Midsagittal section through the upper cervical spine.

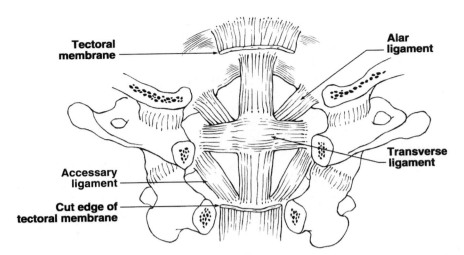

FIG. 3.3. Posterior view of the upper cervical spine. The lamina of C1 and C2, as well as the spinal cord, has been removed to allow visualization of the ligamentous structures.

can occur at 65 degrees of rotation. With transverse ligament disruption, dislocation can occur at 45 degrees of rotation. Finally, the paired alar ligaments also restrict rotary motion, since sectioning of one ligament will increase contralateral rotation (5,15,17–19).

As with the C0-C1 junction, distraction and compressive motion at the C1-C2 junction is indicative of an underlying pathologic process. Compression is limited by the lateral mass articulation of the C1-C2 joints. Unstable atlas ring fractures with disruption of the transverse ligament and erosive conditions of the lateral mass articulations can render the C1 ring incompetent to compressive loads and result in basilar invagination. The tectoral membrane and posterior atlantooccipital membrane limit distraction at the C1-C2 junction.

LOWER CERVICAL SPINE

The middle and lower cervical spine segments have essential similar anatomic and functional characteristics and can be effectively represented by the functional spinal unit (FSU). The FSU is defined as the smallest segment of the spine that exhibits biomechanical characteristics similar to those of the entire spine. It is composed of two vertebral elements, the intervertebral disc, and associated ligamentous and capsular structures (Fig. 3.5).

Compression of the lower cervical spine is resisted by the intervertebral disc, vertebral body, and, depending on the position of the spine, the facet joints. The C3 through C6 vertebral bodies have a concave upper and a convex lower surface. The lateral projections of the upper end plate are called *uncus* ("hook") and form the uncovertebral joints (joints of Luschka) with the corresponding convex lateral surface of the lower end plate of the superior vertebra. These joints support part of the axial load after disc degeneration. The average vertebral body size increases from C2 to C7, with width ranging from 15.6 to 23.4 mm and depth ranging from 15.6 to 18.1 mm. The average pedicle height is 7 mm, and average width is 5 to 6 mm. The angle made by the pedicle decreases from 40 degrees in C3 to 29 degrees in C7 (23). The laminae project posteromedially from the pedicles and form the spinous process in the midline, and the facets laterally. The articular surfaces of the facets

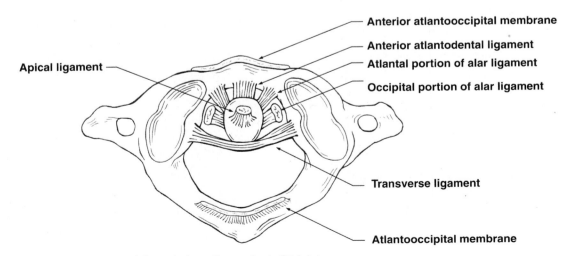

FIG. 3.4. Axial view of the axis from the occiput–C1 joint.

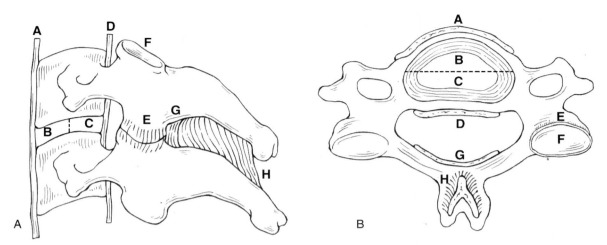

FIG. 3.5. Lateral **(A)** and axial **(B)** views of a functional spinal unit of the middle and lower cervical spine. The important anatomic structures are as follows: anterior longitudinal ligament (*A*), anterior disc and annulus (*B*), posterior disc and annulus (*C*), posterior longitudinal ligament (*D*), facet capsules (*E*), facet joints (*F*), ligamentum flavum (*G*), and interspinous ligament (*H*).

are inclined approximately 45 degrees from the horizontal plane and get steeper in the lower segments. The motion segments are connected and stabilized by the intervertebral disc, the ligaments, and the facet capsules.

Intervertebral Disc

Compressive forces are transferred through the intervertebral disc, the vertebral body, and the facet joints. The intervertebral disc is a viscoelastic material and its mechanical properties are dependent on the rate of loading. At low load rates the disc deforms and is more flexible, but at higher rates the disk becomes stiff (2). Degeneration and dehydration of the disc affect the viscoelastic characteristics (creep and relaxation). A degenerated disc will deform more and faster than a healthy disc, applying greater load to the periphery of the end plate through the annulus. The disc is the major compressive component of the spine, and the ability to tolerate vertical loading in excess of the failure point of the vertebral body is well documented (24,25). The tensile properties of the disc annulus are related to the orientation of the collagen fibers. The annulus is stronger in a direction 15 degrees from horizontal and weakest along the disc axis (26). The disc responds to loading by dehydrating and getting stiffer until a new equilibrium is reached. When the applied stress is reduced, the disc rehydrates accordingly (27).

Vertebral Body

There is an obvious trend toward increased compression strength from upper cervical levels to lower lumbar levels. The basic average value of 1,700 N comes from the classic work of Messerer (28). A similar value of 1,570 N was found in various studies of vertical impact loading with cadavers (29). Bell and colleagues (1) have shown that a 25%

decrease in osseous tissue results in a more than 50% decrease in the strength of a vertebral body. In general, vertebral body strength decreases with age and osteoporosis (30).

The rate of load application (fast or slow) is an important factor in determining the type of fracture. Fast loading rates produce burst-type fractures with gross displacement, whereas slow loading rates produce wedge-shaped fractures. After a fast-loading-rate impact injury (burst fracture), the spine recoils, and the residual canal encroachment can be significantly less than the maximum during impact (31).

Facet Joints

The facet joints aid in resisting compressive loads depending on the position of the spine. The superior articular facets of C2 to C4 face posteromedially and are circular or oval. From T1 and lower, the facets face posterolaterally and have a more transverse orientation. The transition between C4 and T1 can be gradual or sudden. The most frequent site of the transition is at the C5-C6 segment (32).

Zdeblick and colleagues (3,4) studied the role of the facet capsules and joints in resisting flexion. In a nondestructive flexion test, posterior displacement increased 4% after a 25% bilateral capsule resection, 5% after a 50% resection, 32% after a 75% resection, and 22% after complete resection. Flexion-moment testing revealed no significant difference between intact specimens and those treated by laminectomy or by laminectomy with 25% bilateral partial facetectomy. A 50% facetectomy resulted in a 2.5% increase in posterior strain, and 75% or 100% facetectomy resulted in a 25% increase in posterior strain compared with normal.

Zdeblick and colleagues (3,4) have also described the contribution of the facet joints and capsules to torsional stability. Although no gross subluxation was seen, torsional displacement increased 1% after 25% capsular resection,

19% after 50% resection, and 25% after 75% or 100% resection. After 75% and 100% facetectomy, torsional stiffness decreased significantly to 57% and 49% of normal, respectively. The facet capsule is an important stabilizer in acceleration injuries of the cervical spine (33,34). Additional torsional stability is also provided by the intervertebral disc (35).

Uncinate Processes and Uncovertebral Joints

The exact role of the uncovertebral joints is not known. A finite-element model study of the C5-C6 FSU has found that the uncinate processes and the uncovertebral joints are important contributors to the coupled motion of the lower cervical spine. The uncinate processes were found to reduce both the primary and the coupled motion, and surgical resection is expected to increase instability of the FSU (25).

Ligaments

The ligaments of the cervical spine provide passive stability and guide motion. Spinal ligaments are pretensioned, but they tend to lose some of their mechanical properties with increased age. The ligamentum flavum is the tissue with the highest percentage of elastic fibers in the body and has the highest preload (18 N in the young spine and 5 N in the older) (36). This pretension avoids impingement of the cord from ligament bulking. The ligamentum flavum is relatively constant in width (5 mm).

The other spinal ligaments are also pretensioned, but with significantly lower loads (37,38). The anterior longitudinal ligament (ALL) is attached firmly to the bodies and loosely to the discs. The posterior longitudinal ligament (PLL) is firmly attached to the disc but loosely to the body. The anterior and posterior longitudinal ligaments are approximately 7.5 mm wide and 12 mm long at levels C3 through T1 (39). The material properties of the ALL and PLL are the same. The ALL is two times stronger than the PLL because it has double the cross-sectional area (38). The supraspinous ligament is more vertically oriented than the interspinous ligament by 15 to 20 degrees (39). Morphometric and biomechanical studies have found that the ALL and PLL have higher failure stress values (strength) compared with the ligaments of the posterior complex. In contrast, failure strain (elongation to failure) was higher in the posterior ligaments (interspinous ligament, joint capsules, and ligamentum flavum) (40).

The capsule ligaments provide flexion stability to the FSU (2,41). The capsular ligaments are oriented posteriorly at approximately 45 degrees to the transverse plane (39). Zdeblick (4) has found that resection of more than 50% of the facet capsule leads to significant instability. A recent clinical study has compared the magnetic resonance imaging (MRI) findings of patients with unilateral or bilateral facet dislocation. ALL rupture was associated significantly with a bilateral facet dislocation. Damage to the PLL was not a consistent finding in unilateral facet dislocations. Disc disruption was a frequent finding in both injury types (42). In order to produce a unilateral facet dislocation *in vitro*, the ipsilateral facet capsule, annulus fibrosus, and ligamentum flavum had to be disrupted (43).

Lower Cervical Spine Functional Anatomy and Kinematics

The FSU has six degrees of freedom about the three-axis system of coordinates (three rotations and three translations) (10). The load-deformation curve of the FSU is biphasic. At smaller loads, the spine deforms easily, offering little resistance. At higher loads, the spine provides resistance in deformation at an increased rate. Panjabi (44) has termed the first phase of the FSU load-deformation curve the *neutral zone* (NZ), and the second phase the *elastic zone* (EZ). The range of motion (ROM) of the FSU is the sum of the NZ and the EZ. Loads that exceed the EZ result in permanent deformation and represent the phase of plastic deformation leading to catastrophic failure. This is the traumatic ROM (2). The FSU of the lower cervical spine is composed of two vertebral elements, the intervertebral disc, and associated ligamentous and capsular structures.

The primary motion at the lower cervical spine is flexion and extension in the sagittal plane. The average IAR for this rotation has been estimated to lie inside the posterior half of the body of the inferior vertebra, and moves superiorly toward the disc from C2 to C7. As the IAR moves closer to the disc space, the arc of rotation becomes sharper (8). Rotation and lateral bending are coupled motions in the lower cervical spine. This is the result of the inclination of the facet joints. Panjabi and associates (21,45) have found that every 1 degree of axial rotation produces 0.75 degrees of lateral bending in the same direction. Lateral bending produces coupled axial rotation in a ratio of 0.67 at C2 and 0.13 at C7 (21,45). Moroney (46) has found that the ratio of coupled lateral bending to axial rotation was 0.51 and the ratio of coupled axial rotation to lateral bending was 0.32.

Translations are clinically very important in determining the instability of the FSU. The maximum value of normal anterior-posterior translation has been found to be 2.7 mm, with a reported average of 0.5 mm (46) to 2 mm (2,10,45). Lateral translations (one side) were found on average to be 0.14 mm (46) and 1.5 mm (45). Vertical translations were negligible. The differences between the values found were attributed to the different moments applied in these experiments (19.6 N versus 50 N, respectively).

Distraction, be it pure or part of a combined motion of the cervical spine, is resisted by multiple structures. The foremost of these is the annulus of the intervertebral disc. In pure distraction, the entire annulus and other ligamentous structures resist tensile loads (22,47,48). In cervical flexion, the posterior annulus is subject to greater tensile loads; the opposite is true in extension. In extension, the ALL also resists distraction. In flexion, the supraspinous and interspinous ligaments, the ligamentum flavum, and facet capsules aid in resisting distraction. The contribution of the PLL in resisting distraction is dependent on the IAR. In a compressive-flexion injury to the cervical spine, the IAR is slightly anterior to the PLL, and tensile-distraction loads are not realized under the latter stages of this injury. In a distractive-flexion injury, the IAR is further anterior, thus placing the PLL under tension earlier in the injury process (49).

Forward flexion is restrained by multiple anatomic structures in the posterior portion of the functional spinal unit. These include the supraspinous and interspinous ligaments, along with the ligamentum flavum. Zdeblick and colleagues (3,4) studied the role of the facet capsules and joints in resisting flexion. The facet joints are the primary restraints against forward translation in the lower cervical spine. Raynor and associates (50) found that under shear loading conditions, 70% facet resection resulted in facet fracture and specimen failure. With 50% facet resection, the specimen-potting jig failed. Panjabi and colleagues (41) found that while anterior translation increased after sectioning either all anterior or posterior structures, the degree of translation increased significantly after disruption of the facet joints. The exact role of the uncovertebral joints is not known. They are thought to prevent posterior translation and limit lateral bending (11,51). In addition, they may act as a guide mechanism to flexion and extension and play a role in the coupling of rotation with lateral bending.

FUNCTIONAL ANATOMY AND INSTABILITY OF THE CERVICAL SPINE

Determining the stability of the cervical spine as it relates to the functional anatomy is both challenging to the clinician and of significant clinical importance to the patient. Defining *stability* or *instability* is the first step in this important process. White and Panjabi (2,52) defined clinical stability as the ability of the spine, under physiologic loads, to maintain its pattern of displacement so that there is no initial or additional neurologic deficit, no major deformity, and no incapacitating pain. They further defined physiologic loads as loads that are incurred during normal activity. These definitions have been most useful when evaluating afflictions of the cervical spine, be it from trauma, degenerative conditions, tumors, or surgery.

Much of the anatomic, functional, and biomechanical work of the cervical spine has enabled criteria to be developed to evaluate clinical stability. The remaining sections examine the criteria for clinical instability of the upper and lower cervical spine.

Upper Cervical Spine

Instability in the C1-C2 level is more common than at C0-C1 and can be the result of trauma, rheumatoid arthritis, or tumor. As discussed earlier, there is sagittal motion at the C1-C2 level, which accounts for up to 3 mm of anterior translation of C1 on C2, as measured in lateral radiographs. This distance is called the anterior atlantodental interval.

Translation greater than 3 mm indicates that the transverse ligament must be attenuated, and translation greater than 5 mm indicates that the ligament has ruptured (11).

A V-shaped predental space is not indicative of instability (2) and can measure 0 to 18 degrees, with a mean value of 6 degrees in neutral and 9 degrees in flexion (53). In traumatic cases where a V-shaped predental space is discovered, it is possible that the transverse ligament may be attenuated and the anterior ring of the atlas hinges on the anterior atlantodental ligaments, as described by Dvorak and Panjabi (15). Clinical evaluation of the patient will differentiate between a preexisting laxity and a new pathology. With the transverse ligament intact, a complete bilateral dislocation can occur at 65 degrees of rotation. With transverse ligament disruption, dislocation can occur at 45 degrees of rotation (22).

Sagittal plane axial instability is indicative of an underlying pathologic process. Compressive loads are transferred to the lateral mass articulation of the C1-C2 joints. Fractures of the atlas ring with disruption of the transverse ligament or erosive destruction can result in basilar invagination. Total lateral displacement of more than 6.9 mm of the lateral masses of C1 over the masses of C2 as measured in an anteroposterior radiograph is indicative of a burst fracture of the atlas with insufficiency of the transverse ligament (54). Distractive forces acting on the C1-C2 junction are resisted mainly by the tectorial membrane (13). Clinical stability at the C0-C1 and C1-C2 joints is intimately linked through their functional anatomy.

Evaluating instability begins with a careful review of the presenting complaints and a thorough history. Quality cervical radiographs—including a lateral and open-mouth odontoid view as well as lateral flexion-extension views—or computed tomographic (CT) scans, or both, are essential when confirming the presence of clinical instability. Various radiographic criteria have been established to evaluate the upper cervical spine for clinical instability (Table 3.1). These conditions include occipitocervical dislocations, basilar invagination, and rotational or translational instability at either the C0-C1 or C1-C2 joints.

Occipitocervical dislocations can be in the longitudinal, anterior, or posterior directions. The dens–basion distance and Power's ratio are useful in these conditions. The normal distance from the tip of the dens to the basion is less than 5 mm in adults and 10 mm in children; any increase is

TABLE 3.1. *Criteria for Upper Cervical Spine Instability*

>8°	Axial rotation C0-C1 to one side
>1 mm	C0-C1 translation
>7 mm	Overhang C1-C2 (total right and left)
>45°	Axial rotation C1-C2 to one side
>3 mm	C1-C2 translation at the AADI
<13 mm	Posterior atlantodental interval
	Avulsed transverse ligament

AADI, anterior atlantodental interval.
Adapted from White AA, Panjabi MM. *Clinical biomechanics of the spine,* 2nd ed. Philadelphia: JB Lippincott, 1990.

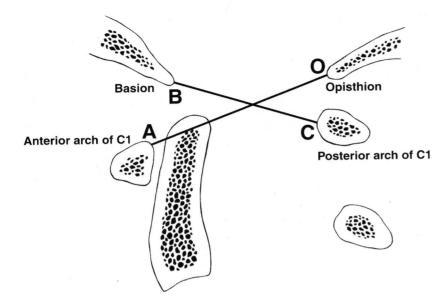

FIG. 3.6. Power's ratio. The ratio of the distance from *BC* to *AO* normally equals 1.0. If the ratio is greater than 1, an anterior occipitoatlantal dislocation may exist. Ratios slightly less than 1 are normal except in posterior dislocations, fractures of the odontoid process or ring of the atlas, or congenital abnormalities of the foramen magnum. In these conditions, the ratio may approach 0.7.

indicative of a possible longitudinal dislocation. Power's ratio (the ratio of the distance from the basion to the posterior arch of the atlas divided by the distance from the opisthion to the anterior arch of the atlas) can be useful in determining translational dislocations (Fig. 3.6) (55). A value greater than 1.0 is indicative of an anterior dislocation. A ratio of less than 1.0 is normal, except in posterior dislocations, where the ratio can approach 0.7. Fractures of the odontoid or ring of C1 and congenital narrowing of the foramen magnum can also yield values less than 1.0. Additional criteria for clinical instability at the C0-C1 joint include more than 1 mm of translation between the dens and basion on flexion-

extension radiographs (2) and greater than 8 degrees of unilateral axial rotation as determined by CT scans (5,6).

Basilar invagination represents vertical or compressive instability at the C0-C1 joint. This occurs most commonly in rheumatoid arthritis but can also occur secondary to tumor or trauma. Numerous bony landmarks at the base of the skull are used to create reference lines by which the degree of basilar invagination can be measured (Fig. 3.7). Because of overlying bony shadows from the skull base, plain lateral tomography or reconstructed CT images of the upper cervical spine are sometimes necessary to determine the appropriate landmarks and the extent of invagination.

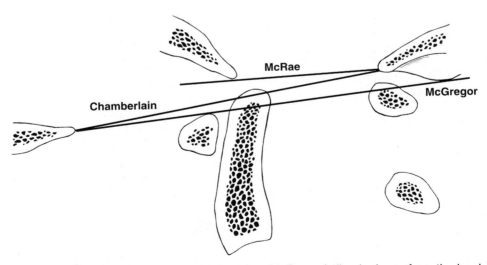

FIG. 3.7. Methods of determining basilar invagination. McGregor's line is drawn from the hard palate to the lowest point of the occiput. Protrusion of the tip of the dens greater than 4.5 mm above this line is abnormal. Chamberlain's line extends from the dorsal margin of the hard palate to the dorsal lip of the foramen magnum. The normal position of the dens is between 1 mm below this line and as much as 0.6 mm above it. McRae's line extends from the basion to the posterior lip of the foramen magnum. Protrusion of the tip of the dens above McRae's line is indicative of basilar invagination. Ranawat's line (not shown) is determined by drawing a line from the midportion of the C2 pedicle silhouette perpendicular to a line along the long axis of C1. Basilar invagination is present if this line is less than 12 mm.

Clinical instability at the atlantoaxial joint involves abnormal translation and rotation. An AADI greater than 3 mm is indicative of injury to the restraints against anterior translation. A posterior atlantodental interval less than 13 mm may also represent anterior translational instability. Posterior translation is rare and is the result of a dens fracture, a congenitally absent dens or anterior ring of C1, or a dens destroyed by tumor or infection.

Rotational displacement between C1 and C2 can be unilateral anterior, unilateral posterior, or unilateral combined anterior and posterior (5–7). The axis of rotation and deficient anatomic restraints determine the type of rotational displacement. Both the unilateral anterior and posterior atlantoaxial dislocations rotate around an axis centered at the contralateral joint. Anterior displacement is more common than posterior displacement and is usually the result of arthritic or infectious conditions that can weaken or disrupt the transverse ligament and dislocated joint's capsule. Posterior displacement is usually the result of a deficient dens, either congenital or acquired.

Unilateral combined anterior and posterior dislocations occur when one lateral mass moves forward and the other backward. The axis of rotation for this condition is the dens as the capsular ligaments are disrupted bilaterally. Stability may be preserved if the dens, the tectorial membrane, and the transverse ligament remain intact.

Lower Cervical Spine

Upper cervical spine kinematics is highly constrained by bony morphology and ligamentous attachments, making the establishment of radiologic criteria easier. In the lower and middle cervical spine, the viscoelastic intervertebral disc and the coupled kinematics make recognition of clinical instability more difficult.

Gross instability can be safely detected with static or dynamic radiographs. Translation and rotation of the FSU can then be compared with the normal values found from kinematic studies in vitro. If one considers 2.7 mm as the highest reported value of anterior translation in vitro (45,46), and an average radiographic magnification to be 30%, then the result is the criterion of 3.5 mm of maximum normal sagittal plane translation proposed by White et al (2). Angular deformity in the sagittal plane can also be compared with the normal values found in vitro. Any increase of sagittal rotation of the injured FSU in dynamic radiographs of more than 11 degrees compared with the presumed intact FSU above or below is indicative of instability (2). An FSU that exhibits more than 20 degrees of sagittal rotation (ROM) in dynamic flexion-extension radiographs is above all normal limits found in both in vivo (7,11) and in vitro studies (2) and is considered unstable. All these criteria have been included in the checklist for the diagnosis of clinical instability created by White and Panjabi (52). The checklist is provided in Table 3.2.

In cases of degenerative painful cervical syndromes, the definition of clinical instability is more difficult. In most of these cases the range of motion of the FSU is found between normal limits and is sometimes even less. Clinical studies have proved that temporary external stabilization of a suspected painful and unstable FSU can satisfactorily predict the expected pain relief offered by an arthrodesis. Panjabi (56) conducted an in vitro study to measure the effects of external fixation on the load-deformation curve

TABLE 3.2. *Checklist of Clinical Instability in the Middle and Lower Cervical Spine*

Element	Point value
Anterior elements destroyed or unable to function	2
Posterior elements destroyed or unable to function	2
Positive stretch test	2
Radiographic criteria	4
A. Flexion-extension x-rays	
1. Sagittal plane translation > 3.5 mm or 20%	2
2. Sagittal plane rotation > 20°	2
OR	
B. Resting x-rays	
1. Sagittal plane displacement > 3.5 mm or 20%	2
2. Relative sagittal plane angulation >11°	2
Abnormal disc narrowing	1
Developmentally narrow spinal canal	1
1. Sagittal diameter < 13 mm	
OR	
2. Pavlov's ratio < 0.8	
Spinal cord damage	2
Nerve root damage	1
Dangerous loading anticipated	1

A total of 5 points or more equals instability.
Adapted from White AA, Panjabi MM. *Clinical biomechanics of the spine,* 2nd ed. Philadelphia: JB Lippincott, 1990.

of the stabilized FSU. He found that the greatest decrease occurred in the neutral zone (69%), with the total ROM losing only 39% of the intact value. These findings led Panjabi to redefine clinical instability as "a significant decrease in the capacity of the stabilizing system of the spine to maintain the intervertebral neutral zones within the physiological limits, so that there is no neurological dysfunction, no major deformity, and no incapacitating pain" (10).

REFERENCES

1. Bell GH, Dunbar O, Beck JS, et al. Variation in strength of vertebrae with age and their relation to osteoporosis. *Calcif Tissue Res* 1967;1:75.
2. White AA, Johnson RM, Panjabi MM, et al. Biomechanical analysis of clinical stability in the cervical spine. *Clin Orthop* 1975;109:85.
3. Zdeblick TA, Zou D, Warden KE, et al. Cervical stability following foraminotomy: a biomechanical *in vitro* analysis. *J Bone Joint Surg Am* 1992;74:22–27.
4. Zdeblick TA, Abitbol JJ, Kunz DN, et al. Cervical stability after sequential capsule resection. *Spine* 1993;18:2005–2008.
5. Dvorak J, Panjabi MM, Gerber M. CT—functional diagnostics of the rotatory instability of the upper cervical spine; an experimental study in cadavers. *Spine* 1987;12:197.
6. Dvorak J, Panjabi MM, Gerber M, et al. CT—functional diagnostics of the rotatory instability of the upper cervical spine. *Spine* 1987;12:726.
7. Dvorak J, Froehlich D, Penning L, et al. Functional radiographic diagnosis of the cervical spine: flexion/extension. *Spine* 1988;13:748.
8. Dvorak J, Panjabi MM, Novotny JE, et al. *In vivo* flexion-extension of the normal cervical spine. *J Orthop Res* 1991;9:824–834.
9. Moroney SP, Schultz AB, Miller JAA. Analysis and measurement of neck loads. *J Orthop Res* 1988;6:713–720.
10. Panjabi MM, Dvorak J, Sandler A, et al. Cervical spine kinematics and clinical instability. In: The Cervical Spine Research Society, eds. *The cervical spine,* 3rd ed. Philadelphia: Lippincott–Raven, 1998.
11. Penning L. Normal movement of the cervical spine. *AJR Am J Roentgenol* 1978;130:317–326.
12. Sherk HH. Developmental anatomy of the normal cervical spine. In: The Cervical Spine Research Society, eds. *The cervical spine,* 3rd ed. Philadelphia: Lippincott–Raven, 1998.
13. Werne S. Studies on spontaneous atlas dislocation. *Acta Orthop Scand* 1957;23:1–150.
14. Wiesel SW, Rothman RH. Occipito-atlantal hypermobility. *Spine* 1979;4:187.
15. Dvorak J, Panjabi MM. Functional anatomy of the alar ligaments. *Spine* 1987;12:183.
16. Panjabi MM, Oxland TR, Parks EH. Quantitative anatomy of cervical spine ligaments. I. Upper cervical spine. *J Spinal Disord* 1991;4:270–276.
17. Dvorak J, Schneider E, Saldinger P, et al. Biomechanics of the craniocervical region: the alar and transverse ligaments. *J Orthop Res* 1988;6:452.
18. Panjabi M, Dvorak J, Crisco JJ 3rd, et al. Effects of alar ligament transection on upper cervical spine rotation. *J Orthop Res* 1991;9:584–593.
19. Panjabi M, Dvorak J, Crisco J 3rd, et al. Flexion, extension, and lateral bending of the upper cervical spine in response to alar ligament transections. *J Spinal Disord* 1991;4:157–167.
20. Lin RM, Tsai KH, Chu LP, et al. Characteristics of sagittal vertebral alignment in flexion determined by dynamic radiographs of the cervical spine. *Spine* 2001;26:256–261.
21. Panjabi M, Dvorak J, Duranceau J, et al. Three-dimensional movements of the upper cervical spine. *Spine* 1988;13:726.
22. Fielding JW, Cochran GVB, Lawsing JF, et al. Tears of the transverse ligament of the atlas: a clinical and biomechanical study. *J Bone Joint Surg Am* 1974;56:1681–1691.
23. Panjabi MM, Duranceau J, Goel V, et al. Cervical human vertebrae. Quantitative three-dimensional anatomy of the middle and lower regions. *Spine* 1993;16:861–874.
24. Hirsch C. The reaction of intervertebral discs to compression forces. *J Bone Joint Surg Am* 1955;37:1188.
25. Virgin W. Experimental investigations into physical properties of intervertebral disc. *J Bone Joint Surg Br* 1951;33:607.
26. Galante JO. Tensile properties of the human annulus fibrosus. *Acta Orthop Scand Suppl* 1967;100.
27. Adams MA, Hutton WC. The effect of posture on the fluid content of lumbar intervertebral disks. *Spine* 1983;8:665–671.
28. Messerer O. *Uber Elasticitat and Festigkeit der Meuschlichen Knochen.* Stutgart: J.G. Cottaschen Buchhandling, 1880.
29. Yoganandan N, Kumaresan S, Pintar FA Geometric and mechanical properties of human cervical spine ligaments. *J Biomech Eng* 2000;122(6):623–629.
30. McBroom RJ, Hayes WC, Edward WT, et al. Prediction of vertebral body compressive fracture using quantitative computed tomography. *J Bone Joint Surg Am* 1985;67:1206.
31. Carter JW, Mirza SK, Tencer AF, et al. Canal geometry changes associated with axial compressive cervical spine fracture. *Spine* 2000;25:46–54.
32. Pal GP, Routal RV, Saggu SK. The orientation of the articular facets of the zygoapophysial joints at the cervical and upper thoracic region. *J Anat* 2001;198:431–441.
33. Panjabi MM, Cholewicki J, Nibu K, et al. Capsular ligament stretches during *in vitro* whiplash simulations. *J Spinal Disord* 1998;11:227–232.
34. Winkelstein BA, Nightingale RW, Richardson WJ, et al. The cervical facet capsule and its role in whiplash injury: a biomechanical investigation. *Spine* 2000;25:1238–1246.
35. Clausen JD, Goel VK, Traynelis VC, et al. Uncinate processes and Luschka joints influence the biomechanics of the cervical spine: quantification using a finite element model of the C5-C6 segment. *J Orthop Res* 1997;15:342–347.
36. Nachemson A, Evans J. Some mechanical properties of the third lumbar interlaminar ligament (ligamentum flavum). *J Biomech* 1968;1:211.
37. Przybylski GJ, Patel PR, Carlin GJ, et al. Quantitative anthropometry of the subatlantal cervical longitudinal ligaments *Spine* 1998;23:893–898.
38. Tkaczuk H. Tensile properties of human lumbar longitudinal ligaments. *Acta Orthop Scand Suppl* 1968;115.
39. Panjabi MM, Oxland TR, Parks EH. Quantitative anatomy of cervical spine ligaments. II. Middle and lower cervical spine. *J Spinal Disord* 1991;4:277–285.
40. Yoganandan N, Sances A, Maiman DJ, et al. Experimental spinal injuries with vertical impact. *Spine* 1986;11:855–860.
41. Panjabi MM, White AA, Johnson RM. Cervical spine mechanics as a function of transection of components. *J Biomech* 1975;8:327.
42. Vaccaro AR, Madigan L, Schweitzer ME, et al. Magnetic resonance imaging analysis of soft tissue disruption after flexion-distraction injuries of the subaxial cervical spine. *Spine* 2001;26:1866–1872.
43. Sim E, Vaccaro AR, Berzlanovich A, et al. *In vitro* genesis of subaxial cervical unilateral facet dislocations through sequential soft tissue ablation. *Spine* 2001;26:1317–1323.
44. Panjabi MM. The stabilizing system of the spine. II. Neutral zone and instability hypothesis. *J Spinal Disord* 1992;5:390–397.
45. Panjabi MM, Summers DJ, Pelker RR, et al. Three-dimensional load displacement curves of the cervical spine. *J Orthop Res* 1986;4:152.
46. Moroney SP, Schultz AB, Miller JAA, et al. Load-displacement properties of lower cervical spine motion segments. *J Biomech* 1988;21:767.
47. Goel VJ, Njus GO. Stress-strain characteristic of spinal ligaments. Presented at the 32nd Transactions of the Orthopedic Research Society, New Orleans, Louisiana, 1986.
48. Myklebust JB, Pintar F, Yoganandan N, et al. Tensile strength of spinal ligaments. *Spine* 1988;13:526–531.
49. Webb JK, Broughton RBK, McSweeney T, et al. Hidden flexion injury of the cervical spine. *J Bone Joint Surg Br* 1976;58:322.
50. Raynor RB, Pugh J, Shapiro I. Cervical facetectomy and its effect on spine strength. *J Neurosurg* 1985;63:278–282.
51. Frykholm R. Lower cervical vertebrae and intervertebral discs. Surgical anatomy and pathology. *Acta Chir Scand* 1951;101:345.
52. White AA, Panjabi MM. *Clinical biomechanics of the spine.* Philadelphia: JB Lippincott, 1990.
53. Monu J, Bohler SP, Howard G. Some upper cervical norms. *Spine* 1987;12:515–519.
54. Spence K, Decker S, Sell K. Bursting atlantal fracture associated with rupture of the transverse ligament. *J Bone Joint Surg Am* 1970;52:543–549.
55. Powers B, Miller MD, Kramer RS, et al. Traumatic atlanto-occipital dislocation with survival. *Neurosurgery* 1979;4:12–17.
56. Panjabi MM. Lumbar spine instability: a biomechanical challenge. *Curr Orthop* 1994;8:100–105.

CHAPTER 4

Cervical Spine Kinematics and Clinical Instability

Manohar M. Panjabi, James J. Yue, Jiří Dvořák, Vijay Goel, Todd A. Fairchild, and Augustus A. White

A more complete understanding of cervical spine stability continues to evolve and be defined. Ultimately, this insight may directly assist the clinician in the often daunting task of evaluating the clinical stability of the cervical spine. The goals of this chapter are to introduce the biomechanical concept of kinematics, or the study of motion of the spine; to define the role of anatomic elements in providing mechanical stability to the spine; and to provide some practical guidelines for determining clinical instability.

BASIC CONCEPTS OF KINEMATICS OF THE CERVICAL SPINE

Kinematics is the study of the motion of bodies without consideration of the influencing forces. The challenge for the clinician is to become familiar with the normal *range of motion* (ROM) and the characteristic *patterns of motion* in the various regions of the spine. The ranges are generally expressed as rotation and translation in three planes. Too much motion may be indicative of structural damage to the spine. Too little motion may accompany stiffness and pain. There may also be irregularity in the pattern of motion. Abnormal motion patterns that have been described include irregular scatters of the instantaneous axes of rotation (IAR), reversed coupling patterns, and rotation of vertebrae in uncharacteristic directions.

The study of kinematics provides a basis for determining when too much or irregular motion may be associated with pain or neurologic impairment. The following metaphor from Lovett's (1) classic work on the mechanism of the normal spine and its relation to scoliosis serves as an excellent introduction to a presentation of the normal kinematics of the cervical spine:

It is as if one undertook, for example, to investigate a railroad accident solely from a study of the wrecked cars. Much could be learned as to the effect and direction of the destructive forces, the amount of force expended, and the kind of damage done, but more could be learned and future accidents could be better prevented by a study of the normal running of the trains, their proper relations to each other at the time of the accident, and by an investigation of the signal system and the routine precautions adopted.

The key to the "normal running of the trains" is the kinematics of the spine. With a thorough knowledge of kinematics, the clinician is more likely to make new discoveries of irregularities and correlate them, when possible, with clinical conditions. That a thorough knowledge of spinal kinematics is helpful in understanding all aspects of the diagnosis and management of spinal pathology is especially true of the cervical spine, for it is the most mobile portion of the spine.

Physiologic Motion and Functions of the Cervical Spine

To analyze, understand, and correct the various malfunctions of the spine, it is essential that we first fully characterize the normal functions. The three functions of the human spine are (a) to support the appendicular skeleton and the trunk, (b) to protect the neural elements, and (c) to allow a substantial amount of complex motion. Certain clinical problems are known to be associated with irregularities in the amount and possibly the type of motion present in the spine. Some of the diseases associated with irregular motion in the spine are well recognized and documented through clinical observations. Other diseases may be associated with motion irregularities even though the full pathology and associated clinical consequences have not yet been fully characterized.

The functions and anatomic designs of the occipitoatlantoaxial complex (C0-C1-C2) and the lower cervical spine (C2 through C7) are dissimilar; therefore, it is advantageous to study the kinematics of each region separately. The occipitoatlantoaxial complex is grouped and labeled the *upper cervical spine*. Because of kinematic (2), kinetic (3), and clinical uniqueness (4,5), the cervical region is further divided into the middle cervical (C3 through C5) and the lower cervical (C6 through T1) regions.

Relevant Biomechanical Terms

Some key kinematic terms are defined here to facilitate further reading (6).

Translation: Motion of a rigid body in which a straight line in the body always remains parallel to itself.

Rotation: Motion of a rigid body in which a straight line does not remain parallel to itself (Fig. 4.1). The angle between the two positions of the straight line (i.e., A1–B1 and A2–B2) is the angle of rotation.

Center of rotation (COR): When a rigid body moves in a plane, there is a point, in the body or some hypothetical extension of it, that does not move. This is the COR of the body for that step of motion (Fig. 4.1). The line perpendicular to the motion plane and passing through the COR is called the IAR. The COR or IAR is obtained by the intersection of the perpendicular bisector of the translation vectors A1–A2 and B1–B2 of any two points (e.g., points A and B).

Degrees of freedom (dof): The number of independent coordinates in a coordinate system required to completely specify the position of an object in space.

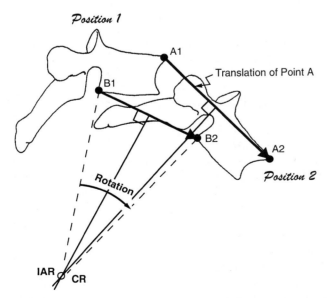

FIG. 4.1. A vertebra is shown in two positions in the sagittal plane. The motion is a rotation about the center of rotation (CR) or about the instantaneous axis of rotation (IAR).

Neutral position: The erect posture of the spine in which the overall internal stresses in the spinal column and the muscular effort to hold the posture are minimal.

Range of motion: The range of physiologic intervertebral motion, measured from the neutral position. It is divided into two parts: neutral zone and elastic zone.

Neutral zone (NZ): That part of the range of physiologic intervertebral motion, measured from the neutral position, within which the spinal motion is produced with minimal internal resistance. It is the zone of relatively high flexibility or laxity.

Elastic zone (EZ): That part of the range of physiologic intervertebral motion, measured from the end of the NZ up to the physiologic limit, in which spinal motion is produced against substantial internal resistance. It is the zone of high stiffness.

Biomechanical Tests

Three types of basic biomechanical tests can be used to analyze an *in vivo* or *in vitro* animal study: strength, fatigue, and flexibility (7). A *strength test* consists of loading an implant or a spinal construct (specimen plus instrumentation) to determine the load (defined by its direction and point of application) carrying capacity. A load is applied until the specimen fails. A *fatigue test* determines the capacity of the spinal construct to carry varying physiological loads until the fusion matures and unloads the implant. The load can be varied but is always less than the failure load. The cyclic load is applied until the specimen fails. A *stability test* determines the capability of the spinal construct to minimize micromovements at the site of fusion to promote initiation of fusion and maturation.

Stability testing can be further divided into flexibility and stiffness testing. To conduct a stability test, the lower mount of the testing apparatus is fixed to the test table, and the upper mount is subjected to a load (force or moment) or to displacement (rotation or translation). In the case of load application, motions or displacements are measured. This is the *flexibility* method. If displacement is applied, then the loads are measured. This is the *stiffness* method.

In Vivo Kinematics

The concept of *in vivo* passive kinematics has been well described in the work of Dvorak and colleagues (8–10). Investigations with functional radiographs have shown that additional motion can be gained by exerting external forces on the "fully" flexed or extended neck, an important finding to bear in mind when evaluating voluntary flexion-extension tests. This also fits with the assertion that the stretch test (passive axial traction) is more likely to show existing pathology than is measurement of active (that is, voluntary) flexion and extension (6).

The differences between active and passive *in vivo* ROM must be considered in the interpretation of laboratory and clinical studies of normal ranges of motion. Considering that in daily clinical routine we do not deal with healthy volunteers but rather with patients who have either injury or painful conditions resulting from ongoing degenerative changes, we must be aware that the patient's active motion may be restricted by motion-induced pain rather than pathology. However, we should be interested, especially when we suspect a segmental instability, in how the motion (both rotation and translation) looks beyond the limit of active motion. In an injured patient population, examination of passive flexion and extension was shown to result in the identification of more hypermobile segments (8,11). Similar observations related to passive motion of the cervical spine have been made with lateral bending (12) and axial rotation (9). Examining the total motion of the cervical spine with a spine motion analyzer (13), it was found that passive tests resulted in larger ROM with smaller associated standard deviation (SD). Active tests showed substantially less motion than passive tests in measurements of lateral bending and axial rotation of the cervical spine.

An Ongoing Field

Much of the research presented herein requires further confirmation and suggests new avenues for investigation. Attempts have been made to distill fact from postulate and to integrate biomechanical research with clinical applications. As in any research field, there are numerous problems to overcome. The kinematics of interest is that of the *in vivo* cervical spine. The experimental techniques for precise, no-risk, *in vivo* measurements are still being refined. To date, only simple motions have been satisfactorily measured *in vivo*. The characteristics of the muscle forces that result in *in vivo* physiological motions have been emulated during experimental motion testing (14). *In vitro* studies have been performed to simulate vertebral motion, but whether the motions produced experimentally are the same as those produced *in vivo* is not known. Obviously, these problems must be addressed. The purpose of this chapter is to present the state of the art in regard to cervical spine kinematics; useful areas of clinical relevance are indicated.

BASIC KINEMATICS OR MOTIONS OF THE CERVICAL SPINE

The measurement of motion in the cervical spine is a routine part of the clinical examination of patients with neck pain resulting from either injury or degenerative changes. Various methods for recording data with varying degrees of accuracy and repeatability are used, ranging from the use of different types of goniometers to visual estimation of motion (5,15–19). Although the value of assessing the ROM is not yet documented, the understanding and knowledge of normal age- and sex-related values of ROM is the basis for analysis of altered and possibly pathologic motion patterns as well as decreased or increased ROM (13,16,20).

To obtain normal values, 150 healthy, asymptomatic volunteers were tested using the CA-6000 spine motion analyzer (OSI, Hayward, CA) (13). In this system, the subject is seated in a specially designed chair, and the device is attached and zeroed. The following motions can then be assessed by asking the subject to perform active motion, which is followed by passive examination by the physician: (a) flexion and extension, (b) lateral bending, (c) axial rotation, (d) rotation out of maximum flexion, and (e) rotation out of maximum extension. In addition to the usual physiological motions of flexion-extension, lateral bending, and axial rotation from the neutral position, axial rotations at full flexion and extension postures were also measured.

The volunteers were divided into groups based on sex and the following age decades: 20 to 29, 30 to 39, 40 to 49, 50 to 59, and 60+ years. The overall tendency was for ROM to decrease as age increased (Fig. 4.2). This proved true in nearly all motions, with the most dramatic decrease in motion occurring between the groups aged 30 to 39 and 40 to 49 years. The only motion that did not decrease with age was the rotation out of maximum flexion, which remained the same or showed a slight increase, on average, as age increased. The average values for age decades and for gender groups for each motion, along with significant differences, are shown in Table 4.1. Substantially less motion was evident in the active tests in comparison of lateral bending and axial rotation. Generally, for passive tests, the SD was lower (Table 4.2).

Women showed greater ROM in all these motions. In the age range of 40 to 49 years, women again showed significantly greater ROM in axial rotation and rotation at maximal flexion. There were no significant differences between gender groups for the group aged 60+ years. The well-established clinical observation that motion of the cervical spine decreases with age (21) has been confirmed in this study (13). An exception to this finding was the surprising observation that the rotation of the upper cervical spine, mainly at the atlantoaxial joint (tested by rotating the head at maximum flexion of the cervical spine, which presumably locks the other levels) did not decrease with age. The measurement data for rotation out of maximum flexion suggest that the rotation of the atlantoaxial joint does not decrease with age but rather remains constant or increases slightly, perhaps to compensate for the reduced motion of the lower segments.

In a clinical study, Mayer and associates (16) used two inclinometers connected to a computer system to measure flexion-extension, lateral bending, and axial rotation. Fifty-eight normal subjects (mean age 32 years) were divided into two groups: the youngest versus the oldest. Using this kind of division of the normal group, the investigators noted no sex- or age-related differences in ROM, possibly due to the small groups or the mean age of the group (32 years, SD = 12.6 years), or both. Comparison with the study by Dvorak showed the dramatic decrease in ROM occurs between the fourth and fifth decades of life, a finding also demonstrated in the pathologic and anatomic studies of Luschka (22) and later confirmed by Töndury and Theiler (23).

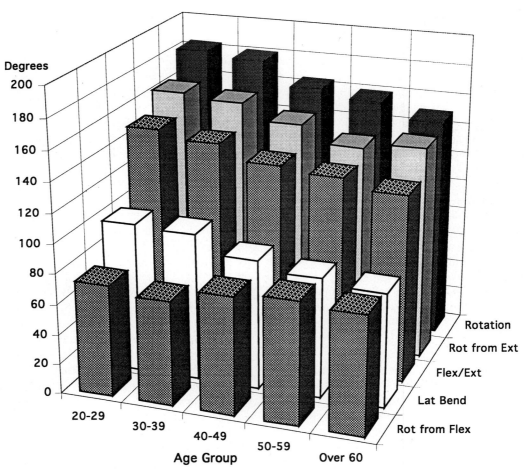

FIG. 4.2. With increase in age, there is an overall decrease in motion due to the normal age-related changes in the cervical spine. In one study, the largest decrease in motion occurred in the age groups of 30 to 39 and 40 to 49 years. Rotation from flexion (axial rotation with cervical spine in full flexion) is the only motion that stayed the same or actually increased slightly with age. (From: Dvorak J, Antinnes JA, Panjabi MM, et al. Age and gender related normal motion of the cervical spine. *Spine* 1992;17: S393–398, with permission.)

TABLE 4.1. *Average (Standard Deviation) Head–Shoulder Rotations in Degrees*

Age decade	Flexion-extension		Lateral bending		Axial rotation		Rotation from flexion		Rotation from extension	
	M	F	M	F	M	F	M	F	M	F
20–29	152.7[a]	149.3	101.1	100.0	183.8	182.4	75.5[a]	72.6	161.8	171.5
	(20.0)	(11.7)	(13.3)	(8.6)	(11.8)	(10.0)	(12.4)	(12.7)	(15.9)	(10.0)
30–39	141.4	155.9[a]	94.7[a]	106.3[a]	175.1[a]	186.0[a]	66.0	74.6	158.4	165.8
	(11.4)[b]	(23.1)	(10.0)[b]	(18.1)	(9.9)[b]	(10.4)	(13.6)[b]	(10.5)	(16.4)	(16.0)
40–49	131.1	139.8	83.7	88.2[a]	157.4	168.2	71.5	85.2	146.2	153.9[a]
	(18.5)	(13.0)	(13.9)	(16.1)	(19.5)[b]	(13.6)	(10.9)[b]	(14.8)	(33.3)	(22.9)
50–59	136.3[a]	126.9	88.3	76.1	166.2[a]	151.9	77.7	85.6	145.8	132.4[a]
	(15.7)	(14.8)	(29.1)[b]	(10.2)	(14.1)	(15.9)	(17.1)	(9.9)	(21.2)[b]	(28.8)
60+	116.3	133.2	74.2	79.6	145.6	154.2	79.4	81.3	130.9	154.5
	(18.7)	(7.6)	(14.3)	(18.0)	(13.1)	(14.6)	(8.1)	(21.2)	(24.1)	(14.7)

[a] Significant difference from cell directly adjacent to the right (i.e., gender within age group difference).
[b] Significant difference from cell directly adjacent below (i.e., age group within gender differentiation).

TABLE 4.2. *Comparison of Means and Standard Deviations in Degrees for Normal Active Cervical Spine Rotations*

Motion	Active (Dvorak)	Active (Lantz)
Flexion-extension	141.3 (15)	116.1 (12.9)
Lateral bending	91.4 (14.4)	84.1 (13.8)
Axial rotation	175 (12)	144.2 (11.9)
Rotation from flexion	81.4 (15.9)	—
Rotation from extension	165 (16.9)	—

Data from Dvorak J, Antinnes JA, Panjabi MM, et al. Age and gender related normal motion of the cervical spine. *Spine* 1992;17:S393–S398; and Lantz CA, Chen J, Buch D. Clinical validity and stability of active and passive cervical range of motion with regard to total and unilateral uniplanar motion. *Spine* 1999;24:1082–1089.

Upper Cervical Spine

Most of the axial rotation and some of the flexion-extension and lateral bending of the head occurs in the upper cervical spine (C0-C1-C2). The highly specialized anatomy of this region is designed to provide seemingly paradoxical attributes: loose enough to allow nearly 50% of the cervical spine axial rotation, sufficiently tight to protect the delicate structures of the spinal cord and vertebral arteries, and strong enough to carry the weight of the head and resist muscle forces. It is therefore a very complicated structure, with motion determined by the orientation of the articular processes and limited by the ligaments (Fig. 4.3).

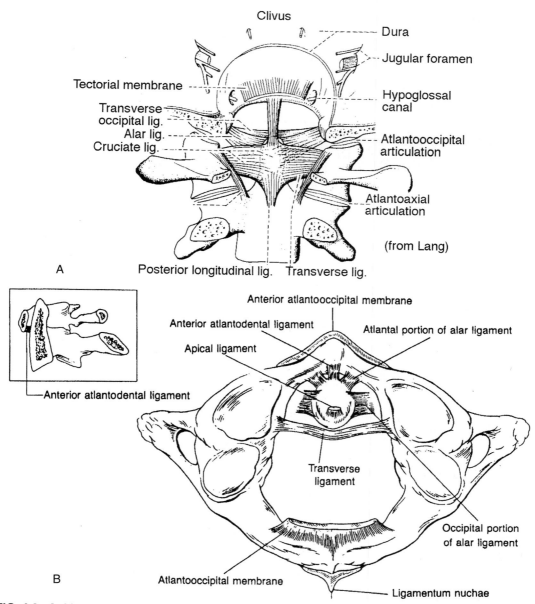

FIG. 4.3. A: Ligaments of the upper cervical spine, posterior view. (From: Lang J. *Kleinische Anatomie aer Halswirbelsäule.* Stuttgart: G. Thieme Verlag, 1991, with permission.) **B:** Top view of the C1-C2 joint. Schematic of the major ligaments involved in the clinical stability of the upper cervical spine.

TABLE 4.3. *Average Rotations in Degrees at the Atlantooccipital (C0-C1) Joint According to Different Investigators*

Study (Ref.)	Flexion (total)	Side bending (one side)	Axial rotation (one side)
Fick, 1904	50	30–40	0
Poirier and Charpy, 1926	50	14–40	0
Werne, 1957 (31)	13	8	0
Penning, 1978 (91)	35	10	0
Dvorak et al., 1985	—	—	5.2
Goel et al., 1988 (26)	23.0	3.4	2.4
Dvorak et al., 1987 (24,25)	—	—	4
Penning and Wilmink, 1987 (40)	—	—	1
Panjabi et al., 1988 (83)	24.5	5.5	7.2

The disparity in the results is mostly due to the differences in the methods used in this mixed group of *in vitro* and *in vivo* studies.

The atlantooccipital (C0-C1) joints are spheroid articulations; that is, they allow motion in the shape of a sphere. The joint capsule connecting them is very tight, serving to limit the possible movements and prevent dangerous hypermotion that could pinch the spinal cord or the vertebral arteries. The dominant movement in the atlantooccipital joint is flexion and extension of approximately 22 to 24 degrees (Table 4.3). The lateral bending is 5 to 10 degrees. The idea of axial rotation in this joint had long been rejected; however, more recent investigators have shown axial rotation in both *in vitro* and *in vivo* studies (24–27).

The atlantoaxial (C1-C2) joint (Table 4.4) consists of four joint spaces: the two atlantoaxial lateral joints, the atlantoaxial median joint (between the anterior arch of the atlas and the dens axis), and a joint between the posterior

TABLE 4.4. *Average Rotations in Degrees at the Atlantoaxial (C1-C2) Joint According to Different Investigators*

Study (Ref.)	Flexion-extension (total)	Side bending (one side)	Axial rotation (one side)
Fick, 1904	0	0	60
Poirier and Charpy, 1926	11	—	30–80
Werne, 1957 (31)	10	0	47
Penning, 1978 (91)	30	10	70
Dvorak et al., 1985	—	—	32.2
Goel et al., 1988 (26)	10.1	42	23.3
Dvorak et al., 1987 (24,25)	—	—	43.1
Penning and Wilmink, 1987 (40)	—	—	40.5
Panjabi et al., 1988 (83)	22.4	6.7	38.9

As in Table 4.3, the differences in the results of the studies are due to the different methods used.

surface of the dens and the transverse ligament, which is connected to the anterior joint space. From the medial part, there is a large synovial fold in the lateral atlantoaxial joint. This joint capsule, in contrast to that of the atlantooccipital joint, is loose, allowing a great deal of motion. It is here that most of the axial rotation occurs, a fact reflected in the anatomy as the vertical dens of the axis (C2) acts as a pivot about which the atlas (C1) rotates.

The motion in the upper cervical spine, especially in the atlantoaxial joint, is mainly limited by the alar ligaments, which connect the dens axis, the occipital condyles, and the anterior arch of the axis (25,28,29) with nonstretchable collagen fibers (30). According to Werne (31), alar ligaments are of great importance in limiting the axial rotation—a belief that has been confirmed by newer investigations (Fig. 4.4) (25,32). In conjunction with the tectorial membrane (the only elastic ligament in the upper cervical spine), the alar ligaments also limit the flexion of the occiput. During lateral bending (Fig. 4.5), the alar ligament is responsible for the forced rotation of the second vertebra (9,31).

The cruciate ligament (Fig. 4.3) has cleverly evolved to restrict potentially dangerous anterior motion of the atlas during flexion movement of the head while still allowing the atlas to turn freely around the dens during axial rotation. It consists of two main parts: the horizontally oriented transverse ligament and the vertically oriented longitudinal fibers. At the level of the dens, there is a thin layer of cartilage covering the transverse ligament (10), which allows the ligament to move more freely during rotation and protects it from friction damage. The transverse ligament consists of collagen fibers with an interesting fiber orientation similar to a folding lattice. This allows extensive stretching of the ligament during axial rotation without damage to the fibers. *In vitro* experiments show failure of the transverse ligament to occur between 170 and 700 N (corresponding to about 17 to 70 kg) (10). The apical ligament has no functional meaning (33).

Middle and Lower Cervical Spine

The anatomic structures of the motion segments of the middle and lower cervical spine (C2 through T1) are somewhat different from those in the upper cervical spine (Table 4.5). Their particularities include the uncovertebral joints, which support part of the axial load once the intervertebral disc loses its elasticity due to age-related transformations (23,33,34). The articular processes of the cervical spine are inclined approximately 45 degrees from the horizontal plane (Fig. 4.6), with steeper inclinations in the lower segments. This inclination allows far less axial rotation than occurs in the upper cervical spine. The transverse processes hide and protect the spinal nerve and the vertebral artery.

The motion segments are connected and stabilized by ligaments—anteriorly by the anterior longitudinal ligament and dorsally by the posterior longitudinal ligament (PLL). The density of nociceptive and mechanoreceptive innervation

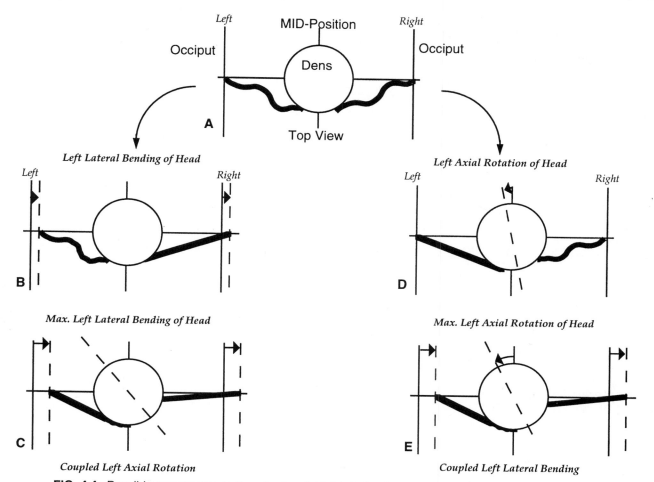

FIG. 4.4. Possible movements in the atlantoaxial joint during lateral bending and axial rotation of the head according to Werne. (From: Werne S. Studies in spontaneous atlas dislocation. *Acta Orthop Scand Suppl* 1957;23, with permission.)

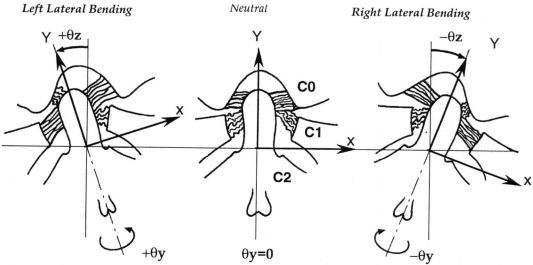

FIG. 4.5. Function of the alar ligaments during side bending of the head. (From: Dvorak J, Panjabi M. Functional anatomy of the alar ligaments. *Spine* 1987;12:183–188, with permission.)

TABLE 4.5. *Average Total Flexion-Extension Rotations (in Degrees) of Healthy Adults in the Middle and Lower Cervical Region*

Region	Dvorak et al., 1988 (8,9) In vivo, active	Dvorak et al., 1988 (8,9) In vivo, passive	White and Panjabi, 1990 (6)	Penning, 1978 (91): In vivo, active
C2-C3	10	12	10	12
C3-C4	15	17	15	18
C4-C5	19	21	20	20
C5-C6	20	23	20	20
C6-C7	19	21	17	15
C7-T1	—	—	9	—

Penning 1960

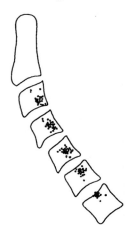

Dvorak et al, 1991

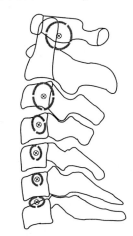

FIG. 4.7. The centers of rotation for the sagittal plane motion. (From: Penning L. *Functional pathology of the cervical spine.* Amsterdam: Excerpta Medica, 1968:1–23; and Dvorak J, Panjabi MM, Novotny JE, et al. *In vivo* flexion-extension of the normal cervical spine. *J Orthop Res* 1991;9:824–834, with permission.)

of the PLL is high in comparison to that of other cervical spine ligaments and the disc. This results in a very sensitive ligament that indirectly controls the innervation of neck muscles through nociceptive and mechanoreceptive reflexes (35). The laminae are connected by the strong ligamentum flavum, which consists almost exclusively of elastic fibers and is a major limiting structure in flexion movement.

The dominant motion in the lower cervical spine is flexion-extension. With use of flexion-extension radiographs, different parameters can be measured, including segmental rotation, translatory movement, and the location of the center of rotation (36–38). Because there is a substantial motion difference between actively and passively performed movements, the use of passively performed radiographs has been recommended in diagnosing segmental instability, such as can occur after trauma (8).

The first description of the center of rotation in healthy adults of which we are aware was derived from Penning's (39) measurements of flexion and extension radiographs (Fig. 4.7). With computer-assisted methods (36–38), the average center of rotation has been determined and has confirmed Penning's findings. Lysell (2) describes the so-called top angle, or arc of motion, as being flat at the level of C2 and steep at the lower cervical spine. The motion

of the upper segments during flexion-extension is therefore fairly horizontal, whereas the motion of the lower segments is more like that of an arc (Fig. 4.8 and Table 4.5). The findings of the centers of rotation (Fig. 4.7) and the top angle (Fig. 4.8) are similar. The center of rotation in the upper region is slightly farther down than in the lower region, where the center of rotation is closer to the moving vertebra. The greater distance of the vertebra to the center of rotation in the upper region produces more flat motion, whereas smaller distance provides a sharper arc of motion.

The lateral bending of the cervical spine is normally coupled with an axial rotation to the same side (6,16). This means that the spinous processes are moving in the direction opposite to that of the motion (Fig. 4.9). This coupled motion is of clinical importance because palpation of the spinal processes can serve as an indirect indicator of disturbed

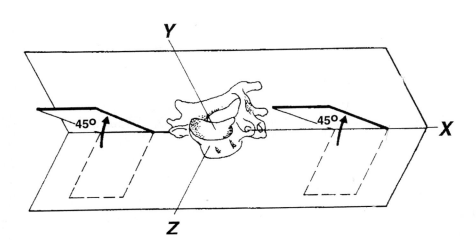

FIG. 4.6. Orientation of the articular processes of the lower cervical spine in the frontal plane.

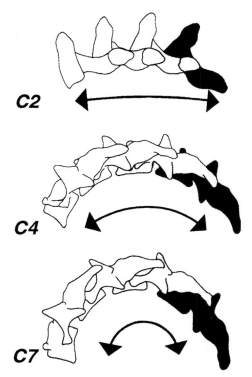

FIG. 4.8. Segmental motion arc according to Lysell (2). The flatter the articular surfaces, the flatter the arc of the motion segments, and vice versa. (From: White AA, Panjabi MM. *Clinical biomechanics of the spine*, 2nd ed. Philadelphia: JB Lippincott, 1990:321, with permission.)

function in motion segments. The lateral bending of the cervical spine below the first cervical vertebra has been variously reported by different researchers. According to Penning and Wilmink (40) the lateral bending is 35 degrees, whereas White and Panjabi (6) report 4 to 10 degrees per motion segment. The axial rotation, as measured with functional computed tomographic (CT) scans (18,24,25), is 3 to 7 degrees, whereas an *in vitro* study (32) showed slightly higher results of 8 to 12 degrees.

FUNCTIONAL ROLE OF THE SPINAL ELEMENTS: SPINAL STABILITY

Instability may arise due to fracture of bony elements or to soft tissue–related disorders, including injuries and dissection during surgery. Determining whether a spine is "stable" is extremely difficult, especially in the comatose or obtunded patient. It would be helpful to document the forces (magnitudes and types) needed to induce spinal injuries and the effects of such injuries and various surgical procedures on the kinematics of the spine. Both *in vivo* investigations in humans and animals and *in vitro* investigations of ligamentous spinal segments have been undertaken to accumulate biomechanical data of clinical importance. This section reviews the biomechanical literature on the functional role of various spinal elements in the cervical spine. The review is primarily based on the *in vitro* data reported in the literature. *In vitro* studies can be performed accurately and under controlled conditions and provide a comparative database for a surgeon's interpretation and decision making.

Upper Cervical Spine

High-speed-impact loads that may be imposed on the spine are one of the major causes of spinal instability in the cervical region, especially in the upper region. To quantify the likely injuries of the atlas, Oda and coworkers (41) subjected upper cervical spine specimens to high-speed axial impact by dropping 3- to 6-kg weights from various heights. The load produced axial compression and flexion of the specimen. Both bony and soft tissue injuries, similar to Jefferson's fractures, were observed. The bony fractures observed were six bursting fractures, one four-part fracture without a prominent bursting, and one posterior arch fracture. The major soft tissue injury involved the transverse ligament. There were five bony avulsions and three midsubstance tears.

The study was extended to determine the three-dimensional load-displacements of fresh ligamentous upper

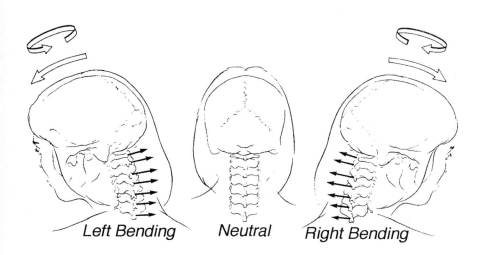

Left Bending   Neutral   Right Bending

FIG. 4.9. Coupled axial rotation during lateral bending of the head. (From: White AA, Panjabi MM. *Clinical biomechanics of the spine*, 2nd ed. Philadelphia: JB Lippincott, 1990:321, with permission.)

cervical spines (C0 through C3) in flexion, extension, and lateral bending before and following the impact loading in the axial mode (42). The largest increase in flexibility due to the injury was in flexion-extension—about 42%. In lateral bending, the increase was on the order of 24%; in axial rotation it was minimal—about 5%. These increases in motion are in concordance with the actual instabilities observed clinically. Jefferson (43) noted that patients with burst fractures of the atlas could not flex their heads, but could easily rotate without pain.

Heller and associates (44) tested the transverse ligament attached to the C1 vertebra by holding the C1 vertebra and pushing the ligament in the middle along the anteroposterior (AP) direction. The specimens were loaded with an MTS Systems (Eden Prairie, MN) testing device at varying loading rates. Eleven specimens failed within the substance of the ligament, and two failed by bone avulsion. The mean load to failure was 692 N (range, 220–1590 N). The displacement to failure ranged from 2 to 14 mm (mean, 6.7 mm). This study, when compared with the work of Oda and colleagues (41,42), suggests that (a) AP translation of the transverse ligament with respect to the dens is essential to produce its fracture; (b) rate of loading affects the type of fracture (bony versus ligamentous) but not the displacement at failure; and (c) even "axial" impact loads are capable of producing enough AP translation to produce a midsubstance tear of the ligament, as reported by Oda and coworkers (41,42).

The contribution to stabilization by the alar ligament of the upper cervical spine is of particular interest in evaluation of the effects of trauma, especially in the axial rotation mode. Goel and associates (27), in a study of occipitoatlantoaxial specimens, determined that the average values for axial rotation and torque at the point of maximum resistance were 68.1 degrees and 13.6 N-m, respectively. They also observed that the value of axial rotation at which complete bilateral rotary dislocation occurred was approximately the point of maximal resistance. The types of injuries observed were related to the magnitude of axial rotation imposed on a specimen during testing. Soft tissue injuries (such as stretch or rupture of the capsular ligaments, or subluxation of the C1-C2 facets) were confined to specimens rotated to or almost to the point of maximum resistance. Specimens that were rotated well beyond the point of maximum resistance also showed avulsion fractures of the bone at the points of attachment of the alar ligament or fractures of the odontoid process inferior to the level of alar ligament attachment. The alar ligament did not rupture in any of the specimens.

Chang and associates (45) extended this study to determine the effects of rate of loading (dynamic loading) on the occipitoatlantoaxial complex. The specimens were divided into three groups and tested until failure at three different dynamic loading rates: 50, 100, and 400 degrees per second, as compared to the quasi-static (4 degrees per second) rate of loading used by Goel and colleagues. The results showed that at the higher rates of loading, (a) the specimens became

stiffer and the torque required to produce "failure" increased significantly (e.g., from 13.6 N-m at 4 degrees per second to 27.9 N-m at 100 degrees per second); (b) the corresponding right-angular rotations (65 to 79 degrees) did not change significantly; and (c) the rates of the alar ligament midsubstance rupture increased, and that of "dens fracture" decreased. No fractures of the atlas were noted. This is another example of the rate of load application affecting the type of injury produced.

The forces required to produce various types of dens fractures have been documented by Doherty and colleagues (46), who harvested the second cervical vertebra from fresh human spinal columns. Force was applied at the tip of the dens until failure occurred. The direction of the applied force was adjusted to exert extension bending or combined flexion and lateral bending on the tip of the dens. Extension resulted in type III fractures, and the combined load led to type II fractures of the dens. Furthermore, dynamic loading modes are essential to produce midsubstance ligament ruptures as opposed to dens fractures, especially in a normal specimen.

The rotation-limiting ability of the alar ligament was investigated by Dvorak (24) and Panjabi (32) and their associates. A mean increase of 10.8 degrees or 30% (divided equally between the occipitoatlantal and atlantoaxial complexes) in axial rotation was observed in response to an alar lesion on the opposite side. Dvorak and Panjabi (47) verified these laboratory findings with a clinical study of 9 healthy adults and 43 patients with cervical spine instability, concluding that axial rotation of the occipitoatlantoaxial complex can increase after trauma-induced lesions of the alar ligaments. Panjabi and coworkers (48) determined the effects of alar ligament transections on the stability of the joint in flexion, extension, and lateral bending modes. Their main conclusion was that the motion changes occurred subsequent to alar ligament transection. The increases, however, were direction dependent.

Crisco and associates (49) compared changes in three-dimensional motion of C1 relative to C2 before and after capsular ligament transections in axial rotation. Two groups of cadaveric specimens were used to study the effect of two different sequential ligamentous transections. In the first group (n = 4), transection of the left capsular ligament was followed by transection of the right capsular ligament. In the second group (n = 10), transection of the left capsular ligament preceded transection of the left and right alar and transverse ligaments. The greatest changes in motion occurred in axial rotation to the side opposite the transection. In the first group, transection of left capsular ligaments resulted in a significant increase in axial rotation ROM to the right of 1.0 degree. After the right capsular ligament was transected, there was a further significant increase of 1.8 degrees to the left and of 1.0 degree to the right. Lateral bending to the left also increased significantly by 1.5 degrees after both ligaments were cut. In the second group, with the nonfunctional alar and transverse ligaments, transection of the capsular ligament resulted in greater increases in

ROM: 3.3 degrees to the right and 1.3 degrees to the left. Lateral bending to the right also increased significantly by 4.2 degrees. Although the matter is more complex than this, in general these studies show that the major function of the alar ligament is to prevent axial rotation to the contralateral side. Transection of the ligament increases the contralateral axial rotation by about 15%.

Middle and Lower Cervical Spine

In the C2 through T1 region of the spine, as in the upper cervical region, instabilities have been produced in a laboratory setting in an effort to understand the dynamics of traumatic forces on the spine (50,51). In one study, fresh ligamentous porcine cervical spine segments were subjected to flexion-compression, extension-compression, and compression-alone loads at high speeds (dynamic/impact loading) (50). The resultant injuries were evaluated by anatomic dissection. The severity of the resulting injuries was related mostly to the addition of bending moments to high-speed axial compression of the spine segment, since compression alone produced the least amount of injury and no definite pattern of injuries could be identified. Similar results have been reported by other investigators (32,51). The relevant studies describing the effects of instabilities produced by traumatic forces or surgical procedures on the spine are reviewed in the following paragraphs.

In vitro studies to determine the feasibility of the "stretch test" in predicting instability of the spine in the cervical region were performed by Panjabi and coworkers (52). Four cervical spines (C1 through T1; age 25 to 29) were loaded in axial tension in increments of 5 kg to a maximum of one-third of the specimen's body weight. The effects of sequential AP transection of soft tissues of a motion segment on the motion in one group and of posterior-anterior transections in another group were investigated. The intact cervical spine went into flexion under axial tension. Anterior transection produced extension. Posterior transection produced opposite results. Anterior injuries creating displacements of 3.3 mm at the disc space (with a force equal to one-third body weight) and rotation changes of approximately 3.8 degrees were considered precursors to failure. Likewise, posterior injuries resulting in 27 mm separation at the tips of the spinous process and an angular increase of 30 degrees with loading were considered unstable. This work supports the concept that spinal failure results from transection of either all the anterior elements or all the posterior plus at least two additional elements.

In a study by Goel and associates (26,53), the three-dimensional load-displacement motion of C4-C5 and C5-C6 as a function of transection of C5-C6 ligaments was determined. Transection was performed posteriorly, starting with the supraspinous and interspinous ligaments followed by the ligamentum flavum and the capsular ligaments. With the transection of the capsular ligaments, the C5-C6 motion segment (injured level) showed a significant increase in motion in extension, lateral bending, and axial rotation. A significant increase in flexion resulted when the ligamentum flavum was transected. Similar results were reported by Zdeblick and coworkers (54). This study also demonstrated increased motion in the segment immediately superior to the level of injury in flexion and lateral bending loading modes.

A major path of loading in the cervical spine is through the vertebral bodies, which are separated by the intervertebral disc. The role of the cervical intervertebral disc has received little attention. *In vivo* "injuries" result in disc degeneration and may produce osteophytes, ankylosed vertebrae, and changes in the apophyseal joints (55). The effects of total discectomy on cervical spine motions are of interest (56). Schulte and colleagues (57) reported a significant increase in motion after C5-C6 discectomy. Motion between C5 and C6 increased in flexion (66.6%), extension (69.5%), lateral bending (41.4%), and axial rotation (37.9%). In previous studies, Martins (58) and Wilson and Campbell (59) could not detect increases in motion roentgenographically and deemed the spines functionally stable. The reasons for this discrepancy in results are not apparent. The experimental designs were quite different, as were the methods of motion measurement. However, the disc obviously is a major structural and functional component of the cervical spine.

Cervical vertebral laminae may transmit loads. Laminectomies result in the removal of part of this loading path and the attachment points for the ligamentum flavum, interspinous ligament, and the supraspinous ligament. It is not surprising that total laminectomy results in significant modifications in the motion characteristics of the cervical spine, especially in children. For example, Bell and associates (60) reported that multiple-level cervical laminectomy can lead to increase in postoperative hyperlordosis or kyphosis in children. However, there was no correlation between diagnosis, sex, location, or number of levels decompressed and the subsequent development of deformity. Postlaminectomy spinal deformity in the cervical spine, however, is rare in adults, probably owing to stiffening of the spine with age and changes in facet morphology. Goel and coworkers (26,53) removed the laminae of multisegmental cervical spines (C2 through T2) at the level of C5 and C6 (total laminectomy). In flexion-extension mode, an increase in motion of about 10% was evident.

In another *in vitro* study, the effects of multilevel cervical laminaplasty (C3 through C6) and laminectomy with increasing amounts of facetectomy (25% and more) on the mechanical stability of the cervical spine were investigated (61). Cervical laminaplasty was not significantly different from the intact control, except for producing a marginal increase in axial rotation. However, cervical laminectomy with facetectomy of 25% or more resulted in a highly significant increase in cervical motion as compared with that of the intact specimens in flexion, extension, axial rotation, and lateral bending. There was no significant change in the coupled motions after either laminaplasty or laminectomy. The researchers recommended that concurrent arthrodesis be performed in patients undergoing laminectomy accompanied by more than 25% bilateral facetectomy. Alternatively, one may use laminoplasty to achieve decompression if feasible. More recently, the effect of laminoplasty on spinal motion using *in vivo* testing protocols has also been investigated (62,63).

Facet joints play an integral part in the biomechanical stability of the cervical spine. Cusick and associates (64) found that total unilateral and bilateral facetectomies decreased compression-flexion strength by 31.6% and 53.1%, respectively. Facetectomy resulted in an anterior shift of the IAR, resulting in increased compression of the vertebral body and disc. This work confirmed the findings of Raynor and coworkers (56,65), who reported that bilateral facetectomy of as much as 50% did not significantly decrease shear strength; however, with a 75% bilateral facetectomy, a significant decrease in shear strength was noted. When exposing an unfused segment, one should take great care to limit facet capsule resection to less than 50%. With resection of more than 50% of the capsule, postoperative hypermobility can occur and may require stabilization.

A SYSTEMATIC APPROACH TO CLINICAL INSTABILITY

"Clinical instability of the spine" is a controversial term, and significant disagreement exists even among experts (66). Clinical instability can occur as a result of trauma, disease, surgery, or some combination of the three. However, certain underlying observations relate the mechanical derangement to clinical problems of pain and neurologic deficit. These various considerations have been combined in the form of the following definition (6): Clinical instability of the spine is "the loss of the ability of the spine under physiologic loads to maintain relationships between vertebrae in such a way that there is neither initial nor subsequent damage to the spinal cord or nerve roots, and in addition, there is neither development of incapacitating deformity nor severe pain." In this definition, *physiologic loads* are those incurred during normal activity of the particular patient being evaluated. *Incapacitating deformity* is defined as gross deformity that the patient finds intolerable. *Incapacitating pain* is defined as pain that cannot be controlled by nonnarcotic analgesic medications.

To systematize the evaluation of clinical instability, we have proposed the use of a checklist (6). This approach ensures that all pertinent factors, both clinical and biomechanical, are considered and reasonably balanced. As in the earlier sections of this chapter, we separate the cervical spine into three regions: upper, middle, and lower.

Stability Evaluation of the Occipitoatlantal Joint

The anatomic and biomechanical characteristics of the occipitoatlantal (C0-C1-C2) joint complex and its specific patterns of instability are very different from those of the middle and lower cervical spine. Presently, no checklist is available for this region of the spine.

Anatomy

The anatomic structures that provide stability for articulation of C0-C1 include the cup-shaped configuration of the occipitoatlantal joints and their capsules, along with the anterior and posterior atlantooccipital membranes (Fig. 4.3). Additional anatomic stability is gained through the ligamentous connections between the occiput and the axis: the tectorial membrane, alar ligaments, and apical ligament (67). We believe that because of its structural characteristics, the occipitoatlantal joint is relatively unstable, at least in children. Its stability may increase in adult life because of a decrease in elasticity of the ligaments.

Biomechanics

Weisel and colleagues (68) showed that the normal range of sagittal plane translation in flexion-extension does not exceed 1 mm. This measurement is made between the basion of the occiput and the tip of the odontoid. The findings of more than 5 mm between the tip of the dens and the basion of the occiput or more than 1 mm of translation in flexion-extension are important and useful criteria for instability (Fig. 4.10).

Symptoms of weakness of the limbs, with or without associated neck and occipital pain, provide additional indications of instability. The criteria are shown in Table 4.6. When any

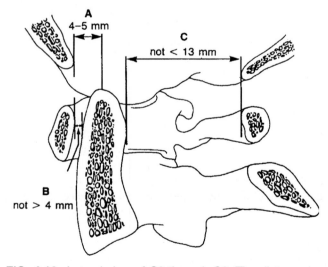

FIG. 4.10. Lateral view of C0 through C2. The distance between the basion of the occiput and the top of the dens is 4 to 5 mm (*A*). An increase of more than 1 mm in this distance in flexion-extension views is believed to indicate instability of C0-C1, if one assumes that the transverse ligament of the atlas is intact. The distance between the anterior border of the dens and the posterior border of the ring of C1 should not be more than 4 mm (*B*). Another important measurement must be considered: the distance between the posterior margin of the dens and the anterior cortex of the posterior ring of C1. This distance is of concern if it is less than 13 mm (*C*). (From: White AA, Panjabi MM. *Cervical biomechanics of the spine*, 2nd ed. Philadelphia: JB Lippincott, 1990, with permission.)

TABLE 4.6. *Criteria for Occipitoatlantal Joint Complex Instability*

>8°	Axial rotation C0-C1 to one side
>1 mm	C0-C1 translation (as measured in Fig. 4.13)
>7 mm	Overhang C1-C2 (total right and left, on anteroposterior radiograph)
>45°	Axial rotation C1-C2 to one side
>4 mm	C1-C2 translation (as in Fig. 4.13)
<13 mm	Posterior body of C2 to posterior ring of C1 (as in Fig. 4.13)
Avulsed transverse ligament	

Data from White AA, Panjabi MM. *Clinical biomechanics of the spine,* 2nd ed. Philadelphia: JB Lippincott, 1990.

of these criteria are present, one should make a comprehensive analysis of the C0-C1-C2 complex for possible clinical instability.

Stability Evaluation of the Atlantoaxial Joint

Anatomy

The most important anatomic structures affecting the clinical stability of the C1-C2 articulation are transverse ligaments, dentate ligaments, the apical and alar ligaments, and joint capsules (32,49,67). The dentate, alar, and apical ligaments are considered secondary stabilizers of the C1-C2 complex. The cruciate ligament, the most well-developed portion of which is the transverse ligament, is the major stabilizing ligament. The atlantooccipital membrane also plays a role in the stabilization of these joints. The importance of the mutual dependence of these major ligaments and an intact normal dens is apparent. If the dens is hypoplastic, congenitally not intact, or fractured, the ligaments cannot provide stability.

Biomechanics

Studies of horizontal translation showed that an anterior dislocation of C1 on C2 can occur with an insufficiency of the transverse ligament only. The alar ligaments and the tectorial membrane did not prevent dislocation after the transverse ligament was transected. The biomechanical studies of Fielding and coworkers (69) on the transverse ligament showed that the structure, although very weak in some subjects, prevented more than 3 mm of anterior translation of C1 on C2 when present. These studies also showed that the alar ligaments deform readily and are not capable of preventing additional displacement under loads that would rupture the transverse ligament.

Stability Evaluation of the Middle and Lower Cervical Spine

A checklist for the middle and lower cervical spine (C2 through T1) has been developed (6) based on biomechanical studies (70,71) and is shown in Table 4.7. Some factors

TABLE 4.7. *Checklist for the Diagnosis of Clinical Instability in the Middle and Lower Cervical Spine*

Element	Point value
Biomechanical considerations	
Anterior elements destroyed or unable to function	2
Posterior elements destroyed or unable to function	2
Positive stretch test	2
Radiographic criteria[a]	4
A. Flexion-extension radiographs[b]	
1. Sagittal plane translation > 3.5 mm or 20%	2
2. Sagittal plane rotation > 20°	2
OR	
B. Resting radiographs[a]	
1. Sagittal plane displacement > 3.5 mm or 20%	2
2. Relative sagittal plane angulation >11°	2
Other considerations	
Abnormal disc narrowing	1
Developmentally narrow spinal canal	1
1. Sagittal diameter < 13 mm	
OR	
2. Pavlov's ratio < 0.8	
Spinal cord damage	2
Nerve root damage	1
Dangerous loading anticipated	1

A total of 5 points or more equals instability.
[a] See Figures 4.13 and 4.14 for information on making these measurements.
[b] See Figure 4.13.
Adapted from White AA, Panjabi MM. *Clinical biomechanics of the spine,* 2nd ed. Philadelphia: JB Lippincott, 1990.

important for the evaluation of clinical instability are presented in this section.

Anatomic and Biomechanical Considerations

A schematic diagram of the anatomy of the middle and lower cervical spine is shown in Figure 4.11. At the level of the intervertebral disc, the annulus fibrosis appears to be the crucial stabilizing structure (6). Bailey (72,73) has emphasized the importance of this structure. Munro (74) performed experimental studies on cadaver spines and concluded that cervical spine stability derives mainly from the intervertebral discs and the anterior longitudinal ligaments and PLL.

Checklist Considerations

White and Panjabi and colleagues (70,71) performed experiments on cervical spine functional spinal units in high-humidity chambers using physiologic loads to simulate flexion and extension. They defined the anterior elements as the PLL and all structures anterior to it. The posterior

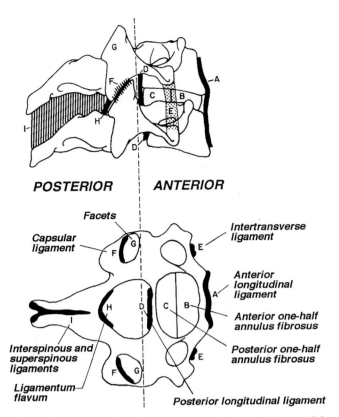

POSTERIOR | **ANTERIOR**

Facets
Capsular ligament
Intertransverse ligament
Anterior longitudinal ligament
Anterior one-half annulus fibrosus
Posterior one-half annulus fibrosus
Interspinous and superspinous ligaments
Ligamentum flavum
Posterior longitudinal ligament

FIG. 4.11. Schematic of ligamentous structures that participate in the stabilization of the middle and lower cervical spine. The components are divided into anterior and posterior elements. Anatomic components posterior to the posterior longitudinal ligament are defined as the posterior elements. The posterior longitudinal ligament and all the anatomic components anterior to it are defined as the anterior elements. In the experiments on clinical stability, ligaments were cut in the alphabetical order indicated in the diagram from anterior to posterior and in reverse alphabetical order from posterior to anterior. (From: White AA, Panjabi MM. *Clinical biomechanics of the spine*, 2nd ed. Philadelphia: JB Lippincott, 1990:321, with permission.)

elements were defined as all structures behind the PLL. On the basis of these studies, it was suggested that if a functional spinal unit (FSU) has all its anterior elements plus one additional structure, or all its posterior elements plus one additional structure, it will probably remain stable under physiologic loads. Therefore, to provide for some clinical margin of safety in the checklist, we suggest that any FSU in which all the anterior elements or all the posterior elements are either destroyed or unable to function should be considered potentially unstable. Two points are given for the loss of each of these anatomic elements.

Controlled, monitored axial traction (the stretch test) may be helpful to evaluate the integrity of the ligamentous structures of the middle and lower cervical spine. Figure 4.12 and Table 4.8 provide a diagrammatic synopsis of this test and the details of the procedure. An abnormal test is indicated by differences either greater than 1.7 mm of interspace

separation or greater than 7.5 degrees of change in angle between vertebrae, comparing the prestretch condition with the condition after application of axial traction equivalent to one-third body weight. This is based on a biomechanical study simulating the stretch test in fresh cadaveric cervical spines (52). Two points in the checklist are given for a positive stretch test.

One final anatomic consideration should be noted. If all other considerations are the same, patients with the anterior elements destroyed or unable to function are more clinically unstable in extension, whereas patients with the posterior elements destroyed or unable to function are more unstable in flexion. These factors should be considered during patient transfers and when a patient's neck is immobilized after injury.

Radiographic Criteria

The measurement of translation and displacement is shown in Figure 4.13. This method takes into account variations in magnification and should be useful when there is a tube-to-film distance of 72 inches. Sagittal plane displacement or translation greater than 3.5 mm on either static (resting) or dynamic (flexion-extension) lateral radiographs should be considered potentially unstable. This value was determined from an experimentally obtained value of 2.7 mm and an assumed radiographic magnification of 30% (71). If the radiographic magnification is not known, the 3.5-mm measurement is equivalent to a translation or displacement of 20% of vertebral body AP diameter. Two points in the checklist are given for abnormal sagittal plane displacement or translation.

Angular measurements are shown in Figure 4.14. There is no magnification problem in measuring rotation or angulation. More than 20 degrees of sagittal plane rotation on dynamic (flexion-extension) radiographs should be considered abnormal and potentially unstable. This value was based on a review of the literature of *in vitro* and *in vivo* cervical spine ROM (6). When dynamic radiographs cannot be obtained (that is, in an acute traumatic setting), a static (resting) lateral radiograph that shows more than 11 degrees of relative sagittal plane angulation should be considered potentially unstable. This value is based on a biomechanical study (70). Note that 11 degrees of relative angulation means 11 degrees more than the amount of angulation at the presumed intact FSU above or below the one in question. This standard of comparison takes into account the normal angulation between FSUs (that is, the normal cervical lordosis). Two points in the checklist are given for abnormal sagittal plane rotation or abnormal relative sagittal plane angulation.

Note that a total of four points in the cervical checklist is given for the radiographic measurements just described: Either dynamic (flexion-extension) or static (resting) radiographs are used in the checklist, not both. When both dynamic and static radiographs have been obtained, the measurements should be made on the dynamic films. Static

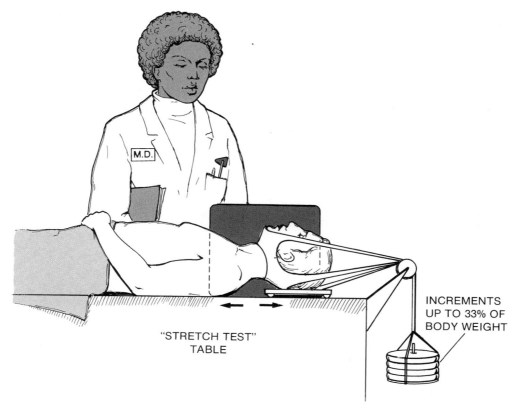

FIG. 4.12. Diagrammatic synopsis of stretch test. A physician knowledgeable about the test is in attendance. The neurologic status is monitored by following signs and symptoms. Incremental loads up to 33% of body weight or 65 pounds are applied. Each lateral radiograph is checked before the axial load is augmented. The neurologic hammer symbolizes neurologic examination; the roller platform under the head reduces friction. (From: White AA, Panjabi MM. *Clinical biomechanics of the spine*, 2nd ed. Philadelphia: JB Lippincott, 1990:321, with permission.)

radiographs should be used in the cervical checklist only when flexion-extension films cannot be obtained.

The radiographic interpretation in general, especially for sagittal plane translation and displacement, is decidedly different in children up to age 7 years (75). It is risky to interpret radiographs of patients in this age group without knowledge of some of the normal findings that may appear to be pathologic to an inexperienced physician.

Two final radiographic considerations should be noted. First, Bailey (73) remarked, and we have observed, that in

TABLE 4.8. *Procedure for Stretch Test to Evaluate Clinical Stability in the Lower Spine*

1. It is recommended that the test be performed under the supervision of a physician.
2. Traction is applied through secure skeletal fixation or a head halter. If the latter is used, a small portion of gauze sponge between the molars improves comfort.
3. A roller is placed under the patient's head to reduce frictional forces.
4. The radiographic film is placed 0.36 m (14 inches) from the patient's spine. The tube distance is 1.82 m (72 inches) from the film.
5. An initial lateral radiograph is taken, carefully evaluating for C0-C1-C2 subluxation. Abnormal displacement in this region should be looked for on each film because it can often be difficult to identify.
6. A 10-pound weight is added. (If the initial weight is 10 pounds, this step is omitted.)
7. Traction is increased by 10-pound increments. A lateral radiograph is taken and measured.
8. Step 7 is repeated until one-third of body weight or 65 pounds is reached.
9. After each additional weight application, the patient is checked for any change in neurologic status. The test is stopped and considered positive should this occur. The radiographs are developed and read after each weight increment. An abnormal separation of the anterior or posterior elements of the vertebrae is the most typical indication of a positive test. An interval of at least 5 minutes should be allowed between incremental weight applications; this will allow for development of the film, performance of the necessary neurologic checks, and creep of the viscoelastic structures involved.
10. The test is contraindicated in a spine with obvious clinical instability.

Data from White AA, Panjabi MM. *Clinical Biomechanics of the Spine,* 2nd edition, Philadelphia: JB Lippincott, 1990.

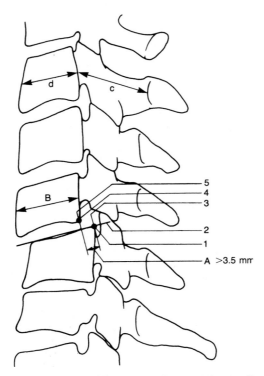

FIG. 4.13. The method for measuring translatory displacement is as follows: (*1*) A point is marked at the posterosuperior angle of the projected image of the vertebral body below the interspace of the functional spinal unit (FSU) being evaluated. (*2*) A line is drawn along the upper vertebral end plate of the vertebra below the interspace of the FSU under analysis. (*3*) At the point where this intersects the mark, at the posterior portion of the end plate, a short perpendicular line is drawn. (*4*) Next, a mark is made at the posteroinferior angle of image of the vertebral body above the interspace of the FSU being evaluated. (*5*) A short line through the second mark and perpendicular to the line on the subjacent vertebral end plate is drawn. The linear distance between the two perpendicular lines is measured. This can be called distance *A*. The anteroposterior sagittal plane diameter at the midlevel of the supraadjacent vertebra is measured. This distance is called *B*. If distance *A* is more than 20% of distance *B*, instability is considered to exist, and should be so entered on the checklist. An alternate method is to simply measure the linear distance *A;* if this is more than 3.5 mm, it is considered suggestive of instability, and two points are entered onto the checklist. Pavlov's ratio is a reliable, accurate method for recognizing a developmentally narrow canal without the variables involved in linear measurements. The measurement *c* is the distance between the midlevel of the posterior aspect of the vertebral body and the nearest point on the corresponding spinolaminar line. The measurement *d* is apparent on lateral radiographs as the anteroposterior distance from the front to the back of the vertebral body measured at the midlevel. The ratio *c/d* is considered normal if it is 1.0 or greater, and abnormal if less than 0.8. These measurements are used in conjunction with the checklist (Table 4.7).

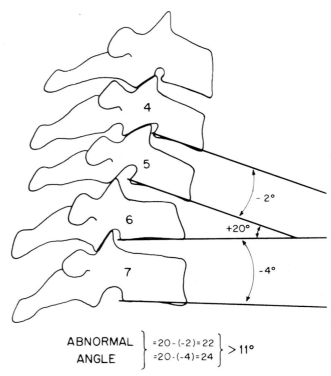

FIG. 4.14. The angulation between C5 and C6 is 20 degrees, which is more than 11 degrees greater than that at either adjacent interspace. The angle at C4 and C5 measures −2 degrees, and that at C6 and C7 measures −4 degrees. This finding of abnormal angulation is based on a comparison of the interspace in question with either adjacent interspace, which allows for the angulation present due to the normal lordosis of the cervical spine. We interpret a difference of 11 degrees or greater as evidence of clinical instability. These measurements are to be used in conjunction with the checklist (Table 4.7). (From: White AA, Panjabi MM. *Clinical biomechanics of the spine*, 2nd ed. Philadelphia: JB Lippincott, 1990:321, with permission.)

the traumatized spine there may be narrowing of the disc at the damaged FSU (72). In patients younger than 35 years, we submit that posttraumatic disc narrowing is suggestive of disruption of the annulus fibroses and of possible instability. Second, if all other considerations are the same,

patients with a developmentally narrow spinal canal are more apt to develop neurologic deficit because less space is available for the spinal cord. A developmentally narrow canal is defined as one measuring less than 13 mm in its AP dimension on a lateral radiograph (76) or with a Pavlov's ratio of less than 0.8 (3,57,77). The 13-mm absolute value accounts for some radiographic magnification, whereas the Pavlov's ratio need not consider magnification because it is the ratio of the AP diameter of the canal to the AP diameter of the vertebral body. One point each in the checklist is given for abnormal disc narrowing or a developmentally narrow canal.

Clinical Considerations

Is the presence of distinct medullary or root damage associated with spinal trauma or disease evidence of clinical instability? This question deserves some discussion. We have suggested that clinical instability concerns the prediction of subsequent neurologic damage. What is the importance of the presence of initial neurologic damage to the probability of subsequent neurologic damage? We believe that if the trauma is severe enough to cause initial neurologic damage, the support structures probably have been altered sufficiently to allow subsequent neurologic damage and that the condition is thus clinically unstable. However, Gosch and colleagues (78) showed that it is possible to produce medullary damage in animals with intact supporting structures. In general, we believe that neurologic deficit is an important consideration in the evaluation of clinical instability. Evidence of root involvement is a weaker indicator of clinical instability. For example, a unilateral facet dislocation may cause enough foraminal encroachment to result in root symptoms or signs but not enough ligamentous damage to render the FSU unstable. Two points in the checklist are given for spinal cord damage, and one point is given for nerve root damage.

Although further intensive clinical studies will be required, the stretch test method has recently been evaluated in preliminary clinical trials by Harris and colleagues (79) in obtunded patients and shown to be a possible method of spinal stability assessment in this patient population.

The final consideration involves the important individual variations in physiologic load requirements. The clinician uses judgment in an attempt to anticipate the magnitude of loads that the particular patient's spine is expected to maintain after injury. Anticipating dangerous loads can be helpful. One point in the checklist is given if dangerous loading is anticipated.

SPINAL INSTABILITY: THE NEUTRAL ZONE

The definition of spinal instability presented previously indicates that a significant "change in the patterns of displacement" may be associated with pain and/or neurologic dysfunction and therefore may be an indicator of spinal instability. This has been the basis for most of the diagnostic indicators used clinically for determination of instability in the last 50 years. Often, the change in the "pattern of displacement" has been interpreted as hypermobility or increased ROM. Knutsson was probably the first to observe that patients with low back pain had increased AP translational ROM. Several similar studies have been made since then, some confirming the hypermobility concept (80) and others showing *decreased* ROM (18) in patients with low back pain. Therefore, hypermobility or a significant increase in ROM may not be as reliable an indicator of clinical instability as once believed. This indicates the need for new interpretation of "change in the pattern of displacement." The neutral zone (NZ) was proposed as an indicator of clinical instability (81).

Measurement Methods

When a spinal specimen is physiologically loaded repeatedly in a particular direction, the specimen does not return to its initial position on release of the load, but exhibits a certain residual displacement. The residual displacements,

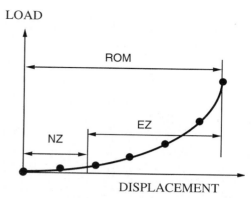

FIG. 4.15. The load-displacement curve of a functional spinal unit or motion segment is generally nonlinear. To document this aspect, neutral zone (NZ) and elastic zone (EZ) are needed in addition to range of motion (ROM). (From: White AA, Panjabi MM. *Clinical biomechanics of the spine*, 2nd ed. Philadelphia: JB Lippincott, 1990:321, with permission.)

measured from the neutral position, present just before the beginning of the third load cycle define the NZ. The elastic zone (EZ) is computed as the difference between the ROM and the NZ (Fig. 4.15). Methods are available to quantify the NZ, EZ, and ROM *in vitro* (81–83). A brief description follows.

The process consists of loading three times to the estimated maximum physiologic load, in several incremental steps. The load-displacement values are recorded during the third load cycle, which begins 30 seconds after removal of the load at the end of the second load cycle, to allow for viscoelastic creep. The process is then repeated by loading in the opposite direction. The residual displacements present between the beginning of the third load cycle in one direction and the third load cycle in the opposite direction constitute the NZ region. The neutral position is the midway point, making the NZ equal to half of the NZ region. The ROM is the maximum motion due to the physiologic load (Fig. 4.15). The EZ is obtained simply as the difference between the ROM and NZ. Average values of NZ, EZ, and ROM for flexion-extension, lateral bending, and axial rotation for the upper cervical spine have been obtained (83) and are shown in Figure 4.16.

Experimental Observations

Neutral zone and ROM empirical measurements were made in a human cadaveric model (18). Detailed data of the upper, middle, and lower cervical spine were recorded (Tables 4.9 and 4.10). These data support the use of *in vitro* studies over *in vivo* studies. With flexion-extension moment loading, coupled translations in the sagittal plane were anteriorly directed for flexion and posteriorly directed for extension at all intersegmental levels. With axial loading, the cervical spine exhibited the largest main rotation at C1-C2 and the largest coupled extension at C0-C1. Coupled lateral bending was present at all levels, in the same direction as the applied torque. Lateral bending moment elicited

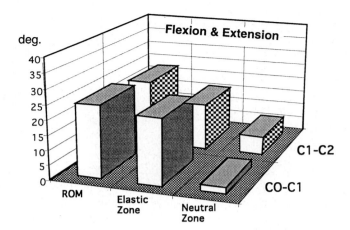

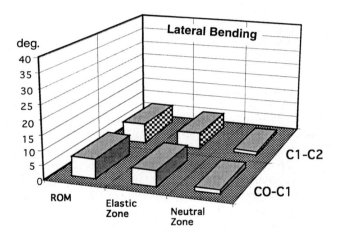

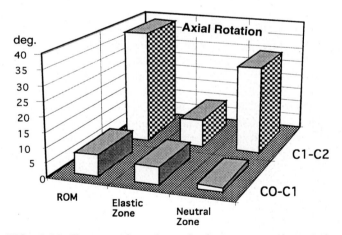

FIG. 4.16. Ranges of motion, elastic zones, and neutral zones for the atlantooccipital (C0-C1) and atlantoaxial (C1-C2) joints for flexion-extension, lateral bending, and axial rotation are shown. (From: Panjabi MM, Dvorak J, Duranceau J, et al. Three-dimensional movements of the upper cervical spine. *Spine* 1988;13:726–730, with permission.)

the largest main lateral bending in the middle region and at C0-C1. Coupled axial rotation was in the same direction as the lateral bending at all intersegmental segments.

Both the NZ and ROM are measures of displacement. Several experimental studies support the view that the NZ is a more sensitive parameter than ROM in characterizing spinal instability. The NZ increases with injury and fractures and decreases with muscle action and spinal fixation. These studies are summarized in the following sections.

Neutral Zone and Spinal Injury

In a high-speed-trauma experiment on porcine cervical spine specimens, both the NZ and ROM increased with the severity of injury (84). However, in a direct comparison between the NZ and ROM, the NZ increases (measured as a percentage of the intact behavior) were larger than the corresponding increases in ROM for the same injury. For example, in extension-compression trauma, the NZ for the axial rotational instability increased by 540%, whereas the corresponding ROM increase was only 240%. In the latest study of this subject in our laboratory, in which spine specimens were subjected to high-speed trauma of increasing severity, we found the increase in flexion-extension NZ to be the first indicator of the onset of injury (82). This was not true of the increases in the corresponding ROM.

Richter and colleagues (85) examined sequential injury to the discoligamentous structures of C5-C6. Load-displacement properties were evaluated (NZ and ROM) and compared with the normal preinjury load-displacement patterns. Compared with the intact functional spinal unit, significant differences were observed in flexion-extension during all stages of sequential injury to the discoligamentous structures. Only the last stage of injury affected axial displacements. Lateral bending was unaffected.

Neutral Zone and Fractures

In another study, instability of experimentally produced fresh cadaveric thoracolumbar compression fractures was measured before and after experimental trauma (86). Physiologic moments were applied in the vertical planes—sagittal plane, frontal plane, and several planes in between—in the presence of 400 N preload. NZ was measured in each plane. Ching and coworkers (86) plotted the neutral zones on a graph, with flexion-extension on the x-axis and lateral bending on the y-axis. Both the intact and postinjury values were plotted. The lines joining the points formed approximate rectangles. The NZ rectangles increased in area as a result of the injury. The rectangles were quantified by the area and the distance of the centroid from the origin. The decrease in height was highly correlated ($r^2 = 0.83$) to the NZ centroidal shift due to the trauma. Furthermore, small height decreases corresponded to large NZ centroidal shifts. Ching and coworkers, interpreting their findings in a clinical setting, suggest that even small height decreases (less than

TABLE 4.9. *Neutral Zones Measured from Multidirectional Flexibility Testing, in Degrees*

	C0-C1	C1-C2	C2-C3	C3-C4	C4-C5	C5-C6	C6-C7
Flexion	3.0 ± 1.0	4.0 ± 2.4	0.7 ± 0.6	0.3 ± 0.5	1.8 ± 1.3	1.8 ± 1.3	1.0 ± 0.7
Extension	13.9 ± 4.1	8.7 ± 6.7	1.0 ± 0.7	1.7 ± 1.7	1.9 ± 1.8	2.1 ± 2.0	1.3 ± 1.0
Axial rotation	2.5 ± 1.6	39.6 ± 7.5	1.1 ± 0.5	1.6 ± 0.5	2.4 ± 0.6	1.7 ± 0.5	0.6 ± 0.3
Lateral bending	3.6 ± 1.5	2.4 ± 1.2	4.1 ± 1.1	4.4 ± 1.2	4.4 ± 1.1	3.0 ± 1.1	2.2 ± 1.0

Values are mean ± standard deviations. Values for axial rotation and lateral bending sum both right and left sides.

50%) should "be considered when assessing compression fracture instability" (86). Therefore, the NZ was shown to be an indicator of another aspect of compression fractures.

Slosar and colleagues (77) produced experimental burst fractures in the laboratory and measured stiffness in flexion, lateral bending, and axial rotation, both before and after the trauma. They reported all load-displacement curves to be bilinear (that is, having two distinct regions of constant stiffness values). In the initial phase, the load-displacement curve showed low stiffness; in the latter phase, it showed high stiffness. These two behaviors are predictable from the concepts of neutral and elastic zones, respectively. For all three motion types, the initial-phase stiffness decreased much more significantly than the latter-phase stiffness. For flexion, lateral bending, and axial rotation, the EZ increased by 20%, 42%, and 61%, respectively. The corresponding increases for the NZ were 49%, 80%, and 87%. This indicates that for all three instability tests the NZ increased much more than the corresponding EZ. Slosar and colleagues (77) further noted that all NZ increases (over the intact values) were statistically significant, whereas none of the EZ increases were significant. Their study clearly shows that the NZ is an important and sensitive parameter in indicating injury.

Neutral Zone and Muscles

In three studies—two *in vitro* experiments (7,84) and the other a mathematical model of the spine (87)—the application of simulated deep muscular forces to the injured spinal specimen was investigated. In all three studies, sequential injuries of the spinal column components resulted in corresponding increases in NZ and ROM. On using a novel muscle force replication system, results similar to *in vivo*

measurements of ROM and load displacement were obtained (Fig. 4.17)(7). Application of an anteriorly and inferiorly directed force vector to the middle of the spinous process decreased the NZ almost to the intact value, but the ROM did not decrease. Therefore, if there were an increase in NZ (e.g., in a clinical setting due to degeneration or trauma), the muscles might be capable of decreasing it and restoring it to near-normal values.

Neutral Zone, Spinal Fixation, and Neck Pain

In a clinical study, a small external fixator was used to stabilize a spinal segment temporarily in the cervical spine (88). The fixator is used as a diagnostic tool, and its successful application in extinguishing the pain at a particular segmental level identifies that segment as the source of pain. Surgical arthrodesis was performed at the level diagnosed as the source of pain. At 10.2-month follow-up, the average pain had decreased (8.3 points preoperatively to 2.6 points postoperatively, on a visual analog pain scale of 0 to 10).

To quantify the underlying motions responsible for the pain in the clinical study of Grob and Dvorak (88), an *in vitro* experiment in fresh cadaveric human cervical spine specimens (89) was conducted. The purpose of the study was to answer several questions. Does the application of the fixator reduce the intervertebral motion? If it does reduce motion, how much reduction occurred in what motion direction? Which parameter was reduced the most: NZ or ROM? The specimen was first tested intact for its three-dimensional flexibility; normal protocols were used for this purpose. The pins were inserted in the lateral masses of C4, C5, and C6 by a standard surgical technique simulating *in vivo* surgery. The fixation was applied to prevent motion

TABLE 4.10. *Ranges of Motion Measured from Multidirectional Flexibility Testing, in Degrees*

	C0-C1	C1-C2	C2-C3	C3-C4	C4-C5	C5-C6	C6-C7
Flexion	7.2 ± 2.5	12.3 ± 2.0	3.5 ± 1.3	4.3 ± 2.9	5.3 ± 3.0	5.5 ± 2.6	3.7 ± 2.1
Extension	20.2 ± 4.6	12.1 ± 6.5	2.7 ± 1.0	3.4 ± 2.1	4.8 ± 1.9	4.4 ± 2.8	3.4 ± 1.9
Axial rotation	9.9 ± 3.0	56.7 ± 4.8	3.3 ± 0.8	5.1 ± 1.2	6.8 ± 1.3	5.0 ± 1.0	2.9 ± 0.8
Lateral bending	9.1 ± 1.5	6.6 ± 2.3	8.6 ± 1.8	9.0 ± 1.9	9.3 ± 1.7	6.5 ± 1.5	5.4 ± 1.5

Values are mean ± standard deviations. Values for axial rotation and lateral bending sum both right and left sides.

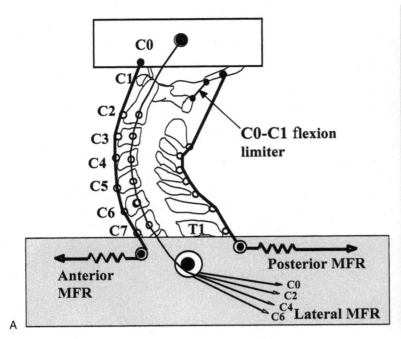
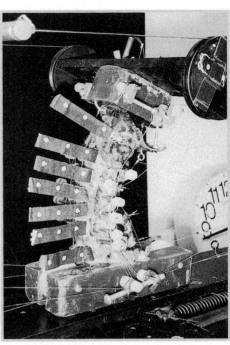

FIG. 4.17. A: The muscle force replication (MFR) system. For the lateral MFR, the cables are anchored at C0, C2, C4, and C6 and are guided to pass through intersegmental centers of rotation. For the anterior and posterior MFR, both cables are anchored at C0 and are guided to pass on the anterior and posterior aspects of each vertebra, respectively. **B:** Flexibility testing of the specimen with MFR. Photograph of the specimen with the MFR system.

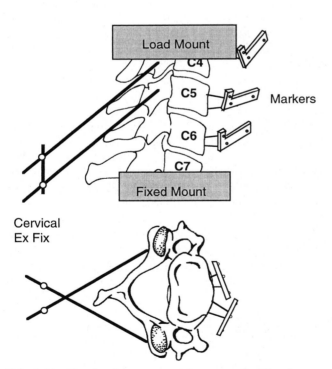

FIG. 4.18. Sketch of the external fixator applied to a human cervical spine specimen. Also shown are the markers, each containing three light-emitting diodes for recording the three-dimensional intervertebral motions with an optoelectronic motion measurement system. (From: Panjabi MM. Lumbar spine instability: a biomechanical challenge. *Curr Orthop* 1994;8:100–105, with permission.)

at C4-C5 or C5-C6 (Fig. 4.18). The specimen was then tested a second time with the same protocol. Results were expressed as the percentage of decreases in motions due to application of the fixator. For ROM, the greatest decreases were in axial rotation, followed by flexion, lateral bending, and extension (Fig. 4.19). All NZ decreases were greater. The greatest decrease was in flexion-extension, followed by axial rotation and lateral bending. On the average, ROM decreased by about 39%, whereas the NZ decreased by 69%.

How do we integrate the combined findings of the *in vivo* clinical study (88), in which the application of the external fixator eliminated the neck pain, and the *in vitro* biomechanical study (89), in which the same fixator decreased the NZ more than the ROM? A free interpretation of these findings, achieved with an innovative use of the load-displacement curve, is provided in the following section.

Neutral Zone and Pain Hypothesis

A typical load-displacement curve showing the NZ and ROM was shown in Figure 4.15. In the NZ, spinal motion is easy, but in the rest of the ROM (that is, the EZ), much more effort is required to produce the motion. Let us consider a ball in a bowl as an analogy of the NZ, EZ, and ROM (Fig. 4.20). The ball moves easily in the shallow part of the bowl (NZ) and requires effort in the steeper part (EZ). The shape of the bowl indicates the magnitude of spinal stability or instability. A shallower bowl (e.g, a soup

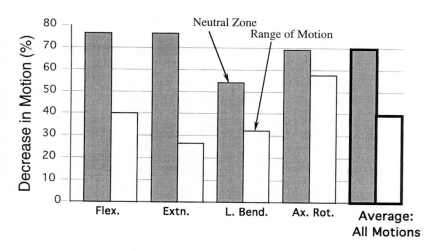

FIG. 4.19. Percentage decreases in neutral zone and range of motion due to application of the external fixator for flexion, extension, lateral bending, and axial rotation. Also shown are the average decreases. (Based on data from Panjabi MM. Lumbar spine instability: a biomechanical challenge. *Curr Orthop* 1994;8: 100–105, with permission.)

plate; Fig. 4.20B) represents a less stable spine, and a deeper bowl (e.g., a wine glass; Fig. 4.20C) may represent a more stable spine.

Having a ball in a bowl as our analogy of stable and unstable spines, we can interpret the previously mentioned motion–pain relation of the cervical spine in the following manner. For each person without such neck pain, there is a normal range of NZ and a pain-free zone (Fig. 4.21). The NZ is smaller than the pain-free zone. In a painful spine, on the other hand, the NZ is larger than the pain-free zone, thus representing a painful condition. With adequate fixation with an external fixator or fusion, the NZ is decreased. When the decrease is sufficient (that is, the NZ is smaller than the pain-free zone), the spine is again pain free.

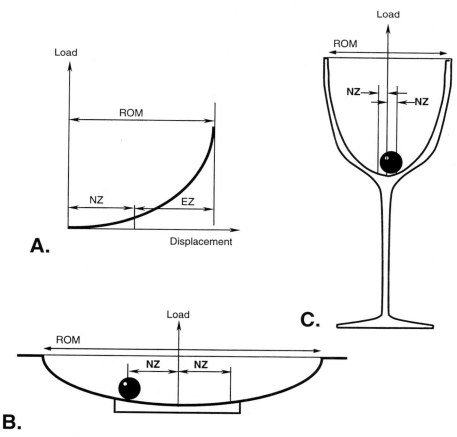

FIG. 4.20. A: An analogy of the load-displacement curve is a ball in a bowl. **B:** A shallow soup plate, with relatively large neutral zone (NZ), represents a spinal segment that is relatively unstable. **C:** A wine glass represents a spinal segment that is relatively more stable because its NZ is relatively much smaller.

Normal

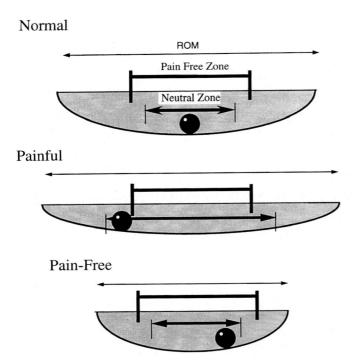

Painful

Pain-Free

FIG. 4.21. An interpretation of a mechanical pain hypothesis. In a normal subject, the neutral zone (NZ) is less than the pain-free zone. In a patient with pain, the NZ is larger than the pain-free zone. With fixation provided either by an external fixator or fusion, the NZ is again brought within the pain-free zone. (From: Panjabi MM. Lumbar spine instability: a biomechanical challenge. *Curr Orthop* 1994;8:100–105, with permission.)

The interactions between the NZ, pain-free zone, and spinal state (injury and fixation) have been explored in a study in which the initial activity of the sternocleidomastoid (SCM) muscle was measured using electromyography in normal volunteers and in patients who had a history of chronic whiplash-associated disorder (90). Surprisingly, the whiplash group showed no evidence of the predicted earlier activation of SCM muscles. Many whiplash patients never reached the point in the ROM where SCM muscle activity rises sharply, as it did in the normal controls. The movements of the whiplash patients remained within the region of low muscle activity, suggesting a restricted ROM secondary to pain or a fear of pain. The interactions between the NZ, pain-free zone, and spinal state (injury and fixation) continue to be confirmed. However, further clinical studies are necessary to validate the hypothesis.

SUMMARY

Kinematics is the division of mechanics that studies the motion of bodies without considering the forces that produced the motion. The study of kinematics provides a basis for determining when too much irregular motion may be associated with pain or neurologic impairment. This chapter presented three aspects of clinically relevant kinematics of the cervical spine.

First, to differentiate the abnormal and normal cervical spine, high-quality normal motion and coupling pattern data are needed. The ROM for flexion, extension, lateral bending, and axial rotation is provided for each intervertebral level based on *in vitro* and *in vivo* studies. Recently, the head motion with respect to the trunk was ascertained *in vivo* in a three-dimensional manner. In studies of patients and normal subjects, the motions produced passively (i.e., with the assistance of the examiner) were shown to be greater in magnitude and to have decreased SD. Among normal subjects, most cervical spine motion decreased with age and was gender dependent. Maximum motion at a single level occurs at C1-C2 in axial rotation. The locations of the centers of rotations (in flexion-extension) vary with the level in the middle and lower cervical spine regions. The centers of rotation are located farther down from the moving vertebra in the middle region of the spine as compared with those in the lower region, resulting in an arc of motion that is flatter in the middle and steeper in the lower region. Strong coupling exists throughout the cervical spine. The coupling patterns are quite different in the upper cervical spine and in the middle and lower cervical regions and are also dependent on the direction of motion and the posture of the cervical spine.

Mechanical stability of the spine is provided by the integrity of the osteoligamentous spine. Several *in vitro* biomechanical studies have been made of the various spinal components. The upper cervical spine, when traumatized at high speed in an experiment, became unstable mostly in flexion-extension, unstable to a lesser degree in lateral bending, and unstable to a very slight degree in axial rotation. The transverse ligament at the C1 level is a major stabilizing element in the upper cervical spine, which is especially important when the spine is loaded in anteriorly directed shear, such as during a fall with the posterior aspect of the head striking the floor. The average strength of the transverse ligament was about 700 N. Rotatory bilateral dislocation at the C1-C2 level occurs when the normal motion (about 40 degrees to one side) is exceeded by an additional 30 degrees of rotation. Transection studies of ligaments (alar, capsular, transverse) and tectorial membrane have documented the role of these elements in the mechanical stability of the upper cervical spine. In the middle and lower cervical spine, similar biomechanical studies have been performed. These data sets have provided the basis for determining cervical spine instability.

The clinically important problem of spinal instability was approached systematically. A clear definition of clinical instability was provided. The checklist for the middle and lower regions of the spine helps determine the clinical instability of a patient in a step-by-step manner. This decision-making process is based on several biomechanical studies that have provided the relevant data. A new hypothesis of clinical instability, based on the concept of the NZ, was presented. The NZ may be thought of as the looseness or laxity of the spine in the vicinity of the neutral position. The hypothesis states that significant increases in the NZ may indicate clinical instability, in contrast to the traditional view in which increases in ROM are interpreted as the signs of clinical instability. Several biomechanical and clinical studies were presented to support this concept. Appropriately conducted prospective clinical studies can prove the validity and determine the usefulness of this new hypothesis.

ACKNOWLEDGMENTS

This work was supported in part by NIH grants AR40166 and AR49019 and the Daniel E. Hogar Fund. We would like to acknowledge Mr. Aaron Sandler's contribution in describing *in vivo* studies in the last edition of this book chapter.

REFERENCES

1. Lovett R. The mechanism of the normal spine and its relation to scoliosis. *Boston Med Surg J* 1905;153.
2. Lysell E. Motion in the cervical spine. An experimental study on autopsy specimens. *Acta Orthop Scand* 1969;123(Suppl):1.
3. Shea M, Edwards WT, Hayes WC, et al. Variation of stiffness and strength along the human cervical spine. *J Biomech* 1991;24:95–107.
4. Torg J, Sennett B, Vegso J, et al. Axial loading injuries to the middle cervical spine segment: an analysis and classification of twenty-five cases. *Am J Sports Med* 1991;19:6–20.
5. Torg JS, Pavlov H, Genuario SE, et al. Neuropraxia of the cervical spinal cord with transient quadriplegia. *J Bone Joint Surg Am* 1986; 68:1354.
6. White AA, Panjabi MM. *Clinical biomechanics of the spine*, 2nd ed. Philadelphia: JB Lippincott, 1990.
7. Panjabi MM, Miura T, Cripton P, et al. Development of a system for *in-vitro* neck muscle force replication in whole cervical spine experiments. *Spine* 2001;26:2214–2219.
8. Dvorak J, Fröhlich D, Penning L, et al. Functional radiographic diagnosis of the cervical spine: flexion/extension. *Spine* 1988;13: 748–755.
9. Dvorak J, Penning L, Hayek J, et al. Functional diagnostics of the cervical spine using computer tomography. *Neuroradiology* 1988;30: 132–137.
10. Dvorak J, Schneider E, Saldinger PF, et al. Biomechanics of the craniocervical region: the alar and transverse ligaments. *J Orthop Res* 1988;6:452–461.
11. Dvorak J, Panjabi MM, Grob D, et al. Clinical validation of functional flexion/extension radiographs of the cervical spine. *Spine* 1993;18: 120–127.
12. Reich C, Dvorak J. The functional evaluation of craniocervical ligaments in sidebending using x-rays. *Manual Med* 1986;2:108–113.
13. Dvorak J, Antinnes JA, Panjabi MM, et al. Age and gender related normal motion of the cervical spine. *Spine* 1992;17:S393–S398.
14. Panjabi MM. Cervical models for biomechanical research. *Spine* 1998;23:2684–2699.
15. Alund M, Larsson S. Three-dimensional analysis of neck motion: a clinical method. *Spine* 1990;15:87–91.
16. Mayer T, Brady S, Bovasso E, et al. Noninvasive measurement of cervical tri-planar motion in normal subjects. *Spine* 1993;18:2191–2195.
17. Miura T, Panjabi, MM, Cripton PA. A method to simulate *in-vivo* cervical spine kinematics using *in-vitro* compressive preload. *Spine* 2002;27:43–48.
18. Panjabi MM, Crisco JJ, Vasavada A, et al. Mechanical properties of the human cervical spine as shown by three-dimensional load-displacement curves. *Spine* 2001;26:2692–2700.
19. Rippstein J. *Poly Goniometer*. Stuttgart: Teufel, 1974:38–56.
20. Dvorak J, Dvorak V, Schneider W, et al.: *Manual medicine diagnostics*, 3rd ed. Stuttgart: Thieme, 2002.
21. Gore DR, Sepic SGG. Roentgenographic findings of the cervical spine in asymptomatic people. *Spine* 1986;11:521–524.
22. Luschka H. *Die Halbgelenke des menschlichen Körpers*. Berlin: Reimers, 1858.
23. Töndury G, Theiler K. *Entwicklungsgeschichte und Fehlbildungen der Wirbelsaule*. Stuttgart: Hippokrates-Verlag, 1990.
24. Dvorak J, Hayek J, Zehnder R. CT—functional diagnostics of the rotatory instability of the upper cervical spine: part 2. An evaluation on healthy adults and patients with suspected instability. *Spine* 1987; 12:726–731.
25. Dvorak J, Panjabi MM, Gerber M, et al. CT—functional diagnostics of the rotatory instability of upper cervical spine: 1. An experimental study on cadavers. *Spine* 1987;12:197–205.
26. Goel VK, Clark CR, Galles K, et al. Moment-rotation relationships of the ligamentous occipito-atlanto-axial complex. *J Biomech* 1988; 21:673–680.
27. Goel VK, Winterbottom JM, Schulte KR, et al. Ligamentous laxity across CO-C1-C2 complex: axial torque-rotation characteristics until failure. *Spine* 1990;15:990–996.
28. Cave AJE. On the occipito-atlanto-axial articulations. *J Anat (Lond)* 1934;68:416.
29. Ludwig K. Ueber das lig alare dentis. *Z Anat Entwichl Gesch* 1962; 116:442–444.
30. Saldinger P, Dvorak J, Rahn BA, et al. Histology of the alar and transverse ligaments. *Spine* 1990;15:257–261.
31. Werne S. Studies in spontaneous atlas dislocation. *Acta Orthop Scand Suppl* 1957;23.
32. Panjabi M, Dvorak J, Crisco JJ, et al. Effects of alar ligament transection on upper cervical spine rotation. *J Orthop Res* 1991;9:584–593.
33. Lang J. *Klinische Anatomie der Halswirbelsäule*. Stuttgart: G. Thieme Verlag, 1991.
34. Töndury G, Theiler K. *Entwicklungsgeschichte und Fehlbildungen der Wirbelsäule*, 1st ed. Stuttgart: Hippokrates, 1958.
35. Wyke BD. Neurology of the cervical spinal joints. *Physiotherapy* 1979;65:72–76.
36. Dvorak J, Panjabi MM, Chang DG, et al. Functional radiographic diagnosis of the lumbar spine: flexion-extension and lateral bending. *Spine* 1991;16:562–571.
37. Dvorak J, Panjabi MM, Novotny JE, et al. *In vivo* flexion/extension of the normal cervical spine. *J Orthop Res* 1991;9:828–834.
38. Dvorak J, Panjabi MM, Novotny JE, et al. Clinical validation of functional flexion/extension x-rays of the lumbar spine. *Spine* 1991; 16:943–950.
39. Penning L. *Functional pathology of the cervical spine*, vol. 59. Amsterdam: Excerpta Medica, 1968:1–23.
40. Penning L, Wilmink JT. Rotation of the cervical spine. A CT study in normal subjects. *Spine* 1987;12:732–738.
41. Oda T, Panjabi MM, Crisco JJ, et al. Experimental study of atlas injuries. II. Relevance to clinical diagnosis and treatment. *Spine* 1991; 16:S466–S473.
42. Oda T, Panjabi MM, Crisco JJ, et al. Multidirectional instabilities of experimental burst fractures of the atlas. *Spine* 1992;17:1285–1290.
43. Jefferson G. Fracture of the atlas vertebra: report of four cases, and a review of those previously recorded. *Br J Surg* 1920;7:407–422.
44. Heller JG, Amrani J, Hutton WC. Transverse ligament failure—a biomechanical study. *J Spinal Disord* 1993;6:162–165.
45. Chang H, Gilbertson LG, Goel VK, et al. Dynamic response of the occipito-atlanto-axial (C0-C1-C2) complex in right axial rotation. *J Orthop Res* 1992;10:446–453.
46. Doherty BJ, Heggeness MH, Esses SI. A biomechanical study of odontoid fractures and fracture fixation. *Spine* 1993;18:178–184.
47. Dvorak J, Panjabi M. Functional anatomy of the alar ligaments. *Spine* 1987;12:183–188.
48. Panjabi M, Dvorak J, Crisco J, et al. Flexion, extension, and lateral bending of the upper cervical spine in response to alar ligament transections. *J Spinal Disord* 1991;2:157–167.
49. Crisco JJ, Takenori O, Panjabi MM, et al. Transections of the C1-C2 joint capsular ligaments in the cadaveric spine. *Spine* 1991;16:S474–S479.
50. Southern EP, Oxland TR, Panjabi MM, et al. Cervical spine injury patterns in three modes of high-speed trauma—a biomechanical porcine model. *J Spinal Disord* 1990;3:316–328.

51. Yoganandan N, Pintar FA, Sances A, et al. Strength and motion analysis of the human head-neck complex. *J Spinal Disord* 1991;4: 73–85.
52. Panjabi MM, White AA, Keller D, et al. Stability of the cervical spine under tension. *J Biomech* 1978;11:189–197.
53. Goel VK, Clark CR, Harris KG, et al. Kinematics of the cervical spine: effects of multiple total laminectomy and facet wiring. *J Orthop Res* 1988;6:611–619.
54. Zdeblick TA, Abitbol JJ, Kunz DN, et al. Cervical stability after sequential capsule resection. *Spine* 1993;18:2005–2008.
55. Lipson JL, Muir H. Proteoglycans in experimental intervertebral disc degeneration. *Spine* 1981;6:194–210.
56. Raynor RB, Moskovich R, Zidel P, et al. Alterations in primary and coupled neck motions after facetectomy. *J Neurosurg* 1987;12: 681–687.
57. Schulte KR, Clark CR, Goel VK. Kinematics of the cervical spine following discectomy and stabilization. *Spine* 1989;14:1116–1121.
58. Martins A. Anterior cervical discectomy with and without interbody bone graft. *J Neurosurg* 1976;44:290–295.
59. Wilson D, Campbell D. Anterior cervical discectomy without bone graft. *Neurosurgery* 1977;47:551–555.
60. Bell DF, Walker JL, O'Connor G, et al. Spinal deformity after multiple-level cervical laminectomy in children. *Spine* 1994;19:406–411.
61. Nowinski GP, Visarius H, Nolte LP, et al. A biomechanical comparison of cervical laminaplasty and cervical laminectomy with progressive facetectomy. *Spine* 1993;18:1995–2004.
62. Lee S-J, Harris KG, Nassif J, et al. *In vivo* kinematics of the cervical spine. I: Development of a roentgen stereophotogrammetric technique using metallic markers and assessment of its accuracy. *J Spinal Disord* 1993;6:522–534.
63. Lee S-J. Three-dimensional analysis of post-operative cervical spine motion using simultaneous roentgen stereophotogrammetry with metallic markers. Doctoral dissertation, University of Iowa, Iowa City, IA, 1993.
64. Cusick JF, Yoganandan N, Pintar F, et al. Biomechanics of cervical spine facetectomy and fixation techniques. *Spine* 1988;13:808–812.
65. Raynor RB, Pugh J, Shapiro I. Cervical facetectomy and its effect on spine strength. *J Neurosurg* 1985;64:278–282.
66. Nachemson A. Lumbar spine instability: a critical update and symposium summary. *Spine* 1985;10:290–291.
67. Hecker P. Appareil ligamenteux occipito-atloïdo-axoïdien: ëtude d'anatomie comparëe. *Arch Anat Hist Embryol* 1923;2:57–95.
68. Weisel H, Kraus D, Rothman RH. Atlanto-occipital hypermobility. *Orthop Clin North Am* 1978;9:969–972.
69. Fielding JW, Cochran GVB, Lansing JF, et al. Tears of the transverse ligament of the atlas: a clinical biomechanical study. *J Bone Joint Surg Am* 1974;56:1683.
70. Panjabi MM, White AA, Johnson RM. Cervical spine mechanics as a function of transection of components. *J Biomech* 1975;8:327.
71. White A, Panjabi M. *Spinal kinematics in the research status of spinal manipulative therapy.* Washington, DC: US Department of Health, Education, and Welfare, 1975.
72. Bailey RW. Fractures and dislocations of the cervical spine: orthopedic and neurosurgical aspects. *Postgrad Med* 1964;35:588.
73. Bailey RW. Observations of cervical intervertebral disc lesions in fractures and dislocations. *J Bone Joint Surg Am* 1963;45:461.
74. Munro D. Treatment of fractures and dislocations of the cervical spine complicated by cervical cord and root injuries: a comparative study of fusion vs. non fusion therapy. *N Engl J Med* 1961;264:573.
75. Cattell HS, Filtzer DL. Pseudo-subluxation and other normal variations of the cervical spine in children. *J Bone Joint Surg Am* 1965;47: 1295.
76. Ferguson RJL, Caplan LR. Cervical spondylitic myelopathy. *Neurol Clin* 1985;3:373.
77. Slosar PJ Jr, Patwardhan A, Lorenz M, et al. The three-dimensional instability patterns of the thoracolumbar burst fracture. *Trans Orthop Res Soc* 1992;17:67.
78. Gosch HH, Gooding E, Schneider RC. An experimental study of cervical spine and cord injuries. *J Trauma* 1972;12:570.
79. Harris MB, Kronlage SC, Carboni PA, et al. Evaluation of the cervical spine in the polytrauma patient. *Spine* 2000;25:2884–2891.
80. Lehmann T, Brand R. Instability of the lower lumbar spine. Presented at a meeting of the ISSLS, Toronto, Canada, June 6–10, 1982.
81. Panjabi MM. The stabilizing system of the spine. II. Neutral zone and instability hypothesis. *J Spinal Disord* 1992;5:390–397.
82. Oxland TR, Panjabi MM. The onset and progression of spinal injury: a demonstration of neutral zone sensitivity. *J Biomechanics* 1992;25: 1165–1172.
83. Panjabi MM, Dvorak J, Duranceau J, et al. Three dimensional movements of the upper cervical spine. *Spine* 1988;13:726–730.
84. Panjabi MM, Duranceau JS, Oxland TR, et al. Multidirectional instabilities of traumatic cervical spine injuries in a porcine model. *Spine* 1989;14:1111–1115.
85. Richter M, Wilke HJ, Kluger P, et al. Load-displacement properties of the normal and injured lower cervical spine *in vitro*. *Eur Spine J* 2000;9:104–108.
86. Ching RP, Tencer AF, Anderson PA, et al. Thoracolumbar compression fractures: a biomechanical comparison of pre- and post-injury stability. *Trans Orthop Res Soc* 1992;17:68.
87. Nolte LP, Panjabi MM. Spinal stability and intersegmental muscle force—a mathematical model. Presented at the meeting of the ISSLS, Kyoto, Japan, May 15–19, 1989.
88. Grob D, Dvorak J. Temporary segmental fixation of the cervical spine. Presented at the meeting of the European Spine Society, Rome, Italy, October 10, 1991.
89. Panjabi MM. Lumbar spine instability: a biomechanical challenge. *Curr Orthop* 1994;8:100–105.
90. Klein G, Mannion A. Trapped in the neutral zone: another symptom of whiplash-associated disorder? *Eur Spine J* 2001;10:141–148.
91. Penning L. Normal movement of the cervical spine. *AJR Am J Roentgenol* 1978;130:317–326.

SELECTED READINGS

Adams M, Hutton WC. Prolapsed intervertebral disc. *Spine* 1982;7:184–191.
Binder L, Villanueva M, Howieson D, et al. The Rey AVLT recognition memory task measures motivational impairment after mild head trauma. *Arch Clin Neurophysiol* 1993;8:137–147.
Burton C. Low-back care: the gravity of the situation. In: Kirkaldy-Willis W, Burton C, eds. *Managing low back pain*, 3rd ed. New York: Churchill Livingstone, 1992:329–336.
Dvorak J, Vadja E, Panjabi M, et al. Normal motion of the lumbar spine as related to age and gender. *Eur Spine J* 1995;4:18–23.
Ettlin T, Kischka U, Reichmann S, et al. Cerebral symptoms after whiplash injury of the neck: a prospective clinical and neuropsychological study of whiplash injury. *J Neurol Neurosurg Psychiatry* 1992;55:943–948.
Genarelli T, Adams J, Graham D. Acceleration induced head injury in monkey. I. The model, its mechanical and physiological constraints. *Acta Neuropathol (Berl)* 1981;7(Suppl):23–25.
Goel VK, Clark CR, McGowan CD, et al. An *in-vitro* study of the kinematics of the normal, injured and stabilized cervical spine. *J Biomech* 1984;17:363–376.
Lee S-J, Harris KG, Goel VK, et al. Spinal motion following cervical fusion—*in vivo* assessment with roentgen stereophotogrammetry. *Spine* 1994;19:2336–2342.
Moroney SP, Schultz AB, Miller JA, Anderson GB. Load displacement properties of lower cervical spine motion segments. *J Biomech* 1988; 21:769–779.
Parnianpour M, Nordin M, Kahanovitz N, et al. The triaxial coupling of torque generation of trunk muscles during isometric exertions and the effect of fatiguing isoinertial movements on the motor output and movement patterns. Volvo Award in Biomechanics. *Spine* 1988;13:982–992.
Pearcy M, Shepard J. Is there instability in spondylolisthesis? *Spine* 1985; 10:175–177.
Shono Y, McAfee PC, Cunningham BW. The pathomechanics of compression injuries in the cervical spine—nondestructive and destructive investigative methods. *Spine* 1993;18:2009–2019.
Torg JS. Pavlov's ratio: determining cervical spinal stenosis on routine lateral roentgenograms. *Contemp Orthop* 1989;18:153.
White AA, Johnson RM, Panjabi MM, et al. Biomechanical analysis of clinical stability in the cervical spine. *Clin Orthop* 1975;109:85.
Yonenobu K, Hosono N, Iwasaki M, et al. Laminoplasty versus subtotal corpectomy—a comparative study of results in multisegmental cervical spondylotic myelopathy. *Spine* 1992;17:1281–1284.

CHAPTER 5

Mechanisms of Injury in the Cervical Spine: Basic Concepts, Biomechanical Modeling, Experimental Evidence, and Clinical Applications

Mark Bernhardt, Willard B. Wong, Manohar M. Panjabi, and Augustus A. White III

By understanding the mechanisms of injury in the cervical spine, one becomes more adept at evaluating, treating, and preventing such injuries. Knowing the mechanisms of injury alerts clinicians to suspect specific injury patterns. This knowledge enables physicians to direct the history and physical examination toward specific signs and symptoms. Imaging studies that are more likely to yield useful information will be obtained, and unnecessary studies can be omitted with greater confidence.

Clinicians who know which anatomic structures are injured and the extent to which they are compromised are better able to treat the injuries and, in many cases, to prevent injuries. Often, a knowledge of the mechanism of injury (MOI) will aid considerably in the analysis. For example, the realization that rear-end vehicle collisions caused hyperextension injuries of the cervical spine led to the development and widespread use of car seat headrests (1). In 1975, the realization that using the head as a battering ram (spearing) in tackle football could result in cervical quadriplegia led to rules forbidding this type of tackling. Subsequent to implementation of such rules, the prevalence of cervical quadriplegia has dramatically decreased (2,3). Another example is illustrated in a study by Hoek Van Dijke and colleagues (4). In response to the observation that pilots of high-performance aircraft frequently sustained cervical spine injuries due to their exposure to high gravitational forces (5), these investigators measured accelerations about the head of an F-16 fighter pilot during simulated air combat maneuvers. With the aid of a spine model, they calculated

the forces on the lower cervical spine and noted that the forces were of the same order of magnitude as failure loads of cervical vertebrae and estimations of maximum cervical spine muscle forces. They further calculated that the forces on the neck could be substantially reduced by decreasing the mass of the pilot's helmet or shifting the center of mass of the helmet posteriorly, thus potentially reducing the risk of cervical spine injury.

In litigation cases, an analysis of the MOI can help determine responsibility for a given cervical spine injury. Evaluating the mechanism of injury thus becomes an important component of medicolegal analysis.

KEY BIOMECHANICAL CONCEPTS

One may observe distinctly different cervical spine injury patterns, such as dens fractures or bilateral facet dislocations, in different persons who have been involved in apparently similar accidents, such as falling from a ladder. Closer examination, however, discloses that what at first appeared to have been similar accidents actually represented several very different circumstances. From a biomechanical perspective, the conditions in which the accident occurs, or the MOI, cannot be adequately described by a simple explanation of the event that led to the injury. A statement such as "The patient fell from a ladder" does not specify the height from which the subject fell, the subject's weight, the point that first contacted the ground, the position of the subject's head and neck at the time of contact, or the characteristics of the

TABLE 5.1. *Variability of Load at Failure of Human Cadaveric Cervical Spines*

Study	Failure load (N)	Load velocity (m/s)	No. of cadavers
Cadaver segments			
Bauze and Ardran (6)	1,420 (maximum)	Slow hand pump	14
McElhaney et al. (7)	960–6,840	0.64	14
Maiman et al. (8)	645–7,440	0.0025–1.52	13
Whole cadavers			
Yoganandan et al. (9)	3,000–14,700	Drop from 0.9–1.5 m	15
Nusholtz et al. (10)	3,200–10,800	4.0–5.9	8
Alem et al. (11)	3,000–17,000	7–11	10

From: The Cervical Spine Research Society, eds. *The cervical spine*, 3rd ed. Philadelphia: Lippincott–Raven, 1998:80, with permission.

surface onto which the patient fell. When one realizes that each of these conditions can differ greatly and that each specific injury pattern is due to a specific set of conditions, one can begin to appreciate the complexities of describing injury mechanisms. Only after all conditions have been considered can one begin to understand the true MOI.

This chapter focuses on seven basic biomechanical concepts that the authors believe characterize the conditions that result in any specific injury of the cervical spine:

1. Magnitude of the force
2. Rate of load application
3. Displacement
4. Direction of the force relative to the subject or spine
5. Point of load application
6. Preposition of the head and functional spinal units
7. Anatomic, material, and structural characteristics of the spine at the site of injury

These concepts address the conditions that should be noted in all studies of the production of cervical spine injuries. Differences in these conditions may account for some of the large variations in loads to failure that have been shown within and between studies on cadaveric cervical spines (Table 5.1).

Magnitude of the Force

Force is defined as any action that tends to change the state of rest or motion of a body to which it is applied. Force is a vector quantity that has magnitude and direction. The unit of measure for the magnitude of force is newtons (N).

Instantaneous failure is failure that results from a single (ultimate) load cycle. *Fatigue failure* is failure that results from the growth of cracks in structures subjected to repetitive load cycles. The lowest load that will cause fatigue failure within a reasonable time is the *fatigue*, or *endurance, limit*. The process of fatigue is documented by fatigue curves. The load is plotted on the ordinate, and the number of load cycles to failure, in a logarithmic scale, is plotted on the abscissa. Generally, a straight line connects the ultimate load and the endurance limit points. (When the load on the ordinate is replaced by stress, then the fatigue curve is called stress–number of cycles to failure or simply an S-N curve.) More

simply, cumulative loading can result in fatigue failure, and the greater the load in excess of the endurance limit, the fewer number of cycles are required to reach failure.

For steel, cyclic loads of magnitudes as low as 20% of the ultimate failure load will cause fatigue failure. Similar failure can occur in cortical bone at 35% of the failure load. However, *in vivo*, the fatigue limit is probably greater than 35% because reparative biological processes may compensate for the propagation of fatigue cracks.

Rate of Load Application

Because biological tissues are sensitive to the rate of loading, changing the load rate may alter the pattern and severity of injury. Consideration of the concept of viscoelasticity is useful.

Viscoelasticity is defined as the time-dependent property of a material to show sensitivity to rate of loading or deformation. Creep and relaxation are two characteristics of viscoelastic materials that can be quantitatively documented. During creep tests, the load is suddenly applied and is kept constant; the resulting displacement is recorded as a function of time. In relaxation tests, a deformation is produced and held constant while the resulting decrease in load is recorded as a function of time.

Bone, ligaments, tendons, and passive muscles demonstrate viscoelastic behavior. Because of this viscoelastic behavior, their stress–strain curves are dependent on the rate of loading. In general, the greater the rate of loading, the steeper the resulting curves become; however, the rate of change of the stress–strain curve slope as a function of increasing rate of loading is not identical for bone, ligaments, tendons, and passive muscles.

Increasing the tensile loading rate of an anterior cruciate bone-ligament-bone preparation increases the probability that ligament failure will occur before bone failure (12). In the cervical spine, increasing the axial compression loading rate increases the probability of single-level vertebral body fractures, whereas quasi-statically loaded cervical spines are more likely to sustain multilevel bony and ligamentous injuries.

Increasing the loading rate also increases the energy absorption to failure (13) and the energy dissipated in the surrounding tissues. Yoganandan and associates (14) characterized the uniaxial dynamic tensile response of human cervical anterior longitudinal ligaments and ligamentum flavum for loading rates at 9 to 2,500 mm/s. They reported that the ultimate tensile failure load and energy-absorbing capacity at failure increased nonlinearly with the logarithm of the loading rate (14). Other investigators have found similar responses in compact bone and ligaments (12,15).

In accidents, energy-absorbing materials positioned at the point of head impact can increase the time over which the spine is loaded, effectively reducing the rate of loading. This reduces the peak impact force but does not necessarily reduce the total energy transferred to the neck or to a cadaver model (10). In some cases, deflection of the head and neck can result in forces being dissipated to the shoulders or chest. Energy-absorbing materials, however, have the propensity to pocket the skull upon impact, preventing it from being deflected out of the path of the load. If the final position of the head or functional spinal unit (FSU) is limited or constrained, tested human cadaveric cervical spines have shown increased energy at failure and increased injury in comparison with unconstrained specimens (13).

These studies indicate that padded surfaces that protect the skull at impact may not reduce and may even increase the risk and extent of cervical spine injury. However, one must recognize the important and proven efficacy of padded surfaces in the prevention of head and facial injuries and the reduction of contusions and fractures in other areas of the body. The authors are not suggesting that padded protective surfaces be eliminated, but believe that the possible increased risk of injury to the cervical spine with padded protective surfaces must be weighed against the notably decreased risk of injury to other areas of the body.

Displacement

Work is the product of force times distance. *Energy* is the work done. The unit of work or energy is the newton-meter (N-m) or joule (J). When a load deforms the body, the corresponding energy is termed *strain energy;* when a load displaces the body, the corresponding energy is termed *potential energy.* If a load imparts motion to the body, the energy is termed *kinetic energy.*

For a given load, greater displacements result in more severe cervical spine injury (16,17). The concept of limiting extremes of motion to prevent injury led to the provision of headrests on car seats and of shoulder neck rolls for football linemen. Seatbelt restraints have been shown to reduce the prevalence of severe cervical spine injuries significantly (18).

The flexibility of the spine varies at different load magnitudes. Studies of the lumbar spine (19–21) have shown that the spine easily deforms at smaller loads. As the load increases, the resistance to deformation increases at an increasing rate. A similar response is assumed in the cervical spine.

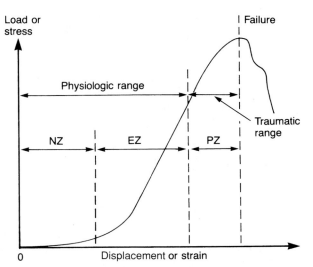

FIG. 5.1. The load-displacement curve of the spine is generally nonlinear. At small loads, there is relatively large displacement; at larger loads, there is relatively less displacement. This load-displacement curve may be divided into physiologic and traumatic ranges. The physiologic range of motion (ROM) may be further divided into two parts. The first part is the neutral zone (NZ), which is the displacement beyond the neutral position due to application of a small force. In the second part, the elastic zone (EZ), more load is required per unit displacement. The traumatic range is defined by the plastic zone (PZ); it is the displacement beyond the elastic zone to failure. (From: White AA, Panjabi MM. *Clinical biomechanics of the spine*, 2nd ed. Philadelphia: JB Lippincott, 1990:21, with permission.)

The Neutral, Elastic, and Plastic Zones

The load-displacement curve for a particular FSU has three regions: the neutral zone (NZ), the elastic zone (EZ), and the plastic zone (PZ). (For zone definitions, see Chapter 4.) The sum of the NZ and EZ constitutes the physiologic range of motion (ROM), whereas the PZ is the region of trauma.

Oxland and Panjabi (22–24) hypothesize that the NZ correlates with other parameters indicative of spinal instability and is probably more sensitive than corresponding changes in ROM (Fig. 5.1). The NZ increases with injury to the spinal column. They further hypothesized that the neuromuscular system can compensate for the increased NZ by increased muscle activity, which may, however, increase the muscle fatigue and risk for further injury. If the neuromuscular system is not able to fully compensate, due to either extensive injury to the spinal column or muscle fatigue, the resultant instability may lead to neurologic injury, deformity, or pain.

Instantaneous Axis of Rotation

Displacement occurs relative to a fixed axis in space. When a rigid body moves in a plane, at every instant there is a point in the body or in some hypothetical extension of it that does not move. An axis perpendicular to the plane of motion and passing through that point is the instantaneous axis (center) of rotation (IAR) for that motion at that instant. Although the spine as a whole is not a rigid body, each vertebra (and the skull) is a relative rigid body, and thus the movement of one vertebra (or the skull) relative to an axis creates an IAR. Differences in the IAR cause differences in injury patterns.

Two separate studies utilizing similar mechanical testing apparatuses with different IARs loaded human cervical spinal segments in flexion and axial compression. McLain and coworkers (25) used a center of rotation anterior to the vertebral bodies and a loading rate of 50 mm/min (0.85 mm/s), to produce a 5 N-m flexion moment. They noted injuries to all posterior soft tissue articulations prior to disruption of the annulus and no fractures. In contrast, Crowell and coworkers (26) used an axis of rotation at the center of the middle vertebrae and a loading rate of 3 to 5 mm/s and failed the specimens at a 7 ± 5 N-m flexion moment. They produced posterior ligament damage in only two of five specimens, but all five sustained intervertebral disc injuries. There was one wedge fracture of a vertebral body.

Direction of Load Relative to the Subject or Spine

The direction of load is an important determinant of mechanism of injury. It can be evaluated either in a uniplanar analysis or more extensively in three dimensions.

Uniplanar Analysis

Most classification systems for cervical spine injuries describe forces occurring in the sagittal or frontal plane. Clearly, uniplanar systems involving single forces or moments (for example, "flexion injuries") do not fully describe the multitude of injury patterns that occur in the cervical spine. However, as a first approximation, the uniplanar sagittal plane analysis is useful. Analysis in the sagittal plane demonstrates a spectrum of injury patterns for which a variety of combinations of compression forces and bending moments describe a "family" of injuries (Fig. 5.2).

Uniplanar analysis limits one to evaluations of load and displacement in three degrees of freedom (dof). For example, in the sagittal plane (the yz-plane in Fig. 5.2), analysis is limited to forces and translations along the z-axis (first of three degrees) and y-axis (second of three degrees) and moments and rotations about the x-axis (third of three degrees).

Analysis in Three Dimensions

A multiplanar coordinate system (Fig. 5.3) allows one to evaluate the possible loads (forces and moments) and corresponding six possible displacements (translations and rotations) along and about three orthogonal axes. This 6-dof analysis allows a more complete description and evaluation of the biomechanical environment.

Coupling

Coupling is a phenomenon in which there is a consistent association of translation or rotation about or along one axis with a translation or rotation about or along a different axis. It has been described in the upper and lower cervical spine (see Fig. 4.9). In the upper cervical spine, the three-dimensional relative motions have been shown to be affected by prepositioning in full flexion, neutral, or full extension (27).

Major Injuring Vector

Although many injuries are viewed in the sagittal plane (such as on lateral radiographs), a spectrum of injuries may be observed in any of the three traditional planes: sagittal (*zy*),

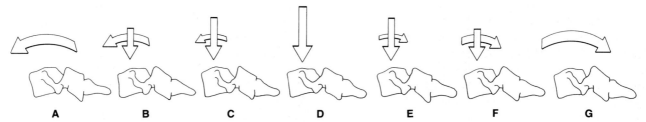

A	B	C	D	E	F	G

FIG. 5.2. Uniplanar analysis of load spectrum for mechanism of injury. This diagram focuses on a sagittal (*yz*) plane analysis. The view is that most injuries in the sagittal plane are the result of some combination of a compression force and a bending moment. The middle vertebra **(D)** is subjected to a pure compression force. To the left **(C, B, A)**, vertebrae are subjected to progressively less compression (−*y*-axis force) and a greater bending moment (+*x*-axis moment). At far left **(A)**, a pure flexion bending moment is shown. The same spectrum of mechanisms is shown **(E, F, G)** in the extension mode (−*y*-axis forces and −*x*-axis moments). Some element of shear is induced in these injuries (not shown). Another aspect of the load combination spectrum is injury pattern. An injury can warn one to suspect other associated injuries. An example is flexion injury, in which there is a major bending moment with a relatively small compression force, which results in a modest wedge compression fracture and extensive disruption of the posterior ligamentous structures, having failed in tension. The families or patterns of injury suggest that when one observes wedge compression fracture, one should suspect disruption of the posterior elements. (From: White AA, Panjabi MM. *Clinical biomechanics of the spine*, 2nd ed. Philadelphia: JB Lippincott, 1990:171, with permission.)

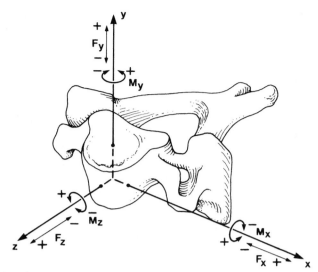

FIG. 5.3. A multiplanar coordinate system with its origin at the center of the vertebral body. The sagittal plane is the *yz*-plane, the frontal (or coronal) plane is the *xy*-plane, and the horizontal (or transverse) plane is the *xz*-plane. Movements are described in relation to the origin of the coordinate system, which is the zero point. Direct forward translation is +*z*; up is +*y*; to the left is +*x*, and to the right is −*x*; down is −*y*; and backward is −*z*. The convention for rotations is determined by imagining oneself at the origin of the coordinate system looking in the positive direction of the axis. Clockwise rotations are positive, whereas anticlockwise rotations are negative. For example, +*x* rotation is roughly flexion. (From: The Cervical Spine Research Society, eds. *The cervical spine,* 2nd ed. Philadelphia: JB Lippincott, 1989:74, with permission.)

more precisely describe the complex forces and moments that occur at each site of injury.

Consideration of the potential difference between the externally applied force and moment and the MIV is necessary when one reviews biomechanical studies that reproduce injury patterns by loading isolated segments containing only one or several FSUs as compared with studies in which entire head-to-T1 specimens are used.

Point of Load Application

Human cadaveric specimens axially loaded posterior to the vertex of the skull fail in extension, and those loaded anterior to the vertex fail in flexion (8). Small (1 cm) variations in anterior-to-posterior distance from neutral in the point of axial load application produce great variations in the resultant fractures (7), as was demonstrated in porcine models (31–33) by dropping a 14.5-kg mass from a height of 1.1 m onto a cylinder placed over a vertebral body. When the cylinder was centered over the geometric center of the vertebral body, the lowest degree of injury was produced— and in no consistent anatomic pattern. Positioning the cylinder 1 cm anterior to the geometric center of the vertebral body produced both the most severe damage to the posterior elements and flexion instability. A cylinder positioned 1 cm posterior to the geometric center produced both the most severe damage to the anterior elements and extension instability.

Nonaxial net forces may result in deflection of the head and neck (13). If this occurs, a sizable portion of the load may be borne by the shoulders instead of the head and neck. (See the discussion of energy-absorbing materials in the section "Rate of Load Application" earlier in this chapter.)

Preposition of Head and Functional Spinal Units

Human cadaveric and calf spine studies demonstrated that the initial head-neck-thorax position and loading conditions dictate the cervical spine response to impact (10,11, 34–36). The response in the sagittal (*yz*) plane includes flexion, buckling, and extension.

A subject buckles under axial centrally applied load if there is sudden "give" or deformation of the structure. This occurs with an axial force when the cervical spine is straight and colinear; it is to be distinguished from bending, which may be caused by an axial load applied to a spine with notable lordosis or kyphosis. In the case of bending, the structure will begin to bend immediately after application of the force. There is no sudden buckling or giving way (Fig. 5.4). Differences in point of load application and direction of the load relative to the spine or subject may also affect the spine's response of bending or buckling.

In human cadaveric testing, prepositioning of the head in a slightly flexed position to eliminate the normal cervical lordosis (thus straightening the spine) results in the least amount of axial deformation under a given axial compression load (Fig. 5.5). This theoretically lessens the ability of the

frontal (*xy*), and horizontal (*xz*) (28). Spinal injury analysis may involve major forces that are not predominantly in the sagittal (*yz*), frontal (*xy*), or horizontal (*xz*) planes (Fig. 5.3).

Any given injury may result from a complex set of external forces and moments applied to the body. Because the site of injury is often different from the points of external force applications, these external forces generate additional moments at the site of injury. The *major injuring vector* (MIV) is a representation of the total (external plus additional) moments and forces at the injury site. The concept of describing the forces and moments experienced at the particular level of injury as opposed to describing these forces and moments in relation to the point of impact of an externally applied load can add a degree of precision to the description of the forces causing a specific injury. Studies of whole spines and cadavers indicate that external mechanical conditions (forces and moments applied to the head) do not always reflect the segmental conditions and patterns of injury at the level of the individual cervical vertebrae (10,16,17,29,30). An axial force applied to a specimen including the occiput to T1 may produce a component of sagittal plane flexion moment at the occipitoatlantal joint while simultaneously producing a component of sagittal plane extension moment in the lower cervical segments. In this case, the MIV can

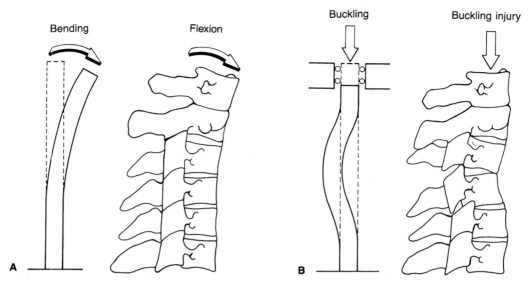

FIG. 5.4. Buckling. **A:** The bending of a beam, analogous to flexion of the cervical spine. There is gradually increasing flexion with increasing load application. **B:** Vertical compression loading results in buckling or sudden give. In the beam model, the convexity of the buckling could proceed in any direction. However, in the cervical spine, the anterior elements, with the discs as the major structure, are more compressible than the posterior elements, which involve the less compressible laminae and facet joints. Therefore, the convexity of the buckling injury is posterior. (From: White AA, Panjabi MM. *Clinical biomechanics of the spine*, 2nd ed. Philadelphia: JB Lippincott, 1990:260, with permission.)

surrounding muscles and ligaments to dissipate the applied energy gradually, as might occur in the case of bending. With a straightened spine, large amounts of energy are absorbed by the spinal column until it buckles, at which point the stored energy is rapidly dissipated to the surrounding soft tissues.

Hamalainen and Vanharanta (37) demonstrated significantly higher cervical erector spinae muscle electromyogram

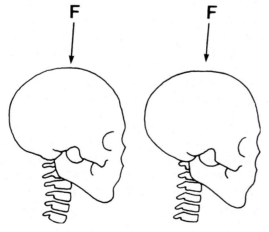

FIG. 5.5. Preposition of head and functional spinal units. **Left:** Axial loading of the initially bent cervical spine will produce bending before failure. **Right:** Axial loading along the straightened cervical spine will result in a buckling mode of failure. (From: The Cervical Spine Research Society, eds. *The cervical spine*, 2nd ed. Philadelphia: JB Lippincott, 1989:74, with permission.)

(EMG) activity in fighter pilots under positive and negative G forces when their necks were flexed or rotated left or right as compared to being in the neutral position. Helleur and coworkers (38) created a mathematical model of the sagittal plane cervical spine and spinal musculature to calculate the effect of high acceleration. They calculated the maximum supportable loads in simulated pilot ejections to be 30, 24, and 15 G for the neutral, flexed, and extended postures, respectively. These studies support the assertion that jet fighter pilots who maintain their heads in neutral position can expect their necks to absorb more energy before failure; that is, if they maintain their necks in a neutral position, injury is less likely to occur.

Cadaver specimens prepositioned in flexion (kyphosis) or extension (lordosis) and then axially loaded failed in flexion or extensions at much lower loads than did the neutral-positioned specimens (8,39). These and other cadaveric studies as well as theoretical mathematical models (9,38,40) suggest that the straightened (rather than lordotic or kyphotic) cervical spine will sustain and withstand the highest externally applied axial load.

Clinically, the importance of the preposition of the head and FSU is exemplified in diving injuries. Recreational diving accounts for 54% to 66% of all sports-related cervical spine injuries (13). Most injuries occur during diving head-first into shallow water with a flexed neck. This results in a "snap-roll" motion on impact with the ground or pool bottom and injuries that include compression and burst fractures and facet dislocations. In contrast, shallow diving with the neck extended results in facial injuries. There is a relatively

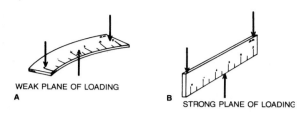

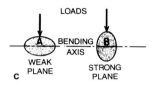

FIG. 5.6. Sectional moments of inertia. Resistance of a structure to bending loads is dependent on its cross-sectional geometry in the plane of bending. **A:** Weak plane of a ruler. **B:** Strong plane of a ruler. **C:** Weak and strong plane of a pedicle. (From: White AA, Panjabi MM. *Clinical biomechanics of the spine,* 2nd ed. Philadelphia: JB Lippincott, 1990:638, with permission.)

low prevalence of serious neck injuries reported with facial-impact diving injuries (13).

Anatomic, Structural, and Material Characteristics

The material and structural properties of objects markedly affect the failure patterns that occur as a result of the various loads applied to them. Considerable difference exists in the individual anatomic variability among subjects. Within the same subject, changes occur in the material and structural properties due to conditions associated with disease and with the normal aging process.

Size and Shape

The sectional or area moment of inertia is a measure of the distribution of a material in a certain manner about its centroid (the point on which the total area may be centered) (Fig. 5.6). This distribution determines the strength in bending.

Objects similar in size and material properties may have large differences in bending strength based on differences in their sectional moment of inertia. The relevance of this concept is demonstrated in interpretations of studies in which the structural properties of surgical constructs or injury patterns are described using animal models with vertebral bodies similar in size but differing in shape from those of humans. Despite similarities in size, differences in shape may affect bending stiffness and patterns of failure, rendering comparisons between certain animal and human models of trauma inaccurate.

Age and Osteoporosis

There is a linear decrease in bone mineral content with increasing age (41). The rate of decrease is not different

between males and females, but the bone mineral content at any age is less in females than in males of the same age.

Lotz and colleagues (42) demonstrated that the compressive strength of trabecular bone is proportional to the square of its apparent density. Bell and coworkers (43) reported that a small loss of osseous tissue produces considerable loss in vertebral bone strength; that is, a 25% decrease in the osseous tissue results in a more than 50% decrease in the strength of the vertebra. This emphasizes the importance of accurate measurement of the bone mineral density of specimens, since a 25% decrease in osseous tissue is not apparent in plain radiographs and yet results in a more than 50% decrease in strength. The implications of the importance of maintaining bone mass to prevent osteoporotic fractures, though uncommon in the cervical spine, are clear.

Age and Ligament Strength

Considerable work has been done to characterize the change in soft tissue related to aging (44). With aging, degenerative changes in soft tissues can weaken them, resulting in injuries from very low-energy trauma. These injuries have been described in the shoulder, knee, and foot (39,44–46). In most studies evaluating age-related changes in ligament strength, the tensile properties of the ligaments of the knee have been examined. Human cadaveric studies of the anterior cruciate ligament reflect decreasing tensile stiffness and ultimate load to failure with increasing age (47,48).

Changes in the ligamentum flavum at the cellular level include decreased cellularity and increased fragmentation of elastic fibers with substitution fibrosus (49). Biomechanically, aging of the ligamentum flavum causes decreased modulus of elasticity and decreased ultimate strength. Little work has been done to evaluate changes in the physical and material properties of other spinal ligaments or facet capsules with age (50).

Studies evaluating age-related changes of the intervertebral disc have concentrated on the lumbar segments. There is a decrease in proteoglycans and water concentration and an increase in noncollagenous protein concentration (44). Structurally, the annulus becomes fissured. These changes alter the load-sharing and dampening properties of the intervertebral disc. In the lumbar spine, this results in less central end-plate fracturing (Schmorl's nodes) and more vertebral body compression fractures with advancing age. Schmorl's nodes and atraumatic compression fractures are rarely noted in the cervical spine; presumably, the relatively lower magnitude of loading accounts for the much lower occurrence of these types of fractures.

Fused Segments (Structural Changes)

Multiple adjacent fused cervical spine segments create a long, stiff lever arm. A condition of increased stress concentration occurs. *Stress concentration* is a sudden change in material or structure, or both, that creates a localized stress peak that cannot be predicted by a simple theory regarding strength of material. This increased stress concentration is due to an abrupt change in modulus, or stiffness, along the spine adjacent to fused segments. When areas of increased stress concentration exist in the cervical spine, major injuries can occur after minor cervical spine trauma. Fusion of multiple cervical spine FSUs can occur congenitally in Klippel-Feil syndrome, developmentally in degenerative ankylosis and ankylosing spondylitis, or iatrogenically after surgical arthrodesis.

Spinal segments adjacent to fused segments may become unstable in patients with Klippel-Feil syndrome. A case of a patient with congenital fusion of several vertebrae who sustained minor trauma (falling back against a car) that resulted in quadriplegia has been reported (51).

In ankylosing spondylitis, the increased stress concentration occurs in the lower cervical spine, where most fractures occur. Mechanisms of hyperextension (52,53) and flexion (54) have been proposed. Major spinal cord compression may occur from bony displacement or epidural hematoma. The difficulty of treating cervical spine fractures involving ankylosing spondylitis relates to the propensity for displacement. This problem is most likely due to the long segment or segments of spine adjacent to the fracture. Despite the loss of elasticity at ankylosed segments, three cases of spinal cord compression from herniated nucleus pulposus have been reported (54).

In 12 of 15 patients whose diagnosis included surgical and congenital fusions of the cervical spine as well as degenerative ankylosis, MacMillan and Stauffer (55) reported posttraumatic instability closely associated with the location of the fusion mass.

Summary of Key Biomechanical Concepts

The specific injury sustained as a result of a load is dependent on the characteristics of that load, the response of the spine or FSU, and the individual anatomic, structural, and material variations existing in each subject. The magnitude of the injuring force and the number of times it is applied determine whether the subject fails instantaneously or in fatigue failure. The rate of load application partly determines the amount of energy absorption to failure and whether the failure occurs primarily through bony or soft tissue elements. The direction of load relative to the spine, the position of the head, and the point of load application determine the response of the spine to axial load. Based on the particular combination of the preceding conditions, the spine will buckle, flex, or extend. Each of the preceding responses will produce a different complex of injuries. The threshold for failure in the cervical spine may be raised or lowered by many variables, including normal anatomic variation and certain diseases that affect material or structural properties or both (56–58).

The seven concepts just discussed may be considered and analyzed under both experimental and clinical conditions.

In studies of cervical spine injury mechanisms, it is worthwhile to consider these concepts and to address them in the experimental design. In the clinical setting, however, the information required for full assessment of these concepts is rarely available. Patients present to the emergency room either comatose or intoxicated or unable to recall the events of the accident. In such cases, a thorough physical examination to detect specific areas of tenderness or contusions and a complete radiographic evaluation can help one deduce the mechanism of injury. For an in-depth analysis of the MOI of a particular injury, it is useful to consider each of the seven concepts and make a determination regarding its applicability or role.

BIOMECHANICAL MODELING

A biomechanical model is a simulator in a laboratory of some aspects of human reality. Several types of models exist, with various advantages and disadvantages. The most common types of biomechanical models are *in vivo* animal, cadaveric, synthetic, and computer models.

The cadaver model may be a whole cadaver, a multiple-vertebrae segment, or an FSU. For biomechanical studies of injuries, all three types of cadaver models have been used. Advantages of these models include faithful reproduction of the anatomy and physical properties of the osteoligamentous spine. Disadvantages include variability from specimen to specimen, lack of availability, and high cost. One can argue that the variability is an asset because it truly represents the reality in the human population. The variability makes it possible to study the effects of age and disease on the physical characteristics of the spine. The variability observed clinically in injuries is thus automatically simulated in experimental trauma using cadaveric models.

Animal cadavers have been used in spine injury research. The obvious disadvantage is the dissimilar anatomy and physical properties. However, availability and greater uniformity in size, internal architecture, and physical characteristics have made them useful for certain types of studies, such as cervical spine trauma (32).

In vivo animal models have been used for spinal injury research, mostly for the study of the effects of healing in ligament and disc injuries and spinal arthrodesis (59–63). Because the anatomy and physical characteristics of animals differ greatly from those of humans, the usefulness of such models in advancing our understanding of injury mechanisms is limited.

Synthetic models of the spine simulate actual spine behavior by incorporating the physical characteristics of the vertebrae, anatomic geometry, and physical characteristics of the soft tissues connecting the vertebrae. Synthetic models, such as Hybrid III car crash dummies, have vertebrae consisting of a hard material such as plastic or steel; the soft tissues are simulated by synthetic rubber of appropriate hardness. The advantages of the synthetic models are that they are highly reproducible and easily obtained. Because they can be used repeatedly without deterioration in their behavior, they are economical. A disadvantage of the present designs is their inability to validly simulate actual spine behavior. For example, the biomechanical response (that is, the load-displacement curve) of the Hybrid III model neck has been documented to be three to five times stiffer than that of the cadaveric cervical spine (64). Another disadvantage of the synthetic models is their lack of anatomic detail. One cannot identify a specific anatomic element, such as the capsular ligament or facet joint. This is necessary if one is interested in the effects of injuries on specific anatomic elements. Another limitation of most of these models is their lack of simulation of the muscular system. To the authors' knowledge, only one model has incorporated muscles (65,66).

The lack of muscle simulation may not be a major disadvantage in the study of injury mechanisms because the reaction time necessary for muscle force generation is too long to be effective in most spinal trauma circumstances; that is, the muscles are too slow to react in a traumatic situation to play a major role in actual injury. Muscle force development time is slow (100 to 200 ms) compared with the rise time (5 to 10 ms) of the loads causing the injury (67,68). Whole cadaveric models incorporate passive muscle properties. Some investigators have included muscle function simulation by applying forces to the cadaveric specimens (69,70).

Computer or mathematical models are sets of equations that incorporate experimentally obtained physical properties of the soft tissues and geometry of the vertebrae (40,71). Mathematical models will be very useful when they can validly incorporate physical characteristics of an osteoligamentous spine and mathematically simulate the muscular forces. Current computer models use finite-element methods, a sophisticated mathematical technique. However, the authors know of no fully validated mathematical models available for the study of injury mechanisms of the cervical spine. Comprehensive validation of these complex mathematical tools is a challenging endeavor.

EXPERIMENTAL AND CLINICAL EVIDENCE OF SPECIFIC INJURY MECHANISMS AND PATTERNS IN THE VARIOUS REGIONS OF THE CERVICAL SPINE

The most common cause of cervical spine and spinal cord injury is motor vehicle accidents (MVAs) (13). Most cervical spine injuries resulting from MVAs are minor sprains and strains caused by rear-end collisions. The rate of severe injuries is nearly the same for crashes from the front as for crashes from the side.

Cervical spine injuries have notably different outcomes based largely on where they occur. At the craniocervical junction, they are often associated with fatalities; in the lower cervical spine, they are typically associated with survival (18).

Major differences in the mechanical properties along the various segments of the cervical spine have been noted (27,29,72). Investigators have described three mechanically distinct regions of the cervical spine: the upper (C0-C1-C2), middle (C2 through C5), and lower (C5 through T1) regions. Awareness of important differences in stiffness in each of the three segments is relevant and helpful in understanding mechanisms of injury in the cervical spine.

Upper Cervical Spine

Fractures of the Occiput

Anderson and Montesano (73) reported a series of six occipital condyle fractures and proposed the following classification system: type I, impacted occipital condyle fracture; type II, occipital condyle fracture associated with a basilar skull fracture; and type III, an avulsion fracture of the occipital condyle. The mechanism of injury suggested for types I and II is a vertical (y-axis) compression. For type III, Anderson and Montesano (73) suggested a combination of anteroposterior (AP) translation (z-axis), axial rotation (y-axis), and lateral bending (z-axis rotation).

Types I and II fractures are considered stable. Type III fractures represent avulsions of a portion of the occipital condyle to which the alar ligament is attached (74). Because the alar ligaments contribute substantially to the stability of the C0-C1 joint (1,75), the authors agree that type III occipital condyle fractures are probably unstable.

Occipitoatlantal Dislocation

Occipitoatlantal (C0-C1) dislocation is more common in children than in adults. Papadopoulos (76) hypothesized that the inherently less stable craniovertebral junction in children as compared with that in adults accounts for the relative higher incidence of this injury in children. The strength of the craniovertebral junction is primarily due to the axiooccipital ligamentous structures. Werne (77) demonstrated that forward flexion of the occiput with respect to the atlas is limited by bony contact of the dens with the anterior foramen magnum. Hyperextension is limited by the tectorial membrane. Sectioning of the alar ligaments and tectorial membrane allows forward translation of the occiput with respect to the atlas.

The mechanism of occipitoatlantal dislocation has not been established. Presumably, there is a major anterior force along the positive z-axis. The skull is translated anteriorly in relation to the atlas. Mainly, this causes a shear type of loading at the atlantooccipital joint, rupturing the articular capsule and causing the dislocation. Bucholz and Burkhead (78), however, who examined 112 victims at postmortem, suggested a hyperextension mechanism. This was based on their associated findings of submental lacerations, mandibular fractures, and lacerations of the posterior mandibular wall. Anderson and colleagues (79) reported five cases of C0-C1 instability associated with traumatic transverse ligament rupture, presumably due to forward flexion or anterior shear forces.

Fractures of the Atlas

Fractures of the Posterior Arch of the First Cervical Vertebra

Fractures of the ring of the first cervical vertebra are believed to result primarily from vertical compression on the posterior aspect of the arch of C1 due to axial compression or hyperextension (80,81). These fractures have been produced by axially loading C0 through C3 cadaveric spine segments (67).

There may be extension of the skull (negative x-axis rotation). The lateral masses of C2 may serve as a fulcrum at the site of injury. The anterior arch of C1 is locked, buttressed, or fixed by these lateral masses, whereas the posterior ring is displaced in the caudad (negative y-axis) direction. This results in tensile failure of the bone in the cephalad surface of the ring in the grooves for the vertebral artery, where these fractures generally appear to begin. This is compatible with the presumed mechanism of injury and the generally accepted maxim that bone fails in tension. This is the weakest point of the ring because it is the thinnest portion and has the lowest area moment of inertia against the type of loading involved. The low area moment of inertia is due to bilateral grooves at the site where the vertebral artery courses from its osseous vertebral canal across the ring of C1 and into the foramen magnum (Fig. 5.7).

Jefferson's Fracture

Jefferson originally described the fracture known by his name as a four-part fracture of the ring of the atlas. The classic four-part fracture pattern, however, is rare. Two- and three-part fractures are much more common (67,82–84). This finding is consistent with the presumption that production of a classic four-part symmetrical Jefferson's fracture would require pure axial loading with the MIV precisely

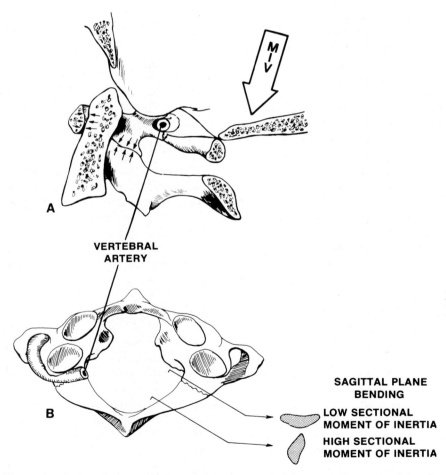

FIG. 5.7. Biomechanical and anatomic factors in a fracture of the posterior arch of the C1 vertebra. **A:** A midsagittal section of the occipitoatlantoaxial complex. The vertebral artery passes across the ring of C1 over a grooved or weakened area of the vertebra. **B:** The top view of the ring of C1 shows the vertebral artery on the left in the region of the fracture on the right. The sectional moment of inertia against bending in the sagittal plane is much smaller where the fracture occurs than it is in the more posterior area. The areas are shown by the cross sections at these two points. (From: White AA, Panjabi MM. *Clinical biomechanics of the spine*, 2nd ed. Philadelphia: JB Lippincott, 1990:195, with permission.)

centered in the *xy*- and *yz*-planes of a neutrally positioned head and neck. Any off-axis loading due to point of load application, direction of load relative to the spine, or prepositioning of the head or spine would result in asymmetric loading. Such noncentered loading would not typically result in the classic four-part Jefferson's fracture, but would produce two- and three-part fractures of the ring of the atlas. Experimental evidence supports this explanation (67).

Fractures of the ring of C1 are the result of axial loading, usually due to a direct blow to the vertex of the head. The spatial orientation of the occipital condyles is such that they act as a wedge when they are driven axially in the caudad direction, causing a bursting effect and tensile fracturing of the ring of the axis.

McElhaney and colleagues (7) produced Jefferson's fractures by axial loading of the essentially straightened cervical spine. In a series of studies, Oda and associates (67,83,84) produced C1 fractures in eight of ten human cadaver cervical spines (C0 through C3) by dropping a 3- to 6-kg mass from 1 m onto the spines, resulting in an axial (negative *y*-axis) high-speed (4.4 m/s) load to the occiput. They positioned the specimens so that the posterior wall of C3 was at a 20-degree angle inclined anteriorly with respect to the frontal plane, which oriented the spine in a straight position. They noted compressive failure force to be less in specimens prepositioned in extension as compared with those prepositioned straight. Transverse ligament avulsions or midsubstance tears resulted in six of the eight specimens. An anterior atlantodental interval greater than or equal to 3 mm correlated with complete disruption of the transverse ligament. Contrary to the common belief that a total lateral mass displacement of less than 7 mm is consistent with an intact transverse ligament, McElhaney and coworkers (7) noted one case of midsubstance transverse ligament tear associated with fracturing of C1 in which the total lateral mass displacement was less than 7 mm. Heggeness and Doherty (34) produced two- and three-part fractures of C1 by rotation (*y*-axis rotation) and postulated that Jefferson's fractures may arise from combination of torsional moments and tension forces.

In view of the preponderance of studies demonstrating Jefferson's fractures resulting from axial loading (*y*-axis) of the vertex of the head, the authors believe this is the most likely MOI. According to Heggeness and Doherty (34), such fractures may be experimentally produced by an MIV of axial rotation, but this is unlikely in a clinical setting. Presumably, increasing upper cervical spine axial rotation leads to increasing incongruence of the lateral mass articulations, causing increased stress concentration in less commonly loaded anatomic regions of the vertebrae. These less commonly loaded anatomic regions may have material properties less able to withstand such loads. An axial moment (around the *y*-axis) together with axial loading (negative *y*-axis) or prepositioning of the upper cervical spine in axial rotation may lower the threshold for fracture.

In the studies of Oda and associates (67,83,84) and Heggeness and Doherty (34) discussed herein, only upper cervical spine segments were used. If the entire cervical spine had been used under the same loading conditions, injuries to other areas of the spine might have occurred first, dissipating the energy and reducing the frequency of the atlas fractures either partially or completely.

Transverse Ligament Disruption

Fielding and colleagues (85) produced ruptures of the transverse ligament in the absence of dens fractures by loading in the horizontal axis in the sagittal plane (MIV in the positive *z*-axis) (Fig. 5.8). Levine and Edwards (86) reported this injury to result from falls and from acute cervical flexion. Panjabi and associates (67) produced midsubstance transverse ligament tears without fractures of the axis in two of ten human cadaveric specimens. A third specimen had a midsubstance transverse ligament tear with associated fracturing of the atlas. An additional five of the ten specimens had bony avulsions of the transverse ligament associated with other fractures of the atlas. Dvorak and coworkers (74)

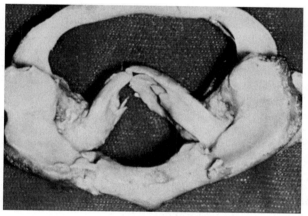

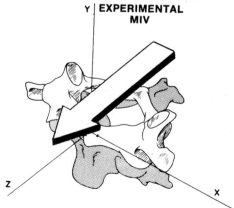

FIG. 5.8. Transverse ligament disruption. Experimental rupture of the transverse ligament. In cadaver studies, this pattern of failure was observed in the absence of fracture. The experimental major injuring vector (MIV) is shown. (From: White AA, Panjabi MM. *Clinical biomechanics of the spine*, 2nd ed. Philadelphia: JB Lippincott, 1990:205, with permission.)

determined the *in vitro* strength of the transverse ligament to be 300 N (compared with a strength of 200 N for the alar ligaments) and considered the alar ligaments to be a "second line of defense" to C1-C2 displacement after the transverse ligament had failed.

Traumatic Atlantoaxial Subluxations and Dislocations

The displacement in atlantoaxial (C1-C2) dislocations and subluxations may be either anterior or posterior (*z*-axis) or axially rotated (*y*-axis). For the anterior dislocation, the MIV is primarily along the positive *z*-axis and is associated with a significant amount of flexion. Posterior fracture-dislocations are due to an MIV in the opposite direction.

The rotatory subluxation of this joint presumably occurs when the force vector is not directly along the *z*-axis, but is actually tangential to the *z*-axis, producing enough torque about the *y*-axis to cause a rotatory subluxation or dislocation.

Myers and associates (87) produced rotatory atlantoaxial dislocation in six of six human cadaveric C0 to T1 specimens by applying a pure axial moment to the base of the skull. Similar testing of the C2 to T1 specimens yielded unilateral facet dislocations at higher torques than are required to produce atlantoaxial dislocations. In the same study, they noted that clinically characteristic injury patterns could not be produced until they allowed for passive changes in length of the spine along the *z*-axis as the axial rotational force was applied. One presumes that not allowing any translation along the *z*-axis while creating substantial moments about the *y*-axis did not allow normal coupling motion characteristic of the spine (see "Direction of Load Relative to the Subject or Spine," earlier in this chapter). This may explain the uncharacteristic injury patterns initially

created when *z*-axis length was held fixed during *y*-axis rotation. The production of completely different injury patterns simply by allowing for passive motion in a direction that was not the same as the major externally applied force emphasizes the importance of analysis of displacement in all planes (see "Displacement" earlier in this chapter).

Fractures of the Axis

Fractures of the Dens

Anderson and D'Alonzo (88) described three types of dens fractures (Fig. 5.9). Fielding and colleagues (85) hypothesized that anterior displacement injuries of the atlas (C2) on the axis are due to flexion and anterior shear and that posterior displacement injuries are due to hyperextension moments and posterior shear forces.

Previous hypotheses have included hyperextension, hyperflexion, and horizontal (*z*-axis) shear as possible mechanisms of dens fractures (89). Altoff (90) showed that dens fractures could not be produced by pure horizontal shear. He was able to produce fractures of the dens by applying combinations of various horizontal (*z*-axis) shear and vertical compression (negative *y*-axis) forces. Anderson and D'Alonzo type III fractures were produced by a combination of compression and shear force applied in the sagittal plane. Moving the experimental force vector 45 degrees out of the sagittal plane (that is, applied from an anterolateral direction) produced a fracture analogous to the type II fracture. When the vector was applied from a direction 90 degrees to the sagittal plane (in the coronal or *xy*-plane), a fracture analogous to type I was produced (Fig. 5.9). A liberal interpretation of this experiment is as follows: As the vector

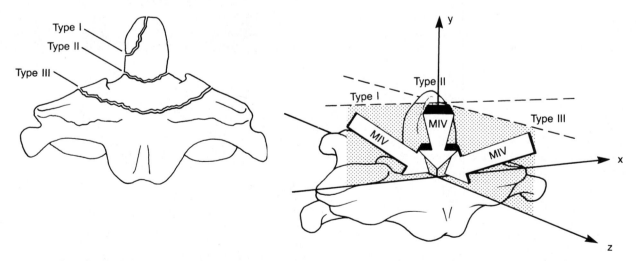

FIG. 5.9. Dens fractures. **A:** The three types of dens fractures as described by Anderson and D'Alonzo (88). **B:** Based on the experimental work of Altoff (90), a significantly different major injuring vector (MIV) could be determined for each of the three types. We present these in an attempt to show the MIV for each of the three fractures. As shown, they all come in an angle about 45 degrees to the vertical. The MIV for type I is mainly in the *xy*-plane, type III is mainly in the *yz*-plane, and type II is in an oblique plane halfway between the other two. (From: White AA, Panjabi MM: *Clinical biomechanics of the spine*, 2nd ed. Philadelphia: JB Lippincott, 1990:198, 200, with permission.)

consisting of compression and shear forces moves out of the sagittal plane and is directed more in the coronal plane, the dens fracture produced is relatively more cephalad.

Somewhat contrary to the experimental studies of Altoff (90), Craig and Hodgson (91), in a clinical review of nine patients with superior facet fractures of the axis, reported five associated type III dens fractures. Because the facet fractures of the axis were frequently unilateral and depressed laterally, Craig and Hodgson (91) postulated the MOI to be a load directed laterally in the xy-plane. These findings reflect the importance of the key biomechanical concept of direction of force relative to the subject or spine in the determination of resultant injury pattern.

Although the issue is somewhat controversial, the origin of os odontoideum is believed more likely to be traumatic than developmental (92–94). The MOI is probably similar to that of a type I or II dens fracture.

Superior Facet Fractures of the Axis

Craig and Hodgson (91) described nine cases of unilateral superior facet fractures of the axis, with associated fracture of the dens in seven of the nine cases. The superior facet fractures occurred in a coronal (xy) or sagittal (yz) plane, sometimes with associated depression of the anterior or lateral portion of the facet. The investigators speculated that the mechanism of injury of the sagittal plane fracture was a laterally directed force with the atlas and axis prepositioned in neutral, whereas the mechanism of injury of the coronal plane fractures was a laterally directed force with the atlas and axis prepositioned in rotation about the y-axis.

Hangman's Fracture and Fracture-Dislocation: Traumatic Spondylolisthesis of the Axis

Hangman's fracture-dislocation (C2-C3) is also known as traumatic spondylolisthesis of the axis. This injury occurs in judicial hangings when placement of the knot of the rope in a submental position causes extreme cervical hyperextension (95,96).

This traditional view of the mechanism of injury was challenged by a study by James and Nasmyth-Jones (97), who examined cervical spines exhumed after judicial hangings that occurred between 1882 and 1945. Only 3 of 34 victims sustained the classic hangman's fracture, and in 2 of these 3 victims, the fractures were nondisplaced. These findings were unexpected. However, James and Nasmyth-Jones did not know the position of the knots in relation to the victims' necks at the time of hanging, and the paucity of hangman's fractures in this study may have been due to "improper" hanging techniques. Furthermore, the presumed MOI of hangman's fractures may be the exception to the rule.

Levine and Edwards (98) reviewed 52 patients with traumatic spondylolisthesis of the axis. They classified the injury patterns into three types and hypothesized MOI for each type. According to their data, type I injuries have a fracture through the neural arch with no angulation and as much as 3 mm of displacement and are due to a hyperextension-axial loading force. Type II fractures have both marked angulation and marked displacement and are due to two sequential forces. Initially, there is hyperextension-axial loading, which is followed by anterior flexion and compression. Type IIa fractures have minimal displacement but severe angulation and are due to flexion-distraction. Type III fractures have bilateral facet dislocations between the second and third cervical vertebrae and a fracture of the neural arch of the axis. This injury pattern is believed to be due to flexion-compression.

Currently, most traumatic spondylolisthesis injuries result from MVAs. Presumably, the MOI in this setting is an extension moment (negative x-axis rotation) with a component of vertical axial compressive force (negative y-axis). This is in distinct contrast to the distractive force (positive y-axis) and extension moment (negative x-axis rotation) that is believed to occur during hangings in which a submental knot position is used. Considering all of the evidence, there appear to be at least two MOIs for traumatic spondylolisthesis, as follows. With the head and neck prepositioned in extension, distractive loading occurs (as in hangings with submental knots) or compressive loading occurs (as in MVAs). Whether the MOI hypothesized by Levine and Edwards (98) of the neck in flexion with an axial or distractive loading produces traumatic spondylolisthesis of the axis is not clear.

Some anatomic considerations of interest are relevant here. The transverse foramina for the vertebral arteries are in the region of the pedicles (isthmus) of C2. Because of these foramina and the configuration of the neural arch, the structure of C2 in this region has a relatively low area moment of inertia to bending in the sagittal plane (see "Anatomic, Material, and Structural Characteristics," earlier in this chapter). This may be a factor in determining the site of failure. In addition, there is another structural consideration. The occipitoatlantoaxial complex has other characteristics that potentiate failure of the pedicle (isthmus). The large extension force creates a bending moment on the dens so that it rotates in the sagittal plane about the negative x-axis. This bending moment is balanced by two forces—a tensile force produced in the anterior longitudinal ligament, the disc, and the posterior longitudinal ligament on one side, and a compressive joint reaction force between the facet joints of C2 and C3 on the other side. These two equal and opposite forces create a balanced bending moment. The effect of all these loads is production of a maximum bending moment in the region of the pars interarticularis. Because the cross section of the bone is small (low area moment of inertia), this site is the weakest and thus the most susceptible to fracture.

Middle and Lower Cervical Spine

Unilateral Facet Dislocation

An appreciation of this injury is linked with the understanding of the normal kinematics of the cervical spine (see

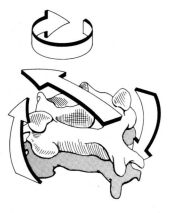

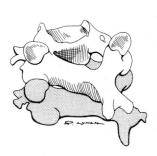

FIG. 5.10. The mechanism of injury (MOI) in a unilateral facet dislocation, an injury that results from an exaggeration of the normal coupling of axial rotation and lateral bending. If a significant vertical compression ($-y$-axis) component is added, there may be a fracture of the left facet. If there is flexion and lateral bending, as shown here, but with a severe torque in the opposite direction ($+y$-axis moment), there may be a fracture of the right facet. (From: White AA, Panjabi MM. *Clinical biomechanics of the spine,* 2nd ed. Philadelphia: JB Lippincott, 1990:221, with permission.)

the section "Coupling" earlier in this chapter). A unilateral facet dislocation is caused by an exaggeration of the normal kinematics of the spine. Physiologic lateral bending is coupled with axial rotation so that the spinous processes tend to move toward the convexity of the physiologic curve. When this is exaggerated in trauma, the facet on one side proceeds too far caudad, and the one on the opposite side proceeds too far cephalad and dislocates (Fig. 5.10) (described in "Magnitude of the Force" and in "Displacement").

Bauze and Ardran (6) produced two unilateral facet dislocations by slowly applying an axial load to whole human cervical spines prepositioned in flexion. The lower segments were stiffened by insertion of a steel rod into the spinal canal. The base of the skull was allowed to translate freely. Unilateral facet dislocations were produced in the two specimens where "considerable rotation and lateral flexion occurred."

Myers and colleagues (87) consistently produced unilateral facet dislocations with and without facet fractures in human cadaveric cervical spines by applying a pure axial torsional (y-axis rotation) force to C2 while the lower cervical segments were fixed. However, they were unable to produce any radiographically evident lower cervical spine injuries by applying the axial torque through the base of the skull because atlantoaxial rotatory subluxations occurred at a statistically significant lower torque than did middle or lower cervical spine unilateral facet dislocations. Therefore, although unilateral facet dislocations can be produced in the laboratory by pure axial torsion, such torsion may not be the MOI in clinical conditions.

Unilateral Facet Fracture-Dislocation

When fracture is associated with dislocation, a large joint-reactive force is created at the fractured facet articulation, with an impingement of the surfaces. This results in failure through the base of the more cephalad facet (inferior articular process), which sometimes propagates into the lamina. This can develop in one of two ways. There is either a major element of axial compression involved with rotation and lateral bending, or there is nonphysiologic association of axial rotation with lateral bending (Fig. 5.10).

Hyperflexion Sprain

Hyperflexion is the anterior subluxation of vertebral body and subjacent articular mass with increase in the interspinous space ("fanning") and reversal of cervical lordosis. This condition is probably caused by the same mechanism that produces bilateral facet dislocations, but presumably with a lower magnitude of force and less displacement (99,100). Other investigators have conceptualized this injury pattern as one of flexion-distraction (101).

In an illustrative case report of hyperflexion sprain, Paley and Gillespie (102) described an Olympic high jumper whose unconventional technique during the landing of the Fosbury flop caused a severe flexion moment about her cervical spine. She presented after two incidents of minor trauma, reporting neck pain stiffness and momentary paresthesias of all four extremities. Her physical examination elicited a positive Lhermitte's sign. A cervical spine lateral radiograph showed increase in the C5-6 interspinous space, 4 mm anterior translation of C5 on C6, and more than 11 degrees of relative sagittal plane angulation at C5-C6 without fracture, consistent with a hyperflexion sprain.

Bilateral Facet Dislocation and Fracture-Dislocation

The MIV is presumed to be a flexion-bending moment (positive x-axis rotation) very near the midsagittal plane. A major asymmetrical application tends to result in lateral bending and axial rotation and unilateral rather than bilateral facet dislocation.

Bauze and Ardran (6) consistently produced purely ligamentous bilateral facet dislocations by slowly axially loading human cadaveric cervical spines prepositioned in flexion. The spines had been stiffened by insertion of a rod into the neural canal of the lower segments. The lower segments were fixed, but the upper segments were allowed to translate forward.

The mechanisms of bilateral facet dislocation were illustrated by Scher (103), who reviewed cervical spine injuries sustained by rugby players. In rugby, the scrum is a period of play in which the front-row players flex their necks and charge forward while the remaining players push from behind.

Of 15 reported cervical spine injuries that occurred during the scrum, 11 were bilateral and 3 were unilateral facet dislocations. Scher (103) reported a patient's description of the unfortunate event. The patient reported that when the scrum collapsed, his forehead struck the ground and the rest of the pack kept pushing from behind. He felt his chin being forced onto his chest, at which stage he clearly heard a "snap" and became completely paralyzed (103). In view of the great limitations on human experiments for MOI studies, these clinical reports, although not controlled, provide some of the best information on the subject.

Some investigators have reported that bilateral facet dislocations can be caused by tensile forces (13,104), but the head is much more commonly loaded in compression. This apparent conflict may be explained by noting that forces applied to the head may not reflect the segmental conditions or MIV at the level of injury (see "Direction of the Force Relative to the Subject or Spine"). Recall that the directional response to an externally applied load can be affected by the direction of force relative to the subject or spine, the point of load application (key biomechanical concept 5), and the preposition of the head and functional

spinal units (key biomechanical concept 6). Perhaps a compressive (negative *y*-axis) load applied to the top of the head in a C0-T1 specimen prepositioned in flexion resulted in a bending moment with an IAR far anterior to the cervical facet joints. This might cause tensile forces at the facet joints, explaining the apparent conflict between the externally applied compressive force and bilateral facet dislocations from tensile forces.

The Full-Nelson Injury

Well-documented *in vivo* injuries provide insight into the MOI for certain injury patterns. For example, a healthy 17-year-old boy engaging in horseplay was held in a full Nelson by one friend while another held one of his arms in abduction and another held the other arm in full extension. Fortunately for the advancement of clinical science, another friend took the picture shown in Figure 5.11A. The subject was able to resist the flexion forces on his neck initially, but then he fatigued. When this occurred, he heard a creaking sound in his neck, followed by a ripping feeling in the anterior part of his throat and the sensation of electric shocks in both

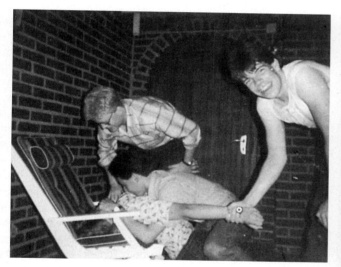

A

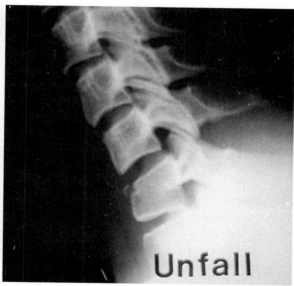

B

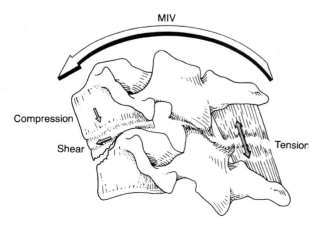

C

FIG. 5.11. Full-Nelson injury. **A:** This landmark photo was taken just at the moment that the young man's neck yielded, cracked, and sustained the injuries shown in the radiograph. **B:** There is slight separation of the posterior elements and slight compression of the body of C7. The small triangular portion of bone has resulted in association with shear failure of the bone. There is slight anterior translatory displacement of the body of C6 on C7. **C:** Diagram of major injuring vector (MIV), mechanism of injury, and the specific structures involved. (Photograph and radiograph courtesy of Professor H. W. Staudte, University of Aachen, West Germany; reprinted from White AA, Panjabi MM. *Clinical biomechanics of the spine*, 2nd ed. Philadelphia: JB Lippincott, 1990:225, with permission.)

arms. Radiographs showed an anterior subluxation of C6 on C7, with a slight compression of C7 involving a fracture of the anterosuperior rim of C7 (Fig. 5.11B). This fracture was probably due to avulsion by the anterior attachment of the annulus fibrosis, which pulled off a rim of bone as a result of shear loading directed anteriorly. There was anterior translation of C6 on C7, separation of the posterior elements, and subluxation of the facet joints (105).

With reference to the key biomechanical concepts, this injury pattern illustrates the importance of the direction of load relative to the spine (key biomechanical concept 4). Specifically, in uniplanar analysis, this represents primarily a flexion bending moment injury among the spectrum of injury patterns occurring in the sagittal or *yz*-plane, which is closely represented by Figure 5.2A. The value of this clinical mishap is to document a mechanism of injury in an *in vivo* human experiment. It shows precisely what can occur when a large bending moment is applied in the flexion mode (positive *x*-axis rotation). It also fits into a spectrum of sagittal plane injury analysis theory and provides a basis for extrapolation to other presumed loading patterns.

Cervical Compression Fractures

The group of cervical compression fractures includes several fracture patterns. These injuries involve vertebral body failure and include simple anterior compression fractures, burst fractures, and teardrop fractures. The different injury patterns are due to differences in magnitude of load, point of load application, preinjury positioning in the *yz* or sagittal plane, and direction of forces and moments in relation to the *x*-axis.

Simple Compression Fractures

Simple compression fractures are probably secondary to an MIV roughly parallel to the *y*-axis, anterior to the injured FSU's IAR in the sagittal plane, producing a slight moment of bending about the *x*-axis (a positive *x*-axis moment or, roughly, a slight flexion force). McElhaney and associates (7) produced anterior compression fractures by applying an axial load 1 cm anterior to neutral. Axial loads applied more than 1 cm anterior to neutral produced buckling rearward and subsequent disc and end-plate failure. This is an example of the importance of the point of load application (key biomechanical concept 5) in determining the final injury pattern.

Teardrop and Burst Fractures

The teardrop fracture is characterized radiographically by a triangular fragment of bone apparent at the anterior/inferior border of the involved vertebra as projected on a lateral radiograph. Seeing this fracture fragment should make one aware of the possible presence of several additional fractures along different injury planes. It is important to recognize that a fracture line may extend sagittally, splitting the vertebral

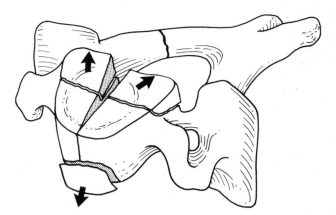

FIG. 5.12. Orientation of common fracture planes and directions of fragment displacements commonly occurring in teardrop fractures. (From: White AA, Panjabi MM. *Clinical biomechanics of the spine*, 2nd ed. Philadelphia: JB Lippincott, 1990:173, with permission.)

body into left and right fragments (Fig. 5.12). These halves may displace posteriorly, causing neural canal encroachment (106,107). Proposed mechanisms of injury include hyperflexion (108), a combination of flexion and compressive loading (93), as well as hyperextension (109).

A fracture of the anteroinferior aspect of a vertebral body could be caused by an axial load (negative *y*-axis translational force) resulting in shear failure or an MIV causing an extension moment (negative *x*-axis rotational force) resulting in a tensile failure (Fig. 5.13).

Torg and associates (2) reported 55 teardrop fractures, 35 of which occurred in football players while tackling. Thirty-one patients had an associated fracture line in the sagittal plane. Twenty-seven of these 51 became permanently quadriplegic. Reviewing the records and game films, Torg and coworkers (2) concluded that the teardrop fracture pattern is due to axial loading at the vertex of the head with the neck prepositioned in flexion, which straightens out the normal cervical lordosis. Similar injuries and mechanisms of injury have been described in ice hockey (110). These injuries exemplify the concepts of point of load application (key biomechanical concept 5) and prepositioning of the head (key biomechanical concept 6).

The clinically observed MOI of teardrop fractures has been confirmed by biomechanical laboratory studies on human cadavers that produced this fracture pattern by axial compression of the neutral and minimally flexed cervical spine (8,11,16). The presence of a sagittal fracture plane has been observed in clinical injuries of this type (106,107, 111). Thus, careful clinical observations and experimental cadaveric studies have established the MOI in teardrop fractures.

Hyperextension Fractures

Marar (112) reviewed 45 patients with severe hyperextension injuries and noted primarily soft tissue failures. His

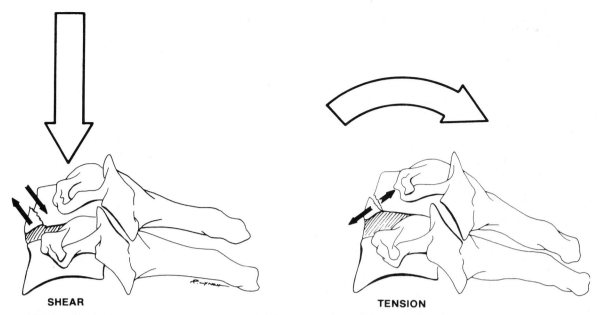

FIG. 5.13. Teardrop fractures. A triangular fragment of bone at the anteroinferior portion of the vertebral body may result from either shear or tensile failure. In compressive loading, there are shear stresses along a line about 45 degrees to the force vector. In extension loading, the same region of bone is subjected to tensile stresses. (From: White AA, Panjabi MM. *Clinical biomechanics of the spine*, 2nd ed. Philadelphia: JB Lippincott, 1990:191, with permission.)

studies included four patients who died of their injuries. The postmortem examinations of these four patients disclosed a complete transverse fracture of the vertebral body at the level of the inferior portion of the pedicles. The spinal cord had been compressed between the upper portion of the fractured vertebra and the lamina of the subjacent vertebra. Spontaneous reduction had taken place, and the fracture could not be visualized on routine radiographs. In these cases, knowledge of the MOI might lead one to suspect the occult injury and prompt further imaging studies, including carefully administered stress radiographs such as a stretch test (72). The hyperextension MOI in the production of vertebral body fractures was further supported by human cadaver studies (113). Marar (113) manually applied a backward rotational force (negative x-axis moment) to produce complete vertebral body fractures in five of seven cadavers.

Clay Shoveler's Fracture

Clay shoveler's fractures are fractures of one or more of the spinous processes in the lower cervical or upper thoracic spine. Clay shoveler's fracture often occurs after repetitive lifting preceded by pain. The classic example is that of an unconditioned worker who has had symptoms of pain between the shoulders for several days or weeks when lifting a shovel full of clay. At one point as the worker is tossing the clay out of the shovel, some of the clay sticks to the shovel, and there may be the sound of a crack, followed by severe pain in the back between the shoulders, which

suggests a fatigue failure mechanism (see "Magnitude of the Force" earlier in this chapter).

This injury is believed to be due to forces transmitted to the spinous processes of the cervical spine from the shoulder girdle through the trapezius, rhomboid, and the posterior serratus muscles. The major vector of force of these muscles is back and forth along the x-axis.

Gershon-Cohen and coworkers (114) proposed an alternative MOI for fractures of the lower cervical spinous processes. They noted fractures resembling clay shoveler's fractures in persons involved in MVAs. These investigators also produced similar fractures by tugging sharply on the heads of supine and prone cadavers, simulating hyperflexion and hyperextension (114).

It has also been suggested that failure could be due to pull through the ligamentum nuchae and supraspinous ligaments (114,115). However, this is unlikely in view of the rather delicate, almost nonexistent nature of the ligamentum nuchae in humans and the rather thin interspinous and supraspinous ligaments in the cervical and thoracic spine (116,117).

Soft Tissue Injuries

The most common cause of cervical spine injury is vehicular accidents, most of which result in soft tissue injuries. In rear-end collision vehicular trauma, cervical spine soft tissue injury may occur either through hyperextension in which the head may first accelerate forward (flexion) and then rotate backward (extension) or through a combination of axial compression and hyperextension as the face or frontal bone strikes the windshield (118,119).

Whiplash

From a biomechanical standpoint, the term *whiplash* does not clearly describe the MOI. From a layman's standpoint, whiplash implies injury to soft tissues of the neck without direct application of force to the head or neck as would occur in acceleration hyperextension injuries. The term *whiplash* applies to a complex and variable set of clinical circumstances and an equally variable symptom complex. There is usually a history of a minor or moderately severe rear-end collision. The patient presents with some combination of a large variety of symptoms, the only common factor being neck pain. Radiographs of the cervical spine are generally normal, except for the possible loss of physiologic cervical lordosis. The soft tissue injuries present include a spectrum of severity ranging from minor sprains to complete tears and avulsions of muscles, ligaments, and intervertebral discs.

Whiplash injuries have been simulated in several experimental studies. Macnab (120) used anesthetized monkeys in a supine position and dropped them from various heights. The monkeys' bodies were supported, but their heads and necks were not. Before hitting the ground, they were suddenly decelerated, simulating a cervical hyperextension whiplash. Clemens and Burrow (121) subjected 15 unembalmed cadavers between the ages of 50 and 90 years to 19 km/h rear-end impacts producing 13 to 16 G. In both these studies, injuries ranged from minor tears of the sternocleidomastoid muscle to partial avulsions of the longus colli and retropharyngeal hematomas. The most common finding was intervertebral disc failures and tears of the anterior longitudinal ligament, which occurred in up to 90% of cases.

More recently, investigators conducting postmortem examinations of accident victims noted injuries similar to those produced under experimental conditions. The studies confirmed that the common whiplash injury may be associated with major soft tissue disruption and even fractures that are usually not evident on plain radiographs.

Taylor and colleagues (119,122,123) sagittally sectioned 105 postmortem cervical spines. The cause of death in 60 of these was fatal head and chest trauma. Among extension injuries, the most frequently damaged structure was the intervertebral disc (96%). Taylor and coworkers identified three patterns of intervertebral disc injury. The first pattern is one of anterior rim lesions consisting of linear clefts of the peripheral cartilage plate through the region where the cartilage plate lamellae are continuous with the lamellae of the annulus fibrosus. The anterior longitudinal ligament is intact, cervical alignment is often normal, and the lesion is not visible on postmortem plain radiographs. The second pattern consists of posterior contusions and herniations of the intervertebral discs, and the third consists of partial or complete avulsions along the disc–vertebral interface, occurring most commonly in children. The anterior rim lesions (first pattern) have been

documented by magnetic resonance imaging (MRI) in patients sustaining whiplash-type injuries (124). Taylor and associates (119,122,123) noted high signal intensity on T2-weighted images paralleling the vertebral end plate. In severe injuries, one or both of the longitudinal ligaments may be torn. At times, there was associated instability and a spinal cord injury. Other common injuries included soft tissue injury of the facet joints (76%), dorsal root ganglia contusions (17%), and damage to the vertebral arteries (9%) (119,122).

In a similar study, Jonsson and colleagues (125) examined cryoplaned sections of 22 traffic accident victims with fatal craniocerebral injuries. The site of impact, or point of load application, varied among the 22 victims. The authors found that all the victims had cervical spine injuries. Two hundred forty-five cervical spine injuries were not detected on optimum radiographs taken before postmortem examination, and only four were detected on reassessment of the radiographs after analysis of the pathoanatomic findings. Commonly injured structures included the facet joints, uncovertebral joints, and intervertebral discs.

Jonsson and associates (126) reviewed 50 consecutive patients with whiplash-type cervical distortions resulting from MVAs. Five patients had cervical instability noted on flexion-extension radiographs, but their MRI scans failed to show any posterior soft tissue injury despite surgically confirmed extensive acute soft tissue injury in both patients who subsequently underwent posterior cervical fusion. Twenty-four patients who had persistent pain 6 weeks after the injury underwent cervical MRI scans, all of which showed reduced signal intensity in 34% of 144 discs and 11 large disc herniations.

Reflecting the recent reported alarming increases in whiplash injuries, several experimental studies, both *in vivo* with volunteers as well as *in vitro* with cadaveric preparations, have been conducted. The major finding of these studies is a proposal for a different injury mechanism than that hypothesized by Macnab in 1964 (120). Panjabi and coworkers (127,128) carried out a set of whiplash trauma to fresh cadaveric whole cervical spine specimens. The occiput-to-T1 specimen was provided with an appropriate surrogate head and was fixed at T1 onto a sled of a benchtop mini-sled model. Increasing horizontal accelerations were applied to the sled, simulating rear-end collision, while motions of the head and each vertebra were monitored using potentiometers, accelerometers, and high-speed cameras. Intervertebral injuries were documented using flexibility tests before and after each trauma, as well as by a function of radiographs. Based on eight specimens, they found the whiplash trauma to induce a biphasic response in the cervical spine. In the first phase, occurring about 75 to 110 milliseconds after the impact, the head was purely translating rearward with respect to T1, resulting in an S-shaped curve in which the upper cervical spine was in flexion while the lower cervical spine was subjected to hyperextension. In the second phase, occurring about 150 to 200 milliseconds after the impact, the head rotated backward and the entire cervical spine went into extension. The flexibility test showed that the injuries were due to hyperextension of the lower cervical spine, and the high-speed movie showed that these occurred in the first phase of whiplash trauma.

This injury mechanism has been confirmed by *in vivo* studies using volunteers (129). In this study, rear-end collision was simulated by a sled on rails moving on an inclined plane. During the trauma, the cervical spine was cineradiographed at 90 frames per second. Kinematics of the spine was documented by analyzing the intervertebral motions. In conclusion, the S-shaped injury mechanism in the first phase of whiplash trauma is a major new discovery that may have a significant effect on the design of car seats and headrests.

Some of the cervical spine injuries noted during postmortem inspection of traffic accident victims have been reproduced in the laboratory setting. Shea and coworkers (130) investigated hyperextension injuries by applying a tensile load at a rate of 5 mm per second to human cadaveric cervical spines prepositioned in extension. They produced anterior longitudinal ligament tears and failures of the intervertebral disc. The most common level of injury was C5-C6, and they noted a correlation between the level of injury and the degree of disc degeneration.

Cervical Spinal Cord Neuropraxia

Torg and colleagues (2,56–58) have reported cervical spinal cord neuropraxias to occur as a result of brief axial loading of a developmentally or congenitally narrowed cervical spine prepositioned in slight flexion. A cervical spine prepositioned in flexion will straighten the alignment of the FSUs and eliminate normal physiologic lordosis.

Initially, a large review of athletes who had experienced stinger symptoms disclosed no increased risk of sustaining a permanent neurologic injury (56,57). Subsequently, however, Torg and colleagues (58) reported four athletes who had experienced stinger symptoms, continued in contact sports, and subsequently experienced an axial load to a flexed cervical spine that resulted in permanent neurologic injury. Torg and colleagues therefore advise against participation in contact sports by players with "spear tackler's spine" who continue to use inappropriate tackling technique. They described spear tackler's spine as arising from circumstances in which a person with a straight and stenotic or degenerated cervical spine has a history of using the crown of his head to make initial contact during tackling. They emphasized that it is the inappropriate tackling technique that imposes the greatest risk of permanent neurologic injury to the player.

GUIDELINES FOR BIOMECHANICAL INTERPRETATION OF RADIOGRAPHS

Background information for proper interpretation of radiographs requires a careful history and physical examination, which should attempt to distill information relative to the seven basic biomechanical concepts discussed earlier in this chapter. Some major injuries may not be apparent on static radiographs (57,112,122,125,131–134). Crowell and coworkers (135) noted that experimentally produced bony and soft tissue failure was sometimes not recognizable on radiographs or even by direct observation of the anatomic specimen unless the mechanism of injury was reproduced. Similar observations were made by Jonsson and colleagues, who studied traffic accident victims (126).

Some guidelines for the biomechanical interpretation of radiographs of the spine after trauma follow. These are not absolute rules, but they are acceptable maxims based on current knowledge.

- Bone tends to fail first along lines of tensile stress; next it may fail as a result of either shear or compression, in that order. The vertebrae are well designed to withstand compressive loads.
- One may assume that, in the cervical spine, the anterosuperior or the anteroinferior triangle of the vertebral body, observed frequently on lateral radiographs, is pulled off by the peripheral annulus fibrous fibers. Thus, the triangular portion of the vertebral body may be pulled off in an extension type of injury, in which the triangular fragment remains with the annular fibers, which remain attached to the intact vertebra, and the fractured vertebra is pulled away by the tensile loads. However, it is also possible in a flexion injury for compressive loading to result in high shear stresses (at a 45-degree angle to the vertical load), causing failure along approximately the same lines in which tensile failure would occur. In this case, a triangular fragment could appear again.
- When a triangular fragment or teardrop is observed, beware of the possibility of an occult sagittal plane fracture of the same vertebral body.
- In compression of an FSU, the vertebral body end plate generally fails first; however, experimental work by Crowell and associates (26) showed occult disc injuries in the absence of vertebral end-plate fractures.
- In the normal anatomy of the FSU, with most loading vectors, the bone tends to fail before the ligamentous structures. There are exceptions, including whiplash-type injuries.
- Where there is wide separation between the anterior and posterior elements, indicating ligamentous rupture, most probably a significant element in the mechanism of injury is axial rotation (torque about the *y*-axis).
- Narrowing between vertebral bodies at a given intervertebral space where there is other evidence of trauma is suggestive of failure of the annulus or its attachment, implicating a mechanism involving shear or tensile loading. Abnormal widening at the disc space has the same implications.
- In whiplash-type injuries, the plain radiographs may be relatively normal despite significant injury to cervical musculature, ligaments, facet joints, and intervertebral discs. These injuries may be better appreciated with an MRI scan, although the precise role of MRI scans in these clinical conditions has yet to be determined. More important

is the recognition of potential major ligamentous injury rendering the spine unstable despite otherwise normal plain radiographs and MRI scans. This logically should be diligently followed by maintenance of appropriate cervical spine immobilization until an evaluation is completed that includes cervical flexion and extension views and/or a stretch test.

- One important variable is time dependent and must be taken into consideration. In any injury to a complex structure such as the spine, changes occur between the onset and completion of the injury. The structure changes its geometric and physical properties. The force vectors of injury change in direction and magnitude. The clinician is challenged to analyze not just one isolated injury occurring instantaneously to one structure, but a series of rapidly changing injury mechanisms affecting a series of rapidly changing structures. Current analyses need not seek this level of complexity. However, the oversimplification involved in the use of a static two-dimension representation of a complicated series of dynamic three-dimensional events should be kept in mind.

SUMMARY

Simple descriptions of an accident, such as "fell off a ladder," do not fully describe the mechanism of injury. An individual injury pattern is the result of a complex set of conditions. The magnitude of displacement is one factor that determines the extent of injury. The direction of the load relative to the spine or subject, the point of load application, and the preposition of the head and FSU determine whether the response of the spine to axial load is to flex, buckle, or extend. Individual anatomic characteristics, including normal anatomic variations and disease processes, affect the material and structural properties of the spine. The rate of load application affects the amount of energy absorption to failure and whether failure occurs predominantly through bony or ligamentous structures. An increased awareness of these concepts continues to improve the precision with which the MOI is defined in both experimental and clinical circumstances.

There is increased awareness of the limitations of biomechanical models in simulating live human spine behavior. Many investigators have conducted biomechanical studies. Among these, Myers and colleagues (87) have investigated the role of torsion in cervical spine trauma. Panjabi, Oda, and Oxland and their associates (21,22,31,69,83,84,136) have examined trauma-induced cervical spine instability and atlas fractures. Shea and colleagues (130) have examined hyperextension injuries in human cadavers, and Yoganandan and Pintar and their coworkers (9,16,17,29,30) have examined the complexity of spinal column responses and injury patterns to axial loading of entire human cervical spines.

Most recognized cervical spine injury patterns have been reproduced in cadavers in laboratories. However, in some cases, such as transverse ligament tears, nearly identical injury patterns have been created under significantly different loading conditions. This observation leads us to believe that experimental loading conditions must be more precisely defined. In certain cases, careful clinical observations, such as those made by Torg and colleagues (2,3,56–58,107) of teardrop and burst-type fractures, help clarify the most clinically relevant mechanism of injury.

Improved imaging techniques as well as extensive cadaveric studies of traffic victims by Taylor and colleagues (119,122) and thorough evaluation of patients by Jonsson and coworkers (125,126) have demonstrated a high prevalence of microscopic and grossly identifiable anatomic lesions in victims of "neck sprains" or whiplash-type injuries.

The wealth of new information contributes to our understanding of the biomechanics of cervical spine trauma and has provided us with a better appreciation of the conditions and mechanisms involved in the creation of specific cervical spine injury patterns. Closer attention paid to experimental loading conditions and accurate measurement of forces and displacements in all planes have allowed more comprehensive descriptions of the MOI of specific injury patterns. However, both laboratory investigators and clinicians must be cognizant of the seven key biomechanical concepts in experimental design and in interpretation of study results.

In experiments involving loading of spine segments, investigators often attempt to minimize the multiple variables involved in an attempt to produce consistent results. To address this, synthetic spine models were developed and continue to be improved. Perhaps of equal importance is the heightened awareness of these models' inability to simulate faithfully the spine's actual behavior and attempts to quantify these differences.

Studies by Torg and colleagues (2,3,56–58,107) in football injuries, McElhaney and associates (7) in diving injuries, and Scher (103) in rugby injuries suggest that valuable information regarding MOI can be gleaned from close observation and documentation of events and injuries occurring to participants of a particular activity.

Although great advances continue to be made in the biomechanics of cervical spine trauma, much work remains to be done, specifically with regard to being aware of and accounting for the seven key biomechanical concepts in the study design.

ACKNOWLEDGMENTS

The authors gratefully acknowledge the support provided by the Daniel E. Hogan Spine Fellowship, Beth Israel Deaconess Medical Center, Boston, Massachusetts; and the Division of Research Support, St. Luke's Hospital, Kansas City, Missouri.

REFERENCES

1. Crisco JJ, Panjabi MM, Dvorak J. A model of the alar ligaments of the upper cervical spine in axial rotation. *J Biomechanics* 1991;24:607–614.

2. Torg JS, Vegso JJ, O'Neill MJ, et al. The epidemiologic, pathologic, biomechanical, and cinematographic analysis of football-injured cervical spine trauma. *Am J Sports Med* 1990;18:50–57.
3. Torg JS, Vegso JJ, Sennett B. The national football head and neck injury registry: 14-year report of cervical quadriplegia (1971–1984). *Clin Sports Med* 1987;6:61–72.
4. Hoek Van Dijke GA, Snijders CJ, et al. Analysis of biomechanical and ergonomic aspects of the cervical spine in F-16 flight situations. *J Biomech* 1993;26:1017–1025.
5. Guill FC. Ascertaining the causal factors for "ejection-associated" injuries. *Aviat Space Environ Med* 1989;60:B44–B71.
6. Bauze RJ, Ardran GM. Experimental production of forward dislocation in the human cervical spine. *J Bone Joint Surg Br* 1978;60:239–245.
7. McElhaney JH, Paver JG, McCracklin HJ. Cervical spine compression responses. In: *Proceedings of the 27th STAPP Car Crash Conference*. Warrendale, PA: Society of Automotive Engineers, 1983:163.
8. Maiman DJ, Sances A, Myklebust JB, et al. Compression injuries of the cervical spine: a biomechanical analysis. *Neurosurgery* 1983;13:254–260.
9. Yoganandan N, Sances A, Maiman DJ, et al. Experimental spinal injuries with vertical impact. *Spine* 1986;11:855–860.
10. Nusholtz GS, Huelke DE, Lux P, et al. Cervical spine injury mechanisms. In: *Proceedings of the 27th STAPP Car Crash Conference*. Warrendale, PA: Society of Automotive Engineers, 1983:179–197.
11. Alem NM, Nusholtz GS, Melvin JW. Head and neck response to axial impacts. In: *Proceedings of the 28th STAPP Car Crash Conference*. Warrendale, PA: Society of Automotive Engineers, 1984.
12. Noyes F, DeLucas J, Torvik P. The biomechanics of anterior cruciate ligament failure: an analysis of strain-rate sensitivity and mechanisms of failure in primates. *J Bone Joint Surg Am* 1974;56:236–253.
13. Myers BS, McElhaney JH. *Cervical spine injury mechanisms: biomechanics and prevention*. New York: Springer-Verlag, 1993:311–361.
14. Yoganandan N, Pintar F, Butler J, et al. Dynamic response of human spine ligaments. *Spine* 1989;14:1102–1110.
15. Peterson R, Woo S. A new methodology to determine the mechanical properties of ligaments at high strain rates. *J Biomech Eng* 1986;108:365–367.
16. Pintar FA, Sances A, Yoganandan N, et al. Biodynamics of the total human cadaveric cervical spine. SAE Technical Paper Series. In: *Proceedings of the 34th STAPP Car Crash Conference*. Warrendale, PA: Society of Automotive Engineers, 1990:55–72.
17. Yoganandan N, Sances A, Pintar F, et al. Injury biomechanics of the human cervical column. *Spine* 1990;15:1031–1039.
18. Yoganandan N, Haffner M, Maiman DJ, et al. Epidemiology and injury biomechanics of motor vehicle related trauma to the human spine. SAE Technical Paper Series. In: *Proceedings of the 33rd STAPP Car Crash Conference*. Warrendale, PA: Society of Automotive Engineers, 1989:223–242.
19. Edwards WT, Hayes WC, Posner I, et al. Variation in lumbar spine stiffness with load. *J Biomed Eng* 1987;109:35–42.
20. Miller JAA, Schultz AB, Warwick DN, et al. Mechanical properties of lumbar motion segments under large loads. *J Biomech* 1986;19:79–84.
21. Panjabi MM, White AA, Southwick WO. Effect of preload on load-displacement curves of the lumbar spine. *Orthop Clin North Am* 1977;8:181.
22. Oxland TR, Panjabi MM. The onset and progression of spinal injury: a demonstration of neutral zone sensitivity. *J Biomech* 1992;25:1165–1172.
23. Panjabi MM. The stabilizing system of the spine. Part I. Function, dysfunction, adaptation and enhancement. *J Spinal Disord* 1992;5:383–389.
24. Panjabi MM. The stabilizing system of the spine. Part II. Neutral zone and instability hypothesis. *J Spinal Disord* 1992;5:390–396.
25. McLain RF, Aretakis A, Mosley TA, et al. Sub-axial cervical dissociation: anatomic and biomechanical principles of stabilization. *Spine* 1994;19:653–659.
26. Crowell RR, Shea M, Edwards WT, et al. Cervical injuries under flexion and compression loading. *J Spinal Disord* 1993;6:175–181.
27. Panjabi MM, Takeori O, Joseph JC III, et al. Posture affects motion coupling patterns of the upper cervical spine. *J Orthop Res* 1993;11:525–536.
28. Sharara KH, Farrar M. Traumatic lateral instability of the cervical spine. *Injury* 1993;24:266–267.
29. Pintar FA, Yoganandan N, Sances A Jr, et al. Kinematic and anatomical analysis of the human cervical spinal column under axial loading. SAE Technical Paper Series. In: *Proceedings of the 33rd STAPP Car Crash Conference*. Warrendale, PA: Society of Automotive Engineers, 1989:191–214.
30. Yoganandan N, Pintar FA, Sances A, et al. Strength and kinematic response of dynamic cervical spine injuries. *Spine* 1991;16:S511–S517.
31. Oxland TR, Panjabi MM, Southern EP, et al. An anatomic basis for spinal instability: a porcine trauma model. *J Orthop Res* 1991;9:452–462.
32. Panjabi MM, Duranceau JS, Oxland TR, et al. Multidirectional instabilities of traumatic cervical spine injuries in a porcine model. *Spine* 1989;14:1111–1115.
33. Southern EP, Oxland TR, Panjabi MM, et al. Cervical spine injury patterns in three modes of high-speed trauma: a biomechanical porcine model. *J Spinal Disord* 1990;3:316–328.
34. Heggeness MH, Doherty BJ. Creation of Jefferson fracture by torsion axis. In: *Proceedings of the 21st Annual Meeting of the Cervical Spine Research Society*. New York: Cervical Spine Research Society, 1993:97.
35. Hodgson VR, Thomas LM. Mechanisms of cervical spine injury during impact to the protected head. In: *Proceedings of the 24th STAPP Car Crash Conference*. Warrendale, PA: Society of Automobile Engineers, 1980:17.
36. Shono Y, McAfee PC, Cunningham BW. The pathomechanics of compression injuries in the cervical spine. *Spine* 1993;18:2009–2019.
37. Hamalainen O, Vanharanta H. Effect of G_z forces and head movements on cervical erector spinae muscle strain. *Aviat Space Environ Med* 1992;63:709–716.
38. Helleur C, Gracovetsky S, Farfan H. Tolerance of the human cervical spine to high acceleration: a modelling approach. *Aviat Space Environ Med* 1984;55:903–909.
39. Hattrup SJ, Johnson KA. A review of ruptures of the Achilles tendon. *Foot Ankle* 1985;6:34–38.
40. Dai QG, Liu YK. Failure analysis of a beam-column under oblique-eccentric loading: potential failure surfaces for cervical spine trauma. *J Biomech Eng* 1992;114:119–128.
41. Hansson T, Roos B. The influence of age, height and weight on the bone mineral content of lumbar vertebrae. *Spine* 1980;5:545.
42. Lotz JC, Gerhart TN, Hayes WC. Mechanical properties of trabecular bone from the proximal femur: a quantitative CT study. *J Comput Assist Tomogr* 1990;14:107–113.
43. Bell GH, Dunbar O, Beck JS, et al. Variation in strength of vertebrae with age: their relation to osteoporosis. *Calcif Tissue Res* 1967;1:75.
44. Buckwalter JA, Woo SLY, Goldberg VM, et al. Current concepts review: soft-tissue aging and musculoskeletal function. *J Bone Joint Surg Am* 1993;75:1533–1548.
45. Brewer BJ. Aging of the rotator cuff. *Am J Sports Med* 1979;7:102–110.
46. Burkhead WZ. The biceps tendon. In: Rockwood CA, Matsen FA, eds. *The shoulder*. Philadelphia: WB Saunders, 1990:791–836.
47. Noyes FR, Grood ES. The strength of the anterior cruciate ligament in humans and rhesus monkeys. Age-related and species-related changes. *J Bone Joint Surg Am* 1976;58:1074–1082.
48. Woo SL, Hollis JM Adams DJ, et al. Tensile properties of the human femur-anterior cruciate ligament-tibia complex. The effects of specimen age and orientation. *Am J Sports Med* 1991;19:217–225.
49. Ramsey RH. The anatomy of the ligamentum flava. *Clin Orthop* 1976;44:129.
50. Nachemson AL, Evans JH. Some mechanical properties of the third human lumbar interlaminar ligament (ligamentum flavum). *J Biomech* 1968;1:211–220.
51. Elster AD, Quadriplegia after minor trauma in Klippel-Feil syndrome—a case report and review of the literature. *J Bone Joint Surg Am* 1984;66:1473.
52. DeWald RL, Ray RD. Skeletal traction for the treatment of severe scoliosis. The University of Illinois halo-hoop apparatus. *J Bone Joint Surg Am* 1970;52:233–238.
53. Murray GC, Persellin RH. Cervical fracture complicating ankylosing spondylitis. A report of eight cases and review of the literature. *Am J Med* 1981;70:1033–1041.
54. Rowed DW. Management of cervical spine cord injury in ankylosing spondylitis: the intervertebral disc as a cause of cord compression. *J Neurosurg* 1992;77:241–246.

55. MacMillan M, Stauffer ES. Traumatic instability in the previously fused cervical spine. *J Spinal Disord* 1991;4:449–454.

56. Torg JS, Pavlov H. Cervical spinal stenosis with cord neurapraxia and transient quadriplegia. *Clin Sports Med* 1987;6:115–133.

57. Torg JS, Pavlov H, Genuario SE. Neuropraxia of the cervical cord with transient quadriplegia. *J Bone Joint Surg Am* 1986;68:1354–1370.

58. Torg JS, Pavlov H, Sennett B, et al. Spear tackler's spine. An entity precluding participation in tackle football and collision activities that expose the cervical spine to axial energy inputs. *Am J Sports Med* 1993;21:640–649.

59. Bueff HU, Panjabi MM, Sonu CM, et al. Functional stability of the canine cervical spine after injury: a three month *in vivo* study. *Spine* 1990;15:1040–1046.

60. Crisco JJ, Panjabi MM, Wang E, et al. The injured canine cervical spine after six months of healing: an *in vitro* three-dimensional study. *Spine* 1990;15:1047–1052.

61. McAfee PC, Farey ID, Sutterlin CE, et al. The effect of spinal implant rigidity on vertebral bone density. A canine model. *Spine* 1991;16(Suppl):S190–S197.

62. Panjabi MM, Pelker R, Crisco J, et al. Biomechanics of healing of posterior cervical spinal injuries in a canine model. *Spine* 1988; 13:803–807.

63. Zdeblick T, Wilson D, Cooke M, et al. Anterior cervical discectomy and fusion. *Spine* 1992;17(Suppl 10):S418–S426.

64. Yoganandan N, Sances A, Pintar F. Biomechanical evaluation of the axial compressive responses of the human cadaveric and mannequin necks. *J Biomech Eng* 1989;111:250–255.

65. Deng YC, Goldsmith W. Response of a human head/neck/upper-torso replica to dynamic loading. I. Physical model. *J Biomech* 1987;20:471–497.

66. Deng YC, Goldsmith W. Response of a human head/neck/upper-torso replica to dynamic loading. II. Analytical/numerical model. *J Biomech* 1987;5:487–497.

67. Panjabi MM, Crisco JJ, Oda T, et al. Experimental study of atlas injuries. I. Biomechanical analysis of their mechanisms and fracture patterns. *Spine* 1991;16:S460–S465.

68. Tennyson SA, Mital NK, King AI. Electromyographic signals of the spinal musculature during G_z impact acceleration. *Orthop Clin North Am* 1977;1:97–119.

69. Panjabi MM, Abumi K, Duranceau J, et al. Spinal stability and inter-segmental muscle forces: a biomechanical model. *Spine* 1989; 14: 194–200.

70. Wilke HJ, Claes L, Schmitt H, et al. A universal spine tester for *in vitro* experiments with muscle force simulation. *Eur Spine J* 1994; 3:91–97.

71. Liu YK, Dai QG. The second stiffest axis of a beam-column: implications for cervical spine trauma. *J Biomech Eng* 1989;3:122–127.

72. White AA, Panjabi MM. *Clinical biomechanics of the spine*, 2nd ed. Philadelphia: JB Lippincott, 1990:318–321.

73. Anderson PA, Montesano PX. Morphology and treatment of occipital condyle fractures. *Spine* 1988;13:731.

74. Dvorak J, Schneider E, Saldinger P, et al. Biomechanics of the craniocervical region: the alar and transverse ligaments. *J Orthop Res* 1988;6:452.

75. Panjabi M, Dvorak J, Crisco J, et al. Effects of alar ligament transection on upper cervical spine rotation. *J Orthop Res* 1991;9:584–593.

76. Papadopoulos SM. Biomechanics of occipito-atlanto-axial trauma. In: Rea GL, Miller CA, eds. *Spinal trauma: current evaluation and management*. AANS Publications, 1993;2:17–23.

77. Werne S. Studies in spontaneous atlas dislocation. *Acta Orthop Scand Suppl* 1957;23:1–50.

78. Bucholz RW, Burkhead WZ. The pathological anatomy of fatal atlanto-occipital dislocations. *J Bone Joint Surg Am* 1979;61:248–250.

79. Anderson PA, Jonsson H, Rauschning W, et al. Traumatic rupture of the transverse ligament associated with occipital cervical instability. In: *Proceedings of the 21st Annual Meeting of the Cervical Spine Research Society*. New York: Cervical Spine Research Society, 1993:42.

80. Sherk H, Nicholson J. Fractures of the atlas. *J Bone Joint Surg Am* 1970;52:1017.

81. Stauffer SE, MacMillan M. *Rockwood and Green's fractures in adults*, 3rd ed. Philadelphia: JB Lippincott, 1991:1329.

82. Alker GJ, Oh YS, Leslie EV, et al. Postmortem radiology of head and neck injuries in fatal traffic accidents. *Radiology* 1975;114:611.

83. Oda T, Crisco JJ, Panjabi MM, et al. Experimental study of atlas injuries. II. Relevance to clinical diagnosis and treatment. *Spine* 1991;16:S466–S473.

84. Oda T, Panjabi MM, Crisco JJ, et al. Multidirectional instabilities of experimental burst fractures of the atlas. *Spine* 1992;17:1285–1290.

85. Fielding JW, Cochran GVB, Lawsing JF, et al. Tears of the transverse ligament of the atlas, a clinical and biomechanical study. *J Bone Joint Surg Am* 1974;56:1683–1691.

86. Levine AM, Edwards CC. Traumatic lesions of the occipitoatlantoaxial complex. *Clin Orthop* 1989;239:53–68.

87. Myers BS, McElhaney JH, Doherty BJ. The role of torsion in cervical spine trauma. *Spine* 1991;16:870–874.

88. Anderson LD, D'Alonzo RT. Fractures of the odontoid process of the axis. *J Bone Joint Surg Am* 1974;56:1663.

89. Schatzker J, Rorabeck CH, Waddell JP. Fractures of the dens (odontoid process): an analysis of thirty-seven cases. *J Bone Joint Surg Br* 1971;53:392.

90. Altoff B. Fracture of the odontoid process. An experimental study. *Acta Orthop Scand Suppl* 1979:177.

91. Craig JB, Hodgson BF. Superior facet fractures of the axis vertebra. *Spine* 1991;16:875–877.

92. Fielding JW, Griffin PP. Os odontoideum: an acquired lesion. *J Bone Joint Surg Am* 1974;56:187.

93. Fielding JW, Hensinger RN, Hawkins RJ. Os odontoideum. *J Bone Joint Surg Am* 1980;62:376.

94. Hukuda S, Ota H, Okabe N, et al. Traumatic atlantoaxial dislocation causing an os odontoideum in infants. *Spine* 1980;5:207–210.

95. Vermooten W. A study of the fracture of the epistropheus due to hanging—with a note on causes of death. *Anat Rec* 1920;20:305–311.

96. Wood-Jones F. The ideal lesion produced by judicial hanging. *Br Med J* 1913;1:53.

97. James R, Nasmyth-Jones R. The occurrence of cervical fractures in victims of judicial hanging. *Forensic Sci Info* 1992;54:81–91.

98. Levine AM, Edwards CC. The management of traumatic spondylolisthesis of the axis. *J Bone Joint Surg Am* 1985;67:217–226.

99. Barquet A, Dubra A. Occult severe hyperflexion sprain of the lower cervical spine. *J Assoc Can Radiol* 1993;44:446–449.

100. Green JD, Harle TS, Harris JH Jr. Anterior subluxation of the cervical spine. *AJNR* 1981;2:243–250.

101. Braakman M, Braakman R. Hyperflexion sprain of the cervical spine: follow-up of 45 cases. *Acta Orthop Scand* 1987;58:388–393.

102. Paley D, Gillespie R. Chronic repetitive unrecognized flexion injury of the cervical spine (high jumper's neck). *Am J Sports Med* 1986;14:92–95.

103. Scher AT. Rugby injuries of the spine and spinal cord. *Clin Sports Med* 1987;6:87–98.

104. Allen BL, Ferguson RL, Lehmann TR, et al. A mechanistic classification of closed, indirect fractures and dislocations of the lower cervical spine. *Spine* 1982;7:1–27.

105. Thiel M, Staudte AW. A momentary documentation of a cervical vertebral fracture. Presented at the European meeting of the Cervical Spine Research Society, Marseilles, France, 1988.

106. Fuentes JM, Bloncourt J, Vlahovitch B, et al. Tear drop fractures. Contribution to the study of its mechanism and of osteo-disco-ligamentous lesions. *Neurochirurgie* 1983;29:129–134.

107. Torg J. *Athletic injuries to the head and face*. Philadelphia: Lea & Febiger, 1982.

108. Schneider RC, Kahn EA. Chronic neurological sequelae of acute trauma to the spine and spinal cord. *J Bone Joint Surg Am* 1956;38:985.

109. Rand RW, Crandall PH. Central spinal cord syndrome in hyperextension injuries of the cervical spine. *J Bone Joint Surg Am* 1962;44:1415.

110. Tator CH. Neck injuries in ice hockey: a recent, unsolved problem with many contributing factors. *Clin Sports Med* 1987;6:101–113.

111. Skold G. Sagittal fractures of the cervical spine. *Injury* 1978;9:294–296.

112. Marar BC. The pattern of neurological damage as an aid to the diagnosis of the mechanism in cervical-spine injuries. *J Bone Joint Surg Am* 1974;56:1648.

113. Marar BC. Hyperextension injuries of the cervical spine. The pathogenesis of damage to the spinal cord. *J Bone Joint Surg Am* 1974; 56:1655.

114. Gershon-Cohen J, Budin E, Glauser F. Whiplash fractures of cervicodorsal spinous processes; resemblance to shoveler's fracture. *JAMA* 1954;155:560–562.

115. Hall RD. Clay-shoveler's fracture. *J Bone Joint Surg* 1940;12:63.

116. Johnson RM, Crelin ES, White AA, et al. Some new observations on the functional anatomy of the lower cervical spine. *Clin Orthop* 1975;111:192–200.

117. White AA. Analysis of the mechanics of the thoracic spine in man. *Acta Orthop Scand Suppl* 1969;127.

118. Severy DM, Mathewson JH, Bechtol CO. Controlled automobile related engineering and medical phenomena. Medical aspects of traffic accidents. In: *Proceedings of Montreal Conference.* 1955: 152.

119. Taylor JR, Finch PM. Neck sprain. *Aust Fam Physician* 1993; 22:1623–1629.

120. Macnab I. Acceleration injuries of the cervical spine. *J Bone Joint Surg Am* 1964;46:1797.

121. Clemens HJ, Burrow K. Experimental investigation of injury mechanism of cervical spine at frontal and rear-front vehicle impacts. In: *Proceedings of the 16th STAPP Car Crash Conference.* New York: Society of Automotive Engineers, 1972:76.

122. Taylor JR, Twomey LT. Acute injuries to cervical joints: an autopsy study of neck sprain. *Spine* 1993;18:1115–1122.

123. Taylor JR, Twomey LT. Disc injuries in cervical trauma. *Lancet* 1991;338:1340–1343.

124. Davis SJ, Teresi LM, Bradley WG Jr, et al. Cervical spine hyperextension injuries: MR findings. *Radiology* 1991;180:245–251.

125. Jonsson H Jr, Bring G, Rauschning W, et al. Hidden cervical spine injuries in traffic accident victims with skull fractures. *J Spinal Disord* 1991;4:251–263.

126. Jonsson H Jr, Cesarini K, Sahlstedt B, et al. Findings and outcome in whiplash-type neck disorders. *Spine* 1994;19:2733–2743.

127. Grauer JN, Panjabi MM, Cholewicki J, Nibu K, Dvorak J. Whiplash produces a bi-phasic curvature of the neck with hyper-extension at lower levels. *Spine* 1997;22:2489–2494.

128. Cholewicki J, Panjabi MM, Nibu K, Babat LB, Grauer JN, Dvorak J. Head Kinematics during *in vitro* whiplash simulation. *Accid Anal and Prev* 1998;30(4):469–479.

129. Kaneoka K, Ono K, Hayashi K. Motion analysis of cervical vertebrae in low-impact, rear-end collisions. Poster presented at AAOS 64th Annual Meeting, San Francisco, February 13–17, 1997.

130. Shea M, Wittenberg RH, Edwards WT, et al. *In vitro* hyperextension injuries in the human cadaveric cervical spine. *J Orthop Res* 1992;10:911–916.

131. Woodring JH, Lee C. Limitations of cervical radiography in the evaluation of acute cervical trauma. *J Trauma* 1993;34:32–39.

132. Mace SE. The unstable occult cervical spine fracture: a review. *Am J Emerg Med* 1992;10:136–142.

133. Sweeney JF, Rosemurgy AS, Gill S, et al. Is the cervical spine clear? Undetected cervical fractures diagnosed only at autopsy. *Ann Emerg Med* 1992;21:1288–1290.

134. Lee C, Woodring J. Sagittally oriented fractures of the lateral masses of the cervical vertebrae. *J Trauma* 1991;12:1638–1643.

135. Crowell RR, Coffee MS, Edwards WT, et al. Cervical ligaments injuries under three dimensional loading. In: *Proceedings of the Cervical Spine Research Society.* New York: Cervical Spine Research Society, 1987.

136. Panjabi MM, White AA, Southwick WO. Mechanical properties of bone as a function of rate of deformation. *J Bone Joint Surg Am* 1973;55:322–330.

CHAPTER 6

Biomechanics of Nonacute Cervical Spine Trauma

Odysseas Paxinos and Alexander J. Ghanayem

The cervical spine is subject to injury from various pathologic conditions other than acute trauma. Degenerative changes, inflammatory disorders, tumor growth, and iatrogenic injury can be the cause of neck pain, instability, deformity, and finally, compression of the neural elements. Each of these disorders affects the biomechanics of the cervical spine in a different way.

Degenerative changes of the cervical spine may be defined as anatomic adaptations to the continuous influence of wear and tear on the involved structures. Stability is achieved by osteophytic formation and disc height reduction in exchange of mobility and space available for the neural tissues. Inflammatory disorders are mediated by a chronic systemic autoimmune response that results in characteristic anatomic changes throughout the body. Rheumatoid arthritis is the most common inflammatory disorder that affects the cervical spine. The inflamed synovium and the release of osteolytic factors result in alteration of the cervical spine's mechanical properties and thus to instability. Tumors of the cervical spine may be benign or malignant, primary or metastatic, and they can affect spine function by mass effect or bone destruction. An important aspect of tumor disease in spine biomechanics is the anticipated destabilization required for partial or complete tumor resection, or the mechanical effects of medical treatment such as radiation therapy. Deformity results from the inability of the spine to maintain alignment under the complex stresses and loads associated with activities of daily living. Stability depends on the nature of the bone, ligaments, muscles, and discs that resist these loads.

Depending on the underlying disease, surgery for nonacute injuries of the cervical spine has two main goals: decompression and stabilization. Because the effects of chronic pathology of the cervical spine can be related to the alteration of the mechanical properties of the tissues, this chapter addresses the biomechanics of nonacute cervical spine injuries and spinal cord impingement, and the role and limitations of surgical treatment options.

INSTABILITY AND NONACUTE TRAUMA

Chronic disorders of the cervical spine can affect both mobility and stability. Information about normal cervical kinematics originates from both *in vivo* and *in vitro* studies. Kinematic data from *in vivo* studies have special clinical interest because they can help distinguish between healthy individuals and patients with cervical disorders (1). Transfer of *in vivo* knowledge to *in vitro* experiments has often been difficult because of problems such as unknown moments and different definitions of neutral posture by different authors (2). On the contrary, *in vitro* data have been used to define the normal range of motion in the various planes and thus to establish clinical criteria of instability (3). Moroney (4) and Panjabi (2) and their associates have provided *in vitro* data on the kinematics and stiffness of the cervical spine. Using pure moments of 1.0 N-m, Panjabi et al. (2) found that the greatest degree of flexion (12.3 degrees) occurred at C1-C2, whereas the greatest degree of extension (20.2 degrees) was observed at C0-C1. With axial moment loading, the greatest rotation (56.7 degrees) was at C1-C2. With lateral bending moments, the average range of motion was 7.9 degrees, with no significant difference between segments (2).

Acute gross instability of the cervical spine can be easily recognized in static radiographs (5). Chronic instability can be detected on dynamic radiographs using data from *in vivo* and *in vitro* kinematic studies as a reference. The upper cervical spine is highly constrained by bony morphology and ligamentous attachments, making the establishment of radiologic criteria easier. Several measurements can be made from radiographs to document deformity and instability of the upper cervical spine and to plan treatment. The anterior atlanto-dental interval (AADI) should be less than 3 mm. Superior migration of the dens can be assessed with McGregor's line. A migration of the tip of the dens of more than 4.5 mm is indicative of vertical settling of the occiput (6).

In the lower cervical spine, the viscoelastic intervertebral disc and the coupled kinematics make recognition of clinical instability more difficult. A functional spinal unit (FSU) that exhibits more than 20 degrees of sagittal rotation in dynamic flexion-extension radiographs is above all normal limits found in *in vivo* (7,8) and *in vitro* studies (2,4) and is considered unstable. Sagittal mobility of an FSU of more than 11 degrees compared with the presumed intact segment above or below is also indicative of instability (3).

Translations, as a component of normal coupling of cervical spine kinematics, occur mainly at the C0-C1 and C1-C2 level and have a posterior direction, with an average value of 11.4 mm (2). This value is well inside the tolerance of the spinal canal space available for the cord (SAC) in the upper cervical spine. In contrast, anteroposterior translations are minimal in the lower cervical spine (average 1.2 mm) (2). Considering 2.7 mm as the highest reported value of anteroposterior translation *in vitro* (2,4,9) and an average radiographic magnification to be 30%, the result is the criterion of 3.5 mm of maximum normal sagittal plane translation proposed by Panjabi and associates (3).

Defining instability in cases of degenerative painful cervical syndromes is more difficult. In most cases a degenerative segment has either normal or decreased range of motion (ROM). The stabilizing effect of neck muscles is difficult to determine from *in vitro* data. Patients with neck pain may have decreased isometric muscle strength (10). Women have about half of the neck strength of men and experience neck pain more frequently (11). Physiotherapy with conditioning of the neck musculature has been shown to improve the symptoms of degenerative disease of the spine.

Clinical studies have shown that temporary external stabilization of a suspected painful and unstable segment can predict the pain relief expected by an arthrodesis with good accuracy (12). Panjabi (13) has introduced the term *neutral zone* (NZ), describing it as the part of the range of motion of a spinal segment at which minimal force application results in large displacement. The same author measured the effects of external fixation on the load-deformation curve of the stabilized segment *in vitro*. He found that the greatest decrease occurred in the neutral zone (69%), with the total ROM losing only 39% of the intact value (12). These findings led Panjabi to redefine clinical instability as follows: "Clinical instability is a significant decrease in the capacity of the stabilizing system of the spine to maintain the intervertebral neutral zones within the physiological limits, so that there is no neurological dysfunction, no major deformity, and no incapacitating pain" (3). The NZ is larger in segments with the greatest range of motion. The larger NZ for flexion occurred in C1-C2 (4.6 degrees), for extension in C0-C1 (13.9 degrees), for axial rotation at

C1-C2 (39.6 degrees), and for lateral bending at C3-C4 and C4-C5 (4.4 degrees at each level) (2).

DEFORMITY AND NONACUTE TRAUMA

The final result of nonacute instability is cervical deformity. Deformity may produce cord or nerve compression and pain. The most frequent cervical deformity is kyphosis, and the most frequent type is iatrogenic, as a result of excessive removal of posterior elements (14,15). Pal and Sherk (16) demonstrated that in the cervical spine 36% of the load is transmitted through the bodies and discs and 64% through the facet joints. The lamina forms a closed ring that increases the stiffness of the articular processes. Disruption of the integrity of this posterior arch–facet complex can cause instability (17,18), shifting the weight-bearing axis anteriorly. The resultant kyphosis requires constant muscular contraction to maintain upright head posture. Eventually, fatigue and pain occur, the deformity progresses, and increased loads are placed on the bodies and discs. The final result is accelerated degeneration and formation of anterior osteophytes. The spinal cord will be then compressed anteriorly on the osteophytes formed in the apex of the kyphotic deformity. The final stage of this process is the evolution of myelopathy. A poorly planned surgical decompression may also aggravate the kyphotic deformity. It is now clear that any preexisting kyphosis significantly increases the risk of deformity after cervical laminectomy (19,20). Kyphotic deformity after posterior surgery is more pronounced in children (21). Increased load shifting from the posterior elements to the anterior column will compress the cartilaginous end plates and will result in wedging of the vertebral bodies (22).

Another frequent cause of cervical spine deformity is the chronic instability produced by the erosive process of inflammatory disorders (Fig. 6.1). A marked deformity of the upper cervical spine is the anterior atlantoaxial subluxation that is present in 45% of patients with rheumatoid arthritis (23–25). The transverse ligament of the atlas has histologic features similar to the articular cartilage and as such is affected early in the development of rheumatoid disease (26). The amount of fibrocartilage present at the level of the atlantodental articulation suggests that the ligament is always under preload and thus is an important stabilizer of the upper cervical spine (26). A finite-element study of the craniovertebral junction found that a 75% reduction in the stiffness of the transverse ligament resulted in atlantoaxial subluxation. Subsequent simulated involvement of the alar ligaments and capsules produced advanced atlantoaxial subluxation and severe deformity (27).

Tumor involvement of the cervical spine will also produce instability, deformity, and neurologic injury. En bloc excision of a tumor as described by Enneking (28) is only rarely possible in the cervical spine due to the small size of the vertebrae, the neurovascular tissues that are in the proximity, and the need for combined anterior and posterior approaches. An intralesional or marginal excision is the only option in most

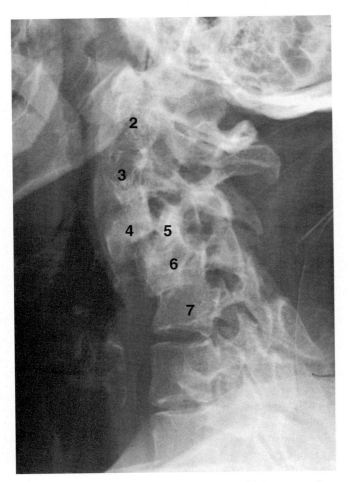

FIG. 6.1. Lateral radiograph of a patient with long-standing rheumatoid arthritis. This demonstrates diffuse instability with multiple levels of spondylolisthesis (stair-step spine).

cases. The margins of excision and tumor aggressiveness are predictors of outcome (29).

BIOMECHANICS OF NONACUTE NEUROLOGIC TRAUMA

In contrast with the volume of information available for the biomechanics of the osseoligamentous structures of the spine, few data exist regarding the physical properties of the spinal cord and the spinal nerves. The spinal cord together with the vascular pia has an elastic strain value of about 10% the original length. This deformation is possible with minimal stress (0.01 N). Further strain is opposed with highly increased stress. Failure stress was found to be about 20 to 30 N (3). The deforming forces acting on the cord produce a variety of compressive, tensile, and shear forces. A bending moment will create tensile stresses on the convex side of the bent spinal cord, and compressive forces on the concave side. These forces may produce ischemia, cell injury, and finally permanent degeneration of the neural tissues. Spinal cord compression may be static or dynamic, but usually both mechanisms coexist, producing myelopathy.

The effect of static cord compression has been well documented by Ogino and associates (30) in a clinicopathologic study. Myelopathic patients were followed clinically until death, and in autopsy the pathologic changes of the cord were investigated. The extent of spinal cord compression correlated well with the severity of pathologic changes in the cord as well as with the clinical symptoms. Static compression is the result of gradual reduction of spinal canal size, which reduces the SAC.

The midsagittal bony diameter from C3 to C7 in Caucasians has been reported to be on average between 14.2 mm (31) and 17 mm (32,33). The semicompressive posterior longitudinal ligament (average width 3.5 mm) and the elastic ligamentum flavum (average width 2.3 mm) normally reduce the effective average canal diameter to 12.7 mm. There are slight variations between sexes and more significant variations between different races, with Asians having reportedly smaller dimensions of the cervical canal (34). The spinal cord measures approximately 10 mm in diameter (range, 8.5–11.5 mm) (35). Several authors have reported on the minimum spinal canal diameter that can be tolerated by the spinal cord. An anteroposterior diameter of less than 12 mm will produce cord compression and symptoms (36,37). Myelopathic changes are more likely to develop in a congenitally narrowed cervical canal, where additional narrowing by spondylotic changes results in spinal cord compression (38). Pavlov's ratio (spinal canal width to vertical body width) should be 1. A ratio less than 0.8 is indicative of spinal stenosis, and an increased risk for cord injury exists (39). In contrast with the lower cervical spine, the upper cervical spine normally has ample SAC. This explains the high tolerance of displacement accepted by the cord in dens fractures and inflammation-induced subluxations.

Dynamic injury to the cord during normal kinematics of the cervical spine is the result of direct impact or ischemia produced by the occlusion of intraspinal vessels as the cord buckles around osteophytes or other canal-occupying lesions. Changes of the transverse dimensions of the normal spinal canal are minimal during the physiologic range of motion. The length of the spinal canal increases with flexion and decreases with extension, imposing a spectrum of compressive, tensile, and shear stresses on the spinal cord during normal kinematics (Fig. 6.2). A bending moment creates tensile stress on the convex side of the spinal cord, and compressive stress on the concave side. The normal spinal cord tolerates these physiologic stresses well. In contrast, when the mechanical properties of the cervical spine are altered, the cord experiences significant deformations. In degenerative spine disease, the ligamentum flavum loses its normal elasticity. As the neck extends, the ligamentum flavum buckles inward (1,7,33,40), which results in significant decrease of the cross-sectional area of the spinal canal. In addition, the spinal cord shortens in extension and its cross-sectional area increases (41). The

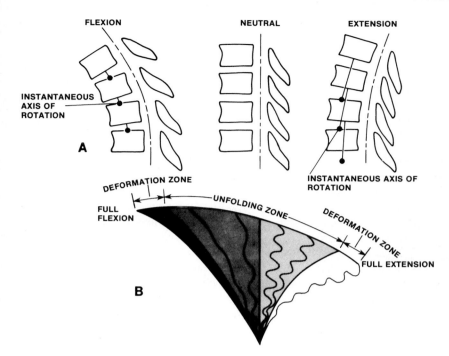

FIG. 6.2. The spinal canal and cord in flexion and extension. **A:** In flexion, the length of the spinal canal increases as compared with that in the neutral position. In extension, the length of the spinal canal decreases. This phenomenon is due to the location of the instantaneous axis of rotation, anterior to the spinal canal. **B:** The spinal cord is required to follow the changes in length and the spinal canal during physiologic motion. This occurs through the mechanisms of unfolding and folding and through elastic deformation of the spinal cord.

combination of reduced transverse dimensions of the canal with increased transverse dimensions of the spinal cord increases the risk for myelopathy from direct repetitive trauma.

Ischemia is another important factor in the development of nonacute injury of the cord. Breig and associates (41) have supported the hypothesis that deformation of the cord in the transverse plane produces selective vessel occlusion as a result of the cord's vascular anatomy. The vessels of the spinal cord are normally able to compensate for deformations during physiologic kinematics. The subarachnoid longitudinal arteries supplying the posterior cord run on the posterior surface on a zigzag course, so they can compensate for the elongation that occurs during cervical spine flexion or anterior compression. The arteries supplying the anterior columns run in an anteroposterior direction, so they relax under anterior cord compression and circulation is not restricted. In contrast, the transverse penetrating vessels arising from the anterior sulcal artery are elongated and occluded as the cord flattens and stretches in the lateral dimension under anteroposterior compression. The resulting ischemia produced by this mechanism affects mainly the medial aspect of the dorsal columns and the lateral corticospinal tracts. Tethering from the dentate ligaments and the cervical roots may affect the vascularity of the cord even more.

Nerve root injury occurs mostly around the intervertebral foramina and can be static or dynamic. Stenosis of the foramina may be the consequence of an intervertebral disc herniation resulting in disc collapse and posterolateral protrusion (42,43) and hypertrophy of the facet joints (44) and the uncinate processes (43). The dimensions of the neural foramina are significantly reduced during extension and ipsilateral bending of the cervical spine, and are increased during flexion and contralateral bending (45,46). The Spurling maneuver is an example of a clinical provocative maneuver that has the intention of reproducing the symptoms of an irritated root by reducing the size of the foramen. The beneficial effect of therapeutic traction under neck flexion is also easily explained in a similar manner (47).

SURGERY FOR NONACUTE TRAUMA

Surgical options in treating nonacute trauma of the cervical spine fall into two main groups: decompression and stabilization. Decompression is indicated when the pathologic changes provoke neurologic deficits. Compression may occur from osteophytes, tumor, and soft tissue such as disc material, ligamentum flavum, hypertrophied joint capsules, inflammatory pannus, tumor mass, hematoma, or abscess. The amount of spinal cord transverse area compression was found to be related to the severity of myelopathy and the outcome after surgical intervention. In animal studies, a compression of the cord over 50% was unlikely to recover after decompression (48). In clinical studies, functional recovery of myelopathic patients after decompression was favorable when the transverse area was greater than 30 mm² and poor if it was less (37,49).

In deciding the appropriate operative approach, the surgeon should consider the site of cord compression and the sagittal alignment of the cervical spine. In patients with normal lordosis, the preferred approach can be either anterior or posterior depending on the site and extent of neural compression. The benefits of the posterior approach are fewer airway complications, less dysphagia and dysphonia, preservation of segmental mobility, and a greater possibility for multilevel decompression. However, the posterior decompression has been linked with increased incidence of kyphotic deformity. A laminectomy with 25% bilateral facetectomies has been shown in clinical studies to induce kyphosis (50–55). Several authors studied the effects of progressive posterior element resection in the stability of the cervical spine in vitro (56–59). Facetectomy of more than 50% caused a statistically significant loss of stability in flexion and torsion. A similar study (58) found that a 50% resection of the facet capsule caused a significant loss of stability. During a posterior approach the neck muscles can be injured. Semispinalis cervicis and capitis muscles are important extensors of the neck and head (16). Although there are no data to document an increased risk of kyphosis with detachment of these muscles, most surgeons prefer to maintain their insertion into the process of C2 when performing a cervical laminectomy. An anterior procedure in patients who have lost the normal cervical lordosis allows the surgeon to address both the deformity as well as the point of compression. An anterior decompression requires fusion, which restricts the mobility of the cervical spine and increases the stresses experienced by the adjacent segments.

Stabilization or arthrodesis of the cervical spine is indicated in the case of primary instability as well as after decompressive procedures. The direction of instability may help dictate the most biomechanically sound method for instrumentation. Posterior ligamentous or bony insufficiency causes an anterior displacement of the instantaneous axis of rotation with a resulting loss of flexural stability. Applying a posterior instrumentation in this situation will stabilize the spine better than an anterior system because it will have a longer moment arm about the anteriorly displaced instantaneous axis of rotation (IAR). In a similar manner, instability in extension caused by anterior insufficiency will create a posterior displacement of the IAR that will better be countered by anterior instrumentation. Understanding the biomechanics of a particular fixation technique is crucial in preventing complications such as implant loosening or failure, loss of alignment, and pseudarthrosis.

Early postoperative implant instability and loosening is usually the result of osteopenic bone or inappropriate instrumentation technique. Bone mineral density is related to screw pull-out strength (60). In clinical studies, implant loosening was more frequent in older patients (61). Anterior fixation systems are generally divided into constrained and nonconstrained systems. Constrained systems anchor the screw to the plate, creating a fixed-angle device that requires unicortical screw fixation. Nonconstrained systems allow for toggling of the screw, and bicortical insertion into the vertebral body is recommended. Biomechanical studies have shown that the constrained constructs are more stiff than the nonconstrained systems initially (62) and after cycling (63). Nonconstrained systems continue to offer good stability in extension after fatigue cycling (64), but they fail in flexion; thus, graft absorption and settling result in failure with a kyphotic deformity.

The length of the anterior plate (61) and the levels of fusion have also been related to an increased incidence of early failure (61,65,66). An oversized plate impinging on the lower healthy disc is usually a source of pain and may require a reoperation for removal (67). Insertion of a screw into the adjacent uninvolved disc is a reason for early loosening (66,68) and should be revised. It is recommended that the caudal screws not be inserted closer than 2 mm to the vertebral end plate (68). Long fibula grafts for multilevel corpectomies stabilized with an anterior buttress plate have a high risk for early implant failure and graft dislodgment (69). Posterior wiring alone with anterior strut graft had a 14% extrusion rate, compared with 0% when utilizing anterior instrumentation as well (70). Circumferential instrumentation after multilevel corpectomies is the most rigid construct biomechanically (71); no graft dislodgment was reported in clinical studies using this technique, but adjacent segment degeneration was a concern (72,73). Posterior lateral mass screw loosening is rare, with a reported incidence of 2.3% to 11.3% (72,74–76). Biomechanical studies have shown that the Magerl technique of screw insertion is stiffer than the Roy-Camille technique (77). The inferior screws of the plate have twice the stiffness of the superior screws (77), and pull-out is more likely to occur superiorly. The clinical significance of a loose lateral mass screw is minor, which is reflected in the low reoperation rate for that reason reported in clinical studies (74,75,77) .

Pseudarthrosis is a common late complication of fusion procedures in the cervical spine. Revision is indicated because of pain, deformity, and neurologic dysfunction. Pseudarthrosis after anterior arthrodesis has been reported to have an incidence of 0% to 29% (61,78–82). Pseudarthrosis is more common (7% to 37%) in noninstrumented arthrodesis (32) than after instrumented procedures (0% to 18%) (67,79,82). In an extensive review of nonautologous interbody fusion materials, Wigfield and Nelson (83) concluded that there is little clinical evidence to justify their general use, whereas others support their use with internal fixation. Pseudarthrosis after posterior plating is rare, and reported fusion rates are between 93% and 100% (40,74–76,84,85). Traditional posterior wiring techniques of the lower cervical spine have a high reported incidence of fusion (98% to 100%), even in revision surgery (86,87). Upper cervical spine pseudarthrosis is more frequent, with a reported incidence between 2.4% and 50% (88). Occipitocervical arthrodesis success rates on the upper ranges vary from 85% to 96% (89–92). If reoperation is decided upon for treating an occipitocervical pseudarthrosis, then plates stabilized with occipital and transarticular screws represent the stiffer construct with the higher chance for fusion (90,93,94). Occipital screws can be inserted unicortically in the midline of the occiput, thus avoiding potential neurologic complications (95).

Reoperation for the treatment of failed instrumented anterior fusion has been proposed with only an anterior approach (96–99), only a posterior approach (86,96,98), or a combined anterior and posterior approach. Fusion rates after anterior revision are reported to range from 45% to 100% (96,97,99,100). Fusion rates after posterior revision surgery are reported to be from 72% to 100% (86,96,100). Combined anterior and posterior instrumentation has the greatest stiffness in biomechanical studies and the best fusion results (100). Loose implants, severe kyphotic deformity with myelopathy, and adjacent segment anterior pathology require anterior or combined anteroposterior revisions (100).

Adjacent segment degeneration following single-level fusion has been reported in 25% of patients after 10 years (101). Long and stiffer constructs such as circumferential fusion have an increased risk of stress concentration in the uninvolved segment that can lead to premature degeneration (100). Degeneration is common after occipitocervical plating, especially in the rheumatoid patient (94). Adjacent segment degeneration that is symptomatic can be treated with extension of the previous fusion. Anterior pathology requires an anterior approach.

CONCLUSION

Nonacute trauma in the cervical spine can produce regional painful syndromes or symptoms from neural compression. A variety of disorders affect the cervical spine and produce chronic injury that manifests as instability or deformity. Surgical options fall into two categories: decompression and stabilization. The ability of the surgeon to decide when to operate, which level or levels to address, and the surgical approach to use depends on a sound understanding of the normal biomechanics and the pathomechanics of each disease process.

REFERENCES

1. Holmes A, Han ZH, Dang GT, et al. Changes in cervical canal spinal volume during *in vitro* flexion-extension. *Spine* 1996;21:1313–1319.
2. Panjabi MM, Crisco JJ, Vasavada A, et al. Mechanical properties of the human spine as shown by three-dimensional load-displacement curves. *Spine* 2001;26:2692–2700.
3. Panjabi MM, Dvorak J, Sandler A, et al. Cervical spine kinematics and clinical instability. In: The Cervical Spine Research Society, eds. *The cervical spine*, 3rd ed. Philadelphia: Lippincott–Raven, 1998.
4. Moroney SP, Schultz AB, Miller JAA, et al. Load-displacement properties of lower cervical spine motion segments. *J Biomech* 1988; 21(9):767.
5. Allen BL, Ferguson RL, Lehmann TR, et al. A mechanistic classification of closed, indirect fractures and dislocations of the lower cervical spine. *Spine* 1982;7:1–27.
6. Reiter MF, Boden SD. Inflammatory disorders of the cervical spine. *Spine* 1998;23:2755–2766.
7. Dvorak J, Panjabi MM, Gerber M, et al. CT—functional diagnostics of the rotatory instability of the upper cervical spine. *Spine* 1987;12:726–730.
8. Penning L. Normal movement of the cervical spine. *Am J Roentgenol* 1978;130:317–326.
9. Panjabi MM, Summers DJ, Pelker RR, et al. Three-dimensional load displacement curves of the cervical spine. *J Orthop Res* 1986;4: 152–155.
10. Vasavada AN, Li S, Delp SL. Three-dimensional isometric strength of neck muscles in humans. *Spine* 2001;26:1904–1908.
11. Mäkelä M, Heliovaara M, Sievers K, et al. Prevalence, determinants and consequences of chronic neck pain in Finland. *Am J Epidemiol* 1991;34:1356–1367.
12. Panjabi MM. Lumbar spine instability: a biomechanical challenge. *Curr Orthop* 1994;8:100–105.
13. Panjabi MM. The stabilizing system of the spine. II. Neutral zone and instability hypothesis. *J Spinal Disord* 1992;4:390–396.
14. Katsumi Y, Honma T, Nakamura T. Analysis of cervical instability resulting from laminectomies for removal of spinal cord tumor. *Spine* 1989;14:1172–1176.
15. Lonstein JE. Post-laminectomy kyphosis. *Clin Orthop* 1977;128:93–100.
16. Pal GP, Sherk HH. The vertical stability of the cervical spine. *Spine* 1988;13:447–449.
17. Raynor RB, Moskovich T, Zidel P, et al. Alterations in primary and coupled neck motions after facetectomy. *Neurosurgery* 1987; 21:681–687.
18. Raynor RB, Pugh J, Shapiro I. Cervical facetectomy and its effect on spine strength. *J Neurosurg* 1985;63:278–282.
19. Mikaw Y, Shikata J, Tamamuro T. Spinal deformity and instability after multilevel cervical laminectomy. *Spine* 1987;12:6–11.
20. Sim FH, Suien HJ, Bickel WH, et al. Swan-neck deformity following extensive cervical laminectomy: a review of twenty-one cases. *J Bone Joint Surg Am* 1974;56:564–580.
21. Bell DF, Walker JL, O'Connor G, et al. Spinal deformity after multiple-level cervical laminectomy in children. *Spine* 1994;4: 406–411.
22. Yasouka S, Peterson HA, Laws ER, et al. Pathogenesis and prophylaxis of postlaminectomy deformity of the spine after multiple level laminectomy: difference between children and adults. *Neurosurgery* 1985;9:145–152.
23. Babic-Naglic D, Nesec-Madavic V, Potocki K, et al. Early diagnosis of rheumatoid cervical myelopathy. *Scand J Rheumatol* 1997; 26:247–252.
24. Clark CR, Goetz DD, Menezes AH. Arthrodesis of the cervical spine in rheumatoid arthritis. *J Bone Joint Surg Am* 1989;71:381–392.
25. Norizono Y, Sakou T, Kawaida H. Upper cervical involvement in rheumatoid arthritis. *Spine* 1987;12:721–725.
26. Mitz S, Schluter T, Putz R, et al. Fibrocartilage in the transverse ligament of the human atlas. *Spine* 2001;26:1765–1771.
27. Puttlitz CM, Goel VK, Clark CR, et al. Biomechanical rationale for the pathology of rheumatoid arthritis in the craniovertebral junction. *Spine* 2000;25:1607–1616.
28. Enneking WF. A system of staging musculoskeletal neoplasms. *Clin Orthop* 1986;204:9–24.
29. Tomita K, Kawahara N, Kobayashi T, et al. Surgical strategy for spinal metastases. *Spine* 2001;26:298–306.
30. Ogino H, Tada K, Okada K, et al. Canal diameter, anteroposterior compression ratio, and spondylotic myelopathy of the cervical spine. *Spine* 1983;8:1–15.
31. Debois V, Herz R, Berghmans D, et al. Soft cervical disc herniations. Influence of cervical canal measurements on development of neurological symptoms. *Spine* 1999;24:1996–2002.
32. Burrows EH. The sagittal diameter of the spinal canal in cervical spondylosis. *Clin Radiol* 1963;14:77–86.
33. Hayashi H, Okada K, Hamada M, et al. Etiologic factors of myelopathy. A radiographic evaluation of the aging changes in the cervical spine. *Clin Orthop* 1987;214:200–209.
34. Lee HM, Kim NH, Kim HJ, et al. Mid-sagittal canal diameter and vertebral body/canal ratio of the cervical spine in Koreans. *Yonsei Med J* 1994;35:446–452.
35. Payne EE, Spitlani JD. An anatomicopathologic study of 70 specimens (using a special technique) with particular reference to the problem of cervical spondylosis. *Brain* 1957;80:571–596.
36. Edwards WC, LaRocca H. The developmental segmental diameter of the cervical spinal canal in patients with cervical spondylosis. *Spine* 1983;8:20–27.
37. Fujiwara K, Yonenobu K, Ebara S, et al. The prognosis of surgery for cervical compression myelopathy. An analysis of the factors involved. *J Bone Joint Surg Br* 1989;71:393–398.
38. Parke WW. Correlative anatomy of cervical spondylotic myelopathy. *Spine* 1988;13:831–837.
39. Pavlov H, Torg JS, Robie B, et al. Cervical spinal stenosis: determination with vertebra body ratio method. *Radiology* 1987;164:771–775.
40. Graham AW, Swank ML, Kinard RE, et al. Posterior cervical arthrodesis and stabilization with a lateral mass plate. Clinical and computed tomographic evaluation of lateral mass screw placement and associated complications. *Spine* 1996;21:323–328.

41. Breig A, Turnbull I, Hassler O. Effects of mechanical stresses on the spinal cord in cervical spondylosis: a study on fresh cadaver material. *J Neurosurg* 1966;25:45–56.

42. Lu J, Ebraheim NA, Huntoon M, et al. Cervical intervertebral disc space narrowing and size of intervertebral foramina. *Clin Orthop* 2000;370:259–264.

43. Giles LG. Mechanisms of neurovascular compression within the spinal and intervertebral canals. *J Manipulative Physiol Ther* 2000;23:107–111.

44. Levine MJ, Albert TJ, Smith MD. Cervical radiculopathy: diagnosis and non operative management. *J Am Acad Orthop Surg* 1996;4:305–316.

45. Nuckley DJ, Konodi MA, Raynak GC, et al. Neural space integrity of the lower cervical spine. *Spine* 2002;27:587–595.

46. Yoo JU, Zou D, Edwards WT, et al. Effect of cervical spine motion on the neuroforaminal dimensions of human cervical spine. *Spine* 1992;17:1131–1136.

47. Humphreys SC, Chase J, Patwardhan A, et al. Flexion and traction effect on C5-C6 foraminal space. *Arch Phys Med Rehabil* 1998;79:1105–1109.

48. Kearney PA, Ridella SA, Viano DC, et al. Interaction of contact velocity and cord compression in determining the severity of spinal cord injury. *J Neurotrauma* 1988;5:187–208.

49. Penning L, Wilmink JT, van Woerden HH, et al. CT myelographic findings in degenerative disorders of the cervical spine: clinical significance. *Am J Roentgenol* 1986;146:793–801.

50. Callahan RA, Johnson RM, Margolis RN, et al. Cervical facet fusion for control of instability following laminectomy. *J Bone Joint Surg Am* 1977;59:991–1002.

51. Epstein JA. The surgical management of cervical spinal stenosis, spondylosis, and myeloradiculopathy by means of the posterior approach. *Spine* 1988;13:864–869.

52. Fager CA. Results of adequate posterior decompression in relief of spondylotic cervical myelopathy. *J Neurosurg* 1973;8:684–692.

53. Herkowitz HN. A comparison of anterior cervical fusion, cervical laminectomy, and cervical laminoplasty for the surgical management of multiple level spondylitic radiculopathy. *Spine* 1988;13:774–780.

54. Mayfield FH. Cervical spondylosis: a comparison of the anterior and posterior approaches. *Clin Neurosurg* 1965;13:181–188.

55. Nowinski GP, Visarious H, Nolte LP, et al. A biomechanical comparison of cervical laminoplasty and cervical laminectomy with progressive facetectomy. *Spine* 1993;18:1995–2004.

56. Cusick JF, Yoganandan N, Pintar F, et al. Biomechanics of cervical spine facetectomy and fixation techniques. *Spine* 1988;13:808–812.

57. White AA, Panjabi MM. Biomechanic considerations in the surgical management of cervical spondylitic myelopathy. *Spine* 1988;13:856–860.

58. Zdeblick TA, Abitbol JJ, Kunz DN, et al. Cervical stability after sequential capsule resection. *Spine* 1993;18:2005–2008.

59. Zdeblick TA, Zou D, Warden KE, et al. Cervical stability after foraminotomy: a biomechanical *in vitro* analysis. *J Bone Joint Surg Am* 1992;74:22–27.

60. Ryken TC, Clausen JD, Traynelis VC, et al. Biomechanical analysis of bone mineral density, insertion technique, screw torque, and holding strength of anterior cervical plate screws. *J Neurosurg* 1995;83:325–329.

61. Majd ME, Vadhva M, Holt RT. Anterior cervical reconstruction using titanium cages with anterior plating. *Spine* 1999;24:1604–1610.

62. Grubb MR, Currier BL, Shih JS, et al. Biomechanical evaluation of anterior cervical spine stabilization. *Spine* 1998;23:886–892.

63. Spivak JM, Chen D, Kummer FJ. The effect of locking fixation screws on the stability of anterior cervical plating. *Spine* 1999;24:334–338.

64. Clausen JD, Ryken TC, Traynelis VC, et al. Biomechanical evaluation of Caspar and cervical spine locking plate systems in a cadaveric model. *J Neurosurg* 1996;84:1039–1045.

65. Shapiro SA, Snyder W. Spinal instrumentation with a low complication rate. *Surg Neurol* 1997;48:566–574.

66. Vaccaro AR, Balderston RA. Anterior plate instrumentation for disorders of the subaxial cervical spine. *Clin Orthop* 1997;335:112–121.

67. Geisler FH, Caspar W, Pitzen T, et al. Reoperation in patients after anterior cervical plate stabilization in degenerative disease. *Spine* 1998;23:911–920.

68. Ripa DR, Kowall MG, Meyer PR, et al. Series of ninety-two traumatic cervical spine injuries stabilized with anterior ASIF plate fusion technique. *Spine* 1991;16:S46–S55.

69. Riew KD, Sethi NS, Devney J, et al. Complications of buttress plate stabilization of cervical corpectomy. *Spine* 1999;24:2404–2410.

70. Epstein NE. The value of anterior cervical plating in preventing vertebral fracture and graft extrusion after multilevel anterior cervical corpectomy with posterior wiring and fusion: indications, results, and complications. *J Spinal Disord* 2000;13:9–15.

71. Panjabi MM, Isomi T, Wang JL. Loosening at the screw-vertebra junction in multilevel anterior cervical plate constructs. *Spine* 1999;24:2383–2388.

72. Swank ML, Sutterlin CE, Bossons CR, et al. Rigid internal fixation with lateral mass plates in multilevel anterior and posterior reconstruction of the cervical spine. *Spine* 1997;22:274–282.

73. Vanichkachorn JS, Vaccaro AR, Silveri CP, et al. Anterior junctional plate in the cervical spine. *Spine* 1998;23:2462–2467.

74. Fehlings MG, Cooper PR, Errico TJ. Posterior plates in the management of cervical instability: long-term results in 44 patients. *J Neurosurg* 1994;81:341–349.

75. Heller JG, Silcox DH, Sutterlin CE. Complications of posterior cervical plating. *Spine* 1995;20:2442–2448.

76. Wellman BJ, Follett KA, Traynelis VC. Complications of posterior articular mass plate fixation of the subaxial cervical spine in 43 consecutive patients. *Spine* 1998;23:193–200.

77. Choueka J, Spivak JM, Kummer FJ, et al. Flexion failure of posterior cervical lateral mass screws. Influence of insertion technique and position. *Spine* 1996;21:462–468.

78. Eleraky MA, Llanos C, Sonntag VKH. Cervical corpectomy: report of 185 cases and review of the literature. *J Neurosurg* 1999;90(Suppl 1):35–41.

79. Geer CP, Papadopoulos SM. The argument for single-level anterior cervical discectomy and fusion with anterior plate fixation. *Clin Neurosurg* 1999;45:25–29.

80. Lowery GL, McDonough RF. The significance of hardware failure in anterior cervical plate fixation. *Spine* 1998;23:181–186.

81. Tuite GF, Papadopoulos SM, Sonntag VK. Caspar plate fixation for the treatment of complex hangman's fractures. *Neurosurgery* 1992;30:761–764.

82. Wang JC, McDonough PW, Kanim LE, et al. Increased fusion rates with cervical plating for three-level anterior cervical discectomy and fusion. *Spine* 2001;26:643–646.

83. Wigfield CC, Nelson RJ. Nonautologous interbody fusion materials in cervical spine surgery: how strong is the evidence to justify their use? *Spine* 2001;26:687–694.

84. Cooper PR, Cohen A, Rosiello A, et al. Posterior stabilization of cervical spine fractures and subluxations using plates and screws. *Neurosurgery* 1988;23:300–306.

85. Nazarian SM, Louis RP. Posterior internal fixation with screw plates in traumatic lesions of the cervical spine. *Spine* 1991;16:S64–S71.

86. Farey ID, McAfee PC, Davis RF, et al. Pseudarthrosis of the cervical spine after anterior arthrodesis. *J Bone Joint Surg Am* 1990;72:1171–1177.

87. Weiland DJ, McAfee PC. Posterior cervical fusion with triple wire strut graft technique: one hundred consecutive patients. *J Spinal Disord* 1991;4:15–21.

88. Smith MD, Phillips WA, Hensinger RN. Complications of fusion to the upper cervical spine. *Spine* 1991;16:702–705.

89. Fehlings MG, Errico T, Cooper P, et al. Occipitocervical fusion with a five millimeter malleable rod and segmental fixation. *Neurosurgery* 1993;32:198–207.

90. Grob D. Application of the occipitocervical plate for occipitocervical and atlantoaxial pathology. In: Fessler RG, Haid RW, eds. *Current techniques in spinal instrumentation.* New York: McGraw-Hill, 1996.

91. McAfee PC, Cassidy JR, Davis RF, et al. Fusion of the occiput to the upper cervical spine. *Spine* 1991;16(Suppl):S490–S494.

92. Mori T, Matsunaga S, Sunahara N, et al. 3 to 11 year follow up of occipitocervical fusion for rheumatoid arthritis. *Clin Orthop* 1998;169–179.

93. Abumi K, Takada T, Shono Y, et al. Posterior occipitocervical reconstruction using cervical pedicle screws and plate-rod systems. *Spine* 1999;24:1425–1434.

94. Huckell CB, Buchowski JM, Richardson WJ, et al. Functional outcome of plate fusions for disorders of the occipitocervical junction. *Clin Orthop* 1999;136–145.

95. Ebraheim NA, Lu J, Biyani A, et al. An anatomic study of the thickness of the occipital bone. Implications for occipitocervical instrumentation. *Spine* 1996;21:1725–1729.

96. Brodsky AE, Khalil MA, Sassard WR, et al. Repair of symptomatic pseudarthrosis of anterior cervical fusion. *Spine* 1992;17: 1137–1143.

97. Coric D, Branch CL, Jenkins JD. Revision of anterior cervical pseudoarthrosis with anterior allograft fusion and plating. *J Neurosurg* 1997;86:969–974.

98. Newmann M. The outcome of pseudarthrosis after cervical anterior fusion. *Spine* 1993;18:2380–2382.

99. Tribus CB, Corteen DP, Zdeblick TA. The efficacy of anterior cervical plating in the management of symptomatic pseudoarthrosis of the cervical spine. *Spine* 1999;24:860–864.

100. Lowery GL, Swank ML, McDonough RF. Surgical revision for failed anterior cervical fusions: articular pillar plating or anterior revision? *Spine* 1995;20:2436–2441.

101. Bohlman HH, Emery LE, Goodfellow DB, et al. Robinson anterior cervical diskectomy and arthrodesis for cervical radiculopathy: long term follow-up of one hundred and twenty two patients. *J Bone Joint Surg Am* 1993;75:1298–1307.

CHAPTER 7

Cervical Orthoses and Cranioskeletal Traction

D. Greg Anderson, Alexander R. Vaccaro, and Kenneth F. Gavin

Cervical spinal orthoses are externally applied devices designed to restrict motion of the spinal column. Forces are indirectly applied to the spine by contacting the soft tissue envelope of the head, neck, and chest. Modern cervical orthoses can be divided into two categories: cervical orthoses and cervicothoracic orthoses. Cervical orthoses contact the head and neck region, whereas cervicothoracic orthoses extend onto the upper chest. Cervical orthoses are generally useful in the treatment of cervical trauma, pain, and instability and in providing postoperative spinal protection (1).

The earliest documented use of cervical orthoses for restricting neck motion and correcting deformities comes from the fifth Egyptian dynasty (2750–2625 BC) (2). The biomechanical principles of modern cervical orthoses can be traced to the devices used by Hippocrates and his successors (2). Today a wide variety of cervical orthoses are available. These devices are often named for their inventors (e.g., Benjamin-Taylor, Thomas, Guilford), the locality where they were designed (e.g., Philadelphia, Yale, Newport, Malibu, Miami) or by a description of the brace (e.g., four-poster, two-poster, sternooccipital mandibular immobilizer).

Cervical orthoses may be prescribed by specifying the specific type of orthosis (e.g., Philadelphia collar) or by specifying the orthosis category (e.g., cervical collar). It is important for the prescribing physician to understand the biomechanical principles of orthosis usage and to communicate to the fitting orthotist the degree and type of instability that is anticipated. Equally important is patient education in the donning, care, and use of the prescribed orthosis and close follow-up.

Advances in materials science and engineering have revolutionized the bracing industry in recent years. Thermoplastic braces are lightweight, relatively comfortable, and durable. Materials that are compatible with magnetic resonance imaging (MRI), such as graphite and titanium, are now commonly used to fabricate halo vest orthoses. Synthetic brace liners such as Ortho-Wick increase patient comfort and compliance. In spite of the advances in orthosis design, many newer braces remain unproven in a clinical setting. Therefore, it is important to thoroughly evaluate an orthosis prior to using the device.

The comfort and motion-restricting properties of cervical orthoses vary widely. When choosing an orthosis for a given condition, the degree and direction of potential instability must be considered along with the level of compliance that is required. Although studies have documented the level of motion restriction of many cervical orthoses in normal spines, the ability of braces to restrict motion in unstable spines has not been well studied. This chapter reviews the biomechanical and clinical features of the commonly used cervical orthoses and discusses the appropriate application of cervical bracing in a clinical setting.

CERVICAL BIOMECHANICS

Although cervical motion has been described in bioengineering terms as having six degrees of freedom (translation and rotation in the x-, y-, and z-planes), clinical cervical motion is usually broken down into flexion-extension, lateral bending, and rotation (3). Cervical range of motion depends on flexibility of the discs, shape and inclination of the facets, ligamentous laxity, and integrity of capsular structures. Kottke and Mundle (4) evaluated cervical motion in a normal population and reported the following averages: flexion, 70 degrees ± 10 degrees; lateral bending in each direction, 45 degrees ± 10 degrees; and axial rotation in each direction, 75 degrees ± 10 degrees. Similar values were reported by Perry and Nickel (5), who described the normal arc of cervical motion to be 145 degrees of flexion-extension, 180 degrees of axial rotation, and 90 degrees of lateral flexion.

Bhalla and Simmons (6) reported that the C4-C5 articulation demonstrated the greatest range of motion, whereas Kottke and Mundle (4) recorded the most mobility at C5-C6. Using cineradiography, Fielding (7) noted that flexion caused a slight anterior translation of the upper cervical vertebral bodies, whereas extension resulted in posterior translation.

SPINAL MOBILITY IN CERVICAL ORTHOTICS

Jones (8) was the first investigator of whom we are aware to report his observations of cervical motion in subjects wearing cervical orthoses. In 1960, he used cineradiography to qualitatively examine the motion of normal subjects wearing soft and rigid collars. Although specific measurements were not made, he concluded that rigid collars restricted motion more than soft collars, but noted that all the collars tested allowed substantial motion of the cervical spine.

A number of studies have attempted to measure cervical motion while wearing various orthotics. Both goniometry (9–12) and radiography (7–9,13–15) have been used to measure cervical motion in normal subjects, cadavers, and mannequins. Fisher and colleagues (9) measured cervical motion using both goniometry and radiography and concluded that goniometry provided an adequate clinical tool to assess the overall motion of the cervical spine in the sagittal plane. Motion control in most cervical orthoses is better for flexion-extension than for lateral bending and axial rotation (3,9,10,14,16,17).

The Camp collar, Philadelphia collar, four-poster brace, and the sternooccipital mandibular immobilizer (SOMI) brace were evaluated by Fisher and associates (9), who studied the cervical motion of ten normal subjects using lateral radiographs. The SOMI brace provided the best restriction to flexion of the upper cervical spine. The four-poster brace provided the best immobilization of the middle and lower cervical spine. Although the Philadelphia collar was rated as most comfortable, it was the least effective at immobilizing all levels, especially the occiput to C2 region. The Camp collar provided the best immobilization of the C1 to C2 region but was noted to be extremely uncomfortable (9,18).

The soft collar, Philadelphia collar, four-poster brace, cervicothoracic brace, and SOMI brace were evaluated in normal volunteers by Johnson and associates (17) using radiography and photographs. In addition, the halo vest orthosis was evaluated in patients following cervical surgery or cervical trauma. The order of stability for flexion-extension (most to least stable) was as follows: halo, cervicothoracic brace, four-poster brace, SOMI and Philadelphia collar (equal), and soft collar. Only the halo orthoses controlled sagittal plane motion (flexion-extension) of the occiput through C2 region. Overall, the halo orthosis provided the best immobilization of all cervical levels. The SOMI orthosis effectively limited C1-C2 flexion (but not extension) and thus was recommended for isolated atlantoaxial flexion instability. Of interest, motion between the occiput and C1 was noted to be increased by the use of a cervical collar.

Kaufman and coworkers (10) measured cervical motion in ten normal subjects wearing the Philadelphia collar, Nec Loc collar, and the soft collar. The Nec Loc collar was the most effective, limiting flexion-extension by 62%, lateral bending by 43%, and axial rotation by 62%. In contrast, the Philadelphia collar limited flexion-extension by 46%, lateral flexion by 25%, and axial rotation by 29%.

In a similar study, Beavis (16) measured cervical motion in normal subjects wearing a soft collar, hard collar, Plastazote collar, and a custom-fit collar. Motion was restricted most by the Plastazote collar, followed by the custom collar and hard collar. The soft collars provided minimal motion restriction.

Podolsky and colleagues (13) evaluated methods of cervical immobilization during trauma extrication and transport. The soft collar, hard collar, Philadelphia collar, extrication collar, bilateral sandbags with tape, and Philadelphia collar combined with sandbags and tape were tested in normal volunteers. Sandbags and tape provided excellent motion restriction except in extension. The addition of the Philadelphia collar helped to further limit extension when combined with sandbags and tape.

Lunsford and coworkers (11) measured cervical motion and skin contact pressure in ten normal subjects wearing the Philadelphia collar, Miami J collar, Malibu collar, and Newport Extended Wear collar (now called the Aspen collar). The Malibu collar provided the best immobilization, restricting lateral bending by 41%, extension by 40%, flexion by 57%, and axial rotation by 61%.

Koch and Nickel (19) evaluated cervical spine mobility in the halo orthosis. Lateral radiographs in various positions were taken of six patients treated in a halo cast for unstable cervical injuries. In addition, compression and traction forces were measured through the upright connectors attaching the halo ring to the cast. So-called snaking of the cervical vertebrae was noted, with some spinal segments assuming a flexed posture and other regions assuming an extended posture. C4-C5 experienced the greatest mobility, which averaged 7.2 degrees. C2-C3 had the highest percentage of normal motion (42% of normal motion). Forces measured at the halo uprights varied widely, from 5 pounds compression to 17 pounds traction. These forces were noted to change dramatically with changes in position or when patients abducted their arms. Neck distraction changed by an average of 3.6 mm with changes in position.

Anderson and associates (20) measured cervical motion using radiographs in 42 patients immobilized in a halo vest for injuries of the cervical spine. Lateral radiographs were taken in a supine and upright position within 5 days of injury. Noninjured levels demonstrated an average 3.9 degrees of angulation, with the greatest motion occurring between the occiput and C1 (8.0 degrees). Injured levels demonstrated an average sagittal plane angulation of 7.0 degrees and translation of 1.7 mm. Fracture site motion greater than 3 degrees of angulation or 1 mm of translation was observed at 77% of the injured levels. The authors recommended obtaining lateral radiographs in both a supine and upright position when treating unstable cervical injuries in a halo so that injuries demonstrating excess motion could be detected and treated by an alternative method.

ORTHOSIS COMFORT

The external forces necessary to control motion vary from the occiput to C7 level within the cervical spine. Forces used to control the spine are applied to the surrounding soft tissues of the neck. Each patient's neck anatomy, flexibility, and soft tissue envelope will vary, thus altering orthosis fit and efficacy. Therefore, a cervical orthosis should be carefully matched to the patient's anatomy. Ideally, the contact area should be maximized to lower contact pressures. Soft or semirigid materials should be used at the sites of skin contact. When possible, so-called breathable materials should be used to minimize perspiration beneath the orthosis. Patient compliance with brace wear is highly related to level of comfort experienced while wearing the brace.

In comatose or insensate patients, skin breakdown due to elevated contact pressure beneath an orthosis remains a significant risk. The risk of skin breakdown can be decreased by trimming or shaving hair beneath the brace and maintaining good skin hygiene. Frequent inspection of skin contact areas is mandatory when using an orthosis for patients with altered sensory function.

Most patients can be successfully fitted with modern, off-the-shelf orthoses, which are available in a wide range of sizes to optimize patient fit. However, in some situations, custom fabrication of an orthosis is necessary to accommodate unusual patient anatomy. With the advent of thermoplastics, custom fabrication is usually a rapid process. In noncompliant patients or those requiring intimate control of neck motion, a plaster or fiberglass body cast may be used in conjunction with a halo ring.

Fisher (18) measured skin contact pressures and cervical motion in eight adults fitted with the SOMI brace. Skin contact pressures were noted to be well in excess of the capillary closing pressure (CCP) with the brace applied in the "usual" fashion. When the braces were refitted to keep the contact pressures at 20 mm Hg (below CCP), there was no substantial increase in the cervical range of motion noted. The authors concluded that with the use of pressure sensors, a cervical orthosis could be applied with less pressure, thus minimizing patient discomfort and lowering the risk of skin breakdown while maintaining an acceptable level of immobilization.

Plaisier and associates (12) measured craniofacial pressures and subjective comfort in 20 normal volunteers wearing the Stifneck collar, Philadelphia collar, Miami J collar, and Newport collar (now called the Aspen collar) in the upright and supine positions. The Stifneck collar exceeded CCP in both the upright and supine positions, while the Philadelphia collar exceeded CCP in the supine position. In contrast, the Newport and Miami J collars were noted to exert pressures below the CCP in both positions. The Newport and Miami J collars were rated as comfortable, whereas the Stifneck collar was rated as uncomfortable.

Unstable cervical conditions often require the use of a cervical orthosis during bathing. In this setting it is useful to provide the patient with a second cervical collar made of Plastazote material, such as the Philadelphia collar, to use during bathing.

When a rigid cervical orthosis is no longer required, weaning should be performed. Weaning is preferable to simply removing the orthosis because it allows the patient an opportunity to gradually regain normal muscle strength and proprioception and lessens the psychological fear many patients have regarding removal of brace protection. During the transition, a schedule of decreasing brace wear can be combined with the use of a soft collar and physical therapy to hasten the return of physiologic neck mobility.

SELECTED ORTHOSES

The soft cervical collar has gained popularity for treating cervical strains and so-called whiplash syndromes. Soft collars are inexpensive and comfortable but provide only minimal motion restriction (Table 7.1). Soft collars provide warmth, promote muscle relaxation, and provide a kinesthetic reminder to patients following minor cervical strains. Soft cervical collars are available in numerous sizes and are well tolerated by patients (Fig. 7.1).

The Philadelphia collar is a two-piece semirigid Plastazote orthosis reinforced with anterior and posterior plastic struts (Fig. 7.2). It is relatively inexpensive and provides better motion control than a soft collar, as detailed in Table 7.1. In addition, the Plastazote construction of the Philadelphia collar makes it a good choice for use during showering and bathing. Due to the absence of a removable liner, the Philadelphia collar is not as optimal for hygiene or comfort with long-term use as the Miami J, Aspen, and Malibu collars.

The Aspen collar (formerly the Newport collar) is a semirigid, two-piece cervical orthosis utilizing an adjustable plastic shell with removable foam pads. It is more expensive and comfortable than the Philadelphia collar and provides better motion restriction (Table 7.1). The Aspen collar includes a relief area for posterior incisions (Fig 7.3). The Aspen collar is also available with a thoracic extension to provide better control of the lower cervical spine and cervicothoracic junction (Fig. 7.4).

The Miami J collar is a similar semirigid two-piece cervical orthosis utilizing a firm plastic shell with removable foam pads (Fig. 7.5). The cost, comfort, and motion restriction are detailed in Table 7.1. The Miami J orthosis provides slightly better motion restriction than the Aspen collar but does not include an optional thoracic extension.

The Malibu brace is a semirigid two-piece orthosis utilizing a firm plastic shell with incorporated inner padding (Fig 7.6 and Table 7.1). The Malibu brace projects farther on the chest and back compared with the Miami J and Aspen collars. This improves motion restriction in the sagittal plane.

TABLE 7.1. *Comparison of Cervical Orthoses*

			Percent motion restriction			
Orthosis	Flexion	Extension	Total sagittal motion	Lateral bending (1 direction)	Axial rotation (1 direction)	Cost[a] ($)
Soft collar	26	26	10	8	17	19.00
Philadelphia collar	74	59	46	26	29	94.00
Aspen collar	59	64	62	31	38	94.00
Miami J collar	85	75	73	51	65	94.00
Malibu collar	57	40	NT	41	61	229.00
Nec Loc collar	NT	NT	62	43	62	94.00
Stifneck collar	73	63	70	50	57	94.00
SOMI	93	42	87	66	66	264.00
Minerva	NT	NT	NT	NT	NT	398.00
Halo	NT	NT	96	96	99	1,916.00

[a]Prices are based on Medicare allowables for the year 2001 (region A). NT, not tested; SOMI, sterno-occipital mandibular immobilizer.

The semirigid cervical collars described herein are similar in concept, but each has unique features that may prove useful in a particular setting. Each of these collars may be used to treat stable cervical fractures and provide postoperative protection. Our preference is to use a semirigid cervical collar with removable pads for patients requiring more than 2 to 3 weeks of immobilization. These collars provide superior comfort and allow cleaning or exchange of the pads for optimal patient hygiene. Patients are also provided with a Philadelphia collar for use during bathing.

Rigid cervical collars are routinely used during prehospital extrication and transport of accident victims. In this setting the ideal collar is inexpensive, provides rigid motion control, is compact for easy storage, and is easy to apply. The Nec Loc and Stifneck collars (Fig. 7.7) fulfill these goals and are commonly used by paramedics and ambulance personnel (Table 7.1). These collars exert relatively high skin pressures and thus should be used only on a short-term basis.

The SOMI orthosis has a rigid anterior chest piece or yoke attached anteriorly to curved, rigid shoulder supports (Fig. 7.8). Straps cross the patient's back and attach the shoulder supports to the lower section of the yoke. Mandibular and occipital supports project from the anterior yoke to control the head. During eating, an optional head piece employing a forehead strap can be used, allowing removal of the mandibular

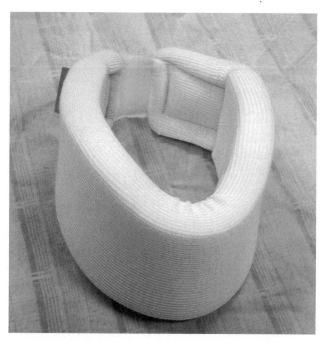

FIG. 7.1. The soft cervical collar has a foam insert housed in a cloth exterior. The collar is fastened with a Velcro strap posteriorly.

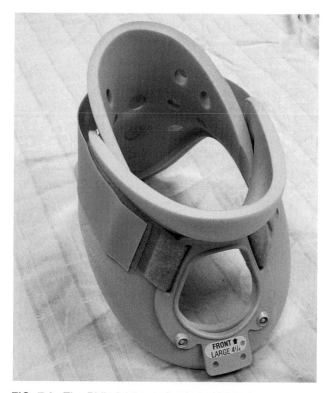

FIG. 7.2. The Philadelphia collar is available with a tracheostomy window as shown. It has a front and back portion with Velcro fasteners on each side.

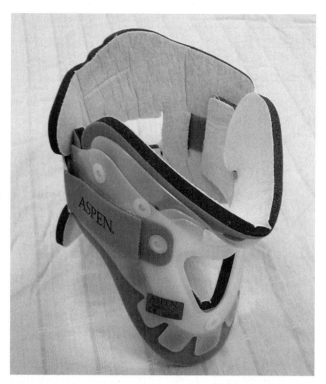

FIG. 7.3. The Aspen collar has removable padded inserts and malleable plastic tabs around the edges of the brace for comfort.

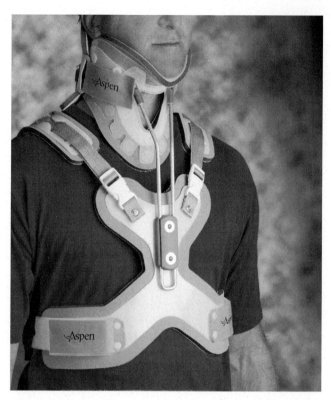

FIG. 7.4. The Aspen cervicothoracic orthosis system uses an Aspen cervical collar attached to an adjustable padded vest for better control of the cervicothoracic junction.

component. The SOMI orthosis can be easily applied to a patient in the supine position. As shown in Table 7.1, the SOMI orthosis provides good restriction to flexion, especially in the upper cervical spine, but is less optimal for control of neck extension (17).

The original Minerva brace was a molded cervicothoracic orthosis that provided fairly rigid control of middle and lower cervical motion at the expense of comfort. The modern Minerva jacket orthosis, however, incorporates a padded, plastic vest component similar to a halo vest and padded extensions to the mandibular region and posterior head, yielding a more comfortable fit (Fig. 7.9). Such a Minerva jacket orthosis was compared with the halo orthosis by Benzel and colleagues (21) in ten patients following cervical surgery or a cervical fracture. The Minerva jacket orthosis was found to allow less sagittal plane segmental motion compared with the halo at all levels except C1 to C2. This phenomenon is attributed to the so-called snaking of the cervical vertebrae within the halo, as described previously. Patients preferred the comfort of the Minerva jacket orthosis to that of the halo orthosis.

Choosing the appropriate treatment for a cervical spine injury involves consideration of a number of factors, such as injury type, severity, neurologic status, risk of displacement, patient body habitus, and patient compliance. Therefore, treatment for each cervical injury should be individualized. The most commonly recommended orthotics used to treat common cervical spine injuries are listed in Table 7.2.

Complications of Cervical Orthotics

Complications of cervical orthoses may include inadequate immobilization, skin rash or breakdown, psychological dependence, muscle atrophy, soft tissue contracture, pain, and decreased pulmonary function (22). Essentially, all cervical orthoses can be modified or adjusted to increase comfort and decrease skin pressure. In general, the risk of complications can be minimized by proper brace selection and fitting and close follow-up.

THE HALO SKELETAL FIXATOR

Perry and Nickel (5) first used the halo orthosis for immobilization of unstable cervical spines in patients with poliomyelitis. The original halo consisted of a complete metal ring that curved upward posteriorly to allow surgical access to the cervical spine. Metal pins inserted through holes in the ring pierced the outer table of the skull, providing secure fixation of the head. The ring attached to a molded body cast by two upright posts. Since its original description, the halo orthosis has been used for stabilization of trauma, tumors, infections, inflammatory conditions, surgical arthrodeses, and congenital malformations involving the cervical spine of both children and adults (1,5,23–31).

Modern halo rings are often composed of radiolucent and nonferromagnetic materials such as carbon fiber and titanium that allow radiographic and MRI studies to be performed in

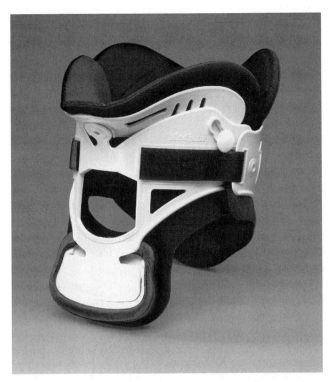

FIG. 7.5. The Miami J collar has comfortable padded inserts and an anterior extension to better control cervical flexion.

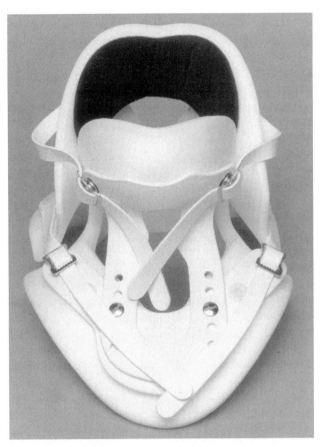

FIG. 7.6. The Malibu collar has a plastic shell with a padded interior. The front and back portion of the collar fasten with adjustable straps.

the halo device. Molded plastic body jackets with padded inserts are available in a wide range of sizes and have replaced the need for body casting in most situations (Fig. 7.10). In spite of these advances, the basic principles and halo application techniques have changed little since their original description. This section reviews the proper application of the halo orthosis and reviews complications related to halo usage.

Application of the Halo Ring

The optimal position for the anterior halo pins is in the anterolateral skull, approximately 1 cm above the orbital rim, below the greatest circumference (equator) of the skull and cephalad to the lateral two-thirds of the eyebrow. This region has been described as the "safe zone" because it lies lateral to the supraorbital and supratrochlear nerves and the frontal sinus and medial to the temporalis fossa. In addition, the halo pin is protected from displacement into the orbit by the supraorbital rim and lies on a relatively flat portion of the skull, preventing superior migration. Posterior halo pin placement is less critical due to the uniform thickness of the skull and lack of critical anatomic structures. The optimal posterior location is at the 4 o'clock and 8 o'clock positions (12 o'clock is the anterior midline), thus lying behind the ears and opposite the anterior pins. With the pins in these positions, the halo ring should lie just above the eyebrows and the upper helix of the ear (24,32). Usually, four halo pins are used for halo application in an adult. Infants younger than

2 years should be treated with six to eight halo pins. Halo pin torque in children should be reduced to 2 to 5 inch-pounds (29,31).

Garfin and colleagues (33) studied skull osteology in cadavers and noted that the anterolateral and posterolateral skull had the most optimal bone for halo pin placement. The temporal fossa, in contrast, was noted to have much thinner cortical bone and little space between the bony tables.

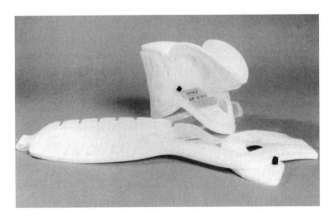

FIG. 7.7. The Stifneck collar flattens for easy storage. This one-piece orthosis is easily applied during accident extrication.

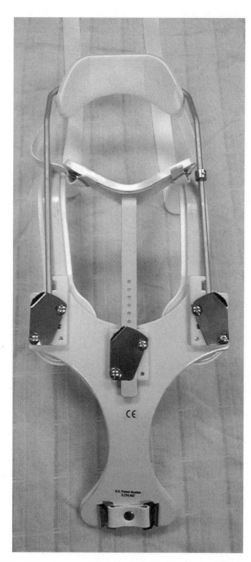

FIG. 7.8. The sternooccipital mandibular immobilizer (SOMI) orthosis has a chest yoke with adjustable chin and occipital supports.

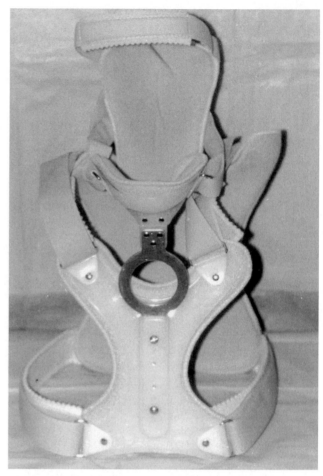

FIG. 7.9. The Minerva vest orthosis has an adjustable vest with chin and posterior head supports.

Pin placement in the temporal fossa may also tether the temporalis muscle, which can cause pain and impede mastication.

Halo pins should be inserted perpendicular to the skull (at the equator) to improve the mechanical strength of the bone–pin interface (34,35). Pin insertions up to 10 inch-pounds (1.13 newton-meters) have been shown to minimally penetrate the outer table of the skull (36). Mechanical testing of the pin–bone interface with cyclic loading and load-to-failure has shown that 8 in-lb (0.9 N-m) of torque significantly improves the mechanical quality of the bone purchase compared with 6 in-lb (0.68 N-m).

A minimum of three individuals should be used to apply a halo device. One person immobilizes the head, while the second and third persons apply the halo ring. Proper sizing of the ring and vest should be undertaken prior to starting the application process. The ring should allow 1 to 2 cm of clearance around the perimeter of the head. Vest sizes are determined by measuring the patient's chest circumference. All materials should be assembled prior to beginning halo application (Table 7.3). A resuscitation crash cart should be available during the procedure.

The patient should be placed in a supine position. Folded towels are placed under the head and shoulders to provide access for halo ring placement. Alternatively, the patient's head may be supported beyond the edge of a gurney. The head should be manually immobilized throughout the halo application process.

Hair is shaved at the posterior pin sites, and the skin is prepared with povidone-iodine solution. The halo ring is placed around the skull in the optimal location and held with positioning pins or a fourth assistant. The skin is then anesthetized with local anesthetic at the site selected for the halo pin insertion. The anesthetic should be injected to the level of the galea.

The pins should be threaded through the halo ring holes and advanced to the point of skin contact. Diagonal opposing pins should then be advanced in small (2 in-lb) increments to allow all the pins to seat evenly. The pins are tightened with a torque screwdriver to the appropriate torque (6 to 8 in-lb). Skin incisions are not required for the halo pins (37). During

TABLE 7.2. *Commonly Recommended Orthotics for Treating Cervical Spine Injuries*

Diagnosis	Orthosis
Occipitocervical dislocation and subluxation	Surgery plus halo
Fractures of the atlas	
Posterior arch	Rigid collar
Jefferson's fractures	
<7 mm displaced	Rigid collar or SOMI
>7 mm displaced	Halo
Ruptured mid-transverse ligament	Surgery
Odontoid fractures	
Type I	Rigid collar
Type II	Halo
If: >4 mm translation, >10-degree angulation,	
or >40 yr old	Consider surgery
Type III	Halo
Atlantoaxial rotatory deformities	
Reducible	Rigid collar/SOMI
Unreducible	Traction or surgery
Hangman's fracture	
Type I	Rigid collar
Type II	Rigid collar/halo
Type III	Surgery
C3 through C7 flexion-compression fractures	
Stable (intact posterior ligamentous complex)	Rigid collar/halo
Unstable	Surgery
C3 through C7 burst fractures	
Neurologically intact/stable fracture pattern	Halo/Minerva/Yale
Neurologic deficit/unstable fracture pattern	Surgery
Facet dislocations	
Unilateral	Halo, then surgery
Bilateral	Halo, then surgery
Distraction-extension injuries	
Intact ligaments/disc	
Without spinal cord compression	Halo/surgery
With spinal cord compression	Surgery
Ruptured ligaments/disc/fracture	Surgery
C3 through C7 compression-extension injuries	
No displacement	Rigid collar/Minerva/Yale
Displaced	Surgery

SOMI, sternooccipital mandibular immobilizer.

tightening of the anterior pins, the patient should be asked to close his or her eyes and relax the forehead to prevent tethering of the skin. Any area of skin tenting around the halo pins after final tightening should be released with a scalpel.

The halo vest should be applied by rolling the patient or elevating the patient's trunk while maintaining in-line traction of the cervical spine. After applying the posterior portion of the halo vest, the patient may return to a supine position. The anterior vest is secured, and then the uprights are assembled to attach the vest and halo ring. Final tightening of all components should be performed. Radiographs of the cervical spine should then be taken to confirm a satisfactory position of the spine. Halo screwdrivers and wrenches should be maintained at the patient's bedside or taped to the halo vest to be used in an emergency.

The pins should be retorqued 24 to 48 hours after the initial halo application. The pin sites should be cleaned every 1 to 2 days with a dilute solution of hydrogen peroxide. Periodic radiographic studies should be taken to ensure that an appropriate position of the cervical spine is maintained.

After halo removal, the use of a comfortable, semirigid cervical orthosis such as a Philadelphia, Aspen, or Miami J collar is recommended to allow the patient to gradually regain muscle strength and confidence. Physical therapy to improve muscle strength, proprioception, and range of motion is beneficial in restoring cervical function and lessening neck pain.

Indications for the Halo Orthosis

The halo orthosis provides the most rigid fixation of the cervical spine and therefore is indicated for injuries or

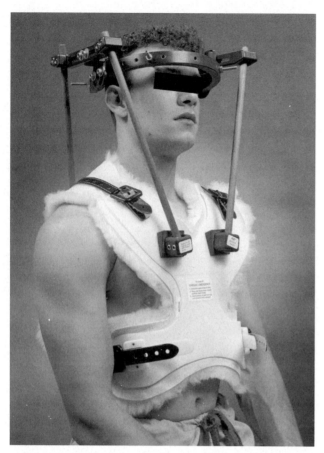

FIG. 7.10. The halo vest orthosis utilizes a rigid ring attached to the skull with pins. The vest portion attaches to the ring with adjustable rigid uprights.

TABLE 7.3. *Materials Necessary for Halo Application*

Halo ring (1–2 cm larger than head)
Sterile halo pins
Torque wrench or "breakaway" wrenches
Halo vest (sized to chest)
Upright connecting rods
Rod-to-ring connector blocks
Wrenches to tighten nuts on halo pins
Razor
Povidone-iodine solution
Sterile gloves
Sterile gauze
Syringe/needle
Local anesthetic
Crash cart

conditions where the level of instability warrants the increased discomfort and risks inherent to the halo orthosis. Cervical fractures commonly treated in a halo orthosis include C1 ring fractures, C2 hangman's fractures, C2 odontoid fractures, and subaxial compressive-flexion or burst fractures with intact posterior ligamentous structures. Facet dislocation injuries are generally associated with rupture of the posterior ligamentous structures and therefore have a high incidence of displacement or failure to heal when treated nonoperatively in a halo vest orthosis (38,39).

The halo orthosis is also useful in providing stability to postoperative constructs where an added measure of stability is required. Cooper and colleagues (26) found that the halo orthosis was a useful adjuvant to a posterior cervical fusion. In contrast, Vaccaro and associates (40) reported that the halo orthosis failed to decrease the rate of graft dislodgement in patients following three-level cervical corpectomies treated with an anterior cervical plate.

Halo Complications

Complications of halo usage include pin loosening, pin-site infections, loss of reduction, severe pin discomfort, swallowing difficulties, dural puncture, pin-site bleeding, nerve injury, severe scarring, skin breakdown under the halo vest, and intolerance by patients (41).

Pin loosening may occur during the course of halo treatment and may precipitate pain at the pin site. New-onset pain at a pin site should lead the physician to suspect pin loosening or infection. Pin loosening may be managed by retightening the pin one time. Resistance should be met within the first two complete rotations of the pin. If no resistance is met, the pin should be replaced. In this case, the new pin should be seated prior to removal of the loose pin. Rizzolo and colleagues (42) evaluated patients prospectively with halo pins torqued to 6 in-lb or 8 in-lb and found no significant difference in the rate of pin loosening or halo complications.

Pin-tract infections are relatively common in patients treated with long-term halo immobilization. If pin drainage develops, bacterial cultures should be taken and the infection should be treated with aggressive pin care and antibiotics. If the infection fails to respond or if cellulitis develops, the pin should be replaced and systemic antibiotics should be administered. The new pin should be placed through an adjacent hole in the ring, as long as it will not result in placement of the pin through an area of cellulitis. The new pin should be placed prior to removing the infected pin to prevent shift of the head within the halo ring.

Swallowing difficulties are often an indication of excessive extension of the neck. Generally, flexing the neck or translating the head anteriorly will result in resolution of the dysphagia symptoms.

Dural puncture is a potentially severe complication of halo usage and may result from a fall while wearing a halo orthosis (41). Dural puncture may lead to an intracranial abscess and should be suspected in a patient who presents with symptoms of headache, photophobia, nausea, and fever. Aggressive treatment is indicated, including head computed tomographic scanning, neurosurgical consult, appropriate debridement, and antibiotics. Dural puncture in the absence of infection should be treated with pin removal, prophylactic antibiotics, and upright positioning. If cerebrospinal fluid drainage is a continued problem, a lumbar subarachnoid drain should be considered.

Garfin and associates (43) reported five patients who developed subdural abscesses associated with halo traction. All infections resolved with removal of the pins, drainage and debridement of the abscess, and parenteral antibiotics. Due to the risk of intracranial infection, long-term halo traction was discouraged.

Pin-site bleeding may occur in patients receiving anticoagulation medication. Continued bleeding is an indication to taper or discontinue the anticoagulation therapy. Packing or dressing the pin sites has been reported to be ineffective in controlling the bleeding (24).

Other miscellaneous complications, including nerve injury, should be avoidable with proper halo application technique. Skin breakdown is minimized by applying a well-fitting vest with ample padding. In older patients with severe thoracic kyphosis or in insensate patients, skin breakdown is a potential complication; close skin monitoring should be performed.

Glaser and coworkers (39) reviewed the complications of halo vest usage in 245 patients treated for cervical spine instability following trauma (203 patients) or after surgery (45 patients). Complications included 1 death, 23 patients with loss of reduction, 24 cases of late instability, 14 pin-tract problems, 2 displacements of an anterior strut graft, 5 premature halo removals, and 7 miscellaneous problems. There were no cases of neurologic deterioration in the halo device. The authors noted that ligamentous cervical injuries had a high incidence of late instability in spite of halo treatment.

Cooper and associates (26) reviewed the use of the halo device in 33 patients with unstable cervical spine injuries, including 7 with incomplete neurologic deficits. No neurologic deterioration occurred while in the halo device. Eighty-five percent of the patients achieved a stable cervical spine with halo immobilization. Complications were primarily related to skin breakdown beneath the vest or pin site infections. The authors recommended caution when using the halo with complete spinal cord–injured patients due to the risk of skin breakdown and respiratory compromise.

Sears and Fazl (38) reviewed 173 patients with subaxial cervical injuries (with and without a neurologic deficit) treated with the halo orthosis. Only 44% of the patients with facet dislocations achieved cervical spine stability with halo treatment, and half of those achieving stability had a "poor" anatomic result. Patients without facet dislocations achieved stability 70% of the time and demonstrated a 75% rate of a "good" anatomic result.

CRANIAL TRACTION

The first use of tongs to apply cranioskeletal traction was reported by Crutchfield in 1933 (44). His traction device was modified from a femoral traction caliper and was applied via burr holes in the skull. Other authors, including McKenzie (45), Barton (46), Blackburn (47), and Vincke (48), have described devices that apply traction to the skull. These devices require cranial burr holes and have been associated with a significant risk of pin dislodgement.

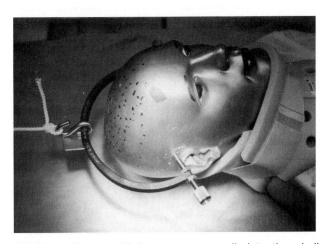

FIG. 7.11. Gardner-Wells tongs are applied to the skull by threading two pins into the outer table of the cranium just superior to the external auditory meatus. This device can then be used to apply longitudinal traction via a rope, pulley, and weights.

Gardner (49) reported the use of the Gardner-Wells tongs in 1973; since that time, this device has gained notable popularity for use in patients requiring cranioskeletal traction. These tongs have a one-piece bow and sharp threaded pins that are easily applied to the skull under local anesthesia. The pins are inserted below the equator of the skull and angle upward to minimize the risk of pin dislodgement. The pins have a spring-loaded indicator that gauges the appropriate pin tension.

The Gardner-Wells tongs are applied to the skull just above the pinna of the ear, in line with the external auditory meatus (Fig. 7.11). To apply a slight flexion or extension moment to the neck, the position of the tongs may be adjusted slightly in a posterior or anterior direction, respectively, relative to the external auditory meatus. The hair at the pin insertion site is shaved and the skin is prepared with povidone-iodine solution. The skin is infiltrated with local anesthetic deep to the galea. The pins are then manually tightened until the indicator protrudes 1 mm. The pins may be retightened 24 hours later to raise the indicator flush with the knurled housing. Pins should be cleaned and cared for in a similar fashion to halo pins.

Gardner-Wells tong traction is infrequently used today for long-term traction in cervical injuries. However, temporary traction stabilization of cervical injuries and reduction of cervical fractures and dislocations remains a popular indication for the use of Gardner-Wells tongs. In addition, some surgeons use Gardner-Wells tongs for intraoperative stabilization and traction during anterior cervical surgery. Traditionally, authors have recommended limiting cervical traction weights to 45 to 80 pounds (50–52). However, cervical traction with weights up to 140 pounds has been safely and successfully used in patients with cervical trauma to obtain a reduction of the spine (53).

Cotler and associates (52,53) have reported a method of reducing cervical dislocations using Gardner-Wells tong traction and serially increasing weights in awake, alert, and cooperative patients. With this method, serial weight applications are applied to the tongs in 10-pound increments, allowing time between each weight application for neurologic examination and radiographs. When the dislocated facet joint reaches the so-called perched position (as seen on a lateral radiograph), gentle extension of the neck is achieved by placing a folded towel beneath the patient's shoulders to allow the facets to reduce. After facet reduction is achieved, the traction weight is reduced to 10 to 20 pounds or the patient is placed in a halo vest. Using Gardner-Wells tong traction, a relatively rapid reduction of a cervical dislocation may be achieved.

Star and colleagues (54) performed a cadaveric study of Gardner-Wells tong traction and reported the result of "high weight reduction" in 53 consecutive patients with facet dislocations. The cadaver study confirmed that the cranial tongs could support over 100 pounds of traction. Using serial weight application to reduce facet dislocations in awake patients, no neurologic deterioration was encountered during the reduction procedure. Thirty-nine patients required more than 50 pounds (the traditional limit) of traction to achieve reduction. Overall, neurologic improvement was achieved in 68% of the patients.

Cotler and coworkers (53) reported the results of 24 patients treated with this method for facet dislocations of the cervical spine. All patients achieved a successful, awake, closed reduction using 10 to 140 pounds of traction. No neurologic deterioration occurred with the reduction procedure. Seventeen patients required more then 50 pounds (the traditional limit) to achieve reduction.

Blumberg and associates (55) evaluated the pull-out characteristics of stainless steel and titanium tongs and pins in cadaver skulls. The titanium tongs and pins were noted to fail by deformation of the pins at lower weights, whereas the stainless steel pins generally failed by producing a skull fracture at very high weights. The authors recommended caution when applying more than 50 pounds of traction to titanium MRI-compatible tongs.

Lerman and colleagues (56) performed a biomechanical evaluation of the pull-out strength of Gardner-Wells tongs after heavy usage. They reported decreased pull-out strength with tongs after heavy usage. This was attributed to under-tightening of the pins caused by wear of the indicator spring. To minimize the risk of tong pull-out or failure, the authors recommended using relatively new tongs when applying high-weight traction.

CONCLUSION

Cervical orthoses are an important adjuvant to the successful treatment of cervical spine conditions where motion restriction is required. The wide array of available orthotics, combined with the limited scientific testing of many of these devices, makes orthotic selection a difficult process. We believe that it is imperative to think in biomechanical terms, considering the type and degree of cervical instability that may be present within the cervical spine. This knowledge will allow the health care practitioner to choose an appropriate orthosis for a given condition.

Although the halo orthosis allows some segmental motion and snaking of the cervical vertebrae, it is the most rigid form of cervical stabilization available. Cranioskeletal traction via Gardner-Wells tongs is a useful means to reduce and stabilize cervical injuries. Tong traction may be safely used in an awake, alert, and cooperative patient in conjunction with serial neurologic examinations and lateral radiographs to reduce facet dislocations. Care should be exercised when applying high-weight traction to titanium or frequently used Gardner-Wells tongs because the risk of tong failure may be increased.

REFERENCES

1. Kostuik JP. Indications for the use of the halo immobilization. *Clin Orthop* 1981;154:46–50.
2. Smith GE. The most ancient splints. *Br Med J* 1908;1:732.
3. White AA, Panjabi MM. *Clinical biomechanics of the spine.* Philadelphia: JB Lippincott, 1978.
4. Kottke FL, Mundle MO. Range of mobility of the cervical spine. *Arch Phys Med Rehabil* 1959;40:379–382.
5. Perry J, Nickel VL. Total cervical spine fusion for neck paralysis. *J Bone Joint Surg Am* 1959;41:37–43.
6. Bhalla SK, Simmons EH. Normal ranges of intervertebral motion of the cervical spine. *Can J Surg* 1969;12:181–187.
7. Fielding JW. Normal and selected abnormal motion of the cervical spine from the second cervical vertebra to the seventh cervical vertebra based on cineradiography. *J Bone Joint Surg Am* 1964;46:1779.
8. Jones MD. Cineradiographic studies of the collar-immobilized cervical spine. *J Neurosurg* 1980;17:633–637.
9. Fisher SV, Bowar JF, Awad EA, et al. Cervical orthoses' effect on cervical spine motion: roentgenographic and goniometric method of study. *Arch Phys Med Rehabil* 1977;58:109–115.
10. Kaufman WA, Lunsford TR, Lunsford BR, et al. Comparison of three prefabricated cervical collars. *Orthot Prosthet* 1986;39:21–28.
11. Lunsford TR, Davidson M, Lunsford BR. The effectiveness of four contemporary cervical orthoses in restricting cervical motion. *J Prosthet Orthot* 1994;6:93–99.
12. Plaisier B, Gabram SG, Schwartz RJ, et al. Prospective evaluation of craniofacial pressure in four different cervical orthoses. *J Trauma* 1994;37:714–720.
13. Podolsky S, Baraff LJ, Simon RR, et al. Efficacy of cervical spine immobilization methods. *J Trauma* 1983;23:461–465.
14. Colachis SC Jr, Strohm BR, Ganter EL. Cervical spine motion in normal women: radiographic study of effect of cervical collars. *Arch Phys Med Rehabil* 1973;54:161–169.
15. Colachis SC Jr, Strohm BR. Radiographic studies of cervical spine motion in normal subjects: flexion and hyperextension. *Arch Phys Med Rehabil* 1965;46:753–760.
16. Beavis A. Cervical orthoses. *Prosthet Orthot Int* 1989;13:6–13.
17. Johnson RM, Hart DL, Simmons EF, et al. Cervical orthoses. A study comparing their effectiveness in restricting cervical motion in normal subjects. *J Bone Joint Surg Am* 1977;59:332–339.
18. Fisher SV. Proper fitting of the cervical orthosis. *Arch Phys Med Rehabil* 1978;59:505–507.
19. Koch RA, Nickel VL. The halo vest: an evaluation of motion and forces across the neck. *Spine* 1978;3:103–107.
20. Anderson PA, Budorick TE, Easton KB, et al. Failure of halo vest to prevent *in vivo* motion in patients with injured cervical spines. *Spine* 1991;16:S501–S505.
21. Benzel EC, Hadden TA, Saulsbery CM. A comparison of the Minerva and halo jackets for stabilization of the cervical spine. *J Neurosurg* 1989;70:411–414.
22. Sypert GW. External spinal orthotics. *Neurosurgery* 1987;20:4.
23. Perry J. The halo in spinal abnormalities. Practical factors and avoidance of complications. *Orthop Clin North Am* 1972;3:69.

24. Botte MJ, Garfin SR, Byrne TP, et al. The halo skeletal fixator. Principles of application and maintenance. *Clin Orthop* 1989;239:12–18.

25. Bucci MN, Dauser RC, Maynard FA, et al. Management of posttraumatic cervical spine instability: operative fusion versus halo vest immobilization. Analysis of 49 cases. *J Trauma* 1988;28:1001–1006.

26. Cooper PR, Maravilla KR, Sklar FH, et al. Halo immobilization of cervical spine fractures. Indications and results. *J Neurosurg* 1979;50:603–610.

27. Lind B, Nordwall A, Sihlbom H. Odontoid fractures treated with halovest. *Spine* 1987;12:173–177.

28. Lind B, Sihlbom H, Nordwall A. Halo-vest treatment of unstable traumatic cervical spine injuries. *Spine* 1988;13:425–432.

29. Mubarak SJ, Camp JF, Vuletich W, et al. Halo application in the infant. *J Pediatr Orthop* 1989;9:612–614.

30. Parry H, Delargy M, Burt A. Early mobilisation of patients with cervical cord injury using the halo brace device. *Paraplegia* 1988;26:226–232.

31. Kopits SE, Steingass MH. Experience with the "halo-cast" in small children. *Surg Clin North Am* 1970;50:935–943.

32. Botte MJ, Byrne TP, Abrams RA, et al. Halo skeletal fixation: techniques of application and prevention of complications. *J Am Acad Orthop Surg* 1996;4:44–53.

33. Garfin SR, Roux R, Botte MJ, et al. Skull osteology as it affects halo pin placement in children. *J Pediatr Orthop* 1986;6:434–436.

34. Ballock RT, Lee TQ, Triggs KJ, et al. The effect of pin location on the rigidity of the halo pin-bone interface. *Neurosurgery* 1990;26:238–241.

35. Triggs KJ, Ballock RT, Lee TQ, et al. The effect of angled insertion on halo pin fixation. *Spine* 1989;14:781–783.

36. Botte MJ, Byrne TP, Garfin SR. Application of the halo device for immobilization of the cervical spine utilizing an increased torque pressure. *J Bone Joint Surg Am* 1987;69:750–752.

37. Botte MJ, Byrne TP, Garfin SR. The use of skin incisions in the application of halo skeletal fixator pins. *Clin Orthop* 1989;246:100.

38. Sears W, Fazl M. Prediction of stability of cervical spine fracture managed in the halo vest and indications for surgical intervention [see comments]. *J Neurosurg* 1990;72:426–432.

39. Glaser JA, Whitehill R, Stamp WG, et al. Complications associated with the halo-vest. A review of 245 cases. *J Neurosurg* 1986;65:762–769.

40. Vaccaro AR, Falatyn SP, Scuder G, et al. Early failure of long segment anterior cervical plate fixation. *J Spinal Disord* 1988;11:410–415.

41. Garfin SR, Botte MJ, Waters RL, et al. Complications in the use of the halo fixation device. *J Bone Joint Surg Am* 1986;68:320–325.

42. Rizzolo SJ, Pizaa MR, Cotler JM, et al. The effect of torque pressure on halo pin complication rates. A randomized prospective study. *Spine* 1993;18:2163–2166.

43. Garfin SR, Botte MJ, Triggs KJ, et al. Subdural abscess associated with halo-pin traction. *J Bone Joint Surg Am* 1988;70:1338–1340.

44. Crutchfield WG. Skeletal traction for dislocation of the cervical spine: report of a case. *South Surg* 1933;2:156–159.

45. McKenzie KG. Fracture, dislocation, and fracture-dislocation of the spine. *Can Med Assoc J* 1935;32:263–269.

46. Barton LG. Reduction of fracture dislocations of the cervical vertebra by skeletal traction. *Surg Gyn Obstet* 1938;67:94–96.

47. Blackburn JD. A new skull traction appliance. *South Surg* 1938;7:16–18.

48. Vincke TH. Treatment of unstable spinal fractures and dislocations. *Clin Neurosurg* 1948;25:193–208.

49. Gardner WJ. The principle of spring-loaded points for cervical traction. *J Neurosurg* 1973;39:543–544.

50. Yashon D, Tyson G, Vise M. Rapid closed reduction of cervical fracture dislocation. *Surg Neurol* 1975;4:513–514.

51. Norrell, H. Treatment of unstable spinal fractures and dislocations. *Neurosurgery* 1978;25:193–208.

52. Cotler HB, Miller LS, DeLucia FA, et al. Closed reduction of cervical spine dislocations. *Clin Orthop* 1987;1(214):185–199.

53. Cotler JM, Herbison GJ, Nasuti JF, et al. Closed reduction of traumatic cervical spine dislocation using traction weights up to 140 pounds. *Spine* 1993;18:386–390.

54. Star AM, Jones AA, Cotler JM, et al. Immediate closed reduction of cervical spine dislocations using traction. *Spine* 1990;15:1068–1072.

55. Blumberg KD, Catalano JB, Cotler JM, et al. The pullout strength of titanium alloy MRI-compatible and stainless steel MRI-incompatible Gardner-Wells tongs. *Spine* 1993;18:1895–1896.

56. Lerman JA, Haynes RJ, Koeneman EJ, et al. A biomechanical comparison of Gardner-Wells tongs and halo device used for cervical spine traction. *Spine* 1994;19:2403–2406.

CHAPTER 8

Pain Mechanisms: Relevant Anatomy, Pathogenesis, and Clinical Implications

Beth A. Winkelstein and James N. Weinstein

Neck pain is a common problem in today's society, affecting an estimated five of every ten people. Although 80% of these people will experience resolution of their pain, the remainder will suffer from persistent and chronic neck pain. Not only is neck pain common, but tremendous cost is associated with its treatment and disability. For example, the cost of whiplash injuries alone has been estimated to be at least $5 billion annually (1). Until we gain a better understanding of the pathomechanisms in neck pain, radiculopathy, and myelopathy, among other painful syndromes in the neck, their treatments will remain somewhat limited.

This chapter describes briefly the anatomy of the cervical spine and its possible sources of pain. Further, we hope to elucidate cogent hypotheses regarding the manifestation of pain symptoms and their mechanisms. In an effort to present these concepts, we begin with a review of the anatomic structures of the cervical spine with a specific focus on their potential for pain generation and relevance to their painful injury risk. Then, a brief discussion of the neurophysiology of pain highlights traditional concepts of injury and pain processing and more recent hypotheses of the central nervous system's neuroimmunologic involvement in persistent pain. The third section of this chapter discusses biomechanical considerations for painful injuries—in particular, facet joint and nerve root injuries. The chapter concludes with a discussion of clinical implications and suggested areas of future work.

It is important to mention at the outset that although this chapter focuses on the mechanisms, pathogenesis, and implications of neck pain, there is at this writing a limited understanding of neck pain mechanisms specifically, with the exception of inferential findings from clinical and mechanical reports. Therefore, much of what is currently known about spinal pain mechanisms comes from literature on low back pain, which provides working hypotheses of potential mechanisms by which the same anatomic tissues may initiate

a pain response in the neck. For example, the discussion on biomechanical factors of nerve root injuries provided in this chapter reflects experimental work with a lumbar radiculopathy model. Given the paucity of basic science research in the area of neck pain, these lumbar studies form a cogent presentation of relevant and important issues that may likely be extrapolated to the cervical spine. Also, much of this chapter deals with whiplash injury mechanisms. This by no means is meant to suggest that whiplash is the only injury mechanism producing painful neck syndromes; however, a large portion of biomechanics research related to neck pain is focused on whiplash injury prevention, mechanism, and pathology, so this literature provides a detailed discussion related to painful injury mechanisms in the neck. Every effort is made here to provide a discussion of each of these topics with specific relevance to the cervical spine and neck pain.

RELEVANT ANATOMIC STRUCTURES: POTENTIAL PAIN SOURCES

Many anatomic structures of the cervical spine have the potential for generating pain. These same structures, by virtue of their biomechanical or physiologic functions, are particularly important in a variety of neck injuries and pathologic syndromes (Fig. 8.1). Potential anatomic pain sources include both hard and soft tissue components, such as the intervertebral disc, muscles, and facet joints. Studies have demonstrated nociceptors to exist in all of these tissues. Equally relevant to pain generation are the neural components themselves, because they can be injured directly during many neck loading scenarios.

Hard and Soft Tissue Components

The cervical intervertebral disc functions to absorb shock and transmit compressive loads through the spinal column.

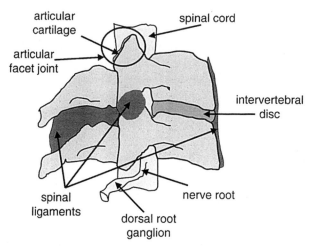

FIG. 8.1. The anatomic structures and tissues of the cervical motion segment and spinal cord that can potentially lead to painful neck syndromes when injured. Both hard and soft tissues, such as the intervertebral disc, ligaments, and articular facet joint, can be injured. Also at risk are the neural components, such as the spinal cord, nerve roots, and dorsal root ganglion.

While its primary function may be viewed as a biomechanical one, its anatomy suggests that it has the capacity to generate pain. The outer annulus of the disc is innervated (2–5). Degeneration or local mechanical loading in the disc annulus can stimulate free nerve fibers to generate a painful response via mechanical or chemical mediators (2,3). Despite these anatomic suggestions of nociceptive mechanisms, no physiologic studies have been performed to document molecular or cellular changes associated with persistent pain from annulus changes in the neck. More catastrophic injury to the cervical disc by direct insult also poses potential risks. Certainly, the effects of degeneration (aging) on the cervical spine, and the disc in particular, present an additional pathway for pain initiation leading to disc changes, annulus stimulation, and overall spinal changes similar to those reported in low back pain.

It is important to recognize that neck musculature plays a unique role in neck pain through the potential for its own injury and by altering the kinematics and kinetics of other structures of the cervical spine, potentially leading to exacerbation of existing loading and painful conditions. Muscles contain nerve fibers, both Aδ and C types (6,7). In fact, in skeletal muscle, as many as half of the neural units have been identified as having nociceptive functions (8). Innervation of neck musculature is provided mostly from the dorsal rami of C2 through C4 (9). Neck muscles have the potential to incite an inflammatory response to their own injury, which in turn can lead to a more severe pain response when they undergo further injury (10).

Muscles are a particularly vulnerable structure for injury in the cervical spine, especially during bending motions; in many neck loading scenarios, the muscles themselves may simultaneously undergo eccentric contraction while also being elongated as a result of head or torso motions. This concomitant lengthening and force exertion makes them particularly susceptible to injury or pain. Uniquely, not only are neck muscles at risk for their own injury, but they also pose a threat to the other tissues in which they insert or with which they are in contact. For example, the facet capsule has been shown to have semispinalis and splenius capitis muscle fibers inserting directly onto it (11), presenting a pathway of direct loading to the capsule when these muscle fibers become activated. Such direct mechanical aggravation via muscles can superimpose additional injury on an already injured or painfully stimulated structure, producing the potential for a more severe mechanism of pain signaling.

The cervical articular facet joint is a complicated joint with a variety of sources for pain generation. Each facet surface is covered with articular cartilage; synovial folds exist in the space between the articulating facet surfaces. Due to their orientation, the articulation of successive articular processes forms a column supporting compressive loads in the cervical spine. The facet capsular ligament, or facet capsule, is thin and loosely encloses the entire joint. As a consequence of its laxity, the facet capsular ligament follows the motions of its surrounding bony vertebrae, lacking the stiffness to alter the overall joint kinematics (12). Cervical facet joints are innervated by the medial branches of the dorsal primary ramus from the two levels surrounding the joint (13). Histologic and anatomic studies have identified mechanoreceptors and unmyelinated nociceptors in the cervical facet joint and its capsule (14–16). Although the size of the receptive fields of these pain fibers remains unknown, it has been speculated that each fiber may innervate an area large enough to collectively cover the entire joint (6). Regardless, anatomic evidence of pain-producing elements in this joint of the cervical spine is convincing and suggests that the facet joint as a whole, and its individual components, has the potential for pain generation. Coupling the neuroanatomy of this joint with the compressive loading of its synovial folds and the tensile loading of its capsule, it is a very likely candidate for pain generation in the neck, particularly given the complicated nature of its biomechanics during many scenarios of neck loading.

Neural Components

Structurally, the spinal cord is surrounded by three membranes: the pia mater, arachnoid, and dura mater, with the pia mater being in closest contact with the cord, and the dura enclosing the entire structure. Cerebrospinal fluid is contained between the arachnoid and pia; the epidural space exists between the dura and the bony walls of the neural canal. The neural canal is formed by the posterior bony elements of each vertebra and the neural arches that connect these posterior elements to the anterior vertebral body. The outer white matter of the spinal cord contains the ascending and descending tracts, which are arranged into bundles with specific functions.

The anterior and posterior rootlets coming off the spinal cord combine to form dorsal and ventral nerve roots, which make up the spinal nerve at each level. The location, direction, and number of nerve rootlets vary for each cervical level. Posterior rootlets making up the dorsal root are the sensory fibers, whereas the anterior ones are the effector fibers. Cell bodies of peripheral nerves are housed in the dorsal root ganglion (DRG). The DRG is particularly sensitive to loading; even slight compression of normal DRGs can produce sustained electrical activity and pain (17,18). The dorsal and ventral roots come together in the region of the neural foramen and continue more distally into the periphery as the spinal nerve, to innervate structures outside the spinal column. Unlike spinal and other peripheral nerves, the nerve roots are not enclosed by a thick epineurial sheath, and as such lack the mechanical strength of their peripheral counterparts, placing roots in a potentially more injurious situation when loaded.

NEUROPHYSIOLOGY OF PAIN

A host of neurophysiologic mechanisms exist whereby injury to any of these anatomic elements can lead to nociception and ultimately to pain. An inciting injury and fiber stimulation initiates a central signaling response. In persistent pain, central nervous system (CNS) signals can result in a hypersensitivity or central sensitization response. In addition to central sensitization, the CNS mounts a neuroimmune response that may further contribute to sensitization and persistent pain symptoms.

Tissue Injury and Neuropathic Pain

A tissue (muscle, disc, ligament, etc.) injury in the periphery sets up a classic pathway of physiologic processes by which the insult (injury or inflammation induced) activates local nociceptors in that tissue. These peripheral Aδ and C fibers in turn become sensitized and have both lower thresholds for firing and increased firing rates when stimulated at levels similar to before injury (6). In the locale of the injured tissue, many chemical mediators are simultaneously released that can directly or indirectly act to further excite or sensitize these nociceptors. Such chemical mediators include, but are not limited to, excitatory amino acids, nitric oxide, bradykinin, prostaglandins, histamine, and substance P (6,19). Cytokines are also released in the periphery in association with tissue injury and inflammation. These proteins, in turn, contribute to the local inflammatory response, while further affecting electrophysiologic responses of pain. For example, peripheral injections of interleukin-1β (IL-1β) produce spontaneous discharges and lowered thresholds of activation in conjunction with pain-associated behavioral hypersensitivity (20,21).

The injured primary afferents terminate in the dorsal horn of the spinal cord, where they communicate with spinal neurons via synaptic transmission. Within the spinal cord, many additional neurotransmitters (e.g., glutamate, N-methyl-D-aspartate, substance P, neurofilament protein, vasoinhibitory peptide) modulate postsynaptic responses, with further transmission to supraspinal sites via the ascending pathways (6). More detailed specific signaling responses of the spinal cord are far too complicated to elaborate further in the limited space of this chapter. The pattern of pain transmission just detailed describes the typical response of an acutely painful episode, in which the balance of injury, repair, and healing is achieved and the cascade of electrophysiologic and chemical events resolves following inflammation and injury. However, for the case of persistent pain, the local, spinal, and even supraspinal responses are undoubtedly altered from those just described (22).

Central Sensitization

Persistent pain is believed to be due to the sensitization of the CNS. Although the exact mechanism by which the spinal cord becomes sensitized or in a "hyperexcitable" state currently remains unknown, many hypotheses have emerged. Again, this section provides only a highlight of these theories; more extensive discussions can be found elsewhere in the literature (23–26). Simply, low-threshold Aβ afferents, which normally do not serve to activate a pain response, become recruited to transmit spontaneous and movement-induced pain (26). This central hyperexcitability is characterized by a "windup" response of repetitive C fiber stimulation, expanding receptive field areas, and spinal neurons taking on properties of wide-dynamic-range neurons (27). Ultimately, Aβ fibers stimulate postsynaptic neurons to transmit pain where these Aβ fibers previously had no effect, all leading to central sensitization. However, this is by no means the only mechanism of central sensitization.

Neuroimmunologic Responses in the Central Nervous System

While central sensitization contributes to physiologic mechanisms of persistent pain, recent research has demonstrated the role of neuroimmune responses in the CNS in contributing to persistent pain (28). For example, many investigations have focused on the role of the immune system and the CNS inflammatory response in generating pain following nerve and nerve root injuries. Immune activation with cytokine production may indirectly induce the expression of many common pain mediators, such as glutamate, nitric oxide, and prostaglandins, in the CNS. These, in turn, can lead to spinal sensitization. Events that induce behavioral hypersensitivity also activate immune cells both centrally and in the periphery.

Substantial support exists for the role of neuroimmune activation and proinflammatory cytokines in the etiology of persistent pain states. CNS immune activation mediates chronic pain; immune cell products, cytokines, and chemokines (*chemo*tactic cyto*kines*) all contribute in the genesis of chronic neuropathic pain (29–31). Cytokines and growth factors have been strongly implicated in the generation of pathologic pain states at both peripheral and central nervous system sites (32,33). In separate studies, the origin of these spinal cytokines has been addressed using *in situ* hybridization, axonal transport blockade, and peripheral macrophage depletion (34–36). From this body of work, a cascade of events in the CNS has been proposed following injury (28): Cells become activated and can release cytokines that can not only lead to further activation, but also to the release of mediators. In conjunction with this neuroimmune activation, a neuroinflammatory response occurs in which immune cells migrate from the periphery into the CNS. This infiltration may lead to further changes in the CNS and potentially to central sensitization.

BIOMECHANICAL CONSIDERATIONS IN PAINFUL CERVICAL INJURY

As a mechanistic picture begins to emerge of the physiologic responses of pain, we turn our attention to the mechanisms by which various structures in the neck may be injured. Although the exact injury mechanisms leading to neck pain remain largely uncharacterized, several hypotheses indicate a consensus agreement on potential sites of injury. Historically, much of the work in this area has been performed in the context of understanding pain mechanisms of whiplash injury. Two such specific injuries include those of the facet joint and of the nerve roots. These will each be discussed here with regard to the biomechanics of their injury and pain generation.

Facet Joint Injury Mechanisms

Clinical studies implicate the facet joint as a site of painful injury in the neck. This joint has been identified as the most common source of neck pain (37,38), with as many as 62% of neck pain cases arising from the facet joint. Medial branch and anesthetic joint blocks and provocative testing have both implicated the facet joint in neck pain, particularly in the case of whiplash sufferers (39,40). Experimental studies in the lumbar spine have provided further evidence to suggest that the facet joint is a likely site of pain generation in the cervical spine. For example, visible stretch of the facet capsule has been reported during spinal loading of the facet joint, suggesting its potential for uncontrolled loading and motion (41). Moreover, mechanical stimulation of lumbar facet capsules in animal models initiates electrical activity consistent with nociception (42,43). Although such experimental work is currently absent in the cervical spine, it strongly suggests loading to the facet capsule as a possible mechanism of injury or nociceptive changes consistent with painful stimulus signals.

Many of the hypotheses of facet-mediated pain imply that "abnormal" motion patterns are developed in the cervical spine, which lead to local injuries. For example, the facet joint injury mechanism for whiplash put forth by Ono and

Kaneoka and associates (44,45) hypothesizes that following impact, the lower cervical spine undergoes extension while the upper portion is in flexion, compressing the facet surfaces together in the posterior portion of the joint, resulting in a bony collision and concomitant stretching of the anterior longitudinal ligament. The hypothesized change in spinal curvature, facet bone impingement, and potential synovial fold pinching in the joint space has also been proposed by Panjabi and co-workers (46,47) and Yoganandan and colleagues (48–50). The proposed pinching mechanism has support as a pain mechanism when recalling that nociceptors exist in the synovial folds of human articular facets (16). Although histologic and mechanical studies suggest this pinching mechanism of painful injury, a definitive mechanism of pain has yet to be addressed and is entirely speculative at present.

Similarly, the potential for loading and painful stimulation also exists for the cervical facet capsules. Using isolated cadaveric motion segment testing, it was determined that gross structural failure of the cervical facet capsule does not occur during normal flexion-extension motions observed in neck loading during whiplash scenarios (51). In fact, maximum capsular strains (103.6%) at failure were approximately nine times those during vertebral bending in whiplash simulations (flexion, 12.1%; extension, 11.6%) (51,52). Siegmund and associates (53) demonstrated that maximum capsular strain (16.8%) in combined posterior shear and extension remained significantly below those strains (94%) at joint failure in shear, further demonstrating that gross joint capsule disruption does not occur in whiplash. Although these studies reflect isolated motion segment behavior, Panjabi and colleagues have also shown, using cadaveric head-neck specimens, that the maximum capsular elongation is 35.4% (46,47), which is less than that observed for capsule failure as reported by Winkelstein and colleagues (51,52). Although these studies show that catastrophic gross failure of the facet capsule does not occur during cervical spine whiplash motions, this work is unable to address the potential for pain generation or nociceptive sensation.

Interestingly, prior to catastrophic facet capsule failures, a subcatastrophic ligament failure was consistently observed in both tension and shear failures of the joint (51,53) (Fig. 8.2). Despite these subcatastrophic failures, the capsular ligament structure is maintained, suggesting small fiber ruptures that may not contribute to the joint's overall strength. The maximum capsule strains in these cases (35% to 65%) were not significantly different from those observed during the combined loading simulations of motion segments (51,53). This strongly suggests a possibility of capsule injury that, although not disrupting the integrity of the joint, may actually present a likely mechanism for nociceptor activation. Unfortunately, such data on loading of this joint, its nerve fibers, and their nociception activation still remain uncharacterized. Although these studies implicate the possibility of a subcatastrophic injury to the facet capsule resulting in pain generation, they remain inferential until further work is performed to understand their physiologic meaning.

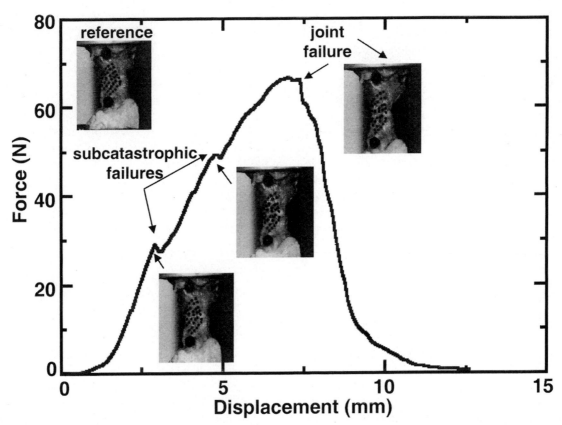

FIG. 8.2. Force-displacement plot of a cervical facet capsule failure in tension, illustrating the joint failure event and subcatastrophic failures. Also shown are images of the joint's configuration at these failures. Of particular interest are the subcatastrophic failures, in which the overall mechanical integrity is maintained and there are no obvious geometric changes or discontinuities in the capsular ligament. Better characterizing the physiologic meaning of these subcatastrophic injuries will help understand the potential for neck pain from loading or injury to this joint.

The close proximity of neck musculature, coupled with its propensity for activation during sudden neck motion, has led to the hypothesis that neck musculature presents an additional mechanism for injuring the facet capsule under certain loading situations. Muscle activation can directly alter spinal kinematics, and consequently loading to specific components such as the facet joint; additionally, direct muscle loading to soft tissue components can occur (12). For example, muscle fibers have been determined to insert on approximately 23% of the C4 through C6 human facet capsules (54). Facet loading by activated muscles during rapid muscle elongation has been estimated to be as large as 44 to 54 N, which is within the range of loads recorded during subcatastrophic failures of the facet joint (54), indicating a potential threat for injurious loading to the capsule via muscle loading. When considering that muscle loading is likely superimposed on other mechanical demands to this joint, the painful injury risk is further increased.

Strong evidence exists by many overlapping research communities suggesting that the facet joint is a likely source of pain in the neck due to its rich neuroanatomic characteristics, the clinical evidence of anesthetic pain relief, its kinematic and kinetic properties in biomechanical studies, and its potential risk for these so-called subcatastrophic injuries.

When taken separately, these findings can only offer speculative information regarding neck pain and the facet joint. Integrating all of these efforts, it is possible to develop a more complete understanding of the facet joint's potential for injury and its subsequent ability to generate pain. However, truly understanding this joint's ability to incite pain in the neck is only possible through an interdisciplinary approach to research that incorporates both biomechanical and physiologic components of injury and pain (Fig. 8.3). Such work would strengthen the existing understanding of the meaning of these subcatastrophic failures in the context of pain and physiologic responses.

Nerve Root Injury Mechanisms

Deformation of cervical nerve roots is also a potential mechanism for neck pain. Painful radiculopathy, although a condition primarily studied in the lumbar spine, can occur in the cervical spine as well. Cervical nerve root compression can result from a number of injury scenarios and anatomic changes: joint dislocation, disc collapse, disc protrusion, and osteophyte formation (55). As such, it is useful to address this class of injuries with particular attention to the role of

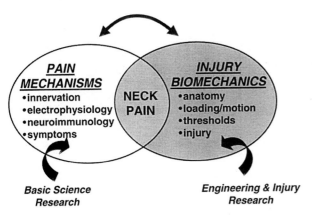

FIG. 8.3. An interdisciplinary approach is required to study the pathogenesis of painful neck injuries. Such an approach incorporates physiologic assessment of nociception and clinically relevant behavioral symptoms with a biomechanical perspective of injury, failure, and loading.

mechanics in the mechanism of pain responses *in vivo*. The potential for nerve root injury certainly exists in the neck, given the amount of flexibility in the cervical spine coupled with the neck's potential for undergoing loading due to head and torso motions. The neural foraminal space can decrease by as much as 20% for cadaveric cervical spine motions within normal ranges of motion (55). Although this study indicates a potential mechanism by which nerve root impingement may occur, it does not address the relation between these violations of foraminal space and physiologic changes of nociception. In fact, because these deformations reflect motions within the neck's normal range of motion, it is inferred that they do not actually produce injury or pain *in vivo*. Regardless, this experimental work provides a foundation by which motions of the neck can present the potential for direct injury to neural tissue.

Aldman (56) hypothesized that pressure gradients from blood flow resistance can occur in the CNS for rapid spine motion and that these gradients can directly load the nerve roots and spinal ganglia, causing their injury. Coupling these pressure wave effects with superimposed mechanical compression and tethered stretching of these structures, the pathomechanisms of painful nerve root injuries in the neck begin to emerge (56,57). However, the pathophysiology of this hypothesis remains unclear; this work in the cervical spine is limited to an *in vivo* porcine model of rapid head and neck extension that produces leaking of the plasma membrane of spinal ganglia nerve cells, suggesting their injury (58). Although suggesting a pathway for injury, this study provided no direct measure of pain due to these injuries. Nonetheless, these collective investigations have offered another potential mechanism by which neck pain can result from nerve root injuries in the neck.

Although work linking nerve root injury of any kind to physiologic pain mechanisms in the neck is currently lacking, it is possible to draw on current research for painful *lumbar* radiculopathy to gain insight into potential mechanisms of

neck pain. Therefore, for the purpose of discussing nerve root mechanics and nociception, the remainder of this section focuses on recent work using biomechanics in *in vivo* models of persistent radicular pain. These studies can help establish a road map for similar work in the neck.

Direct nerve root injury affects pain and its physiologic responses. For example, altered functional responses in porcine models of cauda equina compression include changes in electrical impulse propagation and conduction velocity (59–61). Nerve root compression also significantly reduces blood flow in the region of injury (62). Of particular interest for pain, nerve root compression has been shown to induce repetitive neuronal firing in the dorsal horn of the spinal cord (60), suggesting a direct mechanism of spinal cord plasticity and central sensitization for these mechanical injuries. In conjunction with electrophysiologic changes, functional behavioral testing has revealed decreased ambulation for these injuries (18,63). However, all of these functional changes simply *imply* a connection with pain-associated changes, while not specifically investigating behavioral symptoms of hypersensitivity and nociceptive changes in the CNS.

Therefore, understanding the relation between injury events and pain-related behaviors is a key element for developing an understanding of the pathogenesis of pain. To this end, investigators have implemented simple biomechanical techniques to quantify nerve root tissue deformation in a rodent model of painful lumbar radiculopathy (64,65) (Fig. 8.4). Local mechanics at injury has a distinctive role in modulating behavioral sensitivity: More severe nerve root injuries (with greater degrees of tissue impingement)

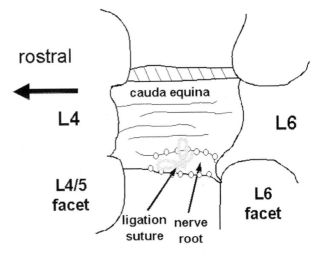

FIG. 8.4. The biomechanical technique of applying image analysis to an *in vivo* lumbar radiculopathy model of persistent pain. In this model, an L5 laminectomy exposes the cauda equina and L5 nerve roots. The L5 dorsal and ventral nerve roots on the left side are ligated with a suture material (shown schematically). Images are acquired prior to and at the time of injury, and the nerve root border is digitized. The nerve root borders are shown here as they would be digitized in the images (*dots*). (Modified from Winkelstein BA, Weinstein JN, DeLeo JA. The role of mechanical deformation in lumbar radiculopathy: an *in vivo* model. *Spine* 2002;27:27–33.)

produce a greater degree of pain-associated behavioral sensitivity than those injuries with lesser tissue compression (of approximately one-half that in the severe group) (64,65). In fact, there is a significant positive correlation in this pain model between behavioral sensitivity and injury magnitude (65). Most simply, the greater the nerve root compression at injury, the worse the clinical symptoms of behavioral sensitivity and pain. Using a simple application of biomechanics in basic science pain research points to the feasibility and extreme utility of this and similar lines of research for delineating the *specific* mechanisms of nerve root injury and other pathologies of the neck, and of the spine in general (Fig. 8.3).

Although defining the relation between injury events and pain behaviors is necessary for developing a cause-and-effect relation, understanding the relation between nerve root injury and its specific and relevant *nociceptive* physiologic responses is crucial for understanding the mechanisms by which such injuries result in persistent pain. For example, as discussed earlier, a host of immune changes occur in the spinal cord that contribute to central sensitization and pathologic correlates of persistent pain. Of interest with regard to persistent pain is the following question: How, if at all, do biomechanics at nerve root injury modulate these immune changes? A statistically significant correlation exists between spinal mRNA levels of pro- and antiinflammatory cytokines (TNFα, IL-1β, IL-6, IL-10) and the degree of nerve root impingement (65). Similarly, spinal expression of the proinflammatory protein IL-1β is greater for qualitatively more "severe" injuries (66), suggesting that any modulatory effects are preserved at both the message and protein levels for these cytokines. Although these findings suggest a modulatory effect of injury severity on one aspect of the neuroimmune cascade for painful radiculopathy, they cannot unilaterally suggest that a series of events occurs following an injury and that the nature of these events is simply greater or less based on the initial magnitude of the injury.

Spinal microglia and astrocytes are likely responsible for the upregulation and release of these inflammatory cytokines (28). As such, it is helpful to understand the relation of mechanics and cellular activation in the spinal cord. As observed with behavioral sensitivity responses and other spinal neuroimmune cascades in animal models, spinal microglial activation shows a greater intensity for greater degrees of nerve root deformation (66,67). However, these responses are not related to the specific pain-related behaviors of these animals. The behavioral sensitivity of individual rats on the day of analysis of activation did not demonstrate a correlative relation (67). Although microglial activation shows a graded response according to injury severity, it cannot explain the pain-associated behavioral responses. Moreover, the degree of spinal astrocytic activation did not show a relation with initial injury. These findings highlight the need for defining the relation of an injury event, its physiologic responses, *and the behavioral symptoms of pain*. Without placing the injury and physiologic findings in

TABLE 8.1. *Factors Affecting Painful Neck Injury Mechanisms*

Mechanical factors
  Magnitude of load
  Magnitude of deformation
  Direction of application
  Rate of application
  Duration of application
  Initial geometry (configuration) of anatomic structure
  Loading frequency (e.g., repetitive or single application)
Physiologic factors
  Responses of specific anatomic structures (e.g., individual tissue responses)
  Anatomic features (e.g., stenosis)
  Inflammation (preexisting)
  Degeneration (preexisting)
  Electrophysiologic sensitivity
  Electrophysiologic preconditioning before injury
  Immunologic preconditioning before injury
Other factors
  Genetics
  Gender
  Age
  Comorbidities
  Psychological factors
  Psychosocial and/or environmental issues

the context of pain-associated behaviors, any work to truly understand pain mechanisms will fall short.

The question remains: Are the mechanisms by which pain is established and/or maintained, given an injury, serial or integrative events? Glial activation suggests that although microglia may become activated according to a dose-response characteristic prescribed by the intensity of the injury event, these physiologic changes may not *necessarily* be the only ones contributing to a clinically observed symptom, such as increased behavioral sensitivity. In this case, for example, it may be possible that some subpopulation or secondary action of the activated CNS cells is the crucial physiologic contributor to pain symptoms. Because it remains undetermined what this action is, continued research is needed to further delineate the *specific* mechanisms of persistent pain and then understand their relation to the injury event. This section has addressed only the effect of injury magnitude, but undoubtedly many factors relating to injury (both mechanical and otherwise) can potentially affect the physiologic responses and pain (Table 8.1).

Other Potential Neck Pain Mechanisms

Although much of this discussion on neck pain mechanisms has focused on facet joint and nerve root injuries as potentiating events, it is recognized that these are by no means the only two anatomic sites of painful injury in the cervical spine. Undoubtedly, direct insult to the spinal cord results in persistent pain along with other sequelae. An extensive review of animal models of painful spinal cord injuries has been provided by Vierck and associates (68). From these models it is reported that incomplete injuries of the cord more often produce behavioral hypersensitivity, which is consistent with the clinical picture. As with painful radicular injuries, spinal cord injuries result in a host of physiologic changes, including chemical, molecular, and inflammatory changes (69). In fact, for these injuries, a secondary spread of injury throughout the spinal cord has been reported and suggested to affect the distribution of pain symptoms (70). In addition, direct electrophysiologic studies document functional neuronal changes in association with cord injuries (69), suggesting the central sensitization phenomenon described earlier.

In addition to direct injury of neural elements of the cervical spine, injury to disc and muscle can provide mechanisms by which nociceptive pain can be initiated. Certainly, anatomic studies implicate these tissues as having nociceptive innervation (4,5,7). Just as the facet joint is at risk for injury during certain motions and loading scenarios of the cervical spine, it is also possible that the intervertebral disc has the potential for mechanical injury. In contrast to facet joint injuries, however, disc injuries sustained in the cervical spine likely result from much more severe loading scenarios, leading to canal impingement, instability, and more gross disruption of the neck structure as a whole. Moreover, while muscle sprains and subcatastrophic injuries also present the possibility of generating nociceptive changes, these often resolve and fail to result in chronic neck pain. However, better understanding the mechanism by which these injuries resolve will certainly help with understanding the difference between acute and chronic pain states in the neck.

Confounding Factors Affecting Neck Pain

Given the extreme complexity of understanding painful injuries in general and neck pain mechanisms in particular, it must be recognized that a variety of factors exist that can affect injury mechanisms. For example, many biomechanical factors have been shown to alter neuronal function, such as rate, loading duration, and load magnitude, among others. Given the complexity of pain mechanisms, the factors that confound the injuries themselves can play a very large role in neck pain (Table 8.1). Among these, the physiologic milieu at the time of injury is believed to modulate (i.e., potentially worsen) painful outcome. For example, it has been shown that the pain-associated behaviors resulting from a second radiculopathy injury are significantly greater than those behavioral responses to the first injury (71). Expanding on these findings, it can be hypothesized that injury following a preexisting "minor" tissue injury may result in a more severe nociceptive response than in the absence of any preexisting damage. It is not unlikely that an initial injury produces the local inflammatory changes discussed earlier, which in turn may lower that tissue's threshold for mechanical injury. In fact, it has been shown that the mechanical insult required to produce behavioral hypersensitivity in the presence of an inflammatory insult is nearly one-half that required in its absence, despite resulting in the same degree of sensitivity (22).

Inferences can be made in light of these findings for whiplash-associated neck pain. Epidemiologic studies indicate that patients with preexisting spinal degeneration at the time of injury experience more severe and longer-lasting symptoms of neck pain (72–74). It is possible that such degeneration can contribute to inflammatory changes in the facet joint that may increase this joint's susceptibility to mechanical injury. Therefore, when it undergoes motions or loading that may not normally elicit nociceptive changes, the nerve fibers may be presensitized and fire under mechanical conditions that are much less severe than previously required to initiate nociception. The same may be true for degenerative changes in other spinal tissues.

Continuing with the whiplash example, a number of other mechanical and anatomic factors have the potential for altering painful injury events. Such features of the injury event include restraint use, collision type, gender, and head position at injury. For example, as many as 57% of whiplash patients suffering from persistent neck pain at 2 years following initial injury reported having their heads axially rotated at the time of injury (75,76). In contrast, of those who were asymptomatic at follow-up, only 28% had their heads rotated, which was significantly less than those experiencing persistent pain. Biomechanical studies have shown that axial rotation of the neck both reduces normal ranges of spinal motion and alters the kinematics of individual tissue components of the cervical spine (12). Spinal torque has been shown to alter facet capsule mechanics and differentially increase capsular strains (51), increasing the overall risk for painful injury to this ligament. As previously described, muscle activation during loading can also serve as a confounding factor of painful injury.

Additional geometric and anatomic factors contributing to neck pain risk are gender, existing spinal degeneration, stenosis, and genetics (9). In the case of whiplash, females experience increased symptom persistence when compared with males (9). The anatomic considerations specifically related to gender, which include decreased neck muscle strength and spinal canal size, add support to the role of neck mechanics in affecting a pain mechanism. Moreover, anecdotal evidence has shown that smaller spinal canal size is associated with more symptomatic responses in whiplash (77). Finally, more recent clinical research into spinal pain in general has shown that genetics may play a key role in pain persistence for a given injury, accounting for many discrepancies observed among different patients having seemingly similar injuries (22). Future research into neck pain mechanisms would be strengthened if it considered the role of genetics in many of the issues discussed in this chapter.

IMPLICATIONS: CLINICAL APPLICATIONS AND FUTURE RESEARCH

From the issues presented in this chapter, we can pull together many aspects that contribute to neck pain. In this context, then, it is possible to synthesize these findings to discuss preventing these injuries and treating and managing them. As continued biomechanical research is performed to determine mechanisms of tissue injury that initiate physiologic responses, it becomes clear that preventive strategies may be developed in the near future to protect some of these structures in the neck from undergoing kinematically and kinetically risky situations.

As the understanding of neck injuries and spinal pain grows, increased research is being focused on development of effective treatment modalities. Although a host of clinical studies point to nerve blocks of facet joints for pain relief (37–40), the exact site of injury often remains elusive in neck pain, making it extremely challenging to act at the structural site of injury for therapy. For this reason, pharmacologic treatment options offer a promising approach for manipulating those aspects of the CNS response that contribute to chronic nociception. For example, global immunosuppressants have been shown to ameliorate pain behaviors in rodent models of both neuropathic and radiculopathic pain (78). Efforts to target more specific elements of the neuroimmune cascade also offer a promising method of more selectively manipulating particular aspects of the CNS's response without using a broad shotgun approach. Pharmacologic antagonists to and inhibitors of particular proinflammatory cytokines, chemokines, and other analgesic mediators (e.g., IL-1, tumor necrosis factor, monocyte chemoattractant protein,

TABLE 8.2. *Suggested Future Work to Delineate Neck Pain Mechanisms: Specific Areas of Investigation and Their Related Fields of Research*

1. Anatomic identification and characterization of sources of pain in the neck
   Identify contributing anatomic structures
   Understand "injury" of the relevant anatomic structures
   Clinical, engineering, and physiology research fields

2. Neck pain research
   Physiologic characterization of neck pain responses
   Clinical and physiology research fields

3. Painful neck injury mechanisms
   In vivo loading to relevant anatomic structures
   Characterization of the physiologic responses of persistent neck pain
   Clinical, engineering, and physiology research fields

4. Treatment and management
   Behavioral hypersensitivity attenuation
   Pharmacologic treatments
   Clinical and physiology research fields

cyclooxygenase-2) have shown effectiveness in animal pain models for attenuating both behavioral hypersensitivity and elements of the CNS neuroimmune cascade (78–82). Indeed, combinations of some of these agents have been shown to have increased effectiveness in reducing pain.

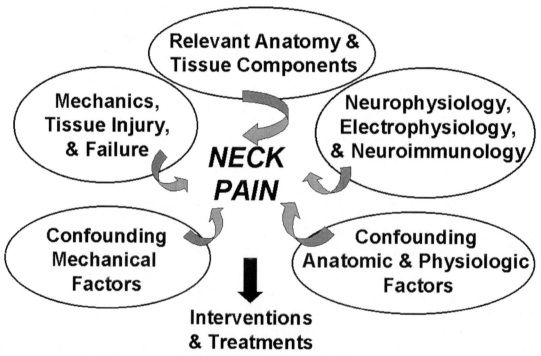

FIG. 8.5. Further requirements needed for development of a truly complete understanding of neck pain and its mechanisms. Such an understanding requires considering the relevant anatomy, biomechanics, and physiology, and the appropriate factors that confound each of these areas. Along with such an integrated understanding will come information useful to the prevention and treatment of painful syndromes of the neck.

As continued research identifies the specific physiologic pathways (both electrophysiologic and immunologic) that are responsible for chronic pain, it will become more feasible and even more tractable to target specific sites along these pathways for selectively manipulating and modulating a persistent pain response. Given the complex nature of these nociceptive responses, there is likely no single agent that offers a cure-all for neck pain. However, with continued integrative efforts, progress will be made in this area.

What clearly emerges from this discussion is a picture of what is missing in this area. Much remains unknown about the specific nature of neck injuries and their development of chronic pain (Table 8.2). Although clinical, biomechanical, and basic science researchers have worked separately to clarify the contributions to pain, injury, and nociceptive responses in each of these areas, it is imperative that these communities begin to work together to develop a more integrative and therefore more complete understanding of neck pain injuries and chronic pain mechanisms (Fig. 8.5 and Table 8.2). The development of a clinically relevant *in vivo* model of neck pain would undoubtedly increase our understanding of neck pain. Also needed are efforts to begin to definitively determine the relation of mechanical injury to many neck structures and their physiologic pain response. Without these efforts, the understanding of neck pain will remain at its current state, which is more inferential than conclusive.

ACKNOWLEDGMENT

This work was supported by the National Institute of Neurological Disorders and Stroke grant NS11161.

REFERENCES

1. National Highway Traffic Safety Administration, Office of Crashworthiness Standards. *Head restraints: identification of issues relevant to regulation, design, and effectiveness.* Washington, DC: US Department of Transportation, 1996.
2. Yoshizawa H, O'Brien JP, Smith WT, et al. The neuropathology of intervertebral discs removed for low-back pain. *J Pathol* 1980;132:95–104.
3. Ashton IK, Roberts S, Jaffray DC, et al. Neuropeptides in the human intervertebral disc. *J Orthop Res* 1994;12:186–192.
4. McCarthy PW, Petts P, Hamilton A. RT97- and calcitonin gene-related peptide-like immunoreactivity in lumbar intervertebral discs and adjacent tissue from the rat. *J Anat* 1992;18:15–24.
5. Kojima Y, Maeda T, Arai R, et al. Nerve supply to the posterior longitudinal ligament and the intervertebral disc of the rat vertebral column as studied by acetylcholinesterase histochemistry. I. Distribution in the lumbar region. *J Anat* 1990;169:237–246.
6. Cavanaugh JM. Neurophysiology and neuroanatomy of neck pain. In: Yoganandan N, Pintar FA, eds. *Frontiers in whiplash trauma: clinical and biomechanical.* Amsterdam: IOS Press, 2000:79–96.
7. Yamashita T, Cavanaugh JM, El-Bohy A, et al. Mechanosensitive afferent units in the lumbar facet joint. *J Bone Joint Surg Am* 1990;72:865–870.
8. Mense S, Meyer H. Different types of slowly-conducting afferent units in cat skeletal muscle and tendon. *J Physiol* 1985;363:403–417.
9. Spitzer WO, Skovron ML, Salmi LR, et al. Scientific monograph of the Quebec task force on whiplash-associated disorders: redefining "whiplash" and its management. *Spine* 1995;20:1S–73S.
10. Siegmund GP, Brault JR. Role of cervical muscles during whiplash. In: Yoganandan N, Pintar FA, eds. *Frontiers in whiplash trauma: clinical and biomechanical.* Amsterdam: IOS Press, 2000:295–320.
11. Kiefer SA, Heitzman ER, eds. *An atlas of cross-sectional anatomy.* Hagerstown, MD: Harper & Row, 1979.
12. Winkelstein BA, Myers BS. The cervical motion segment, combined loading, and the facet joint: a mechanical basis for whiplash injury. In: Yoganandan N, Pintar FA, eds. *Frontiers in whiplash trauma: clinical and biomechanical.* Amsterdam: IOS Press, 2000:248–262.
13. Lang J. *Clinical anatomy of the cervical spine.* New York: Thieme Medical Publishers, 1993.
14. McLain RF. Mechanoreceptor endings in human cervical facet joints. *Spine* 1994;19:495–501.
15. Giles LGF, Harvey AR. Immunohistochemical demonstration of nociceptors in the capsule and synovial folds of human zygapophyseal joints. *Br J Rheumatol* 1987;26:362–364.
16. Inami S, Shiga T, Tsujino A, et al. Immunohistochemical demonstration of nerve fibers in the synovial fold of the human cervical facet joint. *J Orthop Res* 2001;19:593–596.
17. Cavanaugh JM, Ozaktay AC, Yamashita T, et al. Mechanisms of low back pain: a neurophysiologic and neuroanatomic study. *Clin Orthop* 1997;335:166–180.
18. Howe JF, Loeser JD, Calvin WH. Mechanosensitivity of dorsal root ganglia and chronically injured axons: a physiological basis for the radicular pain of nerve root compression. *Pain* 1977;3:25–41.
19. Kawakami M, Weinstein JN. Associated neurogenic and nonneurogenic pain mediators that probably are activated and responsible for nociceptive input. In: Weinstein J, Gordon S, eds. *Low back pain: a scientific and clinical overview.* Rosemont, IL: AAOS, 1986:265–273.
20. Fukuoka H, Kawatani M, Hisamitsu T, et al. Cutaneous hyperalgesia induced by peripheral injection of interleukin-1β in the rat. *Brain Res* 1994;657:133–140.
21. Perkins MN, Kelly D. Interleukin-1β induced desarg9bradykinin-mediated thermal hyperalgesia in the rat. *Neuropharmacology* 1994;33:657–660.
22. DeLeo JA, Winkelstein BA. Physiology of chronic spinal pain syndromes: from animal models to biomechanics. *Spine* 2002;27:2526–2530.
23. Coderre TJ, Katz J, Vaccarino A, et al. Contribution of central neuroplasticity to pathological pain: review of clinical and experimental evidence. *Pain* 1993;52:259–285.
24. Dubner R, Basbaum AI. Spinal dorsal horn plasticity following tissue or nerve injury. In: Wall PD, Melzak R, eds. *Textbook of pain.* Edinburgh: Churchill-Livingstone, 1994:225–241.
25. Woolf CJ. Evidence for a central component of post-injury pain hypersensitivity. *Nature* 1983;306:686–688.
26. Devor M. Pain arising from the nerve root and the dorsal root ganglion. In: Weinstein J, Gordon S, eds. *Low back pain: a scientific and clinical overview.* Rosemont, IL: AAOS, 1986:187–208.
27. Cook AJ, Woolf CJ, Wall PD, et al. Dynamic receptive field plasticity in rat spinal cord dorsal horn following C-primary afferent input. *Nature* 1987;325:151–153.
28. DeLeo JA, Yezierski RP. The role of neuroinflammation and neuroimmune activation in persistent pain. *Pain* 2001;91:1–6.
29. DeLeo J, Colburn R. The role of cytokines in nociception and chronic pain. In: Weinstein J, Gordon S., eds. *Low back pain: a scientific and clinical overview.* Rosemont, IL: AAOS, 1986:163–185.
30. DeLeo J, Colburn R, Nichols M, et al. Interleukin (IL)-6 mediated hyperalgesia/allodynia and increased spinal IL-6 in two distinct mononeuropathy models in the rat. *J Interferon Cytokine Res* 1996;16:695–700.
31. Watkins L, Maier S, Goehler L. Immune activation: the role of proinflammatory cytokines in inflammation, illness responses, and pathological pain states. *Pain* 1995;63:289–302.
32. Lewin G, Rueff A, Mendell L. Peripheral and central mechanisms of NGF-induced hyperalgesia. *Eur J Neurosci* 1994;6:1903–1912.
33. Woolf C, Safieh-Garabedian B, Ma Q, et al. Nerve growth factor contributes to the generation of inflammatory sensory hypersensitivity. *Neuroscience* 1994;62:277–331.
34. Arruda J, Colburn R, Rickman A, et al. Increase of interleukin-6 mRNA in the spinal cord following peripheral nerve injury in the rat: potential role of IL-6 in neuropathic pain. *Mol Brain Res* 1998;62:228–235.
35. Colburn R, DeLeo J. The effect of perineural colchicine on nerve injury-induced spinal glial activation and neuropathic pain behavior. *Brain Res Bull* 1999;49:419–427.

36. Rutkowski M, Pahl J, Sweitzer S, et al. Limited role of macrophages in generation of nerve injury-induced mechanical allodynia. *Physiol Behav* 2000;71:225–235.

37. Aprill C, Bogduk N. The prevalence of cervical zygapophyseal joint pain: a first approximation. *Spine* 1992;17:744–47.

38. Barnsley L, Lord S, Bogduk N. Whiplash injury. *Pain* 1994;58:283–307.

39. Bogduk N, Marsland A. The cervical zygapophyseal joints as a source of neck pain. *Spine* 1988;13:610–617.

40. Barnsley L, Lord S, Bogduk N. Comparative local anaesthetic blocks in the diagnosis of cervical zygapophyseal joint pain. *Pain* 1993;55:99–106.

41. Yang KH, King AI. Mechanism of facet load transmission as a hypothesis for low-back pain. *Spine* 1984;9:557–565.

42. Avramov AI, Cavanaugh JM, Ozaktay AC, et al. Effects of controlled mechanical loading on group II, III, and IV afferents from the lumbar facet: an *in vitro* study. *J Bone Joint Surg Am* 1992;74:1464–1471.

43. Cavanaugh JC, El-Bohy AA, Hardy WH, et al. Sensory innervation of soft tissues of the lumbar spine in the rat. *J Orthop Res* 1989;7:278–288.

44. Ono K, Kaneoka K, Wittek A, et al. Cervical injury mechanism based on the analysis of human cervical vertebral motion and head-neck-torso kinematics during low-speed rear impacts. In: *Proceedings of the 41st STAPP Car Crash Conference.* Warrendale, PA: Society of Automotive Engineers, 1997:339–356.

45. Kaneoka K, Ono K, Inami S, et al. Motion analysis of cervical vertebrae during simulated whiplash loading. Presented at the World Congress on Whiplash Associated Disorders, Vancouver, BC, February 7–11, 1999.

46. Panjabi MM, Cholewicki J, Nibu K, et al. Capsular ligament stretches during *in vitro* whiplash simulations. *J Spinal Disord* 1998;11:227–232.

47. Panjabi MM, Cholewicki J, Nibu K, et al. Simulation of whiplash trauma using whole cervical spine specimens. *Spine* 1998;23:17–24.

48. Yoganandan N, Pintar FA. Facet joint local component kinetics in whiplash trauma. *Adv Bioengineering* 1997;36:221–222.

49. Yoganandan N, Pintar FA, Cusick JF, et al. Head-neck biomechanics in simulated rear impact. In: *42nd Annual Proceedings of the AAAM.* Des Plaines, IA: AAAM, 1998:209–231.

50. Yoganandan N, Pintar FA. Biomechanical assessment of whiplash. In: Yoganandan N, Pintar FA, Larson SJ, et al., eds. *Frontiers in head and neck trauma.* Netherlands: IOS Press, 1998:344–373.

51. Winkelstein BA, Nightingale RW, Richardson WJ, et al. The cervical facet capsule and its role in whiplash injury: a biomechanical investigation. *Spine* 2000;25:1238–1246.

52. Winkelstein BA, Nightingale RW, Richardson WJ, et al. Cervical facet joint mechanics: its application to whiplash injury (99SC15). In: *Proceedings of the 43rd STAPP Car Crash Conference.* Warrendale, PA: Society of Automotive Engineers, 1999:243–252.

53. Siegmund GP, Myers BS, Davis et al. Mechanical evidence of cervical facet capsule injury during whiplash: a cadaveric study using combined shear, compression and extension loading. *Spine* 2001;26:2095–2101.

54. Winkelstein BA, McLendon RE, Barbir A, et al. An anatomic investigation of the cervical facet capsule quantifying muscle insertion area. *J Anat* 2001;198:455–461.

55. Nuckley DJ, Konodi MA, Raynak GC, et al. Neural space integrity of the lower cervical spine. Effect of normal range of motion. *Spine* 2002;27:587–595.

56. Aldman B. An analytical approach to the impact biomechanics of head and neck. In: *Proceedings of the 39th AAAM Conference.* Des Plaines, IA: AAAM, 1986:439–454.

57. Svensson MY, Aldman B, Lovsund P, et al. Pressure effects in the spinal canal during whiplash extension motion—a possible cause of injury to the cervical spinal ganglia. In: *Proceedings of the International IRCOBI Conference.* Eindhoven: SAE, 1993:189–200.

58. Ortengren T, Hansson H, Lovsund P, et al. Membrane leakage in spinal ganglion nerve cells induced by experimental whiplash extension motion: a study in pigs. *J Neurotrauma* 1996;13:171–180.

59. Cornefjord M, Sato K, Ohlmarker K, et al. A model for chronic nerve root compression studies. Presentation of a porcine model for controlled slow-onset compression with analyses of anatomic aspects, compression onset rate, and morphologic and neurophysiologic effects. *Spine* 1997;22:946–957.

60. Hanai F, Matsui N, Hongo N. Changes in responses of wide dynamic range neurons in the spinal dorsal horn after dorsal root or dorsal root ganglion compression. *Spine* 1996;21:1408–1415.

61. Skouen J, Brisby H, Otami K, et al. Protein markers in cerebrospinal fluid experimental nerve root injury. A study of slow-onset chronic compression effects or the biochemical effects of nucleus pulposus on sacral nerve roots. *Spine* 1999;24:2195–2200.

62. Yoshizawa H, Kobayashi S, Kubota K. Effects of compression on intraradicular blood flow in dogs. *Spine* 1989;14:1220–1225.

63. Hu S, Xing J. An experimental model for chronic compression of dorsal root ganglion produced by intervertebral foramen stenosis in the rat. *Pain* 1998;77:15–23.

64. Winkelstein BA, Weinstein JN, DeLeo JA. The role of mechanical deformation in lumbar radiculopathy: an *in vivo* model. *Spine* 2002;27:27–33.

65. Winkelstein BA, Rutkowski MD, Weinstein JN, et al. Quantification of neural tissue injury in a rat radiculopathy model: comparison of local deformation, behavioral outcomes, and spinal cytokine mRNA for two surgeons. *J Neurosci Meth* 2001;111:49–57.

66. Hashizume H, DeLeo J, Colburn R, et al. Spinal glial activation and cytokine expression following lumbar root injury in the rat. *Spine* 2000;25:1206–1217.

67. Winkelstein BA, DeLeo JA. Nerve root tissue injury severity differentially modulates spinal glial activation in a rat lumbar radiculopathy model: considerations for persistent pain. *Brain Res* 2002;956:294–301.

68. Vierck CJ, Siddall P, Yezierski RP. Pain following spinal cord injury: animal models and mechanistic studies. *Pain* 2000;89:1–5.

69. Burchiel KJ, Hsu FPK. Pain and spasticity after spinal cord injury. *Spine* 2001;26:S146–S160.

70. Yezierski RP. Pain following spinal cord injury: pathophysiology and central mechanisms. In: Sadkuhler J, Bromm B, Gebhart GF, eds. *Progress in brain research.* Amsterdam: Elsevier, 2000:429–449.

71. Hunt JL, Winkelstein BA, Rutkowski MD, et al. Repeated injury to the lumbar nerve roots produces enhanced mechanical allodynia and persistent spinal neuroinflammation. *Spine* 2001;26:2073–2079.

72. Miles KA, Maimaris C, Finaly D, et al. The incidence and prognostic significance of radiological abnormalities in soft tissue injuries to the cervical spine. *Skeletal Radiol* 1988;17:493–496.

73. Maimaris C, Barnes MR, Allen MJ. Whiplash injuries of the neck: a retrospective study. *Injury* 1988;19:393–396.

74. Watkinson A, Gargan MF, Bannister GC. Prognostic factors in soft tissue injuries of the cervical spine. *Injury* 1991;22:307–309.

75. Radanov BP, Sturzenegger M, DiStefano G. Long-term outcome after whiplash injury. *Medicine* 1995;74:281–297.

76. Sturtzenegger M, Radanov BP, DiStefano G. The effect of accident mechanisms and initial findings on the long-term course of whiplash injury. *J Neurol* 1995;242:443–449.

77. Petterson K, Karrholm J, Toolanen G, et al. Decreased width of the spinal canal in patients with chronic symptoms after whiplash injury. *Spine* 1995;20:1664–1667.

78. Winkelstein BA, Rutkowski MD, Sweitzer SM, et al. Nerve injury proximal or distal to the DRG induces similar spinal glial activation and selective cytokine expression but differential behavioral responses to pharmacological treatment. *J Comp Neurol* 2001;438:127–139.

79. Arruda J, Sweitzer S, Rutkowski M, et al. Intrathecal anti-IL-6 antibody and IgG attenuates peripheral nerve injury-induced mechanical allodynia in the rat. *Brain Res* 2000;879:216–225.

80. DeLeo J, Hashizume H, Rutkowski M, et al. Cyclooxygenase-2 inhibitor SC-236 attenuates mechanical allodynia following nerve root injury in rats. *J Orthop Res* 2000;18:977–982.

81. Hashizume H, Rutkowski M, Weinstein J, et al. Central administration of methotrexate reduces mechanical allodynia in an animal model of radiculopathy/sciatica. *Pain* 2000;87:159–169.

82. Sweitzer S, Martin D, DeLeo J. IL-1ra and sTNFr reduces mechanical allodynia and spinal cytokine expression in a model of neuropathic pain. *Neuroscience* 2001;103:529–539.

CHAPTER 9

Pharmacologic and Psychological Treatment of Chronic Pain

Bogdan P. Radanov

Different aspects that should be considered in the pharmacologic and psychological treatment of pain are related to the modulation of nociceptive impulses or signals. In addition, if pain becomes chronic, neither pharmacologic nor psychological treatment employed in isolation will lead to results that satisfy the patient. According to clinical experience, a combination of pharmacologic and psychological treatment of chronic pain frequently appears to be the best choice.

To understand the possibilities of pharmacologic and psychological treatment of pain, some knowledge of the basic mechanisms of pain may be necessary. In this regard, the molecular mechanisms involved in generating impulses or signals, referred to as *nociception,* as well as the processes of translation and modulation of these impulses in the central nervous system (CNS), appear of interest. In particular, the considerably complex processes involved in the modulation of nociceptive impulses that may be crucial in developing chronic pain deserve interest. All processes involved in generating and experiencing pain are very complex, and their comprehensive summary is beyond the scope of this chapter. Fortunately, several comprehensive reviews of the biological basis of pain exist, and the interested reader is encouraged to consult these (1–3). Here only a rough summary of the mechanisms will be provided.

THE GENERATION OF PAIN

There are considered to be three different mechanisms of pain: nociceptive, inflammatory, and neuropathic pain (3). The nociceptive impulse or signal originates from the electrical activity (action potential) of the peripheral terminals of unmyelinated C fibers and thinly myelinated Aδ fibers. Although there is no identifiable anatomic structure

in the periphery that would deserve the term *receptor,* these fibers are considered to contain receptors that are indeed ion channels sensitive to mechanical stimuli, protons, cold, or heat. Under circumstances potentially dangerous for tissue, these receptors may generate a nociceptive impulse or signal, which is an action potential perceived as pain. This is referred to as *nociceptive pain.*

Inflammatory pain, in contrast, is the result of a more complex process following tissue damage in which chemical mediators emerge (e.g., histamine, serotonin, bradykinin, prostaglandins, adenosine triphosphate, H$^+$, nerve growth factor, tumor necrosis factor-α, endothelins, interleukins). These chemical mediators are frequently referred to as "inflammatory soup" (1,3). These mediators act on free nerve terminals and generate an action potential (i.e., a nociceptive impulse or signal). In addition, in the inflammatory tissue, a complex reaction of small vessels and the surrounding tissue cells (e.g., mastocytes) occurs to activate or to modify the stimulus response of nociceptor afferents. In summary, tissue lesion due to trauma or inflammation initiates different biological processes that are responsible for generating the nociceptive impulses or signals. Accordingly, acute pain is considered to result from noxious (i.e., potentially harmful) messages arising from the activation of free unmyelinated or thinly myelinated terminals found in cutaneous, muscular, and joint tissues and in certain visceral structures (1).

Finally, neuropathic pain arises from different mechanisms in the peripheral or central nervous system (4). Sensitized nociceptors may induce changes in central processing, which may lead to spinal cord hyperexcitability in which input from mechanoreceptors by the Aβ fibers (e.g., touch) is perceived as pain. This phenomenon explains essential features of neuropathic pain such as hyperalgesia (intensity of pain that is higher than might be expected) and allodynia (pain that is perceived from an influence that is usually not perceived as painful, such as a slight blow on the skin). Reorganization in the dorsal horn, which is considered to result from C-fiber degeneration, seems responsible for allodynia and is provoked by the activity of Aβ fibers. Furthermore, particularly following nerve lesions, the sympathetic system may interact with spinal afferent neurons and further sensitize nociceptors (4,5).

The Role of Prostaglandins in Generating Pain Impulses

One of the central mechanisms in the generation of pain impulses that has been studied in considerable detail and is best understood is the synthesis of prostaglandins (Fig. 9.1). Because this process determines pain treatment in a considerable way, some aspects should be briefly mentioned here.

Damage of the cell's phospholipid membrane leads to a release of eicosanoids (e.g., free arachidonic acid), which are metabolized as shown in Figure 9.1. In this metabolism, prostaglandins are synthesized from phospholipids. As indicated in the figure, the enzyme cyclooxygenase (COX) plays a central role in this process. It is important to note that in the process of metabolism of phospholipids, different chemicals emerge. Some of these are eminently important for functioning of the organism (e.g., renal flow, function of the endothelium, gastric mucosa), whereas others, such as prostaglandins, are involved in the inflammatory reaction.

In acute pain, prostaglandins play a major role due to sensitization of receptors (free nerve terminals of C fibers and Aδ fibers) to the other chemical mediators of which the aforementioned "inflammatory soup" consists (1). Because prostaglandins are involved in the sensitization and activation of free nerve terminals, and because prostaglandins are synthesized by the enzyme COX, COX inhibitors became a frequent choice in the treatment of acute pain. Prostaglandins, in addition, help establish structural

changes in the synapses, thus increasing transmission in the synapses of the CNS, particularly in the dorsal horn of the spinal cord.

In summary, COX is important for pain in the acute phase. However, many of the exact mechanisms remain unknown. In chronic pain—that is, where there is no apparent tissue lesion or where an inflammatory reaction cannot be detected (rheumatoid arthritis may be an exception)—COX may be of limited importance. Accordingly, chronic pain appears to arise from other grounds.

Toward an Understanding of Chronic Pain: Modulation of Nociceptive Impulses

In 1965, Melzack and Wall (6) set a milestone in the understanding of the pain phenomenon with their gate-control theory. This theory was the first to integrate nociceptive impulses and the emotional and cognitive aspects of the experience of pain. Furthermore, gate-control theory offered a framework that contributed to comprehensively understanding how chronic pain may develop. This theory builds on anatomic structures and considers a so-called gate system in the dorsal horn of the spinal cord in which processing and modulation of the nociceptive impulse takes place. To understand this process, the simplified summary that follows may be helpful (Fig. 9.2).

As mentioned earlier, the nociceptive impulse reaches the dorsal horn of the spinal cord through unmyelinated C fibers and thinly myelinated Aδ-fibers, where they are switched to the second neuron (labeled "WDR Neuron" in Fig. 9.2 for wide-dynamic-range neuron, so called because it receives afferent input from different fibers). In addition, C and Aδ fibers simultaneously give collateral impulses to GABAergic and opioidergic neurons of the spinal cord (Fig. 9.2). By their action, GABAergic and opioidergic neurons reduce the excitatory influence on the WDR neuron and elevate stimulus threshold (i.e., the WDR neuron becomes inhibited). Simul-

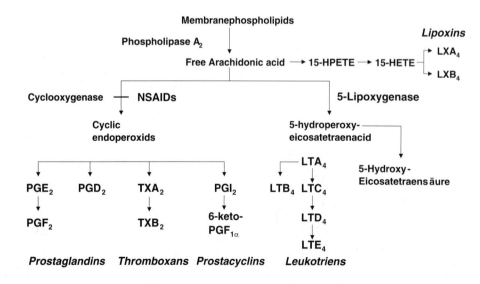

FIG. 9.1. Biosynthesis der eicosanoids. Adopted from K. Brune und B. Hinz (From, Brune K, Hinz B. Nichtopioidanalgetika (antipyretische Analgetika und andere) (German). In: Zenz M, Jurna I, eds. *Lehrbuch der Schmerztherapie.* Stuttgart: Wissenschaftliche Verlagsgesellschaft, 2001: 233–253.).

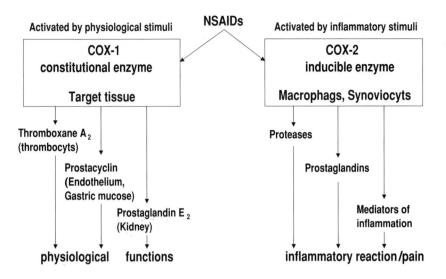

FIG. 9.2. Regulation of prostaglandinsynthesis by COX-1 und COX-2, according to Vane 1994 (From, Vane J. Towards a better aspirin. *Nature* 1994;367:215–216.).

taneously, descending pathways from the midbrain also act on WDR, GABAergic, and opioidergic neurons via norepinephrinergic (NE) and serotoninergic (5HT) pathways. These descending pathways thereby contribute to the inhibition of the WDR neuron. Because of these processes the nociceptive impulses are modified and passed up the spinal cord and through the thalamus to the cerebral cortex, where they are perceived as pain.

Once nociceptive impulses have entered the CNS (i.e., have passed through the gate), this information is spread out in different parts, including the spinal cord, medulla, and cortex. Because of this spreading of the nociceptive impulses, reflex phenomena are triggered (e.g., on the level of spinal cord), and endocrine reactions may follow (e.g., by the hypothalamus). Finally, the same impulses are processed in the brain cortex in terms of triggering cognitive and emotional activity. It is important to note in regard to descending modulation due to NE and 5HT that these neurotransmitters are critically involved in psychological functioning, mainly regulating the emotional and affective status of a person.

From the processes involved in the modulation of pain, the following conclusions may be drawn that appear to be of importance for treatment strategy in chronic pain.

1. The insufficient inhibitory modulation of the centripetal nociceptive impulses is central to the development of chronic pain.
2. Both physiologic and psychological influences execute an inhibitory modulation on the nociceptive impulses by the appropriate pathways and are responsible for the development of chronic pain.

Consequences of Insufficient Inhibitory Modulation: Central Sensitization

The modulation of nociceptive impulses as outlined earlier is indeed a restraining of the nociceptive impulse. Experimental investigations have shown that with therapy-resistant

or chronic pain, inhibitory modulation is insufficient (1). Research has also demonstrated that because of the inadequate inhibitory modulation of the nociceptive impulse, neurobiological changes of the WDR neuron may take place (1,7). These changes may occur in a considerably short time period and can be described briefly as follows.

The nociceptive impulses (e.g., through an inflammation or a peripheral lesion) arise as a result of a peripheral lesion in which chemical mediators mentioned previously in the so-called "inflammation soup" play a role. These mediators generate the nociceptive impulses (C and Aδ fibers), which stimulate the WDR neuron. The sustained nociceptive stimulation of the WDR neuron (mainly by the glutamatergic C fibers) results in a sustained depolarization (i.e., excitation) of this neuron.

In this process, the binding of the C fibers' glutamate on the WDR neuron's N-methyl-D-aspartate (NMDA) receptor is crucial. This receptor is responsible for controlling calcium ion channels. The opening of calcium ion channels, among other actions, sets the second-messenger system in motion, followed by the transcription of the genetic information and an increased gene expression (by the so-called immediate early genes). This expression is followed by an increased reproduction of NMDA receptors on the WDR neuron. This appears to be a biologically meaningful mechanism, which should protect the WDR neuron from excessive stimulation. However, the increased density of NMDA receptors on the WDR neuron can result in changes in the biological characteristics of this neuron. The consequences of this may be as follows:

1. Because there is a higher density of the NMDA receptors on the WDR neuron, many presynaptic impulses (which are numerous) can contribute to the sustained depolarization of this neuron. In relation to chronic pain, the most important consequence is that due to aforementioned changes in the WDR neuron, nonnociceptive impulses may excite this neuron, to be perceived as pain.

2. As a result of the biological changes that have taken place, the WDR neuron shows an unusually high spontaneous discharge, which again is perceived as pain.

The mentioned biological changes are also known as the *windup phenomenon* and represent the basis of central sensitization (1,8). The process of central sensitization is currently thought to have considerable importance in the development of chronic pain. Given central sensitization, and in particular the fact that the described biological changes of the WDR neuron can take place rapidly (7), an important aspect of pain treatment is the prevention of central sensitization or its reversal.

It must be kept in mind that under some circumstances the WDR neuron may change its biological properties to either fire at a higher rate or fire under the influence of many other afferent impulses. In this case, even nonnociceptive impulses may lead to pain (e.g., a simple movement of a limb, slight pressure on tissue). This gives the impression of oversensitivity, in which pain results even from inadequate influences (i.e., those that are usually nonpain-provoking), which may be seen as a psychological problem of the patient. Indeed, this frequent clinical observation is based on a hypersensitivity of the CNS. If a hypersensitivity becomes established, treating pain with only pharmacologic agents may become increasingly problematic.

Conclusions for Treatment of Chronic Pain

Because chronic pain results from changes in the biological properties of the WDR neuron, the principal issue becomes acting on modulation (i.e., down-regulation of the impulse ratio). Careful consideration of previously mentioned facts would indicate that in treating chronic pain the exclusive prescription of prostaglandin synthesis inhibitors will be of limited value. These agents may have some influence on nociceptive impulses if they occur in chronic pain (e.g., in rheumatoid arthritis, where continuous tissue damage may take place). An additional positive effect of COX inhibitors may be in reducing the rate of synaptic transmission in the CNS, which, as mentioned, is under some influence of prostaglandins.

More important to note, treating chronic pain using only pharmacologic agents may fail because the doses required for complete analgesia may be over the toxic level. The benefit of using only nonsteroidal antiinflammatory drugs (NSAIDs) for treatment of chronic pain is limited because they cannot influence down-regulation of the WDR neuron. These considerations indicate that in chronic pain the pharmacologic treatment will have to focus on different pharmaceutical substances, and that nonpharmacologic strategies may be helpful. Given the fact that in many chronic pain syndromes the down-regulation of the WDR neuron is required, opioids rather than NSAIDs may be employed.

PHARMACOLOGIC TREATMENT OF CHRONIC PAIN

Opioids

In acute pain, particularly postoperative or other severe pain, and in moderate to severe chronic pain, opioids appear to be the drug of choice. This is clearly supported by a huge clinical experience. The choice of an opioid, the route of administration, and sometimes changes between the drugs should be carefully considered. Opioids (the name comes from *opium,* which is the Greek term for "juice," that is, the extract from the poppy plant) are a group of morphinelike substances with primarily analgesic properties.

How Opioids Work

The pharmacologic effects of all opioids are based on their interactions with the three opioid receptors—mu (μ), kappa (κ), and delta (δ)—which were discovered in the early 1970s. The mu receptor is the principal structure of opioids' analgesic action. Opioid receptors exist in the periphery, in the spinal dorsal horn, in the brainstem, the thalamus, and the cortex. The effects of opioids include a decrease of presynaptic transmitter release, hyperpolarization of postsynaptic neurons, and disinhibition.

The discovery of opioid receptors introduced the search for endogenous substances that may be responsible for modulation of action. This research identified enkephalins, endorphins, and dynorphins. As a further consequence of this research in the 1980s, precursor molecules of endogenous opioid-receptor agonists were identified: proenkephalin, proadrenocorticotropic hormone (pro-ACTH), ACTH endorphin (proopiomelanocortin), and prodynorphin. The endogenous opioids are localized as follows: Enkephalin is found in the amygdala, hypothalamus, the midbrain periaqueductal gray matter, the rostroventral medulla, and the dorsal horn of the spinal cord; β-endorphin is mainly found in the hypothalamic arcuate nucleus and the midbrain periaqueductal gray matter. Dynorphins have a similar distribution to that of enkephalins (9).

According to the distribution of opioid receptors and endogenous opioids, the main site of action of opioids is at the spinal and supraspinal levels. Spinal and supraspinal mechanisms of opioid action are synergic. In addition, the fact that opioid receptors exist in the periphery suggests that opioids likely act on structures outside the CNS as well. Opioids should be used for moderate or severe nociceptive pain. However, their efficacy in neuropathic pain seems to be poorly supported by clinical experience.

Genetic Variations in Opioid Receptors

It is well established that there are genetic variations of the mu receptor (10), which are considered responsible for differences in the receptor affinity of different opioids and accordingly contribute to their analgesic potential. It has been hypothesized (11), although not proved, that the side effects of opioids (nausea, vomiting, sedation, and in some cases hallucinations) are connected to opioids' different receptor affinity.

Choice of Opioid and Route of Administration

According to their affinity to opioid receptors, opioids are classified into the following groups: agonists, partial agonists (e.g., buprenorphine), agonists/antagonists (e.g., butorphanol, nalbuphine, pentazocine, dezocine), and antagonists (e.g., naloxone, naltrexone, cholecystokinin). Not all substances with opioid-receptor affinity are employed in treatment, which is mainly based on a cost-effectiveness analysis in which the balance between effect and side effects is crucial. The most widely used opioids are summarized in Table 9.1, which includes dosages and some additional comments.

The main advantage of opioids in the treatment of pain is their excellent and quickly realized analgesia in moderate and severe pain. The initiation of opioid treatment, in particular when the parenteral route of administration is preferred, should be performed by an experienced professional using adequate equipment.

There is usually no ceiling effect of opioids (i.e., increased dosage provides increased analgesia). Opioids are available in different forms and can be administered by oral, sublingual, rectal, parenteral, intraspinal, or transdermal application. In severe acute pain, parenteral administration (preferably intravenous, which gives the possibility for better titration) should take place. In chronic pain, the parenteral administration of opioids should be omitted and long-acting opioid forms preferred. Morphine is still a standard, and the belief that drugs other than morphine may act faster, longer, or have fewer side effects seems unsupported based on clinical experience (11). The choice of opioid, tolerance, pain sensitivity to opioids, and the decision of whether to switch one opioid to another or to change the route of administration still remain matters of discussion (11).

Rotation of Opioids

In some patients, the therapeutic potential of one opioid may diminish. In these cases, a change to a different opioid (so-called rotation) may be necessary. This is usually done in the following way. First, an equivalent dosage to the dosage of the opioid that is being replaced should be found according to existing equivalency tables. Equivalencies are based on intramuscular morphine doses in opioid-naive individuals; these may vary considerably in patients treated with opioids over a longer period of time. For this reason, the new opioid should be started at 50% of the equivalent dosage and increased step by step according to its analgesic effect and side effects. However, changing the route of administration has demonstrated improvement in analgesic effect (12), which may make rotation unnecessary.

Disadvantages and Side Effects of Opioid Treatment

The main side effects are nausea and vomiting, obstipation, and CNS activity (euphoria or suppression/inhibition of different kinds). Side effects can be understood by considering that the same opioid receptors (mainly mu and particularly kappa receptors) mediate both analgesia and physiologic phenomena. Some active metabolites may contribute to adverse effects; for example, norpethidine may cause tremor or convulsions, normeperidine has some seizure potential, and morphine-6-glucuronide may be toxic, particularly in patients with impaired renal function. If compared on the basis of the same degree of analgesia, opioids seem not to differ in their adverse effects (11). Constipation is a side effect of all opioids and is based on central and peripheral receptor affinity. Tolerance for this side effect is not confirmed, which requires adequate treatment in patients suffering from it (e.g., stool softeners or laxatives). Furthermore, patients may experience problems in the urinary system (bladder spasm, urinary retention or urgency). Muscular problems such as spasms may cause agitation or anxiety.

The introduction of opioids in the treatment of chronic pain may be compromised by the belief that these drugs may cause respiratory depression and frequently and unavoidably lead to tolerance and dependence. However, there is suggestion that nociceptive input in the respiratory center counterbalances respiratory depressant potential (13), indicating that patients suffering from severe pain may have a lower risk for respiratory depression. Carefully titrated and well-timed doses of opioids of appropriate size prevent respiratory depression (11). (Observation is recommended while using fentanyl intravenously.) Respiratory depression, if it occurs at all, usually occurs within 10 minutes of intravenous administration, 30 minutes of intramuscular administration, or 90 minutes of subcutaneous administration. Respiratory depression is the most dangerous side effect due to depression of the CNS and may be anticipated by other symptoms, such as drowsiness, mental clouding, or severe sedation.

Some of the opioids (e.g., meperidine) may cause excitation or seizures (a possible consequence of its metabolite normeperidine). Other relatively frequent side effects (in particular, with higher doses) are myoclonus or clonic spasm of a single muscle or group of muscles. The emetic side effect usually occurs in the initial phase of treatment, and tolerance to it is observed in most patients (11). Nausea and vomiting are caused by the stimulation of the chemoreceptor trigger zone. They can be managed by antiemetics, but there are a few cases of nonmanageable nausea or vomiting that may require change to another opioid or even discontinuation of opioids.

TABLE 9.1. *Opioids in Treatment of Chronic Pain*

Drug name	Average single dose*	Recommended average 24 hours dose†	Proposed dosing interval	Comment
Opioids for mild to moderate pain				
Codein	15–50 mg	200 mg	4 to 6 hours	Short action, weak analgesic.
Dextropropoxyphen	65 mg	150–300 mg	8 to 12 hours	In some contries, controlled release form available with 12 hours dosing interval.
Dihydrocodein	60–120 mg	120–240 mg	3 to 4 hours (12 hours)	In some contries, controlled release form available with recommended 8 to 12 hours dosing interval.
Tilidin	50–100 mg	200–300 mg	2 to 3 hours (8 to 12 hours)	
Tramadol	50–100 mg	up to 400–600 mg	2 to 4 hours (8 to 12 hours)	Different forms available in some countries (oral, subcutaneous, intravenous, rectal, and controled release). In some contries easilly prescribed because no particular prescription regulations. Potent sedation. Frequent nausea/vomiting.
Opioids for moderate to severe pain				
Buprenorphine	0.2–0.4 mg	?	6 to 8 hours	Doses over 4 mg to not show higher analgesia.
Fentanal	50–100 micrograms		0.5 to 1 hour	Quick onset of action, short half-life. Very potent analgesic. Respiratory depression may not be obvious for minutes. Different application forms.High comfort with transdermal application form in different doses with 72 hours analgesic action. In some patients considerable side effects (e.g. nausea/vomiting).
Hydromorphone	1.5 mg (oral 7.5 mg)		3 to 4 hours	Quick onset of action, short half-life. Very potent analgesic. Different application forms.
Levophanol	2 mg (oral 4 mg)		6 to 8 hours	High analgesic potential. Careful dose titration. May considerably accumulate.
Meperidine	100 mg	300 mg	2 to 3 hours (8 to 12 hours)	Toxic metabolite, which may provoke seizures.
Methadone	10 mg (oral 20 mg)	30–40 mg	6 to 8 hours	Short analgesic action, long half-life. May accumulate with dose increase to cause toxic effect.
Morphium	10 mg (oral 30 mg)		3 to 4 hours	Standard opioid. In many aspects "gold standard" to which analgesic effect of other opioids is compared in terms of equianalgesic potential. Different application forms include controled release with long-term action.
Pethidin	50 mg (oral 150 mg)	recomm. max. 500 mg	3 to 4 hours	Different application forms. Active metabolite Norpethidin is potentially toxic. First-pass efect is significant. Cautious in hepatic failure.
Propoxyphene			3 to 6 hours	Not recommended for routine administration. Toxic metabolite.

Comments: Some of opioids in the table are not available in all coutries. Some of theese drugs exist in different application forms (e.g. for intravenous, rectal, transdermal use or controled release form) of which all forms are not available in all countries. In addition, all countries have specific restrictions for prescription of opioids which are imperative to follow. Furthermore, in every single patient general aspects in prescription using side and adverse effects, development of tolerance and dependence should be taken into consideration and related to the individual patient's disposition. It is highly recommended that treatment with opioids, in particular those with high analgesic potential, is restricted to experienced professionals. This is particularly recommended for initiation of treatment with opioids.

All opioid analgesics should not be taken in combination with monoamino-oxydase inhibitors (MAOI) because of dangerous side effects (e.g. respiratory depression, hypertension) some of which may be lethal.

*Considerable differences in recommended average single dose should be considered in drugs with different application forms, where for example intravenous, subcutaneous or intramuscular dose is usually significantly lower then oral dose.

†Opioids have no ceiling effect. For this reason the recommended average 24 hours dose should be understood relatively.

Tolerance and Dependence

The exact percentage of patients who show tolerance and dependence following prolonged use of opioids is not known. Clinical experience suggests that tolerance to opioids develops more rapidly when using a parenteral route of administration, in particular with substances with a short half-life. In addition, psychological effects may be responsible for development of tolerance and the requirement of higher doses. Patients who develop tolerance usually complain of decreased duration of analgesic effect. Clinical experience indicates that in patients in whom relief of pain has been achieved with opioids, drug-seeking behavior does not occur (14). Rapid discontinuation of opioids will induce a withdrawal syndrome that may include agitation, anxiety, insomnia, tremor, tachycardia, muscle cramps, yawning, lacrimation, fever, and different signs of hyperexcitability of the sympathetic nervous system. Pain insensitive to opioids is not very frequent but may occur in both cancer patients and in noncancer pain (usually nerve compression or nerve destruction).

Nonopioid Analgesics in Treatment of Pain

Nonsteroidal Antiinflammatory Drugs

Because prostaglandins are critically involved in the generation of nociceptive impulses, prostaglandin synthesis inhibitors (i.e., inhibitors of cyclooxygenase) play a key role in the treatment of acute pain. In acute pain (in particular, in mild to moderate pain), many of these substances show excellent analgesic effect, similar to that of weak opioids. The prescription of NSAIDs is not followed by a development of tolerance and subsequent dependence. These substances are easily available and are usually inexpensive (this is particularly true for nonselective COX inhibitors). However, their specific analgesic effect (in particular, in nonrheumatoid pain) is frequently poorly documented because studies with NSAIDs were mainly conducted with patients suffering from rheumatoid arthritis. In these studies, parameters other than pain (e.g., inflammation of joints) were used as the main criteria of effectiveness.

It is well recognized that the antiinflammatory action and analgesic effects of NSAIDs do not have a linear relation (15). This makes it difficult to understand the analgesic effect of NSAIDs as being based mainly on prostaglandin synthesis inhibition. The prescription of NSAIDs in chronic severe pain is likely to need careful reassessment. For example, some studies indicate that the analgesic effect of NSAIDs may result from an action in the CNS (16).

Problems with Prostaglandins and Cyclooxygenase in Pain and Its Treatment

As mentioned earlier, COX appears to have at least two isoenzymes, COX-1 and COX-2, which have different biological properties (Fig. 9.3). COX-1 mainly activates

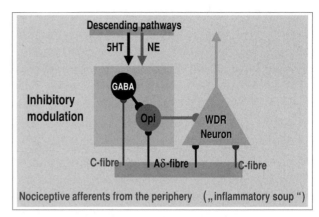

FIG. 9.3. Gate-Control Theory: Scheme of modulation of the nociceptive impulses.

physiologic functions in different tissues, whereas COX-2 is responsible for inflammatory reactions. The adverse effects of traditional NSAIDs and salicylates, which inhibit both COX-1 and COX-2, are related to their inhibition of COX-1, which (among other physiologic functions) synthesizes gastroprotective substances (17,18).

The antiinflammatory and accordingly analgesic effect of NSAIDs used to be connected to the inhibition of COX-2-dependent pathways. This led to development of COX-2 inhibitors, which were introduced for treatment of rheumatoid arthritis. Apart from antiinflammatory action and the assumption that chemical mediators resulting from the inflammatory process are essential in generating pain, COX-2 inhibitors showed fewer of the adverse effects frequently observed with classical NSAIDs, such as effects in the upper gastrointestinal tract (17,18) or bleeding (19). Based on their antiinflammatory action, COX-2-inhibitors were introduced for treatment of different pain conditions as well. It has been thought that selective inhibition of COX-2, which synthesizes prostaglandins, might provide essential advantages in treatment of pain, whereas the possible negative effects resulting from COX-1 inhibition might be prevented. However, selective COX-2 inhibitors (i.e., selective inhibitors of prostaglandin synthesis) did not fulfill expectations; in particular, they did not show superior analgesic effect when compared with nonselective COX inhibitors (20). More recently, it has been suggested that selective COX-2 inhibitors are less analgesic then nonselective COX inhibitors (19–21). The role of selective COX-2 inhibitors in pain may further appear confused by the fact that acetaminophen, a potent analgesic drug, has almost nonexistent ability to inhibit COX-1 or COX-2. In addition, one previously considered advantage of COX-2—namely, its safety in the long term—has become increasingly questioned (22,23).

More recently, a variant of COX-1, COX-3, has been identified as an inducible isoenzyme expressed in the later stages of inflammation (24). Interestingly, acetaminophen, a substance with fair analgesic effect, has some affinity to

TABLE 9.2. *Nonopioid Analgesics in Treatment of Chronic Pain*

Chemical class	Generic name	Average single dose	Recommended dose 24 hours dose	Proposed dosing interval	Comment
Para-aminophenol derivates	Acetaminophen	500–1,000 mg	4,000 mg	4 to 6 hours	Overdosage leads to hepatotoxicity. Careful administration in chronic alcoholism
Salicylates Acetylated	Aspirin	500–1,000 mg	4,000 mg	4 to 6 hours	Inhibition of platelet aggregation. Competes with NSIAD on protein binding with potential toxic effect. Gastrointestinal bleeding and ulceration.
Nonacetylated	Diflunisal	1,000 mg	1,500 mg	12 hours	Gastrointestinal intolerance and bleeding (less then aspirin)
	Salsalate	1,500 mg	2,000–3,000 mg	8 to 12 hours	Usual side effects of NSAID may occur.
Propionic acid derivates	Ibuprofen	400–600 mg	2,400 mg	4 to 6 hours	Usual side effects of NSAID may occur. Better tolerated then aspirin with less gastrointestinal side effects. Low incidence of hepatotoxicity.
Arylacetic acid derivates	Naproxen	250–500 mg	1,250 mg		Usual side effects of NSAID may occur. Long-term safety unknown.
Phenylalcanoid acid derivates	Fenoprofen	200 mg	800 mg	4 to 6 hours	Usual side effects of NSAID may occur.
	Ketoprofen	50–75 mg	300 mg	6 to 8 hours	Usual side effects of NSAID may occur.
	Flurbiprofen	100 mg	200 mg	6 to 8 hours	Usual side effects of NSAID may occur.
Acetic acid derivates	Indomethacin	25–50 mg	100–200 mg	6 to 12 hours	Gastric mucose inflammation, or necrosis with bleeding. Careful administration in positive history of gastric bleeding. In some patients irritation possible.
Pyranocarboxilic acid derivates	Etodolac	300–600 mg	600–1,200 mg		High gastrointestinal toxicity may be observed.
Indene derivates	Tolmetin	200–600 mg	1,800 mg	6 to 8 hours	Usual side effects of NSAID may occur.
	Sulindac	150–200 mg	400 mg	12 hours	Good analgesic, usually well tolerated.
	Diclofenac	50–75 mg	200 mg	6 to 8 hours	Frequently considered first choice NSAID.
Antranilacid derivates Fenamate	Mefenacid	500 mg	500–1,500 mg	6 to 8 hours	May cause upper gastrointestinal problems. If tolerated shows good analgesia.
Keto-enol acid derivates Oxicams	Piroxicam	20 mg	20–40 mg	24 hours	Renal parameters control recommended in cases with longer administration
	Tenoxicam	20 mg	20–40 mg	12 to 24 hours	Upper gastrointestinal tract side effects may be frequent leading to intolerance and complianace problems.
Pirazolidindions	Meloxicam	7.5 mg	7.5–15 mg	12 to 24 hours	Must be avoided in hepatic failure. Careful control of renal parameters may be recommended.
Other derivates	Phenylbutazon	200 mg	200–60 mg	12 hours	Gastrointestinal, renal side effector bronchial spasms may be frequent.
Pyrazolinons	Nimesulid	200 mg	400 mg	12 hours	Should not be taken in patients with positive history of gastro-intestinal bleeding or renal failure.
	Phenazon	200 mg	600–800 mg	4 to 6 hours	Must be avoided in hapatic or renal failure. May cause allergy.
	Propyphenazon	250 mg	500–750 mg	4 to 6 hours	Contraindicated in a number of gastrointestinal problems incl. porphyria (list of disorders to indicate restriction in use should be individually taken into account).
Pyridilcarbamat	Metamizol	500–1,000 mg	4,000 mg	4 to 6 hours	May cause thrombocytopenia, leucopenia or agranulocytose.
	Flupirtin	100 mg	300 mg	6 to 8 hours	
Coxibs (COX-2 inhibitors)	Rofecoxib	12.5–25 mg	25–50 mg	once daily	Different doses for acute or chronic pain are recommended. Advantages emerge mainly from selectivity or lack of inhibition of COX-1 (e.g. gastrointestinal or renal side effects).
	Celecoxib	100 mg	100–200 mg	once daily	May have significant interactions due to blockage of different lines of the cytochrom-P-450-enzymes. Precise information of all medications patients uses is necessary. Advantages of COX-2-inhibitors. Clinical experience may indicate lower analgesic effect. Side effects seen in other coxibs may occur. Caution in renal or hepatic failure.
	Valdecoxib	10–40 mg			

Comments: This table contains the routinely usednon-opioid analgesics, frequently referred to as non-steroidal anti-inflammatory drugs (NSAID). Some of these pharmaceuticals are not available in all countries. In addition, some of this drugs, strictly taken do not belong to the group of NSAID. All probable side or toxic effects cannot not be mentioned. Most possible side effects could be understand if considering the mechanism of action of NSAID (see also figure 9.1—biosynthesis of eicosanoids). Before treatment in cases with history of adverse effects or presumed risk for adverse effects (in particular gastrointestinal or renal problems or asthma) careful choice of the drug and frequent clinical and laboratory controls may be imperative. Particularly careful use of NSAID is recommended in early pregnacy (many of these drugs are recommended to be avoided, for which acetaminophen may be exception). In all NSAID conrol of gastrointestinal, vascular, blood and renal parameters is recommended in particular in chronic use. Coxibs are frequently coinsidered to show little gastrointestinal side effects. Newer research may support the view that coxibs mainly have advantages in patient with a history of gastrointestinal bleeding. Many of substances in this table may cause allergic reaction.

block the COX-3 variant, which gives rise to speculation that this COX variant is considerably involved in pain. In addition, nonselective COX inhibitors (e.g., diclofenac, ibuprofen) show powerful COX-3 inhibition, which further indicates that the inhibition of this COX variant may be considerably important in the treatment of pain. More interesting, this COX variant is expressed both in the tissue and in the brain and spinal cord (25). This may give rise to hypotheses explaining the analgesic effect of nonselective COX inhibitors or acetaminophen.

Advantages of Nonsteroidal Antiinflammatory Drugs for the Treatment of Pain

NSAIDs are rapidly absorbed, highly protein bound, and have a considerably low tissue distribution. NSAIDs are metabolized in the liver and have a very low clearance (26). Salicylates compete with other NSAIDs on protein binding sites and may increase the concentration of some of these drugs, with toxicity as a potential consequence. Toxicity of NSAIDs is poorly documented because most studies were conducted with elderly patients. The influence of physiologic processes in the organism indicates that in chronic prescription of NSAIDs, physiologic parameters—in particular, renal function—should be controlled by laboratory examination from time to time.

Considering some recent critical reviews (3,27) and the biological basis of chronic pain discussed earlier in this chapter, prescription of NSAIDs in cases of chronic pain (apart from rheumatoid arthritis) may be seriously questioned.

Some frequently used NSAIDs are summarized in Table 9.2, which contains some recommendations for dosages and comments regarding substance-specific side effects.

Disadvantages and Side Effects

The most prominent disadvantage of NSAIDs is their toxicity, of which in the long term gastrointestinal intolerance and ulcerations are the most prominent manifestations. This problem, however, is mainly observed with chronic use, usually over months. In addition, the inhibition of COX enzymes by NSAIDs may compromise renal flow, with related consequences. These drugs do not show higher analgesic potential with increasing dosage (i.e., they show a ceiling effect), and their full efficacy usually occurs after several days. Furthermore, NSAIDs are usually not helpful in severe pain.

It is important to note that in contrast to acute pain, in which chemical mediators play an important role, chronic pain does not evidently involve these substances. Prescription of NSAIDs in chronic pain thus appears poorly justified. It should be considered that the lack of therapeutic efficacy may frustrate the patient and contribute to additional problems in treatment.

Acetaminophen and Methimazole

Acetaminophen and methimazole have many advantages. They do not show adverse effects on gastrointestinal tract mucosa, on the kidney, or on platelet aggregation. They may show analgesic effect in chronic pain (in cases with mild, sometimes moderate pain). Both drugs are usually well tolerated, with few side or toxic effects. Possible adverse effects are mentioned in Table 9.2.

Adjuvant Pharmacologic Treatment of Chronic Pain

In adjuvant treatment of chronic pain, a heterogeneous group of pharmaceuticals play a role and, based mainly on clinical observation, are believed to show some beneficial effect. However, recent reviews (27) seriously question the empirical basis of employing some of these pharmaceuticals in treatment of chronic pain. Adjuvant pharmacologic treatment seem to show advantages particularly if taken in combination with other pain-relieving substances.

Antidepressants

Most interest in adjuvant treatment of pain has focused on antidepressants. Introduction of antidepressants in pain treatment may be justified based on the fact that there is considerable involvement of descending (i.e., noradrenergic and serotonergic) pathways in the modulation of nociceptive impulses. Because these neurotransmitter pathways are inherently involved in regulation of patients' emotional status, their involvement may be of particular importance in patients who in addition to pain suffer from affective symptoms. Biologically speaking, these symptoms may indicate a relative insufficiency of descending modulatory neurotransmitter pathways (i.e., serotonin and norepinephrine). However, a systematic review (28) did not confirm benefit in treatment of chronic low back pain with these agents.

Nevertheless, the antidepressants—in particular, tricyclic agents (e.g., amitriptyline, usually in doses lower than used for treatment of clinical depression)—are considered important adjuvant agents in the treatment of chronic pain (29). It is believed that these agents may lead to relief of pain while improving mood, reducing the level of depression (if depression is present), and promoting sleep. It is important to note that sleep is frequently disturbed in chronic pain patients, and sleep disturbance may contribute to the vicious circle. In addition, it has been proposed that tricyclic antidepressants may have a direct effect on nociceptive afferents (e.g., by blocking sodium ion channels) and are particularly effective because they augment the analgesic response to opioids.

Neuropathic Pain Syndromes

A considerably specific treatment may be required for neuropathic pain syndromes (e.g., postherpetic pain, diabetic neuropathy, or pain due to damage of a plexus, nerve root, or single nerves). In neuropathic pain, NSAIDs are usually ineffective and even opioids do not always show sufficient analgesia. Previously these syndromes were treated using classic anticonvulsants (e.g., phenytoin, carbamazepine, clonazepam, gabapentin). In particular, newly developed anticonvulsants (e.g., gabapentin or even more recently developed substances, such as pregabalin) show considerable advantages in treatment of neuropathic syndromes (30). Gabapentin is usually well tolerated, with few side effects (e.g., headache, dizziness) that are mostly of limited duration, and has high efficacy in neuropathic pain. However, the maximum effect requires sufficient dosages (e.g., above 1,600 mg per day; most patients require dosages between 2,400 and 3,600 mg per day). Unfortunately, in clinical routines this caveat is frequently neglected, with the disadvantage that these difficult-to-treat syndromes continue.

Clinical observations indicate that a combination of tricyclics (which may be very effective in diabetic neuropathy), codeine, and newly developed anticonvulsants (e.g., gabapentin) may show a great benefit. Administration of antidepressants, anticonvulsants, and local anesthetics is advocated for neuropathic pain (11).

Muscle Relaxants

A systematic review identified muscle relaxants (either alone or in combination) as effective in treatment of pain associated with muscle spasm (31). However, their effect appears better supported in acute than in chronic musculoskeletal pain (32). Baclofen has recently been shown to be effective in neuropathic pain associated with dystonia (33).

Steroids

Corticosteroids are a further group of substances with analgesic effect that, usually in combination with other potent analgesics, may be used for rather specific indications (27). These indications include bone metastases, spinal cord compression, acute nerve compression, and increased intracranial pressure. Corticosteroids may be further indicated as epidural injections in disc herniation pain, spinal stenosis, or foraminal stenosis (both lumbar and cervical) (27).

Neuroleptics and Benzodiazepines

Previously, antidepressants and neuroleptics were frequently introduced in treatment of chronic pain. Usually, a combination of haloperidol and tricyclic antidepressants (e.g., amitriptyline) was used. This is no longer standard treatment in pain syndromes. Nowadays, neuroleptics or benzodiazepines are rarely introduced in the treatment of pain syndromes. Sometimes, neuroleptics (e.g., haloperidol in individually titrated doses of between 1 and 10 mg

or even more) may be required to help patients gain distance from severe pain, usually cancer pain. Neuroleptics are never used as single substances, but rather are used in combination with highly potent opioids. Benzodiazepines (e.g., alprazolam) may be ordered on a timely limited schedule in patients who suffer from anxiety in combination with their pain.

PSYCHOLOGICAL ASPECTS OF PAIN TREATMENT

According to the International Association for the Study of Pain [IASP (34)], pain is "an unpleasant sensory and emotional experience associated with actual and potential tissue damage, and described in terms of such damage." This definition includes the psychological dimension in both acute or chronic pain. Notwithstanding this definition, in clinical routine the investigation of a patient with pain first entails the search for a possible organic cause. As pointed out previously, pain is frequently considered exclusively as a nociceptive phenomenon (35). Interindividual differences in reporting pain following the same potentially pain-provoking procedure indicate impressively that nociception is not always associated with pain experience. In contrast, pain experience without nociception is a well-acknowledged phenomenon. Indeed, pain is a perceptual phenomenon but involves different CNS mechanisms for which nociception may by no means be necessary. Usually, if an organic cause for pain is not found, an underlying psychological cause is assumed and the patient is referred for psychological or psychiatric treatment.

The IASP definition's introduction of a psychological dimension in the experience of pain highlights that pain cannot be evaluated or treated irrespective of a person's disposition. To understand the person's disposition and to incorporate this aspect into treatment, the person's past and current situation must be focused on. From the patient's past, what is most important are particular circumstances under which emotional development occurred. Furthermore, personality factors (i.e., traits) (36,37) that may establish how the person copes with different difficulties are important. Assessing this, one may understand why current psychosocial disposition (e.g., marital and family situation, job-related factors) is important.

These very specific aspects of pain experience may require the involvement of an experienced psychotherapist, particularly in treatment. Recent studies clearly indicate that cognitive aspects may play the most important role in pain (38), of which focusing of attention appears of particular relevance (39). Based on this observation, distraction of attention is one of the most important psychological interventions in cognitive-behavioral treatment of pain. Distracting attention from pain-related factors may be helpful in acute pain conditions but may be difficult in chronic pain, where a sort of continuous attention distraction is required.

Basis of Psychological Treatment of Pain

To understand the psychological and behavioral aspects of pain in order to integrate them into treatment strategy, the following physical aspects should be briefly summarized: The nociceptive process begins when tissue damage occurs whereby the initial stimulus in the afferent nerve fibres is generated. This process is referred to as transduction. The generated action potential ascends to the cortex, a process that is referred to as transmission. In this process the signal (electrical impulse) first reaches the dorsal horn of the spinal cord. At this site the afferent nerve builds a synapse with the neuron of the spinothalamic tract (below the WDR neuron). In the spinothalamic tract, the signal continues to the thalamus and from there to various areas of the cortex. Once the signal reaches the cortex, pain is perceived, a process referred to as perception.

On different levels in the CNS, the nociceptive signal is modulated under the influence of different structures. Depending on this process of modulation, persons will experience pain in different ways, thus showing various somatic, psychosocial, and functional phenomena. These phenomena will influence behavior, that is, how a person reacts to pain experience (e.g., avoidance, withdrawal) and the manner in which pain and related distress is communicated to others (e.g., shouting, crying). Finally, pain may cause suffering that mainly is a result of the loss of different aspects that are inherently connected with an individual, such as functional ability, social status, or social role. Suffering is indeed a psychological or mainly emotional reaction to pain and may clarify why persons suffering from pain have an exaggeration in their behavior (fatigue, exhaustion, concentration, etc.).

Psychological Interventions

Psychological intervention should be focused on alleviating suffering. The first goal is improvement of emotional status, for which medication may be used. Second, strategies should be used for compensation of the experienced loss (e.g., alternative functions, supporting activities that may provide acknowledgment in the social environment and help to identify new roles and positive experiences). Finally, for patients in whom pain cannot be sufficiently influenced, improvement of the quality of life may become the main focus of psychological therapeutic intervention.

In the first instance, assessment of the emotional status of the patient is necessary. Many chronic pain patients suffer as discussed previously and will develop some sort of emotional or affective disturbance. Many studies indicate that patients suffering from chronic pain do not demonstrate symptoms of clinical depression (40–42) but rather symptoms that may be classified as a chronic form of adjustment disorder with mixed emotions according to the *Diagnostic and Statistical Manual of Mental Disorders,* Fourth Edition (43), which means that the most prominent symptoms are

dysphoria, irritability, anger, and sadness. These affective symptoms appear important to treat because affective disequilibrium may cause additional symptoms, such as vegetative symptoms (i.e., a somatic hypervigilance, sleep disturbances with a nonrestorative sleep, poor concentration, reduced libido). Many of these symptoms may eventually contribute to a vicious circle and lead to a nontreatable chronic disorder. For this reason, pharmacologic treatment of affective problems may be the first step at this stage.

Antidepressants may be the main treatment required. However, the choice of the drug and dosage should be carefully considered in order to avoid side effects in patients who frequently suffer from a severe form of somatic hypervigilance. Tricyclic antidepressants may show anticholinergic effects, and selective serotonin reuptake inhibitors may cause gastrointestinal problems or libido loss by their action on the postsynaptic terminals. Given the fact that clinical depression cannot be detected in a majority of these patients, lower doses of antidepressants may be the treatment of choice. Substances to positively influence sleep (e.g., amitriptyline, trimipramine) may be the best choice to start, in particular because an initial positive effect may strengthen the therapeutic alliance and profoundly influence the course of treatment.

Cognitive-Behavioral Therapy

Apart from treatment with antidepressants and, where necessary, with other psychopharmaceuticals, modern psychological therapy of chronic pain is mainly based on cognitive-behavioral therapy. This therapy considers that pain is not simply a sensory event but that experience of pain includes affective, cognitive, and behavioral aspects. The main goal of cognitive-behavioral therapy is to enable the patient to control pain and its consequences (what was previously referred to as suffering). Achievement of these goals may considerably improve a patient's quality of life.

Therapy is based on experience with chronic pain patients who increasingly believe that they have attempted everything to control their pain, without success, and who consequently are afraid of a serious underlying cause of pain and of a possible worsening. In many patients this fear leads to a minimization of both physical and social activities. A sort of *vita minima* (minimal life activity) is a frequent consequence, which in these cases enhances the suffering. This decrease in activity unavoidably leads to an increasing loss of muscle strength and joint mobility and continuous decrease in fitness. Many of these patients develop a fatalistic attitude and rely on hope that by a miracle their pain may disappear. In this stage, patients focus on themselves in a kind of fearful expectation and have no distractors or positive experiences. In terms of cognitive-behavioral psychology, these individuals show a dysfunctional behavior in which pain controls the patient instead of the patient controlling the pain (38).

Currently, cognitive-behavioral treatment is the standard therapeutic measure for acute and chronic pain. This treatment is summarized in an extensive way in the literature

(44) and will not be dealt with in detail in this chapter. Cognitive-behavioral therapy focuses on disruption of the vicious circle that was roughly outlined earlier. The first requirement is that the patient must learn that pain is manageable, or at least that some improvement of quality of life is possible; this becomes the main goal of treatment instead of focusing on full pain relief. The following paragraphs discuss techniques used in this treatment.

Education is the fundamental part of treatment. In this regard, patients should know the essentials about pain, such as how it is generated and modified and what may improve the modification of pain. In particular, patients should know about factors or activities that may aggravate or alleviate pain. This may enable the patient to analyze his or her own behavior and uncover the activities that may aggravate or alleviate his or her pain in order to foster positive aspects that may be crucial to helping the patient break out from isolation. Possible positive additional effects may be increased participation in physical activities that do not provoke pain, a gain in physical fitness, social reintegration, and gaining distractors that may help the patient not to focus exclusively on the pain experience.

Distraction is the refocusing of attention away from the pain experience (45). The most favorable distractors are those which the patient likes, thus giving the patient some affective benefit as well. The patient should not be given suggestions or prescriptions of what to do for distraction. Instead, an analysis of behavior with the assistance of the therapist is central. This should include analysis of activities that aggravate (to be avoided if possible) or alleviate (to be fostered) symptoms. Distractors should be pleasurable activities or stimuli that match the particular situation. Patients should engage in finding the activity; in cases of positive effect, patients should be encouraged to continue the activity.

Relaxation techniques are widely employed in cognitive-behavioral treatment. Relaxation may help to reduce fear and anxiety and introduce more positive feelings. Many pain patients show a high level of negative effects (such as anxiety and fear), which lead to increased activity of the autonomous nervous system with different potentially pain-provoking consequences. Indeed, many patients are under sustained stress, of which increased muscle tension is one important aspect in promoting pain. The following relaxation techniques can be used: autogenic relaxation training, progressive muscle relaxation, imagery, biofeedback (e.g., muscular, respiratory), or hypnosis. Many of these techniques—in particular, imagery and biofeedback—should be performed with the assistance and supervision of an experienced therapist. Working on different aspects of emotional experience following a relaxation session may be essential for changing behavior. Some authors suggest music as an additional aspect of cognitive-behavioral treatment for pain. Music is believed to have similar effects as other relaxation techniques.

Family or systemic intervention in chronic pain—which mainly means involvement of family members—appears to be very important. Pain affects family life in many ways because it affects patients' social roles. There is limited research experience on this aspect, but personal experience may support this type of intervention.

REFERENCES

1. Besson JM. The neurobiology of pain. *Lancet* 1999;353:1610–1615.
2. Julius D, Basbaum AI. Molecular mechanisms of nociception. *Nature* 2001;413:203–210.
3. Scholz J, Woolf CJ. Can we conquer pain? *Nature Neuroscience* 2002; 5(Suppl):1062–1067.
4. Fields HL, Rowbotham M, Baron R. Postherpetic neuralgia: irritable nociceptors and deafferentation. *Neurobiol Dis* 1998;5:209–229.
5. Baron R. Peripheral neuropathic pain: from mechanisms to symptoms. *Clin J Pain* 2000;16:S12–S20.
6. Melzack R, Wall PD. Pain mechanisms: a new theory. *Science* 1965; 150:971–979.
7. Hoheisel U, Koch K, Mense S. Functional reorganisation in the rat dorsal horn during an experimental myositis. *Pain* 1994;59:111–118.
8. Dickenson AH. Spinal cord pharmacology of pain. *Br J Anaesth* 1995; 75:193–200.
9. Fields HL, ed. *Pain.* New York: McGraw-Hill, 1987.
10. Pasternak GW. Modulation of opioid analgesia: tolerance and beyond. In: Kalso E, McQuai H, Wiesenfeld-Hallin Z, eds. *Opioid sensitivity of chronic noncancer pain. Progress in pain research and management,* vol. 14. Seattle: IASP Press, 1999:83–94.
11. McQuai H. Opioids in pain management. *Lancet* 1999;353:2229–2232.
12. Kalso E, Heiskanen T, Rantio M, et al. Epidural and subcutaneous morphine in the treatment of cancer pain: a double-blind cross-over study. *Pain* 1996;67:443–449.
13. Borgbjerg FM, Nielsen K, Franks J. Experimental pain stimulates respiration and attenuates morphine-induced respiratory depression: a controlled study in human volunteers. *Pain* 1996;64:123–128.
14. Porter J, Jick H. Addiction rate in patients treated with narcotics. *N Engl J Med* 1980;302:123.
15. McCormack K, Brune K. Dissociation between antinociceptive and anti-inflammatory effects of the nonsteroidal anti-inflammatory drugs. A survey of their analgesic efficacy. *Drugs* 1991;41:533–547.
16. Fabbri A, Cruccu G, Sperti P, et al. Piroxicam-induced analgesia: evidence for a central component which is not opioid mediated. *Experientia* 1992;48:1139–1142.
17. Bombardier C, Laine L, Reicin A, et al. Comparison of upper gastrointestinal toxicity of rofecoxib and naproxen in patients with rheumatoid arthritis: VIGOR study group. *N Engl J Med* 2000;343:1520–1528.
18. Silverstein FE, Faich G, Goldstein JL, et al. Gastrointestinal toxicity with celecoxib vs. nonsteroidal anti-inflammatory drugs for osteoarthritis and rheumatoid arthritis: the CLASS study. A randomized controlled trial. *JAMA* 2000;284:1247–1255.
19. FitzGerald GA, Patrono C. The coxibs, selective inhibitors of cyclooxygenase-2. *N Engl J Med* 2001;345:433–442.
20. Mazario J, Gaitan G, Herrero JF. Cyclooxygenase-1 vs. cyclooxygenase-2 inhibitors in the introduction of antinociception in rodent withdrawal reflexes. *Neuropharmacology* 2001;40:937–946.
21. Bensen WG, Fiechtner JJ, McMillen JI, et al. Treatment of osteoarthritis with celecoxib, a cyclooxigenase-2 inhibitor: a randomized control trial. *Mayo Clin Proc* 1999;74:1095–1105.
22. Kaplan-Machlis B, Klostermeyer BS. The cyclooxygenase-2 inhibitors: safety and effectiveness. *Ann Pharmacother* 1999;33:979–988.
23. Spiegel BM, Targownik L, Dulai GS, et al. The cost-effectiveness of cyclooxygenase-2 selective inhibitors in the management of chronic arthritis. *Ann Intern Med* 2003;138:795–806.
24. Willioughby DA, Moore AR, Colville-Nash PR. COX-1, COX-2 and COX-3 and the future treatment of chronic inflammatory disease. *Lancet* 2000;355:646–648.
25. Chandrasekharan NV, Dai H, Roos KL, et al. COX-3, a cycloexygenase-1 variant inhibited by acetaminophen and other analgesic/antipyretic drugs: cloning, structure, and expression. *Proc Natl Acad Sci USA* 2002;99:13926–13931.
26. Denson D, Katz J. Nonsteroidal anti-inflammatory agents. In: Raj PP, ed. *Practical management of pain,* 2nd ed. St. Louis: Mosby, 1992.

27. Curatolo M, Bogduk N. Pharmacologic pain treatment of musculo-skeletal disorders: current perspectives and future prospects. *Clin J Pain* 2001;17:25–32.
28. Turner JA, Denny MC. Do antidepressant medications relieve chronic low back pain? *J Fam Pract* 1993;37:545–553.
29. Watson CPN. Antidepressant drugs as adjuvant analgesics. *J Pain Sympt Management* 1994;9:392–405.
30. Sindrup SH, Jensen TS. Efficacy of pharmacological treatment of neuropathic pain: an update and effect related to mechanism of drug action. *Pain* 1999;83:389–400.
31. Aker PD, Gross AR, Goldsmith CH, et al. Conservative management of mechanical neck pain: systematic overview and metaanalysis. *BMJ* 1996;313:1291–1296.
32. Van Tulder MW, Koes BW, Bouter LM. Conservative treatment of acute and chronic nonspecific low back pain. A systematic review of randomized controlled trials of the most common interventions. *Spine* 1997;22:2128–2156.
33. von Hilten BJ, van de Beek WJ, Hoff JI, et al. Intrathecal baclofen for the treatment of dystonia in patients with reflex sympathetic dystrophy. *N Engl J Med* 2000;343:654–656.
34. International Association for the Study of Pain, Subcommittee on Taxonomy. Part II. Pain terms: a current list with definitions and notes on usage. *Pain* 1979;6:249–252.
35. Turk DC, Okifuji A. Assessment of patients' reporting of pain: an integrated perspective. *Lancet* 1999;353:1784–1788.
36. Engel GL. "Psychogenic" pain and the pain-prone patient. *Am J Med* 1959;26:899–918.
37. Blumer D, Heilbronn M. Chronic pain as a variant of depressive disease. The pain-prone disorder. *J Nerv Ment Dis* 1982;170:381–406.
38. Pincus T, Morley S. Cognitive-processing bias in chronic pain: a review and integration. *Psychol Bull* 2001;127:599–617.
39. Petrovic P, Ingvar M. Imaging cognitive modulation of pain processing. *Pain* 2002;95:1–5.
40. Novy DM, Nelson DV, Berry LA, et al. What does the Beck Depression Inventory measure in chronic pain? A reappraisal. *Pain* 1995;61:261–270.
41. Williams ACC, Richardson PH. What does the BDI measure in chronic pain? *Pain* 1993;55:259–266.
42. Radanov BP, Begré S, Sturzenegger M, et al. Course of psychological variables in whiplash injury: a 2-year follow-up with age, gender and education pair-matched patients. *Pain* 1996;64:429–434.
43. American Psychiatric Association. *Diagnostic and statistical manual of mental disorders,* 4th ed. Washington, DC: American Psychiatric Association, 1994.
44. Turk DC, Meichenbaum D. Cognitive-behavioural approach to the management of chronic pain. In: Wall P, Melzack R, eds. *Textbook of pain,* 3rd ed. London: Churchill Livingstone, 1994.
45. McCaffery M, Beebe A. *Pain: clinical manual for nursing practice.* St. Louis: Mosby, 1989.
46. Brune K, Hinz B. Nichtopioidanalgetika (antipyretische Analgetika und andere) (German). In: Zenz M, Jurna I, eds. *Lehrbuch der Schmerztherapie.* Stuttgart: Wissenschaftliche Verlagsgesellschaft, 2001:233–253.
47. Vane J. Towards a better aspirin. *Nature* 1994;367:215–216.

SECTION II

Neurologic and Functional Evaluation

CHAPTER 10

Evaluation of Patients with Cervical Spine Lesions

Seth M. Zeidman

Appropriate neurologic assessment is critical in the evaluation and treatment of cervical disc herniation and degenerative diseases of the cervical spine. In discussing cervical intervertebral disc lesions and degeneration, precise terminology and definitions are essential. The clinical spectrum of symptomatology for cervical disc disease can be divided into four broad categories: (a) cervical degenerative discogenic (internal disc disruption), (b) cervical radiculopathy, (c) cervical myeloradiculopathy, and (d) cervical myelopathy. Defining where patients fall along this continuum is a necessary prerequisite to providing optimal management.

DEGENERATIVE DISC DISEASE

Cervical disc disease results from disc degeneration, that is, mechanical breakdown of disc integrity. Cervical disc degeneration most commonly results from aging, but the condition is affected by lifestyle, genetics, smoking, nutrition, and physical activity. Radiographic degenerative changes may reflect simple aging and do not necessarily indicate a symptomatic or even a pathologic process. Cervical disc degeneration includes degenerative annular tears, loss of disc height, and nuclear degradation. Disc degeneration often develops insidiously, without overt clinical manifestations. Initial symptoms may reflect mechanical instability and only later denote neural compression. The disc begins to degenerate in the second decade of life. Circumferential tears form in the posterolateral annulus after repetitive use. Several circumferential tears can coalesce into radial tears, which progress into radial fissures. The disc then disrupts with tears passing throughout the disc. Loss of disc height occurs with subsequent peripheral annular bulging. Proteoglycans and water escape through fissures formed from nuclear degradation, resulting in further thinning of the disc space. Vertebral sclerosis and osteophytic formation ultimately result.

With aging, the intervertebral discs desiccate, resulting in disc height loss. Disc degeneration causes instability, resulting in irregular vertebral movement. This puts greater stress on the articular cartilage of the vertebrae and their respective end plates. Osteophytic spurs develop at the margins of these end plates. Cervical instability produces posterior joint strain with consequent axial and referred pain from injured and stressed ligaments and damaged facet joints. Intervertebral disc height collapse forces bony prominences and the uncovertebral joints of adjacent vertebral bodies to approach and ultimately oppose one another, with resultant reactive hyperostosis and osteophyte formation. Osteophytes stabilize adjacent vertebrae whose hypermobility is caused by the degeneration of the disc. Osteophytes increase the articulation surface area, allowing a more equal distribution of compressive forces.

Osteophytes develop along the posterior portion of the vertebrae in association with uncovertebral joint and facet osteoarthritis, which may produce zygapophyseal joint hypertrophy, decreased anteroposterior diameter of the vertebral canal, and neural foraminal encroachment. Osteophytic compression of the intervertebral foramina can occur from either the uncovertebral or the zygapophyseal joint hypertrophy. Compression of the nerve root initially affects the larger, more pressure-sensitive A fibers, resulting in the characteristic radiculopathic syndromes of weakness, numbness, and reflex loss. Uncovertebral and facet hypertrophy can cause epidural adhesions and perineural inflammation. The combination of root compression and inflammation produces pain in a radicular distribution, that is, radiculopathy.

Cervical Internal Disc Disruption and Discogenic Pain

Cervical discogenic and internal disc disruption is a subjective disorder without objective neurologic deficits or testable abnormalities. Internal disc disruption was initially popularized by Crock, who described disc lesions characterized by alteration in internal structure and metabolic functions not associated with rupture or other definable pathoanatomy. A biochemical basis for deficiency was postulated, a hypothesis subsequently based on certain inflammatory-type pathologic features as shown by microscopy, in addition to intraoperative observations suggestive of peridiscal inflammation. Crock cited the often-observed element of increased peridiscal vascularity with sympathetic trunk matting and softening of the vertebral bodies. Clinical features of internal disc disruption are variable; however, Crock pointed out certain universal features that serve to differentiate the condition from others, such as rupture. A constant symptom described as a deep-seated, dull, aching neck pain was invariable. Shoulder girdle or limb pain was typically described as nondermatomal and generalized, in contrast to the more discrete pain characteristic of nerve root compression. A significant association with headache and constitutional symptoms has been noted.

The cardinal lesion rendering a cervical disc painful is internal disc disruption. The characteristic feature of internal disc disruption is a radial fissure extending to the innervated outer third of the annulus fibrosus. As radial fissures extend to the outer third of the annulus, nerve endings are exposed to the inflammatory and algogenic chemicals produced by nuclear degradation. As a radial fissure develops, fewer and fewer lamellae remain intact to bear the load. At some stage, the threshold for mechanical nociception is attained, especially if the nerve endings have been chemically sensitized. Disc stimulation reveals this condition by showing a reduced threshold for mechanical stimulation of the disc.

Cervical Radiculopathy

Classic syndromes of cervical root compression are well defined (Table 10.1). Many tests and signs have been described to complement the physical examination and to define more clearly the nature of a patient's neck and arm pain and its relationship to compression of either nerve roots or the spinal cord. The onset of symptoms with radiculopathy may be insidious, or patients may ascribe their symptoms to some inciting event. Acute trauma can trigger radicular symptoms. Patients with abrupt onset of radicular complaints still may have a soft disc rupture superimposed on cervical degenerative disease. Radiculopathy is the most common symptom that results in cervical disc surgery.

In patients with cervical radiculopathy, the arm pain greatly exceeds mechanical problems in the neck (Fig. 10.1). Radiculopathy is defined as pain and associated neurologic deficits in a nerve root distribution. This results from compression of cervical nerve roots by herniated disc material or degenerative disc disease at or near the vertebral foramen. Discomfort and numbness in a root distribution are often the only symptoms. The pain is related to neck position and worsened by rotation, lateral flexion, or extension of the head. Patients may be roused from sound sleep by severe neck pain. Moving or extending the neck reproduces the arm pain.

The term *radiculopathy* implies consistently reproducible neurologic findings: motor loss, sensory abnormalities, and reflex changes. Radicular symptoms are characterized by proximal pain and distal paresthesias in the distribution of the affected nerve root. In general, symptoms are referable to an individual nerve root. There may be overlap between dermatomes innervated by a particular nerve, and

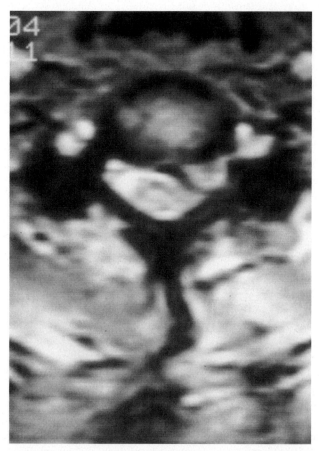

FIG. 10.1. Radiculopathy resulting from disc herniation. Magnetic resonance imaging demonstrated lateral disc herniation in a patient who presented with unilateral radiculopathy.

TABLE 10.1. *Classic Nerve Root Involvement: Radiculopathy*

Root	Sensory change	Motor change	Reflex change
C5	Lateral arm	Deltoid, biceps	Biceps
C6	Thumb, index finger	Biceps, wrist extensors, brachioradialis	Biceps
C7	Middle finger	Triceps, wrist flexors	Triceps
C8	Little finger	Hand intrinsics	None

only rarely are findings isolated to a single dermatome. Likewise, because there is overlap of the innervation to the muscles and reflexes in the upper extremities, clinical localization is not exact.

Isolated numbness may develop, with minimal pain or without pain. Patients occasionally present with a motor deficit without sensory pain or numbness. Usually, the deficit affects a single nerve root and evolves so slowly that the patient is able to compensate with other muscle groups. Only simultaneous symmetric assessment of arm and hand musculature will detect the motor loss. Arm abduction sometimes brings relief to patients with a ruptured cervical disc. Patients occasionally present with an arm draped over the head. Relief is uncommon in patients with spondylosis.

The neck compression test reproduces radicular symptoms with lateral flexion, rotation, and vertical compression of the patient's head. The Spurling sign results in cervical root compression and pain with hyperextension and contralateral rotation of the neck. This has been reported to be present in 25% to 50% of patients with radiculopathy. The Valsalva test creates radicular symptoms with intentional increases in intraabdominal pressure. Radicular symptoms may be improved by 10 to 15 pounds of axial traction or by elevation of the patient's hand over the head while the patient is sitting.

Two thirds of patients with acute radiculopathies remain persistently symptomatic, and only one third obtain long-term relief with medical and physical therapy. In contrast to acute radiculopathy, chronic radiculopathy is generally unaffected by either neck position or motion. The principal manifestation of chronic progressive radiculopathy is atrophy. Older patients with unilateral or bilateral multilevel involvement and atrophic changes often have symptoms that simulate those of other neurologic disease. More chronic radiculopathies with spondylotic disease affecting two or more adjacent levels sometimes involve more than one nerve root. Determination of the levels warranting operative intervention requires careful neurologic examination of the patient.

Cervical Myeloradiculopathy

Myeloradiculopathy is defined as a radiculopathy with myelopathic findings. Myelopathic findings are more common than root symptoms. Motor and reflex changes are observed more often than sensory changes, and analgesia is more common than anesthesia. Motor findings are generally paretic at the lesion level and spastic below that level. Arm findings can be unilateral, but leg findings are typically bilateral. Sensory disturbances can be variable and are typically below the area of compression. Touch is usually preserved, with decreased pain and temperature sensation. Reflex changes typically follow the pattern of motor involvement.

Cervical myeloradiculopathy represents a well-known syndrome in which patients manifest a variety of symptoms. The most common presentation is subtle neck pain in conjunction with radicular complaints. On initial examination, patients exhibit signs of radiculitis and radiculopathy. However, the reflexes in the lower extremities are hyperactive. Careful questioning of the patient elicits their decreased ability to run or to button their clothing. During the initial evaluation, such patients should be asked to run in place in the examination room or to stand on one leg with eyes closed. These maneuvers provoke the subtle signs of myelopathy. The pathologic substrate of myeloradiculopathy is compression of both the spinal cord and nerve root.

It is now known from trauma experiments that as much as 30% of the spinal cord volume can be lost without affecting the neurologic examination. Patients with broad-based disc herniations, typical radiculopathy, and normal neurologic findings in the lower extremities who report improvement in their ability to run and walk after successful anterior decompression have been observed. Hindsight shows that some patients are treated for radiculopathy when they actually also had a subtle myelopathy that was not diagnosed preoperatively.

Cervical Spondylotic Myelopathy

Cervical spondylotic myelopathy (CSM) is a neurologic disorder manifested in its most severe form by spastic gait, clumsy hands with atrophy and sensory impairment, sphincter disturbances, and pain related to the underlying spondylosis of the cervical spine. CSM is a graded process with myriad clinical manifestations. Compressive, ischemic, and dynamic factors all contribute to the pathophysiology. CSM is typically a slowly progressive disorder that ultimately produces significant disability and results from a combination of factors.

ETIOLOGY

Although the clinical manifestations of myelopathy due to spinal cord tumors, abscesses, trauma, and other conditions are similar, our discussion is confined to disorders associated with cervical spondylosis. The common initiating pathology in the production of CSM is spinal cord compression (Fig. 10.2). Chronic or (subacute) myelopathy secondary to cervical spondylosis is a common entity. Myelopathy due to cervical spondylosis was initially recognized in the 1950s.

Degenerative changes, such as a posterior protruding disc, ossification of the posterior longitudinal ligament (OPLL), vertebral osteophytes, facet joint spurs, overriding joint of Luschka, invagination or ossification of the ligamentum flavum, and trauma can contribute to spinal stenosis, which leads to spinal cord compression (Fig. 10.3). The sequelae of spinal cord compression result from the interaction of three synergistic factors: canal narrowing secondary to degenerative disc disease and congenital cervical

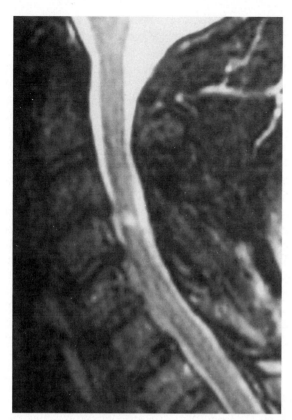

FIG. 10.2. Magnetic resonance imaging showing intrinsic spinal cord hyperdensity supradjacent to disc herniation in a patient with acute myelopathy.

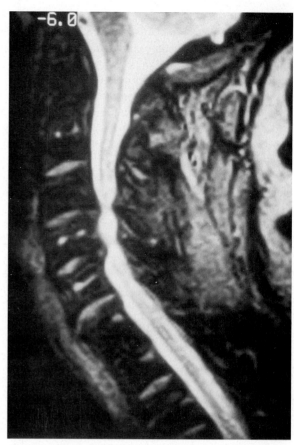

FIG. 10.3. Magnetic resonance imaging in a patient with severe spondylotic disease and myelopathy resulting from stenosis.

stenosis, compromise of cord circulation, and repetitive motion and intermittent mechanical compression of the spinal cord.

Compression may be secondary to disc herniation, degenerative osteophyte production, OPLL, or congenital spinal stenosis with minor degenerative changes. Chronic disc degeneration with osteophyte formation is the most common cause of myelopathy in older patients. Spondylotic myelopathy is the most common cervical cord disorder during and after middle age. Within the cervical cord, there is a gradation of sensitivity to direct compression of the cord, with the most sensitive area being the corticospinal tract, followed by anterior horn cells, anterior funiculus, and posterior funiculus.

The normal spinal canal has a diameter of 17 to 18 mm between C3 and C7. The normal spinal cord anteroposterior (AP) diameter is about 9 mm. There should be a minimum of 1 mm of cerebrospinal fluid (CSF) on each side of the cord and 1 mL of dura. These additional 4 mm, in addition to the 9 mm of cord, demand a space of 13 mm. Therefore, an AP cervical vertebral canal diameter of 13 mm or less results in spinal cord impingement.

The two major components are (a) compressive forces from spinal canal narrowing, and (b) dynamic forces due to cervical spine motion. Although trivial trauma may prompt

recognition of the neurologic deficit, myelopathy is nearly always a progressive process. Repetitive trauma to the spinal cord sustained with movement in a spondylotic canal may be a major cause of progressive myelopathy.

Spinal cord compression may be confined to a single level secondary to disc herniation or to a sizable osteophyte, or it can extend over several segments (Fig. 10.4). When it is multilevel, it is often caused by multilevel degenerative changes or OPLL (Fig. 10.3). Occasionally, diffuse compression occurs over many segments in a patient with a congenitally narrowed canal and mild age-related spondylosis, and the cord has insufficient space.

Pressure on the spinal cord results in vascular compromise, with resultant ischemia. Cervical spinal cord blood flow is dependent on the integrity of both the anterior and posterior spinal arteries, in addition to the radicular supply from the vertebral arteries. The position of the anterior spinal artery is variable and may extend well anterior to the cord. Anterior compressive pathology, including spondylotic ridging and disc compression, may hinder arterial flow, producing focal ischemia. Ischemia can also be secondary to local compression of intramedullary branches. This is more prominent in the gray matter because vascular

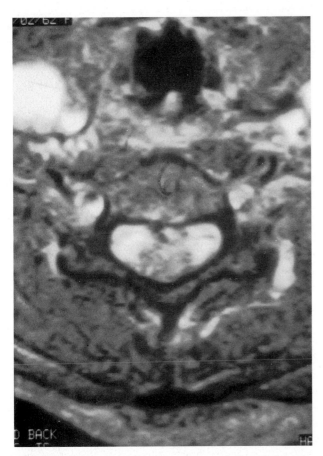

FIG. 10.4. Soft disc herniation of central disc. Axial magnetic resonance imaging of patient with acute development of cervical myelopathy with numb and clumsy hands and lower extremity clonus.

tary movement disorders aggravate the normal cervical spine trauma and may induce premature cervical spondylosis with resultant myelopathy.

The cervical spine normally has a lordotic curvature. Degenerative disc disease results in loss of intervertebral disc height, with obliteration of cervical lordosis and a straightened or even kyphotic spine. Kyphosis may be a cause of cord compression as well. In the presence of underlying spinal cord compression, the natural movements of the cervical spine produce increased pressure on the cord. Extension of the neck causes ligamentum flavum prolapse and buckling, exacerbating preexisting anterior pathology, and can initiate painless loss of neurologic function caudal to the area of compression. Therapy should address this compression and relieve cord impingement. There is no medical therapy to relieve or correct spinal cord impingement. Cervical spine immobilization and nonsteroidal anti-inflammatory drugs (NSAIDs) may reduce the incidence of microtrauma, which can contribute to progression. When one considers that patients live for years after the initial symptoms appear, spinal cord decompression is mandated.

Recent studies have convincingly demonstrated that apoptosis also plays a pivotal role in numerous pathologic processes, contributing to the adverse effects of various diseases and traumatic conditions. A growing body of evidence has implicated apoptosis as a key determinant of the extent of neurologic damage and dysfunction after acute spinal cord injury and in chronic cervical myelopathy. There is now strong evidence to support a significant role for apoptosis in secondary injury mechanisms after acute spinal cord injury as well in the progressive neurologic deficits observed in such conditions as spondylotic cervical myelopathy (1,2).

SIGNS AND SYMPTOMS

The classic presentation of myelopathy is numbness and clumsiness of the hands in association with a stiff, spastic unsteady gait. Patients with CSM generally report neck stiffness; unilateral or bilateral deep, aching neck, arm, and shoulder pain; and possibly stiffness or clumsiness while walking. Patients sometimes report greater difficulty walking at night, owing to reduced proprioceptive input.

CSM usually develops insidiously and with a stepwise "stuttering" progression. In the early stages of CSM, complaints of neck stiffness are common because of the presence of advanced cervical spondylosis. Other common complaints include crepitus in the neck with movement; brachialgia, which is characterized as a stabbing pain in the preaxial or postaxial border of the arm, elbow, wrist, or fingers; a dull, achy feeling in the arm; and numbness or tingling in the hands. Symptoms may be asymmetric, particularly in the legs. Loss of sphincter control or frank incontinence is rare; however, some patients may complain of slight hesitancy on urination.

The clumsiness experienced in the hands reflects the neuroanatomy of the efferent innervation of the hand muscula-

demands of the gray matter are four to five times that of the white matter and it is therefore more sensitive to ischemia. Gray-matter ischemia accounts for the lower motor neuron phenomena observed in many patients. The etiology of the progressive pathology dictates the therapeutic response. If there is marked anterior compression, this pressure may be directly on the anterior spinal artery, accelerating the course of pathologic events. More commonly, the microcirculation of the cord in the area of compression is damaged.

Although the compressive pathophysiology exceeds the vascular changes, in the more advanced stages, it is a combination of both pathologic entities that ultimately leads to spinal cord damage. Development of significant myelopathy secondary to cord compression has three components: degree of cord compression, rate of compression, and constancy or intermittence of the compressive force. Acute CSM can develop in the presence of spondylosis and can occur without an identifiable inciting event. Acute myelopathy can arise in the setting of extreme hyperextension, acute disc herniation with cord compression and torticollis, or other involuntary movement disorders. Patients with torticollis, torsion dystonia, and other involun-

ture. The corticospinal tracts and extrapyramidal system travel down the posterolateral funiculus of the spinal cord to synapse with internuncial neurons two to three segments above the primary motor neuron. For example, intrinsic muscles of the hand are driven by motor fibers descending down the corticospinal tract to end and synapse with internuncial neurons as high as C5 and C6. Here there is an internuncial neuronal pool with a variety of both inhibitory and facilitatory influences from the local afferent input. The internuncial neuronal pool then feeds down the cord to the anterior horn cells at the C8 cord level. Here, the anterior horn cell output is modulated and emerges as the final output from C8 and T1 and goes to the hand. If the internuncial neuronal pool is disrupted, normal coordination and smoothness of hand function is disrupted, and clumsiness appears. With disruption of the neuronal pool higher in the spinal cord, the hand can appear as if it has a lower motor neuron disease. Within the cervical enlargement with its corresponding large quantity of gray matter in the cervical cord, disruption of the internuncial neurons can lead to the classic symptoms of numbness and clumsiness, which are difficult to fit with a single radicular pattern. This is an important part of the myelopathy and is termed *myelopathy hand*. OPLL as high as C2 can present with this clinical finding. Loss of hand dexterity, with painful dysesthesias and difficulty in writing, is common. The syndrome of myelopathy hand may be the most important indicator of a good response to surgery.

In patients with myelopathy, the cord signs and symptoms generally outweigh the focal radicular disorder, and motor loss exceeds sensory loss. Lower motor involvement occurs at the level of the lesion, with atrophy of upper extremity muscles, especially hand intrinsics. Upper motor neuron findings are noted below the level of the lesion, with lower extremity spasticity and hyperreflexia. The sensory fibers are polysynaptic, and the posterior columns remain intact because the circulation is well collateralized, enters from posterior, and is therefore minimally affected. Focal sensory loss is less readily appreciated. Many patients have a subtle loss of sharpness to pinprick on the lower half of the body, with a sensory gradient across the trunk to normal sensation. Analgesia is more common than anesthesia, which is more common than proprioceptive loss. Reflex changes may be present, with relative hyperreflexia in the legs as compared with the arms. Bilateral Hoffman and Babinski signs are commonly present.

Lhermitte sign is the axial shocklike sensation elicited by neck flexion, extension, or axial compression. It is classically produced by pressing down on the top of the head. Lhermitte sign is present in as many as 25% of myelopathic patients. Babinski and Hoffman signs are nonspecific findings with upper motor neuron lesions and can be demonstrated in patients with myelopathy secondary to cervical disc disease. Determination of the range of motion (ROM) of the cervical spine should be performed actively, passively, and against resistance.

Acute myelopathy can occur spontaneously or after minor or major trauma. The common presentation is a central spinal cord syndrome with pain. The neurologic loss is that of lower motor abnormalities in arms and hands with hyperreflexia and with spasticity in the legs. Acute myelopathy after minor trauma can occur without fracture or dislocation. It is often associated with spondylosis or congenital stenosis. Static cord impingement often cannot be demonstrated radiographically. Acute myelopathy also occurs in young people with congenital spinal stenosis or multiple sports traumas. Such patients may develop diffuse cervical spinal stenosis as a result of multiple minor spinal injuries. Patients with congenital or acquired stenosis and an AP diameter of less than 10 mm are vulnerable to acute spinal cord injury when the spine is sufficiently hyperextended. Such patients typically are football players who present after some trivial trauma with what has been described as neurapraxia, stinger, or spinal cord concussion. Cervical spondylosis produces canal narrowing, and hyperextension precipitates acute compression and injury. Dynamic compression of the spinal cord results in neurologic injury, often a central cord syndrome.

The anterior spinal artery syndrome has a variety of causes. Acute quadriparesis and dissociation of sensory loss with preservation of posterior column functions are its hallmarks. Acute soft disc herniation with cord compression can present with myelopathy and requires urgent surgical intervention. This should be suspected in patients whose plain radiographs demonstrate congenital or spontaneous fusion and in patients with previous cervical injury.

Few studies of the natural history of spondylotic myelopathy have been performed, and those that have were small, with dissimilar disability grading systems and with outcomes that are not comparable. Despite these limitations, some information can be gleaned from the available literature. Myelopathy secondary to spondylosis typically has an insidious onset, developing over a prolonged period. The natural history is characterized by long intervals of clinical stability punctuated by short periods of worsening and ultimately intermittent progression. Myelopathy may initially appear as an isolated condition, in conjunction with a severe radiculopathy or as a significant component of myeloradiculopathy. Patients may have very minor degenerative changes and become symptomatic. Their neurologic deficits can be dramatic and anxiety producing, causing patients to present for evaluation. Once myelopathy occurs, complete reversal is rare. Patients with myelopathy often go for long periods of time without development of new or worsening signs and symptoms.

Spondylotic myelopathy may present as a stepwise deterioration (75%), as a relentless downhill slide without plateaus or remissions (20%), or as a downhill course with occasional remissions (5%). In few patients, the myelopathy will reverse with conservative care or no care. Significant reduction in neurologic deficits is unusual. After conservative treatment, most myelopathic patients experience periods of stable disability punctuated by episodes of progressive deterioration. Reported improvements may represent a plateau with lack of progression or with the patients growing accustomed to their disability. After onset of clinical myelopathy,

TABLE 10.2. *Classification System for Myelopathic Gait Abnormalities*

Grade	Root signs	Cord involvement	Gait	Employment
0	Yes	No	Normal gait	Possible
I	Yes	Yes	Normal gait	Possible
II	Yes	Yes	Mild abnormality	Possible
III	Yes	Yes	Severe abnormality	Impossible
IV	Yes	Yes	Only with assistance	Impossible
V	Yes	Yes	Chairbound or bedridden	Impossible

rarely do patients regain neurologic normality, and spontaneous remission of symptoms is unlikely.

Nurick postulated that the degree of disability in cervical myelopathy was established early in the disease process and rarely progressed (3). In a clinical review of 1,355 patients with CSM, Epstein reported that conservative therapy resulted in 36% improvement and 64% nonimprovement. In the group with nonimprovement, 26% of patients significantly deteriorated neurologically.

A subset of patients presents with relentless progression that proceeds to severe disability. Our clinical experience is most similar to that of Symon and Lavender, who reported that more than two thirds of the patients with myelopathy whom they studied displayed relentless deterioration of neurologic function rather than a series of plateaus and downhill progression. Patients presenting with markedly myelopathic findings in association with drastically reduced spinal canal dimensions over several levels can expect progressive deterioration.

Real improvement in patients with myelopathy can be expected after operative cord decompression if symptoms have been present for less than 2 years. When the duration of symptoms exceeds 2 years, demonstrable significant improvement in patients is rare. Age at presentation and duration of disease before treatment are the most important factors affecting prognosis. Increased age is associated with poorer outcome. Age and clinical severity are less important factors than duration of disease and the operation performed. Myelopathy is a treatable condition, and prompt diagnosis improves the likelihood of favorable outcome.

Attempts at grading myelopathy have focused on the effects on patient performance. Patient grading is essential to evaluate the results of various available therapies. A standardized grading system for myelopathy would allow more complete understanding of the natural history of this disorder as well as provide a valid means of comparing the results of the different treatment modalities. Identification of more serious neurologic problems, the rapidity of their progress, and their response to therapy would then dictate the urgency for treatment. Double-blinded, prospective, randomized trials of both anterior and posterior procedures as well as conservative therapy are the best methods for determining the efficacy of the various therapies available today.

Nurick devised a classification system for myelopathy on the basis of gait abnormalities (Table 10.2). His scale involves a grading system of 0 to 5 for progressively worsening myelopathic gait abnormalities (3).

The Japanese Orthopaedic Association (JOA) devised an objective assessment scale quantitating the severity of spondylotic myelopathy (Table 10.3). The scale encompasses four categories: motor dysfunction of the upper extremities, motor dysfunction of the lower extremities, sensory deficits of the extremities and trunk, and sphincter dysfunction. The rating system allows more accurate assessment of postoperative recovery and identifies the more global effects of

TABLE 10.3. *Criteria for Evaluation of the Operative Results of Patients with Cervical Myelopathy by the Japanese Orthopaedic Association (JOA Score)*

I. Upper extremity function
    0. Impossible to eat with either chopsticks or spoon
    1. Possible to eat with spoon, but not with chopsticks
    2. Possible to eat with chopsticks, but inadequate
    3. Possible to eat with chopsticks, but awkward
    4. Normal
II. Lower extremity function
    0. Impossible to walk
    1. Need cane or aid on flat ground
    2. Need cane or aid only on stairs
    3. Possible to walk without cane or aid, but slow
    4. Normal
III. Sensory
    A. Upper extremity
        0. Apparent sensory loss
        1. Minimal sensory loss
        2. Normal
    B. Lower extremity
        0. Apparent sensory loss
        1. Minimal sensory loss
        2. Normal
    C. Trunk
        0. Apparent sensory loss
        1. Minimal sensory loss
        2. Normal
IV. Bladder function
    0. Complete retention
    1. Severe disturbance
        (1) Inadequate evacuation of the bladder
        (2) Straining
        (3) Dribbling of urine
    2. Mild disturbance
        (1) Urinary frequency
        (2) Urinary hesitancy
    3. Normal

myelopathy as regard the arms and sphincters. The maximal score is 17 points. To assess recovery rate after surgical intervention in patients with OPLL-induced myelopathy, Hirabayashi and colleagues devised a score based on the JOA scale. JOA scores less than 7 indicate severe myelopathy, a score between 8 and 12 indicates moderate myelopathy, and scores above 13 indicate mild myelopathy.

The natural history of CSM is poor. As many as 70% of patients have a significant progressive disorder within 1 year. Although much of the literature suggests a smaller percentage, our data do not indicate such good prognosis. Preoperative assessment of patients requires repeated examinations and evaluations. To an objective observer, most patients referred for neurosurgical evaluation are deteriorating. However, patients must be convinced that their condition is worsening. Only when patients appreciate their progressive neurologic condition should operative intervention be recommended. All patients treated on our service were convinced that their condition was worsening. If neurologic examination is consistent with the diagnosis of myelopathy, diagnostic studies can confirm and document the dysfunction. The initial management of such patients is dependent on accurate diagnosis. Patients with myelopathy have a measurable neurologic deficit. The neurologic deficit should be determined and confirmed by repeated examinations. Once disease progression is documented, operative intervention can be discussed. When patients are aware of their condition, their informed consent is more easily obtained. If patients understand the progressive nature of their disease, operative intervention is quite feasible. Informed consent should emphasize that 70% to 80% of patients treated with the appropriate surgical procedure will improve.

In patients in whom hypermobility of the cervical spine can be demonstrated, external immobilization will protect the spinal cord from further trauma. Such immobilization will rarely result in dramatic clinical improvement, but it does provide a useful interim measure while plans for definitive therapy are being completed. Collar treatment resulted in an overall improvement rate of 37% in cases of mild myelopathy. Duration of myelopathic symptoms before treatment with collar immobilization was correlated with outcome. Clinical improvement was noted in 54% of patients with symptom duration of less than 1 year and in 40% of patients with symptom duration of 1 to 2 years. No patients improved with collar immobilization when symptoms had been present for more than 2 years. Nurick's review of 104 patients described in the literature who were treated with a collar showed that 40% improved, 36% were unchanged, and 24% were worse (3).

Symptomatic resolution or even improvement with conservative treatment is rare. Patients with the signs and symptoms of myelopathy will have some degree of permanent disability; most will have disease progression. Close observation should be the rule when conservative care is chosen for a patient with myelopathy. Any patient with moderate or severe myelopathy is a candidate for surgery. Progression of the myelopathy is an indication for surgery.

DIFFERENTIAL DIAGNOSIS

Amyotrophic Lateral Sclerosis

Patients with painless, spontaneous development of atrophy and fasciculations in the upper extremities are more likely to have a motor neuron disease such as amyotrophic lateral sclerosis (ALS). Some researchers consider the presence of fasciculations to be a reliable indicator of motor neuron disease. There is no way to exclude the diagnosis of ALS completely if wasting of hand muscles, upper extremity fasciculations, or hyperreflexia is present. Fasciculations represent a late stage of cervical nerve root compression and are rare in cervical disc disease. Because cases of compressive cervical myelopathy with severe canal stenosis and associated signs of ALS have been documented, clinically a certain diagnosis may not be possible. Unequivocal sensory loss excludes the diagnosis of isolated ALS. Electromyography (EMG) is usually diagnostic, particularly if the lower extremities are involved.

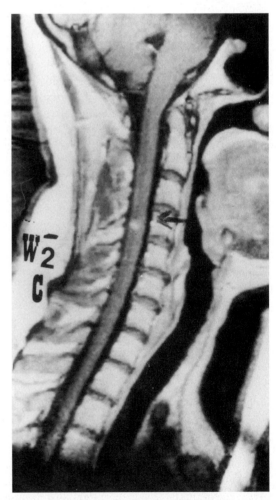

FIG. 10.5. Magnetic resonance imaging (MRI) in a patient who presented with myelopathy. The patient's history disclosed that symptoms were intermittent. MRI and subsequent lumbar puncture confirmed the diagnosis of multiple sclerosis.

Multiple Sclerosis

The diagnostic evaluation of multiple sclerosis (MS) includes magnetic resonance imaging (MRI) with and without gadolinium of the brain and cervical cord, CSF examination, and evoked potentials (Fig. 10.5). If results of all these tests are negative, the chance that a spastic paraparesis is MS is less than 5%. Abnormalities of CSF immunoglobulin G (IgG) and oligoclonal bands are more reliable indicators of MS than is CSF pleocytosis or increased protein (44,70). Subacute combined degeneration can mimic myelopathy.

INTRINSIC SPINAL CORD LESIONS—TUMOR, SYRINGOMYELIA, ARTERIOVENOUS MALFORMATION

Intrinsic spinal cord lesions, which can produce both myelopathic and radiculopathic symptoms, including vascular malformations, syrinxes, and tumors, can be excluded with diagnostic imaging, including computed tomography (CT) and MRI (Fig. 10.6).

Spinal dural arteriovenous fistulas are the most common vascular malformation involving the spinal cord. They are supplied by a dural artery and drain through spinal veins and an arteriovenous shunt in the intervertebral foramen. They are more common in males, with an average age older than 50 years. Initial symptoms are most commonly lower extremity weakness, sensory changes, pain, and bladder dysfunction. The course in most patients is one of progressive neurologic deterioration. Diagnosis is often delayed, with time to diagnosis exceeding 15 months. MRI is the most sensitive imaging modality, with typical findings of increased signal in the cord on T2-weighted images.

DIAGNOSTIC IMAGING

Preoperative evaluation of degenerative disc disease demands precise anatomic localization of the pathologic process, which requires demonstration of both compressive pathology and compressed neural structures. Plain film radiography, CT myelography, and MRI are the commonly available diagnostic modalities. In all patients, plain cervical spine radiographs are needed, in flexion and extension, to evaluate stability. In patients with diffuse arthritic changes, flexion and extension films are particularly important because the hypermobile joint is often the source of the pain even though objective evidence of spinal instability cannot be demonstrated.

Discometric and discogram studies can be used to confirm the diagnosis (Fig. 10.7). When and if a single level is identified that is clearly responsible for most of the patient's pain, anterior cervical discectomy and fusion can help 70%

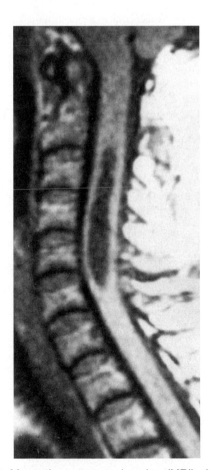

FIG. 10.6. Magnetic resonance imaging (MRI) showing syringomyelia. The patient presented with myelopathy and lower extremity hyperreflexia. MRI demonstrated a cervical syrinx, which was successfully treated with syringopleural shunting.

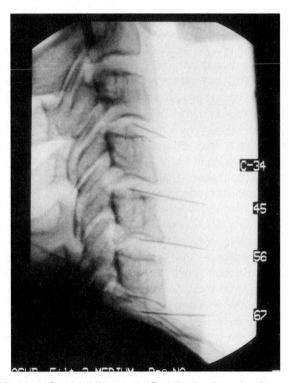

FIG. 10.7. Cervical discogram. Preinjection lateral radiograph showing multiple-needle technique.

to 80% of patients (83). The discometric and discogram studies should be viewed as a confirmatory study. When the physician does not have a firm idea about the vertebral level of the disease before the study, it should not be performed. Even if the study is positive and surgery is performed, the results are seldom good, and fewer than half of patients are helped. To achieve success in treating this group of patients, the patient's signs and symptoms must be convincing, the secondary gains minimal, and the diagnostic studies confirmatory of the clinical impression.

If surgical intervention is anticipated, a more extensive diagnostic evaluation is necessary. Cervical myelography immediately followed by CT scanning (CT myelography) is useful in planning the operative approach. CT myelography permits precise visualization of the spinal cord in the axial plane, clearly demonstrates bony detail and abnormalities, and defines the relationship of the cord and the spinal canal, including deformation or compression of the cord. Spondylotic compression is generally not well defined with MRI, but CT myelography is excellent for assessing the patient with spondylotic myelopathy before surgical intervention. However, it is an invasive study requiring intrathecal contrast.

CT scanning without myelography is of little value in determining the surgical approach to disc disease, but it better defines vertebral structure and bony abnormalities than any other diagnostic modality; therefore, in marked lateral foraminal stenosis from facet and uncovertebral osteoarthritis, it may prove useful. It provides accurate information regarding the dimensions and configuration of the spinal canal and foramina.

The more bony the abnormality on plain films, the more likely that CT will provide definitive diagnosis. If plain films reveal minimal pathology, attention is directed to a soft tissue lesion, for which MRI is the superior imaging modality. MRI scans frequently demonstrate a broad-based centrally herniated disc. If CT is not diagnostic, one should consider MRI and vice versa. In many centers, MRI has nearly eliminated myelography because it is noninvasive and allows precise definition of the pathology.

Soft disc herniations are precisely localized by MRI. The foramina and intervertebral discs are well demonstrated, and nerve root compression can often be appreciated. Sagittal and axial images exclude intrinsic or external symptoms with associated headache compatible with discogenic and arthritic disruption. With surgical correction of the myeloradiculopathy, some of the patients reported relief of their headache. The axial neck pain and subscapular pain were similarly relieved. This generally occurred after anterior cervical discectomy and fusion in which the articulations were mechanically distracted by use of a generous intervertebral bone graft.

Because of the number of patients presenting with this constellation of complaints in the absence of demonstrable neurologic deficit, the provocative discography of Aprill and other investigators has received broader interest for diagnosis.

Some patients present with multilevel discogenic disruption from degenerative disease or flexion-extension injuries. It is difficult to identify a single level responsible for most of the pain. The pain is aggravated by motion or axial loading and relieved by rest and immobilization in a cervical collar. Patients with discogenic symptoms have no objective neurologic findings. They report intermittent chronic pain in the posterior cervical region, shoulder, chest wall, and interscapular region. The painful neck in cervical disc degeneration is frequently tender to palpation of the spinous processes or deep cervical musculature.

Aprill has used provocative discometry and discography in this setting. Needles are placed in the nucleus of the suspected joints, and a small amount of fluid is injected. Reproduction of the patient's pain syndrome constitutes a positive result. Injection of a small amount of local anesthetic agent should then relieve the pain. The idea is logical, and experience suggests that the technique is helpful. However, no studies in the literature prove that surgical treatment of the identified discs is beneficial. The predictive value of discography as an indication for surgery remains to be proved in controlled trials. One injected joint may be more painful in 40% to 50% of patients, whereas in the remainder, pain apparently originates from more than one level.

Patients are often referred in a desperate situation, characterized by incapacitating pain without objective neurologic deficits. Standard imaging studies do not localize a treatable abnormality. Discography is now used to try to identify patients who may benefit from surgery. I now believe that patients with normal radiographs and normal MRI scan should not undergo discometric study. Patients with diffuse, multilevel, arthritic changes without a single level displaying hypermobility or a marked degree of disproportionate collapse with traction osteophytes or spurring should not be subjected to discometry or discography because I have found that operating on these patients is not beneficial.

Ideally, discography should identify a group of patients with one-level disease who can benefit from anterior fusion. This group constitutes about 5% of our current surgical practice.

INITIAL MANAGEMENT

Severe unremitting pain and profound neurologic deficit usually require urgent surgical intervention. Decreasing pain with increasing neurologic deficits also warrants concern and merits prompt diagnosis and treatment. Most patients with symptomatic degenerative disc disease improve at least initially with conservative therapy.

In patients with cervical discogenic and arthritic disruption of a single joint, many of which cases occur after trauma such as a motor vehicle crash, customary initial conservative measures are indicated, including immobilization in a soft cervical collar, physical therapy, and treatment with NSAIDs, muscle relaxants, antidepressants, and non-narcotic analgesics. Many patients improve without further treatment. Therapy for this type of injury is usually administered on an outpatient basis, although brief hospitalization may be required if pain is severe or progression of deficits is uncertain. Traction has proved unrewarding in the relief of pain and in patients with a hard disc may exacerbate the situation. Traction does provide effective immobilization, and in patients with a soft disc, herniation can be helpful. Physical therapy is often effective and can be used in conjunction with deep heat and ultrasound therapy.

Some patients opt for chiropractic or manipulative therapy, which is reportedly effective in some patients, although it poses a certain degree of risk. One to three times a year, I am referred a patient with cervical disc disease who has been severely injured by manipulation therapy.

Medical therapy with medications can be as simple as ingestion of buffered aspirin with each meal. This treatment does carry a 10% to 20% risk for gastritis or gastrointestinal upset in patients. NSAIDs are likewise effective for an acute event. More chronic therapy is possible, but long-term use of NSAIDs, such as naproxen or ibuprofen, is associated with renal injury.

It is difficult to set an arbitrary time after which nonsurgical treatment should be discontinued and surgery considered. Conservative management should continue as long as the patient is improving. Surgery is reserved for more severe and intractable cases that persist in provoking intolerable symptoms for months. Progressive or resistant neurologic deficits may require early operative decompression. The goals of operation are to prevent further damage and to allow remaining neurons to resume functioning. The decision to proceed with operative treatment must be based on a clear demonstration of the site of origin of the pain, weakness, or neurologic deficit.

Cervical discogenic and arthritic disruption represents a rare indication for operation, and the neurosurgeon who does not operate on any such patient may be wise. Anterior cervical discectomy and fusion yield good results if one can identify a specific level responsible for most of the pain. Discectomy without fusion does not help in this group of patients. Discometry may define patients who will benefit from surgery, but this must be proved. In our experience, only a few patients in this category should ever be considered for surgery.

With radiculopathy, the diagnosis is usually clear. Significant motor weakness is an indication for early operation. If the problem is acute or the neurologic deficit progressive, it is essential to repeat the examination in rapid fashion and obtain the appropriate diagnostic studies expeditiously to allow performance of the operative procedure. If the problem is more chronic, a series of examinations will allow full appreciation of the neurologic syndrome.

Most radiculopathies improve in time without surgical treatment, although some residual weakness and pain can persist. If weakness and pain are persistent or increasingly

severe, operative intervention is necessary (Fig. 10.8). Devastating outcomes as a result of untreated radiculopathy are rare, but associated spinal cord problems can occur and are apparently vascular in origin. The primary goal of surgical treatment is improvement in the patient's quality of life. Radicular complaints often force operative intervention. The patients who require operative care generally fall into two distinct groups: younger patients with a herniated disc and older patients with osteoarthritic bony stenosis. The operative procedure I most commonly use is posterior laminoforaminotomy or anterior cervical discectomy and fusion (Fig. 10.9).

In patients with myeloradiculopathy, it is usually the radiculopathy that causes the patient to seek attention, but the myelopathy must be addressed. The goal of therapy is cord decompression and immobilization. The problem is most often a broad-based disc herniation with or without a spondylotic bar associated with spinal canal stenosis. Decompression and immobilization are most appropriately performed by the anterior approach.

Myelopathy patients with progressive signs and symptoms require operative decompression of the cord. With one-level

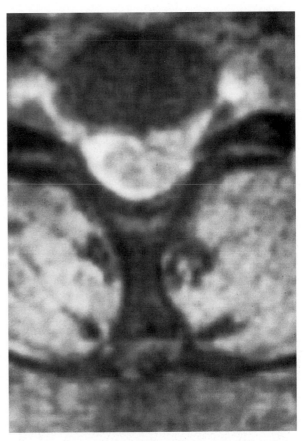

FIG. 10.8. Soft disc herniation of lateral disc. Axial magnetic resonance imaging in a patient with a lateral cervical disc herniation and radiculopathy, which was successfully treated with a posterior laminoforaminotomy and removal of the herniated portion of the disc.

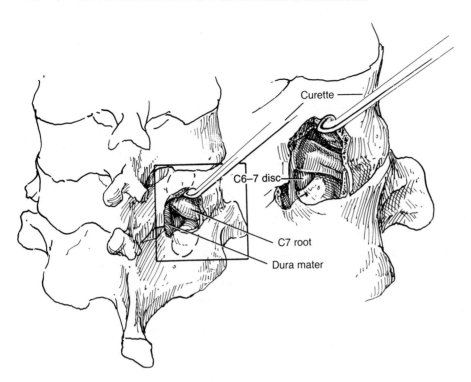

FIG. 10.9. Keyhole foraminotomy and discectomy.

disc herniation, an anterior approach is clearly superior. For multilevel disc herniation and resultant marked degenerative compression, the anterior approach is usually preferred. When congenital spinal stenosis exists with minor degenerative changes or diffuse osteoarthritic changes, a posterior decompressive laminectomy or laminoplasty is effective.

PERIOPERATIVE STEROID MANAGEMENT

In an effort to prevent intraoperative spinal cord injury, I began using perioperative prophylactic steroid administration during performance of all cervical spine surgery. On the basis of the compelling data from NASCIS II, I and my colleagues initiated a program of perioperative dosing of patients operated on for CSM with the intensive intravenous regimen proposed in the study. Although no clinical studies have been performed supporting this course of action, I hope that large intravenous doses of methylprednisolone will exert a therapeutic effect in preventing posttraumatic neuronal degeneration and maximize the potential for recovery should any inadvertent intraoperative spinal cord trauma occur. Typically, length of stay is 1 day.

RESULTS OF SURGERY

Internal Disc Disruption

Whitecloud and Seago, using provocative discography, evaluated the results of surgical intervention in 40 patients with chronic discogenic symptoms (4). They excluded patients with cervical spondylosis, radiculopathy, or myelopathy. Using strict criteria for evaluation of surgical results, they reported 70% good or excellent results after anterior disc excision and fusion. This favorable surgical outcome in a complex and difficult patient population mandates more thorough evaluation of diagnostic disc injection in the evaluation of patients with discogenic pain or radiculitis.

Radiculopathy

Zeidman and Ducker reported 172 patients operated on for cervical radiculopathy (5). Because some patients underwent laminoforaminotomies at multiple levels, 243 levels in all underwent operation. Most of the patients had pathology at C5-C6 and C6-C7. The average age of patients undergoing posterior cervical laminoforaminotomy for radiculopathy was 49 years. In 43 patients (25%), a one-level laminoforaminotomy without discectomy was performed. Sixty patients (35%) required a posterolateral discectomy for herniated disc fragments, again mostly at C5-C6 and C6-C7. Patients operated on for herniated discs were younger (mean age, 43 years) than those without discectomy.

A group of 68 patients (40%) who were slightly older (mean age, 55 years) were operated on at multiple levels. Preoperative diagnostic studies showed multilevel foraminal stenosis due to osteoarthritis. Multilevel foraminotomies were performed to relieve the patients of more diffuse upper extremity symptoms.

In 167 patients (97%) who underwent laminoforaminotomies, radicular pain was relieved; 77% of patients were monitored for 2 years or longer, and the remainder were monitored for 1 year. Radicular pain was not relieved in 5 patients (3%), 4 of whom had undergone operation at multiple levels. Improvement in the motor weakness back to baseline function was achieved in 36 of the 39 (93%) patients with preoperative motor deficits who underwent laminoforaminotomies with discectomy. Patients with C6 and C7 radiculopathy showed rapid and occasionally immediate improvement or recovery of motor function. The 68 patients who underwent multilevel laminoforaminotomies initially presented with pain and weakness and obtained significant relief of their pain but minimal relief of their weakness. Four of these patients (5.8%) obtained substantial relief of their preoperative motor deficits. Almost all patients undergoing laminoforaminotomy with discectomy or one-level laminoforaminotomies had a decrease in preoperative sensory abnormalities. In contrast, the degree of reduction of sensory deficits was not as great in patients who underwent multilevel laminoforaminotomies. No patient regained depressed reflexes. No wound infections occurred in any patient. Four patients had air embolism without clinical sequelae. The only significant morbidity was a central cord syndrome in 1 patient, which resolved within a few months, with some residual deficit.

Many factors determine the selection of either an anterior or posterior approach to cervical radiculopathy secondary to degenerative disc disease. These include the surgeon's training, familiarity with each technique, previous favorable or unfavorable experiences with a particular operation, a concept of pathological mechanisms, and knowledge of the existing literature. Posterior cervical laminoforaminotomy for radiculopathy has been proved to produce good outcomes as compared with anterior cervical discectomy with or without fusion in selected cases.

Some of the problems associated with the posterior approach include a higher incidence of nerve root trauma secondary to nerve root manipulation while removing disc fragments. This is most common at the C4-C5 level because the C5 nerve root is quite sensitive to even minor manipulations. This likely reflects the relatively shorter course of the C5 nerve root and its relatively greater tethering. Depending on the eccentricity of the disc fragment or osteophyte, the posterior procedure may not directly address the area of pathology and provide only indirect nerve root decompression. There is a well-published, higher incidence of recurrence of radiculopathy with the posterior approach compared with the anterior. There is more postoperative pain with the posterior technique compared with anterior discectomy and fusion. Perhaps, newer muscle splitting techniques with microscopic will diminish postoperative pain and spasm. I favor anterior cervical discectomy and fusion over posterior laminoforaminotomy in many cases, for the previously discussed reasons. In selected patients with lateral soft disc herniations, the posterior technique is certainly preferable.

Myelopathy

That surgical treatment of CSM is better than no treatment appears to be fairly well established, although even this assumption continues to be questioned. Rowland contends that the outcome of surgery has not been conclusively proved better than the natural history or nonoperative therapy and notes that there are no clear guidelines for the selection of patients who will benefit from surgery and no standardization of preoperative evaluation, trials of nonoperative therapy, ascertainment of progressive disability, or assessment of outcome and thus recommends a controlled, multicenter trial (6).

Gorter and Epstein extensively reviewed the literature on this issue. Accumulated data on the results of nonoperative therapy for CSM indicate that 3% to 50% of patients can expect to improve without surgical intervention. The remainder will deteriorate further. Surgery for CSM yields better results, irrespective of the approach. Arnasson and colleagues (7) reviewed 114 patients with CSM and reported the results of anterior surgery and posterior surgery; and 69% improved. The results were independent of patient age or duration of symptoms.

The anterior approach is directed toward the degenerative structure, degenerative disc, and osteophytic spurs responsible for cord and root compression. Extensive anterior decompression and arthrodesis procedures allow direct removal of diseased ventral features and eliminate the dynamic forces that may be the cause of CSM. The anterior approach has classically been restricted to patients manifesting disease at either one or two levels, although some proponents of the approach report using the anterior approach for three, four, or five levels of disease. Patients undergoing anterior procedures often have better results in terms of preoperative motor performance than patients who undergo posterior procedures. Treatment for multilevel cervical spinal stenosis has consisted of anterior or posterior decompression approaches. If the spinal cord compression is limited to the disc space at one, two, or, some authors argue, three levels, an anterior approach is indicated. The posterior approach is not indicated for isolated anterior disease. The worst results in laminectomy series have been obtained in patients who have undergone limited laminectomy. Limited laminectomy for one- or two-level disease can produce posterior dural sac "herniation" due to anterior compression. Extended laminectomy allows the thecal sac to float posteriorly off the anterior osteophytes and avoid this complication. However, postoperative MRI confirms that posterior migration of the spinal cord after laminectomy may be inadequate to clear osteophytes in patients with straight or reversed cervical curvature. Spinal anatomy should be considered in the selection of the best surgical procedure and the extent of laminectomy for patients with spondylotic myelopathy.

Multiple discectomies and interbody fusion may be appropriate in patients with spinal cord compression due to disc herniation or osteophytes around the disc margins. Multilevel discectomies with multilevel interbody fusions are associated with an increased risk for pseudoarthrosis, may not adequately address osteophytic cord compression, and may not correct kyphotic deformity. The use of corpectomies is indicated in cases of spinal cord compression due to discs or osteophytes that extend beyond the disc margins. Furthermore, it may reduce the incidence of nonunion and allow more complete and safer removal of osteophytes compressing the spinal cord. In addition, corpectomy is advantageous for patients with CSM who are kyphotic. Performance of an extended procedure for isolated disease is not justified. The anterior approach allows direct spinal fusion, which may eliminate the abnormal forces causing osteophyte production or disc degeneration and which allows treatment of a lordotic curve or kyphotic deformity that, even with posterior spinal cord decompression, can produce myelopathic symptoms. However, the risk for substantial morbidity is increased by the use of corpectomies rather than multilevel discectomies with interbody fusions.

In patients with diffuse spondylosis with cervical stenosis over an extended region and in patients with a congenitally narrowed cervical canal, the posterior approach has many benefits. Laminectomy with foraminotomies not only releases the thecal sac, releasing the spinal cord from mechanical compression, but also decompresses the roots. The procedure is completed rapidly and is not as physiologically demanding on either the patient or the surgeon. Cervical laminectomy enlarges the spinal canal but does not reduce all the dynamic forces, which may actually increase cervical mobility, leading to exacerbation of the myelopathy. Certain patients with CSM demonstrate instability in the upper cervical vertebral column associated with marked narrowing of the lower cervical segments. Such a combination of pathology makes it difficult to use routine surgical procedures, especially in elderly and severely debilitated patients. In patients with diffuse disease and abnormal spinal movement, surgical fusion may be added but often will not alter the pathologic process. The risk for delayed spinal deformity secondary to multilevel laminectomy is low in such patients; consequently, it does not place constraints in this patient population. As indicated by the results of multiple series, paying strict attention to the lateral extent of laminectomy reduces the risk for postlaminectomy instability and kyphosis to nearly zero. Of note, however, is that in younger patients, especially after tumor removal, spinal fusion may be necessary in nearly every case.

In the performance of decompression laminectomy, there is no justification for dural opening and dentate ligament section. Benzel and colleagues evaluated 75 patients who underwent surgical treatment for CSM with laminectomy plus dentate ligament section, laminectomy alone, or anterior cervical decompression and fusion (8). All patients who improved substantially in the laminectomy plus dentate ligament group, as well as in the laminectomy-alone groups, had normal cervical lordosis. The remainder had either normal lordosis or no curve. All patients in the anterior cervical fusion group had either a straight spine or kyphosis. These results implicate spine curvature, in addition to choice of operation, as important factors in determining outcome. Benzel suggested that patients with myelopathy and cervical kyphosis were best treated with anterior cervical fusion and that patients with cervical lordosis were best treated with a posterior procedure. Although selected patients might benefit from dentate ligament section, no criteria are available that differentiate this small subset of patients. Except in the studies of Benzel and colleagues (8) and Crandall and Batzdorf (9), patients undergoing dentate sectioning, especially those with kyphosis, had the poorest results. The greatest incidence of clinical worsening was noted in patients undergoing these procedures, particularly when a limited laminectomy was performed. Although the best results are obtained by surgeons performing extensive laminectomies with foraminotomies and osteophyte removal, I do not recommend this procedure to all surgeons. The excellent results obtained with posterior excision of osteophytes is not something that all surgeons can achieve. A significant portion of the morbidity classically associated with the posterior approach for treatment of CSM derives from early series in which this approach was used.

Goals of obtaining and adequately maintaining the spinal canal decompression prompted development of a variety of decompressive laminectomy techniques. These approaches prevent progressive restriction of the spinal canal by scar retraction after laminectomy and maintain static and dynamic cervical spine stability. Maintenance of canal decompression usually is not a problem after routine laminectomy. I use a small Hemovac drain in such patients in the immediate (24-hour) postoperative period. Preventing the layering of blood products beneath a four-layer muscular closure is important, and none of our patients has had "postlaminectomy membrane." However, structures lateral to the canal must be preserved, including the pedicles and facet joints, if stability is to be maintained after extensive cervical laminectomies. Although concern regarding postoperative subluxation and "swan neck deformity" has been raised, such complications did not occur in our series, possibly because of the strict respect paid to the facet joints laterally and preservation of their integrity throughout the surgical procedure. A 45-degree 1- or 2-mm Kerrison punch can open the foramina by removing the soft tissue and bone in direct contact with the nerve root without destroying joint integrity. With regard to the extent of the laminectomy, I do not typically decompress the spine two levels above and below the area of compression, but remove only enough lamina to relieve cord compression. The laminectomy often extends one level above and below the area of myelographic compression to remove any impedance to the posterior translation of the dural sac. Surgeons performing osteophytectomy by a posterior approach advocate further laminectomy extension to allow adequate spinal cord retraction for safe removal of osteophytes.

The surgical approach to patients with CSM remains controversial. Several series directly comparing the anterior and posterior procedures have been reported. In 1963, Dereymaker compared anterior cervical discectomy with interbody fusion to laminectomy with dural opening: 48% of patients operated on anteriorly showed improvement, as compared with 26% operated on posteriorly (10). Since then, the literature has been replete with articles extolling the virtues of one procedure over another. Mayfield compared the anterior and posterior approaches in 1965 and reported improvement in 80% of patients undergoing laminectomy and in 100% of patients treated with anterior discectomy and fusion. Despite satisfactory results with the posterior approach, concern about a 14% incidence of postoperative instability with subluxation and increased postoperative pain requiring painful rehabilitation in patients undergoing laminectomies prompted Mayfield to abandon the posterior approach.

Reviewing surgical studies between 1966 and 1970, Goner reported a 73% improvement incidence in 345 patients treated with anterior fusion and a 70% improvement rate among 184 patients treated with laminectomies. Epstein, reviewing a larger group of patients, noted similar improvement rates. Crandall reported better results for laminectomy with dural opening (80% improvement) than for an anterior procedure (71%) in 1966 (9). Only 31% of patients with dural closure showed improvement. Kadoya reported improvement in 95% of patients undergoing anterior osteophytectomy (11). Therefore, despite occasional reports to the contrary, surgery appears to produce better results in treatment of CSM than does nonoperative treatment. Nurick reported improvement in 73% of patients treated anteriorly, in 50% of patients treated with a posterior approach, and in only 30% of patients treated conservatively (3).

Gregorius and colleagues reported improvement in 73% of patients treated by the anterior approach, whereas only 33% of patients who underwent laminectomy improved (10). Only percent of patients treated with laminectomy had the dura opened and a graft applied during the procedure. Diffuse disease was treated by laminectomy, whereas focal disease was treated by an anterior discectomy and fusion. Phillips' (12) report of 102 cases treated in 10 years yielded similar results: 73% of 65 patients operated on by anterior approach improved; 53% of 24 receiving laminectomies improved; and 37% of 24 patients treated nonoperatively improved.

Guidetti and Fortuna (13) reported that 82% of patients improved after undergoing an anterior procedure for cervical spondylosis, and 66% to 81% of patients improved after undergoing a posterior procedure. The best results were achieved in patients who underwent extensive laminec-

tomies with foraminotomies. Patients undergoing dentate ligament sectioning had a worse outcome than those who did not. The more severe the initial presenting syndrome, the poorer the long-term outcome. Hukuda and colleagues (14) reported on 191 patients with CSM operated on in a 19-year period with an average follow-up of 31 months. Posterior operations provided better results for transverse lesions, Brown-Séquard syndrome, and motor syndromes, but brachialgia and cord syndrome and central cord syndrome were satisfactorily treated by anterior procedures. Of the three anterior and three posterior techniques used, no one technique showed overall superiority. Although no comparative study shows the posterior approach to be superior to the anterior approach, evidence suggests that the posterior approach may be at least as good for treatment of cervical spondylosis in certain situations. This is particularly true when one considers that the patient groups treated with the two approaches are often dissimilar. Yonenobou and associates (15) compared anterior fusion with extensive laminectomy and laminoplasty to determine the treatment of choice for multilevel CSM. Forty-one patients undergoing subtotal corpectomy and strut grafting and 42 undergoing laminectomy and laminoplasty were followed for at least 2 years postoperatively. Factors affecting surgical prognosis (age at surgery, duration of symptoms, severity of neurologic deficit, anteroposterior canal diameter, transverse area of the cord at the site of maximum compression, number of levels involved) were statistically comparable between the two groups. The difference between the recovery rate and final score between the two groups was not statistically significant.

The initial results 1 year after surgical treatment are quite rewarding. The improvement afforded to patients is often maintained for several years. Within 5 years, about 15% of the patients have recurrence of their signs and symptoms. About half of the patients have new pathology at a different level or an incomplete fusion with a hypertrophic joint. The other half have no obvious reason for their progressive pathology, and diagnostic studies show an atrophic spinal cord. Ten years after operation, an even greater number of patients have deteriorated, with obvious cord atrophy. A disturbing incidence of progression of myelopathy was noted 10 years after surgery. MRI identified many of the causes (e.g., newly developed intervertebral disc herniation and progression of spondylosis associated with spinal malalignment in both cephalad and caudal directions). Other adverse changes were hypertrophy of the yellow ligament and OPLL. Use of improved decompression techniques such as decompression to a width of 16 mm or more with intraoperative ultrasonography and extirpation of the posterior longitudinal ligament may reduce the incidence of late neurologic deterioration. The only diagnostic study correlating with poor results is MRI. If on T2-weighted image, the cord shows edematous or demyelinated areas, it is highly probable that the patient will not improve by undergoing either anterior or posterior decompressive procedures.

No one operation is best. It is therefore prudent to select the appropriate operation. Kurz presented a comparative analysis of the ability of different surgical procedures to address adequately the compressive problems sustained by a patient with symptomatic cervical myelopathy. Anterior decompression discectomy with graft fusion is a safe procedure, but its effectiveness may be limited when the extent of disease is more than three intervertebral disc levels. Anterior corpectomy with graft fusion permits more direct and extensive access to the spinal cord and is the procedure of choice for CSM associated with spinal deformity. Rigid external or internal immobilization is required, but operative morbidity was no greater in our series. Cervical laminectomy may be effective in decompressing the spinal cord when no associated spinal deformity or instability is present, provided that extensive resection of facet joints is avoided.

Based on a review of previous studies, and in my opinion, biomechanical considerations suggest the following guidelines for surgical management of CSM. It is not recommended that the dura mater or the pia mater be opened or that the dentate ligaments be transected in surgical treatment of CSM. Anterior decompression and fusion, preferably with the Smith-Robinson technique, is recommended for patients with anterior impingement of the spinal cord at one or two levels in the absence of a narrow spinal canal. Posterior decompression is recommended when three or more levels are involved and particularly when there is developmental stenosis of the canal [i.e., a developmental anteroposterior diameter (DAD) below 13 mm and a spondylotic anteroposterior diameter (SAD) below 11 mm]. Neurologic outcome of laminectomy and laminoplasty for CSM is not different. If there is evidence of instability or a potential for it, posterior decompression procedures should be accompanied by a facet fusion or, in the case of laminoplasty, some fusion modification. In some circumstances, significant multilevel anterior spur formation and compression in association with a stenotic canal should be treated with anterior and posterior surgery, with appropriate attention paid to maintaining adequate stability. The advantages and disadvantages of these various surgical procedures and their relative appropriateness in various clinical conditions will be gradually clarified through well-designed and executed laboratory and clinical investigations.

Misalignment and instability after cervical laminectomy, performed to treat spondylotic myelopathy, have been described as possible adverse effects. Hansen-Schwartz and colleagues reported on 46 patients who underwent laminectomies (16). Static subluxation was observed in 26% of the patients with an average slip of 3.7 mm; 7% had abnormal intervertebral movement. Seventy-four percent of the patients showed abnormal spinal curvature as judged from radiographs. However, no correlation with outcome was observed. Although some patients develop postural anomaly, laminectomy remains, in terms of instability, a justifiable procedure in the elderly patient with spondylosis.

Houten and Cooper reported their results with multilevel laminectomy and instrumentation with lateral mass plates for CSM (17). They found that this was associated with minimal morbidity, provided excellent decompression of the spinal cord (as visualized on MRI), produced immediate stability of the cervical spine, prevented kyphotic deformity, and precluded further development of spondylosis at fused levels. Neurologic outcomes were equal or superior to those for multilevel anterior procedures, and this procedure prevented spinal deformity associated with laminoplasty or noninstrumented multilevel laminectomies.

Operative procedures on the cervical vertebral column and spinal cord must be individualized for the patient. Most present series suggest that the anterior approach, occasionally corpectomy, may be associated with the highest levels of clinical improvement, but posterior approaches offer significant advantages in treatment of patients with multilevel disease. Laminectomy must be avoided, however, in the presence of curvature reversal of the cervical vertebral column. In certain select cases, consideration of a combined anterior and posterior approach or total stabilization may be considered. Although no consensus exists regarding the exclusivity of a specific surgical procedure, and although all possible approaches should be considered, the final decision should be based on detailed compressive and biomechanical pathology. Complete radiographic and neurophysiologic studies, including evaluation in various dynamic positions of the cervical spine (flexion, extension, and rotation), assist in defining the most efficacious treatment method.

Many options are available for surgical treatment of CSM; each has advantages and disadvantages. I have described my approach to this clinical syndrome and the surgical techniques I prefer for each of its variants. Clear, objective scientific data based on randomized, prospective clinical studies comparing the various surgical alternatives are lacking. The information that exists does not clearly favor any one approach or operative option. It is critical to remember that each surgeon's experience and skill with a given technique have a profound impact on outcome. Contemporary spine surgeons should be well versed in multiple operative techniques and should choose an appropriate approach for each patient based on that patient's clinical presentation, unique anatomy, and pathologic condition, modified by the surgeon's personal experience.

A review of the extensive literature on CSM shows that the clinical picture and pathology are now better defined and the complex pathogenetic mechanisms better understood. Improved monitoring and improved anesthesia technique allow avoidance of intraoperative hypotension. With recent advances in investigative procedures such as CT, MRI, and somatosensory evoked potentials, the diagnosis can be more accurate and the assessment more complete. Careful selection of patients for the appropriate treatment modality (conservative, anterior, or posterior surgery) is crucial to successful management of patients.

Operations do not improve all patients. For reasons not entirely clear, 15% of patients do not obtain significant clinical improvement. Many of these patients report improvement, but objective evidence is lacking. In this group of patients, the progression of the myelopathy is usually halted. In most reported series, 3% to 5% of patients have poor outcomes, almost invariably associated with intraoperative hypotension. Inexplicable deterioration does occasionally occur. Finally, bad results occur, with or without operative care. Some of our selected patients who have undergone myelogram or CT have not obtained good results. In no case have I noted persistent compression. I believe that a bad result does not imply bad surgery (malpractice) even though in the current medicolegal climate, malpractice suits are common. Full audit over 2 years or longer is often more relevant than a single case when assessing bad results.

REFERENCES

1. Fehlings MG, Skaf G. A review of the pathophysiology of cervical spondylotic myelopathy with insights for potential novel mechanisms drawn from traumatic spinal cord injury. *Spine* 1998;23(24):2730–2737.
2. Kim DH, et al. Molecular biology of cervical myelopathy and spinal cord injury: role of oligodendrocyte apoptosis. *Spine J* 2003;3(6):510–519.
3. Nurick S. The pathogenesis of cervical spondylotic myelopathy. *Acta Neurol Belg* 1976;76(5–6):274–275.
4. Whitecloud TS 3rd, Seago RA. Cervical discogenic syndrome. Results of operative intervention in patients with positive discography. *Spine* 1987;12(4):313–316.
5. Zeidman SM, Ducker TB. Posterior cervical laminoforaminotomy for radiculopathy: review of 172 cases. *Neurosurgery* 1993;33(3):356–362.
6. Rowland LP. Surgical treatment of cervical spondylotic myelopathy: time for a controlled trial. *Neurology* 1992;42(1):5–13.
7. Arnasson O, Carlsson CA, Pellettieri L. Surgical and conservative treatment of cervical spondylotic radiculopathy and myelopathy. *Acta Neurochir* (Wien) 1987;84(1–2):48–53.
8. Benzel EC, et al. Cervical laminectomy and dentate ligament section for cervical spondylotic myelopathy. *J Spinal Disord* 1991;4(3):286–295.
9. Crandall PH, Batzdorf U. Cervical spondylotic myelopathy. *J Neurosurg* 1966;25(1):57–66.
10. Gregorius FK, Estrin T, Crandall PH. Cervical spondylotic radiculopathy and myelopathy. A long-term follow-up study. *Arch Neurol* 1976;33(9):618–625.
11. Kadoya S, et al. Anterior osteophytectomy for cervical spondylotic myelopathy in developmentally narrow canal. *J Neurosurg* 1985;63(6):845–850.
12. Phillips DG. Upper limb involvement in cervical spondylosis. *J Neurol Neurosurg Psychiatry* 1975;38(4):386–390.
13. Guidetti B, Fortuna A. Long-term results of surgical treatment of myelopathy due to cervical spondylosis. *J Neurosurg* 1969;30(6):714–721.
14. Hukuda S, et al. Operations for cervical spondylotic myelopathy. A comparison of the results of anterior and posterior procedures. *J Bone Joint Surg Br* 1985;67(4):609–615.
15. Yonenobu K, et al. Choice of surgical treatment for multisegmental cervical spondylotic myelopathy. *Spine* 1985;10(8):710–716.
16. Hansen-Schwartz J, Kruse-Larsen C, Nielsen CJ. Follow-up after cervical laminectomy, with special reference to instability and deformity. *Br J Neurosurg* 2003;17(4):301–305.
17. Houten JK, Cooper PR. Laminectomy and posterior cervical plating for multilevel cervical spondylotic myelopathy and ossification of the posterior longitudinal ligament: effects on cervical alignment, spinal cord compression, and neurological outcome. *Neurosurgery* 2003;52(5):1081–1087; discussion, 1087–1088.

CHAPTER 11

Neurologic Evaluation of the Cervical Spine

Maurice R. Hanson and Nestor Galvez

SYMPTOMS OF CERVICAL DYSFUNCTION

The principal symptom that brings the patient to medical attention is usually pain. Other symptoms may accompany pain, including as weakness, numbness, and paresthesias, but they are not usually the major concerns in the early phases.

Pain of cervical origin can be considered in one or more of five categories: (a) local pain, (b) referred pain, (c) radicular pain, (d) funicular pain, and (d) pain due to myospasm (1) (Table 11.1).

The key discriminating features in this scheme include the mode of onset (acute, subacute, or chronic); nature of the pain (dull, aching, sharp, or stabbing); location of the pain at onset and subsequent spread, if any; factors that alleviate or exacerbate the pain; and potential underlying causes.

Local pain is of a deep, aching quality; it is made worse with loading and movement and usually does not radiate. It is the pain most often encountered in cervical spondylosis with or without muscle tension and is also termed *mechanical pain*. Metastatic disease to the spine often causes local pain that is typically worse at night, with recumbency and rest.

Referred pain accompanies local pain and is usually dull, aching, relatively diffuse, nonradicular, and sometimes segmental, but of little localizing value. A common example is the aching pain in the shoulder and chest from chronic cervical spondylosis. An uncommon cause is the referred pain to the shoulder from disease causing irritation of the diaphragm.

Radicular pain is quite specific in its typical form. It is sharp and stabbing and radiates distally in specific areas of the extremity. It is often associated with other sensory symptoms, such as paresthesias, and is invariably worse with anything that compresses or stretches the inflamed nerve root. Because it arises from irritation of the dorsal root, it has a dermatomal distribution (Fig. 11.1). There may be a superimposed and more diffuse, chronic ache (myotomal pain). Radicular pain is most often encountered in cervical disc disease and less likely in tumors such as metastasis and neurofibromas.

Funicular pain is due to dysfunction of intraspinal sensory pathways, either the spinothalamic tract or the posterior columns. It is characteristically diffuse and burning and sometimes knifelike, is localized on the trunk or extremity, and is frequently provoked by tactile stimulation, flexion of the neck, or anything that distorts ascending pathways. A form of this pain is the electric-like sensation in the limbs that occurs with neck flexion (Lhermitte sign). The most frequent causes of this unusual pain are intramedullary lesions, such as syringomyelia, spinal cord tumors, or myelitis, and compressive lesions, such as cervical spondylosis.

Pain due to myospasm is among the most common causes of neck pain. The onset is gradual or acute. It may remain localized or spread to other areas. It is often associated with muscle tenderness, limited motion, and tender trigger points, as in the myofascial pain syndromes (1).

In addition to pain, other sensory symptoms that are helpful in diagnosis and localization include paresthesias, dysesthesias, and numbness. Paresthesias (pins and needles sensation) and dysesthesias are irritative phenomena and are more frequent and useful in localization than absence of sensation. When present, paresthesias may be clinically diagnostic, especially with digit localization. In radiculopathies, the location of the paresthesias is among the most helpful localizing phenomena (2). Isolated paresthesias of the thumb indicate the C6 root, paresthesias of any combination of digits two to four suggest C7, and paresthesias of digit five suggest the C8-T1 level.

The other major symptom is weakness. This is sometimes a difficult symptom to assess, especially in the pres-

TABLE 11.1. *Classification of Pain of Spinal Origin*

- Local
- Referred
- Radicular
- Funicular
- Pain due to myospasm

(From Byrne et al.)

ence of pain, because of incomplete voluntary effort due to guarding. It is also often less helpful in the diagnosis of radiculopathy because of myotomal overlap. Nonetheless, the pattern may be diagnostic, such as the shoulder girdle weakness and scapular winging that occur after the severe pain of acute brachial plexitis.

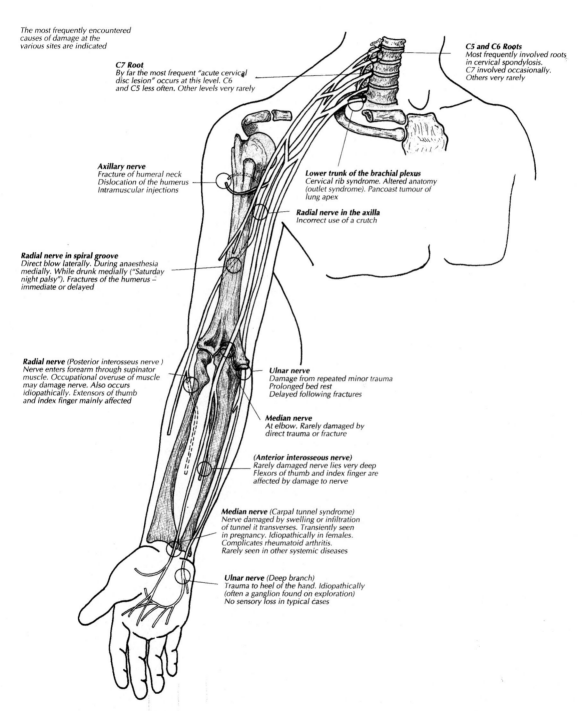

The most frequently encountered causes of damage at the various sites are indicated

C7 Root
By far the most frequent "acute cervical disc lesion" occurs at this level. C6 and C5 less often. Other levels very rarely

C5 and C6 Roots
Most frequently involved roots in cervical spondylosis. C7 involved occasionally. Others very rarely

Axillary nerve
Fracture of humeral neck
Dislocation of the humerus
Intramuscular injections

Lower trunk of the brachial plexus
Cervical rib syndrome. Altered anatomy (outlet syndrome). Pancoast tumour of lung apex

Radial nerve in the axilla
Incorrect use of a crutch

Radial nerve in spiral groove
Direct blow laterally. During anaesthesia medially. While drunk medially ("Saturday night palsy"). Fractures of the humerus – immediate or delayed

Radial nerve (Posterior interosseus nerve)
Nerve enters forearm through supinator muscle. Occupational overuse of muscle may damage nerve. Also occurs idiopathically. Extensors of thumb and index finger mainly affected

Ulnar nerve
Damage from repeated minor trauma
Prolonged bed rest
Delayed following fractures

Median nerve
At elbow. Rarely damaged by direct trauma or fracture

(Anterior interosseous nerve)
Rarely damaged nerve lies very deep
Flexors of thumb and index finger are affected by damage to nerve

Median nerve (Carpal tunnel syndrome)
Nerve damaged by swelling or infiltration of tunnel it transverses. Transiently seen in pregnancy. Idiopathically in females. Complicates rheumatoid arthritis. Rarely seen in other systemic diseases

Ulnar nerve (Deep branch)
Trauma to heel of the hand. Idiopathically (often a ganglion found on exploration) No sensory loss in typical cases

FIG. 11.1. Anatomy of the nerve supply to the arm. (From Patten J. Diagnosis of cervical root and peripheral nerve lesions affecting the arm. In: *Neurological differential diagnosis*, 2nd ed. London: Springer, 1996:282–297, with permission.)

PRINCIPLES OF THE EXAMINATION

The first basic principle is that the examination be tailored to the patient's history. The second basic principle is that the examination be thorough. There is, unfortunately, a growing tendency to minimize this principle in the era of high-resolution imaging. Nowhere is this more treacherous and misleading than in cervical spinal cord disorders.

The examination begins with, or incorporates, a focused general physical examination, beginning with the observation of how the patient holds his or her neck during the history taking and of how freely the neck moves when the patient is distracted.

Observation of the spinal motion includes both passive and active range of motion (ROM). Observe for limited motion in one direction or another and estimate or measure the degree of limitation. Localized muscle tenderness is a useful observation in neck pain, especially if the spontaneous pain can be recreated. At the same time, palpate the supraclavicular fossae for abnormal or firm masses and vascular structures.

In patients with upper limb pain, it is important to exclude local structural limb and joint pathology. This includes use of passive and active ROM of the shoulder, elbow, and wrist (3) as well as careful palpation over the acromioclavicular joint and the ventral aspect of the shoulder for bicipital tendinitis. Consider rotator cuff pathology if attempts to abduct the shoulder result in pain.

In the forearm, radiohumeral bursitis (epicondylitis, "tennis elbow") might be confused with a C6 radiculopathy. The diagnosis of epicondylitis can be suspected by observing the inability to extend fully the elbow actively or passively because of pain. Hand grasp results in pain due to tightening of the extensor wrist tendons as the wrist reflexly extends. Localized tenderness just distal to the radial aspect of the elbow is a useful sign. Disappearance of pain and tenderness with injection of a local anesthetic confirms the diagnosis.

Local wrist pathology may be confused with radicular disease and is sometimes caused by de Quervain synovitis when it radiates into the thumb and forearm. In addition to tenderness over the tendons, pain is increased when the hand is forcibly ulnar-deviated with the thumb flexed and adducted (Finkelstein maneuver) (3).

Special maneuvers of the neck and upper limb can be helpful in situations in which the cause of the limb pain may be obscure. These tests must be interpreted cautiously because of the high frequency of false-positive results in normal individuals.

In the Spurling maneuver, the neck is extended and the chin rotated toward the side of the limb pain along with downward compression of the head. A positive result with the reproduction of the radicular pain is due to nerve root compression (4). Accentuation of the neck pain is not diagnostic. The arm pain must be elicited to be considered useful. The Naffziger sign is another potentially helpful test when a radicular pain source is sought. A positive result consists of digital pressure over the internal jugular veins for several seconds or until the head feels full, reproducing the arm pain. The mechanism is due to increased intracranial and intraspinal pressure resulting in accentuated traction of inflamed nerve roots.

The controversial thoracic outlet syndrome (TOS) is another entity that should be considered in the differential diagnosis of limb pain. The symptoms are neurologic, vascular, or both and tend to relate to the distal limb (forearm and fingers) rather than neck, shoulder, and arm. TOC may be confused with a C8-T1 radiculopathy because of the sensory symptoms on the medial side of the forearm, hand, and fourth and fifth fingers. Ischemic symptoms may be intermittent or chronic and vary from Raynaud phenomenon to ischemic digits, with embolization from mural thrombi developing in the poststenotic dilation of the subclavian artery. Venous occlusion is uncommon. Careful inspection of the upper arm and chest for venous dilation usually is sufficient to exclude it.

If TOS is a consideration, blood pressure recordings in both arms and auscultation for bruit above and below the clavicle is necessary. Careful palpation of the supraclavicular fossa is required, looking for a bony protuberance from a cervical rib, an anomalous first rib, or an enlarged firm mass from lung cancer. Next, the radial pulse is felt during neck extension with the chin rotated toward the side and with full expansion of the chest (Adson maneuver). Another maneuver, the costoclavicular maneuver, involves adduction of the arms to the side and active retraction of the scapulae while palpating both radial pulses. With either maneuver, the result is clinically important only when the appropriate pulse is diminished and the neurologic signs or symptoms are reproduced.

In patients with acroparesthesias, assessment for the carpal tunnel syndrome with the Tinel and Phalen maneuvers is useful, although of limited specificity and sensitivity.

THE NEUROLOGIC EXAMINATION

Cranial and Related Nerves

In patients with neck and arm pain, careful examination of the cranial nerves may yield diagnostic clues as to the cause. Among these is Horner syndrome with ipsilateral ptosis, miosis, and variable anhidrosis. There is both depression of the upper lid and elevation of the lower lid. The anisocoria may be subtle but is more apparent in a darkened room because the intact pupil enlarges in darkness, whereas the affected pupil cannot enlarge. If Horner syndrome develops in the context of cervical disease, it will be at the level of C8-T1 spinal segments, the ciliospinal center, or the preganglionic fibers as they cross to ascend in the cervical sympathetic trunk. The fibers then ascend for their final synapse in the superior cervical ganglion. Neck pain associated with lesions of the superior cervical ganglion and adjacent fibers generally involve skull-based tumors such as metastases, lymphoma, and nasopharyngeal carcinoma. Apical lesions involve the preganglionic fibers.

In the preganglionic intramedullary segment (C8 to T2), conditions that need to be considered are intramedullary or paravertebral tumors, syringomyelia, cervical ribs, subclavian aneurysm, and inflammatory processes such as tuberculosis. Associated signs include atrophy and weakness of the intrinsic hand muscles (C8-T1 spinal cord segment or lower trunk of the brachial plexus). Anhidrosis, if present, is confined to the face. Instillation of hydroxyamphetamine 1% in a patient with suspected Horner syndrome is helpful for localization. Horner syndrome due to preganglionic lesions causes dilation of the pupil, whereas that due to postganglionic lesions does not (5).

Neck and arm pain associated with facial sensory loss may be due to intramedullary spinal lesions as the descending tract of V extends to about C2 in the neck, and sensory loss or other signs in the opposite side may be present.

Ocular movements in neck and arm pain should be thoroughly evaluated. Nystagmus, including downbeat nystagmus on lateral or primary gaze, is sometimes observed with lesions of the craniovertebral junction, including Arnold-Chiari I malformation.

Muscles innervated by the lower cranial nerves, including the pharynx, tongue, and sternocleidomastoid, may be weak or atrophic in patients tumors of the skull base.

Motor Examination

Observations should include muscle bulk and strength, the presence or absence of focal atrophy and fasciculation, and other abnormal involuntary movements, such as tremors, spasms, tics, or myoclonus. Note should be taken of muscle tone, including spasticity.

Certain general principles of muscle evaluation include assessment in a rostrocaudal sequence: neck, shoulder, arm, forearm, hand, chest, abdomen, thigh, leg, foot, then toe, comparing right and left.

An important consideration is the length-strength principle; that is, muscles are strongest when they act from their shortest position and weakest from their longest position. Hence, the most useful information is obtained from the largest muscles by placing them at some disadvantage. For example, the triceps muscle is best examined with the elbow partially flexed, whereas the small hand and finger muscles are best tested while at their full advantage. For example, the first dorsal interosseous is maximally abducted against examiner resistance. When possible, the muscle belly should be palpated during strength testing. For example, in a patient with suspected radial neuropathy, one might miss the fact that the brachioradialis muscle is denervated and atrophic if not palpated even though the elbow flexion power is preserved owing to intact biceps and brachialis muscles.

The evaluation of the shoulder girdle begins with free arm movement extending the arms forward, followed by a lateral abduction and observing for limited scapular motion, including scapular winging. Arm abduction is initiated by the supraspinatus muscle, followed by the deltoid and finally scapular rotation to elevate the arms vertically. Scapular abduction is tested with the hand on the hips, forcing the elbows backward against the examiner's resistance. Elbow flexion is performed with the arm fully supinated (biceps and brachialis muscles), followed by flexion with the arm partially pronated to test the brachioradialis muscle. As emphasized earlier, the triceps are tested from a position of partial elbow flexion designed to put the muscle at a relative disadvantage because it is so powerful in full extension. Wrist extensors and flexors and finger abduction and adduction are usually tested at their maximal muscle contracture, again palpating the bulk (6).

Recall that finger flexion and grip strength depend on partial wrist extension, and any disorder that weakens wrist extension will result in pseudo weakness of grip function. In this case, grip function is examined by passively extending the wrist.

Sensory Examination

In no other aspect of the neurologic evaluation is the conundrum of tailoring the examination to the clinical and historical features more operative. A detailed examination of all portions the limbs and trunk in each patient is time consuming and often unrewarding. The sensory symptoms are often more helpful than objective findings because of the necessary reliance on a subjective response, the complex representation of sensation centrally, and the variability in distribution of peripheral receptors in various parts of the limbs and trunk. There is also a great deal of dermatomal overlap of adjacent roots, as evidenced by the observation that destruction of a single dorsal root rarely results in loss of sensation. A peripheral nerve usually contains fibers from several roots.

The topography of sensory disturbances from a peripheral nerve lesion differs from that of a nerve root lesion. Nerve division produces a loss of all forms of cutaneous sensation within the area surrounded by a partial loss of sensation in which tactile loss exceeds that due to pain and temperature. When examining and mapping an area of sensory loss, it is best to begin in the affected area and to work toward the intact area (7).

Muscle Stretch Reflex

Muscle stretch reflexes (MSRs) are among the most reliable indicators of localization in the neurologic examination of the cervical spine. A unilateral loss of an MSR is supportive of a lesion of the lower motor neuron. Other hallmarks of a lower motor lesion are hypotonic weakness and fasciculations.

It is important to begin the analysis with an assessment of the jaw jerk to gauge the general level of reflex activity above the neck. It is also necessary to observe the movements of the limb distant from the reflex being tested. Pathologic hyperreflexia is often seen as a spread of reflex activity distally or proximally. This takes on more importance when accompanied by clonus of the wrist. An important localizing response is the so-called inverted radial reflex indicative of C5 and C6 dysfunction. Here, the biceps or brachioradialis reflexes are diminished and accompanied by extension of the forearm and flexion of the fingers indicative of an upper motor syndrome below the C5 or C6 segment.

The lower limb reflexes are usually hyperactive, with a positive Babinski sign. The triceps may be normally hypo-active compared with the biceps, and their bilateral diminution does not indicate dysfunction if unsupported by other clinical findings.

The expected response is further highlighted when the segmental roots are discussed in detail.

Diagnosis and Localization of Cervical and Brachial Lesions

There is no sensory root of C1. It functions only as a motor nerve (Figs. 11.1 to 11.4; Tables 11.2 and 11.3). Isolated lesions are rare. There is no segmental representation of the arm above C5. Sensory disturbances of C2, C3, and C4 result in symptoms localized to the dorsal scalp (C2); occiput, upper neck, and jaw (C3); and lower neck

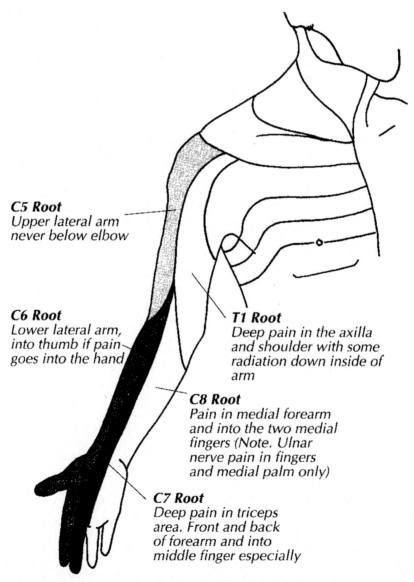

C5 Root
Upper lateral arm never below elbow

C6 Root
Lower lateral arm, into thumb if pain goes into the hand

T1 Root
Deep pain in the axilla and shoulder with some radiation down inside of arm

C8 Root
Pain in medial forearm and into the two medial fingers (Note. Ulnar nerve pain in fingers and medial palm only)

C7 Root
Deep pain in triceps area. Front and back of forearm and into middle finger especially

FIG. 11.2. Distribution of pain and paraesthesias. (From Patten J. Diagnosis of cervical root and peripheral nerve lesions affecting the arm. In: *Neurological differential diagnosis*, 2nd ed. London: Springer, 1996:282–297, with permission.)

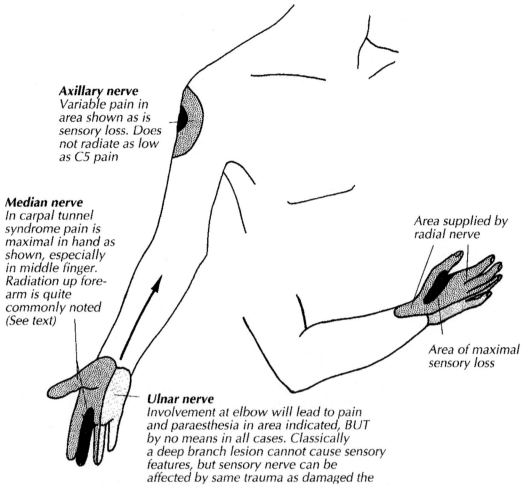

Axillary nerve
Variable pain in area shown as is sensory loss. Does not radiate as low as C5 pain

Median nerve
In carpal tunnel syndrome pain is maximal in hand as shown, especially in middle finger. Radiation up forearm is quite commonly noted (See text)

Area supplied by radial nerve

Area of maximal sensory loss

Ulnar nerve
Involvement at elbow will lead to pain and paraesthesia in area indicated, BUT by no means in all cases. Classically a deep branch lesion cannot cause sensory features, but sensory nerve can be affected by same trauma as damaged the

FIG. 11.3. Distribution of pain and paraesthesias in peripheral nerve lesions. (From Patten J. Diagnosis of cervical root and peripheral nerve lesions affecting the arm. In: *Neurological differential diagnosis,* 2nd ed. London: Springer, 1996:282–297, with permission.)

and upper shoulder region (C4). Motor disturbances affect neck movements of flexion, extension, lateral flexion, and head rotation. Diaphragmatic paresis may also occur because some fibers arise from C3 and C4 (8).

In the cervical region, the named nerve root exits above the lower segment (C5 root exits between the C4-C5 vertebral segment). Lesions of the C5 nerve root cause pain in the shoulder and upper arm as well as medial scapula, but not below the elbow. Sensory loss, if any, is found as an oval patch over the lateral upper arm, whereas the muscles most affected are the infraspinatus, supraspinatus, and deltoids. The MSR principally affected is the biceps tendon jerk.

A C6 radiculopathy results in pain in the lateral forearm, thumb, and index finger, with numbness or paresthesias localized to the thumb. Weakness, when present, is most often observed in the brachialis, biceps, and brachioradialis (elbow flexors). Less often, forearm supination and pronation are involved. The pain may have a similar distribution

to a radial nerve lesion, but the brachioradialis is often atrophic, and some wrist or finger extension weakness is observed in a radial neuropathy.

The principal cause of C5 and C6 radiculopathies, especially when chronic, and particularly when they occur together, is cervical spondylosis. It is advised to look carefully for an inverted radial reflex and signs of spasticity in the legs.

A C7 radiculopathy is the most common radiculopathy (2). The pain tends to be more diffuse and aching, often located in the posterior arm and ventral or dorsal aspects of the forearm. When it does involve the hand, it usually involves the second to fourths digits. The triceps jerk is reliably diminished. It is important to examine several C7 innervated muscles because weakness would be expected to involve the elbow, wrist, and finger extensors, wrist flexors, and sometimes shoulder adduction.

A radial nerve lesion might mimic a C7 radiculopathy, but weakness of wrist flexion argues against a radial neuropathy.

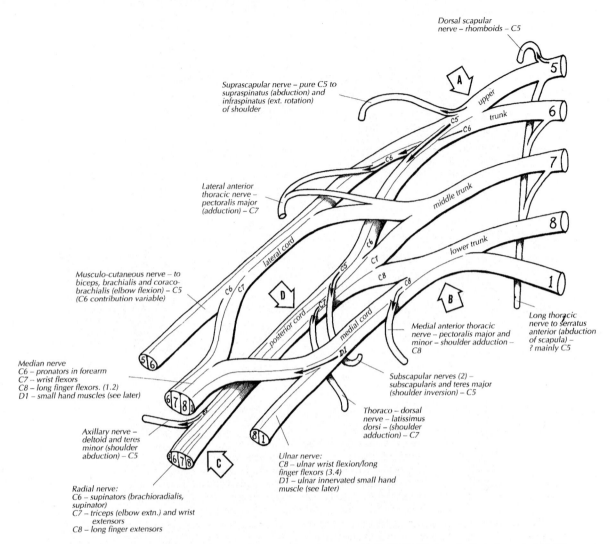

FIG. 11.4. Anatomy of the brachial plexus, showing the eventual destinations of all root components. (From Patten J. Diagnosis of cervical root and peripheral nerve lesions affecting the arm. In: *Neurological differential diagnosis*, 2nd ed. London: Springer, 1996:282–297, with permission.)

Either may inhibit the triceps jerk and may coexist in traumatic injuries.

Carpal tunnel syndrome (CTS) may be confused with C7 nerve root irritation, and both may coexist. Pain in the forearm is not uncommon in CTS, and the paresthesias may be in a similar distribution, but the distribution of the weakness and reflex loss serves to distinguish them.

The most common cause of a C7 radiculopathy is an acutely herniated disc and less likely cervical spondylosis.

C8-T1 radiculopathies are often lumped together because they are usually affected by similar processes and share clinical findings. They are the least common of the cervical radiculopathies.

The pain extends from the elbow to the fifth finger on the medial surface of the forearm (C8) or to the axilla and shoulder (T1). Sensory loss, when present, involves the distal medial forearm and fifth digit. C8 weakness occurs with the long flexors of the thumb and index finger (anterior in-

terosseous) as well as the flexor digitorum profundus to the second and third digits, whereas T1 involves the intrinsic hand muscles, including the thenar group of muscles.

The finger flexor reflex is altered when C8 is involved.

The areas of major confusion for C8-T1 lesions are ulnar mononeuropathies and lower trunk brachial plexopathies. Ulnar neuropathy can be easily excluded if the thenar muscle is involved or if one or more of the long finger flexors are paretic. Sensory loss above the wrist is not consistent with an ulnar neuropathy (9).

A lower trunk lesion is more problematic and may be more reliably diagnosed with an electromyogram and nerve conduction studies showing denervation of the abductor pollicis brevis with a normal distal latency, denervation of other C8-T1 innervated muscles, and a diminished or absent sensory nerve action potential recording the fifth digit with normal distal latencies and no ulnar conduction abnormalities at the elbow. The cause of a C8-T1 or lower trunk

TABLE 11.2. *Comparative Data—Nerve Root Lesions in the Arm*

Roots	C5	C6	C7	C8	T1
Sensory supply	Lateral border upper arm to elbow	Lateral forearm including thumb & index	Over triceps, mid-forearm & middle finger	Medial forearm to include little finger	Axilla down to the olecranon
Sensory loss (Main location)	As above over deltoid	As above over thumb & radial border of hand	Middle fingers Front and back of hand	Little finger Heel of hand to above wrist	In axilla (usually minimal)
Area of pain	As above and medial scapula border	As above esp, thumb and index finger	As above and medial scapular border	As above (up to elbow)	Deep aching in shoulder and axilla to olecranon
Reflex arc	Biceps jerk	Supinator jerk	Triceps jerk	Finger jerk	None
Motor deficit (Muscles most involved and easily tested)	Deltoid Supraspinatus Infraspinatus Rhomboids	Pronators and supinators of forearm Biceps Brachioradialis Brachialis	Triceps Wrist extensors Wrist flexors Latissimus dorsi Pectoralis major	Finger flexors Finger extensors Flexor carpi Ulnaris (Thenar muscles in rare patients)	All small hand muscles (thenar muscles via C8 in rare patients)
Causative lesions	Brachial neuritis Cervical spondylosis Upper plexus avulsion	Cervical spondylosis Acute disc lesions	Acute disc lesions Cervical spondylosis	Rare in disc lesions or spondylosis (See T1 usually affected by same pathology)	Cervical rib Altered anatomy of first rib Pancoast tumour Metastatic carcinoma in deep cervical nodes Outlet syndromes

(*Reprinted with permission from Patten J. Diagnosis of cervical root and peripheral nerve lesions affecting the arm. Table 16.1)

TABLE 11.3. *Comparative Data—Nerve Lesions in the Arm*

Nerves	Axillary	Musculocutaneous	Radial	Median	Ulnar
Sensory supply	Over deltoid	Lateral forearm to wrist	Lateral dorsal forearm and back of thumb & index finger	Lateral palm Index, middle & lateral half ring finger	Medial palm and fifth & medial half ring finger
Sensory loss	Small area over deltoid	Lateral forearm	Dorsum of thumb & index (if any)	As above from skin crease at wrist	As above but often none detectable
Area of pain	Across shoulder tip	Lateral forearm	Dorsum of thumb & index	Thumb index & middle finger. Often spreads up forearm to elbow (reason unknown)	Ulnar supplied fingers & palm distal to wrist. Occasionally pain along course of nerve up to elbow (can be confusing)
Reflex arc	None	Biceps jerk	Triceps jerk & supinator jerk	Finger jerks (flexor digitorum sublimis)	None
Motor deficit	Deltoid (teres minor cannot be evaluated) usually very obvious	Biceps Brachialis (coracobrachialis weakness not detectable)	Triceps Wrist extensors Finger extensors Brachioradialis & supinator of forearm	Wrist flexors Long finger flexors to thumb index & middle finger Abductor pollicis brevis	All small hand muscles excluding abductor pollicis brevis Flexor carpi ulnaris Long flexors of ring & little finger
Causative lesions	Fractured neck of humerus Dislocated shoulder Deep i.m. injections	Very rarely Damaged	Crutch palsy Saturday night palsy Fractured humerus In supinator muscle itself	Carpal tunnel syndrome Direct trauma to wrist Suicide attempt Falling on glass Palmar space infection	Elbow Local trauma Bed rest (resting on elbow) Fractured olecranon Wrist Local trauma Ganglion at wrist joint

(Reprinted with permission from Patten J. Diagnosis of cervical root and peripheral nerve lesions affecting the arm. Table 16.2)

TABLE 11.4. *Entities Which Can Be Confused with Cervical Radiculopathies*

- Parsonage-Turner syndrome
- Suprascapular nerve entrapment
- Thoracic outlet syndrome
- Carpal tunnel syndrome
- Upper limb plexopathy
- Radial neuropathies
- Ulnar neuropathies
- Craniovertebral junction disorders

lesion may be ominous, including a the possibility of a Pancoast tumor.

There are diverse entities of variable causation, some relatively common, and others rare, which can be confused with segmental nerve root pathology. Some have already been noted, including focal peripheral neuropathies (Table 11.4).

Parsonage-Turner syndrome or acute brachial plexitis may masquerade as a C5 radiculopathy. The classic clinical picture of severe shoulder pain followed by weakness as the pain subsides leaves little doubt as to the diagnosis. Sensory loss, if present, is found over the deltoid region. Weakness may involve C5 through C8 ventral roots and may be quite patchy. The presence of a scapular winging due to serratus anterior muscle involvement is quite frequent and fortifies the diagnosis. Of note is the fact that this disorder is bilateral in one third of cases. It may be recurrent, familial, or both.

Another uncommon shoulder neuropathy is the suprascapular nerve entrapment in the suprascapular notch, with weakness of the infraspinatus and supraspinatus muscles, leading to a frozen shoulder. The diagnosis is suspected with severe weakness and atrophy of the spinatus muscles. If the shoulder is so immobile and painful that formal testing is precluded, an electromyogram may show denervation of the spinatus muscles with sparing of the deltoid muscle, which may itself be atrophic from disuse.

The TOC has already been described. This syndrome has markedly declined in terms of frequency of diagnosis because the cervical root syndromes and carpal tunnel syndrome have been better defined. The neurological syndrome is rare. Deep aching in the axilla and medial arm or forearm, weakness of the intrinsic hand muscles, and paresthesias of the fifth finger are hallmarks. Most cases are associated with an enlarged C7 projection, with a tight band compressing the lower trunk of the brachial plexus (10). The more common vascular syndrome is the result of a high

rib displacing the axillary artery upward, causing stenosis and poststenotic dilation.

Finally, a number of lesions can produce an array of confusing signs and symptoms. These are lesions of the cervical–medullary junction and upper cervical spine caused by congenital anomalies, skull base tumors (especially a foramen magnum meningioma), and upper cervical spondylotic myelopathy (C2-C3 and C3-C4 levels). Suboccipital and neck pain associated with Lhermitte phenomena are early symptoms, followed by lower cranial nerve palsies along with unilateral upper limb stiffness and clumsiness, followed by the leg, then contralateral limbs (the "windmill effect"). Unusual dissociated syringomyelic-type sensory loss is observed along with a lower motor neuron type of wasting and weakness of the intrinsic hand muscles attributable to distant "vascular effects." Numb and clumsy hands with four-limb spasticity and distal C8-T1 weakness and wasting are the key features of the upper cervical spondylotic syndrome. These lesions are, in many circumstances, eminently treatable and have a good long-term outlook if recognized early.

These are but a few of the highlights of the clinical examination of the cervical spine. The crucial take-away message is that with a good history, a thorough and focused examination, and a fundamental knowledge of the anatomy, one can accurately arrive at a diagnosis and appropriate treatment in most cases.

REFERENCES

1. Byrne TN, Benzel EC, Waxman SG. Pain of spinal origin. In: *Disease of the spine and spinal cord.* Oxford, New York: Oxford University Press, 2000:94–100.
2. Yoss RE, Corbin KB, MacCarty CS, et al. Significance of symptoms and signs in localization of involved root in cervical disc protrusions. *Neurology* 1957;7:673–683.
3. Burkhalter WE. An organ of movement: basic approach. In: Hale MS, ed. *A practical approach to arm pain.* Springfield, IL: Charles C. Thomas, 1971:3–13.
4. Dawley JA. Cervical radiculopathy as a cause of arm pain. In: Hale MS, ed. *A practical approach to arm pain.* Springfield, IL: Charles C. Thomas, 1971:37–44.
5. Slamovits TC, Glaser JS. The pupils and accommodation. In: Glaser JS, ed. *Neuro-ophthalmology,* 3rd ed. Philadelphia: Lippincott Williams & Wilkins, 1999:43.
6. Demyer WE. Examination of the somatic motor system. In: *Technique of the neurologic examination,* 4th ed. New York: McGraw-Hill, 1994: 209–275.
7. Matthews B. Examination of sensation. In: *Introduction to clinical neurology,* 3rd ed. Baltimore: Williams & Wilkins, 1968:72–85.
8. Brazis PB, Masden JC, Biller J. *Localization in clinical neurology,* 4th ed. Philadelphia: Lippincott William & Wilkins, 2001:95–96.
9. Patten J. Diagnosis of cervical root and peripheral nerve lesions affecting the arm. In: *Neurological differential diagnosis,* 2nd ed. London: Springer, 1996:282–297.
10. Wilbourn AJ. Thoracic outlet syndrome: thoracic outlet syndrome is overdiagnosed. *Muscle Nerve* 1999;22:130–138.

CHAPTER 12

Anatomic Localization

Gordon K. T. Chu and Michael G. Fehlings

Injuries to the cervical spine can cause variable symptoms; the resultant injury encompasses a full spectrum of signs and symptoms from the subtle to the patently obvious. The roles of computed tomography (CT) and magnetic resonance imaging (MRI) cannot be overstated; however, the physical examination of the patient is still of major importance. A complete examination of the patient is necessary not only to ensure an accurate diagnosis but also to note any neurologic deficits that need to be followed closely so that decisions regarding the type and urgency of treatment can be made at the earliest possible time.

Spinal injuries have been known since the time of the ancient Egyptians (1). However, anatomic localization was difficult to achieve because the concept of specialization of the central nervous system was not recognized until the 19th century. The work of Broca and Wernicke demonstrated that neurologic deficits can be traced back to specific regions of the brain (2). Similarly, such ideas could be transferred to spinal cord injuries. Sherrington's work with serial root sections on Rhesus monkeys demonstrated dermatomal innervation of nerve roots (3). He noted that not only did each nerve root innervate a specific dermatome but that the areas of innervation for adjacent nerve roots overlapped each other. In humans, segmental innervation was noted first in herpes zoster infections, which allowed mapping of cutaneous areas to the nerve root ganglion affected. This was followed by Foerster's pioneering work (4), which revealed innervation patterns in humans similar to Sherrington's discoveries.

ANATOMY OF CERVICAL SPINAL CORD

The key to anatomic localization is a thorough understanding of the anatomy of the cervical spinal cord, the nerve roots, and peripheral nerves. The cervical spinal cord consists of eight cervical segments that are surrounded by seven cervical vertebrae. The first cervical root emerges between the atlas and the occiput, the second to seventh roots leave the spinal canal above the corresponding vertebrae, whereas the eighth root emerges between the intervertebral foramina of C7 and T1. There is a cervical enlargement in the lower four segments of the cervical cord and the first segment of the thoracic cord due to the innervation of the upper limbs. The cervical cord contains the largest number of fibers in the white matter because the descending fibers for the lower limbs have not yet left the cord, and the ascending fibers contain both upper and lower limb fibers (5,6). The gray matter is also larger because of innervation of the upper limbs. A cross section of the cervical cord consists of an H-shaped gray matter surrounded by white matter. The gray matter is divided into a dorsal, ventral, and intermediate zone. The white matter can be divided into three funiculi or columns: dorsal, lateral, and ventral.

The dorsal funiculus carries ipsilateral ascending axons from neurons in the dorsal root ganglion and dorsal horn. It is bound by the dorsal horn and dorsal septum and consists of a medial fasciculus gracilis and a lateral fasciculus cuneatus. The dorsal columns contain axons, which are traditionally thought to subserve functions of discriminative touch, vibration, and position sense. However, the functional importance of the dorsal columns is far more complex because surgical lesioning can only produce minimal persistent sensory deficits. Furthermore, other studies have shown that proprioceptive signals from the lower limbs are carried only in the dorsal columns as far as the thoracic cord and then synapse with the dorsal nucleus of Clarke; the pathway then continues rostrally by way of the dorsal spinocerebellar tract in the lateral funiculus. However, clinically, loss of the posterior columns secondary to disease states such as subacute combined degeneration or neurosyphilis still results in loss of position sense with unsteadiness of gait. These columns are also arranged somatotopically as the medial fasciculus gracilis carries impulses from more caudal regions, whereas the lateral cuneatus has the more rostral fibers. There are also other descending axons within the dorsal columns, which have little clinical importance.

The lateral white matter tracts are composed of a multitude of ascending and descending tracts. Of these, only the most clinically important tracts are briefly discussed. The lateral spinothalamic tract carries innervation concerning pain and temperature sensation. The axons originate from laminae I and V of the dorsal horn and initially cross within one or two spinal segments anterior to the central canal in the ventral white commissure and then continue in the spinothalamic tract. The tract is somatotopically arranged with fibers corresponding to the rostral region medially and the caudal regions more laterally. Other ascending tracts include the ventral spinocerebellar tract and the previously described dorsal spinocerebellar tract. The lateral corticospinal tract is also located in the lateral funiculus. This tract consists of axons from the premotor and motor cortex of the contralateral frontal lobe and is responsible for voluntary, discreet, and skilled movements. Similar to other tracts previously described, this tract also has a somatotopic organization with the arrangement with cervical fibers more medial than the lumbar and sacral fibers. Other descending tracts include the rubrospinal tract and the medullary reticulospinal tract.

In the ventral funiculus, there is a ventral corticospinal tract composed of fibers that did not cross the midline at the pyramidal decussation. The anterior spinothalamic tract also runs in the ventral funiculus and carries fibers conveying "light touch" sensation. The vestibulospinal tract is a third tract that is in the ventral funiculus and is responsible for mediating equilibratory reflexes.

The gray matter in the cervical spinal cord, as compared with the other regions of the spinal cord, is similarly divided into the dorsal and ventral horns and the intermediate zone. The dorsal horn contains neurons, which synapse with axons from the dorsal root ganglion and therefore mainly subserve a sensory function. The spinal trigeminal nucleus and tract also descend into the first two to four segments of the cervical cord terminating in the substantia gelatinosa of the dorsal horn and the dorsolateral tract of Lissauer, respectively. The ventral horn contains large motor neurons whose axons leave the spinal cord to synapse on skeletal spinal muscle fibers.

ANATOMIC LOCALIZATION

Cervical injury is not difficult to diagnose, but care must still be taken when patients are examined so as not to miss devastating injuries. Patients who on cursory examination appear to have nothing more than neck pain and radicular symptoms can in reality have compression of the cord secondary to an extrinsic mass. The key to distinguishing these and other pathology is to have a systematic approach to the patient, which must be used each time. The first step to lo-

calization is to distinguish between disease in the central nervous system and that in the peripheral nervous system. Disease in the peripheral nervous system can then be further subdivided into processes that involve the nerve roots, nerve plexuses, or peripheral nerves. This distinction is obviously important because it allows for the proper treatment of these conditions. Sensory symptoms secondary to nerve root pathology normally involve numbness or pain in the specific dermatome distribution, although overlap of adjacent nerve roots prevents complete anesthesia of the dermatome. The pain is usually sharp in nature and is often aggravated by changes in head position or neck motion. The Spurling sign (rotation and lateral bending of the head to the symptomatic side) can be elicited with nerve root pathology secondary to disc herniation (7). Increases in intrathoracic pressure, such as straining or coughing, can also exacerbate the pain. Pain is often a more prominent feature of nerve root pathology than sensory deficits. The area of pain involved may also be more extensive than the nerve root dermatome it sometimes extends to the muscle groups subserved by the root. A C5 nerve root lesion can cause pain from the rhomboids to the biceps. Paresthesias may also occur as a result of nerve root irritation. Of the above sensory symptoms, pain is usually the most obvious from nerve root compression. Peripheral nerve lesions result in a more definitive area of numbness than root lesions, and the area involved is no longer dermatomal in distribution but follows the particular nerve involved. Similarly, nerve root dysfunction affects a different set of muscles when compared with peripheral nerve injury. Injury to a single nerve root may only cause paresis to a group of muscles because of compensation by adjacent roots, whereas complete muscle paralysis may mean multiple nerve roots or peripheral nerve injury. Muscular atrophy may also be masked with single nerve root lesions.

Spinal cord lesions differ from peripheral lesions in that they can present with root symptoms and signs, but they have more generalized effects as well. Cord lesions can cause motor and sensory deficits below the level of injury. In terms of motor deficits, there can be paresis to paralysis of muscle groups below the lesion, which do not occur with peripheral nervous system injuries. Chronically, the affected muscles become spastic in tone with accompanying hyperreflexia. Similarly, sensory deficits due to spinal cord lesions can vary from mild to complete sensory loss of all modalities. The sensory impairment may be subtle, presenting with clumsiness of gait or grasp due to involvement of proprioceptive tracts. Electrical shocklike sensations can radiate up and down the spine, usually as a result of flexion of the neck (Lhermitte sign), and can indicate spinal cord pathology (8), although the causes can vary from multiple sclerosis to central disc herniation. Pain from cord lesions can be different from radicular pain because it is more diffuse and ill defined. Cord lesions also affect the autonomic nervous system, causing loss of bowel and bladder function and loss of regulation of vascular tone. A more complete description of the effects of spinal cord lesions is given in later in this chapter.

Once the pathology has been identified as being localized to the roots, peripheral nerves, brachial plexus, or spinal cord, then other more specific signs and symptoms may point to the exact root, nerve, or cord level involved.

CERVICAL RADICULOPATHY

Cervical radiculopathy at different levels can often be distinguished by specific signs and symptoms. Each cervical nerve root innervates a specific dermatome and muscle group (Figs. 12.1 and 12.2). C1 and C2 radiculopathies are extremely rare. The C1 nerve root subserves no sensory dermatome, and the C2 dermatome includes the posterior aspect of the head behind the ears. C1 and C2 have no specific motor innervation but can contribute to the motor innerva-

tion of cranial nerve 11 and the ansa cervicales. C3 nerve root dysfunction is also quite rare (9). The C3 dermatomal pattern involves the anterior and posterior aspect of the neck. Again, there is no specific motor function with the C3 root, although diaphragmatic paresis may be noted. Patients with C2 or C3 radiculopathy may complain of headache. C4 radiculopathy involves pain over the base of the neck above the clavicle and medial shoulder. Diaphragmatic and shoulder muscle paresis can occur with C4 involvement. Radiculopathy of the C5 nerve root is still uncommon but less so than the above nerve roots. The sensory innervation ranges from the top of the shoulder to the lateral aspects of the arm. A complete examination of shoulder motion is necessary to differentiate from shoulder pathology. The deltoid muscle is mainly innervated by this root, and there may be profound weakness in abduction of the shoulder. This may mimic a rotator cuff tear, but unlike the rotator cuff tear, there should

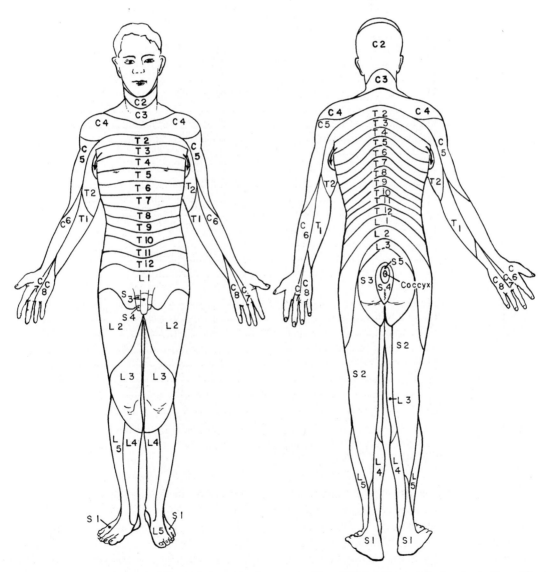

FIG. 12.1. Sensory innervation of the spinal nerves. (Reprinted with permission from Barr ML, Kierman JA. *Spinal cord in the human nervous system: an anatomical view point,* 5th ed. Philadelphia: JB Lippincott, 1988:81.)

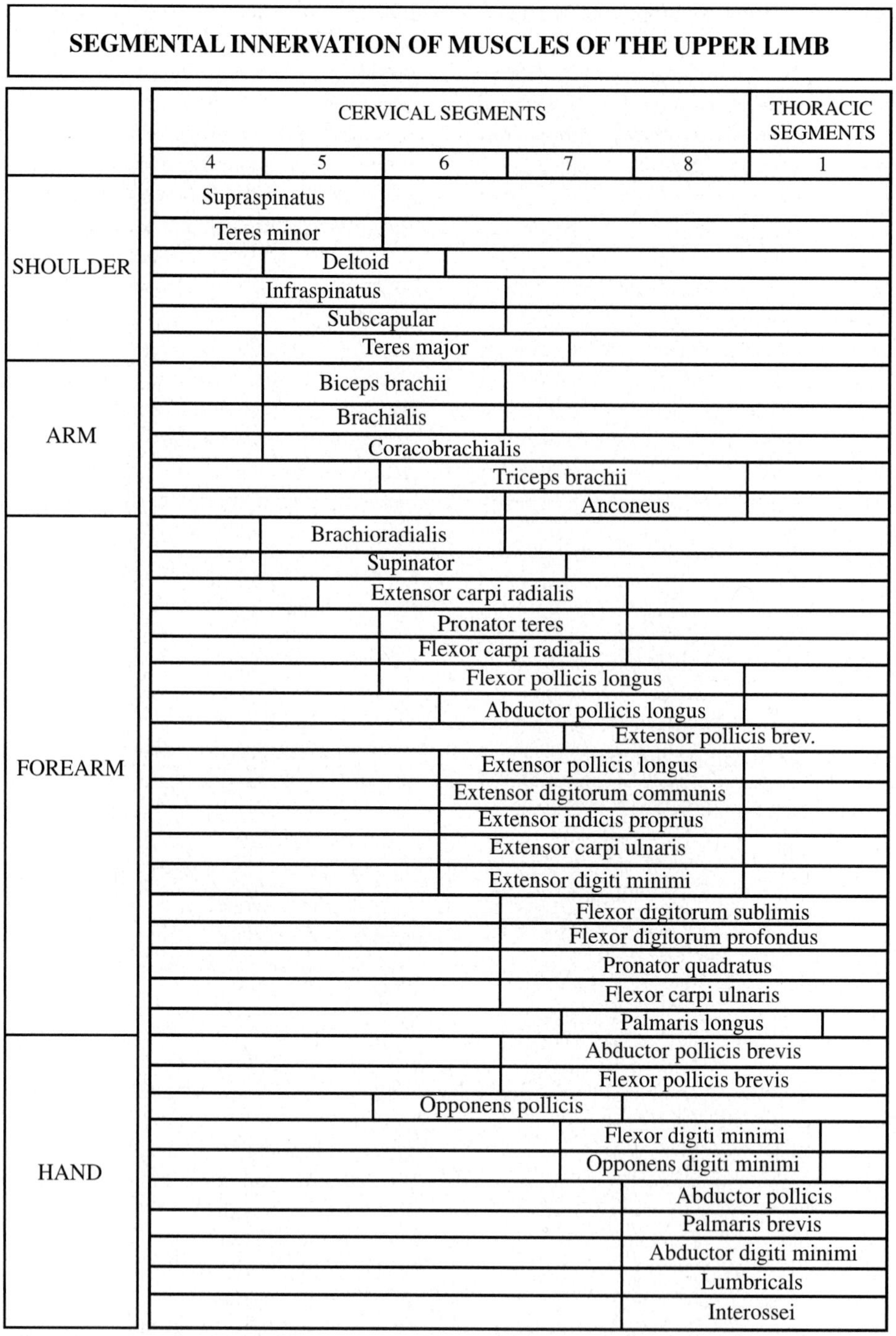

SEGMENTAL INNERVATION OF MUSCLES OF THE UPPER LIMB

Region	Muscle	\[Cervical\] 4	5	6	7	8	\[Thoracic\] 1
SHOULDER	Supraspinatus	X	X				
	Teres minor	X	X				
	Deltoid		X	X			
	Infraspinatus	X	X	X			
	Subscapular		X	X			
	Teres major		X	X	X		
ARM	Biceps brachii		X	X			
	Brachialis		X	X			
	Coracobrachialis		X	X	X		
	Triceps brachii			X	X	X	
	Anconeus				X	X	
FOREARM	Brachioradialis		X	X			
	Supinator		X	X	X		
	Extensor carpi radialis			X	X		
	Pronator teres			X	X		
	Flexor carpi radialis			X	X		
	Flexor pollicis longus			X	X	X	
	Abductor pollicis longus				X	X	
	Extensor pollicis brev.					X	X
	Extensor pollicis longus			X	X	X	
	Extensor digitorum communis			X	X	X	
	Extensor indicis proprius			X	X	X	
	Extensor carpi ulnaris			X	X	X	
	Extensor digiti minimi			X	X	X	
	Flexor digitorum sublimis				X	X	X
	Flexor digitorum profondus				X	X	X
	Pronator quadratus				X	X	X
	Flexor carpi ulnaris				X	X	X
	Palmaris longus				X	X	
HAND	Abductor pollicis brevis				X	X	X
	Flexor pollicis brevis				X	X	X
	Opponens pollicis			X	X	X	
	Flexor digiti minimi				X	X	X
	Opponens digiti minimi				X	X	
	Abductor pollicis					X	X
	Palmaris brevis					X	X
	Abductor digiti minimi					X	X
	Lumbricals					X	X
	Interossei					X	X

FIG. 12.2. Muscles of the upper limb innervated by the cervical spinal nerves. (Reprinted with permission from Parent A. Spinal nerves and peripheral innervation. In: *Carpenter's human neuroanatomy,* 9th ed. Baltimore: Williams and Wilkins, 1996:279.)

be minimal tenderness over the shoulder itself. There may also be weakness in internal and external rotation (supraspinatus and infraspinatus) of the shoulder. These muscle groups are less consistently affected. The biceps brachii muscle can also be weakened, along with a diminution of the biceps reflex. C6 radiculopathy is quite common and often presents with pain radiating from the base of the neck, along the biceps, and down the lateral aspect of the forearm to involve the thumb and pointer finger. There may also be numbness in the first two digits. There may be paresis of the biceps, the brachioradialis, and the wrist extensors. The biceps reflex is often abnormal. C7 radiculopathy is just as common as C6 if not more so. Pain or numbness involving the middle finger is the usual sensory disturbance with possible overlap to the surrounding fingers. The pain may radiate from the posterior shoulder, along the triceps, to the middle finger. The main muscle weakness that is seen with C7 nerve root dysfunction is that of the triceps. Patients can sometimes compensate by internal rotation, and this must be looked for and avoided during the physical examination. The triceps reflex is affected with C7 radiculopathy. Other muscle groups involved include the pronators, finger extensors, latissimus dorsi, and wrist flexors. The C8 nerve root mediates sensation from the ulnar side of the hand, mainly the ring and pinkie fingers; therefore, pain and numbness are mostly in that region. C8 primarily supplies both the digitorum flexor superficialis and profundus and therefore controls finger flexion. There may also be paresis of finger adduction and abduction because C8 and T1 innervate the interossei muscles of the hand. The patient may complain of difficulties grasping objects such as cups. Innervation of the upper limb muscle by the cervical nerve roots is summarized in Figure 12.2.

PERIPHERAL NERVE INJURIES

Peripheral nerve injuries are often due to entrapment at various points along the route the nerve travels. These entrapment injuries are gradual in onset, causing numbness and pain before weakness, in contrast to traumatic nerve injuries, which are quick in onset and present with minimal pain and in which the severity of the injury appears immediately. These entrapment neuropathies are therefore more likely to be mistaken for nerve root dysfunction because of its slow onset and painful presentation. The nerves that are commonly trapped arise from either the trunks or the cords of the brachial plexus.

Dorsal Scapular Nerve

The dorsal scapular nerve is supplied by the C5 nerve root and branches off from the upper trunk of the brachial plexus. It may become entrapped within the scalenus medius muscle, causing paresis with the rhomboids. This entrapment also causes pain within the rhomboid unilaterally. Often, symptoms may be elicited by turning the patient's head toward the painful side and flexing laterally in the opposite direction. This can be distinguished from C5 radiculopathy because there is no deltoid weakness.

Long Thoracic Nerve

The long thoracic nerve arises from the fifth, sixth, and seventh cervical roots. It supplies the serratus anterior and is purely a motor nerve. Dysfunction of this nerve causes winging of the scapula. As radiculopathy of C5, C6, or C7 occurs with sensory symptoms and paresis of muscles in the upper limb; this is easily distinguished from injury to the long thoracic nerve.

Suprascapular Nerve

The suprascapular nerve arises from the upper trunk of the brachial plexus and is a pure motor nerve supplied by C5

and C6. It innervates the supraspinatus and infraspinatus muscles, and its entrapment causes weakness in shoulder abduction and external rotation. It is most commonly trapped at the suprascapular notch. There is no biceps weakness, as can occur with C5 and C6 nerve root dysfunction. The pain is more localized to the shoulder region, and diagnosis can also be made with a nerve block at the suprascapular notch or with electromyography.

Median Nerve

The median nerve arises from the union of branches of the medial and lateral cords of the brachial plexus. It has contributions from the fifth cervical to the first thoracic root. It supplies sensation to the first three and one half digits on the palmar side extending to just beyond the nail beds on the dorsum of the hand. Its muscular innervation is limited to muscles in the forearm and hand (discussed later). It has a major branch just distal to the elbow, the anterior interosseous nerve, which is purely a motor nerve. It further branches just before the flexor retinaculum, giving off a palmar cutaneous branch that is purely sensory and provides sensation to the base of the thenar eminence. Before its first division, the median nerve may become entrapped at four regions as it passes from the arm to the forearm. The first area of entrapment is at the ligament of Struthers. In about 2% of the population, there is a supracondylar process just above the medial epicondyle, and the ligament of Struthers joins the two bony prominences. The median nerve passes underneath it. The next level of entrapment is at the lacertus fibrosus (bicipital aponeurosis) at the elbow joint. The third region is at the pronator teres muscle, and the last area is at the origin of the flexor digitorum superficialis muscle. Entrapment at these locations causes roughly the same constellation of signs and symptoms and is often termed the *pronator syndrome*. This syndrome consists of pain in the forearm and numbness and paresthesias in the sensory distribution of the nerve. The entrapments are all above the level of the branching of the anterior interosseous nerve, so that all the muscles innervated by the median nerve are involved. The muscles in the forearm include the pronator teres, the flexor carpi radialis, the palmaris longus, and the flexor digitorum superficialis. The anterior interosseous nerve innervates the flexor pollicis longus, the lateral part of the flexor digitorum profundus, and the pronator quadratus. In the hand, the median nerve innervates the LOAF muscles (the first two lumbricals, the opponens, the abductor pollicis brevis, and the flexor pollicis brevis). It may be difficult to determine the site of entrapment, but an x-ray may reveal a supracondylar process, which suggests involvement at the ligament of Struthers. Pain with flexion of the elbow and the forearm pronated implies entrapment at the lacertus. If the pronator teres is the origin of the neuropathy, there might be pain in pronation while the wrist is held in flexion. Entrapment at the flexor digitorum superficialis causes pain with resisted flexion of the superficialis to the middle finger. Median nerve entrapment may appear similar to C6 or C7 radiculopathy owing to a similar pattern of sensory disturbance, but it must be remembered that the median nerve does not innervate muscles of the arm, so that there would be no weakness in the biceps or triceps as there would be for C6 or C7 root disturbances. Furthermore, the median nerve does not innervate extensor muscles in the forearm, so that wrist extensors would not be weakened.

The median nerve gives off a branch, the anterior interosseous nerve, beneath the flexor digitorum superficialis; this branch is purely motor and innervates the muscles previously discussed. This branch may become compressed, causing weakness of its innervated muscles. This weakness may be elicited by the pinch sign, wherein the patient attempts to form an O with the thumb and forefinger but the terminal phalanges extend rather than flex. This syndrome is distinct from cervical radiculopathies because there is no sensory loss.

The median nerve can also be compressed at the carpal tunnel, giving rise to the syndrome of the same name. Common symptoms include weakness or clumsiness of the hand along with paresthesias and numbness in the first three and one half fingers, but they often involve the whole hand. These symptoms may be reproduced by percussing over the carpal tunnel (Tinel sign) or by prolonged exaggerated wrist flexion (Phalen test). The sensory symptoms may mimic C6 or C7 radiculopathy, but there is no weakness in the muscles of the arms or forearms, although the two conditions may coexist.

The palmar cutaneous branch of the median nerve may also be injured and have sensory deficits similar to a C6 radiculopathy, but there is no motor component to this nerve.

Ulnar Nerve

The ulnar begins from the medial cord of the brachial plexus and has contributions from the C7, C8, and T1 nerve roots. The ulnar innervates only two muscles in the forearm, the flexor carpi ulnaris and the medial part of the flexor digitorum profundus, and it innervates all the intrinsic muscles of the hand except for the LOAF muscles. Its sensory distribution consists of the medial aspects of the hand, including the medial one and one half fingers. The most common area for entrapment is at the elbow, causing the cubital tunnel syndrome. This syndrome presents with pain from the medial aspects of the elbow radiating down to the small and ring finger. Tinel sign would be positive at the elbow. There may be weakness and atrophy of the muscles innervated by the nerve. This syndrome may mimic C8 or T1 radiculopathy, but the other muscles that either nerve root innervates are not affected, including the flexors of the thumb, forefinger, and middle finger and the thenar muscles.

The ulnar nerve may become entrapped at Guyon canal at the wrist. This leads to numbness only on the palmar side of the hand because the innervation for the dorsum of the hand branches off before entering the canal. There is weakness in the hand muscles supplied by the ulnar nerve. This syndrome is differentiated from C8 or T1 radiculopathy for the same reasons as given earlier. This syndrome can further be distinct from the entrapment at the elbow because of full sensation at the dorsum of the medial aspects of the hand.

Radial Nerve

The radial nerve receives contributions from C5 to T1 and continues from the posterior cord of the brachial plexus. It travels dorsally downward between the long and medial heads of the triceps supplying that muscle and the brachioradialis. It further supplies the wrist extensors and the supinator, then it continues into the forearm as the posterior interosseous nerve supplying the finger extensors and the abductor pollicis longus. Along the route, the radial nerve also gives off several cutaneous branches, which supply sensation along the dorsum of the arm, forearm, and hand, including the first three and one half fingers up to just before the nail beds. There can be compression of the nerve at the axilla, resulting in weakness of the triceps and more distal muscles along with numbness in the sensory distribution of the nerve. This may be mistaken for C6 or C7 radiculopathy except that weakness of wrist extensors resulting in a wrist drop would be uncommon for C7 dysfunction, and C6 radiculopathy would have biceps weakness, which is lacking in radial nerve injuries. The radial nerve can also be injured at the level of the midhumerus, which results in weakness of the wrist and finger extensors but not the triceps. This separates it from C7 injury; similarly, normal strength in the biceps differentiates this from a C6 problem. At the forearm, the nerve may become entrapped, causing pain and aching in the extensor muscles of the forearm, but again there is no triceps weakness. The posterior interosseous may also become trapped, causing weakness in finger extension with no sensory loss; this should also be easily distinguished from C6 or C7 root injury.

BRACHIAL PLEXOPATHY

Brachial plexopathy can present in a variety of ways from stretch injuries to avulsions. Brachial plexus injuries in the upper, middle, or lower trunk may be difficult to distinguish from multiple root injuries. Lower plexus injuries in the cords may mimic peripheral nerve injuries. Often, the history of the injury will allow one to make the distinctions. However, it is beneficial to obtain electrodiagnostic testing to differentiate between plexus and other root or nerve injuries. Brachial neuritis can cause upper extremity weakness along with severe pain. The pain is aggravated with movement. This condition can be distinguished from radiculopathies because the pain precedes the weakness and subsides as the weakness progresses.

CERVICAL SPINAL CORD INJURIES

Spinal cord injuries can be subclassified into complete and incomplete lesions (10,11). Complete and incomplete cervical spinal cord injuries can include all the radicular signs and symptoms at the level of injury; in addition, there will be effects that are more generalized throughout the body. Complete cervical spinal cord injuries include complete loss of motor and sensory function below the level of injury. Initially, there is complete flaccidity of the muscles and areflexia below the lesion. This is known as *spinal shock* (12) and lasts for at least a few weeks; the muscular tone then becomes spastic with hyperreflexia and clonus. Reflexes such as the bulbocavernosus reflex and the anal reflex usually return earlier than the deep tendon reflexes. The superficial or cutaneous reflexes such as the abdominal and cremasteric reflexes disappear, but this is not a consistent finding. There is also a withdrawal response that develops in which the whole leg withdraws secondary to plantar stimulation. The Babinski sign (13) (dorsiflexion of the great toe and fanning of the remaining toes) is also present and can accompany the leg withdrawal. Sensory loss is complete in all modalities below the level of the lesion. A sensory level with light touch and pinprick testing localizes the lesion to an approximate spinal cord level, but cord edema after injury may cause the level to be higher than the actual injury site. Similarly, the flaccidity of certain muscle groups is helpful in localization. Spinal cord injury also results in autonomic changes that would not be observed in root or peripheral nerve injury. After cord injury, the vasomotor control is lost, and a subsequent neurogenic shock may result in hypotension. This can be distinguished from shock secondary to blood loss because neurogenic shock is accompanied by a paradoxic bradycardia as opposed to tachycardia. The diagnosis of neurogenic shock should be a diagnosis of exclusion in trauma situations so as not to overlook other important causes of shock, such as intraabdominal bleeding. Bladder, bowel, and sexual function are also lost with complete cervical cord injury initially. Bladder function can eventually recover to allow reflex emptying; similarly, reflex emptying of the rectum can occur. In cervical cord injury, there is also Horner's syndrome due to interruption of fibers originating in the hypothalamus that travel down the cervical cord to the ciliospinal center at C8, T1, and T2. Horner's syndrome is often less well defined with injury above C8 because the ciliospinal center is more involved at the lower level. Localization on the basis of autonomic dysfunction is difficult because cervical spinal cord injury at all levels results in autonomic dysfunction, but the presence of such dysfunction helps in differentiating between an injury to the cord as opposed to the roots or peripheral nerves. Segmental variation in the cervical cord allows localization based on signs and symptoms after injury.

Complete spinal cord injury at the C1 to C3 levels is almost always fatal unless immediate respiratory support is given. Sensory loss involves the whole body below the head and extends to the occipital area if C2 is involved. Furthermore, there may be sensory loss in the outermost regions of the face secondary to injury of the descending spinal tract of the trigeminal nerve. The spinal tract can descend as far as C4, with the caudal part carrying impulses from the outermost part of the face. Localization is usually not difficult because of the obvious lack of all motor and sensory function below the neck in these patients. Motor function remains in the platysma, sternocleidomastoid, and trapezius, owing to innervation from cranial nerves seven and eleven. Complete injuries at C4 are similar to C1 to C3 injuries, but there may be adequate function of the diaphragm secondary to innervation from a preserved C3 segment. The respiratory rate is increased, and the patient compensates by using the auxiliary muscles such as sternocleidomastoid, trapezius, and platysma. The patient is unable to cough effectively and requires frequent suctioning. Artificial ventilation and tracheostomy are necessary for C1 to C4 injuries. Sensation from a C4 lesion is maintained to the middle of the neck and above.

Complete injuries at C5 still have impaired diaphragmatic function initially, and full function may recover after the spinal shock wears off. Levator scapulae and rhomboids are also partially innervated and, combined with the other auxiliary muscles of respiration mentioned previously, will improve the vital capacity of the lung when compared with C1 to C4 lesions. The supraspinatus and infraspinatus are also paretic, but not paralyzed, so that limited external rotation of the arms is possible. The shoulder may be elevated because of the unopposed action of the trapezius and levator scapulae. The muscles innervated by C5 and below are paralyzed. The reflexes below the lesion are hyperactive, but the deltoid, biceps, and supinator reflexes are decreased or nonexistent. Sensory loss starts below the neck and clavicle. There is also a triangular area of the ventral aspect of the shoulder with sensation.

Patients with a complete C6 injury have intact diaphragmatic function. This injury results in shoulders that are elevated, arms that are abducted, and forearms that are flexed because of the uninhibited actions of deltoid, biceps, and brachioradialis. Care must be taken to avoid flexion contractures at the elbow joints in these patients. The deltoid and biceps reflex may be exaggerated, but the triceps reflex is diminished or absent. There is sensation to the lateral aspects of the arm from C5 innervation, but the rest of the arm and body is numb.

At the C7 level, respiration is normally strong enough without the need for tracheostomy and ventilation support. The position of the arms is similar to that in C6 injury except less marked because of partial innervation of the arm adductors and internal rotators (subscapularis, pectoralis major, teres major, and latissimus dorsi). The triceps muscle can be partially innervated by C6 and therefore can oppose the elbow flexion by the biceps muscle. The more caudal the injury at C7, the stronger the triceps muscle function. Unlike complete C6 lesions, the wrist extensor, extensor carpi radialis longus, is active and causes extension of the wrist with radial deviation. However, there is no finger extension, resulting in a hand position with an extended wrist and flexed fingers, sometimes known as *preacher's hand*. The biceps and brachioradialis reflex are present, whereas the triceps reflex is diminished. The sensory loss includes the inner aspect of the arms and the third to fifth finger.

In complete C8 injuries, adduction and internal rotation are preserved, which eliminates the atypical arm positions seen with C6 and C7 injuries. The triceps is strong enough to extend the forearm against gravity. The radial deviation of the hand is lessened as a result of the action of the extensor carpi radialis brevis. Flexion and extension at the wrist can be normal, and there is partial strength in the finger flexors. However, lumbricals and interossei are paralyzed, which results in a clawed hand deformity. There is a more evident Horner's syndrome, and disturbances of sweating involving the arms and upper trunk may be present. The triceps reflex is still diminished, as is the finger flexor reflex. The sensory loss is similar to C7 injury, except that there is some sensation in the third finger.

The T1 segment is technically not part of the cervical cord, but it is functionally important in cervical injury because of its control of intrinsic hand muscles. T1 injury results in partial paralysis of the adductor pollicis, interossei, lumbricals, and opponens, and there is complete paralysis of the abductor pollicis brevis. Both the finger flexors and extensors are functioning, as is the abductor pollicis longus. All arm reflexes are normal, while reflexes caudal to the lesion are hyperactive. There is a Horner's syndrome. Sensory loss begins on the medial aspects of the arms and continues down the rest of the body.

Incomplete cervical cord injuries can be divided into specific syndromes depending on the area of the cord injured. The syndromes include central cord, anterior cord, posterior cord, and Brown-Séquard syndromes.

The central cord syndrome is commonly described as a result of syringomyelia but can also result from traumatic cord injury secondary to formation of hematomyelia. These conditions cause a central cavitation that can extend through many cervical segments and that results in a syndrome in which the levels of weakness between the arms and the legs are unequal and there is a dissociated sensory loss. Hyperextension of the neck can also result in this syndrome (14). The motor findings can be explained based on the somatotopic organization of the corticospinal tract in the spinal cord, as previously described. The nerve fibers controlling the arm muscles are located medially in the corticospinal tract and are therefore these muscles are affected more severely by the central cavitation initially. The anterior horn cells can be destroyed by the cavity, leading to atrophy and weakness in the small hand muscles. The muscles below the lesion become spastic and hyperreflexic, similar to other types of cord injury. The sensory loss is often in a capelike distribution involving arms, shoulders, and upper thorax. Also, pain and temperature sensations are more affected because of involvement of the anterior commissure. As the cavity enlarges, the sensory loss may be more widespread, but there can still be sacral sparing because, similar to the motor fibers, the sacral sensory fibers are situated more peripherally in the cord.

Anterior cord syndromes (15) usually result from decreased blood supply from the anterior spinal artery. This artery supplies the anterior horns and the ventral and lateral funiculi, but not the dorsal columns. This results in lower motor signs in the cervical segments involved, such as muscle flaccidity and hyporeflexia, whereas there are spasticity and hyperreflexia below the lesion. Bladder and other autonomic functions can be disrupted similarly to other injuries of the cervical cord. There is also loss of pain and temperature sensations, but position sense, vibration sense, and some touch sensations are preserved.

Posterior cord syndromes are possible in the cervical spine through trauma or tumors, but this is rarely confined to the posterior columns. True posterior column syndromes can be caused by tabes dorsalis or subacute combined degeneration, but they are not localized to the cervical spinal cord. There is only loss of the modalities subserved by the dorsal columns.

Brown-Séquard syndrome, also known as *hemisection of the spinal cord*, can be caused by lacerations, tumors, or trauma (16,17). The injury causes ipsilateral loss of dorsal column sensations, ipsilateral weakness, and contralateral loss of pain and temperature sensation. The weakness associated with this syndrome is generally of the upper motor neuron variety caudal to the lesion, but at the level of the lesion, there are lower motor neuron symptoms due to direct damage to the anterior horn cells. Similarly, there is an ipsilateral loss of pain and temperature at the level of injury and one to two levels below, owing to the decussation of the spinothalamic tract within the spinal cord.

Tumors arising at the foramen magnum may at first cause an ipsilateral spastic monoparesis of the arm, followed by the ipsilateral leg, then the contralateral leg, and then the contralateral arm (18).

Incomplete injuries encompass any injury to the spinal cord that does not result in complete loss of motor and sensory function below the level of injury. Therefore, incomplete injuries need not fit neatly into any of the above syndromes to be classified as incomplete. For instance, injuries in patients with sacral sensation (sacral sparing) but with otherwise complete motor and sensory loss are still classified as incomplete, although functionally they may resemble complete cord injuries.

CONCLUSION

Anatomic localization of lesions in the cervical spine requires a meticulous and methodical approach that must be used in every patient in whom this type of injury is suspected. This approach, combined with proper use of imaging and diagnostic equipment, will reduce the likelihood of a missed or mistaken diagnosis.

REFERENCES

1. Hughes JT. The Edwin Smith surgical papyrus: an analysis of the first case reports of spinal cord injuries. *Paraplegia* 1988;26(2): 71–82.
2. Kaitaro T. Biological and epistemological models of localization in the nineteenth century: from Gall to Charcot. *J Hist Neurosci* 2001;10 (3):262–276.
3. Bennett MR, Hacker PM. The motor system in neuroscience: a history and analysis of conceptual developments. *Prog Neurobiol* 2002;67(1): 1–52
4. Tan TC, Black PM. The contributions of Otfrid Foerster (1873–1941) to neurology and neurosurgery. *Neurosurgery* 2001;49(5): 1231–1235.
5. Barr ML, Kiernan JA. Spinal cord. In: Barr ML, Kiernan JA, eds. *The human nervous system,* 5th ed. Philadelphia: JB Lippincott, 1988:63–83.
6. Parent A. Spinal cord: regional anatomy and internal structure. In: Parent A, ed. *Carpenter's human neuroanatomy,* 9th ed. Baltimore: Williams & Wilkins, 1996:325–367.
7. Tong HC, Haig AJ, Yamakawa K. The Spurling test and cervical radiculopathy. *Spine* 2002;27(2):156–159.
8. Woolsey RM, Young RR. The clinical diagnosis of disorders of the spinal cord. *Neurol Clin* 1991;9(3):573–583.
9. Chen TY. The clinical presentation of uppermost cervical disc protrusion. *Spine* 2000;25(4):439–442.
10. Guttman L. Clinical symptomatology of spinal cord lesions. In: Vinken PJ, Bruyn GW, eds. *Handbook of clinical neurology,* Vol 2. Amsterdam: North-Holland, 1969:178–216.
11. Wagner R, Jagoda A. Spinal cord syndromes. *Emerg Med Clin North Am* 1997;15(3):699–711.
12. Atkinson PP, Atkinson JLD. Spinal shock. *Mayo Clin Proc* 1996;71: 384–389.
13. Kumar SP, Ramasubramanian D. The Babinski sign: a reappraisal. *Neurol India* 2000;48:314–318.
14. Schneider RC, Cherry G, Pantek H. The syndrome of acute central cervical spinal cord injury. *J Neurosurg* 1954;11:546–577.
15. Schneider RC. The syndrome of acute anterior spinal cord injury. *J Neurosurg* 1955;12:95–122.
16. Roth EJ, Park T, Pang T, et al. Traumatic cervical Brown-Séquard and Brown-Séquard plus syndromes: the spectrum of presentations and outcomes. *Paraplegia* 1991;29:582–589.
17. Rumana CS, Baskin DS. Brown-Séquard syndrome produced by cervical disc herniation: case report and literature review. *Surg Neurol* 1996; 45:359–361.
18. Adams RD, Victor M. Intracranial neoplasms. In: Adams RD, Victor M, eds. *Principles of neurology,* 5th ed. New York: McGraw-Hill, 1993: 554–598.

CHAPTER 13

Neurologic Examination: Grading Scales

Charles H. Tator

Effective management of patients with acute cervical spinal cord injury (SCI) depends on accurate clinical neurologic examination and subsequent classification and grading of the extent and severity of the neurologic injury (1). Indeed, the most useful classifications have been based on the assessment of the functional neurologic damage as determined by the clinical neurologic examination rather than on other criteria such as electrophysiology or imaging. An accurate system of clinical neurologic assessment and recording permits the development of a rational treatment plan, allows reliable and consistent serial monitoring of the patient during the acute and rehabilitative phases of care, and provides useful data for the early determination of prognosis. Furthermore, the system of neurologic assessment and classification must be sufficiently reliable to allow accurate comparison of serial observations by the same or different observers. Many methods of classifying and scoring the extent and severity of the clinical neurologic deficit have been developed, and this chapter provides a review and critical analysis of the various systems, both simple and complex, that have been used. I emphasize the usefulness of the new system now known as the International Standards for Neurological and Functional Classification of Spinal Cord Injury (ISCSCI-92), which was initially devised in the 1980s by the American Spinal Injury Association (ASIA). Then, in the early 1990s, ASIA convened consensus meetings of representatives from several disciplines and from several countries involved in the management of patients with acute SCI. In 1992, ASIA, along with the International Medical Society of Paraplegia (IMSOP), published the International Standards for Neurological and Functional Classification of Spinal Cord Injury (2). This ISCSCI-92 classification is a considerable improvement over other methods, and it is my opinion that this system should be used by all physicians and surgeons managing patients with acute SCI.

SIMPLE SYSTEMS OF CLASSIFICATION AND SCORING

Complete versus Incomplete Spinal Cord Injury Syndromes

One of the simplest and most useful systems is the grading of cases into complete and incomplete neurologic injuries. Indeed, before the development of the more complex systems, this method was in use for several decades of this century. A complete injury was initially defined as complete loss of voluntary motor function below the level of the injury, complete absence of somatic sensation below the level of the injury, and loss of voluntary control of bowel and bladder function. Later, other features were added to the definition of the complete syndrome, including the presence of abnormal reflexes such as priapism and the early return of the bulbocavernosus reflex. In contrast, a patient was considered to have an incomplete syndrome when there was any residual voluntary motor function or sensation below the level of the injury. As shown in Table 13.1, a large number of incomplete syndromes have been described, generally based on the anatomic site of injury in the transverse plane of the spinal cord.

The major advantages of this method are its simplicity and its ability to provide information useful for determining prognosis. However, the prognostic effectiveness of this simple system relates mainly to complete injuries in which there is virtually no likelihood of major recovery such as return of ambulation. For example, Hansebout (3) showed that only a very small number of complete injuries recover ambulation. He analyzed several large series of acute SCI patients and found that a small percentage of initially complete cases (usually 1% to 2%) had substantial recovery of distal cord function. Even then, it could be argued that complete injuries with subsequent recovery represent misdiagnosis because of factors discussed in detail later, such as inebriation, sedative or other drug effects, spinal shock,

TABLE 13.1. *Complete and Incomplete Neurological Syndromes in Acute Cervical Spinal Cord Injury*

1. Complete Spinal Cord Injury Syndromes—ASIA/IMSOP Grade A
   (a) Unilevel: no zone of partial preservation
   (b) Multilevel: with zone of partial preservation
2. Incomplete Spinal Cord Injury Syndromes—ASIA/IMSOP Grades B, C, or D
   (a) Cervicomedullary syndrome
   (b) Central cord syndrome
   (c) Anterior cord syndrome
   (d) Posterior cord syndrome
   (e) Brown-Séquard syndrome
3. Spinal Cord Injury Without Radiological Abnormality (SCIWORA)—ASIA/IMSOP Grades A, B, C, or D
4. Spinal Cord Injury Without Radiological Evidence of Trauma (SCIWORET)—ASIA/IMSOP Grades A, B, C, or D
5. Reversible or Transient Syndromes
   (a) Cord concussion
   (b) Burning hands syndrome
   (c) Contusion cervicalis
   (d) Hysteria
   (e) Malingering
6. Spinal Cord Trauma Syndromes Without Direct Cord Injury

uncooperativeness, or a concomitant head injury. I believes that about 1% to 2% of patients with complete spinal cord injuries recover substantial distal cord function, even in the absence of all of the factors that can interfere with precise, early classification, and that early appropriate treatment can increase this number. In contrast, in incomplete injuries, the prognosis for recovery is generally much better (4). However, with incomplete injuries, the accuracy of prognostication in individual cases in the early phase is very poor because there is a wide spectrum of possible degrees of recovery ranging from minimal to almost total recovery. In addition to inaccuracy about prognostication, there are other major disadvantages to the simple systems, including lack of precision in describing what constitutes a complete injury. For example, until recently, there was no universally accepted definition of a complete injury. Features were included in the definition of completeness such as the return of the bulbocavernosus reflex, but these are extremely unreliable. Furthermore, the simple system does not allow quantification of the severity of the neurologic deficit in groups of patients and is of minimal value for serial observation in a given patient. Therefore, the simple system cannot be used alone and must be supplemented by one of the complex methods described later.

Incomplete Acute Cervical Spinal Cord Injury Syndromes

Table 13.1 shows the large variety of incomplete acute neurologic syndromes occurring in SCI. In general, these syndromes are named according to the presumed location of the injury in the transverse plane of the spinal cord (5)

(Figs. 13.1 to 13.5). For two reasons, it is useful for practitioners to categorize incomplete patients according to the location of the injury in the cord. First, recognition of the type of incomplete syndrome provides information about the mechanism of injury that is often useful for selection of treatment; second, the various categories of incomplete injury tend to have differing prognoses for recovery.

Cervicomedullary Syndrome

A high proportion of injuries to the upper cervical cord include damage to the medulla as well, in which case the term *cervicomedullary syndrome* (6,7) or *cruciate paralysis* is used (8). These injuries may extend to C4 or even lower in the cord and may extend up to the pons, due to either direct injury or vascular injury to the vertebral arteries.

The essential features are respiratory insufficiency or arrest, hypotension, varying degrees of tetraparesis and sensory changes from C1 to C4, and sensory loss over the face, conforming to the onion-skin or Dejerine pattern. There is often greater arm than leg weakness. Of course, the higher the lesion, the more severe the manifestations, such as in patients with atlantooccipital dislocation. The mechanisms

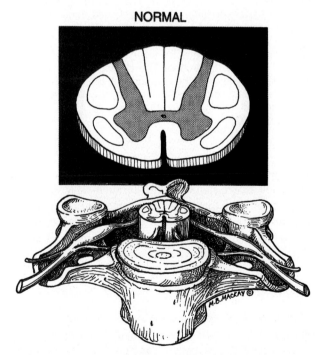

NORMAL

FIG. 13.1. The normal spinal cord and spinal column. The normal relationships between the spinal cord, spinal column, and nerve roots are depicted in the midcervical region. For clarity, the dura mater has been omitted. In the **upper diagram**, the gray matter is *finely stippled*, and the corticospinal and spinothalamic tracts are *outlined*. The intervertebral disc is shown. (From Narayan RK, Wilberger JE Jr, Povlishock JT, ed. *Neurotrauma*. New York: McGraw-Hill: 1996:1059–1073, with permission.)

CENTRAL CORD SYNDROME

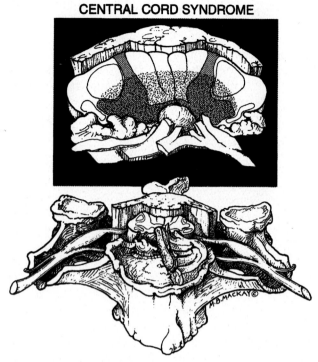

ANTERIOR CORD SYNDROME

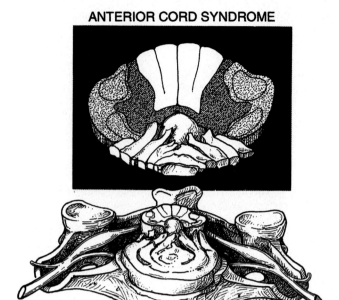

FIG. 13.2. Central cord syndrome. The drawing depicts a case of cervical spondylosis with osteoarthritis of the cervical spine, including anterior and posterior osteophytes and hypertrophy of the ligamentum flavum. Superimposed is an acute hyperextension injury, which has caused rupture of the intervertebral disc and infolding of the ligamentum flavum. The spinal cord is compressed vertically and dorsally. The central portion of the cord, (*rough stippling*) sustained the greatest damage. The damaged area includes the medial segments of the corticospinal tracts presumed to subserve arm function. (From Narayan RK, Wilberger JE Jr, Povlishock JT, ed. *Neurotrauma.* New York: McGraw-Hill: 1996:1059–1073, with permission.)

FIG. 13.3. Anterior cord syndrome. A large disc herniation is shown compressing the anterior aspect of the cord and resulting in damage (*rough stippling*) to the anterior and lateral white-matter tracts and to the gray matter. The posterior columns remain intact. (From Narayan RK, Wilberger JE Jr, Povlishock JT, ed. *Neurotrauma.* New York: McGraw-Hill: 1996:1059–1073, with permission.)

of spinal cord injury also include traction injury from severe dislocation as in atlantoaxial dislocation, anteroposterior compression from burst fracture, odontoid fracture, or ruptured disc. More skillful and prompt first aid has increased the likelihood of survival, and thus there are now more cases of these injuries arriving at hospitals than previously.

Acute Central Cord Syndrome

Schneider et al. described the acute central cervical cord syndrome characterized by a disproportionately greater loss of motor power in the upper extremities than the lower extremities with varying degrees of sensory loss (9). He hypothesized that acute compression was an etiologic factor in many cases (Fig. 13.2). There are many similarities between the central cord syndrome and the syndrome of cruciate paralysis, and clinically, it may be very difficult to make this distinction, as discussed in detail elsewhere (10).

There is recent evidence that the syndromes characterized by greater arm than leg weakness are not due to the

presumed differing locations of the arm and leg fibers in the corticospinal tract, as previously thought (11). There is evidence from careful clinicopathologic and magnetic resonance imaging (MRI) correlations (12) and from evidence that the lateral corticospinal tract subserves mainly distal limb musculature. Thus, the functional deficit is more pronounced in the hands when this tract is primarily the site of damage. Prognosis varies considerably, and many patients remain with substantial weakness and proprioceptive loss, especially in the hands.

Anterior Cord Syndrome

Anterior cord syndrome was also originally described in the setting of acute cervical trauma by Schneider (13), who presented two cases of "immediate complete paralysis with hyperesthesia at the level of the lesion and an associated sparing of touch and some vibration sense." In Schneider's view, this is "a syndrome for which early operative intervention is indicated." The anterior aspect of the cord is damaged, and in severe cases, there may only be sparing of the posterior columns (Fig. 13.3). Less severe cases may have some retention of motor function as a result of sparing of some fibers in the lateral corticospinal tracts.

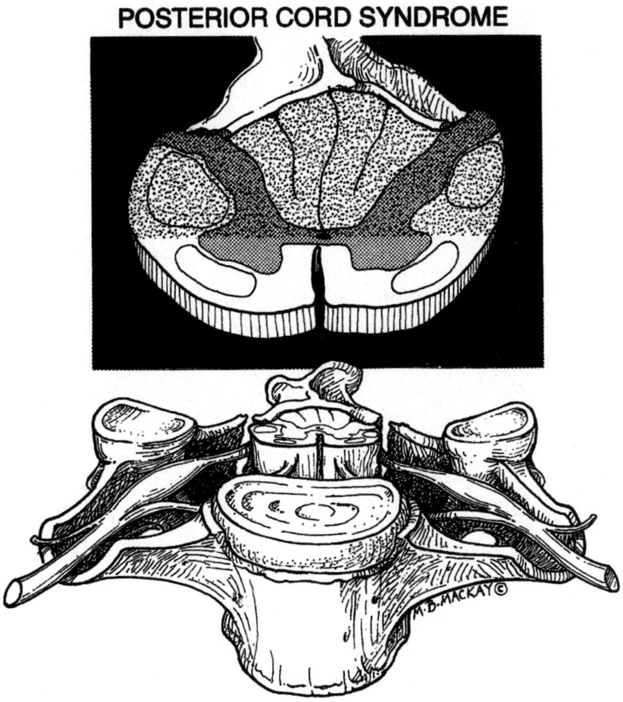

POSTERIOR CORD SYNDROME

BROWN - SÉQUARD SYNDROME

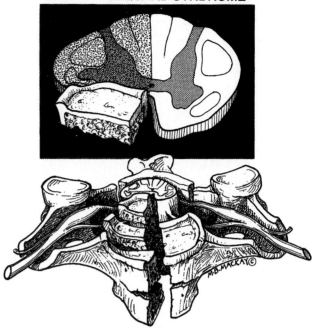

FIG. 13.4. Posterior cord syndrome. A laminar fracture is depicted with anterior displacement of the fractured bone and compression of the posterior aspect of the spinal cord. The damaged area of the spinal cord (*rough stippling* in the **upper diagram**) includes the posterior columns and the posterior half of the lateral columns, including the corticospinal tracts. (From Narayan RK, Wilberger JE Jr, Povlishock JT, ed. *Neurotrauma.* New York: McGraw-Hill: 1996:1059–1073, with permission.)

FIG. 13.5. Brown-Séquard syndrome. A burst fracture is depicted with ventral displacement of bone fragments and disc, resulting in unilateral compression and damage (*rough stippling*) to one half of the spinal cord. (From Narayan RK, Wilberger JE Jr, Povlishock JT, ed. *Neurotrauma.* New York: McGraw-Hill: 1996:1059–1073, with permission.)

Posterior Cord Syndrome

Posterior cord syndrome is an extremely rare type of incomplete syndrome. Many observers, including myself, have doubted its existence. Supposedly, it occurs after major destruction of the posterior aspect of the cord but with some residual functioning spinal cord tissue anteriorly (Fig. 13.4). Thus, clinically, the patient would have retained spinothalamic function but would have lost movement and proprioception because of damage to the posterior half of the cord, including the corticospinal tracts and posterior columns.

Brown-Séquard Syndrome

Brown-Séquard syndrome is caused by a lesion of the lateral half of the spinal cord (Fig. 13.5) and is characterized by ipsilateral motor and proprioceptive loss and contralateral pain and temperature loss. The syndrome can be associated with a variety of mechanisms of injury, most frequently hyperextension, although also with flexion, locked facets, and compression fractures.

Brown-Séquard syndrome may be present from the start or may only become apparent several days after injury as a gradual evolution from a bilateral incomplete injury. Hybrid combinations of Brown-Séquard and other incomplete syndromes may occur. For example, I have seen frequent examples of central cord injuries that are quite asymmetric, with the more severely damaged side of the cord showing features of a Brown-Séquard syndrome.

Spinal Cord Injury without Radiological Abnormality and Spinal Cord Injury without Radiological Evidence of Trauma

In children, the syndrome of SCI without radiologic abnormality (SCIWORA) is more common than in adults and represents a substantial percentage of pediatric SCI (14). Children are more susceptible to these injuries presumably because of the laxity of their spinal ligaments and the weakness of their paraspinal muscles. Children with SCIWORA tend to be less severely injured than those with definite evidence of bony injury, but complete injuries have been described. By definition, the negative radiologic examination includes only plane films and tomography, either conventional or computed tomography (CT). If a negative MRI were included in the definition, the number of cases would diminish dramatically because of the extreme sensitivity of MRI in detecting mild cord injury and spinal column injuries such as torn ligaments and ruptured discs.

True SCIWORA can also occur in adults but is much less frequent than the syndrome of acute spinal cord injury without radiologic evidence of trauma (SCIWORET) (15). Patients with SCIWORET have abnormal radiologic exams, but the x-rays do not show any evidence of trauma. Before the use of CT or MRI in spinal trauma, the prevalence of SCIWORET in adults with SCI was about 14% (5). The addition of CT has reduced the prevalence of SCIWORET to about 5%. A recent analysis of the prevalence of SCIWORET in acute SCI (16) showed that many patients with SCIWORET have demonstrable compression by myelography or MRI and should be considered for early surgical decompression. It is likely that very few SCIs will remain undetected by MRI because of its high sensitivity for detecting mild SCI and nonbony spinal column lesions. Cervical spondylosis is the most commonly associated condition in adults with SCIWORET, but other conditions, including spinal stenosis, ankylosing spondylitis, disc herniation, and nucleus pulposus embolism, may on rare occasion be associated with SCI and not show radiologic evidence of trauma (15).

Reversible or Transient Syndromes

A number of complete or incomplete SCI syndromes (Table 13.1) are reversible or transient, one of the most interesting of which is the burning hands syndrome, which frequently occurs in athletes (17) and is characterized by transient paresthesias and dysesthesias in the upper limbs, especially the hands. It may exist with or without long tract signs, which if present are usually evanescent. Biemond (18) found pathologic changes in the posterior horn of one case and termed the condition *contusio cervicalis posterior*. Braakman and Penning (19) found that hyperextension was the most frequent mechanism of injury. Torg and colleagues (20) described a transient incomplete spinal cord syndrome with sensory and motor deficits lasting up to 48 hours in football players and used the inappropriate term "neurapraxia." All of these patients had radiologic spinal abnormalities, such as ligamentous instability, disc disease, or spinal stenosis. These transient cord injury syndromes

are usually bilateral, which distinguishes them from the other syndrome of "stingers" or "burners" in athletes due to unilateral nerve root or brachial plexus lesions (especially traction injury), most of which are also transient (17).

Spinal cord concussion is a transient loss of motor or sensory function of the spinal cord, which usually recovers within minutes, but always within hours. In almost all instances, the initial clinical examiner is told by the patient that the symptoms are rapidly diminishing and finds a normal neurologic examination. The exact pathophysiology of spinal cord concussion is unknown, but it is most likely due to a biochemical abnormality in the spinal cord such as leakage of potassium from the intracellular to the extracellular space.

Spinal Cord Trauma Syndromes without Direct Spinal Cord Injury

This relatively rare syndrome differs from SCIWORET and SCIWORA in that these patients sustain a lesion of the spinal cord that manifests as an acute spinal cord syndrome and is associated with trauma, but there is no direct trauma to the spine. The syndrome can occur in both children and adults and usually produces the clinical findings of the anterior spinal artery syndrome. Keith (21) described several cases in children with major abdominal, thoracic, or limb trauma and concluded that many of them had sustained an aortic injury that caused occlusion of intercostal or lumbar arteries with subsequent occlusion of medullary arteries and spinal cord infarction. Rarely, penetrating injuries, such as gunshot wounds, can interrupt major arterial feeders to the cord without direct trauma to the spine. Severe hypotension and systemic shock in trauma patients can also result in spinal cord ischemia and infarction, even without concomitant cerebral ischemia.

COMPLEX SYSTEMS OF CLASSIFICATION AND SCORING

Several complex systems have been devised for grading and scoring the neurologic deficit after acute SCI, most of which allow accurate initial and subsequent serial evaluations and varying degrees of quantification (Table 13.2).

TABLE 13.2. *Complex Systems for Classifying and Scoring the Neurological Examination in Acute Spinal Cord Injury*

System	Features	Advantages	Disadvantages
Frankel	5 severity grades	Simple, easy to understand	Cannot quantify recovery Imprecise definitions of grades A, C, and D Ceiling effect
Sunnybrook	10 severity grades 17 neurological changes	More accurate initial grading Allows quantification of recovery in individuals and groups	No numerical scores of motor and sensory function
ISCSCI-92 (ASIA/IMSOP)	5 severity grades	Improved definition of completes Allows quantification of neurological scores	Ceiling Effect
Benzel	7 severity grades Sphincter control		Cannot be used for initial examination

Almost all have been used in one or more clinical trials in SCI (22).

Frankel System

The Frankel system of grading neurologic deficit after acute SCI was first published in 1969 (23). The system was developed in England at the Stoke-Mandeville Hospital started by Ludwig Guttman, one of the first specialized centers for the management of SCI. The system involves classifying the injuries into five grades of deficit, with grade A being a complete injury, grades B to D varying degrees of severity of incomplete injury, and grade E normal neurologic function (Table 13.3). The system permits tracking of individual patients and also comparisons between groups of patients recorded by cross-tabulation. For example, the initial neurologic deficit can be recorded on the horizontal axis, and the follow-up or final neurologic deficit can be recorded on the vertical axis with 25 possible combinations (24). One of the best examples of the use of this system is the National Spinal Cord Injury Database reported by Stover and colleagues (25), which documents the neurologic recovery in almost 10,000 SCI patients compiled by the Model Spinal Cord Injury System Program in the United States at 19 centers during 1973 to 1985. Indeed, the long-term and extensive data accumulated serve as an excellent data bank of the natural history of neurologic recovery from SCI. For example, the data clearly show that most SCI patients experience some neurologic recovery. It is important to recognize that with all the complex systems, neurologic recovery includes recovery of nerve root function at the level of the injury or caudally and spinal cord recovery at the level of the injury or caudally (26). The Frankel system showed that even a small number of neurologically complete cases could recover some caudal neurologic function indicative of cord recovery. Stover and colleagues (25)

found the best recovery in the B and C categories of incomplete injuries, in which 30% to 50% of patients improved one Frankel grade. Currently, 60% of patients with SCI have incomplete injuries (10). Thus, these high rates of natural recovery, especially among patients with incomplete injury who received only the standard of care during the era before the development of the prospective randomized control clinical trials in SCI (22), make it mandatory to employ rigorous study methodology and accurate outcome measures in clinical trials of patients with SCI. The deficiencies of the Frankel system include inability to quantitate neurologic recovery, the ceiling effect (described later), and imprecise definitions of grades, especially C and D. Many of these deficiencies have been rectified in the systems subsequently devised.

Sunnybrook System

I devised the Sunnybrook system in the late 1960s (27). This was the first system for quantifying neurologic recovery in individual patients and between groups of patients. The system comprises 10 grades of neurologic function and 17 types of "neurologic change," including 8 types of neurologic deterioration and 8 types of neurologic improvement (Table 13.4). One of the important differences between the Frankel and Sunnybrook systems is the more precise definitions of grades C and D. In the Frankel System, grades C and D are defined on the basis of the preserved motor function being "useless" in grade C and "useful" in grade D. The Sunnybrook scale defines motor function more precisely on the basis of the Medical Research Council (MRC) muscle grading system, with normal strength graded as 5 and complete paralysis graded as 0. In grades 3 to 5 of the Sunnybrook system, most key muscles below the neurologic level of injury have muscle strength less than MRC 3; and in grades 6 to 8, most key muscles below the neurologic level have muscle strength greater than or equal to MRC 3. Neurologic recovery can be quantitated in several ways, based on the 10 neurologic grades or the 17 neurologic changes. Grade change can be assessed by cross-tabulation comparing the initial and subsequent neurologic grades, similar to the Frankel system (100 possible improvement or deterioration combinations). Changes in grade can also be converted to a percentage of the possible changes that an individual patient could make. For example, a patient who deteriorated from grade 7 to grade 2 deteriorated five grades out of a possible six grades and would be considered to have deteriorated −86% (−5/6 × 100). A patient improving from grade 1 to grade 2 would have improved one grade out of a possible nine grades and would be considered to have improved 11% (1/9 × 100). In this way, the percentage change in grade could be established for each patient between admission and discharge, discharge and follow-up, or admission and follow-up. To calculate the percentage change in selected groups of patients or in the entire population, the individual percentage changes can be summed and averaged. In addition, the

---

TABLE 13.3. *Frankel Classification Grading System*

Grade A	Complete neurological injury—No motor or sensory function clinically detected below the level of the injury.
Grade B	Preserved sensation only—No motor function clinically detected below the level of injury; sensory function remains below the level of injury but may include only partial function (sacral sparing qualifies as preserved sensation).
Grade C	Preserved motor non-functional—Some motor function observed below the level of the injury, but is of no practical use to the patient.
Grade D	Preserved motor function—Useful motor function below the level of the injury; patient can move lower limbs and walk with or without aid, but does not have a normal gait or strength in all motor groups.
Grade E	Normal motor—No clinically detected abnormality in motor or sensory function with normal sphincter function; abnormal reflexes and subjective sensory abnormalities may be present.

TABLE 13.4. *Sunnybrook Scale and Neurological Changes*

A: Neurological grade: Sunnybrook scale of the severity of the neurological injury

Grade	Description	Corresponding Frankel Grade
1	Complete motor loss; complete sensory loss	A
2	Complete motor loss; incomplete sensory loss	B
3	Incomplete motor useless*; complete sensory loss	C
4	Incomplete motor useless*; incomplete sensory loss	C
5	Incomplete motor useless*; normal sensory	C
6	Incomplete motor useful*; complete sensory loss	D
7	Incomplete motor useful*; incomplete sensory loss	D
8	Incomplete motor useful*; normal sensory	D
9	Normal motor; incomplete sensory loss	D
10	Normal motor; normal sensory	E

B: Neurological change method for assessment of neurological improvement or deterioration after acute SCI

Neurological change number	Description of neurological change
1	Deteriorate to complete motor; complete sensory loss
2	Deteriorate to complete motor; incomplete sensory loss
3	Deteriorate to incomplete motor; complete sensory loss
4	Deteriorate to incomplete motor; incomplete sensory loss
5	Deteriorate to incomplete motor; normal sensory
6	Deteriorate to normal motor; incomplete sensory loss
7	Deteriorate to higher level, but grade the same
8	Deteriorate at same level, but grade the same
9	No change
10	Improve at same level, but grade the same
11	Improve at lower level, but grade the same
12	Improve to complete motor; incomplete sensory loss
13	Improve to incomplete motor; complete sensory loss
14	Improve to incomplete motor; normal sensory
15	Improve to incomplete motor; normal sensory
16	Improve to normal motor; incomplete sensory loss
17	Improve to normal

*See text for definitions of useless and useful

percentage of patients improving, deteriorating, or remaining unchanged on the basis of neurologic grade can be determined for further analysis of neurologic recovery. In the Sunnybrook system, neurologic recovery can also be based on the scale of neurologic change, and this provides a more detailed assessment of the neurologic improvement or deterioration than provided by the neurologic grade method. Seventeen possible types of neurologic improvement or deterioration are listed in Table 13.4, representing the most important ways in which neurologic status can change after SCI. The worst deterioration is deterioration to complete motor loss and complete sensory loss and is designated change 1; and the best improvement, improvement to normal, is designated change 17. A numerical value for a patient's change in neurologic status can then be determined by calculating changes as a percentage of the possible change that a patient with that particular neurologic grade can make, beginning at change 9, which is designated "no change." For example, a grade 1 patient (complete motor loss and complete sensory loss) who improved neu-

rologically to a status of incomplete motor loss and normal sensory function would be judged to have improved from change 9 to change 15, an improvement of six out of a possible eight changes, or 75% improvement. Not all of the 17 possible changes are applicable to each of the 10 neurologic grades. For example, a patient who is initially grade 1 with complete motor and complete sensory loss cannot deteriorate by changes 1, 2, 3, 4, 5, or 6 of Table 13.4. Indeed, there are only five possible patterns or sequences of neurologic changes required for evaluating all the possible types of improvements or deteriorations among patients in the 10 neurologic grades. These five patterns are then used to quantify the neurologic change in each patient and in selected groups of patients (27). Note that the second method based on neurologic change is more detailed than the method based on neurologic grade and can identify many types of improvements and deteriorations of insufficient magnitude to produce a change in neurologic grade. Frequent examples are patients who recovered function in a nerve root at the level of injury, such as a patient with complete spinal cord injury at C5 who recovered function in the deltoid and biceps muscles. This recovery would be designated as change 10 (Table 13.4) because there was improvement at the same level of the cord as the injury occurred, and the patient remained the same grade. Such an improvement would not be recognized by the neurologic grades method because the patient's neurologic grade remained the same (grade 1).

The percentage of possible improvement or deterioration implies a complex calculation based on the potential for recovery calculated for each patient. For example, a cervical incomplete injury has the potential to recover more muscle groups than a lumbar incomplete injury. Thus, a cervical injury would have to recover more muscle groups to register a 50% recovery than a lumbar injury. Ideally, the methods used to compute neurologic recovery should be clearly stated, including the statistical tests to assess the significance of the recovery among groups of patients. Although the Sunnybrook system has been used to date in only one randomized prospective controlled trial in acute SCI (28), the same principles of "potential" or "possible" recovery have been incorporated into the assessment methodology of other trials. For example, the NASCIS (National Acute Spinal Cord Injury Study) trials have used similar methodology (29,30), and it is likely that at least some of the controversy about these trials is due to a lack of understanding of the methods used to calculate recovery as a percentage of the possible recovery that could have occurred in a given patient or in groups of patients (31).

American Spinal Injury Association and International Medical Society of Paraplegia System, Currently Known as the International Standards for Neurological and Functional Classification of Spinal Cord Injury

Table 13.5 shows the new ISCSCI-92 grading scale containing five grades of impairment, with grade A denoting a complete injury, grades B to D varying levels of incomplete injury, and grade E a patient with normal motor and sensory spinal cord function (2). Completeness in grade A is now much more precisely defined as absence of sensory and motor function in the lowest sacral segment, as originally described by Waters and associates (32). This represents a major improvement in the definition of a complete SCI and improves

the precision of distinguishing between complete and incomplete injuries. To make this distinction, the clinician must test touch and pinprink sensation in the lowest sacral dermatomes perianally at the mucocutaneous junction as well as deep anal sensation. Also, voluntary motor contraction of the external anal sphincter must be tested by digital examination. The distinction between complete and incomplete is crucial for planning treatment and for predicting outcome. The ISCSCI-92 system also has introduced the concept of the "zone of partial preservation," which applies only to complete cervical injuries and recognizes the frequent clinical situation that the neurologic deficits in complete cervical injuries may extend for more than one cervical cord segment.

The grade B patient in the ISCSCI-92 system has only sensory preservation below the level of injury, as in the Frankel grade B patient and Sunnybrook grade 2 patient. The ISCSCI-92 system adopts the more precise definitions for grades C and D of the Sunnybrook system based on MRC levels of muscle strength. Inherent in the ISCSCI-92 system is the concept of quantitation of motor and sensory function to achieve motor and sensory scores (Fig. 13.6). The motor score is obtained by testing the strength of 10 key muscle groups—5 in the upper extremities and 5 in the lower extremities—based on the MRC grading system as defined previously, with normal strength graded as 5 and complete paralysis graded as 0. The maximum normal motor score obtained by summing both sides of the body is 100. The sensory score is calculated on the basis of pinprick and light touch in 28 dermatomes on each side of the body. Each modality in each dermatome is scored out of 2 with normal sensation scored as 2 and absent sensation scored as 0, and thus the normal sensory score is 112 for pinprick and 112 for light touch. This system has been the most frequently used for clinical trials in acute SCI (22).

The ISCSCI-92 classification also provides more precise definitions of the neurologic level, sensory level, skeletal level, and zone of partial preservation (Fig. 13.6). The neurologic level is defined as the most caudal segment of the spinal cord, with normal sensory and motor function on both sides of the body. Because the level of normal segments may differ on the two sides of the cord after injury, and may also differ in terms of the presence of preserved motor and sensory function, there may be up to four different segments identified in determining the neurologic

---

TABLE 13.5. *International Standards for Neurological and Functional Classification of Spinal Cord (ISCSCI-92) (ASIA/IMSOP)*

Grade A	Complete Injury	No motor or sensory function is preserved in the sacral segments S4-5.
Grade B	Incomplete Injury	Sensory but not motor function is preserved below the neurological level and extends through the sacral segments S4-5.
Grade C	Incomplete Injury	Motor function is preserved below the neurological level, and the majority of key muscles below the neurological level have a muscle grade less than 3 on MRC scale.
Grade D	Incomplete Injury	Motor function is preserved below the neurological level, and the majority of key muscles below the neurological level have a muscle grade 3 or greater on MRC scale.
Grade E	Normal	Motor and sensory function are normal.

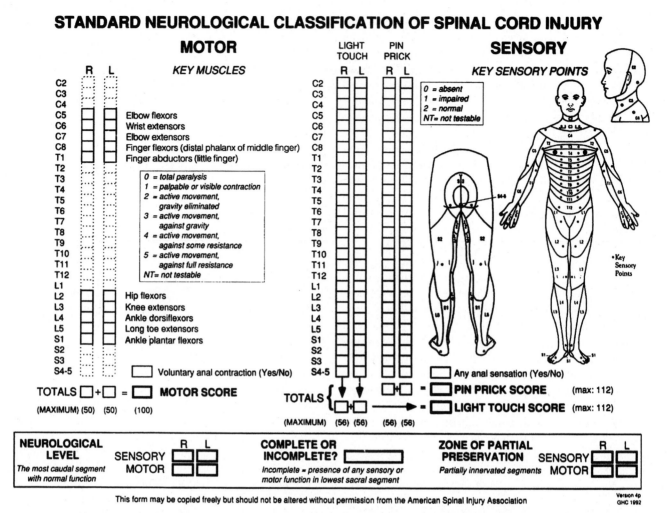

FIG. 13.6. International Standards for Neurological and Functional Classification of Spinal cord Injury (ISCSCI-92). This diagram contains the principal information about motor, sensory, and sphincter function necessary for accurate classification and scoring of acute spinal cord injury. The 10 key muscles to be tested for the motor examination are shown on the **left** along with the Medical Research Council grading system, and the 28 dermatomes to be tested on each side for the sensory examination are shown on the **right**. The system for recording the neurologic levels, the completeness of the injury, and the zone of partial preservation (in complete injuries) are shown at the **bottom**.

level: right sensory, left sensory, right motor, and left motor. These levels are determined by neurologic examination of a key sensory point in each of the 28 right and 28 left dermatomes and of a key muscle in each of the 10 right and 10 left myotomes. A zone of partial preservation may be present in complete injuries and is defined as encompassing those dermatomes and myotomes caudal to the neurologic level that remain partially innervated (Table 13.5 and Fig. 13.6). The vertebral level of an injury is defined as the level of greatest vertebral damage on radiologic examination. It is clear that the vertebral level and the neurologic levels may be similar or may differ by one or more segments.

As noted earlier, the NASCIS trials in which the ISCSCI-92 methods or modifications thereof were employed have aroused considerable controversy about the results

(31). The major concerns relate to the way the results were analyzed and reported. Instead of clearly stating the exact percentage increase in motor or sensory scores for groups of patients, other outcome parameters were emphasized, such as the percentage increase in the potential recovery in an attempt to deal with the differing baseline neurologic status of patients in the trial. Although such manipulations provide a method for evaluating the opportunities for recovery from injuries at different levels and of varying severity, the complex computations and statistical tests were not easily understood by many practitioners. Another concern was that the raw data were not made readily available for others to analyze. To prevent such confusion and uncertainty, reports of clinical trials must contain all the raw and derived data for each outcome measure of neurologic recovery.

TABLE 13.6. *Modified Benzel Classification*

Grade	Description	Comparable ISCSCI-92 grade
I	Complete—No motor or sensory function is preserved in the sacral segments S4-5	A
II	Sensory preservation—Sensory but no motor function is preserved in the sacral segments S4-5	B
III	Motor function is preserved below the neurological level, and the majority of key muscles below the neurological level have muscle grades <3/5. Unable to walk	C
IV	Some functional motor control below the level of injury that is significantly useful (i.e. assist in transfers, etc.). Unable to walk independently	D
V	Motor function allows walking with or without assistance, but significant problems secondary to lack of endurance or fear of falling limit patient mobility. Limited walking	D
VI	Independent ambulation >25 feet but may have difficulties with micturition and/or dyscoordination	D
VII	Neurologically intact with the exception of minimal deficits that cause no functional difficulties	E

Benzel System

The Benzel system was described in 1986 originally for thoracic and lumbar injuries (33) but has also been used in studies of injuries at cervical levels (34). The two GM-1 ganglioside trials organized by Geisler and colleagues used a "modified Benzel classification" that comprises seven grades of function (35,36) (Table 13.6). The first three grades are virtually the same as the ISCSCI-92 system, but grade D of the latter is expanded into three different levels of function based on varying degrees of ability to ambulate. The investigators in this trial emphasized the improved precision of this expanded scale for detecting degrees of recovery that would be considered functionally important by patients with neurologic deficits from SCI. However, with its emphasis on ambulatory function, this classification has the major disadvantage that it cannot be used for the initial pretreatment assessment of neurologic function. Similar to the Frankel system, the data can be displayed in cross-tabulation form, with the five baseline ISCSCI-92 scores on the vertical axis and the seven Benzel scores on follow-up on the horizontal axis. Significant recovery was defined as a two-grade change. For routine use in managing patients with SCI, this system offers no advantages, although there may be some merit for specific study trials.

Other Systems

The Japanese Orthopaedic Association (JOA) has developed several systems for classifying neurologic function in various spinal conditions, although these systems have been applied mainly to nontraumatic myelopathy, especially cervical spondylotic myelopathy. The major advantage of the JOA systems is their usefulness for quantifying overall functional change in SCI patients, including assessment of bladder function. Lucas and Ducker (37) and Bracken and colleagues (38) also devised earlier systems for grading and quantifying acute SCI that have been superseded by subsequent systems.

PITFALLS AND SHORTCOMINGS OF NEUROLOGIC CLASSIFICATION, SCORING, AND ANALYSIS OF NEUROLOGIC RECOVERY

Inaccurate Initial Examination, Including Missed Diagnosis

The diagnosis of SCI may be missed because of an inadequate or incomplete history or physical examination or because multiple factors may obscure the diagnosis (Table 13.7). An example is the inebriated victim of a car crash who was not wearing a seat belt and who sustained a head injury as well as an SCI. The combination of the accompanying head injury and inebriation make it extremely difficult to examine the patient. Also, the presence of multiple trauma may divert the examiner's attention toward more obvious but often less important injuries such as limb fractures. Other difficult situations include patients who are psychologically upset by the injury or who are hypoxic and become restless, uncooperative, or agitated. In all these instances, the practitioner's diagnostic acumen is severely

TABLE 13.7. *Pitfalls and Shortcomings in Neurological Classification and Scoring and Analysis of Neurological Recovery*

1. Inaccurate Initial Examination Including Missed Diagnosis
   (a) Uncooperative Patient
      -Inebriation
      -Cognitive impairment from head injury
      -Mentally challenged
   (b) Hysteria
   (c) Malingering
   (d) Inexperienced Observer
2. Shock-Spinal and Systemic
3. Ceiling Effect
4. Inadequate Follow-up
   (a) Early death
   (b) Travellers
5. Poor Inter-Rater Reliability

taxed. Indeed, the patient's reactions may be so bizarre that the diagnosis of hysteria may be mistakenly made. This diagnosis is extremely dangerous in situations involving trauma. Thus, in the presence of alcohol, multiple trauma, head injury, or bizarre behavior, one must make the "safe assumption" that there is an accompanying spinal injury. With major trauma to the abdomen or chest, one should always suspect that the trauma was sufficient to dislocate the spine.

Spinal Shock and Systemic Shock

Spinal shock is a type of neurogenic shock that occurs in major SCI and can be a source of considerable confusion. Spinal shock implies the loss of somatic motor, sensory, and sympathetic autonomic function due to SCI (39). The more severe the spinal cord injury, and the higher the level of injury, the greater the severity and duration of spinal shock. Thus, spinal shock is most severe in complete, upper cervical cord injuries. The somatic motor component of spinal shock consists of paralysis, flaccidity, and areflexia with respect to deep tendon reflexes and cutaneous reflexes, and the sensory component is anesthesia to all modalities. The autonomic component is systemic hypotension, skin hyperemia and warmth, and bradycardia due to loss of sympathetic function but persisting parasympathetic function (unopposed vagotonia). The exact mechanism of spinal shock is unknown but may be due to temporary, local effects on impulse conduction in the traumatized cord caused by electrolyte or neurotransmitter changes. Thus, hypotension, bradycardia, and warm extremities are manifestations of spinal shock that frequently accompanies major cervical SCI. In contrast, systemic shock usually causes hypotension, tachycardia, and cold extremities. Systemic shock can also occur in SCI, if there is an accompanying injury, such as a ruptured spleen. Thus, in the first few hours and days after SCI, difficulties can arise because there is often a combination of the physiologic, temporary effects of spinal shock and the pathologic, more permanent effects of the SCI, as well as the overall effects of systemic shock.

Another problem is the variable duration of spinal shock. I recommend the following guidelines: (a) the somatic motor and sensory components of spinal shock last only 1 hour or less and thus have terminated by the time most patients are examined in the first hospital reached, which in most countries is now within 1 to 4 hours of injury; (b) the reflex and autonomic components of spinal shock may last days to months, depending on the level and severity of SCI. In practical terms, these guidelines mean that the motor and sensory deficits detected 1 hour or later after SCI are due to physical cord injury rather than to spinal shock. This is certainly a safe course to follow because it eliminates the possible error of missing a serious SCI because the observed deficits were incorrectly attributed to spinal shock.

Ceiling Effect

Most systems for grading neurologic function after SCI have the major shortcoming of being unable to record neurologic improvement or deterioration of insufficient magnitude to produce a change in grade. This limitation is termed the *ceiling effect* and is especially a problem with grade D patients in both the Frankel and ISCSCI-92 systems who have sufficient strength to allow ambulation. For these patients to improve to grade E, they would have to recover fully and achieve a completely normal neurologic examination, which is very rare. Other classifications, such as the Benzel and Sunnybrook systems, provide a larger number of categories (Benzel, 7; Sunnybrook, 10), especially for incomplete injuries, and theoretically would be less subject to the ceiling effect. However, these systems have been used much less often, and there is no definite proof that they would be superior to the ISCSCI-92 system for avoiding the ceiling effect.

Inadequate Follow-up

Unfortunately, many patients are lost to follow-up before an adequate posttrauma interval has elapsed. Neurologic recovery is usually very slow, especially after major SCI, and thus most clinical trials have required at least a 6 months' period of observation before calculating the final neurologic recovery. However, even this interval is too brief for most patients, who continue to recover for at least 12 months. Indeed, it is not uncommon for recovery to continue for 3 to 4 years after major SCI, although most of the recovery occurs within the first 6 to 12 months. There are numerous reasons for incomplete follow-up, including early mortality, incarceration, travel, and residence in another country.

Poor Interrater Reliability

Although the ISCSCI-92 system is the best of the currently available systems, it is recognized the there are still significant shortcomings. Indeed, interrater reliability of some aspects of the system has been shown to be poor (40). There is an ongoing specialist committee in charge of updating and revising the ISCSCI-92 system.

GRADING OF FUNCTIONAL RECOVERY IN THE REHABILITATION AND FOLLOW-UP PHASES AFTER ACUTE SPINAL CORD INJURY

There has been a recent emphasis on determining the effect of SCI and therapy on the overall function of the patient. Initially, attempts were made to use nonspecific functional outcome measures such as the Functional Independence Measure (FIM) that had been developed for other neurologic disorders (41). For example, in the recently completed NASCIS 3 clinical trial of methylprednisolone versus tirilazad, FIM was one of the outcome measures

(30), and in the second GM-1 ganglioside study, recovery of bowel and bladder function was included as an outcome measure (40). Recently, a more specific functional outcome measure of spinal cord function, the Spinal Cord Independence Measure, was developed and tested in patients with spinal cord lesions including SCI (41,42). This measure includes self-care, respiratory and sphincter management, and mobility. The preliminary results were promising, but this measure has not been tested in a large randomized prospective control trial in SCI.

REFERENCES

1. Michaelis L, Braakman R. Current terminology and classification of injuries of spine and spinal cord. In: Vinkin P, Bruyn G, eds. *Handbook of clinical neurology*. Amsterdam: North-Holland, 1976:145–153.
2. American Spinal Injury Association. *Standards for neurological and functional classification of spinal cord injury*, revised ed. Chicago: American Spinal Injury Association, 1992.
3. Hansebout R. Comprehensive review of methods of improving cord recovery after acute spinal cord injury. In: Tator C, ed. *Early management of acute spinal cord injury*. New York: Raven, 1982:181–196.
4. Tator C. Classification of spinal cord injury based on neurological presentation. In Narayan RK, Wilberger JE Jr, Povlishock J, eds. *Neurotrauma*. New York: McGraw-Hill, 1996:1059–1073.
5. Tator CH. Spine-spinal cord relationships in spinal cord trauma. *Clin Neurosurg* 1983;30:479–494.
6. Schneider RC, Thompson JM. The syndrome of the acute central cervical spinal cord injury. *J Neurol Psychiatry Neurosurg* 1958;21:216–227.
7. Schneider RC. Concomitant craniocerebral and spinal trauma, with special reference to the cervicomedullary region. *Clin Neurosurg* 1970;17:266–309.
8. Dickman CA, et al. Cruciate paralysis: a clinical and radiographic analysis of injuries to the cervicomedullary junction. *J Neurosurg* 1990;73(6):850–858.
9. Schneider R, Cherry G, Pantek H. The syndrome of acute central cervical spinal cord injury. J Neurosurg 1954;11:546–577.
10. Tator C. Clinical manifestations of acute spinal cord injury. In: Tator C, Benzel E, eds. Contemporary management of spinal cord injury: from impact to rehabilitation. Park Ridge, IL: American Association of Neurological Surgeons, 2000:21–32.
11. Levi AD, Tator CH, Bunge RP. Clinical syndromes associated with disproportionate weakness of the upper versus the lower extremities after cervical spinal cord injury. *Neurosurgery* 1996;38(1):179–183; discussion, 183–185.
12. Quencer RM, et al. Acute traumatic central cord syndrome: MRI-pathological correlations. *Neuroradiology* 1992;34(2):85–94.
13. Schneider RC. A syndrome in acute cervical spine injuries for which early operation is indicated. *J Neurosurg* 1951;8:360–367.
14. Pang D, Wilberger JE Jr. Spinal cord injuries without radiographic abnormalities in children. *J Neurosurg* 1982;57:114–129.
15. Tator CH. Spinal cord syndromes with physiological and anatomic correlations. In: Menezes AH, Sonntag VKH, eds. *Principles of spinal surgery*. New York: McGraw-Hill, 1996:2847–2859.
16. Saruhashi Y, et al. Clinical outcomes of cervical spinal cord injuries without radiographic evidence of trauma. *Spinal Cord* 1998;36(8):567–573.
17. Wilberger JE, Maroon JC. Occult posttraumatic cervical ligamentous instability. *J Spinal Disord* 1990;3(2):156–161.
18. Biemond A. Contusio cervicalis posterior. *Med T Geneesk* 1964;108:1333.
19. Braakman R, Penning L. Injuries of the cervical spine. In: Vinken PJ, Bruyn GW, eds. *Handbook of clinical neurology,* Vol 25. Amsterdam: North-Holland, 1976:227–380.
20. Torg JS, et al. Neurapraxia of the cervical spinal cord with transient quadriplegia. *J Bone Joint Surg Am* 1986;68(9):1354–1370.
21. Keith WS. Traumatic infarction of the spinal cord. *Can J Neurol Sci* 1974;1(2):124–126.
22. Tator C, Fehlings M. Clinical trials in spinal cord injury. In: Biller J, Bogousslavsky J, eds. *Clinical trials in neurologic practice: blue books of practical neurology*. Boston: Butterworth-Heinemann, 2001:99–120.
23. Frankel HL, et al. The value of postural reduction in the initial management of closed injuries of the spine with paraplegia and tetraplegia. I. *Paraplegia* 1969;7(3):179–192.
24. Tator CH, et al. Comparison of surgical and conservative management in 208 patients with acute spinal cord injury. *Can J Neurol Sci* 1987;14(1):60–69.
25. Stover SL, DeLisa JA, Whiteneck GG. *Spinal cord injury. Clinical outcomes from the model systems.* Gaithersburg, MD: Aspen, 1995.
26. Tator CH. Biology of neurological recovery and functional restoration after spinal cord injury. *Neurosurgery* 1998;42(4):696–707; discussion, 707–708.
27. Tator CH, Rowed DW, Schwartz ML. Sunnybrook cord injury scales for assessing neurological injury and recovery. In: Tator CH, ed. *Early management of acute spinal cord injury*. New York: Raven, 1982:7–24.
28. Pitts LH, et al. Treatment with thyrotropin-releasing hormone (TRH) in patients with traumatic spinal cord injuries. *J Neurotrauma* 1995;12(3):235–243.
29. Bracken MB, et al. A randomized, controlled trial of methylprednisolone or naloxone in the treatment of acute spinal-cord injury. Results of the Second National Acute Spinal Cord Injury Study. *N Engl J Med* 1990;322(20):1405–1411.
30. Bracken MB, et al. Methylprednisolone or tirilazad mesylate administration after acute spinal cord injury: 1-year follow up. Results of the third National Acute Spinal Cord Injury randomized controlled trial. *J Neurosurg* 1998;89(5):699–706.
31. Hurlbert RJ. Methylprednisolone for acute spinal cord injury: an inappropriate standard of care. *J Neurosurg* 2000;93[1 Suppl]:1–7.
32. Waters RL, Adkins RH, Yakura JS. Definition of complete spinal cord injury. *Paraplegia* 1991;29(9):573–581.
33. Benzel EC, Larson SJ. Functional recovery after decompressive operation for thoracic and lumbar spine fractures. *Neurosurgery* 1986;19(5):772–778.
34. Benzel EC, Larson SJ. Functional recovery after decompressive spine operation for cervical spine fractures. *Neurosurgery* 1987;20(5):742–746.
35. Geisler FH, Dorsey FC, Coleman WP. Recovery of motor function after spinal-cord injury—a randomized, placebo-controlled trial with GM-1 ganglioside. *N Engl J Med* 1991;324(26):1829–1838.
36. Geisler FH, et al. Measurements and recovery patterns in a multicenter study of acute spinal cord injury. *Spine* 2001;26[24 Suppl]:S68–86.
37. Kiss Z, Tator C. Neurogenic shock. In: Geller ER, ed. *Shock and resuscitation*. New York: McGraw-Hill, 1993:421–440.
38. Jonsson M, et al. Inter-rater reliability of the 1992 international standards for neurological and functional classification of incomplete spinal cord injury. *Spinal Cord* 2000;38(11):675–679.
39. Keith RA, et al. The functional independence measure: a new tool for rehabilitation. *Adv Clin Rehabil* 1987;1:6–18.
40. Geisler FH, et al. The sygen(r) multicenter acute spinal cord injury study. *Spine* 2001;26[24 Suppl]:S87–98.
41. Catz A, et al. The Catz-Itzkovich SCIM: a revised version of the Spinal Cord Independence Measure. *Disabil Rehabil* 2001;23(6):263–268.
42. Catz A, et al. The spinal cord independence measure (SCIM): sensitivity to functional changes in subgroups of spinal cord lesion patients. *Spinal Cord* 2001;39(2):97–100.

CHAPTER 14

Cervical Radiculopathy: Diagnosis and Differential Diagnosis

Michael P. Steinmetz, William McCormick, and Edward C. Benzel

The earliest descriptions of spinal nerve root compression can be traced to early Egyptian medical writings dating around 3000 BC (1). Mixter and Barr first reported lumbar nerve root compression in 1934 (2). Semmes and Murphey are credited as the first to describe cervical disc disease and cervical radiculopathy, which they published in 1943 (3).

RELEVANT ANATOMY

There are eight pairs of cervical nerves. The nerves exit the spinal cord and enter their respective foramina in a relatively horizontal orientation (4). In the cervical spine, the nerves exit above their numbered vertebral body. For example, the C5 exits at the C4-C5 neuroforamina. A transition occurs at the cervicothoracic junction. At the C8-T1 neuroforamina, the C8 nerve exits. At T1-T2, the T1 nerve exits, and all nerve roots below this level exit caudal to their respective numerical vertebrae.

The cervical nerve root may be compressed from a variety of pathologic conditions. From degenerative disease perspective, osteophytes adjacent to the end plates or soft disc protrusion or bulge may compress the nerve at the medial foramen. Within the foramen, the nerve may be compressed by osteophytes adjacent to the uncovertebral or facet joints or lateral disc herniations.

HISTORY AND PHYSICAL EXAMINATION

Patients often complain of intense, stabbing, or burning pain. The pain often corresponds to a specific dermatome; the patient may be able to localize the pain accurately. Valsalva maneuvers such as coughing may exacerbate the pain. Concomitant paresthesias may precede the occurrence of pain. The paresthesias tend to present more distally, whereas the pain is often more proximal in location and at times more diffuse and less localizing. Weakness may also be evident to the patient, and if long standing, there may be muscle atrophy. In almost all cases, posterior neck pain in present (1).

Careful attention to the location of pain and paresthesias may aid in the localization of the compressive lesion. Yoss and colleagues (5) reported that in a C5 radiculopathy, pain did not occur distal to the elbow, and paresthesias were absent from the hand. With a C6 compression, pain was localized in the radial forearm, and the thumb was paresthetic. In a C7 compression, pain was diffuse in the volar and dorsal forearm, and the middle finger was paresthetic. With C8 involvement, pain was in the ulnar forearm, and paresthesias were localized to the little and ring fingers.

When taking the patient's history, one should make note of shoulder pain with movement, shortness of breath or chest pain, and hand pain or paresthesias, which wake the patient at night. A history of trauma, prior cervical surgery, fevers, night sweats, or cancer should be noted. Problems with gait or bowel and bladder incontinence make the diagnosis of myelopathy more likely.

The physical examination should incorporate motor, sensory, reflex, and gait testing. Shoulder abduction, external rotation, elbow flexion-extension, forearm pronation, wrist extension, grip, and finger abduction should be tested. Sensation to light touch and pinprick should be checked in all upper extremity dermatomes and also in the major lower extremity dermatomes. The biceps, triceps, brachioradialis, and pectoral reflexes should be examined. Lower extremity reflexes should also be tested. Signs of upper motor neuron injury should be sought, including Hoffman sign and the Babinski response. The patient's gait should be assessed; this may be done as the patient enters the examination room. The cervical range of motion should be evaluated, and provocative tests, such as Spurling sign, may be used.

TABLE 14.1. *The Practical Physical Examination Findings in Cervical Radiculopathy*

	Level involved			
	C4-5	C5-6	C6-7	C7-T1
Root involved	5	6	7	8
Weakness	Shoulder abduction external rotation	Elbow flexion, forearm pronation	Elbow extension	Hand intrinsics
Sensory loss	Lateral shoulder	Radial arm, thumb	Volar and dorsal arm, middle finger	Ulnar arm, little and ring finger
Reflex involved	Pectoral	Biceps, brachioradialis	Triceps	No reflex

Yoss et al (5) series demonstrated that C5 compression leads to weakness in the supraspinatus and infraspinatus, deltoid, biceps, and rhomboid muscles. Findings may include weakness of shoulder abduction, external rotation, or pronation of the arm. C6 involvement affected the biceps and brachioradialis, leading to weakness in elbow flexion and arm pronation. A C7 lesion leads to weakness in elbow extension and also wrist and finger extension. Depression of reflexes was less specific in Yoss et al series (5). Although reflexes were found to be less specific, it is generally accepted that with a C5 radiculopathy, there is a diminished or absent pectoral reflex. The reflexes affected for C6 are the biceps and brachioradialis, and for C7, the triceps. Refer to Table 14.1 for a comprehensive review of the signs and symptoms of cervical radiculopathy.

IMAGING

The diagnosis of cervical radiculopathy and the level involved may be gleaned from the history and physical examination. Imaging should be used for confirmation of the clinical findings. Plain radiographs should be obtained first but may contribute little to the diagnosis of cervical radiculopathy. The prevalence of cervical spondylosis is 96% to 100% by age 70 years (6). Therefore, most cervical radiographs show some amount of spondylosis. Despite the limitations, cervical radiographs are able to provide valuable information regarding the presence of deformity, instability, congenital anomalies, infection, and neoplasia (7).

Myelography, computed tomography (CT) myelography, and magnetic resonance imaging (MRI) are all valuable in the diagnosis of cervical radiculopathy. Myelography and CT myelography are invasive and carry some, albeit small, risk to the patient, whereas MRI is noninvasive. Myelography is considered the least sensitive and specific examination after plain radiographs (8). The choice between CT myelography and MRI remains controversial. In a very early comparison, using intraoperative findings as the standard, myelography was accurate in 67% of the cases, and CT myelography was accurate in 85%, whereas MRI was accurate in 74% (9). A later similar retrospective study found MRI to be more accurate than CT myelography (88% versus 81%) (10). These older studies suggest that MRI is comparable to CT myelography, but with MRI, it may be difficult to differentiate among extradural lesions, such as disc, osteophyte, or a combination. Ruggieri (8) has pointed out that these studies are based on outdated technology and that no comparison studies have been performed with new MRI technology. Newer MRI coil technology and sequencing techniques, such as gradient echo and three-dimensional volume acquisition, have eliminated problems with extradural lesion identification and have probably made MRI the modality of choice.

In certain instances, the imaging may be equivocal. Electromyography and nerve conduction studies may be helpful in these circumstances. These tests become more important for evaluating other pathology such as nerve entrapment and neuropathy.

DIFFERENTIAL DIAGNOSIS

The differential diagnosis of radiculopathy is broad, and at times, it may be difficult to differentiate other pathology from cervical radiculopathy. Various categories of the differential diagnosis include conditions of instability, primary or secondary neurogenic conditions (both intrinsic and extrinsic), visceral or vascular problems, primary or secondary osseous pathologies, and psychogenic and sociogenic conditions.

Instability or Malalignment

Instability or loss or normal alignment may produce neck and arm pain. The etiology is often trauma, but other pathologies such as tumor or infection may lead to malalignment. The diagnosis is usually obvious from the radiographs and MRI.

Neurogenic Disease

The list of intrinsic neurogenic conditions is large, including demyelinating conditions such as multiple sclerosis, inflammatory diseases, and neoplastic nerve conditions. Specific peripheral neuropathies also are in this category.

These include amyloidosis, hypothyroidism, and rheumatoid arthritis. Idiopathic brachial plexitis is also a consideration. Extrinsic neurogenic conditions include the entrapment neuropathies, such as carpal tunnel syndrome, entrapment of the ulnar nerve at Guyon canal or the cubital tunnel, and thoracic outlet syndrome. Electromyography and nerve conduction velocity studies are most helpful in distinguishing these entities from cervical radiculopathy.

Carcinomas such as schwannoma and neurofibroma may present with radiculopathy. Tumors of the lung, such as Pancoast tumors, may also present with radiculopathy or painless weakness and atrophy of the hypothenar muscles.

Motor neuron disease or anterior lateral sclerosis may be difficult to distinguish from cervical radiculopathy in the early stage. Patients with motor neuron disease have normal sensation, and there are often abnormalities in other extremities or the facial musculature. Tongue fasciculations suggest involvement of the bulbar musculature.

Visceral and Vascular Disease

Pathology in adjacent organs in the region of the neck may cause neck pain or referred pain in the arm (4). An example is carcinoma of the esophagus. Cerebral vascular insufficiency from carotid or vertebral artery blockage by aneurysm or arterial venous malformation may produce neck pain or radiculopathy (11). Cerebral vascular disease (12,13) and cardiac ischemia may also present with radicular symptoms.

Primary or Secondary Osseous or Ligamentous Pathology

Shoulder pathology should be high on the differential diagnosis list. This may be due to rotator cuff injuries or bursitis. There is usually pain on passive range of motion of the shoulder. Primary or metastatic tumor of the spine may cause symptoms from bone disruption or cervical instability or malalignment. There may also be direct compression of the neural elements. Metabolic, inflammatory, and infectious conditions of the spine may also present with cervical pain and radiculopathy. Such conditions include hyperparathyroidism, rickets, and rheumatoid arthritis (4). Laboratory tests may aid in the diagnosis, such as increased erythrocyte sedimentation rate, increased serum calcium, increased serum alkaline phosphatase, or positive serum rheumatoid factor.

Psychogenic and Sociogenic Conditions

Depression may present with cervical radiculopathy. Radiographic, laboratory, and physical examination workup is usually negative. The patient may have a depressed affect, and there are often trigger points of pain. This is usually a diagnosis of exclusion. Also, if the workup is negative, a consideration of malingering due to compensation from personal injury litigation and work-related disability should be considered. This is again a diagnosis of exclusion.

CONCLUSION

The diagnosis of cervical radiculopathy is often straightforward. The diagnosis is typically made from the history and physical examination. Imaging should be performed to confirm the diagnosis. If the confirmatory examination is equivocal, the diagnosis of cervical radiculopathy is called into question. In these circumstances, ancillary tests may be performed to either include or exclude pathologies from the broad list of differential conditions.

REFERENCES

1. Sweeney PJ. Clinical evaluation of cervical radiculopathy and myelopathy. *Neuroimaging Clin N Am* 1995;5:321–327.
2. Mixter WJ, Barr JS. Rupture of the intervertebral disc with involvement of the spinal canal. *N Engl J Med* 1934;211:210.
3. Semmes RE, Murphey F. Syndrome of unilateral rupture of the sixth cervical intervertebral disc, with compression of the seventh cervical nerve root. *JAMA* 1943;121:1209.
4. Sachs BL. Differential diagnosis of neck pain, arm pain, and myelopathy. In: The Cervical Spine Research Society, ed. *The cervical spine*. Philadelphia: Lippincott-Raven, 1998:741–751.
5. Yoss RE, Corbin KB, MacCarty CS, et al. Significance of symptoms and signs in localization of involved root in cervical disk protrusion. *Neurology* 1960;60:673.
6. Irvine DH, Forster JB, Newell DJ, et al. Prevalence of cervical spondylosis in a general practice. *Lancet* 1965;1:1089–1091.
7. Ahlgren BD, Garfin SR. Cervical radiculopathy. *Orthop Clin North Am* 1996;27:253–263.
8. Ruggieri PM. Cervical radiculopathy. *Neuroimaging Clin N Am* 1995;5:349–366.
9. Modic MT, Masaryk TJ, Mulopulos GP, et al. Cervical radiculopathy: Prospective evaluation with surface coil MR imaging. CT with metrizamide, and metrizamide myelography. *Radiology* 1986;161:753–759.
10. Brown BM, Schwartz RH, Frank E, et al. Preoperative evaluation of cervical radiculopathy and myelopathy by surface-coil MR imaging. *Am J Neuroradiol* 1988;9:859–866.
11. Booth R, Rothman R. Cervical angina. *Spine* 1976;1:28.
12. Blennow G. Anterior spinal artery syndrome. *Pediatr Neurosci* 1987;13:32–37.
13. Foo D, Rossier A. Anterior spinal artery syndrome and its natural history. *Paraplegia* 1983;21:1–10.

CHAPTER 15

Myelopathy: Diagnosis and Differential Diagnosis

Samir Lapsiwala and Gregory Trost

The word *myelopathy* comes from two Greek words: *myelos* meaning "spinal cord" and *pathos* meaning "disorder of." A number of disease processes can disrupt the intrinsic function of the spinal cord, and many of these pathologies are treatable; it is therefore essential to find out the cause of myelopathy. Because spinal cord biopsy is rarely indicated and many cases of myelopathy are inflammatory in nature, proper diagnosis and management rely on the patient's history, physical examination, imaging, and cerebrospinal fluid (CSF) findings. Furthermore, in many noninfectious causes of myelopathy, early high-dose corticosteroids may alter the course of the disease, making expeditious patient evaluation imperative. The variety of imaging modalities useful in diagnosing myelopathy as well as in determining the differential diagnosis of myelopathy are discussed in this chapter.

CLINICAL PRESENTATION

Cervical myelopathy is common in elderly people. Cervical myelopathy has no pathognomonic sign or symptoms, and in its early course, it often has subtle and abstract symptoms.

In 1966, Crandall and Batzdorf (1) classified patients with cervical spondylotic myelopathy into five groups, based on dominant spinal cord syndromes: (a) a syndrome due to transverse lesion; (b) a syndrome due to motor systems lesion; (c) central cord syndrome; (d) Brown-Séquard syndrome; and (e) brachialgia and cord syndromes. In transverse lesions, a complete loss of motor, sensory, and sphincter control is observed below the level of injury. The central cord syndrome, typically as a result of a hyperextension injury, is the most prevalent of the partial cord syndromes. It is characterized by bilateral motor paresis, with upper extremities affected to a greater degree than lower extremities, and with distal muscle groups affected to a greater degree than proximal muscle groups. Sensory impairment and bladder dysfunction are variable (2). In central cord syndrome, injury is typically from an inwardly bulging ligamentum flavum affecting the central gray matter and the central portions of the corticospinal and spinothalamic tracts. The prognosis for patients with the central cord syndrome is quite variable, depending on the degree of injury. Of patients younger than 50 years of age, more than 80% regain bladder continence, and about 90% return to ambulatory status. Of those older than 50 years of age, only 30% regain bladder function, with about 50% regaining ambulation (3).

Brown-Séquard syndrome, first described in 1846, results from an anatomic or functional hemisection of the spinal cord. The syndrome in its pure form is characterized by ipsilateral loss of motor function and proprioception-vibration, with contralateral loss of pain and temperature sensation below the spinal cord level of injury. Because fibers associated with the lateral spinothalamic tract ascend or descend one to two cord segments before crossing to the contralateral side, ipsilateral pain and temperature loss may be noted one or two segments above the lesion. Brown-Séquard syndrome has the best prognosis of any of the incomplete spinal cord syndromes, with 80% to 90% of patients regaining bowel and bladder function, 75% regaining ambulatory status, and 70% becoming independent in their activities of daily living (3).

The anterior cord syndrome is characterized by loss of motor function, pain, and crude touch below the level of the lesion, with preservation of posterior column function, including touch, position, and vibratory sensation. The anterior spinal syndrome is most commonly reported after aortic surgery; it has been also reported after severe hypotension, infection, myocardial infarction, and aortic angiography, and from a cervical hyperflexion injury resulting in a spinal cord contusion (4). Functional recovery is variable, with most improvement made in the first 24 hours, but little improvement thereafter. Overall, about 10% to 20% of patients with this syndrome regain some muscle function; however, they have little strength or coordination (3).

In 1985, Fergusson and Caplan (5) defined clinical syndromes in four categories on the basis of neurologic deficits due to cervical spondylosis: (a) lateral or radicular syndrome, (b) medial or spinal syndrome, (c) combined medial-lateral syndromes, and (d) vascular syndromes. The lateral syndrome is due to nerve root pathology, most commonly a result of compression. Clinical signs and symptoms of spinal cord compression are absent. The medial syndrome is a manifestation of a spinal cord abnormality. It has variable clinical signs that depend on the anatomic location of the pathologic factor and on the severity of its effect on the spinal cord. Combined syndromes have evidence of both nerve root and spinal cord involvement. The vascular syndrome is described as a sudden painless myelopathy, frequently in the absence of trauma, that is usually associated with unimpressive imaging studies.

Generally, cervical myelopathy presents with a subtle gait disturbance, followed by upper extremity involvement (6). Myelopathic gait may appear broad based, spastic, and with loss of smooth rhythmic motion. Sudarsky and Ronthal reported that cervical myelopathy was the most common cause of a gait disorder, accounting for 16% of elderly patients with undiagnosed gait disorders (7). Bowel and bladder dysfunction may occur in cervical myelopathy and are manifestations of upper motor neuron disease. The rate of bowel and bladder dysfunction in patients with previously diagnosed myelopathies is reported to be between 15% and 20% each (8). In the series by Lundsford and colleagues, sphincter disturbance was observed in 49% of patients (6). Autonomic dysfunction, such as dysreflexia and hypotension, are not very common in cervical myelopathy.

PHYSICAL EXAMINATION

The physical findings in cervical myelopathy may vary greatly from patient to patient, depending on factors such as the level of and extent of compression, duration of compression, span of segments compressed, and aggravating factors. On motor examination, both upper and lower motor neuron disturbances are observed. Generally, the lower motor neuron is involved at the level of the clinically ex-

pressed lesion, such as a site of stenosis or syrinx. Upper motor neuron involvement is observed below the site of the lesion. Therefore, in cervical myelopathy, the lower extremities express the upper motor neuron lesion, whereas the upper extremities may express both, depending on the level and nature of compression.

In cervical myelopathy, the sensory examination generally demonstrates involvement of both upper and lower extremities. There is variability in presentation. A patient may experience loss of pain and temperature, proprioception, and vibration sense below the level of the lesion. However, touch sensation is usually preserved. Involvement of a posterior column produces ipsilateral position and vibratory sense disturbance, whereas spinothalamic tract involvement produces a contralateral pain and temperature disturbance at several levels below the site of compression. If nerve roots are involved, radicular symptoms, such as numbness and tingling, are experienced in the appropriate dermatomal distribution.

Paralleling the motor examination, reflexes are generally hyperreflexic below the level of the lesion and hyporeflexic at the level of lesion. In cervical myelopathy, involvement of the upper motor neuron is also characterized by the presence of pathologic reflexes, such as the Babinski reflex in the lower extremity and the Hoffman reflex in the upper extremity. In addition, clonus may be present in the lower extremities. Lhermitte sign (a generalized electric shock sensation associated with neck flexion or extension), a classic sign of cervical myelopathy, may be present.

In the series by Lundsford and colleagues of 32 patients with cervical spondylotic myelopathy, 59% of patients had purely myelopathic symptoms, and 41% had combined myelopathic and radicular syndromes (6). Corticospinal tract dysfunction was noted most frequently with motor weakness in 58% of patients. Lower extremity hyperreflexia and the Babinski response were noted in 87% and 54% of cases, respectively, whereas the Hoffman reflex was noted in 13% of cases, and Lhermitte sign was observed in only two patients (6%).

CLASSIFICATION

Nurick devised a classification system for myelopathy based on severity of gait abnormalities (9). His scale involves a grading system of 0 to 5 for progressively worsening myelopathic gait (Table 15.1). The Japanese Orthopaedic Associ-

TABLE 15.1. *Nurick's Classification System for Myelopathy on the Basis of Gait Abnormalities*

Grade	Root signs	Cord involvement	Gait	Employment
0	Yes	No	Normal	Possible
I	Yes	Yes	Normal	Possible
II	Yes	Yes	Mild abnormality	Possible
III	Yes	Yes	Severe abnormality	Impossible
IV	Yes	Yes	Only with assistance	Impossible

TABLE 15.2. *The Japanese Orthopedic Association Scale: An Objective Assessment Scale Quantitating the Severity of the Spondylotic Myelopathy Based on Four Categories: Motor Function of the Upper Extremities and Lower Extremities, Sensory Changes in the Trunk and Extremities, and Bladder Function.*

I. Upper Extremity Function
    0 Impossible to eat with either spoon or chopsticks
    1 Possible to eat with spoon, but not with chopsticks
    2 Possible to eat with chopsticks, but inadequate
    3 Possible to eat with chopsticks, but awkward
    4 Normal
II. Lower Extremity Function
    0 Impossible to walk
    1 Need a cane or aid on flat ground
    2 Need a cane or aid on stairs
    3 Possible to walk without a cane or aid, but slow
    4 Normal
III. Sensory
    A. Upper Extremity
      0 Apparent sensory loss
      1 Minimal sensory loss
      2 Normal
    B. Lower Extremity
      0 Apparent sensory loss
      1 Minimal sensory loss
      2 Normal
    C. Trunk
      0 Apparent sensory loss
      1 Minimal sensory loss
      2 Normal
IV. Bladder Function
    0 Complete retension
    1 Severe disturbance
    2 Mild disturbance
    3 Normal

ation devised an objective assessment scale to quantitate severity of the spondylotic myelopathy (10–12). This scale encompasses four categories: motor function of both the upper and lower extremities, sensory changes in the trunk and extremities, and bladder function (Table 15.2). This scale assesses the more global effects of myelopathy. A score of less than 7 indicates severe myelopathy, a score between 8 and 12 indicates moderate myelopathy, and a score above 13 indicates mild myelopathy.

NATURAL HISTORY

On review of the natural history of cervical myelopathy, Clark and Robinson found no evidence of a patient ever returning to baseline function. In addition, they found that 75% of patients experienced episodic worsening; 20% showed slow, steady progression; and 5% had a rapid onset followed by lengthy disability. Roberts studied 24 patients with cervical myelopathy for up to 6.5 years and found that about one third improved, one third remained the same, and one third deteriorated (13). Motor symptoms tended to be much more progressive and less likely to improve than sensory abnormalities.

DIAGNOSIS

Radiography

The diagnosis of cervical myelopathy or spinal cord compression depends on precise correlation between clinical history, neurologic findings, and accurate radiologic imaging studies. Obtaining plain cervical spine radiographs is an essential first step. This includes anteroposterior, lateral, oblique, and lateral flexion-extension views. As demonstrated in Figure 15.1, radiographs are evaluated with an emphasis on alignment, disc space height, presence or absence of spurring, foraminal encroachment, and the diameter of the spinal canal. Using a target film distance of 72 inches, a measurement of 13 mm is often considered as the lower limit of normal for the sagittal diameter of the cervical spine. Use of the Pavlov ratio, measuring the spinal canal distance from midbody to the spinal laminar line divided by the width of the cervical body at that level, obviates the need for precision of the 72-inch measurement (14). A ratio value of 1.0 or greater is normal, and 0.8 or less is indicative of cervical spine stenosis.

Although roentgenographic abnormalities represent structural changes in the spine, they may not be clinically important. The presence of degenerative changes within the cervical spine has been shown to be age related and equally present in both symptomatic and asymptomatic individuals. Gore and associates studied the incidence and severity of

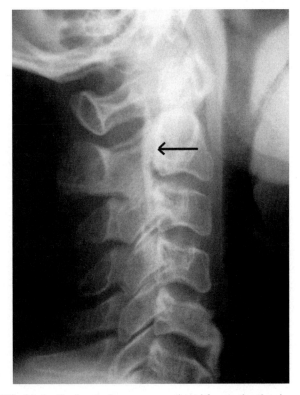

FIG. 15.1. Radiographs are a good tool for evaluating bony anatomy. In this case, an *arrow* identifies calcified posterior longitudinal ligament.

degenerative changes observed on lateral roentgenograms in 200 asymptomatic men and women in five age groups with an age range of 20 to 65 years (15). They found that between ages 60 and 65 years, 95% of the men and 70% of the women had at least one degenerative change on the roentgenogram.

Myelography

Myelography is helpful in the diagnosis of extradural neural compression by visualization of the change in the contour of the contrast-filled thecal sac rather than direct visualization of the compressing structure. The addition of postmyelography computed tomography (CT) greatly enhances the diagnostic capabilities of myelography (Fig. 15.2). It can add considerable anatomic information to the spondylosis workup, especially in visualization of nerve root takeoff. A major advantage of myelography is that it provides visualization of the entire spine up to the foramen magnum. The major disadvantage of myelography is its invasive nature and its lack of specificity. Oil-based contrast agents, such as Pantopaque (ethyl iodophenylundecylate), have been associated with arachnoiditis and a high incidence of adverse reactions. However, since the introduction of nonionic, water-soluble contrast media, a low incidence of adverse effects has been observed. The most common reported adverse effects include headache, nausea, vomiting, and back pain (16).

In one study, 24 of 25 patients with suspected spinal cord compression who underwent iohexol myelography had optimally informative myelogram, and in only one case was the examination semiinformative (17). Similar to plain radiography, myelographic findings must be correlated with clinical findings. Hitselberger and Witten reported a 21%

incidence of cervical spine filling defects in 300 patients undergoing posterior fossa oil-based myelography for suspected acoustic tumors (18). All were asymptomatic for neck or arm pain.

Computed Tomography

Benefits of CT over myelography include direct visualization of the neural structures as well as potential neural compressing structures. Other advantages of CT over myelography include better visualization of lateral pathology such as foraminal stenosis, less invasiveness, ability to perform this test on an outpatient basis, and ability to visualize neural structures below a complete myelographic block. CT myelography is more sensitive than nonintrathecal contrast-enhanced CT and usually yields accurate and specific information on extradural, intradural, and intramedullary lesions. Potential disadvantages of CT include the effects of partial volume averaging and exposure to radiation. CT is better in diagnosing bony abnormalities than magnetic resonance imaging (MRI), but CT does not show neural structures in as great detail as MRI (Figs. 15.3 and 15.4).

Magnetic Resonance Imaging

MRI offers direct imaging in multiple planes, better definition of neural elements, and increased accuracy of evaluation of intrinsic spinal cord disease compared with myelography. MRI is generally considered the procedure of choice in myelopathic patients because neural structures and potential neural compressing structures are visualized in more detail than with CT or CT myelography. In a blinded retrospective review, Brown and coworkers

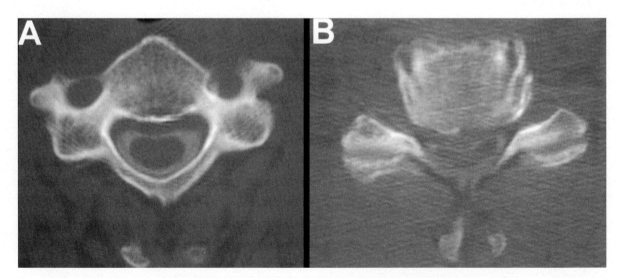

FIG. 15.2. A normal computed tomography (CT) myelogram in which contrast dye is visualized around the spinal cord circumferentially (**A**). Notice how neural structures are still difficult to visualize. CT, however, provides a great deal of information regarding spinal cord size and extra neural compression (**B**).

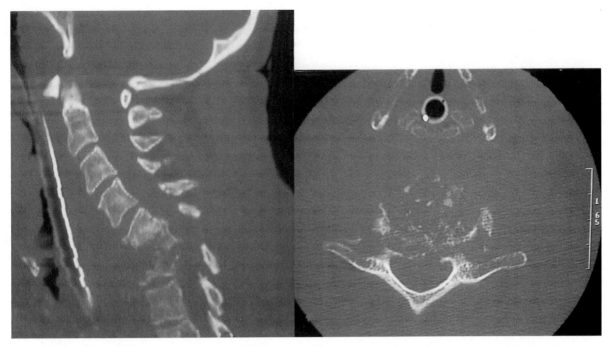

FIG. 15.3. Computed tomography (CT) scans demonstrate osteomyelitis of C5 and C6 with canal compromise in both axial and sagittal reconstructed views. Notice that neural structures are not visualized well.

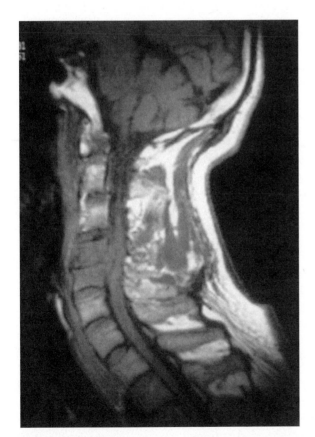

FIG. 15.4. A T1-weighted sagittal magnetic resonance imaging study of the cervical spine in a different patient demonstrates osteomyelitis of C4 and C5 with spinal canal compromise. Notice the detail of anatomy visualized of the spinal column and the spinal cord compared with computed tomography (see Fig. 15.3).

studied 34 patients who underwent cervical spine surgery after MRI (19). MRI correctly predicted 88% of all surgically proven lesions, compared with 81% for CT myelography, 58% for myelography, and 50% for CT.

MRI may reveal degenerative changes of the spine in the absence of clinical symptoms. Boden and colleagues reported that up to 19% of asymptomatic patients had an abnormal MRI of the cervical spine (20). Matsumoto and associates reported the presence of herniated discs on MRI in more than 85% of asymptomatic patients older than 60 years of age (21). In short, MRI is advantageous tool for evaluation of myelopathy and other spinal cord disease; however, the imaging findings must be correlated with clinical findings.

Other Modalities

Nerve conduction studies and electromyography usually do not add value in the workup of patients with myelopathy unless a concomitant peripheral nerve disease is also suspected. Somatosensory evoked potentials on the other hand are helpful to evaluate nervous system function in a number of diseases involving the spinal cord. In patients with myelopathy, both amplitude and latency may be affected.

In patients who have noncompressive myelopathy, a lumbar puncture is essential. With spinal fluid, one can rule out many infectious and inflammatory myelopathies. Also, laboratory evaluation, including blood count, chemistry, liver enzymes, and certain autoantibodies, can aid in diagnosing the cause of the myelopathy.

DIFFERENTIAL DIAGNOSIS

Congenital

Chiari Malformation

In the Chiari malformation type I, the cerebellar tonsils and a variable portion of the cerebellum are displaced through the foramen magnum into the upper cervical canal (Fig. 15.5). Patients with the Chiari malformation may present with a wide variety of symptoms of brainstem, spinal cord, or cerebellar compression. Symptoms of myelopathy may be observed in as many as 30% to 40% of patients with some degree of motor and sensory involvement. Hyporeflexia of the upper extremities, hyperreflexia of the lower extremities, and Babinski reflex are observed in as many as one fourth of patients. A patient with asymptomatic Chiari malformation should undergo suboccipital craniectomy, upper cervical laminectomies, and duraplasty to decompress the foramen magnum. Intradural exploration, lysis of subarachnoid adhesions, and tonsil desertion may also be performed. Prognosis is very good, and most

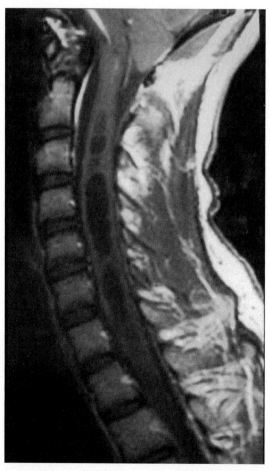

FIG. 15.5. Sagittal magnetic resonance imaging study of the craniocervical junction shows type I Chiari malformation with herniation of the cerebellar tonsils. The patient also has a large septated syrinx in the cervical spine.

patients stabilize or experience improved function, especially if the diagnosis is made early.

Hydromyelia and Syringomyelia

Hydromyelia and syringomyelia can be congenital or acquired (e.g., posttraumatic, postinfectious). They are characterized by cavitation of the spinal cord. The cavity is lined with ependymal cells in hydromyelia but not in syringomyelia. The cervicothoracic region is the most commonly affected region of the spinal cord. At the level of the syrinx, the spinal cord may be of normal transverse size, wider than usual, or occasionally thinner than usual.

Patients with syringomyelia may be asymptomatic or may present with widespread sensory loss and quadriparesis. The clinical presentation is dependent on the location of the syrinx and associated pathologic conditions (e.g., Chiari malformation). The classic presentation of a cervical syrinx includes upper extremity weakness and atrophy, with a suspended and dissociated sensory loss beginning in the hands. As the disease progresses, the long motor and sensory pathways in the spinal cord become involved. This is often accompanied by lower motor neuron weakness of the upper extremities. Patients experience varying degrees of myelopathy, including weakness (30%), sensory disturbances (19%), paresthesias (19%), muscular wasting (5%) and spastic gait (3%) (22).

The treatment varies, depending on the presentation and associated pathologic conditions. Treatment options include observation, treating associated conditions (e.g., suboccipital craniectomy in Chiari malformation), and spinal decompression with or without syrinx drainage operations.

Intraspinal Enterogenous Cysts

Intraspinal enterogenous cysts are rare malformations that lead to spinal cord compression or tethering. Embryologically, these cysts are derived from endoderm that is fused with the developing notochord during the third week of gestation. Although common near the cervicothoracic junction, they may be encountered anywhere from the cerebellopontine angle to the coccyx.

In contrast to many congenital malformations of spinal dysraphism, the clinical symptoms of an intraspinal enterogenous cyst may not be observed until the fourth or fifth decade of life. The symptoms of spinal cord or nerve root compression may mimic other space-occupying lesions of the spinal canal, including disc herniation. Pain is the most common symptom and is often localized to the spinal level of the malformation. In a review by Agnoli and associates of 32 published cases of intraspinal enterogenous cysts, the average patient age was 24 years, with a male to female ratio of 2.3 (23). The most common cyst location was intradural-extramedullary. Each patient had symptoms consistent with myelopathy. Surgery is the definitive treatment for an intraspinal enterogenous cyst.

Atlantoaxial Subluxation

Stability of the atlantoaxial joint is dependent on the transverse atlantal ligament, which prevents excessive ventral translation of the axis while preventing the rotation of the atlas on the axis. Instability due to excessive ventral translation of the atlas can result in compression of the spinal cord between the dens and dorsal ring of the atlas (Fig. 15.6).

Congenital disorders involving the atlantoaxial articulation include hypoplasia or absence of the dens or transverse atlantal ligament. Children with Morquio syndrome (mucopolysaccharidosis type IV), pseudoachondroplasia, spondylometaphyseal dysplasia, Maroteaux-Lamy syndrome, chondrodystrophy calcificans congenital, metamorphic dwarfism, and Pierre Robin syndrome have a high incidence of atlantoaxial instability (24). Instability of the upper cervical spine is associated with the polyarticular form of juvenile rheumatoid arthritis (RA) as well as with juvenile ankylosing spondylitis (24).

The most common genetic disorder associated with atlantoaxial instability is Down syndrome (trisomy 21). Although the estimate of incidence may vary, most studies report that between 7% and 20% of patients with Down syndrome demonstrate atlantoaxial instability (24,25). Pueschel

and Scola examined 404 Down syndrome patients and observed a significant difference in atlanto-dens interval and spinal canal width compared with children without Down syndrome (25). A total of 59 (14.6%) of 404 patients displayed atlantoaxial instability. Fifty-three (13.1%) patients had asymptomatic atlantoaxial instability. Six (1.5%) patients had symptomatic atlantoaxial instability, all of whom underwent surgery to prevent further injury to the spinal cord.

Clinical presentations may vary, and early diagnosis is often difficult. This is due in part to vague presenting complaints and inherent communication difficulties with young children. Because many patients are asymptomatic, only a high level of suspicion by a primary care physician can help establish the diagnosis. The onset of symptoms of cord compression found with atlantoaxial instability is gradual and may be exacerbated by minimal trauma (26). The preferred treatment in symptomatic patient is arthrodesis of C1 to C2 to allow sufficient room for the spinal cord. The treatment of asymptomatic patients, however, is controversial.

Other Pathologies

Myelopathy has also been reported in conditions such as Klippel-Feil anomaly, severe scoliosis, and dystonic cerebral palsy.

Acquired

Spondylotic Myelopathy

The complex process associated with degenerative changes of the cervical spine often begins with the intervertebral disc. The nucleus pulposus loses about 23% of its water content with age, resulting in loss of disc height and elasticity. As the nucleus pulposus is replaced by fibrocartilage, the motion at the disc space is limited. As described by Keyes and colleagues, with these degenerative changes, the ball-bearing movement of the intervertebral disc is replaced by a sliding motion that places stress on the anterior and posterior longitudinal ligaments and vertebrae, resulting in osteophyte formation (27). Degeneration of the disc also leads to tearing of the annulus fibrous and herniation of the disc material into the spinal canal.

A dorsally placed osteophyte can cause spinal cord compression, leading to myelopathy (Fig. 15.7). Depending on the location and the longitudinal length of spinal cord compression, a patient may have any of the previously described clinical syndromes. The lower cervical spine seems to be more vulnerable to spondylosis, mainly owing to extensive mobility. The most important risk factors for developing spondylotic myelopathy seem to be spinal canal size and impairment of blood supply to the spinal cord (28–30). An alternate hypothesis of intermittent compression of the spinal cord during flexion and extension neck movement by a thickened ligamentum flavum has also been proposed (31).

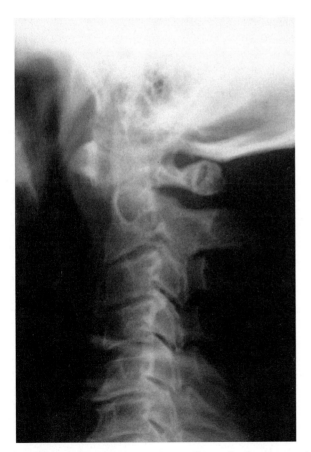

FIG. 15.6. Lateral cervical spine radiograph shows an atlantodental interval of greater than 6 mm in a patient with atlantoaxial subluxation.

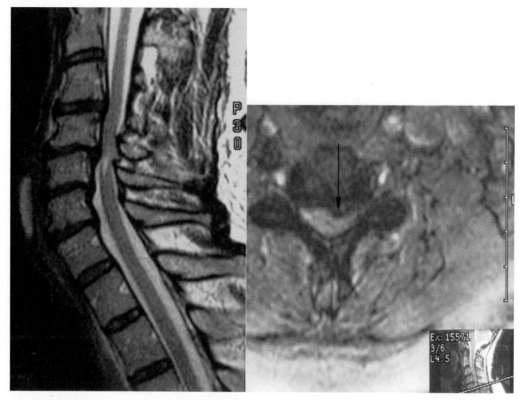

FIG. 15.7. Magnetic resonance imaging of the cervical spine in two different patients shows severe degenerative disc disease. The sagittal image demonstrates diffuse canal compromise and compression of the spinal cord causing signal change within the cord. The axial shows a left-sided herniated disc–osteophyte complex (*arrow*) compressing the spinal cord and the exiting nerve root.

Patients presenting with spondylotic myelopathy often have signs and symptoms of radiculopathy. The most commonly affected age group is 50 to 70 years, and men are affected more frequently than women. The symptoms of myelopathy may develop progressively or in a stepwise fashion and may develop or be aggravated after a trauma. Neck, shoulder, and arm pain are common presenting complaints. Muscle spasms, paresthesias, fasciculation, and weakness in the distribution of affected nerve roots are often encountered. Hyporeflexia of the upper extremities, hyperreflexia of the lower extremities, and pathologic reflexes are often observed. Spastic gait and sphincter problems are often seen.

In general, the pain can be successfully treated with rest, antiinflammatory drugs, and analgesics. First, a conservative approach to treatment, including rest, cervical collar, and neck strengthening exercise are recommended. This is associated with a high success rate. If a patient is moderately or severely disabled or has progressive myelopathy despite conservative management, surgery should be considered.

Arachnoid Cyst

Arachnoid cysts are leptomeningeal diverticula that occur in the extradural or intradural space. Most spinal intradural arachnoid cysts are thought to be congenital, but multiple etiologic theories have been proposed. The rare association of this lesion with neural tube defects and mild vertebral column anomalies supports a congenital etiology. However, numerous authors have postulated that a substantial number of arachnoid intradural cysts are caused by trauma or arachnoiditis (32,33). Patients may be asymptomatic, and cysts are often found incidentally on radiologic studies or at autopsy. They are a rare cause of spinal cord or nerve root compression. Most arachnoid cysts communicate with the subarachnoid space, rather than existing as closed cavities. The location of an arachnoid cyst depends on local abnormalities of tissues and hydrodynamic forces (34).

Extradural arachnoid cysts are herniations of arachnoid space through a defect in the dura mater. They can be congenital or induced by previous trauma. Cysts may cause erosion of the pedicles or other spinal elements and can be appreciated on plain radiographs. Intradural arachnoid cysts, like extradural arachnoid cysts, can be found at any level and are usually dorsal. Signs and symptoms are similar to extradural arachnoid cysts. Clinical signs and symptoms are similar to other space-occupying lesions, including pain, radicular dysfunction, and myelopathic manifestations. Symptoms may differ considerably with change in posture and with change in intrathoracic and intraabdominal pressure. Symptoms may be transient or relapsing and remitting. Surgery is the treatment of choice in symptomatic individuals.

Other Mechanical Compressive Lesions

Myelopathy has also been reported in various conditions such as Paget disease, ossification of the posterior longitudinal ligament (OPLL) (Figs. 15.1 and 15.8), epidural lipomatosis, and hypertrophy of the bone marrow in extramedullary hematopoiesis. Epidural lipomatosis is a rare cause of myelopathy and is most commonly associated with exogenous corticosteroid use (35). It is treated with decompressive laminectomy and fat debulking.

Paget disease of the bone is associated with involvement of the central and peripheral nervous system. The brain, spinal cord, cauda equina, spinal roots, and cranial nerves can be affected in Paget disease because of their anatomic relationship to bone. Neurologic syndromes are uncommon but include headache, dementia, brainstem and cerebellar dysfunction, cranial neuropathies, myelopathy, cauda equina syndrome, and radiculopathies (36). The etiology is believed to be compression of cranial and spinal foramina by expanded bone and basilar invagination due to softened bone. This leads to compression of the brainstem, cerebellum, and lower cranial nerves. Myelopathy and radiculopathy most commonly result from hypertrophy of the spine, with direct spinal cord compression. Spinal stenosis can also result from ossification of extradural structures or pathologic fractures. Ischemia from vascular compression or a steal syndrome has also been described (37).

MRI, CT myelography, and plain radiographs assist in the localization of the lesion and direct the therapy. Treatment options include surgical decompression and medical management with calcitonin or bisphosphonates. The selection of treatment strategies varies, depending on the rate of progression and the severity of the neurologic deficit.

OPLL is a common, well-recognized cause of spinal stenosis and myelopathy in Japan. It is also observed in whites, especially among elderly people, as a cause of myelopathy. Ossification may occur anywhere from C1 to C7, but it occurs most often in the midcervical spine. The age of affected patients ranges from 42 to 75 years, and there is no gender preponderance. The posterior longitudinal ligament is ossified in its superficial layer, but not the deep layer. Clinically, patients may be asymptomatic or have severe myelopathy. Treatment is surgical for symptomatic patients.

Trauma

According to some estimates, there are 10,000 new spinal cord injuries in the United States each year. Patients with acute spinal cord injury may present with either complete or incomplete injury depending on the mechanism and force of the injury. Fracture-dislocation is nearly always present with spinal cord injury. However, spinal cord injuries occurring without concomitant radiologically demonstrable trauma to the skeletal elements or compromise of the spinal canal without fracture are also uncommonly observed. Treatment of incomplete spinal cord injuries is intravenous methylprednisolone, followed by decompression and stabilization.

Progressive posttraumatic myelopathy is also a well-known entity. Often, patients have neurologic deficits long after their spinal cord injury. The reported prevalence is up to 5% of cervical spinal cord injury (38,39). Possible causes include arachnoiditis, spinal column instability, spinal cord compression, spinal cord tethering, cystic myelopathy, and syringomyelia (Fig. 15.9).

Neoplastic

About 15% of primary central nervous system (CNS) tumors are intraspinal. Tumors of the spine are grouped by their location. They are divided in four categories: extradural, intradural, extramedullary, and intramedullary. Intramedullary tumors make up 5% of all spinal tumors and originate from cells of neural tissue, such as astrocytes and ependymal cells. Extramedullary intradural tumors (40%) arise from the leptomeninges, peripheral nerve sheaths, or myelin. Extradural tumors comprise 55% of spinal tumors arise from skeletal or epidural tissues.

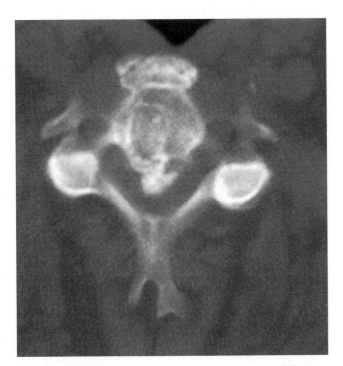

FIG. 15.8. Cervical spine computed tomography (CT) demonstrated an ossified anterior and posterior longitudinal ligament causing narrowing of the spinal canal. (Courtesy of Dr. Daniel K. Resnick.)

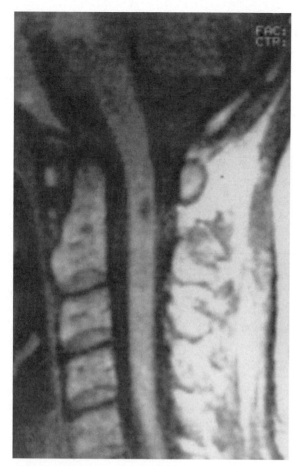

FIG. 15.9. Magnetic resonance imaging of a patient with a history of cervical spine trauma and slowly progressive myelopathy demonstrates a small syrinx at the level of previous injury. Notice that there are no fractures associated with the trauma and no structures compressing the spinal cord.

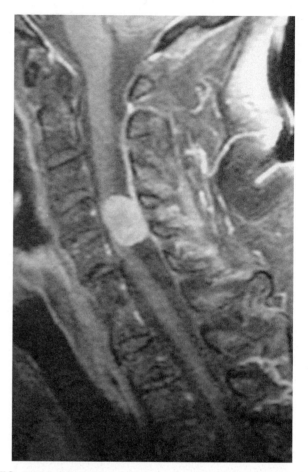

FIG. 15.10. Magnetic resonance imaging shows extramedullary intradural tumor displacing the spinal cord anteriorly in a patient who presented with cervical myelopathy. (Courtesy of Dr. Daniel K. Resnick.)

Common extradural tumors include metastatic tumors, chordomas, osteoid osteoma, osteoblastoma, aneurysmal bone cyst, vertebral hemangioma, and multiple myeloma. Although metastatic tumors can be found in each location, they are usually extradural. Intradural extramedullary tumors include meningioma (Fig. 15.10), schwannoma, neurofibroma, and lipoma. Intramedullary spinal tumors include astrocytoma, ependymoma, dermoid, epidermoid, hemangioblastoma, and lipoma.

Distinguishing among intramedullary, extramedullary, intradural, and extradural on clinical grounds is difficult. Pain is the most common complaint. Pain is usually progressive and increases with Valsalva maneuver or with recumbent position. Pain associated with intramedullary tumors is usually not radicular, but instead bilateral, poorly localized, diffuse, burning, and involving a large area of the body (40). Extramedullary tumors may present initially with a radicular localized pain. A gait disturbance is also common, especially in children. Intradural tumors may have a syringomyelia-like syndrome, including segmental upper extremity weakness and hyporeflexia, lower extremity hyperreflexia, and dissociative anesthesia. Also, long tract signs, such as clumsiness, spasticity, ataxia, muscle atrophy, and fasciculation, are observed. Paresthesia and dysesthesia are common. Sphincter disturbances frequently occur in intramedullary tumors or tumors of the cauda equina. Children may present with scoliosis or a visible mass over the spine.

The diagnosis is made by the aforementioned studies. Treatment and prognosis depend on the type of tumor and its location.

Vascular

Spinal Hemorrhages

Spinal hemorrhage can occur in the substance of the spinal cord itself, subarachnoid space, subdural space, or epidural space (Fig. 15.11). In each case, the presentation is typically sudden pain followed by neurologic signs and symptoms at the level of the hematoma.

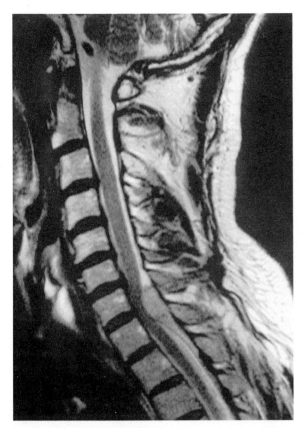

FIG. 15.11. T2-weighted magnetic resonance imaging study of the cervical spine in an acutely myelopathic patient demonstrates acute epidural hematoma at the level of C7 to T2, displacing the spinal cord ventrally.

An intramedullary hemorrhage is commonly due to trauma, a ruptured spinal arteriovenous malformation (AVM), or a neoplasm. Clinically, patients have sudden severe back pain, with or without a radicular component. The hemorrhage may cause a central cord syndrome or a complete spinal cord injury. CSF may show evidence of hemorrhage. Myelography and MRI are usually diagnostic. Treatment of nontraumatic intramedullary hemorrhage is individualized. In a small portion of patients, especially in patients with incomplete spinal cord injury, drainage of the hematoma may be beneficial.

Spontaneous subarachnoid hemorrhage of the spine is associated with spinal AVM, neoplasm, coagulopathy, and infection. The clinical presentation of a spinal subarachnoid hemorrhage is sharp, severe sudden neck and back pain. There are associated radiculopathies and myelopathy. If the blood circulates over the cerebral convexities, the patients may have signs and symptoms of intracranial subarachnoid hemorrhage. CSF analysis is usually diagnostic, and treatment depends on the etiology.

Common etiologies for spinal subdural and epidural hematoma include trauma (lumbar puncture, epidural anesthesia), bleeding diathesis, and ruptured AVM. Although these hematomas may occur at any level of the spine, the thoracic region is most common. They are usually located dorsally. Clinically, patients usually present with back pain. A radicular component is usually the first symptom. Progressive myelopathy is common. Paraplegia, sensory loss, and bladder and bowel disturbance may ensue over several hours. Recovery without surgery is rare. Therefore, surgery is usually the treatment of choice.

Spinal Arteriovenous Malformation

Spinal AVMs are classified in four categories: type I, dural arteriovenous fistula (AVF); type II, intramedullary AVM (glomus AVM); type III, juvenile type intramedullary AVM; and type IV, perimedullary AVF (41). Type I is the most common and type III the least common.

Type I AVMs are predominantly found in the lower thoracic and conus medullaris regions of the spine. The AVM consists of an arterial feeder that enters the dura mater in the region of the nerve root sleeve, and a small cluster of veins inside the dura make up the fistula. The arterial feeder typically does not contribute any blood supply to the spinal cord. Type I spinal AVMs are slow flow and produce venous hypertension within the spinal cord. This leads to spinal cord hypoperfusion, ischemia, and neurologic deficit. Affected patients usually present with symptoms of progressive myelopathy, which are exacerbated by physical exertion. Aminoff and associates reported that only 9% of patients were still capable of unrestricted walking within 3 years of initial presentation (42). Surgery is the first line of treatment. Immobilization is used as an adjunctive therapy.

Type II, III, and IV AVMs typically present in childhood or early adulthood (Fig. 15.12). Signs and symptoms can be caused by hemorrhage, arterial steal, or a space-occupying lesion. Clinical presentation is usually acute. In these AVM types, signs and symptoms of myelopathy depend on the location and the amount of hemorrhage. Treating these AVMs is very difficult. Immobilization and surgery play a major role.

Spinal Epidural Varices

Usually, epidural varices produce signs and symptoms of lumbar and sacral radiculopathies. However, there are several cases reported of myelopathy associated with spinal epidural varices (43). Signs and symptoms probably develop from thrombosis and progressive venous distension with spinal cord compression. Treatment is a decompressive laminectomy.

Medical Myelopathies

Medical myelopathies include noncompressive myelopathies caused by intrinsic disease of the spinal cord. Most of these diseases present clinically with an acute or subacute course. The diagnosis is made through history and physical examination along with imaging findings.

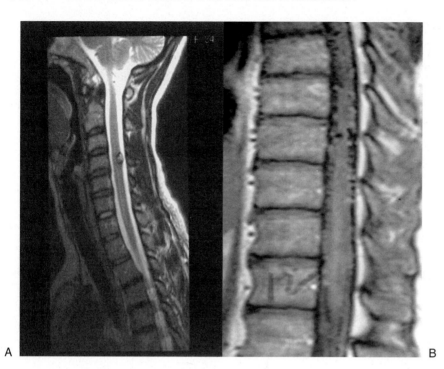

FIG. 15.12. A: A cervical spine cavernous malformation in a patient with progressive myelopathy. The patient's symptom progressions are due to repeated hemorrhages. **B**: A large thoracic spine arteriovenous malformation with multiple dilated veins and diffuse signal change within the spinal cord.

Acute Idiopathic Transverse Myelitis

Before the recent advances in imaging technology, patients presenting with either acute or subacute evolving myelopathy and a negative myelogram for a mass lesion were diagnosed with transverse myelopathy. Ropper and Poskanzer described transverse myelopathy as "an acute intramedullary dysfunction of the spinal cord, either ascending or static, involving both halves of the cord, often over considerable length, and appearing without history of previous neurologic disease" (44). Many different neuropathologic processes, such as infectious, inflammatory, toxic, and metabolic, fall under the term *transverse myelopathy*. Acute idiopathic transverse myelitis is used when no known cause of myelopathy is identified.

Acute idiopathic transverse myelitis most often presents with progressive paresthesias and weakness of the legs. The symptoms generally evolve over 1 to 2 weeks but may develop abruptly. Initially, symptoms may be asymmetric. However, late in the disease, symmetric paraplegia and gross sensory loss are common. Disease may progress to involve the upper extremities and cause bowel and bladder dysfunction.

The differential diagnosis of transverse myelitis includes multiple sclerosis, postinfectious or postvaccination myelitis, toxic myelopathy, and metabolic or vitamin deficiency myelopathy. Workup of patients with transverse myelitis includes obtaining a history of recent viral illness, vaccination, travel, prior syphilis, connective tissue disease, and prior neurologic illness. Blood work should include serum VDRL, vitamin levels, erythrocyte sedimentation rate, and laboratory work for connective tissue disease. A lumbar puncture is usually indicated to rule out infectious causes and multiple sclerosis. MRI of the spinal cord with and without intravenous contrast is the best imaging modality (Fig. 15.13). Miller and coworkers found lesions in the appropriate cervical spine region in 64% patients with multiple sclerosis (45). Choi and colleagues evaluated the MRI characteristic of 17 patients with idiopathic transverse myelitis and found a centrally located hyperintensity occupying more than two thirds of the cross-sectional area of the spinal cord (88%); involvement of three to four vertebral segments (53%), and variable amount of spinal cord expansion (47%) (46).

Although there are no randomized controlled trials establishing efficacy, corticosteroids are used as a primary treatment of acute idiopathic transverse myelitis. In a study by Sebire and associates, five children with severe acute transverse myelopathy were treated with intravenous methylprednisolone and compared with a historical group of 10 patients (47). The results showed that in the methylprednisolone treatment group, compared with the historical group, the median time to walk independently was significantly reduced (23 versus 97 days) and the proportion of patients with a full recovery within 12 months was significantly higher (80% versus 10%). All patients in the treatment group had complete motor recovery within 1 year, in contrast to only 2 of 10 patients in the historical control group. No serious adverse effects were reported.

Multiple Sclerosis

Multiple sclerosis (MS) is an inflammatory relapsing or progressive disorder of CNS white matter and a major cause of disability in young adults. Pathologically, multi-

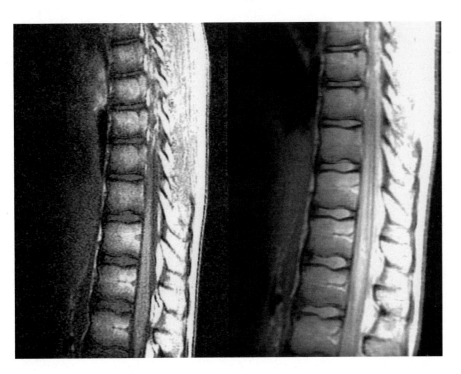

FIG. 15.13. T1- and T2-weighted magnetic resonance imaging (MRI) studies in a patient who presented with subacute myelopathy and who had a negative workup except for thoracic MRI. These images show diffuse signal change within the spinal cord on both sequences. The patient was diagnosed with idiopathic transverse myelitis.

focal areas of demyelination with relative preservation of axons are seen in white matter. MS has a wide range of clinical features. Many signs and symptoms are characteristic, and a few are virtually pathognomonic for the disorder. Spinal cord involvement causing myelopathy as the initial presentation of MS is common. Lumsden found the presence of demyelinating plaques in the spinal cords of most MS patients on postmortem examination (48). Poser and coworkers found that 109 of 1,271 (9%) patients with MS had only a spinal form of MS causing myelopathy (49). However, Liebowitz and colleagues reported that about 25% of patients with MS also had involvement of the spinal cord (50).

Sensory symptoms are the most common presenting manifestation in MS and ultimately develop in nearly all patients. Numbness, paresthesias, dysesthesias, and hyperesthesias are common. These may occur in practically any distribution: one or more limbs, part of a limb, trunk, face, or combinations. Pyramidal tract dysfunction is common in MS and causes weakness, spasticity, loss of dexterity, and hyperreflexia. Motor deficits can occur acutely or in a chronic progressive fashion and are usually accompanied by other symptoms. Paraparesis, quadriparesis, hemiparesis, weakness of one limb, and facial weakness are common manifestations. Urinary urgency, frequency, and urge incontinence (due to detrusor hyperreflexia or detrusor-sphincter dyssynergia) result from spinal cord lesions and are frequently encountered in MS patients.

Although it may be difficult to separate spinal MS from postinfectious myelitis, the evolution of myelopathy in MS frequently occurs over a few weeks rather than over a few days. CSF sometimes shows signs of inflammation with pleocytosis and elevation of proteins. With elevated immunoglobulin G (IgG), oligoclonal bands are often present in the CSF. Patients with MS also have abnormal somatosensory evoked potentials and visual evoked potentials.

Neuromyelitis Optica (Devic Disease)

Neuromyelitis optica (NMO) is an uncommon neurologic illness characterized by the occurrence of optic neuropathy and myelopathy in close temporal relationship (Fig. 15.14). It is considered by many authors to be a variant of MS. NMO may occur with acute disseminated encephalomyelitis, autoimmune disorders, MS, and possibly viral infections. Pathologically, acute spinal cord lesions demonstrate diffuse swelling and softening that extend over several levels or involve nearly the entire spinal cord in a continuous or patchy distribution. In acute lesions, destruction with dense macrophage infiltration, involving white and gray matter, loss of myelin and axons, and lymphocytic cuffing of vessels is observed. In chronic lesions, the spinal cord is atrophic and necrotic, with cystic degeneration and gliosis.

The symptoms of optic neuritis and myelitis develop over hours to days and are often preceded or accompanied by headache, nausea, somnolence, fever, or myalgias. Continued progression of symptoms over weeks or months occasionally occurs. More than 80% of patients develop bilateral optic neuritis. Bitemporal or junctional visual field deficits, indicating chiasm involvement, are sometimes present early in the course of the optic neuritis. Visual impairment is followed within days or weeks by a transverse or ascending

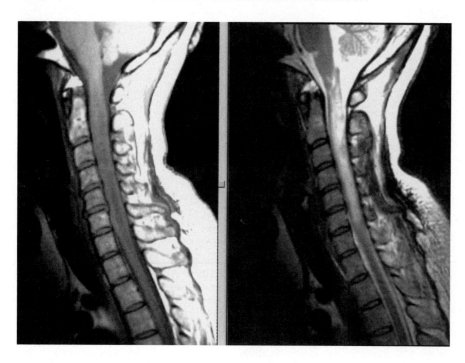

FIG. 15.14. T1- and T2-weighted cervical spine magnetic resonance imaging studies in a patient with Devic disease. Diffuse signal change is appreciated on both T1 and T2 image sequences, indicating diffuse demyelination.

myelitis. Myelopathy symptoms are sometimes heralded by localized back or radicular pain. Lhermitte sign is common. Severe degrees of neurologic deficits are usual, and the degree of recovery is variable.

Myelopathies Due to Connective Tissue Disease

The spinal cord may be the target of a variety of systemic autoimmune diseases, including RA, Sjögren syndrome (SS), systemic lupus erythematosus, polyarthritis nodosa, Wegener granulomatosis, and more. In most cases, there is already evidence of a systemic involvement, and exclusive spinal cord involvement is rare.

Rheumatoid Arthritis

RA is a chronic systemic inflammatory disease predominantly affecting diarthrodial joints and frequently a variety of other organs. RA occurs worldwide in all ethnic groups. Prevalence rates range from 0.3% to 1.5% in most populations (51). The peak incidence of onset is between the fourth and sixth decades, but RA may begin at any time from childhood to later in life. Females are two to three times more likely to be affected than males. RA is believed to be an autoimmune disease. Autoantibodies to the Fc portion of IgG molecules or rheumatoid factors are present in the blood and synovial tissues of 80% of RA patients. High titers of serum rheumatoid factor, typically of the IgM isotype, are associated with more severe disease.

The clinical presentation is highly variable. In most cases, joint pain or stiffness develop slowly over several weeks to months. Usually, one or more small joints of the hands, wrists, shoulders, or knees are the first symptomatic areas. The pattern of joint involvement is typically polyarticular and symmetric, generally with worse symptoms in the morning. Malaise, fatigue, and low-grade fever may accompany musculoskeletal discomfort. Extraarticular involvement includes cardiac, pulmonary, neurologic, or ophthalmologic manifestations.

Neurologic manifestations occur in patients with moderate to severe RA. They may be caused by direct effects of the disease process or by secondary effects from bone or joint involvement. Neurologic manifestations include CNS vasculitis, distal sensorimotor or sensory polyneuropathy, and spine involvement. Destruction of cartilage, bone, tendons, and ligaments from a combination of proteolytic enzymes, metalloproteinases, and soluble mediators and formation of pannus is largely responsible for CNS dysfunction at the cervicomedullary junction. Substantial disease of the cervical spine is present in up to 70% of patients with advanced disease (52). The most common change in the cervical spine includes atlantoaxial subluxation. However, vertebral body erosion and collapse (53), rheumatoid discitis, dural thickening, and fibrosis with spinal cord compression have all been reported. Atlantoaxial subluxation is present in 12% to 37% of patients with rheumatoid cervical disease (52). Cervical subluxation is often asymptomatic. In patients who are symptomatic, myelopathy is a common presentation. The most common and characteristic neurologic features are numbness and paresthesias predominating in the upper extremities, degradation of fine motor task, neck pain, flexor spasms, sphincter disturbances, hyperreflexia, and sensory changes (54). The natural course of atlantoaxial subluxation is relatively benign. In one series, the prevalence of myelopathy increased from 3% to only 10% during 5 years (55).

MRI is useful in identifying pannus formation and craniocervical involvement in RA. For many symptomatic patients, conservative treatment may stabilize symptoms. Surgical decompression and stabilization may be helpful in early symptomatic ambulatory patients, but it is often not helpful and dangerous in nonambulatory patients with advanced disease (56).

Sjögren Syndrome

SS is a chronic immune-mediated inflammatory disorder characterized by lymphocytic infiltration of the exocrine glands, especially the lacrimal and salivary glands. Patients present with dry eyes, dry mouth, and noninflammatory arthritis. Although neurologic disorders have generally been considered rare manifestations of SS, up to 20% of patient with SS develop CNS complications, including mild aseptic meningitis; cognitive, affective, or personality disorders; focal cerebral deficits; and seizures (57). In a study by Alexander and associates, spinal cord involvement, including progressive myelopathy, acute transverse myelitis, or intraspinal hemorrhage, was found in 85% of patients with CNS involvement (57).

Neurosarcoidosis

Sarcoidosis is an inflammatory disease characterized by the presence of noncaseating granulomas in affected tissues. Signs and symptoms of sarcoidosis may occur in almost any organ system. The duration and severity of symptoms associated with sarcoidosis are highly variable, ranging from asymptomatic adenopathy to destruction of vital organs leading to death. Virtually any part of the nervous system can be affected by neurosarcoidosis, and neurologic complications are a major cause of morbidity in sarcoidosis. Cranial nerve palsies are the most commonly reported neurologic manifestations. Polyneuropathy, aseptic meningitis, seizures, optic neuritis, and hypothalamic-pituitary syndromes have been reported. Several cases of myelopathy have also been reported in the literature. Possible causes of myelopathy include granulomatous disease in intramedullary, extramedullary-intradural, or extradural sites causing cord compression. The clinical presentation and severity varies according to the location and extent of disease in the spinal cord. Radiologically and clinically, spinal cord sarcoid is very difficult to distinguish from malignant spinal cord tumor (58). Most patients with neurosarcoidosis have associated extraneurologic abnormalities. The diagnosis is made by a high clinical suspicion in a patient with systemic sarcoid and by having extraneural biopsies. Spinal cord biopsy needs to be considered on case-by-case basis (59). Treatment is with steroids.

Toxic and Metabolic Myelopathies

Subacute Combined Degeneration

Workup of a patient with myelopathy should include evaluation of vitamin levels and liver function. Subacute combined degeneration due to vitamin B_{12} (cobalamin) deficiency is a treatable disease that presents with the insidious progression of paresthesias of the extremities. Vitamin B_{12} deficiency may develop in several ways. The most common cause is the inability to absorb B_{12} because of deficiency of intrinsic factor (pernicious anemia). Other causes include failure to release B_{12} from binding proteins caused by severe deficiency of gastric acid, malabsorption syndromes involving the ileum mucosa, or B_{12} absorption by the ileum. Besides direct damage to ileal mucosa, various causes of vitamin B_{12} malabsorption include bacterial overgrowth in the intestine (blind loop syndrome), infestation by the fish tapeworm, severe pancreatic disease, and interference by certain medications. Finally, there is dietary B_{12} deficiency, which is rare and is found mainly in strict vegetarians.

Subacute combined degeneration of the spinal cord, peripheral nerve dysfunction, and cerebral dysfunction are classic features of the vitamin deficiency. In a review by Healton and colleagues of 143 patients with 153 episodes of cobalamin deficiency, 74% of the episodes presented with neurologic symptoms, including paresthesias, numbness, gait ataxia, fecal incontinence, leg weakness, impaired manual dexterity, impaired memory, and impotence (60). The remaining 26% presented with nonneurologic symptoms classically associated with pernicious anemia, including fatigue, syncope, palpitations, sore tongue, diarrhea, and other bowel disturbances.

Patients are treated with intramuscular (IM) injections of 1,000 μg of cobalamin per day for 5 days, then 500 to 1,000 μg IM every month. Oral replacement is an alternative for patients who cannot tolerate intramuscular injections. The earlier intervention begins, the more likely the patient is to have a complete recovery. In the study by Healton and colleagues, all patients responded, and in 57 of 143 patients (47%), recovery was complete (60). Paresthesias are usually first to improve within several weeks, whereas spinal cord dysfunction may require several months.

Myelopathy Due to Liver Failure

Hepatic myelopathy is a rare complication of cirrhosis and usually occurs in the setting of surgical or spontaneous portocaval shunts. Its pathophysiology is not known. It presents with motor involvement of the lower limbs without clinical sensory abnormality, leading to spastic paraparesis. These neurologic features are related to a symmetric loss of myelin in the lateral corticospinal tracts (61). Usefulness of liver transplantation in this setting has not yet been determined.

Myelopathy Due to Toxins

Myelopathy may occur secondary to exposure to several environmental, industrial, or medical agents. In many cases, signs and symptoms of other organ systems overshadow those of myelopathy. Rarely, a patient undergoing spinal anesthesia, myelogram, or intrathecal injection of other agent can become myelopathic. In the past, penicillin was frequently administered intrathecally for treatment of pneumococcal meningitis, which occasionally caused radiculitis, arachnoiditis, or transverse myelitis (62). Similarly, intrathecal administration of methylene blue to detect the site of CSF leak produced myelopathy in a few cases (63). Myelopathy from spinal anesthesia can be either acute or delayed. It is not clear whether direct neurotoxicity from the anesthetic or carrier agents such as phenols cause the myelopathy. Myelopathy is often permanent and may include paraplegia and sensory and sphincter dysfunction. Use of intrathecal chemotherapeutic agents such as methotrexate, cytosine arabinoside, and thiotepa can cause myelopathy (64,65).

The use of nonionic contrast agents for myelograms has essentially eliminated the complication of associated spinal cord toxicity. Historically, both oil- and water-soluble ionic myelographic agents have been reported to induce arachnoiditis and spinal cord dysfunction.

Orthocresol phosphates, which are used as industrial solvents, are highly toxic to the nervous system when ingested. Although accidental occupational exposure is rare, patients were often exposed by ingesting triorthocresyl phosphates in lieu of ethanol or by ingesting olive oil contaminated with lubricating oil (66). The clinical picture is of an acute peripheral neuropathy developing over a period of weeks, followed by myelopathy. Other toxins such as *Lathyrus sativa* found in chickpeas causes lathyrism, which is seen mainly in India and North Africa. Patients have an acute neurologic syndrome of pain, sensory complaints, and lower extremity weakness that evolves into ataxia and spastic paraplegia (67). The prognosis of recovery is poor.

Paraneoplastic Myelopathies

Metastasis is the usual cause of nervous system dysfunction in patients with cancer. However, cancer also can exert deleterious effects on the nervous system by mechanisms other than metastasis. Paraneoplastic neurologic disorders are defined as disorders of nervous system function that cannot be ascribed to invasion of the nervous system by neoplastic cells or by any other mechanisms related to the presence of cancer, including coagulopathy, vascular disorders, infections, metabolic and nutritional deficits, and toxic effects of cancer therapy (68). Paraneoplastic disorder can affect any part of or any cell type of the nervous system, including the spinal cord. The presence of inflammatory infiltrates in the CNS of patients with paraneoplastic syndromes, coupled with the detection of anti-CNS antibodies, suggests immune-related mechanisms (69).

Several different myelopathies are observed with paraneoplastic syndrome. Subacute motor neuronopathy is observed in patients with Hodgkin disease and other lymphomas. It has a subacute course whereby anterior horn motor neurons are affected. Patients have progressive, painless, asymmetric weakness of the legs and arms with no to very mild sensory loss. Examination reveals involvement of corticospinal tract with extensor plantar (Babinski) reflexes. On pathologic examination, degeneration of anterior horn cells and sometimes demyelination in the white matter of the spinal cord are appreciated. The clinical course is different from most remote effects of cancer in that some patients improve spontaneously, independently of the course of the underlying lymphoma.

Subacute necrotic myelopathy is a condition that affects both gray and white matter equally. The clinical picture is that of rapidly ascending sensory and motor myelopathy, usually to the midthoracic levels. The patient becomes paraplegic and incontinent within hours or days. The neurologic symptoms often precede discovery of the neoplasm, and the illness is clinically and pathologically indistinguishable from idiopathic subacute necrotic myelopathy. The diagnosis is difficult because epidural or intramedullary spinal metastases and arteriovenous spinal cord anomalies may present similarly. MRI scan is essential in diagnosis.

Infectious Myelopathies

Viral Myelitis

Most viruses that invade the spinal cord have a predilection for a specific location in the spinal cord, for example, gray matter versus white matter and anterior horn versus posterior horn (Fig. 15.15). Many different viruses, including human immunodeficiency virus (HIV), human T-cell lymphotrophic virus type I (HTLV-I), poliovirus, and herpesvirus, can cause myelitis.

Human Immunodeficiency Virus

The neurologic complications of HIV infection are both common and varied. Although most neurologic complications occur in the late phase of HIV infection when a patient is immunocompromised, a patient may also manifest certain neurologic afflictions early in infection. A survey of the literature of neurologic manifestations associated with acquired immunodeficiency syndrome (AIDS) shows a broad disease spectrum affecting about one third of the patients in large hospital series (70). Some common complications of HIV infection include opportunistic infection, opportunistic neoplasm, AIDS dementia complex, aseptic meningitis, polyneuropathy, psychotic depression, and myelopathy.

The most common spinal cord affliction in AIDS patients is vacuolar myelopathy. First described by Petito and colleagues, who observed it in 20 of 89 consecutive autopsies of patients with AIDS, it was observed that vacuolar myelopathy was most severe in the lateral and posterior columns of

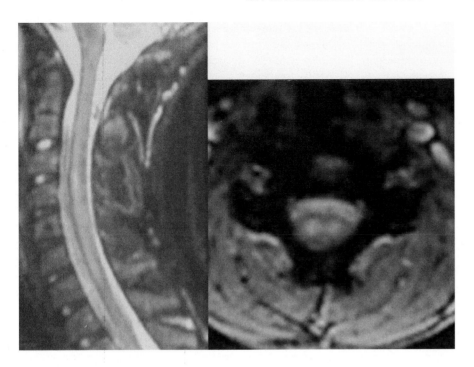

FIG. 15.15. Sagittal and axial magnetic resonance imaging (MRI) studies of the cervical spine in an 11-year-old boy who presented with headaches and nuchal rigidity. Spinal tap showed 86 lymphocytes, and the head MRI was negative. A few days after admission, the patient became myelopathic, and a cervical spine MRI showed diffuse signal changes within the cord. The patient was diagnosed with viral myelitis.

the thoracic spinal cord (71). Histologic examination reveals loss of myelin and microvacuolization of the white matter associated with collection of lipid-laden macrophages. There is relative sparing of axons except in the area of marked vacuolization. The disorder is generally of subacute or gradual onset, and progression with painless gait disturbance is characterized by ataxia and spasticity. Bladder and bowel difficulty usually follow deterioration of gait, and sensory symptoms and signs are less prominent than gait dysfunction unless there is concomitant neuropathy. Patients do not manifest a distinct sensory or motor level as in transverse myelopathies, but rather they have distal loss of large-fiber modalities accompanied by increased deep tendon reflexes and Babinski sign. Vibratory and position senses are disproportionately affected compared with pinprick, temperature, or light touch.

To diagnose myelopathy in an AIDS patient, other causes must be excluded first. The single most useful study is an MRI of the spinal cord. Myelography is not needed if there are no mass lesions. If there is anything unusual in presentation, such as back pain or radicular findings, a more aggressive diagnostic approach should be taken. A lumbar puncture is helpful to rule out other infectious causes and to check for HIV pathogens. The prognosis is poor, and there is no known effective treatment.

Human T Cell Lymphotrophic Virus Type I–associated Myelopathy

HTLV-I, a retrovirus, is the causative agent of a slowly progressive myelopathy called HTLV-I–associated myelopathy (HAM), also known as *tropical spastic paresis*. It is a chronic progressive demyelinating disease that affects the spinal cord and white matter of the CNS. The lifetime incidence of HAM in HTLV-I carriers is estimated to be about 0.25%, and typical time of onset of HAM is in the fourth decade of life, with a female-to-male ratio of 2:1 (72). Clinically, patients present with gait disturbance and weakness and stiffness of the lower extremities. Lower extremities are affected to a much greater degree than upper extremities. Spasticity may be moderate to severe, and low back pain is common. As the disease progresses, bladder and bowel dysfunction can occur (73). Sensory involvement is generally mild and can result in a variable degree of sensory loss and dysesthesias. Disease progression is variable. In one series, after a mean period of 14.4 years (range, 1 to 30 years), 34% of patients could walk with minor difficulty, 40% of patients could walk with difficulty using a cane or crutches, and 26% of patients were bedridden (74).

Workup should include an MRI, which may be normal or may show atrophy of the spinal cord and nonspecific lesions in the brain (73). In the CSF, protein and immunoglobulin levels are moderately elevated, and oligoclonal bands are frequently seen. High antibody titers to HTLV-I in serum and CSF, in addition to atypical lymphocytes resembling adult T cell leukemia cells, may also be found in the CSF and in the peripheral blood (75).

The pathogenesis of HAM has been suggested to be immunologically mediated. Pathologic findings consist of perivascular and parenchymal infiltration of mononuclear lymphoid cells accompanied by myelin and axonal destruction. This leads to degeneration of the white matter, most conspicuously in the thoracic spinal cord (75). Varying degrees of brain parenchymal degeneration have also been described, with reactive astrocytosis and perivascular mononuclear cell infiltration.

There is no effective treatment for HAM. Corticosteroids, plasmapheresis, cyclophosphamide, and interferon-α may produce transient responses. Danazol, an anabolic steroid, has been reported to improve gait and bladder function; its mechanism of action is poorly understood (76).

Poliovirus

Poliovirus, a member of the enterovirus family, can cause myelitis. Fortunately, because of effective vaccination, this illness has become rare in the Western hemisphere. In the United States, 10 to 15 cases are reported annually. Most of these are vaccine associated. Acute anterior poliomyelitis is a febrile illness associated with flaccid paralysis and signs of meningeal inflammation. Most individuals with poliovirus infection have no symptoms or mild gastrointestinal or flulike symptoms. If an effective immune response is not mounted, aseptic meningitis and paralytic poliomyelitis may occur. First, neurologic signs include muscle spasms, headache, and neck pain. Paralysis is usually rapid, occurring in a few hours to days. Weakness is asymmetric and may involve bulbar muscles. Usually, sensory loss is not observed. The patient may have transient urinary retention. CSF studies may show pleocytosis with elevated proteins and normal glucose. There is no effective treatment once patients have paralysis.

Herpesvirus

The herpes family viruses, which includes varicella zoster, herpes simplex, and cytomegalovirus (CMV), cause infections of the CNS of several types: (a) acute encephalitis, (b) benign recurrent lymphocytic meningitis, (c) acute facial nerve paralysis, (d) recurrent ascending myelitis, and (e) neuritis localized to a single sensory nerve. Varicella zoster virus is responsible for chickenpox and shingles. The virus may remain latent within dorsal root ganglia and become activated periodically, spreading centrifugally along the nerve and causing a painful, blistering dermatomal eruption. Rarely, the virus spreads centripetally, resulting in transverse myelitis (77).

Herpes simplex virus (HSV) type 2 mainly causes infection below the umbilicus, whereas HSV type 1 causes infection above the umbilicus. Usually, herpes infection causes recurrent, painful vesicle formation in the affected area. Between active eruptions, the virus lies dormant in the dorsal root ganglia. Both the initial infection and recurrences may be complicated by radicular pain. The latter may result in pain radiating into the buttock, groin, genitalia, or lower extremities. This radicular pain may be misinterpreted as the result of a lumbar disc problem when it occurs as a prodromal symptom (before the outbreak of the blistering rash) or when it occurs in the absence of an obvious rash. HSV type 2 may also be associated with aseptic meningitis, autonomic (bowel, bladder, and sexual) dysfunction, and, rarely, myelitis. These neurologic complica-

tions are more common in the presence of primary genital herpes, but they may also been seen at the time of recurrence. CMV is an opportunistic virus transmitted through bodily fluids and organs. CMV myelitis is well recognized in immunocompromised patients such as those with AIDS. Many cases have been reported of an association of CMV with transverse myelitis (78).

Bacterial Myelopathy

Syphilis

Syphilis is a complex systemic illness with protean clinical manifestations caused by the spirochete *Treponema pallidum*. It is most often transmitted by sexual contact. It is diagnosed by direct darkfield microscopy, immunofluorescence, immunoperoxidase or silver staining, and epidemiologic, serologic, and clinical findings. After exposure, there is an incubation period lasting about 3 weeks followed by a primary stage characterized by a nonpainful skin lesion known as a chancre that is usually associated with regional lymphadenopathy and early bacteremia. A florid secondary bacteremic or disseminated stage follows the primary stage, which is accompanied by generalized mucocutaneous lesions, lymphadenopathy, and protean clinical findings. This is followed by a period of subclinical infection (latent syphilis) detected only by reactive serologic testing and, in a small number of patients, a late or tertiary stage. Tertiary stage infection is characterized by progressive disease involving principally the ascending aorta or the CNS or by the development of a characteristic granulomatouslike lesion known as a *gumma* that can involve virtually any organ.

The spirochetes invade the CNS during the secondary stage, resulting in acute syphilitic meningitis. The tertiary stage in CNS is characterized by meningovascular syphilis, in which pathologically granulomatous Heubner arteritis is observed. If the arteritis involves the spinal cord, patients develop syphilitic meningomyelitis, with an infarct located in the involved territory. Patients may present with a Brown-Séquard syndrome, an anterior spinal artery syndrome, or a variety of other spinal presentations (79). Tabes dorsalis is a parenchymal disease of the nervous system secondary to invasion by *T. pallidum*. It is characterized by lightening pain, ataxia, urinary disturbance, paresthesias or dysesthesias in a radicular distribution, and absent lower extremity reflexes. As the disease progresses, proprioceptive and vibratory sense is lost owing to neuronal degeneration and infiltration of inflammatory cells into the dorsal columns and posterior spinal nerve roots of the spinal cord. Loss of the pupillary reaction to light with preservation of pupillary constriction to accommodation (Argyll-Robertson pupil) may be present. The patient has a broad-based, footslapping gait. The peak incidence for tabes dorsalis is 15 to 20 years after the primary infection (80). Gummatous neurosyphilis is characterized by gumma located in the basal cisterns, leptomeninges, or within the parenchyma. They produce focal neurologic deficits and cranial nerve palsies by exerting pressure on adjacent structures.

Because neurosyphilis of all clinical types is associated with a CSF inflammatory response, the CSF cell count provides the best monitor for the effectiveness of therapy. Penicillin is the drug of choice, and antimicrobial resistance does not occur. Normalization of the spinal fluid is the required end point of antibiotic therapy. After the CSF normalization occurs, clinical relapses usually do not occur.

Other Bacterial Infections

A patient presenting with fever, back pain, and signs and symptoms of myelopathy should be ruled out for an epidural abscess (Figs. 15.3 and 15.4). Infections of the epidural space originate from contiguous spread or through hematogenous routes from a distant source. Cutaneous sites of infection are the most common remote sources, especially in intravenous drug users. Abdominal, respiratory tract, and urinary sources are also common. *Staphylococcus aureus* accounts for most infections, followed by streptococci and gram-negative anaerobes. In high-risk patients, tuberculous abscesses remain common. Diagnosis is made with MRI and blood work, including elevated white cell count, erythrocyte sediment rate, and C-reactive protein. Treatment includes intravenous antibiotics and surgery if the patient has signs of spinal cord compression.

A number of other bacterial infections, such as brucellosis, *Bartonella henselae* (cat-scratch disease), *Burkholderia pseudomallei*, and *Borrelia burgdorferi* (Lyme disease), have been reported to cause myelopathy (81–83).

Other Causes of Myelopathy

Electric Injury

Electrical injuries of the nervous system result from accidental exposure to high-tension currents, lightning, and even electroshock therapy. Although most currents sufficient to cause significant neurologic damage are fatal, some people do survive and are subject to damage throughout the neuraxis. In high-voltage exposures, transient loss of consciousness, confusion, anoxia from cardiac arrhythmias, and seizures are common. Spinal cord injury may result from fractures or ligamentous disruption of the cervical, thoracic, or lumbar spine and from direct injury from the current and heat (84,85). In one series, 5 of 116 electrical accident victims experienced spinal cord involvement (85). These 5 cases were detected from a few days up to 4 weeks after the injury. All patients had incomplete lesions, including 2 with quadriparesis and 3 with paraparesis.

Neurologic damage in patients without evidence of spinal injury seems to follow two patterns: immediate and delayed. Patients with immediate damage have symptoms of weakness and paresthesias that develop within hours of the insult. Lower extremity findings are more common than upper extremity findings. These patients have a good prog-

nosis for partial or complete recovery. Delayed neurologic damage may present from days to years after the insult. The findings usually fall into three clinical pictures: ascending paralysis, amyotrophic lateral sclerosis, or transverse myelitis (84). Motor findings predominate. Sensory findings are also common but may be patchy and may not match the motor levels. Although recovery is reported, the prognosis is usually poor (86).

Radiation Injury

Adverse effects of ionizing radiation on the nervous system are related to the total dose of radiation, the size of each fraction, the total duration over which the dose is received, and the volume of nervous system tissue irradiated (Fig. 15.16). Injury to the spinal cord from radiation is divided into early transient myelopathy and late progressive myelopathy. Early myelopathy is rare with current dosing regiment and follows radiation therapy to the neck or upper part of the thorax. Patients present 6 to 12 weeks after the treatment, and symptoms generally resolve spontaneously within few weeks (87). Radiation injury is characterized by Lhermitte sign. Early radiation syndromes are believed to

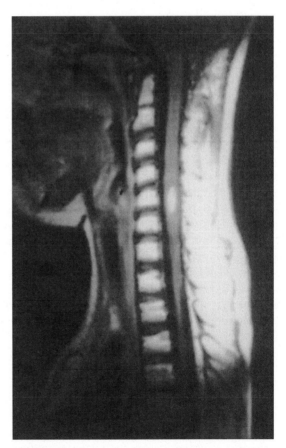

FIG. 15.16. An example of radiation necrosis of the spine in a patient several years after radiation. Notice the signal change of the vertebral body due to fatty replacement of the bone marrow.

result from demyelination, possibly caused by radiation-induced damage to oligodendroglia. Late myelopathy is characterized by progressive paralysis, sensory changes, and sometimes pain 6 to 12 months after completion of the treatment. Sensory deficits are usually more severe than motor deficits, and Brown-Séquard syndrome is often present at onset. Patients often respond transiently to steroids. Although progression of this disorder may plateau, patients generally become paraplegic or quadriplegic. Pathologic changes include necrosis of the spinal cord with degeneration of myelin sheaths and loss of oligodendrocytes.

Barotrauma

After a rapid change in atmospheric pressure, barotrauma to the spinal cord can occur. At higher atmospheric pressures, greater amounts of gases are dissolved in the tissues. When this high atmospheric pressure is diminished rapidly, inert nitrogen gas is released from tissue and occludes small blood vessels. Neurologic decompression sickness can present with a wide spectrum of symptoms, ranging from headache to confusion to a comatose state. In barotrauma-related myelopathy, patients complain of paresthesias and sensory loss in the trunk and extremities, a tingling or constricting sensation around the thorax, ascending leg weakness, pain in the lower back or pelvis, and loss of bowel and bladder control. The thoracic spinal cord is most commonly affected (88). The neurologic examination often reveals monoparesis or paraparesis, a sensory level, and sphincter disturbances.

Pathologic features within the spinal cord include hemorrhagic infarctions, edema, bubble defects, axonal degeneration, and demyelination (89). The diagnosis of neurologic decompression sickness is clinical and should be suspected in any patient with a recent history of diving. Neuroimaging studies may further clarify the diagnosis but should not delay treatment. MRI may demonstrate nonenhancing, high-signal lesions suggesting ischemia, edema, and swelling. The initial management is similar to that of arterial gas embolism and decompression illness. The patient requires transport to a recompression facility emergently. Recompression therapy reduces the size of bubbles, facilitating easier reabsorption and dissipation. Most recreational divers with neurologic decompression sickness have an excellent recovery after prompt recompression therapy (89).

REFERENCES

1. Crandall PH, Batzdorf U. Cervical spondylotic myelopathy. *J Neurosurg* 1966;25(1):57–66.
2. Merriam WF, Taylor TK, Ruff SJ, et al. A reappraisal of acute traumatic central cord syndrome. *J Bone Joint Surg Br* 1986;68(5):708–713.
3. Kirshblum SC, O'Connor KC. Predicting neurologic recovery in traumatic cervical spinal cord injury. *Arch Phys Med Rehabil* 1998;79(11):1456–1466.
4. Gharagozloo F, Larson J, Dausmann MJ, et al. Spinal cord protection during surgical procedures on the descending thoracic and thoracoabdominal aorta: review of current techniques. *Chest* 1996;109(3):799–809.
5. Ferguson RJ, Caplan LR. Cervical spondylitic myelopathy. *Neurol Clin* 1985;3(2):373–382.
6. Lunsford LD, Bissonette DJ, Zorub DS. Anterior surgery for cervical disc disease. 2. Treatment of cervical spondylotic myelopathy in 32 cases. *J Neurosurg* 1980;53(1):12–19.
7. Sudarsky L, Ronthal M. Gait disorders among elderly patients. A survey study of 50 patients. *Arch Neurol* 1983;40(12):740–743.
8. Hukuda S, Mochizuki T, Ogata M, et al. Operations for cervical spondylotic myelopathy. A comparison of the results of anterior and posterior procedures. *J Bone Joint Surg Br* 1985;67(4):609–615.
9. Nurick S. The natural history and the results of surgical treatment of the spinal cord disorder associated with cervical spondylosis. *Brain* 1972;95(1):101–108.
10. Yonenobu K, Abumi K, Nagata K, et al. Interobserver and intraobserver reliability of the Japanese Orthopaedic Association scoring system for evaluation of cervical compression myelopathy. *Spine* 2001;26(17):1890–1894; discussion, 1895.
11. Hirabayashi K, Miyakawa J, Satomi K, et al. Operative results and postoperative progression of ossification among patients with ossification of cervical posterior longitudinal ligament. *Spine* 1981;6(4):354–364.
12. Hukuda S, Mochizuki T, Ogata M, et al. Operations for cervical spondylotic myelopathy. A comparison of the results of anterior and posterior procedures. *J Bone Joint Surg Br* 1985;67(4):609–615.
13. Roberts A. Myelopathy due to cervical spondylosis treated by collar immobilization. *Neurology* 1966;16:951–959.
14. Pavlov H, Torg JS, Robie B, et al. Cervical spinal stenosis: determination with vertebral body ratio method. *Radiology* 1987;164(3):771–775.
15. Gore DR, Sepic SB, Gardner GM. Roentgenographic findings of the cervical spine in asymptomatic people. *Spine* 1986;11(6):521–524.
16. McGann GM, Gleeson FV, Kelly I, et al. The influence of needle size on post-myelography headache: a controlled trial. *Br J Radiol* 1992;65(780):1102–1104.
17. Yadav RK, Sharma A, Mishra DS, et al. An evaluation of myelography with non-ionic water soluble contrast medium-iohexol. *J Indian Med Assoc* 1999;97(1):16–19.
18. Hitselberger WE, Witten RM. Abnormal myelograms in asymptomatic patients. *J Neurosurg* 1968;28(3):204–206.
19. Brown BM, Schwartz RH, Frank E, et al. Preoperative evaluation of cervical radiculopathy and myelopathy by surface-coil MR imaging. *AJR Am J Roentgenol* 1988;151(6):1205–1212.
20. Boden SD, McCowin PR, Davis DO, et al. Abnormal magnetic-resonance scans of the cervical spine in asymptomatic subjects. A prospective investigation. *J Bone Joint Surg Am* 1990;72(8):1178–1184.
21. Matsumoto M, Fujimura Y, Suzuki N, et al. MRI of cervical intervertebral discs in asymptomatic subjects. *J Bone Joint Surg Br* 1998;80(1):19–24.
22. Schliep G. Syringomyelia and syringobulbia. In: Vinkin PJ. Bruyn GW, eds. *Handbook of clinical neurology.* Amsterdam: North-Holland, 1978.
23. Agnoli AL, Laun A, Schonmayr R. Enterogenous intraspinal cysts. *J Neurosurg* 1984;61(5):834–840.
24. Phillips WA. Congenital anomalies of the atlantoaxial joint. In: Clark C, ed. *The cervical spine,* 3rd ed. Philadelphia: Lippincott-Raven, 1998:317–329.
25. Pueschel SM, Scola FH. Atlantoaxial instability in individuals with Down syndrome: epidemiologic, radiographic, and clinical studies. *Pediatrics* 1987;80(4):555–560.
26. Davidson RG. Atlantoaxial instability in individuals with Down syndrome: a fresh look at the evidence. *Pediatrics* 1988;81(6):857–865.
27. Keyes DC, EL C. The normal and pathological physiology of the nucleus pulposus of the intervertebral disc. An anatomical, clinical, and experimental study. *J Bone Joint Surg* 1932;14:897–939.
28. Bohlman HH, Emery SE. The pathophysiology of cervical spondylosis and myelopathy. *Spine* 1988;13(7):843–846.
29. Ogino H, Tada K, Okada K, et al. Canal diameter, anteroposterior compression ratio, and spondylotic myelopathy of the cervical spine. *Spine* 1983;8(1):1–15.
30. Veidlinger OF, Colwill JC, Smyth HS, et al. Cervical myelopathy and its relationship to cervical stenosis. *Spine* 1981;6(6):550–552.
31. Taylor AR. The mechanism of injury to the spinal cord in the neck without damage to the vertebral column. *J Bone Joint Surg Am* 1951;33:543–547.

32. Mirich DR, Hall JT, Carrasco CH. MR imaging of traumatic spinal arachnoid cyst. *J Comput Assist Tomogr* 1988;12(5):862–865.

33. Rabb CH, McComb JG, Raffel C, et al. Spinal arachnoid cysts in the pediatric age group: an association with neural tube defects. *J Neurosurg* 1992;77(3):369–372.

34. Fortuna A, La Torre E, Ciappetta P. Arachnoid diverticula: a unitary approach to spinal cysts communicating with the subarachnoid space. *Acta Neurochir* 1977;39(3–4):.

35. Stern JD, Quint DJ, Sweasey TA, et al. Spinal epidural lipomatosis: two new idiopathic cases and a review of the literature. *J Spinal Disord* 1994;7(4):343–349.

36. Poncelet A. The neurologic complications of Paget's disease. *J Bone Miner Res* 1999;14[Suppl 2]:88–91.

37. Yost JH, Spencer-Green G, Krant JD. Vascular steal mimicking compression myelopathy in Paget's disease of bone: rapid reversal with calcitonin and systemic steroids. *J Rheumatol* 1993;20(6):1064–1065.

38. Lee TT, Alameda GJ, Gromelski EB, et al. Outcome after surgical treatment of progressive posttraumatic cystic myelopathy. *J Neurosurg* 2000;92[2 Suppl]:149–154.

39. Marshall LF, Knowlton S, Garfin SR, et al. Deterioration following spinal cord injury. A multicenter study. *J Neurosurg* 1987;66(3):400–404.

40. Shenkin HA, Alpers BJ. Clinical and pathological features of gliomas of the spinal cord. *Arch Neurol Psychiatry* 1944;52:87–105.

41. Anson JA, Spetzler RF. Classification system of spinal arteriovenous malformations and implications for treatment. *BNI Q* 1992;8(2):2–8.

42. Aminoff MJ, Logue V. The prognosis of patients with spinal vascular malformations. *Brain* 1974;97(1):211–218.

43. Dickman CA, Zabramski JM, Sonntag VK, et al. Myelopathy due to epidural varicose veins of the cervicothoracic junction. Case report. *J Neurosurg* 1988;69(6):940–941.

44. Ropper AH, Poskanzer DC. The prognosis of acute and subacute transverse myelopathy based on early signs and symptoms. *Ann Neurol* 1978;4(1):51–59.

45. Miller DH, McDonald WI, Blumhardt LD, et al. Magnetic resonance imaging in isolated noncompressive spinal cord syndromes. *Ann Neurol* 1987;22(6):714–723.

46. Choi KH, Lee KS, Chung SO, et al. Idiopathic transverse myelitis: MR characteristics. *AJNR Am J Neuroradiol* 1996;17(6):1151–1160.

47. Sebire G, Hollenberg H, Meyer L, et al. High dose methylprednisolone in severe acute transverse myelitis. *Arch Dis Child* 1997;76(2):167–168.

48. Lumsden CE. Multiple sclerosis and other demyelinating diseases. In: Vinkin PJ, Bruyn GW, eds. *Handbook of clinical neurology*. Amsterdam: North-Holland, 1970:217–319.

49. Poser S, Herrmann-Gremmels I, Wikstrom J, et al. Clinical features of the spinal form of multiple sclerosis. *Acta Neurol Scand* 1978;57(2):151–158.

50. Leibowitz U, Halpern L, Alter M. Clinical studies of multiple sclerosis in Israel. 5. Progressive spinal syndromes and multiple sclerosis. *Neurology* 1967;17(10):988–992.

51. Cecil RL, Goldman L, Bennett JC, et al. *Cecil textbook of medicine*, Vol 2. Philadelphia: WB Saunders, 2000.

52. Nadeau SE. Neurologic manifestations of connective tissue disease. *Neurol Clin* 2002;20(1):151–178.

53. Lorber A, Perason CM, Rene RM. Osteolytic vertebral lesions as a manifestation of rheumatoid arthritis and related disorders. *Arthritis Rheum* 1961;4:514.

54. Castro S, Verstraete K, Mielants H, et al. Cervical spine involvement in rheumatoid arthritis: a clinical, neurological and radiological evaluation. *Clin Exp Rheumatol* 1994;12(4):369–374.

55. Weissman BN, Aliabadi P, Weinfeld MS, et al. Prognostic features of atlantoaxial subluxation in rheumatoid arthritis patients. *Radiology* 1982;144(4):745–751.

56. Casey AT, Crockard HA, Bland JM, et al. Surgery on the rheumatoid cervical spine for the non-ambulant myelopathic patient-too much, too late? *Lancet* 1996;347(9007):1004–1007.

57. Alexander EL, Malinow K, Lejewski JE, et al. Primary Sjögren's syndrome with central nervous system disease mimicking multiple sclerosis. *Ann Intern Med* 1986;104(3):323–330.

58. Vinas FC, Rengachary S, Kupsky WJ. Spinal cord sarcoidosis: a diagnostic dilemma. *Neurol Res* 2001;23(4):347–352.

59. Cacoub P, Sbai A, Hausfater P, et al. [Spinal cord involvement revealing systemic sarcoidosis]. *Rev Neurol* (Paris) 2000;156(10):784–788.

60. Healton EB, Savage DG, Brust JC, et al. Neurologic aspects of cobalamin deficiency. *Medicine* (Baltimore) 1991;70(4):229–245.

61. Yengue P, Adler M, Bouhdid H, et al. Hepatic myelopathy after splenorenal shunting: report of one case and review of the literature. *Acta Gastroenterol Belg* 2001;64(2):231–233.

62. Walker AE. Toxic effect of intrathecal administration of penicillin. *Arch Neurol Psychiatry* 1947;58:39–45.

63. Schultz P, Schwarz GA. Radiculomyelopathy following intrathecal instillation of methylene blue. A hazard reaffirmed. *Arch Neurol* 1970;22(3):240–244.

64. Luddy RE, Gilman PA. Paraplegia following intrathecal methotrexate. *J Pediatr* 1973;83(6):988–992.

65. Saiki JH, Thompson S, Smith F, et al. Paraplegia following intrathecal chemotherapy. *Cancer* 1972;29(2):370–374.

66. Smith HV, Spalding JMK. Outbreak of paralysis in Morocco due to ortho-cresyl phosphate poisoning. *Lancet* 1959;2:1019–1021.

67. Dastur DK. Lathyrism. Some aspect of the disease in man and animals. *World Neurol* 1962;3:721–730.

68. Dalmau JO, Posner JB. Paraneoplastic syndromes affecting the nervous system. *Semin Oncol* 1997;24(3):318–328.

69. Wilkinson PC, Zeromski J. Immunofluorescent detection of antibodies against neurones in sensory carcinomatous neuropathy. *Brain* 1965;88(3):529–583.

70. Helweg-Larsen S, Jakobsen J, Boesen F, et al. Neurological complications and concomitants of AIDS. *Acta Neurol Scand* 1986;74(6):467–474.

71. Petito CK, Navia BA, Cho ES, et al. Vacuolar myelopathy pathologically resembling subacute combined degeneration in patients with the acquired immunodeficiency syndrome. *N Engl J Med* 1985;312(14):874–879.

72. Kaplan JE, Osame M, Kubota H, et al. The risk of development of HTLV-I-associated myelopathy/tropical spastic paraparesis among persons infected with HTLV-I. *J Acquir Immune Defic Syndr* 1990;3(11):1096–1101.

73. Gessain A, Gout O. Chronic myelopathy associated with human T-lymphotropic virus type I (HTLV-I). *Ann Intern Med* 1992;117(11):933–946.

74. Roman GC, Roman LN. Tropical spastic paraparesis. A clinical study of 50 patients from Tumaco (Colombia) and review of the worldwide features of the syndrome. *J Neurol Sci* 1988;87(1):121–138.

75. Osame M, Matsumoto M, Usuku K, et al. Chronic progressive myelopathy associated with elevated antibodies to human T-lymphotropic virus type I and adult T-cell leukemialike cells. *Ann Neurol* 1987;21(2):117–122.

76. Harrington WJ Jr, Sheremata WA, Snodgrass SR, et al. Tropical spastic paraparesis/HTLV-1-associated myelopathy (TSP/HAM): treatment with an anabolic steroid danazol. *AIDS Res Hum Retroviruses* 1991;7(12):1031–1034.

77. Celik Y, Tabak F, Mert A, et al. Transverse myelitis caused by Varicella. *Clin Neurol Neurosurg* 2001;103(4):260–261.

78. Miles C, Hoffman W, Lai CW, et al. Cytomegalovirus-associated transverse myelitis. *Neurology* 1993;43(10):2143–2145.

79. Terry PM, Glancy GR, Graham A. Meningovascular syphilis of the spinal cord presenting with incomplete Brown-Séquard syndrome: case report. *Genitourin Med* 1989;65(3):189–191.

80. Roos KL. Neurosyphilis. *Semin Neurol* 1992;12(3):209–212.

81. Haran MJ, Jenney AW, Keenan RJ, et al. Paraplegia secondary to Burkholderia pseudomallei myelitis: a case report. *Arch Phys Med Rehabil* 2001;82(11):1630–1632.

82. Salgado CD, Weisse ME. Transverse myelitis associated with probable cat-scratch disease in a previously healthy pediatric patient. *Clin Infect Dis* 2000;31(2):609–611.

83. Yousif B, Nelson J. Neurobrucellosis—a rare complication of renal transplantation. *Am J Nephrol* 2001;21(1):66–68.

84. Levine NS, Atkins A, McKeel DW Jr, et al. Spinal cord injury following electrical accidents: case reports. *J Trauma* 1975;15(5):459–463.

85. Varghese G, Mani MM, Redford JB. Spinal cord injuries following electrical accidents. *Paraplegia* 1986;24(3):159–166.

86. Clouston PD, Sharpe D. Rapid recovery after delayed myelopathy from electrical burns. *J Neurol Neurosurg Psychiatry* 1989;52(11):1308.

87. Schultheiss TE, Stephens LC. Invited review: permanent radiation myelopathy. *Br J Radiol* 1992;65(777):737–753.

88. Greer HD, Massey EW. Neurologic injury from undersea diving. *Neurol Clin* 1992;10(4):1031–1045.

89. Newton HB. Neurologic complications of scuba diving. *Am Fam Physician* 2001;63(11):2211–2218.

CHAPTER 16

Diagnosis of Cervical Spine Disorders: Neurophysiologic Tests

Jiří Dvořák, Stan Vohanka, and Martin Sutter

Patients with cervical spinal disorders, with or without symptoms and signs, often show discrepancies between clinical and neuroradiologic (magnetic resonance imaging [MRI], computed tomography [CT], myelogram) findings that make it difficult to pinpoint the cause (such as a particular nerve root or spinal cord segment) of the patient's complaints. The common pathology associated with degenerative changes is presented in Figure 16.1 (1).

Neurophysiologic examinations should help answer the following questions in patients with cervical spinal disorders:

- Which neural elements are involved?
- Which spinal segment is responsible for a mechanical or other irritation?
- Is the lesion chronic, acute, or progressing, or has neural function improved?
- Is another disorder present that may be responsible for the patient's complaints (e.g., carpal tunnel syndrome)?
- Are abnormal imaging findings relevant if clinical findings are absent (e.g., detection of subclinical lesion)?

CURRENTLY USED ELECTRODIAGNOSTIC TECHNIQUES

The spectrum of neurophysiologic assessment consists of needle electromyography (EMG), electroneurography (ENG), and evoked potentials. Although the somatosensory evoked potentials (SSEPs) and motor evoked potentials (MEPs) are most helpful in the investigation of the central nervous system pathways, EMG, conventional neurography and F-wave studies are useful for evaluation of the peripheral segments of the sensory and motor pathways. Therefore, the clinical examination determines the

neurophysiologic tests accordingly. To perform all possible tests is not feasible in daily practice because of compliance of the patient and also the time involved with examination performance. The clinician should ask the questions as precisely as possible and indicate the suspected clinical diagnosis in order to facilitate the neurophysiologic examination.

Table 16.1 shows the different neurophysiologic tests together with the neural structures they assess.

SOMATOSENSORY EVOKED POTENTIALS

For spinal cord evaluation, SSEPs are most relevant. These are potentials recorded from the lumbar and cervical spine as well as the first components of scalp recordings.

Generally, the sensitivity of the method in the evaluation of radicular lesions is restricted because localized signal deceleration is diluted (masked) by normal conduction in other parts of the somatosensory pathway.

SSEPs are generally recorded after electrical stimulation of peripheral nerves or skin (dermatomal SSEPs). The nerves used are the posterior tibial, sural, or common peroneal nerves of the lower limbs and the median radial and ulnar nerve for the upper limbs. In radicular and in spinal disease, several nerves, which are supplied by different segments, must be stimulated for a level diagnosis. SSEPs from the tibialis nerve are recommended for the diagnosis of cervical myelopathy (2).

SSEPs from stimulation of the tibial nerve were delayed in cervical spondylosis, particularly the N11 component. However, similar data had also been reported previously in electrical cortical stimulation studies (3,4). The value of SSEPs was extensively studied from a prognostic point of view (5,6).

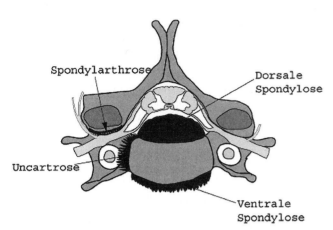

Spondylarthrose

Dorsale
Spondylose

Uncartrose

Ventrale
Spondylose

FIG. 16.1. Schematic drawing of common pathology due to degenerative changes of the cervical spine, possibly leading to compression of neural structures. Appropriate neurophysiologic examinations to assess the function of nerve root and spinal cord. EMG, electromyography; MEP, motor evoked potentials; SEP sensory evoked potentials; F wave. (From Dvorak J, Grob D. *Halswirbelsäule: Diagnostik und Therapie.* Stuttgart, New York: Thieme-Verlag, 1999:1–352, with permission.)

MOTOR EVOKED POTENTIALS

A method of painless magnetoelectric transcranial stimulation of the cerebral cortex was introduced in 1985 by Barker et al (7,8). They applied short magnetic pulses, designed to stimulate peripheral nerves, to the scalp and recorded muscle action potentials from upper and lower limb muscles.

The coil is placed to stimulate the motor cortex, the cervical nerve roots, and the lumbar nerve roots. MEPs are generally recorded at the following muscles: abductor pollicis, adductor minimi, quadriceps, tibialis anterior, gastrocnemius, extensor hallucis, and abductor hallucis (9). The segmental innervation of these muscles is used for a level diagnosis analogous to the segmental distribution of the afferent nerves stimulated for SSEPs. Surface recording electrodes are placed over the motor end plate (9).

For motor root stimulation over the cervical and lumbar spine, the intensity of the stimulator is adjusted so that a po-

tential with a steep negative rise can be recorded. With this, the onset latency is not critically dependent on the positioning of the coil or the stimulation strength (10). The excitation site of the nerve root is most likely in the region of the root exit from the intervertebral foramen and does not differ from that suggested for electric stimulation over the spine (10–12). In patients with a lateral compression of the nerve root, the peripheral nerve latency is not delayed, whereas in patients with more medially localized herniations, a prolonged CML is the most frequent finding (13).

M-WAVE AND F-WAVE EVALUATION FOR THE INTERPRETATION OF MOTOR EVOKED POTENTIALS

M Wave

To judge the MEP waveform, it is also necessary to obtain an M wave or compound muscle action potential (CMAP) recording by means of conventional electrical stimulation. The M wave is the response to a supramaximal stimulus of the peripheral nerve and therefore an electric measure of muscle "size" (14). It is used as a reference signal with which posttranscranial stimulation MEP amplitude and duration are compared (i.e., MEP amplitude and duration are expressed as ratios of M-wave amplitude and duration, respectively).

F Wave

F-wave recordings allow for the determination of total peripheral conduction time, or peripheral latency (PL), from the anterior horn cell to the muscle, which includes the conduction over the motor root to its exit from the intervertebral foramen.

Because the excitability of the spinal motor neuron fluctuates periodically, the appearance, latency, and amplitude of the F wave changes in each record. The difference between the shortest and longest latencies, or the *chronodispersion*, and the number of elicited waves after given number of stimuli, or the *persistence* (expressed as percentage), are routinely evaluated parameters.

TABLE 16.1. *Neurophysiological Techniques Used for Evaluation of Different Neural Structures*

Neurophysiological technique	Neural structures evaluated
Somatosensory evoked potentials (SEPs)	Sensory nerve fibers and dorsal roots, spinal cord dorsal columns
Motor evoked potentials (MEPs)	Corticospinal tract (lateral spinal cord), motor roots and motor nerve fibers
Neurography	Motor and sensory nerve fibers
F-wave	Motor roots, motor nerve fibers
H-reflex	Dorsal and motor roots, sensory and motor nerve fibers
Electromyography (EMG) of limb muscles	Motor roots and motor nerve fibers
Electromyography (EMG) of paraspinal muscles	Motor roots

(From Dvorak et al. 1996.)

The F wave is usually normal in mild cases of radiculopathy. Distinct delay of the F wave or a reduced number of clearly distinguishable F waves after a given number of supramaximal peripheral stimuli, yet normal distal motor conduction studies, is a sign of a proximal lesion. The large delay of F-wave shortest latency is typical for proximal or diffuse demyelinating lesions such as CIDP syndrome or hereditary Charcot-Marie-Tooth neuropathies. Typical findings for compressive-ischemic root lesion are absence or decreased persistence, mild prolongation of short latency, and prolonged chronodispersion. Generally sensitivity of this test in root lesions is low. Despite these limitations, F waves have a diagnostic value for anterior root lesions. When F waves are recorded in a chronic neuropathic process, axonal reflexes must be differentiated (15,16).

ELECTROMYOGRAPHY

Needle EMG examines segmentally affected muscles (chosen on the bases of clinical investigation). The needle is repositioned on 10 different sites in a muscle so as not to miss denervated parts. Increased insertional activity, spontaneous activity (involuntary) such as sharp positive waves, fibrillations, fasciculations, and diminished motor unit recruitment are signs of denervation.

In normal muscles, motor unit action potentials are elicited only in response to neural discharges. Denervated muscle fibers become unstable because they are no longer under neural control, and individual muscle fibers fire in the absence of neural stimuli. These signs of denervation in the EMG can be spotted at the earliest about 8 days after the nerve lesion and are termed *acute signs* of denervation.

EMG performed with needle concentric electrodes is the oldest neurophysiologic method to diagnosis nerve root compression syndrome and is considered the gold standard (17). EMG is claimed to have almost no false-positive results (18). Diagnostic limitations of needle EMG can be summarized as follows: EMG detects reliably acute motor axonal loss (if the reinnervation is considered a sign of chronic root lesion, the diagnostic sensitivity increases, but the rate of the false-positive findings also increases). EMG is not able to diagnose the sensory axonal loss and focal proximal conduction block. The innervation of the cervical paraspinal musculature is poorly localized, but denervation potentials in the paraspinal muscles can indicate lesions that are located at the levels of the nerve root or the spinal cord (19).

EMG is important in the differential diagnosis of cervical spondylosis. It shows degrees of denervation and the number of roots involved, but it has no prognostic value (19).

The increase latency of MEPs is a sensitive sign; however, the specificity is low. The increased central motor latency can be found in the degenerative but also inflammatory diseases of the central nervous system such as multiple sclerosis. Kameyama and associates examined 67 patients with clinically relevant cervical myelopathy and 24 patients with cervical canal stenosis without myelopathy (20) and found a positive correlation for the group of myelopathy patients. De Mattei and co-workers found a sensitivity of MEP in patients with cervical compression myelopathy of 70% for upper extremity muscles and of 95% for lower extremity muscles (21).

The correlation between an imaging method (MRI) and needle EMG was the focus of a paper by Nardin and colleagues (22), who concluded, based on examination of 47 patients with cervical and lumbar radiculopathy, that needle EMG and MRI are complementary diagnostic methods. A good correlation was found among patients with an abnormal neurologic examination, but the confirmation of the mild radiculopathy was poor.

Tanaka and associates examined MEPs in patients with clinically relevant cervical myelopathy who underwent decompressive surgery (23). Patients who presented with central motor latency longer than 15 ms or a polyphasic wave pattern of the potential had worse surgical results than remaining patients.

The differentiation of anterior horn cell disease and the cervical spinal myelopathy comparing the EMG and dermatomal SSEP assessed by Kang (1995) clearly pointed out the superiority of the dermatomal SSEPs, which, as expected, were normal in all 12 patients with amyotrophic lateral sclerosis, whereas in 19 of 20 patients with cervical myelopathy, a pathologic finding was observed.

For cervical myelopathy, Vohanka and Dvorak suggested the routine use of SSEPs from stimulation of the tibial nerve as well as MEPs from upper and lower extremities (2).

SSEPs (especially in combination with MEPs) are a reliable tool in the assessment of subclinical spondylotic cervical cord compression. Normal initial evoked potential findings predict a favorable 2-year clinical outcome (6). On the other hand, in patients with clinical signs of cervical myelopathy (mild to moderate), correlation between clinical postsurgical outcome and evoked potential parameters yielded conflicting data, and authors concluded (5) at longitudinal evoked potentials have limited use in the evaluation of therapy results. The group changes of some SSEP and MEP parameters correlated with the changes in clinical score, but between individuals, the correlation was poor.

REFERENCES

1. Dvorak J, Grob D. *Halswirbelsäule: Diagnostik und Therapie.* Stuttgart, New York: Georg Thieme Verlag, 1999:1–352.
2. Vohanka S, Dvorak J. Motor and somatosensory evoked potentials in cervical spinal stenosis. In: 40th Congress of the Czech and Slovak Neurophysiology, Brno, 1993.
3. Abbruzzese G, et al. Electrical stimulation of the motor tracts in cervical spondylosis. *J Neurol Neurosurg Psychiatry* 1988;51:796–802.
4. Esteban GR, Lagranja AR, Lopez MAC. Delayed short-latency somatosensory evoked potentials in premature diagnosis of medullary disturbances in cervical spondylosis. *Electromyogr Clin Neurophysiol* 1988; 28:361–368.
5. Bednarik J, et al. The value of somatosensory and motor evoked evoked potentials in pre-clinical spondylotic cervical cord compression. *Eur Spine J* 1998;7(6):493–500.

6. Bednarik J, et al. The value of somatosensory- and motor-evoked potentials in predicting and monitoring the effect of therapy in spondylotic cervical myelopathy. Prospective randomized study. *Spine* 1999; 24(15):1593–1598.

7. Barker AT, et al. Magneic stimulation of the human brain. *J Physiol* 1985;369:3P.

8. Barker AT, Jalinous R, Freeston IL. Non-invasive magnetic stimulation of the human motor cortex. *Lancet* 1985;1:1106–1107.

9. Chomiak J, et al. Motor evoked potentials: appropriate positioning of recording electrodes for diagnosis of spinal disorders. *Eur Spine J* 1995;4:180–185.

10. Britton TC, et al. Clinical use of the magnetic stimulator in the investigation of peripheral conduction time. *Muscle Nerve* 1990;13:396–406.

11. Cadwell J. Principles of magnetoelectric stimulation. In: Chokroverty S, ed. *Magnetic stimulation in clinical meurophysiology.* Boston: Butterworths, 1989:13–32.

12. Mills KR, Murray NMF. Electrical stimulation over the human vertebral column: which neuronal elements are exited? *Electroencephalogr Clin Neurophysiol* 1986;63:582–589.

13. Bischoff C. et al. The value of magnetic stimulation in the diagnosis of radiculopathies. *Muscle Nerve* 1993;16(2):154–161.

14. Reiners K, Herdmann J, Freund HJ. Altered mechanisms of muscular force generation in lower motor neuron disease. *Muscle Nerve* 1989; 12:647–659.

15. Kimura J. F-wave velocity in the central segment of the median and ulnar nerves: a study in normal subjects and patients with Charcot-Marie-Tooth disease. *Neurology* 1974;24:539–546.

16. Roth G. Intranervous regeneration of lower motor neuron. II. Study of 1153 motor axon reflexes. Second part: contralateral motor axon reflex crossed facial reinnervation. *Electromyogr Clin Neurophysiol* 1978;18(5):311–350.

17. Shea P, Woods W, Werden D. Electromyography in diagnosis of nerve root compression syndrome. *Arch Neurol Psychiatr* 1950;64:93–104.

18. Wilbourn A, Aminoff M. AAEE Mini Monograph #32: The electrophysiological examination in patinets with radiculopathies. *Muscle Nerve* 1988;11:1011–1014.

19. Negrin P, Lelli S, Fardin P. Contribution of electromyography to the diagnosis, treatment and prognosis of cervical disc disease: a study of 114 patients. *Electromyogr Clin Neurophysiol* 1991;31(3):173–179.

20. Kameyama O, et al. Transcranial magnetic stimulation of the motor cortex in cervical spondylosis and spinal canal stenosis. *Spine* 1995; 20:1004–1010.

21. De Mattei M, et al. Usefulness of motor evoked potentials in compressive myelopathy. *Electromyogr Clin Neurophysiol* 1993;33(4):205–216.

22. Nardin RA, et al. Electromyography and magnetic resonance imaging in the evaluation of radiculopathy. *Muscle Nerve* 1999;22(2):151–155.

23. Tanaka M, et al. The evaluation of motor evoked potentials (MEPs) by magnetic stimulation in cervical spondylotic myelopathy. *Neuro-Orthopaedics* 1999;25:75–89.

CHAPTER 17

Multimodal Intraoperative Monitoring During Cervical Spine Surgery

Martin Sutter and Jiří Dvořák

Injury of the spinal cord and nerve roots is an inherent risk with surgical treatment of the spine and may lead to serious individual, social, and medicolegal consequences. To avoid complications and improve the quality of surgical procedures, the monitoring of the integrity of the central and peripheral nervous system during spinal surgery has become an important tool. In the 1970s, the intraoperative wake-up test was used with corrective surgery of the spine (1). This was subsequently replaced by somatosensory evoked potential (SSEP) testing during the 1980s and 1990s. Both have clearly been shown to provide relatively high false-positive and false-negative values in predicting postoperative neurologic outcome (2,3).

These methods are, therefore, being increasingly replaced by electrophysiologic multimodal intraoperative monitoring (MIOM), which assesses the descending motor as well as the ascending sensory pathways, at various combinations of sites on the neurologic structure at risk.

At Schulthess Clinic in Switzerland, MIOM has been used in surgery of the cervical spine for selected cases on a routine basis since the year 2000. During the period of January 2000 to June 2003, the combined monitoring of motor evoked potentials (MEPs) and SSEPs was used in a total of 514 spinal operations, of which 131 patients had undergone cervical spine and spinal cord surgery. In this chapter, an overview of the methods and techniques are presented. MIOM has become one of the tools that can be used to achieve the surgical goal of safety.

HISTORY

SSEPs were introduced in the 1940s (4) but have only been used in clinical practice since the 1970s (5). SSEP assesses sensory impulse conduction in the dorsal column,

lemniscal pathway, thalamus, and parietal cortex. In a large multicenter survey, intraoperative SSEP monitoring during scoliosis surgery was shown to reduce significantly postoperative neural deficits such as paraparesis and paraplegia (6). However, spinal cord monitoring with SSEP has clear limitations and documented false-negative results (2,3). It reflects only sensory ascending pathways and the dorsal vascular supply of the spinal cord, not the integrity of upper (corticospinal tract) and lower motoneurons (nerve roots) and the anterior spinal artery supply. After basic physiologic research in the 1950s (7), MEPs with spinal cord recordings were introduced for clinical diagnostic examinations (8) and for monitoring scoliosis surgery (9) in the 1980s. The direct spinal cord stimulation and recording technique (spinal cord evoked potentials, SCEPs) had already been introduced in the early 1970s by Tamaki et al (10) and Kurokawa (11). Spinal electrodes allow the simultaneous recording of spinal SSEPs and cortical somatosensory evoked potentials (CSEPs). Corticomuscular and spinomuscular evoked potentials reveal information about the functioning of the upper and lower motoneuron as well as neuromuscular transmission. They are recorded by compound muscle action potentials (CMAPs). This technique has become possible by using modern electrical stimulator techniques. These provide short repetitive trains of single stimuli. The introduction of intravenous anesthesia, as with propofol or ketamine, in combination with short-acting opioids has also facilitated the process (12).

PRINCIPLES OF MOTOR AND SENSORY EVOKED POTENTIALS

The neural structures to be stimulated and recording sites (cortex, spinal cord, nerves, muscles) must be chosen

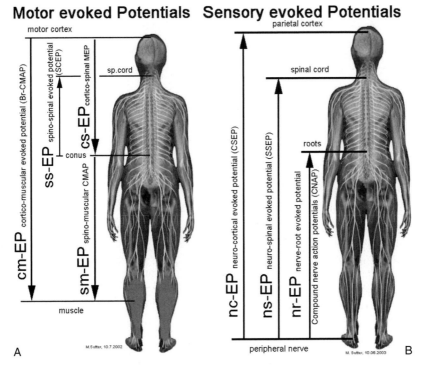

FIG. 17.1. Stimulation and recording sites for motor evoked potential and somatosensory evoked potentials.

at the spinal cord segment that innervates the muscles and nerves of diagnostic interest and the potentials traveling through the neural structures of any anticipated injury (Fig. 17.1). Reliable monitoring should be performed on both the right and left sides and proximal as well as distal to the site of risk, to distinguish systemic changes (e.g., anesthetic, perfusion, temperature) from direct surgery-related changes. The same scalp needle electrodes can be used for transcranial electrical motor stimulation in corticomuscular or corticospinal evoked potentials as well as for recording neurocortical evoked potentials (or CSEPs). The same epidural or subarachnoid spinal electrodes can be used rostrally for recording the neurospinal evoked potentials (or spinal SSEPs) and spinospinal evoked potentials (or SCEPs) and also for stimulating spinomuscular evoked potentials (or spinal motor evoked potentials, SMEPs) and for control recordings in corticospinal evoked potentials. The same distal spinal electrode primarily used for monitoring the corticospinal tract in corticospinal evoked potentials can be used as a control in recording the neurospinal evoked potentials (or spinal SSEPs) and as the stimulation site in spinospinal evoked potentials (or SCEPs). In cervical spine surgery, the recording of CMAPs from peripheral muscles in corticomuscular and spinomuscular evoked potentials in the upper extremities yields information about ventral nerve root innervation and, at the legs, primarily information

of the corticospinal tract. The peripheral nerves and dermatomes are often selected as well.

EQUIPMENT

MIOM requires close collaboration between the neurologist, surgeon, and anesthetist. The neurologist or electrophysiologist performing the MIOM must have a clear understanding of the surgical procedure and its specific risks to accomplish adequate interpretation of the electrophysiologic results. The equipment for MIOM is the same as that used for SSEP monitoring or regular preoperative electrophysiologic examinations. A conventional electromyography (EMG) recording device with a four- or eight-channel amplifier and two stimulators is used for MIOM (Fig. 17.2A). Stimulation of peripheral nerves in SSEP and recording of compound muscle action potentials in MEP is normally done using surface electrodes (Fig. 17.2B). The same monopolar needle electrodes (e.g., 0.7 mm diameter, 30 mm length) (Fig. 17.2C) can be used at C3 and C4 (electroencephalogram, 10–20 system) for cortical motor stimulation and recording of cortical sensory evoked potentials. Bipolar spinal electrodes are placed in the subarachnoid space or epidurally for electrical stimulation or recording. They are introduced either preoperatively by lumbar puncture or intraoperatively by the surgeon (Fig. 17.2D). The mounting of electrodes and cables is carried

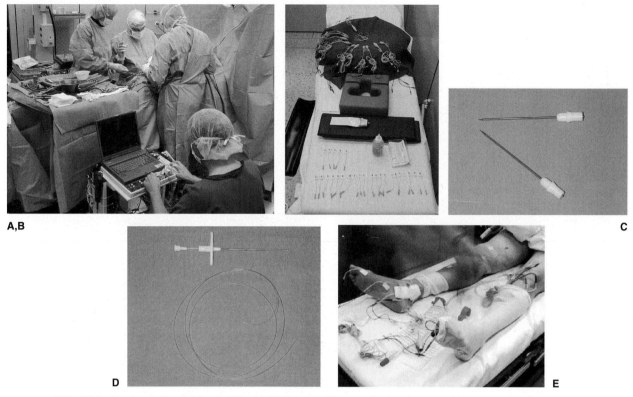

A,B

C

D

E

FIG. 17.2. Equipment used for multimodal intraoperative monitoring (see text).

out at the same time as induction of anesthesia (Fig. 17.2E). With an experienced team, this may prolong the presurgical procedure by up to 15 minutes, depending on whether a spinal electrode is to be used already at the beginning of surgery with a dorsal approach or in procedures with a primarily ventral approach.

DIFFERENT MODALITIES USED IN SPINAL CORD MONITORING

Motor Evoked Potentials

Electrical scalp stimulation can activate the corticospinal tract and evoke a synchronized stable D (direct) wave followed by various I (indirect, transsynaptically activated) waves that are recorded along the spinal cord (7). As a result of general anesthesia, the recording of peripheral muscle activation is more difficult. It is possible, however, after the introduction of a short train of transcranial electrical stimulation (13). The use of intravenous anesthesia is preferred over inhalation anesthetics. This is usually performed with propofol or ketamine, in combination with short-acting opioids (14). Intraoperative MEPs can also be elicited by trains of transcranial magnetic stimulation (15), but electrical stimulation with scalp needle electrodes leads

to much more reliable and reproducible potentials. They are easier to perform as well.

Corticomuscular Evoked Potentials

In corticomuscular evoked potentials (Fig. 17.3), the motor cortex is stimulated transcranially (C3-C4 resp. C4-C3) and is recorded at the contralateral muscles simultaneously. Stimulation is usually performed with trains of five single stimuli, each of 0.2 ms (0.2 to 0.7 ms) duration, 100 mA (50 to 200 mA) intensity, and an interstimulus interval of 2.5 ms (2 to 5 ms). The stimulus trains are repeated one per second (1/s), and two to six evoked CMAPs may be averaged.

Naturally, the monitoring of corticomuscular evoked potentials must be performed without muscle relaxants. Because corticomuscular evoked potentials may lead to significant muscle twitches, the surgeon should be informed before performing this test. For quantitative analysis of CMAP, supramaximal motor stimulations are used.

Corticomuscular evoked potentials should not be performed in patients with a history of epilepsy or acute or subacute stroke because they may provoke seizures. In our collective experience of 514 patients with MIOM, one seizure was observed in a patient who had no history of epilepsy. This was interrupted promptly with a bolus of

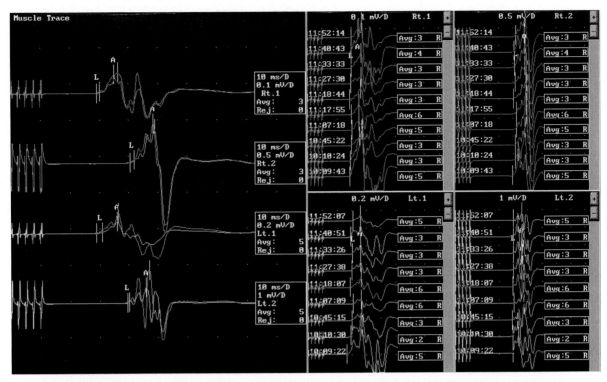

FIG. 17.3. Time course (from bottom to top) of simultaneously recorded corticomuscular evoked potentials of tibial anterior and abductor hallucis muscles. Traces of muscles: Rt.1, tibialis anterior muscle right; Rt.2, abductor hallucis muscle right; Lt.1, tibialis anterior muscle left; Lt.2, abductor hallucis muscle left.

propofol. Two surface electrodes on each peripheral muscle are necessary to record CMAPs. Latency, amplitude, and shape of each CMAP are analyzed. In general, 50-Hz and 3-kHz filters are used for recording, but in computer-assisted surgery, 50-Hz and 0.3-kHz filter settings may be required to reduce dual-current artifacts. For accurate trend analysis, stimulus intensity and recording filters must not be changed during the surgical procedure. To identify surgically related changes, the recording of two to four muscle pairs should be performed simultaneously. Depending on the cervical surgical procedure, three muscle pairs are usually used for monitoring cervical root function, and one muscle pair on the legs is used for monitoring the corticospinal tract. The tests are usually repeated at 5-minute intervals for accurate trend analysis and on surgical demand.

Corticomuscular evoked potentials are highly sensitive for surgical as well as global systemic changes because they always reflect upper and lower motoneuron and neuromuscular transmission. During long surgical procedures, CMAP amplitudes may gradually decline as a result of arterial hypotension, temperature loss, or accumulation of drug metabolites. In patients who already have a severe neurologic deficit, monitoring with corticomuscular evoked potentials may be difficult, even at the beginning of the surgical procedure. Loss of CMAP in spinal surgery indicates a functional deficit of a nerve root or its corticospinal supply.

If signals of corticospinal (D waves) or spinospinal (SCEPs) evoked potentials are unchanged in lower motoneuron dysfunction, as with cervical spine monitoring, the corticomuscular evoked potential recording of different muscle groups, together with corticospinal evoked potentials, allows true level diagnosis of lesions of the corticospinal tract, considering that anterior horn cells are located one half to one level above the cervical spine segment. For corticomuscular evoked potentials, the sternocleidomastoid (C2, C3, C4), deltoid (C4, C5), biceps brachii or brachioradialis (C5, C6), triceps brachii or extensor digitorum communis (C7), and abductor digiti minimi (C8, T1) muscles allow relatively selective nerve root monitoring. In cervical spine surgery, the abductor hallucis (S1, S2), or, if there is concomitant polyneuropathy or radiculopathy, the tibialis anterior (L5, L4) or vastus medialis (L4, L3) muscles may be used for monitoring the corticospinal tract. For nerve root or plexus monitoring, combined medial, ulnar, radial, and musculocutaneus nerve SSEP monitoring may be necessary to identify and localize nerve and root lesions.

Corticospinal Evoked Potentials

In corticospinal evoked potentials, transcranial electrical stimulation is carried out using the same monopolar needle electrodes at C3-C4 as in corticomuscular evoked potentials for the right corticospinal tract and at C4-C3 for the left corticospinal tract (Fig. 17.4). Stimulation with single stimuli of 0.2 ms duration, 100 mA (50 to 200 mA) intensity, repeated 3/s, are usually used to elicit D waves (indicating direct activation of the corticospinal tract). With transcranial electrical stimulation, only few I waves (indicating indirect, transsynaptic activation of corticospinal tract) are elicited.

In Figure 17.4, 5 to 52 potentials have been averaged using a filter setting of 500 Hz and 3 kHz. Caudal to the T12 level, corticospinal evoked potentials show increasing polyphasic and decreasing amplitudes, indicating compound nerve action potentials (CNAPs) of the nerve roots at the level of the conus medullaris and cauda equina. The latency (L) and baseline to negative peak amplitude (A) of the averaged D waves are analyzed for quantitative trend monitoring. Tests of each corticospinal tract are usually repeated at 5-minute intervals for quantitative trend analysis, or on surgical demand. D waves are usually highly stable potentials during the whole surgical procedure and allow monitoring of the corticospinal tracts, even in severe neurologic deficits and when the patient needs intraoperative muscle relaxation (and when corticomuscular evoked potential monitoring is therefore not possible).

Gradual reductions of the amplitude to 50% during long-lasting operations are usually not associated with clinical signs, but sudden changes of as little as 5% to 10% of the amplitude, in combination with deformity of the potential, may indicate postoperative central paresis. Persistent loss of the D waves at the end of the operation usually is associated with limb paraplegia or tetraplegia, depending on the level and laterality of the alteration.

Spinal electrodes for D-wave recording may be placed intraoperatively in the epidural or subarachnoidal space. In ventral surgical procedures, or when there is a need for monitoring the surgical dorsal approach, a subarachnoid spinal electrode can easily be introduced in the subarachnoid space after a lumbar puncture (16). Use of rostral and caudal spine electrodes can help distinguish cortical or systemic involvement from purely spinal cord damage (important in spinal vascular disorders and spinalis anterior syndrome). Corticospinal evoked potentials can be performed without relevant muscle twitches and without disrupting the surgeon.

Spinomuscular Evoked Potentials

Spinomuscular evoked potentials (Fig. 17.5) are elicited by placing an epidural or subarachnoidal bipolar spinal electrode on the spinal cord. The potentials are recorded from the muscles using surface electrodes. For recording pattern, the same is true as for corticomuscular evoked po-

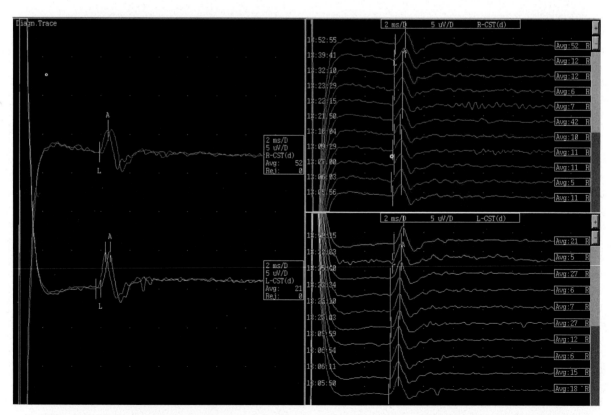

FIG. 17.4. Time course (from bottom to top) of cortical somatosensory evoked potentials showing normal D waves followed by few I waves. R-CST, right corticospinal tract; L-CST, left corticospinal tract.

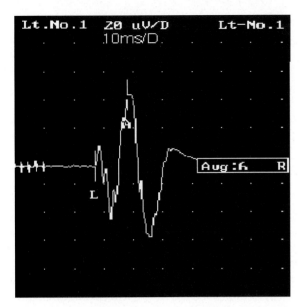

FIG. 17.5. Single spinomuscular evoked potential as elicited from spinal cord at level T10 and recorded from left tibialis anterior muscle.

tentials. Direct stimulation of the spinal cord must be done very carefully. The current is slowly and gradually increased and should be limited to 15 mA because of severe muscle twitches. Spinomuscular evoked potentials should not be performed on the craniocervical junction because of the risk for accidental stimulation of vagus nuclei. Stimulus duration is 0.2 ms for repeated single stimuli, and trains of up to five stimuli are usually repeated 1/s.

Depending on lateral positioning of the spinal electrode, the spinomuscular evoked potential may elicit CMAPs asymmetric to the limbs. Evidence of preserved spinomuscular evoked potentials to the legs is mainly helpful in the differentiation between upper corticospinal tract lesions and systemic or metabolic disorders and, in combination with corticomuscular, corticospinal, spinospinal, and neurospinal evoked potentials, allows true level diagnosis. This spinomuscular evoked potential test setting is also used for selective nerve root, tissue, or pedicle screw stimulation tests done with monopolar needle or bipolar stimulators. Repetition rate of the stimuli in these cases is higher (5.9/s) to obtain faster results.

Continuous Electromyography

Continuous EMG recordings can be made with the same surface muscle recordings and filter settings as corticomuscular or spinomuscular evoked potentials. During intraoperative irritation or compression of a nerve root, the so-called myotonic discharge (repetitive pseudorhythmic firing of motor units) may indicate nerve root damage.

Sensory Evoked Potentials

With cervical spine surgery, sensory evoked potentials are elicited by stimulation of the median, ulnar, and radial nerve trunks or with dermatomal stimulation to prevent intraoperative nerve root and dorsal tract damage. Tibial or peroneal nerve SSEPs are used to monitor the extent of dorsal column pathology. Recording can be accomplished using the same transcranial needles at C3-C4 (resp. C4-C3) as those used for motor stimulation. Spinal subarachnoidal or epidural electrodes are used to establish the affected level and to distinguish systemic changes.

Neurocortical Evoked Potentials

Neurocortical evoked potentials (Fig. 17.6) are recorded transcranially with monopolar needles (C3-C4, resp. C4-C3) after stimulating peripheral nerves, showing typically shaped cortical somatosensory evoked potentials. Peripheral nerve trunk stimulation is carried out using surface electrodes, typically with 10 to 30 mA, a stimulus duration of 0.2 ms, and a repetition rate or 5.9/s to reduce dual-current artifacts. Latencies and amplitudes are measured for trend analysis. In combination with MEPs, SSEPs remain widely used and helpful for monitoring nerve root and spinothalamocortical tract function. The combination of several nerve SSEPs facilitates diagnostics of the affected level.

Neurospinal Evoked Potentials

Neurospinal evoked potentials (Fig. 17.7) are observed after the stimulation of the peripheral nerves and recorded with the spinal electrodes primarily used for corticospinal evoked potentials. They are performed simultaneously with neurocortical evoked potentials. Neurospinal evoked potential recordings assist with sensory level diagnostics, distinguishing root from dorsal tract involvement and helping differentiate systemic from surgically related changes.

Spinospinal Evoked Potentials

In cervical spine surgery, spinospinal evoked potentials (Fig. 17.8) are recorded with the rostral spinal electrode after caudal spinal cord stimulation by the same electrodes used for corticospinal evoked potentials. Because of its high risk, stimulation at the craniocervical site should not be performed. Spinal cord evoked potentials are stable, comparable with D-wave monitoring, although they are thought to be indicative of activity in sensory-related tracts (16). A reduction of amplitude of 50% or more suggests a postoperative spinal cord disorder. Spinospinal evoked potentials have to be performed very carefully, with slowly and gradually increasing stimulation from 0.5 mA to a maximum of 15 mA, usually with a repetition rate of 10/s. Spinospinal evoked potentials can

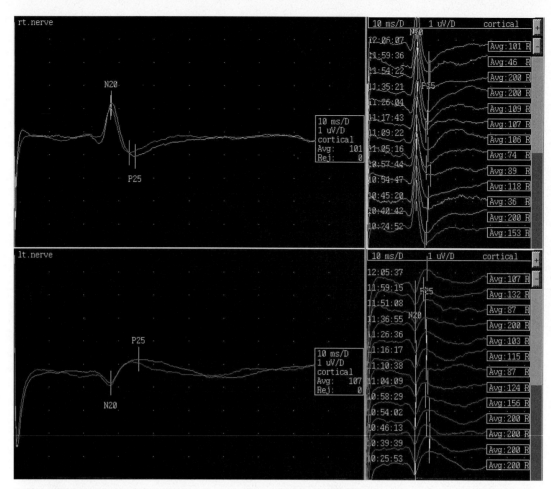

FIG. 17.6. Right and left medial nerve cortical somatosensory evoked potentials (neurocortical evoked potentials of the medial nerve, left, are mirrored for all C3-C4 recordings).

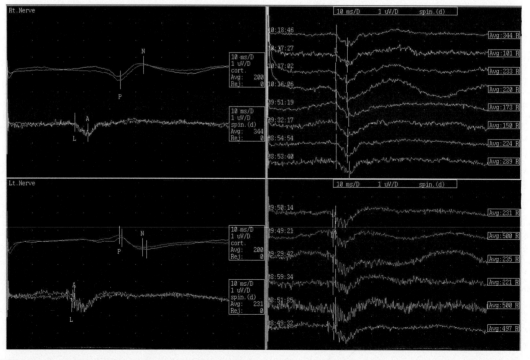

FIG. 17.7. Neurospinal evoked potentials (NSEPs) of the tibial nerves. Time course of NSEP of the tibial nerve, right (**upper right**) and of the tibial nerve, left (**lower right**); simultaneous recording of neurocortical and neurospinal evoked potentials (**left**).

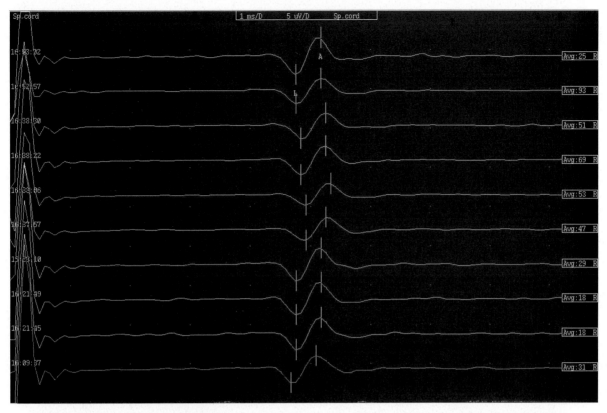

FIG. 17.8. Spinal-spinal evoked potential with epidural stimulation at T12 and epidural recording at T2. SCEP, spinal cord evoked potential.

cause severe tonic muscle contraction and even metabolic acidosis.

CASE REPORTS

Case 1

A 42-year-old man presented with foraminal disc herniation at C6-C7. This caused progressive neuropathic pain and sensorimotor deficits of the left root C7 (Fig. 17.9). Anterior decompression surgery was performed under multimodal intraoperative monitoring, with corticomuscular evoked potentials (Fig. 17.10) and continuous EMG of brachioradialis and triceps muscles and neurocortical evoked potentials of the radial nerve (Fig. 17.11).

During the anterior surgical approach and head extension, a continuous reduction of neurocortical evoked potential amplitude of the left radial nerve was observed (Fig. 17.11A and B). This recovered after correction of the head position. Again during nerve root decompression, a transient alteration of the neurocortical evoked potential of the left radial nerve was observed. This recovered completely after the decompression procedure. Because of fading muscle relaxation (done for previous intubation), continuous increase of all amplitudes of the corticomuscular evoked potential was observed (Fig. 17.10).

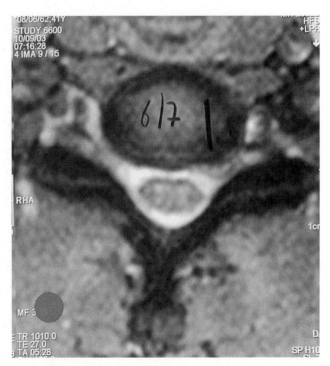

FIG. 17.9. Magnetic resonance imaging showing lateral-foraminal disc herniation C6-C7 left.

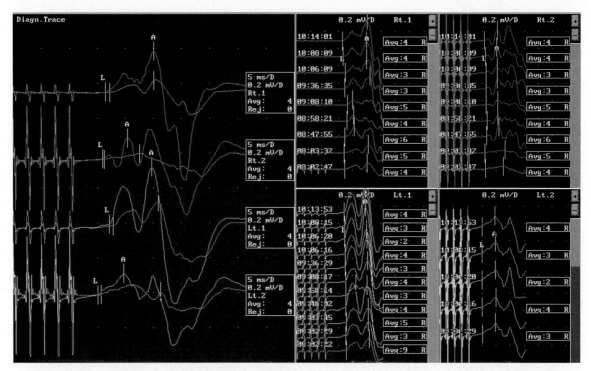

FIG. 17.10. Corticomuscular evoked potentials of brachioradialis and triceps muscles, right (Rt.1, Rt.2; *red traces*) and left (Lt.1, Lt.2, *green traces*) sides.

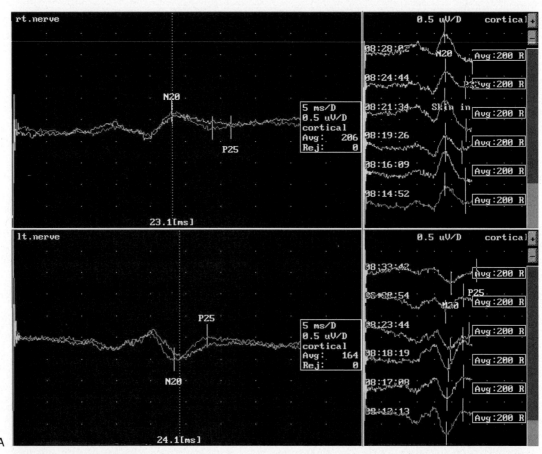

FIG. 17.11. A: Neurocortical evoked potentials of the radial nerves (right nerve—**top**, *blue traces;* left nerve, **bottom,** *green trace* of picture). **B**: Quantitative trend analysis of neurocortical evoked potentials of the radial nerves based on Fig. 17.12A. The **right side** of the picture shows the affected left nerve root. Latencies are shown by the *green traces*, amplitudes by the *yellow traces*. Beginning of operation at the **top**, end of operation at the **bottom** of the picture.

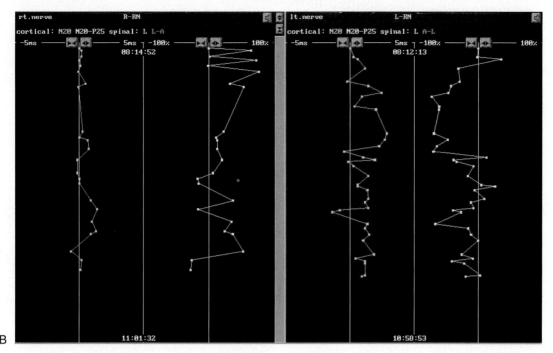

FIG. 17.11. *Continued*

Continuous EMG myotonic discharge of the left triceps muscle was observed during nerve root decompression. Because of the deterioration of sensory function of the left C7 root, the MIOM suggested that the head was incorrectly positioned. After repositioning of the head, there was a full recovery of the electrophysiologic test. During the nerve decompression procedure, a small deterioration was also observed in the neurocortical evoked potential. This subsequently improved after decompression, indicating surgically related nerve root irritation. MIOM proved to be a useful tool for preventing non-surgical postoperative neurologic deficits. Immediately after surgery, the patient had radicular symptoms with no other neurologic changes. The preoperative neurologic deficits improved slowly during the ensuing 3 months.

Case 2

A 55-year-old man presented with spinal stenosis at C1-C2 due to a malformation of the upper cervical spine that caused progressive myelopathy (Fig. 17.12). Before the

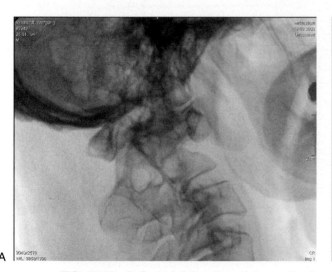

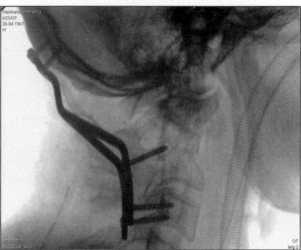

FIG. 17.12. A: Dorsal dislocation of dens with stenosis at C0 to C2. **B**: Transoral decompression and resection of dens, dorsal widening of atlas and foramen magnum with fusion at C0 to C4. Postoperative radiograph.

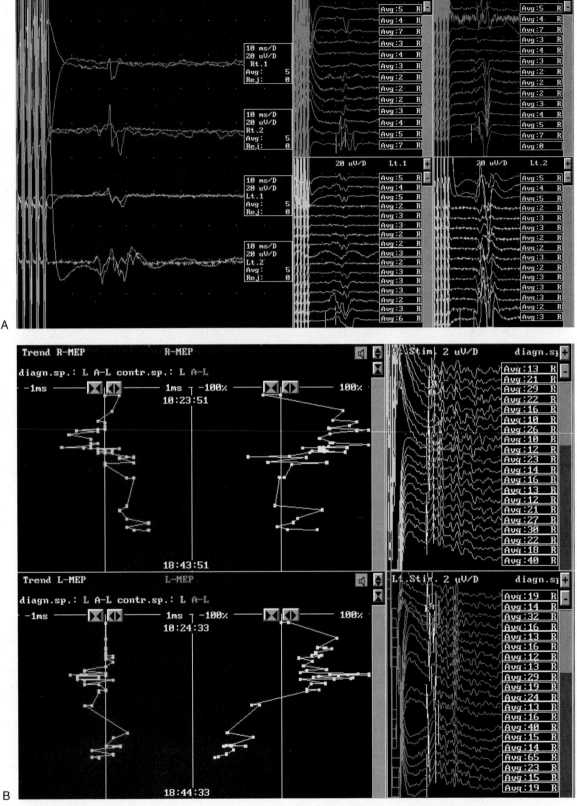

FIG. 17.13. A: Corticomuscular evoked potentials: Rt. 1, brachioradial muscle, right; Rt. 2, abductor digiti minimi muscle, right; Lt. 1. brachioradial muscle, left; Lt. 2, abductor digiti minimi muscle, left. The **right side** of the figure shows the time course; first recording at the **bottom**, last at the **top**. **B**: Cortical somatosensory evoked potentials. **Right**: *Green traces* show D waves of the left corticospinal tract; *red traces* show D waves of the right corticospinal tract. Left: The trend window. *Green traces* show latencies; *yellow traces* show amplitudes. **C**: Neurocortical evoked potentials of the median nerves (*green traces*, right nerve; *red traces*, left nerve). Potentials of the left median nerve are inverted because of the recording position at C3-C4.

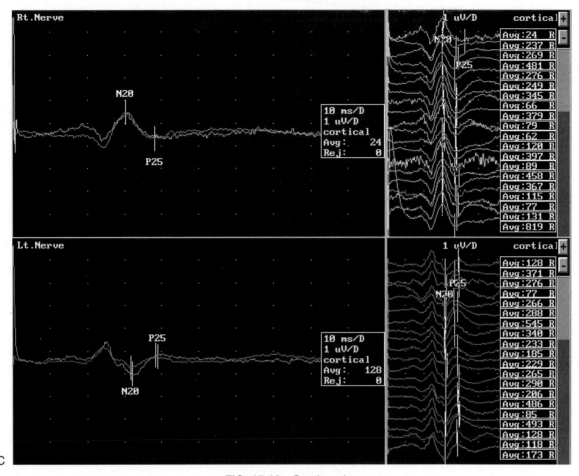

FIG. 17.13. *Continued*

intended dens resection and dorsal fusion at C0-C3, a pathologic delayed CMAP and corticomuscular evoked potentials were observed, especially on the muscles of the right side (Fig 17.13A). D waves demonstrated severe pathologic (polyphasic) patterns on both sides, even at the beginning of the operation (Fig. 17.13B). After the transoral decompression, the patient was turned to the prone position. A deterioration with progressive reduction of the CMAP and D-wave amplitudes (Fig. 17.13A and B) along the right corticospinal tract (up to 80%) was observed. At the beginning of the operation, the neurocortical evoked potentials of the median nerves (Fig. 17.13C) were delayed on both sides. Additionally, deformation of the potentials on the left side was observed. During the operation, no remarkable changes of neurocortical evoked potentials were observed. The deterioration of corticospinal tract function was communicated immediately to the surgeon, but no persistent compression of the spinal cord could be detected at the end of surgical procedure. After the observed MIOM changes, early postoperative extubation and clinical examination were performed. These confirmed an increased spastic tetraparesis. Because of further progression of neurologic deficits, post-

operative edematous swelling or bleeding was suspected, and MRI was performed (Fig. 17.14A and B).

After transoral dens resection and repositioning to the prone position, deterioration of the corticospinal tract function with progression was discovered by MIOM. The cause of this deterioration was not clear and was diagnosed only by the postoperative MRI. This confirmed spinal cord compression at C0-C1 and led to a second dorsal decompression at this level. This case illustrates not only the diagnostic potential of MIOM but also the need for surgical intervention in selected cases.

CONCLUSION

During the period of January 2000 to June 2003, 131 patients underwent cervical spine surgery with multimodal intraoperative monitoring at our institution. This population included intramedullary-extramedullary tumors (21 patients), decompression of multisegmental stenosis (87 patients), correction of deformities (5 patients), and decompression and spinal fusion (18 patients). The mean patient age was 57 years (8 to 87 years). MIOM testing duration was 4.2 hours (0.5 to 10.8 hours), totaling 551 hours by the

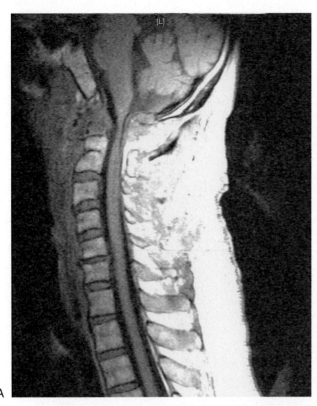

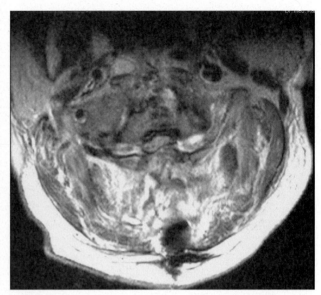

FIG. 17.14. Postoperative magnetic resonance imaging study showing probable persistent dorsal compression. Consecutive extended posterior decompression at C0 and C1 was performed, which led to a gradual improvement of the spastic tetraparesis within 4 weeks.

same neurologist. Eighty-two operations were without significant changes in MIOM (latencies < 10%, reductions of amplitude < 50%). Twenty-four cases had transient systemic changes (e.g., anesthesia, blood pressure). Thirty-two cases were due to the surgical procedure, in which the surgeon or anesthetist was immediately informed and the procedure adapted. Based on MIOM, 18 cases of transient-slight neurologic deficit were predicted (17 true positive, 1 false positive), 107 were negative, 3 were false negative [2 showed radiculopathy of nonmonitored roots, 1 had progressive deterioration due to edema after transoral-dorsal C1-C2 decompression requiring C0-C1 decompression as well (case report 2)]. In 3 cases, no prediction was possible for technical reasons. Based on these data for multimodal intraoperative monitoring in cervical spine surgery, a sensitivity of 85% and a specificity of 97% for prediction of postoperative clinical neurologic status were observed.

MIOM can replace conventional CSEPs or wake-up testing and enables one to observe real-time function of the motor and sensory pathways selectively.

The combined monitoring of ascending and descending long tracts at various sites of interest obtains reliable information of the spinal cord function (17). MIOM is technically demanding; however, it is a reliable method for obtaining relevant online information of neurologic spinal cord and nerve root function during the surgical procedure. Particularly in

procedures such as resection of cervical spinal tumors and correction of deformities, this method, in the hands of experienced neurophysiologists, is potentially beneficial. MIOM is a reliable method for reducing intraoperative complications.

REFERENCES

1. Vauzelle C, Stagnara P, et al. Functional monitoring of spinal cord activity during spinal surgery. *Clin Orthop* 1973;93:173–178.
2. Lesser RP, Raudzens P, et al. Postoperative neurological deficits may occur despite unchanged intraoperative somatosensory evoked potentials. *Ann Neurol* 1986;19:22–25.
3. Deutsch H, Arginteanu M, et al. Somatosensory evoked potential monitoring in anterior thoracic vertebrectomy. *J Neurosurg* 2000;92[2 Suppl]:155–161.
4. Dawson GD. Cerebral responses to electrical stimulation of peripheral nerve in man. *J Neurol Neurosurg Psychiatry* 1947;10:137–139.
5. Nash CL, Brodkey J, et al. A model for electrical monitoring of spinal cord function in scoliosis patients undergoing correction. *J Bone Joint Surg Am* 1972;54:197–198.
6. Nuwer MR, Dawson EG, et al. Somatosensory evoked potential spinal cord monitoring reduces neurologic deficits after scoliosis surgery: results of a large multicenter survey. *Electroencephalogr Clin Neurophysiol* 1995;96(1):6–11.
7. Patton HD, Amassian VE. Single and multiple unit analysis of cortical stage of pyramidal tract activation. *J Physiol* 1954;17:345–363.
8. Merton PA, Morton HB. Stimulation of the cerebral cortex in the intact human subject. *Nature* 1980;285:227.
9. Boyd SG, Rothwell JC, et al. A method of monitoring function in corticospinal pathways during scoliosis surgery with a note on motor conduction velocities. *J Neurol Neurosurg Psychiatry* 1986;49:251–257.

10. Tamaki T, Yamashita T, et al. Spinal cord monitoring. *Jap J Elektraenceph Elektromyogr* 1972;1:196.
11. Kurokawa T. Spinal cord action potentials evoked by epidural stimulation of cord: a human and animal record. *Jap J Elektraenceph Elektromyogr* 1972;1:64–66.
12. Zentner J. Motor evoked potential monitoring during neurosurgical operations on the spinal cord. *Neurosurg Rev* 1991;14(1):29–36.
13. Taylor BA, Fennelly ME, et al. Temporal summation: the key to motor evoked potential spinal cord monitoring in humans. *J Neurol Neurosurg Psychiatry* 1993;56:104–106.
14. Jones SJ, Harrison R, et al. Motor evoked potential monitoring during spinal surgery: responses of distal limb muscles to transcranial cortical stimulation with pulse trains. *Electroencephalogr Clin Neurophysiol* 1996;100(5):375–383.
15. Ubags LH, Kalkman CJ, et al. A comparison of myogenic motor evoked responses to electrical and magnetic transcranial stimulation during nitrous oxide/opioid anesthesia. *Anesth Analg* 1999;88(3):568–572.
16. Tamaki T, Noguchi T, et al. Spinal cord monitoring as a clinical utilization of the spinal evoked potential. *Clin Orthop* 1984;54(184):58–64.
17. Iwasaki H, Tamaki T, et al. Efficacy and limitations of current methods of intraoperative spinal cord monitoring. *J Orthop Sci* 2003;8(5):635–642.

CHAPTER 18

Neurophysiologic Monitoring During Cervical Spine Surgery

Alexander R. Vaccaro and Daniel M. Schwartz

Intraoperative neurophysiologic monitoring (IONM) represents the application of modified electrophysiologic recording techniques to document changes in the functional status of central or peripheral nervous systems that are at risk for injury during surgery. It permits detection of alterations in neural function early enough to initiate interventional measures, thereby minimizing or preventing postoperative neurologic deficit. Although IONM has gained almost universal acceptance as a clinical alternative for assessing spinal cord and nerve root function during instrumented thoracolumbar surgeries, it has yet to receive similar acceptance for cervical spine surgery. With improved surgical techniques and a more comprehensive understanding of the biomechanics of advanced internal fixation methods, the number of patients undergoing cervical spine surgery today has grown by an order of magnitude over that in the past decade. Patients with cervical myelopathy, cervical instability, and metabolic bone disease such as ankylosing spondylitis are clearly at high risk for surgical and nonsurgical intraoperative neural injury. As such, IONM could play a role in the prevention of untoward neural injury in selected cases. These situations are discussed herein.

Among the myriad IONM techniques available, three play a principal role in assessing spinal cord and nerve root function during cervical spine surgery: transcranial electric motor evoked potentials (TceMEPs), mixed-nerve somatosensory evoked potentials (SSEPs), and spontaneous electromyography (spEMG). A fourth, dermatomal evoked potentials (DEPs), is of limited value in a very select population of patients presenting with acute radiculopathy primarily from soft disc herniation.

TRANSCRANIAL ELECTRIC MOTOR EVOKED POTENTIALS

Motor evoked potentials (MEPs) are neuroelectric events elicited from descending motor pathways including the corticospinal tract (CST), spinal cord interneurons, anterior horn cells, peripheral nerves, and skeletal muscles innervated by excited alpha motor neurons following transcranial electric or magnetic stimulation (Fig. 18.1). The CST or pyramidal tract has widespread cells of origin across the premotor, motor, and somatosensory cortices. The CST axons course from the cortex through the internal capsule to the caudal medulla. Here, the CST fibers become pyramidal decussations, forming the lateral CST, to descend into the lateral and anterior funiculi of the spinal cord. CST axons that originate in the premotor and motor cortices enter the spinal cord gray matter, where they interact with spinal interneurons that go on to synapse with alpha motor neurons, which innervate peripheral muscle. Lateral CST fibers that synapse in the cervical segment of the spinal cord are arranged medially and followed laterally by fibers that synapse in the thoracic, lumbar, and sacral regions.

Merton and Morton (1) were among the first investigators to record compound muscle action potentials (CMAPs) from humans following excitation of motor cortex cells to a short-duration (50 μS), high-voltage (2,000 V) electrical pulse delivered to electrodes affixed to the scalp at the vertex (Cz) and 6 cm anterior. Levy and York (2) took this pioneering work one step further by eliciting spinal epidural motor potentials to electrical stimulation between the vertex and hard palate. Since that time, many reports have appeared attesting to the efficacious application of eliciting volleys in corticospinal tract axons following transcranial

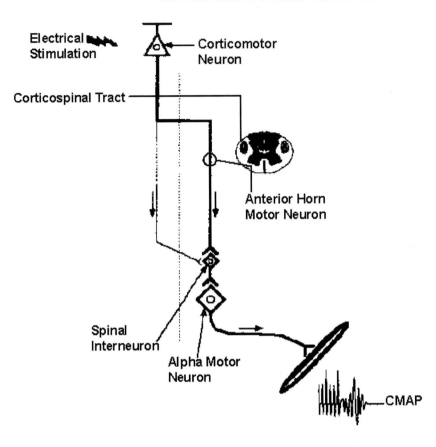

FIG. 18.1. Schematic of the anatomic pathway for elicitation of transcranial electric motor evoked potentials.

activation of motor cortex either from a single electrical pulse or from trains of short-duration electrical stimuli and recording the ensuing response either from the spinal cord or peripheral muscle during spine surgery (3–13). Although transcranial magnetic stimulation to induce current flow in the volume conductive tissue of the cortical mantle has been used successfully to elicit MEPs in the clinical laboratory, numerous shortcomings preclude its use in the operating room (14,15).

The clinical methodology for eliciting TceMEPs involves delivering electrical pulse trains through electrodes either inserted subdermally into the scalp overlying the motor cortex or affixed on the scalp surface. Although there is no particular standard for the type of stimulating electrode best suited for depolarizing cortical motor neurons, our experience has shown the greatest success with commercially available corkscrew electrodes.

In contrast either to SSEPs, peripheral nerve conduction velocity tests, or stimulated EMG, anodal electrical stimulation is considered better than conventional cathodal stimulation for exciting corticomotor neurons. Several different electrode arrays for stimulating the motor cortex have been used. These include (a) a single anode at Cz (American Encephalographic Society) (16) and a cathode at Fz; (b) a pair of electrodes placed respectively over C3-C4 or C1-C2, with anodal stimulation applied to that electrode within the pair that is contralateral to the side of muscle recording (i.e., anodal stimulation applied to C1 with C2 as the cathode would elicit a compound muscle action potential over the right side of the body and vice versa); (c) a circumferential array consisting of five linked cathodes affixed across the forehead and behind each mastoid with the anode at Cz; and (d) anodal electrodes over C3-C4 with Cz as the cathode. Our experience favors the anodal reversal technique with corkscrew electrodes inserted over C1-C2 or C3-C4, with the opposite electrode serving as the cathode and then reversing the polarity for recording a CMAP contralateral to the side of stimulation.

During our exploratory phase with TceMEPs, the circumferential montage advocated by Ubags and associates (17) was studied. Two limiting factors were observed. First, the circumferential montage resulted in not only depolarization of corticomotor neurons but also direct stimulation of the internal capsule and other deep brainstem structures. Second, it was hypothesized that the placement of stimulating electrodes on the earlobe or mastoid area could lead to direct stimulation of the spinal cord such that there is excitation of the collateral 1A afferent sensory fibers. The latter would result in a descending mixed sensorimotor response, thereby offsetting corticospinal tract purity.

At present, the commercially available dedicated transcortical electrical stimulator that has received the most clinical and research attention for eliciting MEPs is the Digitimer D185 Multipulse (Digitimer Corp., Welwyn Garden City, UK). This device permits controlled delivery of a very brief (50 μs), high-voltage electrical pulse either singly or in multiple pulse trains of variable number and interstimulus interval up to 1,200 V. Of particular benefit is that the Digitimer measures the actual current delivered based on alterations in stimulating electrode impedance.

As an alternative to the Digitimer, some professionals involved in intraoperative neurophysiologic monitoring are beginning to use electrical stimulators that are internal to commercially available neurophysiologic monitoring acquisition and recording systems. Such devices are limited to a maximum output of 400 V, in contrast to the high-voltage output D185. By linking two such stimulators in series, however, it is possible to double the output voltage. To achieve even greater electrical power, most users of this approach increase the stimulus duration from 50 μs, indigenous to the Digitimer, to 500 to 1,000 μs.

There are several practical limitations to this modified stimulating paradigm versus using a dedicated transcortical stimulator like the D185. First, simply linking two 400-V maximum electrical stimulators together does not guarantee a combined output of 800 V. Not only does the actual voltage fluctuate, but also the voltage appears to drop for successive pulses in the stimulus train. Moreover, unlike the Digitimer, the internal stimulation technique provides no measure of the actual delivered current. Thus, the user does not know how much overall energy is actually being delivered to the motor cortex. The use of the Digitimer standalone transcortical electrical stimulator results in elicitation of more consistent MEPs than the use of linked internal devices, particularly in patients with significant spinal cord compromise. Furthermore, although the safety and efficacy of TceMEPs have been shown in virtually tens of thousands of patients worldwide using the Digitimer D185, little is known about the safety of linked internal stimulator boxes and long-duration electrical pulse trains to achieve the same result.

TceMEPs from the CST can be recorded from the spinal epidural or subdural space through a catheter-type electrode or peripheral musculature. A bipolar "epidural electrode" can be inserted directly into the epidural space following laminectomy, through a fenestration of the lamina using an 18-gauge angiocatheter, or percutaneously through a Touhy needle. Responses recorded from the epidural space consist of a primary D wave, so called because it represents direct activation of the CST cells. In awake or lightly anesthetized patients, the D wave is followed by a series of I waves, generated indirectly by cortical synapses (Fig. 18.2). These descending cortical volleys then summate to excite anterior horn cells and spinal alpha motor neurons, thereby inducing a compound muscle action potential. In anesthetized patients, I waves are eradicated secondary to depression of the recurrent CST axon-cortical interneuronal synaptic excita-

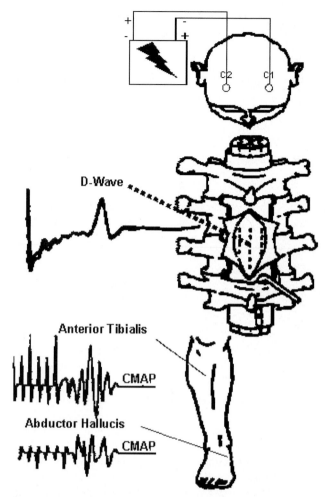

FIG. 18.2. Example of stimulus and recording sites for elicitation of transcranial electric motor evoked potentials.

tion of CST neurons (18). Conversely, the D wave has been shown to be resistant to the effects of total intravenous anesthetics, thereby permitting stable large-amplitude epidural recordings over long time periods (19).

Despite the many advantages of recording D-wave activity to assess CST integrity intraoperatively, it is not without a myriad of disadvantages. First, it requires the placement of two invasive recording electrodes, through either laminectomy, laminocentesis, or percutaneous tap at the low-cervical and midthoracic (T4 to T8) levels. Below T8, the D-wave voltage is too small for monitoring purposes (20). If the surgical approach is ventral, it becomes necessary to thread the electrode percutaneously under radiographic guidance to ensure proper placement in the midline epidural space. Clearly, this results in delay of surgery and carries the risk for epidural complications. Second, the placing of an epidural electrode precisely in midline is virtually impossible. Hence, responses often favor one side of the spinal cord over the other, making it difficult to acquire information about left versus right sides. Third, because the CSTs for the upper and lower extremities pass through the cervical spinal cord in close proximity to one another, it is not possible to provide differential information. Rather, the D wave reflects global CST behavior. Consequently, it is possible to miss an injury to the spinal cord motor fibers responsible for the arm and hand, while sparing lower extremity integrity.

The preferred alternative to using D-wave TceMEPs is to record a CMAP (Fig. 18.2). In contrast to recording D waves, a CMAP reflects not only excitation of the anterior horn cells but also alpha motor neurons innervating peripheral muscle. The appeal here is that essentially all of the aforementioned disadvantages related to recording D waves are eliminated when muscle recording is used. Important to cervical spine surgery is that recording myogenic TceMEPs allows for intraoperative monitoring during neck extension for intubation and for patient positioning, in an effort to identify nonsurgical effects of potential spinal cord compression injury.

CMAPs can be recorded either from subdermal needle electrodes introduced into upper and lower extremity muscle or from self-adhesive surface electrodes affixed over the muscle. In general, we favor the former because it allows the electrode to be inserted closer to the muscle belly and tendon.

Of particular relevance is that myogenic TceMEPs are extremely sensitive to the effects of inhalational anesthetics (18). This is certainly not surprising because such agents depress cortical neuronal and anterior horn cell activity, both of which are critical for eliciting a TceMEP. Hence, it is imperative that only a total intravenous anesthetic protocol be used. In contrast to recording D waves, myogenic TceMEPs are also compromised in the presence of neuromuscular relaxation. Use of partial muscle paralysis is far too unpredictable to be considered; therefore, muscle paralysis should be used sparingly only when absolutely necessary, such as for intubation and during exposure and muscle dissection.

SOMATOSENSORY EVOKED POTENTIALS

The application of SSEPs for monitoring spinal cord function intraoperatively has withstood the test of time on tens of thousands of patients worldwide over the past two decades. Indeed, SSEPs continue to be the primary modality used to monitor spinal cord dorsal column function in many surgical settings. From its beginnings in monitoring during surgical correction of spinal deformity to its current widespread use in surgery of the cervical, thoracic, and thoracolumbar spine, SSEP monitoring has proved acceptably efficacious if the injury is global and if the patient has baseline responses of sufficient amplitude to detect a substantial change. At best, SSEPs serve only as an inferential measure of spinal motor tract function.

Despite their high rate of success, particularly in scoliosis surgery, there are times when SSEPs are either unrecordable or simply unreliable because of small amplitudes and poor waveform morphology. This is true even when careful attention is paid to controlling the anesthetic regimen so as not to compromise response amplitude (21). Patients with severe myelopathy, spinal cord tumor, obesity, or peripheral neuropathy, either alone or in combination, often present with IONM challenges that are beyond the capabilities of SSEPs. Without alternative or complementary monitoring methods, therefore, these patients would be unmonitorable or the interpretation for substantial and real change would be difficult, at best.

Indeed, the potential for neurologic complications associated with cervical spine surgery has increased in recent years. This is due, at least in part, to the use of advanced internal fixation devices (e.g., wires, screws, rods, plates) for correcting complex cervical spine deformities. These breakthrough advances in cervical spine implants not only have broadened the spectrum of spinal disorders amenable to surgical correction but also have heightened the risk for neurologic deficits not readily identified with SSEP monitoring. Because SSEPs reflect the integrity of spinal cord white matter and are mediated through the dorsal columns, they provide no information about the condition of the spinal cord gray matter (22). With SSEPs alone, therefore, there remains a small but definite risk for a false-negative finding, particularly when monitoring patients with preexisting spinal cord compromise, such as those with cervical myelopathy or acute spinal cord injury. In such patients, the vascular supply to both the ventral and lateral aspects of the spinal cord supplied by the anterior spinal artery are vulnerable to hypotension-induced ischemic injury, which often are not manifest in the SSEPs at all or within the critical time necessary to initiate intervention for injury reversal.

ELECTROMYOGRAPHY

Because SSEPs are neither sensitive nor specific for identifying injury to a spinal nerve root, owing to their multiple nerve root mediation, spEMG is used to detect neural trauma to cervical motor nerve roots during decompression, foraminotomy, removal of bony fragments, tumor resection, distraction or traction, and implant placement. Abrupt traction of a spinal nerve root or mechanical contact by a surgical instrument should elicit an intermittent EMG burst or sustained neurotonic activity, respectively. In general, elicitation of brief synchronized burst activity is not considered to indicate an injury-related potential. On the other hand, sustained neural "trains" that mimic motorboat, popcorn, or dive-bomber sounds are warnings of potential nerve root injury.

In addition to cervical nerve root monitoring, spEMG can also be used during ventral approaches to the cervical spine to identify traction injury to the recurrent laryngeal nerve. A special electrified endotracheal tube (Medtronic Xomed, Jacksonville, FL) serves as the recording electrode.

DERMATOMAL EVOKED POTENTIALS

SSEPs elicited by mixed peripheral nerve stimulation are mediated through multiple spinal nerve roots as they enter the cervical or lumbosacral spinal cord. As a result, it is entirely possible to see unchanged SSEPs in the presence of segmental nerve root injury. To circumvent this problem, some surgical neurophysiologists have advocated recording afferent cortical evoked potentials after electrical stimulation of a particular dermatomal field (23–25). In select acute radiculopathic patients undergoing ventral cervical decompression of the cervical nerve roots, DEPs are characteristically reduced in amplitude or prolonged in latency, or are completely absent at baseline. After decompression, it is possible to observe either reemergence of a response from a previously absent baseline or a 50% or greater increase in amplitude (25). Likewise, DEPs can also demonstrate the functional consequences of mechanical nerve root traction in the form of amplitude suppression (10,24,26).

There has been ongoing debate about the value of DEPs in IONM. After a decade of recording intraoperative DEPs to assess the adequacy of cervical or lumbar spinal nerve root decompression, we have concluded that successful recording is dependent two factors: (a) use of a total intravenous anesthetic, and (b) careful patient selection. Because cortical DEPs are quite fragile, any concentration of nitrous oxide or potent inhalational agent precludes reliable recording (21). Moreover, DEPs are only of potential value in patients who are undergoing surgical decompression for acute (≤6 months) radicular symptoms, mostly secondary to soft disc herniation. In patients with myelopathic signs and in those with longer-standing radicular symptoms, DEPs are usually noninformative.

Technically, DEPs are recorded in a similar manner to cortical SSEPs; however, the level of electrical stimulation must be held low (10 to 15 mA) so as not to spread either to another dermatome or to a mixed nerve. Excessive averaging also results in amplitude degradation; therefore, more than 25 averages are inadvisable.

NEUROPHYSIOLOGIC MONITORING DURING CERVICAL SPINE SURGERY

IONM is a dynamic process, and clinically important changes can occur almost any time before or during the operative procedure. A multimodality approach to IONM is necessary to assess functional integrity of the spinal cord, nerve roots, brachial plexus, and at times the recurrent laryngeal nerve and vertebral arteries. Figure 18.3 presents a simplified strategic flow diagram for IONM during cervical

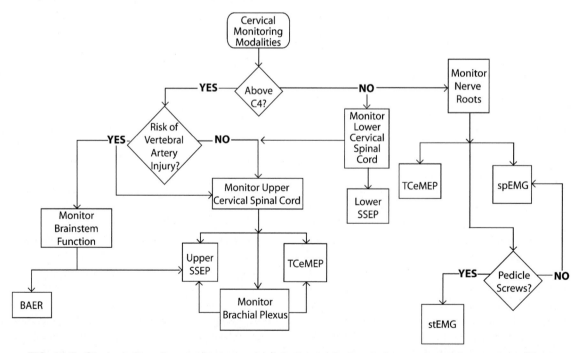

FIG. 18.3. Strategic flow diagram for neurophysiologic monitoring during cervical spine surgery. (From Schwartz DM, Sestokas AK. A systems based algorithmic approach to intraoperative neurophysiological monitoring during spinal surgery. *Semin Spine Surg* (in press), with permission.)

spine surgery. For a detailed discussion of a systems-based approach to neurophysiologic monitoring, see Schwartz and Sestokas' article (27).

Patients such as those with cervical myelopathy, cervical instability, and ankylosing spondylitis are clearly at heightened risk both for surgical and nonsurgical intraoperative neural injury compared with those undergoing one-level or multilevel anterior discectomy with or without internal fixation. Consequently, for these patients, IOMN, if used, must begin immediately after induction for monitoring asleep intubation in order to prevent spinal cord compression secondary to excessive neck extension.

The strategy for monitoring asleep intubation should commence with recording of TcMEPs from upper extremity hand and lower extremity leg and foot muscles before and after placement of the endotracheal tube. Because of the need to record a CMAP, it is best to induce the patient without administering a muscle relaxant. After a preintubation TceMEP baseline is recorded, either a depolarizing short-acting (e.g., succinylcholine) or medium-duration nondepolarizing (e.g., rocuronium) drug is administered in a dosage sufficient to facilitate intubation, but not to obliterate the TceMEP for a long time period. Immediately upon intubation and before the full effect of the neuromuscular blockade, a repeat TceMEP is obtained to ensure preservation of motor function.

Next, an upper extremity cortical and subcortical SSEP is elicited by ulnar nerve stimulation. The ulnar nerve is preferred over the more popular median nerve as a stimulation site for upper extremity SSEPs owing to its lower spinal nerve root entry at C7-T1.

Because of their sensitivity to identifying impending brachial plexopathy (28), ulnar nerve SSEPs may be re-recorded immediately after application of countertraction of the shoulders with adhesive tape for positioning or after the patient is turned prone. If the unilateral ulnar nerve SSEP is noted to change 30% or more after shoulder taping, then the tape should be released immediately and reapplied with less countertraction. TceMEPs also should be reelicited after positioning or the application of weight for neck traction, to ensure corticospinal tract integrity. If a substantial change in TceMEPs is noted, it is imperative first to raise the patient's mean arterial blood pressure (MAP) to 90 mm Hg or higher to improve perfusion to the spinal cord. If the change is secondary to weight placement, then the weight may be removed. After recovery, the amount of weight should be titrated to a tolerable amount.

If TceMEP amplitude changes result from turning the patient from supine to prone, and the response amplitude does not show any signs of improvement within 15 minutes of raising the MAP, a spinal cord injury steroid (NASCIS-2) protocol may be considered. Reevaluation of TceMEPs with intermittent SSEP testing should be conducted over the next 20 minutes. If improvement in TceMEP amplitude of at least 30% is not noted, we recommend not proceeding

with surgery. In this case, the patient should be turned supine and the monitoring continued throughout emergence from anesthesia.

Assuming no untoward changes in neurophysiologic homeostasis with positioning, multimodality monitoring during cervical spine surgery may proceed as follows. When surgery involves the upper cervical spine (i.e., C1 to C4), SSEPs need only include responses to upper extremity stimulation; however, below C4, it is imperative to include lower extremity (posterior tibial or peroneal nerve) SSEPs to monitor the entire neuraxis. In the latter situation, upper extremity SSEPs act to complement their lower extremity counterparts, both as a cross-check of proximal cervical spinal cord integrity and as protection against impending brachial plexus injury. TceMEPs may be used as the primary measure of spinal cord motor tract integrity.

For ventral procedures, TceMEPs may be recorded after placement of vertebral body distracters because the decompression approaches the posterior longitudinal ligament and it involves the spinal cord. TceMEPs also may be recorded before and after application of weight or neck extension (i.e., the "water-ski maneuver") for vertebral body distraction, impaction of interbody fusion graft, and placement of internal fixation devices that either may give rise to spinal cord compression or produce concussive injury.

Surgery of the upper cervical spine in patients with instability either due to fracture or degenerative disease poses particular risk for vascular insult owing in part to the proximity of the vertebral and anterior spinal artery. For these patients, the augmentation of SSEPs with brainstem auditory evoked potentials to provide complete neurophysiologic cover of the dorsal brainstem circulation may be considered.

In our experience, most intraoperative electrophysiologic changes identified during cervical spine surgery are due to blood pressure changes. It is therefore our clinical philosophy to have anesthesia maintained at an MAP of 75 mm Hg or higher.

In addition to iatrogenic spinal cord injury, spinal nerve root palsy remains an unsolved complication after laminectomy or laminoplasty for cervical myelopathy. The cause of the iatrogenic radiculopathy has been attributed to the dorsal migration of the spinal cord after decompression, causing stretching and edema of the affected nerve roots, most commonly C5 and C6. Although most patients recover spontaneously after transient nerve root palsy, some patients require further surgical intervention, including foraminotomy, durotomy, or additional anterior decompression to relieve the tethered nerve roots. Until recently, this complication had gone undetected intraoperatively because of the relative insensitivity of SSEPs and DEPs to such decompression-induced nerve root injuries. Therefore, we have added TceMEP recordings from deltoid and biceps muscles, coupled with spEMG whenever the C5 and C6 nerve roots are at risk for iatrogenic injury (29).

CONCLUSION

In their review of 100 patients who underwent cervical spine surgery, Epstein and coworkers stated that SSEP monitoring helped reduced the prevalence of quadriplegia from 3.7 to 0% (30). Since that time, there have been significant advances in cervical spine instrumentation and surgical technique, thereby affording surgical correction to even the most challenging of cervical disorders. As a result, IONM has had to keep pace by expanding the neurophysiologic armamentarium for assessing the functional integrity of the corticospinal tract, cervical motor nerve roots, and both spinal cord and brainstem vascular supplies. This type of multimodality, algorithmic approach to neurophysiologic monitoring may improve the safety of selected corrective cervical spine surgical procedures.

REFERENCES

1. Merton QA, Morton HB. Electrical stimulation of human motor and visual cortex through the scalp. *J Physiol (Lond)* 1980;305:9–10.
2. Levy WJ, York D. Clinical experience with motor and cerebral evoked potential monitoring. *Neurosurgery* 1987;20:169–182.
3. Boyd SG, Rothwell JC, Cowan JM, et al. A method of monitoring function in corticospinal pathways during scoliosis surgery with a note on motor conduction velocities. *J Neurol Neurosurg Psychiatry* 1986; 49:251–257.
4. Burke D, Hicks RG, Stephen JPH, et al. Assessment of corticospinal and somatosensory conduction simultaneously during scoliosis surgery. *Electroencephogr Clin Neurophysiol* 1992;85:338–396.
5. Burke D, Hicks RG. Surgical Monitoring of motor pathways. *J Clin Neurophysiol* 1998;15:194–205.
6. Stephen JPH, Sullivan MR, Hicks RG, et al. Cotrel-Dubousset instrumentation in children using simultaneous motor and somatosensory evoked potentials monitoring. *Spine* 1996;21:2450–2457.
7. Jones SJ, Harrison R, Koh KF, et al. Motor evoked potential monitoring during spinal surgery: responses of distal limb muscles to transcranial cortical stimulation with electric trains. *Electroencephalogr Clin Neurophysiol* 1996;100:375–383.
8. Morota N, Deletis V, Constantini S, et al. The role of motor evoked potentials during surgery for intramedullary spinal cord tumors. *Neurosurgery* 1997;41:1327–1336.
9. Gjokaslan ZL, Samudrala S, Deletis V, et al. Intraoperative monitoring of spinal cord function using motor evoked potentials via transcutaneous epidural electrode during anterior cervical spine surgery. *J Spin Disord* 1997;10:299–303.
10. Schwartz DM, Sestokas AK, Turner LA, et al. Neurophysiological identification of iatrogenic neural injury during complex spine surgery. *Semin Spine Surg* 1998;10:242–251.
11. Clancie B, Harris W, Broton JG, et al. "Threshold-level" multipulse transcranial electrical stimulation of motor cortex for intraoperative monitoring of spinal motor tracts: description of method and comparison to somatosensory evoked potentials monitoring. *J Neurosurg* 1998; 88:457–470.
12. Drummond DS, Schwartz DM, Johnston DR, et al. Neurologic injury complication surgery for spinal deformity: etiology, prevention and treatment. In: Dewald R, ed. *Fundamentals of spine surgery: a core curriculum.* New York: Thieme, in press.
13. Schwartz DM, Wierzbowski LR, Fan D, et al. Intraoperative neurophysiological monitoring during spine surgery. In: Vaccaro AR, Zeidman S, Betz R, eds. *Principals and practices of spine surgery.* Philadelphia: WB Saunders, in press.
14. Gugino LD, Aglio LS, Potts G. Perioperative use of transcranial magnetic stimulation. *Tech Neurosurg* 2001;7:33–51.
15. Gugino LD, Aglio LS, Segal M. The use of transcranial magnetic stimulation for monitoring spinal cord motor paths. *Semin Spine Surg* 1997;9:315–336.
16. American Encephalographic Society. Guideline thirteen: guideline for standard electrode position nomenclature. *J Clin Neurophysiol* 1994; 11:111–113.
17. Ubags LH, Kalkman CJ, Been HD, et al. The use of a circumferential cathode improves amplitude of intraoperative electrical transcranial myogenic motor evoked responses. *Anesth Analg* 1996;82:1011–1014.
18. Gugino L, Schwartz DM. Monitoring motor evoked potentials. Invited presentation at the Annual Meeting of the Society for Neurosurgical Anesthesia and Critical Care, New Orleans, September 12, 2001.
19. Deletis V. Intraoperative monitoring of the functional integrity of the motor pathways. In: Devinski O, Berie A, Dogali M, eds. *Electrical and magnetic stimulation of the brain and spinal cord. Advances in neurology,* Vol 63. New York: Raven, 1993:201–214.
20. MacDonald DB, Janusz M. *An approach to intraoperative neurophysiologic monitoring of thoracolumbar aneurysm surgery.* (in press).
21. Schwartz DM, Schwartz JA, Sestokas AK, et al. Influence of nitrous-oxide on posterior tibial nerve cortical somatosensory evoked potentials. *J Spinal Dis* 1997;10:80–86.
22. Dimitrijevic MR. Clinical neurophysiology of neural stimulation. In: Ducker TD, Brown RH, eds. *Neurophysiology and standards of spinal cord monitoring.* New York: Springer-Verlag, 1998:11–15.
23. Toleikis JR, Varlvin AO, Shapiro DE, et al. The use of dermatomal evoked responses during surgical procedures that use intrapedicular fixation of the lumbosacral spine. *Spine* 1993;18:2401–2407.
24. Schwartz DM. Intraoperative neurophysiological monitoring during cervical spine surgery. *Oper Tech Orthop* 1996;6:6–12.
25. Owen JH, Toleikis JR. Nerve root monitoring. In: Bridwell KH, Dewald RL, eds. *The textbook of spinal surgery,* 2nd ed. Philadelphia: Lippincott-Raven, 1997.
26. Schwartz DM, Sestokas AK, Turner LA, et al. Neurophysiological identification of iatrogenic neural injury during complex spine surgery. *Semin Spine Surg* 1998;10:242–25.
27. Schwartz DM, Sestokas AK. A systems based algorithmic approach to intraoperative neurophysiological monitoring during spinal surgery. *Semin Spine Surg* (in press).
28. Schwartz DM, Drummond DS, Hahn M, et al. Prevention of positional brachial plexopathy during surgical correction of scoliosis. *J Spinal Dis* 2000;13:178–182.
29. Fan D, Schwartz DM, Vacarro AR, et al. Intraoperative neurophysiological detection of iatrogenic C5 nerve root injury during laminectomy for cervical compression myelopathy (in press).
30. Epstein NE, Danto JD, Nardi D. Evaluation of intraoperative somatosensory evoked potential monitoring during 100 cervical operations. *Spine* 1993;18:737–747.

CHAPTER 19

The Wake-up Test

Daxes M. Banit and Bruce V. Darden

The goal of cervical spinal surgery is to maximize the benefits while minimizing complications. In the current era of increasingly technical interventions often involving instrumentation, the risk for intraoperatively-induced postoperative neurologic deficits is ever increasing (1). In the review of data from the Scoliosis Research Society Morbidity and Mortality Committee, Schmitts reported a 0.5% incidence of spinal cord injuries (2). A 17% incidence of neurologic complications, with a 4% major spinal cord injury rate in instrumented spinal cases, was reported by Wilber and colleagues (3).

The causes of iatrogenic spinal cord injuries are varied, ranging from mechanical to ischemic insults. Preexisting deformities, as well as preexisting neurologic deficits, are known to increase the likelihood of postoperative neurologic injuries. The cord can also be subjected to ischemia from intraoperative hypotension, iatrogenic trauma, or distraction maneuvers. Dolan and coworkers demonstrated spinal cord ischemia with experimental distraction (4). Intraoperative hypotension may also play a role in spinal cord injury. Bradshaw and associates documented evidence of spinal cord insult with lesser degrees of distraction in the setting of hypotension (5).

The goal of any intraoperative spinal cord monitoring is to detect the spinal cord insult early, to allow reversal of any maneuver that may have caused the insult. Some neurologic changes are permanent and will not improve, but many intraoperative injuries are reversible. The efficacy of intraoperative testing and monitoring has increased recently with the advent of new technologies.

Some monitoring techniques are clinically based, requiring a reduction in anesthesia and having the patient follow commands, as with the Stagnara wake-up test (6,7). Another clinically based examination is the ankle clonus test. This test is performed by a forced dorsiflexion maneuver of the foot, followed by holding tension on the foot in the dorsiflexed position. A positive result, indicating intact motor

tracts in the spinal cord, is demonstrated by the rhythmic contraction of the gastrocnemius-soleus muscle. The clonus test is predicated on the different stages of recovery from general anesthesia. The lower motor neuron function returns before the inhibitory upper motor neuron impulses; therefore, there is an excitatory state with the patient not yet responsive to verbal stimuli (8).

The other method of intraoperative monitoring is electrophysiologically based. The exact testing method is dependent on whether sensory or motor function is to be monitored. A somatosensory evoked potential involves a peripheral site of stimulation and recording the signal centrally in the upper cervical spinal cord or cerebral cortex. A motor evoked potential entails magnetic or electrical central stimulation of the motor cortex or spinal cord and recording motor nerve or muscle action potentials. In addition, electrically or mechanically induced electromyograms can be used during transpedicular instrumentation. Electrophysiologic monitoring is well described in the literature (1,9–12).

THE WAKE-UP TEST

The wake-up test was first described by Vauzelle and colleagues in 1973 for monitoring spinal cord function in scoliosis surgery (7). This test consists of awakening the patient intraoperatively. This can be done at any point in the surgery but is usually performed after the completion of spinal instrumentation or manipulation. The surgeon notifies the anesthesiologist 30 to 45 minutes in advance to begin reducing the anesthetic state. When the patient reaches a lightened anesthetic state, he or she is asked to move the hands. When this is accomplished, lower extremity function is verified by asking the patient to move the feet. If the patient is unable to the move the lower extremities, the test is repeated. A second negative response is then addressed by examining possible causes of a neurologic insult and then carrying out a corrective maneuver, such as reversal of deformity correction. Surgery then proceeds after deepening the anesthetic state.

The complications of the wake-up test include pain, air embolism, rod dislocation, accidental extubation, bronchospasm, dislodgment of halo or tong fixation, dislodgment of intravenous lines and catheters, and recall of intraoperative events. A premise of the test is that the function being monitored has been assessed at baseline function for intraoperative comparison. In addition, the wake-up test requires that the patient cooperate with the examination.

The principal advantage of the wake-up test is the lack of expensive equipment or the need for trained personnel. Another benefit of the test is that it assesses motor function. Somatosensory evoked potentials monitor posterior column function, with the supposition that an insult that affects the anterior motor tracts will also affect the posterior tracts and hence will be detected. There are reports of false-negative monitoring during which no disturbance was noted and the patient awoke with a motor deficit (13, 14). It has been reasoned that although a distraction maneuver would affect both the anterior and posterior tracts, a vascular insult involving the anterior arterial system could preferentially affect the anterior motor tracts more than the posterior sensory tracts. With regard to thoracic and lumbar surgery, occasional false-negative results have been reported in the literature for the wake-up test (15,16). This is often the result of delayed-onset paraplegia as a sequela of distraction.

An implicit aspect of all monitoring procedures is that the monitored function must involve the surgical zone, that is, the monitored stimulus must pass through the surgical site. An example of such an oversight is when somatosensory evoked potential monitoring is performed with median nerve stimulation for lower cervical spine surgery (17).

DEFICIENCIES OF THE WAKE-UP TEST

One problem with the use of the wake-up test in cervical spine surgery is that the surgical site involves neurologic tracts to the upper extremities as well as lower extremities. As originally described, the upper extremities served as controls for the test. In cervical spine surgery, the test can demonstrate that the motor tracts are intact if a patient moves his or her hands. If the converse situation occurred with no demonstrable motor function elicited, it would be difficult to assess whether the loss is due to the anesthetic state or to a surgical insult. Another disadvantage of the classic Stagnara wake-up test is that it can only detect a neurologic injury after the completion of instrumentation. A lag time is required in reducing the state of anesthesia before the test can be administered. Given a 30- to 45-minute lag time, the test cannot be performed repeatedly without adding considerable operative time and exposing the patient to the risk for prolonged anesthesia. There have been reports of reducing the lag time to 10 minutes with shorter-

acting anesthetics administered through an infusion (18). In distinction, whereas the electrophysiologic methods of monitoring are also anesthetic dependent, they do allow for continuous monitoring of both sensory and motor tracts. These tests allow for earlier detection of an abnormality and for immediate reversal of the surgical insult. For example, if the initial instrumentation caused a problem, it could be addressed immediately rather than after the completion of all instrumentation, with the cord sustaining a prolonged period of injury (15).

CONCLUSION

In conclusion, a surgeon should be familiar with the complete spectrum of intraoperative monitoring techniques. There are no fail-safe methods; one test can serve as a backup to a primary testing procedure. Currently, with the advancements in electrophysiologic techniques allowing for monitoring of both motor and sensory tracts, the wake-up test is often relegated to a backup role. The surgeon may opt to perform a clinically based test to verify or further assess an electrophysiologic change in complicated cases (19). An important point regarding the use of the wake-up test in the cervical spine is that upper extremity function cannot serve as a control. A negative test with no demonstration of motor function does not rule out a spinal cord injury due to confounding factors such as anesthesia or patient compliance. The wake-up test only provides beneficial information if the patient demonstrates upper extremity motor function.

REFERENCES

1. Owens J, Tamaka T. Application of neurophysiological measures during surgery of the spine. In: Frymoyer JW, ed. *The adult spine: principles and practice*, 2nd ed. Philadelphia: Lippincott-Raven, 1997: 673–701.
2. Schmitts EW. Neurological complications in the treatment of scoliosis: a sequential report of the Scoliosis Research Society, 1971–1979. Reported at the 17th annual meeting of the Scoliosis Research society, Denver, 1981.
3. Wilber RG, Thompson GH, Shaffer JW, et al. Post operative neurological deficits in segmental spinal instrumentation. *J Bone Joint Surg Am* 1984;66:1178–11187.
4. Dolan EJ, Transfeldt EE, Tator CH, et al. Post operative neurological deficits in segmental spinal instrumentation. *J Bone Joint Surg Am* 1984;66:756–764.
5. Bradshaw K, Webb JK, Fraser AM. Clinical evaluation of spinal cord monitoring in scoliosis surgery. *Spine* 1984;9:636–643.
6. Hall JE, Levine CR, Sudhins KG. Intraoperative awakening to monitor spinal cord function during Harrington instrumentation and spine fusion: description of procedure and report of three cases. *J Bone Joint Surg Am* 1978;60:533–536.
7. Vauzelle C, Stagnara P, Jouvinroux P. Functional monitoring of spinal cord activity during spinal surgery. *Clin Orthop* 1973;93:173–178.
8. Dimitrejevic M, Sherwood A, Nathan P. Clonus, peripheral and central mechanisms. In: Desmedt JE, ed. *Neurology*. New York: Krager, 1978: 173–182.
9. Ben-David B. Spinal cord monitoring. *Orthop Clin North Am* 1988; 19:427–448.
10. Cusick JF, Maiman DJ, Hoffman MD. Electrodiagnostic studies in cervical spine disease. In: Frymoyer JW, ed. *The cervical spine*. Philadelphia: Lippincott-Raven, 1998:179–190.

11. Wilborn A. Electrodiagnosis. In: Herkowitz H, Garfin S, Balderston R, et al, eds. *The spine*. Philadelphia: WB Saunders, 1999:135–157.

12. Zeidman SM, Osenbach RK, Marino CJ, et al. Principles of intra-operative monitoring. In: CSRS Editorial Committee, eds. *The cervical spine*. Philadelphia: Lippincott-Raven 1998:191–204.

13. Ben-David B, Haller G, Taylor P. Anterior spinal fusion complicated by paraplegia: a case report of a false negative somatosensory evoked potential. *Spine* 1987;12:536–539.

14. Chatrian G, Berger MS, Wirch AL. Discrepancy between intraopera-tive SSEPs and postoperative function. *J Neurosurg* 1988;69:450–454.

15. Ben-David B, Taylor P, Haller G. Posterior spinal fusion complicated by posterior column injury. A case report of a false negative wake up test. *Spine* 1987;12:540–543.

16. Schmitts EW. Post instrumentation paraplegia and a negative Stagnara wake up test. Reported at the 14th annual meeting of the Scoliosis Research Society, Boston, 1978.

17. Lesser RP, Raudzins P, Luders H, et al. Postoperative neurological deficits may occur despite unchanged intraoperative somatosensory evoked potentials. *Ann Neurol* 1986;19:22–25.

18. Van Beem H, Koopman-van Gemert A, Kruls H, et al. Spinal cord mon-itoring during vertebral column surgery under continuous alfentanil in-fusion. *Eur J Anaesthesiol* 1992;9:287–291.

19. Glassman SD, Johnson JR, Shields CB, et al. Correlation of motor evoked potentials, somatosensory evoked potentials, and the wake up test in a case of kyphoscoliosis. *J Spinal Disord* 1993;6:194–198.

20. Winter RB. Congenital kyphoscoliosis with paralysis following hemi-vertebra excision. *Clin Orthop* 1976;119:116–125.

CHAPTER 20

Nonparalytic Anesthesia and Real-Time Monitoring

William Mitchell, Lee Buono, and Edward C. Benzel

Spine surgery is continuously evolving and becoming increasingly more complex. Surgeons are tackling more difficult pathology on a regular basis. Technical prowess and technologic advancements have made this possible. Adjunctive measures such as steroids and intraoperative monitoring techniques have been present and available for some time, but their use and perceived effectiveness and utility have vacillated. In the pages that follow, the available methods of intraoperative neurophysiologic monitoring for spinal surgery are addressed.

WAKE-UP TEST

A number of methods have been developed for the intraoperative monitoring of spinal cord function. In 1973, Vauzelle and colleagues described the intraoperative wake-up test (1). This enabled the gold standard. With this test, the patient is awoken from general anesthesia to undergo a neurologic examination. Therefore, one can definitively, relatively, and accurately identify significant neurologic deficits that may have occurred as a result of intraoperative manipulation or instrumentation. If a neurologic deficit is identified, corrective measures may be undertaken.

The requirements for the performance of an intraoperative wake-up test are simple. Each patient must be screened preoperatively to assess his or her capacity for tolerance of the technique. The ability to participate may be limited by the patient's underlying demeanor or premorbid personality traits. This assessment is not only difficult but also often an unreliable predictor of the patient's ability to tolerate intraoperative awakening. Nevertheless, a full explanation must ensue. It must describe the procedure and conditions upon awakening (i.e., intubation, confusion, levels of discomfort). Language barriers may be overcome by prerecording commands for examination (2).

The anesthesia technique is critical for patient wakefulness and extent of discomfort. It goes without saying that anesthesia technique is the foremost factor in achieving a successful intraoperative wake-up test. The anesthesiologist must take part in the preoperative screening process in preparation for the patient's unique concerns. Care must be taken during the induction of anesthesia to guard against discomfort from intubation. Topical anesthesia is commonly used during induction to avoid excess discomfort from the endotracheal tube. Great care should be taken to secure the patient with chest and lap belts and with four-point restraints to avoid self-injury, extubation, and loss of intravenous access.

Although anesthetic regimens may vary, there exist general principles that are fundamental to the technique. The introduction of local anesthetic to the pharynx and larynx, either by transcutaneous injection or spray, is paramount for patient comfort upon awakening. Paralytic agents administered during induction must be carefully monitored by muscle twitches. Moreover, communication (about surgical timing to wakefulness) is imperative between the surgeon and the anesthesiologist. Halogenated anesthetics are used sparingly and often are reserved for younger patients with iatrogenic hypertension. Concomitant use of electrophysiologic monitoring may be affected by halogenated anesthesia. An initial loading dose of narcotic is appropriated with continuous infusion, and reservation is given to further boluses. Narcotics and halogenated anesthesia, preferably fentanyl and isoflurane, are discontinued 30 minutes before to awakening. About 10 minutes before awakening, paralytics are reversed and nitrous oxide discontinued. Strict adherence to this regimen should provide a wakeful patient who is able to follow commands in about 5 minutes.

Once awakened, the patient is asked to move the arms and legs. Discovered deficits demand reevaluation of the patient's head position and instrumentation or consideration of vascular compromise. Therefore, both the surgeon and anesthesia team must be prepared for reawakening after their initial assessment.

Although current means of electrophysiologic monitoring may obviate the need for the intraoperative wake-up test, technical difficulties or misinterpretation remain a confounding variable in the indirect assessment. Therefore, although crude, the wake-up test should remain a tool in the surgeon's armamentarium. It provides an assessment of motor function. It is emphasized that the evaluation of sensation is limited.

CURRENT ELECTROPHYSIOLOGIC TECHNIQUES

The utility of the intraoperative wake-up test is limited by patient tolerance. In addition, it only provides a brief view of neurologic status during a surgical procedure. Modern neurophysiologic monitoring provides the benefits of patient comfort and the possibility of indirect continuous assessment of neurologic status.

Current techniques for intraoperative spinal cord monitoring include somatosensory evoked potentials (SSEPs), somatosensory cortical evoked potentials (SCEPs), spinal SSEPs, spinal recording of spinal evoked potentials (SPSEPs), dermatomal evoked potentials (DEPs), motor evoked potentials (MEPs), and electromyography (EMG). From the time of conception to application, continuous neurophysiologic monitoring has become an important tool that may reduce intraoperative morbidity.

Somatosensory Evoked Potentials

First introduced in 1972, the principle of SEP is continuous real-time recording of conduit function (3,4). The spinal cord is the conduit through which stimulation of a selected peripheral nerve provides an afferent signal. It is conducted through the spinal cord and recorded either at the spine cord or cortex. Most of the signal is conducted through the dorsal columns and only a fraction through the ventral tracts (5,6). Therefore, SEP monitoring essentially reflects dorsal column function. Moreover, in part because of this selectivity, false-negative records have been reported. Although reported rates vary, the largest series of 50,000 patients concluded a 0.067% false-negative rate (7). On average, the false-negative rate is less than 2%, whereas the false-positive rate is less than 3% (8–12).

While relying on neurophysiologic monitoring of any kind, one must be aware of the limitations of the technology and take steps to avoid misinterpretation. It is, therefore, considered common practice to secure two separate proximal and distal sights for production of the afferent volley. This aids in the determination of technical failure or neurologic injury. A technical failure commonly produces alterations in the latencies or amplitude in one of two volleys. Alternatively, neurologic injury would affect both volleys.

Moreover, one must realize that following significant surgical manipulation that may affect the spinal cord, changes in SEP signals may be delayed for up to 30 minutes (10). Therefore, it is imperative to continue recording for at least 30 minutes after maneuvers considered of substantial risk for neurologic injury.

SEPs may be recorded either cortically or subcortically. It may be self-evident that when recording an electrical signal through a conduit, reduction in the conduit length reduces noise, resistance, and error. Reduction to lower ordered neurons is beneficial in subcortical recording because of lowered sensitivities to anesthesia and environmental change. During procedures of the cervical spine, median nerve stimulation is appropriate for upper cervical to midcervical levels. However, ulnar stimulation must be instituted for lower cervical levels. In the advent of a severe peripheral neuropathy, it is often necessary to stimulate the paraspinous musculature because of pathologic peripheral conduction blockade.

Currently, there are no universally accepted criteria for interpreting the significance of intraoperative changes in SEP monitoring. However, changes in amplitude greater than 50% or increases in latency greater than 10% should remain a guideline for impending spinal cord injury (13). Because of the shortened volley, latency changes become less important in subcortical recording. Moreover, although changes in velocity may be a sensitive indicator of spinal cord injury, quantification has proved cumbersome and therefore does not play a significant role in SEP monitoring.

Halogen inhalation anesthetics have a consistent dose–response effect in SEP recording (13–16). The effects are poorly understood yet produce a reliable prolongation of latency and reduction of amplitude. Narcotic dosing has also proved to affect signals (14,15). Although more commonly observed with higher doses, bolus dosing of potent narcotics has a varying effect on signal amplitude and latency. Benzodiazepines do not affect the amplitude nor latency, but they have been shown to increase noise from muscle recordings in the periphery (13,15).

Anesthetic regimens should avoid the use of paralytics and rely on nitrous inhalation, as well as continuous infusion without bolus, of narcotic analgesia. The use of halogen anesthetics should be kept to a minimum, especially during cortical recording. The introduction and use of propofol has had a profound neuroanesthetic effect and is an effective regimen without affecting evoked recording (16).

Factors that play a role in the sensitivity of SEPs to anesthetic depression are predominantly twofold. First, recording from lower-order neurons (less synapses) reduces the likelihood of anesthetic depression. Second, previous spinal cord injury has been shown to increases the sensitivity of neurons to anesthetic depression (17).

Other than anesthesia, environmental and physiologic factors play a significant role in signal recording. These factors include 60-Hz noise from other operating equipment (e.g., electric drills, warming blankets, headlights), hypocarbia, hypothermia, and hypotension (16,18). The keys to signal conduction are amplitude and latency. Changes in amplitude or latency are the warning signs of possible neurologic injury. Animal studies have shown susceptibility to neurologic injury during surgical manipulation during periods of hypotension through ischemia (17). This is evident also in humans with decreases in the SEP amplitudes during periods of relative intraoperative hypotension. Although no definitive data exist, maintaining a mean arterial pressure (MAP) of 10% above the patient's baseline MAP is a practical rule in spinal decompression and instrumentation surgery.

SEP may help with deformity surgery as suggested by Nuwer and associates survey of 50,000 monitored spinal surgeries (60% scoliosis, 7.5% fractures, 6.5% kyphosis, and 5.5% spondylolisthesis) (19). The major limitations in using SEP for monitoring the spinal cord are the time delay between injury and manifestation on SEP and the lack of definitive correlation with anterior column function. Motor tracts may be damaged without a change in SEP (8,20,21). Therefore, the surgeon must avoid developing a false sense of security based solely on SEP. If used, they must be considered one instrument in the armamentarium. In addition, the surgeon must be prepared for the false-positive result and its ramifications. The false-positive rate ranges from 9% to 28%, depending on the location and number of channels and recording sites (22,23).

Spinospinal Evoked Potentials

The aforementioned principle of reduction in the number of synapses has significant benefits. Spinal stimulation and recording provide both a reduction in the sensitivity to anesthetic depression and higher baseline amplitudes. In addition, significant peripheral nerve disease may hinder adequate recording with both SEP and SPSEP. This problem is avoided by the use of spinal cord stimulation and recording. Spinal evoked potentials provide a more consistent response when compared with cortical SEP (24, 25). Additionally, more rapid acquisition of responses can be achieved as a result of the need for fewer repetitions, adding to overall efficiency (24,25).

Recording and stimulation electrodes are placed in the epidural or subarachnoid space. Although invasive, reported complications remain exceedingly low by percutaneous implantation or under direct visualization (24). The technical challenge of percutaneous placement remains the ability to achieve midline placement. Paramedian recording or stimulation may result in unilateral monitoring and changes in the spinal potentials (26). Electrodes may migrate during the procedure, which may herald alarming changes in amplitude and latency. Despite shortening the synapses, SPSEP has similar limitations as SEP (Figs. 20.1 to 20.3).

Dermatomal Evoked Potentials

DEP signals reflect function over several levels of spinal cord due to peripheral stimulation of a mixed nerve. Selective recording of regional spinal cord function can only be achieved through isolation of the sensory afferents by dermatomal recording. Although DEP is seldom used in cervical spine monitoring, technologic advancement warrants an overview.

Achievement of proper cutaneous stimulation requires each electrode to be positioned in each targeted dermatome. Baseline recording should include comparative analysis of each side to allow for measurement of between-limb laten-

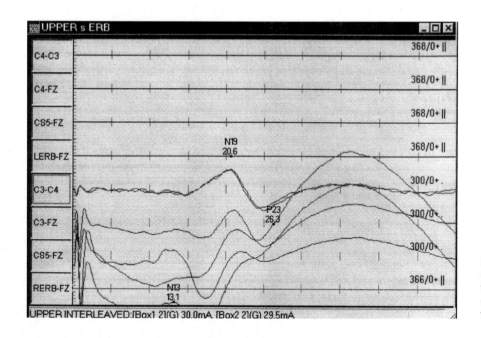

FIG. 20.1. Intraoperative monitoring during intradural left L3 tumor resection. Normal baseline in the right upper extremity somatosensory evoked potential.

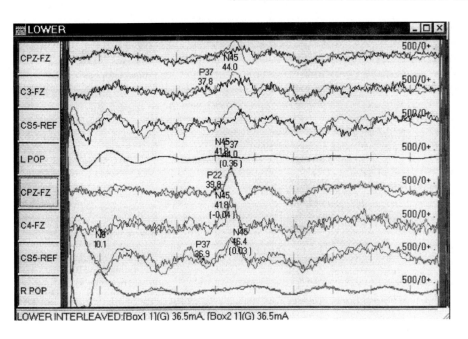

FIG. 20.2. Intraoperative monitoring during intradural left L3 tumor resection. Normal lower extremity intraoperative somatosensory evoked potential.

cies (27). This technique may be useful to monitor C5, which is a more sensitive nerve root. It has a higher injury rate than other cervical roots. Additionally, it may have usefulness in the lumbar spine or when the pathology is at the nerve root level.

Motor Evoked Potentials

The shortcomings of SEP monitoring are that of posterior column selectivity, limitations due to peripheral nerve disease, and time delay. A variable false-negative rate exists with SEP. An undetermined fraction of this is due to unrecorded injury to the ventral spinal cord (13,16).

The need for monitoring of ventral spinal cord function becomes increasingly important with deformity correction and ventral decompressions. Deformation of the ventral spinal cord may have a limited effect on dorsal column function, thereby increasing the false-negative rate of SEP. Furthermore, vascular compromise of the ventral spinal cord will likely spare the posterior columns and thereby not be manifested by changes in SEP. Although used less often, MEP enables assessment of the ventral spinal cord and is associated with a shorter delay between injury and electrophysiologic changes.

First introduced by Levy and York in 1983 (28), intraoperative MEP recording has gained significant interest

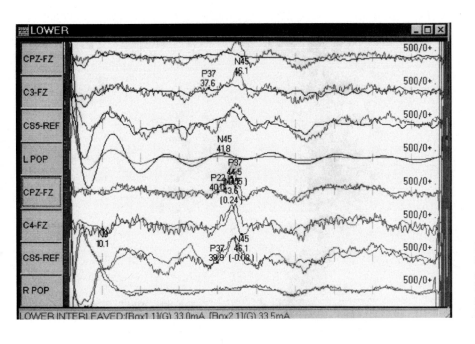

FIG. 20.3. Intraoperative monitoring during intradural left L3 tumor resection. Decreased amplitude of the left lower extremity somatosensory evoked potential (CPZ-FZ to CX5-REF).

within the surgical community. Proximal stimulation in MEPs can be achieved at the cortical, brainstem, or spinal cord level. Distal recordings sites may be located at the spinal level, peripheral nerve, or muscle. As with SEP monitoring, the application of the principles of dual volley recording should be considered.

Transcranial cortical stimulation must overcome the resistance of the skull. As such, current requirements are higher and associated with a significant degree of discomfort (29, 30). A balance must be maintained between quantity of stimulation and anesthetic to control normal physiologic responses to pain. Preinduction baseline recording is therefore not possible because of the discomfort associated with MEP stimulation.

Obvious contraindications to transcranial MEP include awake procedures as well as a previous history of seizure activity. Continued MEP stimulation may result in seizure activity that could remain unrecognized during general or paralytic anesthesia.

Magnetic current induction of the cerebral cortex is now becoming more prevalent for this reason. First introduced in 1985, transcranial magnetic stimulation yields a compound motor action potential without the need for signal averaging (31,32). A magnetic field (usually in the form of a skull cap) is placed over the patient's head and rotated, thereby inducing an electrical current, as first described by Faraday in 1831. In addition, it is painless and provides a more rapid means of signal analysis owing to the obviated need for averaging (33,34). Although expensive and cumbersome, magnetic current induction will no doubt take the place of transcranial stimulation as the technology improves.

There are several significant restrictions on magnetic stimulation, including anesthesia technique, technical difficulties with the cap, and interpretation; the technique was recently approved by the U.S. Food and Drug Administration (FDA).

One can electrically stimulate the spinal cord to record MEP by placing electrodes into the (a) epidural space (35–37); (b) interspinous ligaments outside the surgical field; and (c) lamina (21). Significant amplitude changes range from 20% to 50% (24,37–40); 50% is also recommended for MEP (cortical) (41,42) and SEP (43).

The time delay between injury and changes in MEP is significantly shorter than for SEP. In addition, it enables the surgeon to assess eloquent motor function. It does not rely on posterior column assessment to infer anterior column integrity.

Electromyography

EMG is often used with pedicle screw placement. Electrodes are placed on muscles innervated by nerve roots in question. Recording electrodes are separated by 5 cm, with the active electrode over the belly of the muscle and the reference electrode on the tendon. Subdermal or surface electrodes may be employed. Muscle relaxation must remain constant when recording (two to three twitches out of a train of four). Mechanically and electrically elicited responses can be obtained. Mechanical techniques must assess biphasic response and rule out artifact. Electrical techniques consist of a stimulating cathode electrode that transmits current through device to the anode electrode. If there is no stimulation of adjacent roots manifested by EMG activity, the wall of the pedicle is presumed to be intact. The stimulus can be recorded in milliamperage or volts. Darden and colleagues (44) concluded the following: (a) EMG threshold of more than 7 mA or 30 V (pedicle intact); (b) EMG threshold of less than 7 mA or 30 V (inspect and if appropriate no intervention); and (c) EMG threshold of less than 6 mA or 20 V (pedicle likely breached). The utility of these data is in question because the clinical effect of a fractured pedicle is usually nil (Figs. 20.4 and 20.5).

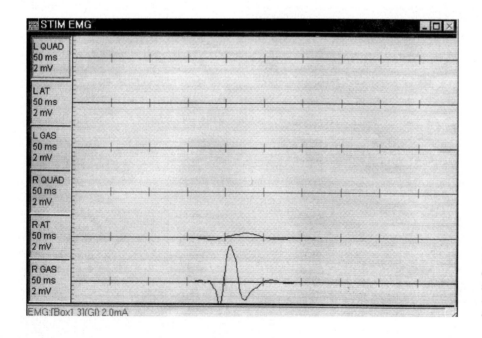

FIG. 20.4. Intraoperative monitoring during lumbar laminectomy and fusion with instrumentation from L3 to S1. Direct S1 nerve root stimulation at 2 mA.

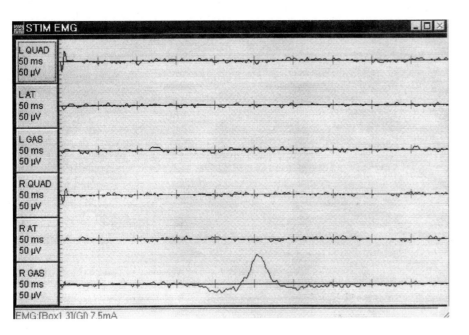

FIG. 20.5. Intraoperative monitoring during lumbar laminectomy and fusion with instrumentation from L3 to S1. Right S1 pedicle screw stimulation at 6.5 mA suggesting breached pedicle.

SUMMARY

Intraoperative electrophysiologic monitoring can be used to the patient's advantage in selected clinical situations. Each of the monitoring strategies is associated with advantages and disadvantages. A multimodality strategy can minimize the disadvantage associated with a single modality approach.

It is emphasized that monitoring techniques cannot replace clinical wisdom and meticulous technique. For many surgeons, the selected use of a carefully chosen monitoring strategy that is superimposed and a solid, clinical decision-making foundation should provide a desirable surveillance paradigm.

REFERENCES

1. Vauzelle C, Stanara P, Jouvinroux P. Functional monitoring of spinal cord activity during spinal surgery. *Clin Orthop* 1973;93:173.
2. Mizutani AR, Drummond JC, Karagianes TG. A less than rude awakening. *Anesthesiology* 1989;69:287.
3. Croft BA, Brod JS, Nuisen FE. Reversible spinal cord trauma: a model for electrical monitoring of spinal cord function. *J Neurosurg* 1972; 36:299.
4. Tomaki T, Yamashita T, Kobayashi H, et al. Spinal cord monitoring. *Jpn J Electroencephalogr Electromyogr* 1972;1:196.
5. Cusick JF, Myklebust JF, Larson SJ, et al. Spinal cord potentials in the primate: neural substrate. *J Neurosurg* 1978;49:551.
6. Giblin DR. Somatosensory evoked potentials in healthy subjects and in patients with lesions of the nervous system. *Ann N Y Acad Sci* 1964; 112:93.
7. Dawson EG, Carlson LG, Kanim LEA, et al. Somatosensory evoked potential spinal cord monitoring reduces neurological deficits after scoliosis surgery: results of a large multicenter survey. *EEG Clin Neurophysiol* 1995;96:6.
8. Dinner DS, Luders H, Lesser RP, et al. Intraoperative spinal somatosensory evoked potential monitoring. *J Neurosurg* 1986;65:807–814.
9. Ginsburg HH, Shetter AG, Raudzens PA. Postoperative paraplegia with preserved intraoperative somatosensory evoked potentials. Case report. *J Neurosurg* 1985;63:296–300.
10. Grundy BL. Monitoring of sensory evoked potentials during neurosurgical operations: methods and applications. *Neurosurgery* 1982;11: 556–575.
11. Jones SJ, Carter L, Edgar MA, et al. Experience of epidural spinal cord monitoring in 410 cases. In: Schramm J, Jones SJ, eds. *Spinal cord monitoring*. Berlin: Springer-Verlag, 1986;215–220.
12. Lesser RP, Raudzens P, Luders H, et al. Postoperative neurological deficits may occur despite unchanged intraoperative somatosensory evoked potentials. *Ann Neurol* 1986;19:22–25.
13. American Electroencephalographic Society Evoked Potentials Committee. American electroencephalographic society guidelines for intraoperative monitoring of sensory evoked potentials. *J Clin Neurophysiol* 1987;4:397–416.
14. Koht A. Anesthesia and evoked potentials: overview. *Int J Clin Monitoring Computing* 1988;5:167–73.
15. McMeniman WJ, Purcell GJ. Neurological monitoring during anesthesia and surgery. *Anesth Intensive Care* 1988;16:358–367.
16. Schramm J. Spinal cord monitoring: current status and new developments. *Central Nerv Syst Trauma* 1985;2:207–227.
17. Dinner DS, Shields RW Jr, Luders H. Intraoperative spinal cord monitoring. In Rothman RH, Simeone FA, eds. *Spine*, Vol II. Philadelphia: WB Saunders, 1992:1801.
18. Kochs E. Electrophysiological monitoring and mild hypothermia. *J Neurosurg Anesthesiol* 1995;7:222–228.
19. Nuwer MR, Dawson EG, Carlson LG, et al. Somatosensory evoked potential spinal cord monitoring reduces neurologic deficits after scoliosis surgery: results of a large multicenter survey. *EEG Clin Neurophysiol* 1995;96:6.
20. Ben-David B, Haller G, Taylor P. Anterior spinal fusion complicated by paraplegia: a case report of false-negative somatosensory evoked potential. *Spine* 1987;12:536.
21. Owen GH, Bridwell KH, Grubb R, et al. The clinical application of neurogenic motor evoked potentials to monitor spinal cord function during surgery. *Spine* 1991;16:S385.
22. Ashkenaze D, Mudiyan B, Boachie-Adjei O, et al. Efficacy of spinal cord monitoring in neuromuscular scoliosis. *Spine* 1993;18:1627–1633.
23. Lubicky JB, Spadoro JA, Yuan HA, et al. Variability of somatosensory evoked potential monitoring during spinal surgery. *Spine* 1989;14: 790–798.
24. Tamaki T, Tsuji H, Inoue S, et al. The prevention of iatrogenic spinal cord injury utilizing the evoked spinal cord potential. *Int Orthop* (SICOT) 1981;4:313–317.
25. Tsuyama N, Tsuzuki N, Kurokawa T, et al. Clinical application of spinal cord action potential measurement. *Int Orthop* (SICOT) 1978;2:39–46.
26. Owen JH. Evoked potential monitoring during spinal surgery. In: Bridwell KH, Dewald RL, eds. *The textbook of spinal surgery*. Philadelphia: Lippincott, 1997;31–64.

27. Katifi HA, Sedgwick EM. Somatosensory evoked potentials from posterior tibial nerve and lumbosacral dermatomes. *Electroencephalogr Clin Neurophysiol* 1986;65:249–259.
28. Levy WJ Jr, York DH. Evoked potentials form the motor tracts in humans. *Neurosurgery* 1983;12:422.
29. Owen JH, Laschinger J, Bridwell K, et al. Sensitivity and specificity of somatosensory and neurogenic-motor evoked potentials in animals and humans. *Spine* 1988;13:1111.
30. Shimuzu H, Shimoji K, Maruyama Y, et al. Human spinal cord potentials produced in lumbosacral enlargement by descending volleys. *J Neurophysiol* 1982;48:1108.
31. Barker AT, Freeston IL, Jalinous R, et al. Magnetic stimulation of the human brain. *J Physiol* 1985;369:3p.
32. Barker AT, Jalinous R, Freeston IL, et al. Noninvasive magnetic stimulation of the human cortex. *Lancet* 1985;2:1106–1107.
33. Mills KR, Murray NMF, Hess CW. Magnetic and electrical transcranial brain stimulation: physiological mechanisms and clinical applications. *Neurosurgery* 1987;20:164–168.
34. Rothwell JC, Day BL, Thompson PD, et al. Some experiences of techniques for stimulation of the human cerebral motor cortex through the scalp. *Neurosurgery* 1987;20:156–163.
35. Machida M, Weinstein SL, Yamada T, et al. Spinal cord monitoring: electrophysiological measures of sensory and motor function during spinal surgery. *Spine* 1985;407.
36. Machida M, Weinstein SL, Yamada T, et al. Dissociation of muscle action potentials and spinal somatosensory evoked potentials after ischemic damage to the spinal cord. *Spine* 1988;13:1119.
37. Tamaki T, Noguchi T, Takano H, et al. Spinal cord monitoring as a clinical utilization of spinal evoked potentials. *Clin Orthop* 1984;185:58–64.
38. Burke D, Hicks R, Stephen J, et al. Assessment of corticospinal and somatosensory conduction simultaneously during scoliosis surgery. *EEG Clin Neurophysiol* 1992;85:388–396.
39. Imai T. A clinical study on intra-operative spinal cord monitoring with spinal evoked potential for scoliosis. *J Jpn Orthop Assoc* 1988;62:511–521.
40. Ohmi Y, Tohno S, Harada S, et al. Spinal cord monitoring using evoked potentials recorded from epidural space. In: Homma S, Tamaki T, eds. *Fundamentals and clinical application of spinal cord monitoring.* Tokyo: Saikon Press, 1984:203–210.
41. Kitagawa H, Itoh T, Takano H, et al. Motor evoked potential monitoring during upper cervical spine surgery. *Spine* 1989;14:1078–1083.
42. Zentner J. Noninvasive motor evoked potential monitoring during neurosurgical operations on the spinal cord. *Neurosurgery* 1989;24:709–712.
43. Jones SJ, Edger MA, Ransford AO, et al. A system for the electrophysiological monitoring of the spinal cord during operations for scoliosis. *J Bone Joint Surg Br* 1983;65:134–139.
44. Calancie B, Klose J, Baier S, et al. Isoflurane induced attenuation of motor evoked potentials caused by electrical motor cortex stimulation during surgery. *J Neurosurg* 1991;74:879.

CHAPTER 21

Diagnostic Blocks

Nikolai Bogduk

Pain is a subjective experience. It is not morphologic. It cannot be palpated. It cannot be seen. It cannot be photographed. Nor can it be x-rayed.

When physicians attribute a patient's neck pain to a lesion seen on a plain radiograph, on computed tomography (CT), or on magnetic resonance imaging (MRI), they rely on inferences. They infer that the lesion that they see is consistently associated with pain. This is not necessarily the case, and few such inferences have been validated. Some are acceptable, although not proven. Others are unacceptable because they contradict available, objective data.

Upon finding a tumor or a fracture, it seems reasonable to attribute the pain to that lesion. Some tumors and fractures, however, may be painless, and despite their presence, the patient's pain could be due to some other cause.

In contrast, spondylosis per se is not a cause of neck pain, nor is osteoarthrosis of the synovial joints of the neck. Cervical spondylosis is essentially equally prevalent in patients with neck pain and in individuals without pain (1,2). Osteoarthritis of the zygapophysial joints of the neck is actually slightly more common in individuals with no neck pain (1). Therefore, finding spondylosis on a radiograph is not tantamount to finding the cause of the pain. Spondylosis is a normal age-related change (3,4) and, in the context of neck pain, constitutes an incidental finding.

In patients with neck pain, radiographic imaging is often nondiagnostic. Tumors and metabolic disorders of the cervical spine are rare, especially in patients with no history or clinical features of such disorders. Even fractures are a relatively rare cause of neck pain. In surveys of emergency departments, fractures are evident in only about 3% of patients presenting with known or suspected neck injury (5).

Two large surveys, each involving more than 1,000 cases, found plain films of the cervical spine to be unproductive investigations. The British study (2) concluded that "there were no unexpected findings of malignancy or infection in any of the films"; and "X-ray examination of the neck should be performed if there is a clinical suspicion of infection or malignancy or after some instances of trauma. . . . In most cases, however, there seems to be little point in requesting films of the neck to find cervical spondylosis." After a 5-year follow-up, the American study (6) concluded that "no medically dangerous diagnoses would have been missed if the cervical spine series had not been done." These data disarm the physician seeking to diagnose neck pain. Radiographic imaging may not provide the answer.

SOURCES OF NECK PAIN

Any of the elements of the cervical spine could, in theory, be a source of pain. These include the bones, ligaments, and muscles of the neck, the cervical intervertebral discs, and the synovial joints. However, there are no reliable or valid clinical tests or investigations by which to incriminate bones, ligaments, or muscles as the source of pain in patients with no suggestion of tumor, fracture, infection, or inflammatory disease. A valid diagnosis of pain from these structures cannot be made.

Some authorities maintain that pain stemming from the cervical intervertebral discs can be diagnosed using disc stimulation and discography (7,8). In the absence of other means of diagnosing or refuting discogenic pain, this notion is attractive, but cervical discography is subject to high false-positive rates (9); and if all discs are studied in a patient, symptomatic discs are often found at multiple levels (10). Such findings are either false positive or indicate that discogenic pain occurs at so many segmental levels that it defies operative management. For this reason, the diagnostic utility of cervical discography lies more in preventing unnecessary surgery than in pinpointing a single, treatable source of pain (10).

Of all the possible sources of idiopathic neck pain, perhaps the most extensively and most rigorously studied are the cervical zygapophysial joints.

CERVICAL ZYGAPOPHYSIAL JOINT PAIN

In normal volunteers, distending the cervical zygapophysial joints with careful, intraarticular injections of contrast medium elicits neck pain and referred pain in characteristic locations (11) (Fig. 21.1). The same patterns have been confirmed using electrical stimulation of the nerves that innervate these joints (12). These so-called pain maps, however, are not diagnostic of zygapophysial joint pain because the same patterns are seen when the intervertebral discs are stimulated (10). What the maps reflect is the segmental innervation of the source of pain. As such, they can be used to indicate at which segmental level investigations should commence. For this purpose, the maps have been found to serve quite well to predict which level is painful (13,14).

DIAGNOSTIC BLOCKS

Because zygapophysial joint pain cannot be seen on x-ray, CT, or MRI, its diagnosis relies on other means, such as controlled diagnostic blocks of the painful joint.

The cervical zygapophysial joints are innervated by the medial branches of the cervical dorsal rami (15) (Fig. 21.2).

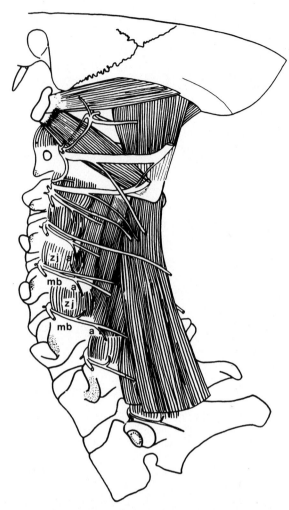

FIG. 21.2. A sketch of a lateral view of the cervical spine showing the course of the medial branches (mb) of the cervical dorsal rami and their articular branches (a) to the cervical zygapophysial joints (zj).

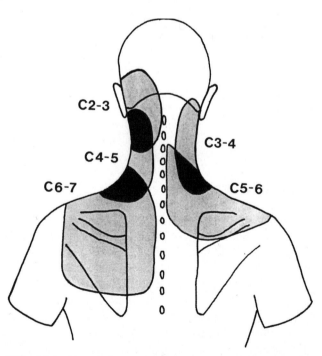

FIG. 21.1. Maps of the distribution of pain produced in normal volunteers by stimulating the cervical zygapophysial joints. The same patterns obtain for pain stemming from the intervertebral discs at corresponding segments.

At typical cervical levels, each joint is supplied by the ipsisegmental medial branches. Thus, the C5-C6 zygapophysial joint, for example, is innervated by the C5-C6 medial branches. The C2-C3 zygapophysial joint is innervated by the third occipital nerve (C3) and a communicating loop from this nerve to the C2 dorsal ramus.

The medial branches of the cervical dorsal rami assume a constant course around the waist of their ipsisegmental articular pillar. The third occipital nerve crosses the C2-C3 joint. This constancy of location allows the cervical zygapophysial joints to be anesthetized using medial branch blocks, in which small volumes (0.3 mL) of local anesthetic can be injected selectively onto the target nerves.

Cervical medial branch blocks have face validity (16). Local anesthetic, injected onto the medial branches in volumes of 0.5 mL or less, does not spread to anesthetize other structures that might feasibly be competing sources of pain. In particular, the local anaesthetic does not spread to the spinal nerves or epidural space. It does not diffuse randomly or widely through the neck muscles. Rather, it spreads only in the cleavage plane between semispinalis capitis and semispinalis cervicis.

Medial branch blocks have construct validity: they accurately identify patients with zygapophysial joint pain. However, a single, diagnostic block has been shown to have a false-positive rate of 27% (17). Consequently, a valid diagnosis of zygapophysial joint pain cannot be made using a single, diagnostic block. To be valid, diagnostic blocks must be controlled.

For research purposes, placebo controls can be used, but these controls can be cumbersome and impractical. They require informed consent for a sham procedure, and necessitate at least three procedures: one active block to find a putatively painful joint, and then two confirmatory blocks in which placebo or an active agent is randomly allocated (18,19).

A more convenient and practical control is a comparative local anesthetic block (19,20). This involves anesthetizing the target joint on each of two separate occasions using local anesthetic agents with different durations of action, under double-blind conditions. The response to such blocks is negative when on each occasion the patient obtains no relief of pain. A concordant positive response is one in which the patient obtains complete relief of pain on each occasion, and the relief is concordant with the expected action of the agent used—that is, long-lasting relief when a long-acting agent is used, but short-lasting relief when a short-acting agent is used. A discordant positive response is one in which the patient obtains complete relief of pain on both occasions but the duration of relief following the shorter-acting agent is paradoxically longer lasting than after the longer-acting agent.

The construct validity of comparative local anesthetic blocks of the cervical zygapophysial joints has been demonstrated (20). It has also been tested against placebo (21). When compared with placebo blocks, concordant responses to comparative blocks are only moderately sensitive but very specific. That means that not all patients with zygapophysial joint pain will necessarily be detected, but those positive responses are unlikely to be false positive. Discordant responses to comparative local anaesthetic blocks are less specific but have higher sensitivity. They detect more patients as possibly positive, but 35% of these results may be false positive. Nevertheless, 65% of discordant responses have been shown to be true positive (21).

Cervical medial branch blocks have predictive validity and therapeutic utility. A positive response to blocks predicts a possible response to treatment (22–24). If diagnosed by controlled blocks, cervical zygapophysial joint pain can be successfully treated by radiofrequency medial branch neurotomy (22–25). In this regard, comparative blocks and placebo-controlled blocks are equally predictive (23).

To my knowledge, no other test for neck pain has been subjected to such rigorous scientific scrutiny as have cervical medial branch blocks. They are the only tests shown to have face validity, construct validity, and predictive validity.

In addition to having scientific and clinical validity, controlled diagnostic blocks have been shown to be cost effective (26). The critical factor is the ratio between the cost of treatment and the cost of performing controlled blocks. Placebo-controlled blocks have been shown to be cost effective whenever this ratio is greater than 8.3.

TECHNIQUE

The standard approach for cervical medial branch blocks requires that the patient lay on a fluoroscopy table, in a lateral position with the target side up. The skin is prepared as for an aseptic procedure. A true lateral view of the cervical spine is imperative (18,19).

For typical cervical medial branches, the target point lies at the intersection of the diagonals of the articular pillar (18, 19) (Fig. 21.3). At C7, the target point is different because the root of the C7 process occupies most of the center of the articular pillar and displaces the nerve cephalad. The target point for the C7 medial branch is the apex of the C7 superior articular process. The third occipital nerve (C3) has a variable course and requires three target points (Fig. 21.4). These lie along an axial line that bisects the C2-C3 zygapophysial joint. The first target point lies on this line opposite the bottom of the C2-C3 intervertebral foramen. The second point lies opposite the apex of the C3 superior articular process, and the third point lies midway between the first two points (18,19).

To anesthetize a typical cervical zygapophysial joint, both medial branches that innervate it need to be blocked.

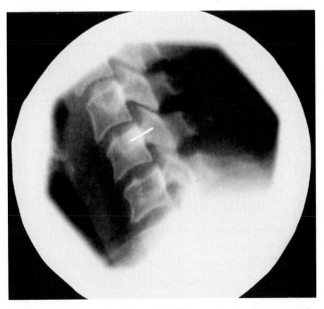

FIG. 21.3. A lateral radiograph of the neck showing a needle in position to block the medial branch of the C5 dorsal ramus.

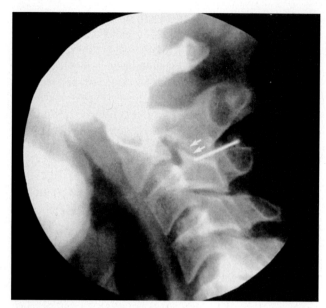

FIG. 21.4. A lateral radiograph of a C2-C3 zygapophysial joint, showing the three target points for blocks of the third occipital nerve.

For the C2-C3 joint, only the third occipital nerve needs to be blocked.

After the target point has been identified, a puncture point on the skin is selected directly overlying the target point. Through the puncture point, a 25-gauge, 90-mm spinal needle is inserted and is progressively advanced to the target point until it strikes bone. Safety is ensured by having the point of the needle never stray beyond the perimeter of the articular pillar on which the target point lies. When the needle is in correct position, no more than 0.3 mL of local anesthetic needs to be injected to anesthetize the target nerve.

INTERPRETATION

If a single zygapophysial joint is the source of a patient's pain, then anesthetizing that joint should completely relieve the pain. The patient's postprocedural visual analog score should be zero and should remain that way for the duration of action of the agent used.

If a patient has bilateral pain, anesthetizing the responsible joint on one side should provide complete relief of pain on that side. Such a response constitutes a positive response for that side. On a separate occasion, the opposite side can be investigated. If painful joints have been identified on both sides, both sides can be anesthetized simultaneously to confirm the responses to blocks and to provide complete relief of pain bilaterally.

If a patient has two painful joints on the same side at consecutive levels, blocking the upper joint should completely relieve the upper half of the pain. On a subsequent occasion, blocking the lower joint should relieve the lower half of the pain. On a third occasion, both joints can be blocked

simultaneously to confirm the response and to provide complete relief of pain.

If a patient has pain from two joints at nonconsecutive levels, each joint can be addressed separately. Blocking one joint should completely relieve the upper part of the patient's pain, whereas blocking the other joint should relieve the lower pain.

In this regard, the common patterns that are often encountered include the following (27,28): a single joint, most commonly at C5-C6 in patients with neck pain and referred pain to the shoulder girdle or at C2-C3 in patients with neck pain and headache; single joints at the same segment bilaterally, most often C5-C6 or C2-C3; two joints at displaced levels, most often C5–6 and C2–3; and two consecutive joints, usually C5-C6 and C6-C7.

The emphasis in interpreting the response to blocks is that the patient must obtain complete relief of pain in the area targeted. Partial relief of pain does not constitute a positive response. The patient may still have pain in other areas—higher up, lower down, or on the other side—but in the area targeted, the patient must report complete relief. Other areas can be investigated subsequently and separately to determine whether another zygapophysial joint or some other source is responsible for any remnant pain.

Most critically, any positive response to an initial diagnostic block must be confirmed on a subsequent occasion using a control block. For this purpose, blocks can be readily undertaken on a double-blind basis, randomly allocating a short-acting agent such as lidocaine or a long-acting agent such as bupivacaine, on each occasion.

Studies on the utility of diagnostic blocks have shown that, on average, no more than two or three blocks are required to establish a diagnosis of cervical zygapophysial joint pain: one or two blocks to find the painful joint, and one more to check the response with a control block (14). If the patient's pain map is carefully interpreted, the responsible joint can usually be pinpointed after the first block. If not, the responsible joint may lie at an adjacent segmental level. If diagnostic blocks at two consecutive levels prove negative, however, proceeding to a third block is very unlikely to prove positive (14); the source of the patient's pain will usually not be found in the zygapophysial joints.

EPIDEMIOLOGY

I am aware of three studies that have determined the prevalence of cervical zygapophysial joint pain in patients with chronic neck pain. One used placebo-controlled blocks (27), and two used comparative blocks (14,29). Their results were uniform. Using a worst-case analysis, the prevalence of zygapophysial joint pain (and 95% confidence limits) were 54% (40% to 68%) (29), 49% (33% to 64%) (27), and 36% (27% to 45%) (14). Essentially, half or nearly half of all patients with chronic neck pain have zygapophysial joint pain. Among vehicle occupants who developed neck pain after a severe so-called whiplash accident, the prevalence was reported to be a mean of 74% (65% to 83%) (30). In patients with neck pain and headache after whiplash, the prevalence of zygapophysial joint pain was reported to be 53% (31). These figures show that diagnostic blocks of the cervical zygapophysial joints are important. They detect a very common source of pain in patients in whom no other investigation has been or can be diagnostic. Unless diagnostic blocks are performed, these patients remain without a diagnosis and without an option for treatment.

THERAPEUTIC UTILITY

I am aware of only one proven treatment for cervical zygapophysial joint pain. Percutaneous radiofrequency medial branch neurotomy has the ability to render patients pain free who have proven cervical zygapophysial joint pain. This procedure has been evaluated in observational studies (23–25,32) and submitted to a randomized, double-blind, placebo-controlled trial (22).

The singular indication for medial branch neurotomy is complete relief of pain after controlled diagnostic blocks of the cervical zygapophysial joints (22,25). In this regard, placebo-controlled blocks and comparative blocks are equally predictive of a response (23).

The response rate of medial branch neurotomy has been shown to be 70%. This implies that 70% of patients can expect to obtain complete relief of pain, accompanied by restoration of activities of daily living and no need for other continuing care (22,23,25). The duration of relief, however, is finite, and amounted to a median period of at least 263 days in one study (23) and 412 days in a longer study (25). Pain recurs ostensibly because the coagulated nerve regenerates. However, if pain recurs, the operation can be repeated to obtain relief. After repeat neurotomy, pain relief has been reported for a median period of at least 218 days (23,25).

In some patients, when pain recurs, it is not of sufficient intensity to warrant repeat neurotomy. These patients can resume a reasonably normal life without requiring reoperation. However, if needs be, the operation can be repeated several times. Patients have undergone as many as six repetitions, with each restoring complete relief of pain and the patient maintaining complete rehabilitation for up to 5 years (23,25).

Cervical medial branch neurotomy is a safe procedure when performed correctly. Its only limitation is that its effects are not permanent.

CONCLUSION

Systematic evaluations have established that cervical zygapophysial joint blocks are a valid diagnostic tool. Moreover, they are epidemiologically relevant. They can provide a diagnosis in about 50% of patients with chronic neck pain.

Zygapophysial joint pain cannot be diagnosed from history alone, by physical examination, or by radiographic imaging. Unless diagnostic blocks are performed, patients with this condition may remain undiagnosed and ineligible for treatment. Radiofrequency neurotomy is a proven treatment for cervical zygapophysial joint pain, but it is not a perfect treatment.

At a fundamental level, the development and application of cervical zygapophysial joint blocks has vindicated a principle: that chronic neck pain can be pinpointed and managed. All that is required is that appropriate and valid tools be used. The zygapophysial joints are only one of the possible sources of neck pain. If appropriate diagnostic tools are developed for other sources of neck pain, their application will serve to reduce the burden of chronic neck pain even further.

REFERENCES

1. Fridenberg ZB, Miller WT. Degenerative disc disease of the cervical spine. A comparative study of asymptomatic and symptomatic patients. *J Bone Joint Surg Am* 1963;45:1171–1178.
2. Heller CA, Stanley P, Lewis-Jones B, et al. Value of x-ray examinations of the cervical spine. *BMJ* 1983;287:1276–1278.
3. Gore DR, Sepic SB, Gardner GM. Roentgenographic findings of the cervical spine in asymptomatic people. *Spine* 1986;1:521–524.
4. Elias F. Roentgen findings in the asymptomatic cervical spine. *N Y State J Med* 1958;58:3300–3303.
5. Roberge RJ, Wears RC, Kelly M, et al. Selective application of cervical spine radiography in alert victims of blunt trauma: a prospective study. *J Trauma* 1988;28:784–788.
6. Johnson MJ, Lucas GL. Value of cervical spine radiographs as a screening tool. *Clin Orthop* 1997;340:102–108.
7. Bogduk N, Aprill C, Derby R. Discography. In: White AH, ed. *Spine care. Volume one: diagnosis and conservative treatment*. St Louis: Mosby, 1995:219–238.
8. Schellhas KP, Smith MD, Gundry CR, et al. Cervical discogenic pain: prospective correlation of magnetic resonance imaging and discography in asymptomatic subjects and pain sufferers. *Spine* 1996;21:300–312.
9. Bogduk N, Aprill C. On the nature of neck pain, discography and cervical zygapophysial joint pain. *Pain* 1993;54:213–217.
10. Grubb SA, Kelly CK. Cervical discography: clinical implications from 12 years of experience. *Spine* 2000;25:1382–1389.
11. Dwyer A, Aprill C, Bogduk N. Cervical zygapophysial joint pain patterns. I. A study in normal volunteers. *Spine* 1990;15:453–457.
12. Fukui S, Ohseto K, Shiotani M, et al. Referred pain distribution of the cervical zygapophyseal joints and cervical dorsal rami. *Pain* 1996;68:79–83.
13. Aprill C, Dwyer A, Bogduk N. Cervical zygapophyseal joint pain patterns. II. A clinical evaluation. *Spine* 1990;15:458–461.
14. Speldewinde GC, Bashford GM, Davidson IR. Diagnostic cervical zygapophysial joint blocks for chronic cervical pain. *Med J Aust* 2001;174:174–176.
15. Bogduk N. The clinical anatomy of the cervical dorsal rami. *Spine* 1982;7:319–330.
16. Barnsley L, Bogduk N. Medial branch blocks are specific for the diagnosis of cervical zygapophysial joint pain. *Reg Anesth* 1993;18:343–350.
17. Barnsley L, Lord S, Wallis B, et al. False-positive rates of cervical zygapophysial joint blocks. *Clin J Pain* 1993;9:124–130.
18. Bogduk N. International Spinal Injection Society guidelines for the performance of spinal injection procedures. 1. Zygapophysial joint blocks. *Clin J Pain* 1997;13:285–302.
19. Bogduk N, Lord SM. Cervical zygapophysial joint pain. *Neurosurg Q* 1998;8:107–117.
20. Barnsley L, Lord S, Bogduk N. Comparative local anaesthetic blocks in the diagnosis of cervical zygapophysial joints pain. *Pain* 1993;55:99–106.

21. Lord SM, Barnsley L, Bogduk N. The utility of comparative local anaesthetic blocks versus placebo-controlled blocks for the diagnosis of cervical zygapophysial joint pain. *Clin J Pain* 1995;11:208–213.

22. Lord SM, Barnsley L, Wallis BJ, et al. Percutaneous radio-frequency neurotomy for chronic cervical zygapophysial-joint pain. *N Engl J Med* 1996;335:1721–1726.

23. McDonald G, Lord SM, Bogduk N. Long-term follow-up of cervical radiofrequency neurotomy for chronic neck pain. *Neurosurgery* 1999; 45:61–68.

24. Lord SM, Barnsley L, Bogduk N. Percutaneous radiofrequency neurotomy in the treatment of cervical zygapophysial joint pain: a caution. *Neurosurgery* 1995;36:732–739.

25. Lord SM, McDonald GJ, Bogduk N. Percutaneous radiofrequency neurotomy of the cervical medial branches: a validated treatment for cervical zygapophysial joint pain. *Neurosurg Q* 1998;8:288–308.

26. Bogduk N, Holmes S. Controlled zygapophysial joint blocks: the travesty of cost-effectiveness. *Pain Med* 2000;1:25–34.

27. Lord S, Barnsley L, Wallis BJ, et al. Chronic cervical zygapophysial joint pain after whiplash: a placebo-controlled prevalence study. *Spine* 1996;21:1737–1745.

28. Lord SM, Bogduk N. The cervical synovial joints as sources of post-traumatic headache. *J Musculoskeletal Pain* 1996;4:81–94.

29. Barnsley L, Lord SM, Wallis BJ, et al. The prevalence of chronic cervical zygapophysial joint pain after whiplash. *Spine* 1995;20:20–26.

30. Gibson T, Bogduk N, Macpherson J, et al. Crash characteristics of whiplash associated chronic neck pain. *J Musculoskeletal Pain* 2000;8:87–95.

31. Lord S, Barnsley L, Wallis B, et al. Third occipital nerve headache: a prevalence study. *J Neurol Neurosurg Psychiatry* 1994;57:1187–1190.

32. Sapir D, Gorup JM. Radiofrequency medial branch neurotomy in litigant and nonlitigant patients with cervical whiplash. *Spine* 2001;26:E268–E273.

CHAPTER 22

Diagnostic Cervical Disc Injection

Seth M. Zeidman

Cervical diagnostic disc injection (discography) remains one of the more controversial areas of spinal surgery. Discography is classically defined as the direct visualization of the intervertebral disc by percutaneous injection of water-soluble iodine solution into the nucleus pulposus with a small-gauge needle. More than 40 years ago in Scandinavia, Hirsch (10) and Lindblom (17) used direct puncture to study the lumbar intervertebral disc to localize symptomatic levels in patients with low back pain (10). Cervical discography was introduced by Smith and Nichols (32) in 1957 and Cloward (2) in 1958. Later, an analgesic-therapeutic component was incorporated into the radiographic and provocative aspects of the study (38).

Proponents of discography contend that it is the best radiologic method to assess anatomy of the intervertebral disc, especially when used in conjunction with computed tomography (CT) (19,23). Discography can demonstrate abnormalities of the cervical disc not appreciated on myelography, plain CT, or magnetic resonance imaging (MRI). Many experienced clinicians use cervical discography as a diagnostic tool in the evaluation of patients with complex cervical symptomatology (6, 8,19). The most important component of the discogram is the use of disc injection for production of pain during injection that accurately reproduces the patient's symptoms (concordant pain). Opponents of discography argue that although the test may be sensitive, it is nonspecific (16,22). Discs with abnormal appearance can frequently be observed in asymptomatic patients. Opponents further contend that surgical intervention based on diagnostic disc injection is, by its very nature, condemned to limited success.

Despite extensive experience with diagnostic cervical disc injection, the role of discography in evaluation of patients with degenerative cervical disc disease and neck pain remains somewhat controversial and incompletely defined (22,36). This chapter briefly reviews some of the historical background of the procedure, delineates the method for its performance, reviews the basic pathophysiology of disco-

genic pain, touches on the potential complications of discography, and outlines some of the arguments for and against diagnostic cervical disc injection.

HISTORY

Early interest in the anatomy, physiology, and pathoanatomy of the intervertebral disc was fostered by the work of Schmorl (28), who described nucleus pulposus herniation into the vertebral body. Schmorl's research stimulated additional investigation of the intervertebral disc, the most significant of which was the contribution of Keys and Compere (14). In the next two decades, there followed an extremely large, diverse literature on disc lesions, notably, disc injury with herniation. Because of the inherent limitations of imaging at the time, the scope of the literature primarily included mechanisms of disc injury, general disc pathology, surgical and nonsurgical treatment of the ruptured disc, and subsequent treatment outcomes.

Aside from a few articles on myelography, relatively little was published before the 1950s regarding the radiographic diagnosis of cervical disc pathology. Lindblom (17) published one of the most significant articles in 1948, reporting the poor sensitivity and specificity of myelography in demonstrating the herniated disc. This opinion was shared by Scoville and colleagues (29). Lindblom, distressed by the unreliability of myelography, conceived direct puncture to study the intervertebral disc (17).

In 1957, Smith and Nichols (32) were the first to use diagnostic disc injection, or discography, as a diagnostic tool for evaluation of cervical intervertebral disc degeneration. Diagnostic cervical disc injection technique was subsequently popularized by both Cloward (2–5) and Smith (31). Working independently, these two investigators developed similar techniques for evaluating chronic discogenic pain. Their premise was based on the observation that injection of a symptomatic disc could reliably produce clinical symptoms and a similar discometric profile. That is, a normal disc accepted a small volume of fluid, and abnormal discs accepted larger fluid volumes. A normal discometric profile was invariably associated with a clinically insignificant, "physiologic" pain response. Furthermore, each investigator stressed the relative importance of the concordant pain response on disc distention as opposed to the qualitative appearance of a discogram that was deemed generally nonspecific. Furthermore, the clinical value of anesthetic disc injection was also evident to both examiners. Ultimately, both Smith (31) and Cloward (2) used diagnostic cervical disc injection technique to facilitate surgical patient selection.

Cloward (2) popularized discography in several articles, advancing the thesis that direct disc puncture provided a greater diagnostic database regarding disc injuries in general and that, as a diagnostic procedure, it was more comprehensive than myelography (2). Furthermore, Cloward wrote that the indications for and chief value of discography were related to its ability to diagnose a discopathic or discogenic basis for a given posttraumatic pain syndrome in the absence of a myelographic defect. Beginning in 1958, Cloward (2) championed discography as a routine diagnostic study. In subsequent years, however, many clinicians began to question the validity of cervical discography as a diagnostic tool.

Holt (11) reported on 50 prisoners at the Missouri state penitentiary who underwent cervical discography without fluoroscopic guidance with large (22-gauge) needles. Injection of sodium diatrizoate produced significant pain in all subjects. Holt concluded that cervical discography was painful, expensive, and without diagnostic value (39). Cloward (1) and other researchers vehemently refuted the evidence presented by Holt, describing it as scientifically inaccurate and based on false premises and conclusions (7). Many subsequent international researchers reported the validity of cervical discography as a diagnostic procedure. Although his study was fundamentally flawed by improper or at least suboptimal technique, Holt's work caused the credibility of discography to undergo intense scrutiny.

In 1976, Roth (38) reemphasized the earlier work of Smith regarding the anesthetic injection of the cervical disc. Again using the positive postanesthetic clinical response as surgical selection criteria for discectomy and anterior cervical fusion, Roth reported a high surgical success rate.

Since then, a dramatic polarization of opinion has developed regarding the efficacy of discography. This in many ways reflects the parallel controversy over the efficacy and role of surgery for discogenic pain (36,37).

NONINVASIVE IMAGING AND DISCOGRAPHY

The late 1970s and early 1980s heralded major advances in imaging technology with enhanced sensitivity and specificity for pathoanatomy (18). In conjunction with intrathecal contrast enhancement, CT and MRI revolutionized diagnostic spinal imaging. Computer-based technologies have significantly advanced overall diagnostic capability, but radiographic appearances may be deceiving. It is impossible to predict the clinical relevance of an imaged intervertebral disc lesion accurately. Correlation of symptoms with imaging data is not sufficiently reliable to allow unequivocal determination of the nature, location, and extent of symptomatic pathology. This is particularly true in the patient population with chronic discogenic pain (27).

MRI and CT are recognized as the primary methods for investigation of disc herniation and degeneration. Investigators have contended that discography adds little to the diagnostic workup when CT and MRI are available (16,27). However, retrospective studies describe a generally poor correlation between MRI and provocative discography in the cervical spine (6,9). The ability of MRI to identify and localize the source of cervical discogenic pain accurately has been limited. Because of its invasive nature, discography introduces the risk for infection and neural injury. Many have proposed that MRI could replace the technique and remove the risk for infection.

Parfenchuck and Janssen (40) attempted to correlate the morphology of sagittal T2-weighted MRI of the cervical spine with provocative discography and CT discograms in 52 patients with discogenic pain. They noted a significant correlation between MRI abnormality and pain response to discography. However, the false-positive and false-negative rates were high. MRI was a useful adjunct to cervical discography, but some MRI patterns could not be considered pathologic, and discography was required to diagnose discogenic pain (12,40). Parfenchuck and Janssen (12,40), after comparing the ability of discography, discography with CT, and MRI in detecting a painful disc, concluded that MRI was the only imaging technique with strong correlation. In light of these studies, cervical discography may have a place in assessing patients with chronic severe neck pain with a presumed discogenic pain generator.

Schellhas and co-workers (41) compared and attempted to correlate MRI and cervical discography in evaluation of patients with discogenic pain. Ten asymptomatic subjects and 10 patients with chronic neck pain underwent cervical discography after MRI. Disc morphology and provoked responses were recorded at each level studied. Discographically normal discs were never painful, whereas intensely painful discs all exhibited tears of both the inner and outer aspects of the annulus. Schellhas and co-workers (41) concluded that MRI was ineffective in detecting significant annular tears and could not reliably identify the source of cervical discogenic pain.

Diagnostic cervical disc injection is an adjunctive diagnostic procedure. High-resolution CT and MRI remain the primary imaging modalities. However, discography may be helpful in delineating symptomatic annular tears and fissures as well as lateral and far-lateral disc herniations, some of which can be missed even on MRI (40). Discography is a reliable means of evaluating the integrity of the intervertebral disc. The normal disc will often accept 0.5 mL of saline or contrast media without difficulty. Considerable force is required to inject any volume of fluid into a healthy disc, and accommodation of 1 mL or more of liquid by a disc is indicative of either degeneration within the nucleus pulposus or extravasation of material through a rent in the annulus fibrosus. Extravasation of contrast material occurs through fissures and tears of the annulus and may be apparent with both degeneration and herniation.

The type and distribution of pain the injection causes should be noted. Testing the patient's response to intradiscal injection as well as to intradiscal local anesthetic agent is termed *provocation-analgesic discography*. Proponents of discography contend that morphologic assessment of the intervertebral disc can be complemented by the critical physiologic induction of pain that is similar or identical to the subjective complaint (concordant pain). The disc or discs that reproduce the patient's symptoms are the ones that may be amenable to efficacious treatment. Provocation-analgesic discography has been used increasingly in evaluation of patients with chronic discogenic symptoms.

Re-creation of pain with saline or contrast injection in some patients but not in others is troubling, all the more troubling when one is faced with a patient with an asymptomatic but dramatic morphologic derangement. Degenerative patterns are often noted and nonspecific pain often elicited in asymptomatic discs, limiting test usefulness. Concordant pain has been postulated to result from the microenvironment in the intervertebral disc and the sensitized state of annular nociceptors.

DISCOGENIC PATHOLOGY AND INDICATIONS FOR DISCOGRAPHY

Regarding symptomatic cervical disc disorders, the following simple classification encompasses most pathology: (a) symptomatic cervical spondylosis; (b) cervical herniation; and (c) internal disc disruption.

Symptomatic Cervical Spondylosis

Symptomatic cervical spondylosis has generally been considered a normal aging process. The pathophysiology begins with disc desiccation and progresses to disc space narrowing, marginal osteophytic spurring, and, finally, degenerative changes at the facet joint level. Clinical features vary, yet they correlate to some degree with discal dehydration. Symptoms range from episodic axial neck discomfort to severe acquired spinal stenosis with nerve root or cord entrapment.

Cervical Herniation

Cervical herniated disc disorders have been well chronicled in modern imaging texts. Sensitivity of MRI for disc prolapse has variably been reported to approach 98%.

Internal Disc Disruption

The final category, internal disc disruption, was initially popularized by Crock (42), who described disc lesions characterized by alteration in internal structure and metabolic functions unassociated with rupture or other definable pathoanatomy. A biochemical basis for deficiency was postulated, a hypothesis subsequently based on certain inflammatory-type pathologic features as shown by microscopy, in addition to intraoperative observations suggestive of peridiscal inflammation. Crock cited the often-observed element of increased peridiscal vascularity with sympathetic trunk matting and softening of the vertebral bodies. Clinical features of internal disc disruption are variable; however, Crock pointed out certain universal features that serve to differentiate the condition from others, such as rupture. A constant symptom described as a deep-seated, dull, aching neck pain was invariable. Shoulder girdle or limb pain was typically described as nondermatomal and generalized, in contrast to the more discrete pain characteristic of nerve root compression. A significant association with headache and constitutional symptoms was also noted.

The cardinal lesion rendering a cervical disc painful is internal disc disruption. The characteristic feature of internal disc disruption is a radial fissure extending to the innervated outer third of the annulus fibrosus. As radial fissures extend to the outer third of the annulus, nerve endings are exposed to the inflammatory and algogenic chemicals produced by nuclear degradation. As a radial fissure develops, fewer and fewer lamellae remain intact to bear the load. At some stage, the threshold for mechanical nociception is attained, especially if the nerve endings have been chemically sensitized. Disc stimulation reveals this condition by showing a reduced threshold for mechanical stimulation of the disc.

Discography has been postulated to provoke pain by either one or some combination of the following mechanisms:

1. Contrast injection into the disc increases intradiscal pressure. In an abnormal disc, stretching of the annular fibers of the disc stimulates nerve endings.
2. The injection may result in some biochemical or neurochemical stimulation that causes pain.
3. The injection may increase pressure at the end plates, or pressure may be transferred to the vertebral body throughout the end plate, resulting in an increase in intravertebral pressure. This theory is supported by studies reporting disc injection resulting in end-plate deflection and increased specimen height.
4. The presence of pain on injection of a seemingly normal disc may be due to transfer of pressure from the injection to an abnormal, symptomatic adjacent disc, thus eliciting a positive pain response.

Pathophysiologic mechanisms evoked include (a) biochemical irritation of adjacent neural structures; (b) spinal instability resulting in adjacent nerve root irritation; (c) leakage of biochemical antagonist, possibly disc protein metabolite, into the general circulation; and (d) autoimmune reaction through the spinal circulation pathway. Crock (43) advocated discography as the preferable diagnostic method; he believed it to be the only diagnostic tool capable of detecting the condition. Recently, many authors have provided the anatomic and histologic proof required for an intervertebral disc to generate pain (15,30,44). They have shown that the outer one third to one half of the annulus is richly innervated with a variety of free and complex nerve endings (24,28,41). Furthermore, Weinstein and colleagues demonstrated the biochemical means by which a disc can be a pain generator (44). They demonstrated the presence of substance P, calcitonin gene-related peptide, and vasoactive intestinal polypeptides in the outer one third of the disc in rats (44). Although the mechanism behind discogenic pain has not yet been proved, there are three proposed hypotheses by which axial pain with and without extremity pain from the disc may occur: mechanical, biochemical, and autoimmune (24,26).

The mechanical model theorizes that the afferent C fibers of the annulus may refer pain both axially and to the extremities. This occurs by the convergence of various primary sensory afferents, serving to innervate different peripheral sites, on dorsal horn neurons of the spinal cord (13). This convergence signal is then relayed to the cells of the anterolateral system, crosses over to the ventral white commissure, courses rostrally in the anterolateral funiculus, and supplies inputs to several thalamic nuclei and finally to the somatic sensory areas of the cerebral cortex (20). Therefore, the brain is unable to differentiate the true origin of the signal received from the myriad potential sites that could be feeding into the incoming signal. Consequently, a misperception in the location of the pain may be referred to a relatively distal axial location or the extremities (58).

The biochemical model proposes that biochemical events may lead to intervertebral disc degradation and, ultimately, to inflammation (45,46). Based on the articular cartilage model, it has been theorized that the disc cells themselves are a source of interleukin-1B (IL-1B) (46). IL-1B has been shown to increase dramatically the biosynthesis of matrix metalloproteinases, nitric oxide, IL-6, and prostaglandin E_2 in normal, nondegenerated discs (46). These biochemical agents are thought to inhibit proteoglycan synthesis and induce matrix degradation, resulting in a net loss of proteoglycans within the intervertebral disc. This leads to a dramatic alteration in the biochemical integrity of the disc, culminating in disc degeneration (25). Disc degeneration has been shown to result in the accumulation of elevated concentrations of phospholipase A_2 (PLA_2). PLA_2 is the enzyme responsible for the liberation of arachidonic acid from cell membranes resulting in the production of prostaglandins and leukotrienes at the site of injury. These chemical mediators serve to initiate and propagate the inflammatory cascade.

The autoimmune theory postulates that nuclear material in the epidural space, as occurs in disc herniations, is recog-

nized by the immune system as an antigen and stimulates reactions leading to inflammation. This occurs because the nucleus pulposus is sheltered from the circulatory system and thus the immune system during normal embryologic development. Autogenous nuclear material injected into the epidural space of dogs has been shown to produce an inflammatory response (46). Many authors have reported the high concentrations of macrophages and migration of mononuclear cells in association with extruded and sequestered discs (31–35). Other inflammatory mediators, such as IL-1α, IL-1β, IL-6, tumor necrosis factor-α, granulocyte-macrophage colony stimulating factor (47), leukotriene B_4, and thromboxane B_2, have also been associated with the inflammatory reactions associated with lumbar disc herniations. Furthermore, in vivo studies have demonstrated increased levels of matrix metalloproteinases, nitric oxide, IL-6, and prostaglandin E_2 in herniated lumbar discs when compared with control discs (23).

In the biochemical and autoimmune hypotheses, exudation of the previously described catabolites known to initiate inflammation has been found in the juxtapositioned epidural and perineural spaces, inciting both axial and extremity symptoms (21,48).

Many investigators have emphasized the difficulty in diagnosing and treating chronic cervical spine disorders. This difficulty again relates primarily to the issue of chronic internal disc disruption syndrome with occult discopathic pain mechanism and protean clinical expression. Anecdotally, I prospectively evaluated 500 patients with chronic cervical pain syndromes; for 3 years, diagnostic imaging with state-of-the art MRI was used to determine imaging sensitivity for the specified chief complaint of neck pain. Other pain features were variables not excluded. A finite structural defect to explain the patient's condition plausibly was determined in only 38% of cases. However, again there exists the dilemma of the clinical relevance of an imaged structural defect. Conventional imaging data are often insufficient because they are not specific enough to predict the site and pathophysiology of a symptomatic cervical spine lesion accurately.

In my personal experience, most clinical indications for diagnostic cervical disc injection include the following:

- Chronic cervical pain syndrome with discopathic clinical features yet nonspecific imaging results (59%)
- Multiple defects demonstrated by imaging to characterize the major discopathic pain generator or generators (17%)
- Discrepant imaging result (defect) to the clinical evaluation (5%)
- Recurrent postsurgical pain disorders related to remote discectomy with anterior fusion (13%)

Discography should be performed only if adequate attempts at conservative (nonoperative) therapy, and noninvasive diagnostic tests, such as MRI, have failed to reveal the etiology of neck pain.

Specific indications for discography include the following:

- Persistent, severe symptoms when other diagnostic tests have failed to clearly confirm a suspected disc as a source of the pain
- Evaluation of abnormal discs or recurrent pain from a previously operated disc
- Assessment of patients in whom surgery has failed, to determine whether pseudoarthrosis or a symptomatic disc could be the source of pain
- Assessment of discs before fusion to determine whether the discs of the proposed fusion segment are symptomatic and whether the discs adjacent to this segment can support a fusion

THE DISCOGRAM

The shape of the nucleus pulposus is variable and is best demonstrated in the lateral projection. The nucleus pulposus appears as a slightly oval mass, often with a horizontal relatively lucent band through its center (Fig. 22.1). The pattern of contrast dispersal is the least important criterion in cervical discography. However, several characteristic patterns of abnormality are evident after contrast injection into cervical discs:

- Rupture of the annulus fibrosus with escape of contrast media beneath the longitudinal ligament or into the epidural space
- Degeneration of the nucleus pulposus, which appears as a collapsed deflated balloon filling the sac space and even extending beyond it
- Fissures of the annulus allowing escape of contrast through the inner fibers annulus, which results in a collar-stud appearance of contrast media
- Intraosseous herniation with escape of contrast through the vertebral end plates
- Contrast leakage beneath an unfused ring epiphysis leading to vertebral edge separation

The normal disc accepts a limited volume of fluid, and gentle distention does not produce significant pain. The volume of the nucleus pulposus in the adult cervical disc is well established. The maximum volume accepted by almost all cervical discs is less than 0.5 mL (18). Discs accepting more than 0.5 mL typically demonstrate posterolateral leakage. Intraoperative pressure-volume measurements demonstrate that normal-appearing discs accept 0.2 to 0.4 mL of

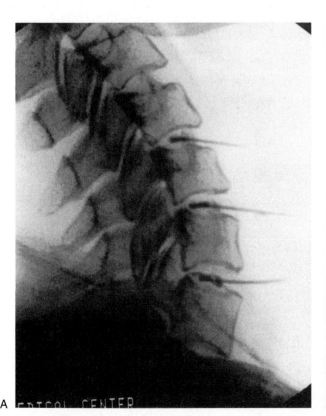
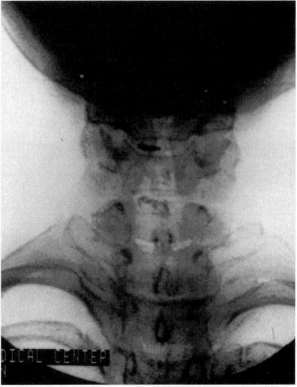

FIG. 22.1. A: Lateral spot film of normal discograms C4 to C7, contrast injection volume of 0.3 to 0.4 mL without concordant pain response. **B:** Anteroposterior radiograph after C4 to C7 disc injection with normal-appearing discograms.

fluid with an elevated infusion pressure. Discs with low pressure and accommodation of 1.5 mL generally have posterolateral extravasation of fluid. Radiographically degenerated discs accept 0.5 to 1.5 mL of fluid with intermediate pressure.

Excessive volume with decreased resistance and the presence of a pain response similar to the presenting symptoms are indications of an abnormal and symptomatic disc. Posterior protrusion and leakage of contrast into the epidural space are significant radiographic findings.

The uncovertebral articulations are relatively attenuated portions of the annulus fibrosus. The thinning of the annulus produces linear clefts, which communicate with the nucleus. These are a normal part of the aging process, and opacification of one or both lateral recesses is common in adults; they are not necessarily considered degenerative changes.

Procedure

Cervical discograms should be performed by an experienced spine specialist using standard aseptic technique in a radiographic suite suitable for performance of myelograms (i.e., with a C-arm fluoroscope). Proper discographic technique mandates the ability to work in both the frontal and lateral planes to ensure safe and efficient needle placement (Fig. 22.2).

It is essential that the discographer be extremely knowledgeable regarding the patient's clinical history, chief symptom and pain complex profile, and clinical indications for diagnostic discography. This preliminary information assessment will serve to optimize the credibility of the ultimate diagnostic data. Such preliminary attention to detail also ensures the appropriateness of the requested examination.

Patients are prepared in the same way as for a cervical myelogram. No prophylactic antibiotics are administered except to patients with beards, diabetes mellitus, or mitral valve prolapse. However, with cervical discography, perhaps the single most important aspect of patient preparation is intravenous sedation. Without optimal patient sedation, valid diagnostic results probably will not be obtained. One technique consists of slowly infused midazolam (Versed). More than 57,000 doses have been administered in a 10-year period without complication. Each dose is titrated to individual patient response; dosages range from 2 to 10 mg. This range reflects considerable variation as a result of individual susceptibility, previous medication regimens most notably including narcotics and tranquilizers, and the age of the patient. The primary purpose is to achieve a level of conscious sedation with subconscious awareness to facilitate the patient's tolerance for the procedural discomfort that will subsequently allow reliable discrimination between significant and insignificant pain.

After conscious sedation is achieved, proper patient positioning is the primary consideration (Fig. 22.3). Essential to this is optimal extension of the patient's neck, which is achieved by buttressing the upper trunk and shoulders with a sponge. This facilitates radiographic disc exposure and subsequent access to needle puncture. The anterior neck is liberally prepared in aseptic fashion. The skin of the anterior and anterolateral neck is prepared with povidone-iodine (Betadine) paint solution. Sterile drapes are applied with their margins overlying the sternomastoid muscles.

Dual-plane fluoroscopy may be achieved either with conventional C-arm fluoroscopy alone or in conjunction with a

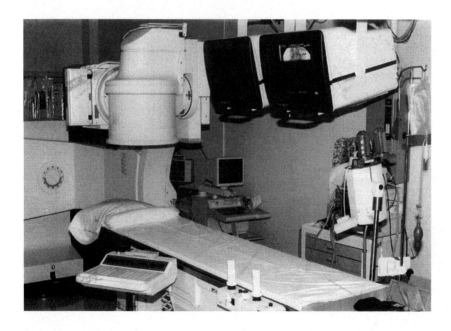

FIG. 22.2. Hospital-based neurointerventional suite with multidirectional C-arm fluoroscopic system. Although quite expensive, the all-purpose C arm affords the most favorable, patient friendly radiographic support for any interventional spinal diagnostic study.

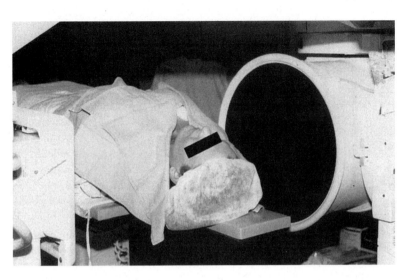

FIG. 22.3. Direct lateral fluoroscopic visualization of the cervical spine before injection of contrast media. We emphasize the need for proper patient positioning to facilitate visualization of lower neck disc spaces.

vertically mounted fluoroscopic system. We use a multidirectional C-arm fluoroscopic system.

A needle approach directed through the right neck is generally used because at the level of the mid and lower cervical spine, the esophagus is midline or slightly to the left of the spine in most patients. A right-sided approach also is slightly technically easier for right-handed discographers.

The levels to be studied are first identified with fluoroscopy. The shoulders may have to be manually depressed to allow adequate visualization of the discs at C5-C6, C6-C7, and especially C7-T1. Sterile draping of the shoulders facilitates sufficient displacement (Fig. 22.4).

The index and middle finger of the left hand serve to identify the space between the trachea and the medial margin of the sternocleidomastoid (SCM) muscle. Digital palpation of the space between the medial edges of the trachea allows identification and retraction of the carotid artery and, with firm pressure applied to the index finger, sweeps the laryngotracheal structures leftward. The anterior surface of the spine and the carotid tubercle are palpable in most patients (Fig. 22.5).

Historically, several needle techniques have been used. I strongly believe that smaller is clearly better in the neck. Specifically, a 25-gauge, single-needle technique is exclusively used in an attempt to maximize validity of diagnostic

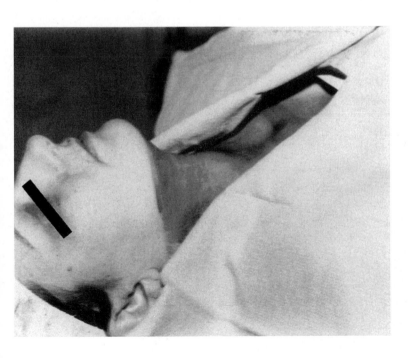

FIG. 22.4. Anteroposterior patient positioning for cervical disc injection. Margin of sterile drape overlies sternocleidomastoid muscle.

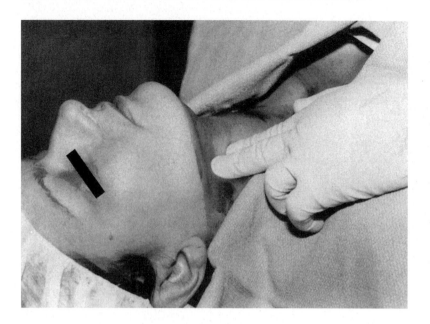

FIG. 22.5. Digital pressure with index and middle fingers applied to space between the trachea and medial margin of the sternocleidomastoid muscle. The index finger then gently yet firmly displaces the laryngotracheal structures to the left.

data and minimize postprocedural discomfort; it is important to avoid puncture of the SCM muscle.

The needle entry point should be just medial to the medial edge of the SCM muscle. The entry site should be slightly lateral at C3-C4 (to avoid puncture of the hypopharynx) and slightly medial at C7-T1 (to avoid the apex of the lung).

Administration of local anesthetic is unnecessary when 25-gauge needles are used (Figs. 22.6 and 22.7).

The needle is directed to the superior aspect of the vertebral body immediately below the disc being studied. Contact with the anterior aspect of the body determines the depth to the most anterior aspect of the spine and facilitates safe

insertion beyond this point. Slight retraction and cephalad redirection guide the needle into the anterior surface of the annulus (Fig. 22.8).

Patients almost invariably report some discomfort at this time because the periosteum and annulus are well innervated. The needle is then advanced into the nucleus pulposus under lateral fluoroscopic guidance. Movements of the needle should be slow and deliberate, not jerky or rapid (Fig. 22.9). Minimal resistance should be encountered. If advancement requires substantial amounts of pressure, then something is wrong—either position, trajectory, or orientation. The clinician should back the needle out and reassess insertion in both the anteroposterior (AP) and lateral

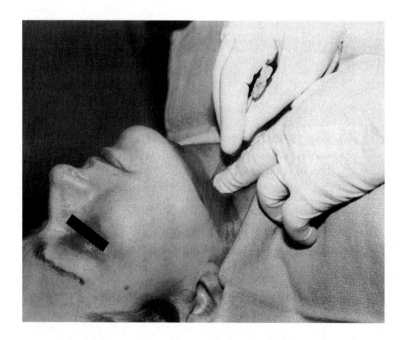

FIG. 22.6. Cervical disc injection at the C3-C4 level. A slightly more lateral approach is used at this level to avoid puncture of the hypopharynx.

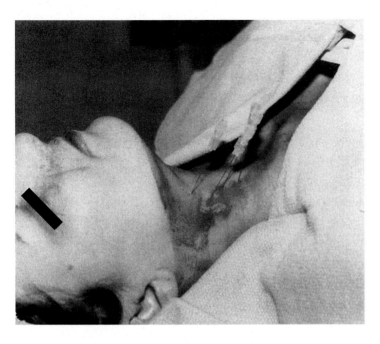

FIG. 22.7. Placement of 25-gauge needles at C3-C4, C4-C5, and C5-C6. The lower needles are placed slightly medial to the C3-C4 entry site.

planes. Needle position should be radiographically confirmed and documented before any contrast agent is injected (Fig. 22.10). This last point is critical. Puncture of the spinal cord is surprisingly well tolerated in many patients, but injection of contrast media is not!

Injection Technique

All injections should be performed under direct lateral fluoroscopic guidance. Standard 3.5-inch, 25-gauge spinal needles are used. Larger needles are more painful and do not add much control. Smaller needles are overly flexible and can get misdirected. A 3.0-mL syringe is used for injection. Larger syringes require too much force to allow the clinician to appreciate differences in injection resistance; tuberculin syringes (1.0 mL) provide an overwhelming hydraulic advantage, making it difficult to detect normal disc resistance.

Three syringes are prepared for disc injection. The first of these consists of normal saline, the second is a nonionic contrast agent, and the third is a long-term anesthetic such as bupivacaine. Injection is performed initially under lateral fluoroscopic visualization.

With standard 3.5-inch, 25-gauge spinal needles, a fraction of 1 mL of normal saline is hand-injected into the intervertebral space. Patients are clinically graded by the extent to which injection reproduces their symptoms (P0, normal; P1, mildly abnormal; P2, grossly abnormal). The volume the disc accepts and the quality of the resistance should be recorded. If saline instillation provokes a painful response, the location, distribution of the pain, and an assessment of its relative intensity are obtained by direct inquiry; 0.5 mL of bupivacaine 0.5% is then instilled and usually reduces the induced pain rapidly. Contrast material (0.5 mL

of Omnipaque-300 nonionic contrast) is instilled for the purpose of discography at each of the selected levels after the local anesthetic has been administered and appropriate radiographs obtained (Fig. 22.11).

The discometric profile for a given disc injection is defined as the volume of solution accepted and the quality of discal resistance to injection. As already noted, a normal

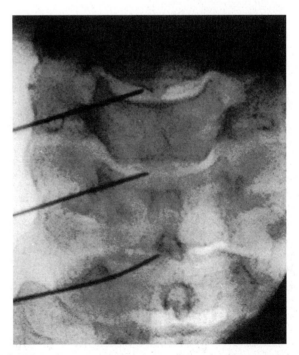

FIG. 22.8. Anteroposterior spot radiograph of lower cervical spine demonstrating preinjection appearance of needle positioning at C4-C7; 25-gauge needles are used.

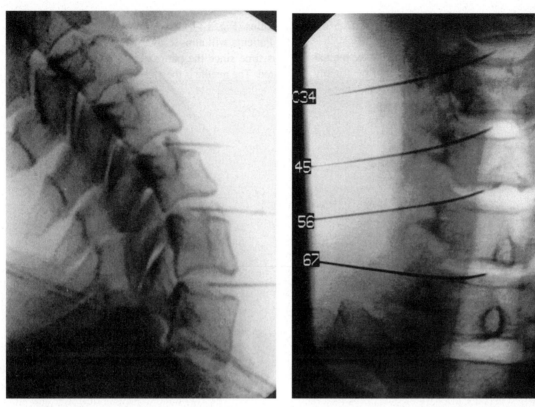

A   B

FIG. 22.9. A: Lateral spot radiograph of 25-gauge needle positioning before injection in the central disc compartments at C4 to C7. **B**: Anteroposterior spot radiograph preinjection, with 25-gauge needle positioning at C3 to C7.

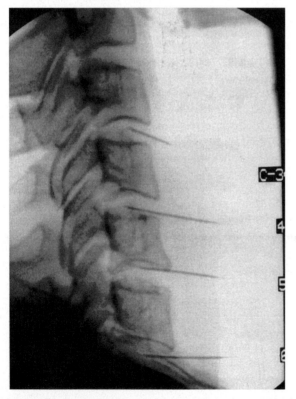

FIG. 22.10. Preinjection lateral radiograph of 25-gauge needle positioning at C3 to C7. Note the somewhat high-riding needle position at C5-C6; the needle was subsequently repositioned.

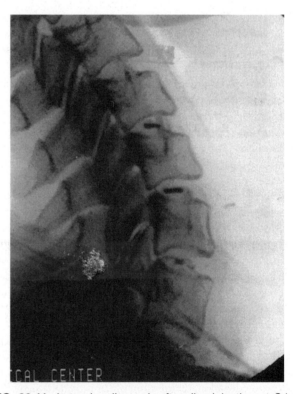

FIG. 22.11. Lateral radiograph after disc injection at C4 to C7 demonstrating normal nucleograms; each disc exhibited intense resistance to hand injection after instillation of 0.3 to 0.4 mL of contrast media without provocation of significant symptoms.

disc accepts 0.2 to 0.4 mL and offers firm resistance. Patient responses vary from no discomfort to a fleeting physiologic pain response easily distinguished from principal symptoms. After the normal saline disc distention, contrast injection further serves to corroborate the painless injection result.

Assessment of the resistance to injection, amount of contrast material injected, reproduction of clinical symptoms, relief with injection of local anesthetic agent, and extent of contrast extravasation should be assessed and recorded for each evaluated level in all patients. With a clinically significant disc distention result, an attempt is made to characterize the pain response by direct patient inquiry regarding location and degree of pain. Often, the characterization is evident through patient verbalization or body language. My clinical team of investigators includes clinical nurse and radiologic technologists who are specifically trained in observing patients for specific pain responses. With experience, the team becomes extremely proficient in distinguishing between discordant and concordant pain response. Finally, a concordant response is followed by an anesthetic disc response.

Postprocedure Care

When the procedure is completed, the patient convalesces for about 1 hour. An ice pack is applied to the neck. When the sedation wears off, the patient is asked to prepare a postprocedure pain diagram along with pain intensity rating.

At discharge, patients receive an instruction form that advises them of typical postprocedural symptoms in addition to signs of possible complication, such as infection. Short-term narcotics are provided to assist in postprocedural pain management. Patients are advised that any progressive increase or sudden change in the severity of their pain or neurologic deficit should arouse suspicion and that further investigation may be warranted. Standard instructions inform patients regarding changes in signs of pain, swallowing, or progression of their typical pain.

Complications

Cervical discography has a comparatively low incidence of complications. However, any meaningful discussion of the role of cervical discography in evaluation of degenerative disc disease must include a determination of the risks inherent in the procedure. We retrospectively analyzed 4,400 cervical disc injections in 1,357 patients performed by an experienced radiologist between 1988 and 1993 to define the morbidity and mortality associated with discography. Significant complications from diagnostic procedures occurred in less than 0.6% of the patients and in 0.16% of the cervical disc injections (48).

More recently, Guyer and colleagues (49) published complication data from 269 cervical disc injections done during 161 cervical discography procedures. They reported a complication rate of 1.49% per cervical disc injection and 2.48% per cervical discography procedure. They concluded that cervical discography can have a low complication rate when performed by those well experienced with cervical disc injections.

The major complications of diagnostic cervical disc injection are neural injury and infection. Neural injury has been reported as the result of direct needle puncture of the spinal cord. However, several cases of spinal cord impalement without neurologic sequelae have also been reported.

Careful deliberate advancement of the needle and proper visualization prevent such technical problems and their potential for catastrophe. However, the occurrence of such problems reemphasizes the necessity to obtain confirmation of appropriate needle placement before any contrast media is injected.

Spinal cord compression is a rare complication of cervical discography. Performing diagnostic cervical disc injections in patients with significant cord compromise can cause clinical catastrophe. Laun and associates (50) reported on a patient in whom quadriplegia with severe radicular pain developed within seconds of contrast medium injection into the intervertebral space. During the injection, the patient reported severe pain in the arm. Subsequent surgery demonstrated sequestered intravertebral disc fragments in the spinal canal. Disc fragments were pushed into the spinal canal during the examination. Neurologic defects resolved slowly after surgery (50). Discography is not advised for patients with congenital spinal stenosis, and myelopathy or cord compression is a contraindication to diagnostic cervical disc injection (48). Discitis, subdural empyema, spinal cord injury, vascular injury, and prevertebral abscess have all been reported as complications of diagnostic cervical disc injections (48,49).

The principal infectious complication is discitis, which is reported to occur in 0.1% to 1% of cases. The typical presentation of postdiscography discitis is a marked increase in axial neck pain, usually delayed in onset. Occasionally a radicular component is present. Laun and associates (50) reported a patient in whom cervical discography resulted in acute bacterial cervical spondylodiscitis 48 hours after the procedure; the symptoms persisted for 15 months.

Generally, an elevated erythrocyte sedimentation rate is the first study to indicate any abnormality and demonstrates significant elevations by 3 weeks after discography. Fever is typical. Guyer and colleagues (49) reported on nine patients with postdiscography discitis. The most consistent sign was the marked exacerbation of neck pain, which was followed by an elevated sedimentation rate at 20 days (mean). Seven patients initially had negative bone scan at 33 days (mean). Seven patients initially had negative bone scans, in 5 patients changes were evident on plain radiographs, and 5 patients had positive MRI results. The source of cervical discitis ranged from 6 to 7 weeks and usually resulted in spontaneous fusion (49).

Various etiologies have been proposed for discitis, including inadequate skin preparation and needle contamination. Cloward (2) postulated that inadvertent esophageal perforation associated with improper needle placement is responsible. The organisms typically cultured are the indigenous mouth and oropharyngeal flora, implicating an esophageal source, transmitted by discography. Epidural, subdural, and retropharyngeal abscesses may occur as sequelae of fulminant disc space infection or as the primary infection after penetration of the esophagus or hypopharynx.

Most cases of cervical discitis are self-limited, with spontaneous resolution. Patients can be treated with antibiotics and bedrest with or without neck bracing, with radiologic evidence of spontaneous fusion developing over several weeks. Cervical discitis often proceeds to spontaneous fusion within 7 weeks.

Major infectious complications such as development of a spinal epidural abscess are rare but dramatic. Epidural or retropharyngeal abscess may occur as sequelae of fulminant disc space infection (pyogenic discitis). Lownie and Ferguson (51) reported a case of spinal subdural empyema after discography. The overall complication rate was 13% (4 of 31), and complications included development of an acute epidural abscess that led to myelopathy and eventual quadriplegia.

ROLE AND EFFICACY OF DISCOGRAPHY IN EVALUATION OF DISCOGENIC PAIN

Controversy exists concerning management of patients who present with axial neck pain with few or no radicular symptoms and who have failed to respond to prolonged nonsurgical treatment methods. Clinical outcome studies of anterior cervical discectomy and fusion (ACDF) following positive provocative cervical discography are rare. Such studies could document the clinical outcome for patients who have undergone anterior cervical discectomy and fusion for the primary indication of neck pain, as diagnosed by discography (52).

The goal of presurgical evaluation is to document objective evidence of specific anatomic lesions that, when treated surgically, yield a measurable and predictable outcome. Cervical discography can serve as an objective test to help select surgical levels. The use of cervical discography still evokes controversy. There are authors who believe that discography can detect the source of the patient's pain. There are others who have noted false-positive results and believe that discography is not useful in determining the source of the patient's pain. Smith and co-workers (53) reported on a prospective correlation of MRI and discography in asymptomatic subjects and in subjects experiencing pain. They reported three false-positive discs out of 40 discs in asymptomatic group, with specificity of 92.5% and positive predictive valve of 86.4%, concluding that provocation of concordant pain rather than morphologic abnormality was the definitive finding.

Ohnmeiss and associates (54) studied 269 cervical discs in 161 patients to assess the correlation between postdiscographic CT-imaged discs and concordant pain responses. They reported that that among the 234 abnormal-appearing discs, 77.8% elicited pain on provocation. Clinical pain was elicited on only 14.3% of the 35 normal-appearing discs. They concluded a significant relation ($p < 0.01$) between the radiographic image of the disc and the elicitation of clinical pain upon provocation.

Diagnostic disc injection has been used as an adjunct in clinical decision making regarding selection of levels for fusion for many years. In 1969, Riley and colleagues (55) used intraoperative cervical discometry and discography to determine the levels for cervical discectomy and fusion in 93 patients. Discometric pressure measures and epidural leakage of contrast media were the primary diagnostic criteria for surgical intervention. They reported 72% good or excellent results for discectomy and fusion.

Provocation-analgesic discography has been used increasingly for evaluation of patients with chronic discogenic symptoms. In 1976, Roth (38) used local anesthetic injection into the cervical discs as an additional component of the discogram. Using relief symptoms as a criterion for determination of the symptomatic levels, he reported a very high success rate for anterior cervical discectomy and fusion.

Whitecloud and Seago (56) retrospectively analyzed 34 patients with chronic discogenic pain and without cervical spondylosis, radiculopathy, or myelopathy who underwent cervical arthrodesis on the basis of positive cervical provocation-analgesic discography. The investigators sought to determine the validity of cervical discography in diagnosis and treatment of patients presenting with cervical discogenic syndrome. Symptomatic cervical levels were selected by reproduction of the patient's symptoms with injection. They reported that 70% of the patients had good to excellent results after anterior cervical discectomy and fusion.

Osler (57) used analgesic discography to confirm the location of the lesion in patients with a discogenic pain syndrome. He concluded that analgesic discography confirms the diagnosis and accurately locates the pain-producing disc. Analgesic discography resulted in an 81% excellent or good result.

Siebenrock and Aebi (58) retrospectively reviewed 27 patients who underwent cervical fusions of 39 cervical levels for discogenic pain. The source of pain in all patients was identified by positive discography, defined as provocation of their characteristic pain. Fusions were performed using a ventral approach and included 22 one-level, 7 two-level, and 1 three-level procedures; iliac bone graft was done in all patients. Overall, 19 patients (73%) had good to excellent results; 6 patients (23%) had a fair outcome; and 1 (3.8%) had a poor result. More good to excellent results (87.5%) were obtained after two-level fusions than after one-level fusions (61.9%). Patients presenting with pain radiation to the arms had a more favorable outcome (58).

Hubach (59) prospectively studied 193 patients who underwent anterior cervical fusion on the basis of cervical discography. Discography was performed at the symptomatic and adjacent levels, and all levels with positive discograms were fused. The overall percentage of excellent and good results was 82% (59).

Motimaya and colleagues performed a retrospective study of 46 patients who underwent cervical disc examination by discography (60). They then evaluated results of 14 of the 16 patients who underwent cervical spine fusion at those levels in accordance with positive results on discogram. The average symptomatic period before discography was 12 months, and cervical disc pain was localized in all 16 patients. After discectomy and anterior fusion, all 14 patients had good to excellent results at 6 months. At a mean follow-up of 6.5 months, 11 patients (78%) had good to excellent results. The authors concluded that cervical discography was helpful in localizing the symptomatic disc levels in patients being considered for surgical intervention.

On the basis of these reports, with their highly favorable outcomes in a patient population with particularly difficult problems, one might conclude that the efficacy of cervical discography is well established. However, in contrast, Merriam and Stockdale (61) concluded that, as a technique to locate symptomatic levels, cervical discography was worthless, but that a normal nuclear image indicated an asymptomatic level. They believed that pain reproduction during injection did not reliably indicate clinical status.

Grubb and co-workers (62) conducted a retrospective study of 807 cervical disc injections in 173 cervical discograms over 12 years. They discovered that 50% of the discs provoked elicited a concordant pain response and that greater than 50% of the patients studied had three or more abnormal disc levels. More than half of the discograms yielded three or more painful discs (more than expected). The authors concluded that treatment decisions based on information from fewer than three discs studied may be tenuous.

Connor and Darden performed a retrospective review of 31 patients with a positive discogram (63). They reported on 22 patients who underwent anterior cervical discectomy and fusion on the basis of cervical discography. One patient had an excellent result (5%), 9 patients had good results (41%), and 6 patients each had a fair and poor results (54%). They concluded that diagnostic cervical discography did not provide sufficient clinical predictive value to substantiate its potential risks and complications.

In a prospective case-control study, Palit and colleagues (64) reported on patients who underwent ACDF based on positive discography findings. They noted a satisfactory outcome in 79% patients with average follow-up of 53 months (range, 24 to 87 months).

Concern exists with false-positive discograms used independently (65). Fifty-six patients had discography and medial branch blocks; a symptomatic disc and Z joint was seen in 41%, a symptomatic disc alone in 20%, and a symptomatic Z joint only in 23%; 17% had neither disc or Z-joint pain. Symptoms after provocative discography could be, at times, eliminated by medial branch blocks, suggesting that other structures provoked. "Interpretation of a positive discogram should be tempered in cases where posterior element blocks have not been performed" (65).

CONCLUSION

Cervical discography, particularly provocation-analgesic discography, is a highly specialized procedure that requires the skill of a highly trained radiologist with special expertise in the procedure. It is a complex procedure with multiple components requiring considerable experience as well as some limited but dramatic associated morbidity. Diagnostic injection of the cervical intervertebral discs may be indicated in evaluation of patients with disabling cervical symptoms without a demonstrable etiology on standard radiographic studies (CT and MRI).

In my practice, cervical discography is employed as a confirmatory study in patients with suspected one- or two-level pathology on the basis of their clinical presentation and examination. Discography is used to confirm the presence of abnormal pathology and to re-create the patient's pain (concordant pain). Discography should never be used to seek something to operate on in patients without a clear clinical picture. By the same token, we have never heard of a patient with a discogram that re-created the patient's pain at three levels who improved with surgical intervention. In summary, cervical discography is a useful tool but has some severe limitations.

REFERENCES

1. Cloward RB. Cervical discography defended. *JAMA* 1975;233:862.
2. Cloward RB. Cervical discography. Technique, indications, and use in the diagnosis of ruptured cervical disks. *AJR Am J Roentgenol* 1958; 79:563–574.
3. Cloward RB. Cervical diskography: a contribution to the etiology and mechanism of neck, shoulder and arm pain. *Ann Surg* 1959;150:1052–1064.
4. Cloward RB. Cervical discography. *Acta Radiol* 1963;1:675–688.
5. Cloward RB. The anterior approach for removal of ruptured intervertebral discs. *J Neurosurg* 1958;15:602–617.
6. Colhoun EI, McCall W, Williams L, et al. Provocation discography as a guide to planning operations on the spine. J Bone Joint Surg Br 1988;70:267–271.
7. Crock HV. A reappraisal of intervertebral disc lesions. *Med J Aust* 1970;1:983–989.
8. Fernstrom U. A discographical study of ruptured lumbar discs. *Acta Chirurg Scand* 1960;258:1–60.
9. Handal J, Schleusner R, Zardus M, et al. Clinical correlation of cervical magnetic resonance imaging and cervical discography. *Orthop Trans* 1991;15:223–227.
10. Hirsh C. An attempt to diagnose level of disc lesion clinically by puncture. *Acta Orthop Scand* 1948;18:132–140.
11. Holt EJ. Fallacy of cervical discography. Report of 50 cases in normal subjects. *JAMA* 1964;188:799–801.
12. Hsu KY, Zucherman JF, Derby R, et al. Painful lumbar end-plate disruptions: a significant discographic finding. *Spine* 1988;13:76–78.
13. Ito S, Yamada Y, Tsuboi S. An observation of ruptured annulus fibrosis in lumbar discs. *J Spinal Disord* 1991;4:462–466.
14. Keyes D, Compere E. Normal and pathological physiology of the nucleus pulposus and intervertebral disc. *J Bone Joint Surg* 1932;14:897–938.
15. Kikuchi S, Macnab I, Moreau P. Localisation of the level of symptomatic cervical disc degeneration. *J Bone J Surg* 1981;63:272–277.
16. Klafta LA. The diagnostic inaccuracy of the pain response in cervical discography. *Cleve Clin Rev* 1969;36:35–39.
17. Lindblom K. Diagnostic puncture of intervertebral disks in sciatica. *Acta Orthop Scand* 1948;17:231–239.

18. Marshall LL, Trethewie ER, Curtain CC. Chemical radiculitis. *Clin Orthop* 1977;129:61–67.
19. Massare C, Bard M, Tristant H. Cervical discography. Speculation on technique and indications from our own experience. *J Radiol* 1974;55: 395–399.
20. McCall IW, Park WM, O'Brien JP, et al. Acute traumatic interosseous disc herniations. *Spine* 1985;10:134–137.
21. McCarron RF, Wimpee MW, Hudkins PG, et al. The inflammatory effect of nucleus pulposus. *Spine* 1987;12:760–764.
22. Meyer RR. Cervical discography. A help or hindrance in evaluating neck, shoulder, arm pain. *Am J Radiol* 1963;90:1208–1215.
23. Murtagh FR, Arrington JA. Computer tomographically guided discography as a determinant of normal disc level before fusion. *Spine* 1992; 17:826–830.
24. Park WM, McCall IW, O'Brien JP, et al. Fissuring of the posterior annulus fibrosus in the lumbar spine. *Br J Radiol* 1979;52:382–387.
25. Pascaud JL, Mailhes F, Pascaud E, et al. The cervical intervertebral disc: diagnostic value of cervical discography in degenerative and post-traumatic lesions. *Ann Radiol* 1980;23:455–460.
26. Riley LJ, Robinson R, Johnson K, et al. The results of anterior interbody fusion of the cervical spine. *J Neurosurg* 1969;30:127–133.
27. Saternus K, Bornscheuer H. Comparative radiologic and pathologic anatomic studies on the value of discography in the diagnosis of acute intervertebral disc injuries in the cervical spine. *ROFO* 1983;139:651–657.
28. Schmorl G. Die Pathalogie der Wirbelsaule. *Dtsch Orthop Ges* 1926; 21:3.
29. Scoville W, Whitcomb B, Mclaurin R. The cervical ruptured disc: report of 115 operative cases. *Trans Am Neurol Assoc* 1951;76:222–224.
30. Shinomiya K, Nakao N, Shindoh K, et al. Evaluation of cervical discography in pain origin and provocation. *J Spinal Disord* 1993;6:422–426.
31. Smith G. The normal cervical diskogram with clinical observations. *AJR Am J Roentgenol* 1959;81:1006–1010.
32. Smith G, Nichols PJ. Technic for cervical discography. *Radiology* 1957;68:718–720.
33. Sneider SE, Winslow OP, Pryor TH. Cervical discography: is it relevant? *JAMA* 1963;185:163–165.
34. Williams JL, Allen MB, Harkess JW, et al. Late results of cervical discectomy and interbody fusion: some factors influencing the results. *J Bone Joint Surg Am* 1968;50:277–286.
35. Yoshizawa H, O'Brien JP, Smith WT, et al. The neuropathology of intervertebral discs removed for low back pain. *J Pathol* 1980;132:95–104.
36. Zucherman J, Derby R, Hsu K, et al. MRI scan does not replace discography. *Orthop Trans* 1989;13:16.
37. Zucherman J, Derby R, Hsu K, et al. Normal magnetic resonance imaging with abnormal discography. *Spine* 1988;13:1355–1359.
38. Roth DA. Cervical analgesic discography. A new test for the definitive diagnosis of the painful-disk syndrome. *JAMA* 1976;235(16):1713–1714.
39. Holt EP Jr. Further reflections on cervical discography. *JAMA* 1975; 231(6):613–614.
40. Parfenchuck TA, Janssen ME. A correlation of cervical magnetic resonance imaging and discography/computed tomographic discograms. *Spine* 1994;19(24):2819–2825.
41. Schellhas KP, Smith MD, Gundry CR, et al. Cervical discogenic pain. Prospective correlation of magnetic resonance imaging and discography in asymptomatic subjects and pain sufferers. *Spine* 1996;21(3): 300–311; discussion, 311–312.
42. Crock HV. Normal and pathological anatomy of the lumbar spinal nerve root canals. *J Bone Joint Surg Br* 1981;63(4):487–490.
43. Crock HV. Applied anatomy of the spine. *Acta Orthop Scand Suppl* 1993;251:56–58.
44. Weinstein J, Claverie W, Gibson S. The pain of discography. *Spine* 1988;13(12):1344–1348.
45. Franson RC, Saal JS, Saal JA. Human disc phospholipase A2 is inflammatory. *Spine* 1992;17[6 Suppl]:S129–132.
46. Matsui Y, Maeda M, Nakagami W, et al. The involvement of matrix metalloproteinases and inflammation in lumbar disc herniation. *Spine* 1998;23(8):863–868; discussion, 868–869.
47. Kitano T, Zerwekh JE, Usui Y, et al. Biochemical changes associated with the symptomatic human intervertebral disk. *Clin Orthop* 1993 (293):372–377.
48. Zeidman SM, Thompson K, Ducker TB. Complications of cervical discography: analysis of 4400 diagnostic disc injections. *Neurosurgery* 1995;37(3):414–417.
49. Guyer RD, Ohnmeiss DD, Mason SL, et al. Complications of cervical discography: findings in a large series. *J Spinal Disord* 1997;10(2): 95–101.
50. Laun A, Lorenz R, Agnoli AL. Complications of cervical discography. *J Neurosurg Sci* 1981;25(1):17–20.
51. Lownie SP, Ferguson GG. Spinal subdural empyema complicating cervical discography. *Spine* 1989;14(12):1415–1417.
52. Garvey TA, Transfeldt EE, Malcolm JR, et al. Outcome of anterior cervical discectomy and fusion as perceived by patients treated for dominant axial-mechanical cervical spine pain. *Spine* 2002;27(17): 1887–1895; discussion, 1895.
53. Smith MD, Kim SS. A herniated cervical disc resulting from discography: an unusual complication. *J Spinal Disord* 1990;3(4):392–394; discussion, 395.
54. Ohnmeiss DD, Guyer RD, Mason SL. The relation between cervical discographic pain responses and radiographic images. *Clin J Pain* 2000;16(1):1–5.
55. Riley LH Jr, Robinson RA, Johnson KA, et al. The results of anterior interbody fusion of the cervical spine. Review of ninety-three consecutive cases. *J Neurosurg* 1969;30(2):127–133.
56. Whitecloud TS 3rd, Seago RA. Cervical discogenic syndrome. Results of operative intervention in patients with positive discography. *Spine* 1987;12(4):313–316.
57. Osler GE. Cervical analgesic discography. A test for diagnosis of the painful disc syndrome. *S Afr Med J* 1987;71(6):363.
58. Siebenrock KA, Aebi M. Cervical discography in discogenic pain syndrome and its predictive value for cervical fusion. *Arch Orthop Trauma Surg* 1994;113(4):199–203.
59. Hubach PC. A prospective study of anterior cervical spondylodesis in intervertebral disc disorders. *Eur Spine J* 1994;3(4):209–213.
60. Motimaya A, Arici M, George D, et al. Diagnostic value of cervical discography in the management of cervical discogenic pain. *Conn Med* 2000;64(7):395–398.
61. Merriam WF, Stockdale HR. Is cervical discography of any value? *Eur J Radiol* 1983;3(2):138–141.
62. Grubb SA, Kelly CK. Cervical discography: clinical implications from 12 years of experience. *Spine* 2000;25(11):1382–1389.
63. Connor PM, Darden BV 2nd. Cervical discography complications and clinical efficacy. *Spine* 1993;18(14):2035–2038.
64. Palit M, Schofferman J, Goldthwaite N, et al. Anterior discectomy and fusion for the management of neck pain. *Spine* 1999;24(21): 2224–2228.
65. Bogduk N, Aprill C. On the nature of neck pain, discography and cervical zygapophysial joint blocks. *Pain* 1993;54(2):213–217.

CHAPTER 23

Outcome Assessment Tools in Cervical Spine Surgery

Steven P. Leon and Isador H. Lieberman

There has been increased interest in the use of outcome tools in clinical research. Outcomes research itself can be thought of as refined and enhanced clinical research, with a focus on patient-based outcomes (1). Several factors—rapidly increasing health care costs; variations in practice patterns, in utilization of health care services, in patient expectations, and in clinical outcomes for related procedures; and the deficiencies in the research literature—have stimulated the rethinking of clinical research methods (1). Outcomes research can be used to justify new medical treatment modalities and health care reimbursements.

Multiple variables must be considered in the measurement of outcomes. These include biologic and physiologic variables as well as physician-derived symptom status. These traditional clinical variables—patient symptoms (e.g., neck pain), physical findings (e.g., weakness), and laboratory investigations (e.g., x-ray, nerve conduction studies)—are prone to reporting biases. More recently, objective outcome measures have been introduced that take into account patients' self-report of their physical function, general health, and overall quality of life, so-called patient-based outcomes (2). These measures may be as or more important than traditional clinical measures because they can reduce or eliminate physician bias and perhaps more directly answer the question, "Is the patient feeling and doing better?" Other measurable variables include work status, patient satisfaction, treatment-related complications, and cost-related variables (3).

One of the more common formats used to gather data to measure patient-based outcomes are questionnaires. It is important that these questionnaires be appropriately crafted as to content, be suitable to the patients or populations being measured, and respond to the purpose for which data are being collected. Patient-based outcomes also have limitations because some questionnaires may only be partially completed or completed by someone other than the patient because of cognitive or physical disabilities the patient may have.

Wilson and Cleary (4) have proposed a conceptual model of five types of outcomes to help answer the question: Which outcome does the researcher want to measure? The first two—biologic and physiologic factors and symptoms—of the five types of outcomes are traditional clinical variables found in most clinical studies and consist of data from physical examinations and laboratory investigations. The next three types of outcomes are patient-based measures: function measures, general health perceptions, and overall quality of life. Function measures assess the ability to perform specific tasks covering physical, social, role, and psychological functions. General health perceptions integrate the various aspects of health as reflected in a patient's subjective rating. The overall quality of life type of outcome is a general measure of a patient's well being. The key to Wilson and Cleary's proposed model is that the various types of outcomes are distinct concepts that may or may not track together as a patient improves. For example, the level of pain (a symptom) may not correlate with radiographic film changes (a biologic factor). As one works through the various types of outcomes in the model, outcomes are increasingly influenced by individual and social factors (4).

In this chapter, we review the traditional and patient-derived outcome measurement tools that are helpful when conducting clinical research related to cervical spine surgery.

TRADITIONAL CLINICAL OUTCOME MEASURES IN CERVICAL SPINE RESEARCH

A variety of traditional outcome measures have been reported in studies pertaining to the cervical spine. For example, several grading or classification schemes have been used to report the outcomes of cervical spine surgery in patients with cervical myelopathy secondary to conditions such as rheumatoid arthritis, cervical spondylosis, and ossification of the posterior longitudinal ligament (OPLL). Although a number of classification systems for myelopathy have been reported, perhaps the most commonly used are the Ranawat classification (5), Nurick classification system (6), and Japanese Orthopaedic Association (JOA) score (7).

The Ranawat classification scale was originally devised to evaluate the neurologic function of patients undergoing cervical spine arthrodesis for rheumatoid involvement of the cervical spine (5). Class I is normal or intact. Patients with subjective weakness with hyperreflexia and paresthesias are class II. When patients develop objective weakness with long tract signs, they are categorized as class III. Class III is further subdivided into IIIA, which includes patients who are ambulatory, and IIIB, comprising patients who are nonambulatory (Table 23.1).

The American Rheumatism Association (ARA) functional grading system developed by Steinbrocker has been used to evaluate the overall functional status of patients with rheumatoid arthritis (8) (Table 23.2). The ARA functional grading system is not a spine-specific instrument but rather is used to assess the physical function of patients with rheumatoid arthritis, taking into account their overall disease burden from rheumatoid arthritis. Although this scale has been used to report postoperative improvement (9,10), the ARA classification system is so crude that it has largely been dismissed by present-day rheumatologists (11). The problem with the ARA functional grading system and, to a lesser degree, the Ranawat neurologic classification system is that they both lack sensitivity to change—they fail to differentiate quite significant clinical changes between classes II and III—and they are also subject to great interobserver error.

Nurick originally proposed a grading scheme to measure the degree of walking difficulty in patients with myelopathy secondary to cervical spondylosis (6). The Nurick grading scheme expands the grades from four on the Ranawat classification scheme to six (Table 23.3). It adds two additional grades (grades 3 and 4) to better differentiate the degree of walking dysfunction. These two additional grades further distinguish between grades IIIA and IIIB in the Ranawat scheme. Grade 3 in the Nurick scale describes the individual who cannot work inside or outside the home because of walking difficulty, and grade 4 describes a patient requiring some form of assistance to ambulate. This expansion in the Nurick scheme increases its sensitivity while maintaining simplicity and ease of use. This has resulted in the widespread use of this outcome measure by many investigators. Several other classification systems, based on variations of the Nurick grading system, have also been used to measure the degree of walking disability (12–14).

The JOA score is probably the most comprehensive of the traditional measures quantifying the degree of impairment secondary to myelopathy. It is objective in nature and measures both upper and lower extremity motor and sensory dysfunction as well as bladder function. A total of 17 points can be scored (7,15) (Table 23.4). Lower scores indicate worse function; higher scores, better function. Although the JOA score is the most comprehensive, it has several limitations. When comparing its grading of lower extremity function with the Nurick grade, it is less sensitive and less descriptive. The JOA uses five scores instead of six in the Nurick scheme, and the three intermediate scores all assume the need for an assistive device (Nurick grade 4). One might also argue that the score is perhaps too heavily weighted with respect to sensory dysfunction, with 6 out of 17 total points used to measure it. Finally, measurement of upper extremity function, although an excellent principle to include, would require some translation or cross-cultural adaptation for more widespread use across other populations because in the JOA score, grading is based on the ability or inability to use chopsticks. Modifications of the JOA scheme have been devised for non-Asians.

Other examples of traditional clinical measures that have been used to measure outcomes in the area of spinal cord injury are the Frankel Neurological Performance Scale and the American Spinal Injury Association (ASIA) motor scoring system (16,17). These measures have been applied to all

TABLE 23.1. *Ranawat Classification*

Class I: No neurological deficit
Class II: Subjective weakness with hyperreflexia
Class IIIA: Objective findings of weakness and log tract signs, ambulatory
Class IIIB: Quadriparetic and nonambulatory

TABLE 23.2. *ARA Functional Grades*

Grade 1: Complete ability to perform all usual duties without handicaps
Grade 2: Adequate for normal activities despite handicap of discomfort or limited motion of one of the joints
Grade 3: Limited to few or none of the duties of usual occupation or self-care
Grade 4: Incapacitated, largely or wholly bed-ridden or confined to a wheelchair with little or no self-care

TABLE 23.3. *Nurick Grading Scheme*

Grade 0: Signs and symptoms of root involvement but without evidence of spinal cord disease
Grade 1: Signs of spinal cord disease but no difficulty in walking
Grade 2: Slight difficulty in walking, which did not prevent full-time employment
Grade 3: Difficulty in walking, which prevented full-time employment or the ability to do all housework, but was not so severe as to require someone else's help to walk.
Grade 4: Able to walk only with someone else's help or with the aid of a frame
Grade 5: Chairbound or bedridden

TABLE 23.4. *Criteria of Evaluation of the Operative Results of Patients with Cervical Myelopathy by the Japanese Orthopedic Association*

I. Upper extremity function	II. Lower extremity function	III. Sensory	IV. Bladder function
0. Impossible to eat with either chopsticks or spoon	0. Impossible to walk	A. Upper extremity	0. Complete retention
1. Possible to eat with spoon, but not with chopsticks	1. Need cane or aid on flat ground	0. Apparent sensory loss	1. Severe disturbance
2. Possible to eat with chopsticks, but inadequate	2. Need cane or aid only on stairs	1. Minimal sensory loss	(1) Inadequate evaluation of the bladder
3. Possible to eat with chopsticks, but awkward	3. Possible to walk without cane or aid, but slow	2. Normal	(2) Straining

4. Normal	4. Normal	B. Lower extremity
		  0. Apparent sensory loss
		  1. Minimal sensory loss
		  2. Normal
		C. Trunk
		  0. Apparent sensory loss
		  1. Minimal sensory loss
		  2. Normal
			(3) Dribbling of urine
			2. Mild disturbance
			  (1) Urinary frequency
			  (2) Urinary Hesitancy
			3. Normal

From, Japanese Orthopedic Association Score. With permission from Wada E, Suzuki S, Kanazawa A, Matsuoka T, Miyamoto S, Yonenobu K. Subtotal Corpectomy versus Laminoplasty for Multilevel Cervical Spondylotic Myelopathy. *Spine* 2001;26:144, with permission.

areas of the spine including, but not limited to, injuries of the cervical spine.

PATIENT-BASED OUTCOME MEASURES

Although the field of patient-based outcome measures is relatively young, the number and types of outcome measures are growing exponentially, making it confusing for the investigator to select one type of outcome measure over another. According to Bombardier, a core set of measures for spine-related outcomes research should include the following five domains: back-specific function, generic health status, pain, work disability, and patient satisfaction. Some of the key questions that an investigator should ask when planning an outcome study are summarized in Table 23.5. Patient-based outcome measures can be categorized into those that are generic measures of health status and those that are disease specific—one for almost every disease, condition, and body part (2).

Generic Health Measures

Generic health status measures are designed to assess broadly the concepts of health, disability, and quality of life and are applicable to patients with different types of conditions. These measures provide a more comprehensive picture of the patient health status than disease-specific measures (18). A generic measure is particularly important in populations with comorbidities because disabilities from comorbidities may influence the patients' response to treat-

ment (19). Despite these advantages, generic health measures are often less responsive to changes in specific disease conditions than disease-specific instruments. Perhaps for these reasons, it is generally recommended that two outcome measures (one generic and one disease specific) be used to gather data. Examples of generic health measuring instruments include the Sickness Impact Profile (SIP) (20), Nottingham Health Profile (NHP) (21), Duke Health Profile (22), COOP/WONCA charts (23), and SF-36 Health Survey (24).

The SIP is a well-established, standardized questionnaire that indicates changes in a patient's behavior due to sickness. It measures the performance of specific behavior, rather than making judgments of capacity, and assesses dysfunction without a positive formulation of health (18).

The NHP is a brief self-administered questionnaire originally designed for use in primary care settings. It asks more directly about feelings and emotional states than about behavioral changes (18).

The Duke profile is a revised and shortened version of the Duke University of North Carolina Health Profile and is also designed for use in primary care settings. It measures physical, mental, social, and perceived health as well as self-esteem and dysfunctions such as anxiety, depression, pain, and disability (18).

The COOP/WONCA charts focus on physical fitness, feelings (mental well-being), daily or usual activities, social activities, overall health, and changes in health.

The SF-36 has been widely adopted because of its brevity and its comprehensiveness. Although these are two competing goals, the SF-36 appears to have achieved a

TABLE 23.5. *A Proposed Set of Patient-Based Outcome Measures for Use in Spinal Disorders*

Domain	Instrument	# Of items (response options)	Score (best to worse)	Time to complete	Dimensions
Back specific function	Roland–Morris	24 (yes/no)	0–24	5 minutes	Physical activities; housework; mobility; dressing; getting help; appetite; irritability; pain
	or Oswestry	10 (6 levels)	0–100	5 minutes	Pain intensity; personal care; lifting; walking; sitting; standing; sleeping; sex life; social life; travelling
Generic health status	SF-36 version 2.0	36 (variable)	8 dimensions: 100–0 each or norm-based: Mean: 50; SD: 10	10 minutes	Eight dimensions: physical function; role physical; bodily pain; general health; vitality; social function; role emotional; and mental health Can be aggregated into two components: Physical and mental health
Pain	Bodily Pain Scale of SF-36	2 (variable)	100–0 or norm-based: mean: 50; SD: 10	2 minutes	Pain intensity; pain interference with work and housework
	(optional) Chronic Pain Grade	7 (11 pt NRS) + number of days in pain		5 minutes	Current, worse, and average pain; disability days; interference with usual activities; recreational, social and family activities; and work (incl. housework)
Work disability*	Work status	10 categories	Nominal scale	1 minute	Employed at usual job, on light duty, or some restricted work assignment, paid leave/sick leave; unpaid leave; unemployed because of health problems; unemployed because of other reason; student, keeping house/homemaker, retired, on disability
	Days off work and days of cut down work†	# of days		2 minutes	
	Time to return to work	# of days		2 minutes	
Satisfaction: back specific	*Satisfaction with care:* Patient Satisfaction Scale	17 (5 levels)			Information; caring; effectiveness of treatment; and others
	Satisfaction with treatment outcome: Global question	1 (7 levels)	1–7	1 minute	Extremely, very, somewhat satisfied; mixed, somewhat, very, extremely dissatisfied

NRS = Numerical Rating Scale.

*The SF-36 physical and mental role scales refer to all roles (work as well as housework). The reader specifically interested in work-related disability would need to modify these scales to refer to work roles only.

†The U.S. National Health Interview Survey asks about days off work and cut down activity both from usual work and other role activities. The reader specifically interested in work-relatedness would need to modify these questions to refer to work roles only.

From, Bombardier C. Outcome Assessments in the Evaluation and Treatment of Spinal Disorders. *Spine* 2000;25:3100–3103, with permission.

compromise between them (18). The SF-36 can be administered in 5 to 10 minutes with a high degree of acceptability and data quality. It has been translated for use in more than 40 countries (25). Figure 23-1 illustrates the taxonomy of items and concepts underlying the construction of the SF-36 scales and summary measures. The SF-36 contains 36 questions and yields an eight-scale profile of scores as well as physical and mental health summary scores (25). The taxonomy has three levels: (a) items, (b) eight scales that aggregate 2 to 10 items each, and

(c) two summary measures that aggregate scales. All but 1 of the 36 items are used to score the eight SF-36 scales. Each item is used in scoring only one scale. The eight scales form two distinct higher-ordered clusters according to the physical and mental health variance that they have in common (25).

Criteria used for evaluating any health status measure include practicality, precision, validity, and responsiveness. For practicality, health status measures should be as brief as possible to minimize the burden to respondents and the

Items   Scales   Summary Measures

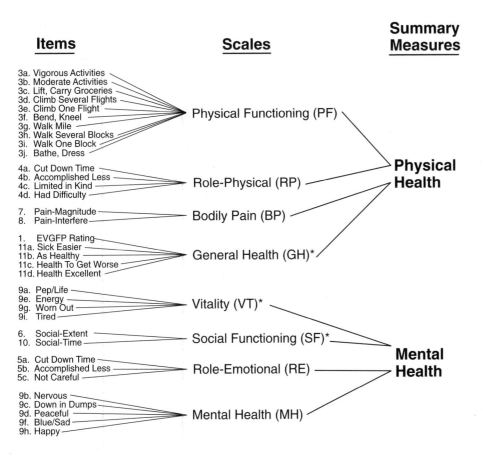

FIG. 23.1. SF-36 measurements model. *Asterisk* indicates significant correlation with other summary measure. (From, Ware JE. SF-36 health survey update. *Spine* 2000;25:3130–3139, with permission.)

cost of data collection and management. A precision measurement, also termed *reliability*, is a measure of how well the measure agrees with itself. McHorney and Carlov reviewed reliability data for the SF-36, NHP, Duke, and COOP charts and found that internal consistency was highest for the SF-36, intermediate for the NHP, and lowest for the DUKE and COOP measures, which is inversely related to the length of each questionnaire. Validity refers to the degree to which the health status measure actually measures health. Responsiveness refers to the ability of a health status measure to detect change when it has occurred. In general, the SF-36 has been identified as being somewhat more responsive than the other measures, which are fairly similar to each other (18).

The SIP, NHP, Duke, and COOP/WONCA charts have been reasonably well studied in terms of their reliability and validity and have been used to some extent in the study of patients with back pain. All these health status measures appear to measure similar concepts of health. Although the SIP is the most extensively tested for reliability, validity, and responsiveness, it has practical limitations because of its length. The NHP is of medium length and easy to complete with simple "yes" and "no" responses, but it appears to have substantial psychometric limitations compared with the SF-36. The Duke Health Profile is brief and shows reasonable validity with other health measures, but its relatively poor reliability makes

it less attractive than the other measures. The COOP/ WONCA charts have the advantage of being very brief and widely available in multiple languages. They have not, however, been as extensively tested in patients with back pain as some of the other measures, and further work is needed to clarify its performance, especially in its responsiveness to this population. Overall, the SF-36 has been identified as having several advantages over the other generic measures and should probably be used, unless the particular setting lends itself to one of the other measures. The Medical Outcome Study (MOS) SF-36 and a shorter version (the SF-12) have been widely adopted in general population surveys and clinical trials and are highly recommended as the generic health measure of choice for spine related research (18).

For a more detailed review with comparisons between these generic health measures, refer to McDowell and Newell (26).

Disease-Specific Outcome Measures

The hallmark of a disease-specific outcome measure is the attribution of symptoms and functional limitations to a specific disease or condition. In a disease-specific measure, only those aspects of health that tend to be affected by the disease are measured, for example, "Because of your neck pain, how long can you read?" This tends to result in high relevance, sensitivity, and responsiveness of the instrument (27).

Several questionnaires are available for assessing functional outcomes related to low back pain (27) (Table 23.6), with the Roland-Morris Disability Questionnaire and the Oswestry Disability Questionnaire being the most widely used and recommended for use in back-related research (28), but there are only a few instruments designed specifically for the cervical spine—the Neck Disability Index (NDI) and the Northwick Neck Questionnaire. The NDI represents a modification based on the Oswestry Low Back Pain Index to assess the activities of daily living of sufferers of disabling neck pain. The NDI consists of five scales from the original Oswestry Index, two being revised considerably, and five new scales with greater relevance for patients suffering disabling neck pain (reading, headaches, concentration, and work) (29) (Table 23.7). The reliability and validity of the NDI have been demonstrated (29,30). In a study comparing the SF-36 (a generic measure) and the NDI (a disease-specific measure) in patients with a variety of disorders of the cervical spine, the NDI was shown to have construct validity (the extent to which the measurement corresponds to theoretical concepts, or constructs, concerning the phenomenon under study) and responsiveness and sensitivity to change. The authors felt there was substantial overlap between the two measures and therefore recommended that both measures were probably not necessary (31).

The Functional Rating Index combines the concepts of the Oswestry Low Back Disability Questionnaire and the NDI and claims to improve on their practicality, requiring an average time of 78 seconds per administration (32).

A scale for measuring symptoms related to degenerative diseases of the cervical spine that includes measures of functional disability and pain and psychological distress has also been proposed (33). Twenty typical symptoms are listed (e.g., neck pain, dysesthesia, and reduced mobility).

Responses are assessed using a six-point scale ranging from "did not have symptom" to "had symptom and suffered very strongly." Psychometric analysis showed good reliability and validity. This scale was developed in Germany and, as far as we know, has yet to be translated. Both this scale and the Functional Rating Index appear to be promising alternatives to the NDI; however, replication of the results in other patient samples by other research teams and direct comparisons with the NDI still need to be carried out.

A patient-based questionnaire to measure the degree of functional disability from myelopathy has also been developed and termed the *Myelopathy Disability Index* (MDI) (11). It was designed specifically in an attempt to improve on the Ranawat and ARA grading systems using a patient-based, self-administered format. The MDI is a short, self-administered questionnaire used to evaluate upper and lower limb functions in patients with myelopathy. It was derived mathematically from the Stanford Health Activity Questionnaire. Its validity and responsiveness have been demonstrated. It has been used by the same group to report surgical outcomes of patients with myelopathy (9). The patient responds to 10 questions on function and graded on a four point scale. The final score is expressed as a percentage. Aside from practical advantages over the Ranawat and ARA grading schemes, the MDI allows for better differentiation of disease status and sensitivity to change with expansion of grades from 4 points on Ranawat to 30 points on the MDI.

RECOMMENDATIONS FOR CERVICAL SPINE SURGERY CLINICAL RESEARCH

Although some advocate the use of one outcome measure (31), we recommend the use of two outcome measures. This represents our existing protocol. Numerous studies have adopted this strategy and have illustrated the advantages of such supplementation (25). This philosophy helps capture the disease specific issues and the generic health and comorbidity issues. It is always easier to collect more data and then eliminate what is not necessary at the end of the study, than to complete the study and not have the appropriate data available for analysis. We use the SF-36 health survey in conjunction with the NDI for our clinical outcome studies involving the cervical spine. Depending on the goals of the study, we supplement with one or more of the following: the ASIA score, visual analog pain scale, work status, and treatment satisfaction status.

By adherence to appropriate outcome tool selection, data collection, and data analysis, we will be able to advance the treatment of cervical spine pathology and provide unrefutable evidence justifying certain treatments while addressing medical-economic concerns.

TABLE 23.6. *Selected Back-Specific Functional Instruments*

Oswestry Low Back Pain Disability Questionnaire (ODQ)
Million Visual Analogue Scale (MVAS)
Roland–Morris Disability Questionnaire (RMDQ)
Waddell Disability Index (WDI)
Low Back Outcome Score (LBOS)
Clinical Back Pain Questionnaire (Aberdeen Low Back Pain Scale) (CBPQ)
Low Back Pain Rating Scale (LBPRS)
Quebec Back Pain Disability Scale (QBPDS)
North American Spine Society Lumbar Spine Questionnaire (NASS LSQ)
Resumption of Activities of Daily Living Scale (RADL)

From, Kopec JA. Measuring Functional Outcomes in Persons with Back Pain. *Spine* 2000;25:3110–3114, with permission.

TABLE 23.7. *Neck Disability Index*

This questionnaire has been designed to give the doctor information as to how your neck pain has affected your ability to manage in everyday life. Please answer every section and mark in each section by checking the ONE item which applies to you. We realize you may consider that two of the statements in any one section relate to you, but please just mark the one that most closely describes your problem.

Section 1 - Pain Intensity
_____ I have no pain at the moment.
_____ The pain is very mild at the moment.
_____ The pain is moderate at the moment.
_____ The pain is fairly severe at the moment.
_____ The pain is very severe at the moment.
_____ The pain is the worst imaginable at the moment.

Section 2 - Personal Care (Washing, Dressing etc.)
_____ I can look after myself normally without causing extra pain.
_____ I can look after myself normally but it causes extra pain.
_____ It is painful to look after myself and I am slow and careful.
_____ I need some help but manage most of my personal care.
_____ I need help every day in most aspects of self care.
_____ I do not get dressed, I wash with difficulty and stay in bed.

Section 3 - Lifting
_____ I can lift heavy weights without extra pain.
_____ I can lift heavy weights but it gives extra pain.
_____ Pain prevents me from lifting heavy weights off the floor, but I can manage if they are conveniently positioned, for example on a table.
_____ Pain prevents me from lifting heavy weights, but I can manage light to medium weights if they are conveniently positioned.
_____ I can lift very light weights.
_____ I cannot lift or carry anything at all.

Section 4 - Reading
_____ I can read as much as I want to with no pain in my neck.
_____ I can read as much as I want to with slight pain in my neck.
_____ I can read as much as I want with moderate pain in my neck.
_____ I can't read as much as I want because of moderate pain in my neck.
_____ I can hardly read at all because of severe pain in my neck.
_____ I cannot read at all.

Section 5 - Headache
_____ I have no headaches at all.
_____ I have slight headaches which come infrequently.
_____ I have moderate headaches which come infrequently.
_____ I have moderate headaches which come frequently.
_____ I have severe headaches which come frequently.
_____ I have headaches almost all the time.

Section 6 - Concentration
_____ I can concentrate fully when I want to with no difficulty.
_____ I can concentrate fully when I want to with slight difficulty.
_____ I have a fair degree of difficulty in concentrating when I want to.
_____ I have a lot of difficulty in concentrating when I want to.
_____ I have a great deal of difficulty in concentrating when I want to.
_____ I cannot concentrate at all.

Section 7 - Work
_____ I can do as much work as I want to.
_____ I can only do my usual work, but no more.
_____ I can do most of my usual work, but no more.
_____ I cannot do my usual work.
_____ I can hardly do any work at all.
_____ I can't do any work at all.

Section 8 - Driving
_____ I can drive my car without any neck pain.
_____ I can drive my car as long as I want with slight pain in my neck.
_____ I can drive my car as long as I want with moderate pain in my neck.
_____ I can't drive my car as long as I want because of moderate pain in my neck.
_____ I can hardly drive at all because of severe pain in my neck.
_____ I can't drive my car at all.

Section 9 - Sleeping
_____ I have no trouble sleeping.
_____ My sleep is slightly disturbed (less than 1 hr. sleepless).
_____ My sleep is mildly disturbed (1–2 hrs. sleepless).
_____ My sleep is moderately disturbed (2–3 hrs. sleepless).
_____ My sleep is greatly disturbed (3–5 hrs. sleepless).
_____ My sleep is completely disturbed (5–7 hrs. sleepless).

Section 10 - Recreation
_____ I am able to engage in all my recreation activities with no neck pain at all.
_____ I am able to engage in all my recreation activities with some pain in my neck.
_____ I am able to engage in most, but not all of my usual recreation activities because of pain in my neck.
_____ I am able to engage in a few of my usual recreation activities because of pain in my neck.
_____ I can hardly do any recreation activities because of pain in my neck.
_____ I can't do any recreation activities at all.

Adapted from, The Neck Disability Index (Menezes AH, van Gilder JC, Clark CR, et al. Odontoid upward migration in rheumatoid arthritis. An analysis of 45 patients with "cranial settling." *J Neurosurg* 1985;63:500–509.).

REFERENCES

1. Keller RB. Outcomes research in orthopedics. *J Am Acad Orthop Surg* 1993;1:122–129.
2. Bombardier C. Introduction: outcome assessments in the evaluation of treatment of spinal disorders. *Spine* 2000;25:3097–3099.
3. Keller RB, Maine AA, Rudicel SA, et al. Outcomes research in orthopedics. *J Bone Joint Surg Am* 1993;75:1562–1574.
4. Wilson IB, Cleary PD. Measures of outcome in quality of life (QOL) model. *JAMA* 1995;273:59–65.
5. Ranawat CS, O'Leary P, Pellici P, et al. Cervical spine fusion in rheumatoid arthritis. *J Bone Joint Surg Am* 1979;61:1003–1010.
6. Nurick S. The pathogenesis of spinal cord disorder associated with cervical spondylosis. *Brain* 1972;95:87–100.
7. Hirabayashi K, Watanabe K, Wakano K, et al. Expansive open-door laminoplasty for cervical spinal stenotic myelopathy. *Spine* 1983;8:693–699.
8. Steinbrocker O, Traeger CH, Batterman RC. Therapeutic criteria in rheumatoid arthritis. *JAMA* 1949;140:659–662.
9. Casey ATH, Crockard HA, Stevens J. Vertical translocation. II. Outcomes after surgical treatment of rheumatoid cervical myelopathy. *J Neurosurg* 1997;87:863–869.
10. Menezes AH, van Gilder JC, Clark CR, et al. Odontoid upward migration in rheumatoid arthritis. An analysis of 45 patients with "cranial settling." *J Neurosurg* 1985;63:500–509.
11. Casey ATH, Bland JM, Crockard HA. Development of a functional scoring system for rheumatoid arthritis patients with cervical myelopathy. *Ann Rheum Dis* 1996;55:901–906.
12. Harsh GR, Sypert GW, Weinstein PR, et al. Cervical spine stenosis secondary to ossification of the posterior longitudinal ligament. *J Neurosurg* 1987;67:349–357.
13. Kumar VGR, Rea GL, Mervis LJ, et al. Cervical spondylotic myelopathy: functional and radiographic long-term outcome after laminectomy and posterior fusion. *Neurosurgery* 1999;44:771–778.
14. Onari K, Akiyama N, Kondo S, et al. Long-term follow-up results of anterior interbody fusion applied for cervical myelopathy due to ossification of the posterior longitudinal ligament. *Spine* 2001;26:488–493.
15. Wada E, Suzuki S, Kanazawa A, et al. Subtotal corpectomy versus laminoplasty for multilevel cervical spondylotic myelopathy. *Spine* 2001;26:1443.
16. American Spinal Injury Association. *Standards for neurological classification of spinal injury patients.* 1982.
17. Frankel H, Hannock DO, Hyslop G, et al. The value of postural reduction in the initial management of closed injuries of the spine with paraplegia and tetraplegia. I. *Paraplegia* 1969;7:179–192.
18. Lurie J. A review of generic health status measures in patients with low back pain. *Spine* 2000;25:3125–3129.
19. Bombardier C. Outcome assessments in the evaluation and treatment of spinal disorders. *Spine* 2000;25:3100–3103.
20. Bergner M, Bobbitt RA, Carter WB, et al. The Sickness Impact Profile: development and final revision of a health status measure. *Med Care* 1981;19:787–805.
21. Hunt SM, McEwen J, McKenna SP. Measuring health status: a new tool for clinicians and epidemiologists. *J R Coll Gen Pract* 1985;35:185–188.
22. Parkerson GR, Broadhead WE, Tse CK. The Duke Health Profile: a 17-item measure of health and dysfunction. *Med Care* 1990;28:1056–1072.
23. Kinnersley P, Peters T, Stott N. Measuring functional health status in primary care using the COOP-WONCA charts: acceptability, range of scores, construct validity, reliability and sensitivity to change. *Br J Gen Pract* 1994;44:545–549.
24. Ware JE, Sherbourne CD. The MOS 36-item Short Form Health Survey (SF-36). *Med Care* 1992;30:473–483.
25. Ware JE. SF-36 Health Survey Update. *Spine* 2000;25:3130–3139.
26. McDowell I, Newell C. *Measuring health: a guide to rating scales and questionnaires.* Oxford, UK: Oxford University Press, 1996.
27. Kopec JA. Measuring Functional Outcomes in Persons with Back Pain. *Spine* 2000;25:3110–3114.
28. Roland M, Fairbank J. The Roland-Morris disability questionnaire and the Oswestry disability questionnaire. *Spine* 2000;25:3115–3124.
29. Vernon H, Mior S. The Neck Disability Index: a study of reliability and validity. *J Manipulative Physiol Ther* 1991;14:409–415.
30. Hains F, Waalen J, Mior S. Psychometric properties of the neck disability index. *J Manipulative Physiol Ther* 1998;21:75–80.
31. Riddle DL, Stratford PW. Use of generic versus region-specific functional status measures on patients with cervical spine disorders. *Phys Ther* 1998;78:951–963.
32. Feise RJ, Menke MJ. Functional rating index: a new valid and reliable instrument to measure the magnitude of clinical change in spinal conditions. *Spine* 2001;26:78–86.
33. Koller M, Kienapfel H, Hinder D, et al. A scale for measuring symptoms related to degenerative diseases of the cervical spine. A reference in determining indications and evaluating surgical outcome. *Chirurg* 1999;70:1364–1373.

SECTION III

Radiographic Evaluation

CHAPTER 24

Plain Radiographic Evaluation of Cervical Spine Injury

Lourens Penning

INITIAL RADIOGRAPHY AND RADIOGRAPH EVALUATION

In radiography for cervical spine injury, the first aim is to obtain a lateral radiograph of the cervical spine. It should preferably be made with the patient still on the transportation stretcher, all handling being postponed until the results of the radiographic examination are known. If handling is necessary, the patient should be lifted "as one piece" by at least four persons. Pressure sores are easily produced in patients with cord lesions and should be prevented by the use of a foam rubber mattress and pads of soft material between the knees and ankles and underneath the calves. Any source of harmful pressure—for example, hard objects in the pocket—should be removed. Suction, insertion of nasal or tracheal tubes, and so forth should be undertaken without moving the head or neck.

Care should be taken to ensure that the lower part of the cervical spine is depicted on the film; superimposition of shoulders must be overcome by traction on arms (Fig. 24.1) (1,2). If pulling on the arms proves unsuccessful, the flying angel projection may be tried (Fig. 24.2) (2). Experience has shown that most fractures and luxations are missed at the lower end of the cervical spine (3).

If performed correctly, the lateral radiograph will disclose most lesions, including those causing dangerous instability. In unconscious patients and patients with multiple injuries, fractures of the cervical spine are easily overlooked because they are not expected (Fig. 24.3). It is a good rule to examine the cervical spine radiologically in every case of head injury. Head injuries often produce abnormal movements of the cervical spine, which

are capable of causing fractures or luxations. If the cervical spine injury is overlooked, endotracheal intubation, suction, and so forth may inflict irreparable damage upon the spinal cord (4).

After it has been ascertained that all seven vertebrae are depicted on the radiograph, the outlines of the bony spinal canal are studied. They reflect the topographic relations among the vertebrae and indicate possible endangering of the spinal cord. Normally, they form a funnel-like figure with a smoothly curved spout. In cases of fractures or luxations, the figure may be deformed in several ways; examples are given in Figure 24.4. Any abnormality in the outlines of the bony spinal canal indicates a need for further examination to determine its cause, which could be interlocking of articular facets or a compression fracture of a vertebral body, for example.

Next, the prevertebral space is evaluated. Widening (by hematoma) indicates injury to the cervical spine and may draw attention to the possibility of certain fractures that might otherwise be missed (Fig. 24.5 and Table 24.1). This is especially true for small anterior avulsions of vertebral bodies, cartilaginous rims, or spondylotic spurs due to distractive hyperextension, and for odontoid fracture without displacement. Demonstration of prevertebral swelling is useful to the anesthetist considering intubation. It also may help explain respiratory distress or difficulties in swallowing. Absence of prevertebral hematoma, however, does not exclude injury to the cervical spine.

An attempt should be made to explain the mechanism of injury, which may give an idea of the localization and the extent of soft tissue injury, reveal possible instability, and indicate therapeutic measures to be taken. A distinction

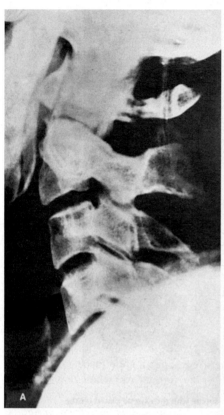

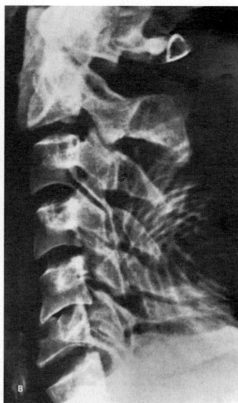

FIG. 24.1. Superimposition of the shoulders on fracture of C6 in a 44-year-old man who fell from a platform 7 m high. (Clinical examination disclosed Brown-Séquard syndrome). **A:** Radiograph disclosing fracture of the posterior arch of atlas. The shoulders are superimposed on the lower cervical vertebrae. **B:** Downward traction on the arms shows an additional compression fracture of the vertebral body of C6. Artifacts overlying the spinous processes are due to support placed under the neck to maintain the lordotic curve.

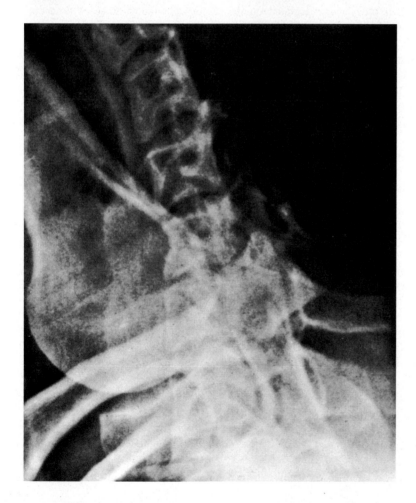

FIG. 24.2. Flying angel projection (swimmer's view). The patient is supine with the cassette placed on the lateral aspect of the shoulder. The arm on the same side as the cassette is raised above the head while the opposite arm is pulled toward the feet to depress the shoulder. The tube is centered on the head of the humerus at the level of the acromion process. Care must be taken that the film and the tube are parallel. (Technique from Scher A, Vambeck V. An approach to the radiological examination of the cervicodorsal junction following injury. *Clin Radiol* 1977;28:243–246.)

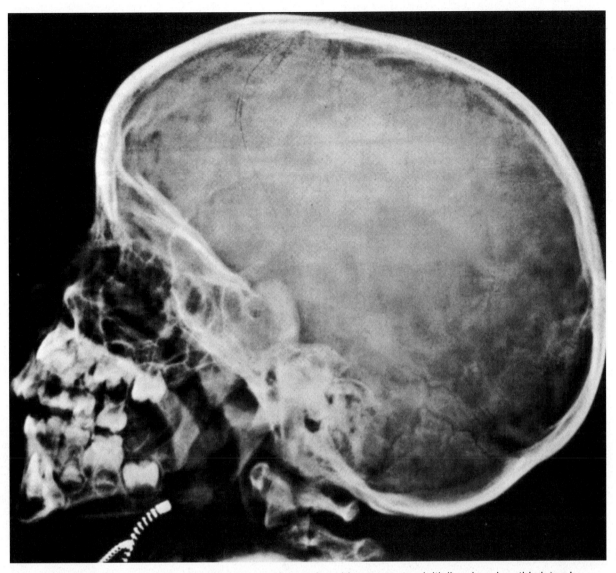

FIG. 24.3. The diagnosis of epiphysiolysis of the odontoid process was initially missed on this lateral skull film of a 4-year-old boy knocked down by a car. After laparotomy, performed because of a battered kidney and hematoma of the liver, respiration had to be maintained artificially; complete cord lesion below the level of C1-C2 was diagnosed. Cervical spine films then drew attention to the epiphysiolysis. The cord lesion proved to be permanent.

can be made between compressive and distractive forces, which may act during hyperflexion or hyperextension (Figs. 24.6 and 24.7). Occasionally, compression and disruption may act together, with the head moving through an arc as suggested by Whitley and Forsyth (Fig. 24.8) (5). Lateral flexion and rotational forces may play an additional role, especially in unilateral lesions. Hyperrotation is important in the production of atlantoaxial rotation luxation (Fig. 24.9).

Sometimes, parallel displacement of the head with respect to the trunk, or vice versa, best explains the type of neck injury produced. This movement causes opposite motions at the upper and lower cervical spine (e.g., hyperextension at the upper cervical region and hyperflexion at the lower cervical region) if the head moves forward with respect to the trunk (Fig. 24.10). It may explain the simultaneous occurrence of a hyperextension fracture of the posterior arch of the atlas and a hyperflexion luxation of the lower cervical spine, for example. Severe disruptive lesions at the craniovertebral junction have been described in parallel movement of the head in deceleration experiments (6). Fractures of the odontoid process are generally explained

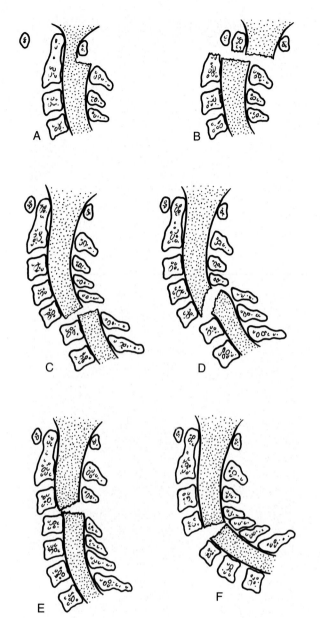

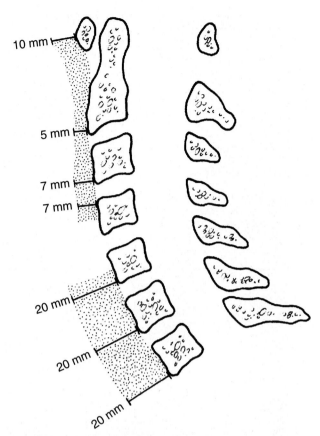

FIG. 24.5. Radiologic width of the prevertebral space: the upper limits of normal width (see Table 24.1 for the range of normal width). Measurements (in mm) are indicated along lines perpendicular to the air shadow of the pharynx and trachea. Larger measurements in injury are considered evidence of prevertebral widening due to hematoma. Note that normal retropharyngeal space is markedly smaller than retrotracheal space (the latter incorporates the esophagus).

FIG. 24.4. Outlines of the spinal canal in several types of injury. Outlines of the bony canal are represented by lines drawn along the posterior borders of the vertebral bodies and the anterior margins of the spinous processes. The canal itself is accentuated by shading. **A:** Anterior pure atlantoaxial luxation, with narrowing of the spinal canal between the odontoid process and the posterior arch of the atlas. **B:** Posterior atlantoaxial luxation due to odontoid fracture (or os odontoideum). Note narrowing of the canal between the odontoid process and the posterior arch of the axis. **C:** Hyperflexion luxation of C5-C6. There is no fracture of the arch of C5. Note narrowing of the canal between the arch of C5 and the body of C6. **D:** Hyperflexion luxation of C5-C6 with fracture of arch C5 ("cord-saving fracture"). There is no narrowing of the spinal canal. **E:** Kyphotic angulation due to hyperflexion injury with disruption of the posterior ligaments. **F:** Lordotic angulation due to hyperextension injury with disruption of the anterior longitudinal ligament and the intervertebral disc.

by sudden forward or backward movement of the head with respect to the trunk (7).

A somewhat controversial subject is the so-called whiplash injury; in our experience, plain radiography is usually negative. The primary movement of the head in this type of injury is backward hypertranslation (8). Demonstration of prevertebral hematoma is important in proving (hyperextensive) laceration of the anterior longitudinal ligament, but the sign will be missed if the first radiographs are not made within 1 to 2 weeks of the injury. Sometimes calcification of the anterior longitudinal ligament occurs weeks or months after a neck injury (Fig. 24.11).

Finally, assessment of spinal instability should be undertaken. Instability in fresh injury cases may be defined

TABLE 24.1. *Normal Prevertebral Soft Tissue Width*

Level	Flexion, mm (range)	Midposition, mm (range)	Extension, mm (range)
C1	5.6 (2–11)	4.6 (1–10)	3.6 (1–8)
C2	4.1 (2–6)	3.2 (1–5)	3.8 (2–6)
C3	4.2 (3–7)	3.4 (2–7)	4.1 (3–6)
C4	5.8 (4–7)	5.1 (2–7)	6.1 (4–8)
C5	17.1 (11–22)	14.9 (8–20)	15.2 (10–20)
C6	16.3 (12–20)	15.1 (11–20)	13.9 (7–19)
C7	14.7 (9–20)	13.9 (9–20)	11.9 (7–21)

The midposition widths were measured on lateral radiographs of 50 noninjured patients, who were normal except for varying degrees of cervical spondylosis in some; their average age was 46 years (range, 15 to 78 years). Widths in flexion and extension were measured in 20 patients with normal prevertebral widths in midposition; their average age was 31 years (range, 16 to 67 years). The sites of measurement are shown in Figure 24.5. No correction has been made for radiologic magnification (about 1.3).

(From: Penning L. Prevertebral hematoma in cervical spine injury: incidence and etiological significance. *Neuroradiol* 1980;1:557–565, with permission.)

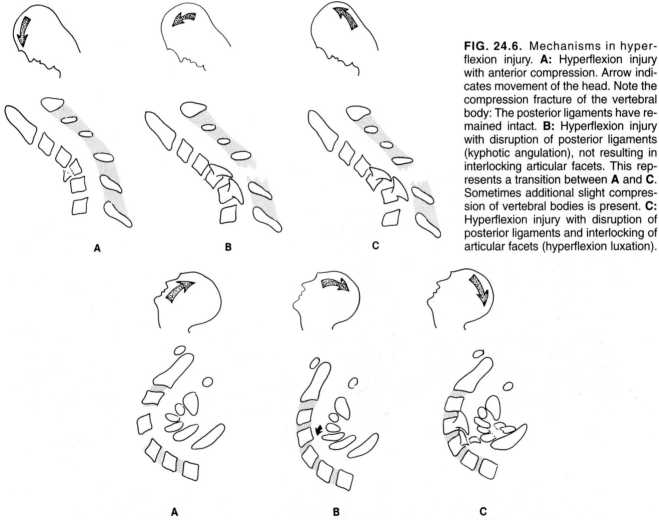

FIG. 24.6. Mechanisms in hyperflexion injury. **A:** Hyperflexion injury with anterior compression. Arrow indicates movement of the head. Note the compression fracture of the vertebral body: The posterior ligaments have remained intact. **B:** Hyperflexion injury with disruption of posterior ligaments (kyphotic angulation), not resulting in interlocking articular facets. This represents a transition between **A** and **C**. Sometimes additional slight compression of vertebral bodies is present. **C:** Hyperflexion injury with disruption of posterior ligaments and interlocking of articular facets (hyperflexion luxation).

FIG. 24.7. Mechanisms in hyperextension injury. **A:** Hyperextension injury with anterior distraction. The arrow indicates movement of the head. Note rupture of the discs and the anterior longitudinal ligament. Avulsions of anterior edges, apophyseal rims, or spondylotic spurs of vertebral bodies may be present. There are no compression fractures of posterior elements. After injury the spine may return to a normal position. **B:** Hyperextension injury with or without rupture of the anterior longitudinal ligament and no posterior compression. Preexisting retrolisthesis and stenosis of the spinal canal will result in a pincers mechanism compressing the spinal cord, even in trivial injury (*small arrow*). **C:** Hyperextension injury with posterior compression. The arrow indicates movement of the head. There are compression fractures of the posterior elements, but no disruption of the anterior longitudinal ligament.

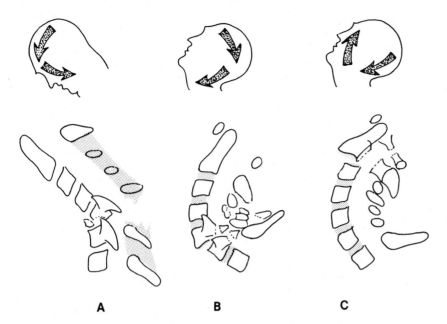

FIG. 24.8. Mechanisms of injury in movement of the head through an arc. **A:** Hyperflexion fracture luxation with anterior compression and posterior distraction, resulting in a compression fracture of the vertebral body and local disruption of articular joints and posterior ligaments. The head moves through an arc as indicated by the arrows. **B:** Hyperextension fracture luxation with anterior disruption and posterior compression, resulting in local disc rupture with massive vertebral displacement and fractures of articular and spinous processes. The head moves through an arc as indicated. **C:** Hangman's fracture (through pedicles of axis with additional anterior displacement of axial body and fracture of posterior arch of atlas) due to hyperextension with anterior distraction and posterior compression. According to Whitley and Forsyth (5), the head moves through an arc, as indicated by the arrows.

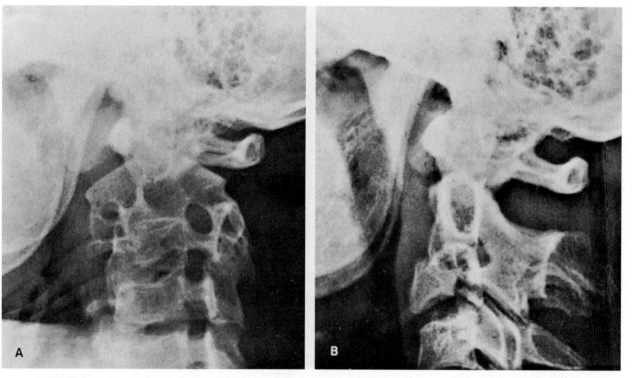

FIG. 24.9. Atlantoaxial rotation luxation in a 21-year-old woman who was in an automobile accident. Incomplete transverse lesion. The head was rotated to the right, and it was impossible to turn it to the normal position. **A:** Radiograph with the head strictly lateral (superimposition of both lower jaws), the atlas lateral, and the axis in an oblique projection: The estimated atlantoaxial rotation is about 50 degrees. **B:** After skull traction, there was rapid reduction of the luxation. Note the block vertebrae C2 and C3 with fracture of their anteroinferior part.

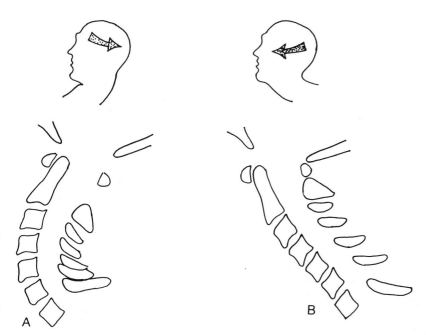

FIG. 24.10. Mechanisms of injury in parallel movement of the head with respect to the trunk. **A:** Backward movement of the head causes hyperflexion of the upper cervical region and hyperextension of the lower cervical region. **B:** Forced forward movement of the head causes hyperextension of the upper cervical region and hyperflexion of the lower cervical region.

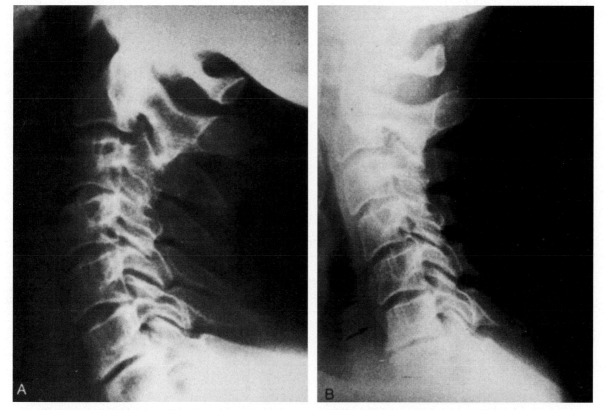

FIG. 24.11. A 50-year-old man had been involved in a head-on car collision, resulting in brain concussion and laceration of the top of the skull. During ambulation 10 days after the injury, he began to report neck pain. **A:** Radiographs of the cervical spine were negative except for anterior spondylosis and degenerative disc narrowing at C6-C7 **B:** Repeat radiography 9 months later, however, showed the presence of local calcification of the anterior longitudinal ligament at C5-C6. This was considered evidence of laceration of this ligament at the time of injury (hyperextension injury most probable).

as the chance of damage to the cord and roots caused by movements of the head and neck. Dangerous instability is especially to be expected in odontoid fractures, interlocking of articular facets, hyperflexion and hyperextension fracture luxation, and lordotic angulation (distractive hyperextension) (9). In such cases, further radiographic examination is deferred until adequate immobilization (e.g., by skull traction) is obtained. Dangerous instability is even more prevalent in elderly patients because of additional weakening of discs and ligaments by aging and spondylosis.

ADDITIONAL RADIOGRAPHY

The anteroposterior (AP) radiograph may provide some useful additional information. Normally, the spinous processes are projected in a vertical row at more or less equal distances. Local widening of the interspinous distance

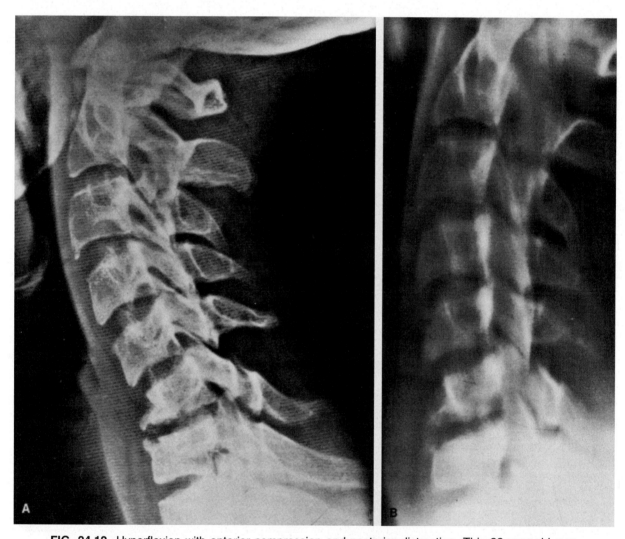

FIG. 24.12. Hyperflexion with anterior compression and posterior distraction. This 22-year-old man collided with a halting truck while riding on a moped, resulting in fracture of the arch through the articular processes. He sustained an incomplete and transient neurologic deficit. **A:** Lateral radiograph showing compression fractures of the body of C6 and, to a lesser degree, C7. Arch C6 is displaced downward. **B** and **C:** Fractures of the articular processes analyzed by tomography. On the right side, note the fracture with diastasis **(B)**, and on the left side, the fracture without diastasis **(C)**. Note normal notching of articular process C7. **D:** Anteroposterior radiograph showing diastasis of spinous processes C5 and C6 due to local rupture of interspinous ligaments. The probable mechanism of injury is hyperflexion with anterior compression and posterior distraction.

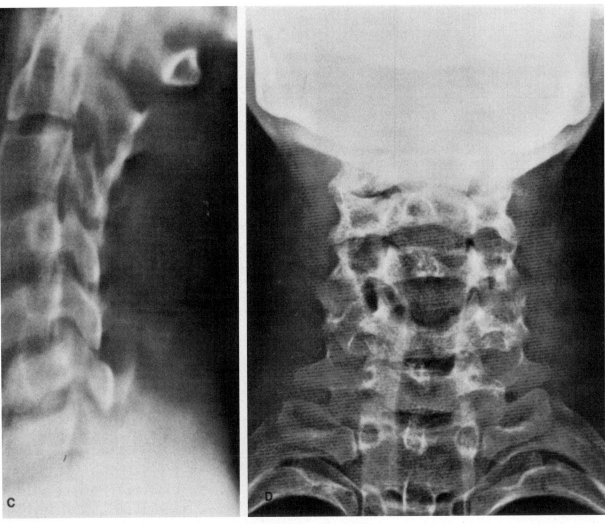

FIG. 24.12. *Continued*

(more than 1.5 times the interspinous distances above and below the widening) indicates the presence of interlocking of articular facets or hyperflexion sprain (Fig. 24.12) (10). The sign is especially useful if the corresponding region has remained obscured by the shoulders in the lateral projection. Scoliotic angulation is observed in unilateral interlocking or unilateral compression of articular facets (Fig. 24.13). Traumatic tilting of an articular process is well disclosed by AP radiography (Fig. 24.14). Open-mouth views may provide additional information in fractures of the atlas, odontoid process, or lateral masses of the axis (Fig. 24.15).

As a rule, oblique views are made at an angle of about 45 degrees, but less rotation (e.g., 15 degrees out of lateral projection) may provide a better view of the articular processes [a semi-oblique or off-lateral view (Fig. 24.16)] (11).

With a patient in skull traction, oblique views are best made with a transportable x-ray apparatus with a C-arch, the patient remaining supine (Fig. 24.17). In other cases, the patient is slightly rotated by raising one shoulder. Oblique views are essential in evaluation of the apophyseal joints [e.g., to determine the side of the lesion in unilateral interlocking (Fig. 24.15)] or in radiographic checking of reposition of interlocking.

Before the advent of computed tomography (CT), classical tomography was sometimes helpful—for example in odontoid fracture without displacement or in fracture of an articular process (Fig. 24.12). During the first stages of its development, CT was especially useful in demonstrating fractures running perpendicular to the (axial) plane of investigation. Fig. 24.16 shows fractures of the vertebral arch not visualized by plain radiography. Although the fractures around the articular process

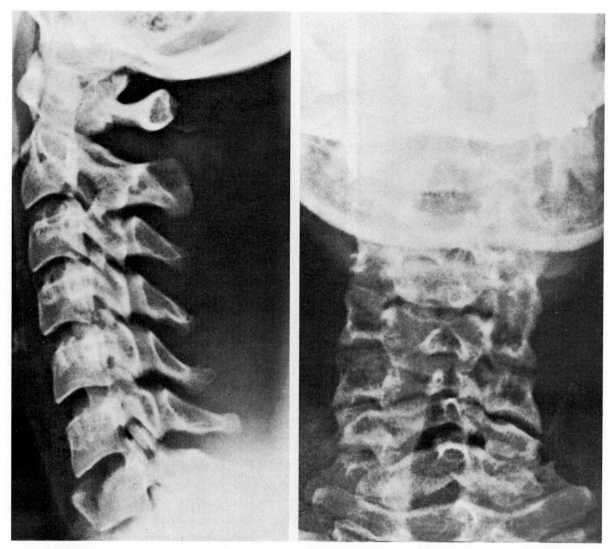

FIG. 24.13. A 24-year-old woman fell from the seventh floor of a building into a shallow pond. She had Brown-Séquard syndrome below C6. **A:** Lateral projection: compression fracture of the body of C7. The condition of the articular processes and the apophyseal joints of C6-C7 is not clear. **B:** Anteroposterior projection: note that the apophyseal joints at C6-C7 are evident. **C:** This oblique view shows that there is interlocking of articular processes C6-C7 on the left side. **D:** An oblique view of the right side shows that the row of articular processes is more or less in line at C6-C7.

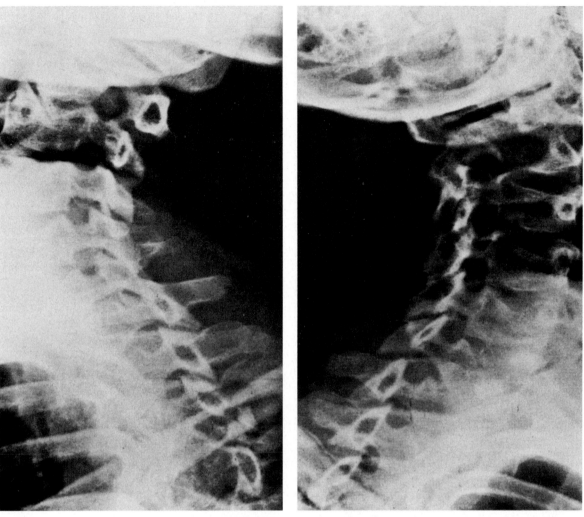

FIG. 24.13. *Continued*

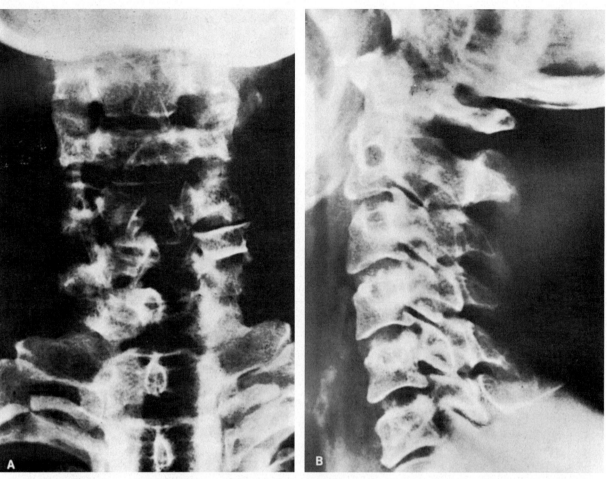

FIG. 24.14. Traumatic tilting of the articular process. **A:** An anteroposterior radiograph discloses end-on projection of joint surfaces of the left-sided articular process of C6 due to traumatic tilting; this is not well visualized on the lateral radiograph **B:** Radiographs of a 37-year-old man who reported neck pain and restricted movements after a car accident. Probable mechanism of injury: compressive hyper-extension and lateral flexion to the left.

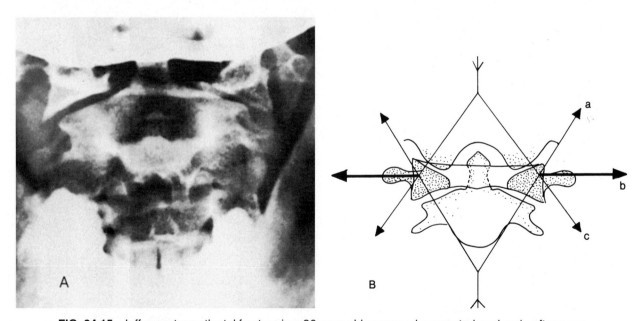

FIG. 24.15. Jefferson-type atlantal fracture in a 36-year-old woman who reported neck pain after a car accident. **A:** Anteroposterior radiograph through the open mouth shows an outward spread of both lateral atlantal masses. A diagnosis of bursting fracture of Jefferson was made. **B:** Mechanism of injury as presented by Jefferson in 1920. (*a*) and (*c*) represent the component force vectors acting on the atlas. The resultant of these forces (*b*) is more or less horizontal and "spreads" the atlas laterally.

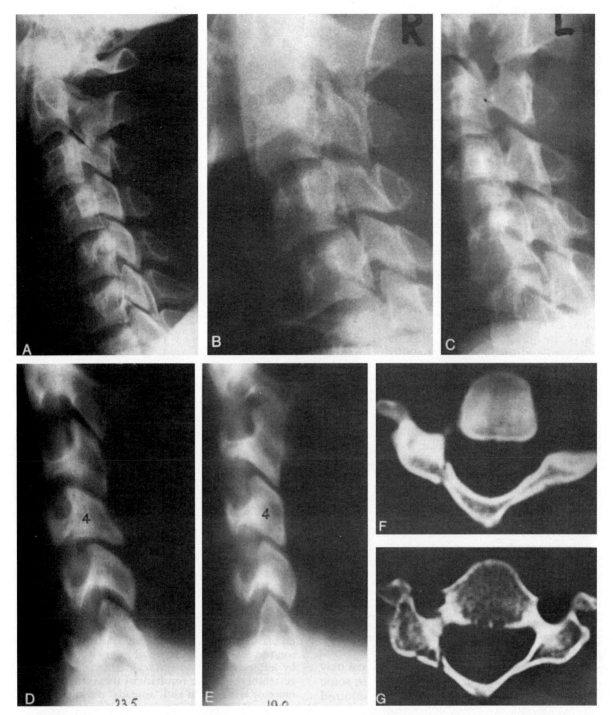

FIG. 24.16. Fracture of the right-sided articular process of C4. **A:** The lateral projection of the cervical spine of this 18-year-old man, who was thrown out of a car during a skid, is puzzling. Anterolisthesis of C3 to C4 draws attention to the articular processes, which are visualized by an off-lateral projection on the right **(B)** and left **(C)**. The right-sided articular process of C4 is tilted, with the inferior articular surface having adopted a more horizontal course. The deformation of the articular process is also visible on a lateral tomogram (right side, **D**; left side, **E**). Additional computed tomographic investigation showed the presence of fractures of the arch around the tilted articular process of C4 **(F).** Surprisingly, similar fractures were present around the right-sided articular process of C3 **(G).** The most probable mechanism of injury is lateral hyperflexion to the right.

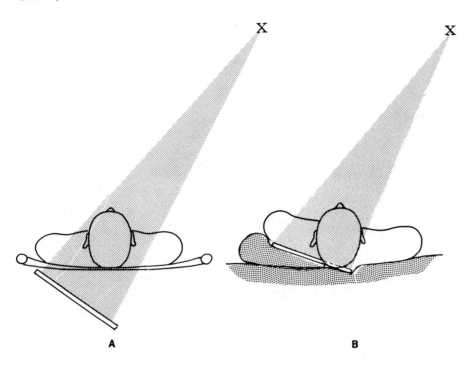

FIG. 24.17. Positioning for oblique views of the cervical spine in patients with acute injury. **A:** Cassette (kept in place by appropriate holder) below the stretcher or frame. **B:** Cassette underneath the neck and raised shoulder of a patient lying on a mattress.

of C4 had already been made likely by plain radiography and classical tomography, the fractures around the articular process of C3 were not expected. Nowadays high-resolution multislice CT with multiplanar reconstruction has become the method of choice in detailed analysis of cervical spine fractures. Nevertheless, in this author's opinion, plain radiography remains a basic method of investigation, able to provide important global information on extent, type and mechanism of cervical spine injury.

PITFALLS IN RADIOGRAPH INTERPRETATION

Congenital or Developmental Anomalies

Anomalies in the context of cervical spine radiography are important for two reasons. They may cause difficulties in interpretation and lead to a false diagnosis of fracture or luxation. They also predispose to severe subjective or objective symptomatology after even minor injuries. This is due to the abnormal anatomic relationship, with less "play" for the nervous system to escape traumatic occurrences.

Congenital Basilar Impression

A high position of the odontoid process above Chamberlain's line is due as a rule to congenital malformation of the base of the skull with occipitalization of the atlas or

hypoplasty of the occipital bone (Fig. 24.18; the differential diagnosis is provided in Fig. 24.19). Conditions that predispose to neurologic damage after injury are a sharpened clivoaxial angle, atlantoaxial luxation, constriction of the foramen magnum, and the presence of tonsillar ectopy (Arnold-Chiari malformation). Trauma is the precipitating factor in the onset of chronic neurologic symptomatology in about half of the cases; as a rule, it is not severe and does not always result in immediate onset of symptoms (12).

Os Odontoideum

The clinical significance of os odontoideum relates to the mobility between the ossicle and the body of the axis (Fig. 24.20). In acute trauma, os odontoideum must be differentiated from fracture of the odontoid process. This should not be difficult because the os is rounded and does not match up with the body of the axis, as is true in an odontoid fracture (13). In chronic cases, differentiation from pseudoarthrosis of the odontoid process may be difficult or impossible, especially because some researchers consider os odontoideum always an acquired lesion (14). Evidence in favor of os odontoideum as a congenital malformation includes shortening of the AP diameter of the atlantal ring, overdevelopment or absence of the anterior arch of the atlas, and the presence of additional anomalies such as the Klippel-Feil anomaly and partial fusions of the bodies of C1, C2, or C3.

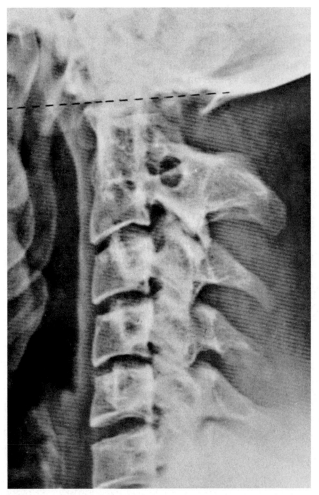

FIG. 24.18. Congenital basilar impression in a 31-year-old man who reported unsteadiness of gait and suboccipital pain after a moped injury that resulted in brain contusion and fracture of the left clavicle. Neurologic investigation showed nystagmus, ataxia, dysarthria, dysmetria, and some loss of appreciation of vibration in the legs. There were no pyramidal signs. Lateral radiograph of the cervical spine showed congenital atlantooccipital fusion, anterior atlanto-axial luxation (anterior atlantodental interspace, 10 mm), ascent of odontoid process 11 mm above Chamberlain's line, and block vertebrae C2-C3.

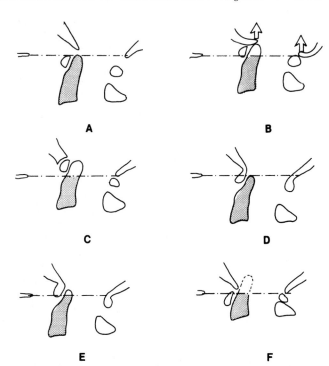

FIG. 24.19. Differential diagnosis of high position of the odontoid process above Chamberlain's line. **A:** The tip of the odontoid process should rise not more than 5 mm above Chamberlain's line (between the dorsal rim of the foramen magnum and the hard palate). The average height of the tip is 1 mm below Chamberlain's line. **B:** Basilar impression is due to weakening of the skull base due to bone diseases (e.g., morbus Paget, osteomalacia). **C:** Congenital basilar impression due to hypoplasia of the basiocciput. **D:** Congenital atlantooccipital fusion without hypoplasia of the basiocciput, which need not result in abnormal position of the odontoid process. Anterior atlantoaxial luxation may be present. **E:** Congenital basilar impression with hypoplasia of the occiput and atlantooccipital fusion. Hypoplasia of the odontoid process and anterior atlantoaxial luxation may be present. **F:** Basilar erosion with destruction of the atlantooccipital and atlantoaxial joints, resulting in ascent of the odontoid process through the atlantal ring into the posterior fossa.

Partial Absence of the Posterior Atlantal Arch

Like numerous other anomalies in the occipitocervical region (15), partial absence of the posterior atlantal arch usually has no clinical significance, although it may be mistaken for a fracture (Fig. 24.21). However, occasionally it has given rise to intermittent paresthesias in all four extremities, with episodes of quadriparesis. This is considered to be caused by forward motion of the posterior tubercle of the atlas on certain movements of the head and neck, with resultant compression of the spinal cord (16).

Spondylolisthesis of the Cervical Spine

Spondylolisthesis of the cervical spine mostly occurs at C6, but occasionally has been described at C2 and C4 (17). Spondylolisthesis of the axis should be differentiated from hangman's fracture (Fig. 24.22) (18). Criteria for differentiation are additional congenital anomalies, such as fusion of parts of C2 and C3, and difficulties in matching the parts of the ostensible fracture. As in os odontoideum, the congenital origin of the defect is debatable; owing to the congenital fusion of the arches, abnormal stress on the pedicles of the arches may have resulted in fracture.

An example of spondylolisthesis of C6 is shown in Figure 24.23. Other defects of pedicles or arches do occur and should not be mistaken for fractures (19).

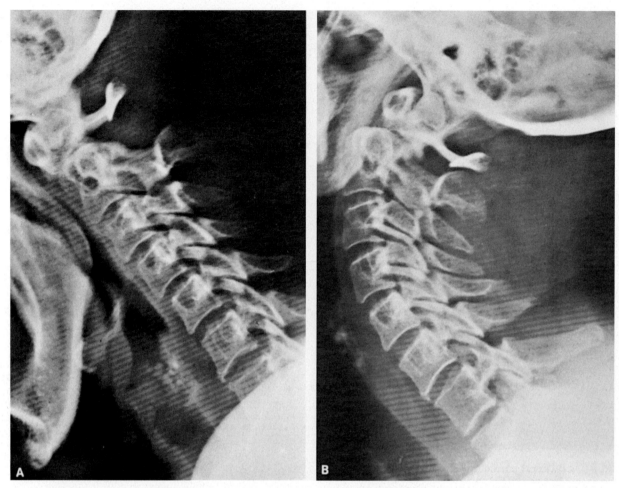

FIG. 24.20. Os odontoideum in a 41-year-old woman who experienced radiating pains and loss of strength in both arms for 1 year. Apart from a fall from a bicycle, there was no history of injury. Lateral radiographs in flexion **(A)** and extension **(B)** show marked atlantoaxial instability due to a mobile os odontoideum. Its congenital origin is suggested by a hypoplastic and stenotic atlantal arch. The diameter of the bony spinal canal between the os and the posterior arch of the atlas was 11 mm (normal, 17–30 mm). In extension, the posterior arch of the atlas and the spinous process of C2 are aligned. In flexion, the os and the axial body are aligned, the spinal canal being narrowed between the axial body and the atlantal arch.

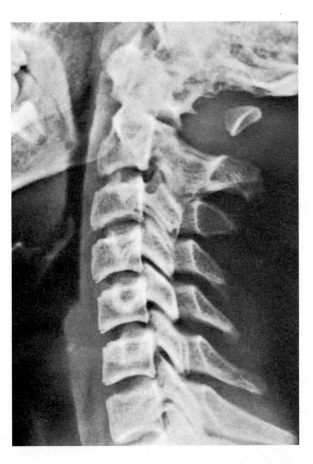

FIG. 24.21. Bilateral partial aplasia of the bony atlantal ring in a 17-year-old girl, which was accidentally discovered during radiography of her jaws for dental correction. Note the epiphyseal rims at the anteroinferior and anterosuperior edges of the vertebral bodies, which appear in the second decade of life and subsequently fuse with vertebral bodies (see also Fig. 24.30).

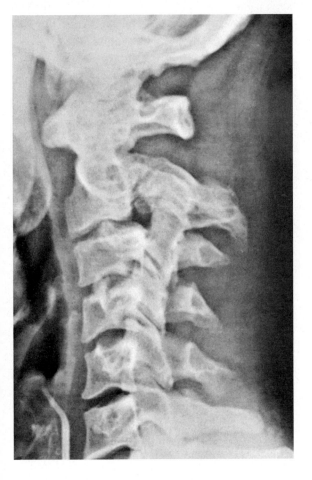

FIG. 24.22. Lateral radiograph of a 41-year-old man with a history of radiating pains in the left arm shows spondylolisthesis of C2 with linear defect (lysis) in the arch of the axis. Apophyseal joints C2-C3 are placed far posteriorly. The posterior arch of the axis is open (no cortical delineation of the anterior margin of the spinous process of C2). Note platyspondylia of C3; the articular pillars of the vertebrae are unusually high. All deformities described are considered to be of developmental origin.

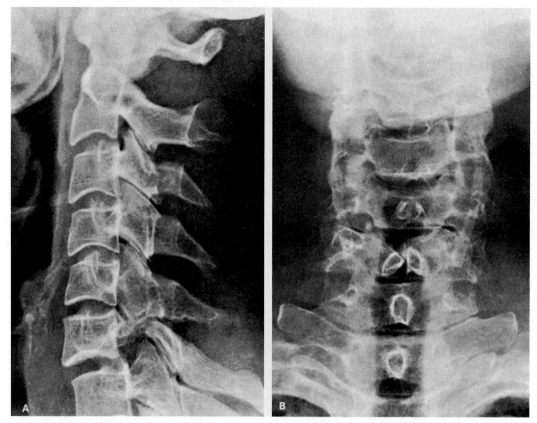

FIG. 24.23. Spondylolisthesis of C6 in a 40-year-old man with no history of injury and with vague symptoms of dysphagia. **A:** Lateral radiograph shows spondylolisthesis of C6 with separation of articular pillars at the interarticular portion. **B:** An additional developmental anomaly is a bifid spinous process, best evident on an anteroposterior radiograph.

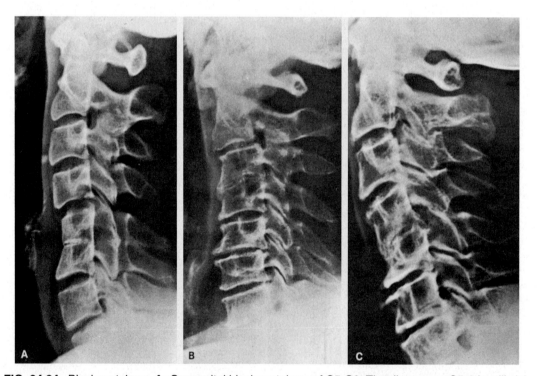

FIG. 24.24. Block vertebrae. **A:** Congenital block vertebrae of C5-C6. The disc space C5-6 is still visible in vestigial form, with local wasting of vertebral block. Note the fusion of articular pillars C5 and C6, with disappearance of joint space and fusion of the posterior arches. Poor visibility of joint space C2-3 is a normal finding owing to inclination of joint surfaces. **B:** Spondylotic block vertebrae of C3-C4, broadening at disc level. Note the normal apophyseal joints and arches. There is marked spondylarthrosis of other parts of the cervical spine. **C:** Traumatic block vertebrae of C4-C5, 4 years after hyperflexion injury. Fusion occurred spontaneously. There is a kyphotic angulation of 15 degrees.

Congenital Block Vertebrae

Congenital block vertebrae, like other anomalies, predispose to neurologic implications after even minor injuries. Block vertebrae C2-C3 may occur in association with congenital basilar impression (Fig. 24.18). Block vertebrae of congenital origin are characterized by wasting at the level of the fusion, with the disc often remaining visible in vestigial form (Fig. 24.24). Such wasting is absent in secondary fusion due to spondylarthrosis, rheumatoid arthritis, or ankylosing spondylitis (Fig. 24.25). In congenital block vertebrae, parts of arches or processes are also fused. Fusion secondary to trauma as a rule is associated with a marked degree of kyphotic angulation (Fig. 24.24C). Fusion may also be the result of anterior spondylodesis (20).

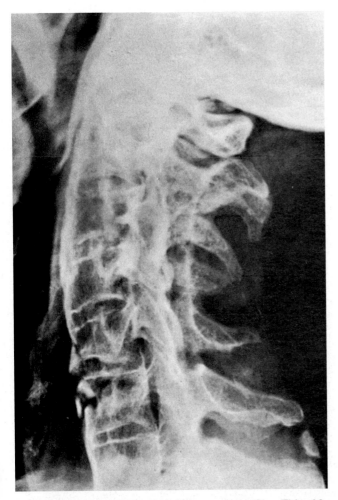

FIG. 24.25. Fracture in ankylosing spondylitis. This 66-year-old man, known to have ankylosing spondylitis for many years, fell from a bicycle. He experienced neck pain owing to a bilateral nerve root lesion of C6. Lateral radiograph shows a fracture of the calcified interior longitudinal ligament at C5-C6 and wedge compression of the body of C5. There is partial ossification of the supraspinous ligament at C6-C7.

Superimposition of Normal Structures

Mach bands are optical phenomena in which dark and light lines appear at the borders of structures of different radiodensity in radiographs (21). They may be especially disturbing at the level of the odontoid or uncinate processes, producing the illusion of fractures (Figs. 24.26 and 24.27). In contrast to fractures, Mach bands do continue and may be followed outside the bony structure allegedly fractured.

Superimposition of teeth or air in the vocal fissure may suggest vertical fractures of the odontoid process or vertebral bodies (Fig. 24.28).

Degeneration of the uncovertebral joints causes a distinct horizontal lucent line over the vertebral body (Fig. 24.29).

Variations of Normal Anatomy

Vertebral Bodies

A slight wedge shape may be incidentally found without a history of injury. Flattening of vertebral bodies is encountered in spondylarthrosis (Fig. 24.29). The end-on projection of uncovertebral joints or apophyseal joints on vertebral bodies in the lateral view should not be mistaken for fractures (Fig. 24.29). Ossifying epiphyseal end plates of vertebral bodies are a normal finding during the second decade of life; they may be avulsed in hyperextension injury (Figs. 24.21 and 24.30) (22,23). Ossifications within the anterior longitudinal ligament may suggest broken spondylotic spurs (Fig. 24.31).

Articular Processes and Apophyseal Joints

In the midcervical region, the articular processes usually have a rhomboid form in lateral projection. However, the frequency of variation from the rhomboid form is rather high, especially at C6 and C7. The articular process of C7 often is notched on its back and elongated so that the posterior edge of the inferior process lies backward in relation to the posterior edges of the other cervical articular processes (Fig. 24.32) (24).

Arthrotic changes of the apophyseal joint may flatten and elongate the articular processes, giving a false impression of compression. A high incidence of apparent compression is found if special projections are used, for example, anteroposterior views with a 20- to 30-degree caudal direction of the central ray. In patients without a history of trauma, unilateral "compression" was noted in nearly half (25). To reduce the chance of a false-positive diagnosis in doubtful cases, tomography is preferred to these special projections.

In the lateral projection, all apophyseal joint spaces are clearly visible, except those between C2 and C3; this is due to slight inclination of the joints in the lateral direction (Fig. 24.27A).

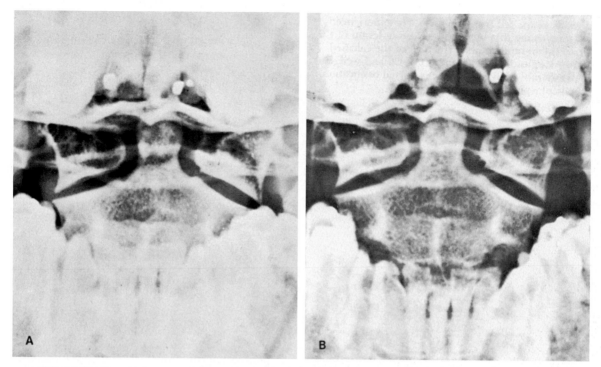

FIG. 24.26. Pseudofracture of the odontoid process. **A:** Open-mouth view suggests a fracture of the odontoid process. **B:** Repeat exposure at a slightly different angle shows a normal odontoid process. The pseudofracture is due to a Mach line produced by the posterior arch of the atlas.

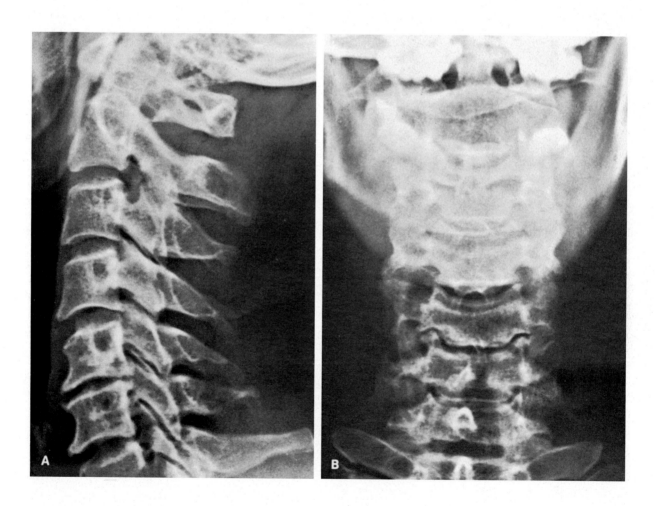

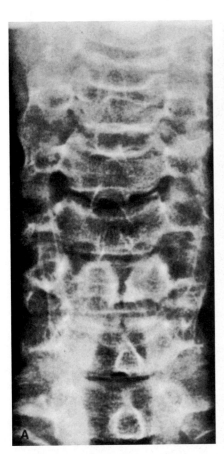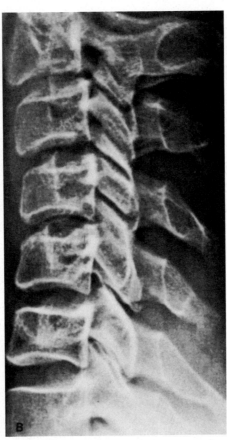

FIG. 24.28. Pseudofracture of C6. **A:** Anteroposterior radiograph shows vertical lucency of the body of C6 which, although it suggests a fracture, is produced by vocal fissure. **B:** Lateral radiograph shows a normal body of C6.

FIG. 24.27. Cervical spondylosis, retrolisthesis of C5-C6, and pseudofractures of the uncinate processes of C6. This 41-year-old woman with neck pain had no history of injury but showed marked spondylarthrotic changes at C5 through C7. **A:** Lateral radiograph shows retrolisthesis of C5-C6 due to disc narrowing. **B:** Anteroposterior radiograph shows marked carthrosis of the uncovertebral joint of C5-C6 producing a horizontal dark line on the body of C5 **(A)**, which should not be taken for a fracture. Pseudofractures of the uncinate processes of C6 **(B)** are due to the Mach effect caused by the inferior edge of the arch of C5. The apophyseal joint spaces of C2-C3 are poorly visible on the lateral radiograph **(A)** owing to normal inclination of the joint surfaces.

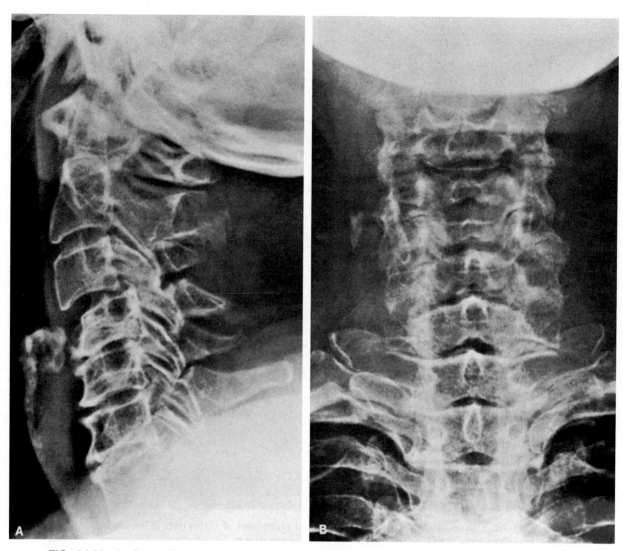

FIG. 24.29. A: Spondylarthrotic anterolisthesis, retrolisthesis, and platyspondylia. This 73-year-old woman with no history of injury showed marked spondylarthrotic changes of the cervical spine. Note the anterolisthesis of C3-C4 due to arthrosis of apophyseal joints (posterior spurring, disappearance of cartilaginous joint space). The retrolisthesis of C4-C5 is due to disc narrowing; the apophyseal joint spaces are normal. **B:** Anteroposterior radiograph showing marked uncarthrosis at this level, producing a horizontal lucent line on the body of C5 in the lateral radiograph **(A).** The same is true of C5-C6, although to a lesser extent. There is spondylarthrotic flattening (platyspondylia) of vertebral bodies C4, C5, and C6 (compare with C3 and C7).

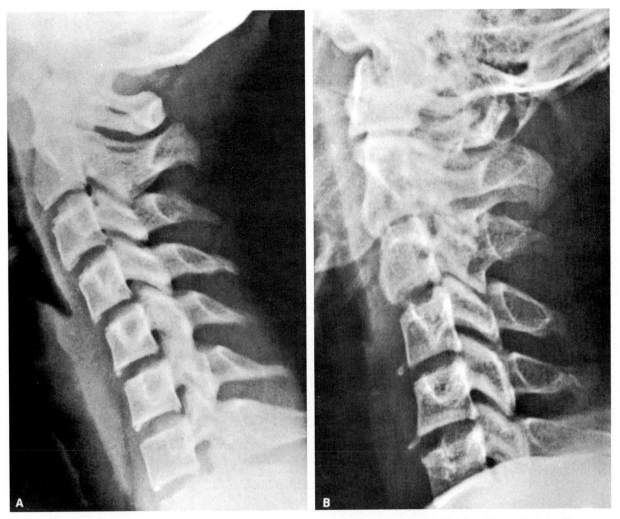

FIG. 24.30. Traumatic avulsion of the epiphyseal end plates of the vertebral bodies ("vertebral rims"). **A:** Normal epiphyseal end plates in a girl aged 12 years. **B:** Traumatic avulsion of epiphyseal end plates at the lower borders of C4 and C5 in an 18-year-old man. Note the slight prevertebral widening at C4 (9 mm). This patient sustained a cerebral contusion, multiple facial fractures, and skin lacerations as a result of a frontal collision with a tractor. There were no signs of cervical cord lesion. Probable mechanism: hyperextension with anterior distraction.

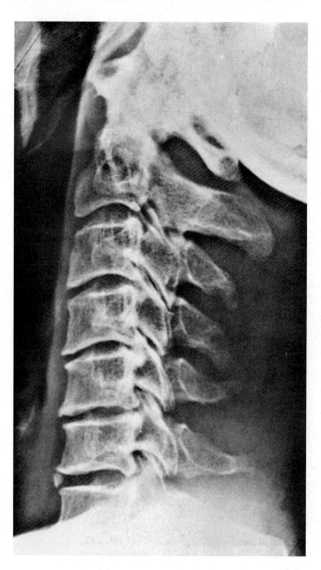

FIG. 24.31. Ossification of the anterior longitudinal ligament at C6-C7 in a 69-year-old man with progressive myelopathy, most probably caused by stenosis of the cervical spinal canal. The bony diameter at C5 was 14 mm (normal, 12–21 mm); additional narrowing was caused by posterior spondylosis of vertebral bodies C4 to C6. Incidental findings included ossification of the anterior longitudinal ligament at C6-C7 and persisting apophysis of the spinous process of C7.

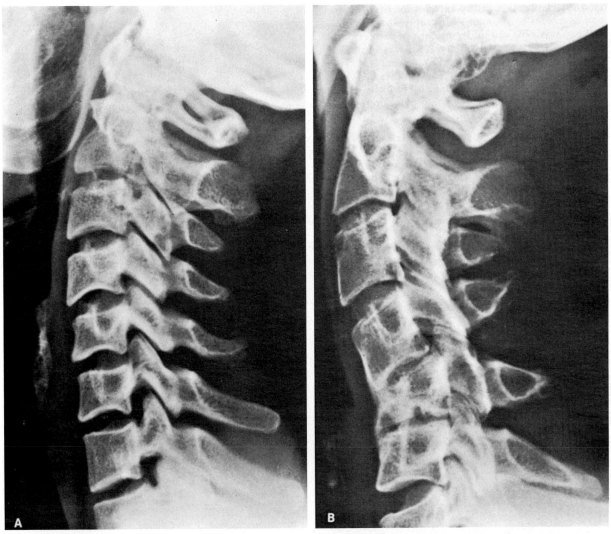

FIG. 24.32. Notching of the articular processes. **A:** Notching of articular processes of C6 and C7 in a normal person. Note the lengthening of the articular pillars of C6 and C7 as compared with C5 and C4. Apophyseal joint spaces C7-T1 are located more posteriorly than joint spaces C6-7 or C5-6. **B:** Old compression fracture of C5 in a 21-year-old man caused by a head-on dive into shallow water; no neurologic symptoms were evident. Note the fusion of C4, C5, and C6 in kyphotic angulation. Normal notching of the articular processes of C7 should not be considered a sign of compression.

Normal and Abnormal Relationships between Vertebrae

Variations in Posture, Angulations, and Torticollis

Normally, in midposition with the patient sitting or standing, the cervical spine shows a slight lordotic curvature. However, there are many variations, including a straight spine and even a slightly kyphotic curvature (22). Curvatures are partly influenced by posture as a whole. In a lying position, and especially in comatose patients, the spine may sag and assume a kyphotic position.

In kyphotic angulation, the cervical spine as a whole is in midposition with one segment more or less flexed. Slight kyphotic angulation is often encountered in spondylarthrosis, notably at the C5-C6 level. Marked kyphotic angulation after trauma is due to local disruption of the posterior ligaments as the result of hyperflexion injury, with or without interlocking of articular facets (Fig. 24.33) (26). Compres-

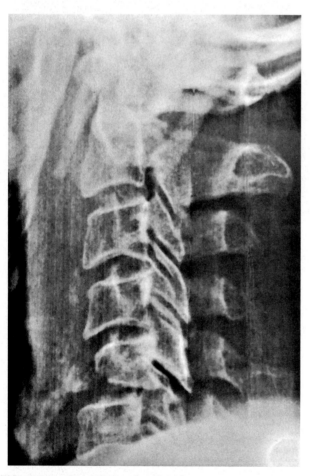

FIG. 24.33. Hyperflexion luxation fracture in a 57-year-old man due to a fall down a flight of stairs. Apart from tingling in the fingers of both hands, he had no neurologic signs. This lateral radiograph shows a compression fracture of the vertebral body of C5 with marked retrolisthesis and diastasis of the apophyseal joint spaces of C5-C6. Note the prevertebral hematoma. Mechanism of injury: hyperflexion with anterior compression and posterior distraction.

sion fractures of vertebral bodies may also produce local kyphosis, which has a tendency to progress. Scoliotic angulation is found in unilateral compression of an articular process or in unilateral interlocking at that level.

In torticollis, the spine may show a variable degree of kyphosis, scoliosis, or rotation. This causes puzzling radiographic images that may lead to misinterpretation. Projections should therefore be standardized as much as possible (for example, by using a strictly lateral or AP view of the trunk on the head). Radiography should be repeated after the torticollis has subsided. Torticollis is most often observed in atlantoaxial lesions; it does not appear in fractures and luxations of the lower cervical spine. In young adults, torticollis may follow trivial injury, usually after a free interval of several hours. It is produced by reflex spasm of paraspinal muscles. Rotation is usually marked; attempts at correction meet with painful resistance. It is important to rule out anterior atlantoaxial luxation (widened anterior atlantodental interspace) due to infection of the upper respiratory tract. In this so-called spontaneous atlantoaxial luxation, a variable degree of atlantoaxial rotation may be present (see Fig. 24.36D) (27,28).

Luxation, Subluxation, and Pseudosubluxation

A luxation, or dislocation, may be defined as the complete and lasting disruption of the articular facets of a synovial joint. In the lower cervical spine (C2 through C7), this applies to the apophyseal joints only, not to the intervertebral discs. The latter may slip, causing anterolisthesis or retrolisthesis of vertebral bodies (see the following section, "Retrolisthesis and Anterolisthesis"). A luxation is present in the interlocking of articular facets and in marked diastasis [as in hyperflexion fracture luxation (Figs. 24.8A and 24.33)].

The designation *subluxation* should be avoided because it is often abused to express uncertainty about the presence of pathology, and may wrongly suggest it. For example, the step formation along the posterior borders of the vertebral bodies in flexed or kyphotic spines in children, especially at the C2-C3 and C3-C4 levels, has repeatedly led to a diagnosis of subluxation (Fig. 24.34). It is now recognized as a normal variation or pseudosubluxation (29,30). Telescoping subluxation is a nontraumatic condition caused by approximation of vertebrae due to disc degeneration, with concomitant telescoping of articular processes without disruption of joint surfaces (Fig. 24.35C) (31).

Atlantoaxial luxations are divided into anterior, posterior, and rotational types (Fig. 24.36). The luxation is termed *pure* if the odontoid process has remained intact and if anterior displacement of more than 2 to 3 mm in adults and 4 to 5 mm in children is due to rupture of the transverse ligament. Such traumatic rupture may occur, but usually the odontoid fractures before the ligament tears (32,33). In pure luxation, preexisting conditions such as congenital basilar impression, rheumatoid arthritis, or ankylosing spondylitis should be excluded. In children, spontaneous pure atlanto-

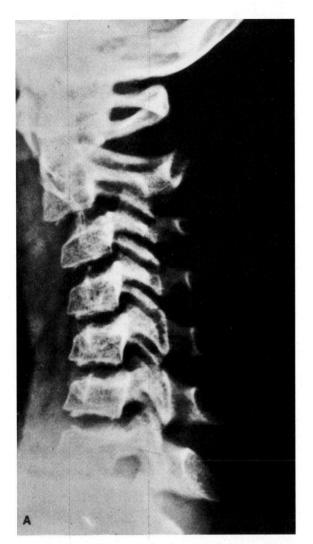 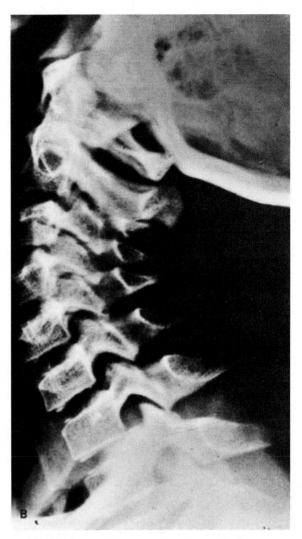

FIG. 24.34. This 9-year-old girl with no history of injury showed pseudosubluxations of the cervical spine in a flexed position. **A:** In a flexed position, the cervical spine shows marked step formation (anterolisthesis) of the posterior borders of the vertebral bodies. **B:** In extension, reverse step formation is evident. These findings are normal in children and should not be diagnosed as subluxation. In adults, step formation is less obvious owing to the more vertical position of the apophyseal joints and lesser mobility, resulting in relatively less gliding movement of the vertebrae. (Courtesy of H. Scheier, Zurich.)

axial luxation may be encountered in infections in the upper part of the neck (27,28). In rheumatoid arthritis, there is often simultaneous erosion of the odontoid process; sometimes the odontoid process has moved upward owing to destruction of the lateral atlantoaxial and atlantooccipital joints (Fig. 24.37).

Traumatic pure atlantoaxial luxation in the posterior direction is extremely rare (34,35). Anterior or posterior luxation, possibly combined with some degree of lateral luxation, is a common finding in fresh and old nonunited fractures of the odontoid process and in os odontoideum.

Rotatory luxation may be diagnosed if rotation exceeds 45 degrees and the articular facets are shown to be interlocked on CT scans. Radiography with the head in the lateral position will show the atlas to be in the same lateral

position, because rotation between occiput and atlas is virtually impossible. However, the axis and lower cervical spine will have rotated more than 45 degrees, presenting themselves as in oblique projection (Fig. 24.10). Smaller degrees of atlantoaxial rotation (less than 40 degrees) are within the physiologic range of movement and may not be called luxation or subluxation. Their occurrence is evident from the rotated position of the head during radiography (e.g., as the result of muscle spasm). In the absence of head rotation, atlantoaxial (counter) rotation may be compensatory for rotation of the lower cervical spine in scoliosis or in unilateral interlocking or unilateral articular mass compression. In the lateral radiograph, C2 rotation is evidenced by projection of a lateral mass anterior to the axial body (Fig. 24.36).

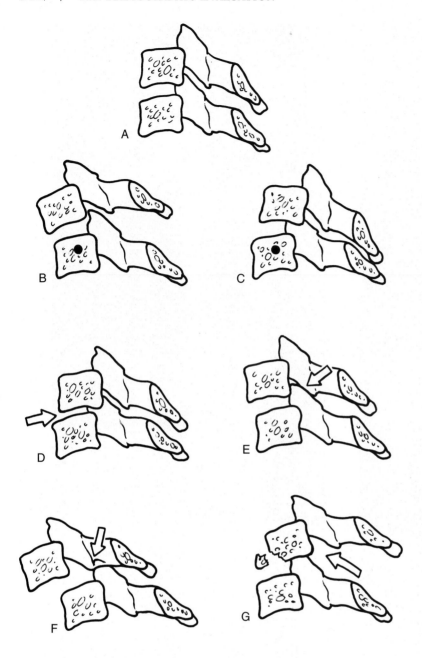

FIG. 24.35. Relationships in apophyseal joints. **A:** Normal vertebral relationship in lateral view. **B** and **C:** Normal flexion-extension movement (*dot* indicates instantaneous axis of movement). Note anterior gliding in flexion and posterior gliding in extension, not to be confused with retrolisthesis and anterolisthesis, which occur in midposition. **D:** Retrolisthesis due to disc narrowing. The oblique course of the apophyseal joints forces the upper vertebra in a posteroinferior direction (*arrow*). The designation *telescoping subluxation of apophyseal joints* should not be used because it might wrongly suggest a traumatic genesis. **E:** Anterolisthesis due to disappearance of joint cartilage owing to arthrosis or arthritis. The upper vertebra slips anteriorly (*arrow*). **F:** Traumatic interlocking as the result of hyperflexion with posterior distraction. **G:** Traumatic diastasis of apophyseal joint space in hyperflexion fracture luxation with anterior compression and posterior distraction.

Asymmetric position of the odontoid process between the lateral masses of the atlas in the AP view, or lateral overriding (offset) of the atlantoaxial joint edges, is no sign per se of injury to the upper cervical region. We believe that the margins of normalcy should be rather wide to avoid pitfalls. However, bilateral atlantal overriding is an indication of atlantal burst fracture (Jefferson's fracture) with bilateral atlantal spread, or anterior atlantoaxial luxation, in which the ostensible atlantal spread is caused by relatively large radiologic magnification (Fig. 24.15) (36, 37). It has also been described in simultaneous anterior and posterior spina bifida of the atlas (38).

Differences in interspace between the posterior arch of the atlas and the occiput on the one hand and the spinous

processes of the axis on the other hand have no pathologic significance and do not indicate posterior ligament rupture, as may be the case in the C2 to C7 region.

Retrolisthesis and Anterolisthesis

In retrolisthesis, a vertebral body slips posteriorly in relation to the vertebrae below. In spondylarthrosis, retrolisthesis is a common finding in disc narrowing in the midcervical region (C3 through C6) (Figs. 24.27 and 24.29). It is explained by the oblique position of the intervertebral joints, which forces the upper vertebral body slightly backward in approaching the vertebral body below. Retrolisthesis is often seen below block vertebrae, especially C2 and C3.

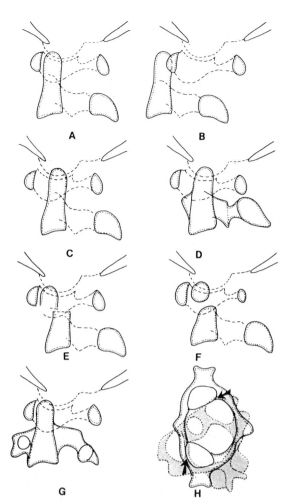

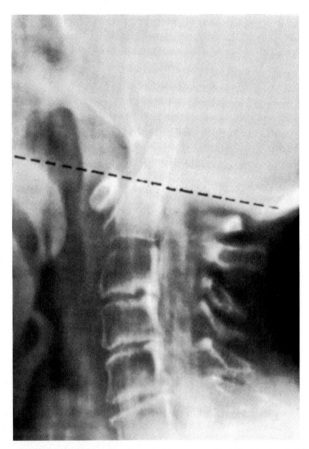

FIG. 24.37. Basilar erosion in rheumatoid arthritis in a 38-year-old woman with a history of rheumatoid arthritis for 20 years and headache. Neurologic examination showed the presence of the extrapyramidal syndrome. This midline tomogram shows the ascent of the axial body through the atlantal ring due to rheumatoid destruction of atlantoaxial and atlantooccipital joints (probably old and long-standing). The interrupted line is Chamberlain's line. Note the rheumatoid changes of vertebral end plates.

FIG. 24.36. Schematic representation of several types of atlantoaxial luxation. **A:** Normal atlantoaxial relationship, that is, anterior atlantodental interspace not exceeding 2 mm in adults and 5 mm in children. **B:** Pure posterior atlantoaxial luxation. **C:** Pure anterior atlantoaxial luxation. Note the pathologically enlarged anterior atlantodental interspace. Further anterior luxation is counteracted by the check-rein effect of the alar ligaments (film). **D:** Atlantoaxial luxation with rotation as it occurs spontaneously in infections of the upper respiratory tract. Atlantoaxial rotation remains within the normal limit of 30 to 45 degrees. **E:** Anterior atlantoaxial fracture luxation (odontoid fracture). Luxation may also occur in a posterior or lateral direction. Intermittent luxation may be the result of nearthrotic or pseudoarthrotic healing. **F:** Anterior atlantoaxial luxation due to os odontoideum. Luxation may also occur in the posterior direction. Luxation, as a rule, is intermittent (atlantoaxial instability), depending on the position of the head. Note the shortening of the atlantal anteroposterior diameter and deformation of the anterior and posterior arches. **G** and **H:** Atlantoaxial rotation luxation. Rotation markedly exceeds the normal limit of 45 degrees because of interlocking of the articular facets (*arrows*). There is no rotation between the atlas and the occiput. (Measurements of normal atlantoaxial rotation are from Penning L, Wilmink JT. Rotation of the cervical spine: a CT study in normal subjects. *Spine* 1987;12:732–738.)

Retrolisthesis in disc narrowing without fracture of the corresponding vertebral body should not be considered the result of injury, but of preexisting spondylarthrosis. Retrolisthesis with fracture is a common finding in hyperflexion injury with compression (Fig. 24.33). Retrolisthesis is the cause of extra narrowing of the spinal canal in retroflexion. In congenital or acquired stenosis of the canal, this may cause pinching of the cord even in mild hyperextension injuries.

Anterolisthesis (forward slipping of a vertebral body) is produced by arthrotic or arthritic changes of the intervertebral joints (Fig. 24.29). It also occurs in spondylolisthesis (Figs. 24.22 and 24.23). Trauma may cause anterolisthesis through the interlocking of articular facets in hyperflexion injury or through compression of articular facets in hyperextension injury. At C2-C3, marked anterolisthesis may be encountered in hangman's fracture. Anterolisthesis in the presence of arthrotic or arthritic changes without evidence of fracture should not be considered the result of injury.

An extensive review of false-positive interpretations of radiographs in cervical spine injury is presented by Kim and associates (39). The most common causes of error were degenerative disorders (retrolisthesis or anterolisthesis diagnosed as traumatic subluxation; uncovertebral joint degeneration; platyspondylia; ossification of the anterior longitudinal ligament) and congenital anomalies (block vertebrae, asymmetry at the base of the odontoid, os odontoideum).

REFERENCES

1. Lodge T, Higginbottom E. Fractures and dislocations of the cervical spine. *X-ray Focus* 1966;7:2.
2. Scher A, Vambeck V. An approach to the radiological examination of the cervicodorsal junction following injury. *Clin Radiol* 1977;28:243.
3. Paakkala T, Keski-Nisula L, Lektinen E. Fehl-befundung in der Röntgendiagnostik der Halswirbelsäulenverletzungen. *Fortschr Rontgenstr* 1978;128:550.
4. Kapp JP. Endotracheal intubation in patients with fractures of the cervical spine. *J Neurosurg* 1975;42:731.
5. Whitley JR, Forsyth HF. Classification of cervical spine injuries. *AJR Am J Roentgenol* 1960;83:633.
6. Unterharnscheidt F. Neuropathology of rhesus monkeys undergoing −Gx impact acceleration. In: Ewing CL, Thomas DJ, Sances A, et al., eds. *Impact injury of the head and spine.* Springfield, IL: Charles C Thomas, 1983:94–176.
7. Howorth MB, Petrie JG. *Injuries of the spine.* Baltimore: Williams & Wilkins, 1964.
8. Penning L. Acceleration of the cervical spine by hypertranslation of the head. *Eur Spine J* 1992;1:1–19.
9. Holdworth FW. Fractures, dislocations, and fracture-dislocations of the spine. *J Bone Joint Surg Am* 1970;52:1534.
10. Naidich JB, Naidich TP, Garfein C, et al. The widened interspinous distance: a useful sign of anterior cervical dislocation in the supine frontal projection. *Radiology* 1977;123:113.
11. Buetti-Bäuml C. *Funktionelle Röntgendiagnostik der Halswirbelsäulle.* Stuttgart: Georg Thieme, 1964.
12. Schmidt H, Sartor K, Heckl L. Bone malformations of the craniovertebral region. In: *Handbook of clinical neurology*, vol. 32. Amsterdam: Excerpta Medica, 1977:1–98.
13. Minderhoud JM, Braakman R, Penning L. Os odontoideum: clinical, radiological and therapeutic aspects. *J Neurol Sci* 1969;8:521.
14. Fielding JW, Griffin PP. Os odontoideum: an acquired lesion. *J Bone Joint Surg Am* 1977;59:37.
15. Wackenheim A. *Roentgendiagnosis of the craniovertebral region.* New York: Springer-Verlag, 1974.
16. Richardson EG, Boone SC, Reid RL. Intermittent quadriparesis associated with a congenital anomaly of the posterior arch of the atlas. Case report. *J Bone Joint Surg Am* 1975;57:853–854.
17. Charlton DP, Gehweiler JA, Morgan CL, et al. Spondylolysis and spondylolisthesis of the cervical spine. *Skeletal Radiol* 1978;3:79.
18. Gehweiler JA, Martinez S, Clark WM, et al. Spondylolisthesis of the axis vertebra. *AJR Am J Roentgenol* 1977;128:682.
19. Liliequist B. Absent cervical pedicle. *Acta Neurochir* 1977;38:125.
20. Braunstein E, Hunter LY, Bailey RW. Long-term radiographic changes following anterior cervical fusion. *Clin Radiol* 1980;31:201.
21. Daffner RH. Pseudofracture of the dens: Mach bands. *Am J Roentgenol* 1977;128:607.
22. Bailey DK. The normal cervical spine in infants and children. *Radiol Clin North Am* 1952;59:712.
23. Keller RH. Traumatic displacement of the cartilaginous vertebral rim: a sign of intervertebral disc prolapse. *Radiology* 1974;110:21.
24. Kattan KR. The notched articular process of C7 (dorsalization of C7). *Am J Roentgenol* 1976;126:612.
25. Vines FS. The significance of "occult" fractures of the cervical spine. *Am J Roentgenol* 1969;107:493.
26. Lidstrom A. Injuries in the cervical spine. *Acta Chir Scand* 1954;106: 212.
27. Fielding JW, Cochran GVB, Lawsing JF, et al. Tears of the transverse ligament of the atlas. *J Bone Joint Surg Am* 1974;56:1683.
28. Watson JR. Spontaneous hyperaemic dislocation of the atlas. *Proc R Soc Med* 1932;25:586.
29. Cattel LHS. Filtzer DL. Pseudosubluxation and other normal variations of the cervical spine in children. *J Bone Joint Surg Am* 1965;47:1295.
30. Zeitler E, Markuske H. Roentgenolgische Bewegungsanalyse der Halswirbelsäule bei gesunden Kindern. *Fortschr Roentgenstr* 1962;96:87.
31. Hadley LA. *The spine: anatomico-radiographic studies, development and the cervical spine.* Springfield, IL: Charles C Thomas, 1964.
32. Davis D, Bohlman H, Walker AE, et al. The pathological findings in fatal craniospinal injuries. *J Neurosurg* 1971;5:603.
33. Fielding JW, Hawkins RJ. Atlantoaxial rotatory fixation. *J Bone Joint Surg Am* 1977;59:37.
34. Haralson RH, Boyd HB. Posterior dislocation of the atlas on the axis without fracture. *J Bone Joint Surg Am* 1969;51:561.
35. Patzakis MJ, Knopf A, Elfering M. et al. Posterior dislocation of the atlas on the axis: a case report. *J Bone Joint Surg Am* 1974;56:1260.
36. Jefferson G. Fracture of atlas vertebra: report of four cases and review of those previously reported. *Br J Surg* 1920;7:407.
37. Spense KF, Decker S, Sell KW. Bursting atlantal fracture associated with rupture of transverse ligament. *J Bone Joint Surg Am* 1970;52: 543.
38. Budin E, Sondheimer F. Lateral spread of the atlas without fracture. *Radiology* 1966;87:1095.
39. Kim KS, Rogers LF, Regenbogen V. Pitfalls in plain film diagnosis of cervical spine injuries: false positive interpretation. *Surg Neurol* 1986; 25:381–392.

CHAPTER 25

Computed Tomography and Myelography of the Cervical Spine

Christopher G. Ullrich

The first computed tomography (CT) scanner became commercially available in 1972. It was capable of scanning only the head. The machine revolutionized neuroradiology. The first whole-body CT scanner was marketed in 1974. The thin-section capability (1.5 mm) necessary for high-quality cervical spine CT evaluation was introduced in 1977. Two-dimensional multiplanar reconstruction imaging was developed in the late 1970s. Two-dimensional CT images are produced by reprocessing axial CT image data into other tomographic projections, typically sagittal and coronal views. Creation of curved two-dimensional CT reconstruction images became possible in the mid-1980s. Three-dimensional CT image technology was pioneered in the 1980s as well. Three-dimensional CT images are computer graphic displays that integrate axial CT image data into lifelike images (Fig. 25.1). This technique is directly related to the prior development of computer-aided design and manufacturing (CAD/CAM) systems for industrial applications. Continuous-rotation CT scanners, commonly called helical or spiral CT scanners, were widely produced in the early 1990s. The first commercial helical 4-channel multidetector CT (MDCT) was introduced in 1998. This was followed by the availability of 8- and 16-channel MDCT systems; 32- and 64-channel MDCT systems are being actively developed. These MDCT machines allow rapid volumetric acquisition of CT data and are ideally suited to two- and three-dimensional CT image processing. CT remains a very important modality for cervical spine studies.

Myelography is a term that denotes imaging techniques involving the injection of a contrast agent into the subarachnoid space to provide visualization of the spinal cord and intrathecal nerve roots. Air myelography was introduced in 1920; combined with conventional tomography, it was quite capable of demonstrating the outline of the spinal cord well. Iophendylate (Pantopaque) was developed in 1940. This material was insoluble in spinal fluid and quite dense. It required removal at the end of the imaging procedure, a process that was often unpleasant for the patient. Pantopaque provided a good assessment of the cervical spinal cord and nerve roots and was the preferred myelographic examination agent until the early 1980s. In 1978, metrizamide (Amipaque) became the first water-soluble myelographic agent available. It came in a lyophilized form and had to be reconstituted immediately before the myelogram was performed. Unlike Pantopaque, it did not require removal from the subarachnoid space at the end of the procedure. More important, it was suitable for concurrent use with CT. Iohexol (Omnipaque) and iopamidol (Isovue) are second-generation water-soluble myelogram agents, both introduced in 1986. They are stable in mixed form and less neurotoxic than metrizamide. The combination technique of CT with myelography (CTM) remains a powerful method for evaluating the cervical spine today.

The basic technology of CT imaging and the derivation of two- and three-dimensional CT reconstruction images are reviewed in this chapter. Myelography, with emphasis on its combined use with CT, is discussed. Imaging principles are illustrated. A brief review of clinical applications of CT concludes the chapter.

BASIC COMPUTED TOMOGRAPHY TECHNOLOGY

The axial CT image is defined by a cartesian coordinate system called a *matrix*. Values for x and y, respectively, denote the horizontal and vertical edges of the axial CT

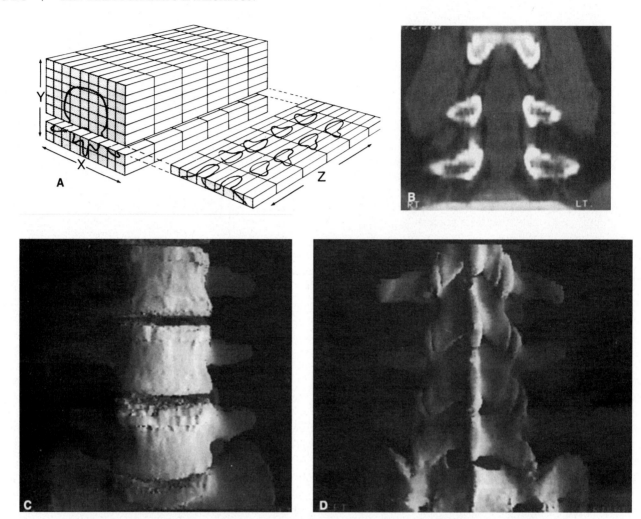

FIG. 25.1. The basic concept of two- and three-dimensional computed tomographic (CT) reconstruction images. **A:** Six consecutive axial CT images of the lumbar spine are shown. Each rectangular block represents a voxel. A consecutive series of axial CT images is a three-dimensional array of voxels or Hounsfield number data whose spatial locations are defined by the matrix, the CT image thickness, and the CT table movement. The computer selection of appropriate voxels to produce a two-dimensional CT coronal reconstruction image (*xz*-plane of voxels) is shown. **B:** This typical two-dimensional CT coronal reconstruction image of the lumbar spine from L3 to S1 through the midpedicle area clearly shows the nerve roots exiting into the neural foramina. This image retains the tissue-density discrimination of the original axial CT images. **C:** The voxels defining the surface of the vertebral body are identified, a reference light source is assumed, and the same basic CT data are now a three-dimensional CT image. This anteroposterior view clearly demonstrates the anatomic relationship between the vertebral bodies. Osteophytes are also identified, but all the adjacent soft tissue structures are absent. **D:** The posteroanterior view (180-degree rotation) beautifully demonstrates the alignment of the facet joints in a fashion unobtainable with two-dimensional CT techniques and with a clarity seldom achieved with conventional radiography. The lifelike quality of these three-dimensional images is striking.

matrix. The *pixel* (picture element) is the basic unit of a matrix. The *voxel* (volume element) is the volume of tissue defined by the pixel and the CT image thickness. The matrix position of each voxel is mathematically described by *x* and *y* coordinate numbers. Based on the detected x-ray attenuation data, the CT scanner calculates and assigns an appropriate Hounsfield number to each voxel. By designating shades of gray for various Hounsfield number values,

the familiar CT video image display is created. The *z*-axis mathematically describes the movement of the CT scanner table and therefore defines the spatial relationships among successive axial CT images. A consecutive series of axial CT images may be considered a three-dimensional array of voxel or Hounsfield number data for which spatial locations are defined by the matrix, the CT image thickness, and the CT table position at which each successive axial

CT image is obtained. The computer precisely identifies the spatial location of each voxel by x, y, and z coordinate numbers.

Two-dimensional CT multiplanar reconstruction images are produced by selecting the appropriate voxel data from each successive axial CT image to create a "new" tomographic view. Selecting voxel data in the yz-plane produces a sagittal view; xz-plane data represent a coronal view (Fig. 25.1). These images can be no better than the quality of the axial CT image data from which they are derived. "Targeted" algorithms produce the best axial CT images of the cervical spine. The two-dimensional CT reconstruction images have the same contrast resolution as the original axial CT images; they also retain the spatial resolution of the axial CT images along the x- and y-axes. However, spatial resolution along the z-axis, which is only subtly evident on the axial CT images, is prominently displayed on the two-dimensional CT reconstruction images. The z-axis spatial resolution, which is directly related to the CT image thickness and the CT table incrementation, is usually inferior to the spatial resolution obtained along the x- and y-axes of the original axial CT image. As a general principle, the quality of a two-dimensional CT reconstruction image is dramatically improved by use of thinner axial CT images and smaller CT table increments. If the CT gantry is angled for the axial images, a software correction must be used; otherwise, the reconstruction image will be spatially distorted.

Three-dimensional CT images are commonly produced by a surface contour method. Simply described, the voxels in each CT image that define the edge of the structure to be displayed are identified. The computer does this by identifying all voxels that have Hounsfield numbers above or below a threshold value selected by the system operator. By drawing a line connecting each edge-defining voxel, the contour (outline) of the surface anatomy is obtained. Because the relationship between successive axial CT images is also known, a spatial or three-dimensional array of data describing the anatomical outline is defined. If a reference light source is assumed, shading is introduced to the data, and the visual perception of three dimensions is created (Fig. 25.1C). Unlike two-dimensional CT images, these contour three-dimensional CT images provide no density discrimination beyond locating the surface-defining voxels based on the selected threshold Hounsfield number value. Once created, these three-dimensional CT images may be rotated to allow evaluation from many perspectives (Fig. 25.1D). The images may be sectioned or edited to reveal internal surface details (Fig. 25.2E). Color coding may be used to highlight anatomic relationships. The technical factors that improve two-dimensional CT reconstruction images have a similar impact on three-dimensional CT images. The three-dimensional images add no new information, but they do display certain aspects of the axial CT data to better advantage.

Volumetric three-dimensional CT image processing classifies tissues into different ranges of CT values. It preserves the range of CT values within the classified tissue. In a sense, it maintains tissue texture rather than merely defining its surface as does contour processing. Volumetric processing requires more complicated computer computations and therefore tends to require more time to perform than contour methods. It also requires a more sophisticated operator. However, it allows a variety of additional image processing techniques to be used, including variable transparency and ray projection imaging. Images resembling conventional radiographs or CT angiograms can be produced from the CT data. If bone surface displays are used, the contour and volumetric techniques yield images of very similar appearance. All the three-dimensional CT images that illustrate this chapter were produced using volumetric processing. A detailed discussion of this topic is beyond the scope of this chapter.

Until the advent of helical CT scanners, all CT data were acquired as discrete "slices" localized in space by the patient table position where the image was made. Helical CT produces a seamless volume of CT data by combining a continuously rotating CT x-ray source with a smoothly advancing CT patient table. Typically, the CT x-ray tube rotates 360 degrees every second. The CT patient table advances continuously at a constant velocity measured in millimeters per second. *Pitch* is the term that describes the relationship between the speed of the CT table and the thickness of the acquired CT images. If the image thickness is 3 mm and the table velocity is 3.0 mm/s, the pitch is 1.0. If the image thickness is 3 mm and the table velocity is 6.0 mm/s, the pitch is 2.0. For most cervical spine applications, a pitch of 1.0 or 1.5 is used with image thicknesses of 1.0 to 3.0 mm.

MDCT involves the simultaneous acquisition of four or more images per CT gantry rotation, thus allowing rapid high-resolution scanning over large anatomic areas. Data acquisition times of less than 10 seconds for the entire cervical spine are possible with 16-channel MDCT systems. This seamless volume of CT data may be calculated as consecutive CT images or at intervals as close as 0.5 mm. This "interpolated" CT image series is equivalent to multiple overlapping images; it is obtained much faster and at a lower x-ray dose than would occur with conventional CT imaging. Patient motion is minimized by the rapid helical data acquisition. The combination of reduced patient motion and overlapping images produced by helical CT is very favorable for generating high-quality two- and three-dimensional CT reconstruction images.

There are some important differences between helical and conventional single-slice CT images. Mathematical corrections must be made to compensate for the table motion and slight obliquity of the helical data. This results in

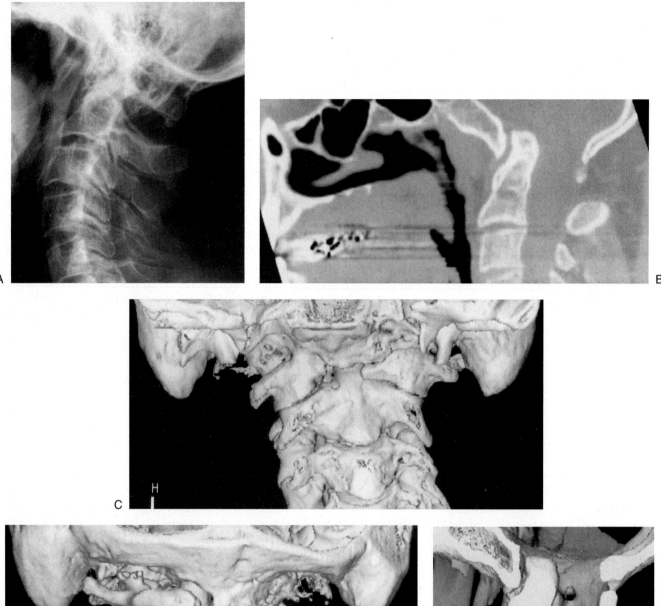

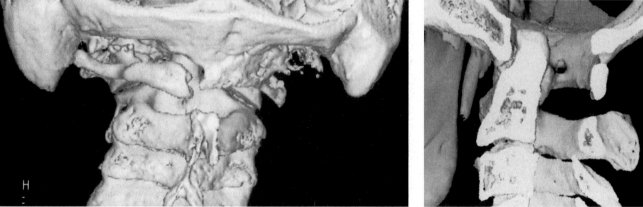

FIG. 25.2. In a 42-year-old quadriparetic man, magnetic resonance imaging (MRI) examination showed compression of the cervicomedullary junction by the odontoid process. **A:** A lateral radiograph of the cervical spine shows unusual anatomy at C0-C1. The odontoid process and the arches of C1 are indistinct. **B:** A midline sagittal two-dimensional computed tomographic (CT) reconstruction image shows that the anterior arch of C1 is assimilated to the clivus. The occipital margin of the foramen magnum appears low in position, and the posterior arch of C1 is abnormal. A well-formed odontoid process lies in the foramen magnum. **C:** An anteroposterior three-dimensional reconstruction image shows the entire anterior arch of C1 assimilated to the inferior margin of the clivus. The lateral masses of C1 and the C1-C2 facet joints are more normally developed. **D:** A posterior three-dimensional CT reconstruction image demonstrates that the right posterior arch of C1 is fused to the occiput; the left posterior arch is more normally segmented. A small midline gap is apparent in the posterior arch of C1. **E:** A split sagittal three-dimensional CT reconstruction image looking into the right side of the spinal canal clearly shows C0-C1 assimilation with a foramen for the right vertebral artery to pass through the fused occiput and C1 segments. Trying to understand and convey to other clinicians this complex bony segmentation anomaly through use of axial and two-dimensional CT images alone is much more difficult than viewing properly processed three-dimensional CT images.

an effective increase in the nominal helical image thickness of as much as 25% (i.e., a selected 2-mm image thickness may actually represent 2.5 mm of tissue). Beam-hardening image artifacts within the spinal canal caused by dense bone are slightly more prominent on helical images. Low-contrast resolution is reduced and image noise is increased because lower radiation doses are used to obtain helical images than are used in conventional single-slice techniques. For many clinical applications, however, the benefits of helical scanning outweigh these disadvantages.

Improved image processing methods and applications are the subject of very active research. Frameless stereotaxic surgery spatially registers axial, two-dimensional, and three-dimensional CT images to operating room instruments and the patient. Such systems allow real-time interaction between the surgeon and the image data in the operating room. The precise location of a surgical instrument is continuously displayed in relation to the patient images, providing a virtual reality that, it is hoped, will eliminate uncertainty. Computer-simulated surgery can be performed before the actual procedure. Stabilization implants can be sized and selected preoperatively with greater accuracy. Lifelike solid models can be manufactured. Image-guided computer-assisted spinal surgery is now becoming a reality. All of these amazing developments are dependent on high-quality CT or magnetic resonance data, powerful computers, and sophisticated software. They are best performed using a team approach, combining the skills of the technologist, radiologist, and surgeon.

COMPUTED TOMOGRAPHY WITH AND WITHOUT INTRAVENOUS CONTRAST

The primary clinical indications for unenhanced CT of the cervical spine are the evaluation of congenital segmentation anomalies (Fig. 25.2), fractures (Figs. 25.3 to 25.7), bony deformities and destructive lesions, bony fusion integrity, central and neuroforamen spinal stenosis, ossification of the posterior longitudinal ligament, and osteoid osteoma. A CT image thickness of 3 mm or less should be used. Helical CT is frequently used for these studies; excellent studies can also be obtained with conventional CT. Two-dimensional CT reconstruction images are routinely prepared in most cases. Three-dimensional CT reconstruction images are used for complicated anatomic circumstances.

The role of CT in the evaluation of patients with significant cervical spine trauma deserves additional comment. The traditional teaching has been to perform a five-view cervical spine radiographic examination: lateral, anteroposterior (AP), AP open-mouth, and oblique views. If a fracture or questionable finding was identified, a focused CT study would be undertaken. This approach is time consuming. The radiographs obtained by portable technique are frequently suboptimal. Delays in clearing the cervical spine are common. Important cervical spine fractures are occasionally missed, particularly at C0-C1 and C7-T1. Recognizing these limitations, some trauma centers have been evolving new imaging protocols that consist of an initial lateral radiograph followed by "whole cervical spine" helical CT studies. This produces a rapid complete evaluation for cervical fractures and dislocations, but isolated nondisplaced ligamentous injuries may still go undetected. This approach is not only time efficient but also relatively cost effective.

C1-C2 instability, subluxation, and fixation can be investigated by performing successive CT studies with the patient in the following positions: head neutral, head turned to the right, and head turned to the left. Three-dimensional CT images (360-degree views at 30-degree intervals) of each position are prepared, along with sagittal and coronal two-dimensional CT reconstruction images oriented to the C2 vertebral body. In children, up to 95% of the inferior articular facet of C1 can extend forward of the C2 superior articular facet and be considered normal when the head is turned. In adults, this forward movement of C1 on C2 rarely exceeds 80%. The adult atlantoaxial distance should not exceed 3 mm in any position. Rotational movement to the right and left is expected to be symmetric. Torticollis is the most common indication for doing this type of examination.

The most common indication for CT with intravenous enhancement is the evaluation of cervical radiculopathy. Epidural veins surround the cervical nerve root in the neuroforamen in a predictable pattern. Displacement, splaying, or effacement of these veins in the neuroforamen is a very sensitive indication of nerve root compression in the neuroforamen from herniated disc or other etiologies (Fig. 25.8). A herniated disc confined within the neuroforamen may be missed by unenhanced CT due to the lack of fat in the neuroforamen and the similar CT density of the native veins, nerve root, and herniated disc. For best results, these intravenous contrast-enhanced CT studies must be performed with a CT image thickness of 2 mm or less. If image noise is high at C7-T1 due to the patient's shoulders, CT images 3 mm thick made at 2-mm increments will produce a better study at this level.

The appropriate use of helical CT for this examination is less established because maximum image quality is required for successful examination. Intravenous contrast-enhanced CT is now a secondary procedure to magnetic resonance imaging (MRI) for imaging epidural tumor, infection, and spinal cord lesions (Fig. 25.9). MRI and intravenous contrast-enhanced CT are generally equal for the diagnosis of herniated disc in the spinal canal, but I consider intravenous contrast-enhanced CT somewhat better than MRI for identifying herniated disc confined to the neuroforamen (Fig. 25.10). Present disadvantages of MRI are that some pulse sequences

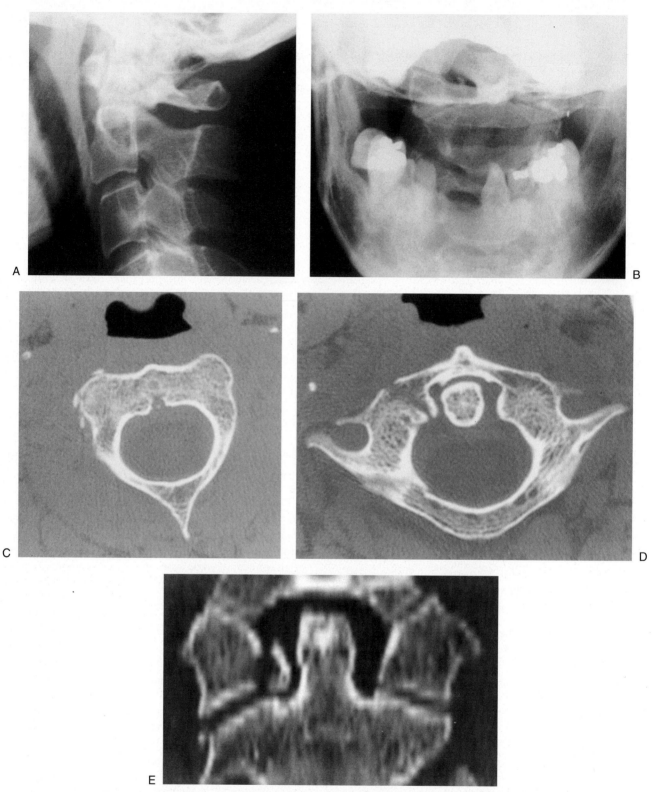

FIG. 25.3. A 45-year-old male patient reported neck pain after being involved in a motor vehicle accident. **A:** The lateral radiograph shows a subtle discontinuity of the posterior arch of C1. This finding was not apparent on two other lateral radiographs. The absence of prevertebral soft tissue swelling at C1 does not exclude an acute fracture. **B:** The anteroposterior open-mouth odontoid view shows a subtle misalignment of the right lateral mass of C1 relative to C2. A small avulsion fracture of the lateral margin of the right C2 superior articular facet is also evident. **C:** Bone algorithm technique axial computed tomographic (CT) scan at upper C2 confirms the right articular facet fracture. **D:** Bone algorithm technique axial CT at C1 shows fractures of the right anterior and posterior arches of C1. The atlantoaxial distance and the prevertebral soft tissues are normal. **E:** A two-dimensional CT coronal reconstruction image shows the right lateral mass C1 and C2 fractures with slight displacement better than the radiograph **(B)** does. The odontoid process is intact. When a cervical fracture is not demonstrated unequivocally on plain radiographs, further evaluation by CT with two-dimensional CT reconstruction images is usually appropriate.

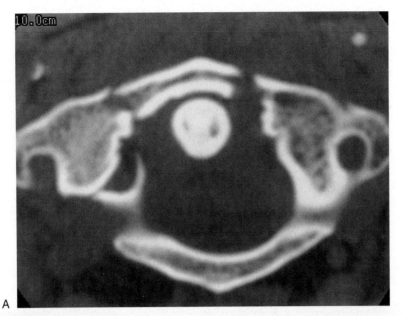

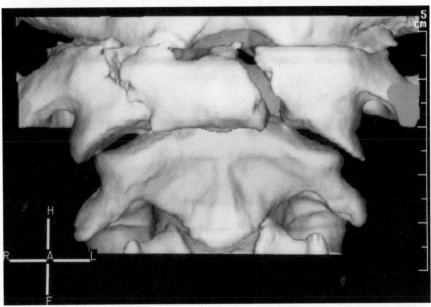

FIG. 25.4. A 24-year-old man reported neck pain after being involved in a motor vehicle accident. No neurologic deficits were evident. **A:** An axial computed tomographic (CT) scan at C1 shows fractures of the right and left anterior arches of C1. The midportion of the anterior arch of C1 remains aligned with the odontoid process. The nondisplaced posterior arch of C1 fracture was better shown on other axial CT images. **B:** Three-dimensional CT nicely demonstrates the lateral displacement of the lateral masses of C1 relative to C2. The C1 anterior arch fractures are easily identified. This Jefferson-type C1 fracture is usually the result of an axial force vector.

require image thicknesses of 3 mm or greater and that MRI produces confusing signals in the neuroforamen. Newer pulse sequences are showing promise for reducing these MRI problems.

The presence of cervical stabilization hardware presents challenges for both CT and MRI. In general, MRI is more severely degraded than CT. Titanium implants are less problematic than stainless steel devices. In the presence of large implants, postmyelogram CT may be the only successful technique for postsurgical evaluation. CT can be an excellent method for evaluating surgical fusion integrity; thin axial images with two-dimensional multiplanar

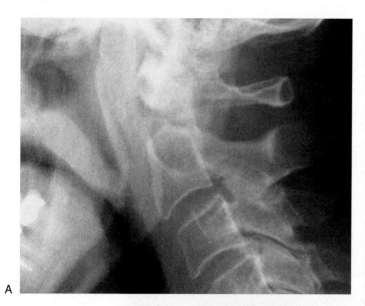

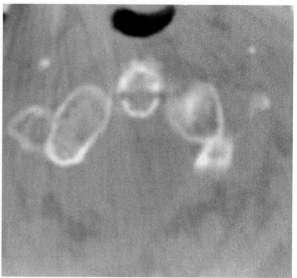

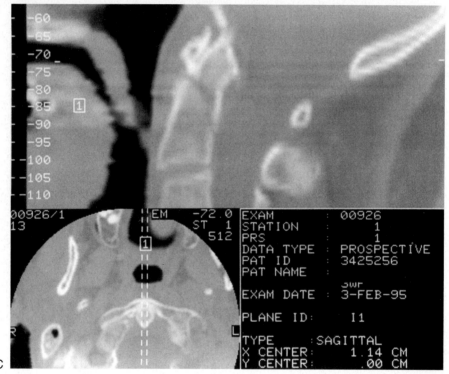

FIG. 25.5. A 73-year-old woman reported neck pain after falling at home. **A:** The lateral radiograph shows an ill-defined lucency at the base of the odontoid process. The odontoid process angles backward relative to the C2 vertebral body. The bones are osteoporotic. **B:** An axial computed tomographic (CT) scan shows a fracture at the base of the odontoid. **C:** A midline two-dimensional CT reconstruction image shows the odontoid fracture and displacement best. CT with two-dimensional CT reconstruction images should be routinely used to complete the radiographic evaluation of cervical spine fractures.

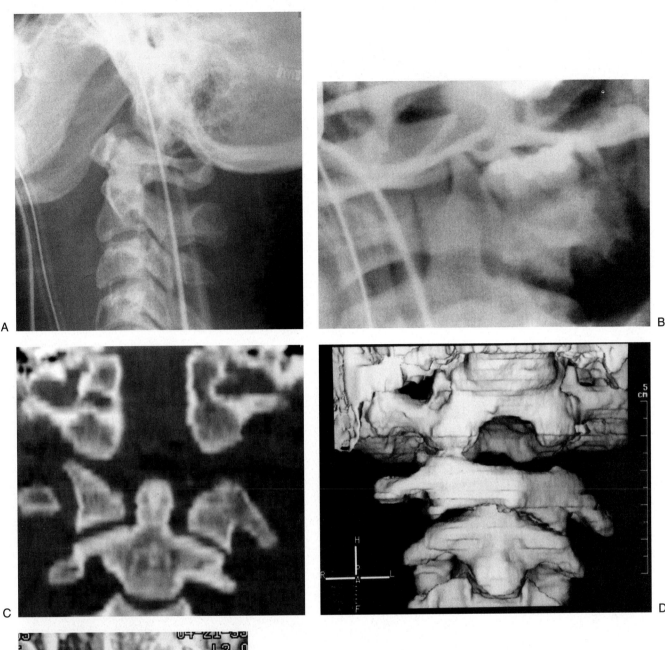

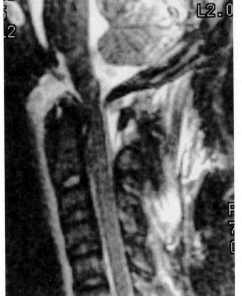

FIG. 25.6. A 19-year-old woman was struck by a motor vehicle. **A:** The lateral radiograph shows a normal atlantoaxial distance, but the occipital condyles appear distracted from C1. **B:** An anteroposterior view shows widening of the right C1-C2 joint. The C0-C1 relationship is difficult to evaluate. A two-dimensional computed tomographic (CT) coronal reconstruction image **(C)** and a three-dimensional CT reconstruction image **(D)** confirm a C0-C1 dislocation, more severe on the left than on the right. The right C1-C2 joint space is widened. **E:** A sagittal inversion recovery magnetic resonance imaging (MRI) scan shows extensive soft tissue edema in the upper cervical area. The spinal cord appears narrowed at C1. MRI is superior to CT in identifying spinal cord and paraspinal soft tissue injuries. A posterior occipitocervical fusion was performed. The woman survived, but had extensive neurologic deficits.

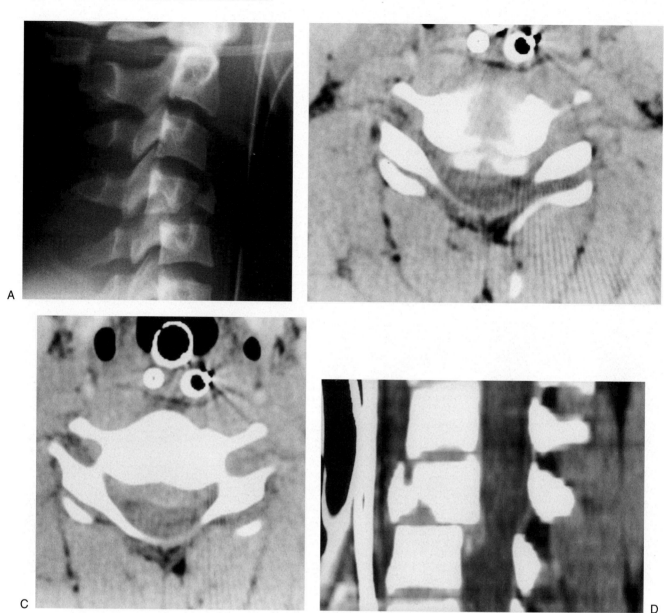

FIG. 25.7. A 20-year-old man presented with quadriparesis after being involved in a motor vehicle accident. **A:** The lateral radiograph shows a C4-C5 fracture dislocation. The C4-C5 facet joint spaces and posterior spinous process distances are widened. **B:** Axial computed tomographic (CT) images at the C4-5 disc space and 1.5 mm lower **(C)** show the C4 retrolisthesis, and indicate that the left C4-C5 facet joint is widened more than the right, but no facet fracture is apparent. This is an unstable fracture. Axial CT image **(C)** and sagittal two-dimensional CT reconstruction image **(D)** show an extruded disc fragment and probable hemorrhage behind the upper C5 vertebral body. The soft tissue injuries as well as the bony fractures must be examined. If a CT bone algorithm is used, a separate CT image series calculated with a soft tissue (standard) algorithm should also be obtained to detect associated disc herniations or epidural hematoma. In most cases, the standard-algorithm CT images suffice for complete CT evaluation.

reconstruction images are required for thorough assessment of the fusion.

MYELOGRAPHY WITH COMPUTED TOMOGRAPHY

Cervical myelography is now usually performed as an outpatient procedure. With fluoroscopy, a lumbar or lateral cervical puncture with a 22-g spinal needle is performed to access the subarachnoid space. Water-soluble contrast, typically a 300 mg/mL concentration, is injected under fluoroscopic observation. For lumbar injections, the contrast is advanced into the cervical spine by briefly tilting the head of the patient's table downward, and then resuming a neutral table position once the contrast material is in the cervical subarachnoid space. Radiographs are obtained in AP,

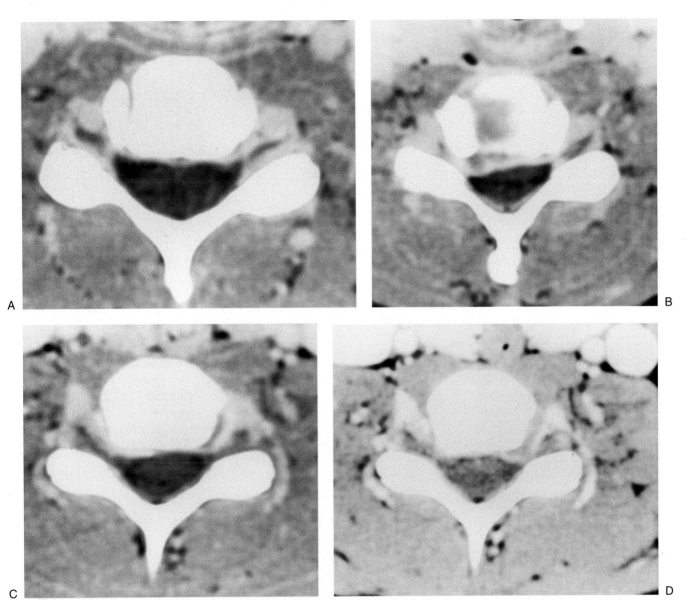

FIG. 25.8. Computed tomography with intravenous contrast enhancement (CT-IV) for evaluating cervical radiculopathy is shown, with serial CT examinations in the same patient. All of the axial CT images are 1.5 mm thick. Intravenous contrast enhancement was produced by either rapid drip or power injector methods. **A:** A CT-IV axial image at C4-C5 demonstrates normal opacified epidural veins that lie anterior and posterior to the low-density C5 nerve root in the neuroforamen. The anterior vein is closely applied to the posterior margin of the uncovertebral joint. **B:** In January 1992, the patient presented with right C6 radiculopathy. An axial CT-IV image at the C5-6 disc space shows a herniated disc in the central and right lateral aspect of the spinal canal compressing the right C6 nerve root. The left C5-C6 neuroforamen is normal. **C:** An axial CT-IV image at C6-C7 recorded on the same day as that shown in **B** demonstrates a small asymptomatic disc herniation on the left confined to the neuroforamen. Note the venous displacement as compared with that in the right neuroforamen. **D:** A posterior discectomy at C5-C6 had relieved the patient's right C6 radiculopathy. In October 1992, the patient presented with new left C7 radiculopathy. An axial CT-IV image at C6-C7 shows a larger disc herniation than that in **C,** compressing the left C7 root. The herniated disc displaces the epidural vein away from the posterior margin of the vertebral body. The patient's pain was relieved after left posterior discectomy at C6-C7. **E:** An axial CT-IV image at C5-C6 shows normal postoperative appearance. A laminectomy defect is present on the right. The C6 root is the low-density structure in the neuroforamen. The right epidural vein is now normal in caliber and lies against the posterior margin of the C5 vertebral body. **F:** In September 1994, the patient presented with recurrent left C7 radiculopathy. An axial CT-IV image at C6-C7 shows a recurrent left C6-7 disc herniation compressing the left C7 nerve root. A normal laminectomy defect is evident.

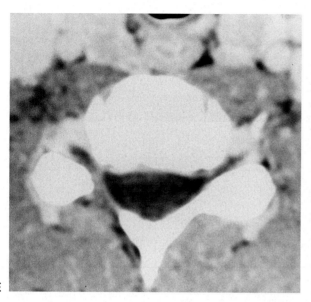

E

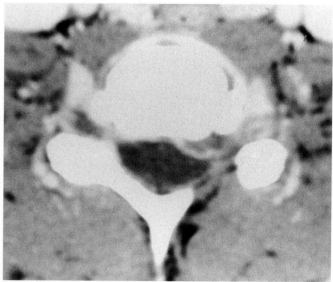

F

FIG. 25.8. *Continued*

oblique, and lateral projections with the neck in extension or neutral position. Lateral erect flexion and extension views may be obtained at the end of the procedure. Care must be taken not to allow the contrast to rapidly enter the basal cisterns of the brain. Rapid entry of contrast greatly increases the chances of side effects, which include con-

fusion and seizures. In patients with cervical spinal stenosis or myelopathy, the spine should not be maintained in a hyperextended position. Maintenance of the spine in such a position can induce a spinal cord infarct and subsequent quadriplegia. Such patients should be explicitly instructed to tell the physician if they notice changes in sensation

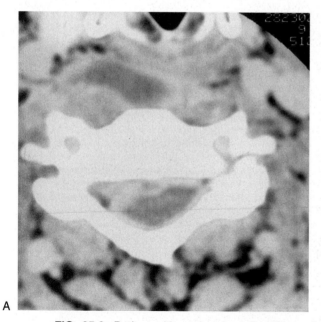

A

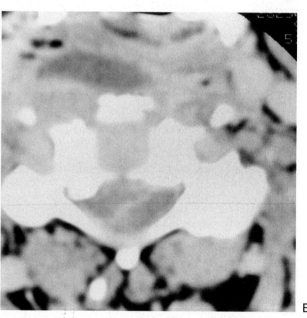

B

FIG. 25.9. Patient with neck pain and stiffness, fever, and dysphagia. Axial computed tomography scans with intravenous contrast enhancement (CT-IV) at the mid-C5 vertebral body level **(A)** and at the C4-5 disc space **(B)** show a prevertebral abscess and an intraspinal epidural abscess. The epidural abscess at C4-5 **(B)** resembles a disc herniation displacing the spinal cord backward and to the left. The diffuse epidural enhancement at mid-C5 **(A)** is consistent with infection. Magnetic resonance imaging with gadolinium enhancement is the preferred imaging method when epidural abscess is clinically suspected, but CT-IV imaging can also make this diagnosis effectively in many cases.

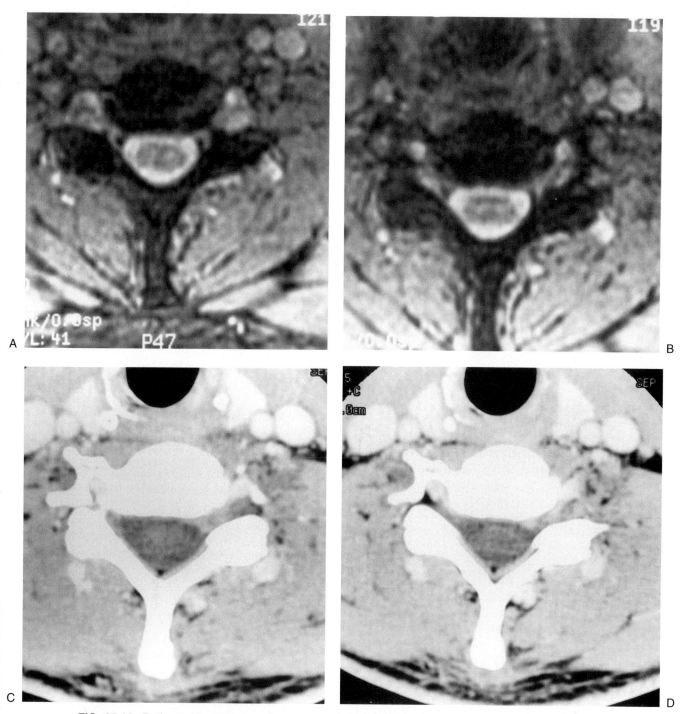

FIG. 25.10. Patient with clinically well-defined left C7 radiculopathy. **A** and **B:** Consecutive axial T2-weighted volume-acquisition gradient-echo magnetic resonance imaging (MRI) scans, 2 mm thick, made at C6-C7 do not show a definite lesion. **C** and **D:** Consecutive axial computed tomography with intravenous contrast enhancement (CT-IV) images, 1.5 mm thick, made at C6-C7 clearly demonstrate a small left disc herniation confined to the neuroforamen. The epidural vein shows segmental effacement, whereas the adjacent veins appear dilated. The right C6-C7 neuroforamen appears normal. The patient made an excellent recovery after a left C6-C7 microdiscectomy. CT-IV images are often better than MRI for the diagnosis of disc herniation confined to the neuroforamen because the images have a predictable appearance. Gradient-echo MRI scans often produce confusing signals in the neuroforamen, making confident diagnosis very difficult. Volume-acquisition, fast spin echo MRI scans may reduce this problem. MRI and CT-IV images are equally effective in identifying disc herniations in the cervical spinal canal.

or motor strength during the examination so that prompt corrective action can be taken before disaster strikes. With good technique, such tragedy is usually avoidable. Cervical myelography is an excellent survey examination; it is often the only study that incorporates a dynamic component in the evaluation of spinal cord and nerve root compression (Figs. 25.11 and 25.12).

Cervical myelography is usually very well tolerated. In patients who are kept well hydrated, remarkably few side effects occur on the day of the study. The most troublesome problem is postlumbar puncture headache. In patient surveys conducted in our department, fewer than 5% of patients report significant headache problems on the day after undergoing myelography. Most patients recover with conservative treatment. Persistent postural headaches are effectively treated with an epidural blood patch.

Cervical myelography is now rarely performed without a postmyelogram CT (CTM). CTM provides improved characterization of myelographic defects by clearly showing osteophytes, disc herniations, and the spinal cord contour (Figs. 25.11 and 25.12). CT demonstrates lesions not well appreciated by myelography alone. CT imaging is best performed within 2 hours of completion of the myelogram; this ensures that good contrast will be present and minimizes the reduced discrimination of the spinal cord due to contrast staining. Immediately before the CT examination, the intrathecal contrast must be thoroughly mixed with the spinal fluid to produce a uniform distribution. This is accomplished by having the patient roll over three times before lying down on the CT scanner table. For the diagnosis of radiculopathy, it is critical to use CT images 2 mm thick or less. Myelopathy can be adequately studied with 3-mm consecutive images. In complex anatomic cases, two- and three-dimensional reconstruction images are prepared from the axial CT data.

A primary CTM technique has also been described. It involves injecting a reduced dose of water-soluble contrast, followed by immediate CT imaging. A conventional myelogram is not performed. This reduces the study cost but sacrifices the dynamic component of the myelogram. It does not avoid the postmyelogram headache but does diminish other near-term side effects of the contrast agent. This technique is best used to define or reexamine an already recognized lesion.

Many patients have cervical root sleeves that do not extend well out into the neuroforamen. In patients with clinical cervical radiculopathy symptoms and a negative or equivocal cervical myelogram, I often use intravenous contrast enhancement during the CTM. I term this combined study the "double-contrast CT myelogram" (DCCTM). By opacifying the epidural veins as well as the subarachnoid space, DCCTM allows a more confident exclusion of a herniated disc confined completely to the neuroforamen (Figs. 25.13 and 25.14). In my experience of more than 20 years, this technique has been extremely reliable. It is not commonly practiced.

MAGNETIC RESONANCE IMAGING, COMPUTED TOMOGRAPHY, AND COMPUTED TOMOGRAPHY WITH MYELOGRAPHY

MRI, CT, and CTM should not be viewed as competitive modalities so much as complementary ones. They are imaging tools to be used to solve specific diagnostic problems. The choice of test is governed by factors such as suspected diagnosis, cost, availability, and local expertise. In most cases, more than one of these methods can provide the correct diagnosis. The relationship between MRI, CT, and CTM is extensively discussed in Chapter 26, "Magnetic Resonance Imaging of the Cervical Spine and Spinal Cord."

CTM is a great diagnostic improvement over myelography alone. The advent of CT with intravenous contrast enhancement significantly reduced the need for myelography to evaluate cervical radiculopathy. MRI, with its ability to image the spinal cord, epidural soft tissues, and bone marrow directly, further reduced the need for myelography. CTM, however, remains an excellent presurgical evaluation because of its dynamic component, reliability, accuracy, and ease of interpretation. Additional imaging tests are seldom required after CTM has been performed. CTM is still preferred by many surgeons. It remains my procedure of choice for presurgical evaluation of patients with multilevel cervical spondylosis.

It is important to bear in mind that a "good" diagnostic imaging test is correct 90% of the time, as usually defined by review of cases for a specific diagnosis such as herniated disc. In practice, when all diagnostic possibilities are considered, the correct percentage is probably somewhat lower. This also means that the results of these imaging tests may be incorrect up to 10% of the time. If a patient has a clinical history and symptoms highly suggestive of surgical disease and a negative or noncorrelating MRI or CT scan, cervical CTM is often warranted before one decides that a correlating anatomic lesion amenable to surgery does not exist.

ACKNOWLEDGMENT

This chapter is dedicated to the memory of Dr. George Alker, Jr., who authored the chapter on CT in the first two editions of this book. His professional life was committed to teaching, research, and patient care. He was an enthusiastic member of the Cervical Spine Research Society. He is remembered and missed by everyone who knew and worked with him.

The manuscript was prepared with the diligent assistance of Mrs. Jane Shaeffer of Charlotte Radiology, P.A. None of this could have been possible without the excellent work and cooperation of the staff of the Departments of Radiology and Medical Photography at the Carolinas Medical Center. The emotional support and understanding of my wife, Betsy, were essential to the completion of this task.

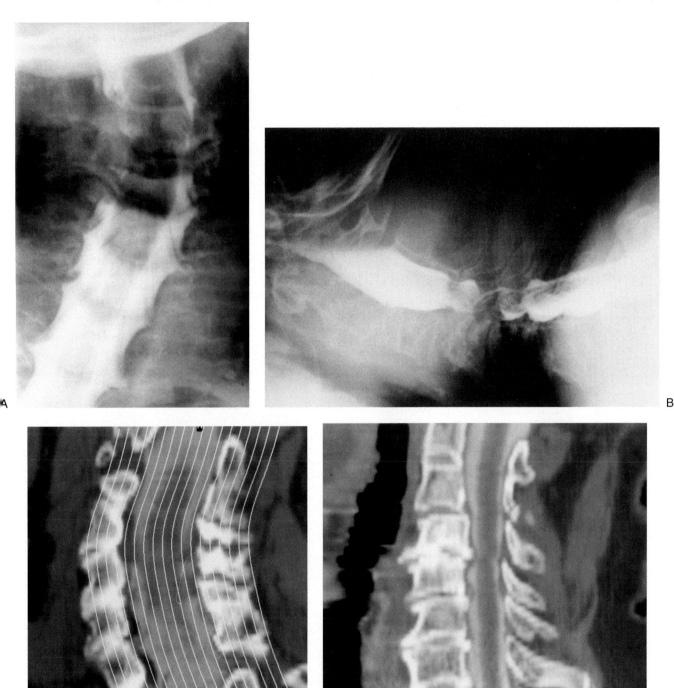

FIG. 25.11. A 69-year-old woman presented with clinical signs of myelopathy. Anteroposterior **(A)** and lateral cervical myelographic **(B)** radiographs show definite spinal cord compression at C3-C4, C4-C5, and C5-C6 due to spinal stenosis. Prominent posterior impressions on the thecal sac are due to the ligamentum flavum. **C:** A localization image uses a coronal two-dimensional computed tomographic (CT) reconstruction image to show the curved path for the sagittal two-dimensional CT reconstruction image **(D)**. The curved image plane compensates for the patient's scoliosis. **D:** A midcervical curved sagittal two-dimensional CT reconstruction image shows mild spinal cord atrophy at C4-C5 associated with degenerative disc disease and spinal stenosis. Spinal cord compression is not evident at C3-C4 and C5-C6. In comparison with appearance on the lateral cervical myelogram **(B)**, ligamentum flavum impressions are almost absent on the posterior thecal sac. The CT images are produced with the patient supine and with the neck in neutral position. The dynamic component observed on the myelogram is vital in appreciating the full extent of disease in this patient.

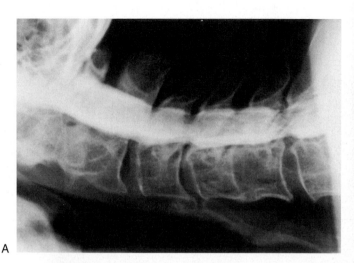

A

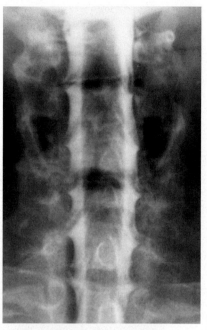

B

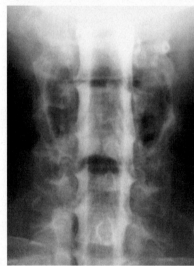

C

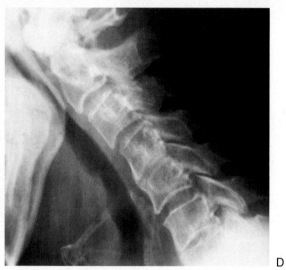

D

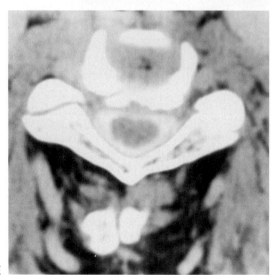

E

FIG. 25.12. A patient who previously underwent anterior interbody fusion at C4-C5 with good clinical result reported new right neck and shoulder pain; clinical attention was directed toward the right C4 nerve root. **A:** The lateral cervical myelogram shows a C4-C5 interbody fusion. A clinically asymptomatic mild central spinal stenosis is evident at C5-C6. A mild central spinal stenosis at C3-C4 associated with a slight retrolisthesis of the C3 vertebral segment on C4 is also evident. **B:** An anteroposterior (AP) cervical myelogram made with the spine *in extension* shows a definite right C3-C4 root sleeve defect; the right C4 nerve root is compressed. The right C5 through C8 nerve roots show no evidence of compression. **C:** An AP cervical myelogram made with the spine in *neutral position* shows a reduction in the right C4 nerve root compression. **D:** Comparison of this erect flexion lateral cervical spine radiograph with the lateral cervical myelogram **(A)** shows mild instability at C3-C4. No instability is evident at C5-C6. **E:** A postmyelogram axial CT scan at C3-C4 shows a small amount of degenerative gas in the disc space. The spinal stenosis evident on the lateral myelogram **(A)** is not identified here. An uncovertebral spur narrows the right C3-C4 neuroforamen but underestimates the right C4 nerve root compression evident on the AP extension myelogram **(B)**. The dynamic aspect of the cervical myelogram was critical to correct identification of the immediate clinical problem of this patient. A C3-C4 anterior interbody fusion produced a good clinical result. Although asymptomatic now, the central spinal stenosis at C5-C6 in this patient will probably require surgery in the future.

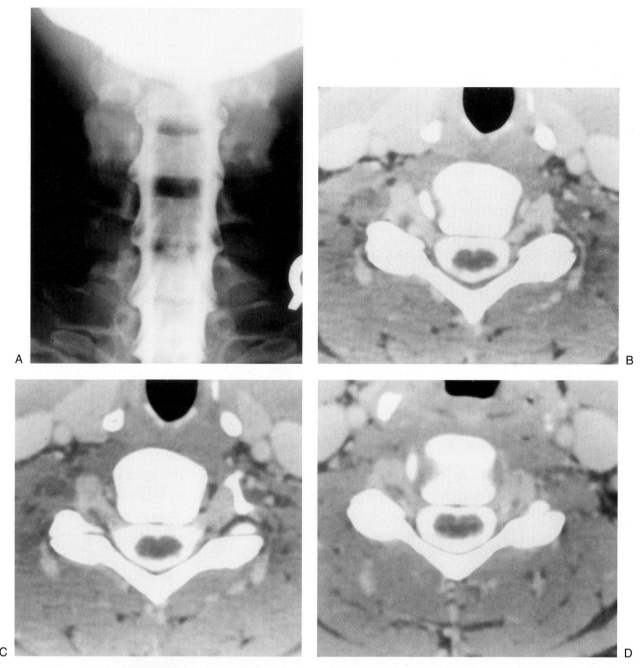

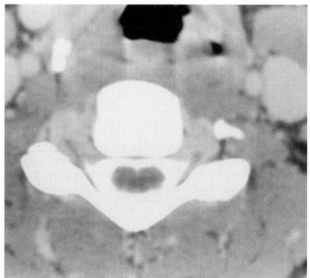

FIG. 25.13. A 35-year-old woman reported left arm pain. A clinical diagnosis of left C6 radiculopathy was made. **A:** An anteroposterior (AP) cervical myelogram shows no evidence of left or right C5 through C8 nerve root compression. Because the clinical diagnosis was C6 radiculopathy and the myelogram appeared normal, intravenous contrast enhancement (IV) was provided during the postmyelogram CT scan to ensure that a disc herniation was not overlooked. I term this combined IV/intrathecal CT technique the double-contrast CT myelogram (DCCTM). **B** and **C:** Consecutive axial DCCTM images 1.5 mm thick were obtained at C6-C7. **C** is 1.5 mm cephalad to **B**. **D** and **E:** Consecutive axial DCCTM images 1.5 mm thick were obtained at C5-C6. **E** is 1.5 mm cephalad to **D**. The enhanced epidural veins are easily distinguished from the intrathecal contrast in the root sleeves. The root sleeves in this patient do not extend very far out into the neural foramina. DCCTM combines the best aspects of both the IV and postmyelogram CT techniques, allowing a more confident diagnosis. This is a normal DCCTM study. There is no evidence of mechanical nerve root compression in the cervical spine as the cause of this woman's left arm pain.

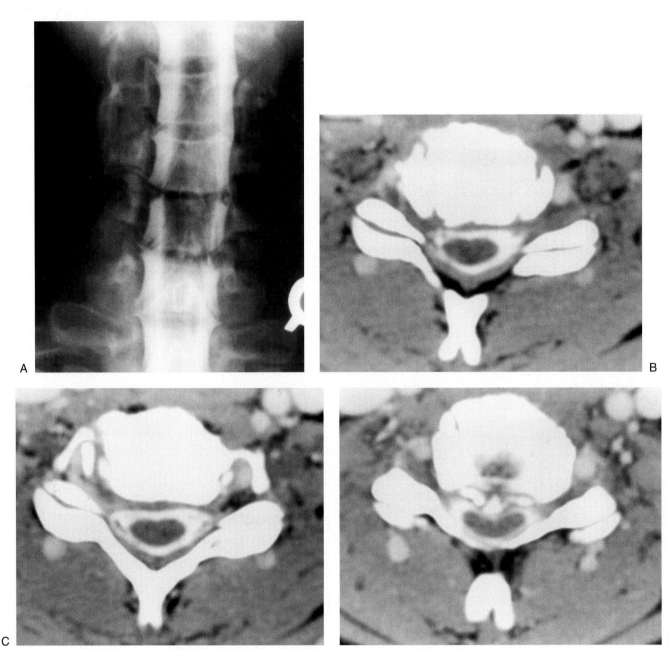

FIG. 25.14. A 50-year-old woman presented with new right arm and neck pain consistent with a right C7 distribution. **A:** An anteroposterior (AP) cervical myelogram shows splaying of the spinal cord, indicating compression at C5-C6. Prominent root sleeve defects are present on the left at C5-C6 and on the right at C6-C7. There is a minor root sleeve defect on the right at C5-C6. **B:** A double-contrast computed tomographic myelogram (DCCTM) image 1.5 mm thick at C6-C7 shows displacement of the veins in the right neuroforamen and subtle effacement of the right C7 root sleeve as compared with the left. **C:** A DCCTM image 1.5 mm thick made 3 mm above image **B** shows displacement of epidural veins in the right neuroforamen and normal anatomic findings in the left neuroforamen. Images **B** and **C** are diagnostic of a herniated disc confined to the right C6-C7 neuroforamen, compressing the right C7 nerve root. Without use of intravenous contrast enhancement and thin-section CT images, a definite diagnosis of a soft disc herniation on the right at C6-C7 would have been much more difficult on the postmyelogram CT. This finding corresponded well with the patient's clinical presentation. This disc herniation was surgically confirmed. **D:** A DCCTM image 1.5 mm thick at C5-C6 shows a chronic calcified central disc herniation deforming the spinal cord. Uncovertebral spurs are causing a moderate left and mild right neuroforamen stenosis. This CT scan correlates well with the myelogram findings at C5-C6 in **A**.

SELECTED READING

Acheson MB, Livingstone RR, Richardson ML, et al. High resolution CT scanning in the evaluation of cervical spine fractures: comparison with plain film examinations. *Am J Roentgenol* 1987;268:1179–1185.

Badami JP, Norman D, Barbaro NM, et al. Metrizamide CT-myelography in cervical myelopathy and radiculopathy: correlation with conventional myelography and surgical findings. *Am J Neuroradiol* 1985;6:59–64.

Baleriaux D, Noterman J, Ticket L. Recognition of cervical soft disk herniation by contrast-enhanced CT. *Am J Neuroradiol* 1983;4:607–608.

Barba CA, Taggert J, Morgan AS, et al. A new cervical spine clearance protocol using computed tomography. *J Trauma* 2001;51:652–656; discussion 656–657.

Bartlett RJ, Hill CR, Gardiner E. A comparison of T2 and gadolinium enhanced MRI with CT myelography in cervical radiculopathy. *Br J Radiology* 1998;71:11–19.

Berne JD, Velmahos GC, El-Tawil Q, et al. Value of complete cervical helical computed tomographic scanning in identifying cervical spine injury in the unevaluable blunt trauma patient with multiple injuries: a prospective study. *J Trauma* 1999;47:896–902; discussion 902–903.

Blackmore CC, Mann FA, Wilson AJ. Helical CT in the primary trauma evaluation of the cervical spine: an evidence-based approach. *Skeletal Radiol* 2000;29:632–639.

Blackmore CC, Ramsey SD, Mann FA, et al. Cervical spine screening with CT in trauma patients: a cost-effectiveness analysis. *Radiology* 1999;212:117–125.

Blease GC III, Wippold FJ II, Bae KT, et al. Comparison of CT myelography performed in the prone and supine positions in the detection of cervical spinal stenosis. *Clin Radiol* 2001;56:35–39.

Bonnier L, Ayadi K, Vasdev A, et al. Three-dimensional reconstruction in routine computerized tomography of the skull and spine: experience based on 161 cases. *J Neuroradiol* 1991;18:250.

Breidahl WH, Low V, Khangure MS. Imaging the cervical spine: a comparison of MR with myelography and CT myelography. *Australas Radiol* 1991;35:306.

Clayman DA, Sykes CH, Vines FS. Occipital condyle fractures: clinical presentation and radiologic detection. *Am J Neuroradiol* 1994;15:1309–1315.

Cowan IA, Inglis GS. Atlanto-axial rotatory fixation: improved demonstration using spiral CT. *Australas Radiol* 1996;40:119–124.

Crim JR, Moore K, Brodke D. Clearance of the cervical spine in multitrauma patients: the role of advanced imaging. *Semin Ultrasound CT MR* 2001;22:283–305.

Houser OW, Onofrio BM, Miller GM, et al. Cervical disc prolapse. *Mayo Clin Proc* 1995;70:939–945.

Houser OW, Onofrio BM, Miller GM, et al. Cervical neural foraminal canal stenosis: computerized tomographic myelography diagnosis. *J Neurosurg* 1993;79:84–88.

Houser OW, Onofrio BM, Miller GM, et al. Cervical spondylotic stenosis and myelopathy: evaluation with computed tomographic myelography. *Mayo Clin Proc* 1994;69:557–563.

Keats TE, Dalinka MK, Alazraki N, et al. Cervical spine trauma. American College of Radiology Appropriateness Criteria. *Radiology* 2000;215 (Suppl):243–246.

Keenan HT, Hollingshead MC, Chung CJ, et al. Using CT of the cervical spine for early evaluation of pediatric patients with head trauma. *Am J Roentgenol* 2001;177:2605–2609.

Leone A, Cerase A, Colosimo C, et al. Occipital condylar fractures: a review. *Radiology* 2000;216:635–644.

Maigne JY, Deligne L. Computed tomographic follow-up study of 21 cases of nonoperatively treated cervical intervertebral soft disc herniation. *Spine* 1994;19:189–191.

Newton TH, Potts DG. *Modern neuroradiology, volume 1: computed tomography of the spine and spinal cord.* San Anselmo: Clavadel Press, 1983.

Noble ER, Smoker WR. The forgotten condyle: the appearance, morphology, and classification of occipital condyle fractures. *Am J Neuroradiol* 1996;17:507–513.

Osborne AG. Spine and spinal cord. In: *Diagnostic Neuroradiology.* St. Louis: Mosby-Year Book, 1994:785–918.

Penning L, Wilmink JT, VanWoerden HH, et al. CT myelographic findings in degenerative disorders of the cervical spine: clinical significance. *Am J Neuroradiol* 1986;7:793–801.

Ramsey RG. Spine and spinal cord. In: *Neuroradiology.* Philadelphia: WB Saunders, 1994:786–943.

Reul J, Gievers B, Weis J, et al. Assessment of the narrow cervical spinal canal: a prospective comparison of MRI, myelography and CT-myelography. *Neuroradiology* 1995;37:187–191.

Rothman SLG, Glenn WV Jr. *Multiplanar CT of the spine.* Baltimore: University Park Press, 1985.

Russell EJ. Cervical disk disease. *Radiology* 1990;177:313–325.

Russell EJ. Computed tomography and myelography in the evaluation of cervical degenerative disease. *Neuroimaging Clin N Am* 1995;5:329–348.

Russell EJ, D'Angelo CM, Zimmerman RD, et al. Cervical disk herniation: CT demonstration after contrast enhancement. *Radiology* 1984;152:703–712.

Sener RN, Ripeckyj GT, Otto PM, et al. Recognition of abnormalities on computed scout images in CT examinations of the head and spine. *Neuroradiology* 1993;35:229.

Shafaie FF, Wippold FJ II, Gado M, et al. Comparison of computed tomography myelography and magnetic resonance imaging in the evaluation of cervical spondylotic myelopathy and radiculopathy. *Spine* 1999;24:1781–1785

Shanmuganathan K, Mirvis SE, Levine AM. Rotational injury of cervical facets: CT analysis of fracture patterns with implications for management and neurologic outcome. *Am J Roentgenol* 1994;163:1165–1169.

Silberstein M, Tress BM, Hennessy OF. Prediction of neurologic outcome in acute spinal cord injury: the role of CT and MR. *Am J Neuroradiol* 1992;13:1597.

Smoker WRK. Craniovertebral junction: normal anatomy, craniometry, and congenital anomalies. *Radiographics* 1994;26:255.

Ullrich CG, Binet EF, Sanecki MG, et al. Quantitative assessment of the lumbar spinal canal by computed tomography. *Radiology* 1980;134:137–143.

Veres R, Bago A, Fedorcsak I. Early experiences with image-guided transoral surgery for the pathologies of the upper cervical spine. *Spine* 2001;26:1385–1388.

Vezina JL, Fontaine S, Laperriere J. Outpatient myelography with fine needle technique: an appraisal. *Am J Roentgenol* 1989;153:383–385.

Weidner A, Wabler M, Chiu ST, et al. Modification of C1-C2 transarticular screw fixation by image-guided surgery. *Spine* 2000;25:2668–2673; discussion 2674.

Welch WC, Subach BR, Pollack IF, et al. Frameless stereotactic guidance for surgery of the upper cervical spine. *Neurosurgery* 1997;40:958–963; discussion 963–964.

Yousem DM, Atlas SW, Hackney DB. Cervical spine disk herniation: comparison of CT and 3DFT gradient echo MR scans. *J Comput Assist Tomogr* 1992;16:345.

Zinriech SJ, Rosenbaum AE, Wang H, et al. The critical role of 3-D CT reconstruction for defining spinal disease. *Acta Radiol* 1986;369:699–702.

CHAPTER 26

Magnetic Resonance Imaging of the Cervical Spine and Spinal Cord

Christopher G. Ullrich

Magnetic resonance imaging (MRI) is based on the physical phenomenon of nuclear magnetic resonance (NMR). Physicists Edward M. Purcell of Harvard University and Felix Bloch of Stanford University independently described NMR in 1946 and received the 1952 Nobel Prize for this achievement. Since then, NMR spectroscopy has become a powerful analytic technique for studying the chemistry and physical structure of molecules. Attempts to apply NMR techniques to medical imaging began around 1970. Working at the State University of New York (SUNY) Downstate Medical Center, Raymond Damadian's research team produced the first whole-body human image on July 3, 1977. Images of much smaller objects had previously been obtained by Damadian and by other research groups, including Paul Lauterbur at SUNY Stonybrook and Peter Mansfield, Waldo Hinshaw, and E. Raymond Andrews at the University of Nottingham. Although crude, Damadian's image demonstrated that a powerful medical imaging device was possible. Intense commercial development followed, with the first Food and Drug Administration (FDA) market approvals for MRI devices granted in 1984. Magnetic resonance imaging technology continues to rapidly evolve.

This chapter briefly reviews the technical concepts related to MRI. The characteristic appearance of these images is described, and specific clinical applications in the cervical spine and spinal cord are illustrated. The relationship between MRI and computed tomography (CT) of the cervical spine is a focus of this chapter. Finally, speculation is made concerning future development and medical applications of MRI.

PHYSICS OF NUCLEAR MAGNETIC RESONANCE

Although a detailed physics explanation of NMR is well beyond the scope of this chapter, a basic understanding of the underlying physical phenomenon involved in NMR is essential to understanding MRI. Simply stated, atoms whose nuclei contain an odd number of protons and neutrons resemble a continually spinning top and behave as a small bar magnet. In nature, these atoms are randomly aligned and no magnetic forces are apparent. When an external magnetic field is applied, its force tends to align the magnetic poles of the spinning nuclei. Most of the nuclei will be in a low-energy state, in alignment with the external magnetic field. High-energy nuclei align themselves against the external magnetic field.

The spinning nuclei precess around the vector of the external magnetic field, resembling wobbling tops. Each nucleus precesses (wobbles) at its own specific frequency, called the *Larmor* or *resonant frequency*, and is determined by the strength of the "bar magnet" of the nucleus and the externally applied magnetic field. If a radio wave at the exact resonant frequency is beamed at right angles to the magnetic field, some low-energy nuclei will absorb energy, undergo a "spin flip," and convert to the high-energy state. This absorbed energy is emitted at the same radio frequency when the nucleus returns to the low-energy state. This characteristic absorption and release of specific radio frequencies is descriptively termed *nuclear magnetic resonance*.

The character of the high-energy nucleus can also be described by the time it takes to return to the low-energy state. The spin-lattice relaxation time T1 is determined by the interaction between the nucleus and its environment (*lattice*). The spin–spin relaxation time T2 describes the interaction between adjacent nuclei. Therefore, the same high-energy nucleus will emit its characteristic radio signal at different times depending on what surrounds it. These properties (resonant frequency, T1, and T2) form the basis of NMR spectroscopy and make it a powerful technique for analyzing molecules and their environment.

MAGNETIC RESONANCE IMAGING

The terms NMRI and MRI are equivalent, but the latter term is preferred in the diagnostic radiology literature because of the prevalent public phobia about anything identified as "nuclear" and also to distinguish this method from nuclear medicine techniques involving radioactive isotopes.

Magnetic field strength is measured in tesla (T) units. MRI devices are broadly categorized as low field (less than 0.3 T), midfield (0.3–0.9 T), and high field (1.0 T or greater). The MRI devices that are 3.0 T are the highest field strength currently approved by the FDA. A superconducting magnet is used most commonly in midfield and high-field systems. These devices produce an extremely uniform magnetic field, a highly desirable feature. They are costly to build and operate. These high-field MRI systems can support the high power gradients and radio frequency switching speeds necessary to implement rapid imaging sequences, including echo planar MRI and MR spectroscopy. They can reliably perform the thin-section imaging needed for excellent MRI of the cervical spine. The MRIs used to illustrate this chapter were produced with 1.5-T MRI systems.

MRI systems are developing along several pathways. Open-design MRI systems using superconducting magnets with field strengths of 0.7 T to 1.0 T have become available. These units can produce adequate thin-section images that are essential for good-quality cervical spine studies. The maximum field of view is usually limited to no more than 40 cm, which can make total spine examinations tedious. New 1.5-T MRI systems using short-bore magnet designs seem less confining to patients than the older magnets. Improved coil and gradient design along with sophisticated pulse sequences are further improving image quality and reducing examination times. Recently approved 3.0-T MRI systems promise to deliver still higher resolution images and even more rapid image acquisitions. Pulsation, magnetic susceptibility, and chemical shift artifacts are significant technical challenges to good cervical spine imaging at 3.0 T. Rapid technical changes are likely to continue for the next few years.

Resistive magnets, used in low-field systems, produce a less stable magnetic field. Permanent magnets, used in low-field or midfield systems, produce a stable magnetic field. Magnetic field uniformity comparable to that of superconducting magnets is difficult to achieve with either permanent or resistive magnet designs. These magnets are used primarily in low-cost imagers because the magnets are less expensive to manufacture, site, and maintain. They are also adaptable to wide-aperture or open-imager designs. The primary limitations of these low-field systems for cervical spine imaging are their common inability to perform thin (2-mm) images and their long data-acquisition times. Regardless of the magnet or magnetic field strength used, diagnostic cervical spine images can be obtained if proper imaging techniques are used.

The NMR instrument obtains its signal from the entire sample volume. To mathematically reconstruct an image, the MRI signal must be localized within the object being imaged. This localization is usually obtained using a gradient technique. A *gradient* is a small secondary magnetic field that has a known variable strength. Magnetic field strength influences the exact resonant frequency. With a gradient applied, the slightly different radio frequencies detected determine where the signal arises. This information, in combination with the shape and orientation of the radio frequency pulse, determines the precise location of the signal and permits mathematical image reconstruction. Most machines use two-dimensional (2D) Fourier transformation mathematics to calculate the MRI from the detected signal in a manner similar to radiographic CT.

Two time variables describe how the machine functions and determine the nature of the image obtained. The repetition time interval between radio frequency input pulses is termed *TR*. After the input pulse, the time at which the echo (emitted resonant radio frequency signal) is detected is termed *TE*. These time values are expressed in milliseconds.

At present, virtually all clinical MRI is performed using the hydrogen nuclei signal (proton imaging). Hydrogen, as a constituent of water, is the most abundant resonant nucleus in soft tissues and therefore provides the strongest signal. Other nuclei, such as sodium and phosphorus, may be imaged using high-field-strength systems, but the image quality is low owing to the weak signals obtained. Well-described practical clinical applications for these additional nuclei remain to be developed.

The methods for acquiring MRI data are termed *pulse sequences*. Spin-echo (SE), inversion recovery (IR), gradient-echo (GRE), and fast or turbo spin echo (FSE) are some of the techniques used. Spin-echo pulse sequences are described by TR and TE values. By varying these factors, different tissue-contrast relationships are obtained (Fig. 26.1). If a short TR/TE technique (e.g., SE = 500/30) is used, the image is termed *T1 weighted* because most of the detected echo signals reflect the T1-governed nuclear interactions (*spin lattice*). The resulting image shows a low signal from cortical bone owing to a paucity of water molecules. The cerebrospinal fluid (CSF) is hypointense, relative to muscle and spinal cord, because of its short T1 value. Fat has an increased signal relative to the spinal cord, whereas most lesions are either low or isointense compared with the spinal cord (Fig. 26.2). These T1-weighted images tend to have the best spatial resolution because the strongest signal is obtained with such pulse sequences.

Long TR/TE techniques (e.g., SE = 2,500/120) are termed *T2-weighted* images because most of the detected signal is determined by the T2 (*spin–spin*) interactions of the nuclei.

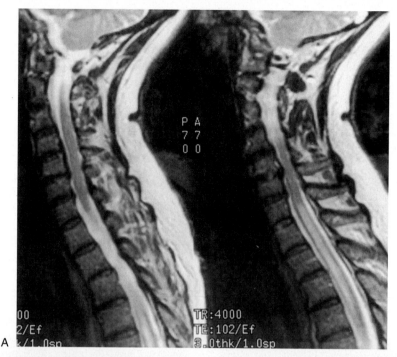

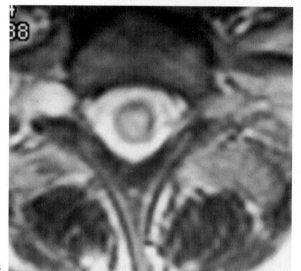

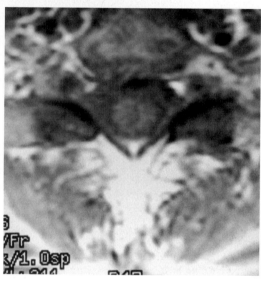

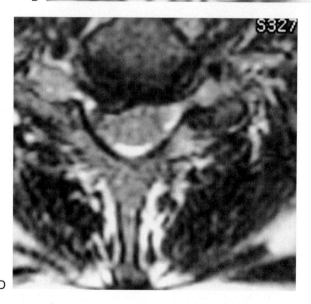

FIG. 26.1. This 56-year-old woman suddenly developed weakness in both legs 1 week after the onset of a flulike illness. **A:** A pair of sagittal T2-weighted fast spin echo (FSE) images depict an enlarged spinal cord with extensive increased T2 signal extending from the C7-T1 to the T6 vertebral level. **B:** An axial T2-weighted FSE magnetic resonance image (MRI) made at the first thoracic vertebral level confirms a diffuse central increased T2 signal within an enlarged spinal cord. Some sparing of the peripheral white matter is noted. **C:** An axial T1-weighted spin-echo (SE) MRI made at the first thoracic vertebral level shows no evidence of a syrinx or abnormal gadolinium enhancement. MRI is superior to other imaging techniques for showing intrinsic spinal cord lesions. A presumptive diagnosis of viral myelitis was made. The patient gradually improved with medical therapy. **D:** An axial T1-weighted SE MRI made at the C6-C7 level shows an asymptomatic right C6-7 herniated disc. The lesion is also seen on the sagittal T2-weighted MRI **(A).**

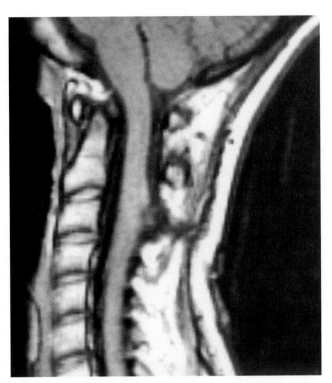

FIG. 26.2. This 16-year-old girl had vague neck pain complaints and a cutaneous dimple on the posterior neck. The sagittal T1-weighted spin-echo image shows a tract from the posterior neck into the spinal canal at C3. The spinal cord is expanded, and epithelial tissue is visible along the posterior aspect of the spinal cord. Magnetic resonance imaging is the procedure of choice for the initial evaluation, but it does not demonstrate the associated posterior bony dysraphism well. The radiographic diagnosis of dorsal dermal sinus with epidermoid tumor in the spinal cord was confirmed at surgery.

The emitted signal resulting from T1-governed events has already dissipated. The term *T2*-weighted* is used for GRE images because GRE T2 values differ somewhat from SE T2 values. The CSF now demonstrates greater intensity than the spinal cord, producing the so-called *pseudomyelogram effect*. The bone signal remains quite low compared with the spinal cord, whereas fat continues to show an increased signal. Pathologic processes tend to show an increased signal compared with the spinal cord because in most cases they are associated with increased tissue water (Fig. 26.1). Small lesions lying in the spinal fluid or adjacent to it can be obscured when both the spinal fluid and the lesion demonstrate an increased signal.

Images produced using long-TR and short-TE technique (e.g., SE = 2,500/30) are termed *balanced* because relatively equal contributions of T1- and T2-governed echoes are involved. In the cervical spine, this technique may allow pathologic processes to have a high signal while the spinal fluid remains isointense or hypointense relative to the spinal cord. Lesions that may be masked on a more heavily T2-weighted image might now be apparent.

Gadolinium compounds can be used for intravenous enhancement in MRI in a manner similar to the use of iodine contrast agents for CT. Gadolinium shortens T1 relaxation time, producing a brighter T1 signal. It has little impact on T2-weighted images and does not cross the intact blood–cord barrier. It will accumulate in areas of infection, inflammation, and tumors (Fig. 26.3), making these sites more conspicuous on T1-weighted images. Unlike iodine intravenous contrast for CT, it is relatively ineffective as an agent for arterial opacification because of both the small volume of injection and its rapid clearance from the bloodstream. Veins often show some "brightening." Injected gadolinium contrast is generally well tolerated; allergic reactions are rare. Because of issues of cost and time, gadolinium is used selectively when an appropriate clinical diagnosis is considered.

Normal fat produces a relatively bright signal on both T1- and T2-weighted images, which can obscure gadolinium enhancement on T1-weighted images and abnormal T2 signal on T2-weighted images. This bright fat signal can be reduced or eliminated by adding a fat-suppression pulse to the standard SE pulse sequence; IR pulse sequences also produce fat suppression. Inversion recovery images resemble fat-suppressed T2-weighted SE images and are quite useful in patients with trauma (Fig. 26.4), infection, or bony metastases. Most centers use these fat-suppressed images electively in the appropriate clinical setting.

Data acquisition in MRI is usually performed with a 2D technique in which multiple adjacent images are obtained simultaneously. A small gap is often present between these successive images. Direct axial, coronal, and sagittal image planes are produced without moving the patient, but separate data acquisitions must be performed for each image plane. It is often possible to obtain two or more TE values simultaneously (so-called *dual* or *multiecho* techniques), particularly when a long TR is employed in the pulse sequence.

Volume imaging techniques are also feasible. Unlike 2D image methods, in which each image is separately encoded, volume techniques encode the entire imaging area as one seamless data set. Once obtained, any desired image plane can be extracted from the volume data set, thus eliminating separate data acquisitions. Volume data sets are ideal for three-dimensional (3D) image processing. Two types of volume data acquisitions are possible. *Isotropic acquisitions* take longest to perform but produce equal resolution in all three orthogonal imaging planes (axial, coronal, and sagittal). *Anisotropic acquisitions* are quicker and therefore more commonly used. The primary imaging plane will have the best spatial resolution; the two other orthogonal planes will have somewhat reduced spatial resolution. Volume acquisitions using conventional SE pulse sequences take 20 minutes or longer and are not practical. GRE anisotropic volume acquisitions, which take less than 6 minutes, are commonly used to obtain thin-section axial MR images of the cervical spine. Two-millimeter-thick T2-weighted axial images with no spatial gaps can be obtained from the C2 to

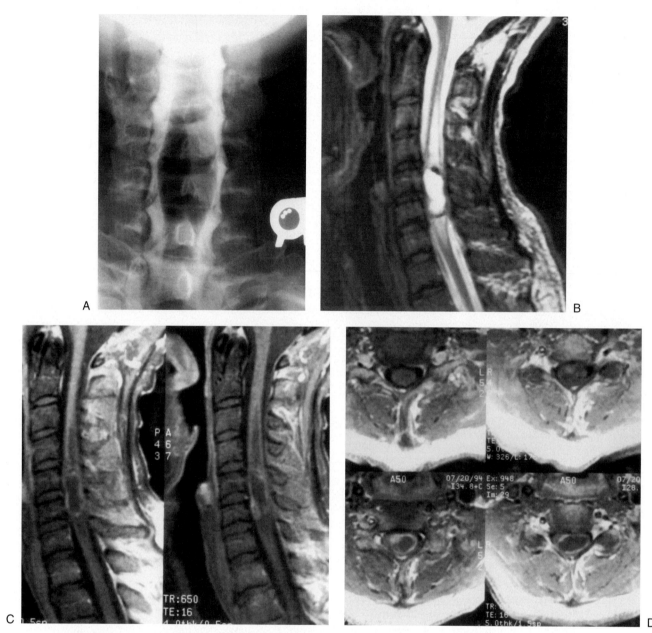

FIG. 26.3. This 33-year-old man presented with a clinical history and findings of slowly progressive cervical myelopathy. **A:** An anteroposterior myelogram shows an expansile intraaxial lesion at the C5-C6 levels. Myelography is unable to classify this abnormality further. **B:** A midsagittal T2-weighted fast spin echo (FSE) image confirms a well-defined intraaxial lesion at C5-C6. It has very high T2 signal, with focal areas of low signal along the margin. Increased T2 signal extends above and below the lesion, consistent with spinal cord edema. **C:** Two adjacent post-gadolinium-enhanced sagittal T1-weighted spin-echo (SE) magnetic resonance images. **D:** Four consecutive post-gadolinium-enhanced axial T1-weighted SE magnetic resonance images at C5-C6 show a low-T1-signal central cyst with faint enhancement along most of the cyst wall. A focal enhancing nodule in the cyst wall is noted inferiorly and to the right. The radiographic diagnosis of hemangioblastoma was surgically confirmed. For examining the spinal cord, magnetic resonance imaging is superior to all other imaging techniques.

T1 vertebral levels in one acquisition. Presently, 2D slice techniques are limited to a thickness of 3 mm and require at least 0.5-mm gaps between images to maintain image quality. Interleaved 2D image acquisition techniques can eliminate the spatial gaps between images but double the image acquisition time.

A variety of different imaging coils are used for MRI. These coils are antennas that detect the emitted resonance signal. Optimized coil design has a real impact on the quality of the image obtained. The head coil is designed for imaging the brain. It usually can produce high-quality images of the foramen magnum and cervical spine down to the

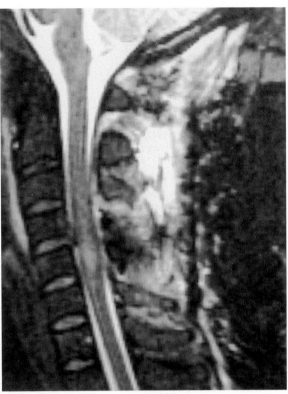

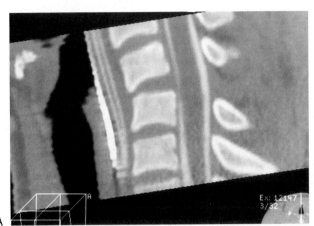

FIG. 26.4. This 35-year-old woman suffered a C4-C5 fracture with quadriplegia in a motor vehicle accident. **A:** A midsagittal two-dimensional computed tomographic (CT) reconstruction image made from a primary CT myelogram performed the day of the accident. The spinal cord is enlarged at C5, consistent with a contusion. There is no internal detail of the spinal cord by CT. The spinal cord is not mechanically compressed. The posterior aspect of the C4-5 disc space is distracted, but no effacement of the intrathecal contrast behind the C4-5 disc space is seen. A kyphotic deformity centered at C4-C5 is noted. The posterior interspinous process distance at C4-5 is widened, indicating ligamentous disruption. **B:** A midsagittal inversion recovery magnetic resonance image (MRI) made 5 days after the CT examination. The kyphotic deformity seen in **A** has been reduced. A small disc herniation now projects into the spinal canal that was not seen in **A**. The migration of the C4-5 disc fragment presumably occurred in association with the fracture-dislocation reduction. Neither the C4-5 disc herniation nor a small hematoma behind the C4 vertebral body is significantly compressing the spinal cord. The spinal cord contusion, along with extensive posterior paraspinal soft tissue injuries, is now directly visualized by MRI. Migrating disc fragments associated with fracture reduction on rare occasions have produced spinal cord compression and significant new neurologic deficits. These disc fragments and epidural blood can be seen with high-resolution CT, but they often have similar CT densities. On MRI, as in this case, the blood and disc fragments often have slightly different signal characteristics.

C2-C3 level. Most MRI systems have a surface coil that is designed for spinal imaging. These coils allow the entire cervical spine to be examined at high resolution in a single field of view. Phased-array coils are multiple-surface coils that can be operated together to obtain better image quality over a larger field of view (Fig. 26.5). The MRI body coils are designed for thoracic and abdominal imaging and usually provide poor images of the spine and spinal cord; generally speaking, they should not be used for cervical spine examinations.

Many other technical factors contribute to better quality in cervical spine MRI examinations. Properly placed saturation pulses can reduce imaging artifacts related to physiologic motion. Cardiac gating is sometimes helpful. The direction of phase and frequency encoding gradients can be important in reducing image artifacts. Physiological motion and magnetic susceptibility artifacts remain significant challenges for MRI of the cervical spine and spinal cord. A detailed examination of these factors is beyond the scope of this chapter. Also beyond the scope of this chapter are physics discussions of many other advanced MRI techniques, such as MR angiography without or with gadolinium enhancement, echoplanar MRI, cerebrospinal fluid flow measurements using magnitude or phase contrast encoding, perfusion and diffusion MRI, time-resolved imaging, cortical activation functional MRI, and MR spectroscopy. So too are image processing techniques such as ray and maximum-intensity projection imaging, image segmentation, multimodality image fusion, volumetric 3D visualization and model manufacturing, and image-guided surgery and simulation.

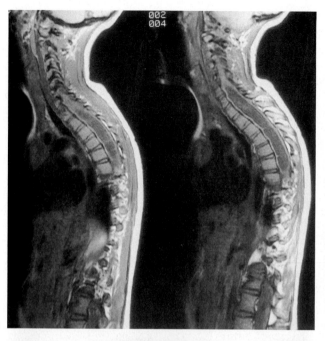

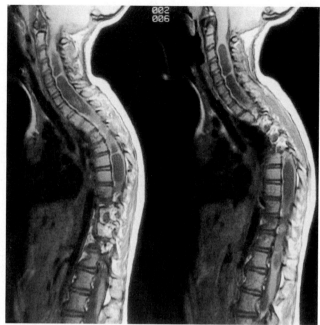

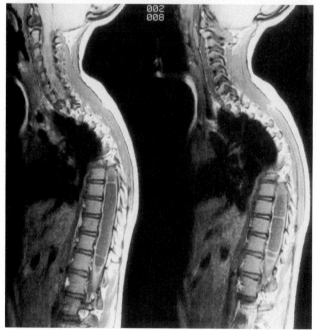

FIG. 26.5. An 8-year-old girl with a levoscoliosis of the dorsal spine. **A–C:** Six consecutive sagittal T1-weighted spin-echo images made from left to right demonstrate a multiseptated syrinx extending from C2-C3 to the conus. A Chiari II malformation with a large quantity of cerebellar tissue at C1 is present, best seen in **B**. Simultaneous examination of the cervical and thoracic spine was accomplished with phased-array magnetic resonance imaging coils. Magnetic resonance imaging is the procedure of choice for screening examinations of the spine and spinal cord.

In summary, MRI is performed by placing the patient in an external uniform and stable magnetic field. A radio frequency pulse is beamed into the patient to induce the NMR phenomenon. A receiver coil detects the emitted radio frequency as the nuclei revert to a low-energy state within the magnetic field. Gradients produce slight local variations in the strength of the magnetic field and permit spatial localization of the emitted resonant frequency. This detected signal is mathematically processed using 2D Fourier transformation into the MR image. By varying TR and TE factors, spin-echo images that are T1 or T2 weighted are produced. The T1 images have the best spatial resolution; T2 images tend to accentuate pathology.

ADVANTAGES AND LIMITATIONS OF MAGNETIC RESONANCE IMAGING

MRI involves the use of nonionizing radiation and is considered biologically safe by current testing standards. No known deleterious effects are produced in a normal subject. Because of its excellent spatial and contrast resolution, MRI exhibits high lesion sensitivity. By skillful use of the many available pulse sequences, normal and diseased tissues can be identified and characterized accurately; intravenous gadolinium contrast agents also assist in this process. Gadolinium is well tolerated by patients; anaphylactic reactions are rare. With the patient supine, MRI allows direct sagittal, coronal, axial, and oblique images to be obtained. Volume-acquisition imaging techniques are feasible as well. With high-field MRI systems, patient examination times of 30 minutes or less are common. These capabilities have made MRI a major modality for the evaluation of the cervical spine.

Not all patients can be examined successfully by MRI. Patients with cardiac pacemakers or implanted defibrillators should not be examined because the magnetic field will disrupt operation of these devices. A variety of medical implants are potentially incompatible with safe MRI examinations, including some heart valves, lens implants, cochlear implants, infusion pumps, and older cerebral aneurysm clips. Patients with medical implants (e.g., orthopedic rods and plates, joint prostheses, and permanent dental work) can be safely examined. Usually there is a loss of image detail around the site of these materials as a result of distortion of the local magnetic field. The remainder of the image often looks unaffected, but subtle image distortion and artifacts may be present, which can affect the perceived diagnosis. If the area of interest is adjacent to metal, MRI is probably not going to be clinically satisfactory. Patients should be questioned carefully about metal and medical devices in the body before MRI examinations are done. MRI centers maintain lists of devices that can pose problems. If necessary, the medical-device manufacturer can be contacted for advice before MRI. Occasionally, a patient must be disqualified for MRI because of traumatically acquired metal in the body.

The aperture diameter of most superconducting magnets is 60 cm; the bore of the magnet appears as a long, narrow tube to the patient. About 5% of patients are claustrophobic when placed in such magnets; most such patients can tolerate the examination by using oral medications. Intravenous or general anesthesia is rarely needed in adults. Some obese patients cannot physically fit into these systems.

The low-field-strength, open-aperture MRI systems more easily accommodate claustrophobic, obese, and critically ill patients. Problems related to medical devices and metal are also less significant than when a high-field-strength MRI system is used; however, examination times tend to be much longer, and image quality is often marginal for good cervical spine studies. In many, but not all, such cases, a high-resolution CT scan or CT myelogram would be a better choice for the patient.

CLINICAL APPLICATIONS OF MAGNETIC RESONANCE IMAGING IN THE CERVICAL SPINE

Many other chapters in this book review specific clinical cervical spine problems in great detail, and numerous well-documented MRIs are presented. This section is devoted to

discussing the principles of MRI evaluation and the appropriate relationships between MRI and CT. Rather than consider MRI, CT, and CT myelography as modalities in conflict, they should be viewed as complementary diagnostic imaging tools to be used to solve specific clinical problems. With a thorough understanding of each technique and knowledge of its local availability, appropriate clinical choices can be reliably made.

In its ability to examine the spinal cord, MRI is unsurpassed. No other imaging technique permits direct evaluation of intrinsic abnormalities of the spinal cord (Fig. 26.1). The basic MRI examination consists of sagittal T1-weighted and sagittal and axial T2-weighted SE images. The T2-weighted GRE images are somewhat less sensitive to increased T2 signal in the spinal cord, but they do produce a good pseudomyelogram effect. If tumor (Fig. 26.3), sarcoid, infection, or inflammatory disease is suspected, intravenous gadolinium enhancement with sagittal and axial T1-weighted SE imaging is performed. Tumors often expand the spinal cord and show a focal enhancement within an area of diffuse increased T2 signal (Fig. 26.3). Infection, inflammatory lesions, and acute infarction tend to show a more diffuse nonfocal enhancement within an area of increased T2 signal. The size of the spinal cord may be normal in this situation. A specific diagnosis depends on the clinical history and CSF laboratory studies.

Acute multiple sclerosis plaques may sometimes resemble spinal cord tumor or infectious lesions. An MRI examination of the brain showing characteristic periventricular white matter or corpus callosum lesions confirms the diagnosis of multiple sclerosis. A negative MR brain study does not exclude this diagnosis.

Hemorrhage into the spinal cord may be associated with trauma, tumor, or a vascular malformation. Acute bleeding has a variable MRI appearance, which sometimes can be extremely confusing. The spinal cord is usually expanded (Fig. 26.4). Gadolinium administration is almost always unrewarding in the presence of acute blood. If hemosiderin deposition is detected, prior hemorrhage has occurred. Vascular malformations may produce increased T2 signal in the spinal cord without having bled. MR angiography can sometimes identify the abnormal vessels of these malformations, but conventional angiography remains the standard for definitive diagnosis of these lesions.

Cervical spondylosis is the most frequent clinical cause for compressive cervical myelopathy. Radicular symptoms are often concurrently present. The basic MRI examination is similar to that for intrinsic spinal cord disease. If radiculopathy is a consideration, a volume-acquisition T2-weighted GRE axial image series is added to provide thin-section images of the neuroforamina. Volume-acquisition T2-weighted FSE imaging may also be used for this purpose. Some centers add oblique sagittal T1-weighted images to improve assessment of the neuroforamina. Satisfactory MRI evaluation of the cervical spine requires sagittal images 3 to 4 mm thick. Axial and oblique sagittal images to evaluate the neuroforamina need to be 2 mm thick or less. Axial images to assess spinal cord compression can be 3 to 5 mm thick. Most high-field and midfield MRI systems can produce this level of performance, but many low-field-strength MRI systems use thicker image planes to improve the signal-to-noise ratio of their images. Although this produces better-looking images, it can easily lead to partial volume-averaging problems in the cervical spine studies that are performed. The result will be missed small but symptomatic disc herniations, inadequate assessment of the neuroforamina, and other similar problems.

Estimating the degree of spinal stenosis is best done from the axial, not the sagittal, images. The GRE images have a definite tendency to exaggerate the severity of stenosis due to "blooming" of the apparent edge of the bone related to magnetic susceptibility effects (Fig. 26.6). The worse the degenerative stenosis, the more pronounced this error becomes. Although T2-weighted SE images are less affected, the problem of overestimation of stenosis can still occur. If the spinal cord itself exhibits increased T2 signal, assessment of spinal cord size and compression is often better made from axial T1-weighted images.

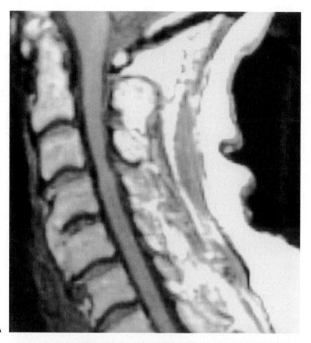

A

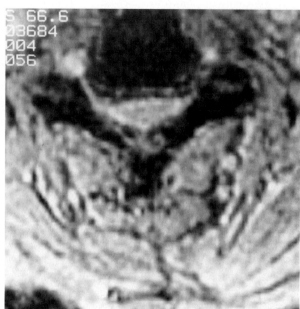

B

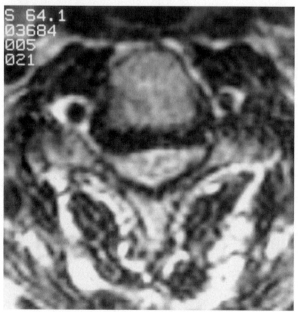

C

FIG. 26.6. A 76-year-old man was sent with a request to evaluate cervical myelopathy. **A:** A midsagittal T1-weighted spin-echo image displays a focal spinal cord compression at C3-C4 due to a degenerative spinal stenosis. A large bridging osteophyte at C4-C5 has effectively fused that segment. **B:** An axial T2-weighted gradient-echo (GRE) image at C3-C4 seems to indicate a more severe stenosis than the T2-weighted fast spin echo (FSE) image (**C**). **C:** An axial T2-weighted FSE magnetic resonance image (MRI) at C3-C4 also shows central degenerative spinal stenosis. Increased T2 signal is present in the spinal cord itself but was not apparent with the GRE technique. A magnetic susceptibility artefact in the GRE image causes a subtle "blooming" of the bony cortical margins of the spinal canal, resulting in a more severe appearance to this patient's spinal stenosis. Overestimation of spinal stenosis and a poor resolution of intrinsic spinal cord signal abnormalities are common problems with GRE MRI techniques.

Cervical myelography with CT is still preferred over MRI by many surgeons for the preoperative assessment of cervical myelopathy in the presence of multisegmental degenerative spondylosis. This preference relates to the dynamic examination component seen with myelography along with the accurate assessment of the bony cervical spine and spinal stenosis that CT provides. Myelography with CT is not a screening study, but it is an excellent preoperative planning study; additional presurgical imaging studies are almost never needed. With or without intravenous enhancement, CT will also provide a good assessment of cervical spinal stenosis; however, CT studies cannot match the ability of MRI to image the spinal cord itself (Fig. 26.4).

Compressive cervical myelopathy also may result from epidural tumor, infection, or blood (Fig. 26.7), and MRI is the procedure of choice in these cases. Intravenous (IV) gadolinium enhancement with sagittal and axial T1-weighted images with or without fat suppression is preferred if tumor or infection is suspected (Fig. 26.3). Inversion recovery images are useful for depicting bony metastasis or infection as well as for epidural blood (Figs. 26.4 and 26.8), tumor, or abscess. For those patients who are unable to undergo MRI,

CT with IV enhancement can also provide the correct diagnosis in almost all of these cases. CT may also be needed prior to operative intervention if extensive bone involvement is identified.

In regard to patients who present only with acute radiculopathy, CT and MRI are generally equivalent in the diagnosis of disc herniation into the spinal canal; CT with intravenous enhancement is better than or equal to MRI for identifying herniated discs confined to the neuroforamen. In this situation, MRI is disadvantaged by the sometimes confusing signals seen in the neuroforamen on GRE thin-section images and by the 3 mm or greater image thickness typically needed to perform T2-weighted FSE imaging. Image "blooming" can exaggerate apparent neuroforamen stenosis as well. Both MRI and CT have a small percentage of technically unsatisfactory examinations: CT may suffer from increased image noise at the base of the neck due to prominent shoulders, and MRI is easily degraded by patient motion, magnetic susceptibility effects, and pulsation artifacts. Patients who weigh more than 300 pounds are difficult to examine satisfactorily with either MRI or CT.

When spinal cord injury has occurred, MRI is the imaging procedure of choice. The primary reason for doing MRI

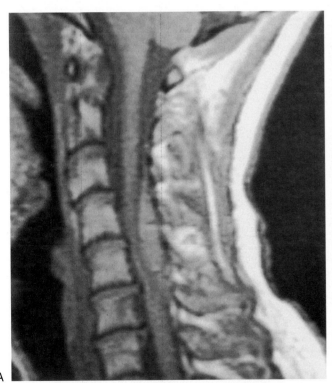
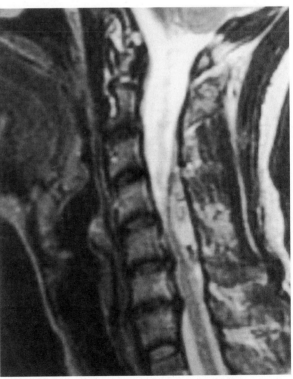

A   B

FIG. 26.7. A spontaneous left posterior epidural hematoma at C3 through C5 developed in this 38-year-old woman. **A:** Midsagittal T1-weighted spin-echo image (TR: 450; TE: 11). **B:** Midsagittal T2-weighted fast spin echo image (TR: 2,769; TE: 128). When acute, these lesions are typically isointense to spinal cord on T1-weighted magnetic resonance imaging (MRI) and hyperintense on T2-weighted MRI, as seen here. Occasionally it is difficult to distinguish epidural hematoma from epidural abscess and tumor by MRI criteria alone.

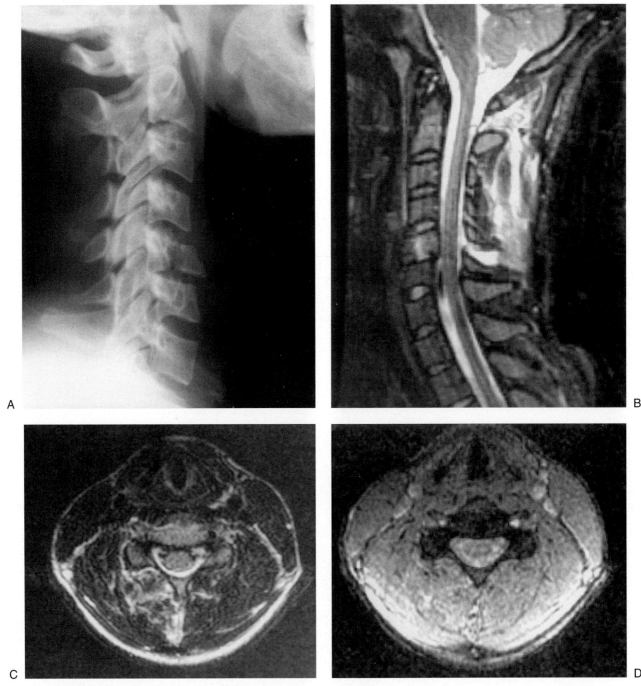

FIG. 26.8. This 25-year-old woman was injured in a motor vehicle accident. She was neurologically intact. **A:** A lateral cervical spine radiograph exhibits a C5 vertebral body fracture with a slight posterior displacement of C5 on C6. The interspinous process distance at C5-C6 is widened, indicating ligament injury. The probable mechanism is a flexion force. **B:** A midsagittal inversion recovery (IR) magnetic resonance image (MRI) shows extensive posterior paraspinal soft tissue injury denoted by the diffuse high signal from C5-C6 to C1. The interspinous process ligament at C5-C6 shows high signal, consistent with disruption. The other interspinous process ligaments have a normal signal, as does the spinal cord. The C5 vertebral body fracture is identifiable, but it would be seen better by computed tomography. Also noted is injury to the anterior C4-5 disc space, slight posterior displacement of C5 on the C6 vertebral body, and a small hematoma behind the C6 vertebral body. No disc herniation is observed. Because IR technique suppresses high signal from normal fat while still detecting edema and blood, it is an excellent sequence for studying trauma patients. **C:** An axial T2-weighted fast spin echo MRI made at C4 shows right posterior paraspinal hemorrhage and edema. **D:** An axial T2-weighted gradient-echo MRI also made at C4 does not show the soft tissue damage seen in **C**. The correct choice of pulse sequences is critical to successful MRI examinations.

is to identify cord compression by herniated disc, bone, or hematoma (Fig. 26.4). Identification of either intrinsic spinal cord hemorrhage or edema spanning more than two vertebral segments is associated with poor clinical recovery, but it has almost no impact on immediate patient management. Ligamentous injuries can be well demonstrated by IR or fat-suppressed T2-weighted MRI but only if performed within several days of the acute injury (Fig. 26.8). Chronic ligamentous injuries are not consistently demonstrated by MRI, even when impressive clinical symptoms are present. Patients with stable posttraumatic spinal cord deficits who develop a clinical deterioration in spinal cord function should be evaluated with MRI to exclude the late onset of a cyst or syrinx (Fig. 26.9). Plain radiographs and CT are better than MRI for characterizing the associated bone injuries and, in acute trauma, usually precede MRI. Flexion and extension radiographs remain the best way to assess cervical spinal stability.

There is clinical controversy about when MRI should be performed in alert patients who have cervical spine fracture-dislocations and are neurologically intact. The most cautious opinion is that MRI should be obtained prior to closed reduction, but many reputable surgeons feel that closed reduction with clinical monitoring is safe in these patients without performing an MRI study. For patients with impaired consciousness or spinal neurologic deficit, MRI is generally performed prior to closed reduction. The further loss of even one additional functional neurologic level in a patient with spinal cord injury has a profound impact on that patient's long-term rehabilitation status.

At the foramen magnum, upward migration of the odontoid process can cause mechanical compression of the lower medulla and upper cervical spinal cord. Congenital bony segmentation anomalies with partial or complete assimilation of the C1 vertebral segment to the occiput result in a high position for the odontoid. Basilar invagination related to Paget's disease and other causes has a similar effect. Genetic disorders, including the mucopolysaccharidoses (Morquio's syndrome, Hurler's syndrome, and others) and achondroplasia, may be associated with a foramen magnum that is "too small." Rheumatoid arthritis produces a fibrous proliferation around an eroded odontoid. This fibrous material, termed *pannus*, may become large enough to compress the spinal cord. C1-C2 subluxation due to connective tissue disease, odontoid insufficiency, or disruption of the atlantoaxial ligaments results in mechanical spinal cord compression between the posterior arch of C1 and the back of the C2 vertebral body (Fig. 26.10).

The Chiari malformation involves the downward displacement of cerebellar tissue into the upper cervical spinal canal. In the Chiari I malformation, the cerebellar tonsils extend below the foramen magnum. In the Chiari II malformation, both elements of the cerebellum and medulla are in the upper cervical spinal canal. Symptomatic mechanical compression of the cervicomedullary junction may occur. A spinal cord syrinx also may be associated with the Chiari

malformation (Fig. 26.5). Rarely, a tumor such as meningioma or neurofibroma arises at the foramen magnum, compressing the cervicomedullary junction. In this area, MRI should be performed in axial and sagittal planes. Gadolinium enhancement is useful primarily when tumor is suspected. Magnetic resonance angiography is helpful for evaluating the position and patency of the vertebrobasilar arteries. Although MRI produces an excellent image of the soft tissue abnormalities and is the initial imaging procedure of choice in the foramen magnum region, the bony anatomy may be difficult to fully appreciate. In such cases, CT with two- and three-dimensional reconstruction images is helpful for understanding the deranged bony structures that are present (Fig. 26.10).

Quantitative MRI measurement of CSF velocity, flow direction, and flow rates in the upper cervical spine and foramen magnum areas may be noninvasively determined using phase contrast or magnitude MRI techniques. The data are usually related to the cardiac cycle. Some surgeons believe that this type of data can help decide which patients with equivocal cervicomedullary junction compression related to the Chiari malformation would benefit from occipitocervical decompression surgery. Interpretation of this type of data remains problematic because the reproducibility of the data is somewhat variable, the definition of normal is fairly broad, and the correlation with clinical symptoms is imprecise.

Usually, MRI and CT studies are performed with the patient supine and the neck in a neutral position. Myelography has revealed many lessons about the dynamic mechanical aspects of cervical spine disease. The term *kinematic MRI* identifies a group of image acquisition techniques in which still images are made with the cervical spine in different positions. These individual images are then played in a movie loop, recreating a sense of motion. The images are typically acquired as single slices using a rapid acquisition technique such as GRE or FSE. Echo planar MRI will allow real-time image acquisition as the patient is actually moving (*MR fluoroscopy*). The cervical spine is taken through a range of motion, such as flexion to extension or the head turning from right to left. Spinal cord motion, dynamic stenosis, and instability that is not apparent in the usual spine-neutral position may be appreciated with such maneuvers. Although interesting anecdotal pathological cases have been shown, high-quality normative data using standardized MRI techniques have not been well defined. Pathological criteria remain loosely established, as do the clinical indications for when kinematic MRI should be performed. These "movies" can be entertaining and occasionally useful; however, they tend to be tedious and technically demanding to produce, and therefore are not commonly used in most imaging centers. Even the advocates of kinematic MRI use these techniques only in a very select group of their patients.

Recognition that most cervical spinal stenoses are most pronounced in the neck-extended position used for myelography has led some radiologists to suggest that cervical CT and MRI should be routinely performed with the patient

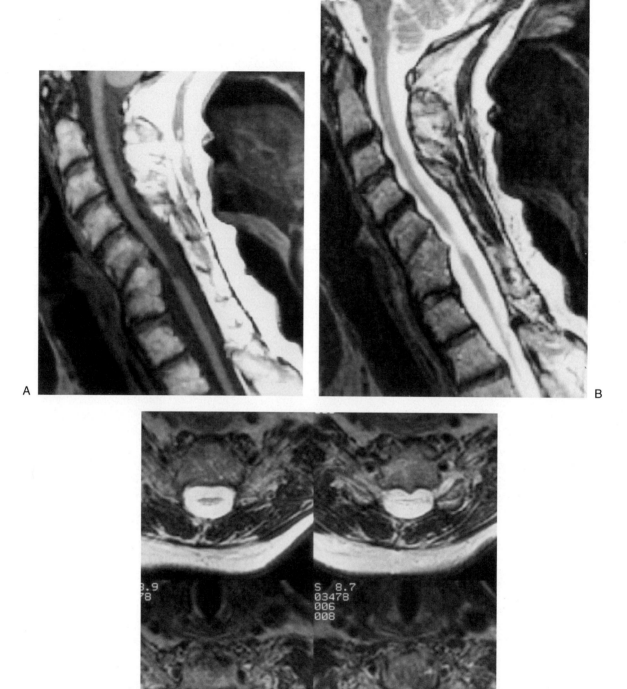

FIG. 26.9. This 54-year-old quadriplegic man has known posttraumatic spinal cord atrophy due to an old C5 to C7 spinal fracture. Because of a recent decline in neurologic function, a request was made to evaluate him for a syrinx. **A:** Sagittal T1-weighted spin-echo magnetic resonance imaging (MRI) shows posttraumatic spinal cord atrophy that is most severe at the C6 level. Prior laminectomies from C4 to C7 are somewhat difficult to appreciate. **B:** Sagittal T2-weighted fast spin echo (FSE) MRI reveals increased T2 signal in the atrophic spinal cord at C6. No other spinal cord lesions are evident. No mechanical compression of the spinal cord is noted. **C:** Four consecutive axial T2-weighted FSE magnetic resonance images made from C6 to C5 vertebral levels confirm the spinal cord atrophy and that the increased T2 signal is in the spinal cord itself. There is no evidence of a syrinx or expansile cyst. Axial images almost always should be obtained if a syrinx is clinically suspected or a focal cord lesion is seen in the sagittal images.

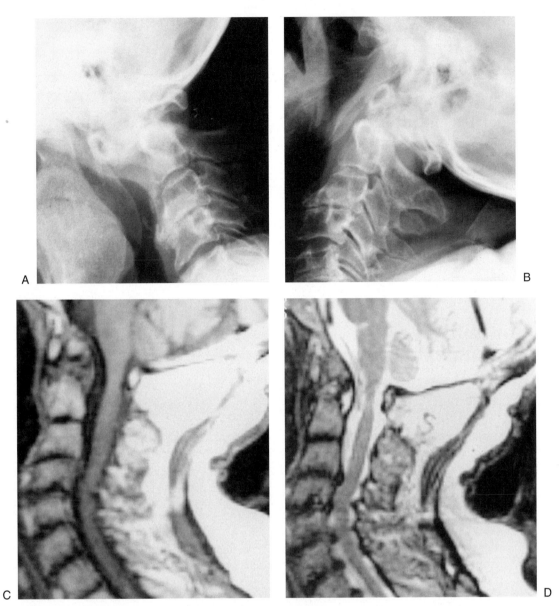

A

B

C

D

FIG. 26.10. A 67-year-old woman with rheumatoid arthritis has slowly progressive quadriparesis. **A** and **B:** Lateral flexion and extension erect cervical spine radiographs exhibit marked instability at C1-C2. The odontoid process appears fractured at its base and is moving in concert with the anterior arch of C1. A severe spinal stenosis occurs in flexion at C1-C2 due to the close approximation of the posterior arch of C1 to the posterior aspect of the C2 vertebral body. **C** and **D:** Sagittal T1-weighted spin-echo (SE) and T2-weighted fast spin echo magnetic resonance images made the day after **A** and **B** confirm the separation of the odontoid from the body of C2, presumably because of the erosion by rheumatoid pannus and then fracture. The T1 image shows a mild focal narrowing of the spinal cord at C1, with the T2 image showing definite increased T2 signal **(D)**, indicating cord injury due to the C1-C2 instability. Rheumatoid arthritis–associated degenerative changes in the midcervical region are causing a mild spinal stenosis at C3-C4 and C4-C5 without abnormal T2 signal in the spinal cord. The patient was offered surgery for her instability, but she refused. **E:** Ten months later, the patient was reexamined because her neurologic function had significantly deteriorated. Comparison of this new midsagittal T1-weighted SE magnetic resonance image (MRI) with image **C** shows a more severe spinal stenosis at C1-C2 with much greater spinal cord compression. The odontoid remnant is now subluxed forward relative to C2. The midcervical abnormalities are similar to **C**. **F:** Sagittal two-dimensional computed tomographic (CT) reconstruction image obtained the day after the MRI in **E** shows the odontoid remnant displaced in front of C2. The deformity was now fixed rather than unstable as seen in **A** and **B**. The bones are osteoporotic, an observation difficult to make on MRI. **G:** A sagittal split three-dimensional (3D) CT reconstruction image looking into the right side of the spinal canal shows the same displacement of the odontoid seen in **F**. The subluxed right lateral mass of C1 is clearly visible anterior to the C2 vertebral body margin. A normal atlantoaxial distance is preserved. The slitlike residual spinal canal at C1-C2 is graphically depicted on the 3D CT image. The patient underwent decompression and stabilization surgery but recovered very little neurologic function. The CT and MRI are complementary studies in this case. MRI is best for spinal cord and pannus evaluation. CT is superior to MRI for assessing the bony abnormalities in this patient.

347

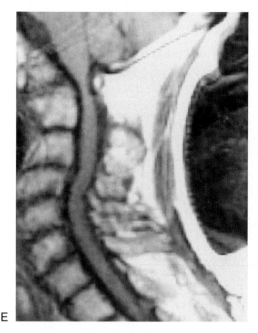

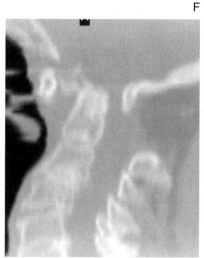

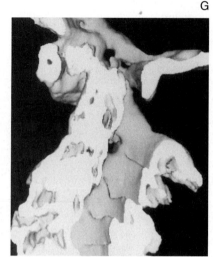

FIG. 26.10. *Continued*

placed in a neck-extended position. Trying to do this presents several practical technical challenges. This position is uncomfortable for many patients, leading to patient motion degradation during the examination. For those patients with good extension, adequate angulation of the axial imaging plane becomes difficult for CT and increases the MRI examination time. Patients with compressive myelopathy are at risk for spinal cord injury when placed in extension for a prolonged period of time. Any imaging protocol that requires repositioning the patient during the study is time consuming. At present, these types of techniques have not been widely employed in daily medical practice.

Postoperative evaluation is an important clinical concern and can be a radiological challenge. Unlike the lumbar spine, there is much less of a practical problem distinguishing between epidural scar and recurrent disc herniation in the cervical area. MRI gadolinium enhancement remains very useful for evaluating postoperative tumor, infection, and inflammation or infarction of the spinal cord. The integrity of bony fusion is more effectively investigated using high-resolution CT than MRI due to the poor MR signal produced by cortical bone. Postsurgical spinal cord injury is usually best demonstrated by MRI. Titanium implants cause minor CT and mild MR imaging artifacts. Metal debris from surgical burrs as well as stainless steel spinal implants causes severe MRI artifacts; CT is variably affected, usually less severely than MRI. In some cases, a myelogram followed by CT is the only imaging study that will succeed in patients with extensive or bulky spinal implants. Kinematic MRI techniques have not been commonly adopted for evaluating fusion integrity. Flexion and extension radiographs are still frequently used for this purpose.

The association of spinal trauma with vertebral artery injury has long been recognized. Conventional catheter angiography is rarely undertaken to identify these injuries due to the risk, cost, and lack of treatment options even when vascular injuries can be demonstrated. MR angiography (MRA) can noninvasively find these vertebral artery injuries. CT angiography (CTA), which requires IV contrast injection, is also diagnostically effective. Even though definite identification of vertebral artery injury is now much easier, little improvement in treatment for these vascular injuries has so far been developed.

Several well-recognized advanced MRI capabilities that have been developed for brain evaluation have yet to be successfully applied to the cervical spinal cord. MR perfusion imaging qualitatively measures tissue blood flow, and MR diffusion imaging provides an indication of cell viability. This information would be very useful in assessing spinal cord trauma and infarction. MR spectroscopy (MRS) techniques provide noninvasive *in vivo* direct measurement of adenosine triphosphate (ATP), *N*-acetylcholine, and other metabolic substrate levels. MRS data may allow better biochemical characterization of tumors, multiple sclerosis plaques, infarction, and inflammatory lesions. Functional MRI (fMRI) denotes a group of MRI techniques that can temporally resolve local changes in neural tissue related to functional activity. Normal neural tissues become metabolically active when stimulated or carrying out tasks. When active, local blood flow and oxygen consumption increase, and MRI can detect these changes related to time. For example, if the right hand were purposefully moving, numerous motor neural cells in the right side of the cervical spinal cord from C4 to C8 would be actively discharging. If a stimulus were applied to the right hand, the sensory cells in the right side of the cervical spinal cord would become active. By carefully designing stimulation and activity testing paradigms, spinal cord function could be mapped. All of these advanced MRI techniques are limited in their application to the cervical spinal cord by factors such as the small size of the cervical spinal cord, its intrinsic pulsation, the adjacent pulsation of the cerebrospinal fluid and vertebral arteries, and magnetic susceptibility issues related to nearby bone and air. For present practical purposes, these advanced MRI techniques will remain areas for future clinical development in the cervical spine.

ACKNOWLEDGMENTS

The manuscript was prepared with the diligent assistance of Mrs. Jane Shaeffer of Charlotte Radiology, P.A. None of this could have been possible without the excellent work and cooperation of the staff of the Departments of Radiology and Medical Photography at the Carolinas Medical Center. The emotional support and understanding of my wife, Betsy, were essential to the completion of this task.

SUGGESTED READING

Algra PR, Bloem JL, Tissing H, et al. Detection of vertebral metastases: comparison between MR imaging and bone scintigraphy. *Radiographics* 1991;11:219.

Backes WH, Mess WH, Wilmink JT. Functional MR imaging of the cervical spinal cord by use of median nerve stimulation and fist clenching. *Am J Neuroradiol* 2001;22:1854–1859.

Barlett RJ, Hill CR, Gardiner E. A comparison of T2 and gadolinium enhanced MRI with CT myelography in cervical radiculopathy. *Br J Radiol* 1998;71:11–19.

Benitah S, Raftopoulos C, Baleriaux D, et al. Upper cervical spinal cord compression due to bony stenosis of the spinal canal. *Neuroradiology* 1994;36:231.

Breidahl WH, Low V, Khangure MS. Imaging the cervical spine: a comparison of MR with myelography and CT myelography. *Australas Radiol* 1991;35:306.

Brunberg JA, DiPietro MA, Venes JL, et al. Intramedullary lesions of the pediatric spinal cord: correlation of findings from MR imaging, intraoperative sonography, surgery, and histologic study. *Radiology* 1991;181:573.

Bulas DI, Fitz CR, Johnson DL. Traumatic atlanto-occipital dislocation in children. *Radiology* 1993;188:275.

Casselman JW, Jolie E, Dehaene I, et al. Gadolinium-enhanced MR imaging of infarction of the anterior spinal cord. *Am J Neuroradiol* 1991;12:561.

Chamberlain MC, Sandy AD, Press GA. Spinal cord tumors: gadolinium-DTPA-enhanced MR imaging. *Neuroradiology* 1991;33:469.

Cornelius RS. Imaging of acute cervical spine trauma. *Semin Ultrasound CT MR* 2001;22:108–124.

Crim JR, Moore K, Brodke D. Clearance of the cervical spine in multitrauma patients: the role of advanced imaging. *Semin Ultrasound CT MR* 2001;22:283–305.

Curati WL, Kingsley DPE, Kendall BE, et al. MRI in chronic spinal cord trauma. *Neuroradiology* 1992;35:30.

Davis PC, Reisner A, Hudgins PA, et al. Spinal injuries in children: role of MR. *Am J Neuroradiol* 1993;14:607.

Davis SJ, Teresi LM, Bradley WG Jr, et al. Cervical spine hyperextension injuries: MR findings. *Radiology* 1991;180:245.

Deliganis AV, Baxter AB, Hanson JA, et al. Radiologic spectrum of craniocervical distraction injuries. *Radiographics* 2000;20(Suppl):S237–250.

Egelhoff JC, Bates DJ, Ross JS, et al. Spinal MR findings in neurofibromatosis types 1 and 2. *Am J Neuroradiol* 1992;13:1071.

Elster AD, Chen MYM. Chiari I malformations: clinical and radiologic reappraisal. *Radiology* 1992;183:347.

Eschelman DJ, Beers GJ, Naimark A, et al. Pseudoarthrosis in ankylosing spondylitis mimicking infectious diskitis: MR appearance. *Am J Neuroradiol* 1991;12:1113.

Falcone S, Quencer RM, Green BA, et al. Progressive posttraumatic myelomalacic myelopathy: imaging and clinical features. *Am J Neuroradiol* 1994;27:747.

Flanders AE, Spettell CM, Tartaglino LM, et al. Forecasting motor recovery after cervical spinal cord injury: value of MR imaging. *Radiology* 1996;201:649–655.

Friedman DP. Herpes zoster myelitis: MR appearance. *Am J Neuroradiol* 1992;13:1404.

Friedman DP, Tartaglino LM. Amyotrophic lateral sclerosis: hyperintensity of the corticospinal tracts on MR images of the spinal cord. *Am J Roentgenol* 1993;160:604.

Gero B, Sze G, Sharif H. MR imaging of intradural inflammatory diseases of the spine. *Am J Neuroradiol* 1991;12:1009.

Golash A, Birchall D, Laitt RD, et al. Significance of CSF area measurements in cervical spondylitic myelopathy. *Br J Neurosurg* 2001;15:17–21.

Goldberg AL, Baron B, Daffner RH. Atlantooccipital dislocation: MR demonstration of cord damage. *J Comput Assist Tomogr* 1991;27:174.

Hackney DB, Ford JC, Markowitz RS, et al. Experimental spinal cord injury: imaging the acute lesion. *Am J Neuroradiol* 1994;27:960.

Hofmann E, Warmuth-Metz M, Bendszus M, et al. Phase-contrast MR imaging of the cervical CSF and spinal cord: volumetric motion analysis in patients with Chiari I malformation. *Am J Neuroradiol* 2000;21:151–158.

Holtas S, Basibuyuk N, Fredriksson K. MRI in acute transverse myelopathy. *Neuroradiology* 1993;35:221.

Humphreys SC, Hodges SD, Patwardhan A, et al. The natural history of the cervical foramen in symptomatic and asymptomatic individuals aged 20–60 years as measured by magnetic resonance imaging. A descriptive approach. *Spine* 1998;23:2180–2184.

Keats TE, Dalinka MK, Alazraki N, et al. Cervical spine trauma. American College of Radiology Appropriateness Criteria. *Radiology* 2000;215(Suppl):243–246.

Kochran JP, Quencer RM. Imaging of cystic and cavitary lesions of the spinal cord and canal: the value of MR and intraoperative sonography. *Radiol Clin North Am* 1991;29:867.

Kricun R, Shoemaker EI, Chovanes GI, et al. Epidural abscess of the cervical spine: MR findings in five cases. *Am J Roentgenol* 1992;278:1145.

Levi AD, Choi WG, Keller PJ, et al. The radiographic and imaging characteristics of porous tantalum implants within the human cervical spine. *Spine* 1998;23:1245–1250; discussion 1251.

Levi LM. Functional MR imaging evaluation of spinal cord function by use of neurophysiological stimuli. *Am J Neuroradiol* 2001;22:1811–1812.

Martich V, Ben-Ami T, Yousefzadeh DK, et al. Hypoplastic posterior arch of C-1 in children with Down syndrome: a double jeopardy. *Radiology* 1992;183:125.

Mascalchi M, Salvi F, Piacentini S, et al. Friedreich's ataxia: MR findings involving the cervical portion of the spinal cord. *Am J Roentgenol* 1994;163:187.

Matsumoto M, Fujimura Y, Suzuke N, et al. MRI of cervical intervertebral discs in asymptomatic subjects. *J Bone Joint Surg Br* 1998;80:19–24.

Morio Y, Teshima R, Nagashima H, et al. Correlation between operative outcomes of cervical compression myelopathy and MRI of the spinal cord. *Spine* 2001;26:1238–1245.

Muhle C, Metzner J, Weinert D, et al. Classification system based on kinematic MR imaging in cervical spondylitic myelopathy. *Am J Neuroradiol* 1998;19:1763–1771.

Muhle C, Wiskirchen J, Weinert D, et al. Biomechanical aspects of the subarachnoid space and cervical cord in healthy individuals examined with kinematic magnetic resonance imaging. *Spine* 1998;23:556–567.

Narita Y, Watanabe Y, Hoshino T, et al. Myelopathy due to large veins draining recurrent spontaneous caroticocavernous fistula. *Neuroradiology* 1992;34:433.

Neuhold A, Stiskal M, Platzer C, et al. Combined use of spin-echo and gradient-echo MR-imaging in cervical disk disease: comparison with myelography and intraoperative findings. *Neuroradiology* 1991;33:422.

Numaguchi Y, Rigamonti D, Rothman MI, et al. Spinal epidural abscess: evaluation with gadolinium-enhanced MR imaging. *Radiographics* 1993; 13:545.

Pfirrmann CW, Binkert CA, Zanetti M, et al. MR morphology of alar ligaments and occipitoatlantoaxial joints: study in 50 asymptomatic subjects. *Radiology* 2001;218:133–137.

Quencer RM. Spinal epidural abscess: evaluation with gadolinium-enhanced MR imaging: invited commentary. *Radiographics* 1993;13:559.

Quencer RM, Bunge RP, Egnor M, et al. Acute traumatic central cord syndrome: MRI-pathological correlations. *Neuroradiology* 1992;34:85.

Quencer RM, Nunez D, Green BA. Controversies in imaging acute cervical spine trauma. *Am J Neuroradiol* 1997;18:1866–1868.

Rahmouni A, Divine M, Mathieu D, et al. Detection of multiple myeloma involving the spine: efficacy of fat-suppression and contrast-enhanced MR imaging. *Am J Roentgenol* 1993;160:1049.

Ramsey RG. Spine and spinal cord. In: Ramsey RG, ed. *Neuroradiology.* Philadelphia: WB Saunders, 1994:786–943.

Reul J, Gievers B, Weis J, et al. Assessment of the narrow cervical spinal canal: a prospective comparison of MRI, myelography and CT-myelography. *Neuroradiology* 1995;37:187–191.

Salazar JL, Misra M, Bloom D, et al. MRI artifacts following anterior cervical diskectomy. *Surg Neurol* 1997;48:23–29.

Schick RM. Normal age-related changes in bone marrow in the axial skeleton at MR imaging. *Radiology* 1991;179:877.

Schubeus P, Schorner W, Hosten N, et al. Spinal cord cavities: differential-diagnostic criteria in magnetic resonance imaging. *Eur J Radiol* 1991; 12:219.

Schweitzer ME, Hodler J, Cervilla V, et al. Craniovertebral junction: normal anatomy with MR correlation. *Am J Roentgenol* 1992;278:1087.

Sengupta DK, Kirollos R, Findlay GF, et al. The value of MR imaging in differentiating between hard and soft cervical disc disease: a comparison with intraoperative findings. *Eur Spine J* 1999;8:199–204.

Shafaie FF, Wippold FJ II, Gado M, et al. Comparison of computed tomography myelography and magnetic resonance imaging in the evaluation of cervical spondylotic myelopathy and radiculopathy. *Spine* 1999; 24:1781–1785.

Shen W-C, Lee SK, Ho Y-J, et al. MRI of sequela of transverse myelitis. *Pediatr Radiol* 1992;22:382.

Singh A, Crockard HA, Platts A, et al. Clinical and radiological correlates of severity and surgery-related outcome in cervical spondylosis. *J Neurosurg* 2001;94(Suppl 2):189–198.

Sklar EM, Post JM, Falcone S, et al. MRI of acute spinal epidural hematomas. *J Comput Assist Tomogr* 1999;23:238–243.

Stabler A, Eck J, Penning R, et al. Cervical spine: postmortem assessment of accident injuries—comparison of radiographic, MR imaging, anatomic, and pathologic findings. *Radiology* 2001;221:340–346.

Stabler A, Reiser MF. Imaging of spinal infection. *Radiol Clin North Am* 2001;39:115–135.

Sze G, Kawamura Y, Negishi C, et al. Fast spin-echo MR imaging of the cervical spine: influence of echo train length and echo spacing on image contrast and quality. *Am J Neuroradiol* 1993;14:1203.

Tien RD, Buxton RB, Schwaighofer BW, et al. Quantitation of structural distortion of the cervical neural foramina in gradient-echo MR imaging. *J Magn Reson Imaging* 1991;1:683.

Toro VE, Goodrich A, Lundy DW, et al. MR artifacts after anterior cervical diskectomy and fusion: cadaver study. *J Comput Assist Tomogr* 1993;17:696.

Vaccaro AR, Falatyn SP, Flanders AE, et al. Magnetic resonance evaluation of the intervertebral disc, spinal ligaments, and spinal cord before and after closed traction reduction of cervical spine dislocations. *Spine* 1999;24:1210–1217.

Vaccaro AR, Klein GR, Flanders AE, et al. Long-term evaluation of vertebral artery injuries following cervical spine trauma using magnetic resonance angiography. *Spine* 1998;23:789–794; discussion 795.

Vaccaro AR, Madigan L, Schweitzer ME, et al. Magnetic resonance imaging analysis of soft tissue disruption after flexion-distraction injuries of the subaxial cervical spine. *Spine* 2001;26:1866–1872.

Van de Kelft E, van Vyve M, Selosse P. Postsurgical follow-up by MRI of anterior cervical discectomy without fusion. *Eur J Radiol* 1992;27:196.

Volle E, Assheuer J, Hedde JP, et al. Radicular avulsion resulting from spinal injury: assessment of diagnostic modalities. *Neuroradiology* 1992; 34:235.

Wallace SK, Cohen WA, Stern EJ, et al. Judicial hanging: postmortem radiographic, CT, and MR imaging features with autopsy confirmation. *Radiology* 1994;193:263.

Wang P-Y, Shen W-C, Jan J-S. MR imaging in radiation myelopathy. *Am J Neuroradiol* 1992;13:1049.

Weller SJ, Rossitch E Jr, Malek AM. Detection of vertebral artery injury after cervical spine trauma using magnetic resonance angiography. *J Trauma* 1999;46:660–666.

Woodard EJ, Leon SP, Moriarty TM, et al. Initial experience with intraoperative magnetic resonance imaging in spine surgery. *Spine* 2001;26: 410–417.

Yousem DM, Atlas SW, Hackney DB. Cervical spine disk herniation: comparison of CT and 3DFT gradient echo MR scans. *J Comput Assist Tomogr* 1992;16:345.

CHAPTER 27

Nuclear Medical Evaluation of the Cervical Spine

Kazuo Yamashita and Yoshihisa Hasegawa

During the past 50 years, the development of nuclear medical imaging apparatuses and bone-seeking radiopharmaceuticals has markedly advanced, and the image quality of bone scintigrams has continuously improved. Plain roentgenograms, tomograms, computed tomographic (CT) scans, and magnetic resonance imaging (MRI) provide detailed information regarding the morphologic changes occurring in the bone. Bone scintigraphy using technetium-99 (^{99m}Tc) phophonate compounds, which reflects biochemical changes in the bone, is often more sensitive in the detection of bone lesions and easier to apply in the examination of the whole body than other modalities. Presently, bone scintigraphy is the most frequently performed nuclear medical examination and is used widely in both the diagnosis and investigation of bone disease, including benign and malignant tumors, infections, trauma, joint diseases, and metabolic bone diseases.

PHYSICAL AND BIOLOGICAL PRINCIPLES OF SCINTIGRAPHY

Imaging Instruments

The first nuclear medical imaging apparatus ever developed was the rectilinear scanner built in 1950 by Cassen and Curtis (1). This was a moving-detector imaging system. Radiopharmaceutical-emitted gamma rays passed through the holes of a collimator and interacted with the scintillator [NaI(T1)], losing energy due to the photoelectric effect and Compton effect, and *scintillations*, or flashes of light, were emitted. The scintillations were converted into electrical pulses and enhanced by an optically coupled photomultiplier tube (PMT). The output pulse passed through the preamplifier–amplifier system, and only the pulses selected by a pulse-height analyzer arrived at the recording devices.

The detector scanned over the target organ, and the recording device, which moved with the detector, produced dots on the recording medium with a density related to the distribution of radioactivity in the organ.

The scintillation camera, developed in 1957 by Anger (2), has replaced the rectilinear scanner. It is the most widely used instrument today for nuclear medical imaging. It is a stationary-detector imaging system. Gamma rays interact with a large, flat, round plate scintillator [NaI(T1)], and light flashes are emitted. The location of each light flash is determined with multiple PMTs and an electronic system, and a dot of light is produced on the face of a cathode ray tube in corresponding position. The image of the dots of light may be recorded on either film or paper media. The signals may also be digitalized and processed by computer.

Various apparatuses have been developed to obtain tomographic images of the distribution of radioactivity at different depths in the body (3,4). Among them, single-photon emission computed tomography (SPECT) is widely used today. In the rotation-type scintillation camera SPECT machine, one or more scintillation detectors are mounted on a gantry and rotate 360 degrees around the patient. The data collected are reconstructed by computer into multidimensional tomograms. The advantages of this technique are that multiple transverse tomographic images can be simultaneously obtained, and tomograms from any other desired angle as well as three-dimensional images can be constructed. This equipment also can be used for routine planar imaging. Instruments with as many as two or three scintillation cameras in one unit specifically designed for SPECT use are commercially available.

Another tomographic acquisition technique is positron emission tomography (PET). This method began to attract attention in the mid-1970s with the successful development of PET scanners and the synthesis of [^{18}F]fluoro-2-deoxy-D-glucose (FDG) (5). The emitted positron is annihilated by immediately binding with an electron, resulting in the simultaneous release of two 5.10-MeV photons at an angle 180 degrees from each other. Using coincident detection techniques, tomographic images mapping the metabolic distribution of the PET agent are produced. Maximum resolution is 3 to 4 mm. Because of the need for a cyclotron to produce the positron-emitting agents, most of which have a short half-life, the high installation and operational costs of the apparatus, and the need for specialized personnel, PET has not yet become widely available.

Radioactive Tracer Selection

The first artificial radioisotope used as a tracer in metabolic studies was ^{32}P, an element localized in the bone, prepared by Chiewitz and Havesy (6) in 1935. Various other radioisotopes have been historically used in studies of bone metabolism, including ^{85}Sr, ^{87m}Sr, ^{47}Ca, and ^{18}F; ^{99m}Tc tripolyphosphate, introduced by Subramanian and McAfee (7) in 1971, was superior to any of these preceding radionuclides for diagnostic bone imaging with respect to both its metabolic and physical properties. Further bone imaging improvements were obtained with the subsequent development of ^{99m}Tc polyphosphate (^{99m}Tc-PPx), ^{99m}Tc pyrophosphate (^{99m}Tc-PPi), ^{99m}Tc hydroxyethylidene diphosphonate (^{99m}Tc-HEDP), ^{99m}Tc methylene diphosphonate (^{99m}Tc-MDP), and ^{99m}Tc hydroxymethylene diphosphonate (^{99m}Tc-HMDP). Today, ^{99m}Tc-MDP and ^{99m}Tc-HMDP are regarded as the best radionuclides and are widely used.

The mechanism of accumulation of ^{99m}Tc phosphate and diphosphonate has not yet been elucidated. Increased vascularity, bone mineralization (particularly on the increased hydroxyapatite surface), immature collagen or osteoid, and enzyme systems are assumed to influence uptake (8–10). Nakashima and associates (11) investigated ^{99m}Tc-MDP concentration in mouse osteosarcoma and found that autoradiographs showed the concentration of the tracer in new bone laid down in response to tumor growth. Thus, the mineralization of the bone matrix was considered to play a significant role in ^{99m}Tc uptake.

Several tracers other than the bone-seeking radioisotopes are used in studies of infectious diseases and tumors of bone. Ramanna and associates (12) reported that ^{201}Tl chloride is useful for the assessment of response to preoperative chemotherapy in bone sarcoma. Gallium-67 (^{67}Ga) citrate is reported to be useful in the detection of osteomyelitis, especially in neonates, an age group in which poor results are obtained using ^{99m}Tc phosphate scans alone (13).

The PET radiopharmaceutical most frequently used today for cancer studies is the glucose analogue FDG. Because aerobic glycolysis is enhanced in malignant cells, malignant tumors are detected by PET using FDG because of their increased metabolic rate of glucose. This method has been reported to be useful in the diagnosis of osteosarcoma (14), bone metastases of breast cancer (15), head and neck cancers, lung cancer, and chronic musculoskeletal infections, especially those involving the spine (16). Positron

emitter–labeled amino acids and thymidine also are used for PET studies of cancer; their increased uptake is thought to be related to the increased protein synthesis and nucleic acid metabolism of malignant tumors.

Immunoscintigraphy is a method of studying the localization of antigens using radiolabeled antibodies. Since the method of preparation of monoclonal antibodies was developed by Koehler and Milstein (17) in 1975, highly pure and homogeneous antibodies that recognize a single antigenic determinant have become readily available. Immunoscintigraphy using monoclonal antibodies against tumor-related antigens is expected to allow a more specific diagnosis than other imaging techniques; however, the antibodies examined to date cannot yet be applied in routine clinical use because of both the low accumulation rates in tumors and the high background activity. The production of human antimouse antibody (HAMA) (18) resulting from the use of mouse-produced monoclonal antibodies is another problem of this technique. Attempts are in progress to develop methods of increasing the accumulation rates of monoclonal antibodies in tumors, decreasing the background activity, and controlling the production of HAMA.

Imaging Technique

Bone scintigraphy is performed 3 to 4 hours after intravenous injection of 555 to 740 MBq of ^{99m}Tc-MDP or ^{99m}Tc-HMDP. It is necessary for the patient to urinate before scanning to minimize radioactivity in the bladder and to facilitate detection of a lesion in the pelvis. Three-phase scintigraphy (19) may be performed in some conditions. Perfusion images are obtained every 2 to 5 seconds beginning immediately after injection, blood pool images after 1 to 5 minutes, and bone scintigrams after 3 to 4 hours. This technique is useful in the differential diagnosis of osteomyelitis.

The scintillation camera device allows scanning of the whole body with movement of either the bed or the detector and is useful for whole-body imaging in bone scintigraphy. The spatial resolution of the scinticamera in the scan mode is somewhat inferior to that of spot images; spot views should be taken for close examination of any suspicious regions detected with whole-body scanning.

Magnified imaging using a pinhole collimator (20,21) and SPECT (22,23) are reported to be useful in the close evaluation of sites of abnormal accumulation detected using conventional bone scintigrams. SPECT is considered to be effective in the evaluation of the spine, pelvis, hip joints, knee joints, and facial bones. SPECT of the cervical spine provides good discrimination of the anterior vertebral body, the trachea, and thyroid cartilage. These structures are superimposed on routine planar images, making accurate interpretation difficult (24).

INDICATIONS FOR SCINTIGRAPHY

Bone scintigraphy is highly sensitive to quantitative changes in the skeleton, but it is not sufficiently specific to define the quality of disease or pathologic condition. The greatest value of bone scintigraphy is in the evaluation of bone tumors, particularly in the detection of bone metastases. Bone scintigraphy has proved valuable in the evaluation of various pathologic conditions of the spine (25,26):

1. Metastatic spine tumors
   a. Detection of bone metastases
      (i) Diagnosis of symptomatic lesions
      (ii) Detection of occult lesions
      (iii) Assessment of the extent of bone metastases
   b. Staging the disease, particularly in prostate cancer, breast cancer, lung cancer, Ewing's sarcoma, and osteogenic sarcoma
   c. Planning of radiotherapy fields
   d. Location of suitable biopsy sites
   e. Assessment of response to therapy
   f. Differentiation of pathological from traumatic fracture
   g. Determination of the distribution of bone metastases from different primary tumors
2. Primary spine tumors
   a. Location of lesion
   b. Assessment of extent of lesion
   c. Differentiation of benign from malignant lesion
   d. Assessment of stage of disease
   e. Assessment of progress of disease
3. Inflammatory diseases
   a. Early diagnosis
   b. Assessment of distribution
   c. Assessment of response to therapy
4. Metabolic bone diseases
   a. Assessment of extent of skeletal involvement, particularly of associated pathological fractures
   b. Assessment of response to therapy
5. Assessment of bone graft incorporation

THE NORMAL BONE SCINTIGRAM

Normal whole-body scans using ^{99m}Tc-MDP and ^{67}Ga citrate are shown in Figure 27.1. In ^{99m}Tc scans, increased uptake of tracer is generally localized in the epiphyseal plates and the osteochondral junctions of the ribs in children. In adults, the sternum, the sternoclavicular junctions,

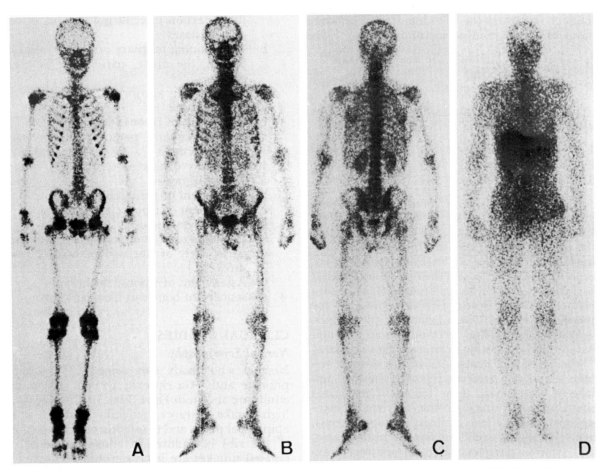

FIG. 27.1. A: Normal bone scan of a 9-year-old boy, anterior view. High uptake of ^{99m}Tc-MDP is localized at the epiphyses or apophyses of the skeleton. **B:** Normal bone scan with ^{99m}Tc-MDP of a 50-year-old man, anterior view. **C:** Posterior view of the same patient as in **B**. **D:** Normal scintigraphy with ^{67}Ga citrate of a 32-year-old man, anterior view. High uptake of the tracer in the liver is normal.

the acromion, and the anterior superior iliac spine show up as areas of increased uptake in an anterior view. The pedicles and spinous processes of the thoracic and lumbar spine, the inferior angles of the scapulae, and the sacroiliac joints show normal increased uptake in a posterior view. Increased uptake is frequently seen in the cervical area as a result of calcification of the tracheal and laryngeal cartilages in the anterior view, particularly in older adults. Ossicles in the ligamentum nuchae are also positive. Occasionally, increased uptake is seen in the thyroid gland as a result of accumulation of free pertechnetate. Bone-seeking isotopes are excreted in the urine, usually resulting in normal increased activity in the kidneys and bladder.

In ^{67}Ga scans, occasional visualization of the thymus in children and increased uptake in the liver, intestine, colon, and bone are normal. The spinal column is situated posteriorly; therefore, a posterior view is more useful to detect or assess spinal diseases than an anterior view. In diagnosing spinal disorders, it should be remembered that increased uptake of tracer in the bladder (^{99m}Tc) and liver or colon (^{67}Ga) often masks spinal lesions.

In general, the intensity of the radioactivity of a lesion should be evaluated in comparison to the surrounding soft tissues, normal adjacent areas, or contralateral bone. For quantitative measurements, Simon and Kirchner (27) proposed a rating system for bone scans using ^{99m}Tc in which increased uptake by sacroiliac joints on posterior imaging in whole-body scans was defined as a base. For ^{67}Ga scans, a similar scale was proposed based on the intensity of the liver.

THE ABNORMAL BONE SCINTIGRAM

Most pathological conditions of bone result in an increased accumulation of the bone-seeking isotope. This increased uptake is nonspecific, but very sensitive. Any abnormality associated with increased new bone formation will cause a localized increased concentration of bone-seeking isotope. The following cause a localized increased uptake in the spine:

1. Malignant diseases
   a. Primary spine tumors
   b. Metastatic spine tumors
   c. Paraspinal tumors invading the spine
2. Benign lesions
   a. Benign spine tumors
   b. Infection
   c. Fracture
   d. Degenerative conditions such as spondylosis, articular facet osteoarthritis, or ankylosing spinal hyperostosis (Forester's disease)
   e. Postfusion pseudoarthrosis
   f. Metastatic calcification
   g. Paget's disease

It is impossible to make a definitive diagnosis of the lesion corresponding to the area of increased uptake of the bone-seeking isotope from the skeletal scintigram alone. Comparative studies that include roentgenograms, CT scans, MRIs, or bone biopsy are needed.

Occasionally, the bone scan shows an abnormal area of decreased uptake of the bone-seeking isotope (a "cold" or "photopenic" lesion). The following are causes of decreased uptake in the spine (26):

1. Artefact
   a. Extrinsic: Pendants, belt, buckles, coins, splints, etc.
   b. Intrinsic: Metal rods, plates, prostheses, etc.
2. Irradiation
3. Spine tumors that do not evoke an osteoblastic response
4. Avascularity

Metastatic Spine Tumors

Detection of bone metastases is the most important indication for bone scintigraphy. Many studies comparing bone scintigraphy and radiography in the detection of bone metastases confirm that bone scintigraphy is much more sensitive than conventional radiography (28). At least 50% of bone mineral content must be lost before a metastatic lesion in the trabecular bone can be seen radiographically (29). Positive bone scans can predate radiographic detection of bone metastases (30). In our series of spinal metastases, 201 patients with breast cancer were examined by bone scintigraphy using ^{99m}Tc-MDP for the purpose of detecting spinal metastases. Of these 201 patients, 57 had spinal metastases. Detection by bone scintigraphy was obtained earlier than by plain radiography in 9 (15.8%) of 57 patients. Spinal metastases were detected later by bone scintigraphy in only 1 patient (1.8%), whereas in 47 patients (82.5%) they were detected simultaneously. In the early-detection bone scan group of 9 patients, all of whom were asymptomatic, radiographic changes were found after an interval of 2 to 11 months (average 5.3 months) following scintigraphic detection.

Since the introduction of ^{99m}Tc phosphate and diphosphonate as a tracer in the early 1970s (7), bone scintigraphy has been considered the most sensitive modality for the detection of bone metastases. Studies comparing bone scintigraphy and MRI in detecting spinal metastases have shown MRI to be more sensitive than bone scintigraphy (31,32). MRI is capable of depicting metastases in the spinal marrow space that are difficult to detect by bone scintigraphy. Whole-body MRI is not practical at this time primarily because of long examination times and cost. Considering bone scintigraphy's high sensitivity in the detection of bone metastases, its widespread availability, and its ease of imaging the entire skeleton, it remains the preferred imaging modality for screening for bone metastases. MRI is an excellent complementary imaging modality in further assessing patients with suspected spinal metastases in whom scintigraphic findings are inadequate for answering clinical suspicion. MRI is superior for demonstrating epidural masses and paravertebral extension of the tumor.

Although scintigraphic findings are nonspecific, recognizable patterns of scintigraphic abnormalities suggesting spinal metastases are commonly seen. Bone metastases usually appear as asymmetrically distributed multiple foci of increased uptake of tracer on bone scan (Fig. 27.2). A bone metastasis can occasionally occur as a single lesion. More commonly, a single focus of increased uptake on bone scan is related to benign disease (33,34). Although a bone scan with five or more new abnormalities always reflected the presence of bone metastases in the follow-up of patients with breast cancer, there was a low prevalence of bone metastases in a bone scan with four or fewer new abnormalities: 11% for solitary and 38% for two to four new abnormalities (35).

In planar images, the vertebral body is superimposed on the posterior elements, where a variety of small lesions can occur in different sites. In SPECT examinations of the spine, lesional contrast is improved, permitting not only improved detection but also, by displaying the slices in transaxial, coronal, and sagittal projections, a perception of three-dimensional anatomy that improves localization and more exact delineation of the lesion (36). The improved diagnostic accuracy in metastatic spine tumors arises from the ability of SPECT to achieve an accurate image of a body section at a prescribed depth (Fig. 27.3).

Where there are extensive bone metastases, diffusely increased uptake of tracer by almost every bone can occur. This is the so-called superscan phenomenon of malignancy, which occurs most often in prostate cancer. The distribution of increased uptake is so uniform that the bone scan can be falsely interpreted as negative. In this situation, uptake in the kidneys and bladder is faint or absent. An absent renal uptake alerts the clinician to the possibility of extensive bone metastases; however, a diagnosis of superscan by an absent renal uptake may be misleading. A false-positive superscan may occur in patients with renal failure or some metabolic bone diseases.

When metastatic spine lesions do not evoke an osteoblastic response, a false-negative study may occur. This situation may occur with rapidly growing, highly destructive lesions. In extreme cases, the large, destructive lesions may appear as cold areas on bone scan. Cold lesions arise most frequently from breast cancer, lung cancer, neuroblastoma, and multiple myeloma.

Bone scintigraphy is also the most useful diagnostic modality for determination of the distribution of bone metastases. Analysis of 112 bone scans from patients with metastatic breast cancer revealed that the rank order of skeletal regions by number of metastatic bone lesions corresponded well with the relative distribution of active bone marrow in the adult skeleton (Table 27.1). Information obtained from skeletal scintigraphy has helped us understand the pathways of bone metastases. There are two different lines of thought among researchers concerning the distribution of bone metastases on bone scans and whether there are any differences in this respect between prostate cancer and other cancers. Some researchers (39,40) reported that the difference was not significant; they propose that the pathway of spread of prostate cancer and other cancers is identical. Others (41,42) reported that the difference was significant; they propose that prostate cancer metastasizes to specific skeletal sites by retrograde venous spread via Batson's vertebral plexus.

Staging patients with bone metastases according to the extent of the disease is needed (43). Efforts to evaluate the extent of bone metastases have been made. Semiquantitative analyses of bone scans based on the number of lesions or skeletal areas on the scan have been attempted in patients with metastatic prostate cancer, and these methods have been used as a stratification variable in clinical practice (44,45). Patients with metastatic prostate cancer and fewer than six bone metastases had a favorable prognosis (46). The value of the distribution of bone metastases on the bone scan relative to survival time in patients with metastatic prostate cancer was emphasized in our study (47). Those with bone metastases exclusively in the pelvis and the lumbar spine had a favorable prognosis.

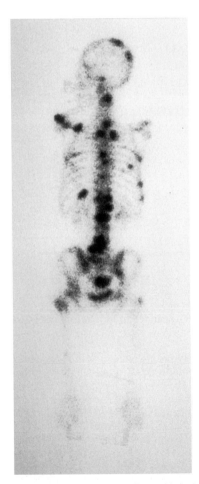

FIG. 27.2. A 31-year-old woman with multiple bone metastases from breast cancer. The posterior view of a ^{99m}Tc-MDP scintigram shows asymmetrically distributed multiple foci of increased uptake, a characteristic pattern associated with bone metastases.

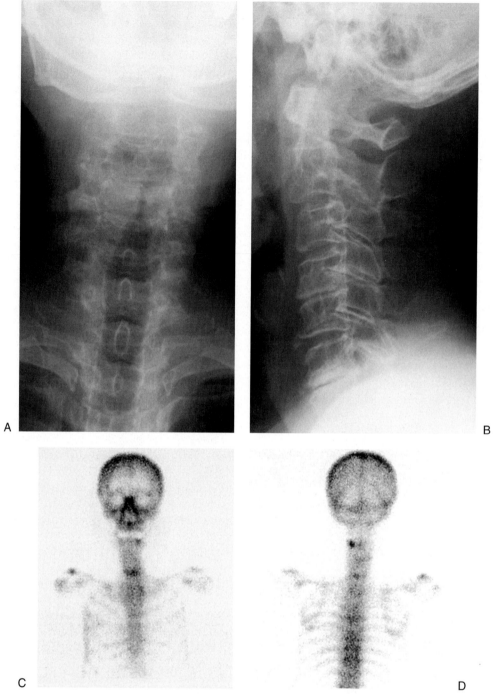

FIG. 27.3. An 83-year-old woman with cervical spine metastasis from breast cancer. **A:** An anteroposterior roentgenogram shows osteosclerosis of the left articular pillar of the C3 vertebra and bony prominences of the uncovertebral articulation in the lower cervical spine. **B:** A lateral roentgenogram shows loss of height of disc space, irregularity of the vertebral margin, and bone sclerosis of the subchondral zone at the C4-5, C5-6, and C6-7 interspaces. **C:** An anterior view of a conventional ⁹⁹ᵐTc-HMDP bone scintigram shows increased uptake in the lower cervical spine. **D:** A posterior view of a conventional ⁹⁹ᵐTc-HMDP bone scintigram shows increased uptake in the upper cervical spine on the left. **E:** Single-photon emission computed tomography (SPECT) sagittal images show the uptake to be localized in the cervical spine. No extraskeletal accumulation is seen. **F:** SPECT coronal images show a hot spot in the upper cervical spine on the left and bands of increased uptake in the lower cervical spine. The former is thought to be caused by metastasis, and the latter by spondylotic change.

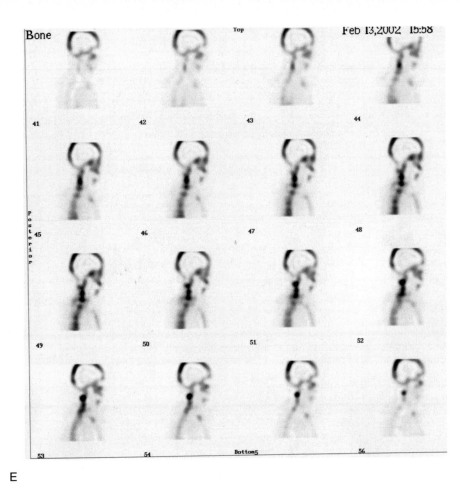

E

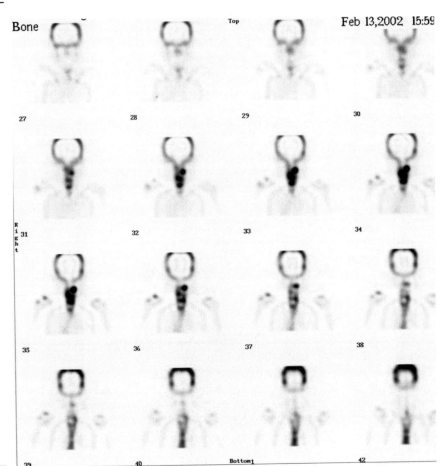

F

FIG. 27.3. *Continued*

TABLE 27.1. *Distribution of Metastatic Bone Lesions Detected by Bone Scintigraphy Using ^{99m}Tc-MDP in 112 Patients with Breast Cancer when Bone Metastasis was First Diagnosed, and the Relative Distribution of Active Bone Marrow in the Adult Skeleton*

Skeletal region	Metastatic bone lesions No. on bone scan[a]	Active bone marrow Percentage (%) in total weight[b]
Skull	28	9.2
Cervical spine	21	4.6
Clavicles	4	0.8
Scapulae	4	2.6
Humeri, upper halves	4	2.3
Thoracic spine	140	16.4
Ribs	158	15.8
Sternum	20	3.3
Lumbar spine	119	12.3
Pelvis, including sacrum	60	26.1
Femora, upper halves	24	6.7
Total	609	100

[a] versus [b], r (Spearman's coefficient of rank correlation) = 0.9266 ($p < 0.0001$).
[b] Woodard's analysis (37; Table I, females) excluded the limb bones. The percentages given here, except the humeri and femors, were adjusted to include the limb bones. Humeral and femoral percentages are from Cristy (38). The clinical course of the 112 patients was published in Yamashita K, Koyama H, Inaji H. Prognostic significance of bone metastasis from breast cancer. *Clin Orthop* 1995;312:89–94.

Primary Spine Tumors

Bone scintigraphy remains an important part of the diagnosis of primary spine tumors. Primary spine tumors are infrequent and usually benign. Among benign spine tumors, osteoid osteoma is one of the most scintigraphically active bone lesions (Fig. 27.4). Osteoid osteoma is associated with increased uptake of bone-seeking isotope as a result of new bone formation and high vascularity. In the cervical spine, osteoid osteoma is usually found in the pedicles and the posterior elements. Osteoblastoma, aneurysmal bone cyst, and osteochondroma (Fig. 27.5) are three other benign spine disorders that produce an active bone scan. These tumors usually affect the posterior elements of the cervical spine. Eosinophilic granuloma, when associated with a collapsed vertebra, also shows a hot lesion. All these primary benign tumors and tumorous conditions of the cervical spine appear as hot lesions, and skeletal scintigraphy cannot differentiate one from another. Roentgenograms and CT scans can differentiate them and delineate the anatomic localization and extent.

The most common primary malignant tumor of the cervical spine in the adult is multiple myeloma. A false-negative scan may occur with multiple myeloma because of its purely lytic nature and the lack of an osteoblastic response (Fig. 27.6). Primary malignant tumors of the cervical spine other than multiple myeloma are rare. Any primary malignant tumor of the cervical spine other than multiple myeloma has markedly increased uptake of bone-seeking isotope. Osteosarcoma appears as a hot lesion because of new bone produced by the tumor itself. The other primary malignant tumors have increased uptake due to reactive new bone produced by the host tissue. The latter reactive bone formation varies, resulting in a marked variation in uptake of bone-seeking isotope within primary malignant tumors. Bone scintigraphy cannot accurately differentiate primary malignant from benign tumors (48). In our series using ^{99m}Tc-MDP, there proved to be no significant differences in the positive ratio between malignant (overall, 94.4%; primary, 93.3%; metastatic, 94.7%) and benign tumors of the spine (85.7%) (Table 27.2). The positive ratio for ^{67}Ga showed a greater differentiation between malignant (overall, 58.7%; primary, 50%; metastatic, 61.1%) and benign tumors (11.1%). Thallium-201 has been proposed as a better agent than ^{67}Ga for distinguishing malignant from benign lesions (49). Both agents are inferior to ^{99m}Tc-MDP for overall lesion detection.

Infection and Miscellaneous

Increased uptake of ^{99m}Tc diphosphonate is also noted in patients with infectious spondylitis, which includes tuberculous spondylitis, pyogenic vertebral osteomyelitis (Fig. 27.7), and discitis, and patients with noninfectious spondylitis, which includes ankylosing spondylitis and seronegative spondyloarthropathy (Fig. 27.8). Spinal osteomyelitis and accompanying soft tissue infection can be diagnosed accurately by ^{67}Ga scintigraphy with SPECT (50). Scintigraphy using ^{111}In-labeled leukocytes has been shown to be of limited value in the diagnosis of spine infection (51).

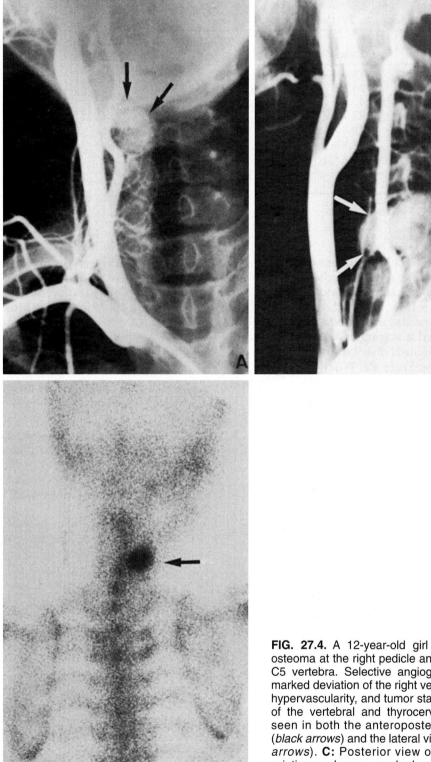

FIG. 27.4. A 12-year-old girl with osteoid osteoma at the right pedicle and body of the C5 vertebra. Selective angiography shows marked deviation of the right vertebral artery, hypervascularity, and tumor stain in the area of the vertebral and thyrocervical arteries, seen in both the anteroposterior view **(A)** (*black arrows*) and the lateral view **(B)** (*white arrows*). **C:** Posterior view of ⁹⁹ᵐTc-MDP scintigram shows a marked accumulation in the same area (*black arrows*).

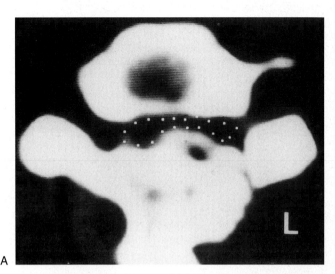

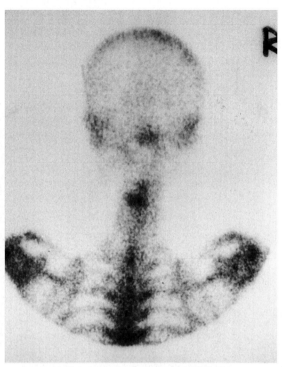

A

B

FIG. 27.5. A 15-year-old boy with osteochondroma of the C3 vertebra. **A:** Computed tomographic myelogram shows spinal cord compression (*dotted line*) due to an irregularly shaped bony protrusion of the C3 lamina. **B:** A posterior view of a ^{99m}Tc-MDP scintigram showing increased uptake in the upper cervical spine, more to the left than the right side.

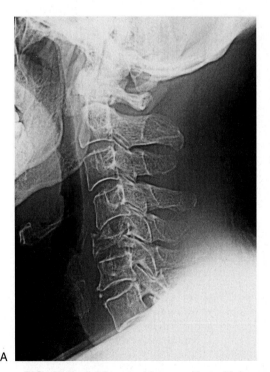

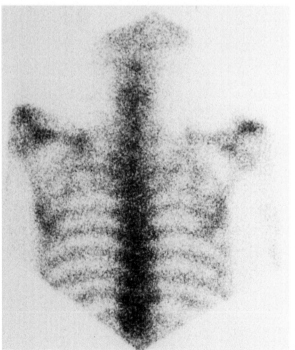

A

B

FIG. 27.6. A 62-year-old man with multiple myeloma and a pathological fracture of the C5 vertebral body. **A:** A lateral roentgenogram shows collapse of the C5 vertebral body. **B:** A posterior view of a ^{99m}Tc-MDP scintigram shows no abnormality in the cervical spine. Highly lytic processes may have a negative bone scan.

TABLE 27.2. *Positive Ratio of ^{99m}Tc-MDP and ^{67}Ga Citrate in Various Diseases of the Spine*

	No. of patients	^{99m}Tc scintigraphy (%)	^{67}Ga scintigraphy (%)
Malignant spinal tumors	92	85/90 (94.4)	27/46 (58.7)
Primary[a]	15	14/15 (93.3)	5/10 (50.0)
Metastatic[b]	77	71/75 (94.7)	22/36 (61.1)
Benign spinal tumors and tumorous conditions[c]	22	18/21 (85.7)	1/9 (11.1)
Spinal cord tumors	22	0/20 (0)	0/10 (0)

[a]Primary malignant spinal tumors: osteosarcoma, myeloma, malignant fibrous histiocytoma, chondrosarcoma, chordoma, hemangioendothelioma, and malignant lymphoma of bone.

[b]Sources of metastatic spinal tumors: lung, stomach, breast, uterus, prostate, kidney, rectum, liver, thyroid, skin, and others.

[c]Benign spinal tumors and tumorous conditions: osteochondroma, giant cell tumor, chondroblastoma, hemangioma, bone cyst, osteoid osteoma, eosinophilic granuloma, osteoblastoma, and desmoplastic fibroma.

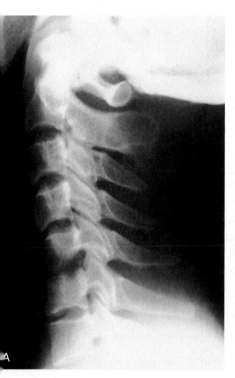

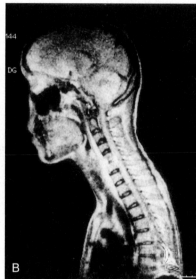

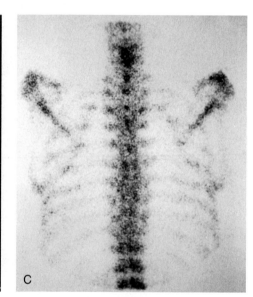

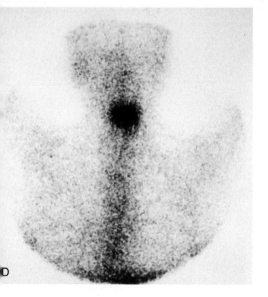

FIG. 27.7. A 35-year-old man with pyogenic vertebral osteomyelitis at the C5-C6 level. **A:** A lateral roentgenogram shows narrowing of the C5-6 interspace with irregularity of the vertebral end plates. **B:** A midsagittal T2-weighted magnetic resonance image shows an increase in signal intensity of the C5-6 intervertebral disc and the adjacent vertebral bodies. A high-signal-intensity epidural and prevertebral mass contiguous to the intervertebral disc is evident. **C:** A posterior view of a ^{99m}Tc-MDP scintigram shows increased uptake in the lower cervical spine. **D:** A posterior view of a ^{67}Ga citrate scintigram shows markedly increased uptake in the same area.

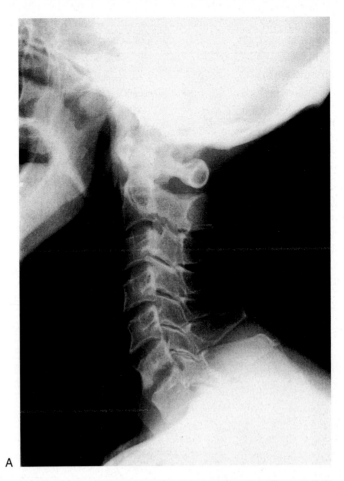

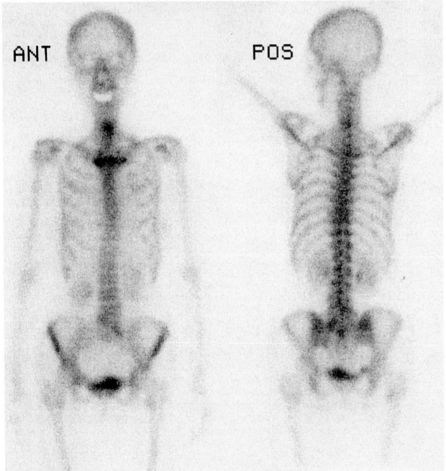

FIG. 27.8. A 71-year-old woman with spondyloarthropathy associated with pustulosis (acne-pustulosis-hyperostosis-ostitis). **A:** A lateral roentgenogram shows erosions of the C6-C7 end plates with subchondral sclerosis. **B:** An anterior view of a ⁹⁹ᵐTc-MDP scintigram shows increased uptake in the lower cervical spine and in the clavicles and sternum.

Metabolic bone diseases such as renal osteodystrophy, osteomalacia, and primary hyperparathyroidism are characterized by diffuse increased uptake of ^{99m}Tc diphosphonate throughout the skeleton. Scintigraphic features of metabolic bone disease include prominent uptake in the calvarium and mandible, beading of the costochondral junctions, the so-called tie sternum sign, and absent or faint renal excretion. These findings are not specific for any particular metabolic bone disease. The degree of scintigraphic abnormality is related to the severity of the disease.

Bone scintigraphy has no role in the initial diagnosis of osteoporosis. The scintigraphic appearance of osteoporosis is usually normal, except when vertebral fractures occur. The scintigraphic appearance of a vertebral fracture due to osteoporosis is intense linear increased uptake. Skeletal scintigraphy is helpful in assessing patients with known osteoporosis who present with spinal pain to clarify whether further vertebral fractures have occurred. It should always be remembered that the scintigraphic appearance of a vertebral fracture is not specific to osteoporosis; other possibilities, including spinal metastases or multiple myeloma, must be considered. The increased uptake in a vertebral fracture due to osteoporosis gradually resolves over the following 6 to 24 months (52). When multiple vertebral fractures are present, skeletal scintigraphy may show different stages of resolution of the increased uptake. This pattern may help differentiate vertebral fractures due to osteoporosis from metastatic spine tumors. SPECT of the cervical spine is useful in the diagnosis of occult fractures (53) and pseudarthrosis (54).

It is of little value to apply scintigraphy to spinal cord tumors, even with hypervascularity such as occurs in hemangioblastoma, or to a spinal arteriovenous malformation. A group of 22 patients with spinal cord tumor were assessed by scintigraphy using ^{99m}Tc diphosphonate and ^{67}Ga citrate. The bone scan showed no uptake in the lesions (Table 27.2).

REFERENCES

1. Cassen B, Curtis L, Reed C, et al. Instrumentation of I-131 used in medical studies. *Nucleonics* 1951;9:46–50.
2. Anger HO. Scintillation camera. *Rev Sci Instr* 1958;29:27–33.
3. Freedman GS, Putman CE, Potter GD. Critical review of tomography in radiology and nuclear medicine. *Crit Rev Clin Radiol Nucl Med* 1975;6:253–294.
4. Budinger TF, Derenzo SE, Gullberg GT, et al. Emission computer assisted tomography with single-photon and positron annihilation photon emitters. *J Comput Assist Tomogr* 1977;1:131–145.
5. Muehllehner G, Karp JS. Positron emission tomography imaging technical considerations. *Semin Nucl Med* 1986;16:35–50.
6. Chiewitz O, Hevesy G. Radioactive indicators in the study of phosphorus metabolism in rats. *Nature* 1935;136:754–755.
7. Subramanian G, McAfee JG. A new complex of Tc-99m for skeletal imaging. *Radiology* 1971;99:192–196.
8. Francis MD. The inhibition of calcium hydroxyapatite crystal growth by polyphosphonates and polyphosphates. *Calcif Tissue Res* 1969;3:151–162.
9. Zimmer AM, Isitman AT, Holmes RA. Enzymatic inhibition of diphosphonate: a proposed mechanism of tissue uptake. *J Nucl Med* 1975;16:352–356.
10. Guillemart A, Besnard JC, Pape A, et al. Skeletal uptake of pyrophosphate labeled with technetium-95m and technetium-96, as evaluated by autoradiography. *J Nucl Med* 1978;19:895–899.
11. Nakashima H, Ochi H, Yasui N, et al. Uptake and localization of Tc-99m-methylene diphosphonate in mouse osteosarcoma. *Eur J Nucl Med* 1982;7:531–535.
12. Ramanna L, Waxman A, Binney G, et al. Thallium-201 scintigraphy in bone sarcoma: comparison with gallium-67 and technetium-MDP in the evaluation of chemotherapeutic response. *J Nucl Med* 1990;31:567–572.
13. Neuman RD, Hoffer PB. Gallium-67 scintigraphy for detection of inflammation and tumors. In: Freeman LM, ed. *Freeman and Johnson's Clinical Radionuclide Imaging*, 3rd ed., vol. 2. Orlando: Grune and Stratton, 1984:1319–1364.
14. Kern KA, Brunetti A, Norton JA, et al. Metabolic imaging of human extremity musculoskeletal tumors by PET. *J Nucl Med* 1988;29:181–186.
15. Minn H, Soini I. Fluoro [F-18]-deoxyglucose scintigraphy in diagnosis and follow-up of treatment in advanced breast cancer. *Eur J Nucl Med* 1989;15:61–66.
16. De Winter F, Van de Wiele C, Vogelaers D, et al. Fluorine-18 fluorodeoxyglucose-positron emission tomography: a highly accurate imaging modality for the diagnosis of chronic musculoskeletal infections. *J Bone Joint Surg Am* 2001;83:651–660.
17. Koehler G, Milstein C. Continuous culture of fused cells secreting antibody of predefined specificity. *Nature* 1975;256:495–497.
18. Shawler DL, Bartholomew RM, Smith LM, et al. Human immune response to multiple injections of murine monoclonal IgG. *J Immunol* 1985;135:1530–1535.
19. Maurer AH, Chen DCP, Camargo EE, et al. Utility of three-phase skeletal scintigraphy in suspected osteomyelitis: concise communication. *J Nucl Med* 1981;22:941–949.
20. Bahk YW, Kim OH, Chung SK. Pinhole collimator scintigraphy in differential diagnosis of metastasis, fracture, and infections of the spine. *J Nucl Med* 1987;28:447–451.
21. Kosuda S, Kawahara S, Ishibashi A, et al. Usefulness of pinhole collimator in differential diagnosis of metastatic disease and degenerative joint disease in the vertebrae: evaluation by receiver operating characteristics (ROC) analysis. *Ann Nucl Med* 1989;3:119–124.
22. Collier BD, Hellman RS, Krasnow AZ. Bone SPECT. *Semin Nucl Med* 1987;17:247–266.
23. Murray IP, Dixon J. The role of single photon emission computed tomography in bone scintigraphy. *Skeletal Radiol* 1989;18:493–505.
24. Yui N, Togawa T, Kinoshita F, et al. Usefulness of bone SPECT of the cervical spine: with special reference to separate visualization of the trachea and thyroid cartilage. *Ann Nucl Med* 1993;7:223–230.
25. Malmud LS, Charkes ND. Bone scanning: principles, technique, and interpretation. *Clin Orthop* 1975;107:112–122.
26. Galasko CSB. Tumors. In: Galasko CSB, Weber PA, eds. *Radionuclide scintigraphy in orthopaedics*. Edinburgh: Churchill Livingstone, 1984:65–109.
27. Simon MA, Kirchner PT. Scintigraphic evaluation of primary bone tumors: comparison of technetium-99m phosphonate and gallium citrate imaging. *J Bone Joint Surg Am* 1980;62:758–764.
28. Galasko CSB. Detection of skeletal metastases. In: Galasko CSB, ed. *Skeletal metastases*. London: Butterworths, 1986:52–87.
29. Edelstyn GA, Gillespie PJ, Grebell FS. The radiological demonstration of osseous metastases: experimental observations. *Clin Radiol* 1967;18:158–162.
30. Osmond JD, Pendergrass HP, Potsaid MS. Accuracy of Tc99m-diphosphonate bone scans and roentgenograms in the detection of prostate, breast, and lung carcinoma metastases. *Am J Roentgenol Radium Ther Nucl Med* 1975;125:972–977.
31. Frank JA, Ling A, Patronas NJ, et al. Detection of malignant bone tumors: MR imaging vs scintigraphy. *Am J Roentgenol* 1990;155:1043–1048.
32. Algra PR, Bloem JL, Tissing H, et al. Detection of vertebral metastases: comparison between MR imaging and bone scintigraphy. *Radiographics* 1991;11:219–232.
33. Corcoran RJ, Thrall JH, Kyle RW, et al. Solitary abnormalities in bone scans of patients with extraosseous malignancies. *Radiology* 1976;121:663–667.
34. Tumeh SS, Beadle G, Kaplan WD. Clinical significance of solitary rib lesions in patients with extraskeletal malignancy. *J Nucl Med* 1985;26:1140–1143.
35. Jacobson AF, Stomper PC, Jochelson MS, et al. Association between number and sites of new bone scan abnormalities and presence of skeletal metastases in patients with breast cancer. *J Nucl Med* 1990;31:387–392.

36. Murray IPC. Bone scintigraphy: the procedure and interpretation. In: Murray IPC, Ell PJ, eds. *Nuclear medicine in clinical diagnosis and treatment*, vol. 2. New York: Churchill Livingston, 1994:909–934.

37. Woodard HQ. The relation of weight of haematopoietic marrow to body weight. *Br J Radiol* 1984;57:903–907.

38. Cristy M. Active bone marrow distribution as a function of age in humans. *Phys Med Biol* 1981;26:389–400.

39. Dodds PR, Caride VJ, Lytton B. The role of vertebral veins in the dissemination of prostatic carcinoma. *J Urol* 1981;126:753–755.

40. Morgan JWM, Adcock KA, Donohue RE. Distribution of skeletal metastases in prostatic and lung cancer: mechanism of skeletal metastases. *Urology* 1990;36:31–34.

41. Styles C. The distribution of bone metastases as shown on isotope scanning: proposed modes of spread. *Australas Radiol* 1989;33:226–228.

42. Cumming J, Hacking N, Fairhurst J, et al. Distribution of bony metastases in prostatic carcinoma. *Br J Urol* 1990;66:411–414.

43. Stoll BA. Natural history, prognosis, and staging of bone metastases. In: Stoll BA, Parbhoo S, eds. *Bone metastasis: monitoring and treatment*. New York: Raven Press, 1983:1–20.

44. Soloway MS, Hardeman SW, Hickey D, et al. Stratification of patients with metastatic prostate cancer based on extent of disease on initial bone scan. *Cancer* 1988;61:195–202.

45. Knudson G, Grinis G, Lopez-Majano V, et al. Bone scan as a stratification variable in advanced prostate cancer. *Cancer* 1991;68:316–320.

46. Ishikawa S, Soloway MS, Van der Zwaag R, et al. Prognostic factors in survival free of progression after androgen deprivation therapy for treatment of prostate cancer. *J Urol* 1989;141:1139–1142.

47. Yamashita K, Denno K, Ueda T, et al. Prognostic significance of bone metastases in patients with metastatic prostate cancer. *Cancer* 1993; 71:1297–1302.

48. Sneppen O, Heerfordt J, Dissing I, et al. Numerical assessment of bone scintigraphy in primary malignant bone tumors and tumor-like conditions. *J Bone Joint Surg Am* 1978;60:966–969.

49. Nadel HR. Thallium-201 for oncological imaging in children. *Semin Nucl Med* 1993;23:243–254.

50. Love C, Patel M, Lonner BS, et al. Diagnosing spinal osteomyelitis: a comparison of bone and Ga-67 scintigraphy and magnetic resonance imaging. *Clin Nucl Med* 2000;25:963–977

51. Whalen JL, Brown ML, McLeod R, et al. Limitation of indium leukocyte imaging for the diagnosis of spine infections. *Spine* 1991;16: 193–197.

52. Matin P. The appearance of bone scans following fractures, including immediate and long-term studies. *J Nucl Med* 1979;20:1227–1231.

53. Seitz JP, Unguez CE, Corbus HF, et al. SPECT of the cervical spine in the evaluation of neck pain after trauma. *Clin Nucl Med* 1995;20:667–673.

54. Coric D, Branch CL, Jenkins JD. Revision of anterior cervical pseudarthrosis with anterior allograft and plating. *J Neurosurg* 1997; 86:969–974.

CHAPTER 28

Angiography of the Cervical Spine and Spinal Cord

Katsuyuki Nakanishi, Christopher G. Ullrich, Hironobu Nakamura, and Keiro Ono

Angiography of the cervical spine and spinal cord is an infrequently performed neuroradiological procedure. Modern developments in contrast agents, catheters, image acquisition, and vascular interventional techniques have both improved the safety of these procedures and broadened their applications. This chapter reviews the indications for cervical angiography. A brief technical overview is provided, and potential complications are presented. A knowledge of cervical vascular anatomy is vital to the appropriate selection and interpretation of these procedures. Both normal and abnormal vascular findings are discussed.

INDICATIONS FOR ANGIOGRAPHY

The following are the most common indications for angiography of the cervical spine and spinal cord:

- *To identify and characterize a primary vascular lesion.* This is almost always undertaken as a secondary procedure after the possibility of such a vascular lesion has been raised either by clinical findings, such as unexplained subarachnoid hemorrhage, or because of magnetic resonance imaging (MRI) or occasionally myelographic evidence of a vascular lesion. These are rare lesions.
- *To delineate the vascularity and vascular blood supply of an already identified lesion or the relationship between a lesion and nearby normal blood vessels.* These angiographies usually are obtained in the context of preoperative planning. It is an uncommon practice to try to distinguish benign from malignant masses using angiographic criteria. Direct percutaneous biopsy is the preferred diagnostic method in most cases involving the bony vertebrae. Spinal cord lesions are generally examined by MRI and dealt with by open surgical procedures.

- *In association with embolization procedures.* Embolizations are most commonly performed within 48 hours of surgery to devascularize lesions and reduce operative blood loss. However, embolization can constitute the primary lesion treatment. Such embolization procedures may be either curative or may provide substantial palliation.

PATIENT PREPARATION

Careful patient preparation is a key factor in successful arteriographic examinations and for avoiding complications. A careful preprocedure medical history and examination is obtained for each patient. Present medications should be identified and appropriately maintained. Adequate hydration is continued throughout the day of the procedure. There are no absolute contraindications for arteriography. Relative contraindications include compromised renal function, multiple myeloma, sickle cell anemia, iodine allergies, hypocoagulation and hypercoagulation states, and severe hypotension or hypertension.

Compromised renal function is not uncommon, particularly in elderly patients. Serum blood urea nitrogen (BUN) and creatinine values are routinely obtained before angiography. In patients with elevated values, hydration before and after angiography, judicious use of contrast media, and the administration of diuretic agents during and after the procedure will usually prevent subsequent renal complications. These patients usually have serum BUN and creatinine values checked the day after angiography to assess any changes in renal function. Patients with multiple myeloma and sickle cell disease are handled in a similar fashion to minimize the risk of renal impairment. Persons dependent on renal dialysis should undergo dialysis soon after the angiogram.

Iodine contrast allergy is usually a manageable problem. Oral or intravenous steroids are administered 24 hours before and after the procedure. Cimetidine and diphenhydramine are given before the procedure. This regimen is quite effective in suppressing most allergic reactions. Nonionic contrast agent is used during the procedure because it is less allergenic. Appropriate resuscitative facilities should be readily available in the angiographic suite at all times. Anesthesia standby is warranted for patients with a history of severe respiratory or cardiovascular reactions. Patients with a history of multiple major allergies are treated in a similar fashion.

Coagulopathies should be routinely corrected before angiography. Impaired coagulation is most commonly the result of medication or hepatocellular dysfunction. These patients are at increased risk for bleeding at the vascular puncture site and are less suitable candidates for embolization and surgical procedures. Hypercoagulopathy causes an increased risk of intravascular thrombus formation and unintended vascular obstruction.

Patients whose diastolic blood pressure exceeds 110 mm Hg also have an increased prevalence of hematoma formation at the vascular access site during and after arteriography. Therefore, the blood pressure should be pharmacologically controlled if possible before the procedure. Hypotensive patients are poor candidates for arteriography until their blood pressure has been stabilized at a normotensive level.

TECHNIQUE

A detailed discussion of spinal angiography technique is beyond the scope of this chapter. Readers who require more specific information are referred to the works by Abrams (1), Djindjian and colleagues (2,3), and Doppman and associates (4–6).

Djindjian and co-workers (2,3) perform spinal angiography with the patient under general anesthesia. This helps produce technically excellent angiograms but does not allow assessment of a developing neurologic deficit during the procedure. We favor the approach of Doppman and associates (4–6), who perform the study with the patient lightly sedated. Using this approach allows early detection of adverse events and reduces the cost of the procedure.

Angiography is performed under strict sterile conditions. Vascular access is usually via the femoral artery. Small-caliber (4 or 5 Fr) catheters are often best for the selective injection of the arteries that provide the blood supply to the spine and spinal cord. A nonionic contrast agent is used because it is less neurotoxic as well as less allergenic. Heparinized saline is used to flush catheters and syringes to reduce the risk of blood-clot formation.

Two methods can be used to obtain the angiogram images: (a) conventional film-screen magnification radiography with manually produced subtraction films or (b) digital subtraction angiography (DSA). The conventional method requires the use of mechanical film changers. Intensifying screens in the changers allow rapid film exposures to be made. Multiple film images are sequentially obtained during injection of the nonionic contrast agent. To get maximum detail, an x-ray tube with a small focal spot is used and geometric magnification is performed. These images have the highest spatial resolution obtainable. Overlapping bone and soft tissue densities can obscure small but important vascular details.

Subtraction films may overcome this difficulty by displaying the contrast-filled vascular system devoid of its surrounding structures. To facilitate the film subtraction process, the first radiograph in any sequence is timed so that no contrast media are present. A reversal film, termed the *mask,* is prepared from this first radiograph. The subtraction film then is produced by rephotographing this mask film superimposed on the contrast angiogram film. Preexisting bone and soft tissue densities are thus "subtracted," leaving only the contrast-media-opacified vascular system visible on the resulting subtraction film. Acceptable subtraction films require exact registration between the mask and the angiogram film. Patient motion degrades the quality of the subtraction. These derived images are extremely helpful for the correct interpretation of the angiogram. Unfortunately, manual film subtraction is a slow, tedious process. Subtraction films are often not available until after the actual angiogram procedure is completed. These film-based angiographic techniques are of excellent quality, but are now obsolete. The now-dominant digital imaging techniques are extensions of this work.

High-resolution intraarterial DSA is now the standard technique for angiography of the cervical spine and spinal cord. The digital image data are acquired either directly from flat panel detector plates or by analog-to-digital conversion of an image intensifier image. Compared with film, a large improvement in contrast resolution is obtained at the expense of somewhat lower spatial resolution. This reduced spatial resolution is seldom critical to clinical diagnosis.

Selective catheterization arterial DSA offers several major advantages over film-based techniques: DSA provides rapid access to both contrast angiogram and subtraction images during the actual procedure, thus shortening procedure time and potentially improving decisions made during the procedure. The superior contrast resolution of DSA allows the use of either more dilute contrast media or a smaller volume of contrast media, which improves patient comfort and lessens the risk of neurotoxicity and nephrotoxicity. Many DSA systems support vascular roadmapping. This capability allows a previously obtained angiographic image to be superimposed on the active fluoroscopic image, facilitating difficult catheterizations and possibly helping to reduce catheter manipulation in small vessels, thereby decreasing the risk of direct vascular injury by the catheter or its guidewire. The primary digital images may also be postprocessed to compensate for patient motion, create dynamic video displays, three-dimensional angiographic images, and so on. Network-accessible computer storage of these DSA images and their radiographic interpretation allows immediate access to this patient data within the entire hospital, the local medical community, and around the world as needed.

Intravenous DSA methods have been extensively described in the literature, particularly in the early 1980s. This technique has virtually no role in angiography of the spine and spinal cord because of the frequent overlapping of vessels and the high rate of poor-quality images. Two other intravenous enhancement technologies deserve brief mention here. Computed tomography angiography (CTA) has been making great improvements in both spatial resolution and image quality. Submillimeter near-isotropic volumetric CT imaging is possible with recently introduced 16-channel multidetector CT scanners. The recently introduced 3.0-T MRI scanners are producing intravenous gadolinium–enhanced angiographic images that approach the quality of DSA imaging. Both CTA and magnetic resonance angiography (MRA) lack the isolated vascular imaging characteristics of selective catheter DSA, which can sometimes be very important to vascular diagnosis. The combination of good image quality, low or no x-ray exposure, ease of image acquisition, and low patient risk inherent in CTA and MRA will reduce the need for catheter diagnostic angiography for many patients. Interventional radiology angiographic procedures will become more important as new embolic and chemotherapy infusion treatments become clinically available.

INTERVENTIONAL RADIOLOGY

Embolization is the most common angiographic type of interventional radiology procedure performed in the spine. Percutaneous biopsy, discectomy, and fusion procedures are not within the scope of this chapter. Indications for embolization include the following:

- Preoperative lesion decompression to facilitate operative resection
- Devascularization to control or avoid excessive operative blood loss
- Palliation of unresectable or advanced lesions

Embolization is not indicated as an alternative to surgery for resectable lesions or in mixed arteriovenous malformations (AVMs) where there is considerable risk of damage to the normal spinal cord.

Various types of material are available for embolization procedures:

- Detachable balloons
- Stainless steel, platinum, or titanium coils
- Particulates such as Gelfoam (Fig. 28.1)
- Polyvinyl alcohol (PVA) foam
- n-Butyl cyanoacrylate (n-BCA)
- Ethanol
- Embosphere microspheres (Biosphere Medical, Rockland, MA)

The choice of embolic agent is based on the lesion to be treated and the desired therapeutic effect. A detailed discussion of the choice of embolization materials is beyond the scope of this chapter. When embolization is being undertaken as a primary treatment or for palliation, permanent agents such as PVA, microspheres, and coils are often used. For preoperative bleeding control, particulate Gelfoam has

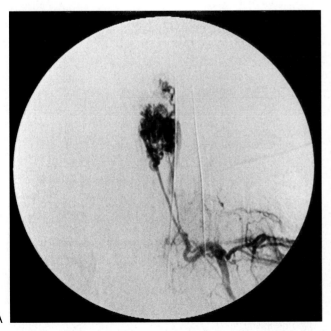
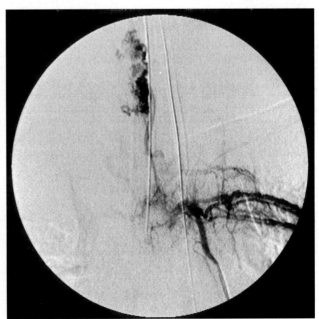

A

B

FIG. 28.1. A 30-year-old woman with an arteriovenous malformation (AVM). **A:** Selective left vertebral artery injection reveals an AVM arising from the left vertebral artery. **B:** After embolization with Gelfoam particles, the AVM shows a decrease in size.

been extensively used in Osaka. Good control of bleeding is obtained when surgery occurs within 48 to 72 hours after Gelfoam embolization. No adverse effects on the spinal cord have occurred in Osaka using Gelfoam. Embolization has been ineffective for controlling venous vascular plexus bleeding in the spinal canal.

Selective catheterization chemotherapy infusion treatment for head and neck cancers has shown patient benefit. This selective infusion permits a much higher local dose of chemotherapy than could be systemically tolerated by the patient. These infusion treatments are often performed in conjunction with either surgery or radiation therapy. Similar infusion chemotherapy for primary and metastatic vertebral body tumors may become available in the future.

COMPLICATIONS OF ARTERIOGRAPHY

The best available data on angiography complications come from the cerebral angiography literature. Variations in patient populations studied and the use of different definitions for complications make direct comparison between published series difficult. Major angiographic complications include death, permanent neurologic deficit, and arterial occlusion requiring surgery or thrombolysis. Minor complications include transient neurologic deficit, hematoma, and urticaria. One well-documented series of 5,000 catheter angiography procedures by Mani and associates (7) reported a 0.16% major complication rate. Another series, reported by Bradoc and Oberson (8), described a 0.13% major complication rate in 6,000 studies performed from 1971 to 1978 and a 0.02% major complication rate in 1,500 studies performed from 1978 to 1982. This improvement was attributed to better patient selection and increased experience with angiography. Minor complications occurred in the range of 1% to 4% in these studies. Risk factors predisposing to complications include long procedure times, large contrast doses, angiographer inexperience, large catheters, and multiple catheter exchanges. Patients with advanced cerebrovascular occlusive disease, recent stroke, subarachnoid hemorrhage, migraine, and posttraumatic and postoperative conditions tended to have more complications.

The angiogram should be discontinued immediately whenever a neurologic complication is identified. Embolization of atherosclerotic debris or thrombi formed on the catheter or an intimal flap due to catheter trauma to the vessel are the most common causes of neurologic deficit. Contrast neurotoxicity is a much rarer cause. Anticoagulation therapy may be helpful when an intimal flap occurs, but it is of no proven benefit with atherosclerotic debris embolization. Thrombi can sometimes be successfully treated with intravascular thrombolysis.

Angiographic complications can be minimized by careful patient preparation and monitoring, meticulous attention to technique, and prudent judgment by the angiographer regarding selective catheterization. There is no substitute for the availability of good angiographic equipment and an experienced angiographic team when performing spinal angiographic procedures.

NORMAL VASCULAR ANATOMY

The blood supply of the spinal cord is categorized by the major feeding vessels to the anterior spinal artery. Three broad territories are defined: cervical, thoracic, and thoracolumbar (Fig. 28.2). The cervical territory is supplied by the paired anterior spinal arteries arising from the fourth portion of the vertebral arteries, which then join to form a single midline anterior spinal artery. Additional blood supply arises from radicular branches of the vertebral artery, which usually accompany the C3 spinal nerve root; from one or more radicular arteries arising from the deep cervical artery at C6; and from radicular arteries de-

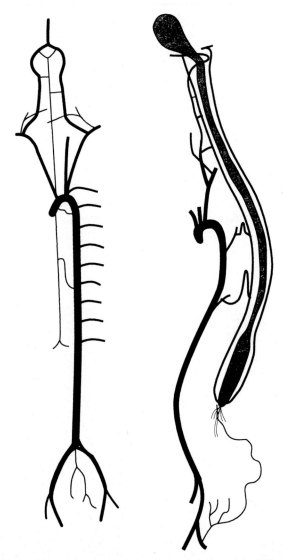

FIG. 28.2. Anteroposterior **(left)** and lateral **(right)** diagrams of the blood supply to the spinal cord. Note the multiple cervical feeders from vertebral and costocervical arteries. There is a single thoracic feeder at T5 and a large artery of Adamkiewicz at T9. Note the anastomotic loop around the conus. (Modified from Doppman JL. Spinal angiography. In: Abrams HL, ed. *Angiography,* 3rd ed. Boston: Little, Brown, 1983.)

rived from the costocervical trunk that accompany the C8 spinal nerve root. A radicular artery also may arise from the ascending cervical artery of the thyrocervical trunk.

The thoracic segment includes the T1 to T7 neurologic levels and is generally perfused by a single dominant radiculomedullary artery arising at T4 or T5. The thoracic anterior spinal artery is smaller than in the cervical or thoracolumbar areas, and angiographic discontinuities are not unusual. It provides blood flow to the adjacent regions only when pathologic conditions are present.

The thoracolumbar territory consists of T8 to the conus. The artery of Adamkiewicz is a large radiculomedullary feeder that arises between T8 and L2 85% of the time, but it occasionally occurs as high as T5. It gives off both cephalad and caudal branches to the anterior spinal artery. It is characterized by a hairpinlike turn before it joins the anterior spinal artery. Disruption of this artery produces a profound paraplegia. The artery of Adamkiewicz arises on the left in 80% of patients. In the cervical and thoracic territories, the radiculomedullary vascular levels are fairly constant, but their side of origin will vary.

The posterior spinal arteries are paired vessels lying on the back surface of the spinal cord medial to the posterior nerve root origins from the cord. They are formed by ascending and descending branches of the posterior radiculomedullary arteries. These arteries parallel the spinal nerve roots and arise in a sequential fashion defined by the vertebral segments.

The blood flow in the spinal cord is bidirectional (Fig. 28.3). Cephalad and caudal flow is governed by local hemodynamic conditions. The venous drainage of the spinal cord follows a segmental pattern that mirrors the arterial anatomy. Radiculomedullary veins from the spinal cord drain into the epidural and paravertebral venous network.

The blood supply of the vertebral column follows the bony segmentation pattern. Branches of local major arteries give rise to radicular arteries, which then provide branches to the vertebral bodies and paraspinal soft tissues as well as the spinal cord (Fig. 28.4). Generous anastomotic vascular

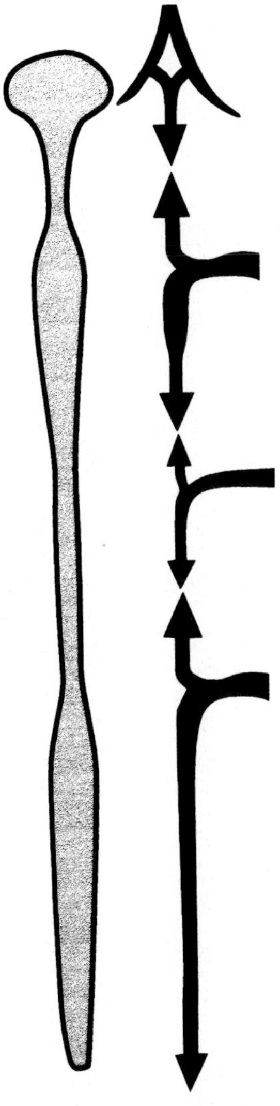

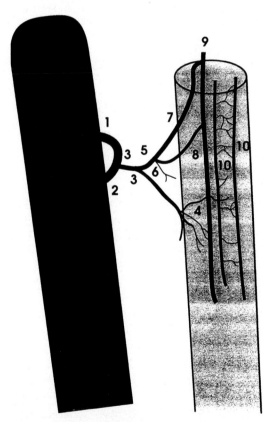

FIG. 28.3. This diagram depicts the bidirectional blood flow along the anterior spinal artery. (Modified from Doppman JL. Spinal angiography. In: Abrams HL, ed. *Angiography,* 3rd ed. Boston: Little, Brown, 1983.)

FIG. 28.4. An idealized drawing of the anterior and posterior radiculomedullary feeders from an intercostal artery: (1) intercostal artery, (2) anterior branch, (3) posterior branch, (4) muscular branch, (5) artery to spinal cord, (6) ganglionic branch, (7) anterior radiculomedullary branch, (8) posterior radiculomedullary branch, (9) anterior spinal artery, (10) posterior spinal artery. (Modified from Doppman JL. Spinal angiography. In: Abrams HL, ed. *Angiography,* 3rd ed. Boston: Little, Brown, 1983.)

TABLE 28.1. *Guide for the Selection of the Appropriate Vessel for Angiography*

Level	Spinal cord	Spine and surrounding tissues
Cervicodorsal region (C1–T2 segments)[a]	1. Vertebral a. Basilar a. Anterior spinal a. Radicular a. accompanying the C3 nerve root 2. Vertebral a. or deep cervical a. radicular a. accompanying the C6 nerve root (artery of the cervical enlargement)[b] 3. Costocervical trunk or 1st intercostal a. radicular a. accompany the C8 nerve root	1. Thyrocervical trunk ascending cervical a. 2. Costocervical trunk deep cervical a. 3. Segmental branches of the vertebral a. 4. 1st intercostal a.
Middorsal region (T1–T7 segments)[c]	Intercostal a.; radicular a. accompanying T4 or T5 nerve root	1. Costocervical trunk 2. Intercostal a.

Dorsolumbosacral region (T8 to conus terminalis)	1. Intercostal a. or lumbar a. arteria radicularis anterior magna (Adamkiewicz) accompanying a nerve root between T9-L2
	2. One or two arteries accompanying the filaments of the cauda equina
	    Lumbar a.
	    Iliolumbar a.
	    Middle and lateral sacral a.
		1. Intercostal a. or lumbar a.
		2. Iliolumbar a.
		3. Middle and lateral sacral a. superior gluteal a. or hypogastric a.

[a]The C1–C4 segments are unique in blood supply; they are supplied by the anterior spinal artery and generally have little or no radicular inflow. The artery is originally supplied by the suboccipital anastomotic confluence formed by the anastomosis of the vertebral, the occipital, and the ascending and deep cervical arteries. The atlantoaxial complex is supplied by the medial branch of the vertebral artery arising from the C3 segment, the anastomotic derivatives of the carotid artery, and a number of direct branches of the vertebral artery that arches over the posterior arch of the atlas (Lazorthes et al., 1958; Lazorthes et al., 1973; Lazorthes et al., 1971; and Parke, 1975).
[b]Lazorthes 1958.
[c]T1, T2 segments are supplied by the extension of the anterior spinal artery of the cervical enlargement.

connections between adjacent spinal segments are common. Except at their outer margins, the disc spaces are nearly avascular.

A knowledge of the normal vascular anatomy is critical to performing the appropriate angiographic procedure. Table 28.1 is a guide to vessel selection based on Djiandjian's study of the blood supply of the spinal cord (2) and Parke's study of the nutrient arteries of the spinal column (9). The work of Lazorthes (10) and Dommisse (11) differs slightly in detail from what is presented in Table 28.1.

PATHOLOGICAL ANGIOGRAPHIC FINDINGS

Before the advent of computed tomography (CT), MRI, and improved percutaneous biopsy and cytology tech-

niques, angiography was used as a primary diagnostic tool in the spine more than it is today. In the past, attempts were made to classify tumors as benign or malignant by angiographic criteria (Table 28.2). Malignant tumors tend to manifest hypervascularity (Fig. 28.5), with a prolonged tumor blush or stain that persists well into the venous phase of the study (Fig. 28.6). Arteriovenous shunting with associated large draining veins occurs in some malignant lesions. Rapidly growing malignant tumors display bizarre, irregular, tangled vessels (Fig. 28.7). Sinusoidal collections of contrast, called *blood pools*, also may be present. Unfortunately, some benign tumors exhibit one or more of these angiographic findings, making confident differentiation by angiographic criteria possible in only about 70% of cases. As stated earlier, the appropriate

TABLE 28.2. *Principal Abnormalities and Their Incidence in Selective Angiography of Spine Tumors, Tumorous Conditions and Spinal Cord Tumor*

	No. of patients	Deviation (%)	Hypervascularity (%)	Tumor vessel (%)	Tumor stain (%)	Dilatation (%)
Malignant spine tumor	27	21 (77.8)	18 (66.7)	25 (92.6)	25 (92.6)	18 (66.7)
Primary	7	5 (71.4)	6 (85.7)	6 (85.7)	6 (85.7)	4 (57.1)
Metastatic	20	16 (80.0)	12 (60.0)	19 (95.0)	19 (95.0)	14 (70.0)
Benign spine tumor, tumorous condition	12	6 (50.0)	5 (41.7)	8 (66.7)	8 (66.7)	4 (33.3)
Spinal cord tumor	6	5 (83.3)	3 (33.3)	2 (33.3)	2 (33.3)	2 (33.3)

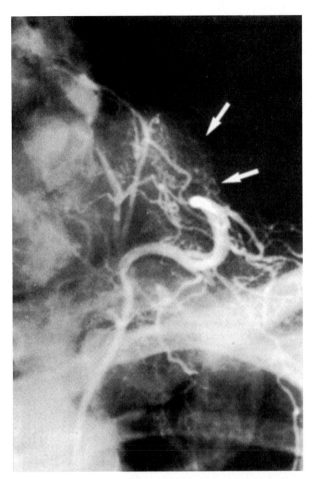

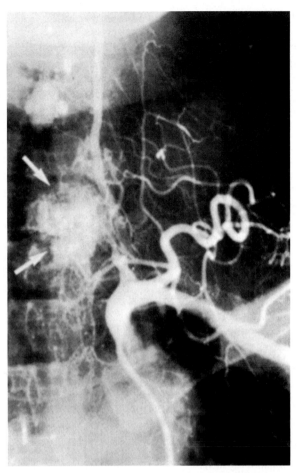

FIG. 28.5. Selective angiography of a 40-year-old woman with osteosarcoma involving the C4 to C7 vertebrae. Note the hypervascularity, tumor stain, and typical tumor vessels (*arrows*) suggesting malignancy, mainly in the territory of the left thyrocervical artery.

FIG. 28.7. Angiography of a 58-year-old woman with a renal cancer metastasis affecting the C7 vertebra. Note the hypervascularity, tumor stain, and tumor vessels, mainly in the territory of the thyrocervical artery.

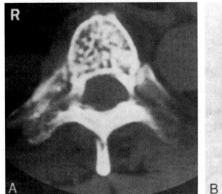
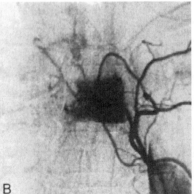
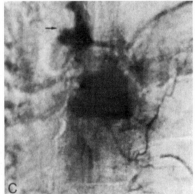

FIG. 28.6. A 59-year-old man with hemangioendothelioma in the T6 vertebra. **A:** Computed tomography shows polka-dot densities in the vertebral body, lytic changes of the transverse processes and ribs, and surrounding soft tissue masses between the pleura and vertebral body. **B:** Note marked hypervascularity, tumor vessels, and tumor stain, fed mainly by the left sixth intercostal artery in the arterial phase. **C:** Further tumor stain was visualized in the adjacent proximal area in the arteriovenous phase (*arrow*).

role for angiography of tumors today is either as a pre-operative planning procedure or as part of an embolization procedure.

The identification and characterization of AVMs and fistulae remains the most widely accepted indication for angiography of the spinal cord. These vascular lesions involve the rapid shunting of blood from the arterial to the venous system without passage through a capillary bed. Arterial blood is thus present in the venous system. Both the involved arteries and veins tend to enlarge because of the high volume flow that occurs. Usually, AVMs are more prominent on the dorsal side of the spinal cord than on the ventral surface. These rare lesions are more frequent in the thoracic than the cervical spinal cord. The term *nidus* is used to describe the focal portion of the AVM where the actual abnormal connection exists. The goal of angiography is to map the involved vessels and precisely identify the nidus. Embolization therapy is sometimes possible as well.

Doppman and associates (5) proposed classifying AVMs into three morphologic types (Fig. 28.8):

1. Type 1 AVMs are characterized by one or two tightly coiled continuous vessels spread along a large longitudinal section of the spinal cord.
2. Type 2 AVMs have a localized plexus or aggregation of vessels into which single or multiple arterial feeders converge and from which one or several draining veins depart. The draining veins can be quite long, extending all the way up to the endocranium or down to the pelvic vessels.
3. Type 3 AVMs have multiple large arterial feeders supplying voluminous malformations that often appear to fill the spinal canal. These are more common in children.

Vasoocclusive disease of the spinal cord is now rarely studied with angiography. Atherosclerotic vascular disease may cause blockage of radicular vessels. Spinal fracture and dislocation, infection, spinal surgery, and thoracic or abdominal aorta surgery can damage the blood supply of the spinal cord. The resulting spinal cord infarction is more readily demonstrated by MRI because of associated spinal cord edema. In such cases, the patient experiences a major neurologic deficit.

Hemangioblastoma is a highly vascular tumor that can occur in the brain or spinal cord. It may be associated with a spinal cord cyst (Fig. 28.9). By angiography, it can closely resemble an AVM; preoperative vascular mapping is occasionally warranted for these tumors. With the possible exception of hemangioblastoma, today angiography has virtually no role in the evaluation of spinal cord tumors. For spinal cord tumor assessment, MRI is vastly superior to angiography and is the procedure of choice for most patients in whom a spinal cord lesion is clinically suspected.

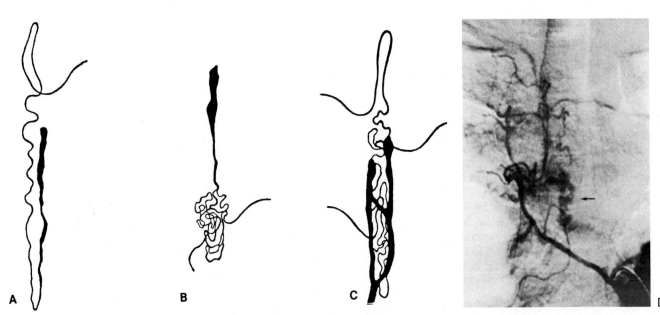

FIG. 28.8. Schematic representation **(A, B, C)** and photograph **(D)** of three types of spinal cord arteriovenous malformations. **A:** Type 1, plain arteriovenous fistula. **B:** Type 2, glomus. **C:** Type 3, juvenile. **D:** A 53-year-old woman with type 1 arteriovenous malformation. The nidus is indicated by an arrow. (Reprinted with permission from Doppman JL, Di Chiro G, Ommaya AK. Percutaneous embolization of spinal cord arteriovenous malformations. *J Neurosurg* 1971;34:48.)

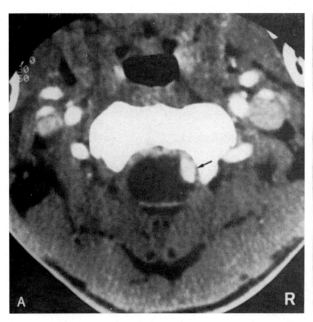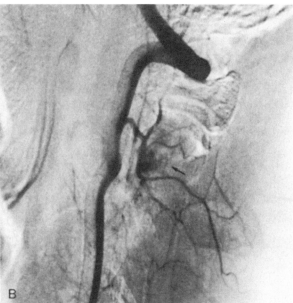

FIG. 28.9. A 29-year-old man with hemangioblastoma at the C2 and C3 level of the spinal cord. **A:** Enhanced computed tomography shows a high-intensity lesion in the spinal cord in association with syringomyelia (*arrow*). **B:** Selective angiography via the left vertebral artery shows hypervascularity and tumor stain (*arrow*).

ACKNOWLEDGMENT

We thank Mrs. Jane Shaeffer for her assistance with manuscript preparation and our families for their emotional support throughout this project.

REFERENCES

1. Abrams HL, ed. *Angiography,* 3rd ed. Boston: Little, Brown, 1983.
2. Djindjian R, Hurst M, Houdart R. *Langiographic de la moelle epinere.* Baltimore: University Park Press, 1970.
3. Djindjian R, Cophignon J, Heron J, et al. Embolization by superselective arteriography from the femoral route in neuroradiology: review of 60 cases. 1. Technique indications, complications. *Neuroradiology* 1973;6:20.
4. Doppman JL, Di Chiro G, Ommaya AK. *Selective arteriography of the spinal cord.* St. Louis: Warren H. Green, 1969.
5. Doppman JL, Di Chiro G, Ommaya AK. Percutaneous embolization of spinal cord arteriovenous malformations. *J Neurosurg* 1971;34:48.
6. Doppman JL. Spinal angiography. In: Abrams HL, ed. *Angiography,* 3rd ed. Boston: Little, Brown, 1983.
7. Mani RL, Eisenberg RL, McDonald EJ Jr, et al. Complications of catheter cerebral angiography: analysis of 5000 procedures. I. Criteria and incidence. *Am J Roentgenol* 1978;131:861–865.
8. Bradoc GM, Oberson R. *Angiography and computed tomography in cerebro-arterial occlusive diseases,* 2nd ed. New York: Springer-Verlag, 1982.
9. Parke WW. Applied anatomy of the spine. In: Rothman RH, Simeone FA, eds. *Spine,* vol. 19. Philadelphia: WB Saunders, 1975:52.
10. Lazorthes G. La vascularisation arterielle de la moelle: recherches anatomiques et application a la pathologie medullaire et a la pathologie aortique. *Neurochirurgie* 1958;4:3.
11. Dommisse GF. *The arteries and veins of the human spinal cord from birth.* Edinburgh: Churchill Livingstone, 1975.

SUGGESTED READING

Atkinson JLD, Miller GM, Krauss WE, et al. Clinical and radiographic features of dural arteriovenous fistula, a treatable cause of myelopathy. *Mayo Clin Proc* 2001;76:1120–1130.
Beaujeux R, Laurent A, Wassef M, et al. Trisacryl gelatin microspheres for therapeutic embolization. II. Preliminary clinical evaluation in tumors and arteriovenous malformations. *Am J Neuroradiol* 1996;17:541–548.
Bemporad JA, Sze G. Magnetic resonance imaging of spinal cord vascular malformations with an emphasis on the cervical spine. *Neuroimaging Clin N Am* 2001;11:111–129.
Bettmann MA, Morris TW. Recent advances in contrast agents. *Radiol Clin North Am* 1986;24:347.
Biondy K, Merland JJ, Hodes JE, et al. Aneurysms of spinal arteries associated with intermedullary arteriovenous malformations 1, 2. *Am J Neuroradiol* 1992;13:913.
Di Chiro G, Wener L. Angiography of the spinal cord: a review of contemporary techniques and applications. *J Neurosurg* 1973;39:1.
Dick HM, Bigliani Lu, Michelsen WJ, et al. Adjuvant arterial embolization in the treatment of benign primary bone tumors in children. *Clin Orthop* 1979;139:133.
Do HM, Jensen ME, Cloft HJ, et al. Dural arteriovenous fistula of the cervical spine presenting with subarachnoid hemorrhage. *Am J Neuroradiol* 1999;20:348–350.
Erdmann MWH, Davies DM, Jackson JE, et al. Multidisciplinary approach to the management of head and neck arteriovenous malformations. *Ann R Coll Surg Engl* 1995;77:53–59.
Eskridge JM. Interventional neuroradiology. *Radiology* 1989;172:991.
Feldman F, Casarella WJ, Digk HM, et al. Selective intra-arterial embolization of bone tumors. A useful adjunct in the management of selected lesions. *Am J Roentgenol Radium Ther Nucl Med* 1975;128:180.
Gonzalez CF. The nervous system. In: Schwarz ED, ed. *The radiology of complications in medical practice.* Baltimore: University Park Press, 1984:1.
Gonzales CF, Doan HT, Han SS, et al. Extracranial vascular angiography. *Radiol Clin North Am* 1986;24:419.

Goyal M, Willinsky R, Montanera W, et al. Paravertebral arteriovenous malformations with epidural drainage: clinical spectrum, imaging features, and results of treatment. *Am J Neuroradiol* 1999;20:749–755.

Hida K, Iwasaki Y, Goto K, et al. Results of the surgical treatment of perimedullary arteriovenous fistulas with special reference to embolization. *J Neurosurg* 1999;90(Suppl 4):198–205.

Hilal SK, Keim HA. Selective spinal angiography in adolescent scoliosis. *Radiology* 1972;102:349.

Hilal SK, Michelsen JW. Therapeutic percutaneous embolization for extraaxial vascular lesions of the head, neck, and spine. *J Neurosurg* 1975;43:275.

Hoffman MG, Gomes AS, Pais SO. Limitations in the interpretation of intravenous carotid digital subtraction angiography. *Am J Roentgenol* 1984;142:261.

Lazorthes G, Gouaze A, Djindjian R. *Vascularisation et pathologie vasculaire de la moelle epiniere*. Paris: Masson, 1973.

Lazorthes G, Gouaze A, Zaden JD, et al. Arterial vascularization of the spinal cord: recent studies of the anastomotic substitution pathways. *J Neurosurg* 1971;35:253.

Leopoine J, Montaut J, Picard L, et al. Embolization prealabel a lexerese dum hemangiome du rachis dorsal. *Neurochirurgie* 1973;19:173.

Newton T, Adams JE. Angiographic demonstration and nonsurgical embolization of spinal cord angioma. *Radiology* 1968;91:873.

Patel D, Grothers O, Harris WH, et al. Arterial embolization for radical tumor resection. *Acta Orthop Scand* 1977;48:353.

Pia HW, Djindjian R. *Spinal angiomas*. Berlin: Springer-Verlag, 1978.

Robb GP, Steinberg I. Visualization of the heart, the pulmonary circulation and the great blood vessels in man: a practical approach. *Am J Roentgenol* 1939;41:1.

Seeger JF, Carmody RF. Digital subtraction angiography of the arteries of the head and neck. *Radiol Clin North Am* 1985;23:193.

Seldinger S. Catheter replacement of the needle in percutaneous arteriography: a new technique. *Acta Radiol* 1953;139:368.

Van Dijk JM, TerBrugge KG, Willinsky RA, et al. Multidisciplinary management of spinal dural arteriovenous fistulas: clinical presentation and long-term follow-up in 49 patients. *Stroke* 2002;33:1578–1583.

Westphal M, Koch C. Management of spinal dural arteriovenous fistulae using an interdisciplinary neuroradiological/neurosurgical approach: experience with 47 cases. *Neurosurgery* 1999;45:451–457; discussion 457–458.

Widlus DM, Murray RR, White RI Jr, et al. Congenital arteriovenous malformations: tailored embolotherapy. *Radiology* 1988;169:511–516.

Willinsky RA, Terbrugge K, Montanera W, et al. Spinal epidural arteriovenous fistulas: arterial and venous approaches to embolization. *Am J Neuroradiol* 1993;14:812.

Yonezawa M, Naruse A. *Spinal angiography* [in Japanese]. Osaka, Japan: Shering, 1978.

CHAPTER 29

Clearing the Cervical Spine in Trauma Patients

Ronald W. Lindsey and Zbigniew Gugala

An accurate assessment of the cervical spine is one of the highest priorities in the initial evaluation of trauma patients who present to an emergency center (EC). In the United States, approximately 10,000,000 patients present annually for trauma care; in all of these patients, the possibility of a cervical spine injury must be considered (1). Cervical spine injury has been estimated to occur in 1% to 3% of all blunt trauma patients (2–4), although these projections can vary depending on the injury mechanism. In major motor vehicle accidents, a major cervical spine injury has been reported for every 300 victims; if the occupant has been ejected from the automobile, a severe cervical spine injury was noted to occur for every 14 victims (5). Past literature has demonstrated that 33% of cervical spine injury patients could suffer a delay in either diagnosis or treatment if not appropriately evaluated (6).

The liberal use of plain radiography has historically been accepted as the routine modality for emergency cervical spine evaluation in the trauma patient (7). Many physicians have become solely dependent upon screening cervical radiography, almost to the exclusion of establishing clinical parameters for cervical spine injury or developing valid clinical indicators for obtaining these imaging studies. The most common etiology of missed cervical spine injury has not been failure to obtain x-rays, but the clinician's willingness to accept roentgenograms that are inadequate or inconclusive, and/or the clinician's failure to interpret the x-rays correctly (8). In the United States, it is estimated that approximately 800,000 cervical spine radiographic examinations are annually performed in the EC for patients with blunt trauma (9). This liberal use of x-rays produces a large number of predominantly normal or inadequate cervical spine x-rays, creates frequent delays in the patient's emergency workup and subsequent treatment, and results in enormous costs in both personnel time and institutional resources (10–12). Additionally, both the patient and the physician are often subjected to unnecessary radiation exposure (9,13).

Despite the numerous problems associated with indiscriminate plain radiography in the trauma setting, this practice has been difficult to restrict. Although the history and physical examination are integral components of the cervical spine evaluation, among physicians there is no consensus on how to prioritize the impact of these clinical components on the diagnostic process. When cervical spine injury is missed or its treatment delayed, subsequent patient morbidity can be devastating, and the cost to society enormous. Finally, for many physicians the potential liability for a missed cervical spine injury more than justifies routine x-ray imaging.

Because of the very low prevalence of positive x-ray findings, the clearance process is extremely inefficient when it is solely dependent on radiography. In a retrospective review of routine cervical spine radiography obtained in 1,686 consecutive trauma patients, Lindsey and associates (14) identified only 32 patients (1.9%) with cervical spine injuries. Moreover, the majority of the cervical spine injuries detected were nonthreatening to the patient's spinal stability or neurologic integrity. These findings suggest that the concept of a specific clinical protocol to better select patients who warrant imaging has enormous merit. The perils of nonselective cervical imaging have been best expressed by Vandemark (15), who stated that "the impact of unnecessary or overly exhaustive cervical spine examinations on patients in the Emergency Department should not be trivialized, and indiscriminate ordering practices must be prevented."

This chapter explores the complex and controversial topic of clearing the cervical spine in trauma patients. Among the issues addressed are (a) the definition of cervical spine clearance, (b) its objectives, (c) which clinical and diagnostic factors determine clearance, (d) which patients must be cleared, and (e) determining acceptable costs of time and resources for the clearance process to be both efficient and accurate. The components of cervical spine clearance are also reviewed to determine the merits of and indications for plain radiography, dynamic imaging, computed tomography (CT), or magnetic resonance imaging (MRI). Finally, existing cervical spine clearance guidelines are analyzed. Although these guidelines have yet to be validated, the pertinent components of each management protocol are synthesized by the authors into a new comprehensive cervical spine clearance algorithm. Although 100% sensitivity is theoretically the ultimate objective, this new algorithm recognizes that the maximum efficiency of a practical guideline may never realize this level of sensitivity.

CLEARANCE

The overwhelming majority of blunt trauma victims presenting to an EC do not have a cervical spine injury. Among the 34,069 patients prospectively analyzed by the National Emergency X-Radiography Utilization Study (NEXUS), cervical spine injury was not present in 33,251 (97.6%) patients (9). To reliably and effectively identify the patients who are injury free, the phrase *clearance of the cervical spine* has recently been introduced to emergency medicine. *Clearance* can be defined as the determination of the absence of cervical spine injury in a particular patient when cervical injury does not exist. The emphasis of clearance is placed on ruling out the presence of injury, but not its precise detection, diagnosis, or classification. Clearance is achieved through a thorough clinical evaluation and those acute adjunctive imaging modalities that are necessary to reliably and efficiently exclude the presence of cervical spine injury. Definitive confirmation of the absence of injury establishes clearance and terminates the cervical spine clearing process.

Cervical spine clearance can only be achieved when the clinician is able to perform a thorough clinical examination. Therefore, the first priority in the clinical assessment of the cervical spine is to determine the patient's level of alertness. For patients with impaired levels of consciousness, the clinical evaluation is inconclusive. Despite all imaging studies being negative for injury, these patients should remain uncleared until they become fully alert. Based on these principles, all blunt trauma patients presenting to the EC with suspected cervical spine injury can be categorized into three major groups:

1. *Patient group I:* Patients who can reliably be cleared by clinical examination without the need for any imaging studies. To qualify for this category, patients must meet all five of the following criteria: (a) full alertness, (b) the absence of intoxication, (c) no midline tenderness, (d) no focal neurologic deficit, and (e) no major distracting injury. Distracting injury is defined as any major injury above the shoulder girdle or any long bone fractures, thoracic or lumbar fracture, pelvic fracture, severe soft tissue injures, or peritonitis (2). Hoffman and colleagues (9) from the NEXUS group prospectively validated these five criteria, and their combined sensitivity approached 99.6%.
2. *Patient group II:* Patients who can be acutely cleared when diagnostic imaging is combined with the clinical examination in the evaluation process. This group includes all the patients who are alert and nonintoxicated but fail one or more of the remaining three clinical criteria. Negative imaging studies are necessary to clear these patients.
3. *Patient group III:* Patients who cannot be cleared at the time of EC presentation. Definitive clearance is not feasible in this group due to the patient's medical instability, inability to undergo a reliable clinical examination, or inconclusive results of the initially performed diagnostic studies. The majority of patients in this group present with an impaired level of consciences due to head injury or intoxication, which inhibits the clearance process. Acute imaging in this group can detect obvious cervical injury, but it cannot definitively rule out its presence. Patient group III requires repeat clinical assessment after patients have become fully alert.

Assigning all blunt trauma victims to one of these three patient groups enhances the efficiency of identifying those patients who are free of cervical spine injury.

The inability to clinically clear a patient is not equivalent to the presence of injury, and always requires the use of adjunctive imaging. Unfortunately, most imaging modalities are more sensitive for injury detection than they are specific for its exclusion. Therefore, the true challenge for imaging in clearing of the cervical spine is to enhance specificity without compromising sensitivity.

The specificity of a diagnostic protocol is defined as its ability to rule out the existence of an injury if the injury is not truly present. Assuming that the sensitivity is high, specificity is the major determinant of an efficient clearance protocol. The specificity of recently reported cervical clearance instruments can vary (12.9% for NEXUS; 42.5% for Canadian C-Rule), but all remain very low (9,16). Even small improvements in clearance specificity will substantially improve a protocol's efficiency. The reduction of superfluous or inconclusive studies in a patient population that is mostly injury free is the desired outcome of optimal clearance specificity. Another method for improving specificity is the development of more complex screening algorithms. However, the continued dilemma in cervical spine clearance is how to provide high sensitivity and specificity while remaining useful for clinical practice. Therefore, apart from high sensitivity and specificity, the clearance protocol should include high "sensibility" (17). The sensibility of a clearance protocol is characterized by the inclusion of clinically reasonable assessment parameters; simple, straightforward structure; and ease of application. These qualities determine the protocol's usefulness, and therefore its acceptance among trauma physicians.

PATIENT MANAGEMENT PRIOR TO AND DURING CLEARANCE

Clearance should begin in the EC (18). Prior to the patient's hospital presentation, cervical spine injury precautions should be initiated in all trauma patients and maintained during this prehospital period (19). These precautions include the initial evaluation, resuscitation, immobilization, extrication, and safe transportation of the victim to the EC. Understandably, most trauma patients will present to the EC with some type of temporary cervical immobilization. However, the presence of cervical precautions upon EC presentation is routine; this alone should not affect the clinician's judgment on the appropriate cervical spine assessment of the patient.

Initial cervical spine screening begins with the assignment of each patient to one of the three patient groups following a brief clinical examination. The majority of the published clearance guidelines address the oriented and alert patient (patient groups I and II) (9,16,20–24), whereas in the obtunded patient (patient group III), the initial evaluation protocols are controversial (25–29). In patient group I, reliable clinical clearance of the cervical spine can be achieved for patients presenting without symptoms or a history suggestive of cervical spine injury (2,14,21). In an alert patient who presents with symptoms indicating possible cervical spine injury (patient group II), clearance will require adjunctive imaging that is negative.

Because of its availability and relative low cost, plain radiography is usually the first imaging modality for patients who cannot be cleared solely by clinical assessment (3, 4,7,14,30–33). The effectiveness of plain radiography is dependent on the number and type of views obtained (7), the technical adequacy of the study (8), and the interpretive

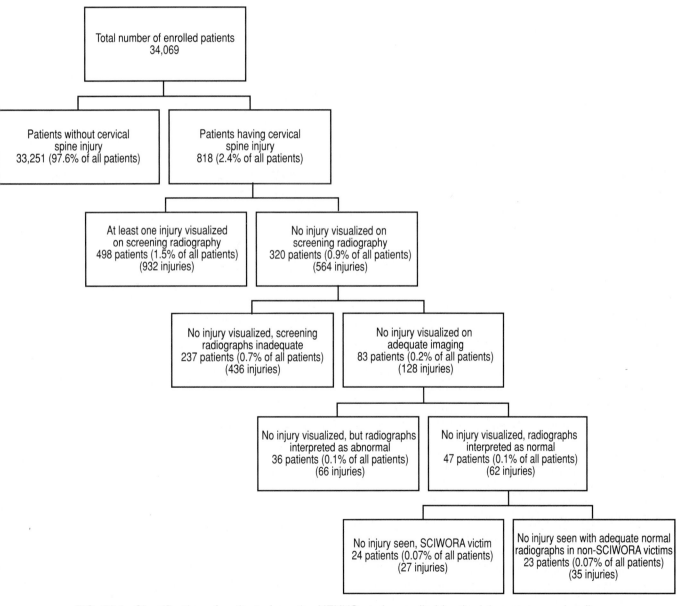

FIG. 29.1. Classification of patients from the NEXUS study enrolled by the injury status and radiographic findings. (Adapted from Mower WR, Hoffman JR, Pollack CV, et al. Use of plain radiography to screen for cervical spine injuries. *Ann Emerg Med* 2001;38:1–7.)

skills of the clinician. It has been suggested that cervical x-rays are not very specific for cervical spine injury, and some clinicians advocate a variety of views or more sophisticated adjunctive imaging. However, Mower and associates (20) from the NEXUS group demonstrated that plain radiography in conjunction with a thorough clinical examination in alert and nonintoxicated patients can result in a very small (0.07%) prevalence of false-negative results (Fig. 29.1).

In patients with impaired consciousness due to head trauma (patient group III), imaging is routinely employed to detect brain injury. Because of the high risk for cervical spine injury in these patients, a CT cervical spine study can be performed along with the CT brain study (21,34).

THE CLINICAL COMPONENTS OF CLEARANCE

History

The EC cervical spine evaluation of the trauma patient begins with a detailed history of the traumatic event. The history should document the nature or mechanism of the patient's injury, and the patient's subjective complaints of discomfort in the cervical spine, head, or upper torso. It is important to document the events immediately following the accident and leading up to the patient's presentation in the EC. A past medical history should identify preexisting cervical spine disorders and their treatment.

The history should provide a clear description of the mechanism of injury. When direct trauma is sustained, it is important to know the energy involved and the direction of its application. If a fall has occurred, the height of the fall should be determined. In the case of a motor vehicle accident, the history must document whether the patient was restrained at the time of the injury.

In a study designed to determine the clinician's ability to clinically predict cervical spine injury, Jacobs and Schwartz (35) identified multiple subjective variables that correlated positively with cervical spine injury (Table 29.1). The most predictive variables included motor vehicle accidents and falls of more than 10 feet. Aspects of the history that correlated less well with cervical spine injury were falls of less than 10 feet, low-energy trauma injury, drugs or alcohol, and loss of consciousness. Although these variables are helpful in establishing the clinician's initial index of suspicion, they are not sufficient to establish the presence or absence of cervical spine injury by themselves.

The first priority in the clinical assessment is to establish the level of the patient's consciousness and whether that level of alertness has been maintained throughout the postinjury period. Clearly, the most complete history is obtained directly from the patient if his or her mental state permits. However, critical details pertaining to the accident can also be obtained from passengers, law enforcement personnel, emergency medical technicians, or witnesses at the scene.

TABLE 29.1. *Variables Positively Correlating with Cervical Spine Injury*

Variable	P value
Motor vehicle accident	0.052
Fall > 10 feet	0.007
Neck tenderness	0.002
Numbness	0.001
Loss of sensation	0.001
Weakness	0.001
Neck spasm	0.001
Loss of muscle power (0–5)	0.001
Decreased sensation	0.001
Loss of anal tone/wink	0.001
Fall < 10 feet	0.083
Low-energy injury	0.700
Drug/alcohol intoxication	0.400
Flexion/extension	0.400
Compression/torsion	0.960
Head trauma	0.370
Neck pain	0.140
Headache	0.140
Loss of consciousness	0.382
Bradycardic hypotension	0.760

(Adapted from Jacobs LM, Schwartz R. Prospective analysis of acute cervical spine injury: a methodology to predict injury. *Ann Emerg Med* 1986;15:44–49.)

Physical Examination

The physical examination can be especially challenging in the emergency setting. A valid physical examination requires that the patient be fully alert and oriented without evidence of intoxication. Ideally, patients should exhibit a class I level of consciousness as defined by Ransohoff and Fleischer (36) (Table 29.2), which requires the patient to be alert, respond immediately to questions, and, although there may be some disorientation or confusion, able to follow complex commands. Any degree of drowsiness, inability to follow simple commands, stupor, or coma would render the physical examination invalid.

TABLE 29.2. *Ransohoff Classification of Consciousness Levels*

Class	Description
I	Alert; responds immediately to questions; may be disoriented and confused; follows complex commands
II	Drowsy, confused, uninterested; does not lapse into sleep when undisturbed; follows simple commands only
III	Stuporous; sleeps when not disturbed; responds briskly and appropriately to noxious stimuli
IV	Deep stupor; responds defensively to prolonged noxious stimuli
V	Coma; no appropriate response to any stimuli; includes decorticate and decerebrate responses
VI	Deep coma; flaccidity; no response to any stimuli

(Adapted from Ransohoff J, Fleischer A. Head injuries. *JAMA* 1975;234:861–864.)

The elements of the physical examination that are major positive predictors for cervical spine injury include neck tenderness, numbness, loss of sensation, weakness, neck spasm, loss of power, decreased sensation, and loss of anal tone/wink. The physical examination for cervical spine injury in trauma patients must also assess for the presence of symptoms attributable to the head and neck and include a thorough, documented neurologic examination. In fact, the presence of any degree of neurologic deficit strongly suggests the possibility of a cervical spine injury until proven otherwise.

The cervical spine examination should determine the patient's neck posture, the presence of focal tenderness, and associated head, face, or neck trauma. The patient is then assessed for full voluntary asymptomatic neck motion in flexion-extension, lateral bending, and rotation. Alternating axial stretching and compressing can be applied to the neck manually through the skull. The presence of a major distracting injury (open fracture, an acute abdomen, or a chest injury) could alter the patient's perception of neck symptoms and invalidate the physical examinations. Clearance in these patients would require a more objective cervical assessment (i.e., imaging) or a delay until consciousness has improved.

In the trauma setting, most clinicians doubt the merits of the history and physical examination as the only screening instrument for cervical spine injury. This concern has been substantiated by studies that demonstrate the clinician's inability to accurately predict cervical spine injury based on the clinical assessment alone (35). This apprehension has been further supported by other reports suggesting the superiority of x-rays over clinical assessment in the clearance process (37). Furthermore, in a review of the clinical presentation of patients with acute cervical spine injury, Walter and colleagues (10) concluded that a cervical spine injury can be more subtle than many clinicians appreciate. In this series, 18% of the patients with cervical spine injury had no complaints of neck pain, a phenomenon that has also been reported by others (38,39).

Ersoy and associates (40) questioned whether mandatory cervical spine x-rays were indicated in all blunt trauma patients and retrospectively demonstrated that radiographs were not necessary in all fully conscious and alert blunt trauma patients who were nonintoxicated, without neurologic deficit, and without neck pain or tenderness. Edwards and colleagues (22) prospectively demonstrated that indiscriminate cervical radiography without clinical indicators resulted in 31% of x-rays being redundant. These authors concluded that using a clinical decision protocol was not only good practice but cost effective.

It appears that the impact of the history and physical examination is primarily dependent on how it is used in the clearance process. Jacobs and Schwartz (35) demonstrated that clinicians were only 11% effective in predicting cervical spine injury using only clinical parameters; the same physicians were 92% effective in determining which patients did not have an injury. The concept that the history and physical examination alone can be exclusively used to clear the cervical spine has had considerable support (9).

In one clinical series it was noted that no alert patients with cervical spine injuries were without symptoms of neck injury, and that therefore the absence of neck symptoms would constitute a reasonable exclusion criterion (41). In another study, Fischer (42) broadened this criterion by demonstrating that no patient with Ransohoff's class I level of consciousness without symptoms of neck pain or tenderness, and without neurologic symptoms attributable to the cervical cord, had sustained a significant cervical spine injury. Lindsey and associates (14) used Fischer's criteria to prospectively evaluate a group of 597 consecutive trauma patients, of whom 17 (2.8%) had suspected cervical spine injury; ultimately, only 5 were true positives. In this series, all false-positive and true-positive patients met Fischer's clinical criteria for radiography, further suggesting that clinical parameters could be used to effectively screen patients.

Therefore, the principal benefit of the history and physical examination in the cervical spine assessment of blunt trauma patients is its ability to identify patients at low risk for cervical spine injury and to permit clearance without other evaluation modalities. Diliberti and Lindsey (30) proposed that while performing the initial history and physical examination, clinicians should not ask the question "Who needs an x-ray?" but instead "Who does not need an x-ray?"

The specificity of the history and physical examination and its use as the only clearance tool has been challenged because of a number of clinical reports of occult cervical spine injury (9,17). These reports often convey the image of patients with cervical spine injury who are alert yet without signs or symptoms of pain or tenderness, who have full cervical spine mobility, and no evidence of neurologic deficit. However, when reviewed more closely, the literature suggests a somewhat different conclusion. Maull and Sachatello (38) suggested that cervical spine injury could be missed in the conscious, sober patient with an otherwise negative history and physical examination, but they fail to document the basis for this conclusion. Bresler and Rich (39) described an occult C4-C5 cervical fracture dislocation in an ambulatory patient who had been ejected from a car. Although the cervical spine injury was thought to be occult, this patient had been drinking prior to the accident, lost consciousness afterward, and was found to have had "mild" tenderness on palpation of the neck. Walter and colleagues (10), in a retrospective review of 67 patients diagnosed with cervical spine injury, reported 12 patients (18%) who had no spontaneous complaints of neck pain in the EC. However, upon closer review, 4 of these patients had tenderness to palpation, and 7 had presented with impaired consciousness (alcohol intoxication, frontal lobe hematoma). Therefore, it seems more accurate to state that the typical report of an "occult" cervical spine injury is not an asymptomatic or unsuspected injury that remains undetected, but rather a symptomatic or suspected injury that is not properly diagnosed.

TABLE 29.3. *Odds Ratios of a Clinical Variable Predicting Clinically Significant Cervical Spine Injury*

Variable	Odds ratio (95% CI)
Dangerous mechanism[a]	5.2 (3.7–7.3)
Age ≥ 65 yr	3.7 (2.4–5.6)
Paresthesias in extremities	2.2 (1.4–3.3)
Ambulatory at any time after injury	1.0 (0.7–1.5)
Sitting position in emergency center	0.61 (0.3–1.2)
Delayed onset of neck pain	0.4 (0.3–0.7)
Absence of midline neck tenderness	0.5 (0.3–0.8)
Able to rotate neck 45 degrees left and right	0.04 (0.01–0.3)
Simple rear-end MVA[b]	0.08 (0.03–0.2)

CI, confidence interval; MVA, motor vehicle accident.

[a]Fall from 1 m or higher; axial load to the head; high-speed MVA, rollover, or ejection; bicycle collision; recreational motorized vehicle collision.

[b]Excludes vehicle pushed into oncoming traffic, hit by bus or large truck, rolled over, or hit by high-speed vehicle; collision.

(Adapted from Stiell IG, Wells GA, Vandemheem KL, et al. The Canadian C-spine Rule for radiology in alert and stable trauma patients. *JAMA* 2001;286:1841–1848.)

The utilization of a purely clinical decision instrument to screen select patients has proven difficult primarily because of the clinician's fear of missing a cervical spine injury. Yet, despite this anxiety, clinicians will tend to accept a technically inadequate x-ray; this has been shown to be the single most common cause for missed injuries (8). Clearly, the solution is to carefully select clinical indicators that can be scientifically validated and then appropriately applied. Recently, the NEXUS group (9) prospectively established five clinical criteria that could obviate the need for cervical x-rays in trauma patients: (a) normal alertness, (b) no intoxication, (c) the absent of midline cervical tenderness, (d) no neurologic deficit, and (e) no painful distracting injury. After reviewing 34,069 patients, this clinical decision instrument identified all but 8 of the 818 patients with cervical spine injury, with a sensitivity approaching 99.6%. The missed 0.4% consisted of 2 patients who were falsely identified as injury free using these criteria: One had insignificant injury that healed untreated; the second presented with major injury, but had fracture of the clavicle that could be defined as a distracting injury. Using this decision instrument, radiography could have been avoided in 4,309 (12.6%) of the 34,069 patients studied (9).

An attempt to identify predictive clinical parameters and correlate them with the presence of cervical spine injury was the objective of another multicenter, perspective, cohort study (Canadian C-Rule) (13). Clinical parameters analyzed were similar to those of NEXUS, but also included mechanism of injury (i.e., high-speed MVA, vehicle rollover, passenger ejection, bicycle collision, etc.), patient's age, and presence of parasthasia (Table 29.3). The Canadian C-Rule study predictive criteria were more comprehensive and resulted in 100% sensitivity and 42.5% specificity (3½ times that of NEXUS) (16).

THE IMAGING COMPONENTS OF CLEARANCE

Plain Radiography

Cervical spine clearance of patient group II is dependent on adjunctive imaging. The imaging options include routine radiography, stress flexion-extension radiography, CT, and MRI. In the acute setting, plain radiography is usually employed; although it is readily available, relatively inexpensive, quick, and sensitive for cervical spine injury, there are currently no validated guidelines for its use in trauma patients (16,43).

Patient group II includes trauma victims without pronounced neurologic deficit attributable to the cervical spine. The first x-ray to be obtained is a single cross-table lateral view (CTLV) (3,4,7,30–33). The CTLV alone is considered to be insufficient (7,33,37), although some emergency physicians rely almost exclusively on this view (44). Among patients with cervical spine injury, the sensitivity of the single CTLV ranges from 74% to 86% (7,31–33,45). The major limitation of the CTLV is its inability to delineate the cervicothoracic junction and C1-2 in many patients.

In a retrospective study, Shaffer and Doris (4) reported that 21% of all cervical spine injuries were missed with a CTLV alone. MacDonald and associates (7) not only found that the CTLV missed 16 of 92 cervical spine injuries, but also that in 18 cases the CTLV was falsely read as positive. Currently, the accepted standard consists of a full cervical series (FCS), which includes a CTLV, an anteroposterior open-mouth view (OM), and a complete anteroposterior cervical view (AP) as the minimum views necessary for maximum specificity and sensitivity. Many radiologists also advocate right and left oblique views as part of an FCS.

The efficacy of cervical x-rays is highly dependent on the quality of the views obtained, and emergency cervical radiographs are frequently inadequate. In a study by Davis and colleagues (8), 94% of the errors leading to missed or delayed diagnosis of cervical spine injuries were the result of the failure to simply obtain adequate cervical spine radiographs. Ross and associates (3) reported that a technically adequate FCS could increase the diagnostic accuracy of plain radiography to 100%; if the FCS is not technically adequate, cervical spine clearance cannot occur without additional imaging.

The effectiveness of the radiographic clearance directly correlates with the quality of the imaging study being interpreted. In a series of 740 cervical spine injuries, Davis and colleagues (8) noted that missed or delayed diagnosis occurred in 34 patients (4.6%) due to inadequate or inconclusive x-rays. Other reports suggest that radiographic assessment failed to detect 8% to 20% of cervical spine injuries as a result of technically inadequate studies (27, 46). However, even when x-rays were optimal, a substantial amount of all errors (47%) were due to x-ray misinterpretations by trauma surgeons and EC physicians that were later corrected by radiologists.

Even when the FCS is of adequate quality and properly interpreted, significant cervical spine injuries may occasionally go undetected. Some authors recommend the standard addition of two oblique views to provide better information regarding spinal alignment and the integrity of the facets and pedicles (47,48). The swimmer's view, which provides better visualization of the cervicothoracic junction, has also been suggested (49). However, the practice of using additional x-ray views in the trauma setting leads to escalating costs in time and resources. Freemyer and associates (50) prospectively compared the three-view versus the five-view cervical spine series and noted that the latter did not increase injury detection but allowed for more specific diagnosis. Therefore, for the purposes of screening, the three-view FCS should suffice. If further imaging is still required, more sophisticated modalities are preferred.

Dynamic Radiography

Despite the adequacy of the studies obtained, static cervical spine radiographs may fail to detect an unstable cervical spine injury (20,51). Dynamic lateral flexion-extension views should be considered in alert patients with a negative FCS and persistent pain who can voluntarily perform the study. The efficacy of lateral flexion-extension views in the acute setting is controversial. In a retrospective review, Lewis and colleagues (52) reported that flexion-extension views in the EC detected cervical spine instability in approximately 8% of patients otherwise cleared by FCS. None of these patients experienced adverse neurologic sequelae, and the authors recommended the use of flexion-extension views in the acute setting. On the other hand, the NEXUS group (51,53) reported that flexion-extension films obtained acutely added little to the screening process for the risk involved. Anglen and associates (54) included flexion-extension films in the acute evaluation of 837 trauma patients and concluded that they were not cost effective because they did not detect significant injury that was not detected by other modalities. These authors recommended that other modalities (i.e., MRI, CT) be used in the acute setting and that flexion-extension films be reserved for the delayed setting.

Dynamic Fluoroscopy

Lateral flexion-extension views are indicated in the alert patient with persistent pain and negative static x-rays. Dynamic views, however, are thought to be hazardous in the obtunded patient who is without the normal protective reflexes. In obtunded patients, Cox and associates (55) reported that dynamic fluoroscopy was an effective modality that did not miss injuries and did not compromise the patient's neurologic status. This was further supported by Brooks and Willett (25), who noted that dynamic fluoroscopy was a quick way to identify more subtle cases of cervical spine instability without reported neurologic complications. Sees and associates (56) also reported that fluoroscopy was both safe and effective in the assessment of the cervical spine.

In the acute setting, dynamic fluoroscopy has its detractors as well. Davis and colleagues (57) reported that isolated ligamentous injuries of the cervical spine without fractures are rare, and in their reported series such patients comprised only 0.04% of all trauma patients. In the 2 patients identified with isolated ligamentous injury without fracture, the cervical spine was stable in both and did not require surgical consideration. These authors concluded that routine dynamic lateral flexion-extension imaging was not indicated to clear obtunded trauma patients because its potential risks exceeded any potential benefits.

Computed Tomography

Plain radiographs, static or dynamic, may fail to detect many cervical spine injuries and can also fail to accurately depict the full extent of a cervical spine injury (3,58). CT is indicated in patients who have negative x-rays but continue to have symptoms, in patients with questionable radiographic abnormalities, or in patients with plain radiography depicting prevertebral swelling that can be suggestive of cervical spine trauma.

Woodring and Lee (23) retrospectively reviewed 216 consecutive patients with cervical spine injury who were all evaluated with an FCS and CT. The FCS failed to identify 61% of the fractures and 36% of the subluxations/dislocations. Barba and associates (26) studied a cervical spine clearance protocol that liberally utilized CT. Patients requiring head CT received only a CTLV and then a full cervical spine CT; all other patients received an FCS with selective CT. By using this protocol, these authors demonstrated that the combination of FCS plus CT scanning increased the accuracy of injury detection from 54% to 100%. Schenarts and colleagues (59) reported that CT can be especially effective in providing a thorough evaluation of the upper cervical spine (occiput through C3). In their series of 70 cervical spine injuries in obtunded patients, plain radiography identified only 55% (38 of 70) of these injuries, compared with 96% (67 of 70) of injuries identified with CT. Berne and co-workers (60) found CT to be efficacious in imaging intensive care patients; the sensitivity of x-rays was only 60%, in comparison with 90% for CT scans. In a study of 120 patients, 93% could be cleared within 24 hours by CT without missing a single injury (58).

The disadvantages of CT include its greater expense, increased radiation exposure, and limited availability (compared with plain radiography). Additionally, CT is ineffective in detecting some ligamentous injuries. CT is best utilized in conjunction with plain radiography to increase both the accuracy and the sensitivity of the clearance process (60).

Magnetic Resonance Imaging

Magnetic resonance imaging has proven to be an effective noninvasive imaging tool for the detection of neural, ligamentous, or disc injury. MRI is primarily indicated for those patients who present with neurologic deficit. In this setting, MRI is an effective and safe method for evaluating the spinal cord because it can depict (a) intraaxial hematoma, (b) spinal cord edema, and (c) spinal cord compression; as a result, MRI is preferable to CT in the assessment of trauma patients with neurologic deficit (61). In select cases, MRI can obviate the need for flexion-extension x-rays or prolonged immobilization (62). The ability of MRI to detect soft tissue or ligamentous injury in the early postinjury period has particular clinical appeal. Benzel and associates (61) studied 174 patients with neck symptoms, a negative neurologic exam, and negative FCS. In this group, MRI detected soft tissue injury in 62 patients (36%), including 27 patients with disc disruption and 35 patients with isolated ligamentous injury.

Perhaps the greatest appeal of MRI is its ability to assess for cervical spine injury in the comatose or obtunded trauma patient. MRI is capable of providing sagittal images of the entire cervical spine that include the spinal cord and extradural soft tissue without stressing or manipulating the spine. D'Alise and co-workers (63) obtained MRI in 120 obtunded patients with negative FCS within 24 hours of their injuries. Thirty-one (26%) of these patients demonstrated injury to the paravertebral structures, disc, or bony spine despite negative plain radiography. These authors concluded that MRI is a valuable imaging modality in the assessment of the cervical spine for nonapparent injury.

EXISTING CLEARANCE ALGORITHMS

The abundance of clinical literature on cervical spine clearance in trauma patients is a testimony to the controversial nature of this issue. Although there are no universally accepted guidelines for establishing cervical spine clearance, there is an enormous need for such an algorithm because of the following reasons:

1. The overwhelming majority of trauma patients requiring cervical spine clearance are injury free.
2. The variation in physicians' cervical clearance practices results in an inefficient utilization of EC resources.
3. A scientifically based clearance guideline would minimize the likelihood of a missed cervical spine injury.
4. An accepted standardized algorithm would permit its validation and refinement.
5. A guideline would assist in organizing and directing physicians in a consistent EC cervical spine assessment.

A number of clearance guidelines have been developed due to the lack of a generally accepted algorithm. Many of these guidelines consist of institutional algorithms that are usually tailored to the available resources of a particular institution or patient population and are influenced by the practice bias of a small group of regional physicians. These institutional algorithms typically recommend nonvalidated assessment criteria, permit a wide range of subjective decision making, and are rarely strictly adhered to. The recognition of the shortcomings of institutional algorithms has commenced the vital task of organizing the various clinical and radiographic components of posttraumatic cervical spine assessment. Additionally, the majority of these institutional guidelines initiated the concept of clinical clearance without routine radiography.

A considerable number of clinical studies focus on segments of the clearance problem (e.g., cervical spine clearance of the obtunded patient, or correlation of the mechanism of injury and presence of cervical spine injury) or the efficacy of a single imaging modality used in clearance (e.g., stress views, CT, MRI). The major contribution of these studies is to create the scientific building blocks from which a more comprehensive algorithm can be developed. In recent years, many of these clinical studies have consisted of prospective randomized efforts from which valid conclusions can be derived.

However, the majority of clinical series are small, single-institution series that are poorly controlled. These studies are usually not well coordinated, and many of them focus on the same issues and often produce inconsistent results. Independent studies not only fail to address all of the relevant aspects of the problem, but also fail to provide the comprehensive data necessary to formulate a more meaningful algorithm. In select cases, the clearance issues investigated by these independent studies are only specific to a particular institution.

Recently, well-coordinated, more comprehensive, multicenter, controlled studies have been reported. Some of these studies exist as prospective observational investigations (e.g., NEXUS, Canadian C-spine study), whereas some others exist as a large consensus of expert opinion. Representative of the latter is the metaanalysis for practice management guidelines for trauma from the Eastern Association for the Surgery of Trauma (EAST) (34). Although these guidelines encompass more than simply management of the cervical spine, their recommendations are evidence based and account for geographic variations in practice patterns.

At the time of its publication, the EAST guidelines recognized that there were no class I scientific studies available on cervical spine clearance upon which to recommend treatment (34). These authors utilized existing papers and formulated their recommendations with a panel of experts. The experts addressed the most controversial issues associated with cervical spine clearance, ranging from which patients required x-rays and what views to use to when to employ stress views or more sophisticated imaging (e.g., CT scan). The EAST guidelines incorporated clinical criteria for excluding imaging, specified the minimum number and type of radiographs to be obtained in the indicated patients, established specific criteria for obtaining CT, and recognized the benefit of lateral flexion-extension stress views in select patients. The EAST guidelines also encouraged the prompt use of MRI in all trauma patients in whom neurologic deficit could be documented. The principle disadvantage of these guidelines is their lack of clinical validation.

NEXUS was a 34,069-patient, multicenter, prospective observational study of the correlation of clinical parameters and imaging modalities in the detection of cervical spine injury. The objective of the study was to determine the clinical criteria that could be used for constructing a comprehensive cervical spine clearance protocol. The study provided multiinstitutional epidemiologic data on patients presenting to the EC with suspected cervical spine injuries (64,65). NEXUS confirmed that the majority of blunt trauma patients do not sustain a cervical spine injury, and that clinical criteria could be used to reliably exclude the need for imaging in the screening process (9). NEXUS established that clearance of the cervical spine can be reliably and efficiently achieved based solely on clinical parameters, thereby defining patient group I (9). In the NEXUS study (9), the clinical parameters for all patients were carefully documented, and all patients received an FCS. In 34,069 prospectively studied patients, only 2 patients with cervical spine injury would have been inappropriately excluded from diagnostic imaging using the clinical criteria. One of these patients had a clavicle fracture that could be designated as a distracting injury; the second patient had an acute extension teardrop fracture of C3 that was thought to be a preexisting injury.

The principle disadvantage of NEXUS is that of the 97.3% of injury-free patients, only 12.9% were excluded from imaging by the required clinical criteria. This low specificity for exclusion was due in part to the inability of many of the enrolled patients to meet all of the five clinical criteria. Also, NEXUS was a prospective validation of the preestablished clinical clearance criteria verified with radiography that was applicable to the selected patients presenting to the EC with suspected cervical spine trauma. NEXUS did not include patients with impaired consciousness, or conscious patients presenting with clinical symptoms. The study assessed the efficiency of plain radiographs and noted that 2.3% of cervical spine injuries could not be detected by plain radiography (20). NEXUS also established that flexion-extension radiography is not efficacious in the emergency setting (51,53). It is important to recognize and accept that no practical clinical system can be expected to be 100% effective.

The Canadian C-Rule study (16) was also a large, multicenter, prospective cohort study focused on clinical data and their correlation with cervical spine injury. The principle advantage of the Canadian study was the high specificity (42.5%) of the clinical criteria used as compared with the NEXUS study (12.9%) (Table 29.4). In addition to the inclusion of the clinical parameters reviewed in the NEXUS study (neck pain, neurologic deficit, alertness, and/or distracting injury), the Canadian C-Rule study also incorporated parameters such as dangerous mechanism of injury, axial load to the head, high-speed motor vehicle accident, a motor vehicle rollover or passenger ejection, bicycle and motorcycle accidents, patient age, and paresthesia. The Canadian C-Rule provided comprehensive criteria upon which to make a clinical decision to include or exclude radiographic imaging in the alert, stable trauma patient.

The principle disadvantage of the Canadian C-Rule is that it, too, was not a clinical validation of the clearance guidelines but a prospective observational study to identify predictive clinical parameters. The Canadian C-Rule study identified a set of multiple clinical factors that should be taken into consideration in the clearance of cervical spine injuries without imaging. Despite the complex nature and multiplicity of these clinical criteria, which imposes the

TABLE 29.4. *Comparison of NEXUS and Canadian C-Rule Studies*

Variable	NEXUS	Canadian C-rule
Total patients	34,069	6,185[a]
Positive for cervical injury	818	151
Sensitivity (%)	99.6	100
Specificity (%)	12.9	42.5

[a]Patients who underwent radiographic examination of the cervical spine.

question of their practical usefulness, the Canadian study established that only 42.5% of the enrolled patients could be reliably excluded from radiographic imaging.

THE AUTHORS' ALGORITHM

The authors have compiled a new comprehensive algorithm to direct and organize the process of cervical spine clearance (Fig. 29.2). The algorithm has been formulated from currently available literature on cervical spine clearance with the objective of organizing the process of cervical spine clearance.

The algorithm begins with maintaining a high level of suspicion for cervical spine injury and following the appropriate Advanced Trauma Life Support (ATLS) guideline for initial clinical evaluation. Critical to the clinical assessment of the cervical spine is whether the patient's level of consciousness will permit an accurate history and physical examination. It is important to appreciate that even if x-rays are negative, the cervical spine cannot be reliably cleared until the patient is alert and receptive to an accurate history and physical examination.

If the patient is alert and oriented (patient group I), a comprehensive physical examination can be performed to determine if clinical symptoms are present. In the absence of neck pain, tenderness, neurologic deficit, or a distracting injury, these patients can be fully cleared clinically without the need for imaging.

Imaging is indicated in all patients symptomatic for cervical spine injury (patient group II). Initial cervical spine imaging should consist of three-view cervical spine series. The radiographs must be technically adequate and permit visualization of the entire cervical spine before clearance is achieved; when the plain radiographs are inconclusive or inadequate, a CT of the cervical spine is always indicated.

Patients who present with neurologic deficit require emergent MRI to evaluate the injury and direct appropriate treatment. When clinical symptoms include neck pain or tenderness, or a major distracting injury is present without neurologic deficit, the patient should undergo a standard three-view cervical spine series. If the FCS is negative and the patient's symptoms resolve, clearance is achieved; if the FCS is negative but the patient's symptoms persist, dynamic radiography consisting of lateral flexion-extension stress views or fluoroscopy is indicated. According to this

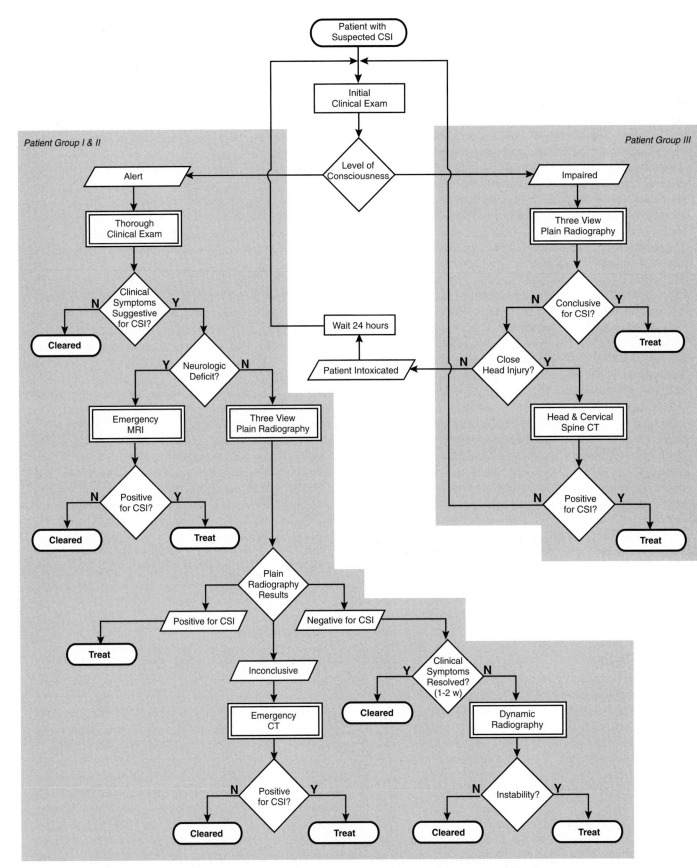

FIG. 29.2. The comprehensive algorithm for clearing the cervical spine proposed by the authors.

guideline, flexion-extension views are not recommended acutely, but preferably 1 to 2 weeks after initial presentation of the patient's persistent symptoms. If dynamic radiography is negative and symptoms remain unresolved, MRI is indicated.

The most difficult patient to complete the clearance process for is one who presents with an impaired level of consciousness (patient group III). Past guidelines have failed to clearly address this subset of patients because of the obvious challenge in providing a thorough workup. In this algorithm, all patients with impaired consciousness should first receive an FCS. If the radiographic assessment is positive for injury, the injury is appropriately treated. However, if the FCS is negative or inconclusive, the clinician must determine the presence or absence of patient intoxication. The intoxicated patient must reenter the beginning of the algorithm until a normal level of consciousness has returned. These patients can only be cleared when they are alert and a reliable physical examination can be performed. In patients with a negative FCS and impaired consciousness due to head trauma, a CT scan of the head with extension to include the cervical spine is warranted. Finally, if the CT is negative, MRI may be appropriate depending on the patient's presentation. If CT and MRI are both negative for injury, these patients still must regain normal consciousness before being cleared.

The inability to establish clearance for whatever reason requires that the patient be treated as if an injury existed. The authors recognize that no algorithm can exhibit 100% sensitivity and be practical for clinical use. The proposed clearance algorithm is comprehensive and straightforward in its ability to address all patient issues. It is based on the existing current scientific evidence, and it minimizes clinician subjectivity or bias in the initial management of trauma patients. Its limitations include a lack of objective clinical validation; although the guidelines for alert patients are supported by the multicenter prospective studies, the management of the patient with impaired alertness is based only upon a consensus of experts' opinions.

REFERENCES

1. Hoffman JR, Schriger DL, Mower W, et al. Low-risk criteria for cervical spine radiography in blunt trauma: a prospective study. *Ann Emerg Med* 1992;21:1454–1460.
2. Velmahos GC, Theodorou D, Tatevosian R, et al. Radiographic cervical spine evaluation in the alert asymptomatic blunt trauma victim: much ado about nothing? *J Trauma* 1996;40:768–774.
3. Ross SE, Schwab CW, David ET, et al. Clearing the cervical spine: initial radiologic evaluation. *J Trauma* 1987;27:1055–1060.
4. Shaffer MA, Doris PE. Limitation of the cross table lateral view in detecting cervical spine injuries: a retrospective analysis. *Ann Emerg Med* 1981;10:508–513.
5. Huelke D, O'Day J, Mandelsohn RA. Cervical injuries suffered in automobile crashes. *J Neurosurg* 1981;54:316–322.
6. Bohlman H. Acute fractures and dislocations of the cervical spine. *J Bone Joint Surg Am* 1979;61:1119–1142.
7. MacDonald RL, Schwartz ML, Mirich D, et al. Diagnosis of cervical spine injury in motor vehicle crash victims: how many x-rays are enough? *J Trauma* 1990;30:392–397.
8. Davis JW, Phreaner DL, Hoyt DB, et al. The etiology of missed cervical spine injuries. *J Trauma* 1993;34:342–346.
9. Hoffman JR, Mower WR, Wolfson AB, et al. Validity of a set of clinical criteria to rule out injury to the cervical spine in patients with blunt trauma. *N Engl J Med* 2000;343:94–99.
10. Walter J, Doris PE, Shaffer MA. Clinical presentation of patients with acute cervical spine injury. *Ann Emerg Med* 1984;13:512–515.
11. Cadoux CG, White JD. High-yield radiographic considerations for cervical spine injuries. *Ann Emerg Med* 1986;15:236–239.
12. Spain DA, Trooskin SZ, Flancbaum L, et al. The adequacy and cost effectiveness of routine resuscitation-area cervical-spine radiographs. *Ann Emerg Med* 1990;19:276–278.
13. Huda W, Bews J. Population irradiation factors (PIFs) in diagnostic medical dosimetry. *Health Phys* 1990;59:345–347.
14. Lindsey RW, Diliberti TC, Doherty BJ, et al. Efficacy of radiographic evaluation of the cervical spine in emergency situations. *South Med J* 1993;86:1253–1255.
15. Vandemark RM. Radiology of the cervical spine in trauma patients: practice pitfalls and recommendations for improving efficiency and communications. *Am J Roentgenol* 1990;155:465–472.
16. Stiell IG, Wells GA, Vandemheen KL, et al. The Canadian C-spine rule for radiography in alert and stable trauma patients. *JAMA* 2001; 286:1841–1848.
17. Stiell IG, Wells GA. Methodologic standards for the development of clinical decision rules in emergency medicine. *Ann Emerg Med* 1999; 33:437–447.
18. Meldon SW, Brant TA, Cydulka RK, et al. Out-of-hospital cervical spine clearance: agreement between emergency medical technicians and emergency physicians. *J Trauma* 1998;45:1058–1061.
19. Soderstrom CA, Brumback RJ. Early care of the patient with cervical spine injury. *Orthop Clin North Am* 1986;17:3–13.
20. Mower WR, Hoffman JR, Pollack CV, et al. Use of plain radiography to screen for cervical spine injuries. *Ann Emerg Med* 2001;38:1–7.
21. Roberge RJ, Wears RC, Kelly M, et al. Selective application of cervical spine radiography in alert victims of blunt trauma: a prospective study. *J Trauma* 1988;28:784–788.
22. Edwards M, Frankema S, Kruit MC, et al. Routine cervical spine radiography for trauma victims: does everybody need it? *J Trauma* 2001; 50:529–534.
23. Woodring JH, Lee C. Limitations of cervical radiography in the evaluation of acute cervical trauma. *J Trauma* 1993;34:32–39.
24. McNamara RM, Heine E, Esposito B. Cervical spine injury and radiography in alert, high-risk patients. *J Emerg Med* 1990;8:177–182.
25. Brooks AR, Willett KM. Evaluation of the Oxford protocol for total spinal clearance in the unconscious trauma patient. *J Trauma* 2001;50: 862–867.
26. Barba CA, Taggert J, Morgan AS, et al. A new cervical spine clearance protocol using computed tomography. *J Trauma* 2001;51:652–657.
27. Gerrelts BD, Petersen EU, Mabry J, et al. Delayed diagnosis of cervical spine injuries. *J Trauma* 1991;31:1622–1626.
28. Chiu WC, Haan JM, Cushing BM et al. Ligamentous injuries of the cervical spine in unreliable blunt trauma patients: incidence, evaluation, and outcome. *J Trauma* 2001;50:457–564.
29. Mirvis SE. Fluoroscopically guided passive flexion-extension views of the cervical spine in the obtunded bunt trauma patient: a commentary. *J Trauma* 2001;50:868–870.
30. Diliberti T, Lindsey RW. Evaluation of the cervical spine in the emergency setting: who does not need an x-ray? *Orthopedics* 1992;15:179–183.
31. Mace SE. Emergency evaluation of cervical spine injuries: CT versus plain radiographs. *Ann Emerg Med* 1985;14:973–975.
32. Harris JH. Radiographic evaluation of spinal trauma. *Orthop Clin North Am* 1986;17:75–86.
33. Kassel EE, Cooper PW, Rubinstein JD. Radiology of spine trauma—practical experience in a trauma unit. *Can Assoc Radiol J* 1983;34: 189–203.
34. Pasquale M, Fabian TC. Practice management guidelines for trauma from the Eastern Association for the Surgery of Trauma. *J Trauma* 1998;44:941–957.
35. Jacobs LM, Schwartz R. Prospective analysis of acute cervical spine injury: a methodology to predict injury. *Ann Emerg Med* 1986;15: 44–49.
36. Ransohoff J, Fleischer A. Head injuries. *JAMA* 1975;234:861–864.

37. Williams CF, Bernstein TW, Jelenko C. Essentiality of the lateral cervical spine radiograph. *Ann Emerg Med* 1981;10:198–204.
38. Maull K, Sachatello C. Avoiding a pitfall in resuscitation: the painless cervical fracture. *South Med J* 1977;70:477–478.
39. Bresler MJ, Rich GH. Occult cervical spine fracture in an ambulatory patient. *Ann Emerg Med* 1982;11:440–442.
40. Ersoy G, Karcioglu O, Enginbas Y, et al. Are cervical spine x-rays mandatory in all blunt trauma patients? *Eur J Emerg Med* 1995;2:191–195.
41. Bachulis BL, Long WB, Hynes GD, et al. Clinical indications for cervical spine radiographs in the traumatized patient. *Am J Surg* 1987;153:473–477.
42. Fischer RP. Cervical radiographic evaluation of alert patients following blunt trauma. *Ann Emerg Med* 1984;13:905–907.
43. Graber MA, Kathol M. Cervical spine radiographs in the trauma patient. *Am Fam Physician* 1999;59:331–342.
44. Gupta KJ, Clancy M. Discontinuation of cervical spine immobilisation in unconscious patients with trauma in intensive care units—telephone survey of practice in south and west region. *BMJ* 1997;314:1652–1655.
45. Blahd WH, Iserson KV, Bjelland JC. Efficacy of the post-traumatic cross table lateral view of the cervical spine. *J Emerg Med* 1985;2:243–249.
46. Reid DC, Henderson R, Saboe L, et al. Etiology and clinical course of missed spine fractures. *J Trauma* 1987;27:980–986.
47. Turetsky DB, Vines FS, Clayman DA, et al. Technique and use of supine oblique views in acute cervical spine trauma. *Ann Emerg Med* 1993;22:685–689.
48. Doris PE, Wilson RA. The next logical step in the emergency radiographic evaluation of cervical spine trauma: the five-view trauma series. *J Emerg Med* 1985;3:371–385.
49. Jenkins MG, Curran P, Rocke LG. Where do we go after the three standard cervical spine views in the conscious trauma patient? A survey. *Eur J Emerg Med* 1999;6:215–217.
50. Freemyer B, Knopp R, Piche J, et al. Comparison of five-view and three-view cervical spine series in the evaluation of patients with cervical trauma. *Ann Emerg Med* 1989;18:818–821.
51. Knopp R, Parker J, Tashjian J, et al. Defining radiographic criteria for flexion-extension studies of the cervical spine. *Ann Emerg Med* 2001;38:31–35.
52. Lewis LM, Docherty M, Ruoff BE, et al. Flexion-extension views in the evaluation of cervical-spine injuries. *Ann Emerg Med* 1991;20:117–121.
53. Pollack CV, Hendey GW, Martin DR, et al. Use of flexion-extension radiographs of the cervical spine in blunt trauma. *Ann Emerg Med* 2001;38:8–11.
54. Anglen J, Metzler M, Bunn P, et al. Flexion and extension views are not cost-effective in a cervical spine clearance protocol for obtunded trauma patients. *J Trauma* 2002;52:54–59.
55. Cox MW, McCarthy M, Lemmon G, et al. Cervical spine instability: clearance using dynamic fluoroscopy. *Curr Surg* 2001;58:96–100.
56. Sees DW, Rodriguez-Cruz LR, Flaherty SF, et al. The use of bedside fluoroscopy to evaluate the cervical spine in obtunded trauma patients. *J Trauma* 1998;45:768–771.
57. Davis JW, Kaups KL, Cunningham MA, et al. Routine evaluation of the cervical spine in head-injured patients with dynamic fluoroscopy: a reappraisal. *J Trauma* 2001;50:1044–1047.
58. Borock C, Gabram S, Jacobs L, et al. A prospective analysis of a two-year experience using computed tomography as an adjunct for cervical spine clearance. *J Trauma* 1991;31:1001–1004.
59. Schenarts PJ, Diaz J, Kaiser C, et al. Prospective comparison of admission computed tomographic scan and plain films of the upper cervical spine in trauma patients with altered mental status. *J Trauma* 2001;51:663–668.
60. Berne JD, Velmahos GC, El-Tawil Q, et al. Value of complete cervical helical computed tomographic scanning in identifying cervical spine injury in the unevaluable blunt trauma patient with multiple injuries: a prospective study. *J Trauma* 1999;47:896–903.
61. Benzel EC, Hart BL, Ball PA, et al. Magnetic resonance imaging for the evaluation of patients with occult cervical spine injury. *J Neurosurg* 1996;85:824–829.
62. Albrecht RM, Kingsley D, Schermer CR, et al. Evaluation of cervical spine in intensive care patients following blunt trauma. *World J Surg* 2001;25(8):1089–1096.
63. D'Alise MD, Benzel EC, Hart BL. Magnetic resonance imaging evaluation of the cervical spine in the comatose or obtunded trauma patient. *J Neurosurg* 1991;91(Suppl 1):54–59.
64. Lowery DW, Wald MM, Browne BJ, et al. Epidemiology of cervical spine injury victims. *Ann Emerg Med* 2001;38:12–16.
65. Goldberg W, Mueller C, Panacek E, et al. Distribution and patterns of blunt traumatic cervical spine injury. *Ann Emerg Med* 2001;38:17–21.

SECTION IV

Pediatric Conditions

CHAPTER 30

The Use of Cervical Orthoses, Halo Devices, and Traction in Children

Lawson A. B. Copley and John P. Dormans

The orthotic device that perfectly immobilizes the pediatric cervical spine does not exist. Numerous studies have shown that all of the currently available devices, including the most restrictive, allow some residual motion of all cervical vertebral levels in all planes (1–19). The orthoses and techniques that these studies have evaluated demonstrate a spectrum of ability to restrict cervical motion. A particular immobilization technique or collar may be effective in limiting a particular segment of the cervical spine, but relatively ineffective in limiting motion in other cervical regions.

Although cervical orthoses are not able to completely eliminate cervical motion, the appropriate selection of a device may allow adequate immobilization for a specific purpose. The decision as to which device or technique should be used in a given clinical situation should be guided by a knowledge of the relative ability of that device or technique to adequately restrict undesirable motion. The purpose of this chapter is to briefly review the evolution of modern cervical spine immobilization techniques as well as categorize and evaluate the effectiveness of currently available forms of cervical immobilization for children.

HISTORY OF CERVICAL IMMOBILIZATION

Several milestones have laid the foundation for the development of modern cervical orthoses. In 1910, Gauvain reported the use of plaster of Paris in the treatment of tuberculosis disease of the spine, which laid the foundation for the modern Minerva cast (20). Although Gauvain considered this to be a very efficient form of immobilization, he noted its limitations to include difficulty in chewing, jaw deformity in young children, and severe facial irritation in bearded men (20). This led to the modifications of the "Fillet" plaster, a device that resembled the modern halo cast (20,21).

Crutchfield developed an invasive form of skeletal traction to stabilize the cervical spine with tongs applied to the cranium (Fig. 30.1A) (22). His report of this technique to treat a patient with a cervical spine dislocation in 1933 rapidly led to its widespread use for posttraumatic cervical instability. Several modifications eventually led to the development of the Gardner-Wells tongs (Fig. 30.1B), which has served in this capacity since shortly after 1973 (23).

The modern halo was preceded by a three-pin "tiara" used during World War II by Bloom, a plastic surgeon, to treat severe maxillofacial trauma with this external stabilization device, which allowed for mobilization of the patient and wound care of severe facial burns (24). Recognizing the potential of this technique, Jacquelyn Perry and Vernon Nickel introduced the concept of the halo device in 1959 in the treatment of neck paralysis in patients with poliomyelitis (25). Soon this technique was commonly used to allow for early restoration of mobility for patients with cervical spine injuries, thereby decreasing the length of time needed for skull traction following injury (26).

Initially the halo was considered to be the best form of immobilization of the cervical spine and thought to be associated with relatively few complications (24). In 1986, however, Garfin reported a high complication rate with halo use (27). These complications included pin-loosening (36%), pin-site infection (20%), severe pin discomfort (18%), pressure sores (11%), cosmetically disfiguring scars (9%), dysphagia (2%), and dural penetration (1%) (27). His experience subsequently was substantiated by other reports and led to attempts to modify the halo apparatus and technique of application in order to reduce the number of complications (28–35). Among these modifications are pin design, angle of pin insertion, number of pins, location of pin insertion, insertion torque, and vest design (36–56). It is still to

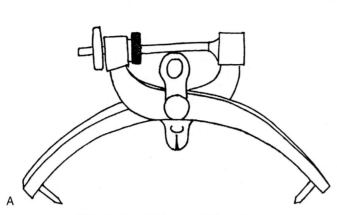
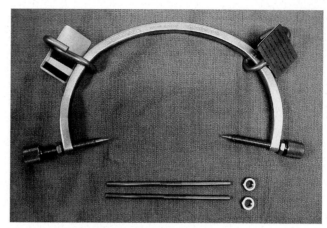

FIG. 30.1. A: Diagram of Crutchfield tongs. **B:** Photograph of Gardner Wells tongs.

be determined whether these modifications have substantially altered the halo from its original design and use.

Another important milestone in the history of cervical immobilization involved the work of White and associates in the biomechanical analysis of the stability of the cervical spine and radiographic evaluation of cervical motion at Yale in the 1970s (11,57). These studies laid the groundwork for numerous comparative studies of different forms of cervical immobilization (1–5,7–19). Additionally, they provided objective criteria to assist in defining significant instability and selecting treatment methods for certain injury patterns (57).

CLASSIFICATION OF CERVICAL IMMOBILIZATION DEVICES

General categories of cervical immobilization devices used in children include: cervical orthoses (CO), cervicothoracic orthoses (CTO), noninvasive traction devices, invasive traction devices, and halo immobilization. These broad categories cover the spectrum of devices available on the market that have grown rapidly in the past few decades with the advent of lightweight plastic materials that can be prefabricated to fit most patients. For many of these products, comparison studies have been performed to indicate their relative efficacy in immobilizing the cervical spine (1–5,7–19). Some have been evaluated to determine closing capillary wedge pressure, which might have a role in decubitus ulcer formation in unconscious patients requiring prolonged immobilization (1,3,6,58–60).

Overall, COs are less restrictive than CTOs. Although CTOs are generally less restrictive than the halo ring and vest, some studies have shown their comparative efficacy in children (4,14,18,61,62). CTOs tend to limit motion in the middle and inferior cervical regions well, but are less effective in limiting the upper cervical spine. The halo tends to limit motion well in the upper cervical region but allows

some paradoxic motion in the lower cervical spine. In general, those devices that have the greatest restriction on cervical motion are associated with higher complication rates (27–29,63).

In addition to off-the-shelf devices, the pediatric cervical spine may be immobilized with custom-fabricated orthoses. Sometimes this is necessary for those with an unusual body habitus or deformity. Generally this is more expensive and time consuming, requiring close communication with a trained orthotist. Another technique that should not be overlooked is direct application of Minerva or halo cast (20,21, 62). This also is time consuming and requires experience as well as capable assistance.

BIOMECHANICAL CONSIDERATIONS

The cervical spine can be analyzed according to motion segments or anatomic region. The motion of each segment from the occipitocervical junction to the cervicothoracic junction can be evaluated in each of three planes including flexion-extension, lateral bending and axial rotation. Further consideration may be given to anteroposterior translation or side-to-side translation at each motion segment. This is useful methodology for biomechanical and radiographic analyses of cervical motion. Also it is relevant clinically when considering the relative motion of an injured segment compared to proximal and distal noninjured segments.

The most relevant work in this area was performed by White and associates (57). They concluded that the normal adult spine should not permit horizontal motion greater than 2.7 mm between vertebrae (3.5 mm with radiographic magnification) or angular displacement greater than 10.7 degrees (commonly rounded to 11 degrees) relative to adjacent vertebrae (57). They also determined that the anterior elements, comprised of the anterior longitudinal ligament, costotransverse ligaments, annulus fibrosus, vertebral body, and posterior longitudinal ligament, were most useful in stabilizing the spine in extension (57). Their cadaveric studies illustrated that the spine would be stable in extension until essentially all of the anterior elements were destroyed or unable to function (57). The posterior elements, comprised of the facet joint capsules, facet joints, ligamentum flavum, and interspinous and supraspinous ligaments, functioned to stabilize the spine in flexion (57). Again, White and associates demonstrated that the spine would be stable in flexion until essentially all of the posterior elements were destroyed (57). Although similar research has not been performed in children, these data are nonetheless useful in evaluating cervical instability in older children and adolescents (older than 8 years) who demonstrate anatomic features and injury patterns similar to adults.

An organized approach to evaluating cervical spine motion segments by radiographic analysis was introduced by Johnson and colleagues in 1977 (11). With this methodology, it became possible to objectively compare various cervical immobilization devices with other devices using volunteers with normal cervical spines. Sagittal-plane motion was measured on lateral cervical spine films in neutral, flexion, and extension. Lateral bending was measured on anteroposterior films during the extreme of this motion. Rotation was measured using overhead photographs of the head and shoulders. This methodology has been repeated in a number of studies comparing other forms of cervical immobilization that were introduced following Johnson's initial comparison of the soft cervical collar, Philadelphia collar, SOMI (sternooccipital-mandibular immobilizer) brace, four-poster brace, cervicothoracic brace, and halo with plastic body vest (1,2,4,5,7,8,10,11,13,14,18,19). Although these studies share similar methodology, it is not possible to compare them directly because not all studies indicate the unrestricted range of motion of the controls.

Other methods of comparative evaluation of cervical immobilization devices include goniometry and cineradiography (3,9,12,15–17). Goniometry has been shown to have a high correlation with radiographic techniques and has the obvious advantage of avoiding radiation exposure (7). However, the precision of this method is limited and it does not give information on the degree of motion at individual vertebral levels (7).

Besides segmental motion analysis, another means of evaluating the cervical spine so as to understand injury and healing patterns is by anatomic region. Most clinical outcome studies that compare different forms of treatment of cervical injuries consider upper cervical injuries separately from subaxial injuries (64–81). Many further divide the upper cervical injuries based on specific fracture type such as atlas (Jefferson), dens (Types I, II, and III), and axis (hangman) fractures (68,70,71,73,75,77,78). It is likely that the biomechanical properties and response to the forces of injury of these different areas are substantially affected by their unique anatomic features. Therefore, such regional anatomic evaluation is helpful in predicting the natural history

of a specific injury and the likelihood of successful outcome with conservative versus operative treatment.

COMPARISON AND EVALUATION OF NONINVASIVE CERVICAL IMMOBILIZATION DEVICES

Cervical Orthoses

Symptomatic Support Collars

A soft collar provides negligible cervical stabilization and has no role in the management of the potentially unstable pediatric spine. In most studies the restricted motion with soft or hard collars is less than 5% (3,9,11,12). This device is used mainly for treatment of minor cervical muscle strains and mild so-called whiplash injuries. The symptomatic relief provided by the soft collar is thought to result from its warming effect on the underlying soft tissues as well as the reminder it serves to the patient to voluntarily limit neck motion during the period of myofascial healing. Patient compliance is high because of the comfort of the device. Hard collars made with supplemental plastic are similar in function to soft collars (Fig. 30.2). They do not add substantially to cervical stabilization.

Prehospital Extrication Collars

The rationale behind the use of prehospital immobilization is to prevent the initiation or propagation of spinal cord injury (SCI) in individuals with high energy trauma who are at risk for underlying cervical spine injury. The mechanism of most cervical spine injury involves motor vehicle accidents, falls, and sporting injuries. With the advent of modern prehospital resuscitation technology, the use of careful cervical immobilization has become the standard of care (1, 5,8,15–17,19,67).

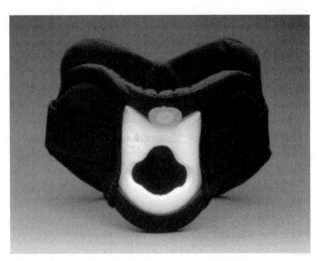

FIG. 30.2. Soft cervical orthosis (Jerome Medical, Moorestown, NJ).

Numerous devices and supplemental immobilization techniques are available. Each has its own advantages and disadvantages. The decision as to which device will be used is largely in the hands of the emergency medical transport services and technicians who are the immediate responders to trauma in the field. However, physician leadership and direction is necessary to prevent patients from presenting to the hospital with suboptimal cervical protection or malalignment caused by improper positioning.

Ideally, a prehospital collar allows for adequate immobilization to prevent further injury and possesses the following features: easy to apply while maintaining in-line cervical immobilization, inexpensive, comfortable for the patient (preventing anxiety or resistance), has small storage space requirements, adjustable to fit a variety of patient sizes and shapes, and creates a low rate of decubitus ulceration of the mandible or occiput with extended use during early hospital evaluation and transportation (especially in unconscious individuals) (1,5,8,15–17,67). Because the exact amount of acceptable residual motion of the spinal cord that prevents initiation or propagation of cervical spine injury is not known, it is necessary to supplement all collars, regardless of their comparative efficacy to competitive brands, with additional techniques of cervical alignment and immobilization. Spine board or short board techniques are the most effective supplemental methods (8,82). These involve head bolsters and taping to prevent the excessive rotational movement that cervical collars allow. Special attention is necessary in the pediatric population in order to maintain neutral cervical alignment. Anthropometric data have shown that the head circumference and sagittal diameter increase at a logarithmic rate during childhood, whereas the thoracic height increases at a linear rate (83). The resulting mismatch creates a situation in which immobilization on a flat spine board produces excessive flexion of the cervical spine (82–86). In this situation, it is necessary to provide supplemental padding under the thorax or an occipital recess for the spine board. Because the exact amount of padding necessary to align the cervical spine may vary substantially from child to child, the thoracic padding technique has the advantage of being adjustable (84–86). The clinical method for establishing a neutral cervical position in the field is to achieve alignment of the external auditory meatus with the shoulder (85).

Padding of the spine board as a whole has been shown to reduce patient discomfort while maintaining similar cervical immobilization to unpadded boards (60). Unfortunately, transcutaneous oxygen tension of the sacrum is not improved with spine board padding (60). The risk of decubitus ulcers from the spine board and prehospital immobilization collars requires the treating physician to make every effort to remove these devices as soon as possible (59,87). In unconscious patients who may require prolonged collar use, alternative techniques to clear the cervical spine may be considered such as fluoroscopy or MRI (87). Consideration also may be given to adopting a meticulous skin care protocol

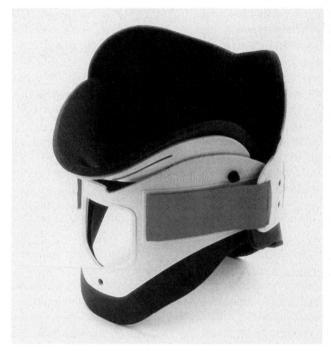

FIG. 30.3. Prehospital extrication immobilization collar (NecLoc; Jerome Medical, Moorestown, NJ).

or evaluating alternative collars, which may have a lower incidence of decubitus formation (58,59). Examples of extrication collars include: the Philadelphia collar (Philadelphia Collar Co., Philadelphia), NecLoc collar (Jerome Medical, Moorestown, NJ) (Fig. 30.3), Stiffneck collar (Laerdal Medical Corp., Armonk, NY), Aspen collar (International Healthcare Devices, Long Beach, CA), Jobst Vertebrace collar (Jobst Institute, Inc., Toledo, OH), and Vacuum Splint cervical collar (Germa, Sweden; supplied by Med-Tech, Loveland, CO).

Ambulatory Immobilization Collars

There are several devices available in this category. Unfortunately, they do not provide adequate immobilization of the cervical spine to be used reliably as a method of treatment for the potentially unstable spine. A study of cervical collars used in rheumatoid atlantoaxial subluxation showed that none of the collars evaluated were effective in limiting anterior subluxation of the atlas in maximum flexion (88). Another study compared the rate of healing of Type II dens fractures treated with a Philadelphia collar to those treated in a halo and demonstrated bony union in 74% of halo patients compared with only 53% of collar patients (78). Indications for the use of these devices include symptomatic treatment for cervical strain or spasm and supplemental immobilization following surgical stabilization in selected cases. One study demonstrated that isolated stable burst fractures of the atlas can be effectively treated with a rigid cervi-

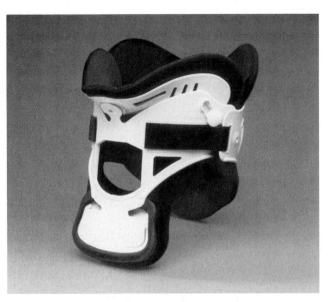

FIG. 30.4. Ambulatory immobilization collar for children (Miami Junior; Jerome Medical, Moorestown, NJ).

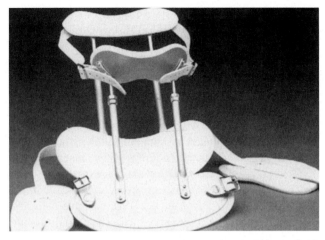

FIG. 30.6. Four poster brace (Seattle-Systems, a USMC company, Poulsbo, WA). (Photographs compliments of Seattle Systems. All rights reserved.)

cal collar (Fig. 30.4), the Miami-J collar (Jerome Medical, Moorestown, NJ) (73).

Some of these devices are well padded and provide a higher degree of patient comfort and compliance. Generally they are more expensive than the prehospital extrication collars. Examples of this type of collar include the Miami J collar (Fig. 30.4), Philadelphia cervical collar, and Aspen collar.

The treatment of children with cervical collars requires one to find a device that takes into account the variability commonly seen in children including posterior occipital prominence, which progressively diminishes with age and relative neck length; this increases into adolescence and then diminishes into adulthood. Unfortunately, many devices and techniques that have been used in children have been scaled-down versions of similar products designed for adult use. As a result of research and improved technology, dedicated pediatric products are available to substantially improve the endeavor to safely and effectively immobilize the pediatric spine. The Miami Junior collar (Jerome Medical, Moorestown, NJ) (Fig. 30.4) was created with these design features in mind. The design of this collar accounts for the anthropometric data that shows an increased occipital size and short neck length in children up to age 2 years but decreasing occipital size and relatively increased neck length in children between 6 and 12 years (Fig. 30.5).

Cervicothoracic Orthoses

There are a variety of devices in this category with pediatric sizing including the two and four poster braces (Fig. 30.6),

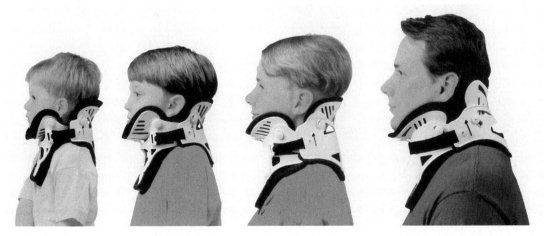

FIG. 30.5. Cervical collar adaptations for anthropometric variations in pediatric and adolescent cervical and occipital development. (Reproduced with permission from Jerome Medical, Moorestown, NJ.)

sternooccipital-mandibular immobilizer (Fig. 30.7) (SOMI, Zinco Industries, Pasadena, CA), Yale brace (Orthomedics, Brea, CA), Johnson CTO, and Minerva braces (Figs. 30.8 and 30.9) (both Seattle-Systems, Seattle, WA). A spectrum of capability to immobilize certain regions of the spine has been reported. Although these braces are more restrictive than cervical collars, careful consideration must be given to the indications for their use. The most relevant concern is whether or not the degree of immobilization achieved with these devices is adequate to allow complete healing of the traumatized spinal segment. Some studies favorably compare certain devices in this category to more invasive forms of immobilization, such as the halo ring and vest (4,10,14). However, concern exists whether CTOs can capably immobilize the occiput and C1 (18).

Suggested uses for these devices include supplemental immobilization of the surgically stabilized spine in highly unstable situations, treatment of SCI without radiographic abnormality (SCIWORA) in children, and definitive treatment of relatively stable cervical fractures at levels in which the device is shown to have efficacy. This somewhat varies between devices. The highly unstable situations that

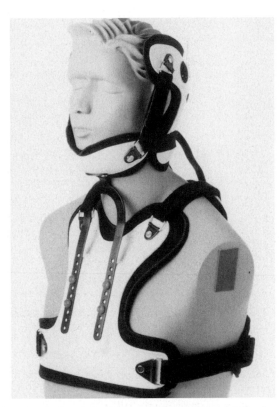

FIG. 30.8. Cervicothoracic orthosis (Johnson C.T.O.; Seattle-Systems, a USMC company, Poulsbo, WA). (Photographs compliments of Seattle Systems. All rights reserved.)

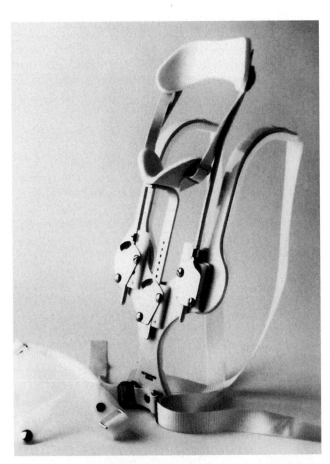

FIG. 30.7. Sterno-occipital-mandibular immobilizer (SOMI; Seattle-Systems, a USMC company, Poulsbo, WA). (Photographs compliments of Seattle Systems. All rights reserved.)

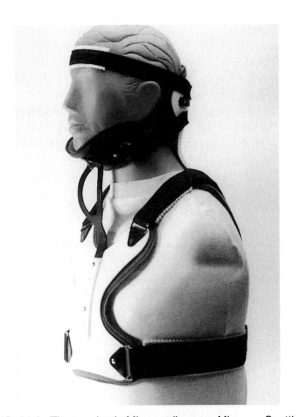

FIG. 30.9. Thermoplastic Minerva (Lerman Minerva; Seattle-Systems, a USMC company, Poulsbo, WA). (Photographs compliments of Seattle Systems. All rights reserved.)

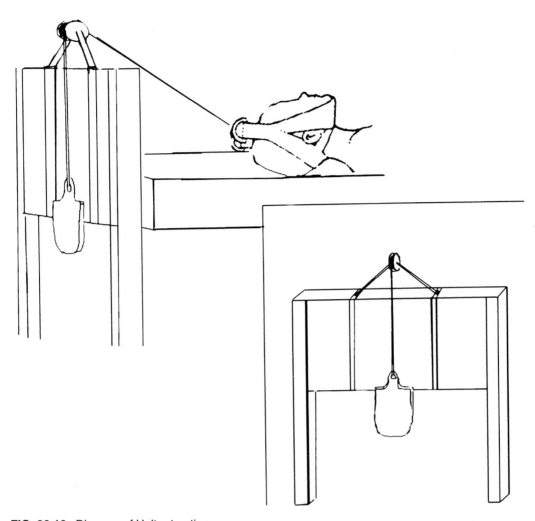

FIG. 30.10. Diagram of Halter traction.

often require surgery include Type II fractures of the dens with subluxation greater than 3 mm and delayed diagnosis (>7 days after injury), and subaxial injuries with severe vertebral body injury (SVBI) or severe ligamentous injury (SLI) (68,70,74,78). The criteria of White and associates remain useful in determining instability of the subaxial cervical spine that likely require surgical intervention in children with mature spinal anatomy (>8 years of age) (57). The use of cervicothoracic orthoses or halo immobilization alone to treat such injuries has been shown to have a high rate of failure (68,70,74,78).

Halter Traction

The use of halter traction is relatively limited in orthopedics (Fig. 30.10). The most common indication is in the treatment of atlantoaxial rotary displacement during the acute inflammatory period (1 to 2 weeks) in an attempt to rest the cervical spine and restore normal alignment before fixed deformity (atlantoaxial rotary fixation) occurs (89). Another use includes that of a prescribed modality during

physical therapy to alleviate cervical strains and muscle spasm. This must be used with caution and should be discontinued if the patient's symptoms worsen or fail to improve after a limited trial (3 to 5 days). The weight limitation of halter traction is 5 to 10 pounds and is often limited by the resultant pain across the temporomandibular joint, mandible, and skin.

INVASIVE CERVICAL IMMOBILIZATION TECHNIQUES

Gardner-Wells tong traction is the most commonly available invasive traction method. This form of traction often is used in the acute trauma setting to accomplish reduction of cervical injuries, particularly facet joint dislocations and fractures with displacement. Skull-based fixation techniques allow sequential addition of traction weight up to 60 or 70 pounds. The device can be applied with local anesthesia. Pin sites are selected 1 cm above the pinna of the auricle of the ear in line with the external auditory meatus. The pin site may be varied 1 cm anterior or 1 cm posterior in order to apply extension or flexion moments, respectively. The starting traction amount is 5 pounds in children and up to 10 pounds in adolescents (65). When reduction of a dislocation is necessary, weight is added in increments of 2 to 5 pounds (depending on patient size), with each addition followed by a lateral radiograph of the cervical spine and careful neurologic examination of the patient. Once reduction is accomplished, the weight is reduced until definitive treatment is completed. If an invasive traction device is necessary to achieve a reduction, then surgery is most likely necessary to establish and maintain long-term stability of the injured segment. This is particularly true for bilateral facet dislocations or other injuries resulting in SLI or SVBI. Conversely, dens fractures and Jefferson fractures in children may be reduced with invasive traction and then maintained with halo immobilization to achieve adequate healing.

Possible complications associated with the use of these invasive traction devices include superficial skin infection around the pin sites and dislodgement of the device (90). Deep infections, including osteomyelitis and cerebral abscess formation, also have been reported (90–92). When applying Gardner-Wells tong traction in older children (>8 years) or adolescents, the pins should be tightened until 1 mm of the spring-loaded stylet protrudes, thus applying 25 pounds of force (44). This results in a mean pull-off strength of 134 ± 34 pounds, which is adequate for nearly all traction loads during reduction and stabilization (44).

Extreme caution should be used in younger children who are at risk for penetration because of decreased skull thickness. Currently there are no clearly defined guidelines as to how much load can be safely applied using this device in small children. If the device is to remain in place for an extended time period, the pins should be retightened 24 hours after the initial application. Periodic radiographs are recommended to evaluate the inner table of the skull and detect pin penetration (91).

Alternatives to Gardner-Wells traction include immediate application of the halo ring with traction applied through the ring itself. The halo may be used as a traction device with modifications to include halo-pelvic traction, halo-femoral traction, halo-Ilizarov traction, and halo-suspension traction with an overhead rod attached to a walker or wheelchair allowing for ambulatory or mobile suspension of the patient from a spring or fish scale during daytime activity (93–95). Complications associated with halo-pelvic traction have been reported to be high, leading to a recommendation that the apparatus be reserved for severe deformities when other means are inadequate (94).

Halo Ring and Vest

Indications for use of the halo ring and vest (Fig. 30.11) include supplemental stabilization of the cervical spine in selected postsurgical patients and stabilization of selected

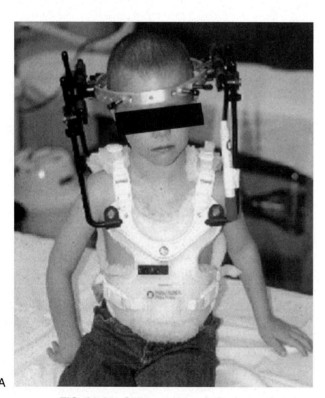
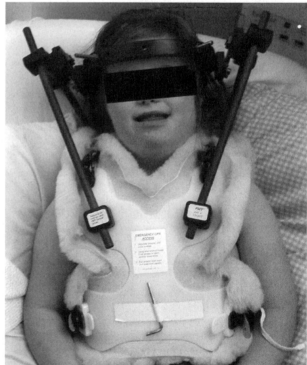

A   B

FIG. 30.11. Child wearing a halo ring and vest.

TABLE 30.1. *Dens Fractures Treated with Halo Immobilization*

Series	Patients at follow-up	Success rate	Failure factors
Ekong, 1981	17	59% II and III	Age >55, >3 mm, II
Clark, 1985	96	68% II	II, displacement, angulation
Dunn, 1986	74	67% II; 100% III	Age >65, >3 mm, II
Lind, 1986	10	90% II	II, gap >5 mm
Mandabach, 1993	9	67% II	Not listed
Szabo, 1996	38	90% II; 100% III	Age >60, >5 mm

acute cervical injuries. More specific indications as to which forms of cervical trauma in older children with adult patterns of injury will likely respond well to halo vest immobilization as definitive treatment can be partly derived from the literature pertaining to treatment outcomes. This information is best divided into those studies dealing predominantly with upper cervical spine (C1-2) and subaxial cervical (C3-7) injuries.

Several trends are noted when reviewing composite data from series involving halo vest management of dens fractures (Table 30.1). Union rates ranged from 59% to 100%, but overall were 73% in 244 patients who completed follow-up in all series (68,70,71,75,77,78). Factors associated with nonunion included age greater than 55 to 65 years, Type II fracture pattern with fracture displacement greater than 3 mm or posterior displacement of the dens, and greater than 1 week time lapse from injury to diagnosis (68,70,71,75, 77,78). Union rates were considered acceptable and an advantage over surgical management in patients who did not demonstrate the factors associated with nonunion (68,70,71, 75,77,78).

Reviewing composite data from series involving halo vest management of subaxial cervical injuries (Table 30.2), the success rate ranged from 58% to 90%, with an overall success of 76% in 746 patients who completed follow-up (64,65,66,69,74,79–81). The most common factor associated with failure was facet dislocation or subluxation (65,66,69,74,80,81). Additional factors included complex fracture dislocations, difficult reduction, advanced stage flexion compression fractures, severe ligamentous injury (including positive stretch test, >20% vertebral body width translation, or >15 degrees of angulation), and severe verte-

bral body injury (loss of vertebral body height of 40%) (64, 65,69,74,76,79–81). The rate of successful outcome was considered acceptable and an advantage over surgery if factors leading to failure were recognized early to prevent prolonged treatment before surgery. One outcome study evaluated 67 patients 2 to 7 years following halo immobilization treatment (76). Although 80% of patients reported neck stiffness and pain at the extremes of neck motion at follow-up, the symptoms were mild and did not have a major impact on return to work or leisure activities (76). The patients demonstrated a significant decrease of rotation (18%) and side bending (18%), but had normal flexion and extension (76).

Halo immobilization generally follows a period of traction that allows for reduction of the fracture or dislocation and resolution of the spasm of injury in the acute setting. This also allows for the evaluation of all nonneurologic injuries while maintaining cervical immobilization. One study advocates acute stabilization of the cervical spine by halo vest application in the emergency department for multiple trauma patients (96). This allows for stabilization of the patients' neurologic status and facilitates diagnosis and treatment of life-threatening injuries (96).

Indications for use of the halo in young children (≤8 years) include stabilization of selected traumatic injuries and supplemental stabilization following surgical treatment of selected cervical spines. It is important to know that not all cervical traumas in young children respond to halo immobilization alone. Atlantoaxial instability from transverse ligament rupture and late instability in os odontoideum require posterior fusion. Children with severe vertebral body flexion-compression fractures of the lower

TABLE 30.2. *Subaxial Cervical Injuries Treated with Halo Immobilization*

Series	Patients at follow-up	Success rate (%)	Failure factors
Cooper, 1979	33	85	Translation, angulation
Chan, 1983	150	89	Facet dislocation
Bucci, 1988	20	60	Complex fracture/dislocation
Lind, 1988	67	90	>20% Translation
Bucholz, 1989	109	85	Locked/perched facets
Sears, 1990	173	60	Hyperflex/subluxation
Rockswold, 1990	99	78	Severe ligamentous injury, severe vertebral body injury
Lemons, 1993	38	58	Flex/compression fractures
Romanelli, 1996	57	79	Facet subluxations

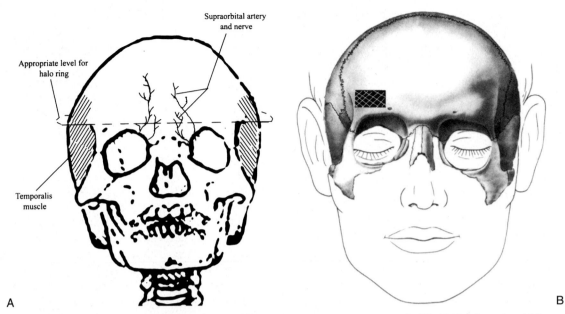

FIG. 30.12. Diagram showing proper placement of halo ring and pins. **A:** The halo ring should be placed at the equator of the skull. **B:** Anterior pins should be placed over the lateral eyebrow. It is important to avoid the supraorbital nerve and arteries and frontal sinus medially and the temporal bone and temporalis muscle laterally. The box (shaded) area indicates a safe placement location for anterior pins.

cervical spine may require anterior interbody fusion to correct or prevent posttraumatic cervical kyphosis (97). In children with anomalous vertebrae and deformity who may have systemic disorders and diminished potential to form a solid arthrodesis of the upper cervical spine, postoperative halo immobilization may provide reliable support to facilitate healing (98). Another occasional use of the halo is in cases of atlantoaxial rotary fixation that have occurred from delayed presentation of torticollis or failure to respond to less aggressive treatment (89). Posterior cervical arthrodesis frequently is necessary in these children as well (89). An advantage of the halo in this instance is to appropriately position the head during the fusion process so as to prevent drifting into recurrent deformity, which might occur with less aggressive forms of postoperative immobilization.

Complications associated with halo use have been reported at variable rates (24,27–29,63). Studies that have been designed purposefully to evaluate for complications have reported higher rates, particularly of superficial pin site infections and loosening. Various other minor complications that have been reported include pressure sores, nerve injury, dysphagia, severe scars, and severe pin discomfort. The most serious events that have been reported include cranial osteomyelitis, cerebral abscess formation, halo dislodgement, and loss of fracture alignment or reduction (30–35,63,92,99,100–103). Although these more serious complications are rare, they require the physician who manages patients with halo immobilization to pay meticulous attention to detail with close follow-up of these pa-

tients and careful instructions as to signs or symptoms that might indicate a problem. An even greater level of attention must be given to quadriplegic or ventilator-dependent children or adolescents. A vigorous nursing and respiratory care treatment protocol has been generated for these patients and has been shown to substantially reduce the otherwise high incidence of complications (104). A number of modifications of halo design and application technique have been studied in an effort to reduce the complication rate associated with halo ring and vest use (36–56).

Halo application (Figs. 30.12 and 30.13) in very young children requires unique modifications. Recommenda-

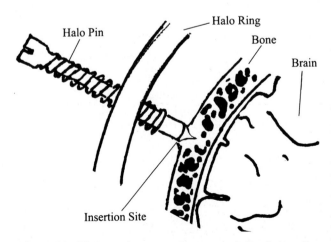

FIG. 30.13. Diagram demonstrating proper halo pin insertion.

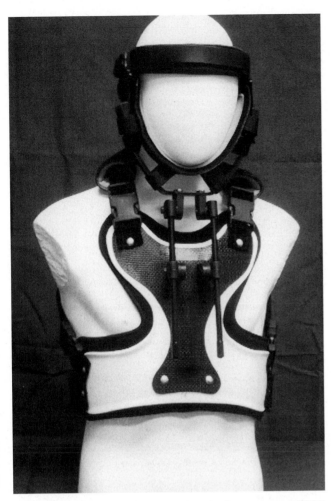

FIG. 30.14. Noninvasive halo (Seattle-Systems, a USMC company, Poulsbo, WA). (Photographs compliments of Seattle Systems. All rights reserved.)

tions include multiple pin constructs (eight to 10 pins), decreased application torque (1 inch pound of torque per year up to age 5), custom molded vests or casting when prefabricated devices are unavailable, and prehalo computer tomography to evaluate skull thickness in the safe areas (21,62,72, 105–110). The rate of complications in children has been shown to be significantly greater than that seen in adults (68% versus 36%) but does not appear to solely result from the fact that more pins are used (28,29). Noninvasive halo devices have been introduced in an effort to reproduce halo immobilization without the risks associated with halo pin insertion (Fig. 30.14).

SPINAL CORD INJURY WITHOUT RADIOGRAPHIC ABNORMALITY

A unique finding in pediatric trauma is the phenomenon of SCIWORA. This is thought to occur from a combination of factors, including ligamentous laxity, horizontal facet orientation, and greater ability of the adult spinal column to elongate compared with the spinal cord in young children. The resulting injury can range from transient cervical cord neurapraxia (CCN) to complete SCI. The treatment for this condition involves immobilization and protection of the cervical spine until it can be adequately proved by flexion and extension lateral radiographs and magnetic resonance imaging (MRI) that no instability from underlying ligamentous disruption exists. The device for immobilization should be as restrictive as possible without resorting to halo immobilization. Typically, this involves a Minerva or other cervicothoracic orthosis (61). Once an adequate time for soft-tissue healing has elapsed (4 to 6 weeks) and the spine is proved radiographically stable, then the immobilization is removed.

SUMMARY

A variety of devices and techniques are available to assist in immobilization of the cervical spine in individuals of all ages. Even the most restrictive devices and techniques are unable to completely immobilize the vertebral segments of the cervical spine. Care must be taken in selecting a device based on the level and type of injury that is encountered. It is important to have specific knowledge as to which types of injury have a significantly lower success rate compared with operative management in order to properly counsel patients and their families.

In the prehospital setting, supplemental techniques must be used in addition to extrication collars in order to ensure that the spine is adequately immobilized to prevent the occurrence or worsening of neurologic injury. Cervical orthoses have limited stabilizing properties and are useful for symptomatic relief or supplemental support following surgical procedures. Cervicothoracic orthoses demonstrate favorable immobilization of the middle and lower cervical spine and may be useful for selected, stable traumatic injuries, SCIWORA and supplemental support following surgery. When a halo vest is chosen for cervical immobilization, meticulous attention to detail and careful follow-up are necessary to reduce the incidence of complications. Children have unique anatomic and developmental traits and should be afforded careful consideration as to the accommodations necessary to safely and adequately immobilize their cervical spines.

CREDITS AND ACKNOWLEDGMENTS

The authors thank Julia Lou for her help in the completion of this chapter. Photographs courtesy of Seattle Systems, a USMC company (Poulsbo, WA) and Jerome Medical (Moorestown, NJ). All rights reserved.

REFERENCES

1. Alberts RA, Mahoney CR, Neff JR. Comparison of the Nebraska collar, a new prototype cervical immobilization collar, with three standard models. *J Orthop Trauma* 1998;12(6):425–430.
2. Askins V, Eismont FJ. Efficacy of five cervical orthoses in restricting cervical motion. *Spine* 1997;22(11):1193–1198.
3. Beavis A. Cervical orthoses. *Prosthet Orthot Int* 1989;13:6–13.
4. Benzel EC, Hadden TA, Saulsbery CM. A comparison of the Minerva and halo jackets for stabilization of the cervical spine. *J Neurosurg* 1989;70:411–414.
5. Cline JR, Scheidel E, Bigsby EF. A comparison of methods of cervical immobilization used in patient extrication and transport. *J Trauma* 1985;25(7):649–653.
6. Fisher SV. Proper fitting of the cervical orthosis. *Arch Phys Med Rehabil* 1978;59:505–507.
7. Fisher SV, Bowar JF, Awad EA, et al. Cervical orthoses effect on cervical spine motion: roentgenographic and goniometric method of study. *Arch Phys Med Rehabil* 1977;58:109–115.
8. Graziano AF, Scheidel EA, Cline JR, et al. A radiographic comparison of prehospital cervical immobilization methods. *Ann Emerg Med* 1987;16:1127–1131.
9. Hartman JT, Palumbo F, Hill BJ. Cineradiography of the braced normal cervical spine. *Clin Orthop* 1975;109:97–102.
10. Johnson RM, Hart DL, Owen JR, et al. The Yale cervical orthosis, an evaluation of its effectiveness in restricting cervical motion in normal subjects and a comparison with other cervical orthoses. *Phys Ther* 1978;58(7):865–870.
11. Johnson RM, Hart DL, Simmons EF, et al. Cervical orthoses, a study comparing their effectiveness in restricting cervical motion in normal subjects. *J Bone Joint Surg* 1977;59-A(3):332–339.
12. Kaufman WA, Lunsford TR, Lunsford BR, et al. Comparison of three prefabricated cervical collars. *Orthot Prosthet* 1986;39(4):21–28.
13. Lau YC, Chang RK, Cheng YC, et al. Study of low-temperature thermoplastic modified custom-molded cervical orthosis for cervical spine fixation. *J Spinal Disord* 1994;7(6):504–509.
14. Maiman D, Millington P, Novak S, et al. The effect of the thermoplastic Minerva body jacket on cervical spine motion. *Neurosurgery* 1989;25(3):363–368.
15. McGuire RA, Degnan G, Amundson GM. Evaluation of current extrication orthoses in immobilization of the unstable cervical spine. *Spine* 1990;15(10):1064–1067.
16. Podolsky S, Baraff LJ, Simon RR, et al. Efficacy of cervical spine immobilization methods. *J Trauma* 1983;23(6):461–465.
17. Rosen PB, McSwain NE, Arata M, et al. Comparison of two new immobilization collars. *Ann Emerg Med* 1992;21:1189–1195.
18. Sharpe KP, Rao S, Ziogas A. Evaluation of the effectiveness of the Minerva cervicothoracic orthosis. *Spine* 1995;20(13):1475–1479.
19. Solot JA, Winzelberg GG. Clinical and radiological evaluation of vertebrae extrication collars. *J Emerg Med* 1990;8:79–83.
20. Gauvain HJ. The use of plaster of Paris in the mechanical treatment of tuberculosis disease of the spine. *Practitioner* 1913;90:190–202.
21. Marks DS, Roberts P, Wilton PJ, et al. A halo jacket for stabilization of the paediatric cervical spine. *Arch Orthop Trauma Surg* 1993;112:134–135.
22. Crutchfield WB. Skeletal traction for dislocation of the cervical spine: report of a case. *South Surg* 1933;2:156.
23. Gardner WJ. The principle of spring-loaded points for cervical traction. *J Neurosurg* 1973;39:543–544.
24. Perry J. The halo in spinal abnormalities, practical factors and avoidance of complications. *Orthop Clin North Am* 1972;3(1):69–80.
25. Perry J, Nickel VL. Total cervical-spine fusion for neck paralysis. *J Bone Joint Surg* 1959;41-A(1):37–60.
26. Nickel VL, Perry J, Garrett A, et al. The halo, a spinal skeletal traction fixation device. *J Bone Joint Surg* 1968;50-A(7):1400–1409.
27. Garfin SR, Botte MJ, Waters RL, et al. Complications in the use of the halo fixation device. *J Bone Joint Surg* 1986;68-A(3):320–325.
28. Baum JA, Hanley EN, Pullekines J. Comparison of halo complications in adults and children. *Spine* 1989;14(3):251–252.
29. Dormans JP, Criscitiello AA, Drummond DS, et al. Complications in children managed with immobilization in a halo vest. *J Bone Joint Surg* 1995;77-A(9):1370–1373.
30. Kameyama O, Ogawa K, Suga T, et al. Asymptomatic brain abscess as a complication of halo orthosis: report of a case and review of the literature. *J Orthop Sci* 1999;4:39–41.
31. Lammens J, Hoogmartens MJ, Fabry G, et al. Meningoencephalitis and cerebral abscess as a complication of the halo device. *Acta Orthop Belg* 1988;54(3):360–362.
32. Rizzolo SJ, Piazza MR, Cotler JM, et al. The effect of torque pressure on halo pin complication rates, a randomized prospective study. *Spine* 1993;18(15):2163–2166.
33. Rosenblum D, Ehrlich V. Brain abscess and psychosis as a complication of a halo orthosis. *Arch Phys Med Rehabil* 1995;76:865–867.
34. Vertullo CJ, Duke PF, Askin GN. Pin-site complications of the halo thoracic brace with routine pin re-tightening. *Spine* 1997;22(21):2514–2516.
35. Williams FH, Nelms DK, McGaharan KM. Brain abscess: a rare complication of halo usage. *Arch Phys Med Rehabil* 1992;73:490–492.
36. Ballock RT, Lee TQ, Triggs KJ, et al. The effect of pin location on the rigidity of the halo pin-bone interface. *Neurosurgery* 1990;26(2):238–241.
37. Botte MJ, Byrne TP, Garfin SR. Application of the halo device for immobilization of the cervical spine utilizing an increased torque pressure. *J Bone Joint Surg* 1987;69-A(5):750–752.
38. Botte MJ, Byrne TP, Garfin SR. Use of skin incisions in the application of halo skeletal fixator pins. *Clin Orthop* 1989;246:100–101.
39. Copley LA, Pepe MD, Tan V, et al. A comparison of various angles of halo pin insertion in an immature skull model. *Spine* 1999;24(17):1777–1780.
40. Copley LA, Pepe MD, Tan V, et al. A comparative evaluation of halo pin designs in an immature skull model. *Clin Orthop* 1998;357:212–218.
41. Fleming BC, Krag MH, Huston DR, et al. Pin loosening in a halo-vest orthosis, a biomechanical study. *Spine* 2000;25:1325–1331.
42. Garfin SR, Botte MJ, Woo SLY, et al. Reliability after repeated use of a torque screwdriver employed for halo pin fixation. *J Orthop Res* 1985;3(1):121–123.
43. Garfin SR, Lee TQ, Roux RD, et al. Structural behavior of the halo orthosis pin-bone interface: biomechanical evaluation of standard and newly designed stainless steel halo fixation pins. *Spine* 1986;11(10):977–981.
44. Krag NH, Byrt W, Pope M. Pull-off strength of Gardner-Wells tongs from cadaveric crania. *Spine* 1989;14(3):247–250.
45. Letts M, Girouard L, Yeadon A. Mechanical evaluation of four-versus eight-pin halo fixation. *J Pediatr Orthop* 1997;17:121–124.
46. Letts M, Kaylor D, Gouw G. A biomechanical analysis of halo fixation in children. *J Bone Join Surg* 1988;70-B(2):277–279.
47. Lind B, Sihlbom H, Nordwall A. Forces and motions across the neck in patients treated with halo-vest. *Spine* 1988;13(2):162–167.
48. Mirza SK, Moquin RR, Anderson PA, et al. Stabilizing properties of the halo apparatus. *Spine* 1997;22(7):727–733.
49. Pliaser B, Gabram SG, Schwartz RJ, et al. Prospective evaluation of craniofacial pressure in four different cervical orthoses. *J Trauma* 1994;37(5):740–720.
50. Smith MD, Johnson LJ, Perra JH, et al. A biomechanical study of torque and accuracy of halo pin insertional devices. *J Bone Joint Surg* 1996;78-A(2):231–238.
51. Triggs KJ, Ballock RT, Byrne T, et al. Length dependence of a halo orthosis on cervical immobilization. *J Spinal Disord* 1993;6(1):34–37.
52. Triggs KJ, Ballock RT, Lee TQ, et al. The effect of angled insertion on halo pin fixation. *Spine* 1989;14(8):781–783.
53. Voor MJ, Khalily C. Halo pin loosening: a biomechanical comparison of experimental and conventional designs. *J Biomech* 1998;31:397–400.
54. Walker PS, Lamser D, Hussey RW, et al. Forces in the halo-vest apparatus. *Spine* 1984;9(8):773–777.

55. Wang GJ, Moskal JT, Albert T, et al. The effect of halo-vest length on stability of the cervical spine. *J Bone Joint Surg* 1988;70-A(3):357–360.

56. Whitesides TE, Mehserle WL, Hutton WC. The force exerted by the halo pin, a study comparing different halo systems. *Spine* 1992;17(105):S413–416.

57. White AA, Johnson RM, Panjabi MM, et al. Biomechanical analysis of clinical stability in the cervical spine. *Clin Orthop* 1975;109:85–96.

58. Black CA, Budarer NMF, Blaylock B, et al. Comparative study of risk factors for skin breakdown with cervical orthotic devices: Philadelphia and Aspen. *J Trauma Nursing* 1998;5(3):62–66.

59. Blaylock B. Solving the problem of pressure ulcers resulting from cervical collars. *Ostomy Wound Manag* 1996;42(4):26–33.

60. Walton R, DeSalo JF, Ernst AA, et al. Padded vs unpadded spine board for cervical spine immobilization. *Acad Emerg Med* 1995;2:725–728.

61. Gaskill SJ, Marlin AE. Custom fitted thermoplastic Minerva jackets in the treatment of cervical spine instability in preschool age children. *Pediatr Neurosurg* 1991;16:35–39.

62. Kopits SE, Steingass MH. Experience with the "halo-cast" in small children. *Surg Clin North Am* 1970;50(4):935–943.

63. Glaser JA, Whitehill R, Stamp WG, et al. Complications associated with the halo-vest. *J Neurosurg* 1986;65:762–769.

64. Bucci MN, Dauser RC, Maynard FA, et al. Management of posttraumatic cervical spine instability: operative fusion versus halo vest immobilization. Analysis of 49 cases. *J Trauma* 1988;28(7):1001–1006.

65. Bucholz RD, Cheung KC. Halo vest versus spinal fusion for cervical injury: evidence from an outcome study. *J Neurosurg* 1989;70:884–892.

66. Chan RC, Schweigel JF, Thompson GB. Halo-thoracic brace immobilization in 188 patients with acute cervical spine injuries. *J Neurosurg* 1983;58:508–515.

67. Chandler DR, Nemejc C, Adkins RH, et al. Emergency cervical-spine immobilization. *Ann Emerg Med* 1992;21:1185–1188.

68. Clark CR, White AA. Fractures of the dens, a multicenter study. *J Bone Joint Surg* 1985;67-A(9):1340–1348.

69. Cooper PR, Maravilla KR, Sklar FH, et al. Halo immobilization of cervical spine fractures, indications and results. *J Neurosurg* 1979;50:603–610.

70. Dunn ME, Seljeskog EL. Experience in the management of odontoid process injuries: an analysis of 128 cases. *Neurosurgery* 1986;18(3):306–310.

71. Ekong CEU, Schwartz ML, Tator CH, et al. Odontoid fracture: management with early mobilization using the halo device. *Neurosurgery* 1981;9(6):631–637.

72. Ewald FC. Fracture of the odontoid process in a seventeen-month-old infant treated with a halo, a case report and discussion of the injury under the age of three. *J Bone Joint Surg* 1971;53-A(8):1636–1640.

73. Lee TT, Green BA, Petrin DR. Treatment of stable burst fracture of the atlas (Jefferson fracture) with rigid cervical collar. *Spine* 1998;23(18):1963–1967.

74. Lemons VR, Wagner FC. Stabilization of subaxial cervical spinal injuries. *Surg Neurol* 1993;39:511–518.

75. Lind B, Nordwall A, Sihlbom H. Odontoid fractures treated with a halo-vest. *Spine* 1987;12(2):173–177.

76. Lind B, Sihlbom H, Nordwall A. Halo-vest treatment of unstable traumatic cervical spine injuries. *Spine* 1988;13(4):425–432.

77. Mandabach M, Ruge JR, Hahn YS, et al. Pediatric axis fractures: early halo immobilization, management and outcome. *Pediatr Neurosurg* 1993;19:225–232.

78. Polin RS, Szabo T, Bogaev CA, et al. Nonoperative management of types II and III odontoid fractures: the Philadelphia collar versus the halo vest. *Neurosurgery* 1996;38:450–457.

79. Rockswold GL, Bergman TA, Ford SE. Halo immobilization and surgical fusion: relative indications and effectiveness in the treatment of 140 cervical spine injuries. *J Trauma* 1990;30(7):893–898.

80. Romanelli DA, Dickman CA, Porter RW, et al. Comparison of initial injury feature in cervical spine trauma of C3-C7: predictive outcome with halo-vest management. *J Spinal Disord* 1996;9(2):146–149.

81. Sears W, Fazi M. Prediction of stability of cervical spine fracture managed in the halo vest and indications for surgical intervention. *J Neurosurg* 1990;72:426–432.

82. Huerta C, Griffith R, Joyce SM. Cervical spine stabilization in pediatric patients: evaluation of current techniques. *Ann Emerg Med* 1987;16:1121–1126.

83. Herzenberg JE, Hensinger RN, Dedrick DK, et al. Emergency transport and positioning of young children who have an injury of the cervical spine. *J Bone Joint Surg* 1989;71-A(1):15–22.

84. Curran C, Dietrich AM, Bowman MJ, et al. Pediatric cervical-spine immobilization: achieving neutral position. *J Trauma Injury Infect Crit Care* 1995;39(4):729–732.

85. Nypaver M, Treloar D. Neutral cervical spine positioning in children. *Ann Emerg Med* 1994;23:208–211.

86. Treloar DJ, Nypaver M. Angulation of the pediatric cervical spine with and without cervical collar. *Pediatr Emerg Care* 1997;13(1):5–8.

87. Chendraskhar A, Moorman DW, Timberlake GA, et al. An evaluation of the effects of semirigid cervical collars in patients with severe closed head injury. *Am Surgeon* 1998;64(7):604–606.

88. Althoff B, Goldie IF. Cervical collars in rheumatoid atlanto-axial subluxation: a radiographic comparison. *Ann Rheum Dis* 1980;39:485–489.

89. Phillips WA, Hensinger RN. The management of rotatory atlanto-axial subluxation in children. *J Bone Joint Surg* 1989;71-A(5):664–668.

90. Celli P, Palatinsky E. Brain abscess as a complication of cranial traction. *Surg Neurol* 1985;23:594–596.

91. Feldman RA, Khayyat GF. Perforation of the skull by a Gardner-Wells tong, case report. *J Neurosurg* 1976;44:119–120.

92. Kaye AH, Briggs M. Brain abscess after insertion of skull traction. *J Bone Joint Surg* 1982;64-B(4):500–502.

93. Graziano GP, Herzenberg JE, Hensinger RN. The halo-Ilizarov distraction cast for correction of cervical deformity, report of six cases. *J Bone Joint Surg* 1993;75-A(7):996–1003.

94. Kalamchi A, Yau AC, O'Brien JP, et al. Halo-pelvic distraction apparatus, an analysis of one hundred and fifty consecutive patients. *J Bone Joint Surg* 1976;58-A(8):1119–1125.

95. Kostuik JP. Indications for the use of the halo immobilization. *Clin Orthop* 1981;154:46–50.

96. Heary RF, Hunt CD, Krieger AJ, et al. Acute stabilization of the cervical spine by halo vest application facilitates evaluation and treatment of multiple trauma patients. *J Trauma* 1992;33(3):445–450.

97. Schwarz N, Genelin F, Schwarz AF. Posttraumatic cervical kyphosis in children cannot be prevented by non-operative methods. *Injury* 1994;25(3):173–175.

98. Koop SE, Winter RB, Lonstein JE. The surgical treatment of instability of the upper part of the cervical spine in children and adolescents. *J Bone Joint Surg* 1984;66-A(3):403–411.

99. Dennis GC, Clifton GL. Brain abscess as a complication of halo fixation. *Neurosurgery* 1982;10(6):760–761.

100. Garfin SR, Botte MJ, Triggs KJ, et al. Subdural abscess associated with halo pin traction. *J Bone Joint Surg* 1988;70-A(9):1338–1340.

101. Humbyrd DE, Latimer FR, Lonstein JE, et al. Brain abscess as a complication of halo traction. *Spine* 1981;6(4):365–368.

102. Victor DI, Bresnan MJ, Keller RB. Brain abscess complicating the use of halo traction. *J Bone Joint Surg* 1973;55-A(3):635–639.

103. Whitehill R, Richman JA, Glaser JA. Failure of immobilization of the cervical spine by the halo vest. *J Bone Joint Surg* 1986;68-A(3):326–332.

104. Browner CM, Hadley MN, Sonntag VKH, et al. Halo immobilization brace care: an innovative approach. *J Neurosci Nurs* 1987;19(1):24–29.

105. Garfin SR, Botte MJ, Centeno RS, et al. Osteology of the skull as it affects halo pin placement. *Spine* 1985;10(8):696–698.

106. Garfin SR, Roux R, Botte MJ, et al. Skull osteology as it affects halo pin placement in children. *J Pediatr Orthop* 1986;6:434–436.

107. Gaufin LM, Goodman SJ. Cervical spine injuries in infants, problems in management. *J Neurosurg* 1975;42:179–184.

108. Loder RT. Skull thickness and halo-pin placement in children: the effects of race, gender and laterality. *J Pediatr Orthop* 1996;16:340–343.

109. Mubarak SJ, Camp JF, Vuletich W, et al. Halo application in the infant. *J Pediatr Orthop* 1989;9:612–614.
110. Wong WB, Haynes RJ. Osteology of the pediatric skull, considerations of halo pin placement. *Spine* 1994;19(13):1451–1454.
Clayman DA, Murakami ME, Vines FS. Compatibility of cervical spine braces with MR imaging: a study of nine nonferrous devices. *Am J Neuroradiol* 1990;11:385–390.

Krag MH, Beynnon BD. A new halo-vest: rationale, design and biomechanical comparison to standard halo-vest designs. *Spine* 1988;13(3): 228–235.
Schriger DL, Larmon B, LeGassick T, et al. Spinal immobilization on a flat backboard. Does it result in neutral position of the cervical spine? *Ann Emerg Med* 1991;20:878–881.

CHAPTER 31

Evaluation of the Cervical Spine in Children

B. David Horn and John P. Dormans

Evaluation of the cervical spine in infants, children, and adolescents poses unique challenges to the practitioner. A thorough understanding of the developmental anatomy and features of the growing spine is required to properly evaluate and treat disorders of the immature cervical spine. Disorders present in children are often congenital or developmental in nature and may be seen infrequently in adults. In addition, children (particularly those who are preverbal, nonverbal, frightened, or in pain) may be difficult to examine and unable to describe their symptoms or localize pain. Radiographic standards and techniques used to evaluate the cervical spine primarily have been described in and derived from adult studies, and must be interpreted in light of the special features of the growing cervical spine. For these reasons, evaluation of the cervical spine in infant children and adolescents differs from that of adults and requires a thorough understanding of the anatomy, growth, and development of the pediatric cervical spine.

DEVELOPMENTAL ANATOMY

The developmental anatomy of the cervical spine is best understood through its embryology. By the third week of gestation, the notochord is formed from mesenchymal tissue (1). Adjacent and parallel to the notochord lies the paraxial mesoderm, which eventually differentiates into segmented somites (1,2). By week three, four cranial and eight cervical somites develop from the mesoderm (1–4). During the fourth week of gestation, these somites further differentiate into sclerotomes and myodermatomes; sclerotomes are the precursors of the spinal column (1–3). The sclerotomes undergo a process known as resegmentation, where each somite divides into a cranial and caudal portion. The cranial half of each somite then fuses with the caudal portion of an adjacent somite, forming a prevertebra (1,2,5).

Ventrally, sclerotomal cells form the vertebral bodies, discs, and costal processes. Dorsally, they form the pedicles and lamina of the vertebrae. The apical and alar ligaments of the atlantoaxial articulation as well as the nucleus pulposus of the intervertebral discs form from the notochord. Spinal growth occurs by endochondral ossification that is preceded by mesenchymal chondrification during weeks five and six.

THE ATLAS

The atlas (Fig. 31.1) develops from three ossification centers (6,7). At birth, the two primary ossification centers are the lateral masses, which have already ossified. A secondary ossification center for the body of the atlas is present by 1 year of age. The posterior arches fuse by 3 to 4 years of age, whereas the neurocentral synchondroses between the lateral masses and the body of C1 fuse by about age 7. As a result, the final internal diameter of the atlas is present by about age 7 years, whereas further growth of the external diameter of the atlas occurs through appositional bone deposition.

THE AXIS

The axis (Fig. 31.2) develops from five primary ossification centers (8,9). The odontoid has two separate ossification centers, which generally fuse in the midline by the seventh month of prenatal development. Persistence of the two halves of the odontoid is known as a dens bicornis. A separate ossification center comprises the body (centrum), whereas two ossification centers make up the right and left lateral masses (neural arches). There are also two secondary ossification centers present in the immature axis (8). One forms the tip of the odontoid, which appears at 3 to 6 years of age. This generally fuses with the body of the odontoid

Atlas

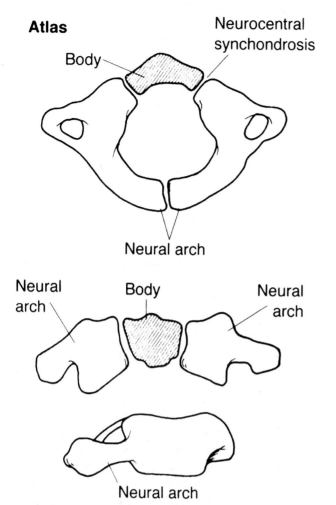

FIG. 31.1. Diagrammatic drawings of the atlas (C1) showing bird's eye, anterior, and lateral views. (From: Copley LA, Dormans JP. Cervical spine disorders in infants and children. *J Am Acad Orthop Surg* 1998;6:205.)

Axis

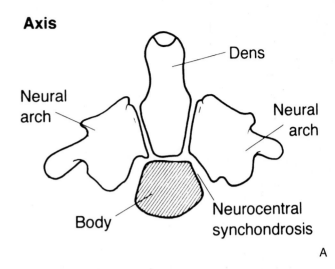

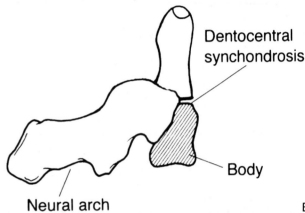

FIG. 31.2. Diagrammatic drawings of the axis (C2) showing **(A)** anterior and **(B)** lateral views. (From: Copley LA, Dormans JP. Cervical spine disorders in infants and children. *J Am Acad Orthop Surg* 1998;6:205.)

by age 12, but may occasionally persist as a separate ossification center. This is termed an ossiculum terminale and is considered a normal anatomic variant (8). The inferior apophyseal ring also contains a secondary ossification center that generally appears at puberty and fuses with the body of the axis by age 25 (8).

The neurocentral synchondrosis between the body of the axis and odontoid generally fuses between 3 and 6 years of age. A remnant of this may be radiographically visible up to age 12. This synchondrosis is positioned caudal to the level of the superior articular facets of C2 and contributes to the height of the odontoid process. Its appearance on an anteroposterior (AP) radiograph has been described as being similar to a "cork in a bottle" and may be present in 50% of children 5 years of age. Its presence can be misinterpreted as a fracture. The synchondrosis is absent in most children by 6 years of age (2,6,8). The synchondroses connecting the

neural arches and the body and odontoid generally fuse at 3 to 6 years of age, whereas the synchondroses between the spinous process usually fuse by 3 years of age (8).

LOWER CERVICAL VERTEBRAE (C3-7)

The vertebrae of the lower cervical spine (Fig. 31.3) each ossify from three ossification centers: one ossification center for the body and two for the neural arches (10). There are two secondary ossification centers present, the superior and inferior ring apophyses. These apophyses ossify during late childhood and contribute to vertebral body height. These fuse with the vertebral bodies by 25 years of age (10). The neurocentral synchondroses between the body and neural arches generally fuse between 3 and 6 years of age. The spinous process synchondrosis located between the two neural arches generally fuse by 3 years of age (10).

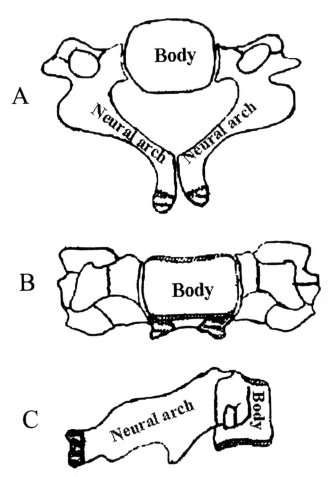

FIG. 31.3. Diagrammatic drawings of vertebrae of the lower cervical spine showing **(A)** bird's eye, **(B)** anterior, and **(C)** lateral views.

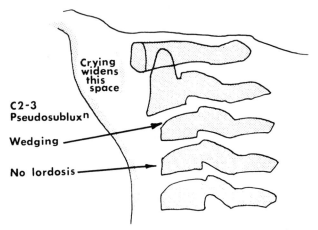

FIG. 31.4. Unique features of the child's spinal column. (From: Rang M. *Spine and spinal cord in children's fractures*, 2nd ed. Philadelphia: JB Lippincott, 1983.)

THE IMMATURE CERVICAL SPINE: HOW IS THE CHILD DIFFERENT?

Anatomic and developmental factors result in many of the unique characteristics of the immature cervical spine (Fig. 31.4). These differences generally occur in children younger than 8 years of age, at which time the cervical spine approaches adult morphology and size (11). Children younger than 8 years of age have increased neck motion compared to adults for several reasons (12,13). The facet joints in the immature cervical spine are horizontally oriented and become more vertical with growth. The facet orientation from C5-7 increases from approximately 55 to 70 degrees during growth, whereas the facets in the upper cervical spine increase vertical orientation from 30 to 70 degrees during growth (12–14). Younger children and infants have generalized ligament laxity and weaker neck muscles compared with older children, and the head accounts for a greater proportion of body weight in young children than adults (13). Incomplete ossification of the cervical spine, particularly in the subaxial region, may give

the vertebral bodies a wedge-shaped appearance on plain radiographs (8,11,14). In addition, incomplete ossification accounts for differences between children and adults in radiographic measurements that are commonly used to evaluate the cervical spine.

These unique anatomic and developmental factors allow for injuries and injury patterns in children not seen in adults. Spinal cord injury without radiographic abnormality (SCIWORA) occurs in children because of a relative mismatch between the elasticity of the vertebral column and spinal cord (6,15–17). In the cervical spine, the spinal column in children can be stretched as much as 2 inches before failure, whereas the spinal cord itself only tolerates about 0.25 inches of stretching before injury (16,18). Ligamentous laxity is thought to account for the high incidence of multilevel spinal injuries seen in children when compared with adults (19). The disproportionate weight of the head compared to the body mass in young children also accounts for the difference in spinal cord injury patterns seen in children younger than 8 years compared to older children. Children in the younger age group are more likely to have injuries of the third cervical vertebrae or higher and have an increased risk of death from their spinal cord injury. Children older than 8 years of age have an adult-type injury pattern, with most injuries occurring caudal to the fourth cervical vertebrae (20).

A commonly seen consequence of the increased mobility of the cervical spine in young children compared to adults or older children is the presence of physiologic cervical spine subluxation (pseudosubluxation) on lateral spine radiographs. This finding is termed pseudosubluxation when it is noted without true subluxation or pathology (Fig. 31.4) (11,14,21). This is a normal physiologic variation and does not need treatment (Table 31.1). Pseudosubluxation occurs most commonly between the second and third cervical vertebrae and between the third and fourth cervical vertebrae

TABLE 31.1. *Cervical Spine Mobility According to Age*

Age (yr)	1	2	3	4	5	6	7	8	9	10	11	12	13	14	15	16	Total (1–16 yr) (n)	(%)	Total (1–7 yr) (n)	(%
Anterior displacement C2-3 (marked)	4	1	3	1	2	2	0	0	1	1	0	0	0	0	0	0	15	9	13	19
Anterior displacement C2-3 (moderate)	1	2	1	3	2	2	4	1	1	2	3	1	1	0	0	0	24	15	15	21
Anterior displacement C2-3 (total)	5	3	4	4	4	4	4	1	2	3	3	1	1	0	0	0	39	24	28	40
Measured anteroposterior movement, 3 mm and over	5	4	5	2	5	6	5	2	4	5	4	6	7	4	4	3	71	44	32	46
Number of children with measured anteroposterior movement over 3 mm and observed anterior displacement at C2-3	4	3	3	1	3	4	3	0	1	3	1	1	1	0	0	0	28	18	21	30
Anterior displacement C3-4[a]	3	2	1	1	2	4	1	0	2	2	2	1	1	0	0	0	22	14	14	20
Overriding of anterior arch of atlas relative to odontoid (extension views)[b]	2+	4++	3++	1	1+	3	0	1	0	0	0	0	0	0	0	0	14	9	14	20
Wide space between anterior arch of atlas and odontoid (flexion views)	2	2	3	2	2	2	1	0	0	0	0	0	0	0	0	0	14	9	14	20
Total (5–11 yr)																				
Presence of apical odontoid epiphysis	0	0	0	0	3	2	3	1	4	1	4	0	0	0	0	0	15	9	18	26
Total (1–5 yr)																				
Presence of basilar odontoid cartilage plate	10	9	9	6	4	0	0	0	0	0	0	0	0	0	0	0	48	30	38	76
Angulation at single level	1	4	1	1	3	3	2	0	1	2	1	2	2	1	2	0	25	16		
Absent lordosis in neutral position	3	0	0	0	0	0	0	1	2	1	3	2	2	5	1	2	22	14		
Absent flexion curvature C2-7 in flexion view	1	2	1	6	4	1	0	0	2	3	1	1	1	1	2	0	26	16		

[a] Twenty of 22 children with anterior displacement at C3-4 also had displacement at C2-3.
[b] Presence of wide atlantoodontoid space in same child (each + represents one child).
From: Cattell HS, Filtzer DL. Pseudosubluxation and other normal variations in the cervical spine in children: a study of one hundred and sixty children. *J Bone Joint Surg* 1965;47:1295–1309.

(11,14,21). This is seen in up to 40% of children under age 8 and may account for as much as 4 mm of anterior-posterior incongruity between the second and third cervical vertebrae with the spine in flexion (12,14). The posterior spinolaminar line of Swischuk (Fig. 31.5) can help differential between pseudosubluxation and true subluxation. This line is drawn along the posterior arch from the first cervical vertebrae to the third and should pass within 2 mm of the posterior arch of the second cervical vertebrae. If this line passes more than 2 mm posterior to the anterior cortex of the posterior arch of C2, the line is disrupted and true subluxation is present (14).

Children also may lack the normal cervical lordosis (Fig. 31.4) seen in adults. This cervical kyphosis or straightening can occur normally in up to 14% of children less than 16 years of age. In children without an injury, cervical lordosis is restored with neck extension (12). The C3 vertebral body also may be wedged (Fig. 31.4) in about 7% of young children (1,11). Computed tomography (CT) or magnetic resonance imaging (MRI) can help differentiate this normal variant from a compression fracture.

HISTORY AND PHYSICAL EXAMINATION

The evaluation of the cervical spine in children should always include a thorough history and physical examination. A history of a difficult or breech delivery, delayed motor development, hypotonia, or later hypertonia may indicate perinatal injury to the upper cervical spine (22,23). A history of injury also may be present in children presenting for evaluation of the neck. Minor trauma that results in neurologic symptoms may be indicative of preexisting pathology such as basilar impression (24). High-energy trauma

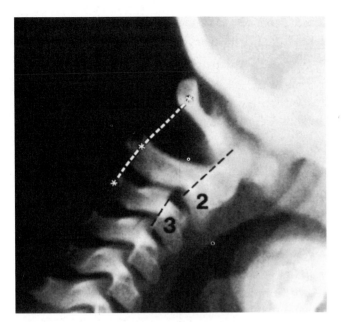

FIG. 31.5. Swischuk's line *(white line)* drawn on a lateral plain radiograph of the cervical spine helps differentiate physiologic versus pathologic subluxation in a child. A pseudosubluxation at C2-3 is shown *(black line)* with a normal Swischuk's line. (From: Loder RT. The cervical spine. In: Morrissy RT, Weinstein SL, eds. *Lovell and Winter's pediatric orthopaedics,* 5th ed. Philadelphia: Lippincott Williams & Wilkins, 2001:799–840.)

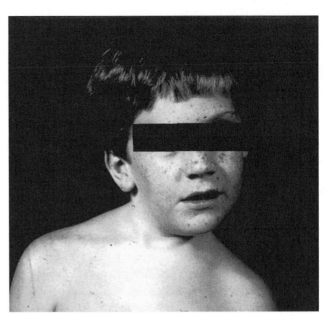

FIG. 31.6. Child with right muscular torticollis showing the head tilted to the right side and rotated to the left.

associated with head or facial injuries, including loss of consciousness, altered mental status, or a neck injury may be consistent with a spinal cord injury (25,26). Generalized developmental or congenital conditions such as Morquio disease, spondyloepiphyseal dysplasia, osteogenesis imperfecta, juvenile arthritis, diastrophic dwarfism, and Down syndrome also may point to underlying cervical spine pathology (27–29). Recent upper respiratory tract infections (e.g., laryngitis or tonsillitis) or surgery (e.g., tonsillectomy) also should be determined in the history because these may precede atlantoaxial rotary subluxation or lead to the development of postsurgical infections that may cause torticollis (Fig. 31.6) (30,31). Symptoms of neck problems may include neck or occipital pain, neck snapping or popping, upper extremity paresthesias, pain, weakness, headaches, seizures, syncope, and torticollis (32–34). Cranial dysfunction also may be present, particularly in pathology involving the brain stem (24). Respiratory distress in infants and newborns also may indicate upper cervical instability and resultant spinal cord compression, whereas a history of decreased exercise tolerance or easy fatigability may be a subtle indicator of cervical myelopathy (35).

A thorough physical examination should be performed while evaluating children for cervical spine disorders. Limitation of motion, stiffness, upper or lower extremity weakness, reflex changes, torticollis and cervical muscle spasm may all be present in cervical spine pathology and should be noted on the physical examination (32–35). Neck webbing,

shortening, and torticollis also may indicate underlying congenital spine anomalies (36,37). A complete neurologic examination also should be performed, including cranial nerve testing, gait evaluation, and upper and lower extremity evaluation (24).

PHYSICAL EXAMINATION

A thorough examination should be performed when evaluating children for a cervical spine disorder. Examination of the infant and child can be much more challenging and difficult than that of an adult. The examination of an infant should be done in a warm examination room and in a quiet and calm atmosphere. If the child is upset or crying, often it is best to wait 5 to 10 minutes while the parents comfort the child before attempting an examination. Infants should be fed and relaxed prior to examination. It may be most effective to examine infants and toddlers while on the lap of a parent or caregiver. In older children, the examination may be complicated by the child's difficulty in following directions and describing relevant signs secondary to the physical examination.

The initial portion of the examination consists of observation. In ambulatory children this should include the child's gait as well as any posturing or abnormal position of the upper extremities that may be exhibited while walking. Any head tilt, rotation, or guarding of neck motion should be noted. Following this general observation the next step is to more specifically observe the position of the head upright. Any tilt or rotation of the head in relationship to the body should be noted. In muscular torticollis the chin is rotated away from the affected side, whereas the head is tilted toward the involved side. The face and skull should be inspected for facial asymmetry or plagiocephaly. Observing the child from the front, rear, and top while supine, helps detect minor degrees of asymmetry that otherwise may not be apparent. In older children, a short neck or low hairline may be indicative of underlying congenital anomalies such as, Klippel-Feil syndrome. Holding the head in a "hanging head" position has been associated with the presence of brain stem and upper cervical spine tumors (38).

Neurologic screening can be performed by observing the patient's gait and checking the patient's ability to toe walk and heel walk. This is a screen for plantar flexion and dorsiflexion strength as well as balance. A rounding test may be used to assess the brain stem and cerebellar function.

The next portion of the examination usually involves palpation of the head and neck region. In younger children, the head should be palpated for the presence of any masses. The anterior fontanelle of infants should be palpated as well. Any fullness should be noted because this may indicate hydrocephalus. In addition, premature closure may suggest craniosynostosis. The anterior fontanelle normally closes between 4 and 26 months of age. The cervical region posteriorly then should be palpated for any masses or areas of tenderness. The cervical paraspinal muscles similarly can be palpated for any areas of tenderness or spasm. The anterior neck as well should be evaluated for any areas of swelling or tenderness and the sternocleidomastoid muscle should be palpated for spasm, fibrosis, or masses. Pseudotumors of the sternocleidomastoid muscles may be noted in congenital muscular torticollis.

The neck then should be checked for active and passive range of motion. Active flexion/extension, rotation, and lateral bending should be evaluated. Passive range of motion also should be gently measured and any guarding, pain, or limitation of motion should be noted.

The cranial nerves may be involved in upper cervical spine disease. Cranial nerves III through VIII, which originate from the brain stem, should be tested. The III, IV, and VI cranial nerves control ocular function. Pupillary reaction to light should be tested as well as extraocular movement. Remember that the IV cranial nerve (trochlear) controls the superior oblique muscle of the eye only. The V cranial nerve (trigeminal) can be tested by checking sensation on the face as well as the corneal reflex. The VII cranial nerve (facial) can be tested by observing for facial symmetry as well as by testing facial muscle strength. The VIII cranial nerve (acoustic) can be tested by a hearing screening. The IX and X cranial nerves (glossopharyngeal and vagus) can be assessed by evaluating the patient's voice for hoarseness, looking for deviation of the uvula, and testing for the gag reflex. The XI cranial nerve is the spinal accessory nerve. This provides motor power to the trapezius muscles and can be tested by assessing shoulder shrug strength. The XII cranial nerve, the hypoglossal, can be evaluated by listening to speech articulation as well as inspecting the tongue. With tongue protrusion, asymmetry or deviation may be indicative of a XII cranial nerve lesion.

The motor system then should be evaluated. Muscle bulk and tone should be assessed for atrophy. Hypertonicity or spasticity may indicate myelopathy from a cervical spine disorder.

Motor and sensory examinations then should be performed for the upper and lower extremities. In children less than 4 years of age it may be difficult to perform manual strength testing. In this situation, observing the child walking, running, crawling, or playing may provide clues regarding the upper and lower extremity neuromuscular function. The biceps motor strength assesses C5 and C6. The biceps reflex, although it involves nerve roots from C5 and C6, primarily assesses the C5 root. Sensation for C5 is the axillary nerve over the lateral deltoid muscle. The integrity of C6 can be assessed by checking the strength of the wrist extensors and brachioradialis reflex. C6 sensory region is over the lateral forearm, thumb, and index finger. Triceps and wrist flexion strength check the C7 motor function. The C7 reflex is the triceps tendon reflex, whereas the sensory testing for C7 is accomplished by testing the sensation over the middle finger, although this is variable and may not be reliable. Finger flexor strength evaluates the C8 motor strength. There is no reflex for C8 sensory examination; this root is over the medial forearm, and the ring and middle finger of the hand. Motor testing for T1 is the interossei muscles, whereas sensory testing of T1 is the medial portion of the arm.

Examination of the spine also should include neurologic evaluation of the lower extremities. Hip flexion strength can be used to assess T1-L3. Quadriceps strength tests L2, L3, and L4. L4 motor testing can be accomplished by testing the strength of the tibialis anterior muscle, assessing the patellar tendon reflex, and checking sensation in the medial aspect of the foot. The L5 nerve root is best tested by the strength of the extensor digitorum longus muscle and sensation of the dorsum of the foot. S1 is best tested through peroneal muscle strength testing as well as gastroc-soleus muscle strength testing. The Achilles tendon reflex also tests S1, as does sensation on the lateral side of the foot. Perianal sensation can be used to assess S2, S3, and S4 root levels.

RADIOGRAPHS

Initial radiographic evaluation should include high-quality cross-table lateral, AP, and open-mouth odontoid process radiographs of the cervical spine. A lateral flexion and extension view also may be helpful to evaluate cervical stability. In cases of suspected traumatic injury, the flexion/extension films should be performed after the static films have been evaluated and the examination should be performed under supervised conditions. Care should be taken to visualize the disc space between the seventh cervical and first thoracic vertebra. This may require specialized radiographic views in order to image the area. In some cases, CT may be indicated in order to evaluate this region adequately.

Analysis of the radiographs typically begins with the assessment of four lines (Fig. 31.7). These are lines connecting: (1) the tips of the spinous processes; (2) the spinolaminar line; (3) the posterior margins of the vertebral bodies; and (4) the anterior margins of the vertebral bodies. All of these lines should follow a smooth, even contour (39). The facets should be inspected for parallelism and interspinous distances also should be evaluated (21). A widening of more than 10 mm between the spinous processes and the first and second cervical vertebrae on the lateral radiograph may indicate an underlying posterior soft-tissue injury with potential spinal cord injury.

In adults, the retropharyngeal and retrotracheal spaces are commonly assessed and measured on the lateral neck radiographs. Children may have increased measurements for these spaces because less of their cervical spine is ossified. Therefore, radiographic interpretation may be difficult.

In general, the retropharyngeal space in children should be less than 7 mm, whereas the retrotracheal space in children should measure less than 14 mm (40). The anterior ring in C1 may not be ossified in children younger than 1 year of age and may cause the anterior arch of the atlas to appear that it overrides the odontoid process (12). In addition, the odontoid process normally may be posteriorly angulated in up to 4% of children (41). Subtle findings suggestive of an injury to the cervical spine include disc space widening, avulsion fractures of the vertebral end plates, and spinous process fractures (Fig. 31.8).

Several other measurements have been described for the upper cervical spine. Many of these help describe the relationship between the base of the skull, first cervical vertebra, second cervical vertebra, and spinal cord.

McGregor's line (Fig. 31.9) is useful for detecting basilar impression (42). This line is drawn from the superior surface of the posterior edge of the hard palate to the most caudal point of the occiput. The distance from the tip of the

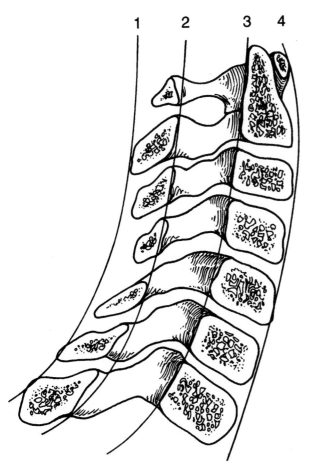

FIG. 31.7. Four-line analysis of cervical spine radiographs. These are lines connecting the (1) tips of the spinous processes; (2) spinolaminar line; (3) posterior margins; and (4) anterior margins of the vertebral bodies of the vertebral bodies. All of these lines should follow a smooth, even contour. (From: Copley LA, Dormans JP. Cervical spine disorders in infants and children. *J Am Acad Orthop Surg* 1998;6:205.)

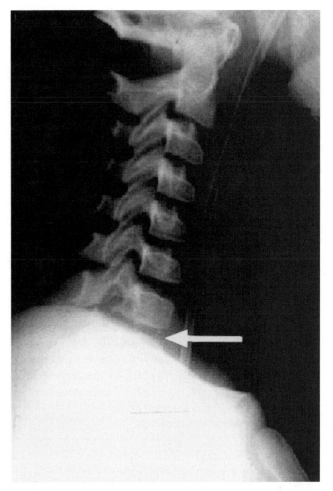

FIG. 31.8. Radiograph demonstrating subtle findings suggestive of unstable injury, such as subtle disc space narrowing at C7-T1 *(large arrow)* and asymmetries of spinous process distances. This child had an occipitocervical SCIWORA (spinal cord injury without radiographic abnormality) injury.

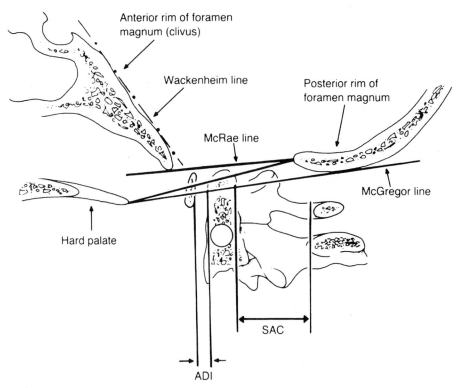

FIG. 31.9. Schematic drawing showing measurements used to describe the relationship between the base of the skull, the first cervical vertebra, second cervical vertebra, and spinal cord. (From: Copley LA, Dormans JP. Cervical spine disorders in infants and children. *J Am Acad Orthop Surg* 1998;6:205.)

occiput to this line is measured. If the tip of the odontoid process lies more than 4.5 mm above McGregor's line, the finding is considered consistent with basilar impression.

McRae's line (Fig. 31.9) defines the opening of the foramen magnum extending from the posterior rim of the foramen magnum, anteriorly to the tip of the clivus (43). Projection of the tip of the odontoid above this line is another radiographic sign of basilar impression.

The Rothman-Weisel method (Fig. 31.10) of measuring anteroposterior translation of the atlantooccipital joint consists of drawing an initial line between the anterior portion of the anterior arch of the atlas and posterior portion of the posterior spinous process of the atlas (44). Then two lines are drawn perpendicular to this line: One is located at the posterior margin of the anterior arch of the atlas, whereas the second line intersects the basion. The distance between these two perpendicular lines should not vary by more than 1 mm with flexion and extension.

Power's ratio (Fig. 31.11) also can be used to evaluate atlanto-occipital instability (45). This is derived by first measuring a line drawn between the basion and posterior margin of the atlas. A second line is drawn from the opisthion to the anterior arch of the atlas, then measured. To obtain Power's ratio, the length of the first line is divided by the length of the second line. A ratio greater than 1 suggests atlantooccipital instability.

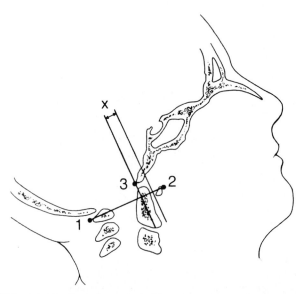

FIG. 31.10. Rothman and Wiesel method of measuring atlantooccipital instability. There should be less than 1 mm translation. (From: Copley LA, Dormans JP. Cervical spine disorders in infants and children. *J Am Acad Orthop Surg* 1998;6:205.)

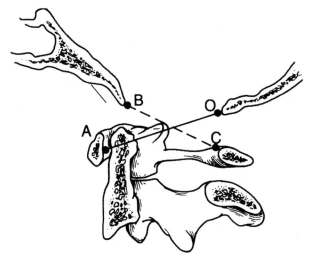

FIG. 31.11. Power's ratio is used to evaluate atlantooccipital instability. (From: Copley LA, Dormans JP. Cervical spine disorders in infants and children. *J Am Acad Orthop Surg* 1998;6:205.)

The middle half of the odontoid process lies directly beneath the basion at an average distance of 5 mm on the lateral radiograph (6,40). Because of incomplete ossification, this distance may be increased to up to 1 cm in children younger than 8 years of age (40). The basion-axial interval, the distance between the basion and posterior axial line, also has been evaluated in occipital cervical instability. This should not measure more than 12 mm in children younger than 13 years of age (46).

The atlantodens interval and the space available for the cord are commonly used measurements in the assessment of the region of the upper cervical spine (Fig. 31.12). The atlantodens interval is the space between the anterior border of the dens and the posterior edge of the anterior ring of the atlas. It should be less than 4 mm in children who are younger than 8 years of age and less than 3 mm in older children. This measurement normally may be larger (up to 5 mm) in children with Down syndrome (21,47).

Steel's "rule of thirds" is a useful guideline in evaluating the space available for the spinal cord at the level of the first cervical vertebrae and remains valid throughout skeletal growth (48,49). At C1, one-third of the space is occupied by the odontoid process and one-third of the space is free space and allows for a safety zone in cases of instability between the first and second cervical vertebrae. This free space constitutes a safety zone in situations where there is instability between the first and second cervical vertebrae. When the atlantoodontoid interval exceeds 10 to 12 mm, both the transverse ligament and alar ligaments (which normally provide stability to the articulation between the odontoid and the axis) have failed; this greatly diminishes the space available for the cord (50). The space available for the cord also may be directly measured by drawing a line from the posterior margin of the odontoid to the anterior margin of

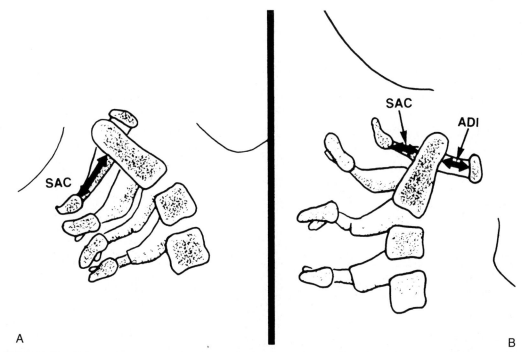

FIG. 31.12. Schematic drawing of the upper cervical spine demonstrating the atlantodens interval (ADI) and space available for the cord in **(A)** extension and **(B)** flexion. The ACI should not exceed 4 mm in a child. (From: Loder RT. The cervical spine. In: Morrissy RT, Weinstein SL, eds. *Lovell and Winter's pediatric orthopaedics,* 5th ed. Philadelphia: Lippincott Williams & Wilkins, 2001:799–840.)

TABLE 31.2. *Sagittal Diameter of the Bony Cervical Spinal Canal in 120 Normal Children: Relation to Age*

Age Group	3–6 (yr)			7–10 (yr)			11–14 (yr)		
Sex	Boys	Girls	Total	Boys	Girls	Total	Boys	Girls	Total
n	20	20	40	20	20	40	20	20	40
Location	Mean (mm)	Mean (mm)	Mean/SD mm	Mean (mm)	Mean (mm)	Mean/SD mm	Mean (mm)	Mean (mm)	Mean/SD mm
C1	20.2	19.6	19.9 ± 1.3	20.5	20.6	20.6 ± 1.3	21.2	21.4	21.3 ± 1.4
C2	18.2	17.6	17.9 ± 1.3	18.8	18.9	18.8 ± 1.0	19.3	19.5	19.4 ± 1.1
C3	16.3	15.8	16.0 ± 1.3	17.3	17.2	17.2 ± 1.0	17.8	17.7	17.8 ± 1.0
C4	16.0	15.6	15.8 ± 1.3	17.0	16.9	16.9 ± 0.9	17.3	17.2	17.3 ± 0.9
C5	15.9	15.5	15.7 ± 1.3	16.7	16.6	16.7 ± 0.9	17.1	16.9	17.0 ± 0.9
C6	15.8	15.3	15.6 ± 1.2	16.5	16.3	16.4 ± 0.9	16.8	16.6	16.7 ± 0.9
C7	15.6	15.0	15.3 ± 1.1	16.1	15.9	16.0 ± 0.9	16.3	16.2	16.2 ± 0.9

From: Markuske H. Sagittal diameter measurement of the bony cervical spinal canal in children. *Pediatr Radiol* 1977;6:129–131.

the posterior ring of C1. A measurement of less than 13 mm indicates spinal cord compression and possible neurologic impingement (Tables 31.2 and 31.3) (51).

SPECIAL STUDIES

The unique challenges of imaging the spine of children often require special imaging studies. Oblique radiographs may be useful in showing the facet joint detail. Tomography may be used to further visualize the cervical spine. These may be useful to further evaluate the anatomy in the upper cervical region, although this method has been supplanted largely by CT. Cineradiographs using fluoroscopy also may be obtained to obtain a dynamic view of the cervical spine motion. These typically are obtained with continuous fluoroscopy with the patient actively flexing and extending the neck. These may be useful in finding patterns of instability not seen on static flexion/extension radiographs, although they have a disadvantage of providing a relatively high radiation dose to the patient (52,53). CT allows a three-dimensional visualization of the cervical spine. This may be particularly useful to define the bony anatomy, because

ligaments and soft tissue do not visualize well with this technique. Two- and three-dimensional reconstructions are useful to visualize spinal anatomy optimally (54). Cases of atlantoaxial rotary displacement may be evaluated with dynamic CT with images taken in neutral and in left and right rotation. Myelography and computer tomography myelography have largely been replaced by MRI, but still may be of value, particularly to demonstrate dural bands or compression of the occipital cervical region.

MRI is widely used to evaluate the cervical spine in children. This technique allows visualization of the brain stem, spinal cord, soft tissue, and bony elements, and also detects for swelling and hemorrhage. MRI is the study of choice for evaluation of the spinal cord in children and is more sensitive than plain radiographs or CT for evaluation of soft tissue, ligaments, discs, and cartilage (Fig. 31.13). This is particularly useful when plain radiographs or CT are equivocal and is useful in evaluating the intubated or uncooperative child. Its major disadvantages include cost and the need for sedation or general anesthesia. Flexion and extension cervical MRIs also can be obtained to assess spinal cord compression secondary to instability (55). This may be useful

TABLE 31.3. *Sagittal Diameter of the Bony Cervical Spinal Canal in 120 Normal Children: Relation to Height*

Height (cm)	Age (yr)	n (Boys and girls)	C1 Mean (mm)	C2 Mean (mm)	C3 Mean (mm)	C4 Mean (mm)	C5 Mean (mm)	C6 Mean (mm)	C7 Mean (mm)
91–100	2.84–4.41	12	19.0	17.2	15.3	15.0	14.9	14.8	14.6
101–110	3.13–5.78	13	19.9	17.7	15.9	15.6	15.5	15.4	15.3
111–120	4.04–7.48	16	20.6	18.5	16.8	16.5	16.4	16.1	15.7
121–130	5.44–10.50	20	20.5	18.8	17.2	16.9	16.6	16.4	16.0
131–140	7.79–11.51	18	20.7	18.9	17.3	17.0	16.7	16.4	16.1
141–150	8.83–13.50	19	21.2	19.2	17.6	17.2	16.9	16.6	16.0
151–160	11.22–14.39	14	21.3	19.5	17.8	17.2	17.1	16.8	16.5
161–170	13.09–14.48	8	21.4	19.6	17.9	17.5	17.2	16.9	16.4

From: Markuske H. Sagittal diameter measurement of the bony cervical spinal canal in children. *Pediatr Radiol* 1977;6:129–131.

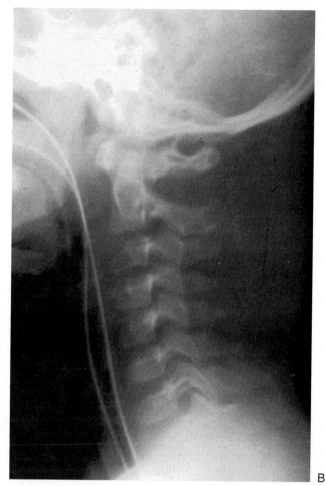

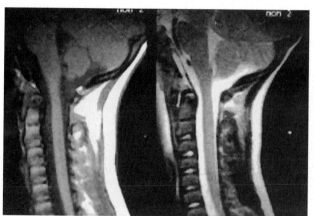

FIG. 31.13. A: Magnetic resonance imaging scans showing posterior bleeding in a 6-year-old patient with cervical spine injury. **B:** The child's plain radiographs were normal.

in identifying cord compromise and helping to select patients for surgical stabilization.

Additional studies also may be required to fully evaluate the cervical spine in infants, children, and adolescents. These may include, a three-phase bone scan with Technetium 99, particularly where osteomyelitis or tumors are suspected. Flexion/extension somatosensory evoked potentials also may be helpful in determining spinal cord function in cases of suspected cervical instability (56).

Evaluation of the cervical spine in infants, children, and adolescents differs from that of an adult. Children, particularly those less than 8 years of age, have substantially different anatomy and pathology than adults. Knowledge of the embryology, development, radiographic anatomy, and use of advance imaging techniques are needed for optimal evaluation of the cervical spine in infants, children, and adolescents.

CONCLUSION

Evaluation of the cervical spine in infants, children, and adolescents differs significantly from that of adults. Children

typically present with traumatic, congenital, or developmental disorders that may only rarely be seen in adults. When obtaining the history of an infant with a neck problem, attention must be paid to perinatal factors such as a difficult or breech delivery. Screening for developmental delays also should be performed and consideration must be given to genetic conditions as well as syndromes. Imaging of the immature cervical spine differs significantly from that of the adult spine. This results from the unique characteristics of the immature skeleton with increased cartilage, increased ligamentous laxity, and differences in the morphology of the spine when compared to adults. Consideration of these factors helps provide an accurate and optimal evaluation of the cervical spine in infants, children, and adolescents.

REFERENCES

1. Keynes RJ, Stern CD. Segmentation and neural development in vertebrates. *Trends Neurosci* 1985;8:220–223.
2. Tachdijian MO. *Pediatric orthopaedics,* 2nd ed. Philadelphia: WB Saunders, 1990.
3. Dormans JP. Evaluation of children with suspected cervical spine injury. *J Bone Joint Surg Am* 2002;84-A:124–132.

4. O'Rahilly R, Meyer DB. The timing and sequence of events in the development of the human vertebral column during the embryonic period proper. *Anat Embryol (Berl)* 1979;157:167–176.

5. Sensenig EC. The development of the occipital and cervical segments and their associated structures in human embryos. *Contrib Embryol Carnegie Inst* 1957;36:141.

6. Sullivan JA. *Fractures of the spine in children.* Philadelphia: WB Saunders, 1994.

7. Ogden JA. Radiology of postnatal skeletal development. XI. The first cervical vertebra. *Skeletal Radiol* 1984;12:12–20.

8. Ogden JA. Radiology of postnatal skeletal development. XII. The second cervical vertebra. *Skeletal Radiol* 1984;12:169–177.

9. Ogden JA, Murphy MJ, Southwick WO, et al. Radiology of postnatal skeletal development. XIII. C1-C2 interrelationships. *Skeletal Radiol* 1986;15:433–438.

10. O'Rahilly R, Müller F, Meyer DB. The human vertebral column at the end of the embryonic period proper. 1. The column as a whole. *J Anat* 1980;131:565–575.

11. Swischuk LE, Swischuk PN, John SD. Wedging of C-3 in infants and children: usually a normal finding and not a fracture. *Radiology* 1993; 188:523–526.

12. Cattell HS, Filtzer DL. Pseudosubluxation and other normal variations in the cervical spine in children. A study of one hundred and sixty children. *J Bone Joint Surg Am* 1965;47:1295–1309.

13. Penning L. Normal movements of the cervical spine. *Am J Roentgenol* 1978;130:317–326.

14. Swischuk LE. Anterior displacement of C2 in children: physiologic or pathologic. A helpful differentiating line. *Radiology* 1977;122:759.

15. Flynn JM, Dormans JP. Spine trauma in children. *Semin Spine Surg* 1998;10:7–16.

16. Grabb PA, Pang D. Magnetic resonance imaging in the evaluation of spinal cord injury without radiographic abnormality in children. *Neurosurgery* 1994;35:406–414; discussion 414.

17. Pang D, Pollack IF. Spinal cord injury without radiographic abnormality in children—the SCIWORA syndrome. *J Trauma* 1989;29:654–664.

18. Leventhal HR. Birth Injuries of the spinal cord. *J Pediatr* 1960;56: 447–453.

19. Hadden WA, Gillespie WJ. Multiple level injuries of the cervical spine. *Injury* 1985;16:628–633.

20. Nitecki S, Moir CR. Predictive factors of the outcome of traumatic cervical spine fracture in children. *J Pediatr Surg* 1994;29:1409–1411.

21. Pennecot GF, Gouraud D, Hardy JR, et al. Roentgenographical study of the stability of the cervical spine in children. *J Pediatr Orthop* 1984;4:346–352.

22. Hillman JW, Sprofkin BE, Parrish TF. Birth injury of the cervical spine producing a "cerebral palsy" syndrome. *Am Surg* 1954;20:900.

23. Towbin A. Central nervous system damage in the human fetus and newborn infant. *Am J Dis Child* 1970;119:529.

24. Teodori JB, Painter MJ. Basilar impression in children. *Pediatrics* 1984;74:1097.

25. Lally KP, Senac M, Hardin WDJ. Utility of the cervical spine radiograph in pediatric trauma. *Am J Surg* 1989;158:540.

26. Rachesky I, Boyce WT, Duncan B. Clinical prediction of cervical spine injuries in children: radiographic abnormalities. *Am J Dis Child* 1987;141:199.

27. Harkey HL, Crockard HA, Stevens JM. The operative management of basilar impression in osteogenesis imperfecta. *Neurology* 1990;27:782.

28. Yamada H, Nakamura S, Tajima M. Neurological manifestations of pediatric achondroplasia. *J Neurosurg* 1981;54:49.

29. Wong VCN, Fong CF. Basilar impression in a child with hypochondroplasia. *Pediatr Neurol* 1991;7:62.

30. Parke WW, Rothman RH, Brown MD. The pharyngovertebral veins: an anatomical rationale for Grisel's syndrome. *J Bone Joint Surg Am* 1984;66:568.

31. Mathern GW, Batzdorf U. Grisel's syndrome: cervical spine clinical, pathologic and neurologic manifestations. *Clin Orthop* 1989;244:131.

32. Michie I, Clark M. Neurological syndromes associated with cervical and craniocervical anomalies. *Arch Neurol* 1968;18:241.

33. Greenberg AD. Atlantoaxial dislocation. *Brain* 1968;91:655.

34. Wadia NH. Myelopathy complicating congenital atlantoaxial dislocation (a study of 28 cases). *Brain* 1967;90:449.

35. Ferguson RL, Putney ME, Allen BLJ. Comparison of neurologic deficits with atlantodens intervals in patients with Down syndrome. *J Spinal Disord* 1997;10:246.

36. Bharucha EP, Dastur HM. Craniovertebral anomalies (a report on 40 cases). *Brain* 1964;87:469.

37. McRae DL, Barnum AS. Occipitalization of the atlas. *Am J Roentgenol* 1953;70:23.

38. Whitmer GG, Davis RJ, Bell DF. Hanging head sign as a presenting feature of spinal cord neoplasms: a report of four cases. *J Pediatr Orthop* 1993;13:322–324.

39. Williams CF, Bernstein TW, Jelenko C 3rd. Essentiality of the lateral cervical spine radiograph. *Ann Emerg Med* 1981;10:198–204.

40. Wholey MH, Bruwer AJ, Baker HLJ. The lateral roentgenogram of the neck (with comments on the atlanto-odontoid-basion relationship). *Radiology* 1958;71:350–356.

41. Swischuk LE, Hayden CKJ, Sarwar M. The posteriorly tilted dens: a normal variation mimicking a fractured dens. *Pediatr Radiol* 1979; 8:27.

42. McGregor M. Significance of certain measurements of skull in diagnosis of basilar impression. *Br J Radiol* 1948;21:171.

43. McRae DL. Bony abnormalities in the region of the foramen magnum: correlation of the anatomic and neurologic findings. *Acta Radiol* 1960; 40:335.

44. Gabriel KR, Mason DE, Carango P. Occipito-atlantal translation in Down's syndrome. *Spine* 1990;15:997–1002.

45. Powers B, Miller MD, Kramer RS, et al. Traumatic anterior atlanto-occipital dislocation. *Neurosurgery* 1979;4:12–17.

46. Harris JH, Carson GC, Wagner LK. Radiologic diagnosis of traumatic occipitovertebral dissociation: 1. Normal occipitovertebral relationships on lateral radiographs of supine subjects. *Am J Roentgenol* 1994; 162:881–886.

47. Locke GR, Gardner JI, van Epps EF. Atlas-dens interval (ADI) in children: a survey based on 200 normal cervical spines. *Am J Roentgenol* 1966;97:135.

48. Steel HH. Anatomical and mechanical considerations of the atlanto-axial articulations. *J Bone Joint Surg Am* 1968;50:1481.

49. Jauregui N, Lincoln T, Mubarak S. Surgically related upper cervical spine canal anatomy in children. *Spine* 1993;18:1939.

50. Fielding JW, Cochran GB, Lawsing JF 3rd, et al. Tears of the transverse ligament of the atlas. A clinical and biomechanical study. *J Bone Joint Surg Am* 1974;56:1683–1691.

51. Spierings ELH, Braakman R. The management of os odontoideum. *J Bone Joint Surg Br* 1982;64:422.

52. Fielding JW. Normal and selected abnormal motion of the cervical spine from the second vertebra to the seventh cervical vertebra based on cineroentgenography. *J Bone Joint Surg Am* 1964;46:1779.

53. Fielding JW. Cineroentgenography of the normal cervical spine. *J Bone Joint Surg Am* 1957;37:1280.

54. McAfee PC, Bohlman HH, Han JS, et al. Comparison of nuclear magnetic resonance imaging and computed tomography in the diagnosis of upper cervical spinal cord compression. *Spine* 1986;11:295–304.

55. Weng MS, Haynes RJ. Flexion and extension cervical MRI in a pediatric population. *J Pediatr Orthop* 1996;16:359.

56. Scarrow AM, Levy EI, Resnick DK, et al. Cervical spine evaluation in obtunded or comatose pediatric trauma patients: a pilot study. *Pediatr Neurosurg* 1999;30:169–175.

CHAPTER 32

Congenital Malformations of the Base of the Skull, Atlas, and Dens

Károly M. Dávid and Alan Crockard

Congenital malformations of the base of the skull, atlas, and dens have great diversity; they may cause acute or progressive neurologic deterioration and may be difficult to treat. Knowledge of the regional development and its genetic control is essential to understand various congenital malformations, which may eventually lead to preventive and therapeutic measures. The first part of this chapter provides a brief description of the normal development of this region based on recent advances in understanding its genetic control. The second part discusses definitions, possible genetic and embryonic background, and clinical findings of the more common osseous and associated neural malformations of this region.

DEVELOPMENT OF THE CRANIOVERTEBRAL JUNCTION AND CERVICAL SPINE AND ITS GENETIC CONTROL

The formation of an ectodermal thickening, called the primitive streak (Carnegie stage 6; 13 to 15 days), in the posterior two-thirds of the bilaminar embryo is the first indication of a rostrocaudal body axis of the human embryo (1). Epiblast cells invaginate through the primitive groove (arising on the primitive streak), forming the intraembryonic mesoderm between the ectoderm and endoderm. Thus, the three-layered embryo is formed during this process called gastrulation. The notochord, a rodlike structure, arises from the primitive node (the rostral thickened endpoint of the primitive streak) growing rostrally in the midline between the ectoderm and endoderm (Carnegie stage 7; 15 to 17 days). The notochord induces the overlying ectoderm to become the neural plate, which later forms the neural tube (2).

Paraxial mesodermal cells (the part of the mesoderm that lies on either side of the notochord) segment into epithelial spheres called somites that appear first in the occipital and

cervical regions (Carnegie stages 9 to 10; 20 to 23 days) (3). Somatogenesis progresses rostrocaudally and, for the first time, imposes a segmental organization on the rostrocaudal body axis. The craniovertebral junction and cervical spine derive from the five occipital and seven cervical somites. It has been suggested that the first occipital somite disappears very early in human development.

Beginning rostrally, the ventromedial parts of the somites lose their epithelial structure and form the sclerotomes, whereas the dorsolateral parts retain epithelial arrangement and form the dermatomes and myotomes. Four occipital sclerotomes are visible in the human embryo at Carnegie stage 14 (31 to 35 days), the first three of which are already fused (4). It is important to make a distinction between the development of axial (central) and lateral vertebral components. The lateral part of each sclerotome shows a division to loose cranial and dense caudal halves in Carnegie stage 13 (28 to 32 days). Cells within the caudal half of the lateral part of sclerotome form the neural arches, whereas the less cell-dense cranial halves contain the spinal nerves, dorsal root ganglia, and intersegmental vessels (5). The loose half of a sclerotome and the dense half of the sclerotome (cranial to it) fuse to form a vertebra during the process of resegmentation. Despite previous controversy on the concept of resegmentation, labeling and transplantation experiments have confirmed that one somite always contributes to two adjacent vertebrae (6). The only exceptions to this rule are the occipital somites, which unite to form the basioccipital. In the occipital region, no ganglia develop and loose sclerotome-halves of only the third and fourth occipital sclerotomes contain hypoglossal nerve fibers. These rootlets unite to form two hypoglossal stems during Carnegie stage 14. The exoccipital (bilateral to basioccipital) develops from only lateral components such as the neural arches of the cervical vertebrae (4).

The axial (perinotochordal) area is still cell-free during the first steps of lateral development. The notochord is surrounded by extracellular matrix, which consists of radially oriented microfibrils and interstitial bodies. By Carnegie stage 13 (28 to 32 days) sclerotome cells immigrate to the perichordal zone, giving rise to the perinotochordal cellular sheath. This sheath also shows zones of high and low cell density at somewhat later stages than in lateral development (Carnegie stages 14 to 15; 32 to 38 days). The high–cell-density zones correspond to intervertebral discs, whereas the low-density areas develop into the centra of vertebrae. The basioccipital also develops from the perinotochordal sheath, but this part does not have dense areas; therefore, no separations by discs happen normally in this area (5,7).

Laterally, the rostral half of the C1 sclerotome assimilates into the occipital condyles. In lower vertebrates the rostral half of the C1 sclerotome persists as a separate bone called the proatlas. Axially, the centrum of C1 becomes separated from the rest of C1 and, as part of the axis, develops into the base of the odontoid process. Certain members of the extinct reptilian group, from which mammals evolved, possessed both an odontoid process and atlas body (centrum of C1). The odontoid process evolved as an addition to the atlas body when the mammalian atlantoaxial articulation became specialized for rotational movement. Therefore, the odontoid process is not homologous with the atlas body (centrum of C1) (8). The ascending chondrification pattern of the odontoid process from the C1 centrum in human embryos (Carnegie stages 20 to 23) supports this observation (Fig. 32.1) (9).

Chondrification of the axial skeleton begins in the sixth week postfertilization (Carnegie stage 17) after mesenchymal formation of the basioccipital and cervical vertebrae is completed (4). Cartilage formation in the vertebral column and basioccipital is believed to be induced by the notochord and neural tube. Prenatal movement also is essential for the proper development of the vertebral column (10). The chondrification centers first appear in the lateral masses and neural arches and in the centra of the vertebrae. The body of the axis chondrifies from the centra of C1 and C2, the former giving rise to the base of the odontoid process. The subdental synchondrosis is equivalent to the rudimentary disc between the embryonic centra of C1 and C2 and is often seen on radiographs and scans postnatally. The anterior arch and tubercle of C1 chondrifies from another midline chondrification point (9). The cartilaginous centra of the cervical vertebrae are relatively wide from side to side and narrow dorsoventrally (11).

The primary ossification centers appear in the vertebral bodies and bilaterally in the neural arches during the ninth week postfertilization. In addition to these, the axis has two lateral ossification centers for the odontoid process and an apical ossification center that develops postnatally. The atlas has two lateral and an anterior primary ossification center to form the lateral masses, posterior arches, and

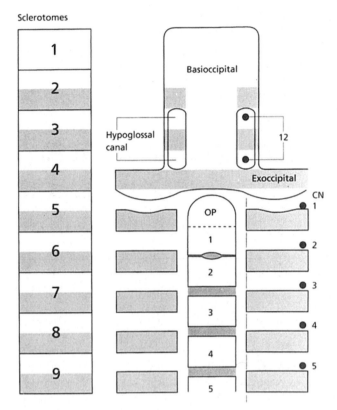

FIG. 32.1. Schematic illustration of vertebral development in the occipitocervical region. The basiocciput develops mainly from the axial primordium of the four occipital somites, whereas the exocciput and lateral portions of the basiocciput derive from the lateral components, such as the neural arches of the cervical vertebrae. Loose halves of the lateral part of only the third and fourth sclerotomes contain nerves: the two hypoglossal stems. Laterally, the cranial half of the C1 sclerotome assimilates into the occipital condyles. Axially, the centrum of C1 (1) separates from the rest of C1 and, as part of the axis vertebra, develops into the base of the dens. The odontoid process evolves as an addition to the centrum of C1 because of rotational movement of the mammalian atlantoaxial articulation (CN, cervical nerve; 12, hypoglossal nerve). (From: Müller F, O'Rahilly R. Occipitocervical segmentation in staged human embryos. *J Anat* 1994;185:251–258.)

anterior arch, respectively. Postnatally, secondary ossification centers appear in the vertebral epiphyses; eventually, the ossification centers unite to form the final shape of the vertebrae (12).

Genetic Control: *Hox* and *Pax* Genes

The precise genetic control of primary segmentation (i.e., the formation of segmental somites from the paraxial mesoderm during the third and fourth weeks of gestation) is unknown. However, two families of regulatory genes have been implicated: the *Hox* and *Pax* genes.

Hox genes encode transcription factors that are used to regionalize the mammalian embryo. Human and mouse, and probably all mammals, contain 39 highly conserved

Hox genes distributed on four linkage groups on different chromosomes, the *Hox* A, B, C and D clusters (Fig. 32.2). They have been demonstrated to have a fundamental role in determining the *identity* of each vertebra (13). This morphogenetic specification of vertebral phenotype along the embryonic axis is an early event controlled by the *Hox* genes.

Expression of individual *Hox* genes is characterized by distinct anterior limits, or "cutoffs." Genes from the more 3′ locations in the *Hox* clusters are expressed earlier and have more rostral expression domains on the body. Different combinations of *Hox* genes expressed within each primordium have led to the concept of a "vertebral column *Hox* code" (14). A specific *Hox* code is involved in the rostrocaudal specification of a mesodermal segment and the determination of vertebral identities and becomes translated into a specific vertebral anatomy. Mutations in *Hox* genes and teratogen-induced disturbance of *Hox* gene expression can both cause alterations of the number and identity of the

cervical vertebrae forming at or near the anterior limit of the expression domain of these *Hox* genes. For example, inactivation of gene *Hox-d3* results in mutant mice with atlas assimilation to the basioccipital (15). Thus, by losing the function of a *Hox* gene, the first cervical vertebra is transformed into a more rostral identity; this is called an "anterior homeotic transformation." Conversely, extension of an expression domain rostrally can transform structures into a more caudal identity, a phenomenon known as "posterior homeotic transformation." This is exemplified by the "gain-of-function" transgenic mutation of *Hox-d4*, in which the occipital region of the skull is changed into cervical vertebral phenotypes, leaving the cervical spine itself unchanged (16). Given this sensitivity of the craniovertebral junction to perturbation by changes in *Hox* gene expression, such genetic changes might prove to be underlying causes of malformations in this part of the human body.

Pax genes (except *Pax-1* and *-9*) contribute to early development of the nervous system. The two exceptions of

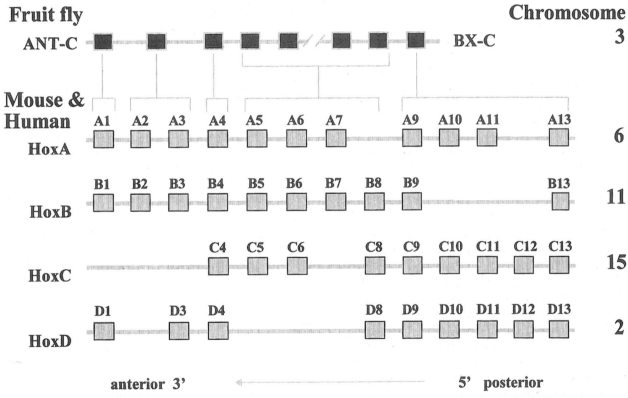

FIG. 32.2. Chromosomal organization of *Hox* genes in the mouse and human and its derivation from an ancestral complex equivalent to that found in *Drosophila*, the fruit fly. There are four clusters (Hox-A, -B, -C and -D) on chromosomes 6, 11, 15 and 2, respectively. The so-called paralogous groups, defined vertically across the clusters and consisting of up to four genes, each on a different chromosome, are linked by common origin from an ancestral gene and identified by a common number (thus, *Hox-A9*, *-B9*, *-C9*, and *-D9* are paralogs). Some paralogs have been lost during the course of evolution. The expression of the genes along the anteroposterior body axis of the embryo corresponds with their sequence within the cluster and along the 3′ to 5′ axis of the chromosome. Thus, *Hox-A2* has a more anterior limit to its expression domain than does *Hox-A9*. (From: David KM, Crockard HA. The early development of the craniovertebral junction and the cervical spine, 3. In Crockard A, Hayward R, Hoff JT, eds. *Neurosurgery: the scientific basis of clinical practice*, 3rd ed. Oxford: Blackwell Science, 1999, with permission.)

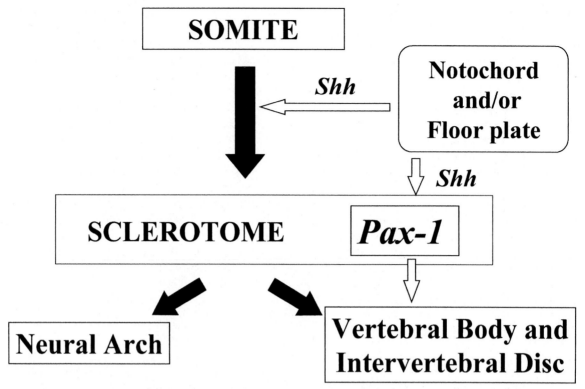

FIG. 32.3. Diagram depicting the range and sequence of tissue interactions that underlie the cell-signaling events necessary to build a vertebral body. Initially, expression of the regulatory gene, *Pax-1,* is involved in primary segmentation of the paraxial mesoderm into somites (not shown here; see text). Subsequently, a peptide signal encoded by the *Shh* gene, emanating from the notochord and the ventral floor plate of the neural tube, acts on the somite to induce sclerotome differentiation. The sclerotome itself then differentially expresses *Pax-1,* with expression ventrally reflecting the dorsoventral specification of each vertebra. Within this ventral expression domain of the sclerotomes, much more intense expression is demonstrated at those axial levels at which the intervertebral discs will form; this appears to function in the resegmentation of the vertebrae (see text for further details). (From: American Association of Neurological Surgeons. The dysmorphic cervical spine in Klippel-Feil syndrome. *Neurosurg Focus* 1999;6:1–11, with permission.)

the *Pax* family act as regulatory genes to independently control the establishment of intervertebral boundaries of the sclerotomes. In particular, the *Pax-1* gene has been found to be pivotal in the reorganization of the sclerotome (17). Signaling from the intact notochord and/or the floor plate of the neural tube is necessary for sufficient *Pax-1* gene expression in somites and sclerotomes during primary segmentation. *Pax-1* gene expression, in turn, is required for the formation of the ventral (axial) parts of the vertebrae. During chondrification of the vertebrae this gene also is strongly expressed in the developing discs (Fig. 32.3) (18). *PAX-1,* the human homolog (19), is expressed in the human vertebral column in the intervertebral disc primordia as early as 7 weeks of development (20). As with the *Hox* homeoproteins, the identity of the downstream target genes (i.e., those whose expression is regulated by the *Pax* proteins) is largely unknown.

Reduced or absent *Pax-1* expression correlates with fusions between adjacent vertebral primordia; however, it is associated also with normally occurring fusions. It has been shown in chick embryos that the fusion of the five occipital

somites to form the basioccipital and the fusion of the dens primordium with the axis are both normal developmental events coincident with a down-regulation of *Pax-1* (Fig. 32.4) (7).

INDIVIDUAL OSSEOUS MALFORMATIONS

The clinical presentation of congenital malformations of the craniovertebral junction is varied and, in the majority, it is impossible to correlate an individual osseous malformation to specific clinical symptoms and signs. In some cases, there are no signs and symptoms at all, or only very minor ones. In others, severe neurologic deficit may develop. Symptoms may be occipital and neck pain, giddiness, and vertigo often related to movements of the head. More common clinical signs are nystagmus, ataxia, dysmetria, lower cranial nerve palsy, and long tract signs, including tetraparesis, spinothalamic and posterior column dysfunctions, and occipital neuralgia. Altered states of consciousness and transient confusion may result from vertebral artery compromise (21). In some cases external

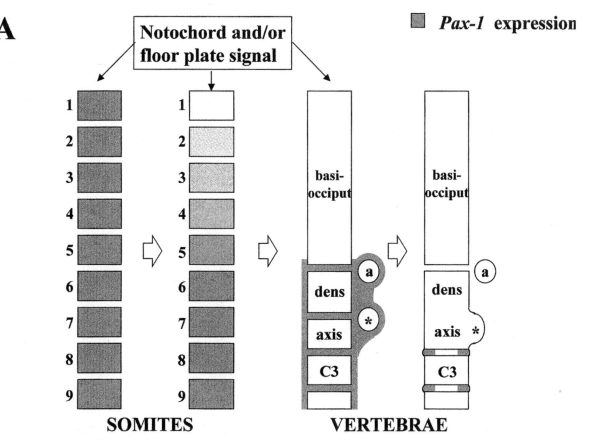

FIG. 32.4. Schematic illustration of normal *Pax-1* gene expression in the craniovertebral region during development. *Pax-1* gene is expressed in each somite evenly. Later, the first five somites (chick embryo) start to switch off the gene in the caudal direction resulting in a fused basiocciput and dens-axis complex. *, Second hypochordal arch; a, atlas. (From: Wilting J, Ebensperger C, Müller TS, et al. Pax-1 in the development of the cervico-occipital transitional zone. *Anat Embryol (Berl),* 1995;192:221–227, and David KM, Crockard HA. The early development of the craniovertebral junction and the cervical spine, 3. In Crockard A, Hayward R, Hoff JT, eds. *Neurosurgery: the scientific basis of clinical practice,* 3rd ed. Oxford: Blackwell Science, 1999.)

features such as torticollis, short broad neck, high scapula, low hairline, and limitation of neck movements may be detected (22). In a small but significant number of patients, there is rapid neurologic deterioration followed by sudden death (23).

Basilar Invagination

Primary basilar invagination consists of occipital hypoplasia with shortening of the basiocciput (clivus) and the upward deformity of the bone of the skull base with protrusion of the odontoid into the foramen magnum. This results in narrowing of the foramen magnum and reduction of the volume of the posterior fossa (22). It is often associated with other occipitocervical malformations, such as all degrees of assimilation of the atlas, remnants of occipital vertebra, anterior and posterior spina bifida of the atlas, Klippel-Feil deformity, Chiari I malformation, and syringomyelia (Fig. 32.5) (24,25). Basilar invagination may be secondary (basilar impression) to some form of bone softening condition; for example, Paget disease, osteogenesis imperfecta

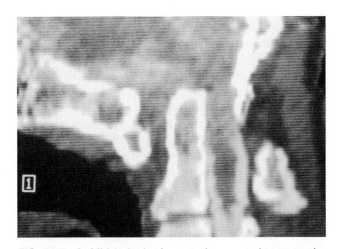

FIG. 32.5. A: Midsagittal reformatted computed tomography myelogram obtained in a patient in whom atlas assimilation into occiput, basilar invagination, C2-3 anterior and posterior fusion, and atlantoaxial subluxation causing anterior medullary compression were revealed. **B:** Line diagram showing the fusion pattern. O, occiput. (From: American Association of Neurological Surgeons. The dysmorphic cervical spine in Klippel-Feil syndrome. *Neurosurg Focus* 1999;6:1–11, with permission.)

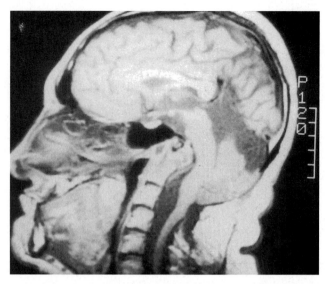

FIG. 32.6. Midsagittal T1-weighted magnetic resonance image of a patient with osteogenesis imperfecta, severe basilar impression, and anterior compression of the brain stem.

(Fig. 32.6), achondroplasia, and rheumatoid arthritis. An excessive amount of granulation tissue may build up around the odontoid process if chronic instability is present, as is seen with assimilation of the atlas and subsequent invagination. This, in itself, may act as a space-occupying mass in the anterior portion of the foramen magnum. In addition, fibrous bands and dural adhesions are common in the posterior cervicomedullary junction and around the cerebellar tonsils in both primary and secondary basilar invagination (23,26).

Etiology

An insufficient amount of paraxial mesoderm may lead to underdevelopment of the occipital somites, subsequent shortening of the clivus, and anteroposterior enlargement of the foramen magnum (27). During the chondrification phase of vertebral development, the cartilaginous odontoid process temporarily can reach as high as the anterior rim of the foramen magnum and it may form an occipitoaxial joint (third occipital condyle) by the end of the embryonic period (11). This configuration is reminiscent of that seen postnatally in basilar invagination, where the upper cervical vertebrae are shifted cranially and the odontoid process moves into the plane of the foramen magnum (22). Normally, the odontoid process later descends relative to the basioccipital and foramen magnum during the fetal period. This is most probably to the result of growth and development of the occipital condyles and lateral masses of C1. If this descent is incomplete for some reason, then basilar invagination may persist and cause ventral neuraxial compression at a later stage.

Clinical Findings

Goel and associates (25) analyzed the cases of 190 surgically treated patients with basilar invagination. In 88 patients without associated Chiari malformation, common presenting signs and symptoms were muscle weakness (100%), neck pain (59%), only posterior column dysfunction (39%), bowel and bladder disturbance (28%), and paraesthesia (25%). These patients also presented with localized signs of torticollis (69%), restricted neck movements (59%), low hairline (48%), webbed (47%), and short neck (41%).

Radiologic Findings

Basilar invagination is defined radiologically by the amount of protrusion of the tip of the odontoid process into the foramen magnum. On lateral radiographs, this protrusion is more than 5 mm beyond McGregor's line (from the hard palate to the lowest point of the occiput) and more than 2.5 mm beyond Chamberlain's line (from the hard palate to the posterior rim of the foramen magnum) (Fig. 32.7). Normally, the tip of the odontoid process should lie below McRae's line (from the anterior to the posterior rim of the foramen magnum), which is now best appreciated on magnetic resonance imaging (MRI) together with possible associated neural compression and canal compromise. According to McRae, sagittal reduction of the foramen magnum to less than 19 mm produces neurologic deficits (28).

Treatment

Goel and associates (25) reported clinical and radiologic improvement following traction in 82% of patients with basilar invagination not associated with Chiari I malformation. If traction reduces anterior compression of the brain stem by the odontoid process, surgical treatment may be posterior occipitocervical stabilization alone. Transoral decompression is performed in patients with irreducible anterior compression followed by posterior stabilization in most cases (23). In patients with associated Chiari I malformation, decompression of the foramen magnum was found to be appropriate, and rarely required a fixation procedure (25).

Assimilation of Atlas to Occiput

There may be varying degrees of bony fusion between atlas and occiput; complete and partial assimilation are

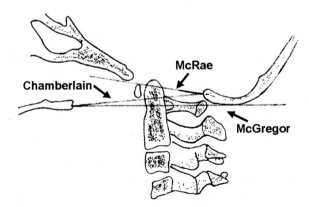

FIG. 32.7. Lateral craniometric lines used to determine basilar impressions. (See text for definitions.)

described. In the majority of cases, assimilation occurs between the anterior arch of the atlas and the anterior rim of the foramen magnum, and it is associated with other skeletal malformations such as basilar invagination, occipital vertebra, spina bifida of atlas, or fusion of the second and third cervical vertebrae (Klippel-Feil syndrome) (Fig. 32.5) (21,28,29). A combination of assimilation of the atlas and segmentation failure between the second and third cervical vertebrae results in progressive laxity of the atlantoaxial joints with development of subluxation between the atlas and axis in childhood. The instability causes progressive proliferation of granulation tissue that, combined with the abnormal clivus and odontoid invagination, leads to progressive anterior neuraxial compromise (23,30).

Etiology

Atlas assimilation is defined as failure of segmentation between the last occipital and first cervical sclerotome. Given the described genetic background, revealed by experimental analysis of transgenic mice model systems, assimilation of atlas into the occiput might be interpreted as an anterior homeotic transformation.

Clinical Findings

Most patients with assimilation of the atlas to the basiocciput have clinical findings that resemble Klippel-Feil syndrome (31). They usually have a low hairline, short neck, and restricted neck movements with occasional torticollis (24,28). When the odontoid process encroaches into the foramen magnum, anterior neuroaxial compression and associated neurologic problems are common. A posterior dural band at the level of the atlas also may be found in association with assimilation of the atlas that may cause symptoms referable to the posterior columns of the cervical spinal cord (loss of proprioception, light touch, and vibration sense). Nystagmus, headache, and occipital neuralgia in the greater occipital nerve distribution also may be present.

Radiologic Findings

Cervical radiographs usually demonstrate assimilation of the atlas to the basiocciput and flexion-extension views may detect instability at C1-2 articulation, especially in cases with associated C2-3 fusion. MRI scan and/or computed tomography myelography (Fig. 32.5) are essential in the evaluation of the amount of granulation tissue in cases of C1-2 instability, degree of neuroaxial compression, and confirmation of osseous malformations.

Treatment

Atlas assimilation into the occiput is not usually symptomatic; however, associated malformations such as basilar invagination, C2-3 fusion with C1-2 instability, and granulation tissue may require treatment. In these cases the initial treatment aims to reduce the deformity with traction and subsequent surgical decompression or posterior stabilization is carried out as discussed.

Anterior and Posterior Spina Bifida of Atlas

Anterior spina bifida is often very narrow and may be median or paramedian. It is much less frequent than defects in the posterior arch, which may be total aplasia, hemiaplasia, and more often, median clefts (22). Congenital hypoplasia of the posterior arch with abnormal segmentation of the cervical spine also has been reported (32).

Etiology

Congenital diseases affecting the connective tissue, such as Morquio syndrome, other mucopolysaccharidoses, and Down syndrome can be associated with severe atlantoaxial subluxation. Considering that the embryo is capable of head movements as early as 6.5 weeks (33), it is perhaps not surprising that in these disorders with ligamentous laxity, there is a high incidence of anterior and posterior spina bifida of C1 (Figs. 32.8 and 32.9), os odontoideum, or apparent hypoplasia of the dens (apparent because ossification has not spread from the centrum of C1 into the cartilaginous dens) (26,34,35). As observed in models of chondrifying human craniovertebral junction (9), the anterior arch of C1 starts to chondrify at about 50 to 53 days and it may be that because of abnormal excessive movements, this process is impaired at an early embryonic stage in these disorders, resulting in anterior and later posterior spina bifida of C1.

Clinical Findings

Anterior and posterior spina bifida of the atlas usually is not clinically symptomatic except when associated with other malformations and atlantoaxial subluxation, as in the mentioned syndromes.

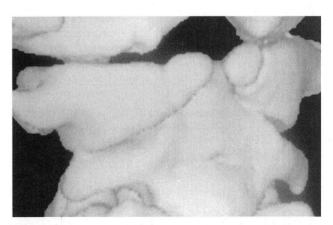

FIG. 32.8. Anterior spina bifida of the atlas causing atlantoaxial instability in 5-year-old girl with Down syndrome. Three-dimensional reconstruction computed tomography scan. (Courtesy of Dominic Thompson.)

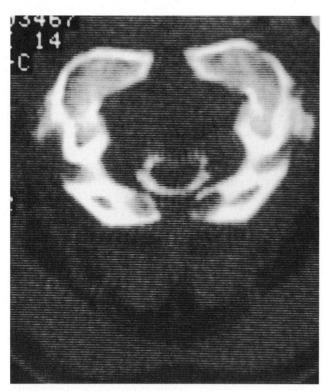

FIG. 32.9. Computed tomography myelogram of a child with Morquio syndrome demonstrating wide anterior and posterior spina bifida of the atlas.

Radiologic Findings

Clefts of the posterior arch have been reported with prevalence of 4% and of the anterior arch of only 0.1%. Of the posterior clefts, 97% are median; only 3% are lateral just behind the lateral masses. Clefts of the anterior arch are nearly always very narrow; they may be median or paramedian (22). Anterior clefts may be detected on anteroposterior view with opened mouth and posterior clefts on lateral views; however, computed tomography scan with bony window is the best diagnostic tool to identify these anomalies.

Treatment

Anterior and posterior spina bifida of the atlas is usually not clinically important and rarely requires treatment. Surgical treatment may be necessary in cases where there are associated malformations such as Klippel-Feil syndrome, basilar invagination, atlantoaxial subluxation, and assimilation of atlas into the basiocciput.

Os Odontoideum

Os odontoideum is a separate bone with smooth, rounded cortical margins that lies cranial to the axis in place of the dens, leaving a variable gap between itself and the small odontoid process. Clinically, it usually is associated with atlantoaxial instability (Fig. 32.10).

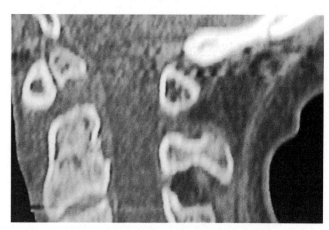

FIG. 32.10. Midsagittal reformatted computed tomography scan of a patient with os odontoideum and atlantoaxial subluxation. (Courtesy of James Kellerman.)

Etiology

The pathogenesis of os odontoideum has been debated; many still believe that, at least in some cases, it is congenital and represents the centrum of either the proatlas (corresponding with the ossiculum terminale) or atlas (C1) (30, 36,37). Os odontoideum in identical twins (38) and familial os odontoideum with C2-3 fusion (39) also have been reported and discussed in support of the congenital theory-based etiology. Intrauterine fracture, especially that caused by increased movements adjacent to fused cervical segments, may be an explanation in favor of the acquired origin. However, most investigators interpret os odontoideum as an acquired malformation, a chronic ununited fracture of the odontoid process (40–42). A chronic ununited fracture of the odontoid and "congenital" os odontoideum cannot be distinguished reliably on any morphologic criteria (35). Furthermore, in patients with connective tissue disorders, it has been shown that surgery for occipitocervical fusion results in spread of ossification from the centrum of C1 into the cartilaginous dens to form a normal-looking odontoid process (26). The cartilaginous odontoid process reaches as high as the anterior rim of the foramen magnum by the end of the embryonic period proper (Carnegie stage 23) (9). Secondary to the abnormal excessive movements and repeated minor trauma in the mentioned disorders, the gracile cartilaginous odontoid process may be fractured or transected, thus producing an os odontoideum and atlantoaxial instability after ossification. This mechanism also has been suggested on clinical grounds (35,43).

Clinical Findings

The prevalence of os odontoideum is unknown. Symptomatic patients who undergo radiographic studies or patients following head or neck trauma may have os odontoideum identified (40). Patients with this abnormality may demonstrate no symptoms, symptoms resulting from local mechanical irritation (neck pain and torticollis) or progressive myelopathy, or transient neurologic symptoms secondary to vertebral artery compression. Cranial nerve impairment typically is absent in association with os odontoideum (44).

Radiologic Findings

The os odontoideum may be in the normal position of the odontoid process (orthotopic), displaced cranially (dystopic) or fused to the clivus (22,31). The line separating an os odontoideum from the body of the axis usually is cranial to the level of the superior articular facets of the axis. Flexion-extension cervical spine radiographs usually demonstrate instability and movement between the os and body of axis. An anteroposterior open-mouth view, CT with bony window, and two- or three-dimensional reconstruction readily identifies the abnormality. An MRI allows visualization of the cervical spinal cord and myelomalacia secondary to atlantoaxial instability.

Treatment

Atlantoaxial instability, if present, requires some form of posterior stabilization. The best fusion rates have been reported with C1-2 transarticular screw fixation. In the presence of os odontoideum, even minor trauma may produce symptoms and upper cervical cord compromise; therefore, preventive stabilization should be considered. Patients with radiographic evidence of cord compression, narrowed upper cervical spinal canal (≤13 mm), history of myelopathy, or progressive neurologic changes should be considered for surgical stabilization of the atlantoaxial complex (40). Anterior decompression may be necessary in patients with irreducible subluxation with basilar invagination or chronic granulation tissue acting as a mass (23).

Ossiculum Terminale Persistens

The ossiculum terminale fuses with the dens by adolescence (before the twelfth year) (45). Very rarely it remains separate in adulthood; then it is called ossiculum terminale

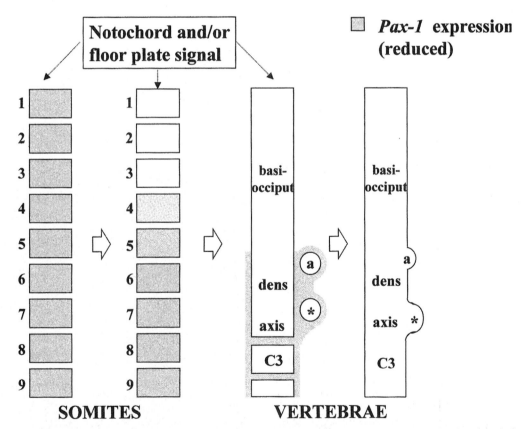

FIG. 32.11. Schematic illustration of reduced *Pax-1* gene expression in the craniovertebral region during development. Reduced *Pax-1* expression may occur either through an absent or insufficient signal from the notochord or floor plate or through a faulty gene product. Given the correlation between reduced *Pax-1* expression and vertebral fusion (see text), this would eventually lead to further fusions in the caudal direction including fusion between the basiocciput and dens. *, Second hypochordal arch; a, atlas. (From: Wilting J, Ebensperger C, Müller TS, et al. Pax-1 in the development of the cervico-occipital transitional zone. *Anat Embryol (Berl),* 1995;192:221–227, and David KM, Crockard HA. The early development of the craniovertebral junction and the cervical spine, 3. In Crockard A, Hayward R, Hoff JT, eds. *Neurosurgery: the scientific basis of clinical practice,* 3rd ed. Oxford: Blackwell Science, 1999.)

persistens. It has no clinical significance because it does not cause atlantoaxial instability (22).

Etiology

It is widely believed that the ossiculum terminale develops from the centrum of the proatlas; however, it is more likely to represent one of the secondary ossification centers that appear at about the time of puberty (10,35,45).

Failure of Upper Cervical Segmentation

A varying degree of C2-3 fusion was the most common level of failure of segmentation in the cervical spine reported in a cohort of 30 patients with Klippel-Feil syndrome (29). The lateral radiograph of a very young child may appear to be normal until ossification of preexisting cartilage occurs to disclose the real extent of a congenital malformation (21,29). Failure of segmentation may rarely happen at C1-2 or C0-2 (46).

Etiology

Impaired or reduced *PAX-1* expression results in local or widespread atypical fusion between the sclerotomal primordia. The phenotypic consequence is vertebral fusions, even through the craniovertebral junction (i.e., failure of segmentation in the midline between clivus and tip of the odontoid process), as rarely seen (Fig. 32.11) (47). The possibility that genetic or environmental influences might disturb expression of *PAX-1*, leading to disorders of primary segmentation, must be considered. A close resemblance of the shape of unsegmented cervical vertebrae in Klippel-Feil syndrome to the narrow and wide cartilaginous vertebrae in the embryo suggests that this failure of segmentation occurs before or during the chondrification of the vertebrae (9). The exact causes of Klippel-Feil syndrome are unknown although genetic factors for C2-3 (autosomal dominant) and C5-6 (autosomal recessive) fusions have been suggested (48) and environmental factors such as alcohol also may have a role (49).

Clinical Findings

Today, the term Klippel-Feil syndrome identifies a phenotype with failure of segmentation in the cervical spine although the classic clinical triad is only present in about half of the cases with cervical fusion (50,51). The prevalence of the syndrome has been estimated to be 1 in 42,000 individuals (48). Klippel-Feil syndrome usually occurs with a number of different anomalies, the frequency of which is largely dependent on patient selection. The most common abnormalities associated with Klippel-Feil syndrome are skeletal anomalies (Sprengel deformity, basilar invagination, skull asymmetry, scoliosis, etc.), impairment of hearing, congenital heart diseases, ocular malformations, cranial and facial asymmetry, cleft palate (50,52), genitourinary

malformations (53), and mirror movements (51,54,55). Other rare associations reported with Klippel-Feil syndrome include partially or completely split cervical cord (56), anomalous rib (57), neurenteric cyst (58), neurenteric fistula causing recurrent meningitis (59), and dermoid cyst (60,61). A detailed description of Klippel-Feil syndrome is given elsewhere in this volume.

ASSOCIATED NEURAL MALFORMATIONS

Chiari I Malformation

Basilar invagination, atlantooccipital fusion, Klippel-Feil syndrome, and spina bifida occulta are common accompaniments of Chiari I malformation. Because a number of these malformations are not manifest until adult life, they are easily misdiagnosed as an acquired progressive neurologic disease.

Etiology

Morphometric study of the posterior fossa, as well as clinical and radiologic findings for symptomatic patients suggest that Chiari I malformation is most likely produced by underdevelopment of the posterior cranial fossa (possibly because of underdevelopment of the occipital somites originating from paraxial mesoderm). Overcrowding in the smaller posterior cranial fossa secondarily induces a downward herniation of the tonsils, as well as an upward shift of the tentorium (Fig. 32.12). Associated basilar invagination caused by a more severe underdevelopment further exacerbates overcrowding (see the preceding) (27,62–64).

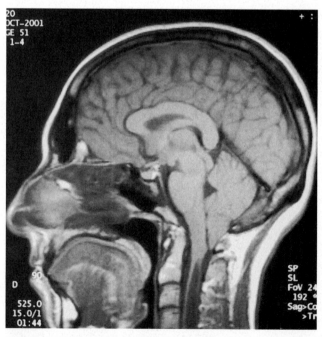

FIG. 32.12. Midsagittal T1-weighted magnetic resonance image of a patient with Chiari I malformation and syringomyelia.

Clinical Findings

Most patients present with headache, limb pain, ataxia, and evidence of sensory loss. The clinical picture develops slowly, and spinal cord abnormalities are accentuated. Hydrocephalus is rare. An early symptom is loss of pain sensation in the cervical dermatomes caused by central cavitation of the spinal cord. Atrophy and weakness of the upper extremities resulting in central cord syndrome follow. Cerebellar ataxia, nystagmus and lower cranial nerve abnormalities also may occur (21).

Radiologic Findings

The extent of cerebellar tonsillar herniation is best demonstrated on sagittal MRI by drawing a line between the basion and opisthion (the plane of the foramen magnum) (Fig. 32.12).

Treatment

In patients with Chiari I malformation, decompression of the foramen magnum was found to be the appropriate treatment (25).

Split Cervical Cord with Klippel-Feil Syndrome

Complete or partial split of the cervical cord rarely occurs; however, when it does, it is often associated with extensive segmentation failure of the cervical vertebrae and craniovertebral junction. Although the phenotype (i.e., complete or partial split of the cervical cord with Klippel-Feil syndrome) has been recognized (56), the relationship between the genes and other embryonic mechanisms resulting in failure of segmentation and split in the spinal cord is not yet known.

CONCLUSION

With increasing knowledge of the embryonic events and their genetic control in vertebral development, revealed mainly by chick and mouse experimental model systems, some human congenital malformations of the craniovertebral junction and cervical spine might be better understood. Further molecular genetic research is necessary to validate these experimental results to human diseases. Besides emphasizing the developmental anatomy and the genetic control, this chapter also covers many of the clinical aspects of these malformations.

REFERENCES

1. O'Rahilly R, Müller F. *Developmental stages in human embryos.* Washington, DC: Carnegie Institute of Washington Publication, 1987: 637.
2. Larsen WJ. *Human embryology,* 2nd ed. New York: Churchill Livingstone, 1997:54–56.
3. Keynes RJ, Stern C. Mechanisms of vertebrate segmentation. *Development* 1988;103:413–429.
4. Müller F, O'Rahilly R. Occipitocervical segmentation in staged human embryos. *J Anat* 1994;185:251–258.
5. Christ B, Wilting J. From somites to vertebral column. *Ann Anat* 1992; 174:23–32.
6. Bagnall KM, Higgins PF, Sanders EJ. The contribution made by cells from a single somite to tissues within a body segment and assessment of their integration with similar cells from adjacent body segments. *Development* 1989;107:931–943.
7. Wilting J, Ebensperger C, Müller TS, et al. *Pax-1* in the development of the cervico-occipital transitional zone. *Anat Embryol (Berl)* 1995; 192:221–227.
8. Jenkins FA. The evolution and development of the dens of the mammalian axis. *Anat Record* 1969;164:173–184.
9. David KM, McLachlan JC, Aiton JF, et al. Cartilaginous development of the human craniovertebral junction as visualised by a new three-dimensional computer reconstruction technique. *J Anat* 1998;192: 269–277.
10. O'Rahilly R, Müller F. The skeletal system and the limbs. In: O'Rahilly R, Müller F, eds. *Human embryology and teratology,* 2nd ed. New York: John Wiley & Sons, 1996:334.
11. O'Rahilly R, Müller F, Meyer DB. The human vertebral column at the end of the embryonic period proper. 2. The occipitocervical region. *J Anat* 1983;136:181–195.
12. Dietrich S, Kessel M. The vertebral column. In: Thorogood P, ed. *Embryos, genes and birth defects.* Chichester, UK: John Wiley and Sons, 1997:281–302.
13. Hunt P, Krumlauf R. *Hox* codes and positional specification in vertebrate embryonic axes. *Annu Rev Cell Biol* 1992;8:227–256.
14. Kessel M, Gruss P. Homeotic transformation of murine vertebrae and concomitant alteration of *Hox* codes induced by retinoic acid. *Cell* 1991;67:1–20.
15. Condie BG, Capecchi MR. Mice homozygous for a targeted disruption of *Hoxd-3* (*Hox-4.1*) exhibit anterior transformations of the first and second cervical vertebrae, the atlas and the axis. *Development* 1993;119:579–595.
16. Lufkin T, Mark M, Hart CP, et al. Homeotic transformation of the occipital bones of the skull by ectopic expression of a homeobox gene. *Nature* 1992;359:835–841.
17. Deutsch U, Dressler GR, Gruss P. *Pax-1,* a member of a paired box homologous murine gene family, is expressed in segmented structures during development. *Cell* 1988;53:617–625.
18. Koseki H, Wallin J, Wilting J, et al. A role for *Pax-1* as a mediator of notochordal signals during the dorsoventral specification of vertebrae. *Development* 1993;119:649–660.
19. Balling R. The undulated mouse and the development of the vertebral column. Is there a human *PAX-1* homologue? *Clin Dysmorphol* 1994; 3:185–191.
20. Smith CA, Tuan R. Human *PAX* gene expression and development of the vertebral column. *Clin Orthop Rel Res* 1994;302:241–250.
21. Bland JH. Congenital anomalies. In: Bland JH, ed. *Disorders of the cervical spine. Diagnosis and medical management.* London: WB Saunders, 1987:303–306.
22. von Torklus D, Gehle W. Anomalies and malformations. In: von Torklus D, Gehle W, eds. *The upper cervical spine.* Stuttgart: Thieme, 1972:14–53.
23. Menezes AH. Congenital and acquired abnormalities of the craniovertebral junction. In: Youmans JR, ed. *Neurological surgery,* 4th ed. Philadelphia: WB Saunders, 1996;1035–1089.
24. Spillane JD, Pallis C, Jones AM. Developmental abnormalities in the region of the foramen magnum. *Brain* 1957;80:11–47.
25. Goel A, Bhatjiwale M, Desai K. Basilar invagination: a study based on 190 surgically treated patients. *J Neurosurg* 1998;88:962–968.
26. Stevens JM, Kendall BE, Crockard HA, et al. The odontoid process in Morquio-Brailsford's disease. *J Bone Joint Surg* 1991;73-B:851–858.
27. Marin-Padilla M. Cephalic axial skeletal-neural dysraphic disorders: embryology and pathology. *Can J Neurol Sci* 1991;18:153–169.
28. McRae DL, Barnum AS. Occipitalization of the atlas. *Am J Roentgenol* 1953;70:23–46.
29. David KM, Stevens JM, Thorogood P, et al. The dysmorphic cervical spine in Klippel-Feil syndrome: interpretations from developmental biology. *Neurosurg Focus* 1999;6:1–11.
30. Greenberg AD. Atlanto-axial dislocations. *Brain* 1968;91:655–684.
31. Hensinger RN. Osseous anomalies of the craniovertebral junction. *Spine* 1986;11:323–333.

32. Chigara M, Kaneko K, Mashio K, et al. Congenital hypoplasia of the arch of the atlas with abnormal segmentation of the cervical spine. *Arch Orthop Trauma Surg* 1994;113:110–112.
33. Bagnall KM, Harris PF, Jones PRM. A radiographic study of the human fetal spine. 1. The development of the secondary cervical curvature. *J Anat* 1977;123:777–782.
34. Menezes AH, Ryken TC. Craniovertebral abnormalities in Down's syndrome. *Pediatr Neurosurg* 1992;18:24–33.
35. Stevens JM, Chong WK, Barber C, et al. A new appraisal of abnormalities of the odontoid process associated with atlanto-axial subluxation and neurological disability. *Brain* 1994;117:133–148.
36. Hensinger RN, Fielding JW, Hawkins RJ. Congenital anomalies of the odontoid process. *Orthop Clin North Am* 1978;9:901–912.
37. Truex CR, Johnson CH. Congenital anomalies of the upper cervical spine. *Orthop Clin North Am* 1978;9:891–900.
38. Kirlew KA, Hathout GM, Reiter SD, et al. Os odontoideum in identical twins: perspectives on etiology. *Skeletal Radiol* 1993;22:525–527.
39. Morgan MK, Onofrio BM, Bender CE. Familial os odontoideum. Case report. *J Neurosurg* 1989;70:636–639.
40. Fielding WJ, Hensinger RN, Hawkins RJ. Os odontoideum. *J Bone Joint Surg* 1980;62-A:376–383.
41. Hawkins RJ, Fielding JW, Thompson WJ. Os odontoideum: congenital or acquired. A case report. *J Bone Joint Surg* 1976;58-A:413–414.
42. Ricciardi JE, Kaufer H, Louis DS. Acquired os odontoideum following acute ligament injury. Report of a case. *J Bone Joint Surg* 1976;58-A:410–412.
43. Crockard HA, Stevens JM. Craniovertebral junction anomalies in inherited disorders: part of the syndrome or caused by the disorder? Review. *Eur J Paediatr* 1995;154:504–512.
44. Pizzutillo PD, Horn BD. Congenital anomalies of the odontoid. In: Clark CR, ed. *The cervical spine,* 3rd ed. Philadelphia: Lippincott-Raven, 1998:334.
45. Ogden JA, Murphy MJ, Southwick WO, et al. Radiology of postnatal skeletal development. XIII. C1-C2 interrelationships. *Skeletal Radiol* 1986;15:433–438.
46. Jeanneret B, Magerl F. Congenital fusion C0-C2 associated with spondylolysis of C2. *J Spinal Disord* 1990;3:413–417.
47. David KM, Thorogood P, Stevens JM, et al. The one bone spine: a failure of notochord/sclerotome signalling? *Clin Dysmorphol* 1997;6:303–314.
48. Gunderson CH, Greenspan RH, Glaser GH, et al. The Klippel-Feil syndrome: genetic and clinical reevaluation of cervical fusion. *Medicine* 1967;46:491–512.
49. Schilgen M, Loeser H. Klippel-Feil anomaly combined with fetal alcohol syndrome. *Eur Spine J* 1994;3:289–290.
50. Gunderson CH, Solitare GB. Mirror movements in patients with Klippel-Feil syndrome. Neuropathologic observations. *Arch Neurol* 1968;18:675–679.
51. Hensinger RN, Lang JR, MacEwen GD. Klippel-Feil syndrome. A constellation of associated anomalies. *J Bone Joint Surg* 1974;56-A:1246–1253.
52. Nagib MG, Maxwell RE, Chou SN. Identification and management of high-risk patients with Klippel-Feil syndrome. *J Neurosurg* 1984;61:523–530.
53. Ramsey J, Bliznak J. Klippel-Feil syndrome with renal agenesis and other anomalies. *Am J Roentgenol* 1971;113:460–463.
54. Schott GD, Wyke MA. Congenital mirror movements. *J Neurol Neurosurg Psychiatry* 1981;44:586–599.
55. Whittle IR, Besser M. Congenital neural abnormalities presenting with mirror movements in a patient with Klippel-Feil syndrome. Case report. *J Neurosurg* 1983;59:891–894.
56. David KM, Copp AJ, Stevens JM, et al. Split cervical spinal cord with Klippel-Feil syndrome: seven cases. *Brain* 1996;119:1859–1872.
57. Rock JP, Spickler EM. Anomalous rib presenting as cervical myelopathy: a previously unreported variant of Klippel-Feil syndrome. Case report. *J Neurosurg* 1991;75:465–467.
58. Whiting DM, Chou SM, Lanzieri CF, et al. Cervical neurenteric cyst associated with Klippel-Feil syndrome: a case report and review of the literature. *Clin Neuropathol* 1991;10:285–290.
59. Gumerlock MK, Spollen LE, Nelson MJ, et al. Cervical neurenteric fistula causing recurrent meningitis in Klippel-Feil sequence: case report and literature review. *Pediatr Infect Dis J* 1991;10:532–535.
60. Roberts PA. A case of intracranial dermoid cyst associated with the Klippel-Feil deformity and recurrent meningitis. *Arch Dis Child* 1958;33:222–225.
61. Diekmann-Guiroy B, Huang PS. Klippel-Feil syndrome in association with a craniocervical dermoid cyst presenting as aseptic meningitis in an adult: case report. *Neurosurgery* 1989;25:652–655.
62. Milhorat TH, Chou MW, Trinidad EM, et al. Chiari I malformation redefined: clinical and radiographic findings for 364 symptomatic patients. *Neurosurgery* 1999;44:1005–1017.
63. Nishikawa M, Sakamoto H, Hakuba A, et al. Pathogenesis of Chiari malformation: a morphometric study of the posterior cranial fossa. *J Neurosurg* 1997;86:40–47.
64. Badie B, Mendoza D, Batzdorf U. Posterior fossa volume and response to suboccipital decompression in patients with Chiari I malformation. *Neurosurgery* 1995;37:214–218.

CHAPTER 33

Treatment of Cervical Spine Instability in the Pediatric Patient

Denis S. Drummond and Harish S. Hosalkar

Pediatric cervical spine instability results from a large spectrum of conditions with a wide range of congenital and acquired etiologies often presenting with an acute or insidious pattern. This chapter focuses on the presentation, evaluation, and treatment of cervical instability in children. The most frequently encountered causes of cervical spine instability in children can be categorized etiologically (Table 33.1).

BIOMECHANICAL FEATURES

Biomechanical features of the pediatric spine play a key role in cervical spine injury patterns. Spinal cord injury without radiographic abnormality (SCIWORA) occurs in young children because of ligamentous laxity. The pediatric spinal column can withstand higher tension force than the spinal cord. The physes and apophyses in the pediatric spine provide sites susceptible to separation, altered growth, and deformity following an injury. There is a high prevalence of injuries occurring between the occiput and C2 in children. This has been explained on a biomechanical basis. The fulcrum for injury is more cephalad in the pediatric cervical spine because children have large heads relative to the rest of their bodies (1).

TRAUMA

Cervical spine injury occurs in approximately 1% of all incidences of pediatric trauma (2,3). However, the fatality rate in these pediatric injuries is double that of adults (2–4). Cervical spine injuries in young children (Table 33.2) are more likely to be associated with neurologic involvement (5).

CONGENITAL

Congenital causes of cervical spine instability are complex because congenital vertebral anomalies of the cervical spine arise from defective somatogenesis. The anomalous vertebral development commonly narrows the spinal canal, causing a focal stenosis, reduction of the space available for the spinal cord, and instability. Congenital anomalies of the cervical spine often occur in clusters, which further

TABLE 33.1. *Classification of Cervical Instability*

Causes	Subtypes
Congenital	Vertebral, ligamentous, or combined anomalies found at birth as an element of somatogenic aberration
	Syndromic disorders (e.g., Down syndrome, Klippel-Feil syndrome, Marfan syndrome, Ehlers-Danlos syndrome)
Acquired	Trauma
	Infection (pyogenic/granulomatous)
	Tumor
	Inflammatory conditions (e.g., juvenile rheumatoid arthritis)
	Storage disorders (e.g., mucopolysaccharidoses)
	Miscellaneous (e.g., postsurgery, skeletal dysplasias)

TABLE 33.2. *Common Cervical Spine Injuries in Children*

Occiput–C1 injuries
Atlantoaxial rotary subluxation
Dens fractures
Hangman fractures
Lower cervical spine fractures
Spinal cord injury without radiographic abnormality

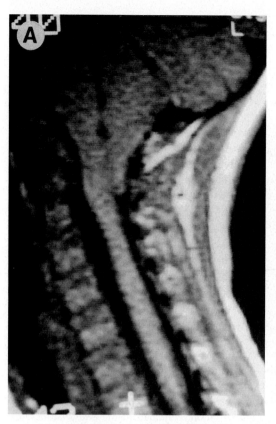
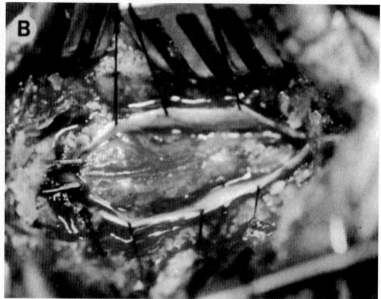

FIG. 33.1. Arnold Chiari I malformation. **A:** T1-weighted magnetic resonance image shows cerebellar tonsil herniation. **B:** Intraoperative pictures after suboccipital craniectomy, removal of the arch of the atlas, and opening of the dura; the herniation is confirmed. (From: Drummond DS. Pediatric cervical instability. In: Wiesel SW, Boden SD, Wisneski RJ, eds. *Seminars in spine surgery.* Philadelphia: WB Saunders, 1996:292–309, with permission.)

complicates these cases because more than one congenital anomaly can exist in the same patient (6). For example, segmental spinal instability associated with focal spinal stenosis greatly increases the risk for myelopathy. Additionally, the radiographic examination is often difficult to interpret in children because of the dynamic process of growth and ossification of the developing spine.

The diagnosis of congenital cervical spine instability is often delayed, suggesting that the neurologic sequelae occur progressively (7). Thus, myelopathy may not be evident initially. Nevertheless, acute onset quadriparesis has been reported in the literature (7).

Defective development of cervical vertebrae frequently is associated with anomalies of the brain stem, such as Arnold Chiari malformations. A caudally displaced brain stem and cerebellum through the foramen magnum characterize these malformations (Fig. 33.1). The occurrence of brain stem anomalies risks further compression of the brain stem and may disturb the flow of cerebrospinal fluid leading to an obstructive hydromyelia. This situation frequently is associated with progressive scoliosis (8–11).

Congenital anomalies often are observed elsewhere in the spine and spinal cord, including the thoracic spine and neural tube. Defective development may coexist in other parts of the musculoskeletal system as well as in other organ systems. Therefore, the need for a thorough investigation in search of associated problems is necessary.

SYNDROMES

The most common syndromes giving rise to cervical instability in children are Down syndrome and Klippel-Feil syndrome.

Instability of the C1-2 level is found in up to 40% of children with Down syndrome (12–17). Further, atlantooccipital instability is now believed to be common in this population (12).

Klippel-Feil syndrome was first described in the early 20th century and is now recognized to be associated with a wide variety of anomalies within the spine and other organ systems (18). Instability may occur at the interface between the normal spine and fused segments or between two fused segments (Fig. 33.2). The syndrome results from defective development of the cervical spine and is marked by a short neck, low hairline, and limited range of motion in the cervical spine (Fig. 33.3) (7,19).

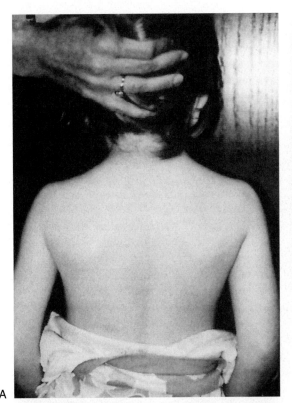

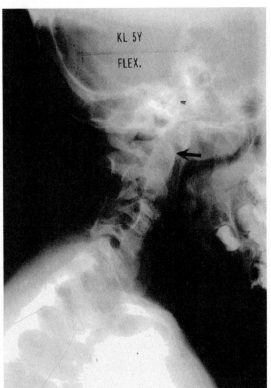

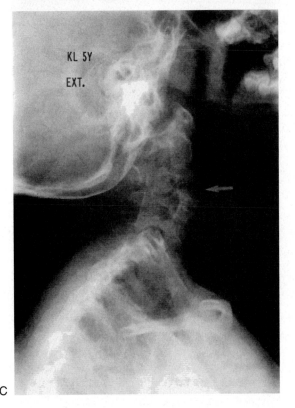

FIG. 33.2. A 5-year-old girl with Klippel-Feil syndrome, occipitalization of the atlas, and a hypoplastic odontoid. **A:** Klippel-Feil may not be immediately obvious on the clinical photograph. **B:** A lateral radiograph in flexion shows a small and rounded odontoid process *(black arrow)*. **C:** Focal instability *(white arrow)* is evident on a lateral radiograph in extension. (From: Drummond DS. Pediatric cervical instability. In: Wiesel SW, Boden SD, Wisneski RJ, eds. *Seminars in spine surgery.* Philadelphia: WB Saunders, 1996:292–309, with permission.)

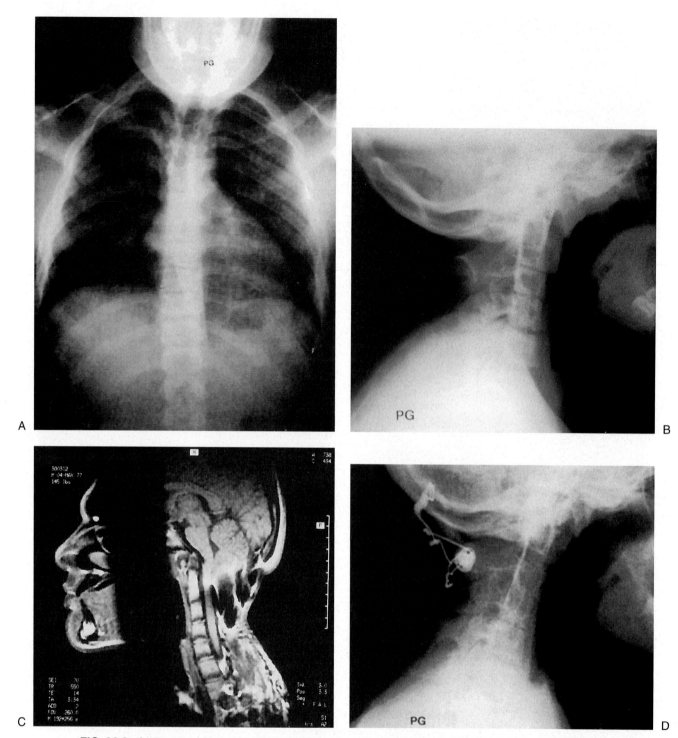

FIG. 33.3. A 17-year-old boy with Klippel-Feil syndrome presented with difficulty in phonation and long tract signs. **A:** An anteroposterior radiograph shows the short neck and bilateral Sprengel deformities. **B:** Lateral radiograph shows the multiply fused vertebrae and basilar impression. **C:** Sagittal T2 magnetic resonance image shows the Chiari I malformation, basilar impression, and a small space available for the cord. **D:** Stability following occipito-cervical arthrodesis. (From: Drummond DS. Pediatric cervical instability. In: Wiesel SW, Boden SD, Wisneski RJ, eds. *Seminars in spine surgery.* Philadelphia: WB Saunders, 1996:292–309, with permission.)

INFECTIONS

Pyogenic infections commonly have an acute presentation and rarely give rise to instability. However, instability may occur secondary to surgical drainage of pyogenic infections, particularly in otolaryngeal surgeries (20).

Chronic granulomatous infections, such as tuberculosis, can give rise to gradual vertebral destruction and instability because of the insidious nature of the disease process. However, tuberculosis occurs more commonly in underdeveloped regions of the world where malnutrition and overcrowding are prevalent (21–23).

TUMORS

Common benign and malignant lesions of the spine are listed in Table 33.3. Primary tumors of the spinal column in children are rare, accounting for less than 5% of all skeletal tumors in children (24). Both benign (expanding or collapsing) and malignant (invasive or destructive) tumors of the pediatric spine can give rise to spinal instability. Often, instability occurs after aggressive tumor treatment, such as a laminectomy over several segmental levels and particularly when the facet joints are included in the resection (25). Arthrodesis for stabilization may be indicated in these cases.

INFLAMMATORY

The most common types of cervical spine involvement in rheumatoid arthritis are (in decreasing frequency) atlantoaxial subluxation, atlantoaxial subluxation combined with subaxial subluxation, subaxial subluxation, and superior migration of the odontoid process combined with any of the first three abnormalities (26). However, cervical spine instability, although documented in adult rheumatoid arthritis, is not commonly found in the juvenile variant.

STORAGE DISEASES

Children with storage diseases, such as Morquio syndrome, may present with atlantoaxial instability. Odontoid hypoplasia,

TABLE 33.3. *Common Benign and Malignant Lesions of the Pediatric Spine*

Tumor	Type
Benign	Osteoblastoma
	Osteochondroma
	Osteoid osteoma
	Aneurysmal bone cyst
	Giant cell tumor
	Hemangioma
Malignant	Metastatic
	Ewing sarcoma
	Chordoma
	Osteosarcoma

rather than transverse ligament incompetency, usually is the cause of instability (27). Myelopathy secondary to instability also is common in these cases.

MISCELLANEOUS

Posterior column resection (postlaminectomy) can proceed to give rise to spinal instability. Similarly, skeletal dysplasias, such as osteogenesis imperfecta, neurofibromatosis, and spondyloepiphyseal dysplasias, may be associated with spinal instability on rare occasions.

COMMON CAUSES OF INSTABILITY BY ANATOMIC ZONES

Atlantoaxial Instability

Atlantoaxial instability is commonly attributed to a congenital etiology, trauma, or Down syndrome.

Atlantoaxial instability associated with congenital vertebral anomalies is complex because of the possibility of multiple coexisting pathologies. These may reduce the space available for the cord and further the risk for myelopathy. For example, focal spinal stenosis complicates instability.

Atlantoaxial rotary subluxation may result from minor trauma and also is common after surgery or infection.

Dens fractures are thought to be the most common cervical spine fractures in children that can be associated with instability. The site of fracture is commonly through the synchondrosis at the base of the dens (Fig. 33.4). Often, there is a strong anterior periosteum that remains intact and provides some stability. Thus, nonunion of pediatric dens fractures is rare (1).

Hangman fractures (C2 spondylolysis) are much less common in children than adults. However, these fractures should be included in the workup for children with a history of motor vehicle accidents because of their etiologic association with seat belt–related injuries.

Agenesis of the dens is extremely rare in children.

Hypoplasia, which has been observed with a higher frequency recently, is a common feature of some of dysmorphic conditions, such as Morquio syndrome and spondyloepiphyseal dysplasia congenita. The dens appears short and stubby in patients with these conditions. Recently, hypoplasia of the dens in the 22q-deletion syndrome has been observed.

Ossification of the dens occurs through three centers of ossification, one on either side of the midline and one at the tip (Fig. 33.5).

Os odontoideum was believed to have a congenital etiology (28). However, it is now accepted that it results from trauma occurring early in life (29–32). The dens presents as a free ossicle that is separated widely from the body of the axis in patients with os odontoideum (Fig. 33.6). Although not a congenital lesion, it remains in the differential diagnosis of both congenital and acquired atlantoaxial instability in young patients.

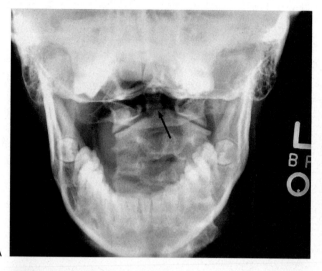

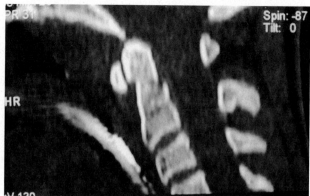

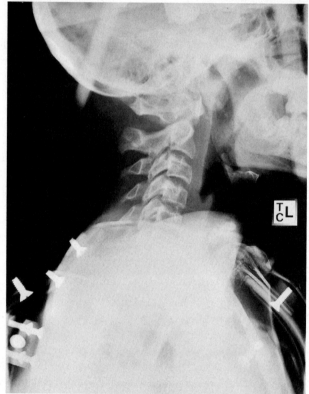

FIG. 33.4. Dens fracture in a 14-year-old girl following trauma. **A:** Open-mouth view showing odontoid fracture *(arrow)*. **B:** Computed tomography scan sagittal cut demonstrating the fracture line with displacement. **C:** Postreduction lateral cervical spine radiograph in halo vest. The fracture proceeded to union uneventfully. (Images courtesy of Denis Drummond.)

Atlantooccipital Instability

Atlantooccipital instability is commonly attributed to congenital causes, trauma, and Down syndrome.

Congenital atlantooccipital instability arises from defective development of the occipital condyles and the lateral masses of the atlas, ligament incompetency, or a combination of the two. Previously it was believed that instability resulting from defective development of the condylar-lateral mass joints was uncommon (33). However, recent ongoing studies by the senior author have determined that this anomaly is a frequent finding of the 22q-deletion syndrome. It appears that when the shape and size of these

structures are altered, smooth condylar motion is prevented and a rocking phenomenon occurs accompanied by translation (Fig. 33.7).

Occipitocervical trauma causing significant disruption usually is a serious and even lethal injury. It is disrupted more frequently in pediatric than adult injuries because of the relatively large size of children's craniums. Hyperextension, lateral rotation, or forward flexion may be the mechanism of injury. Almost 20% of patients with atlantooccipital instability are free of major neurologic injuries, although some may experience cranial nerve injury, vomiting, headache, torticollis, or minor weakness (34–36). The diagnosis may be masked or overlooked in patients with concomitant

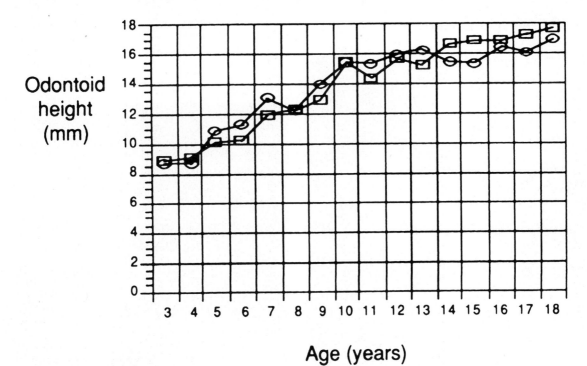

FIG. 33.5. Graph demonstrating the expected age-related ossification of the odontoid as measured from lateral radiographs. Early examination can lead to an erroneous impression of hypoplasia. (From: Drummond DS. Pediatric cervical instability. In: Wiesel SW, Boden SD, Wisneski RJ, eds. *Seminars in spine surgery*. Philadelphia: WB Saunders, 1996:292–309, with permission, and Elliott S. The odontoid process in children. Is it hypoplastic? *Clin Radiol* 1988;39(4):391–393.)

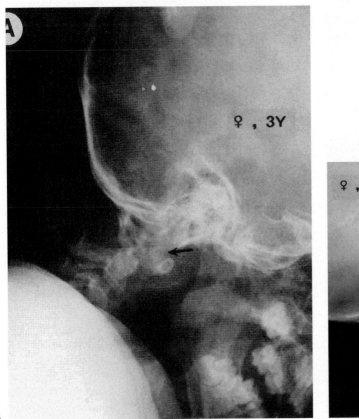

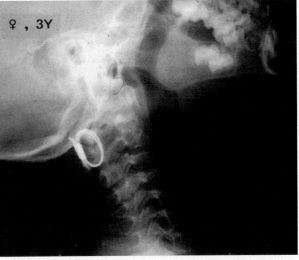

FIG. 33.6. Os odontoideum in a 3-year-old presenting with early signs of cord compression. **A:** A lateral radiograph shows Os odontoideum *(black arrow)* and C1-2 instability. **B:** After halo-gravity traction and reduction, a Brooks interposition arthrodesis was successfully performed, leading to complete neurologic recovery. Note the use of cable to achieve arthrodesis. (From: Drummond DS. Pediatric cervical instability. In: Wiesel SW, Boden SD, Wisneski RJ, eds. *Seminars in spine surgery*. Philadelphia: WB Saunders, 1996:292–309, with permission.)

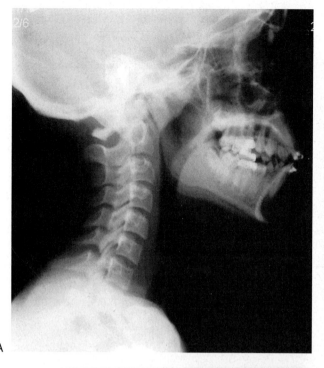

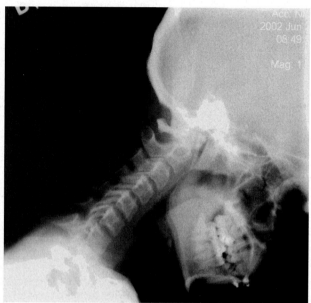

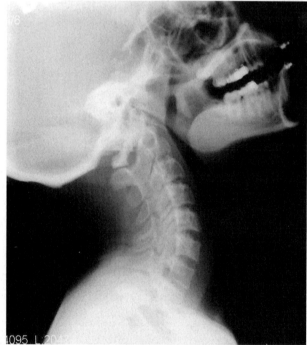

FIG. 33.7. A 14-year-old girl with 22q11.2 deletion syndrome, lateral x-rays of cervical spine: **(A)** neutral, **(B)** flexion, and **(C)** extension radiographs showing evidence of platybasia, occipitocervical, and atlantoaxial instability.

brain injury. One should be alert for clues to cord injury, such as spinal shock and urinary retention in cases of complete cervical lesions, as well as neck pain, tingling, or spasticity out of proportion to cognitive impairment in partial lesions (37). Occipitocervical injuries may remain undeclared for weeks until the spine is manipulated for imaging or traction is placed, or they may reduce spontaneously (38).

The classic example of ligamentous incompetence is observed in children with Down syndrome (Fig. 33.8). Instability of the cervical spine occurs frequently in these children at the atlantooccipital as well as the atlantoaxial level (12), although this is commonly asymptomatic in childhood.

Subaxial Instability

Subaxial instability may be caused by trauma and ligamentous laxity. Lower cervical spine injuries are rare in children. However, injuries to posterior ligaments should be evaluated with flexion and extension lateral cervical spine radiographs. The site of injury typically is the cervicothoracic junction (1).

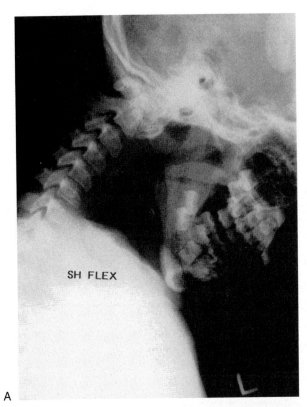

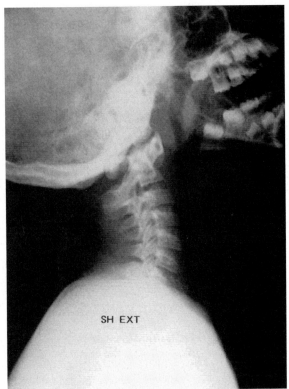

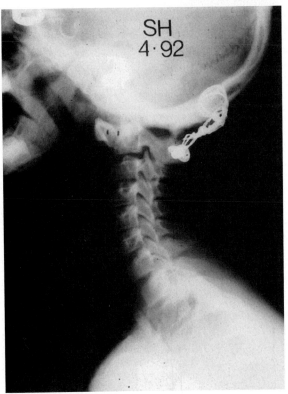

FIG. 33.8. Down syndrome. Lateral radiographs in **(A)** flexion and **(B)** extension show atlantooccipital hypermobility and fixed atlantoaxial subluxation. **C:** Instability and symptoms were relieved by an occipitoaxial arthrodesis. (From: Drummond DS. Pediatric cervical instability. In: Wiesel SW, Boden SD, Wisneski RJ, eds. *Seminars in spine surgery.* Philadelphia: WB Saunders, 1996:292–309, with permission.)

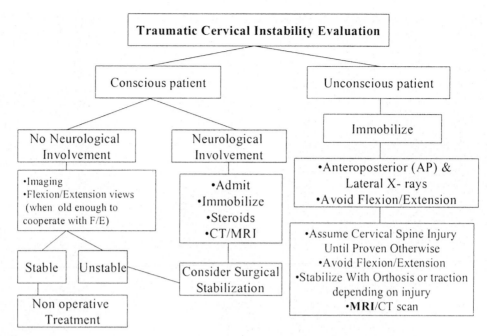

FIG. 33.9. Algorithm for management of traumatic cervical instability.

EVALUATION

Evaluation of the cervical spine is more difficult in children than adults. Head or facial trauma may be a clue to the presence of cervical spine injuries. An unconscious child should be treated presumptively for a cervical spine injury (Fig. 33.9).

A thorough physical examination of the child should be performed with particular attention to the upper cervical spine. The patient may have more than one level of neck injury (2). Tenderness is highly suggestive, but not an essential marker of cervical spine injury (39). SCIWORA and transverse ligament injuries are not readily detectable; hence, a child with major trauma should be protected from excessive neck movement (40,41).

Localizing pain to a precise point may be difficult in children. Therefore, clinical signs are extremely important. Torticollis after trauma may indicate a C1-2 rotatory subluxation or a minor spinal cord injury. Spasm of the sterno-cleidomastoid muscle may be suggestive of spinal injury. The "seat belt sign," a transverse patch of skin contusion across the abdomen, should alert the clinician to associated injuries to abdominal viscera and lumbar spine. Detailed neurologic examination is essential and should include assessment of the bulbocavernous reflex as well as testing of active flexion/extension at all major joints.

The correct approach to an alert (conscious) patient presenting with nontraumatic cervical spine instability is outlined in Figure 33.10. General examination should include assessment of associated presenting features in patients presenting with an insidious onset of stability. Multiple joint

involvement with systemic signs should be assessed in patient with juvenile rheumatoid arthritis (JRA). Detailed evaluation of previous surgical procedures should be performed in postsurgical cases, such as postlaminectomy. A mental status examination should be performed with evaluation of the features of storage diseases in patients with

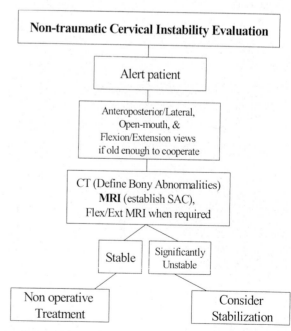

FIG. 33.10. Algorithm for management of traumatic cervical instability.

mucopolysaccharidosis, blue sclera, dentition, and multiple fractures (suggestive of osteogenesis imperfecta). A thorough assessment for other systemic anomalies should be performed in patients with Down syndrome and Klippel-Feil syndrome.

DIAGNOSING INSTABILITY

A cervical spine radiograph is mandatory in all patients presenting with a history of major trauma or unconsciousness. Open-mouth or odontoid assessment views are difficult to obtain in young children and are of questionable benefit (42). Flexion/extension views are indicated when static films are suspicious for a cervical spine injury. They should be done when the child is old enough to cooperate and instability is suspected. Computed tomography (CT) scans are indicated for patients with atlas ring fractures or atlantoaxial rotary subluxation. Dynamic CT scanning may help elaborate the nature of instability and document fixed subluxation. Magnetic resonance imaging (MRI) with static or dynamic (i.e., flexion/extension; only if old enough to cooperate) scans are need when neurologic insult is present or suspected.

Atlantoaxial Instability

Plain radiographs help define the problem. It is important to remember that the growth of the dens may be underestimated as only the ossified (not the cartilaginous odontoid) can be observed by standard radiographs. Figure 33.5 shows the progressive ossification process. The tip of the dens does not reach the upper edge of the ring of the atlas until an average of age 9 in normal children. Therefore, odontoid hypoplasia may be overdiagnosed.

Atlantooccipital Instability

Plain radiographs (anteroposterior [AP] and lateral along with flexion/extension views when feasible) help in the primary evaluation. A CT is useful to demonstrate the exact location of the occipital condyles and can offer a sagittal reconstruction. MRI is helpful in imaging the atlantooccipital interval and can assess the edema in occipitocervical facet capsules (43), basocervical ligaments, and cervicomedullary angulation.

The occipital-C1 level often is difficult to observe because reliable cranial reference points frequently are hard to discern. The occipital condyles normally should rest in the depressions of the atlas facets and the facet–condyle interval should be less than 5 mm (44). The interval between the basion (anterior cortical margin of the foramen magnum) and the tip of the dens should be less than 10 mm (37,45). The Powers' ratio is the most widely used method for

diagnosis of atlantooccipital instability. It is the ratio of a segment drawn from the basion to the posterior arch of the atlas, and the opisthion to the anterior arch of the atlas (46). The published norm for the upper limit for atlantooccipital translation is 1 mm in adults (33,46,47). Two millimeters of translation or less is considered normal for children, and 4 mm is accepted in patients with Down syndrome. Measurements outside these ranges are suggestive of atlantooccipital instability.

It is necessary to determine the space available for the cord (SAC) in patients with an atlantooccipital translation of 5 mm or more. A relatively narrow canal is associated with greater risk for injury than a capacious one.

Also, it is important to observe any pathologic motion, such as a hinged motion or opening at the atlantooccipital articulation (Fig. 33.11). This suggests defective development of the condyle articulation.

Atlantodens Interval

The important radiographic test for instability is the lateral flexion/extension radiograph where translation can be measured by the atlantodens interval (ADI). The ADI is greater in children than adults. Up to 4.5 mm is considered normal (30,48–51). This interval should be measured from the posterior–inferior cortex of the body of the atlas along a line perpendicular to its posterior surface (45). In extension, the anterior arch of the atlas may slide up on the dens. The absence of soft-tissue swelling does not rule out atlantoaxial instability.

MRI is helpful to evaluate the SAC and a flexion/extension MRI can reveal a more dynamic appreciation of the space at this level. Steel, who defined the SAC, observed that a good rule of thumb is that one-third of the space of the cross-sectional diameter can be available for the dens, one-third for the spinal cord, and one-third is needed as available space (52).

Unique Pediatric Diagnostic Features

Retropharyngeal soft-tissue space in children is 6 mm or less at C3, and is less than 14 mm at C6 (44,51). However, these findings are inconclusive in a crying child when the retropharyngeal space may appear spuriously enlarged. The pediatric cervical spine may also demonstrate a unique phenomenon termed pseudosubluxation. The C2-3 vertebrae may translate up to 3 mm in flexion in patients with pseudosubluxation (51). Swischuk's line, drawn between C1 and C3 laminae can help to assess this phenomenon (discussed in Chapter X). Normally, the lamina of the atlas does not fall more than 1 mm forward of this line. It is helpful to be aware of the unique radiographic features of the pediatric spine, including the vertebral variants and developmental patterns while evaluating radiographs (Table 33.4) (45).

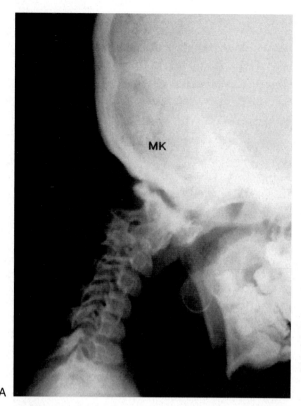

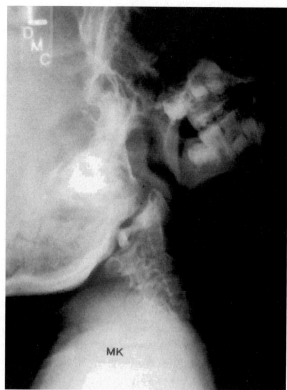

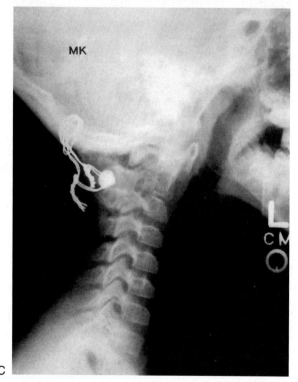

FIG. 33.11. Congenital atlantooccipital instability. **A and B:** Lateral radiographs show translation and a pathologic hinged motion in an otherwise normal 6-year-old boy who presented with intermittent pain. Further imaging showed a reduction of the space available for the cord. **C:** Same patient 1 year after an occipital to C2 arthrodesis. (From: Drummond DS. Pediatric cervical instability. In: Wiesel SW, Boden SD, Wisneski RJ, eds. *Seminars in spine surgery.* Philadelphia: WB Saunders, 1996:292–309, with permission.)

TREATMENT OF CERVICAL INSTABILITY

General Treatment Principles

A sound knowledge of principles and exhibition of great care is required to guide the decisions of management of cervical spine instability in children. Assessment of general condition and neurologic involvement is important during initial stabilization of the patient especially in trauma cases. Radiographs help define the problem. The discrepancy in head size (i.e., larger head in young children) may lead to increased flexion while taking radiographs on a flat board. Therefore, it is important to elevate the body in relationship

TABLE 33.4. *Unique Features of the Pediatric Spine*

Unique features of the pediatric spine	
General features	Secondary centers of ossification of the spinous processes may mimic fractures
	Rounding of anterior vertebral body may give the appearance of a wedge compression fracture
	Horizontal facets and ligamentous laxity allow greater intersegment mobility
	Decreased cervical lordosis
	Wider prevertebral soft tissues may mimic swelling
Special features	
	C1 multiple ossification centers may mimic fractures
	C1-2 atlantodens interval may be up to 4.5 mm in normal children
	C2 normal posterior angulation of odontoid (4% of children) may mimic fracture
	Ossiculum terminale may be confused with a fracture
	Basilar synchondrosis may be confused with a fracture
	C2-3 pseudosubluxation can be mistaken for instability

From: Bulas DI, Fitz CR, Johnson DL. Traumatic atlanto-occipital dislocation in children. *Radiology* 1993;188:155–158.

to the head (with a spacer or sandbag), or modify the standard adult spinal back board (by placing a recess over the occiput area) so as to allow the enlarged head of a child (<6 years old) to rest lower than the thorax (46).

A plaster or thermoplastic body jacket may be an effective way of immobilizing the cervical spine in very young children after fracture, trauma, or in cases of severe instability. Although this technique avoids the pin complications associated with halo use, it is often fraught with skin problems of the head or neck as well as feeding and talking difficulties. Pediatric hard collars often are used to initially immobilize the cervical spine during evaluation, but are rarely used in cases of major cervical spine injury. In such cases a cast brace, or more often a halo vest immobilization, is required. In cases of cervical trauma with acute spinal cord injury immediate stabilization should be achieved with an orthosis such as a halo vest. This provides time for maximum recovery. Systemic steroids may be helpful to control edema while the patient is being evaluated and prepared for surgery (47,48). No attempts at acute reduction should be done when a translation deformity is identified in the initial radiographic assessment because it carries a considerable risk of further neurologic deterioration or permanent cord injury.

Halo Application

Halo stabilization is an important adjunct to the management of problems in the pediatric cervical spine. The main advantages include ease of application, superior immobilization

and positioning of the cervical spine, easy access to wounds of the neck and scalp, few skin complications, free mandibular motion, early mobilization, and shorter hospitalization.

There are a few details that are important with regard to halo placement in children. The pediatric skull is thinner and more porous than the adult skull, and the risk for dural penetration is greater. There is no reliable "safe area" in children for pin placement because the ossification process for the calvarium occurs irregularly from patient to patient (53). Accordingly, CT is advised prior to pin placement in young children to determine the ideal locations for insertion. The procedure should be modified based on the patient's age, because pin loosening with secondary infection is common in this age group. Eight pins at 2 to 4 in/lb torque is recommended in patients under age 6. Four pins at 4 to 6 in/lb is recommended in children between 6 and 8 years; and four pins at 6 to 8 in/lb torque is recommended for those close to adult age (54,55). A customized halo ring, 2 cm larger than the outer diameter of the skull, and a customized bivalve polypropylene vest may be necessary in young children. Vest application may be performed under anesthesia in children and young adolescents to avoid anxiety and lack of cooperation. Newer halo ring designs that offer a variable pin angle prove helpful in addressing challenging situations.

Despite adhering to all these principles, problems and complications with halo immobilizations do occur. A prospective study carried out at our institution in children 3 to 16 years old revealed that pin site infection was the most common complication. There were no complications related to the vest part of the halo vest. Younger patients who had a halo construct with more than four pins (multiple-pin constructs) had a similar rate of complications compared with patients who were managed with a standard four-pin halo construct. In spite of problems and complications, the treatment with halo ring and vest was successfully carried to completion in all patients in this series (56).

(Chapter X further outlines halo application and additional orthoses.)

TREATMENT OF SPECIFIC INJURY PATTERNS ASSOCIATED WITH CERVICAL SPINE INSTABILITY

Atlas (Jefferson) Fractures

Atlas fractures are rare in children and can be confused with synchondroses based on their location and appearance. The pediatric atlas may fracture its ring at a single point, hinging on the opposite synchondrosis or plastically deforming the ring. CTs define the injury better than plain films. Lateral mass widening (>7 mm) beyond the borders of the axis is suggestive of a transverse ligament injury.

Treatment consists of immobilization with an orthosis such as a Philadelphia collar. In case of significant widening (>7 mm), surgical arthrodesis or stabilization with a halo vest may be indicated (57,58).

Dens Fractures

Dens fractures are the most common fractures of the cervical spine in children younger than 11 years old. These fractures usually occur through the synchondrosis in children younger than 6 years of age (2,59,60). The dens is anteriorly displaced in most cases, suggesting an intact periosteal sleeve on the anterior surface. Extending or slightly hyperextending the neck usually achieves reduction (at least 50% apposition provides adequate contact). The intact periosteal sleeve provides excellent healing potential in most cases if a satisfactory degree of immobilization is achieved (61). The spine may be immobilized by a Minerva cast or halo vest for 6 to 8 weeks depending on age.

Atlantoaxial Rotatory Subluxation

Atlantoaxial rotatory subluxation is a unique situation that occurs in children. Fixation of the atlantoaxial joint occurs in a malrotated position secondary to trauma or inflammation. Subluxation also can occur after retropharyngeal abscess, tonsillectomy, or pharyngoplasty. Pharyngeal space inflammation may lead to attenuation of the synovial capsules, transverse ligament, or both, resulting in instability (62).

Fielding and Hawkins have separated the components of rotation and translation in their classification of this disorder into three types (49) (Table 33.5). Type III variants present the greatest concern for instability. Posterior atlantoaxial arthrodesis is recommended for cases that fail halter or halo traction.

Transverse Ligament Disruption

The transverse ligament of the atlas arises within the ring of C1 medial to the facets. It is the primary stabilizer of the dens and works against forward displacement. The secondary stabilizers, the apical and alar ligaments, arise from the tip of the dens and pass to the base of the skull stabilizing the atlantooccipital joint indirectly (63). The upper limit of normal C1-2 translation in children is 4.5 mm. Higher values may suggest disruption of the transverse ligament (45). Acute rupture of the transverse ligament is rare (2).

Plain films may show minimal or no thickening of the retropharyngeal space, whereas CT may show a fleck of bone at one of the origins of the transverse ligament.

Treatment by immobilization usually is successful (50). Failed cases or cases presenting with serious neurologic

TABLE 33.5. *Fielding and Hawkins' Classification of Atlantoaxial Rotatory Subluxation*

Fielding and Hawkins' classification of atlantoaxial rotatory subluxation	
Type I	Unilateral facet subluxation with an intact transverse ligament
Type II	Unilateral facet dislocation with incompetent transverse ligament

symptoms at the outset may require atlantoaxial arthrodesis. Chronic atlantoaxial instability also may occur because of preceding injury or JRA and syndromes such as Down syndrome. Instability also may be seen in certain skeletal dysplasias, such as spondyloepiphyseal dysplasia, and in storage disorders, such as mucopolysaccharidoses. Recommendations for surgical arthrodesis usually involve cases with 8 mm and greater of translation, whereas lesser degrees may be managed on individual evaluation.

Spondylolysis (Pars Interarticularis Fracture) of the Axis

Spondylolysis of the axis and hangman fracture also occur in children. These conditions result from forced hyperextension and usually occur in children younger than 2 years of age (64–66). Radiographs may show forward subluxation of C2 on C3. CT can help demonstrate the exact defect. Treatment of a symptomatic lesion should include immobilization in a Minerva or halo vest for 8 to 12 weeks. If union does not occur and the translation remains excessive, an anterior fusion of the second to the third cervical vertebra should be performed.

ATLANTOAXIAL ARTHRODESIS

Positioning

For most of the arthrodesis techniques described here, the patient is positioned prone following the application of a halo device. When there is an associated spinal instability, great care in the transport of the patient is required. Spinal cord monitoring also should be used throughout this maneuver. Serial lateral radiographs should be acquired to confirm the reduction and position of the cervical spine. The halo should be then fixed to the Mayfield frame.

Gallie Technique

In the Gallie technique (Fig. 33.12), exposure is accomplished via a midline incision between the occiput and C3. The bifid spinous process of C2 and tubercle of the occiput are identified by palpation. It is important to avoid overexposure to prevent inadvertent fusion of adjacent levels. The posterior arch of the atlas is identified in the deeper layers and periosteum incised and elevated for passage of sublaminar wires or cables. The vertebral artery can be avoided by not exposing more than 1 cm lateral from the midline in children and 1.5 cm in adults. An 18- or 20-gauge wire or cable to be used later in securing the graft can be passed around the arch at this point. A Mersiline suture can be used as a leader in difficult situations. A bicortical graft is now harvested from the posterior iliac crest and shaped to fit against the posterior aspect of the atlas and around the spinous process of the axis. With the graft in position the wire loop is folded over the graft and around the spinous process

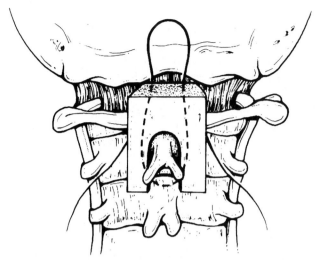

FIG. 33.12. Modified Gallie technique for atlantoaxial arthrodesis. The corticocancellous graft has been cut and shaped to fit the posterior arch of the atlas and the spinous process and laminae of the axis. The loop of wire shown has been passed under the posterior arch of C1. After insertion of the graft, the wire loop is pulled in a caudal direction over the graft and around the spinous process of the axis. The free ends of the wire then are crossed over the graft, and twisted tightly to secure it and provide stability. (From: Drummond DS. Pediatric cervical instability. In: Wiesel SW, Boden SD, Wisneski RJ, eds. *Seminars in spine surgery.* Philadelphia: WB Saunders, 1996:292–309, with permission.)

of the axis. The free ends of the wire are then brought together from the lateral edge of the graft and twisted in the midline, thus securing it and providing cervical stability. Continuous spinal cord monitoring and intraoperative imaging to ascertain the reduction and graft position are important. The authors' prefer the routine use of halo vest to protect arthrodesis construct.

BROOKS ARTHRODESIS

The exposure for the Brooks arthrodesis (Fig. 33.13) is the same as that described in the preceding. The fixation differs as a double 18-gauge wire is passed around the arch of the atlas and lamina of the axis. The authors suggest the use of a braided cable wire because it is soft and relatively safe to pass, resists fatigue well, and provides excellent fixation. Two rectangular grafts 1.25 × 3.5 cm are harvested from the iliac crest and the cancellous surface is prepared to fit into the C1-2 interval. The grafts help to prevent hyperextension and contribute to the stability of the Brooks procedure.

The senior author has modified the Gallie technique by using similar interval grafts under the onlay Gallie graft to achieve improved stability of the construct and increased distribution of autogenous graft. This now is the authors' preferred procedure for younger and small patients.

OCCIPITOCERVICAL INSTABILITY

Treatment of traumatic atlantooccipital disruption consists of reduction using gentle skull traction and stabilization in a halo vest. Care should be taken not to overdistract. Decompression may be necessary for major hematomas at the cervicomedullary junction. Systemic steroids can be useful to reduce edema. Reduction should be confirmed radiographically and stability achieved either by immobilization alone or arthrodesis. Stability should be confirmed with radiographs after the halo is removed. Exact definition of stability at this level has not been documented, although more than 1 mm of translation is abnormal, and 5 mm or greater should be considered for stabilization.

Imprecise definitions of stability and the devastating consequences of reinjury force some surgeons to choose fusion for stabilization. Fusion can be restricted from occiput

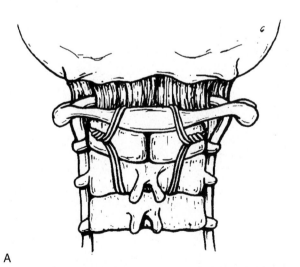

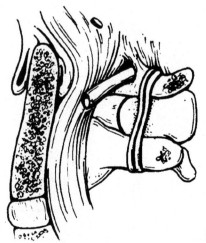

A   B

FIG. 33.13. Brooks interposition atlantoaxial arthrodesis. **A:** The wires have been passed under the arch of C1 on both sides and under the laminae of C2. **B:** The importance of shaping the grafts, which prevent hyperextension and iatrogenic subluxation, is shown. (From: Drummond DS. Pediatric cervical instability. In: Wiesel SW, Boden SD, Wisneski RJ, eds. *Seminars in spine surgery.* Philadelphia: WB Saunders, 1996:292–309, with permission.)

to C1 or C2 in the neurologically intact patient to maximize movement. Bone grafts may be taken from the rib or the iliac crest. However, rib grafts can be readily contoured to span two or more segments. In late cases of unreduced dislocation, reduction should not be forcefully attempted. In such cases, fusion *in situ* with a suboccipital craniectomy (to relieve posterior impingement) can be attempted.

OCCIPITOCERVICAL ARTHRODESIS

Precautions in positioning are the same as described in the preceding. The exposure is an extension of that described for atlantoaxial arthrodesis. The midline incision extends from the occiput to the spinous process of C3.

The senior author has successfully used two techniques for arthrodesis of the occiput to C2 or lower. With both procedures the fixation wires or cables are passed through cranial burr holes that are made as two pairs on either side of the midline.

The first of these procedures was described in 1995 (Fig. 33.14) (67). This technique has been successfully used in more than 40 patients. It is based on a shaped structural graft harvested from the iliac crest. This is fixed by wire or cable to a trough prepared at the base of the occiput and fits over the spinous process of the axis.

The second technique was described in 2001 (Fig. 33.15) (68). It differs from the first in that the structural graft used is rib rather than autogenous iliac crest. Paired autogenous

rib grafts are harvested and fixed to the occiput and axis by sublaminar wires or braided cable. The natural curve of the rib has the advantage of fitting closer to the anatomy of the cervical spine and fusion bed. This procedure appears to be better tolerated and the stability is as good or better than that provided by the iliac on-lay technique. This technique has been successful in seven patients. The postoperative management is the same for both techniques. The patient is immobilized in a halo vest or a four-postcervical orthosis.

SUBAXIAL INJURIES

These injuries represent only 25% of all pediatric cervical spine injuries (69). Fractures and subluxations in the lower cervical spine become more common in older childhood and adolescence. Treatment should follow the principles for adult injury. Despite the slightly improved prognosis for ligament healing in children, those with subluxation and dislocation should be tested by flexion and extension views after immobilization to verify healing.

SUBAXIAL ARTHRODESIS

When internal fixation is limited by the patient's size, specifically in small children, the Dewar procedure (Fig. 33.16) appears to work well. The authors have never been comfortable passing threaded k-wires though the skin and soft tissues, the base of spinous process, and the soft tissue on the

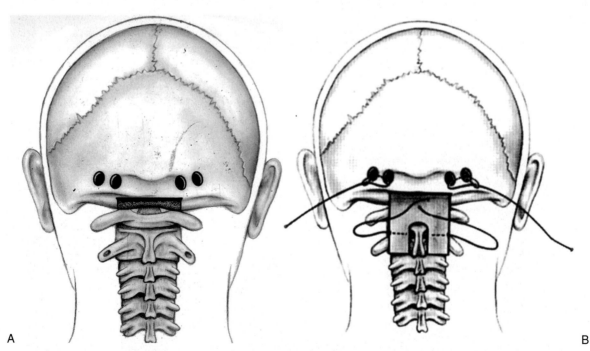

A   B

FIG. 33.14. The authors' technique for occipital-C2 arthrodesis. **A:** After exposure, the occiput is prepared by burr holes on either side of the midline and a trough is made at the base of the occiput with a shape to accept an autograft from the iliac crest. **B:** The graft in place, wire loops are lassoed between the burr holes on each side. The button-wire implants are in place. Joining and twisting the wires secures the graft. (From: Dormans JP, Drummond DS, Sutton LN, et al. Occipitocervical arthrodesis in children. A new technique and analysis of results. *J Bone Joint Surg Am* 1995;77:1234–1240, with permission.)

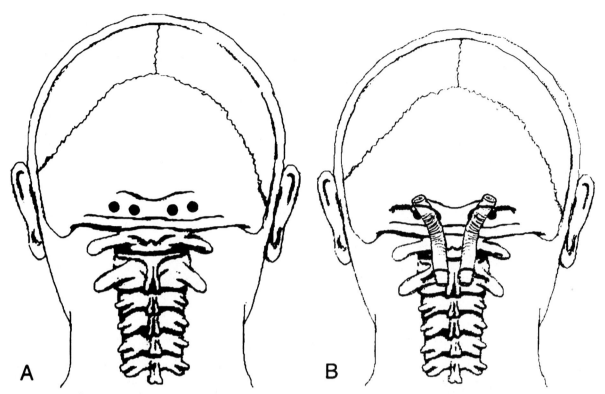

FIG. 33.15. A: Four burr holes are placed into the occiput in transverse alignment, with two on each side of the midline, leaving a strong osseous bridge between the two holes of each pair. **B:** Cranially, a 16-gauge wire is passed through each burr hole pair. Caudally, wires are passed under the lamina on each side of the midline at the second cervical vertebra or at the first vertebra that is both below the level of instability and that has an intact posterior arch. The rib graft is secured into place by twisting the wires.

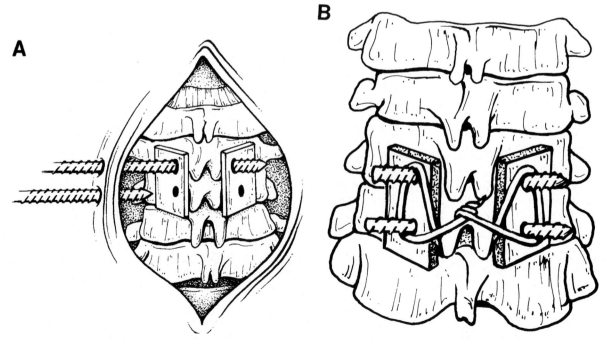

FIG. 33.16. Dewar technique for arthrodesis of the lower cervical spine. **A:** The corticocancellous grafts have been cut and shaped to lie against the spinous processes of the vertebrae to be fused. Threaded K-wires are being inserted through the bases of spinous process. **B:** Stable fixation after securing the wires. (From: Drummond DS. Pediatric cervical instability. In: Wiesel SW, Boden SD, Wisneski RJ, eds. *Seminars in spine surgery.* Philadelphia: WB Saunders, 1996:292–309, with permission.)

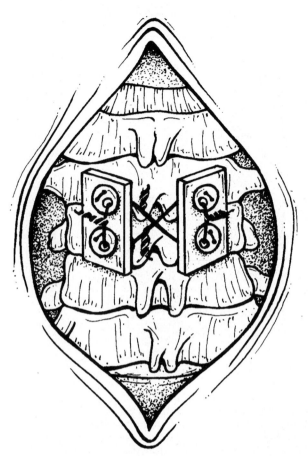

FIG. 33.17. The authors' technique for the modified Dewar arthrodesis of the lower cervical spine. The key to this technique is the button-wire implant. The implants are inserted in pairs at each segmental level to be fused. The beaded wire passes through the two grafts and the base of the spinous process as well as the hold in the face of the opposite button. After cutting all of the wire loops, one loop is twisted to the adjacent ipsilateral wire and the other is joined by crossing to the opposite and contralateral wire. (From: Drummond DS. Pediatric cervical instability. In: Wiesel SW, Boden SD, Wisneski RJ, eds. *Seminars in spine surgery*. Philadelphia: WB Saunders, 1996:292–309, with permission.)

contralateral side. Accordingly, the senior author has modified the procedure using the button-wire implants developed for scoliosis correction (65,66). The Modified Dewar technique is shown in Fig. 33.17. Patients usually are immobilized in a cervical collar for 6 to 8 weeks following surgery.

OTHER SURGICAL TECHNIQUES OF SPINAL STABILIZATION

Interspinous Wire Fixation

Segmental fixation of the lower cervical spine can be satisfactorily performed by interspinous wiring (Fig. 33.18). This is achieved using a 2-mm high-speed burr to create a hole on either side of the base of spinous process. A single motion segment or multiple segments may be fixed in this manner.

Lateral Mass Plate Fixation

Fixation with lateral mass screws and plates can be considered instead of the techniques described in the preceding in older and larger patients (Fig. 33.19). Posterior plate fixation may also include the C1-2 motion segment. The advantage of this type of fixation is that halo vest extended immobilization may not be needed. The authors' experience is derived mainly from older children where screws provided adequate fixation to avoid prolonged orthotic management.

Transarticular Fixation

Transarticular fixation for fusion of C1-2 may be indicated rarely for failed arthrodesis or in case of defective posterior elements. The fixation may be performed from the posterior or lateral approach. Screw placement is critical and good intraoperative imaging in necessary because the margin for error is very small.

Anterior Cervical Instrumentation

Anterior cervical plating is not routinely used in the pediatric spine. It may have a role in larger patients in the presence of significant instability following vertebrectomy. A postulated advantage would be that posterior stabilization not be required. Immediate and good stabilization also could be achieved after multilevel arthrodesis.

COMPLICATIONS OF SURGICAL MANAGEMENT

Progressive deformity of the spine may occur with growth following multiple laminectomies in a pediatric spine. Lonstein reported significant spinal deformities after laminectomy in as many as 50% of cases in their series (25). Risk factors for deformity are extensive laminectomy, neurologic involvement, and younger age at surgery. Hence, laminectomy should be avoided in the pediatric spine or concurrent fusion advocated at the time of laminectomy or shortly thereafter.

CONCLUSION

Cervical spine problems in children differ substantially from those of adults. A clear and comprehensive understanding of the anatomy, physiology, and biomechanics of the pediatric cervical spine is of paramount importance in the treatment of patients with cervical spine instability. A careful and thorough clinical and neurologic evaluation and appropriate radiographic assessment are essential to make an accurate diagnosis, understand the pathogenesis, and outline the appropriate management.

Surgical treatment of cervical spine instability in children may be indicated to protect the neural structures (axis and nerve roots) from insult or damage. Occasionally, arthrodesis

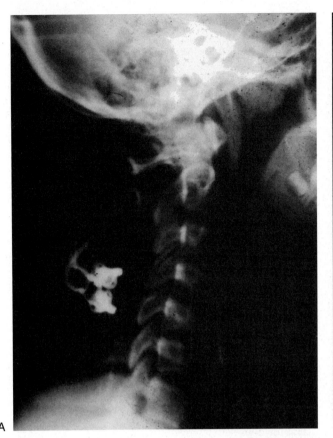
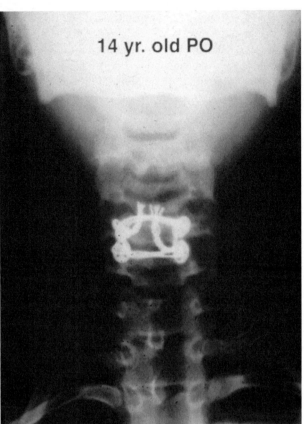

14 yr. old PO

FIG. 33.18. A: Anteroposterior and **(B)** lateral demonstrating intraspinous wire fixation in an 11-year-old patient with cervical instability at C4-5 interval using interspinous button wires.

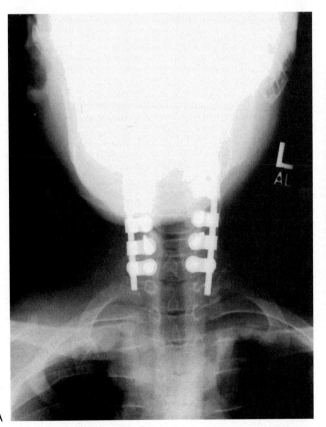
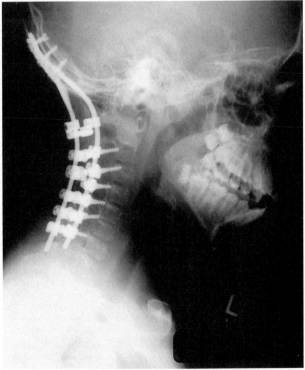

FIG. 33.19. A 10-year-old boy with neurofibromatosis type I and neurologic deficit secondary to cord compression in view of cervical instability. Subsequent to tumor excision and decompression, cervical fusion was performed with lateral mass fixation as demonstrated on postoperative **(A)** anteroposterior and **(B)** lateral radiographs. (Images courtesy of JP Dormans.)

may be necessitated to stabilize the spine. Stabilization allows early mobilization and rehabilitation. Further, the recovery of a single nerve root during decompression and stabilization may go a long way in improving function and overall quality of life for a patient.

REFERENCES

1. Flynn JM. Spine trauma in the pediatric population. In: DS Drummond, ed. *Strategies in the pediatric spine.* Philadelphia: Hanley & Belfus, 2000:249–262.
2. McGrory BJ, Klassen RA, Chao EY, et al. Acute fractures and dislocations of the cervical spine in children and adolescents. *J Bone Joint Surg Am* 1993;75:988–995.
3. Patel JC, Tepas 3rd JJ, Mollitt DL, et al. Pediatric cervical spine injuries: defining the disease. *J Pediatr Surg* 2001;36:373–376.
4. Evans DL, Bethem D. Cervical spine injuries in children. *J Pediatr Orthop* 1989;9:563–568.
5. Hadley MN, Zabramski JM, Browner CM, et al. Pediatric spinal trauma. Review of 122 cases of spinal cord and vertebral column injuries. *J Neurosurg* 1988;68:18–24.
6. Drummond DS, Tahernia AD, Delfico A, et al. Congenital anomalies of the upper cervical spine: Identifying patients at risk for myelopathy. Annual Meeting of the Pediatric Orthopaedic Society of North America. Banff, Alberta, 1997.
7. Scolville WB, Sherman IJ. Platybasia, report of 10 cases. *Ann Surg* 1951;133:496–502.
8. Vandertop WP, Asai A, Hoffman HJ, et al. Surgical decompression for symptomatic Chiari II malformation in neonates with myelomeningocele. *J Neurosurg* 1992;77:541–544.
9. Muhonen MG, Menezes AH, Sawin PD, et al. Scoliosis in pediatric Chiari malformations without myelodysplasia. *J Neurosurg* 1992;77: 69–77.
10. Menezes AH. Chiari I malformations and hydromyelia—complications. *Pediatr Neurosurg* 1991;17:146–154.
11. Isu T, Chono Y, Iwasaki Y, et al. Scoliosis associated with syringomyelia presenting in children. *Childs Nerv Syst* 1992;8:97–100.
12. Tredwell SJ, Newman DE, Lockitch G. Instability of the upper cervical spine in Down syndrome. *J Pediatr Orthop* 1990;10:602–606.
13. Cremers MJ, Ramos L, Bol E, et al. Radiological assessment of the atlantoaxial distance in Down's syndrome. *Arch Dis Child* 1993;69: 347–350.
14. Cremers MJ, Bol E, de Roos F, et al. Risk of sports activities in children with Down's syndrome and atlantoaxial instability. *Lancet* 1993;342:511–514.
15. S, O'Connell E, Blake NS, Ward OC. Atlantoaxial instability in Down's syndrome: clinical and radiological screening. *Ir Med J* 1989;82:64–65.
16. Selby KA, Newton RW, Gupta S, et al. Clinical predictors and radiological reliability in atlantoaxial subluxation in Down's syndrome. *Arch Dis Child* 1991;66:876–878.
17. Van Dyke DC, Gahagan CA. Down syndrome. Cervical spine abnormalities and problems. *Clin Pediatr (Phila)* 1988;27:415–418.
18. RN, Lang JE, MacEwen GD. Klippel-Feil syndrome: a constellation of associated anomalies. *J Bone Joint Surg Am* 1974;56:1246–1253.
19. Klippel M, Feil A. Un ca d'Absence des vertebres cervicales avec thoracique remonant jusqu'a la base du crane. *Nouv Icon Salpetiere* 1912; 25:223–250.
20. Copley LA, Dormans JP. Cervical spine disorders in infants and children. *J Am Acad Orthop Surg* 1998;6:204–214.
21. A 10-year assessment of a controlled trial comparing debridement and anterior spinal fusion in the management of tuberculosis of the spine in patients on standard chemotherapy in Hong Kong. Eighth report of the Medical Research Council Working Party on Tuberculosis of the Spine. *J Bone Joint Surg Br* 1982;64:393–398.
22. Five-year assessments of controlled trials of ambulatory treatment, debridement and anterior spinal fusion in the management of tuberculosis of the spine. Studies in Bulawayo (Rhodesia) and in Hong Kong. Sixth report of the Medical Research Council Working Party on Tuberculosis of the Spine. *J Bone Joint Surg Br* 1978;60-B:163–177.
23. Martin NS. Tuberculosis of the spine. A study of the results of treatment during the last twenty-five years. *J Bone Joint Surg Br* 1970;52: 613–628.
24. Dormans JP, Pill SG. Benign and malignant tumors of the spine in children. In: DS Drummond, ed. *Strategies in the pediatric spine.* Philadelphia: Hanley & Belfus, 2000:263–279.
25. Lonstein JE. Post-laminectomy kyphosis. *Clin Orthop* 1977;93–100.
26. Simmons EH. The cervical spine in ankylosing spondylitis. In: Bridwell KH, DeWald RL, eds. *The textbook of spinal surgery,* 2nd. Philadelphia: Lippincott-Raven, 1997:1129–1158.
27. Beighton P, Craig J. Atlanto-axial subluxation in the Morquio syndrome. Report of a case. *J Bone Joint Surg Br* 1973;55:478–481.
28. Wolin DJ. The os odontoideum: separate odontoid process. *J Bone Joint Surg Am* 1936;45:1459–1471.
29. Fielding JW. Disappearance of the central portion of the odontoid process. *J Bone Joint Surg Am* 1965;47:1228–1230.
30. Fielding JW, Griffin PP. Os odontoideum: an acquired lesion. *J Bone Joint Surg Am* 1974;56:187–190.
31. Freiberger RH, Wilson PD, Nicholson JA. Acquired absence of the odontoid process. *J Bone Joint Surg Am* 1962;47:1231–1236.
32. Hawkins RJ, Fielding JW, Thompson WJ. Os odontoideum: congenital or acquired? A case report. *J Bone Joint Surg Am* 1976;58:413–414.
33. Georgopoulos G, Pizzutillo PD, Lee MS. Occipito-atlantal instability in children. A report of five cases and review of the literature. *J Bone Joint Surg Am* 1987;69:429–436.
34. Harmanli O, Koyfman Y. Traumatic atlanto-occipital dislocation with survival: a case report and review of the literature. *Surg Neurol* 1993; 39:324–330.
35. Hosono N, Yonenobu K, Kawagoe K, et al. Traumatic anterior atlanto-occipital dislocation. A case report with survival. *Spine* 1993;18:786–790.
36. Papadopoulos SM, Dickman CA, Sonntag VK, et al. Traumatic atlantooccipital dislocation with survival. *Neurosurgery* 1991;28:574–579.
37. Kenter K, Worley G, Griffin T, et al. Pediatric traumatic atlanto-occipital dislocation: five cases and a review. *J Pediatr Orthop* 2001; 21:585–589.
38. DiBenedetto T, Lee CK. Traumatic atlanto-occipital instability. A case report with follow-up and a new diagnostic technique. *Spine* 1990;15: 595–597.
39. Rachesky I, Boyce WT, Duncan B, et al. Clinical prediction of cervical spine injuries in children. Radiographic abnormalities. *Am J Dis Child* 1987;141:199–201.
40. Orenstein JB, Klein BL, Ochsenschlager DW. Delayed diagnosis of pediatric cervical spine injury. *Pediatrics* 1992;89:1185–1188.
41. Pang D, Wilberger JE Jr. Spinal cord injury without radiographic abnormalities in children. *J Neurosurg* 1982;57:114–129.
42. Buhs C, Cullen M, Klein M, et al. The pediatric trauma C-spine: is the 'odontoid' view necessary? *J Pediatr Surg* 2000;35:994–997.
43. Bundschuh CV, Alley JB, Ross M, et al. Magnetic resonance imaging of suspected atlanto-occipital dislocation. Two case reports. *Spine* 1992;17:245–248.
44. Pennecot GF, Gouraud D, Hardy JR, et al. Roentgenographical study of the stability of the cervical spine in children. *J Pediatr Orthop* 1984;4:346–352.
45. Bulas DI, Fitz CR, Johnson DL. Traumatic atlanto-occipital dislocation in children. *Radiology* 1993;188:155–158.
46. Powers B, Miller MD, Kramer RS, et al. Traumatic anterior atlanto-occipital dislocation. *Neurosurgery* 1979;4:12–17.
47. Wadia NH. Myelopathy complicating congenital atlanto-axial dislocation. (A study of 28 cases). *Brain* 1967;90:449–472.
48. Fielding JW, Hensinger RN, Hawkins RJ. Os odontoideum. *J Bone Joint Surg Am* 1980;62:376–383.
49. Fielding JW, Hawkins RJ. Atlanto-axial rotatory fixation. (Fixed rotatory subluxation of the atlanto-axial joint.) *J Bone Joint Surg Am* 1977;59:37–44.
50. de Beer JD, Hoffman EB, Kieck CF. Traumatic atlantoaxial subluxation in children. *J Pediatr Orthop* 1990;10:397–400.
51. Cattel HS, Filtzer DL. Pseudosubluxation and other normal variation in the cervical spine in children. *J Bone Joint Surg Am* 1965;47:1295–1309.
52. Apple JS, Kirks DR, Merten DF, et al. Cervical spine fractures and dislocations in children. *Pediatr Radiol* 1987;17:45–49.
53. Wong W, Haynes R. Pediatric halo considerations. Annual meeting of the Pediatric Orthopaedic Society of North America. Phoenix, AZ, 1994.
54. Letts M, Kaylor D, Gouw G. A biomechanical analysis of halo fixation in children. *J Bone Joint Surg Br* 1988;70:277–279.

55. Mubarak SJ, Camp JF, Vuletich W, et al. Halo application in the infant. *J Pediatr Orthop* 1989;9:612–614.

56. Dormans JP, Criscitiello AA, Drummond DS, et al. Complications in children managed with immobilization in a halo vest. *J Bone Joint Surg Am* 1995;77:1370–1373.

57. Birney TJ, Hanley EN Jr. Traumatic cervical spine injuries in childhood and adolescence. *Spine* 1989;14:1277–1282.

58. Lee TT, Green BA, Petrin DR. Treatment of stable burst fracture of the atlas (Jefferson fracture) with rigid cervical collar. *Spine* 1998;23: 1963–1967.

59. Seimon LP. Fracture of the odontoid process in young children. *J Bone Joint Surg Am* 1977;59:943–948.

60. Sherk HH, Nicholson JT, Chung SM. Fractures of the odontoid process in young children. *J Bone Joint Surg Am* 1978;60:921–924.

61. Diekema DS, Allen DB. Odontoid fracture in a child occupying a child restraint seat. *Pediatrics* 1988;82:117–119.

62. Parke WW, Rothman RH, Brown MD. The pharyngovertebral veins: an anatomical rationale for Grisel's syndrome. *J Bone Joint Surg Am* 1984;66:568–574.

63. Hohl M, Baker HR. The atlanto-axial joint: roentgenographic and anatomical study of normal and abnormal motion. *J Bone Joint Surg Am* 1964;46:1739–1752.

64. Fardon DF, Fielding JW. Defects of the pedicle and spondylolisthesis of the second cervical vertebra. *J Bone Joint Surg Br* 1981;63B:526–528.

65. Francis WR, Fielding JW, Hawkins RJ, et al. Traumatic spondylolisthesis of the axis. *J Bone Joint Surg Br* 1981;63-B:313–318.

66. Pizzutillo PD, Rocha EF, D'Astous J, et al. Bilateral fracture of the pedicle of the second cervical vertebra in the young child. *J Bone Joint Surg Am* 1986;68:892–896.

67. Dormans JP, Drummond DS, Sutton LN, et al. Occipitocervical arthrodesis in children. A new technique and analysis of results. *J Bone Joint Surg Am* 1995;77:1234–1240.

68. Cohen MW, Drummond DS, Flynn JM, et al. A technique of occipitocervical arthrodesis in children using autologous rib grafts. *Spine* 2001;26:825–829.

69. McLain RF, Clark CR, el-Khoury GY. C6-7 dislocation in a neurologically intact neonate. A case report. *Spine* 1989;14:125–127.

CHAPTER 34

Klippel-Feil Syndrome

Peter D. Pizzutillo

Naturally occurring variations of normal biological development have captivated human interest and imagination for centuries and have stimulated the search for their primary cause. In 1912, Klippel and Feil expressed their belief that each newly recognized variant should be reported in precise detail in the hope of discovery of clues that would yield greater insight into the process of human evolution. To that end, Klippel and Feil published the clinical and anatomic description of L. Joseph, a 46-year-old man with a past medical history of abdominal complaints, suggestive of appendicitis or ileitis, and recurrent bouts of pleural effusions in early adulthood (1). On December 13, 1911, L. Joseph presented with pleurisy, pulmonary congestion, and nephritis. Physical examination revealed an extremely short neck (Fig. 34.1) with a low hairline and marked limitation of neck motion. He expired 1 month later after the development of albuminuria, an enlarged heart, and tachycardia. Autopsy observations revealed a spinal column consisting of only 12 vertebrae. The four most cephalad vertebrae were combined in an ill-defined fusion mass with rudimentary ribs. The occipitocervical articulation was anomalous and allowed a single plane of motion in flexion and extension.

Klippel and Feil interpreted their findings as a congenital absence of the neck with ribs arising from the base of the skull as a "cervical thorax." The remainder of the spinal column displayed dorsal kyphosis and dorsolumbar scoliosis. These observations constitute the first detailed description of failure of segmentation of cervical vertebrae.

The oldest example of congenital fusion of the cervical spine was observed in an Egyptian mummy (circa 500 b.c.) and reported by Smith in 1908 (2,3). Herodotus wrote of an ancient race in western Libya, the Acephala, whose heads seemed to rest on their trunks because of the apparent absence of the neck. In the sixteenth century, Aldrovani

explained the existence of a similar "monstrosity" by stating that the individual's neck was absent. In 1743, Haller reported his observation of five cervical vertebrae in an anencephalic fetus (2,4). Three years later, Morgagni described an elderly man with occipitoatlantal and C2-3 fusions and a second anencephalic fetus with cervical anatomy similar to that noted in Haller's fetus (2). In 1850, Rokitansky reported congenital fusion from C2 to C7 in a 70-year-old tailor. Although the previous reports were based on autopsy dissections, the introduction of radiography allowed Sick to observe images of congenital fusion of the cervical spine and concomitant Sprengel's deformity in a live 4-year-old girl (2).

Feil's review of medical literature yielded thirteen related cases (5) that served as the basis for his classification of deformity. He defined Type I anomaly as mass fusion of multiple cervical and upper thoracic vertebrae, whereas fusion at one or two disc spaces defined Type II anomalies, and cervical fusion in combination with lower thoracic or lumbar vertebral fusion comprised Type III.

Early investigations of the Klippel-Feil syndrome were isolated to stillborn infants with multisystem congenital anomalies, anencephaly, iniencephaly, occipitalization of the atlas, vertebral fusions, hemivertebrae, and platyspondylia (2,6–10). Although occipital and cervical anomalies occur with increased frequency in individuals with the Klippel-Feil syndrome, it is the congenital failure of segmentation of cervical vertebrae that defines the syndrome (11). Klippel and Feil's index patient displayed not only failure of segmentation of the entire cervical axis but also impaired pulmonary and renal systems. The term Klippel-Feil syndrome refers to individuals with at least one level of failure of segmentation in the cervical spine (Fig. 34.2). The severity of anomalous involvement of the cervical spine or the presence of congenital anomalies of other organ systems do not impact on the appropriateness of the term Klippel-Feil syndrome.

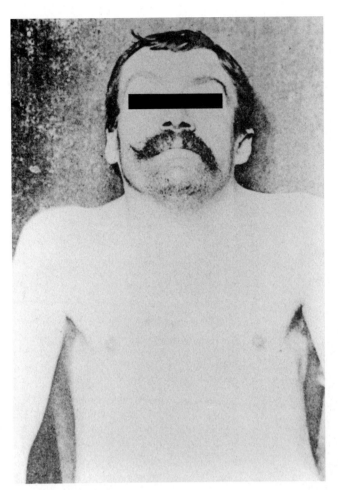

FIG. 34.1. Frontal photograph of L. Joseph.

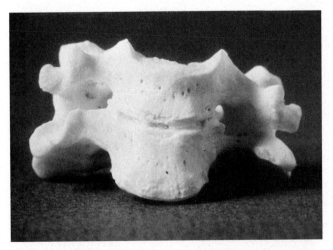

FIG. 34.2. Single-level congenital fusion of cervical vertebrae.

CLINICAL FINDINGS

The patient with Klippel-Feil syndrome may exhibit the "classic" triad of short neck, low hairline, and limited range of neck motion (Fig. 34.3) when the majority of cervical vertebrae are involved. This triad is observed in very few patients with Klippel-Feil syndrome; the majority of involved individuals have a normal appearance (2,12). The latter group is usually diagnosed through incidental radiographic findings or in the comprehensive evaluation of the patient with congenital scoliosis. When few vertebral segments are involved, clinical examination alone is not a reliable diagnostic tool.

The presence of torticollis or webbing of the neck, with or without facial asymmetry, increases the index of suspicion for the existence of cervical spine anomalies but are noted in only 20% of patients with Klippel-Feil syndrome (2,13–15). When torticollis is observed, it is important to define its etiology. Although patients with congenital muscular torticollis may be successfully treated by soft-tissue stretching or surgical release of contracted neck muscles in those who do not respond to stretching, the presence of congenital anomalies

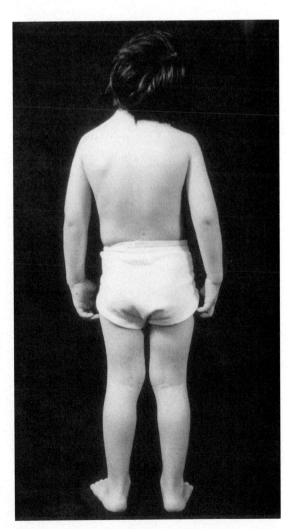

FIG. 34.3. The patient with Klippel-Feil syndrome exhibits a short neck and low posterior hairline.

of the upper cervical spine or occipitoatlantal junction may severely limit the results of stretching exercises or of soft-tissue surgical releases.

The most consistent clinical finding in individuals with segmentation defects of the cervical spine is limitation of neck motion. Flexion and extension of the neck may appear normal even in the presence of complex segmentation defects of the cervical spine. Hensinger and associates (14) reported patients with Klippel-Feil syndrome who demonstrated normal flexion and extension of the neck through

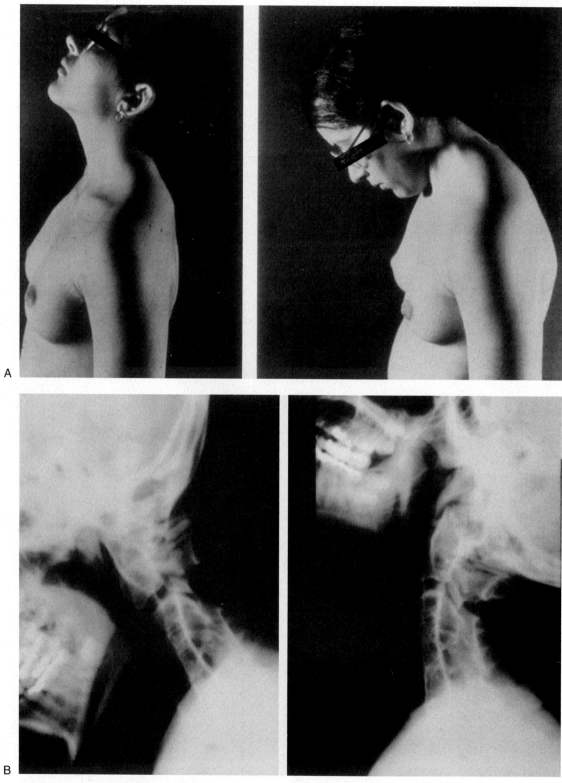

FIG. 34.4. Clinical photographs **(A)** and lateral flexion-extension radiographs **(B)** demonstrate apparent full flexion and extension through one open interspace.

one unfused subaxial interspace (Fig. 34.4). With increased segmental involvement of the cervical spine, lateral bending of the neck becomes substantially compromised. Limitation of sidebending of the neck appears to be the most sensitive clinical test for the presence of congenital anomalies of the cervical spine. The total absence of neck motion is rare and is associated with global involvement of the occipitoatlantal junction as well as the remainder of the cervical spinal axis.

Iniencephaly must be suspected in the presence of a low posterior hairline and fixed hyperextension of the neck (16). Iniencephaly involves malformation of the base of the occiput with exposed brain and spinal cord because of cervical rachischisis and failure of segmentation of the vertebral bodies. The cervical spine is typically positioned in hyperlordosis with compensatory cervicothoracic kyphosis. Posterior surgical approach to the cervical spine is treacherous because the dura is adherent to the skin and subcutaneous tissue.

RADIOLOGIC FINDINGS

Routine radiography, tomography, cineradiography, computed tomography (CT), and magnetic resonance imaging (MRI) have enhanced our understanding of congenital cervical anomalies in patients with Klippel-Feil syndrome. Initial radiographic evaluation of the cervical spine, including anteroposterior, anteroposterior open-mouth, and lateral flexion and extension views, aids in defining the extent of congenital involvement of the cervical spine, coexistent occipitalization of the atlas, stability of the atlantoaxial joint, congenital cervical stenosis, and subaxial stability.

Radiographic images of the cartilaginous cervical spine in the infant with Klippel-Feil syndrome initially may appear to be normal. Progressive ossification of vertebral elements gradually clarifies the congenital changes. With increasing bone maturity, radiographs reveal progressive obliteration of apparent disc spaces. Occasionally rudimentary disc spaces persist in the mature spine. Lateral flexion and extension radiographs of the cervical spine allow identification of segmentation defects in the partially ossified spine and are essential for the detection of intersegmental instability in the more mature spine (Fig. 34.5).

Failure of segmentation of the posterior elements of the spine heralds the presence of segmentation defects of anterior spinal elements in the child (Fig. 34.6) (14). Lateral radiographs of congenitally involved vertebrae reveal vertebral bodies that appear narrow in width when compared with adjacent normal vertebral bodies (17). When the anteroposterior radiographic view of the cervical spine suggests enlargement of the spinal canal, syringomyelia, hydromyelia, or Arnold-Chiari malformation must be considered (18). Although spina bifida occulta is common, complete spinal dysraphism is rare.

The presence of multiple levels of segmentation defects of the cervical spine, either alone or in combination with

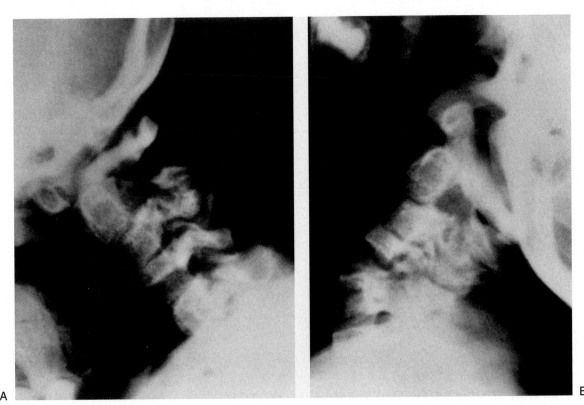

A   B

FIG. 34.5. Lateral flexion-extension radiographs are essential in diagnosing and monitoring intersegmental vertebral instability. **A:** Flexion. **B:** Extension.

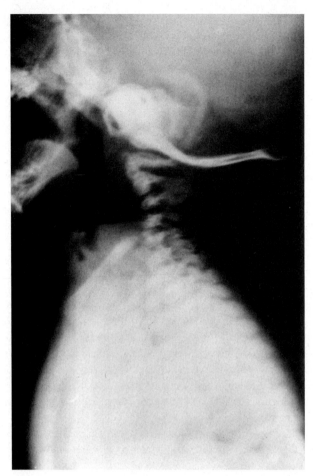

FIG. 34.6. Bony union of posterior elements of the spine may be seen at an early age and herald the existence of congenital fusion of the anterior spinal elements.

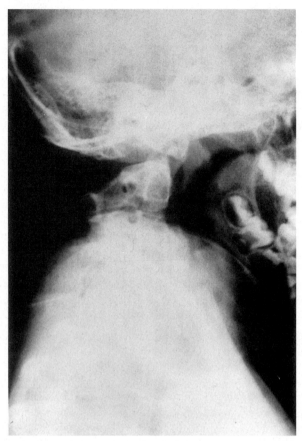

FIG. 34.7. Overlapping shadows from the mandible, occiput, or shoulder may preclude adequate evaluation of the cervical spine by routine radiography.

other congenital changes, such as hemivertebrae, may make the interpretation of routine radiographs confusing and difficult. Malrotation or tilting of the neck, in addition to overlapping shadows from the mandible, occiput, or shoulder, obscure the radiographic details of cervical spine anatomy (Fig. 34.7)(14). AP and lateral flexion/extension tomography of the cervical spine, as well as CT with three-dimensional reconstructions, clarify the anatomic detail of the cervical axis.

Cineradiography provides a dynamic technique that allows precise positioning of the head and neck to critically evaluate axial rotation, lateral bending, and flexion/extension of the cervical spine. Intersegmental instability of the cervical spine or instability of the occipitocervical junction are suggested by sudden translation of one vertebral segment on its adjacent vertebral level, sudden translation of the occiput on the cervical axis, or severe anterior gaping of subaxial disc with cervical extension. Mobility of the immature cervical spine must be evaluated cautiously and not be compared with that of the mature cervical spine. No standard exists for normal motion at the occipitoatlantal junction in children under the age of 10 years. Pseudosubluxation at

C2-3 or C3-4 is common in children less than 8 years of age (19).

CT myelography or MRI provides precise evaluation of anomalies of the brain stem and spinal cord as well as the effects of stenosis of the cervical canal. Ulmer and associates (20) employed CT myelography or MRI to evaluate the cervical spine of 24 patients, between 2 months and 69 years of age, who had radiographic evidence of Klippel-Feil syndrome. The investigators observed subaxial cervical spine degeneration in 10 patients, Chiari I malformation in two patients, mixed anomalies of the cord (dorsal cord cleft to diastematomyelia) in five patients, and normal brain and spinal cord in seven patients.

The evaluation of the cervical spine in patients with congenital anomalies of the thoracic or lumbar spine or with congenital rib deformities results in the identification of segmentation defects of the cervical spine in a substantial segment of this population (21).

EMBRYOLOGY

During the first 3 weeks of fetal life, development of the human blastema results in the formation of a neural tube. The neural tube lies dorsal to the notochord and is surrounded by mesenchymal condensations that differentiate and form a lateral column of somite segments on either side of the neural tube. Somatogenesis produces 44 pairs of mesodermal somites that contribute to the formation of the base of the skull and to the cervical, thoracic, lumbar, sacral, and coccygeal vertebrae. Although the most caudal somites undergo a process of cellular degeneration, the remaining somites differentiate further into an outer dermatome, an inner myotome, and a medial sclerotome (22). Each sclerotome develops a central cleft, the fissure of von Ebner, that separates a cranial collection of loosely packed cells from a caudal dense cellular mass. Cells from the fissure of von Ebner migrate to and around the notochord and act as the precursor of the intervertebral disc. As the cranial cell collection of a given sclerotome migrates and unites with the caudal dense cell mass of its adjacent sclerotome, the stage of resegmentation concludes (23).

Failure of segmentation of the cervical spine has been produced in laboratory animals with the use of teratogenic agents and induction of maternal hypotension. The etiology of segmentation defects of the cervical spine in humans has not yet been elucidated. Gardner (24) suggested that overdistention of the neural tube in the precartilaginous sclerotome stage may adversely influence notochord development and result in apparent congenital fusion. Failure of the development of the fissure of von Ebner prior to the stage of resegmentation (23) has also been offered as a theory. Maternal alcoholism has been suggested as a major factor in the production of segmentation defects of the cervical spine (25,26) but has little supporting data.

With the exception of a small number of families with single-level segmentation defects of the cervical spine, the genetic transmission of failure of segmentation of cervical vertebrae has not been observed in humans. Defects in the Notch signaling pathway including genes Notch 1, delta-like 1 (Dll 1), delta-like 3 (Dll 3), presenilin 1 (Psen 1), lunatic fringe (Lfng), recombining binding protein suppressor of hairless (Rbpsuh), mesoderm posterior 2 (Mesp 2), and mesogenin (Msgn 1) have been identified in the mouse (27) and human (28) with spondylocostal dysostosis. These individuals exhibit short stature, scoliosis, and hemivertebral defects but do not exhibit segmentation defects of the cervical spine that are characteristic of those associated with Klippel-Feil syndrome.

The Homeobox, or *Hox* genes are a family of genes that regulate the differentiation and segmentation of the embryonic axial skeleton and have been identified in *Drosophila melanogaster* and mammals. Because *Hox* genes may either activate or repress DNA sequences that affect the development of the axial skeleton, mutation of the *Hox* genes then may result in congenital anomalies of the axial skeleton.

The regulation of *Hox* gene expression has been extensively examined in the mouse model. Mice with targeted deletions of the *Hoxd-3* gene exhibit reduction in size of the atlas with areas of fusion of its anterior arch to the basioccipital bone. Double mutants of *Hoxd-3* with *Hoxa-3* show complete deletion of the atlas (29).

Clarke and associates (30) reported a family in which 71% of living family members demonstrated radiographic evidence of apparent fused cervical vertebrae. All affected members had a paracentric inversion on chromosome 8q and 90% of affected members had notable vocal impairment ranging from soft, hoarse voice quality to ineffective soft whisper. The findings in the members of this family may yield clues regarding the etiology of Klippel-Feil syndrome, but differ from prior reported individuals with Klippel-Feil syndrome who exhibited no evidence of vocal impairment.

NATURAL HISTORY

Individuals with Klippel-Feil syndrome infrequently develop neurologic impairment or intersegmental instability of the cervical spine. Nonspecific pain involving the neck, occiput, shoulders, or chest may develop but is not accompanied by neurologic deficits and is successfully managed with symptomatic treatment. The most common age of onset of symptoms is between the second and third decades of life (2,14). A review of the literature reveals more than 100 patients with the Klippel-Feil syndrome who have developed neurologic problems as a consequence of occipitocervical anomalies, late intersegmental instability, disc disease, or degenerative joint disease. The spectrum of reported problems includes cervical radiculopathy, spasticity, pain, quadriplegia, and sudden death (31–48). Two-thirds of neurologically compromised individuals had single level segmentation defects of the upper cervical spine, primarily involving the second and third cervical vertebrae. Individuals with normal upper cervical anatomy but varied patterns of segmentation defects of the subaxial cervical spine infrequently experienced neurologic loss. This suggests that force concentration at the occipitoatlantal junction or at the atlantoaxial junction may result in instability at those levels with subsequent neural compromise.

Lateral flexion and extension radiographs of the cervical spine in individuals with Klippel-Feil syndrome were kinematically evaluated and compared with established standards for range of motion of vertebral segments by Pizzutillo and associates (49). The cervical spine was divided into upper and lower segments using MacGregor's line and the inferior borders of the vertebral bodies at C2 and C7. Using lateral flexion and extension radiographs, the total arc of motion of each segment as well as the motion per unfused interspace in both the upper and lower segments were calculated. When compared to controls, 20 degrees of motion per unfused disc space proved to be one standard deviation greater than the mean for normal populations. On this basis, pathologic hypermobility was defined as more than 20 degrees of motion per unfused disc space. Using this standard, the lateral flexion and extension radiographs of 100 individuals with Klippel-Feil syndrome were evaluated. After evaluation of patients and radiographic studies, the authors concluded that neurologic deficits develop in individuals with basilar impression, iniencephaly, or hypermobility at the upper segment. Hypermobility of the lower segment did not correlate with the development of neural deficits but did correlate with the development of degenerative disc disease. Within the study group, one-third were considered at risk for neurologic impairment and one-third were at risk for development of degenerative changes of the subaxial spine (49).

ASSOCIATED PROBLEMS

Cross-sectional studies of the 28- to 30-day human embryo reveal marked proximity of the lower cervical somites to the paired dorsal aorta, pronephric ducts, upper limb buds, and developing mesonephros (22,50). Insult to the embryo at this stage could affect the developing cervical spine, its contiguous neural structures and nearby developing organ systems with the potential for major clinical consequences. Numerous medical reports have confirmed the association of multisystem congenital anomalies with segmentation defects of the cervical spine (14,40). Facial development has been affected with cleft lip, cleft palate, high-arched palate, coloboma, ptosis, Duane contracture of the lateral rectus muscle, lateral rectus palsy, and facial nerve palsy (44,51–55).

Jalladeau reported a 30% prevalence of deafness in 20 patients with Klippel-Feil syndrome (56). Wildervanck later associated deafness with Klippel-Feil syndrome, abducens nerve palsy, and retraction of the eyeball (cervicooculoacoustic syndrome) (23). Deafness may be the result of ankylosis of the ossicles, footplate fixation, absent external auditory canal, or sensorineural deficit (2,46,57–61). Audiometric evaluation of the young patient with Klippel-Feil syndrome is indicated to detect hearing deficits, facilitate language development, and avoid impediments in the educational process.

Stapedectomy is a common surgical treatment for stapes footplate fixation; however, stapes gusher is a serious complication of the procedure and arises from a congenital anomaly linking the subarachnoid and perilymphatic spaces. When the stapes footplate is drilled, a sudden and profuse flow of cerebrospinal fluid (CSF) occurs that causes immediate deafness and requires fascial graft for definitive control. Danilides and associates reported the result of 650 stapedectomy procedures and noted two cases of stapes gusher, one of which occurred in a patient with Klippel-Feil syndrome. Two other patients have been reported with Klippel-Feil syndrome and subarachnoid tympanic fistula who experienced recurrent meningitis (21,57).

The association of cardiovascular anomalies with Klippel-Feil syndrome has been well established. Gray observed 13 of 418 individuals with Klippel-Feil syndrome with congenital anomalies of the cardiovascular system, whereas Nora reported cardiovascular anomalies in five of eight patients with Klippel-Feil syndrome (2,62). Ventricular septal defect, alone or in combination with other defects, is the most frequently occurring cardiac anomaly. In addition,

mitral insufficiency, coarctation of the aorta, right-sided aorta, patent ductus arteriosus, pulmonic stenosis, dextrocardia, atrial septal defect, truncus arteriosus, aplasia of the parietal pericardium, patent foramen ovale, single atrium, single ventricle, and bicuspid pulmonic valve have been reported in association with Klippel-Feil syndrome (2,51, 60–65). Pulmonary anomalies have also been reported in patients with Klippel-Feil syndrome and include failure of lobe formation, ectopic lung, or "restrictive chest cage disease" resulting from shortened trunk, scoliosis, rib absence, rib fusions, and deformation of the costovertebral joints (66,67).

Individuals with Klippel-Feil syndrome may exhibit anomalies of the central nervous system with malformation of the brain stem, disturbance of CSF dynamics, or bony impingement on the brain stem that may alter respiration (68). The coexistence of central nervous system anomalies may render the individual with Klippel-Feil syndrome more susceptible to neural or neurovascular injury as the result of surgical interventions at the cervical spine or in the surgical treatment of scoliosis.

Synkinesia, or mirror motions, may be observed in normal children under the age of 5 years and in 20% of individuals with Klippel-Feil syndrome (14,69). Synkinesia is a disorder of motor control in which the voluntary motion of one limb is involuntarily mirrored by the same part of the opposite limb. Although mirror motions have been reported in both upper and lower extremities, it is more frequent in the upper extremity and more predictably elicited on examination by testing discrete finger motions rather than gross arm motions. Mirror motions are usually less distinct and weaker than the corresponding voluntary motions of the opposite limb (24,64).

Although synkinesia may be pronounced and hamper bimanual activities in the younger child, it becomes muted with advancing age and is infrequently elicitable after the second decade of life. Occupational therapy may be helpful in promoting improved bimanual dexterity in the young child with synkinesia. Mirror motions in individuals with cerebral palsy, basilar impression, occipitalization of the atlas, and hemiparkinsonism tend to persist.

The association of synkinesia and Klippel-Feil syndrome was first reported by Bauman in 1932. Avery and Rentfro (70) and Gunderson and Solitare (71) published the autopsy reports of two individuals with Klippel-Feil syndrome and noted incomplete decussation of the pyramidal tracts in the upper cervical cord with no osseous compromise of the neural structures. Gunderson and Solitare suggest that incomplete decussation of the pyramidal tracts requires alternate and less specific extrapyramidal pathways to control motion of the upper limbs. The repetitive use of secondary pathways could explain the diminished quality of mirror motions over time. Electromyographic evaluation of limbs in individuals with Klippel-Feil syndrome reveals electrical activity consistent with synkinesia that persists even in those in whom observable mirror motion can no longer be elicited (24,72,73). The neurophysiologic mechanism of synkinesia is unknown.

The urogenital system originates from the pronephric ducts that form from mesoderm in proximity to cervical somites. At 28 to 30 days of embryologic life, the pronephric ducts induce the formation of the mesonephros and ureteral buds that develop into the renal system. At 44 to 48 days, the pronephric ducts induce müllerian duct formation, which gives rise to the ovaries, fallopian tubes, uterus, and vagina. An insult to the embryo between the fourth and eighth week of life could result in failure of resegmentation of cervical somites and significant anomalies of the urogenital system. Urogenital anomalies have been observed in 30% of patients with Klippel-Feil syndrome; the most common expression is unilateral absence of the kidney (14,74,75). Other anomalies include absence of the hemitrigone, absence of both kidneys, absence of the ureter, hydronephrosis, ectopic kidney, horseshoe kidney, and congenital fusion of renal pelves in two distinct kidneys (21,50,76,77). Anomalies of the male genitalia include dysplastic and undescended testes. Genital anomalies most frequently occur in females and include absent vagina, duplication of the uterus, absent or rudimentary uterus, unilateral agenesis of the uterus, absent fallopian tube, and ovarian agenesis (50,78–80). Duncan reported that 14 of 167 female patients (8%) with normal cervical spine anatomy exhibited unilateral absence of the kidney and unilateral or total absence of the uterus. He further noted that nine of 10 of female patients (90%) with Klippel-Feil syndrome had unilateral absence of the kidneys and absent uterus (50). The high prevalence of both uterine and renal agenesis in individuals with Klippel-Feil syndrome emphasizes the possibility of a single insult to the embryologic cervical somites and adjacent pronephric ducts as the likely cause for development of the observed anomalies. The group of patients reported by Duncan also demonstrated concomitant Sprengel's deformity, deafness, and anomalies of the upper extremity.

The high prevalence of renal anomalies in individuals with Klippel-Feil syndrome indicates the necessity for ultrasonic imaging of the renal system. If structural or positional abnormalities are noted, intravenous pyelography provides more information for complete evaluation. If unilateral renal agenesis is documented in a female patient, ultrasonic evaluation of the ovaries, fallopian tubes, and uterus is indicated to confirm their status.

Congenital anomalies of the upper extremity that include syndactyly, hypoplasia of the thumb, absent thumb, hypoplasia of the thenar eminence, supernumerary digits, absent ulna, and Sprengel's deformity have been observed in 20% of individuals with Klippel-Feil syndrome (9,12,14,45,46, 48,61,70,81). Sprengel's deformity is the result of failure of descent of the scapula from the embryologic cervical level to its normal position caudal to the first rib. It may be unilateral or bilateral and usually presents a cosmetic rather than functional problem. At 31 days of life, the embryologic scapula is located at the C4 level and slowly descends to a level caudal to the first rib by 42 days of life (17). The time of descent of the scapula coincides with the critical period of cervical somite resegmentation and a single insult to the embryo during this time could result in anomalies of the cervical spine as well as the Sprengel deformity.

Scoliosis, either alone or in combination with kyphosis, has been noted in more than half of reported patients with Klippel-Feil syndrome (2,14,74,75). Congenital anomalies may involve any level of the thoracic and lumbar spine. Orthoses may influence compensatory spinal curvatures in segments that are anatomically normal but have no effect on anomalous segments. Many patients exhibit progressive scoliosis that requires surgical stabilization (12). When surgical intervention is indicated, the concern for neurologic compromise and malalignment that exists in the treatment of congenital scoliosis is compounded by the presence of structural cervical anomalies and potential instability at the occipitocervical or atlantoaxial junctions. Furthermore, the use of spinal instrumentation must be critically analyzed to avoid neurologic compromise, truncal decompensation, or sagittal plane imbalance.

TREATMENT

The complex nature of cervical spine anomalies in conjunction with concomitant anomalies of the remainder of the spine and other organ systems requires a comprehensive evaluation of each patient with continued serial evaluation throughout growth. Physical examination of involved individuals includes the musculoskeletal system in addition to detailed neurologic assessment. Radiographic evaluation of the cervical spine details the nature and severity of anomalous development. Lateral flexion and extension radiographs of the cervical spine document the degree of stability at the occipitocervical and atlantoaxial junctions as well as at open disc spaces between congenitally fused segments. Serial radiographic evaluation of the cervical spine (e.g., every 3 to 5 years) is indicated in the immature individual to rule out developing instability. This is especially important in those with congenital anomalies of the upper cervical spine. Radiographic evaluation of the remainder of the spine is recommended to rule out the existence of congenital anomalies of the thoracic and lumbar spine and to document the degree of existing scoliosis.

The frequent association of nonskeletal anomalies in individuals with Klippel-Feil syndrome suggests the need for comprehensive evaluation of this patient population. Cardiac evaluation, renal ultrasound, or intravenous pyelography, and audiometric evaluation are indicated to rule out the existence of frequently occurring associated anomalies.

Lateral flexion and extension radiographs of the cervical spine aid in defining anatomy and determining the presence and degree of cervical stability. Individuals with no radiographic evidence of basilar impression or iniencephaly and with normal kinematics of the cervical spine have no known increased risk for the development of neurologic compromise or degeneration. Individuals with basilar impression, iniencephaly, or hypermobility of the upper cervical segment do have an increased risk for the development of neurologic compromise. This population requires annual clinical evaluation of cervical instability and neurologic status and should avoid involvement in high impact loading of the neck, such as collision sports. When instability at the occipitocervical or atlantoaxial junction develops and results in neurologic compromise, surgical stabilization is indicated to prevent increased neurologic damage and foster neurologic recovery. Posterior cervical arthrodesis is the most common surgical intervention in these patients and frequently includes the occipitocervical level.

Patients with Klippel-Feil syndrome who demonstrate hypermobility of the subaxial cervical spine are not at significant risk for the development of instability or neurologic compromise but do have an increased risk for degenerative changes. Diminished motion is noted in the lower cervical segment with progression of degenerative disc disease. Pain that occurs in association with degenerative disease is most commonly managed by symptomatic nonsurgical interventions. Occasionally, degenerative changes in conjunction with congenital stenosis of the cervical canal may result in myelopathy and require surgical decompression of the canal and surgical stabilization (49). Surgical interventions involving the cervical spine in patients with Klippel-Feil syndrome primarily are directed at decompression of stenotic spinal canal segments and stabilization of intersegmental instability. Surgical resection of ribs to improve cosmesis and realignment osteotomy of the cervical spine pose substantial risks to the patient and may result in neurologic catastrophe (4). Bracing of the neck to improve alignment has been universally ineffective.

SUMMARY

Patients with Klippel-Feil syndrome exhibit failure of segmentation of cervical elements with apparent congenital fusion of vertebrae. Anomalous involvement of the upper cervical segment or the presence of basilar impression, iniencephaly or occipitalization of the atlas suggest a substantial risk for the development of neural compromise. Congenital fusion involving subaxial cervical spine elements do not share in the high risk for development of neurologic compromise but does suggest substantial risk for the development of degenerative changes. Instability of the upper cervical segment is not common but when present is an indication for surgical stabilization. Bracing of neck deformity is ineffective and resection of upper ribs for improved cosmesis in not indicated.

Coexisting skeletal anomalies include scoliosis, Sprengel deformity, and hypoplasia or absence of the thumb. Scoliosis in association with Klippel-Feil syndrome is most commonly congenital and progressive, and frequently requires surgical intervention. Sprengel deformity may be cosmetically displeasing but does not commonly interfere with functional motion of the shoulder. When shoulder motion is compromised, surgical realignment of the scapula with excision of an omovertebral connection restores functional shoulder motion. Thumb hypoplasia usually does not require treatment; however, absence of the thumb may be treated with pollicization of the index finger.

Frequently occurring anomalies involving nonskeletal systems include deafness as well as urogenital and cardiovascular anomalies. Comprehensive evaluation is indicated to determine the existence of associated anomalies and allow effective treatment interventions.

REFERENCES

1. Klippel M, Feil A. Un cas d'absence des vertebras cervicales avec cage thoracique remontant jusqu'a base du craine. *Nouv Icon Salpetriere* 1912;25:223.
2. Gray SW, Romaine CB, Skandalakis JE. Congenital fusion of the cervical vertebrae. *Surg Gynecol Obstet* 1964;118:373.
3. Turner EL, Shoulders HS, Scott LD. Klippel-Feil syndrome with unusual clinical manifestations. *Am J Roentgenol Rad Ther* 1938;40:43.
4. Bonola A. Surgical treatment of the Klippel-Feil syndrome. *J Bone Joint Surg Br* 1956;38:440.
5. Feil A. *L'absence et la diminution des vertebras cervicales (etude clinique et pathogenique): le syndrome de reduction numerique cervicale.* Theses de Paris, 1919.
6. Bauman GI. Absence of the cervical spine: Klippel-Feil syndrome. *JAMA* 1932;98:129.
7. Bertolotti M. Le anomalie congenite del rachide cervicale. *Chirurgia Degli Organi di Movimento* 1920; 4:395.
8. Bertolotti M. Gli uomini senza collo (Aplasia e fusione del rachide cervicale con spina bifida). *Minerva Med* 1950;41:481.
9. Critchley M. Sprengel's deformity with paraplegia. *Br J Surg* 1926–1927;14:243.
10. Dikshit SK, Agarwal SP, Gupta RC, et al. Klippel-Feil syndrome. *Ind J Pediatr* 1969;36:245.
11. Von Torklus D, Gehle W. *The upper cervical spine.* New York: Grune & Stratton, 1972:38–43.
12. Gunderson CH, Greenspan RH, Glaser GH, et al. Klippel-Feil syndrome: genetic and clinical reevaluation of cervical fusion. *Medicine* 1967;46:491.
13. Frawley JM. Congenital webbing. *Am J Dis Child* 1925;29:799.
14. Hensinger RN, Lang JR, MacEwen GD. Klippel-Feil syndrome: a constellation of associated anomalies. *J Bone Joint Surg* 1974;56A:1246.
15. Stark EW, Borton TE. Hearing loss in the Klippel-Feil syndrome. *Am J Dis Child* 1972;123:233.
16. Sherk HH, Nicholson JT. Cervico-oculo-acusticus syndrome. *J Bone Joint Surg* 1972;54A:1776.
17. Dolan KD. Developmental abnormalities of the cervical spine below the axis. *Radiol Clin North Am* 1977;15:167.
18. Dolan KD. Expanding lesions of the cervical canal. *Radiol Clin North Am* 1977;15:203.
19. Cattell HS, Filtzer DL. Pseudosubluxation and other normal variations in the cervical spine in children. *J Bone Joint Surg Am* 1965;47:1295.
20. Ulmer JL, Elster AD, Ginsberg LE, et al. Klippel-Feil syndrome. CT and MR of acquired and congenital abnormalities of cervical spine and cord. *J Comput Assist Tomogr* 1993;17:215–24.
21. Richards SH, Gibbin KP. Recurrent meningitis due to congenital fistula of stapedial foot plate. *J Laryngol* 1977;91:1063.
22. Arey LB. *Developmental anatomy: a textbook and laboratory manual of embryology,* 7th ed. Philadelphia: WB Saunders, 1965:404–407.
23. Wildervanck LS. Klippel-Feil syndrome associated with abducens paralysis, bulbar retraction, and deaf mutism: case. *Ned Tijdschr Geneeskd* 1952;96:27–52.
24. Gardner WJ. Klippel-Feil syndrome, iniencephalus, anencephalus, hind-brain hernia, and mirror movements. Overdistention of the neural tube. *Child's Brain* 1979;5:361.

25. Lowry RB. The Klippel-Feil anomalad as part of the fetal alcohol syndrome. *Teratology* 1977;16:53.
26. Neidengard L, Carter TE. Klippel-Feil malformation complex in fetal alcohol syndrome. *Am J Dis Child* 1978;132:929.
27. Saga Y, Takeda H. The making of the somite: molecular events in vertebrate segmentation. *Nature* 2001;2:835.
28. Bulman, MP, Kusumi K, Frayling TM, et al. Mutations in the human delta homologue, DLLE, cause axial skeletal defects in spondylocostal dysostosis. *Nat Genet* 2000;24:438.
29. Condle BR, Capecchi MR. Mice with targeted disruptions in the paralogous genes hoax-3 and hoxd-3 reveal synergistic interactions. *Nature* 1994;370:304–307.
30. Clarke RA, Kearsley JH, Walsh DA. Patterned expression in familial Klippel-Feil syndrome. *Teratology* 1996;53:152–157.
31. Bucy PC, Ritchey H. Klippel-Feil's syndrome associated with compression of the spinal cord by an extradural hemangiolipoma. *J Neurosurg* 1947;4:476.
32. DuToit F. A case of congenital elevation of the scapula (Sprengel's deformity) with defect of the cervical spine associated with syringomyelia. *Brain* 1931;54:421.
33. Epstein JA, Carras R, Epstein BS, et al. Myelopathy and cervical spondylosis with vertebral subluxation and hyperlordosis. *J Neurosurg* 1970;32:421.
34. Giannini V, Paterno M. Sindromi neurologiche associate o complicanti il morbo di Klippel-Feil. *G Psichiat Neuropat* 1960;88:955.
35. Illingsworth RS. Attacks of unconsciousness in association with a fused cervical vertebra. *Arch Dis Child* 1956;31:8
36. Kirkham TH. Cervico-oculo acusticus syndrome with pseudopapilledema. *Arch Dis Child* 1969;44:504.
37. Lee ZK, Weiss AB. Isolated congenital cervical lock vertebrae below the axis with neurological symptoms. *Spine* 1981;6:118.
38. List CF. Neurologic syndromes accompanying developmental anomalies of occipital bone, atlas and axis. *Arch Neurol Psychiatr* 1941;45:577.
39. Michie I, Clark M. Neurological syndromes associated with cervical and craniocervical anomalies. *Arch Neurol* 1968;18:241.
40. Mosberg WH Jr. Klippel-Feil syndrome. Etiology and treatment of neurologic signs. *J Nerv Ment Dis* 1953;117:479.
41. Peters JJ. Two cases of Klippel-Feil syndrome associated with severe mental subnormality. *Radiography* 1962;28:316.
42. Rinvik R. A case of the Klippel-Feil syndrome. *Acta Paediatr Iatr* 1944;31:417.
43. Sava GM, Dohn DF, Rothner AD. Anterior decompression for progressive brainstem compression in the Klippel-Feil syndrome. *Cleve Clin Q* 1978-1979;45:325.
44. Sherk HH, Dawoud S. Congenital os odontoideum with Klippel-Feil anomaly and fetal atlantoaxial instability: a report of a case. *Spine* 1981;6:42.
45. Sherk HH, Shut L, Chung S. Iniencephalic deformity of the cervical spine with Klippel-Feil anomalies and congenital elevation of the scapula. *J Bone Joint Surg* 1974;56A:1254.
46. Smith GE. Significance of fusion of the atlas to the occipital bone and manifestations of occipital vertebrae. *BMJ* 1908;2:594.
47. Southwell RD, Reynolds AF, Badger VM, et al. Klippel-Feil syndrome with cervical cord compression resulting from cervical subluxation in association with an omovertebral bone. *Spine* 1980;5:480.
48. Strakx TE, Baran E. Traumatic quadriplegia associated with Klippel-Feil syndrome: discussion and case reports. *Arch Phys Med Rehabil* 1975;56:363.
49. Pizzutillo PD, Woods M, Nicholson MS, et al. Risk factors in Klippel-Feil syndrome. *Spine* 1994;19:2110–2116.
50. Duncan PA. Embryologic pathogenesis of renal agenesis associated with cervical vertebral anomalies (Klippel-Feil phenotype). *Birth Defects* 1977;8:91.
51. Awan KJ. Association of ocular, cervical, and cardiac malformations. *Ann Ophthamol* 1977;9:1001.
52. Brik M , Athayde A. Bilateral Duane's syndrome, paroxysmal lacrimation and Klippel-Feil anomaly. *Ophthalmologica* 1973;167:1.
53. Cooper JC. Klippel-Feil syndrome: a rare cause of cervico-fascial deformity. *Br Dent J* 1976;140:264.
54. Kauffman RL, McAllister WH, Ho C, et al. Familial studies in congenital heart disease. *Birth Defects* 1973;8:82.
55. Thomson J. A case of the Klippel-Feil syndrome. *Arch Dis Child* 1937;12:127.

56. Jalladeau J. *Malformations congenitales associees au syndrome de Klippel-Feil.* Theses de Paris, 1936.
57. Danilides J, Maganaris T, Dimitriadis A, et al. Stapes gusher and Klippel-Feil syndrome. *Laryngoscope* 1978;88:1178.
58. Jarvis JF, Sellars SL. Klippel-Feil deformity associated with congenital, conductive deafness. *J Laryngol Otol* 1979;88:285.
59. McLay K, Maran AGD. Deafness and the Klippel-Feil syndrome. *J Laryngol* 1969;83:175.
60. Palant DI, Carter BL. Klippel-Feil syndrome and deafness. *Am J Dis Child* 1972;123:218.
61. Shoul MI, Ritvo MP. Clinical and roentgenologic manifestations of the Klippel-Feil syndrome (congenital fusion of the cervical vertebrae, brevicollis): report of eight additional cases and review of the literature. *AJR* 1952;68:369.
62. Nora JJ, Cohen M, Maxwell GM. Klippel-Feil syndrome with congenital heart disease. *Am J Dis Child* 1961;102:858.
63. Falk RH, MacKinnon J. Klippel-Feil syndrome associated with aortic coarctation. *Br Heart J* 1976;38:1220.
64. Ford FR. *Diseases of the nervous system in infancy, childhood and adolescence,* 5th ed. Springfield, IL: Charles C Thomas, 1966:167–170.
65. Morrison SG, Perry LW, Scott LP. Congenital brevicollis (Klippel-Feil syndrome) and cardiovascular anomalies. *Am J Dis Child* 1968;115:614.
66. Baga N, Chusid EL, Miller A. Pulmonary disability in the Klippel-Feil syndrome. *Clin Orthop* 1969;67:105.
67. Chaurasia BD, Singh MP. Ectopic lungs in a human fetus with Klippel-Feil syndrome. *Anat Anz* 1977;142:205.
68. Krieger AJ, Rosomoff HL, Kuperman AS, et al. Occult respiratory dysfunction in a cranovertebral anomaly. *J Neurosurg* 1969;31:15.
69. Erskine CA. An analysis of the Klippel-Feil syndrome. *Arch Pathol* 1946;41:269.
70. Avery LW, Rentfro CC. The Klippel-Feil syndrome: a pathologic report. *Arch Neurol Psychol* 1936;36,1068.
71. Gunderson CH, Solitare BH. Mirror movements in patients with the Klippel-Feil syndrome: neuropathic observations. *Arch Neurol* 1968;18:675.
72. Baird PA, Robinson CG, Buckler WSJ. Klippel-Feil syndrome: a study of mirror movement detected by electromyography. *Am J Dis Child* 1967;113:546.
73. Notermans SLH, Go KG, Boonstra S. EMG studies of associated movements in a patient with Klippel-Feil syndrome. *Psychiatr Neurol Neurochir* 1970;73:257.
74. MacEwen GD, Winter RB, Hardy JH. Evaluation of kidney anomalies in congenital scoliosis. *J Bone Joint Surg* 1972;54A:1451.
75. Moore WB, Matthews TJ, Rabinowitz R. Genitourinary anomalies associated with Klippel-Feil syndrome. *J Bone Joint Surg* 1975;57A:355.
76. Duncan PA, Shapiro LR, Stangel JJ, et al. The Mircs Association: müllerian duct aplasia, renal aplasia, and cervico-thoracic somite dysplasia. *J Pediatr* 1979;95:399.
77. Ramsey J, Bliznak J. Klippel-Feil syndrome with renal agenesis and other anomalies. *Am J Roentgenol* 1971;113:460.
78. Baird PA, Lowry RB. Absent vagina and the Klippel-Feil anomaly. *Am J Obstet Gynecol* 1974;118:290.
79. Mecklenburg RS, Krueger PM. Extensive genitourinary anomalies associated with Klippel-Feil syndrome. *Am J Dis Child* 1974;128:92.
80. Park IJ, Jones HW Jr. A new syndrome in two unrelated females: Klippel-Feil deformity, conductive deafness and absent vagina. *Birth Defects* 1971;311.
81. Chemke J, Nisani R, Fischel RE. Absent ulna in the Klippel-Feil syndrome: an unusual associated malformation. *Clin Genet* 1980;17:167.

SUGGESTED READINGS

Albright JA, Brand RA. *The scientific basis of orthopaedics.* New York: Appleton-Century-Crofts, 1979:51–58.
Born CT, Petrik M, Freed M, et al. Cerebrovascular accident complication Klippel-Feil syndrome. *J Bone Joint Surg* 1988;70A:1412–1415.
Brown MW, Templeton AW, Hodges FJ III. The incidence of acquired and congenital fusion in the cervical spine. *AJR* 1964;92:1255.
Eisemann ML, Sharma GK. Wildervanck syndrome: cervico-occulo-acoustic dysplasia. *Otolaryngol Head Neck Surg* 1979;87:892.

Forney WR, Robinson SJ, Pascoe DJ. Congenital heart disease, deafness, and skeletal malformations: a new syndrome. *J Pediatr* 1966;68:14.

Gehring GG, Shenasky JH. Crossed fusion of renal pelves and Klippel-Feil syndrome. *J Urol* 1976;116:103.

Gupta M, Singh RN. The Klippel-Feil syndrome: a case report. *Ind Pediatr* 1978;15:437.

Juberg RC, Gershanik JJ. Cervical vertebral fusion (Klippel-Feil) syndrome with consanguineous parents. *Med Genet* 1976;13:246.

Ross CA, Curnes JT, Greenwood RS. Recurrent vertebrobasilar embolism in an infant with Klippel-Feil syndrome. *Pediatr Neurol* 1987;3:181–183.

Singh SP, Rock EH, Shulman A. Klippel-Feil syndrome with unexplained apparent conductive hearing loss. A case report. *Laryngoscope* 1969;79:113.

Zook EG, Salmon JH. Anomalies of the cervical spine in the cleft-palate patient: an operative danger. *Plast Reconstr Surg* 1977;60:96.

CHAPTER 35

The Cervical Spine in Skeletal Dysplasia

William G. Mackenzie, Suken A. Shah, and Masakazu Takemitsu

Cervical spine disorders in skeletal dysplasia patients are very common. The wide spectrum of pathology is not clearly described in the sparse literature on these disorders. Careful evaluation of the cervical spine in each individual, with attention to the most typical abnormality, results in safe and effective care.

For example, foramen magnum stenosis is present commonly in neonates with achondroplasia, but seen rarely in other disorders. The stenosis can be severe, resulting in upper cervical cord compression with hypotonia, quadriparesis, and apnea. Other pathologic features in the development of the cranium, nasopharynx, and chest wall can aggravate the respiratory abnormalities and result in significant morbidity. Upper cervical spine instability is rare in achondroplasia but common in other forms of skeletal dysplasia, such as spondyloepiphyseal dysplasia and its variants, pseudoachondroplasia, metatropic dysplasia, Morquio syndrome, and metaphyseal chondrodysplasias. Many of these disorders have osseous abnormalities, such as odontoid hypoplasia or aplasia and os odontoideum as well as nonosseous abnormalities such as ligamentous hyperlaxity or soft-tissue deposits. Upper cervical stenosis may be dynamic owing to instability or stable owing to a congenital abnormality or fixed translation. Rotatory fixation is uncommon. Children with metatropic dysplasia can develop severe cervical deformity after surgical decompression without fusion and inadequate immobilization.

Subaxial cervical spine disorders include kyphosis, stenosis, and instability. Kyphosis is seen in children with diastrophic dysplasia, camptomelic dysplasia, and Larsen's syndrome. The kyphosis in diastrophic dysplasia can have associated spina bifida, an important factor when planning operative management. Kyphosis can develop after a laminectomy without fusion.

The following section reviews the cervical spine disorders in the various skeletal dysplasias and is summarized in Table 35.1.

ACHONDROPLASIA

Craniocervical stenosis secondary to a narrow foramen magnum and upper cervical stenosis is seen in 60% or more of children with achondroplasia (Fig. 35.1) (1). The foramen magnum is smaller than normal at all ages and this does not correlate with the circumference size of head (2). One-third of patients with craniocervical stenosis have symptoms of cord compression. Symptoms including apnea, hypotonia and quadriparesis can progress and be lethal (2), but may be alleviated with suboccipital decompression. In a report by Wang and associates (3), patients who required suboccipital decompression had foramen magnum measurements of less than 20 mm in the sagittal diameter, 15 mm in the coronal diameter, and a cross-sectional area of 239 mm². The reported cross-sectional area is approximately one-half of the normal controls. The rate of foramen magnum growth is impaired during the first year of life (4). The prevalence of sudden death in children with achondroplasia under 1 year of age is markedly higher than children in the general population (5). Assessment of the child should include a careful neurologic examination during infancy, a sleep study, computed tomography (CT) (6), and magnetic resonance imaging (MRI) (7). Short-latency somatosensory evoked potentials are described as useful for neurologic evaluation (1,8).

Surgical decompression is effective for symptomatic patients (1,6,9). In addition to the bony procedure, duraplasty is often required for adequate decompression in some patients who have fibrous constriction band. The patients have

TABLE 35.1.

Diagnosis of skeletal dysplasia	Cervical problems
Achondroplasia	Craniocervical stenosis (1–7) Developmental cervical subaxial stenosis (12)
Spondyloepiphyseal dysplasia	Atlantoaxial instability due to odontoid hypoplasia or os odontoideum and ligamentous laxity (13–17)
Spondylometaphyseal dysplasia	Atlantoaxial instability due to odontoid hypoplasia and ligamentous laxity (18)
Pseudoachondroplasia	Atlantoaxial instability due to odontoid hypoplasia and ligamentous laxity (14)
Kniest's dysplasia	Atlantoaxial or occipitoatlantal instability (18–2)
Metaphyseal chondrodysplasia	Atlantoaxial instability due to ligamentous laxity (21,22)
Metatropic dysplasia	Atlantoaxial instability due to odontoid hypoplasia or lateral mass defect of C2 (23,24)
Chondrodysplasia punctata	Atlantoaxial instability due to os odontoideum (Conradi-Hunermann type) (22) Coronal clefts or hypoplasia of the vertebral bodies (26) Subaxial canal stenosis (Rhizomelic type) (25)
Diastrophic dysplasia	Kyphosis due to hypoplasia of vertebral bodies, hypotonia and/or spina bifida (28,29) Atlantoaxial instability due to dysmorphism of the odontoid process (30)
Camptomelic dysplasia	Excessive lordosis and/or kyphosis (33,34)
Mucopolysaccharidosis	
Type 1-Hurler's syndrome	Odontoid dysplasia (36) Abnormal soft tissue formation around the tip of the odontoid (36,37)
Type 2-Hunter's syndrome	Cervical canal stenosis with thickening of the soft tissue (dura) posterior to the odontoid (38,39)
Type 4-Morquio's syndrome	Atlantoaxial instability due to odontoid hypoplasia or os odontoideum with soft tissue thickening (40–47)
Oculoauricular vertebral dysplasia	Atlantoaxial instability due to odontoid hypoplasia Occipital-C1 instability Occipitalization of C1 Failure of segmentation or formation of vertebrae (48)
Osteopathin striata	Kyphosis due to dysplasia and hypotonia (49)
Pyknodysostosis	Kyphosis due to C2 and/or C3 spondylolysis (50,5)
Thanatophoric dysplasia	Platyspondyly Atlantoaxial instability due to odontoid hypoplasia (52)
Multiple epiphyseal dysplasia	Atlantoaxial instability due to os odontoideum (53)
Osteopetrosis	Spondylolysis (54)
Osteopoikilosis	Canal stenosis (55)
Cleidocranial dysostosis	Basilar impression with enlarged foramen magnum (56)
Spondyloepimetaphyseal dysplasia	Atlantoaxial instability due to odontoid hypoplasia and ligamentous laxity (57)

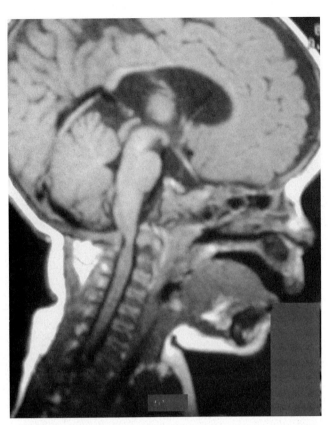

FIG. 35.1. Foramen magnum stenosis in a child with achondroplasia. The small sagittal diameter of the foramen magnum and spinal cord kinking are demonstrated on magnetic resonance imaging. Hydrocephalus is highly associated with the foramen magnum stenosis.

abnormal cerebrospinal fluid (CSF) dynamics and postoperative CSF leaks are common (9).

There are a few case reports of cervical instability in patients with achondroplasia, but this is a rare finding (10,11).

Developmental subaxial cervical stenosis can occur in adults with achondroplasia (12). Myelopathy or radiculopathy can be presenting findings. Posterior laminoplasty is the treatment for subaxial stenosis.

SPONDYLOEPIPHYSEAL DYSPLASIA

Atlantoaxial instability resulting from ligamentous laxity, odontoid hypoplasia or os odontoideum is commonly seen in patients with spondyloepiphyseal dysplasia (13,14). This instability may not be present at birth and appear later (Fig. 35.2). The prevalence of this instability may be different among the types of spondyloepiphyseal dysplasia. The congenital form (spondyloepiphyseal dysplasia congenita; SEDC) has a very high incidence of instability (13,16,17). Atlantoaxial instability is also commonly seen in spondylometaphyseal dysplasia.

PSEUDOACHONDROPLASIA

Ligamentous laxity and odontoid hypoplasia are seen in patients with pseudoachondroplasia. Instability at the atlantoaxial level can result in neurological impairment and require operative intervention (Fig. 35.3)(14).

KNIEST DYSPLASIA

Atlantoaxial and occipitoatlantal instability secondary to odontoid hypoplasia and lack of ligamentous integrity at the occipitoatlantal level are reported in Kniest dysplasia (18–20).

METAPHYSEAL CHONDRODYSPLASIA

Odontoid hypoplasia and ligamentous laxity with atlantoaxial instability is seen in the McKusick type of metaphyseal chondrodysplasia (21,22).

METATROPIC DYSPLASIA

Atlantoaxial subluxation resulting from odontoid hypoplasia is common in patients with metatropic dysplasia (23). Rotatory fixation can develop after decompression surgery at the C1-2 articulation without fusion and inadequate immobilization. Subaxial instability secondary to C2 dysplasia is reported (24). Cervical canal stenosis without instability can be seen in these children.

CHONDRODYSPLASIA PUNCTATA

Atlantoaxial instability resulting from os odontoideum or cervical stenosis can result in cervical cord compression. Kyphosis with subluxation has also been reported (25). As the vertebrae are severely dysplastic (26), anterior fusion combined with posterior fusion is recommended for subaxial kyphosis.

DIASTROPHIC DYSPLASIA

Cervical kyphosis resulting from vertebral body wedging, ligamentous laxity, or spina bifida is seen in many children with diastrophic dysplasia (27–29). Atlantoaxial instability also is reported (30). The kyphosis develops in the neonate and spontaneous resolution of this malalignment is observed in the majority of these children before the age of 6 years if the kyphosis was less than 60 degrees at the first radiographic evaluation (Fig. 35.4) (29). The kyphosis can progress resulting in quadriplegia and death, but this is rare (31). Progressive kyphosis with a normal neurologic examination and no cord compression can be managed by posterior fusion surgery. Some correction of the kyphosis can be

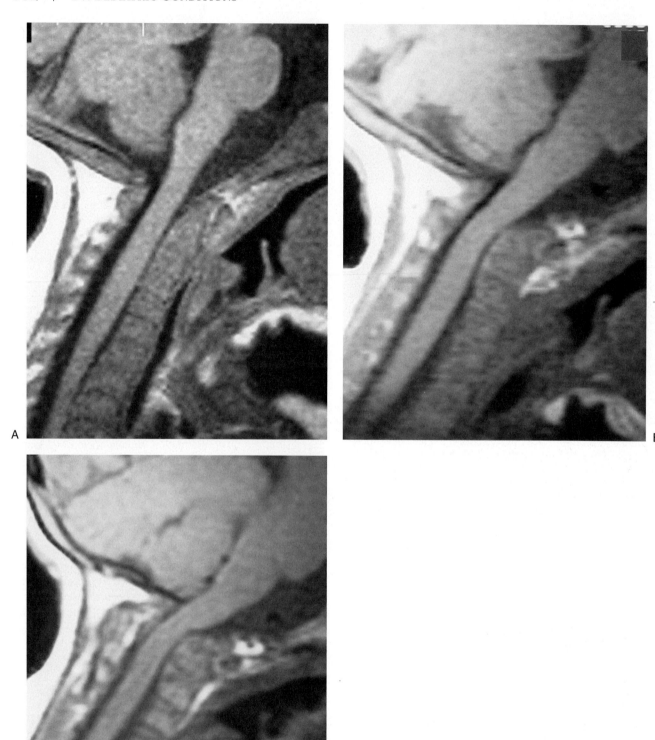

FIG. 35.2. Development of atlantoaxial instability in spondyloepiphyseal dysplasia congenita is demonstrated by magnetic resonance imaging at 3 months **(A)**, 3 years **(B)**, and 7 years of age **(C)**.

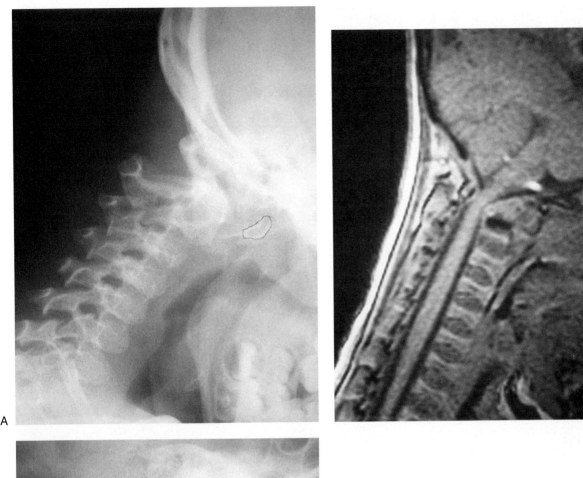

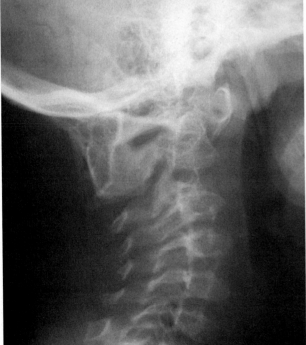

FIG. 35.3. A: Atlantoaxial instability in pseudoachondroplasia. **B:** Spinal cord compression is demonstrated on magnetic resonance imaging. **C:** O-C2 posterior fusion is seen after onlay autologous bone grafting and halo immobilization.

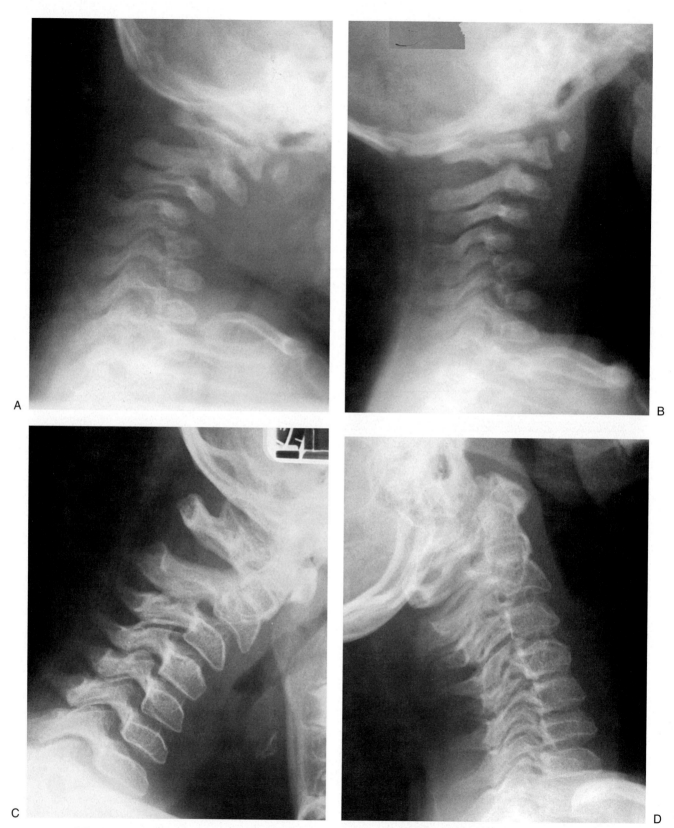

FIG. 35.4. Spontaneous correction of the cervical kyphosis in diastrophic dysplasia. Lateral cervical radiographs at 3 months (**A:** flexion; **B:** extension) and 5 years of age (**C:** flexion; **D:** extension).

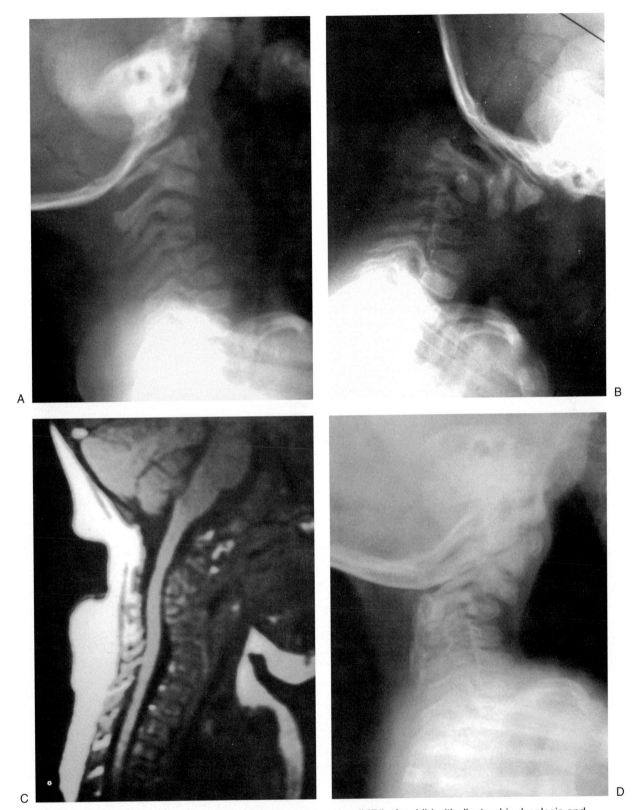

FIG. 35.5. Radiographs and magnetic resonance imaging (MRI) of a child with diastrophic dysplasia and cervical kyphosis treated with posterior cervical fusion. Cervical kyphosis at 1 year of age before surgery (**A:** extension; **B:** flexion; **C:** MRI). Correction of the kyphosis is seen on serial radiographs after posterior fusion and halo immobilization (**D:** 6 months; **E:** 3 years; **F:** 14 years after the surgery) (continued).

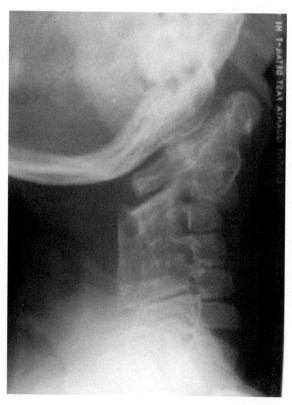
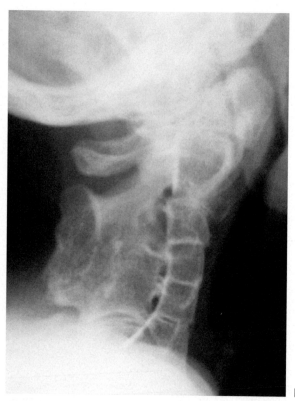

E   F

FIG. 35.5. *Continued*

observed because of continued growth of the anterior column of the cervical vertebrae and tethering posteriorly by the fusion (Fig. 35.5). Severe kyphosis with cord compression requires anterior decompression, strut grafting, and posterior fusion. During exposure, care must be taken because spinal dysraphism is common.

Cervical spondylosis is seen in diastrophic dysplasia after the second decade (32). Long-term follow-up is essential.

CAMPTOMELIC DYSPLASIA

Cervical kyphosis is a characteristic deformity of camptomelic dysplasia. The kyphosis is caused by vertebral malformation, spondylolisthesis, cartilaginous dysplasia, and hypotonia (33,34). The deformity and neurologic manifestations may be progressive, even after a spinal fusion.

MUCOPOLYSACCHARIDOSES

Type 1: Hurler Syndrome

Odontoid dysplasia resulting in atlantoaxial instability is occasionally seen in patients with Hurler syndrome (35). Abnormal soft-tissue formation around the tip of the odontoid can result in myelopathy, and resorption of the soft tissue is reported after bone marrow transplantation (36,37).

Type 2: Hunter Syndrome

Spinal cord compression by thickened soft-tissue posterior to the odontoid can be a problem (38). Decompression from the foramen magnum to the subaxial cervical spine combined with duraplasty is recommended treatment because of deposition in the peridural tissue (39).

Type 3: Morquio Syndrome

Abnormal development at the craniovertebral junction consisting of odontoid hypoplasia and soft-tissue thickening are characteristic findings in patients with this syndrome (8, 40–43). Anterior extradural soft tissues at the craniovertebral junction consisting of reactive ligamentous tissue with or without deposition of mucopolysaccharide can narrow the spinal canal and is compounded by atlantoaxial instability (44). Progressive myelopathy, traumatic quadriplegia, or sudden death by respiratory arrest can result from cord compression (45). The myelopathy becomes evident typically between 4 and 6 years of age. The severity of neurologic manifestations is strongly related to the thickened soft tissue at the craniovertebral junction, not to the type of odontoid hypoplasia or subluxation pattern. Flexion/extension cervical spine radiographs and MRI should be done at an early age. Prophylactic decompression and arthrodesis, if required, has been recommended for children in the first decade with atlantoaxial instability because of the high incidence of neurologic

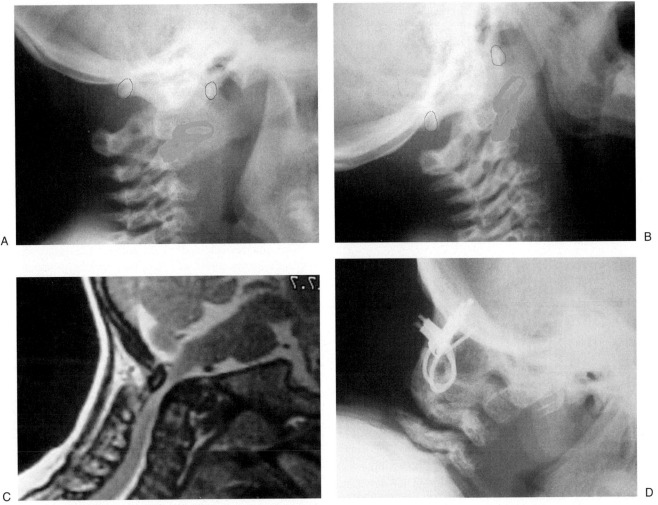

FIG. 35.6. Atlantoaxial instability in Morquio syndrome (**A:** flexion; **B:** extension). Cervicomedullary cord compression and intrinsic cord signal abnormalities are seen on magnetic resonance imaging (**C**). Postoperative x-ray film after C1 decompression, autologous bone graft, occiput-C2 fixation with titanium cables, and halo immobilization (**D**).

injury and poor recovery of established cervical myelopathy after stabilization (Fig. 35.6) (45,46). Anterior transoral decompression has been recommended with significant anterior cord compression (44), but the abnormal soft tissues have been seen to absorb after stabilization by fusion (47).

OCULOAURICULAR VERTEBRAL DYSPLASIA

Atlantoaxial instability resulting from odontoid hypoplasia or junctional instability between unsegmented vertebrae has been reported (48).

OSTEOPATHIA STRIATA

Patients with osteopathia striata typically require no orthopedic intervention. However, there is a case report of a girl who presented with cranial sclerosis, osteopathia striata, and a severe cervical kyphosis with a dysplastic cervical spine resulting in cord compression (49).

Pyknodysostosis

Spondylolysis of the C2 similar to a "hangman fracture" are reported (50,51). There may be potential for spontaneous healing, because the pathogenesis is likely a stress fracture.

Thanatophoric Dysplasia

Platyspondyly is one of the characteristic radiologic findings in patients with thanatorophic dysplasia. Diminished ossification is seen at the area surrounding the foramen magnum (52).

Multiple Epiphyseal Dysplasia

Odontoid dysplasia in multiple epiphyseal dysplasias is documented in a case report (53).

Osteopetrosis

A patient with spondylolysis of C2 and C3 who had posterior fusion surgery was described (54).

Osteopoikilosis

Cervical canal stenosis is reported in a patient with osteopoikilosis (55).

Cleidocranial Dysostosis

Marked basilar impression is seen in a patient with cleidocranial dysostosis because of the enlarged foramen magnum (56)

Spondyloepimetaphyseal Dysplasia

Atlantoaxial instability resulting from odontoid hypoplasia is documented (57).

ASSESSMENT

A careful history can often provide important clues to the presence of a cervical spine disorder. Discomfort is a very uncharacteristic complaint. Children with chronic cervical myelopathy can present with decreased endurance, difficulty with stairs, and progressive weakness. One must be careful to differentiate between decreased function owing to cervical myelopathy or progressive lower extremity valgus seen in children with Morquio syndrome and spondyloepiphyseal dysplasia. The patients must be questioned about bladder and bowel dysfunction.

A careful neurologic examination must be done including upper and lower extremity major muscle group power, reflexes, and sensation. Proprioception or vibration abnormalities can be early findings of myelopathy. Upper motor neuron signs such as clonus, hyperreflexia, and positive Babinski signs must be documented at each evaluation. Limb deformities and contractures can make the neurologic examination difficult and often young children do not cooperate. Subtle weakness can be observed by holding toys above the children's head to reach for and watching these children get up off the floor or out of a chair and walk and run. Serial evaluations are often very helpful in determining the progression of a subtle cervical myelopathy.

MEDICAL IMAGING

Plain Radiographs

Anteroposterior and lateral radiographs of the cervical spine should be obtained initially. These should be obtained sitting or standing, but this may not be possible in the young child.

These films are useful for assessing the osseous abnormalities present in skeletal dysplasias such as platyspondyly present in the spondyloepiphyseal dysplasias and in some children with pseudoachondroplasia. Odontoid hypoplasia or os odontoideum often are seen on the plain radiographs. If there is significant deformity, it is difficult to determine the exact skeletal anatomy of the upper cervical spine. Fixed translational deformities and stenosis are also seen on the plain radiographs. Oblique radiographs are rarely useful.

Flexion/extension lateral radiographs of the cervical spine centered at the occipitocervical junction are important radiographs. A discussion with the family and child explaining that maximum flexion/extension are required for these radiographs often result in more satisfactory films. Often there is concern that positioning of the neck can result in neurologic injury, which is of little concern in the awake patient. The radiology staff may wish a physician to be present for the radiographs.

The anterior atlantodens interval (AADI) is routinely measured but a more important measurement is the space available for the cord (SAC) or the posterior atlantodens interval (PADI). The normal sagittal diameter of the spinal canal at C2 in the average stature infant is 13 mm (58), at 3 to 6 years is 17.9 ± 1.3 mm, at 7 to 10 years is 18.8 ± 1 mm, and at 11 to 14 years is 19.4 ± 1.1 mm (59). In children the ratio of the sagittal spinal cord width to subarachnoid space width at C2 is 0.57 (60). Normal children can have an AADI of 4 mm, pseudosubluxation in flexion at C2-3 and mild kyphosis in flexion. These findings result from facet anatomy, viscoelastic properties of the immature spine, and physiologic laxity.

Computed Tomography

CT provides excellent visualization of the bony anatomy of the upper cervical spine and the size of the canal. It is very useful when planning transarticular screw fixation at C1-2, and lateral mass screws subaxially. These studies can be done quickly and even young children may not need sedation. The cervical spine can be imaged in different positions including flexion, extension, and rotation for more information.

Magnetic Resonance Imaging

MRI requires more time than CT and most children need sedation or a general anesthetic. MRI provides excellent information about the cervical spinal cord and is very accurate in detecting cord compression and intrinsic cord abnormalities. Evaluation of CSF flow can help determine the degree of compression. MRI of the neck in flexion, neutral, and extension assesses the dynamic cord compression and the presence of fixed stenosis.

The positioning of the child for these studies is very important. When children are lying on a flat surface, the cervical spine is typically in a flexed position because of the size of the head relative to the body. The cervical spine is in a neutral position when the external auditory meatus is in line with the shoulder. This position can be achieved by elevating the thorax with a pad or providing a depression in the surface under the occiput. Flexion is achieved by putting padding under the occiput and extension by padding under the thorax. The protocol at the authors' institution is to image the sedated child in neutral or extension initially and only proceed to flexion if no cord compression is observed. CSF flow studies can provide information about the severity of cord compression. MR angiography can be used to evaluate the vertebral and cranial blood flow.

Evoked Potentials

Somatosensory evoked potentials can be done on an outpatient basis in an awake child but have limited clinical usefulness (1,8). Somatosensory and motor evoked potentials can be done under an anesthetic with the neck in flexion/extension to assess the degree of cervical cord compromise.

Urodynamics

Urodynamics can be used to detect the presence of subtle cervical myelopathy.

Ultrasound

Incomplete ossification of the posterior elements of the spine early in life allows visualization of the spinal canal and contents (61,62). In children without skeletal dysplasia, satisfactory visualization of the cord often can be achieved up to about 6 months of age. The ultrasound can be useful for a noninvasive evaluation of spinal cord tethering, syringomyelia or lipomeningocele, or other congenital anomalies.

All of these studies must be interpreted with careful consideration being given to the complete neural axis. For example, in children with metatropic dysplasia and achondroplasia, there can be areas of stenosis in the thoracolumbar spine, which may complicate the neurologic examination.

TREATMENT

A child with skeletal dysplasia and a normal neurologic examination with no evidence of cervical instability or stenosis should be recommended to follow-up with routine biannual or annual visits. There are no established follow-up criteria. Follow-up should include a careful neurologic examination and yearly flexion/extension lateral cervical spine radiographs. If there has been a change in the neurologic examination with or without instability on the lateral cervical spine, radiographs, and MRI should be performed.

Few restrictions are required when a child has a normal neurologic examination and imaging studies. The difficulty arises when the child has a normal neurologic examination and mild upper cervical instability with no cord compression on the flexion/extension MRI. Activity restrictions, such as

staying off the upper level of the adventure playground, avoiding tumbling, diving, and contact sports are reasonable and usually well tolerated by these short-statured children. Use of a firm cervical collar in the car may provide some protection.

Indications for surgical management can be divided into those that are absolute and those that are relative. Absolute indications would be a neurologic examination indicative of cervical myelopathy, progressive kyphosis, anterior atlantoaxial instability greater than 8 to 10 mm with a space available for the cord that is not adequate in flexion or extension, or intrinsic cord abnormalities.

Relative indications may include children with a normal neurologic examination and a stable but severe cervical kyphosis, anterior atlantoaxial instability of 5 to 8 mm or a flexion/extension MRI scan that demonstrates a very limited space available for the cord in full flexion. Prophylactic cervical arthrodesis for an asymptomatic child should not be approached lightly, because this surgery is frequently associated with complications.

Options for surgical management include decompression or arthrodesis alone and decompression and arthrodesis. Decompression is done for stenosis without instability and in the absence of cervical kyphosis. This procedure is most commonly done in children with achondroplasia who have foramen magnum and upper cervical stenosis. These children can be decompressed both at the foramen magnum and the posterior arch of C1 and do not require an occipital cervical fusion (9,12). Subsequent instability is rare.

Arthrodesis without decompression is performed in the presence of cervical instability without fixed stenosis. The unstable segment must be able to be reduced to the point that there is adequate space available for the cervical spinal cord and stabilized (14,24,63).

Decompression and arthrodesis is performed for stenosis and instability. As mentioned, progressive instability is typical of the natural history of SEDC and metatropic dysplasia as well as other disorders. Decompression without arthrodesis in these children without adequate postoperative immobilization can result in severe upper cervical deformities, most commonly postlaminectomy kyphosis (64,65). Lonstein (64) reported a 50% incidence of kyphosis or swan neck deformity in children who underwent cervical laminectomies without fusion. The management of severe kyphosis with cord compression, such as those patients with Larsen's syndrome or diastrophic dwarfism, requires an anterior decompression with multilevel carpectomies, anterior strut grafting, and a posterior stabilization (Fig. 35.7) (28).

The surgical management of these patients requires an experienced, multidisciplinary team. The anesthesiologist must be facile in fiberoptic intubations, because forceful head and neck manipulation cannot be performed for endotracheal intubation (17,66,67). A report described tetraplegia occurring in an 8-year-old girl with Morquio syndrome after manipulation of the neck during general anesthesia (42). Other anesthetic considerations include small airways, lower lung volumes, poor chest compliance, hypothermia,

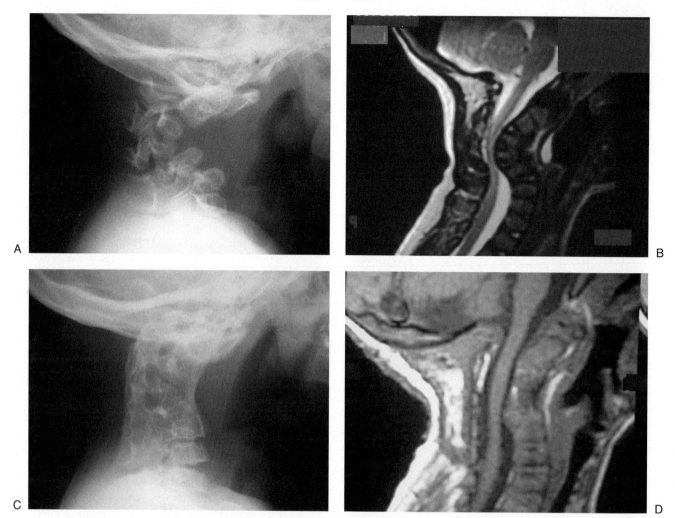

FIG. 35.7. Cervical kyphosis in a child with a familial but undescribed skeletal dysplasia. Lateral cervical x-ray film **(A)** and magnetic resonance imaging (MRI) **(B)** before the surgery at 3 years of age demonstrating severe kyphosis with symptomatic cord compression. Anterior corpectomy and strut grafting with posterior fusion and halo immobilization were performed. Postoperative radiograph **(C)** and MRI **(D)**.

and difficulty with prone positioning. Optimal neurophysiologic monitoring requires avoidance of hypotension, inhaled gases, and muscle relaxants. Somatosensory evoked potentials and transcranial motor evoked potentials should be the standard of care in these cases in which the myelopathic spinal cord may have little reserve for further insult. The surgeon and scrub team should be experienced in order to avoid unnecessary delays and complications.

The technique of arthrodesis of the cervical spine in children is well documented, and certain principles must be followed. Arthrodesis has a high likelihood of success with meticulous exposure of the elements to be fused, decortication, use of autologous bone graft from the iliac crest, ribs, occiput, or proximal tibia, and rigid postoperative immobilization. Koop (24), Dormans (68), and Rodgers (69) have provide detailed descriptions of their respective fusion techniques for the upper cervical spine, and demonstrate that favorable results can be obtained with adherence to the preceding principles.

The use internal fixation is becoming more common in the pediatric cervical spine, and though the anatomy of short-statured patients may preclude the use of some implants, instrumentation is an important part of the surgeon's armamentarium (10,71). Techniques previously described employed wires that could be passed through the occiput via burr holes to assist in immobilization of the occipitocervical junction (Fig. 35.6). Hall added a threaded Kirschner wire to the distal spinous process for stability, and 22 of 23 patients achieved a successful arthrodesis, which was far better than historical cohorts (69). Wires can be used in the subaxial spine, but are prone to pull-out and breakage. Sublaminar wires or cables offer rigid control of a spinal segment, when used in a Brooks or modified Gallie wiring, but cannot be used after a C1 laminectomy or with significant canal stenosis.

The authors' preferred method of stabilization of the atlantoaxial complex in children requiring a C1-2 arthrodesis is the transarticular screw (Fig. 35.8). Anatomic factors

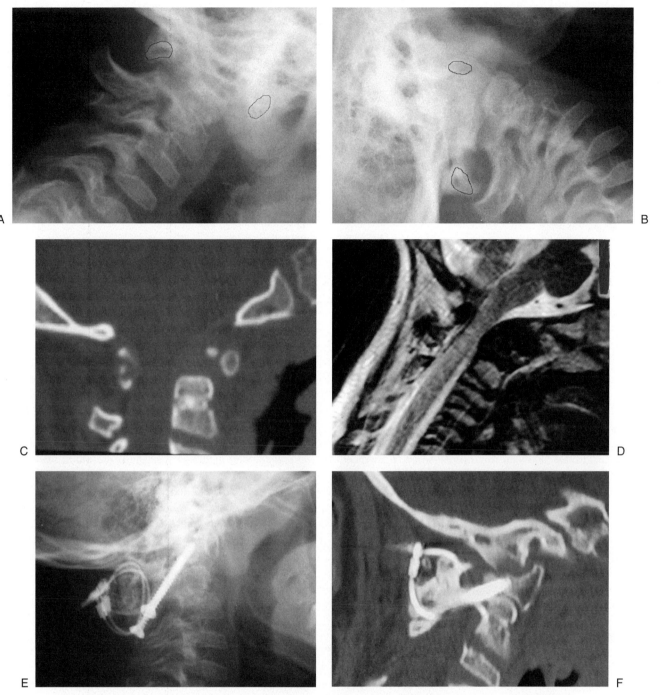

FIG. 35.8. X-ray images of a patient with spondyloepiphyseal dysplasia congenita. Atlantoaxial instability is seen in the lateral cervical view with flexion **(A)** and extension **(B)**. A small ossification center of the os odontoideum is seen on the reconstructed sagittal computed tomographic image **(C)**. Cervical canal stenosis and cord compression is caused by the anterior displacement of C1 **(D)**. Posterior fusion was performed using C1-2 transarticular screws and autologous iliac bone graft with Brooks' wiring technique at 10 years of age. Anatomic reduction and ideal screw position is demonstrated on a plain film **(E)** and reconstructed computed tomographic images **(F,G,H)** (continued).

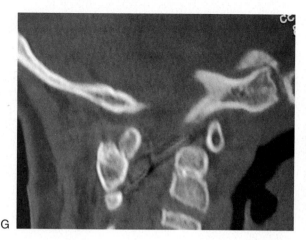

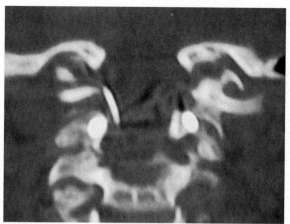

G   H

FIG. 35.8. *Continued*

limit the use of this technique in some children, and other alternative techniques used in these children include; onlay bone grafting and wiring techniques described in the preceding (Fig. 35.9). Transarticular screws are biomechanically superior in various failure modes, but are technically challenging (71–75). The vertebral artery anatomy and lateral mass morphology should be studied by fine-cut CT scans and multiplanar reconstructions through the area preoperatively, and intraoperative fluoroscopy or navigation can facilitate and confirm proper screw placement (72). The atlantoaxial articulation should be reduced prior to screw fixation. Methods of open reduction include manipulation of the spinous processes with towel clips or passing a wire or cable under the posterior arch of C1 and applying traction for reduction (75). Brockmeyer and colleagues (76) reported on 31 patients from 4 to 16 years of age in whom transarticular screws were placed with no vascular or neurologic complications. They concluded that C1-2 transarticular screw fixation technically is possible in a large proportion of pediatric patients with atlantoaxial instability.

Instrumentation for fusions above C1 to the occiput is a useful adjunct for this challenging problem, and may decrease the pseudarthrosis rate. We have found both contoured Luque (77) or unit rods with wires and the newer occipital plate-rod systems for proximal anchorage to the occiput effective in stabilization of this area for fusion (Fig. 35.10). Distal fixation in the subaxial cervical spine can be achieved with lateral mass or pedicle screws, hooks, wires, or cables.

Severe, complex cervical deformities, such as torticollis, can be managed by gradual spinal correction with the halo-Ilizarov distraction cast and subsequent instrumentation and fusion (78). This technique allows gradual, safe, three-dimensional correction of the deformity with the patient in an outpatient setting.

POSTOPERATIVE CARE

The pediatric intensive care unit (PICU) is ideal for the initial postoperative care in these children. Issues such as excess fluid shifts, preexisting restrictive lung disease, and difficult situations with reintubation of a small airway in a patient in a halo often result in the endotracheal tube being maintained for several days postoperatively.

The type of postoperative immobilization is dictated by several factors, including the age of the child, stability of the cervical spine, shape of the trunk, restrictive pulmonary disease, and skin conditions.

Temporary or prolonged cervical traction is rarely required in these children, except in cases of severe kyphosis, or staged anteroposterior procedures. Immobilization usually is achieved with a halo cast or vest or in the older children, with rigid internal fixation a SOMI brace or rigid collar is adequate.

The children are measured preoperatively for the halo. The halo ring is typically of carbon fiber with titanium instrumentation, compatible with postoperative MRI. These children typically have small, stiff thoraces with a pectus carinatum or excavatum and are difficult to fit with the commercial vests; usually a cast is required. Typically, the child is placed into a halo at the beginning of the surgical procedure and the halo is connected to a Mayfield apparatus with a halo adapter. A preoperative CT scan of the equator of the skull is helpful in pin placement to gauge skull thickness and suture location, especially in young children. These children usually require six to eight screws inserted at a lower torque (1 to 4 ft/lb) than adults.

At the conclusion of the procedure, the body cast or vest is applied and the superstructure fixed to the cast. Generous trim lines and a large abdominal window are made, because these children are typically abdominal breathers and require room for abdominal expansion.

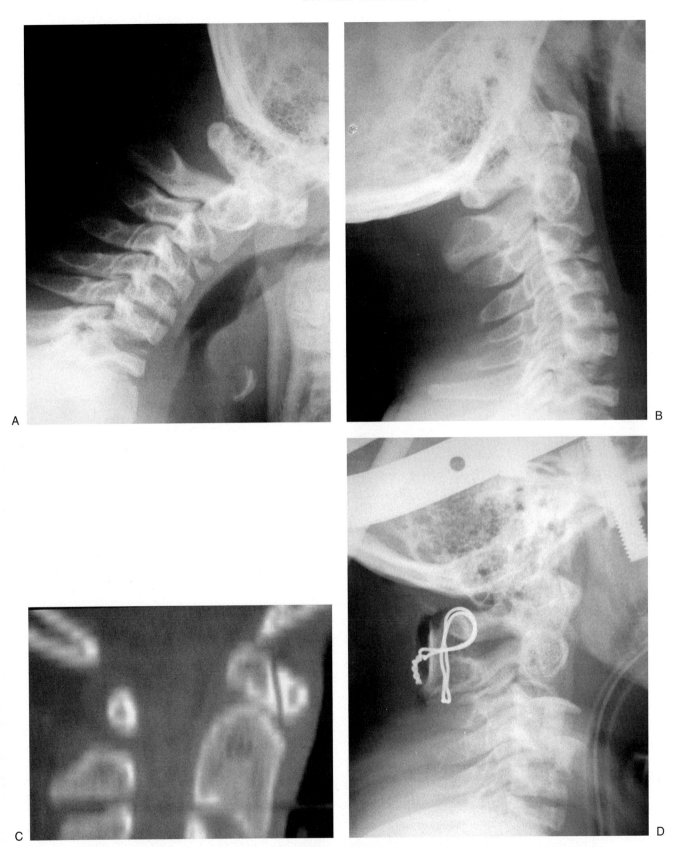

FIG. 35.9. A patient with an unknown skeletal dysplasia treated using Gallie's technique. Atlantoaxial instability with os odontoideum is demonstrated in flexion **(A)** and extension **(B)** radiographs and a sagittal reconstruction computed tomographic image **(C)**. **D:** C1-2 fusion was performed using Gallie's technique at 17 years of age. **E:** Some displacement of C1 on C2 was detected during the immobilization. **F:** Bony fusion was achieved (continued).

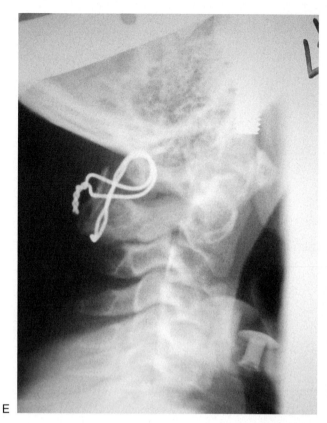

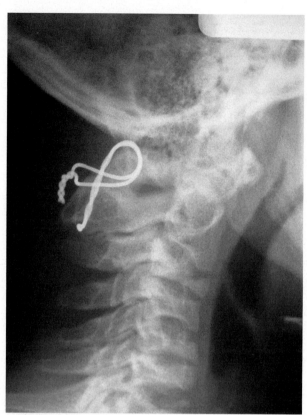

FIG. 35.9. *Continued*

Immobilization is continued until there is evidence of a satisfactory arthrodesis. This typically requires 8 to 12 weeks. Evaluation is done with plain radiographs, including oblique views of the upper cervical spine. If these radiographs demonstrate a satisfactory fusion mass, the halo and body cast are left on and the superstructure removed to allow flexion/extension lateral cervical spine radiographs. If there is no motion and evidence of bridging trabecular bone, the halo and body cast are removed. A SOMI brace or a semirigid cervical orthosis is used for several months postoperatively.

COMPLICATIONS

The most common early complication is respiratory difficulty. The common underlying restrictive lung disease in these patients aggravated by the halo vest or body cast can result in prolonged intubation and secondary problems. Aspiration pneumonia associated with gastroesophageal reflux can be seen occasionally. Satisfactory padding allowing chest expansion and a large abdominal window extending out over the rib margin decreases these problems. The use of supportive ventilation techniques such as nasal noninvasive positive pressure ventilation (NPPV) (BiPAP Respironics Inc., XX) intermittently or continuously may be needed during the time of immobilization. Aggressive pulmonary therapy and rapid mobilization decrease pulmonary complications.

Prolonged drainage from the wound can result from a CSF leak (9,69). A meticulous deep muscle and fascial closure and a watertight skin closure limit this complication. Dural patches and lumbar shunt diversion may be required (69).

Neurologic injury in the upper cervical spine most commonly results from direct trauma, such as during passage of a sublaminar wire or screw. Ransford and associates (46) caution that sublaminar wire passage at C1 and C2 can be unsafe in Morquio syndrome. Neurologic injury may occur even without sublaminar wire passage. In Rodgers and associates' series, a 5-year-old girl with SEDC and atlantoaxial instability had a C1 laminectomy and fusion with wire fixation from occipital drill holes to the C2 spinous process and sustained a neurologic injury (69). She awoke with quadriplegia, which resolved in 48 hours. It was not reported whether intraoperative neurophysiologic monitoring was used or if steroids were given.

Pseudarthrosis rates vary depending on the arthrodesis technique. Key factors in achieving a high rate of arthrodesis include the use of autologous bone graft and internal fixation (Fig. 35.11). An onlay grafting technique with allograft and halo immobilization for occipitocervical fusions in SEDC has a 50% pseudarthrosis rate (79). Stabler and colleagues reported a 100% pseudarthrosis rate in seven children after cervical arthrodesis done with allograft and a variety of techniques (80). Pseudarthrosis rates are low when autologous

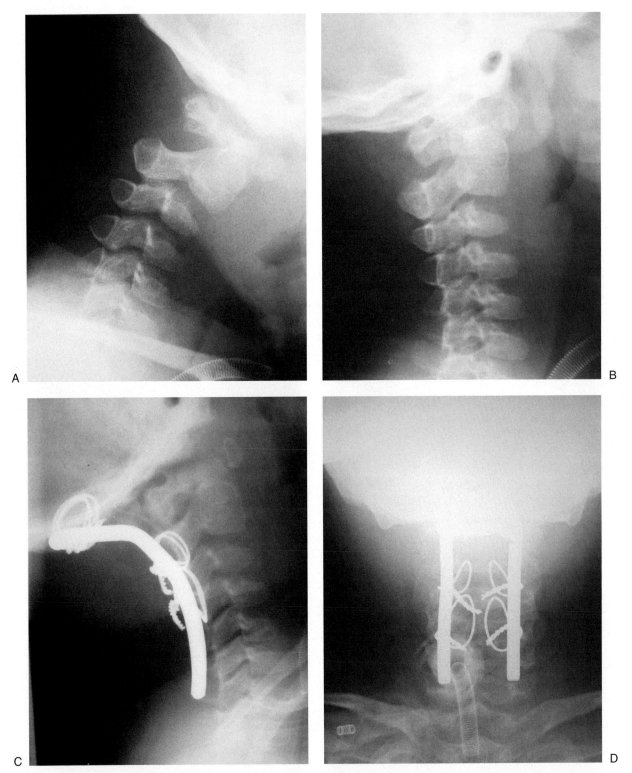

FIG. 35.10. Occipitocervical fusion using the upper end of a unit rod for internal fixation. A child with metatropic dysplasia presented with cervical myelopathy. A C1 decompression without fusion was done at 1 year of age. Radiographs in flexion **(A)** and extension **(B)** at 3 years of age showed odontoid hypoplasia, atlantoaxial instability, and canal stenosis resulting in cervicomedullary cord compression. The instability was stabilized with the occipitocervical fusion using the upper end of a unit rod at 4 years of age **(C,D)**.

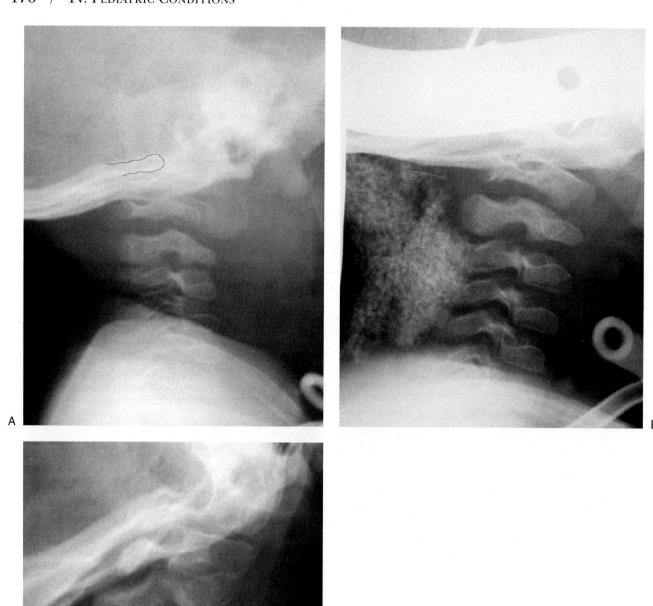

FIG. 35.11. Pseudarthrosis in spondyloepiphyseal dysplasia congenita after posterior occipitocervical arthrodesis at 3 and 7 years of age using onlay allograft and halo immobilization. Preoperative **(A)** and postoperative **(B)** radiographs at 3 and at 9 years of age **(C)**.

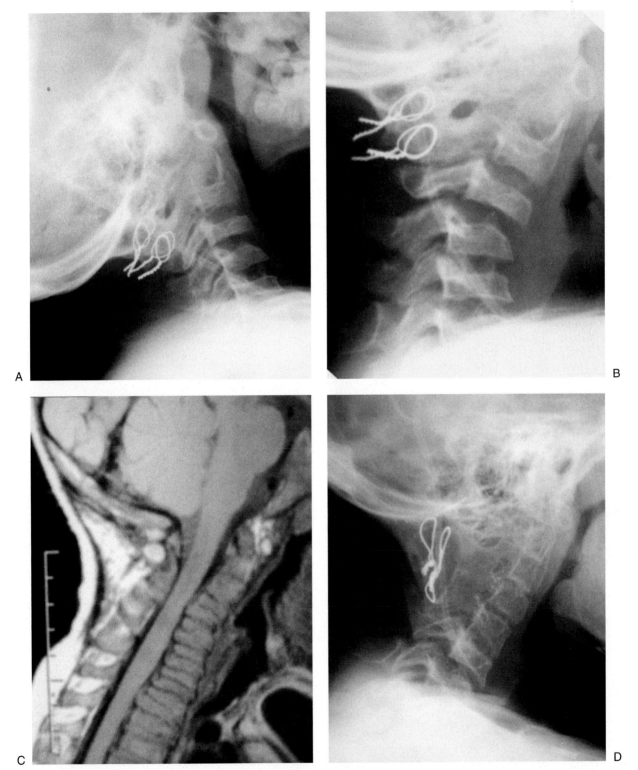

FIG. 35.12. Junctional instability is seen below an occipitocervical fusion in a 14-year-old boy with spondyloepiphyseal dysplasia congenita (**A:** flexion; **B:** extension). Cervical canal stenosis is demonstrated on magnetic resonance imaging (**C**). Posterior fusion was extended to C5 with wire fixation and halo immobilization (**D**).

bone graft is used with a variety of surgical techniques. Onlay autologous bone graft and halo immobilization resulted in 100% fusion rates in 10 children with various types of skeletal dysplasias (14,24). One of these studies used an occipital periosteal flap, which may be of some benefit (24). Two different techniques of occipitocervical wire fixation and autologous bone graft also have low rates of pseudarthrosis and reduce the time of halo immobilization (68,69). Farey and colleagues (72) reported 27 patients with atlantoaxial instability who underwent C1-2 arthrodesis using two techniques; a modified Gallie's technique with postoperative halo immobilization and transarticular screw fixation in addition to the modified Gallie technique with soft collar immobilization. Successful fusion rates were 58% after the modified Gallie's technique with halo, and 100% after the transarticular screw fixation. Atlantoaxial subluxation may not be stabilized by the modified Gallie's technique (Fig. 35.9).

Junctional instability can occur in the midcervical spine below an upper cervical fusion (Fig. 35.12). This can be associated with stenosis and cervical myelopathy.

Complications related to the halo are discussed elsewhere in this publication and are common in these patients (14,45,68). Usually pin tract infections are managed

successfully with increased pin care and oral antibiotics. Occasionally, a screw needs to be inserted into an adjacent site and the offending screw removed. Migration of the screw through the inner table of the skull can occur but is an uncommon complication (Fig. 35.13).

In summary, although patients with skeletal dysplasias can display varied abnormal anatomy and develop complex instability patterns, certain disorders have characteristic problems. Recognition of the patients at risk, thorough imaging, preoperative planning, and meticulous surgical technique result in safe, successful treatment of these individuals and significant improvement in quality of life.

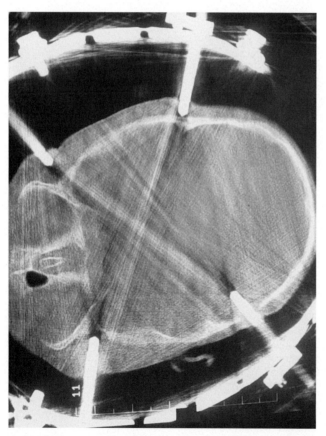

FIG. 35.13. A halo screw *(arrow)* penetration through the inner table in a patient with spondyloepiphyseal dysplasia congenital.

REFERENCES

1. Reid CS, Pyeritz RE, Kopits SE, et al. Cervicomedullary cord compression in young children with achondroplasia: value of comprehensive neurologic and respiratory evaluation. *Basic Life Sci* 1988;48: 199–206.
2. Hecht JT, Nelson FW, Butler IJ, et al. Computerized tomography of the foramen magnum: achondroplastic values compared to normal standards. *Am J Med Genet* 1985;20(2):355–360.
3. Wang H, Rosenbaum AE, Reid CS, et al. Pediatric patients with achondroplasia: CT evaluation of the craniocervical junction. *Radiology* 1987; 164(2):515–519.
4. Hecht JT, Horton WA, Reid CS, et al. Growth of the foramen magnum in achondroplasia. *Am J Med Genet* 1989;32(4):528–535.
5. Pauli RM, Scott CI, Wassman ER Jr, et al. Apnea and sudden unexpected death in infants with achondroplasia. *J Pediatr* 1984;104(3): 342–348.
6. Pauli RM, Horton VK, Glinski LP, et al. Prospective assessment of risks for cervicomedullary-junction compression in infants with achondroplasia. *Am J Hum Genet* 1995;56(3):732–744.
7. Thomas IT, Frias JL, Williams JL, et al. Magnetic resonance imaging in the assessment of medullary compression in achondroplasia. *Am J Dis Child* 1988;142(9):989–992.
8. Nelson FW, Goldie WD, Hecht JT, et al. Short-latency somatosensory evoked potentials in the management of patients with achondroplasia. *Neurology* 1984;34(8):1053–1058.
9. Aryanpur J, Hurko O, Francomano C, et al. Craniocervical decompression for cervicomedullary compression in pediatric patients with achondroplasia. *J Neurosurg* 1990;73(3):375–382.
10. Gulati DR, Rout D. Atlantoaxial dislocation with quadriparesis in achondroplasia. Case report. *J Neurosurg* 1974;40(3):394–396.
11. Hammerschlag W, Ziv I, Wald U, et al. Cervical instability in an achondroplastic infant. *J Pediatr Orthop* 1988;8(4):481–484.
12. Frigon VA, Castro FP, Whitecloud TS, et al. Isolated subaxial cervical spine stenosis in achondroplasia. *Curr Surg* 2000;57(4):354–356.
13. Spranger JW, Langer LO Jr. Spondyloepiphyseal dysplasia congenita. *Radiology* 1970;94(2):313–322.
14. Svensson O, Aaro S. Cervical instability in skeletal dysplasia. Report of 6 surgically fused cases. *Acta Orthop Scand* 1988;59(1):66–70.
15. Kopits SE. Orthopedic complications of dwarfism. *Clin Orthop* 1976; (114):153–179.
16. Wynne-Davies R, Hall C. Two clinical variants of spondylo-epiphysial dysplasia congenita. *J Bone Joint Surg Br* 1982;64(4):435–441.
17. Redl G. Massive pyramidal tract signs after endotracheal intubation: a case report of spondyloepiphyseal dysplasia congenita. *Anesthesiology* 1998;89(5):1262–1264.
18. Bethem D, Winter RB, Lutter L, et al. Spinal disorders of dwarfism. Review of the literature and report of eighty cases. *J Bone Joint Surg Am* 1981;63(9):1412–1425.
19. Merrill KD, Schmidt TL. Occipitoatlantal instability in a child with Kniest syndrome. *J Pediatr Orthop* 1989;9(3):338–340.
20. Rimoin DL, Siggers DC, Lachman RS, et al. Metatropic dwarfism, the Kniest syndrome and the pseudoachondroplastic dysplasias. *Clin Orthop* 1976;(114):70–82.

21. Herring JA, ed. *Tachdjian's pediatric orthopedics*, 3rd ed. Philadelphia: WB Saunders, 2002:1549.
22. Lachman RS. The cervical spine in the skeletal dysplasias and associated disorders. *Pediatr Radiol* 1997;27(5):402–408.
23. Shohat M, Lachman R, Rimoin DL. Odontoid hypoplasia with vertebral cervical subluxation and ventriculomegaly in metatropic dysplasia. *J Pediatr* 1989;114(2):239–243.
24. Koop SE, Winter RB, Lonstein JE. The surgical treatment of instability of the upper part of the cervical spine in children and adolescents. *J Bone Joint Surg Am* 1984;66(3):403–411.
25. Khanna AJ, Braverman NE, Valle D, et al. Cervical stenosis secondary to rhizomelic chondrodysplasia punctata. *Am J Med Genet* 2001;99 (1):63–66.
26. Wells TR, Landing BH, Bostwick FH. Studies of vertebral coronal cleft in rhizomelic chondrodysplasia punctata. *Pediatr Pathol* 1992; 12(4):593–600.
27. Herring JA. The spinal disorders in diastrophic dwarfism. *J Bone Joint Surg Am* 1978;60(2):177–182.
28. Forese LL, Berdon WE, Harcke HT, et al. Severe mid-cervical kyphosis with cord compression in Larsen's syndrome and diastrophic dysplasia: unrelated syndromes with similar radiologic findings and neurosurgical implications. *Pediatr Radiol* 1995;25(2):136–139.
29. Remes V, Marttinen E, Poussa M, et al. Cervical kyphosis in diastrophic dysplasia. *Spine* 1999;24(19):1990–1995.
30. Richards BS. Atlanto-axial instability in diastrophic dysplasia. A case report. *J Bone Joint Surg Am* 1991;73(4):614–616.
31. Bethem D, Winter RB, Lutter L. Disorders of the spine in diastrophic dwarfism. *J Bone Joint Surg Am* 1980;62(4):529–536.
32. Remes V, Tervahartiala P, Poussa M, et al. Cervical spine in diastrophic dysplasia: an MRI analysis. *J Pediatr Orthop* 2000;20(1): 48–53.
33. Ray S, Bowen JR. Orthopaedic problems associated with survival in camptomelic dysplasia. *Clin Orthop* 1984;(185):77–82.
34. Coscia MF, Bassett GS, Bowen JR, et al. Spinal abnormalities in camptomelic dysplasia. *J Pediatr Orthop* 1989;9(1):6–14.
35. Thomas SL, Childress MH, Quinton B. Hypoplasia of the odontoid with atlanto-axial subluxation in Hurler's syndrome. *Pediatr Radiol* 1985;15(5):353–354.
36. Tandon V, Williamson JB, Cowie RA, et al. Spinal problems in mucopolysaccharidosis I (Hurler syndrome). *J Bone Joint Surg Br* 1996; 78(6):938–944.
37. Hite SH, Peters C, Krivit W. Correction of odontoid dysplasia following bone-marrow transplantation and engraftment (in Hurler syndrome MPS 1H). *Pediatr Radiol* 2000;30(7):464–470.
38. Parsons VJ, Hughes DG, Wraith JE. Magnetic resonance imaging of the brain, neck and cervical spine in mild Hunter's syndrome (mucopolysaccharidoses type II). *Clin Radiol* 1996;51(10):719–723.
39. O'Brien DP, Cowie RA, Wraith JE. Cervical decompression in mild mucopolysaccharidosis type II (Hunter syndrome). *Childs Nerv Syst* 1997;13(2):87–90.
40. Langer LO Jr, Carey LS. The roentgenographic features of the KS mucopolysaccharidosis of Morquio (Morquio-Brailsford's disease). *Am J Roentgenol Radium Ther Nucl Med* 1966;97(1):1–20.
41. Blaw ME, Langer LO. Spinal cord compression in Morquio-Brailsford's disease. *J Pediatr* 1969;74(4):593–600.
42. Beighton P, Craig J. Atlanto-axial subluxation in the Morquio syndrome. Report of a case. *J Bone Joint Surg Br* 1973;55(3):478–481.
43. Taccone A, Tortori Donati P, et al. Mucopolysaccharidosis: thickening of dura mater at the craniocervical junction and other CT/MRI findings. *Pediatr Radiol* 1993;23(5):349–352.
44. Ashraf J, Crockard HA, Ransford AO, et al. Transoral decompression and posterior stabilisation in Morquio's disease. *Arch Dis Child* 1991; 66(11):1318–1321.
45. Lipson SJ. Dysplasia of the odontoid process in Morquio's syndrome causing quadriparesis. *J Bone Joint Surg Am* 1977;59(3):340–344.
46. Ransford AO, Crockard HA, Stevens JM, et al. Occipito-atlanto-axial fusion in Morquio-Brailsford syndrome. A ten-year experience. *J Bone Joint Surg Br* 1996;78(2):307–313.
47. Stevens JM, Kendall BE, Crockard HA, et al. The odontoid process in Morquio-Brailsford's disease. The effects of occipitocervical fusion. *J Bone Joint Surg Br* 1991;73(5):851–858.
48. Healey D, Letts M, Jarvis JG. Cervical spine instability in children with Goldenhar's syndrome. *Can J Surg* 2002;45(5):341–344.
49. Kondoh T, Yoshinaga M, Matsumoto T, et al. Severe cervical kyphosis in osteopathia striata with cranial sclerosis: case report. *Pediatr Radiol* 2001;31(9):659–662.
50. Currarino G. Primary spondylolysis of the axis vertebra (C2) in three children, including one with pyknodysostosis. *Pediatr Radiol* 1989; 19(8):535–538.
51. Edelson JG, Obad S, Geiger R, et al. Pyknodysostosis. Orthopedic aspects with a description of 14 new cases. *Clin Orthop* 1992;(280): 263–276.
52. Horton WA, Rimoin DL, Hollister DW, et al. Further heterogeneity within lethal neonatal short-limbed dwarfism: the platyspondylic types. *J Pediatr* 1979;94(5):736–742.
53. Goldberg MJ. Orthopedic aspects of bone dysplasias. *Orthop Clin North Am* 1976;7(2):445–456.
54. Martin RP, Deane RH, Collett V. Spondylolysis in children who have osteopetrosis. *J Bone Joint Surg Am* 1997;79(11):1685–1689.
55. Borman P, Ozoran K, Aydog S, et al. Osteopoikilosis: report of a clinical case and review of the literature. *Joint Bone Spine* 2002;69(2): 230–233.
56. Labauge R, Marty-Double C, Pages M, et al. Cleido-cranial dysostosis with malformation of the cervico-occipital junction. *Rev Neurol (Paris)* 1982;138(4):327–336.
57. Tsirikos AI, Mason DE, Scott CI Jr, et al. Spondyloepimetaphyseal dysplasia with joint laxity (SEMDJL). *Am J Med Genet* 2003; 119A(3):386–390.
58. Naik DR. Cervical spinal canal in normal infants. *Clin Radiol* 1970; 21(3):323–326.
59. Markuske H. Sagittal diameter measurements of the bony cervical spinal canal in children. *Pediatr Radiol* 1977;6(3):129–131.
60. Boltshauser E, Hoare RD. Radiographic measurements of the normal spinal cord in childhood. *Neuroradiology* 1976;10(5):235–237.
61. Cramer BC, Jequier S, O'Gorman AM. Sonography of the neonatal craniocervical junction. *AJR Am J Roentgenol* 1986;147(1):133–139.
62. Harlow CL, Drose JA. A special technique for cervical spine sonography. Illustrated by a patient with meningoencephalocele, Dandy-Walker variant, and syringomyelia. *J Ultrasound Med* 1992;11(9):502–506.
63. LeDoux MS, Naftalis RC, Aronin PA. Stabilization of the cervical spine in spondyloepiphyseal dysplasia congenita. *Neurosurgery* 1991; 28(4):580–583.
64. Lonstein JE. Post-laminectomy kyphosis. *Clin Orthop* 1977;(128): 93–100.
65. McLaughlin MR, Wahlig JB, Pollack IF. Incidence of postlaminectomy kyphosis after Chiari decompression. *Spine* 1997;22(6):613–617. Erratum in: *Spine* 1997;22(11):1276.
66. Roberts W, Henson LC. Anesthesia for scoliosis: dwarfism and congenitally absent odontoid process. *AANA J* 1995;63(4):332–337.
67. Auden SM. Cervical spine instability and dwarfism: fiberoptic intubations for all. *Anesthesiology* 1999;91(2):580.
68. Dormans JP, Drummond DS, Sutton LN, et al. Occipitocervical arthrodesis in children. A new technique and analysis of results. *J Bone Joint Surg Am* 1995;77(8):1234–1240.
69. Rodgers WB, Coran DL, Emans JB, et al. Occipitocervical fusions in children. Retrospective analysis and technical considerations. *Clin Orthop* 1999;(364):125–133.
70. Brockmeyer D, Apfelbaum R, Tippets R, et al. Pediatric cervical spine instrumentation using screw fixation. *Pediatr Neurosurg* 1995;22(3): 147–157.
71. Meyer B, Vieweg U, Rao JG, et al. Surgery for upper cervical spine instabilities in children. *Acta Neurochir (Wien)* 2001;143(8):759–765.
72. Farey ID, Nadkarni S, Smith N. Modified Gallie technique versus transarticular screw fixation in C1-C2 fusion. *Clin Orthop* 1999; (359):126–135.
73. Wang J, Vokshoor A, Kim S, et al. Pediatric atlantoaxial instability: management with screw fixation. *Pediatr Neurosurg* 1999;30(2):70–78.
74. Tokuhashi Y, Matsuzaki H, Shirasaki Y, et al. C1-C2 intra-articular screw fixation for atlantoaxial posterior stabilization. *Spine* 2000; 25(3):337–341.
75. Low HL, Redfern RM. C1-C2 transarticular screw fixation for atlantoaxial instability: a 6-year experience, and C1-C2 transarticular screw fixation—technical aspects. *Neurosurgery* 2002;50(5):1165–1166.
76. Brockmeyer DL, York JE, Apfelbaum RI. Anatomical suitability of C1-2 transarticular screw placement in pediatric patients. *J Neurosurg* 2000;92(1 Suppl):7–11.

77. Chen HJ, Cheng MH, Lau YC. One-stage posterior decompression and fusion using a Luque rod for occipito-cervical instability and neural compression. *Spinal Cord* 2001;39(2):101–108.

78. Graziano GP, Herzenberg JE, Hensinger RN. The halo-Ilizarov distraction cast for correction of cervical deformity. Report of six cases. *J Bone Joint Surg Am* 1993;75(7):996–1003.

79. Shah SA, Taliwal RT, Mason DE, et al. *The treatment of cervical instability in children with skeletal dysplasia.* Proceedings of the 27th annual meeting of the Cervical Spine Research Society. 1999.

80. Stabler CL, Eismont FJ, Brown MD, et al. Failure of posterior cervical fusions using cadaveric bone graft in children. *J Bone Joint Surg Am* 1985;67(3):371–375.

CHAPTER 36

Miscellaneous Conditions of the Cervical Spine

Neurofibromatosis, Juvenile Rheumatoid Arthritis, and Rickets

Alvin H. Crawford and Mohammed J. Al-Sayyad

Knowledge of such pediatric cervical spine disorders as neurofibromatosis, juvenile rheumatoid arthritis, and rickets is essential for the pediatric orthopedist and the spine surgeon. Detailed evaluation and appropriate early management may prevent potential serious neurologic damage and other complications related to the cervical spine.

NEUROFIBROMATOSIS

Neurofibromatosis is a spectrum of diseases involving not only neuroectoderm and mesoderm but also endoderm. It presents with a wide range of clinical manifestations that have in common the presence of schwannomas, neurofibromas, or café au lait spots, or a combination of these (1). Clinically, this multisystemic, hereditary disease may manifest as abnormalities of the skin, nervous tissue, bones, and soft tissues. The primary abnormality is believed to be a hamartomatous disorder of neural crest derivation.

Akenside (2), in 1768, described a patient with multiple neurofibromatosis; however, first credit is most frequently given to Wilhelm G. Tilesius von Tilenau for his 1793 clinical description of a patient with neurofibromatosis (3). In 1882, Frederick Daniel von Recklinghausen (4) coined the term *neurofibroma* and was able to demonstrate that a small cutaneous nerve was connected to each of the cutaneous and subcutaneous tumors. Thus, von Recklinghausen, with his clinical and pathologic description, was the first to associate the origin of the disorder with tumors from arising nerve sheaths (4).

This chapter deals with the primary and secondary effects of neurofibromatosis on the pediatric spine.

Diagnostic Problems

Most investigators now accept four clinical forms of neurofibromatosis (NF): peripheral (NF1), central (NF2), segmental, and mixed. A variety of eponyms have been used to describe all forms, although subsequent information has made these names technically inaccurate or incomplete. The most common type, peripheral neurofibromatosis (NF1), was previously known as von Recklinghausen's neurofibromatosis and is an autosomal dominant disorder affecting about 1 in 4,000 persons; multiple hyperpigmented areas (café au lait macules) and neurofibromas are characteristic.

The 1987 Consensus Development Conference of the National Institutes of Health on neurofibromatosis concluded that the diagnosis of von Recklinghausen's neurofibromatosis (NF1) was established when two or more of the following diagnostic criteria were found (5):

1. Six or more café au lait macules greater than 5 mm in widest diameter in prepubertal children and more than 15 mm in widest diameter in postpubertal individuals
2. Two or more neurofibromas of any type or one plexiform neurofibroma
3. Freckling in the axillary or inguinal regions
4. Optic glioma
5. Two or more Lisch nodules (iris hamartomas)

6. A distinctive osseous lesion such as sphenoid dysplasia or thinning of a long bone cortex with or without pseudarthrosis
7. A first-degree relative (parent, sibling, or offspring) with von Recklinghausen's disease identified by these criteria

Other disorders of pigmentation such as McCune-Albright or Watson's syndrome can be confused with von Recklinghausen's neurofibromatosis.

Genetics

Neurofibromatosis is the most common human single-gene disorder. It affects at least one million people throughout the world and is seen in all racial and ethnic groups. Approximately half of all people with NF1 will suffer serious medical and social complications.

In 1990, the gene locus for NF1 in humans was cloned and its protein product, neurofibromin, was identified (6). The NF1 gene is very large and has been linked to the long arm of chromosome 17. The NF2 locus is probably linked to the long arm of chromosome 22; this genetic linkage is useful for the accurate diagnosis in families that have a high risk for neurofibromatosis. Given the fact that several hundred families with NF1 have shown linkage to DNA markers on 17q (7,8), prenatal diagnosis for NF1 is possible. For the time being, NF1 prenatal diagnosis requires the genetic linkage approach, which means that only families in which two or more generations are already involved can use this aspect of health care (9). Continued rapid scientific progress is expected in molecular genetics for both NF1 and NF2. Such studies should lead to the development of a direct diagnostic test for NF1, which would be especially helpful in establishing the diagnosis in uncertain cases, such as young children with only café au lait spots. This will directly influence classification, patient care, counseling of families, and research.

Clinical Findings

Café au Lait Spots

Café au lait spots are present in well over 99% of all patients with neurofibromatosis. The pigmentation is tan, macular, and melanotic in origin and is located in and around the basal layer of the epidermis; the lesions may vary in shape, size, number, and location (Fig. 36.1A). In neurofibromatosis, these spots are frequently found in areas of the skin not exposed to the sun. The presence of one café au lait spot may be normal.

Lisch Nodules

Lisch nodules, or iris-pigmented hamartomas, are present in 94% of patients with neurofibromatosis who are 6 years of age or older; 28% of younger patients have them (10). They increase in number with age (11), but they do not become symptomatic. The lesions appear to be specific for NF1; they are not seen in normal persons or in patients with central acoustic neurofibromatosis or segmental neurofibromatosis. These nodules are not associated with other manifestations of neurofibromatosis or with the degree of severity, but they are helpful in establishing the diagnosis.

Neurofibromas

Neurofibromas mostly involve the skin, but they may be seen in deeper peripheral nerves. They may be nodular and discrete, or diffuse with interdigitation with surrounding tissues. Highly vascular plexiform neurofibromas may cause segmental or localized hypertrophy. Puberty or pregnancy may cause an increase in the size and number of the lesions (12). It is quite rare for neurofibromas to be present in the absence of café au lait spots (9).

Cutaneous Neurofibroma

Cutaneous neurofibromas, formerly called fibroma molluscum, are found in subcutaneous tissues after puberty. They are usually manifestations of long-standing or adult disease and do not occur with any frequency (12%) in childhood (13) (Fig. 36.1B). These tumors may grow under, be flush with, or be raised above the level of the skin; although they are usually the color of normal skin, early lesions may be violaceous. Recent electron microscopy studies have demonstrated that axons and Schwann cells are present in these tumors; therefore, it is appropriate that they be included under the term *dermal neurofibroma* (14).

Elephantiasis

Frequently, large soft-tissue masses are seen in neurofibromatosis. These masses have been termed *pachydermatocele* or *elephantiasis neuromatosa* and are characterized by a rough, raised, villous type of skin hypertrophy presenting an unmistakable appearance. Although more frequently occurring in adult life, they have been seen in children with varying degrees of involvement. Weiss (15) described this finding as characteristic of neurofibromatosis. There is usually dysplasia of the underlying bone when the lesion occurs in an extremity.

Pigmented Nevi

Eight percent of all patients presenting with neurofibromatosis have pigmented nevi, some presenting with geographic descriptions (e.g., nevus lateralus and "bathing trunk" nevi) (Fig. 36.1C). The nevus lateralus can be described as dark brown, pigmented skin over half the abdominal wall or back, with an abrupt change of pigmentation occurring along the midline. Nevi or hyperpigmentation may be present in up to 6% of children with neurofibromatosis (13), some of which are quite sensitive. The sensitivity is often related to an underlying subcutaneous plexiform neurofibroma.

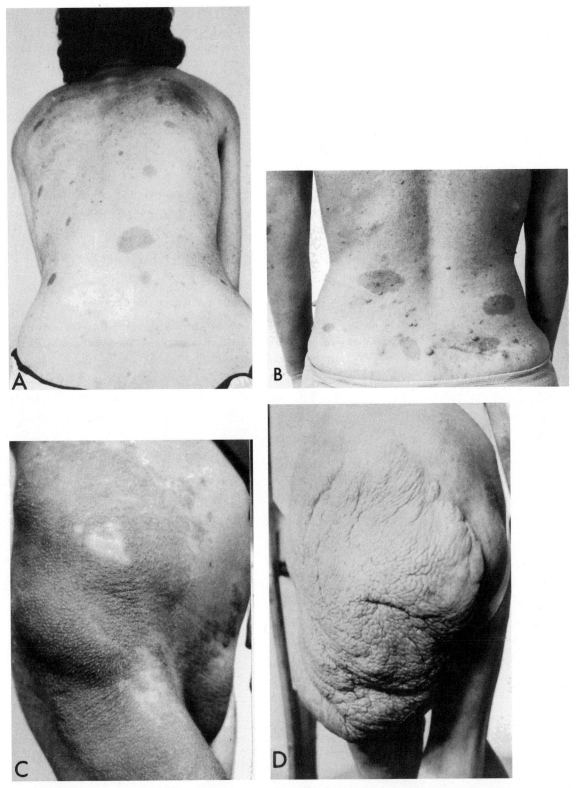

FIG. 36.1. Cutaneous lesions of neurofibromatosis seen in children include café-au-lait spots, fibroma molluscum, pigmented nevi, and verrucous hyperplasia. **A:** Multiple café-au-lait spots in a young patient with scoliosis. Note the variation in size and shape of lesions. These lesions tend to increase in size and number as the child matures. **B:** Multiple café-au-lait spots in an older patient who also has subcutaneous nodules (fibroma molluscum); that is, pedunculated lesions that occur in the postpubescent adolescent. This patient also has several subcutaneous neurofibromas of the intercostal nerves, which are sessile. **C:** This large nevus occurring on only one side of the trunk is the nevus lateralis. It can be quite sensitive, and several patients who had spinal curvatures could not tolerate external corrective devices (e.g., Milwaukee brace or Orthoplast jacket) because of this extreme sensitivity, which is believed to be related to an underlying plexiform neurofibroma. **D:** Verrucous hyperplasia of the skin over the left buttocks. This is the most grotesque of all cutaneous lesions. (From: Crawford AH. Neurofibromatosis in the pediatric patient. *Orthop Clin North Am* 1978;9:11–23.)

Plexiform Neurofibroma

Plexiform neurofibromas are subcutaneous neurofibromas that have a ropy, "bag of worms" feeling. Their cutaneous involvement may cause decreased sensation, causing sores to develop under a brace or cast without the patient's knowledge, or they may be hypersensitive. When a plexiform neurofibroma is found underlying an area of dorsal cutaneous hyperpigmentation, especially when the pigmentation approaches or crosses the midline of the body, it appears that the tumor will be aggressive and may originate from the spinal canal. The plexiform neurofibroma has the potential for malignant degeneration (13).

Optic Gliomas

Although optic gliomas account for only 2% to 5% of all brain tumors in childhood, as many as 70% of cases are found in persons with NF1. In many NF1 patients these tumors change little in size over many years, but a small percentage of such tumors may enlarge rapidly, leading to exophthalmos and visual impairment.

Verrucous Hyperplasia

Verrucous hyperplasia is an infrequent but definite cutaneous lesion of neurofibromatosis. There is tremendous overgrowth of the skin, with thickening of a velvety-soft papillary quality (Fig. 36.1D). Many crevices form and tend to break down easily, with some weeping occurring in the skin folds. The sites often become superficially infected and may give rise to a foul odor. The lesion presents most often unilaterally and can be considered one of the most grotesque lesions of neurofibromatosis.

Axillary and Inguinal Freckling

Freckles—diffuse, small, hyperpigmented spots up to 2 to 3 mm in diameter—found in the armpits and inguinal

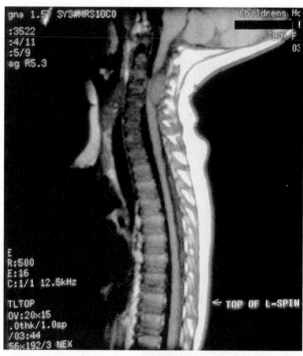

A

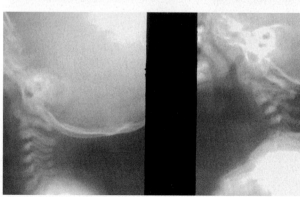

C

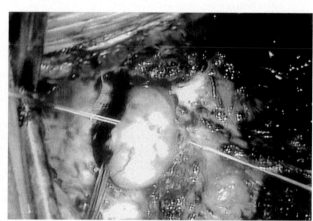

B

FIG. 36.2. This 8-year-old child was noted to have instability of the cervical spine at the C4-5 region. There were dystrophic changes in the vertebral bodies. There is significant deformity of the posterior elements of C2, C3, and C4, and they appear to be absent. Although the instability is similar to that seen following laminectomy, no surgery had been performed. **A:** True lateral radiograph of cervical spine in upright position. Note the apparent absence of the posterior elements of C3-5 and the forward subluxation of C4 on C5. **B:** True lateral radiograph of cervical spine in flexion. Note the severe flexion angle at C4-5 and the marked dystrophic changes in the vertebral bodies. **C:** Oblique view of cervical spine illustrating marked widening of neuroforamina and elongation of the pedicles. (From: Crawford AH. Neurofibromatosis. In: *The pediatric spine: principles and practices.* New York: Raven Press, 1992:619–647.)

region (areas not usually exposed to sunlight) are helpful diagnostic criteria for neurofibromatosis. Freckling and an occasional dermal fibroma may be the only physical findings in the parent of a child who shows all the criteria required for the diagnosis of neurofibromatosis.

Spinal Deformities

Spinal deformities have been noted to occur only in peripheral neurofibromatosis (NF1). The deformities include nondystrophic and dystrophic changes. The dystrophic changes may be intrinsic or associated with spinal canal anomalies secondary to abnormalities of the spinal cord dura mater.

The relative prevalence of spinal deformities in neurofibromatosis is unknown. In a general orthopedic clinic, 2% of the scoliosis population will have neurofibromatosis; in a scoliosis clinic population, approximately 3% will have it. In a neurofibromatosis population, the percentage of patients having some disorder of the spine will vary from 2% to 36% (16,17). According to most authors, the scoliosis associated with neurofibromatosis is usually in the thoracic area and tends to produce a short-segmented, sharply angulated curvature; it usually includes four to six vertebrae and is progressive.

Recent investigators have suggested that there is no standard pattern of spinal deformity in neurofibromatosis; the types of curvature found are variable. Cobb (18) was one of the first to recognize the seriousness of the spinal deformity and especially the deleterious effect of laminectomy in a patient with neurofibromatosis and scoliosis. He also believed that a high proportion of scoliosis classified as idiopathic was possibly secondary to neurofibromatosis.

Radiographic Findings

On plain radiographs, careful attention should be directed to the sagittal plane for evidence of abnormal lordosis, kyphosis, or dystrophic changes. Anteroposterior and lateral radiographs of the cervical spine are recommended at the time of original evaluation of all spinal deformities in patients with neurofibromatosis. If dystrophic changes are noted, oblique radiographs to rule out so-called dumbbell lesions (enlargement of neuroforamina due to intraspinal meningoceles, solitary tumors, or interstitial hypertrophic neuritis) and lateral flexion and extension radiographs to rule out instability should be obtained (Fig. 36.2). One should be suspicious of posterior scalloping of the vertebral bodies or of an increase in the size of the neural foramina, indicating the presence of a spinal canal lesion. These lesions may cause substantial compression to the spinal cord, and their removal has presented considerable technical difficulties. Multiple-view radiographs of the cervical spine are necessary before general anesthesia or halo traction to rule out dystrophic deformity and possible instability.

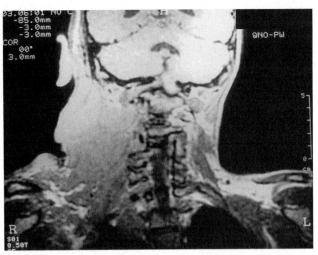

FIG. 36.3. Neck pain and neurological symptoms in this 3-year-old child was evaluated by magnetic resonance imaging (MRI). A tumor was noted in the upper cervical region abutting the spinal cord. She underwent a cervical hemilaminectomy to remove the neurofibroma and developed kyphosis within a 6-month period. **A:** Lateral MRI showing large neurofibroma abutting spinal cord from posterior. **B:** Intraoperative clinical photograph of tumor at time of removal. **C:** lateral cervical spine radiographs dated March 1998 and September 1998, before and after hemilaminectomies to remove and extradural neurofibroma. This was rapid development of kyphosis with 6 months.

Computed tomography (CT) has been used extensively to identify the occasional abnormal structure of the spine in neurofibromatosis; it allows one to assess the spinal canal, its contents, and the associated anatomy. Three-dimensional reconstruction enhances the explicitness of the bony detail. The addition of contrast myelography to CT has allowed the surgeon to identify lesions found in and about the spinal canal. Magnetic resonance imaging (MRI) can be utilized to determine the internal contents of the spinal canal and will show the presence of lesions within and about the spinal cord itself (Fig. 36.3). There are occasional problems interpreting magnetic resonance images of severe deformities because of distortion brought on by the complex three-plane deformity of kyphoscoliosis (19) (Fig. 36.4).

Management of Deformities

Cervical Deformities

The cervical spine deformity is usually kyphosis. Until recently, only casual references to the cervical spine have been evident in studies of other manifestations of neurofibromatosis. Many patients with cervical spine deformities are asymptomatic and show no clinical signs. Even so, curves in this area are more frequently associated with dysplastic lesions than in other areas of the spine (20).

Yong-Hing and associates (21) reviewed 56 patients with neurofibromatosis specifically for abnormalities of the

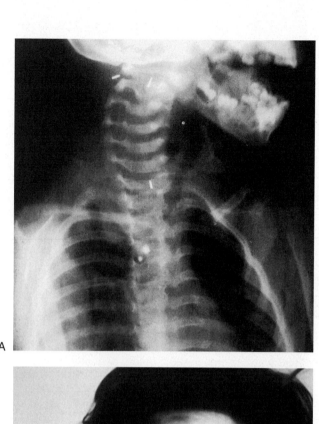

A

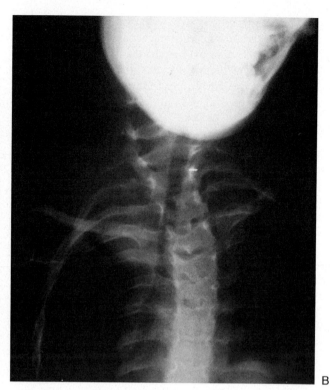

B

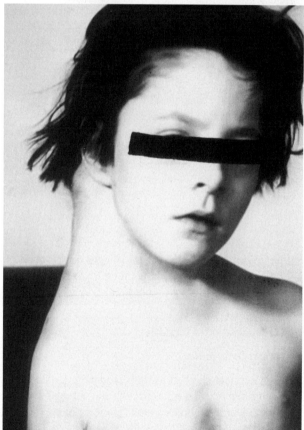

C

FIG. 36.4. Sixteen-year-old child with large plexiform neurofibroma and verrucous hyperplasia of the skin over the right side of her neck. The frontal magnetic resonance image shows tremendous soft-tissue overgrowth with heterogenous changes in the cervical nerve roots and erosions of the vertebrae.

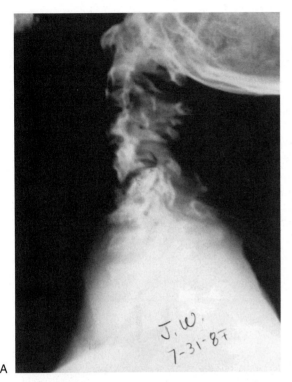

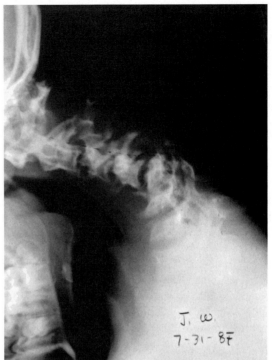

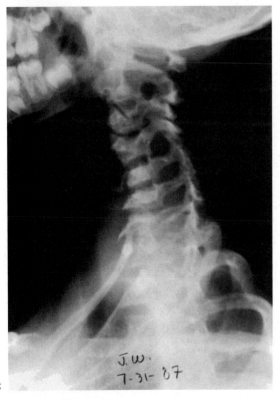

FIG. 36.5. Young child who presented with torticollis and cervical mass. She was noted to have a plexiform neurofibroma over right side of her neck. She underwent with partial reduction but the mass continued to grow. **A:** Frontal radiograph of cervical spine following multiple attempts at reduction of the neurofibromas. Note vascular clips. **B:** Frontal radiograph of cervical spine 3 years later showing widening of neuroforamina increase in soft-tissue shadows and progression of her torticollis. **C:** Clinical photo at 5 years old. Note torticollis and fullness of neck consistent with cervical plexiform neurofibroma.

cervical spine and found 17 to have lesions. Of 37 patients who had thoracic scoliosis or kyphosis, 15 (44%) had cervical spine lesions; many of these patients were asymptomatic. Adkins and Ratvich (22) reviewed 85 patients with von Recklinghausen's neurofibromatosis and found that head and neck masses were responsible for 22% of the patients' complaints. Five cases of atlantoaxial dislocation have been reported in patients with neurofibromatosis, two of whom were noted to have neurofibromas between the odontoid and anterior arch of C1 (21,23,24).

The clinical consequences of cervical NF1 tend to be less marked than in other regions because the cord versus canal diameter is commonly less critical. Because of its generally asymptomatic nature, the problem is probably underreported. However, these lesions should not be disregarded because the tendency of the disease to progress has led to severe neurologic deficits in several cases (25,26).

Any evidence of bony deformity noted on cervical spine radiographs requires orthopedic consultation. Other reasons for consulting an orthopedist and obtaining cervical spine radiographs in a patient with NF1 include torticollis and dysphagia (Fig. 36.5). Both conditions may be related to intraspinal as well as extraspinal neurofibromas.

Posterior spinal arthrodesis is recommended for a severe cervical spine deformity with instability. Autologous bone graft and halo immobilization is usually adequate, and a solid fusion can be expected. If there has been previous surgery such as laminectomy, it may be necessary to perform anterior surgery as well. With the use of laser technology, neurofibromas in this region can now be removed without compromise to the spinal cord. Because of the amount of bone removal required to completely excise the tumor and the resulting instability, posterior spinal fusion should always be carried out (Figs. 36.6 and 36.7). The level of instability will often require an occipitocervical arthrodesis. More recently, the use of pedicle screws into the cervical lateral masses and occiput to enable rod support has improved surgical stabilization when the posterior elements are absent (Fig. 36.8). A halo-assisted orthosis may be utilized to stabilize the occipitocervicothoracic area until fusion takes place.

Paraplegia

Most articles on neurofibromatosis and spinal deformities have included an incidence of paraplegia (27–29). It is

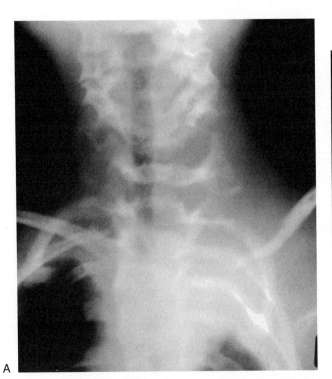
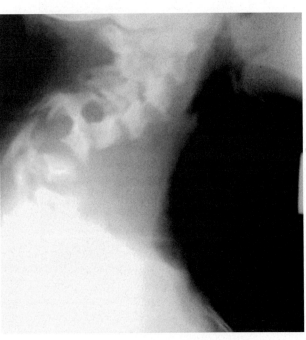

A

B

FIG. 36.6. Thirteen-year-old child's anteroposterior and lateral radiographs following multiple laminectomies without stabilization. There was a large unilateral plexiform mass interdigitating with the cervical nerve roots and extending into the chest wall. No attempts at fusion were carried out following laminectomies. **A:** Frontal radiograph of cervical spine showing dysplastic changes in the vertebra with widening of the neuroforamina. The changes are unilateral in the cervical spine as well as upper ribs and clavicle. The soft-tissue density is indicative of underlying large plexiform neurofibromas. **B:** Lateral cervical spine radiograph showing significant kyphosis and virtual unhinging of the C5-7 posterior elements.

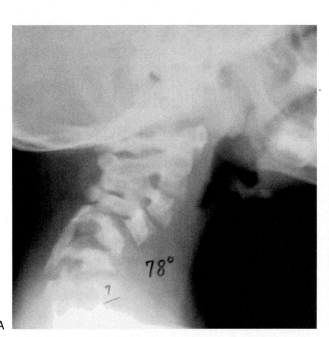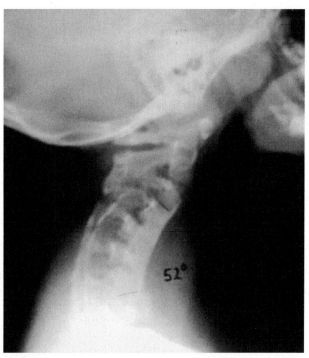

A

B

FIG. 36.7. This child underwent multiple laminectomies for cervical tumors, resulting in destabilization and kyphosis. He underwent an uninstrumented anterior and posterior fusion and was seen 15 months later. **A:** Lateral cervical spine radiograph showing kyphosis of the lower cervical spine, widened neuroforamina, and absence of the posterior elements C4-7. **B:** Fifteen months later there is improvement of the kyphosis following anteroposterior fusion from C4-T2.

possible that neurologic compromise may be related to tumor, structural instability of the vertebral column complex, dural ectasia, vertebral destruction, neurofibromas, neurosarcomas, fibrofatty tissue reaction, severe kyphosis, vertebral subluxation, dislocation, protrusion of ribs into the spinal canal, or progressive dystrophy of the bony elements of the spine. A neoplasm is usually responsible for paraplegia in older patients, whereas spinal malalignment or ribs displacing into the spinal canal are the most common causes in younger individuals. Kyphosis contributes more than scoliosis to neurologic impairment. Rockower and associates (30) reported two patients who, because of vertebral body instability and displacement secondary to neurofibromatous tissue encroachment, developed paraplegia; the problem was solved by carefully monitored traction and spinal arthrodesis. Traction should be used very rarely when the deformity is mostly kyphotic. Traction should be used only with *flexible* kyphosis—never if the kyphosis is rigid. If the kyphosis is rigid, an anterior release, disc excision, and fusion followed by posterior spinal fusion is recommended.

Major and Huizenga (31), Flood and colleagues (32), and Tredwell (33) reported cases of spinal cord compression caused by ribs protruding into the spinal canal. In Major and Huizenga's report, one of the patients had transient paraplegia

following trauma and the other two were investigated and diagnosed prospectively based on the first experience (31). Using CT, these authors were able to demonstrate that the rib heads had penetrated the enlarged neuroforamina, entered the spinal canal, and compressed the thoracic spinal cord. It could be speculated that occult rib penetration into the spinal canal with spinal cord compromise could be a source of paraplegia that, prior to current imaging technology (CT, MRI), was thought to be the natural course of neurofibromatosis with kyphoscoliosis.

With the advent of hardware systems that can apply considerable force to the spine, there is a clear risk of neurologic injury in the presence of instability of the rib end and potential spinal canal protrusion. When contemplating operative treatment in these patients, or if there is a neurologic deficit, the surgeon should carefully evaluate preoperative MRI scans or high-volume CT myelograms, looking for protruding rib ends (31).

For those patients with paraplegia and neurofibromatosis, one must first rule out an intraspinal lesion (tumor, meningocele) as opposed to kyphotic angular cord compression (34). Those with severe spinal curvatures without major kyphosis and with evidence of paraplegia should be assumed to have intraspinal lesions until proved otherwise. An MRI or high-volume CT myelogram done in the prone,

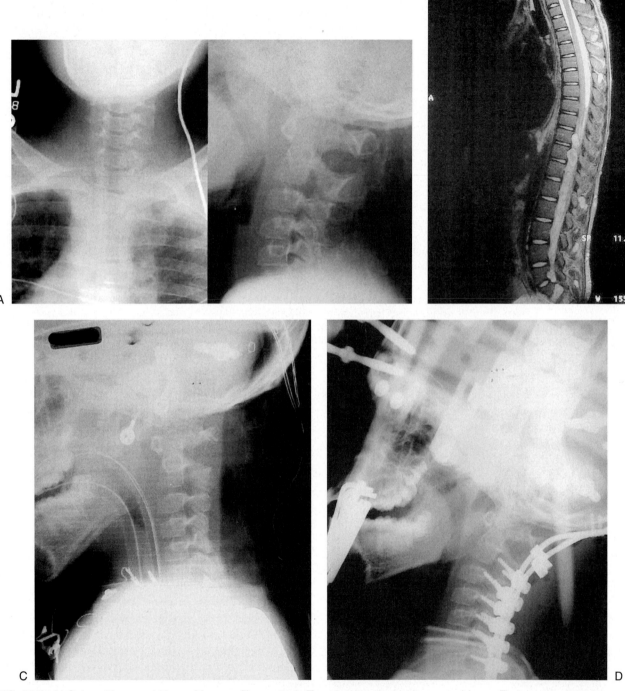

FIG. 36.8. M.S. is a 10-year-old boy with neurofibromatosis Type I who noted balance problems. Two months later he was no longer able to walk. Three weeks later he had a loss of bowel and bladder control and lacked antigravity strength in his proximal muscles. Magnetic resonance imaging revealed a lesion abutting the cervical cord. He underwent wide posterior element release followed by transpedicular fixation, which tended to resolve his neuropathy. **A:** anteroposterior and lateral views of the cervical spine showing no obvious abnormality. **B:** The midsagittal magnetic resonance image shows the invasion of the neurofibroma into the spinal canal. Note the high signal lesion behind the fourth cervical vertebra compressing the spinal cord. Other neurologic lesions can be identified in the soft tissue about the spinous process of T12 and L2. Note the dumbbell lesions appearing to exit at levels T9-10, T10-11, and L5-S1. **C:** Lateral view of the cervical spine showing C1-C6 laminectomy and resection of numerous neurofibromas. **D:** Lateral view of the cervical spine showing the posterior spine fused from occiput to C7 with instrumentation and iliac crest bone graft. The patient is immobilized in a halo vest. **E:** Anteroposterior and lateral view of the cervical spine illustrating stable construct and early fusion.

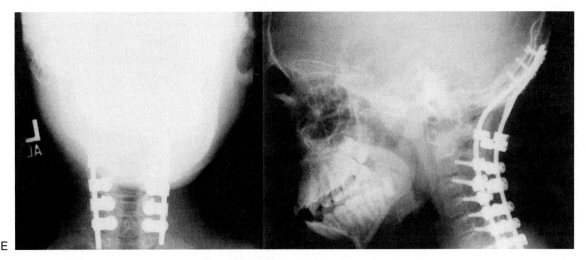

FIG. 36.8. *Continued*

lateral, and supine positions or three-dimensional CT will better elucidate the anatomy of severe spinal deformities (Fig. 36.9). This author has not been able to perform adequate MRI studies in patients with severe deformities because of distortion. If the kyphosis is mobile and no intraspinal tumor is present, the patient should be placed in halo-assisted traction; this must be done with extreme caution and neurologic monitoring. This procedure should definitely not be performed if the kyphosis is rigid. Even if the kyphosis is mobile and there is paraplegia, the author recommends that somatosensory evoked potentials be monitored during traction. If a tumor is anterior, immediate anterior excision, spinal cord decompression, and arthrodesis should be carried out; if the lesion is posterior, a hemilaminectomy with tumor excision and posterior spinal arthrodesis should be performed. If total laminectomy is required, posterior spinal arthrodesis is mandatory. The posterior arthrodesis should be performed with the addition of segmental spinal instrumentation if possible; if not, a halo cast should be applied. Deep wound drainage is necessary in all patients having spinal canal exploration because of the substantial bleeding that may occur once the patient is normotensive. The patient should be observed carefully for development of pseudarthrosis, and augmentation of the fusion mass should be carried out directly if such evidence is present.

Spinal instrumentation and arthrodesis in the face of unrecognized intracanal neurofibroma or structural instability of the laminae due to dural ectasia can cause serious neurologic compromise. Therefore, preoperative neuroradiographic evaluation of the spinal canal is warranted. Winter and associates (35) reported two cases of paralysis due to contusion of the spinal cord by the subperiosteal elevation during exposure of the posterior elements in patients who had unsuspected areas of laminar erosion due to dural ectasia.

Problems Related to Soft Tissue Involvement

Dural Ectasia

A finding unique to neurofibromatosis and Marfan's syndrome is an expansion of the dural sac, which often causes deformity of the adjacent spinal canal and vertebral bodies (36). It expands the spinal canal at the expense of the bony and ligamentous elements (Fig. 36.10). This wide expanse of the spinal canal may explain why, despite the severe progressive deformities of the spine seen in NF1, the spinal cord is rarely injured. The same does not hold true if a neurofibroma develops in the spinal canal, where it can provoke medullary compression, as can any space-occupying lesion. This expansion is responsible for the destabilization of the vertebra, giving rise to spontaneous dislocation (30) of the vertebra as well as penetration of the canal by ribs that have separated from the costotransverse ligaments (31,32). The continuation of this expanding dural sleeve more than likely gives rise to meningocele.

Intrathoracic Meningocele

Intrathoracic meningocele is relatively rare; no more than 88 cases have been reported in the English-language literature (37–40). Pohl (41) reported the first case of a meningocele associated with neurofibromatosis. A meningocele in this instance is a protrusion of the spinal meninges through an intervertebral foramen or bony defect of the vertebra; it contains an extension of the subarachnoid space filled with cerebrospinal fluid.

Meningocele in association with neurofibromatosis can occur at any level of the spine. A posterior mediastinal mass in a patient with neurofibromatosis, particularly if associated with kyphoscoliosis, is most likely a lateral meningocele. With contrast myelography, ultrasonography, or MRI, a well-demarcated soft tissue cystic mass is seen protruding

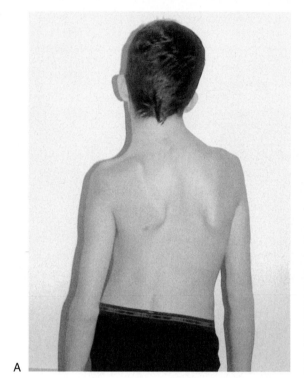
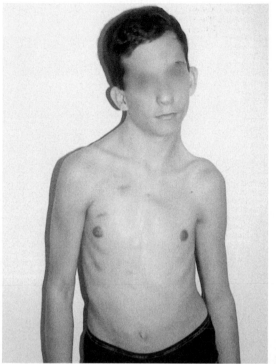
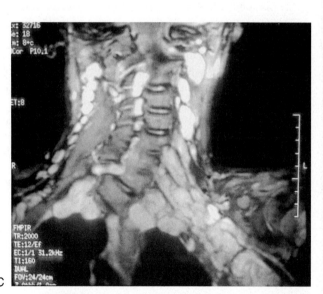
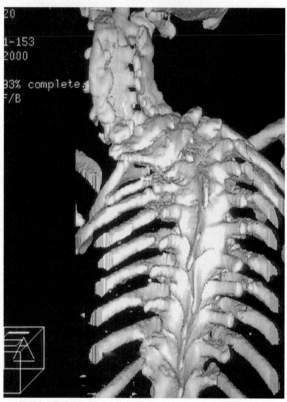

FIG. 36.9. J.S. a 17-year-old patient with neurofibromatosis Type 1 noted to have cervical plexiform neurofibromas, cervical lordosis, and congenital kyphoscoliosis of the upper thoracic spine. He had undergone multiple partial laminectomies of the cervical spine and presented for treatment of scoliosis. **A:** Clinical photograph from posterior showing right dorsal scoliosis truncal imbalance with elevation of right shoulder. **B:** Frontal clinical photograph showing elevation of right shoulder, torticollis, and cervical as well as thoracic scoliosis. **C:** Magnetic resonance image of cervical spine illustrating hypertrophic nerve roots with plexiform neurofibromatous changes exiting the neuroforamina. **D:** Posterior view of three-dimensional (3-D) reconstructed cervical and upper thoracic spine. Note changes of cervical partial laminectomies with absence of ring of C1 and a hemivertebra with two extra transverse processes and ribs on the right T2-3 vertebra. **E:** Anterior view of 3-D reconstructed computed tomography of cervical and upper thoracic spine. Note congenital kyphoscoliosis of upper thoracic spine.

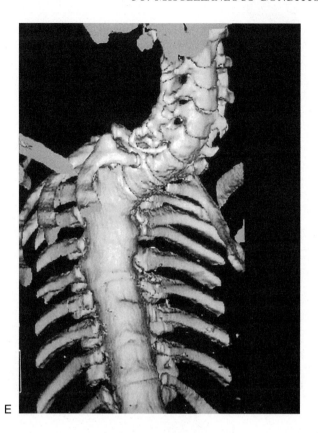

FIG. 36.9. *Continued*

from the spinal canal into the posterior mediastinum. It is often associated with kyphoscoliosis as well as other localized dystrophic bone changes and is usually found at the apex of the kyphoscoliosis on the convex side (39,42). Structural defects in the pedicles, enlargement of the intervertebral foramina, rib deformities including costotransverse dislocation, and scalloping of the vertebral bodies may accompany the mass. Several etiologies for the condition have been implicated, including nerve root sleeve elongation (43) (similar to a hernia of the meninges through the neuroforamina), cystic degeneration in a neurofibroma (44), trauma (45), dural dysplasia, bone dysplasia, regional dystrophy, and congenital derangement. The more likely explanation is that regional dysplasia affecting both bone and meninges is responsible for the formation of the meningocele (46,47).

The posterior scalloping of the vertebral bodies, with deformities of the pedicle and widening of the intervertebral foramina, could be caused either by the presence of a dumbbell tumor (intraspinal neurofibroma) or by saccular dilatations of the dura (dural ectasia). There is a distinct potential instability due to the loss of supporting bone structure when associated with kyphoscoliosis. It is possible that neurofibromatous meningoceles and dural ectasia are variations of the same phenomenon, with the meningocele being more localized and possibly related to its exit through the neuroforamina, and the dural ectasia being more diffuse. Thoracic and sacral meningoceles in patients with NF1 may develop secondary to the growth of ectatic dural outpouchings through preexisting bony deformities, such as enlarged neuroforamina, when exposed to changing cerebrospinal fluid pressures (48).

Most meningoceles (60%) are discovered incidentally on routine radiologic examination of the chest. Pain, though not a characteristic feature, was noted by Miles and associates (39) in 23% of cases; in all but one of the cases, kyphoscoliosis was noted.

Neurologic abnormalities are uncommon (6%) with meningocele, except for those associated with kyphoscoliosis. Pulmonary symptoms (cough 10%, dyspnea 11%) have been associated only with massive intrathoracic lesions.

Because intrathoracic meningoceles are often symptomless, the question of treatment is difficult. If it is a chance radiologic finding and causes no symptoms, the right course would be observation. If there is definite progressive enlargement, an initial attempt should be made to ligate the sac. It may be feasible to occlude the neck of the sac by plicating sutures via video-assisted thoracoscopy. Excision of the lesion is indicated for progressive excavation of the vertebra, neurologic injury, or respiratory distress or if there is evidence of rapid progression in size.

Dumbbell Lesions

A dumbbell lesion is one in which the neurofibroma is constricted as it exits the neuroforamina, giving it the

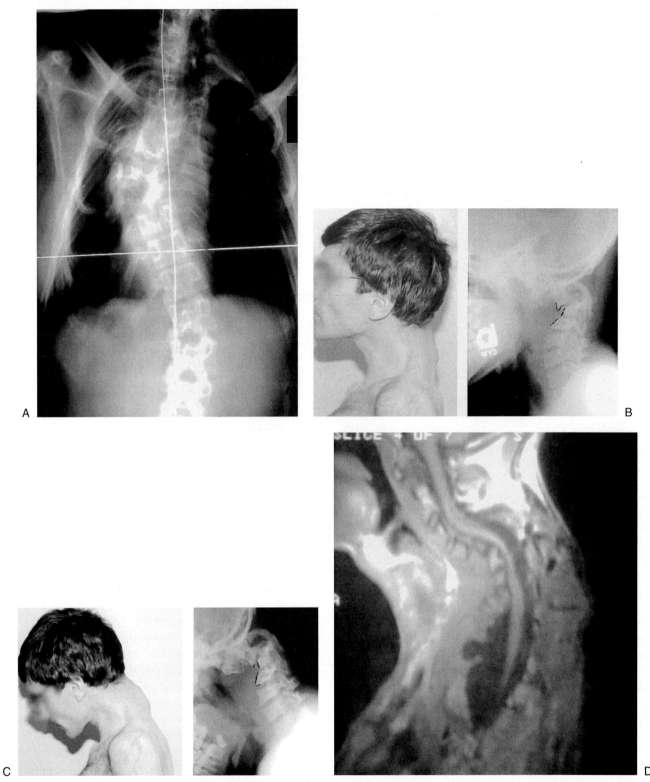

FIG. 36.10. Thirty-nine-year-old man with multiple cervical neurofibromas and thoracic scoliosis. The cervical spine lesion was right sided and extended into the chest. He underwent multiple laminectomies with excision of the cervical neurofibroma 5 years ago. The presence of dural ectasia was noted coincidentally on the cervicothoracic magnetic resonance imaging (MRI) extending into the vertebral bodies. **A:** Coronal thoracolumbar spine radiograph showing right thoracic scoliosis. Note the dysplastic changes of the right rib cage with widening of the intercostal spaces. **B:** Clinical and radiographic lateral view of cervical region. There is obvious clinical and radiographic kyphosis with absence of the posterior elements of the upper four vertebrae. **C:** Clinical and radiographic lateral flexion view of cervical region. There is obvious increase in clinical kyphosis with subluxation of the C3 area. **D:** Sagittal MRI reveals kyphosis with erosive changes of dural ectasia in the vertebral bodies of the upper thoracic spine in addition to the pos laminectomy soft-tissue changes.

494

appearance of a weight lifter's dumbbell. Love and Dodge (49) defined dumbbell neurofibroma of the spine as a benign neoplasm that arises from a nerve root and grows in such a way that two or more portions of the tumor are connected by a narrow stalk through an intervertebral foramen, through the interlaminar space of the vertebra, or through the dura mater. They may be intradural and extradural, intradural, extradural, or extradural and extraspinal. Prior to CT and MRI, this lesion had been identifiable by the widening of the neuroforamina seen primarily on oblique views (Fig. 36.11). It was once thought that central erosion of the vertebral body was by dural ectasia, whereas lateral erosion of the foramina was from a neurofibroma. The tumors may occur at any level of the cord, but the cervical and thoracic levels are most often involved. The tumors may present as nodules arising from the sheath along the nerve, or they may actually invade the nerve. If the tumor invades the nerve with consequent interstitial hypertrophy, then "the nerve becomes the tumor and the tumor becomes the nerve." In this case, resecting the tumor results in a neurologic deficit. The prevalence of malignant degeneration of peripheral neurofibromas is unknown.

We reviewed 260 pediatric patients with NF1 and noted that 9 patients (3.5%) had extrapleural thoracic tumors (50). Ninety-five of these patients were primarily screened by chest radiographs, and many patients might have asymptomatic thoracic tumors that have yet to be diagnosed. All patients were 6 years of age or older. Six were asymptomatic, and 3 presented with respiratory symptoms. A clue to thoracic involvement in 2 patients was the presence of a visible plexiform neurofibroma in the neck, which later was found to have extended into the chest. Focal scoliosis was a major clue to an underlying tumor in 4 patients, and bony changes such as narrowing of ribs were often seen in the area of tumor involvement. Malignant transformation of a benign plexiform neurofibroma occurred in 1 patient. Signs on physical examination that should raise suspicion of an underlying thoracic tumor include a plexiform neurofibroma of the neck or a focal area of scoliosis. When reviewed retrospectively, 8 of the 9 patients had either a symptom or sign on physical examination that was a clue to the underlying tumor. Surgical management of these tumors can be difficult because of frequent involvement of nerves and blood vessels (51).

Vertebral Column Dislocation

Complete dislocation of the spine in neurofibromatosis is rare. In one review of 55 patients who had neurofibromatosis and spinal deformity, only 2 had a lateral subluxation or dislocation of the spine (52); one of the dislocations involved a thoracic vertebra and posterior arch with destruction of the latter, and the other patient had destruction of the articular part of the apophysis. In another study of eight patients who had neurofibromatosis and paraplegia, five patients had a vertebral subluxation or dislocation (28).

Involvement of the cervical spine by neurofibromatosis was noted in one study in which five patients had subluxation of a cervical vertebral body (53). In a second study of 56 patients, 17 had abnormal cervical spines; 1 patient had a fixed subluxation of the second cervical vertebra on the third, and another had an atlantoaxial rotatory instability (21). Isu (54) reported on three patients (two with hemiparesis) who had atlantoaxial dislocation due to neurofibromatosis. He pointed out that laxity of capsular and ligamentous structures in patients with neurofibromatosis may contribute to a predisposition to instability of the cervical spine. Scott's (55) study of scoliosis associated with neurofibromatosis showed a cervical thoracic dislocation, but no details were provided of the history and physical findings. Rockower and colleagues (30) reported two cases of spinal dislocation after minor trauma in children who had neurofibromatosis. One patient had a dislocation of the fourth thoracic vertebra on the fifth and no neurologic deficit. At surgery, neurofibromatous tissue was found to envelop the vertebral bodies anteriorly but not posteriorly. The second patient had a dislocation of the sixth cervical vertebra on the seventh and was quadriparetic. Stone and associates (56) reported a 9-year-old child with neurofibromatosis who had complete dislocation of the first thoracic vertebra on the second anteriorly, with the body of the seventh cervical vertebra situated completely anterior to that of the second thoracic vertebra following a 2-day history of pain in the lower part of the neck. Complete reduction following traction and manipulation was not successful. Surgery resulted in the child having a solid union with no neurologic deficits (56).

Substantial subluxation or dislocation of the spine in patients who have neurofibromatosis can occur with little radiographic or clinical warning because the osseous erosion is so extensive. This diagnosis should be considered in any patient who has neurofibromatosis and unexplained pain in the neck or back. Although similar erosion of bone can be caused by tumor tissue, with diagnostic techniques such as CT, myelography, and especially MRI, one can easily distinguish between tumor and ectasia. The mechanism of dural expansion and osseous erosion is unknown. When seen at operation, the dura in the area of ectasia is extremely thin and fragile. Therefore, every effort should be made to avoid entry into the region of the dural ectasia. Aggressive surgical stabilization should be carried out when radiographic examination reveals instability of the spine, which may precede dislocation (57).

Plexiform Venous Channels

McCarroll (58) pointed out that a plexiform type of venous anomaly may be encountered in the soft tissues; these may surround the spine, impeding the operative approach to the vertebral bodies. In one of Hsu's patients with angular kyphosis, the venous anomalies were so dense that the anterior approach to the internal kyphos had to be abandoned

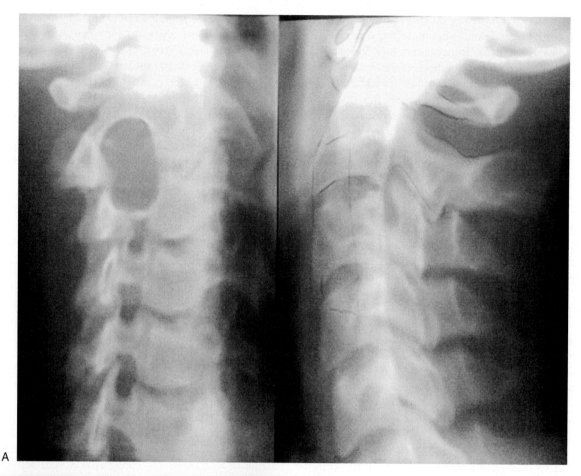

A

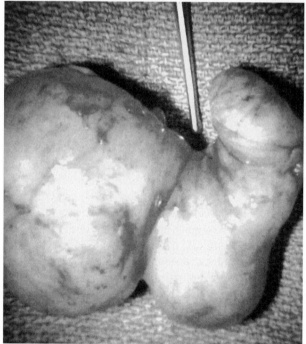

B

FIG. 36.11. A: Oblique and lateral cervical spine radiograph revealing expanded single C2-3 neuroforamina. This is the classic characteristic change seen with a solitary "dumbbell" neurofibroma of the cervical spine. It represents the exit of a neurofibroma through the neuroforamina. **B:** Dumbbell tumor was removed from the neural foramen. The dumbbell appearance refers to the conscription of the neurofibroma that occurs at the neural foramen, where the lesion exits the spinal canal. (From: Crawford AH, Schorry EK. Neurofibromatosis in children: the role of the orthopaedist. *J Am Acad Orthop Surg* 1999;7:217–230.)

because of excessive bleeding (59). Greene and associates (60) classified vascular neurofibromatosis in two categories according to the diameter of the vessel; the larger vessels (greater than 1 mm, such as the aorta, carotid, and proximal renal arteries) that are surrounded by or involved with neurofibromatous tissue reveal intimal hypertrophy, fragmentation of the medial and elastic laminae, and a fibrous adventitial reaction leading to stenosis or aneurysm formation. This author has not experienced excessive venous bleeding while performing anterior removal of neurofibromatous tissue and strut grafting, but warns the reader of the possibility. Wound hematomas following surgery have not been a problem; however, meticulous hemostasis and wound drainage should be carried out.

Pseudarthrosis

Pseudarthrosis occurs more commonly following attempted spinal arthrodesis for both dystrophic and nondystrophic curvatures than for idiopathic ones. The prevalence is higher in those associated with kyphosis of greater than 50 degrees. Prior to the use of segmental spinal instrumentation and anterior-posterior combined surgeries, reexploration was routine for patients with neurofibromatous spinal deformities. The best results are obtained by planning a double arthrodesis right from the start. Even the increased strength of the new spinal column instrumentation may be insufficient to obtain stability at the time of surgery when dealing with deformed dystrophic posterior elements. Use of postoperative orthoses or antigravity casts following anterior and posterior fusions using autogenous bone graft is crucial. Sirois and Drennan (61) speculated that future MRI refinement may permit identification of pseudarthrosis, because calcium ions in the fusion do not return MRI signals. The author has no experience with this technique.

Summary

Careful attention should be paid to the vertebral body shapes on the posteroanterior and lateral spine radiographs. When one sees scalloping and indentation of vertebral bodies, a careful investigation should be carried out for intraspinal pathology such as dural ectasia, meningocele, or dumbbell lesion. The scalloping has been associated with intraspinal neurofibromatosis as well as with the expansion of the dural sac, suggesting dural ectasia or a meningocele. Scalloping can exist only with one of the aforementioned eroding factors. The implication that the deformity is primarily a vertebral or developmental defect associated with neurofibromatosis and not dependent on pressure erosion is incorrect. Because some intraspinal myelography studies have shown that the contrast material does not conform to the posterior scalloped surfaces of the vertebrae, there is a suggestion of an intervening intradural mass. These masses have been clearly elucidated by modern diagnostic technologies such as CT, myelography, and especially MRI.

The vertebral scalloping and dysplasia represent an indirect manifestation of a proximal tumor. Because of the possibility of an intraspinal tumor or dural ectasia, it is strongly recommended that contrast CT or MRI be performed on those patients with dystrophic vertebral bodies and curvatures requiring instrumentation and fusion (62). The author recommends MRI assessment of any areas demonstrated by CT myelogram to be suspicious, as well as any areas that are poorly demonstrated. Three-dimensional CT is currently being used to further delineate the anatomy of severe deformities. The improvement of CT software promises to enhance the value of this technology.

Careful evaluation of the cervical spine is indicated prior to instrumentation of the thoracic or lumbar spine. The most dangerous situation for the neurologically intact neurofibromatosis patient and the surgeon is instrumentation and manipulation of the spine in the presence of unrecognized intraspinal lesions. More often than not, the patient will present to the spinal surgeon with a significant deformity with or without an intraspinal tumor or expansive dura, with no evidence of a neurologic disorder or paraplegia. This author currently utilizes four methods of spinal cord monitoring: short-latency somatosensory evoked potential (SSEVP), neurogenic motor evoked potential (NMEP), electromyography, and the "wake-up" test.

Although correction is the goal of the spine surgeon in idiopathic scoliosis, halting the progression of the deformity, even with a small correction, can be considered a good result in the case of NF1 spinal deformities. The surgeon's responsibility is to stabilize the spine in the most expedient, permanent, and safest way without causing permanent neurologic injury.

JUVENILE RHEUMATOID ARTHRITIS

Juvenile rheumatoid arthritis (JRA) is a systemic disease of childhood characterized by chronic synovitis and is often accompanied by extraarticular disease. JRA is the most common rheumatic disease of childhood and is one of the most common chronic illnesses occurring in children. The annual incidence ranges from 10 to 14 per 100,000 (63,64). The overall prevalence of JRA in the United States has been estimated to be between 57 and 113 per 100,000 children younger than 16 years (65). The etiology of JRA is unknown. It is likely that multiple initiating factors are involved, including infection, trauma, and autoimmunity, all in conjunction with a genetic predilection for arthritis. Involvement of the cervical spine in JRA is common and occurs in 50% of patients who have the polyarticular and systemic onset types (66–68). Ansell suggested that the neck may be the initial site of involvement in 2% of patients with early JRA (68).

Diagnostic Problems and Types of Juvenile Rheumatoid Arthritis

In North America, the most frequently used criteria for making the diagnosis have been those of the American

TABLE 36.1. *America College of Rheumatology Criteria for the Diagnosis of Juvenile Arthritis*

Age at onset	Less than 16 years
Arthritis	One or more joints
Duration of disease	6 Weeks or longer
Onset type	In the first 6 months
Polyarthritis: five or more joints	
Oligoarthritis: fewer than five joints	
Systemic: arthritis with characteristic fever at onset	
Exclusion	Other forms of juvenile arthritis

From: Smith RW. *A treatise on the pathology, diagnosis, and treatment of neuroma.* Dublin: Hodges and Smith, 1849.

College of Rheumatology (Table 36.1) (69). These criteria define the subtypes of JRA according to the mode of onset, with each group having diagnostic and prognostic significance. The International League of Associations of Rheumatologists (ILAR) proposed (70) and revised (71) criteria for the diagnosis and classification of juvenile arthritis, known as the Durban criteria (Table 36.2). The term *juvenile idiopathic arthritis* (JIA) has been proposed to replace JRA and encompasses all juvenile arthritides lasting longer than 6 weeks that are of unknown cause.

The classes according to the American College of Rheumatology are as follows:

1. *Oligoarticular onset (pauciarticular onset):* Defined as arthritis affecting one to four joints during the first 6 months of disease. It is the most frequently encountered subgroup, comprising 40% to 60% of children with JRA. The peak age of onset is 2 years. Girls are affected four times more frequently than boys (72). Cervical spine involvement is rare.

2. *Polyarticular onset:* Defined as arthritis affecting five or more joints during the first 6 months of disease. It is the next most common form of JRA, found in 30% to 40% of children with JRA. Girls predominate. There are two peak ages of onset: 1 to 3 years of age and early adolescence. Symmetric involvement of both knees, wrists, and ankles is most characteristic. Involvement of the cervical spine, hips, and temporomandibular joints is not uncommon. In most patients the onset is insidious, although in a few the disease begins with low-grade fever and acute polyarthritis.

   There are two distinct subgroups of polyarthritis: those with and without the presence of rheumatoid factor (RF). RF-negative polyarthritis can occur at any age (73). This group is associated with an increased incidence of uveitis (5%) (74). RF-positive polyarthritis occurs predominantly in older girls (>8 years). These children are more likely to have a symmetric small joint arthritis, rheumatoid nodules, and early erosive synovitis with chronic course (75,76). However, these children rarely develop uveitis.

3. *Systemic onset:* Defined as JRA that begins with high, spiking fevers greater than 39.4°C (103°F). It is the least

TABLE 36.2. *Durban Criteria*

Age at onset: before 16th birthday
Arthritis in one or more joints
Duration of disease: at least 6 weeks
Onset type:

Systemic arthritis
Arthritis with or preceded by daily fever of at least 2 weeks' duration, accompanies by one or more of the following:
1. Evanescent, nonfixed erythematous rash
2. Generalized lymph node enlargement
3. Hepatomegaly or splenomegaly
4. Serositis

Polyarthritis (rheumatoid factor-negative)
Arthritis affecting five or more joints during the first 6 months of disease; tests for rheumatoid factor are negative

Psoriatic arthritis
1. Arthritis and psoriasis, or
2. Arthritis and at least two of:
   a. Dactylitis
   b. Nail abnormalities (pitting or onycholysis)
   c. Family history of psoriasis confirmed by a dermatologist in at least one first-degree relative

Other arthritis
Children with arthritis of unknown cause that persists for at least 6 weeks, but that either:
1. Does not fulfill criteria for any of the other categories, or
2. Fulfills criteria for more than one of the other categories

Oligoarthritis
1. Persistent oligoarthritis: no more than four joints involved
2. Extended oligoarthritis: affect a cumulative total of five or more joints after the first 6 months of disease

Polyarthritis (rheumatoid factor-positive)
Arthritis affecting five or more joints during the first 6 months of disease, associated with positive rheumatoid factor tests on two occasions at least 3 months apart

Enthesitis-related arthritis
Arthritis and enthesitis, or arthritis or enthesitis with at least two of:
1. Sacroiliac joint tenderness and/or inflammatory spinal pain
2. Presence of HLA-B27
3. Family history of HLA-B27–associated disease in at least one first- or second-degree relative
4. Anterior uveitis that is usually associated with pain, redness, or photophobia
5. Onset of arthritis in a boy after the age of 8 years

common form of JRA, affecting about 20% of children with JRA, girls and boys about equally. Typically, systemic onset JRA begins between 5 and 10 years of age. Cervical spine stiffness is common and can mimic meningismus, although severe neck pain and torticollis are rare. Other systemic manifestations include myocarditis, generalized lymphadenopathy, hepatosplenomegaly, vasculitis, and iritis.

Many children with oligoarticular and polyarticular arthritis will have a normal erythrocyte sedimentation rate and C-reactive protein level. The frequency of antinuclear antibody positivity is greatest in younger girls with oligoarticular arthritis and represents an increased risk for anterior uveitis (77). All children with confirmed arthritis should have a routine ophthalmologic exam with slit lamp. Rheumatoid factor is an autoreactive antibody, usually IgM. RF positivity is infrequent in children with arthritis, and rarely occurs in children under 7 years of age.

Espada and associates (78) reported that children with atlantoaxial subluxation were more frequently seropositive for RF: 10 (45%) of 22 patients with atlantoaxial subluxation and 18 (20%) of 91 patients without atlantoaxial subluxation were seropositive. Hensinger and colleagues (79) studied 121 patients with JRA, with an average follow-up of 6.9 years (range, 1–21 years). None of the 57 patients with pauciarticular onset JRA had cervical symptoms or signs, and only one had minor radiographic changes of disease in the cervical spine. In contrast, clinical stiffness and radiographic changes in the cervical spine occurred commonly in the 51 patients with polyarticular onset disease and in the 13 patients with systemic onset disease. Fried and associates (80) reported that of 92 patients treated for JRA, only 29 had cervical involvement; of the 15 patients who were available for review, 11 had polyarticular arthritis, 3 had systemic JRA, and 1 had pauciarticular disease.

Genetics

The majority of the associations of JRA have been with the human leukocyte antigen (HLA) class II antigens, which are restricted to cells of lymphoid origin. In oligoarticular arthritis, there is an increased association with HLA-DR8, HLA-DR6, and HLA-DR5, with relative risks of 2 to 27, meaning that a child who carries one or more of these genes has a 2- to 27-fold increased risk of developing the disease, compared with the population as a whole. The presence of uveitis is correlated with HLA-DR5 (81). Polyarticular onset arthritis with positive rheumatoid factor is associated with HLA-DR4, whereas HLA-DR7 seems protective. RF-negative polyarticular disease is associated with HLA-DR8, HLA-DPw3, and HLA-DQw4, with relative risk factors of 3 to 10. Systemic onset disease has overlapping risk factors, showing an association with HLA-DR4, HLA-DR5, and HLA-DR8, with relative risks ranging from around 2 to 7 (82).

Polymorphism in the *IL-1α* gene was found to be associated with uveitis and pauciarticular arthritis in Norwegians (83). Children who have an *IL-6* genotype, which has a relatively higher transcription rate when stimulated, may be at greater risk for systemic arthritis (84).

Clinical Findings and Cervical Spine Deformities

Except for rare cases, patients present with peripheral arthritis first and cervical spine involvement later. When obtaining the history, ask patients and parents about neck pain, morning stiffness, trauma history, subjective weakness, gait changes, and urinary incontinence; enquiry about other joint involvement and eye symptoms should follow. The sequence of joint involvement should also be recorded. Detailed cervical spine examination should include documentation of neck range of motion and a thorough neurologic assessment, looking particularly for signs of myelopathy. Limitation of extension is the first and most easily documented involvement of the cervical spine. Loss of lateral flexion is also noted early. Loss of flexion is less significant clinically. Red flags in the history and physical examination should include incoordination, sensory changes, urinary incontinence, persistent torticollis, progressive or acute paresis, weakness, change in deep tendon reflexes, and spasticity.

Cervical stiffness is the most common finding and has been reported in 46% to 64% of patients (66,85). Hensinger and associates (79) evaluated 27 patients in their first year of illness; a 34% incidence of limitation of cervical motion was documented in the first month, and this incidence increased to 64% by the end of the first year.

Neck pain has been reported in only 2% to 17% of patients (85). Neither severe neck pain nor torticollis, occurring either separately or concomitantly, is frequently found in these patients, and its presence may suggest an intercurrent problem. Only 12 of the 121 patients reported by Hensinger and associates (79) complained of pain in the neck. As a rule, patients between 6 and 11 years old who have JRA do not complain of pain and tend not to describe the involved joints as painful (86,87). Older patients, between 12 and 17 years old, tend to report painful sensations more frequently, which may account for the apparent later onset of symptoms.

Torticollis is commonly seen in children with cervical spine involvement; rarely, patients may present with rapid-onset torticollis. This was reported in 1 of 121 patients discussed by Hensinger and colleagues (79). Uziel and associates (67) reported a 6-year-old girl who developed nontraumatic acute torticollis that had been treated with a soft collar for 2 weeks. This patient was then admitted with high-grade fever and severe torticollis; imaging studies revealed atlantoaxial rotatory fixation and atlantoaxial subluxation. On the fifth day of hospitalization, she developed symmetrical arthritis of her elbows, wrists, hips, knees, and ankles. This patient with systemic onset JRA was treated with traction, indomethacin, and corticosteroids. Uziel and colleagues (67) suggested that inflammation of the bursa between the odontoid process and transverse ligament may cause transverse ligament laxity and that the atlas then slides anteriorly. Ansell (68) reported two patients with persistent torticollis.

Lateral mass collapse of the first cervical vertebra resulting in head tilt without rotation has been reported (79).

Atlantoaxial Subluxation

There have been only two reports of early instability in which the onset of axial subluxation was the first indication of JRA, and polyarthritis subsequently developed in both children (88,89). Nathan and associates (89) reported a

6-year-old girl who presented to the Mayo Clinic with neck pain, restriction of neck motion, and an extensor plantar response. Radiographs showed atlantoaxial subluxation, and C1-C2 arthrodesis was carried out. On postoperative day seven, the patient developed acute arthritis of the left knee, and further testing led to the diagnosis of JRA (89).

Fried and colleagues (80) also reported on 2 patients (of 92 patients with JRA) who developed myelopathy. In one patient, a 5-year-old girl with pauciarticular disease, long tract signs, and the atlantoaxial subluxation resolved spontaneously at the age of 11 years; the other patient was a 17-year-old girl in whom the disease had started at the age of 2.5 years and who had hyperreflexia and clonus secondary to atlantoaxial subluxation. Taseski and associates (90) reported on four children with JRA who developed atlantoaxial subluxation, two of whom had long tract signs, and concluded that a preventive treatment can be performed to prevent neurologic complications.

Subaxial Instability

Symptoms or signs of nerve root impingement or myelopathy have been an infrequent finding in children with JRA (80). Ferlic and associates (91) reported the case of a 14-year-old boy with instability at the articulation of the sixth and seventh cervical vertebrae in whom paresthesia of the hands and pain in the neck developed. He required stabilization of the cervical spine and had a solid fusion; his neck pain resolved. Isaacson (129) reported a case in which the cervical spine was fused solidly above C5 and also fused below C6, with the disc between C5 and C6 remaining open; the child developed early nerve root and cord compression symptoms necessitating fusion.

Swan-neck deformity develops as a result of multiple dislocation levels in the cervical spine. Fracture of the odontoid process occurs due to attenuation of the odontoid from the inflammatory reaction resulting in patients presenting with neck pain and stiffness.

Juvenile Rheumatoid Arthritis in Conjunction with Down Syndrome

JRA in conjunction with Down syndrome is unusual and can combine the most serious hazards of each condition. Spontaneous atlantoaxial dislocation in the presence of JRA and Down syndrome was reported by Thalmann and associates (93). Their patient did not have myelopathy and was treated by posterior cervical fusion (93). Andrews (94) reported the case of a 14-year-old girl with myelopathy due to atlantoaxial dislocation; the child had both JRA and Down syndrome. The subluxation in Andrews's case was stabilized with posterior cervical fusion, using wire and autogenous bone graft. Following surgery, the neck pain and torticollis resolved, but the patient remained wheelchair bound. Fried and colleagues (80) reported two patients with Down syndrome and JRA who developed atlantoaxial

subluxation and quadriparesis; both cases died suddenly. Sherk and associates (95) reported a 10-year-old patient with Down syndrome in whom a fixed rotatory displacement of the first cervical vertebra on the second developed approximately 4 years after the onset of polyarticular JRA and was treated with C1-C2 fusion. Four years later the patient developed swan-neck deformity of the cervical spine with dislocation of the fusion mass (C1-C3) on C4. Reduction and posterior fusion from C1 to C6 was carried out. The patient died 6 weeks after surgery, and autopsy showed thromboembolism of the pulmonary artery and vein to be the cause of death (95).

Radiographic Findings

Radiographic changes in JRA are not seen as frequently as in adult rheumatoid arthritis (RA). Radiographic evidence of cervical spine abnormalities in JRA was reported in 27% to 80% of patients in different series (96,97). According to Cassidy, atlantoaxial subluxation is the most characteristic abnormality of the cervical spine in JRA (98). Other investigators consider cervical interapophyseal joint fusion to be the most frequent and characteristic change (78,97–99). The radiographic manifestations of JRA that differ most from adult RA include the following (100,101):

- Relatively late destruction of articular cartilage and bone
- Growth disturbance
- Spondylitis of the cervical spine with associated vertebral subluxation and ankylosis of the apophyseal joint
- Micrognathia

Radiographs are obtained at the onset of JRA as a baseline. In symptomatic patients, assessment includes anteroposterior, open-mouth, lateral, and supervised lateral flexion-extension views. To evaluate for neurologic impingement, CT with myelography or MRI is indicated; to evaluate patients for cervical spine fracture, radionuclide scans, and CT scans are helpful.

Martel (100) and Martel and associates (101) have described five areas of change in the cervical spine. Hensinger and colleagues (79) expanded their classification to seven areas to better reflect the evolution of changes in the odontoid process and in the articulation of the first and second cervical vertebrae. The areas of change are as follows:

1. Anterior erosion of the odontoid process, which is defined as a change in the normal contour of the anterior aspect of the odontoid process at its articulation with the ring of the first cervical vertebra.
2. Anterior-posterior erosion of the odontoid process (the so-called apple core odontoid process). This describes the appearance of the combination of anterior and posterior erosion of the odontoid process due to synovitis. The location of the erosion is due to the position of the synovial joints adjacent to the odontoid process, specifically, its articulation posteriorly with the transverse atlantal

ligament as well as anteriorly with the ring of the first cervical vertebra (100,102). Hensinger and associates (79) reported on two patients with JRA seen in consultation for fracture of an attenuated odontoid process.

3. Subluxation of the first cervical vertebra on the second, which was considered to be present if the distance between the posterior aspect of the anterior ring of the first cervical vertebra and the anterior cortical margin of the odontoid process, measured on radiographs made in flexion, was more than 4 mm. Using this criterion, whenever an apple core odontoid process or extensive anterior erosion of the odontoid process was present, the patient was considered to have subluxation of the first cervical vertebra on the second. This narrowing of the odontoid process permits more movement and a relative increase in the distance (more than 4 mm) between the first cervical vertebra and the odontoid process with flexion. The latter is considered hypermobility rather than a true subluxation.

Swischuk (103) defined the posterior cervical line as a guide in evaluating physiological displacement of the second cervical vertebra on the third. He noted that in normal children, with forward flexion of the cervical spine, the second cervical vertebra slides forward so that its posterior arch comes into a straight-line relationship with the posterior arches of the first and third cervical vertebrae. An intact posterior cervical line indicates that the transverse atlantal ligament and capsular structures are still competent and capable of maintaining the integrity of the articulation of the first and second cervical vertebra. When this line is disrupted, it suggests true subluxation of the first cervical vertebra on the second, with either failure of the soft tissue structures or fracture of the odontoid process or both.

4. The leading edge of the anterior aspect of the ring of the first cervical vertebra is a focal soft tissue calcification appearing adjacent to the ring of the first cervical vertebra, in the anterior atlantooccipital membrane and the atlantoaxial ligament. The etiology of calcification in this area is unknown, but may reflect excessive traction producing osteophytes secondary to hypermobility of the first cervical vertebra relative to the second cervical vertebra and the occiput.

5. Ankylosis of the apophyseal joint was recorded when fusion of the posterior elements was identified. Spontaneous fusion occurred initially in the posterior elements and only later involved the vertebral bodies and disc spaces. Fried and associates (80) reported ankylosis of the facet joints in 4 of 15 cases studied radiographically. Ankylosis of the zygapophyseal joints between the second and third cervical segments is considered particularly characteristic of JRA by some investigators (78, 97,99) (Figs. 36.12, 36.13, and 36.14).

6. Growth abnormalities, change in the longitudinal and circumferential growth between adjacent vertebral bodies, and decreased disc height were preceded by posterior fusion.

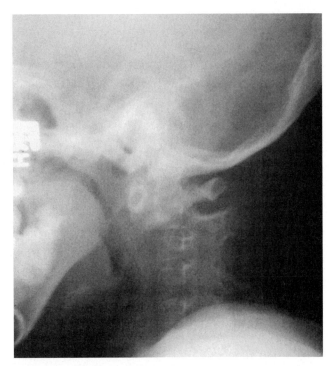

FIG. 36.12. This 12-year-old child with juvenile rheumatoid arthritis underwent undergone spontaneous arthrodesis of the cervical spine below C1. Her clinical motion was surprisingly good in spite of the radiographic findings.

7. Subaxial subluxation between the second and the seventh cervical vertebrae was defined as any change in the relationship between the body or the facet joints of the vertebrae below the second cervical vertebra. This is often associated with ankylosis of the facet joints above or below the area of the subluxation; patients with severe ankylosis often had dramatic subluxation.

Espada and associates (78) reported on the radiographic findings of the cervical spine in 120 patients with JRA. Fifty-seven patients (47%) had polyarticular onset disease, 32 (27%) had pauciarticular onset disease (when followed, only 5 patients had a pauciarticular course), and 31 (26%) had systemic onset disease. Seventy-eight of the 120 patients had a persistent and progressive disease pattern. Twenty-four patients had an atlantodens interval of more than 4.5 mm, and 4 had an atlantodens interval of more than 7 mm; no symptoms or signs of nerve root impingement or myelopathy were found. Erosions of the odontoid occurred in 13% of patients; only 2 patients had the apple core odontoid process. Apophyseal joint fusion was found in 62 patients. C2-C3 fusion was more frequent and was present in 59 of these 62 patients. In 8 patients bony ankylosis involved the entire cervical spine. Various types of perispinal calcifications were observed in 35 of the 120 patients. Twelve patients had linear soft tissue calcifications around the atlas. Posterior longitudinal ligament calcifications were found in 8 patients, and slight anterior longitudinal ligament calcifications were simultaneously present in 3 patients. Growth

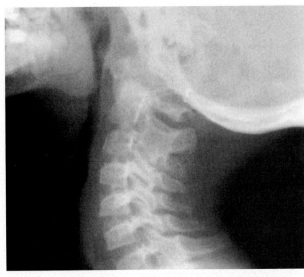
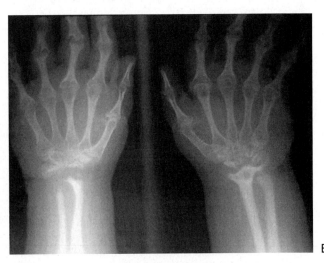

FIG. 36.13. This 15-year-old girl with juvenile rheumatoid arthritis underwent spontaneous fusion of the C2-3 vertebral joints. She has severe extremity involvement. **A:** Lateral cervical spine radiographs revealing C2-3 fusion. **B:** Right and left wrist following multiple carpectomy excisional arthroplasty changes.

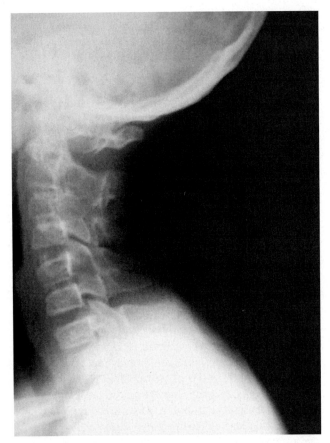

FIG. 36.14. This 14-year-old boy with systemic juvenile rheumatoid arthritis of 11 yrs. Duration was noted to have erosive arthritis of multiple extremity joints and chronic neck pain with limitation of motion. The lateral cervical spine radiograph showed noncontiguous posterior fusions of C2-4 and C5-6.

disturbance, with decreased vertical and anteroposterior diameters of the vertebral bodies and decreased height of the intervertebral discs, was observed in 22% of patients (78).

Children with growth disturbance had an earlier age of disease onset, with an average of 4 years (78). Hensinger and colleagues (79) noted that in general, children with polyarticular disease exhibited more destructive changes in the upper part of the cervical spine, whereas those with systemic onset disease more often had ankylosis of the apophyseal joints.

Management of Cervical Spine Involvement in Juvenile Rheumatoid Arthritis

Nonoperative

Virtually all patients with JRA will be started on a nonsteroidal antiinflammatory drug (NSAID) for control of symptoms. Several selective inhibitors of cyclooxygenase-2 have been marketed and have been used for children who cannot tolerate the usual NSAIDs. These agents have less gastrointestinal toxicity but can cause hepatic and renal side effects (104). Short courses and low doses of glucocorticoids can be useful for rapid and sustained control of inflammation.

The past decade has seen major advances in the treatment of chronic inflammatory arthritis, and simultaneous use of several pharmacologic agents is possible. Medications include methotrexate, leflunomide, hydroxychloroquine, etanercept and sulfasalazine. Methotrexate in a low dose is a major advance in the treatment of JRA; it is given weekly either as an oral dose or subcutaneously (105). If no substantial improvement is observed within a few months of starting the methotrexate, other antirheumatic agents such as sulfasalazine and hydroxychloroquine can be added. The most promising drug to emerge recently is etanercept (106). Etanercept is a biological agent, a tumor necrosis factor (TNF) receptor. In essence, it decreases the amount of available TNF, which in turn decreases the inflammatory response.

Hot packs and range of motion exercises can help prevent deformity (84). Attention to posture, adjusting chair or table height when studying, use of wide mirrors when driving, and avoidance of carrying heavy loads are important. A fitted cervical spine collar tailored so that the chin just rests on the top of the collar can provide excellent pain relief and help maintain a good head position, avoiding the tendency toward increasing flexion. Collars can be especially helpful during long study periods, while watching TV, or when traveling in the car. Patients with involvement of the odontoid process or subaxial subluxation are instructed to use a cervical collar whenever they are in an automobile or in transit.

Operative

Surgical treatment should be reserved for those patients with severe instability, progressive neurologic deterioration, and intractable pain. Procedures include laminectomy, decompression of nerve roots or spinal canal, and spinal fusion. The choice of procedure, anatomical location, and timing of the specific surgical intervention should be individualized and based on the child's symptoms, signs, and radiographic findings. The outcome is generally favorable, and early identification of neurologic impingement and prompt surgical treatment provide the best outcome (79,107).

Neck stiffness, loss of cervical lordosis, and micrognathia can make intubation difficult in patients with JRA, which must be kept in mind during preoperative planning. Care must be taken in handling the neck of these patients to avoid fracture of an already compromised odontoid process.

Summary

The inflammatory process in the cervical spine in patients with JRA is similar to that in the peripheral joints. The normal cervical spine has 32 synovial articulations. The three most common lesions that result in cervical instability are atlantoaxial subluxation, basilar invagination, and subaxial subluxation. Children have less pain and a much lower incidence of neurologic compromise and complications compared with adults with RA. If severe pain or torticollis or both develop in a patient with JRA, one should suspect that there is an additional problem such as infection, fracture, or tumor, rather than assume that these findings are manifestations of JRA. Stiffness of the cervical spine is a common early finding in patients with polyarticular and systemic onset JRA. Newer therapies are available to help control the disease so that joint damage is minimal and function is maintained, but we need to remember that the natural course of JRA is extremely variable. Most children do well with early recognition and management.

RICKETS

Although there are numerous etiologic pathways, all the disease states grouped under the label *rickets* have as their pathogenic mechanism a relative decrease in calcium, phosphate, or both, which is of such magnitude that it interferes with the process of epiphyseal growth and normal mineralization of the skeleton of the growing child.

Diagnostic Problems

Numerous factors are involved in the pathogenesis of rickets (Table 36.3). The symptoms, signs, and radiographic findings rarely provide clues as to the cause of the disease, with the exception of renal osteodystrophy. In general, changes associated with nutritional rickets appear earlier and are milder than those of vitamin D–resistant rickets (108). Patients with chronic renal disease have findings consistent with secondary hyperparathyroidism. It is essential to consider the pathogenesis of the particular type of rickets before starting a treatment plan. Deficiency rickets primarily include vitamin D deficiency, possibly calcium deficiency, phosphate deficiency, and the presence of chelators in the diet.

Children with deficiency rickets usually show low to low-normal serum calcium and phosphorus levels, elevated levels of alkaline phosphatase, elevated parathyroid hormone, and low concentration of 25-hydroxyvitamin D and 1,25-hydroxyvitamin D. Gastrointestinal causes are more common in most settings in the United States and mostly involve hepatic and bowel disease; these patients will have altered hepatic function tests and diminished absorptive capacity. Vitamin D–resistant rickets may be acquired or genetic in origin.

TABLE 36.3. *Causes of Rickets and Osteomalacia*

Deficiency diseases
Vitamin D deficiency
Chelates in the diet
Phosphorus deficiency
Gastrointestinal disorders
Gastric rickets
Hepatobiliary disease
Enteric disorders
Vitamin D–resistant rickets (acquired or genetic)
Phosphate diabetes
Decrease in 1,25-dihydroxyvitamin D production
End-organ insensitivity
Renal tubular acidosis
Unusual forms of rickets
Rickets with fibrous dysplasia
Rickets with neurofibromatosis
Rickets with soft-tissue bone tumors
Rickets with anticonvulsant medication
Renal osteodystrophy

Genetics

Hereditary forms of rickets include pseudo vitamin D–deficiency rickets (PDDR) with mutation in the coding sequence for 25-hydroxyvitamin D-1α-hydroxylase; it has an autosomal recessive inheritance (109). Other inherited forms include hereditary vitamin D–resistant rickets with mutation in coding for vitamin D receptor; it has an autosomal recessive inheritance, and close to 20-point mutation in the vitamin D receptor has been described (110). The most common type of rickets related to renal tubular defect is hypophosphatemic vitamin D–resistant rickets, which is inherited as an X-linked dominant trait. Occasionally, however, autosomal dominant inheritance is observed.

Clinical Manifestation and Cervical Spine Involvement

Children with rickets are described as being apathetic and irritable, often with a short attention span. The height of children with rickets is often under the third percentile. These patients may show bowing of one or both tibias; in addition, they may have thickened wrists and ankles. In florid cases the spine can be affected and presents as smooth dorsal kyphosis and occasionally slight to moderate scoliosis. There might be some flattening of the vertebral body end plates (Fig. 36.15). In young children, flattening of the skull, delayed dentition, and enlargement of the costal cartilages can be seen.

Secondary basilar invagination may occur. This is a deformity of the osseous structures that form the base of the skull at the margin of the foramen magnum. The tip of the odontoid is located more cephalad in its position. In rickets, it is a developmental condition that is usually attributed to softening of the osseous structures at the base of the skull, with the deformity developing later in life (111,112). This complication is rare, but is discussed in textbooks frequently (albeit briefly) in sections dealing with causes of basilar invagination. These patients will frequently have a short neck. Many patients with secondary basilar invagination have been discovered with severe invagination and no neurologic symptoms or signs. If symptoms occur, they are usually related to crowding of the neural structures at the level of the foramen magnum, particularly the medulla oblongata. If posterior encroachment predominates, the presenting symptoms may be those of raised intracranial pressure. Nystagmus seems particularly common with basilar invagination. Impingement on the pyramidal tracts is associated with weakness, hyperreflexia, and spasticity.

Spinal cord compression from ossification of the posterior longitudinal ligament (OPLL) has been reported by Yoshikawa and associates (113). They reported on tetraplegia occurring in two untreated adults with hypophosphatemic vitamin D–resistant rickets from compression of the spinal cord by an OPLL-like process. This is the only available report on such a problem.

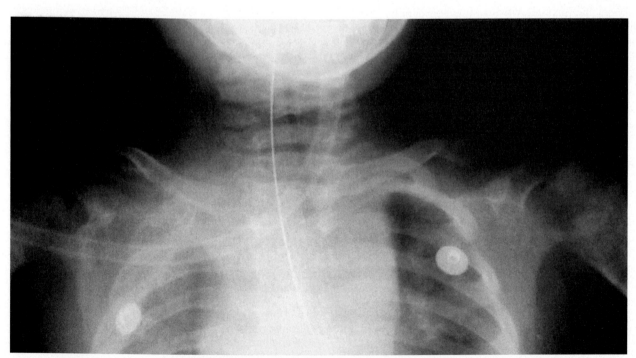

FIG. 36.15. A 4 + 7-year-old boy with oncogenic rickets (with multiple nevi). Anteroposterior radiograph shows the poor definition of endplates of the vertebral bodies of the cervical spine. The end plates in childhood are zones of provisional calcification, which therefore remain soft-tissue dense rather than calcified in active rickets. (Case contributed by Alan Oestreich from Cincinnati Children's Hospital Medical Center.)

Radiographic Findings

Basilar impression is difficult to evaluate radiologically, and many measurement techniques have been proposed (113–117). Discussion of the specifics of these lines is beyond the scope of this chapter, but it is worth mentioning that of the different radiographic lines, McRae's line (117) is most practical and defines the opening of the foramen magnum. It was derived from McRae's clinical observation that if the tip of the odontoid lies below the opening of the foramen magnum, patients will probably be asymptomatic (117); the accuracy of this observation has since been substantiated by Hink and associates (118) and Fielding and colleagues (119). Computed tomography and magnetic resonance imaging have made identification of the condition easier and can clearly detect the site of neural element compression.

Management

The authors have no personal experience in treating patients with rickets who had cervical spine involvement. No reports in the literature of which we are aware discuss the treatment of basilar invagination secondary to rickets, presumably because of its benign course. The very rare symptomatic case requires a multidisciplinary approach (orthopedics, neurosurgery, metabolic bone specialist, and neuroradiology) (120). The primary treatment is surgical, and each case should be considered individually. If the symptoms are caused by posterior impingement, suboccipital decompression and often upper cervical laminectomy are needed. Posterior stabilization should be performed.

REFERENCES

1. Calzavara PG, Carlino A, Anzola GP. Segmental neurofibromatosis. Case report and review of the literature. *Neurofibromatosis* 1988;1: 318–322.
2. Akenside M. Observation on cancers. *Med Trans Coll Phys Lond* 1768;1:64.
3. Tilesius von Tilenau W. *Historia pathologica singularis cutis turpitudinus.* Leipzig: SL Crusius, 1793.
4. von Recklinghausen F. *Uber die multiplen fibrome der haut und ihre beziehung zu den multiplen neuromen.* Berlin: Hirschwald, 1882.
5. National Institutes of Health Consensus Development Conference. Neurofibromatosis. *Neurofibromatosis J* 1988;1:172–178.
6. Goldberg NS, Collins, FS. The hunt for the neurofibromatosis gene. *Arch Dermatol* 1991;127:1705–1707.
7. Fialkow PJ, Sagebiel RW, Gartler SM, et al. Multiple cell origin of hereditary neurofibromas. *N Engl J Med* 1971;284:298–300.
8. Collins FS, Ponder BA, Seizinger BR, et al. The von Recklinghausen neurofibromatosis region on chromosome 17—genetic and physical maps come into focus. *Am J Hum Genet* 1989;44:1–5.
9. Riccardi VM. Neurofibromatosis update. *Neurofibromatosis* 1989;2: 284–291.
10. Lubs ML, Bauer MS, Formas ME, et al. Lisch nodules in neurofibromatosis type 1. *N Engl J Med* 1991;324:1264–1266.
11. Lewis RA, Riccardi VM. Von Recklinghausen neurofibromatosis. Incidence of iris hamartoma. *Ophthalmology* 1981;88:348–354.
12. Crawford AH. Neurofibromatosis. In: Morrissy RT, ed. *Lovell and Winters pediatric orthopaedics,* 3rd ed. Philadelphia: JB Lippincott, 1990.
13. Riccardi VM. Von Recklinghausen neurofibromatosis. *N Engl J Med* 1981;305:1617–1627.
14. Harkin JC, Reed RJ. Tumors of the peripheral nervous system. In: *Armed Forces Institute of Pathology, 2nd series, fascicle 3.* Washington, DC, 1969.
15. Weiss RA. Curvature of the spine in von Recklinghausen's disease. *Arch Dermatol Syphilol* 1921;3:144.
16. Akbarnia BA, Gabriel KR, Beckman E, et al. Prevalence of scoliosis in neurofibromatosis. *Spine* 1992;17:S244–S228.
17. Schorry EK, Stowens DW, Crawford AH, et al. Summary of patient data from a multidisciplinary neurofibromatosis clinic. *Neurofibromatosis* 1989;2:129–134.
18. Cobb J. Outline for the study of scoliosis. *AAOS Instructional Course Lectures* 1948;4:261–275.
19. Betz RR, Iorio R, Lombardi AV, et al. Scoliosis surgery in neurofibromatosis. *Clin Orthop* 1989;245:53–56.
20. Kim HW, Weinstein SL. Spine update. The management of scoliosis in neurofibromatosis. *Spine* 1997;22:2770–2776.
21. Yong-Hing K, Kalamchi , MacEwen GD. Cervical spine abnormalities in neurofibromatosis. *J Bone Joint Surg Am* 1979;61:695–699.
22. Adkins JC, Ravitch MM. The operative management of von Recklinghausen's neurofibromatosis in children, with special reference to lesions of the head and neck. *Surgery* 1977;82:342–348.
23. Samoto T, Wantanabe Y, Suda A. Atlantoaxial dislocation with neurofibromatosis: a case report. *Orthop Traumatol Surg (Japan)* 1981; 24:289.
24. Toyohido I, Miyasaka K, Hiroshi A. Atlantoaxial dislocation associated with neurofibromatosis. *J Neurosurg* 1983;68:451.
25. Haddad FS, Williams RL, Bentley G. The cervical spine in neurofibromatosis. *Br J Hosp Med* 1995;53:318–319.
26. Goffin J, Grob D. Spondyloptosis of the cervical spine in neurofibromatosis: a case report. *Spine* 1999;24:587–890.
27. Miller A. Neurofibromatosis with reference to skeletal changes, compression myelitis and malignant degeneration. *Arch Surg* 1936;32:109.
28. Curtis BH, Fisher RL, Butterfield WL, et al. Neurofibromatosis with paraplegia. Report of eight cases. *J Bone Joint Surg Am* 1969;51: 843–861.
29. Lonstein JE, Winter RB, Moe JH, et al. Neurologic deficits secondary to spinal deformity. A review of the literature and report of 43 cases. *Spine* 1980;5:331–355.
30. Rockower S, McKay D, Nason S. Dislocation of the spine in neurofibromatosis. A report of two cases. *J Bone Joint Surg Am* 1982;64: 1240–1242.
31. Major MR, Huizenga BA. Spinal cord compression by displaced ribs in neurofibromatosis. A report of three cases. *J Bone Joint Surg Am* 1988;70:1100–1102.
32. Flood BM, Butt WP, Dickson RA. Rib penetration of the intervertebral foraminae in neurofibromatosis. *Spine* 1986;11:172–174.
33. Tredwell S. Personal communication, 1992.
34. Robin GC. Scoliosis in neurologic disease. *J Med Sci* 1983;9:578.
35. Winter RB, Lonstein JE, Anderson M. Neurofibromatosis hyperkyphosis: a review of 33 cases with hyperkyphosis with 80 degrees or greater. *J Spinal Disorders* 1988;1:39.
36. Ahn NU, Sponseller PD, Ahn UM. Dural ectasia is associated with back pain in Marfan syndrome. *Spine* 2000;25:1562–1568.
37. Davis F. Neurofibromatosis: a historical perspective. National Neurofibromatosis Foundation, Inc., Newsletter No. 1983, 1940;6:8.
38. O'Neil P, Whatmore WJ, Booth AE. Spinal myelomeningocele in association with neurofibromatosis. *J Neurosurg* 1983;13:82–84.
39. Miles J, Pennybacker J, Sheldon P. Interthoracic meningocele: its development and association with neurofibromatosis. *J Neurol Neurosurg Psychiatry* 1969;32:99–110.
40. Klatte EC, Franken EA, Smith JA. The radiographic spectrum in neurofibromatosis. *Semin Roentgenol* 1976;11:17–33.
41. Pohl R. Menigokele im brustraum unter bilde eines intrathcrakazen rundschattens. *Roentgenpraxis* 1933;5:747–749.
42. Yadeau RE. Intrathoracic meningocele. *J Thorac Cardiovasc Surg* 1965;49:202–209.
43. Sengpiel JW, Ruzicka FF, Lodmell EA. Lateral interthoracic meningocele. *Radiology* 1948;50:515–520.
44. Nanson EM. Thoracic meningocele associated with neurofibromatosis. *Thorac Surg* 1957;433:650–652.
45. Cross JO, Reavis JR, Saunders WB. Lateral interthoracic meningocele. *J Neurosurg* 1949;6:423–432.

46. Salerno NR, Edeiken, J. Vertebral scalloping in neurofibromatosis. *Radiology* 1970;97:500–510.

47. Casselman ES, Mandell GA. Vertebral scalloping in neurofibromatosis. *Radiology* 1979;131:89–94.

48. Angtuaco EJ, Binet EF, Flanigan S. Value of computed tomographic myelography in neurofibromatosis. *Neurosurgery* 1983;13:666–671.

49. Love J, Dodge H. Lumbar (hourglass) neurofibroma affecting the spinal cord. *Surg Gynecol Obstet* 1952;94:161–172.

50. Crawford AH, Schorry EK. Neurofibromatosis in children: the role of the orthopaedist. *J Am Acad Orthop Surg* 1999;7:217–230.

51. Schorry EK, Crawford AH, Egelhoff JC. Thoracic tumors in children with neurofibromatosis-1. *Am J Med Genet* 1997;74:533–537.

52. Savini R, Fasenzi L. Le deforimita del rachide nella neurofibromatosi. Studio clinico e radiografico. *J Orthop Trauma* 2:37–50.

53. Heard G, Holt J, Naylor B. Cervical vertebral deformities in von Recklinghausen disease of the nervous system. A review of necropsy findings. *J Bone Joint Surg Br* 1962;44:880–885.

54. Isu T. Atlantoaxial dislocation with neurofibromatosis. *J Neurosurg* 1953;58:451–453.

55. Scott J. Scoliosis in neurofibromatosis. *J Bone Joint Surg Br* 1965;47:240.

56. Stone JW, Bridwell KH, Shackelford GD, et al. Dural ectasia associated with spontaneous dislocation of the upper part of the thoracic spine in neurofibromatosis. A case report and review of the literature. *J Bone Joint Surg Am* 1987;69:1079–1083.

57. Winter RB. Spontaneous dislocation of a vertebra in a patient who had neurofibromatosis. Report of a case with dural ectasia. *J Bone Joint Surg Am* 1991;73:1402–1404.

58. McCarroll H. Clinical manifestations of congenital neurofibromatosis. *J Bone Joint Surg Am* 1950;32:601–617.

59. Hsu LC, Lee PC, Leong JC. Dystrophic spinal deformities in neurofibromatosis. Treatment by anterior and posterior fusion. *J Bone Joint Surg Br* 1984;66:495–499.

60. Greene JF Jr, Fitzwater JE, Burgess J. Arterial lesions associated with neurofibromatosis. *Am J Clin Pathol* 1974;62:481–487.

61. Sirois JL 3rd, Drennan JC. Dystrophic spinal deformity in neurofibromatosis. *J Pediatr Orthop* 1990;10:522–526.

62. Crawford AH. Pitfalls of spinal deformities associated with neurofibromatosis in children. *Clin Orthop* 1989;245:29–42.

63. Kaipiainen-Seppanen O, Savolainen A. Incidence of chronic juvenile rheumatic diseases in Finland during 1980–1990. *Clin Exp Rheumatol* 1996;14:441–444.

64. Peterson LS, Mason T, Nelson AM. Juvenile rheumatoid arthritis in Rochester, Minnesota 1960–1993. Is the epidemiology changing? *Arthritis Rheum* 1996;39:1385–1390.

65. Singsen BH. Rheumatic diseases of childhood. *Rheum Dis Clin North Am* 1990;16:581–599.

66. Cassidy JT, Petty RE. *Textbook of pediatric rheumatology.* Philadelphia: WB Saunders, 1995.

67. Uziel Y, Rathaus V, Pomeranz A, et al. Torticollis as the sole initial presenting sign of systemic onset juvenile rheumatoid arthritis. *J Rheumatol* 1998;25:166–168.

68. Ansell BM. Joint manifestations in children with juvenile chronic polyarthritis. *Arthritis Rheum* 1977;20:204–206.

69. Cassidy JT, Levinson JE, Bass JC, et al. A study of classification criteria for a diagnosis of juvenile rheumatoid arthritis. *Arthritis Rheum* 1986;29:274–281.

70. Fink CW. Proposal for the development of classification criteria for idiopathic arthritides of childhood. *J Rheumatol* 1995;22:1566–1569.

71. Petty RE, Southwood TR, Baum J, et al. Revision of the proposed classification criteria for juvenile idiopathic arthritis: Durban, 1997. *J Rheumatol* 1998;25:1991–1994.

72. Sherry DD. Pauciarticular-onset juvenile chronic (rheumatoid) arthritis. In: Maddison PJ, Isenberg DA, Woo P, Glass DN, eds. *Oxford textbook of rheumatology.* Oxford, UK: Oxford University Press, 1993:711.

73. Symmons DP, Jones M, Osborne J. Pediatric rheumatology in the United Kingdom: data from the British Pediatric Rheumatology Group National Diagnostic Register. *J Rheumatol* 1996;23:1975–1980.

74. Kanski JJ. Uveitis in juvenile chronic arthritis: incidence, clinical features and prognosis. *Eye* 1988;2:641–645.

75. Schaller JG. Juvenile rheumatoid arthritis: series 1. *Arthritis Rheum* 1977;20:165–170.

76. Stillman JS, Barry PE. Juvenile rheumatoid arthritis: series 2. *Arthritis Rheum* 1977;20:171–175.

77. Rosenberg AM. Uveitis associated with juvenile rheumatoid arthritis. *Semin Arthritis Rheum* 1987;16:158–173.

78. Espada G, Babini JC, Maldonado-Cocco JA, et al. Radiologic review: the cervical spine in juvenile rheumatoid arthritis. *Semin Arthritis Rheum* 1988;17:185–195.

79. Hensinger RN, DeVito PD, Ragsdale CG. Changes in the cervical spine in juvenile rheumatoid arthritis. *J Bone Joint Surg Am* 1986;68:189–198.

80. Fried JA, Athreya B, Gregg JR, et al. The cervical spine in juvenile rheumatoid arthritis. *Clin Orthop* 1983;179:102–106.

81. Malagon C, Van Kerckhove C, Giannini EH, et al. The iridocyclitis of early onset pauciarticular juvenile rheumatoid arthritis: outcome in immunogenetically characterized patients. *J Rheumatol* 1992;19:160–163.

82. De Inocencio J, Giannini EH, Glass DN. Can genetic markers contribute to the classification of juvenile rheumatoid arthritis? *J Rheumatol Suppl* 1993;40:12–18.

83. McDowell TL, Symons JA, Ploski R, et al. A genetic association between juvenile rheumatoid arthritis and a novel interleukin-1 alpha polymorphism. *Arthritis Rheum* 1995;38:221–228.

84. Martin K, Woo P. Juvenile idiopathic arthritides. In: Isenberg DA, Miller JJ, eds. *Adolescent rheumatology.* London: Martin Dunitz, 1999.

85. Reiter MF, Boden SD. Inflammatory disorders of the cervical spine. *Spine* 1998;23:2755–2766.

86. Scott PJ, Ansell BM, Huskisson EC. Measurement of pain in juvenile chronic polyarthritis. *Ann Rheum Dis* 36: 1977;186–187.

87. Beales JG, Keen JH, Holt PJ. The child's perception of the disease and the experience of pain in juvenile chronic arthritis. *J Rheumatol* 1983;10:61–65.

88. Nathan FF, Bickel WH. Spontaneous axial subluxation in a child as the first sign of juvenile rheumatoid arthritis. *J Bone Joint Surg Am* 1968;50:1675–1678.

89. Werne S. Spontaneous dislocation of the atlas (as a complication in rheumatoid arthritis). *Acta Rheumat Scand* 1957;3:101–107.

90. Taseski B, Zeskov P, Skarica R. [Spontaneous atlanto-axial dislocation in juvenile chronic arthritis]. *Reumatizam* 1978;25:82–90.

91. Ferlic DC, Clayton ML, Leidholt JD, et al. Surgical treatment of the symptomatic unstable cervical spine in rheumatoid arthritis. *J Bone Joint Surg Am* 1975;57:349–354.

92. Lipscomb PR, Calabro JJ, Eyring EJ. The role of the orthopaedist in the management of juvenile rheumatoid arthritis. *AAOS Instructional Course Lectures* 1974;23:25–52.

93. Thalmann H, Scholl H, Tonz O. Spontaneous atlas dislocation in a child with trisomy 21 and rheumatic arthritis. *Helv Paediat Acta* 1972;27:391–403.

94. Andrews LG. Myelopathy due to atlanto-axial dislocation in a patient with Down's syndrome and rheumatoid arthritis. *Dev Med Child Neurol* 1981;23:356–360.

95. Sherk HH, Pasquariello PS, Watters WC. Multiple dislocations of the cervical spine in a patient with juvenile rheumatoid arthritis and Down's syndrome. *Clin Orthop* 1982;162:37–40.

96. Barkin RE, Stillman S, Potter T. The spondylitis of juvenile rheumatoid arthritis. *N Engl J Med* 1955;253:1107–1110.

97. Grokoest A, Snyder A, Ragen CH. Some aspects of juvenile rheumatoid arthritis. *Bull Rheum Dis* 1957;3:147–148.

98. Cassidy JT, Martel W. Juvenile rheumatoid arthritis: clinicoradiologic correlations. *Arthritis Rheum* 1977;20:207–211.

99. Ziff M, Contreras V, McEwen C. Spondylitis in postpubertal patients with rheumatoid arthritis of juvenile onset. *Ann Rheum Dis* 1956;15:40–45.

100. Martel W. The occipito-atlanto-axial joints in rheumatoid arthritis and ankylosing spondylitis. *Am J Roentgenol* 1961;86:233–240.

101. Martel W, Holt JF, Cassidy JT. Roentgenologic manifestation of juvenile rheumatoid arthritis. *Am J Roentgenol* 1962;88:400–423.

102. Cabot A, Becker A. The cervical spine in rheumatoid arthritis. *Clin Orthop* 1978;131:130–140.

103. Swischuk LE. Anterior displacement of C2 in children: physiologic or pathologic. *Radiology* 1977;122:759–763.

104. Sherry DD. What's new in the diagnosis and treatment of juvenile rheumatoid arthritis. *J Pediatr Orthop* 2000;20:419–420.

105. Giannini EH, Brewer EJ, Kuzmine N, et al. Methotrexate in resistant juvenile rheumatoid arthritis. Results of the U.S.A.-U.S.S.R.

double-blind, placebo-controlled trial. The Pediatric Rheumatology Collaborative Study Group and The Cooperative Children's Study Group. *N Engl J Med* 1992;326:1043–1049.

106. Lovell DJ, Giannini EH, Reiff A, et al. Etanercept in children with polyarticular juvenile rheumatoid arthritis. Pediatric Rheumatology Collaborative Study Group. *N Engl J Med* 2000;342:763–769.

107. Rawlins BA, Girardi FP, Boachie-Adjei O. Rheumatoid arthritis of the cervical spine. *Rheum Dis Clin North Am* 1998;24:55–65.

108. Rudolf M, Arulanantham K, Greenstein RM. Unsuspected nutritional rickets. *Pediatrics* 1980;66:72–76.

109. Labuda M, Morgan K, Glorieux FH. Mapping autosomal recessive vitamin D dependency type I to chromosome 12q14 by linkage analysis. *Am J Hum Genet* 1990;47:28–36.

110. Malloy PJ, Pike JW, Feldman D. The vitamin D receptor and the syndrome of hereditary 1,25-dihydroxyvitamin D-resistant rickets. *Endocr Rev* 1999;20:156–188.

111. Hensinger RN. Osseous anomalies of the craniovertebral junction. *Spine* 1986;11:323–333.

112. Chakrabarti AK, Johnson SC, Samantray SK. Osteomalacia, myopathy and basilar impression. *J Neurol Sci* 1974;23:227–235.

113. Yoshikawa S, Shiba M, Suzuki A. Spinal-cord compression in untreated adult cases of vitamin-D resistant rickets. *J Bone Joint Surg Am* 1968; 50:743–752.

114. Chamberlain WE. Basilar impression (platybasia): a bizarre developmental anomaly of the occipital bone and upper cervical spine with striking and misleading neurologic manifestation. *Yale J Bio Med* 1939;11:487–496.

115. McGreger M. The significance of certain measurement of the skull in the diagnosis of basilar impression. *Br J Radiol* 1948;21:171–181.

116. Fishgold H, Metzger J. Etude radiotomographique de 1-impression basilaire. *Rev Rheum* 1952;19:261–264.

117. McRae DL, Barnum AS. Occipitalization of the atlas. *Am J Roentgenol* 1953;70:23–46.

118. Hink VC, Hopkins CE, Savara BS. Sagittal diameter of the cervical spinal canal in children. *Radiology* 1962;79:97–108.

119. Fielding J W, Hensinger RN, Hawkins RJ. Os odontoideum. *J Bone Joint Surg Am* 1980;62:376–383.

120. Van Gilder JC, Menezes AH. Craniovertebral junction anomalies. In: Wilkins RH, Rengachary SS, eds. *Neurosurgery*. New York: McGraw-Hill, 1985:2097–2210.

CHAPTER 37

Cervical Spine Injuries in Children

Paul D. Sponseller

Successful treatment of pediatric cervical spine fractures demands the recognition of patterns of injury. Also needed is knowledge of the least invasive means of effective treatment for children. Recent developments in this field have included not only new treatments, but also a better understanding of the epidemiology and prevention of these injuries.

CONCEPTS AND PRINCIPLES

Epidemiology

Fractures and dislocations of the cervical spine are less common in children than adults. They represent only about 2% of all spine trauma, or about seven injuries per 100,000 population per year (1). Cervical spine injury occurs in about 1% of pediatric trauma (1,2). The fatality rate in children's cervical spine trauma (7% to 13%) is double that of adults (1–3). Injuries in young children tend to involve primarily the upper three segments of the spine, in contrast to adults, who more commonly incur injuries of the lower cervical spine. The transition between patterns of injury occurs at about age 11 (Fig. 37.1) (1,2). Cervical spine injuries in young children are more likely to be associated with neurologic damage (4). The reasons for the differences between younger and older groups appear to involve the relatively larger head size (5) in proportion to the rest of the body, as well as delay in muscular control of the head and protective reflexes. Ligamentous laxity is greater in children, and the cervical facets are more horizontal, allowing a greater range of physiologic flexion and extension (6). Children are also vulnerable to spinal cord injury without any radiographic abnormality (SCIWORA).

The most common mechanism of injury across all ages is a motor vehicle accident, whether the injured is an occupant, pedestrian, or cyclist (2). The etiology of younger children's injuries is more likely to include falls or being struck as a pedestrian by a motor vehicle (1,7). Other causes unique to this age group include birth trauma and nonaccidental injury (8,9). Breech presentation may predispose to a traction injury that affects the lower cervical or thoracic spine (9,10). Cephalic presentation more rarely accompanies spinal cord injury; when it does it more often involves the upper cervical spine (10). Older children and adults, by contrast, are more likely to suffer cervical spine injury during sports, such as football, trampoline use, and diving (1,11,12). Gunshot wounds have shown a steady increase in frequency over the past decade (13). Although the thoracic spine is the most common region affected by gunshot injury, the cervical spine also may be injured; these injuries usually involve teenagers.

Normal Development and Anatomy

It is important to have an understanding of the growth of the child's cervical spine in order to interpret injury patterns and distinguish them from normal variants. The atlas develops from three ossification centers: a single anterior center for the body and paired posterior centers for the neurocentral arches (Figs. 37.2 and 37.3A). Ossification centers in the posterior arch are present after the seventh fetal week, but the anterior arch may not ossify until after birth. The posterior synchondrosis between the two halves of the neural arch may fail to fuse and may even be bifid. This common variation has obvious implications for surgical dissection. The canal of the atlas is exceptionally large to accommodate the extensive physiologic degree of rotation that occurs at this joint as well as some forward translation (14). The vertebral arteries run horizontally in a groove on the superior surface of the atlas, about 2 cm from the midline.

The axis normally develops from at least four ossification centers: one for the dens, one for the body, and two for the neural arches (Figs. 37.3B and 37.4). A small secondary ossification center also contributes to development of the cranial tip of the odontoid. The synchondrosis between the dens and body (dentocentral or basilar) is often referred

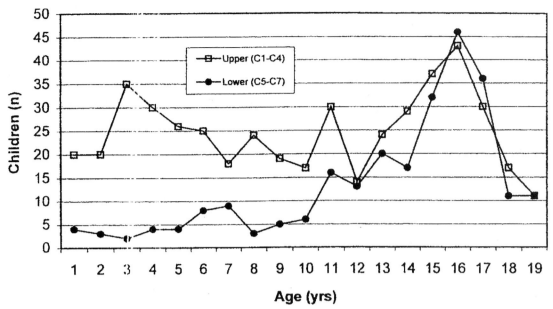

FIG. 37.1. Age distribution of fractures and dislocation at various levels of the cervical spine from a series of 143 fractures in patients aged less than 16 years. The change in injury distribution in adolescence is evident. (From: Patel JC, Tepas JJ, Mollitt, et al. Pediatric cervical spine injuries: defining the disease. *J Pediatr Surg* 2001;36(2):373–376.)

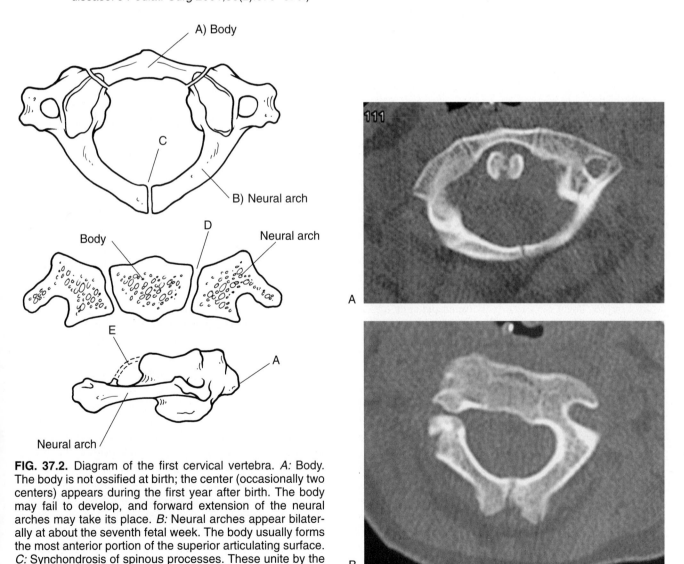

FIG. 37.2. Diagram of the first cervical vertebra. *A:* Body. The body is not ossified at birth; the center (occasionally two centers) appears during the first year after birth. The body may fail to develop, and forward extension of the neural arches may take its place. *B:* Neural arches appear bilaterally at about the seventh fetal week. The body usually forms the most anterior portion of the superior articulating surface. *C:* Synchondrosis of spinous processes. These unite by the third year. Union may rarely be preceded by the appearance of a secondary center within the synchondrosis. *D:* Neurocentral synchondrosis. This fuses about the seventh year.

FIG. 37.3. Radiographic appearance of growth centers *(arrows)* of upper cervical vertebrae. **A:** Atlas. **B:** Axis.

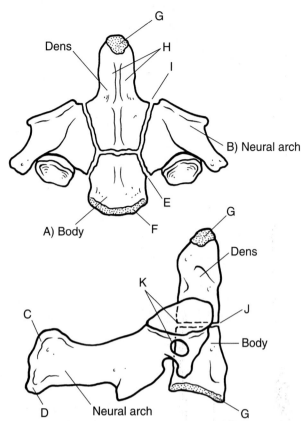

FIG. 37.4. Diagram of the second cervical vertebra. *A:* Body. One center (occasionally two) appears by the fifth fetal month. *B:* Neural arches. These appear bilaterally by the seventh fetal month. *C:* Neural arches. These fuse posteriorly by second or third year. *D:* Bifid tip of spinous process. *E:* Neurocentral synchondrosis. This fuses at 3 to 6 years. *F:* Inferior epiphyseal ring. *G:* "Summit" ossification center for the odontoid by 12 years. *H:* Odontoid (dens). Two separate centers appear by the fifth fetal month and fuse with each other by the seventh fetal month. *I:* Synchondrosis between odontoid and neural arch. This fuses at 3 to 6 years. *J:* Synchondrosis between odontoid and body. This fuses at 3 to 6 years.

to as a *physis*, but it closes early, between the ages of 3 to 6 years. It is recessed below the superior articular facets of the axis. Small, secondary centers of ossification also develop in the tips of the spinous processes.

The interval between the dens and the posterior cortex of the arch of the atlas is termed the atlantodens interval. It may be normally up to 4.5 mm in children, compared with 3 mm in adults (Fig. 37.5). This difference appears to result from unossified cartilage in these structures, as well as greater physiologic ligamentous laxity.

The bodies of the vertebrae below C2 are normally wedge-shaped until about age 8 to 10 years. Apophyseal rings (secondary ossification centers) develop on the superior and inferior surfaces at age 10 to 12 years and fuse by maturity. Displacement of these ring ossification centers beyond the confines of the vertebral body may be a sign of physeal injury (15).

Physical Examination and Acute Care

Neck injuries in children are usually the result of major trauma. Head or facial trauma may be a clue to the presence of cervical spine fractures. The unconscious patient should be treated presumptively for a cervical spine fracture. Tenderness is a highly suggestive but not completely sensitive (84%) marker of cervical spine injury (16). The whole neck should be examined, as a patient may have more than one level of neck injury (1). A pediatric victim of major trauma should be protected from extreme flexion until tenderness of the cervical spine can be ruled out. This is important because some injuries in children are not readily detected by plain radiographs (17–19) such as SCIWORA and transverse ligament injury of the axis. The screening neurologic examination should include, at a minimum, testing of active flexion–extension at all major joints, as well as sensation in all extremities.

Radiographic Examination

A combination of a lateral radiograph and a physical examination for neck tenderness was able to detect 100% of pediatric neck injuries in one series (16). A cervical spine radiograph should be obtained in all children with serious injury, unconsciousness, or head or facial abrasions. In young children, indications for oblique films are unclear because subaxial subluxations are rare in this group. The most helpful studies are the anteroposterior (AP) and lateral radiograph. Open-mouth or odontoid radiographs are difficult to obtain in young children, may require stenting of the mouth, and are of questionable benefit (20). Flexion/extension views are helpful in assessing stability if the static film is abnormal, but two large series have shown no additional benefit if the static films are normal (21,22). Computed tomography (CT) is indicated for patients with suspected atlas ring fractures or rotatory subluxation. Dynamic CT scanning of the atlantoaxial interval may document fixed subluxation.

Normal Values

The occipitoatlantal interval is the most difficult to assess because of the lack of discrete, reproducible landmarks on the lateral films. The occipital condyles should rest in the depressions of the facets of the atlas. The interval between the condyles and facets should be less than 5 mm (23). The basion is the anterior cortical margin of the foramen magnum. The interval between it and the tip of the dens should be less than 10 mm (24,25). The basion is not always visible, however. Powers' ratio (Fig. 37.5) assesses the relative position of the skull base and the atlas: the distance BC (from the basion to the anterior cortex of the C1 lamina) divided by the distance OA (from the opisthion to the posterior cortex of the C1 arch) should be less than 1. A greater value suggests an anterior dislocation of this joint, the usual type. Figure 37.5 shows the normal values for this and other levels of the pediatric cervical spine. Further

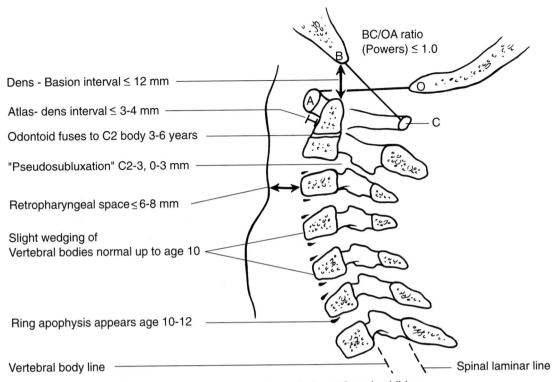

BC/OA ratio
(Powers) ≤ 1.0

Dens - Basion interval ≤ 12 mm

Atlas- dens interval ≤ 3-4 mm

Odontoid fuses to C2 body 3-6 years

"Pseudosubluxation" C2-3, 0-3 mm

Retropharyngeal space ≤ 6-8 mm

Slight wedging of
Vertebral bodies normal up to age 10

Ring apophysis appears age 10-12

Vertebral body line

Spinal laminar line

FIG. 37.5. Normal alignment and relationships of cervical vertebrae in children.

helpful imaging of the atlantooccipital interval may include magnetic resonance imaging (MRI), which can illustrate injury here by showing edema in the occipitocervical facet capsules (26) and basocervical ligaments as well as an acute cervicomedullary angulation. A CT image can be used to show whether the occipital condyles are located in the C1 facets by superimposing them or obtaining a sagittal reconstruction. The anterior cortex of the posterior cervical laminae should form a smooth line or curve (27), whether or not the cervical spine is lordotic. A substantial number of normal children do not have lordosis in the cervical spine (14).

The atlantodens interval is greater in children than adults. Up to 4.5 mm is considered normal (14,17,28–30). This interval should be measured from the posteroinferior cortex of the body of the atlas along a line perpendicular to its posterior surface (24). In extension, the anterior arch of the atlas may slide up on the dens. The absence of soft-tissue swelling does not rule out atlantoaxial instability.

The normal retropharyngeal soft-tissue space in children is 6 mm or less at C3, and the retrotracheal space is less than 14 mm at C6 (14,23). The C2-3 vertebrae may translate up to 3 mm in flexion (14). This phenomenon is termed *pseudosubluxation*. It can be confirmed as a normal variant by examining Swischuk's line, which is drawn between the C1 and C3 laminae, and noting that the lamina of the atlas does not fall more than 1 mm forward of this line.

As many as one of every 10 to 20 spinal cord–injured children may have normal spine radiographs (4,31). This is the phenomenon of SCIWORA, which was brought to light

by Pang and Wilberger (19). It is more common in children under age 10. Some cases even have a normal MRI of the bony and ligamentous elements of the spine adjacent to an obviously injured cord, possibly because the cord was injured by a degree of distraction that is tolerated by the bony and ligamentous elements. It also may represent an ischemic injury in some cases. Finally, in other cases, it may represent a physeal failure through the cartilaginous vertebral end plates. Aufdermaur (32) showed that fracture may occur throughout the hypertrophic zone of the pediatric vertebral end plate in trauma specimens that he examined at necropsy. In a small number of cases with SCIWORA, there are reports that the spinal injury may be exacerbated by improper handling before the diagnosis is made. Therefore, the unconscious trauma victim should be treated carefully even if radiographs are normal until he or she awakens or an MRI is done. The ideal algorithm for evaluating these patients is still evolving. They should be protected with a cervical collar as well as by avoidance of extreme flexion, extension, or rotation, until cleared. SCIWORA is discussed further in Chapter 38.

TREATMENT OF SPECIFIC INJURIES

Atlantooccipital Instability

The joint between the atlas and occiput is a condylar articulation allowing approximately 15 degrees of flexion and extension but minimal rotation. The primary stabilizers

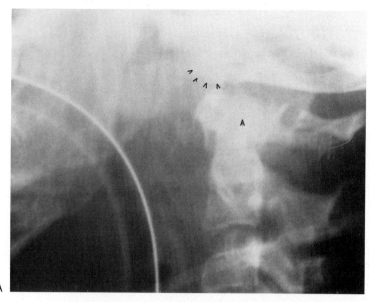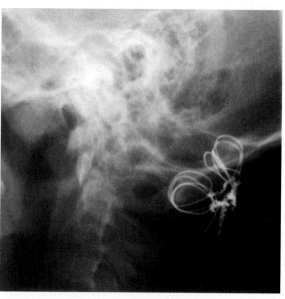

A   B

FIG. 37.6. Traumatic atlantooccipital dislocation. This 12-year-old girl was thrown from a horse. She was neurologically normal. **A:** This first radiograph was taken because she developed right upper extremity weakness 2 days after fixing her femur fracture with an intramedullary rod. Note the displacement of the occipital condyles *(arrowheads)* forward of the facets of the atlas *(arrow).* **B:** The dislocation was reduced with gentle traction, and an atlantooccipital fusion was performed. Her neurologic signs resolved.

of this joint are the paired alar ligaments and tectorial membrane, a continuation of the posterior longitudinal ligament (24,33). It is more frequently disrupted in pediatric than adult trauma because of the relatively large size of the child's cranium. The mechanism of injury is believed to be one of hyperextension in most cases, although lateral rotation or even forward flexion also may be involved. Instability at this level is an increased risk in persons with Down syndrome as well as in those with high cervical fusions below the axis. Dislocation at this level often results in cardiorespiratory arrest secondary to injury of the respiratory centers of the brain stem, C3-5. Skilled resuscitation teams are more and more often saving these patients. Other patients may have an asymmetric partial quadriparesis. Twenty percent of patients with atlantooccipital instability are free of major neurologic injury, although some may experience cranial nerve injury, vomiting, headache, torticollis, or minor weakness (20,24,26,33–38). Some symptoms of brain stem injury may result from vertebrobasilar vascular insufficiency. There are case reports of patients whose diagnoses were not made for weeks after injury (39). The diagnosis of atlantooccipital instability may be masked or overlooked in patients with concomitant brain injury. The clinician should be alert for clues to cervical cord injury in the presence of brain injury. These include spinal shock and urinary retention in cases of complete cervical lesions, as well as neck pain, diffuse tingling, or spasticity out of proportion to cognitive impairment in partial lesions (25).

Radiographic features hinge on demonstrating displacement (usually anterior) of the base of the skull on the atlas, which may include displacement of the condyles on the

facets of the atlas, a Power ratio greater than 1, and an increased dens-basion interval greater than 1 cm (24,40) (Fig. 37.6). It is important to look for fractures of the occipital condyles (41). An MRI may be helpful in diagnosing atlantooccipital dislocation by showing an abnormal cervical cranial angle or soft-tissue edema (42).

Treatment consists of reduction using gentle skull traction, using care not to overdistract. If a significant hematoma is seen at the cervicomedullary junction on MRI, Papadopoulos considers it important to decompress it if the patient has a partial neurologic lesion (38). After reduction is obtained, it is confirmed radiographically. Long-term stability has been achieved either by immobilization alone or arthrodesis. Farley and associates (43) and Georgopoulos and colleagues (44) each reported cases where stability was restored by 8 weeks of treatment in a halo. Stability should be confirmed with flexion/extension views after the halo is removed. One problem is that a precise definition of stability at this level has not been given, although 5 to 10 mm of translation has been proposed as an upper limit (44); Stein and colleagues (45) assessed stability based on whether the occipital condyles appeared to be contained within the facets of the atlas.

Because the diagnosis of stability is not precise and the consequences of reinjury at this level may be devastating, some surgeons prefer to stabilize the articulation by arthrodesis. This arthrodesis can be of the occiput to C1 in the neurologically intact patient, sparing the C1-2 articulation to maximize movement (Fig. 37.6). Although some authors have expressed reservations about the chance of success in obtaining fusion in the narrow atlantooccipital interval, there have been several reports of successful arthrodesis

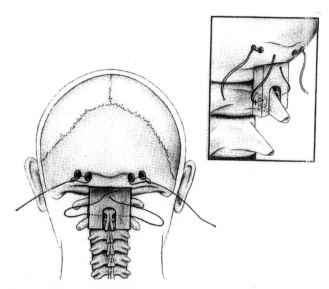

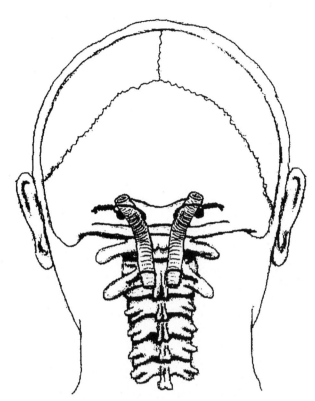

FIG. 37.7. Occipitocervical arthrodesis may be performed using iliac crest anchored in a trough in the occiput, using wires for stabilization. Rigid fixation may allow earlier removal of the halo. (From: Dormans JP, Drummond DS, Sutton LN, et al. Occipitocervical arthrodesis in children. *J Bone Joint Surg* 1995;77(A):1234–1239.)

FIG. 37.8. Occipitocervical arthrodesis may be performed using a rib graft, which has a shape matching the needed contours. (From: Cohen MW, Drummond DS, Flynn JM, et al. A technique of occipitocervical arthrodesis in children using autologous rib grafts. *Spine* 2001;26(7):825–829.)

(44,46). In the patient with pentaplegia, there is less to lose by a trial of closed treatment, except the duration of external immobilization. If arthrodesis becomes necessary, it may be extended down from the occiput to C2 or C3 without ill effects in the pentaplegic patient because there is minimal or no active motor control of the neck. There are numerous means of occipitocervical arthrodesis in children. Bone graft may be taken from the rib or iliac crest (Fig. 37.7). Rib graft may be readily contoured to span several segments, as described by Cohen and colleagues (47) (Fig. 37.8).

Reduction should not be pursued forcefully for the patient who presents very late with an unreduced dislocation. Dibenedetto and Lee (39) recommend arthrodesis *in situ* with a suboccipital craniectomy to relieve posterior impingement.

Atlas (Jefferson) Fractures

Atlas (Jefferson) fractures occur more rarely in children than adults, usually as a result of axial loads. Care must be taken to distinguish between fractures and synchondroses based on their location and appearance. The pediatric atlas may fracture its ring in children in one location, hinging on the opposite synchondrosis, or plastically deforming the ring. CT shows the ring injury more readily than plain films because the ring of the atlas is a transversely oriented structure. If the two lateral masses are widened greater than 7 mm beyond the borders of the axis, it is presumed that there is an injury to the transverse ligament: either rupture of the ligament or avulsion from bone.

Treatment consists of immobilization in an orthosis such as a Philadelphia collar (48,49). If excessive widening

(>7 mm) is seen, surgical arthrodesis or traction followed by halo application is recommended.

Atlantoaxial Subluxation

Transverse Ligament Disruption

The transverse ligament of the atlas arises within the ring of C1, medial to the facets. It is the primary stabilizer of an intact odontoid against forward displacement. The secondary stabilizers, the apical and alar ligaments, arise from the tip of the dens and pass to the base of the skull and stabilize the atlantooccipital joint indirectly (50). The upper limit of normal C1-2 translation in children is 4.5 mm by the method of Locke (24). Greater values suggest attenuation or disruption of the transverse ligament. According to Steel, the anteroposterior diameter of the ring of C1 may be divided with three regions using the so-called rule of thirds: one-third each for the dens, cord, and free space (51).

Acute rupture of the transverse ligament is a rare injury. It comprised less than 10% of pediatric cervical spine injuries in the classic work of McGrory and associates (1), although it was the second most common type of upper cervical spine dislocation in children in another report (17). CT may show a fleck of bone at one of the origins of

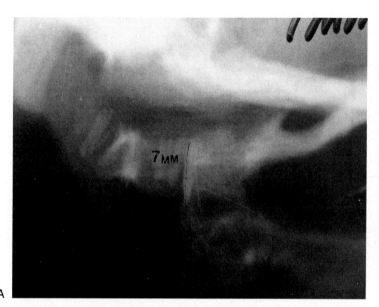

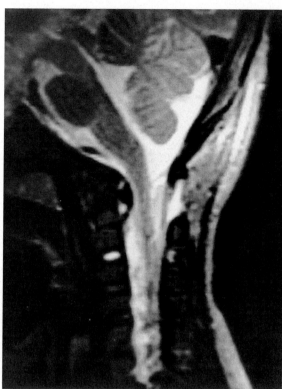

A

B

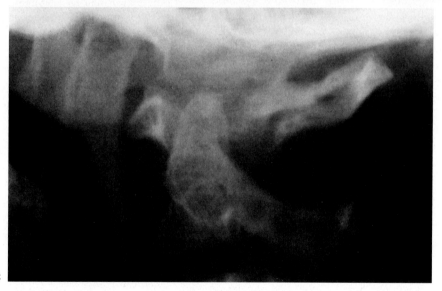

C

FIG. 37.9. Transverse ligament rupture was diagnosed in this 4-year-old boy who had neck pain after a motor vehicle accident. **A:** Plain films at rest showed a 7-mm atlantodens interval. **B:** Magnetic resonance imaging confirmed transverse ligament injury, showing swelling and edema about this structure. **C:** After 8 weeks of immobilization in extension in a Minerva cast, his atlantodens interval decreased to 4 mm in flexion, and he remained stable at 2-year follow-up. (Case courtesy of J. David Thompson.)

the transverse ligament, and plain films may show minimal or no thickening of the retropharyngeal space. An active flexion view may be required to demonstrate the instability in a patient with unexplained neck pain or neurologic findings.

Treatment by immobilization to allow ligament healing has been successful in some but not all cases (Fig. 37.9). De Beer and colleagues (17), for example, had success in all of three children who received nonoperative treatment. Good results were obtained both with bracing in extension

in an orthosis as well as with a Minerva cast for 8 weeks. Some patients had a slight increase in the atlantodens interval on flexion and extension (3.4 to 6 mm) but remained stable neurologically. Their fourth patient had a serious neurologic injury at presentation and underwent immediate atlantoaxial arthrodesis, the most reliable means of achieving stability.

Chronic atlantoaxial instability also may occur from prior trauma or Down syndrome or juvenile rheumatoid arthritis. It also may be seen in certain skeletal dysplasias, such as spondyloepiphyseal dysplasia, Kniest syndrome, and mucopolysaccharidoses. Patients with chronic C1-2 instability greater than 5 mm may need to be advised of restrictions in contact sports and other high-impact activities. Fusion is recommended if the translation is greater than 8 to 10 mm.

Atlantoaxial Rotatory Subluxation

Half of the rotation in the cervical spine occurs at the atlantoaxial level. A unique phenomenon of childhood is that children are more prone to develop fixation of this articulation in a malrotated position: This problem has been termed *atlantoaxial rotatory subluxation*, fixation, or displacement. The etiology may be trauma or inflammation. Pediatricians commonly observe a wryneck, or stiff neck, after an upper respiratory infection, which usually resolves. This syndrome has been given the eponym Grisel syndrome (27,52). Subluxation also has been reported after retropharyngeal abscess, tonsillectomy, or pharyngoplasty. Parke and colleagues (53) demonstrated anastomosis and potential for free flow between veins draining the pharyngeal space and the periodontic plexus as well as direct anastomoses with lymphatics. Any resultant inflammation could lead to attenuation of the synovial capsules, transverse ligament, or both, with resulting instability. Another potential pathogenetic factor is the shape of the superior facets of the axis in children. A study by Kawabe and associates demonstrated that the facets were smaller and more steeply inclined in children, potentially leading to instability (54) (Fig. 37.10). They also demonstrated a meniscus within the

C1-2 joint that could prohibit reduction after displacement occurred.

Fielding and Hawkins emphasized the separate components of *rotation* and *translation* in their classification of this disorder into three types (29). Type I is a unilateral facet subluxation with an intact transverse ligament. Type II is a unilateral facet dislocation with an incompetent transverse ligament. Type III is bilateral facet dislocation with an incompetent transverse ligament, which results in the greatest degree of narrowing of the space available for the cord at the atlantoaxial level. Type I is by far the most common type.

Radiographic diagnosis may be difficult. The plain anteroposterior radiograph should be taken with the shoulders flat and the head in the most neutral position possible. The lateral mass that has rotated forward appears wider. The distance between lateral masses and dens is asymmetrical. The chin is rotated. The lateral view shows a wide, atypical profile of the C1 arch as well as compensatory rotation of the subaxial vertebrae. CT has been a major advance in understanding and diagnosing this problem and also should be done with the head and body in a position as close to neutral as possible. Several tomographic cuts show superimposition of C1 on C2 in the rotated position so that the degree and direction of malrotation may be quantified (Fig. 37.11). Some experts argue that the isolate neutral-position CT can lead to false-positive diagnosis of atlantoaxial

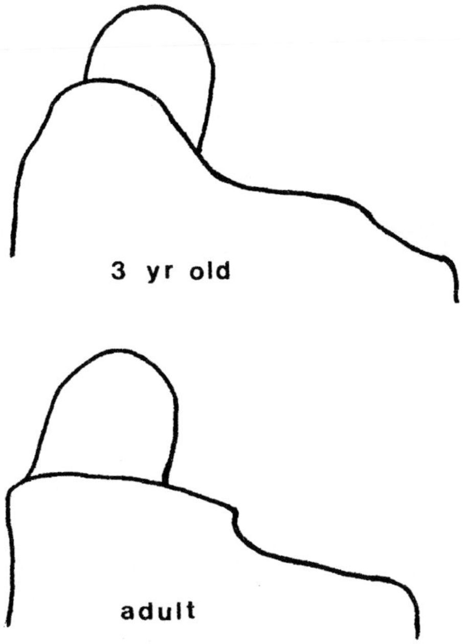

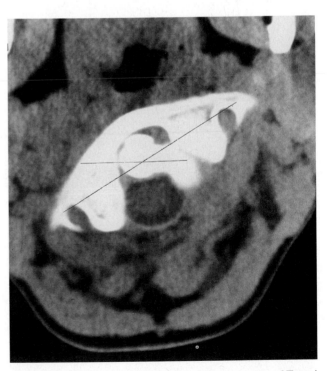

FIG. 37.10. Shape of the superior facet of the axis in the infant versus the mature adult. Notice the smaller, more steeply curved facet in the infant.

FIG. 37.11. Computed tomographic demonstration of Type I atlantoaxial rotatory subluxation. Because of the downward subluxation of the atlas, certain cuts show both vertebrae superimposed.

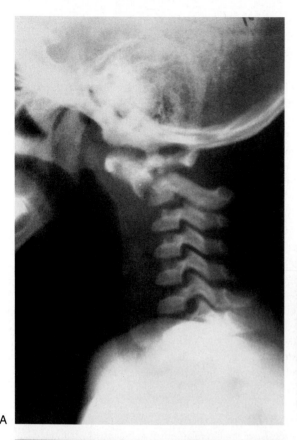

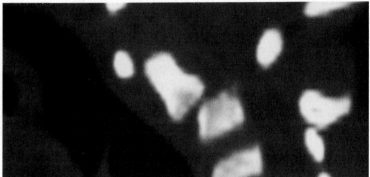

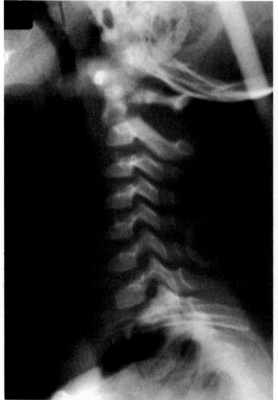

FIG. 37.12. Odontoid fracture in a 3-year-old child after a motor vehicle accident. He was neurologically normal. **A:** Plain lateral film shows displaced odontoid fracture. **B:** Computed tomogram, although ordered unnecessarily, shows that the plane of fracture is at level of the synchondrosis. **C:** The fracture was reduced with extension and held using a halo vest.

rotatory subluxation, in that one can have malrotation in a neutral position with guarding from a soft-tissue injury. They recommend right- and left-rotation (dynamic) CT scans to diagnose rotatory fixation. However, in most cases the malrotation seen on the single best transverse CT image showing the two vertebrae while the patient is in a "neutral" position is adequate to prove fixation and guide treatment.

Clinical findings include neck pain, headache, and the so-called "cock-robin" position of rotation to one side and lateral flexion to the other. If it occurs early in childhood and is long-standing, some plagiocephaly may be noted, which is best seen when looking down on the head from above. Neurologic abnormalities are extremely rare, although there have been a few reports (55). Differential diagnoses include torticollis caused by ophthalmologic problems, sternocleido-mastoid muscle tightness (congenital muscular torticollis), brain stem tumor, vertebral anomalies (hemivertebra) (56,57), and abscess or infection of the vertebral column.

Treatment depends on the duration of symptoms (58). If the rotatory subluxation has been present for a week or less, a soft collar and exercise program (to increase right and left rotation) is indicated. If this fails to produce improvement or if symptoms have been present for longer than a week, halter traction should be added. This may be carried out either at home or in the hospital, depending on the home situation and the severity of symptoms. If the subluxation has been present for longer than 1 month, successful reduction is much less likely (34); however, treatment with halo traction still reduces subluxation in some cases. The halo allows increased traction weight to be used without interfering with opening the jaw or causing skin pressure under the mandible. While the weight is applied to the halo, active rotation to the right and left should be practiced. Involvement of a physical therapist at this stage is helpful. Improvement may be estimated by the increase in the patient's rotation to the previously limited side. Placing the television and other attractions on the side to which the child has difficulty turning may ensure a more frequent stretching effort. Once clinical symmetry is restored, reduction may be confirmed by repeat CT scan. If reduction is not obtained, posterior atlantoaxial arthrodesis is recommended. Some surgeons prefer to perform an open reduction prior to fusion. However, even if the rotational alignment of the atlas and axis is not restored, successful fusion should result in an appearance of normal alignment of the head by relieving the muscle spasm that was occurring in response to the malrotation.

Dens Fracture

Dens fractures are the most common fractures of the cervical spine in children less than 11 years old (1). Usually the fracture line occurs through the basilar or dentocentral synchondrosis (Fig. 37.12), distal to the base of the odontoid, although this is not always the case (59,60). Usually the dens is anteriorly displaced, suggesting an intact periosteal sleeve on the anterior surface of the vertebral body extending up to the dens. This provides excellent healing in most cases, provided a satisfactory degree of immobilization is achieved (61). The growth potential of the dens is preserved after the fracture. This particular physis normally closes at age 3 to 6 years; therefore, further growth is presumed to be appositional. Plain radiographs usually provide the diagnosis, and further imaging is not needed unless an unexplained neurologic deficit occurs.

Extending or slightly hyperextending the neck usually achieves reduction. Although complete reduction of the translation is not necessary, one should strive for at least 50% apposition to provide adequate contact. The spine may be immobilized by a Minerva cast in children under the age of 3 or a halo for older children. A halo also may be used in children of any age in whom reduction is difficult and requires adjustment. The duration of immobilization is approximately 6 weeks in younger children and 8 weeks in older children. Immobilization may be discontinued when there is demonstration of adequate bony healing. Flexion/extension lateral radiographs then should be done to confirm stability and rule out concomitant ligamentous injury.

Os Odontoideum

Os odontoideum is thought to be acquired rather than congenital in most cases. Fielding and Griffin (28) and Fielding and associates (30) reported nine cases, each of whom had documentation of a prior normal odontoid. Schuler and coworkers, in an instructive case report, documented the natural history of one child as an os odontoideum evolved (62). This 2-year-old girl fell out of a crib and would not rotate her head. Initial radiographs appeared normal, and four radiographs over the ensuing year documented resorption of the waist of the dens and development of a typical os odontoideum. Interestingly, the defect was well proximal to the physis, and the axis developed a tuft of bone projecting toward the os. The fracture was believed to be causing interruption of the vascular supply ascending from the body, with the ossicle retaining its vascularity through the apical and alar ligaments. Additional evidence of trauma was shown by Kuhns and colleagues, who found discontinuity of the nuchal cord on MRI of four patients with os odontoideum, which was suggestive of trauma (63).

At initial presentation of a patient with os odontoideum, flexion and extension views should be taken to document the presence or absence of stability (Fig. 37.13). If translation of more than 5 mm is seen, some authors recommend reduction and immobilization after an acute injury to encourage healing. This immobilization should consist of 8 to 12 weeks in a Minerva cast or halo vest in the reduced position. If stability is not achieved, posterior fusion of the atlas to the axis should be carried out for patients with translation greater than 10 mm.

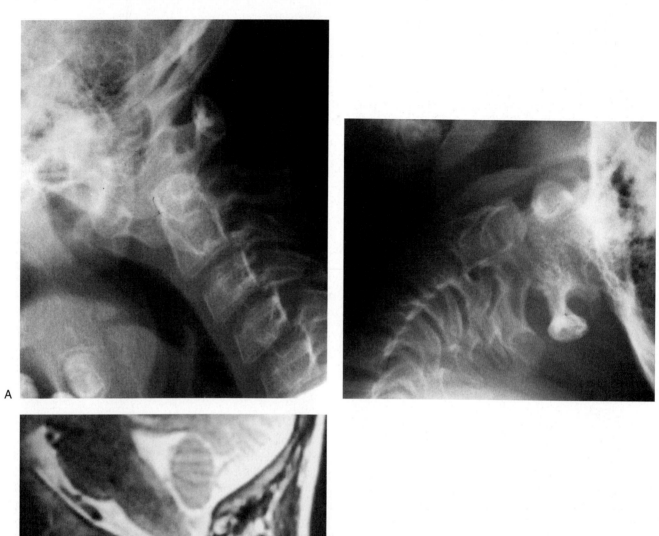

FIG. 37.13. Os odontoideum was discovered in this 12-year-old boy when he developed transient numbness in all four extremities in a wrestling headlock. Flexion **(A)** and extension **(B)** films showed 17-mm translation of C1 on C2. **C:** Magnetic resonance imaging showed no extra space around the cord even at rest. Atlantoaxial arthrodesis was carried out.

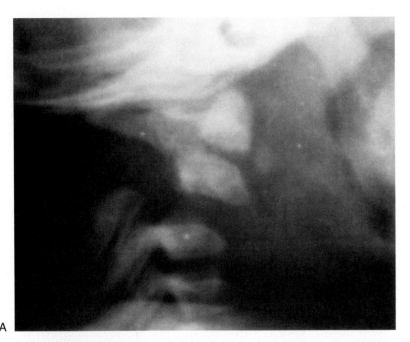

A

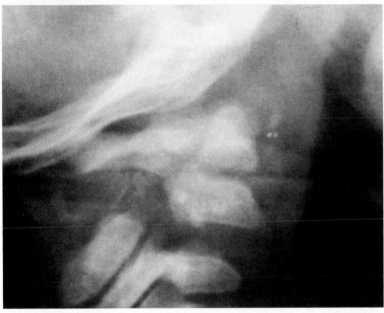

B

FIG. 37.14. This 18-month-old girl had neck pain and stiffness. **A:** Radiograph demonstrated a spondylolysis of the axis. **B:** Films 1 month later demonstrated early callus. The fracture healed after 8 weeks in a Minerva jacket.

Spondylolysis (Pars Interarticularis Fracture) of the Axis

Spondylolysis of the axis (Fig. 37.14) and hangman fracture (Figs. 37.15 and 37.16) also may occur in children. These conditions result from forced hyperextension and usually occur in children under age 2 years (6,64–66). The reasons for this young age predilection may include the relatively large head, poor muscle control, hypermobility normal for this age, and possibility of birth trauma or abuse (shaking).

The radiographs of a patient with spondylolysis of the axis show lucency well anteriorly in the pedicles of the axis, usually with some forward subluxation of C2 on C3. Matthews and associates (67), Nordstrom and coworkers

(68), and Smith and colleagues (69) by contrast, reported similar cases; however, Smith and colleagues called these *persistent synchondroses of the axis* because they thought that the CT showed the defect to be at the level of the neurocentral synchondrosis. Interestingly, later films showed some ossification within the synchondrosis gap. On study of the anatomy of the synchondrosis of the axis vertebra (Figs. 37.3, 37.4B, and 37.15), it can be seen that the synchondrosis is anterior and medial to the vertebral foramen, whereas all of the cases mentioned show the defect in C2 posterior to the vertebral foramen. Because the superior articular process of C2 (for the atlantoaxial joint) is much farther anterior than the inferior articular process, the pars interarticularis region of C2 is also more anterior than it is

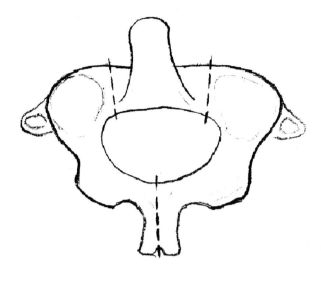

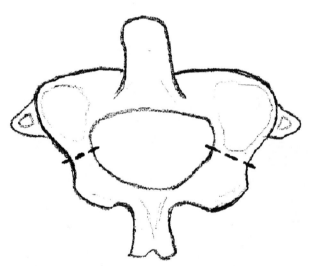

FIG. 37.15. Diagram illustrating the location of the synchondroses of the atlas (a), in comparison to the location of spondylolytic defects in this vertebra reported in children. Note that the synchondrosis is anteromedial to the vertebral foramen, whereas the spondylolytic defects are posterior to them. (From: Howard AW, Letts RM. Cervical spondylolysis in children: is it posttraumatic? *J Pediatr Orthop* 2001;20(5):677–681.)

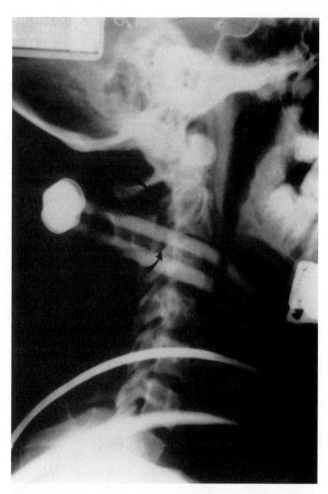

FIG. 37.16. Typical Hangman's fracture in a 14-year-old boy shows a fracture line slightly more posterior than the defect in Figure 37.12.

in other vertebrae. This may lead to the mistaken impression that it is at the level of the synchondrosis. Howard and Letts point out that the embryology favors a traumatic etiology for these defects, rather than attributing them to a persistent synchondrosis (70). Treatment of a symptomatic lesion should be immobilization in a Minerva or halo jacket for 8 to 12 weeks. Pizzutillo and associates (6) reported 80% healing. If union does not occur and the translation remains excessive, an anterior fusion of the second to the third cervical vertebra should be done.

Subaxial Injuries

These injuries represent only one-fourth of all pediatric cervical spine injuries, in contrast to the majority in adults (71). Jones and Hensinger (72) reported the case of a 2-year-old child with hypotonia and motor delay resulting from true C2-3 subluxation whose motor function improved with arthrodesis. Howard and Letts reported bilateral spondylolysis of C4 in a 14-year-old gymnast (70). Fractures and subluxations in the lower cervical spine become more common in older childhood and adolescence. Treatment should follow the principles for adult injury. Despite the slightly improved prognosis for ligament healing in children, those with subluxation and dislocation should be tested by flexion and extension views after immobilization to verify healing.

Spinal Cord Injuries

Partial spinal cord injuries in children have a good prognosis for substantial recovery of function (73); however, if

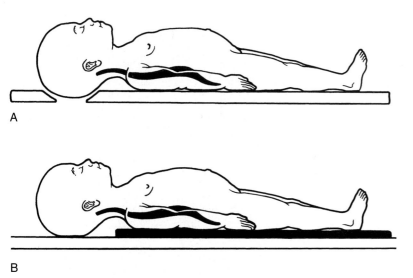

FIG. 37.17. Because of the relatively large head of the small infant, horizontal positioning may result in cervical flexion, which can be overcome by recessing the head **(A)** or elevating the trunk 25 mm **(B)**.

neurologic injury is complete or near complete even after spinal shock has passed, the prognosis for recovery is poor, as in adults. Steroid dosing acutely at the time of injury is usually recommended (as in adults). Late sequelae may include autonomic dysreflexia, development of decubiti, and postlaminectomy kyphotic deformity. Also, any child less than 10 years old with a high-level spinal paralysis has nearly a 100% chance of developing scoliosis. Therefore, follow-up should be arranged to detect and treat this early and arrange appropriate bracing or surgery before the curve becomes severe. (Spinal cord injury in children is further discussed in Chapter XX.)

Immobilization

Acute immobilization of children in whom a neck injury has not been ruled out should be on a backboard with the head taped and sandbags on either side. Herzenberg and associates (5) showed that because of their relatively large heads, children are in relative cervical flexion when placed on a horizontal surface. Therefore, the head should be recessed or the trunk should be elevated by about 25 mm until age 8 years (74) (Fig. 37.17). Definitive immobilization of most unstable pediatric cervical fractures requires control of the upper cervical spine and is best achieved by a Minerva cast or halo jacket (75,76). There are several special considerations when applying a halo for children. The cranium is thinner in children, but its thickness increases progressively with time, reaching adult proportions by age 12 (77,78). The cranial suture lines should be avoided in very young children; they are located at points 4:30 and 7:30 on the cranial circumference as viewed downward from above (Fig. 37.18). The best locations (for pin placement, thickest bone) are the same in children as in adults (79). Pin torque

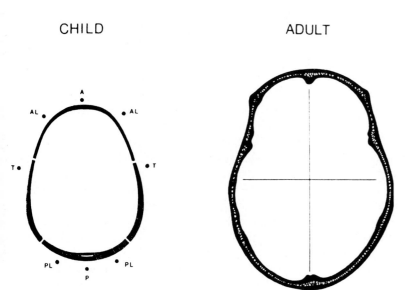

FIG. 37.18. Location of suture lines in infants. Relative thickness of skull in an infant versus an adult.

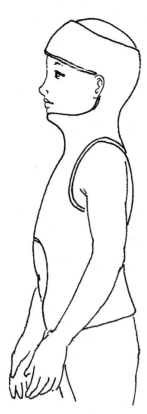

FIG. 37.19. Minerva cast is useful in young children with injuries that do not require detailed visualization or complex reduction.

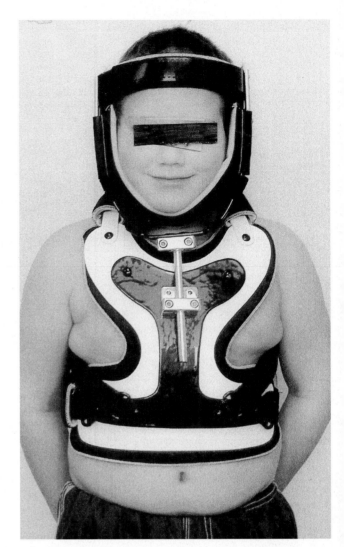

FIG. 37.20. A pinless halo-Minerva orthosis is a useful alternative to a halo with pins in children. (Illustration courtesy of David Skaggs.)

should be 2 in/lb in infants and 4 to 6 in/lb in children (as opposed to 8 in adults) (24). Because of the thinner bone and lower torque, it is recommended to add two to four extra pins in very young children to prevent loosening. The durability of the halo is less well documented in children less than 2 years old. A Minerva cast is an attractive option for younger children, especially those who do not require adjustment of neck position or detailed visualization (Fig. 37.19). A pinless halo orthosis also is available (Fig. 37.20). It is noninvasive yet provides nearly the control and adjustability of a halo vest. A Philadelphia collar may be used for more stable injuries, such as Jefferson fractures with intact transverse ligament or atlas spondylolisthesis without disc disruption.

Surgical Considerations

Surgery is rarely indicated for cervical spine fractures in children; however, several generalizations may be made in cases where fusion is required. The fusion rate is high, and rigid internal fixation often is not needed (80). McGrory and Klassen (81), for example, reported only a 2% rate of nonunion in arthrodesis of pediatric cervical fractures, but over one-third (38%) had unintended extension of the

fusion to an adjacent vertebra. This problem may be prevented by exposing only the levels necessary after localizing them with a radiograph. While making exposure, it is important to be aware of the possibility of an atlas vertebra with a bifid arch or persistent synchondrosis. Allograft bone produces a high rate of pseudarthrosis, even in children, and therefore should not be used (82). The hypermobility of the pediatric spine leads to relatively little limitation of motion after arthrodesis. In the series of McGrory and Klassen (37), however, 29% had some signs of arthrosis at adjacent vertebrae, such as sclerosis and osteophyte formation, a mean of 17 years after arthrodesis.

Subjects pertaining to cervical spine injuries in children which need further work include clarifying protocols for radiographic diagnosis in pediatric trauma as well as guidelines for spinal stability in SCIWORA. Work in these areas is hampered by relatively small series of children with cervical spine injuries. Prospective multicenter studies are needed to answer these questions.

REFERENCES

1. McGrory BJ, Klassen RA, Chao EYS, et al. Acute fractures and dislocations of the cervical spine fractures in children and adolescents. *J Bone Joint Surg Am* 1993;76:988–995.
2. Patel JC, Tepas JJ, Mollitt, et al. Pediatric cervical spine injuries: defining the disease. *J Pediatr Surg* 2001;36(2):373–376.
3. Evans DL, Bethem D. Cervical spine injuries in children. *J Pediatr Orthop* 1985;9:563–568.
4. Hadley MN, Zabranski JM, Browne CM, et al. Pediatric spinal trauma: review of 122 cases of spinal cord vertebral column injuries. *J Neurosurg* 1988;68:481–484.
5. Herzenberg JE, Hensinger RN, Dedrick DK. Emergency transport and positioning of young children who have an injury of the cervical spine. *J Bone Joint Surg Am* 1989;71:1–9.
6. Pizzutillo PD, Rocha EF, D'Astous J, et al. Bilateral fractures of the pedicle of the second cervical vertebra in a young child. *J Bone Joint Surg Am* 1986;68:892–896.
7. Conry BG, Hall CM. Cervical spine fractures and rear car seat restraints. *Arch Dis Child* 1987;62:1267–1268.
8. Caffey J. The whiplash shaken infant syndrome. *Pediatrics* 1974;54: 396–403.
9. Swischuk LE. Spine and spinal cord trauma in the battered child syndrome. *Radiology* 1969;92:73.
10. Shulman ST, Madden JD, Esterly JR, et al. Transection of spinal cord. *Arch Dis Child* 1971;46:291–293.
11. Brown PG, Lee M. Trampoline injuries of the cervical spine. *Pediatr Neurosurg* 2000;32:170–175.
12. Tog J, Das M. Trampoline and minitrampoline injuries to the cervical spine. *Clin Sports Med* 1985;4:45–60.
13. Haffner DL, Hoffer MM, Wiedebusch R. Etiology of children's spinal injuries at Rancho Los Amigos. *Spine* 1993;18:679–684.
14. Cattel HS, Filtzer DL. Pseudosubluxation and other normal variations in the cervical spine in children. *J Bone Joint Surg Am* 1965;47: 1295–1309.
15. Lawson JP, Ogden JA, Bucholz RW, et al. Physeal injuries of the cervical spine. *J Pediatr Orthop* 1987;7:428–435.
16. Rachesky I, Royce WT, Duncan B, et al. Clinical prediction of cervical spine injuries in children. *Am J Dis Child* 1987;141:199–201.
17. deBeer J, Hoffman EB, Kieck CF. Traumatic atlantoaxial subluxation in children. *J Pediatr Orthop* 1990;10:397–400.
18. Orenstein JB, Klein BL, Oschenschlager DW. Delayed diagnosis of pediatric cervical spine injury. *Pediatrics* 1992;89:1185–1188.
19. Pang D, Wilberger JE. Spinal cord injury without radiographic abnormalies in children. *J Neurosurg* 1982;57:119–129.
20. Bus C, Cullen M, Klein M, et al. The pediatric trauma C-spine: is the odontoid view necessary? *J Pediatr Surg* 2000;35(6):994–997.
21. Dwek JR, Chung C. Radiography of cervical spine injury in children: are flexion-extension radiographs useful for acute trauma? *AJR* 2000; 174:1617–1619.
22. Woods W, Brady W, Pollock D, et al. Flexion-extension cervical spine radiography in pediatric blunt trauma. *Emerg Radiol* 1998;5:381–384.
23. Pinnecot GF, Leonard P, Peynot S, et al. Roentgenographic study of the stability of the cervical spine in children. *J Pediatr Orthop* 1984;4: 346–352.
24. Bulas DI, Fitz CR, Johnson DL. Traumatic atlanto-occipital dislocation in Children. *Radiology* 1993;188:155–158.
25. Kenter K, Worley G, Griffin T, et al. Pediatric traumatic atlanto-occipital dislocation: five cases and a review. *J Pediatr Orthop* 2001; 21:585–589.
26. Bundschuh CV, Alley JB, Ross M, et al. Magnetic resonance imaging of suspected atlanto occipital dislocation. *Spine* 1992;17:245–248.
27. Wetzel FT, LaRocca H. Grisel's syndrome: a review. *Clin Orthop* 1989;240:141–152.
28. Fielding JW, Griffin PP. Os odontoideum: an acquired lesion. *J Bone Joint Surg Am* 1974;56:187–190.
29. Fielding JW, Hawkins RJ. Atlanto-occipital rotatory fixation. *J Bone Joint Surg Am* 1977;59:37–44.
30. Fielding JW, Hensinger RN, Hawkins RJ. Os odontoideum. *J Bone Joint Surg Am* 1980;62:376–383.
31. Hamilton MG, Myles ST. Pediatric spinal injury: review of 61 deaths. *J Neurosurg* 1992;77:705–708.
32. Aufdermaur M. Spinal injuries in juveniles: necropsy findings in twelve cases. *J Bone Jt Surg Br* 1974;56:573–579.
33. Bucholz RW, Burkhead WZ. The pathological anatomy of fatal atlanto-occipital dislocations. *J Bone Joint Surg Am* 1979;61:248–250.
34. Burkus JK, Deponte RJ. Chronic atlantoaxial rotatory fixation: correction by cervical traction, manipulation and bracing. *J Pediatr Orthop* 1986;6:631–635.
35. Collalto PM, DeMuth WW, Schwentker EP, et al. Traumatic atlanto occipital dislocation. *J Bone Joint Surg Am* 1986;68:1106–1109.
36. Harmanli O, Kaufman Y. Traumatic atlanto-occipital dislocation with survival. *Surg Neurol* 1993;39:324–330.
37. Hosono N, Yonenobu K, Kazuyoshi K, et al. Traumatic anterior atlanto-occipital dislocation. *Spine* 1993;18:786–790.
38. Papadopoulos SM, Dickman CA, Sonntag VKH, et al. Traumatic atlanto-occipital dislocation with survival. *Neurosurgery* 1991;28: 574–579.
39. DiBenedetto T, Lee CK. Traumatic atlanto-occipital instability: a case report with follow-up and a new diagnostic technique. *Spine* 1990;15: 595–597.
40. Powers B, Milber MD, Kramer RS, et al. Traumatic anterior occipital dislocation. *Neurosurgery* 1979;4:12–17.
41. Ehara S, El-Khoury GY, Sato Y. Cervical spine injury in children: radiologic manifestations. *AJR* 1988;151:1175–1178.
42. Betz RR, Gelman AJ, DeFilipp GJ, et al. Magnetic resonance imaging in the evaluation of spinal cord injured children and adolescents. *Paraplegia* 1987;25:92–99.
43. Farley FA, Graziano GP, Hensinger RN. Traumatic atlanto-occipital dislocation in a child. *Spine* 1992;17:1539–1541.
44. Georgopoulos G, Pizzutillo PD, Lee MS. Occipito-atlantal instability in children. *J Bone Joint Surg Am* 1987;69:429–436.
45. Stein SM, Kirchner SG, Horev G, et al. Atlanto-occipital subluxation in Down syndrome. *Pediatr Radiol* 1991;21:121–124.
46. Sponseller PD, Cass J. Atlanto-occipital arthrodesis for instability with neurologic preservation *Spine* 1997;22(3):344–347.
47. Cohen MW, Drummond DS, Flynn JM, et al. A technique of occipito-cervical arthrodesis in children using autologous rib grafts. *Spine* 2001;26(7):825–829.
48. Birney TJ, Hanley EN. Traumatic cervical spine injuries in childhood and adolescence. *Spine* 1989;14:1277–1282.
49. Lee TT, Green BA, Petrin DR. Treatment of stable burst fracture of the atlas (Jefferson fracture) with rigid cervical collar. *Spine* 1998;23(18): 1963–1967.
50. Hohl M, Baker HR. The atlanto-axial joint: roentgenographic and anatomical study of normal and abnormal motion. *J Bone Joint Surg Am* 1964;46:1739–1752.
51. Apple JS, Kirks DR, Merten DF, et al. Cervical spine fractures and dislocations in children. *Pediatr Radiol* 1987;17:45–49.
52. Grisel P. Enucleation de l'atlas et torticollis nasopharyngien. *Presse Med* 1930;38:50.
53. Parke WW, Rothman RH, Brown MD. The pharyngovertebral veins. *J Bone Joint Surg Am* 1984;66:568–574.
54. Kawabe N, Hirotoni H, Tanaka O. Pathomechanism of atlanto-axial rotatory fixation in children. *J Pediatr Orthop* 1989;9:569–574.
55. Wilson MJ, Michele A, Jacobson E. Spontaneous dislocation of the atlanto-axial articulation including a report of a case with quadriplegia. *J Bone Joint Surg Am* 1940;22:698.
56. Dawson EG, Smith C. Atlanto axial subluxation in children due to vertebral abnormalities. *J Bone Joint Surg Am* 1979;61:582–587.
57. Dubousset J. Torticollis in children caused by congenital abnormalities of the atlas. *J Bone Joint Surg Am* 1986;68:178–188.
58. Phillips WA, Hensinger RN. The management of rotatory atlanto-axial subluxation in children. *J Bone Joint Surg Am* 1989;71:664–668.
59. Seimon LP. Fracture of the odontoid process in young children. *J Bone Joint Surg Am* 1977;59:943–948.
60. Sherk HH, Nicholson JT, Chung SMK. Fractures of the odontoid process in young children. *J Bone Joint Surg Am* 1978;60:921–924.
61. Diekema DS, Allen DB. Odontoid Fracture in a child occupying child restraint seat. *Pediatrics* 1988;87:117–119.

62. Schuler TC, Kurz L, Thompson DE, et al. Natural history of os odontoideum. *J Pediatr Orthop* 1991;11:222–225.

63. Kuhns LR, Loder RT, Farley FA, et al. Nuchal cord changes in children with os odontoideum: evidence for associated trauma. *J Pediatr Orthop* 1998;18:815–819.

64. Fardon DF, Fielding JW. Defects of the pedicle and spondylolisthesis of the second cervical vertebra. *J Bone Joint Surg Br* 1981;63:526–528.

65. Francis WR, Fielding JW, Hawkins RJ, et al. Traumatic spondylolisthesis of the axis. *J Bone Jt Surg Br* 1981;63:313–318.

66. Ruff SJ, Taylor TKF. Hangman's fracture in an infant. *J Bone Joint Surg Br* 1986;68:702–703.

67. Matthews LS, Vetter LW, Tolo VT. Cervical anomaly simulating hangman's fracture in a child. *J Bone Joint Surg Am* 1982;64:299–300.

68. Nordstrom REA, Lahdenrants TV, Kaitila II, et al. Familial spondylolisthesis of the axis is vertebra. *J Bone Joint Surg Br* 1986;68:704–706.

69. Smith T, Skinner SR, Shonnard NH. Persistent synchondrosis of the second cervical vertebra simulating a hangman's fracture in a child. *J Bone Joint Surg Am* 1993;75:1228–1230.

70. Howard AW, Letts RM. Cervical spondylolysis in children: is it posttraumatic? *J Pediatr Orthop* 2001;20(5):677–681.

71. McClain RF, Clark CR, El-Khoury GY. C6–C7 dislocation in a neurologically intact neonate. *Spine* 1989;14:125–127.

72. Jones ET, Hensinger RN. C2–C3 dislocation in a child. *J Pediatr Orthop* 1981;1:419–422.

73. Osenbach RK, Menezes AH. Pediatric spinal cord and vertebral column injury. *Neurosurgery* 1992;30:385–390.

74. Nypaver M, Treloar D. Neutral cervical spine positioning in children. *Pediatrics* 1994;23:208–211.

75. Letts M, Kaylor D, Gouwn D. A biomechanical study of halo fixation in children. *J Bone Joint Surg Br* 1988;70:277–279.

76. Marks DS, Roberts P, Wilton PJ, et al. A halo jacket for stabilization of the pediatric cervical spine. *Arch Orthop Trauma Surg* 1993;112:134–135.

77. Botte MJ, Byrne TP, Garfin SR. Application of the halo device for immobilization of the cervical spine utilizing an increased torque pressure. *J Bone Jt Surg Am* 1985;69:750–752.

78. Mubarak SJ, Camp JT, Vuletich W, et al. Halo application in the infant. *J Pediatr Orthop* 1989;9:612–614.

79. Garfin SR, Roux R, Botte MJ, et al. Skull osteology as it affects halo pin placement in children. *J Pediatr Orthop* 1986;6:424–436.

80. Koop SE, Winter RB, Lonstein JE. The surgical treatment of instability of the upper part of the cervical spine in children and adolescents. *J Bone Joint Surg Am* 1984;66:403–411.

81. McGrory BJ, Klassen RA. Arthrodesis of the cervical spine for fractures and dislocations in children and adolescents. *J Bone Joint Surg Am* 1994;76:86.

82. Stabler CL, Eismont FJ, Brown MD, et al. Failure of posterior cervical fusion using cadaveric bone graft in children. *J Bone Joint Surg Am* 1985;67:375–385.

83. Dormans JP, Drummond DS, Sutton LN, et al. Occipitocervical arthrodesis in children: *J Bone Joint Surg* 1995;77(A):1234–1239.

SUGGESTED READINGS

Ballock RT, Lee TQ, Triggs KJ, et al. The effect on pin location on the rigidity of the halo pin-bone interface. *Neurosurgery* 1990;26:238–241.

Bresnan MF, Abrams IF. Neonatal spinal cord transection secondary to intrauterine hyperextension of the neck in breech presentation. *J Pediatr* 1974;84:734–737.

Dormans JP. Evaluating the child with a cervical spine injury. Instructional Course Lecture. *J Bone Joint Surg* 2002;84A:124–132.

Patrick DA, Bensard DD, Moore EE. Cervical spine trauma in the injured child: a tragic injury with potential for salvageable functional outcome. *J Pediatr Surg* 2000;35(11):1151–1155.

Swischuk LE, Hayden CK Jr, Sawar M. The dens-arch synchondrosis versus the hangman's fracture. *Pediatr Radiol* 1979;8:100–102.

CHAPTER 38

Pediatric Spinal Cord Injury

Randal R. Betz, M.J. Mulcahey, and David H. Clements

From an orthopedic standpoint, the comprehensive care of a child with a spinal cord injury (SCI) is an ongoing process beginning at the time of injury and lasting not only through the rehabilitation and discharge phases, but for the remainder of the patient's life.

The concept of early rehabilitation has led to the development of hospitals and hospital units that specialize in treating patients with SCI. As a result of a patient's early transfer to one of these specialty units (preferably the day of the injury), the number of complications and days spent in the hospital are greatly reduced (1). If at all possible, a child or adolescent with an SCI should undergo rehabilitation in a pediatric rehabilitation facility, where health care providers are specifically trained to address their ever-changing needs.

DEMOGRAPHICS

Prevalence

There are roughly 200,000 people presently living in the United States with some degree of spinal cord impairment resulting from trauma (2,3). It is estimated that there are 7,800 to 11,000 new cases of spinal cord injury each year (4), and that 4% to 14% of such injuries occur in patients less than 15 years of age (5,6). Forty percent have tetraplegia and 60% have paraplegia. Thirty percent to 40% have incomplete lesions.

Etiologies for pediatric spinal cord injury include motor vehicle accidents in approximately 40% of patients, diving in 13%, other sports in 24%, gunshot wounds in 8%, falls in 8%, transverse myelitis in 4% (7), and spinal cord tumors in 3% (8). Etiologies unique to the pediatric population include birth injury (9,10), child abuse, high cervical injuries secondary to skeletal dysplasias, Down syndrome, and juvenile rheumatoid arthritis. With improvements in medical technology, a child with paraplegia or tetraplegia may now survive through normal adulthood (11–13).

Brain injury concomitant with SCI occurs in 25% to 50% of patients (14,15). Careful history of the injury should be obtained, because unrecognized brain injury can substantially affect the rehabilitation process. Patients with both brain and spinal cord injuries may have perceptual deficits, speech deficits, and other associated disabilities that may affect the rehabilitation course.

Lap belt injuries mandate a high index of suspicion for a lumbar distraction injury (Fig. 38.1A,B).

CLASSIFICATION OF SPINAL INJURY

Most spinal cord lesions are initially described as complete (no function or sensation below the level of injury) or incomplete (partial function/sensation below the level of injury). The potentially affected muscles that are tested for function at each level of the spinal cord are listed in Table 38.1. The use of this motor classification system allows for a calculation of total motor index, which then allows for accurate comparison of neurologic recovery from either natural history or surgical intervention (Table 38.2). A system promoted by the American Spinal Injury Association (ASIA) to describe a patient's functional level of injury defines the level of function as that at which there is a minimal muscle power of Grade 3 and intact sensation to pinprick (16), and the next proximal muscle must be Grade 5. In addition, patients are classified by the ASIA Impairment Scale A through E. With the ASIA Impairment Scale, A is complete, B: sacral sparing plus preserved sensation only; C: sacral sparing plus motor function distal to the level of injury but nonfunctional; D: sacral sparing plus motor preservation and functional; and E is normal. This is similar to the old Frankel grading system, but now to be classified as incomplete, there must be evidence of sacral sparing either by perianal sensation or voluntary anal contraction.

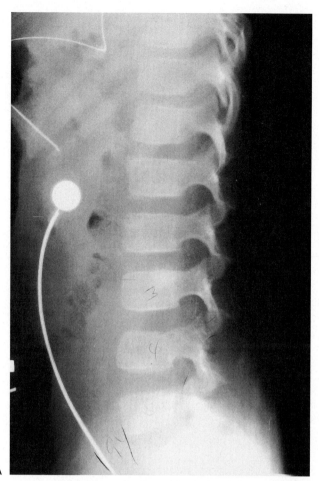
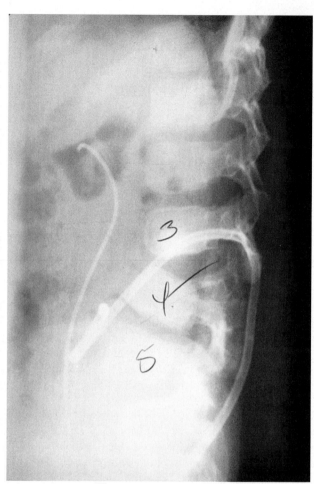

A   B

FIG. 38.1. A: Lateral lumbar radiograph of a 4-year-old child who was involved in a motor vehicle accident. She was in a lap belt in the back seat at the time of impact. She was hemodynamically unstable and was rushed to the operating room for repair of retroperitoneal lacerations. The lateral radiograph shows some suggestion of injury at L3-4. **B:** Lateral radiograph of the same patient 24 hours after the film in **(A)** was taken. Despite careful attempts at positioning this child because of suspected spinal injury, the fracture was displaced further. This flexion-distraction injury then was stabilized using posterior interspinous wiring between L3 and L4.

TABLE 38.1. *Key Muscles for Motor Level Classification*

Motor level	Muscles
C5	Elbow flexors (biceps, brachialis, brachioradialis)
C6	Wrist extensors (extensor carpi radialis longus and brevis)
C7	Elbow extensors (triceps)
C8	Finger flexors: flexor digitorum profundus to the middle finger
T1	Small finger abductors (abductor digiti minimi)
L2	Hip flexors (iliopsoas)
L3	Knee extensors (quadriceps)
L4	Ankle dorsiflexors (tibialis anterior)
L5	Long toe extensors (extensor hallucis longus)
S1	Ankle plantar flexors (gastrocnemius, soleus)

TABLE 38.2. *Motor Examination: Required Elements*

0	Total paralysis
1	Palpable or visible contraction
2	Active movement, full range of motion (ROM) with gravity eliminated
3	Active movement, full ROM against gravity
4	Active movement, full ROM against moderate resistance
5	(Normal) active movement, full ROM against full resistance
NT	Not testable

SPINAL CORD INJURY WITHOUT RADIOGRAPHIC ABNORMALITIES

Introduction

Virtually unique to pediatrics is spinal cord injury without radiographic abnormalities (SCIWORA). These children sustain traumatic myelopathy with no radiographic evidence of bony injury. The incidence may be as high as 67% of all pediatric spinal cord injuries (17). It is thought that the anatomy and pathophysiology of pediatric spines, especially those under 8 years old, may be responsible for this potentially devastating injury. Identification of cervical spine injuries requires a knowledge of the normal variants of the pediatric spine (Figs. 38.2A,B and 38.3). magnetic resonance imaging (MRI) can be very helpful in areas that are difficult to radiograph, such as C7 to T5 (Fig. 38.4). It is rare to diagnose SCIWORA in the 16 and over age group, when the spine has matured to its adult morphology. It is theorized that the inherent elasticity of the immature discs, ligaments, and joint capsules allows significant displacement resulting in spinal cord damage, with subsequent apparently normal realignment.

Mechanism of Injury

There are four primary mechanisms of spinal cord injury: flexion, extension, longitudinal distraction, and ischemia (17–19). Generally, there is no correlation between mecha-

nism and severity of injury. Children 6 months to 8 years have more severe neurologic injuries, and their upper cervical and thoracic spine is more susceptible to injury. Flexion injuries combine with the unique anatomy of the under 8-year-old upper cervical (C1-4) spine to result in cord injury without bony or ligamentous injury. The combination of horizontal orientation of the facets and wedge-shaped vertebrae permits significant anterior motion. Adding the large head and underdeveloped neck musculature into the equation makes the possibility of intervertebral subluxation of sufficient magnitude to cause cord injury a realistic possibility. Extension of the cervical spine may result in anterior folding of the intralaminar ligaments, and spinal cord injury with equal severity at any level (17). In addition, the anterior longitudinal ligament may rupture, with tearing of the intervertebral disc, resulting in injury to the cord. Longitudinal distraction of the elastic pediatric spine may exceed the inelastic cord ability to adapt, also resulting in injury with no obvious radiographic findings. This mechanism may occur in high-speed motor vehicle accidents with a restrained child. Finally, the elasticity of the occiput–C1-2 complex may result in kinking or stretch injury to the vertebral arteries, with subsequent cord ischemia.

Delayed and Recurrent Injury

The onset of neurologic deficit resulting from a spinal cord injury may be delayed from 30 minutes to 4 days (19).

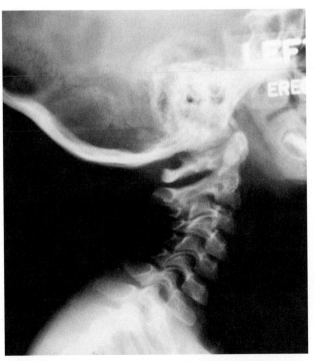
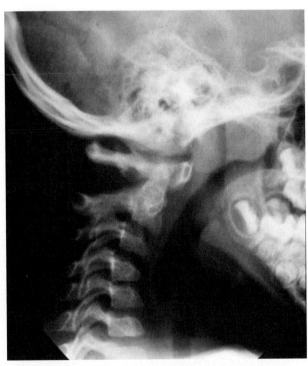

A   B

FIG. 38.2. A: Lateral extension radiograph of the cervical spine. **B:** Lateral flexion radiograph shows pseudosubluxation of the anterior vertebral body of C2-3. The posterior intralaminar line (line of Swischuk) is intact. (From: Swischuk LE. Anterior displacement of C2 in children: physiologic or pathologic? A helpful differentiating line. *Radiology* 1977;122:759–763.)

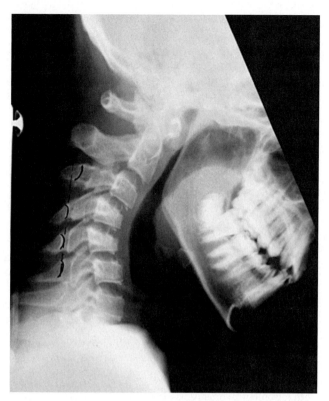

FIG. 38.3. Lateral flexion cervical radiograph shows subluxation after C3-4. The posterior intralaminar line is disrupted to confirm that this is true instability.

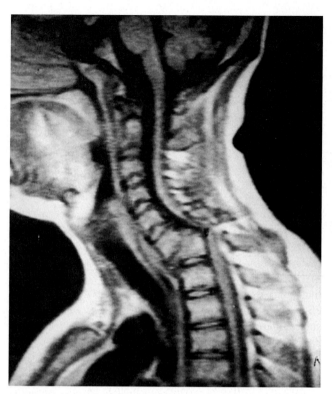

FIG. 38.4. Sagittal cervical magnetic resonance image of a football player with a T7 complete spinal cord injury. Radiographs were indeterminate in defining the spinal column injury.

This phenomenon may be signaled by initial symptoms of subjective distal paralysis, paresthesias, and shooting shocks down the spine with neck movement.

It has been theorized that excessive intervertebral displacement resulting in tearing the restraining structures of the neck may predispose to severe instability even with trivial neck movements (19). This occult instability also may result in recurrent injury in a patient who initially presented with mild neurologic injury but then sustains a second, more severe deficit after subsequent insignificant neck trauma. Protective neck spasm early on, followed by rapid remission of the presenting symptoms without protective immobilization, may help explain this phenomenon.

Thoracic Spinal Cord Injury without Radiographic Abnormalities

Although the rib cage may be expected to protect the thoracic cord against flexion or extension injuries, distraction-type mechanisms may still result in cord damage that is not shown on radiographic studies (17). It has been postulated that the mechanism of injury involves a crush injury to the prone chest, causing an anterior bowing effect on the elastic spine, which results in stretch injury to the cord (17). This mechanism is not seen in supine chest injuries, where the thoracic and abdominal contents protect the spine and pin it in a neutral alignment.

Diagnosis

As implied by its name, SCIWORA is not apparent on conventional cervical spine films (even flexion/extension laterals), tomograms, or CT scans (19). Fortunately, magnetic resonance imaging (MRI) may be useful in both diagnosis and prognosis. Ligament and disc injury may or may not initially be seen on MRI, but if apparent is usually correlated with the mechanism of injury. Isolated examples of physeal injury also have been reported (20–22).

An MRI of the spine should be done in children with suspected SCIWORA to rule out a displaced ring apophysis. Normal MRI findings in the cord usually are associated with an excellent prognosis for recovery. MRI evidence of cord edema with minor or no hemorrhage may offer recovery but suggests the possibility of residual deficits. Major cord hemorrhage or cord discontinuity is correlated with permanent severe cord injury (23). The neurologic level in most children with complete lesions and SCIWORA does not improve (24).

Treatment

Unfortunately, the only successful treatment for SCIWORA is preventive. However, treatment of SCIWORA with rigid immobilization of the neck once the diagnosis is made can be effective. Treatment has been recommended to continue a minimum of 12 weeks to allow ligamentous healing, and a rigid device such as a Guilford brace preferred over a Philadelphia collar (17).

MEDICAL PROBLEMS

Deep Venous Thrombosis

Kewalramani (25) noted a 50% risk of thrombosis in children with spinal cord injury but only a rare occurrence of pulmonary embolus. Most cases of deep venous thrombosis (DVT) occur during the first 3 months after injury, but should be considered a risk whenever a patient is kept at bed rest following plastic surgery for decubitus or any subsequent spinal column surgery. Preventive measures include antiembolism stockings, compression boots, subcutaneous heparin, or low-dose Coumadin.

Immobilization Hypercalcemia

Hypercalcemia is a risk for any patient who is immobilized, but especially for children at bed rest following SCI (26,27). Nand and Goldschmidt (28) reported a 19.8% incidence of hypercalcemia as defined by a serum calcium level of greater than 10.6 dL. Symptoms include nausea, vomiting, abdominal cramps (if the patient has sensation), and distinct personality changes. Diagnosis is confirmed with a high serum calcium level, but must be differentiated from primary and secondary hyperparathyroidism by a parathyroid hormone assay. Treatment consists of intravenous hydration and early mobilization of the patient. A temporary diet with less than 400 mg of calcium per day also may help. Additional treatment aimed at retarding any osteoclastic-mediated bone resorption includes biphosphates and calcitonin (29).

Autonomic Dysreflexia

Patients with injuries above T6 are at risk for autonomic dysreflexia as a result of the traumatic sympathectomy. Autonomic dysreflexia is triggered by noxious afferent stimuli to the skin and viscera below the level of the SCI. The sympathetic reactions cannot be modulated by higher levels of the central nervous system, because their response is blocked at the level of the spinal cord lesion. The autonomic reflex via the lateral horn cells in the spinal cord below the level of injury remains intact and unchecked; this causes reflex arteriolar spasm and blood pressure elevation. The hypertension is recognized by baroreceptors in the carotid sinus, aortic arch, and cerebral vessels. These receptors send impulses to the vasomotor center in the brain stem via the ninth and tenth cranial nerves. The vasomotor center sends efferent vagal stimulus to slow the heart rate and cause dilation of the skin vasculature, which can occur only above the level of injury (30).

Signs and symptoms include hypertension, bradycardia, pounding headaches, vasodilation, flushing, blotching of the skin, and cold sweating above the level of the spinal cord lesion. Anxiety is the major differential diagnosis. If the pulse is elevated instead of decreased, the episode is more likely an anxiety attack. If there is evidence of bradycardia, it is most likely autonomic dysreflexia.

The mainstay of treatment is elimination of the irritation, such as bladder emptying or bowel evacuation. Failing that, medication may be needed.

Respiratory Insufficiency

Depending on the level of injury, respiratory inefficiency of tetraplegia and high-level paraplegia can occur. Decreased inspiratory ventilation is the result of lost intercostal muscles. Decreased expiratory pressure occurs because the diaphragm cannot be passively pushed upward by the contracting abdominal muscles. These patients are at risk for aspiration pneumonia and bronchopneumonia. Prevention of respiratory infections, including pneumococcus and yearly influenza vaccines, is crucial. Postural maneuvers and breathing exercises are essential to train accessory muscles to assist in breathing and help clear secretions.

Cardiovascular Problems

Bradycardia is the primary cardiac problem in patients with tetraplegia. It results from the loss of sympathetic control of the vagovagal reflex (31). In the acute setting, this can account for 66% of mortality in adult patients with cervical SCI. However, the cardiovascular system readjusts itself within 3 to 5 weeks, and the patient does not require a pacemaker. If needed, vagolytic therapy with either atropine or propantheline is effective (32). Hypotension in patients with tetraplegia can occur when they attempt to sit. The use of an abdominal binder can decrease venous pooling and help control this phenomenon.

Vertebral Artery Injury

Although rare, vertebral artery injury can occur with cervical spine trauma. Phenomena not ordinarily associated with cervical trauma, such as altered consciousness, nystagmus, swallowing difficulties, ataxia, and dysarthria should arouse suspicion for this injury (33).

Urologic Problems

The major goals of urologic management of children with SCI are continence and the prevention of urogenital complications, primarily urinary tract infections, urolithiasis, and renal damage. A bladder management program must accommodate the physical and psychosocial development of children and should be convenient and economical, foster independence, and allow adequate privacy.

Fever of Unknown Origin

Fever is a common problem in children with SCI. Evaluation for cause includes acquiring patient history

TABLE 38.3. *Differential Diagnosis of Fever of Unknown Origin*

Most common possibilities
Urinary tract infection
Upper respiratory infection
Atelectasis
Pneumonia
Deep venous thrombosis
Extremity fracture
Early heterotopic ossification
Viral gastroenteritis
Grade III pressure ulcers
Otitis media
Wound infection
Thermoregulator insufficiency

Less common possibilities
Drug fever
Hepatitis
Pancreatitis
Cholecystitis
Appendicitis
Perforated ulcer
Autonomic dysreflexia
Abscess

(e.g., checking for recent urine culture and sensitivity, and recent surgery), performing a physical examination (e.g., routine thigh and calf measurements for swelling, crepitus in the extremity, and skin lesions), ordering laboratory studies (e.g., urinalysis, urine C&S, complete blood count with differential, sedimentation rate, chest radiograph, bilirubin, liver enzymes, and sometimes amylase), and reviewing other studies (e.g., radiographs of extremities and abdomen, bone scan, and venous imaging study of the lower extremities). A sample differential diagnosis is listed in Table 38.3.

ORTHOPEDIC PROBLEMS

Halo Fixators

As with adults, proper halo ring application in children is critical in preventing complications, including pin loosening and infection. Anterior pins should be placed superior and over the middle or lateral one-third of the orbit (to avoid the supraorbital and supratrochlear nerves) and below the greatest circumference of the cranium (34). For the patient older than 12 years, pins should be torqued to 8 in/lb, which has been shown to reduce pin loosening and infection as compared to 5 to 6 in/lb (35). If a pin starts to drain fluid, a culture should be obtained, antibiotics started, and the torque on the pin checked. The pin should tighten within three turns; if it does not, it should be removed and a new one inserted (34).

Younger children (<12 years old) present a unique problem with halo fixation. Multiple pins (10 as compared with four in the adult) with low torque (2 in/lb) have been shown to be safe in infants (Fig. 38.5) (36). For children 2 to 12 years of age, the torque may range from 4 to 6 in/lb. For children

under 6 years of age, computed tomography (CT) scanning of the skull is recommended for pin placement because of the great variability in skull thickness (37,38). When halo fixation fails because of loosening or infection, a Minerva-type cervicothoracolumbosacral orthosis (CTLSO) is effective.

Use of Crutchfield tongs in patients younger than 12 years old is associated with skull penetration and dural fluid leaks. Use of the halo ring for traction, using the principles outlined in the preceding, can be an effective alternative.

Halo vests can cause severe pressure ulcers in a paralyzed patient. Frequent skin inspection beneath the entire halo vest by the nursing staff initially and then by the care provider at home is essential.

Bracing for Spinal Instability

Data on bracing the cervical spine are available for adults and extrapolated to children, but no actual pediatric data are available (39). Recommended bracing by level of injury reported by Johnson and colleagues (39) is listed in Table 38.4. For thoracic and lumbar injuries, a custom thoracolumbosacral orthosis (TLSO) is the preferred choice for bracing.

Spasticity

Spasticity is present whenever an upper motor neuron SCI exists. Spasticity is a condition of excessive reflex activity associated with involuntary movements and clonus accompanied by increased muscle tone. It becomes apparent at about 6 weeks postinjury and seems to plateau after 6 months. A higher incidence of patients with flaccid rather than spastic paralysis is unique to pediatrics. In a review of 169 pediatric patients (40), only 74% had spasticity, with 26% being flaccid. Of adults with SCI, most (>90%) have spasticity. This may result from a more severe SCI secondary to the flexible condition of a child's spinal column. Although spasticity may be annoying to the patient, it is thought to preserve muscle mass, which may aid in preventing pressure ulcers. Spasticity may increase with nociceptive complications such as urinary tract infections, kidney stones, pressure ulcers, bowel impactions, tight clothes, or underinflated wheelchair cushions.

The mainstay of treatment is range of motion. In addition, medication usually is necessary. A baclofen pump can be effective in cases refractory to medication or if side effects are troublesome.

Heterotopic Ossification

Heterotopic ossification occurs in 16% to 53% of patients of all ages with SCI and is most commonly seen at the hips, knees, elbows, and shoulders (41). It can develop up to 14 months after injury in children as compared with 6 months in adults (42), and is most common in patients with tetraplegia. Heterotopic ossification may present subtly

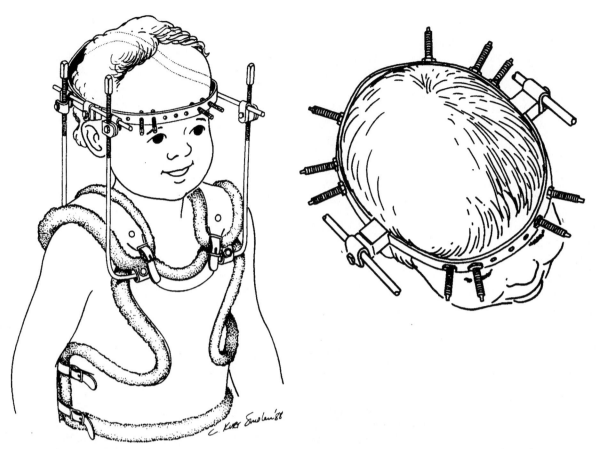

FIG. 38.5. Schematic of halo placement in an infant. Note the increased number of pins, from four to eight or 10. Use 2 pounds per inch of torque instead of 8. (From: Pezeshki C, Brooker AF Jr. Immobilization hypercalcemia. Report of two cases treated with calcitonin. *J Bone Joint Surg Am* 1977;59: 971–973.)

as an inflammatory reaction of increased redness, warmth, swelling, and gradual loss of joint motion. In pediatrics, the only finding commonly seen is decreased range of motion (42), although several patients have presented with knee and hip joint effusions. Three-phase bone scans are often positive 4 to 6 weeks before there is evidence of ossification on plain radiographs (43). Treatment involves maintaining

TABLE 38.4. *Rigid Conventional Braces that Provide the Best Control of Flexion and Extension at Different Levels of the Cervical Spine*

Segmental levels	Brace	Mean motion allowed (degrees)
C1-2	Halo	3.4
	Halo	2.4
C2-3	Four poster	3.7
	Cervicothoracic	3.8
Middle (C3-5)	Cervicothoracic	4.6
Lower (C5-T1)	Cervicothoracic	4.0

From: Johnson RM, Hart DL, Simmons EF, et al. Cervical orthoses. A study comparing their effectiveness in restricting cervical motion in normal subjects. *J Bone Joint Surg Am* 1977;59:332–339.

range of motion and indomethacin. Didronel (etidronate disodium) can be effective, but the dose must be 20 mg/kg per day (initially intravenously). Didronel should be used with caution in children because it may cause growth abnormalities (44). Radiation therapy has been effective in adults, but is not used in children, unless there is a second occurrence, because of the risk of sarcomatous changes.

Heterotopic ossification can be a substantial problem, especially at the hips, as it can prevent a patient from sitting (Fig. 38.6). It appears to become mature after approximately 18 months and can be assessed by bone scan and alkaline phosphatase. The timing of surgery is important. In the past, it was believed that an abnormal serum alkaline phosphatase and an abnormal three-phase bone scan were predictors of recurrence (45). As a result, it was recommended that the bone scan and alkaline phosphatase be repeated and surgery delayed until they returned to normal. However, Garland (46) strongly recommends resecting the HO at 1.5 years after SCI. Waiting any longer for the bones scan and alkaline phosphatase to return to normal risks the development of severe intraarticular fibrosis and femoral neck osteoporosis, which prevent return of hip motion or risk hip fracture during surgery.

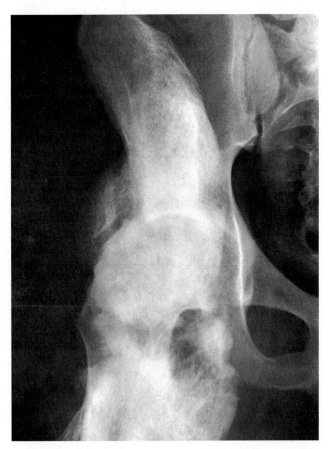

FIG. 38.6. Anteroposterior radiograph of an 18-year-old patient with quadriplegia and severe heterotopic ossification of the right hip. The patient's hip was fixed in 20 degrees of flexion.

Spine Deformity

There is a high prevalence of spine deformity in children and adolescents with SCI. A child injured more than a year before reaching maturity has a 98% chance of developing scoliosis and a 67% chance of requiring surgery (47–49). In contrast, if an adolescent is injured less than 1 year before reaching maturity, there is only a 20% chance that he or she will develop scoliosis, with a 5% risk of progressing to surgery (47).

Prophylactic bracing in the form of a lightweight TLSO may be effective in delaying or preventing surgery. In a comparison series reported by Lieberman and Betz, 24 patients who underwent prophylactic bracing showed an 80% success rate in maintaining their curvature versus 20% failure, progressing over 50 degrees. In comparison, a group of five patients never having been braced showed four of the five (80%) progressing past 50 degrees and requiring surgery. In that study, further analysis of the data showed that starting a brace prior to a curve progressing over 20 degrees or within 1 year postinjury had an excellent success rate for maintaining a curvature as compared to those with later bracing having a much higher rate of progression.

Prior to skeletal maturity, a child should be seen every 3 months for observation of paralytic spine deformities. For children older than 10 years of age, surgery is recommended when curves progress past 40 degrees. For those younger than 10 years, curves up to 80 degrees are tolerated if they are somewhat flexible and temporarily decrease while in a brace; otherwise, surgery is recommended regardless of age.

Dislocated or Subluxated Hips

In an unpublished review of pediatric patients with SCI, there was a 43% prevalence of nonseptic subluxated or dislocated hips in growing children followed a minimum of 3 years. Age at injury correlated with hip deformities, with a 100% prevalence of instability in those injured under 5 years of age and 83% of those injured under 10 years of age. It appears to be equally prevalent in patients with tetraplegia and paraplegia and in males and females. Onset of hip instability following SCI varies, from 7 months to 15 years postinjury. Hip instability has been seen in patients with spastic and flaccid SCI. Several skeletally mature patients have been seen at our center with rapid onset of noninfected hip subluxation.

If left untreated, these unstable hips can develop into a Charcot joint. As the hip dislocates and relocates with spasticity, a vicious circle is created; increased fragmentation of the joint results in further spasticity, until the hip socket is totally destroyed (Fig. 38.7A,B).

In the past, the hips of children with SCI have not routinely been treated. One report of a small series notes no functional deficits in children with SCI with subluxated or dislocated hips (50), but diminution in sitting tolerance has been reported (51). With the development of functional neuromuscular stimulation for computerized standing and walking and the future potential for spinal cord regeneration, more aggressive treatment of hip deformities must be considered. Prophylactic abduction bracing starting at the onset of injury should be instituted in all patients younger than 5 years of age to help prevent subluxation or dislocation. To the authors' knowledge, no reports are yet available on this treatment.

Treatment of a patient with a subluxated or dislocated hip is complex. Spasticity needs to be addressed with medication, nerve blocks, a baclofen pump, or rhizotomies (thermal or open). Soft-tissue contractures must be released. Once the spasticity and contractures are addressed, bony stability should be achieved. The hip instability is usually posterior; therefore, a posterior capsulorrhaphy and an acetabular augmentation posteriorly (52) or a Chiari osteotomy should be considered.

Pain

Chronic pain after SCI can be disabling and can have negative effects on successful school, work, and social interactions (53). Pain can originate from the area of trauma,

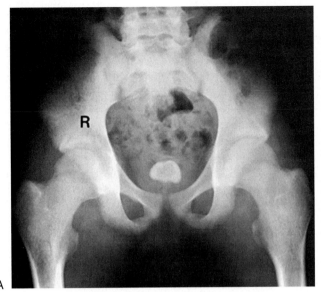
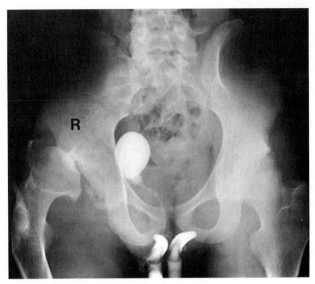

FIG. 38.7. A: This 17-year-old boy with T8 complete paraplegia had severe flexor and adductor spasms. He was instructed to do range-of-motion exercises, sleep prone with a pillow between the legs, and take antispasmodic medication. The patient refused to use the recommendations and did not follow up. **B:** He was seen 9 months later with the right hip dislocated posteriorly with no evidence of sepsis. Fragmentation of the joint confirmed the diagnosis of a Charcot joint.

either in a radicular pattern (specifically from compression of the nerve root at the level of injury) or from mechanical instability of an unhealed fracture, or it can consist of central pain (also known as spinal cord pain or dysesthesia) (54).

Spinal cord dysesthesias constitute a perplexing problem involving numbness, tingling, burning, and pain felt below the level of injury similar to phantom pain after amputation. The dysesthesias are diffuse and do not conform to any dermal distribution. The prevalence of dysesthesias in patients with SCI ranges from 82% to 94% (55) and are influenced by many factors, including depression, anxiety, weather, smoking, alcohol, exercise, and fatigue. Drugs are occasionally effective, including nonsteroidal antiinflammatory agents, amitriptyline (Elavil), carbamazepine (Tegretol), phenytoin (Dilantin), and gabapentin (Neurontin). A transcutaneous electrical nerve stimulation (TENS) unit can be helpful on occasion (54).

Upper extremity pain is common (31% to 55%) in patients with tetraplegia, especially at the C5 level (56,57). This can occur because of muscle deconditioning and shortening, overuse, or cervical radiculopathy. Treatment most often requires muscle strengthening and stretching (58) and alternative ways of performing functional tasks (57).

Reflex Sympathetic Dystrophy

Reflex sympathetic dystrophy has been seen in patients with tetraplegia who complain of diffuse pain, swelling, and stiffness in their upper extremity. A prospective series by Gellman and colleagues (59) showed a prevalence of 12% in adults. Three-phase bone scan is considered the most

sensitive and specific diagnostic study (60), and the diagnosis is confirmed by a response to a stellate ganglion block.

Carpal Tunnel Syndrome

Another study by Gellman and associates (61) reported that 38 of 77 (49%) of patients with paraplegia whose level of injury was at or caudad to the second thoracic vertebrae were found to have signs and symptoms of carpal tunnel syndrome.

Osteopenia

Osteopenia occurs in all patients with SCI. It starts immediately and seems to plateau anywhere between 6 months and 1 year postinjury. Children and adolescents with SCI appear to have bone density that is approximately 60% of that in normal age- and sex-matched controls.

Fractures Secondary to Osteopenia

The prevalence of pathologic fractures occurring secondary to osteopenia patients with SCI ranges from 10% to 20% (22,62–65). In a review of 176 children and adolescents with SCI (40), 25 patients had 54 pathologic fractures. The etiology in 40% included gait training, range-of-motion exercises, and minor trauma. Sixty percent presented with no etiology, and presentation included fever of unknown origin or redness and swelling about the lower extremities. The most frequent locations of secondary fracture were the supracondylar region of the femur and the proximal tibia. Fractures also occurred at the hip and ankle.

Posttraumatic Syrinx

Posttraumatic syrinx following spinal cord injury has been reported (66,67). In the past, the prevalence was thought to be very low (2% to 3%), and diagnosis by CT myelography was required (67). However, studies with MRI report an incidence averaging 50% (66). Therefore, because the cysts are extremely common, it is essential that a patient's symptoms be established and related to a progressive cyst before decompression is considered. Symptoms that may necessitate decompression of a cyst include ascending neurologic level, increasing pain, increased spasticity, and change in bladder management and hyperhidrosis. Surgical treatment may include aspirations or shunting via a catheter into either the intrapleural or intraperitoneal cavity (67). Recent work has shown detethering the scarred area with dural patching to be helpful (68).

Brachial Plexus Palsy

A brachial plexus injury may be seen concomitant with a spinal cord injury (69). The clinical features suggesting associated brachial plexus palsy include lower motor neuron paralysis, absent reflexes, variable sensory changes, and occasionally Horner syndrome.

RESEARCH

A large portion of research is working toward minimizing the trauma at the time of the acute injury. Trauma alone rarely causes the anatomic transection of the spinal cord (<15% of cases) (70). The neurologic deficits caused by microscopic physical disruption of the axons transversing the injury site are compounded by local infarction, microhemorrhages, or edema. Laboratory studies of chronically injured spinal cords indicate that even a few remaining intact axons (5% to 18%) support functional recovery (71,72). However, in some instances remaining axons may be dysfunctional, which is probably owing to demyelination (73).

To minimize secondary damage following the trauma, high-dose methylprednisolone (30 mg/kg of body weight followed by an infusion of 5.4 mg/kg per hour for 23 hours started within 8 hours of injury) is used (74). However, no patients under 13 years of age have been reportedly studied. Gangliosides (Sygen) present in central nervous system cell membranes augment neurite outgrowth *in vitro* and induce regeneration and sprouting of neurons (75,76). Geissler and associates have reported results of a randomized, prospective study of Sygen in approximately 1,000 patients. They showed no change in neurologic status of patients classified ASIA A and slight improvement (without functional significance) in patients classified as ASIA B. In those classified ASIA C and D, earlier neurologic improvement was noted as compared to the control group; however, at 6 months the neurologic status of the two groups was comparable.

Research in regeneration of injured spinal cords has focused on ways to stimulate axonal growth. Brain-derived neurotrophic factor and Schwann cells from peripheral nerves in tissue culture have been found to stimulate neurite outgrowth in a rat model (77). The axonal proteins that appear to inhibit regeneration of the spinal cord in contrast to peripheral nerve regeneration have been identified (78,79). Attempts in laboratories to modulate these protein productions have been through immunologic manipulation (80) and enzymatic alteration, both of which appear to be promising. In animal studies, electrical stimulation of regenerating axons has been performed (81), as has embryonic transfer of fetal tissue (82,83).

Research not only continues to improve and further the potential for spinal cord injury recognition and treatment but also enables better understanding of problems of children with SCI and suggests improvement in functional enhancements and, as a result, quality of life.

REFERENCES

1. Devivo MJ, Kartus PL, Stover SL, et al. Benefits of early admission to an organised spinal cord injury care system. *Paraplegia* 1990;28:545–555.
2. Devivo MJ, Fine PR, Maetz HM, et al. Prevalence of spinal cord injury: a reestimation employing life table techniques. *Arch Neurol* 1980;37:707–708.
3. Harvey C, Rothschild BB, Asmann AJ, et al. New estimates of traumatic SCI prevalence: a survey-based approach. *Paraplegia* 1990;28:537–544.
4. National Spinal Cord Injury Association. Fact Sheet #2: spinal cord injury statistical information. *Spinal Cord Injury: The Facts and Figures,* 1986.
5. Burke DC. *Handbook of clinical neurology,* New York: 1976.
6. Gehrig R, Michaelis LS. Statistics of acute paraplegia and tetraplegia on a national scale. Switzerland 1960–1967. *Paraplegia* 1968;6:93–695.
7. Dunne K, Hopkins IJ, Shield LK. Acute transverse myelopathy in childhood. *Dev Med Child Neurol* 1986;28:198–204.
8. Shriners Hospitals. *Shriners Hospitals Annual Statistical Report for the Shrine Units,* 1991.
9. Abroms IF, Bresnan MJ, Zuckerman JE, et al. Cervical cord injuries secondary to hyperextension of the head in breech presentations. *Obstet Gynecol* 1973;41:369–378.
10. Gordon N, Marsden B. Spinal cord injury at birth. *Neuropadiatrie* 1970;2:112–118.
11. Bracken MB, Collins WF, Freeman DF, et al. Efficacy of methylprednisolone in acute spinal cord injury. *JAMA* 1984;251:45–52.
12. Devivo MJ. *Life expectancy and causes of death for persons with spinal cord injuries.* Research Update. Birmingham, AL: University of Alabama, 1990.
13. Devivo MJ, Stover SL, Black KJ. Prognostic factors for 12-year survival after spinal cord injury. *Arch Phys Med Rehabil* 1992;73:156–162.
14. Davidoff G, Morris J, Roth E, et al. Cognitive dysfunction and mild closed head injury in traumatic spinal cord injury. *Arch Phys Med Rehabil* 1985;66:489–491.
15. Schueneman AL, Morris J. Neuropsychological deficits associated with spinal cord injury. *SCI Digest* 1982;35–36.
16. American Spinal Injury Association. *Standards for neurologic classification of spinal injury patients.* Atlanta, GA: ASIA, 1991.
17. Pang D, Pollack IF. Spinal cord injury without radiologic abnormality in children–the SCIWORA syndrome. *J Trauma* 1989;29:654–664.
18. Kriss VM, Kriss TC. SCIWORA (spinal cord injury without radiographic abnormality) in infants and children. *Clin Pediatr Phila* 1996;35:119–124.
19. Pang D, Wilberger JE, Jr. Spinal cord injury without radiographic abnormalities in children. *J Neurosurg* 1982;57:114–129.

20. Keller RH. Traumatic displacement of the cartilaginous vertebral rim: a sign of intervertebral disc prolapse. *Radiology* 1974;110:21–24.

21. Lawson JP, Ogden JA, Bucholz RW, et al. Physeal injuries of the cervical spine. *J Pediatr Orthop* 1987;7:428–435.

22. Nottage WM. A review of long-bone fractures in patients with spinal cord injuries. *Clin Orthop* 1981;155:65–70.

23. Grabb PA, Pang D. Magnetic resonance imaging in the evaluation of spinal cord injury without radiographic abnormality in children. *Neurosurgery* 1994;35:406–414.

24. Anderson JM, Schutt AH. Spinal injury in children: a review of 156 cases seen from 1950 through 1978. *Mayo Clin Proc* 1980;55:499–504.

25. Kewalramani LS. Neurogenic gastroduodenal ulceration and bleeding associated with spinal cord injuries. *J Trauma* 1979;19:259–265.

26. Christofaro RL, Brink JD. Hypercalcemia of immobilization in neurologically injured children: a prospective study. *Orthopedics* 1979;2: 486–491.

27. Lawrence GD, Loeffler RG, Martin LG, et al. Immobilization hypercalcemia. Some new aspects of diagnosis and treatment. *J Bone Joint Surg Am* 1973;55:87–94.

28. Nand S, Goldschmidt JM. Hypercalcemia and hyperuricemia in young patients with spinal cord injury. *Arch Phys Med Rehabil* 1976;57:553.

29. Pezeshki C, Brooker AF Jr. Immobilization hypercalcemia. Report of two cases treated with calcitonin. *J Bone Joint Surg Am* 1977;59: 971–973.

30. Shea JD, Gioffre R, Carrion H, et al. Autonomic hyperreflexia in spinal cord injury. *South Med J* 1973;66:869–872.

31. Carter RE. Medical management of pulmonary complications of spinal cord injury. *Adv Neurol* 1979;22:261.

33. Lyness SS, Simeone FA. Vascular complications of upper cervical spine injuries. *Orthop Clin North Am* 1978;9:1029–1038.

34. Garfin SR, Botte MJ, Waters RL, et al. Complications in the use of the halo fixation device. *J Bone Joint Surg Am* 1986;68:320–325.

35. Botte MJ, Byrne TP, Garfin SR. Application of the halo device for immobilization of the cervical spine utilizing an increased torque pressure. *J Bone Joint Surg Am* 1987;69:750–752.

36. Mubarak SJ, Camp JF, Vuletich W, et al. Halo application in the infant. *J Pediatr Orthop* 1989;9:612–614.

37. Garfin SR, Roux R, Botte MJ, et al. Skull osteology as it affects halo pin placement in children. *J Pediatr Orthop* 1986;6:434–436.

38. Letts M, Kaylor D, Gouw G. A biomechanical analysis of halo fixation in children. *J Bone Joint Surg Br* 1988;70:277–279.

39. Johnson RM, Hart DL, Simmons EF, et al. Cervical orthoses. A study comparing their effectiveness in restricting cervical motion in normal subjects. *J Bone Joint Surg Am* 1977;59:332–339.

40. Shriners Hospitals. Shriners Hospitals annual pediatric SCI statistical report for the Shrine units. Birmingham, AL: 1998.

41. Venier LH, Ditunno JF Jr. Heterotopic ossification in the paraplegia patient. *Arch Phys Med Rehabil* 1971;52:475–479.

42. Garland DE, Shimoyama ST, Lugo C, et al. Spinal cord insults and heterotopic ossification in the pediatric population. *Clin Orthop* 1989; 245:303–310.

43. Campbell J, Bonnett C. Spinal cord injury in children. *Clin Orthop* 1975;112:114–123.

44. Stover SL, Hahn HR, Miller JMI. Disodium etidronate in the prevention of heterotopic ossification following spinal cord injury. *Paraplegia* 1976;14:146–156.

45. Tibone J, Sakimura I, Nickel VL, et al. Heterotopic ossification around the hip in spinal cord-injured patients: a long-term follow-up study. *J Bone Joint Surg Am* 1978;60:769–775.

46. Garland DE. A clinical perspective on common forms of acquired heterotopic ossification. *Clin Orthop* 1991;263:13–29.

47. Dearolf WW 3d, Betz RR, Vogel LC, et al. Scoliosis in pediatric spinal cord-injured patients. *J Pediatr Orthop* 1990;10:214–218.

48. Lancourt JE, Dickson JH, Carter RE. Paralytic spinal deformity following traumatic spinal-cord injury in children and adolescents. *J Bone Joint Surg Am* 1981;63:47–53.

49. Mayfield JK, Erkkila JC, Winter RB. Spine deformity subsequent to acquired childhood spinal cord injury. *J Bone Joint Surg Am* 1981;63: 1401–1411.

50. Rink P, Miller F. Hip instability in spinal cord injury patients. *J Pediatr Orthop* 1990;10:583–587.

51. Baird RA, DeBenedetti MJ, Eltorai I. Non-septic hip instability in the chronic spinal cord injury patient. *Paraplegia* 1986;24:293–300.

52. Betz RR, Mulcahey MJ, Smith BT, et al. Implications of hip subluxation for FES-assisted mobility in patients with spinal cord injury. *Orthopedics* 2001;24:181–184.

53. Brittell CW, Mariano AJ. Chronic pain in spinal cord injury. *Phys Med Rehabil* 1991;5:71–82.

54. Farkash AE, Portenoy RK. The pharmacological management of chronic pain in the paraplegic patient. *J Am Paraplegia Soc* 1986;9:41–50.

55. Davis R. Pain and suffering following spinal cord injury. *Clin Orthop* 1975;112:76.

56. Bayley JC, Cochran TP, Sledge CB. The weight-bearing shoulder. The impingement syndrome in paraplegics. *J Bone Joint Surg Am* 1987;69: 676–678.

57. Sie IH, Waters RL, Adkins RH, et al. Upper extremity pain in the postrehabilitation spinal cord injured patient. *Arch Phys Med Rehabil* 1992;73:44–48.

58. Sheldon GM. Treatment options for shoulder pain in quadriplegia. *J AOTA* 1988;11:1–3.

59. Gellman H, Eckert RR, Botte MJ, et al. Reflex sympathetic dystrophy in cervical spinal cord injury patients. *Clin Orthop* 1988;233:126–131.

60. McKinnon SE, Holder LE. The use of three-phase radionuclide bone scanning in the diagnosis of reflex sympathetic dystrophy. *J Hand Surg* 1984;9:556.

61. Gellman H, Chandler DR, Petrasek J, et al. Carpal tunnel syndrome in paraplegic patients. *J Bone Joint Surg Am* 1988;70:517–519.

62. Comarr AE, Hutchinson RH, Bors E. Extremity fractures of patients with spinal cord injuries. *Am J Surg* 1962;103:732–739.

63. McMaster MJ, Stauffer ES. The management of long bone fracture in the spinal cord injured patient. *Clin Orthop* 1975;112:44–52.

64. Meinecke FW, Rehn J, Leitz G. Conservative and operative treatment of fractures of the limbs in paraplegia. *Proc Annu Clin Spinal Cord Inj Conf* 1967;16:77–91.

65. Tricot A, Hallot R. Traumatic paraplegia and associated fractures. *Paraplegia* 1968;5:211–215.

66. Backe HA, Betz RR, Mesgarzadeh M, et al. Post-traumatic spinal cord cysts evaluated by magnetic resonance imaging. *Paraplegia* 1991;29: 607–612.

67. Rossier AB, Foo D, Shillito J, et al. Post traumatic cervical syringomyelia. Incidence, clinical presentation, electrophysiological studies, syrinx protein, and results of conservative and operative treatment. *Brain* 1985; 108:439–461.

68. Falci SP, Lammertse DP, Best L, et al. Surgical treatment of post-traumatic syringomyelia and tethered spinal cords. *J Spinal Cord Med* 1999;22:173–181.

69. Grundy DJ, Silver JR. Combined brachial plexus and spinal cord trauma. *Injury* 1983;15:57–61.

70. Bohlman HH. Acute fractures and dislocations of the cervical spine. An analysis of three hundred hospitalized patients and review of the literature. *J Bone Joint Surg Am* 1979;61:1119–1142.

71. Blight AR. Cellular morphology of chronic spinal cord injury in the cat: analysis of myelinated axons by line-sampling. *Neuroscience* 1983;10:521–543.

72. Blight AR, Decrescito V. Morphometric analysis of experimental spinal cord injury in the cat: the relation of injury intensity to survival of myelinated axons. *Neuroscience* 1986;19:321–341.

73. Blight AR, Young W. Central axons in injured cat spinal cord recover electrophysiological function following remyelination by Schwann cells. *J Neurol Sci* 1989;91:15–34.

74. Bracken MB, Shepard MJ, Collins WF, et al. A randomized, controlled trial of methylprednisolone or naloxone in the treatment of acute spinal-cord injury. Results of the Second National Acute Spinal Cord Injury Study. *N Engl J Med* 1990;322:1405–1411.

75. Gorio A, DiGiullo AM, Young W, et al. *Gm1 effects on chemical, traumatic, and peripheral nerve induce lesions to the spinal cord. Development and plasticity of the mammalian spinal cord.* Padua, Italy: 1986.

76. Gorio A, Ferrari G, Fusco M, et al. Gangliosides and their effects on rearranging peripheral and central neural pathways. *Cent Nerv Sys Trauma* 1984;1:29–37.

77. Guest JD, Rao A, Olson L, et al. The ability of human Schwann cell grafts to promote regeneration in the transected nude rat spinal cord. *Exp Neurol* 1997;148:502–522.

78. Caroni P, Schwab ME. Codistribution of neurite growth inhibitors and oligodendrocytes in rat CNS: appearance follows nerve fiber growth and precedes myelination. *Dev Biol* 1989;136:287–295.

79. Schwab ME, Caroni P. Oligodendrocytes and CNS myelin are nonpermissive substrates for neurite growth and fibroblast spreading in vitro. *J Neurosci* 1988;8:2381–2393.
80. Schnell L, Schwab ME. Axonal regeneration in the rat spinal cord produced by an antibody against myelin-associated neurite growth inhibitors. *Nature* 1990;343:269–272.
81. Borgens RB, Blight AR, McGinnis ME. Behavioral recovery induced by applied electric fields after spinal cord hemisection in guinea pig. *Science* 1987;238:366–369.
82. Bregman BS, Kunkel-Bagden E. Fetal tissue transplants promote functional recovery in rats. *Prog Res* 1990;11.
83. Lindvall O, Bjorkland A. Fetal tissue implant in Sweden leads to significant recovery in Parkinson's disease. *Prog Res* 1990;23:5.
84. Winslow EB, Lesch M, Talano JV, et al. Spinal cord injuries associated with cardiopulmonary complications. *Spine* 1986;11:809–812.

CHAPTER 39

Discitis, Osteomyelitis, and Intervertebral Disc Calcification in Children

John M. Flynn and John P. Dormans

Cervical discitis, vertebral osteomyelitis, and disc calcification are very rare conditions in children. Although neck pain is a rare presenting complaint, the cause of such pain for the vast majority of children is injury of muscle, bone or ligaments, torticollis, or referred pain. Most reported cases of cervical spine infection are in adults, who have predisposing risk factors such as penetrating trauma, previous infections, diabetes, or a history of intravenous drug abuse. Most primary infections of the spine in children involve the thoracic and lumbar spine. The discussion in this chapter, to some degree, must be extrapolated from the adult literature and studies of pediatric thoracolumbar spine infections. On the other hand, cervical disc calcification, although rare, has been the subject of many case series, lending more data to management decisions.

The past several decades have brought substantial advances in the diagnosis and understanding of spinal infections in children. Better antibiotics and superior diagnostic imaging techniques are available. Today, the mortality rate from spinal infection is less than 5% (1). Despite this encouraging statistic, spinal infections still can have devastating consequences.

DISCITIS AND OSTEOMYELITIS

Cervical infections are rare but potentially dangerous. Although more than 90% of spine infections in all age groups involve the thoracolumbar spine (2,3), cervical infections have the highest rate of neurologic compromise and the greatest potential for causing disability. In a series of 41 cases of pediatric disc space infection reported by Wenger and associates (4), there was only one case of cervical discitis (caused by *Staphylococcus aureus*). Eismont (5) published a series of four systemically ill infants (2 to 13 weeks of age) with vertebral osteomyelitis. All patients in this series had thoracic and lumbar osteomyelitis. The vertebral bodies of all patients showed severe destruction, whereas the adjacent end plates appeared normal. The authors reported good results when patients were treated with long-term antibiotics. In a series that included 14 cases of vertebral osteomyelitis, Fernandez and associates (6) report one 6-year-old child who had cervical osteomyelitis cause by *Bartonella henselae*. Malik and associates (7) reported the case of a 7-year-old girl who developed a swan neck deformity after infection of the posterior elements of C2, 3, and 4. Cultures were negative. She was treated with débridement and posterior fusion from C1-5. An and Munk (8) presented a case of infection in the same region in a 2-month-old child. Again, cultures were negative. Treatment was by débridement and antibiotics. The result was good at the 24 month follow-up. Sharma and colleagues (9) reported a 6-week-old child with a cervical abscess, C6 vertebral osteomyelitis, and Erb palsy. Cultures grew *Staphylococcus aureus*. Treatment was by débridement and antibiotics.

Disc space infection and vertebral osteomyelitis should be considered as related conditions in a spectrum of disease (4,10). Unique anatomic and developmental features explain the similar etiology and pathophysiology of discitis and vertebral osteomyelitis (11). Although avascular, the nucleus pulposus is metabolically active (12), receiving nutrients from diffusion across the end plates and from the blood vessels in the annulus fibrosis (12,13). In the developing spine, the end plate has an orderly arrangement of cartilage canals. After birth, the cartilaginous end plates become progressively thinner. Thus, bacteria can move directly into the nucleus pulposus in children through the cartilage canals, allowing infection to begin spontaneously in the disc and then spread to adjacent bone. Most of the vessels of the cartilage canals are obliterated by adulthood

(14,15). Hematogenous vertebral osteomyelitis typically begins in the area of the vertebral end plate, just as osteomyelitis of the long bones typically starts in the juxtaphyseal metaphysis. Bacteria arrive through the bloodstream and multiply in the end plate region, then spread secondarily to the disc or vertebral body. If an untreated infection advances, the vertebral and disc tissue can be destroyed, the purulent material can generate pressure on the neural elements, or a septic thrombus can compromise the blood supply to the spinal cord.

Clinical Presentation

The most common presenting complaint is pain (16), usually noted for days to weeks before the time of initial evaluation. The pain frequently radiates to the shoulder and upper back. Patients occasionally complain of radicular pain. When the infection is complicated by an epidural abscess, patients may have signs of radiculopathy or myelopathy. Atypical symptoms, such as headache, chest pain, dysphasia, meningeal irritation, or respiratory problems occur in about 15% of patients (3,17,18). Rarely, patients present with signs of septicemia (19). As might be expected from the anatomic features described, the mean age of presentation for children with discitis is younger than for vertebral osteomyelitis (3 versus 8 years of age) (6). The duration of symptoms is typically longer in children with vertebral osteomyelitis than those with discitis (6). Infants generally have a more acute presentation than other subgroups of patients (3,5,20,21). About 50% of patients in a review of 148 patients reported in the literature had a fever (3).

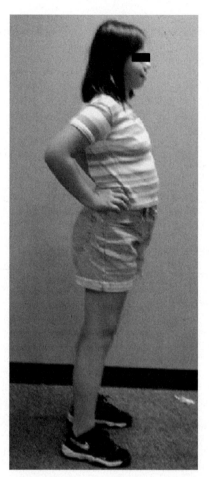

FIG. 39.1. Presentation of a child with disc space infection showing hyperextension and resistance to flexion.

Physical Findings

The most common finding on physical examination is tenderness to palpation of the posterior neck region. Spasm, limited motion, and torticollis also may be present (22,23). Neurologic deficits have been described with vertebral osteomyelitis, typically in older patients with epidural extension. Depending on the series (principally adult patients) the prevalence of neurological deficits in cervical vertebral osteomyelitis ranges form 17% to 82% (3,18,24). Patients with disc space infection often resist flexion and position the spine preferentially in a position of extension (Fig. 39.1).

Laboratory Findings

When a child presents with a possible diagnosis of cervical spine infection, the laboratory evaluation should include: complete blood count (CBC) with differential, erythrocyte sedimentation rate (ESR), C-reactive protein (CRP), blood cultures, and possibly tissue culture (discussed in the following). The white blood cell count is increased in only 42% of cases overall, and is usually normal in patients with chronic infections (3,25). Because it rises quickly in the face of infection and falls quickly with treatment, the CRP has become more useful than ESR in diagnosing and following the effects of treatment in many types of pediatric musculoskeletal infections. However, both ESR and CRP are nonspecific. In one series, blood cultures were positive in 24% of patients with pyogenic spinal infection (3).

Imaging

As in the evaluation of other musculoskeletal infections, plain radiograph should be ordered as the initial imaging study, but there are rarely positive findings until at least 2 weeks after the onset of the infection (2,25–28). The earliest finding on plain radiograph is narrowing of the disc space and abnormal prevertebral soft-tissue contours. Between 3 and 6 weeks, destructive changes in the end plates (Fig. 39.2) and the anterior aspect of the vertebral body are noted. Much later, reactive bone formation, fracture, collapse, and kyphosis are seen (3). In one study, 79% of cases involved at least two vertebrae (2).

Technetium-99 bone scans (Figs. 39.3 and 39.4) and other radionuclide studies are good tests to localize pathology and allow early detection of spinal infections before plain film

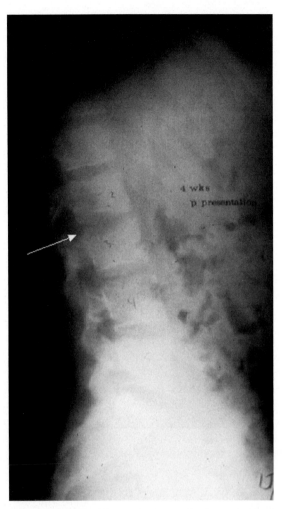

FIG. 39.2. A lateral radiograph shows the irregularity of vertebral end plates *(arrow)* common in disc space infection. Note that disc narrowing may not be seen for 3 weeks.

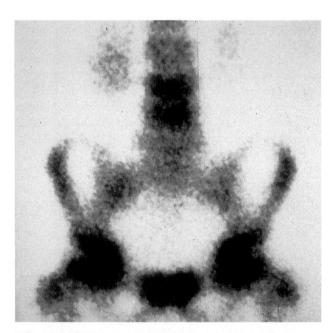

FIG. 39.3. Bone scans can be used to detect disc space infection, although some false-negatives occur. Bone scans are useful early to localize pathology.

changes are seen (29–31). Single-photon emission computed tomography (SPECT) is more sensitive than planar scintigraphy and has better contrast resolution; it also allows three-dimensional localization (32). One study found the sensitivity of planar technetium scintigraphy to be 74% compared with 92% for the SPECT study (33). Gallium scans show evidence of infection earlier in the course of the disease than technetium scans (29,34). In a scenario in which it is important to monitor the response to treatment with imaging, Gallium scans are more useful because they become normal during resolution of the infection; technetium scans remain positive for many months after the disease has resolved (35). Gallium scans have slightly higher specificity than technetium scans (85% versus 78%). Both studies have about 90% sensitivity and 85% accuracy (29,30). Gallium planar scintigraphy had a sensitivity of 69% compared with 92% for the SPECT study. Indium scans alone are not particularly helpful in the evaluation of spinal infections because of low sensitivity. The specificity is 100%, but the sensitivity is only 17% and the accuracy 31% (36).

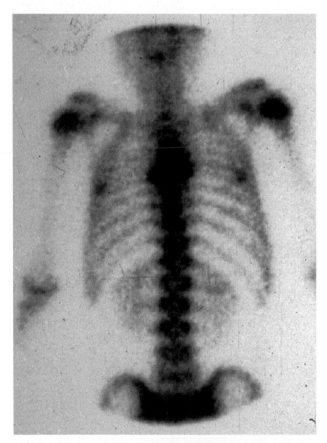

FIG. 39.4. Bone scan showing osteomyelitis of the spine. The origin of infection is arterial, not venous (Batson's plexus), and most patients respond to nonsurgical treatment including antibiotic therapy and immobilization. Long-term antibiotics may be required.

Magnetic resonance imaging (MRI) has largely replaced the computed tomography (CT) scan and is the advanced imaging study of choice in discitis and vertebral osteomyelitis. Although CT scanning shows bone destruction and soft-tissue abscesses well (37–39), MRI provides superior anatomic detail, especially of the disc, ligaments, and other soft-tissue elements, and also eliminates the need for intrathecal injection (Figs. 39.5, 39.6, and 39.7) (40, 41). Modic and associates (30) found that in detecting vertebral osteomyelitis, MRI has 96% sensitivity, 93% specificity, and 94% accuracy. In most cases, MRI can be used to distinguish tumor from infection. In vertebral osteomyelitis, the soft-tissue mass usually surrounds the spine anteriorly, in contrast to neoplasms, which are more likely to have a partial paravertebral soft-tissue mass (sarcoma) or no extension beyond the vertebrae (Fig. 39.7A). Certain neoplasms such as osteoid osteoma, osteoblastoma, aneurysmal bone cysts, and metastasis are more likely to involve the posterior elements than infections and may be osteoblastic (osteoid osteomas, osteoblastoma) compared with the osteolytic appearance of infection (39). Tumors rarely involve the disc spaces and do not have the typical T1- and T2-weighted changes described for infection. Contiguous vertebral involvement is seen more frequently in infections than in tumors; however, contiguous involvement may be seen with aneurysmal bone cyst. Fat planes often are obscured diffusely as a result of edema with infection, whereas they are often intact or only focally altered with most nonaggressive tumors (42). With discitis, the signal intensity in the peridiscal area on T1-weighted sequences is decreased and the junction between the disc and the vertebral body is indistinct. On T2-weighted sequences, the signal intensity is higher than normal in the disc. Gadolinium enhances the disc space and allows better delineation of epidural abscesses (Fig. 39.5) (43). Over time, the T1-weighted sequences revert from a hypointense signal in the vertebral body to a hyperintense fat signal, and the hyperintense signal on T2 diminishes. In the healed stage, the disc space is narrowed or obliterated and spontaneous fusion is common (44,45).

Pathoanatomy of Disc Space Infection

Song and associates (46) examined MRI scans of 16 patients with contiguous discitis and osteomyelitis and defined the anatomic extent of the vertebral and soft-tissue involvement. Altered signal changes were evident in the disc, adjacent vertebra, end plate, and metaphyseal equivalent regions in the anterior prevertebral tissues (Fig. 39.8). Major posterior spread and disc herniation were not evident. Only two of the 16 patients had cervical vertebral involvement. By comparing serial roentgenograms, the mean decrease of disc space height after the acute episode was 43% (range, 51% to 61%). There was no restitution of normal disc space height at latest follow-up in any of the patients (average follow-up 4 years, 5 months). A study of histologic specimens elucidated the vascular anatomy of these immature vertebra, further explaining the disease characteristics (Fig. 39.9).

Biopsy

In most cases, the diagnosis of discitis in children can be made with reasonable certainty based on a careful history and physical examination, laboratory tests, and diagnostic imaging, and confirmed with close follow-up. Usually, antibiotics can be started empirically (or based on blood culture results) and progress can be monitored using improvement

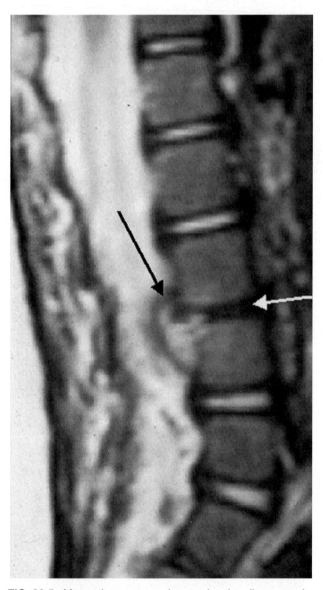

FIG. 39.5. Magnetic resonance image showing disc space infection. Destruction of the end plate is apparent *(white arrow)*. Look for associated abscesses *(black arrow)* in older individuals using gadolinium to differentiate abscesses from phlegmon on magnetic resonance studies.

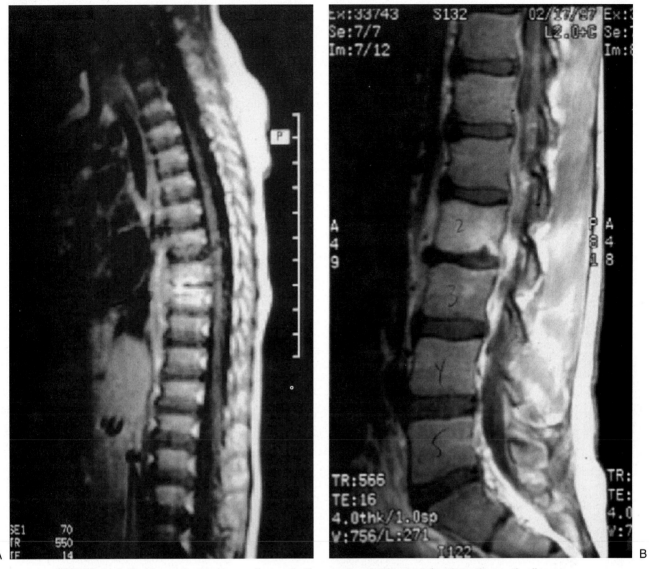

FIG. 39.6. A,B: Magnetic resonance image is the most sensitive test for detecting early disc space infection.

of clinical and laboratory findings as a guide. Thus, although it is ideal to treat such an infection based on the bacteriologic or histologic examination of involved tissue, a biopsy usually is not required or indicated. Biopsy is warranted in rare cases; such as an immunocompromised host, worsening clinical course despite treatment, advanced cases (vertebral osteomyelitis), or rapidly deteriorating status (especially progressive neurologic deficit). Infections in the cervical spine are more likely to lead to instability and neurologic compromise than involvement of the thoracolumbar region. A major or progressive neurologic deficit is an emergency. If the cervical spine is unstable, it should be immobilized (MRI-compatible Gardener-Wells tongs and cervical traction are most commonly used), and an MRI or CT should be obtained.

Some patients need a biopsy. Today, traditional open surgical biopsy has been largely replaced by needle biopsies in the interventional radiology suite (Fig. 39.10). Almost any vertebral body or disc can be safely accessed by needle biopsy (47). Studies report a definitive diagnosis from closed-needle biopsy in only 68% to 86% of cases (3,25,48,49). Open biopsies may have lower false-negative rates because the surgeon is able to select grossly abnormal tissue and provide the pathologist with a larger tissue sample (3). In the cervical spine, open biopsy is often performed as part of the definitive surgical procedure. To summarize, when a biopsy is needed, needle biopsy is usually the best first line option for patients who would not otherwise need surgical management of their cervical spine infection. If the interventional needle biopsy does not provide the diagnosis, and

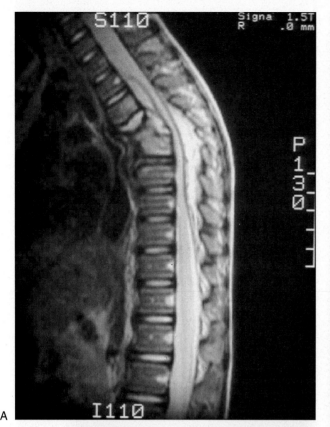

A

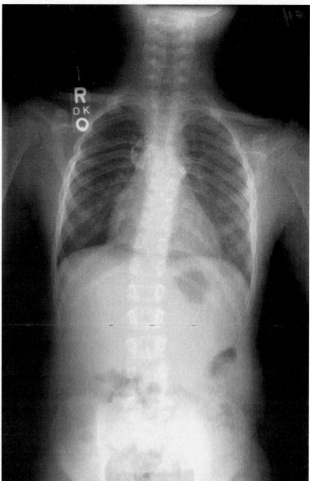

B

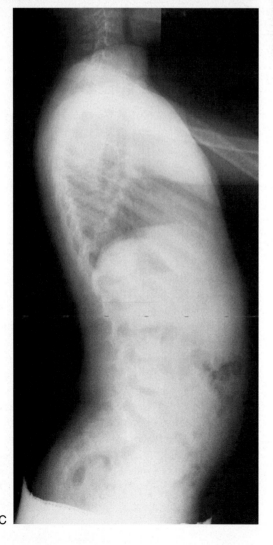

C

FIG. 39.7. A: Magnetic resonance image showing signs of osteomyelitis. Osteomyelitis of the spine is less common than primary disc infection in children. Patients with osteomyelitis of the spine usually present differently because they usually are systemically ill and have an increased temperature and white blood count. The infection is usually caused by *Staphylococcus aureus*. Anteroposterior **(B)** and lateral **(C)** radiographs of same patient 3 years after initial diagnosis. Note the satisfactory alignment of the spine. The patient was asymptomatic and had a normal neurologic examination.

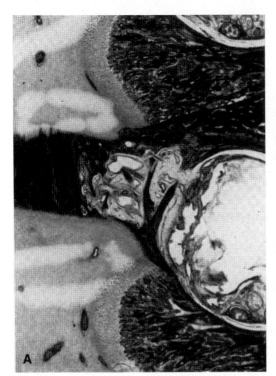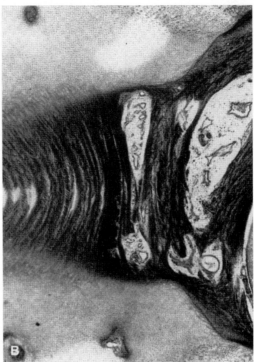

FIG. 39.8. A: Posterior thoracic disc. **B:** Posterior lumbar disc region. In both situations, there is vascular continuity between the posterior vertebral plexus as it courses across the foraminal region and peripheral disc vasculature. In **(B)**, note the contiguous cartilage canals and proximity of some of the physeal and metaphyseal tissues to the disc. (From, Song KS, Ogden JA, Ganey T, et al. Contiguous discitis and osteomyelitis in children. *J Pediatr Orthop* 1997;17:470–477, with permission.)

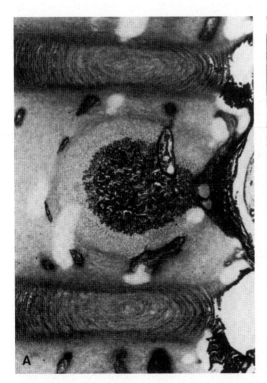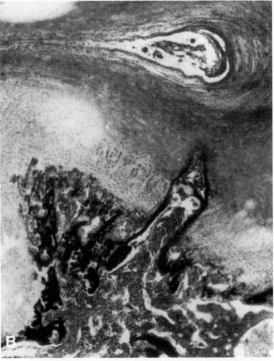

FIG. 39.9. A: Vertebral centrum development (1 year). Note the vascular cartilage canals throughout the nonossified centrum. These are comparable to cartilage canals in the epiphyseal cartilage of long-bone epiphyses. A large vessel crosses the transphyseal region of the primary centrum ossification center, traveling toward the superior disc region. Specimen from a 6-year-old boy who died of traumatic injury. A transphyseal vascular process extends toward the superior disc and its vessels. (From, Song KS, Ogden JA, Ganey T, et al. Contiguous discitis and osteomyelitis in children. *J Pediatr Orthop* 1997;17:470–477, with permission.)

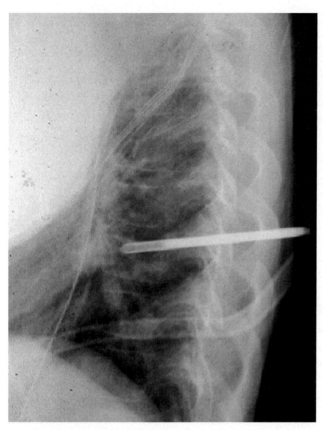

FIG. 39.10. Lateral radiograph showing in-progress biopsy, which can be done with computed tomographic guidance or in the operating room with fluoroscopic imaging. Indications for biopsy include a lack of early response to antibiotics, older patients, patients with past history of drug abuse, and patients with an atypical presentation, including additional destructive findings.

there is no improvement with medical management, a definitive open surgical biopsy is often warranted.

Microbiology

Staphylococcus aureus is the most common pathogen, accounting for 50% of all spinal infections (3). The most frequent gram-negative pathogens (reported in series that contain predominantly adult subjects) are *Pseudomonas*, *Escherichia coli*, and *Proteus* spp., which are common sources of urinary tract infections (25,50–52). Anaerobic infections are uncommon and generally are associated with open fractures, infected wounds, human bites, foreign bodies, or diabetes (3,53). *Salmonella* osteomyelitis is rarely encountered and has a tendency to infect sites of preexisting disease (28,54).

Treatment

The goals of treatment are to establish the diagnosis, prevent or reverse neurologic deficits, eradicate the infection, relieve pain, maintain or establish spinal stability, and prevent relapses. Most disc space infections can be managed effectively with antibiotics and immobilization. Antibiotics are usually administered intravenously for 4 to 6 weeks, followed by an oral course of antibiotics until the signs and symptoms resolve. The CRP is valuable to monitor the success of treatment. In some series, parenteral therapy for less than 4 weeks resulted in a higher rate of treatment failure (2,3,24,50).

On rare occasions, in cases of bacterial cervical vertebral osteomyelitis in children, surgical treatment may be required in addition to antibiotic therapy. There are several indications for surgery. If a patient presents with a clinically important abscess often associated with spiking fevers or worsening course, surgical drainage of the abscess is advised (Fig. 39.11). Additionally, cases refractory to nonoperative treatment (persistently increased CRP or persistent pain) require a surgical resolution. Surgical decompression of neural elements in the presence of a neurologic deficit is sometimes necessary. Finally, surgical intervention is required to prevent or correct spinal deformity or instability (2,24,55,56).

When there is bony collapse and deformity (vertebral osteomyelitis), preoperative traction may be indicated temporarily for spinal realignment and indirect spinal cord decompression. In most cases, the spine should be approached anteriorly to provide direct access to the infected tissues and allow adequate débridement. In cases of epidural extension, the posterior longitudinal ligament should be excised to ensure that the neural elements are decompressed and the infected tissue is removed. In aggressive or untreated infections, bone destruction can extend laterally to the foramen transversarium, placing the vertebral artery at risk during débridement (57). Further, instability (actual or potential) should be addressed surgically. Anterior exposure allows stabilization with autogenous iliac crest strut grafting, which promotes rapid healing without collapse and facilitates rehabilitation (24,58–60). The graft should extend from healthy bone above to healthy bone below (24,55,59,61). When débridement requires more than a two-level corpectomy, a fibular graft may be used (62). Anterior plate stabilization also can augment the structural graft. Laminectomy is contraindicated in most cases because it may lead to neurologic deterioration and increased instability (24,63,64). In cases of major kyphotic deformity, anterior reconstruction with autogenous bone grafts should be done as a first stage after débridement (58,59, 62,65). A combined approach with additional posterior stabilization and fusion (wiring or lateral mass plates) may be indicated in cases of more severe kyphosis, spinal instability, or when postoperative bracing is not possible (62, 63,66).

Immobilization is an important part of the management of vertebral infections in children. In the cervical spine, immobilization is indicated as an adjunct to surgical débridement and grafting, in any case with potential instability, and

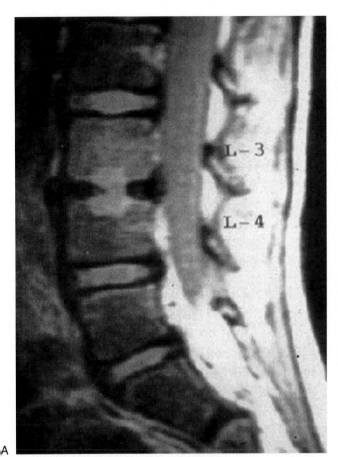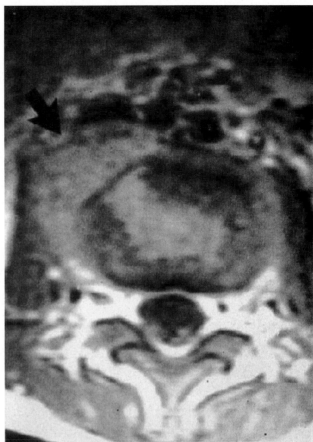

FIG. 39.11. A,B: Indications for surgery for disc space infection include neurologic involvement, severe destruction, and epidural abscess *(arrow)*.

for comfort in stable cases managed with medical treatment alone. The cervical spinal is best stabilized with a halo ring and vest (67), whereas more stable lesions in the lower cervical spine usually can be managed in a cervicothoracic orthosis or hard collar.

Prognosis

Because cases of pediatric vertebral osteomyelitis and are so rare, the literature offers little data regarding prognosis or recurrence rates. The prognostic information that follows is based on literature comprised primarily on teenagers and adults. Relapse of infection is reported to occur in up to 25% of cases, but is much less common if antibiotics are administered for more than 28 days (3,24). Eismont and associates (5) stress the importance of long-term antibiotic treatment to prevent recurrence of infection. The mortality rate is less than 5%; healthy children are expected to be at less risk than elderly patients (3,24), although infants with vertebral osteomyelitis have a poor prognosis and high recurrence rate (5,20). Fewer than 7% of patients overall have residual neurologic deficits (3). Spontaneous fusion occurs in approximately 50% of all patients treated nonoperatively for vertebral osteomyeli-

tis (3,50,68). Infections in the upper cervical spine are reported to have a higher the rate of spontaneous fusion. Almost all cases of cervical infection fuse spontaneously (64,69).

TUBERCULOSIS

Although it is common in developing countries, *Mycobacterium tuberculosis* infection in the cervical spine is rare compared to its incidence in the thoracic spine. There have been several thorough reviews of this subject (70–72). Cleveland reported on 203 patients over a 15-year period. He noted that the majority of infections occurred in the lower spine and that involvement of the cervical and upper thoracic spine was rare (70). Adendorff and associates found similar results (1). In a study of 100 patients by Doub and Badgley, 12% of patients were under the age of 10 and 14% were between 11 and 20 years of age. Children with upper cervical spine involvement usually present with neck pain and stiffness (73). Torticollis also may be present, along with headaches and constitutional symptoms. Neurologic symptoms may vary from none to severe quadriparesis. Lower in the cervical spine, presenting symptoms also can include dysphagia, asphyxia, inspiratory stridor, and kyphosis. In children younger than 10 years of age, more diffuse and extensive involvement is seen with large abscesses, but there is a decreased prevalence of paraplegia and quadriplegia. The neurologic symptoms have a gradual onset over a period of 4 to 8 weeks. Sinus formation is not a prominent feature because of the thick cervical prevertebral fascia, which contains the abscess. Osteolytic erosions are seen in almost every case (Fig. 39.12); in some cases, an increased width of the retropharyngeal soft-tissue space is visible. Instability at the C1-2 level can be seen in some children; rarely is there a fixed C1-2 rotatory subluxation (74). A kyphosis is present in one-fourth of patients with lower cervical spine involvement. Cord compression may occur from the abscesses or the kyphosis. Cultures and biopsies are not always positive. Because the infection usually is located in

the anterior column, many progress to spinal cord compression and paralysis if left untreated.

Treatment

The treatment of patients with acute spinal tuberculosis depends on the resources available and the presence or absence of a neurologic deficit and severe deformity (72). Very little is written about the treatment of tuberculous involvement of the cervical spine in children. To extrapolate from literature in other populations and other regions of the spine, one can support a position that radical débridement and arthrodesis produces better results than radical débridement alone (75–77). In particular, involvement at the cervicothoracic junction presents increase risk for kyphosis.

After the disease has been controlled with medication, the end plates can continue to grow and children may have up to a 50% reduction in the kyphotic deformity with time (72). Thus, prophylactic posterior arthrodesis of the spine in a growing child is not indicated after adequate anterior decompression and arthrodesis (78). Generally, an anterior operative débridement is recommended, because it allows an anterior decompression of the spinal cord and full removal of the abscess and dead bone (72). A posterior approach is used in the rare situation in which the posterior elements are more involved or if posterior stabilization is needed before anterior decompression and arthrodesis are performed (79). Posterior stabilization with metallic implants allows earlier mobilization and does not appear to increase the risk of prolonged infection (80). Surgery performed within about 9 months of acute paraplegia reliably leads to resolution of the neurologic deficit (72). However, Ho and Leong (81) found that operative intervention later than 1 year did not reliably lead to recovery of neurologic deficits.

INTERVERTEBRAL DISC CALCIFICATION

Intervertebral disc calcification in children is a mysterious disorder in its presentation, pathophysiology, and resolution. Hypotheses about its etiology include antecedent trauma or upper respiratory infection (82,83). Since the first report in 1924 (84), over 100 cases have been described in the literature. Boys are affected at a slightly higher rate than girls (1.5:1) (83,85). Most cases occur in school-aged children; considering all cases reported in the literature, the average age at presentation is 8 years (range 8 days to 13 years) (83,85). The process can affect more than one disc. The number of calcified discs averages 1.4 per child (83).

The onset of symptoms is rapid and about 40% of children present with neck pain and about 40% have torticollis (Fig. 39.13) (83). Decreased cervical motion is also common. Neurologic signs and symptoms are rare, only occurring after local symptoms have been present for some time (83). Myelopathy has been reported in 3 of 127 cases in the literature (86). Radiographically, calcified deposits are seen

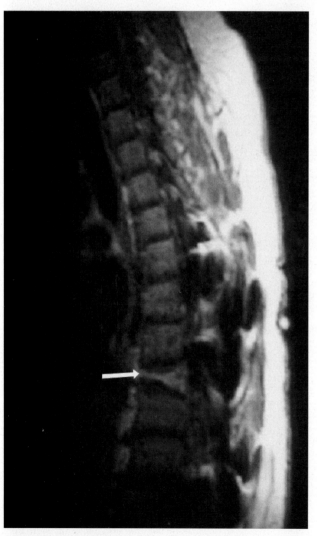

FIG. 39.12. Magnetic resonance image showing evidence of tuberculosis. The differential diagnosis for disc space infection includes eosinophilic granuloma, primary bone tumors, and leukemia (both with preservation of disc space). Tuberculosis is distinguishable by increased destruction with adjacent vertebral involvement *(arrow)*.

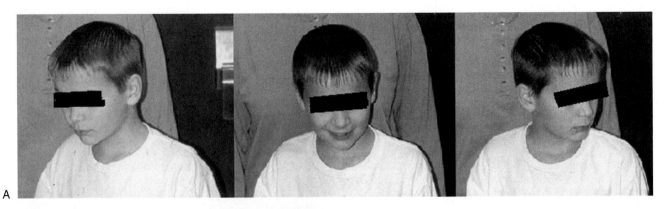

A

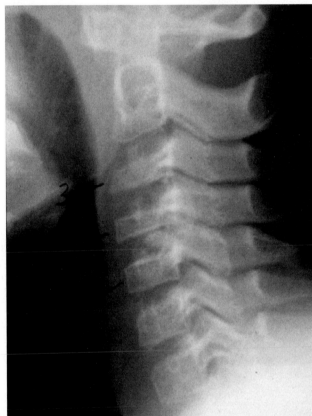

B

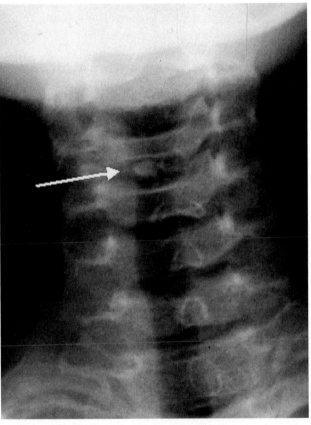

C

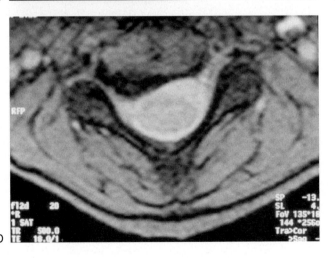

D

FIG. 39.13. A: A 9-year-old-boy presented with neck pain and torticollis. The patient had no neurologic signs or symptoms. The patient was placed in a cervical orthosis during the day with night time cervical traction for several weeks. Pain eventually diminished and the patient achieved increased range of neck motion (ROM). At 1 month follow-up, the patient no longer experienced neck pain and had 90% of normal neck ROM. Plain radiographs revealed disc calcification at the C5-6 level. Lateral **(B)** and posteroanterior **(C)** plain radiographs show flattening of multiple vertebral bodies. Calcification *(arrow)* is visible in the intervertebral discs. **D:** A transverse magnetic resonance image (MRI) scan reveals abnormalities of the cervical disc of C4-5. **E:** Sagittal and parasagittal MRI scans abnormalities of C2-3, C3-4, and C4-5. Cervical end plates are intact and there is no evidence of tumor or an infectious process. The patient was asymptomatic at 1-year follow-up.

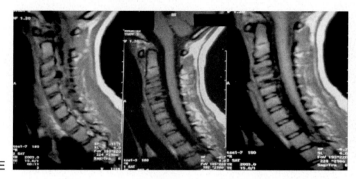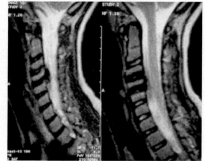

E

FIG. 39.13. *Continued*

delineating the nucleus pulposus (Fig. 39.13). No protrusions were seen in the asymptomatic group of a study by Sonnabend, but 38% of the symptomatic children had detectable protrusions (87) (Fig. 39.13). Recent reports also have shown vertebral body involvement on MRI (71).

The natural history is one of resolution. Without treatment, two-thirds of the children in Sonnabend's study were free of symptoms within 3 weeks, and 95% by 6 months (87). The radiographs showed regression or disappearance of the calcific deposits in 90%. About half of the radiographic improvement occurs within 6 months (87). Children who are asymptomatic may not show radiographic regression even when followed for long periods (88). Children with multiple lesions show variable rates of regression at different disc levels.

Because of the natural history, the treatment is symptomatic unless there is spinal cord compression (82). A short trial of nonsteroidal antiinflammatory medications and a soft cervical collar generally is helpful. Analgesics and cervical traction also can be used, depending on the severity of symptoms (85). Contact sports should be avoided until signs and symptoms resolve. Surgical intervention is rarely needed.

CONCLUSION

Although uncommon, infants and children may develop discitis, osteomyelitis, tuberculosis, or intervertebral disc calcification. Familiarity with presenting signs and symptoms, current imaging modalities, and the natural history of the given disorder as well as appropriate treatment protocols allows the treating medical team to make appropriate decisions and is associated with successful outcomes in the majority of cases.

REFERENCES

1. Adendorff JJ, Boeke EJ, Lazarus C. Tuberculosis of the spine: results of management of 300 patients. *J R Coll Surg Edinb* 1987;32:152–155.
2. Malawski SK, Lukawski S. Pyogenic infection of the spine. *Clin Orthop* 1991;58–66.
3. Sapico FL, Montgomerie JZ. Pyogenic vertebral osteomyelitis: report of nine cases and review of the literature. *Rev Infect Dis* 1979;1:754–776.
4. Wenger DR, Bobechko WP, Gilday DL. The spectrum of intervertebral disc-space infection in children. *J Bone Joint Surg Am* 1978;60:100–108.
5. Eismont FJ, Bohlman HH, Soni PL, et al. Vertebral osteomyelitis in infants. *J Bone Joint Surg Br* 1982;64:32–35.
6. Fernandez M, Carrol CL, Baker CJ. Discitis and vertebral osteomyelitis in children: an 18-year review. *Pediatrics* 2000;105:1299–1304.
7. Malik GM, Crawford AH, Halter R. Swan-neck deformity secondary to osteomyelitis of the posterior elements of the cervical spine. Case report. *J Neurosurg* 1979;50:388–390.
8. An HS, Munk R. Osteomyelitis of the posterior elements of the cervical spine in an infant. *Orthopedics* 1993;16:618–620.
9. Sharma RR, Sethu AU, Mahapatra AK, et al. Neonatal cervical osteomyelitis with paraspinal abscess and Erb's palsy. A case report and brief review of the literature. *Pediatr Neurosurg,* 2000;32:230–233.
10. Currier BL, Eismont FJ. Infection of the spine. In: Rothman RH, Simeone FA, eds. *The spine,* 3rd ed. Philadelphia: WB Saunders, 1992:1319–1380.
11. Copley LA, Dormans JP. Cervical spine disorders in infants and children. *J Am Acad Orthop Surg* 1998;6:204–214.
12. Brown MD, Tsaltas TT. Studies on the permeability of the intervertebral disk during skeletal maturation. *Spine* 1976;1:240.
13. Hassler O. The human intervertebral disc. A micro-angiographical study on its vascular supply at various ages. *Acta Orthop Scand* 1969;40:765–772.
14. Coventry MB, Ghormley RK, Kernohan JW. The intervertebral disk: its microscopic anatomy and pathology. Part 1: Anatomy, development and physiology. *J Bone Joint Surg* 1945;27:105.
15. Rudert M, Tillmann B. Lymph and blood supply of the human intervertebral disc. Cadaver study of correlations to discitis. *Acta Orthop Scand* 1993;64:37–40.
16. Sapico FL, Montgomerie JZ. Vertebral osteomyelitis. *Infect Dis Clin North Am* 1990;4:539–550.
17. Puig Guri J. Pyogenic osteomyelitis of the spine: differential diagnosis through clinical and roentgenographic observations. *J Bone Joint Surg* 1946;28:29.
18. Stone DB, Bonfiglio M. Pyogenic vertebral osteomyelitis: a diagnostic pitfall for the internist. *Arch Intern Med* 1963;112:491.
19. Barron MM. Cervical spine injury masquerading as a medical emergency. *Am J Emerg Med* 1989;7:54–56.
20. Pritchard AE, Thompson WAL. Acute pyogenic infections of the spine in children. *J Bone Joint Surg Br* 1960;42:86–89.
21. Sapico FL, Montgomerie JZ. Vertebral osteomyelitis in intravenous drug abusers: report of three cases and review of the literature. *Rev Infect Dis* 1980;2:196–206.
22. Visudhiphan P, Chiemchanya S, Somburanasin R, et al. Torticollis as the presenting sign in cervical spine infection and tumor. *Clin Pediatr Phila* 1982;21:71–76.
23. Zigler JE, Bohlman HH, Robinson RA, et al. Pyogenic osteomyelitis of the occiput, the atlas, and the axis. A report of five cases. *J Bone Joint Surg Am* 1987;69:1069–1073.
24. Eismont FJ, Bohlman HH, Soni PL, et al. Pyogenic and fungal vertebral osteomyelitis with paralysis. *J Bone Joint Surg Am* 1983;65:19–29.

25. Garcia AJ, Grantham SA. Hematogenous pyogenic vertebral osteomyelitis. *J Bone Joint Surg Am* 1960;42:429.
26. Onofrio BM. Intervertebral diskitis: incidence, diagnosis and management. *Clin Neurosurg* 1980;27:481.
27. Ross PM, Fleming JL. Vertebral body osteomyelitis: spectrum and natural history. A retrospective analysis of 37 cases. *Clin Orthop* 1976; 190–198.
28. Sandiford JA, Higgins GA, Blair W. Remote salmonellosis: surgical masquerader. *Am Surg* 1982;48:54.
29. Bruschwein DA, Brown ML, McLeod RA. Gallium scintigraphy in the evaluation of disk-space infections:concise communication. *J Nucl Med* 1980;21:925–927.
30. Modic MT, Feiglin DH, Piraino DW, et al. Vertebral osteomyelitis: assessment using MR. *Radiology* 1985;157:157–166.
31. Staab EV, McCartney WH. Role of gallium 67 in inflammatory disease. *Semin Nucl Med* 1978;8:219–234.
32. Swayne LC, Dorsky S, Caruana V, et al. Septic arthritis of a lumbar facet joint: detection with bone SPECT imaging. *J Nucl Med* 1989; 30:1408–1411.
33. Feiglan D, Modic M, Piraino D, et al. Evaluation of MRI and nuclear medicine in spinal infections reappraisal. *J Nucl Med* 1985;26:672.
34. Norris S, Ehrlich MG, McKusick K. Early diagnosis of disk space infection with 67 Ga in an experimental model. *Clin Orthop* 1979;293–298.
35. Ono K, Yonenobu K, Fuji T, et al. Atlantoaxial rotatory fixation. Radiographic study of its mechanism. *Spine* 1985;10:602.
36. Whalen JL, Brown ML, McLeod R, et al. Limitations of Indium leukocyte imaging for diagnosis of spine infections. *Spine* 1991;16: 193.
37. Golimbu C, Firooznia H, Rafii M. CT of osteomyelitis of the spine. *AJR Am J Roentgenol* 1984;142:159–163.
38. Kattapuram SV, Phillips WC, Boyd R. CT in pyogenic osteomyelitis of the spine. *AJR Am J Roentgenol* 1983;140:1199–1201.
39. Van Lom KJ, Kellerhouse LE, Pathria MN, et al. Infection versus tumor in the spine: criteria for distinction with CT. *Radiology* 1988; 166:851–855.
40. Bruns J, Maas R. Advantages of diagnosing bacterial spondylitis with magnetic resonance imaging. *Arch Orthop Trauma Surg* 1989;108:30–35.
41. Post MJ, Quencer RM, Montalvo BM, et al. Spinal infection: evaluation with MR imaging and intraoperative US. *Radiology* 1988;169:765–771.
42. An HS, Vaccaro AR, Dolinskas CA, et al. Differentiation between spinal tumors and infections with magnetic resonance imaging. *Spine* 1991;16:S334–S338.
43. Post MJ, Sze G, Quencer RM, et al. Gadolinium-enhanced MR in spinal infection. *J Comput Assist Tomogr* 1990;14:721–729.
44. Sharif HS. Role of MR imaging in the management of spinal infections. *AJR* 1992;158:1333.
45. Van Tassel P. Magnetic resonance imaging of spinal infections. *Top Magn Reson Imaging* 1994;6:69.
46. Song KS, Ogden JA, Ganey T, et al. Contiguous discitis and osteomyelitis in children. *J Pediatr Orthop* 1997;17:470–477.
47. Ottolenghi CE. Aspiration biopsy of the spine. Technique for the thoracic spine and results of twenty-eight biopsies in this region and over-all results of 1050 biopsies of other spinal segments. *J Bone Joint Surg Am* 1969;51:1531–1544.
48. Brugieres P, Revel MP, Dumas JL, et al. CT-guided vertebral biopsy. A report of 89 cases. *J Neuroradiol* 1991;18:351–359.
49. Ghelman B, Lospinuso MF, Levine DB, et al. Percutaneous computed-tomography-guided biopsy of the thoracic and lumbar spine. *Spine* 1991;16:736–739.
50. Frederickson B, Yuan H, Olans R. Management and outcome of pyogenic vertebral osteomyelitis. *Clin Orthop* 1978;160–167.
51. Genster HG, Andersen MJ. Spinal osteomyelitis complicating urinary tract infection. *J Urol* 1972;107:109–111.
52. Redfern RM, Cottam SN, Phillipson AP. Proteus infection of the spine. *Spine* 1988;13:439.
53. Incavo SJ, Muller DL, Krag MH, et al. Vertebral osteomyelitis caused by *Clostridium difficile*. A case report and review of the literature. *Spine* 1988;13:111–113.
54. Carvell JE, Maclarnon JC. Chronic osteomyelitis of the thoracic spine due to *Salmonella typhi*: a case report. *Spine* 1981;6:527–530.
55. Emery SE, Chan DP, Woodward HR. Treatment of hematogenous pyogenic vertebral osteomyelitis with anterior debridement and primary bone grafting. *Spine* 1989;14:284–291.
56. Forsythe M, Rothman RH. New concepts in the diagnosis and treatment of infections of the cervical spine. *Orthop Clin North Am* 1978; 9:1039–1051.
57. Smith NM, Emery SE, Dudley A, et al. Vertebral artery injury during anterior decompression of the cervical spine. A retrospective review of ten patients. *J Bone Joint Surg Br* 1993;75:410–415.
58. Fang D, Cheung KM, Dos Remedios ID, et al. Pyogenic vertebral osteomyelitis: treatment by anterior spinal debridement and fusion. *J Spinal Disord* 1994;7:173–180.
59. Kirkaldy-Willis WH, Thomas TG. Anterior approaches in the diagnosis and treatment of infections of the vertebral bodies. *J Bone Joint Surg Am* 1965;47:87.
60. Southwick WO, Robinson RA. Surgical approaches to the vertebral bodies in the cervical and lumbar regions. *J Bone Joint Surg* 1957;39: 631.
61. Liebergall M, Chaimsky G, Lowe J, et al. Pyogenic vertebral osteomyelitis with paralysis. Prognosis and treatment. *Clin Orthop* 1991; 142–150.
62. Graziano GP, Sidhu KS. Salvage reconstruction in acute and late sequelae from pyogenic thoracolumbar infection. *J Spinal Disord* 1993; 6:199–207.
63. Kemp HB, Jackson JW, Shaw NC. Laminectomy in paraplegia due to infective spondylosis. *Br J Surg* 1974;61:66–72.
64. Messer HD, Litvinoff J. Pyogenic cervical osteomyelitis. Chondro-osteomyelitis of the cervical spine frequently associated with parenteral drug use. *Arch Neurol* 1976;33:571–576.
65. Rajasekaran S, Soudarapandian S. Progression of kyphosis in tuberculosis of the spine treated by anterior arthrodesis. *J Bone Joint Surg Am* 1989;71:1314.
66. Torpey BM, Dormans JP, Drummond DS. The use of MRI-compatible titanium segmental spinal instrumentation in pediatric patients with intraspinal tumor. *J Spinal Disord* 1995;8:76–81.
67. Dormans JP, Criscitiello AA, Drummond DS, et al. Complications in children managed with immobilization in a halo vest. *J Bone Joint Surg Am* 1995;77:1370–1373.
68. King DM, Mayo KM. Infective lesions of the vertebral column. *Clin Orthop* 1973;96:248–253.
69. Collert S. Osteomyelitis of the spine. *Acta Orthop Scand* 1977;48: 283–290.
70. Cleveland M. Tuberculosis of the spine: a clinical study of 203 patients from Sea View and St. Luke's Hospital. *Am Rev Tuberculosis* 1940;41:215.
71. Doub HP, Badgley CE. The roentgen signs of tuberculosis of the vertebral body. *AJR* 1932;27:827.
72. Watts HG, Lifeso RM. Tuberculosis of bones and joints. *J Bone Joint Surg Am* 1996;78:288–298.
73. Akhaddar A, Gourinda H, Gazzaz M, et al. Craniocervical junction tuberculosis in children. *Rev Rhum Engl Ed* 1999;66:739–742.
74. Dormans JP. Evaluation of children with suspected cervical spine injury. *J Bone Joint Surg Am* 2002;84:124–132.
75. A controlled trial of anterior spinal fusion and debridement in the surgical management of tuberculosis of the spine in patients on standard chemotherapy: a study in Hong Kong. *Br J Surg* 1974;61:853–866.
76. Medical Research Council Working Party on Tuberculosis of the Spine. Five-year assessments of controlled trials of ambulatory treatment, debridement and anterior spinal fusion in the management of tuberculosis of the spine. Studies in Bulawayo (Rhodesia) and in Hong Kong. Sixth report of the Medical Research Council Working Party on Tuberculosis of the Spine. *J Bone Joint Surg Br* 1978;60-B:163–177.
77. Upadhyay SS, Saji MJ, Sell P, et al. Longitudinal changes in spinal deformity after anterior spinal surgery for tuberculosis of the spine in adults. A comparative analysis between radical and debridement surgery. *Spine* 1994;19:542–549.
78. Versfeld GA, Solomon A. A diagnostic approach to tuberculosis of bones and joints. *J Bone Joint Surg Br* 1982;64:446–449.
79. Travlos J, du Toit G. Spinal tuberculosis: beware the posterior elements. *J Bone Joint Surg Br* 1990;72:722–723.
80. Oga M, Arizono T, Takasita M, et al. Evaluation of the risk of instrumentation as a foreign body in spinal tuberculosis. Clinical and biologic study. *Spine* 1993;18:1890–1894.
81. Ho EK, Leong JC. Tuberculosis of the spine. In: Weinstein SL, ed. *The pediatric spine. Principles and practice.* New York: Raven Press, 1994;837–849.

82. Bradford R, Rice-Edwards M, Shawden H. Herniation of a calcified nucleus pulposus in a child: case report. *Br J Neurosurg* 1989;3:699–703.

83. Dias MS, Pang D. Juvenile intervertebral disc calcification: recognition, management, and pathogenesis. *Neurosurgery* 1991;28:130–135.

84. Baron A. Uber eine neue Erkrankung der Wirbelsafile. *Jahrb Kinderheilk* 1924;104:357–360.

85. Hahn YS, McLone DG, Uden D. Cervical intervertebral disc calcification in children. *Childs Nerv Syst* 1987;3:274–277.

86. Knupfer M, Rieske K, Pulzer F, et al. Incipient spinal cord compression syndrome due to a herniation of calcified intervertebral disk in a young girl. *Klin Pediatr* 2000;212:117–120.

87. Sonnabend DH, Taylor TKF, Chapman GK. Intervertebral disc calcification syndromes in children. *J Bone Joint Surg Br* 1982;64:25–31.

88. Morris IM, Sheppard L. The persistence of clinical and radiological features after intervertebral disc calcification of childhood. *Br J Rheumatol* 1986;25:219–221.

CHAPTER 40

Torticollis in Children

William C. Warner

Derived from the Latin words, *tortus* and *collum,* the term literally means twisted neck. There are multiple causes and clinical presentations of torticollis in children as well as varying degrees of rotational deformity and tilting of the head. Congenital muscular torticollis is the most common type; however, there are many nonmuscular causes (1) that must be considered before treatment is initiated. The natural history and treatment for nonmuscular causes of torticollis are different from that of congenital muscular torticollis.

CONGENITAL MUSCULAR TORTICOLLIS

Etiology

Congenital muscular torticollis was first described by Hippocrates over 2,000 years ago (2). Alexander the Great was believed to have congenital muscular torticollis and its associated facial deformities (3). In 1643, Minnius was the first to attempt surgical treatment of this condition (4). Anderson gave a more detailed description of this deformity in an article in 1893 (5). In that same year Warren published the first known case report of surgical release in the United States (2).

The deformity is caused by a contracture of the sternocleidomastoid muscle that results in tilting of the head to the involved side and rotation of the head and neck away from the involved muscle (Fig. 40.1). The family usually consults a physician because of the cosmetic deformity associated with this condition. Often a child has a misshapen skull or plagiocephaly, and the torticollis is unnoticed until it is brought to the parents' attention.

The reported prevalence of congenital muscular torticollis varies from 0.084% to 2.1% (6–8). The exact etiology is unknown, but there are several theories. Volkman, in 1885 suggested that torticollis is the result of an intrauterine infection that results in myositis and fibrosis of the sternocleidomastoid muscle. This theory is of historical interest only, because no evidence of underlying infection has been found on histologic examination of the sternocleidomastoid muscle, and there have been no reports of isolating an infecting organism in patients with muscular torticollis.

Stromeyer described a birth trauma theory in which the sternocleidomastoid muscle is torn during a difficult labor and delivery, resulting in bleeding, hematoma formation, fibrosis, and contracture (2,3,9). Although this has been a popular theory, it is not supported by histologic studies, which have failed to show evidence of acute bleeding, hematoma formation, or chronic blood breakdown products (3). Also, this theory does not explain the occurrence of congenital muscular torticollis in patients delivered by cesarean section (10).

Tang and associates proposed a cellular cause for torticollis (11). They found myoblasts and fibroblasts in varying stages of differentiation and degeneration in sternocleidomastoid pseudotumors. The source of these myoblasts and fibroblasts are unknown. However, after birth, environmental changes stimulate the cells to differentiate and a sternocleidomastoid tumor develops. The occurrence of torticollis depends on the fate of the myoblasts. No persistent torticollis occurs if the myoblasts continue normal development and differentiation. If the myoblasts begin degeneration, the remaining fibroblasts produce large amounts of collagen, producing a scarlike contraction of the sternocleidomastoid muscle resulting in torticollis (10,11).

Genetic causes or predisposition for congenital muscular torticollis also have been suggested (12,13). Thompson and colleagues reported congenital muscular torticollis in five related female patients (three of the five were sisters) (12). Although genetics may have some role in the etiology of this condition, reports of a positive family history are rare.

A primary neurogenic theory is supported by findings of progressive denervation and reinnervation on histopathologic specimens of an involved sternocleidomastoid muscle (14). Initial trauma may cause a primary myopathy that

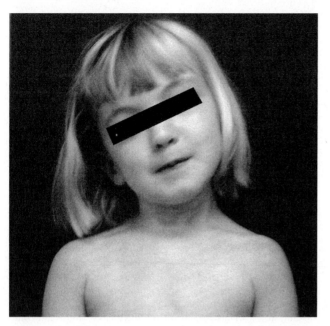

FIG. 40.1. Clinical photo of female patient with torticollis.

unequally involves the two heads of the sternocleidomastoid muscle. With continuing fibrosis of the sternal head, the branch of the spinal accessory nerve to the clavicular head of the muscle can become trapped, leading to a progressive torticollis deformity (10,14).

The most popular theory is one of compartment syndrome of the sternocleidomastoid muscle caused by compression of the neck at the time of birth and delivery. This is supported by surgical histopathology section studies that suggest venous occlusion of the sternocleidomastoid muscle, which may lead to localized ischemia of the muscle and result in edema, degeneration of muscle fibers, and muscle fibrosis resulting in torticollis (15). Using cadaver dissections, Davids and associates demonstrated a definite muscle compartment for the sternocleidomastoid (3). This compartment was defined by the external investing fascia of the neck, a substantial structure that completely envelops the sternocleidomastoid muscle. The compartment was further documented by radiopaque injection studies (3). Manipulation of the head and neck into a position of forward flexion, lateral bending, and lateral rotation caused the ipsilateral sternocleidomastoid muscle to kink in its midsubstance similar to what occurs as a child passes through the birth canal (3). Davids and colleagues also obtained magnetic resonance imaging (MRI) studies on 10 infants with muscular torticollis that showed signal changes similar to those seen in compartment syndromes of the muscles of the forearm or leg (3). This mechanism of localized kinking of the sternocleidomastoid muscle can lead to ischemia, reperfusion, and neurologic injuries to the muscle similar to those that occur in compartment syndrome elsewhere. Although this theory is the most attractive etiology for congenital muscular torticollis, it does not explain why children who

are born by cesarean section develop this deformity or why there is a familial tendency (10,12,16,17).

All of the theories have some merit, but the compartment syndrome theory appears to be the most plausible. This theory is further supported by the association of torticollis with primiparous birth, breech positioning, hip dysplasia, metatarsus adductus, and club feet (17–20). These point to a primary "packing" problem that makes a compartment syndrome more likely to occur.

Clinical Presentation

The clinical presentation of congenital muscular torticollis is variable. Often patients have only a mild deformity with a simple head tilt and slight rotation and minimal restriction of neck motion. In others, the deformity is severe with marked restriction of neck motion and associated deformity of the skull and facial bones, or plagiocephaly (Fig. 40.2). The torticollis usually is detected in the first 2 months of life. A mass may be palpable in the neck during the first 2 to 6 weeks of life. In a report by MacDonald, this mass occurred in 50 of 152 patients (17). However, Coventry reported that a sternocleidomastoid mass was found in only 20% of patients with torticollis (21).

If an infant with congenital muscular torticollis sleeps prone, the affected side is the lower side, which leads to asymmetric pressure on the growing cranium, causing progressive deformity of the skull and facial bones. Recession of the ipsilateral zygoma and forehead and reduction of vertical facial height may occur (22). If an infant sleeps supine, molding occurs on the contralateral side of the skull, which

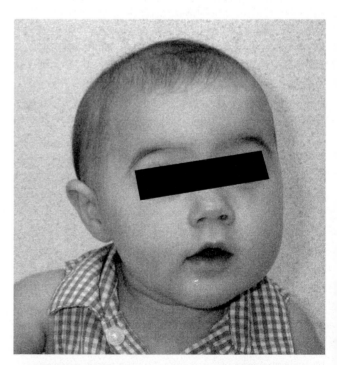

FIG. 40.2. Clinical photo of baby with plagiocephaly.

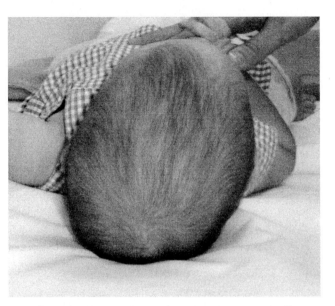

FIG. 40.3. Clinical photo of older child with torticollis.

is known as plagiocephaly (Figs. 40.2 and 40.3). In older children, a thick fibrous band often can be palpated along the sternocleidomastoid muscle (Fig. 40.4). The level of the eyes and ears over time may become unequal and apparent elevation of the ipsilateral shoulder may occur.

Patients with congenital muscular torticollis have an increased prevalence of associated musculoskeletal disorders such as metatarsus adductus, developmental hip dysplasia, and talipes equinovarus (3,19–21). The rate of associated hip dysplasia has been quoted to be as high as 20%, but more recent studies have reported the incidence to be about 8% (18–20,23).

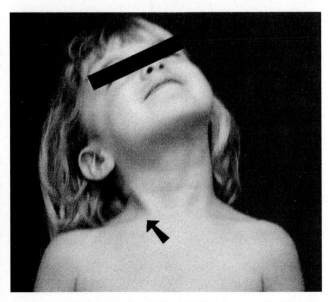

FIG. 40.4. Clinical photo of older child demonstrating fibrotic sternocleidomastoid muscle.

Radiographic Evaluation

Anteroposterior (AP) and lateral radiographs of the cervical spine should be obtained to determine if there are any vertebral anomalies that may be the cause for the torticollis. Computed tomography (CT) scans may be needed to better assess the occiput to C1 region for anomalies if plain radiographs suggest an abnormality. Magnetic resonance imaging has been used as a research tool and demonstrates signal changes within the sternocleidomastoid muscle consistent with fibrosis. Ultrasound also has been used to try quantify the amount of fibrosis in the sternocleidomastoid muscle (24,25). Lin and Chou found that the amount of fibrosis seen on ultrasound tended to decrease with time. Patients in whom the fibrosis did not decrease were more likely to require surgery (24).

Diagnosis

Congenital muscular torticollis can be classified into three clinical groups.

1. A sternomastoid mass group (patients with a clinically palpable sternomastoid mass),
2. Muscular torticollis group (patients with clinical thickening and tightness of the sternocleidomastoid muscle),
3. Postural torticollis group (patients with postural head tilt and clinical features of torticollis but without tightness or mass of the sternocleidomastoid muscle) (26).

The severity of the torticollis can be graded based on the decreased passive range of rotation of the neck on the side of the torticollis compared with that on the normal side. In grade I torticollis, range of motion is symmetrical; in grade II, the motion deficit is 1 to 15 degrees; in grade III, it is 15 to 30 degrees; and in grade IV, it is more than 30 degrees (26–28).

Differential Diagnosis

The list of differential diagnoses of torticollis is varied and long (Table 40.1). Ballock and Song found that almost 20% of their patients with torticollis had nonmuscular causes (1). The diagnosis of torticollis from a nonmuscular cause is probably one of the most important aspects in the treatment of a child with torticollis. The classic picture of a head tilt and rotation combined with a palpable mass in the sternocleidomastoid muscle is not always present or may be equivocal. To establish a cause, it must first be determined whether the deformity was present at birth or acquired and whether or not it is painful. Causes then can be subdivided into osseous versus nonosseous etiologies.

Nonmuscular torticollis caused by osseous malformations usually is not painful. These vertebral anomalies are discussed elsewhere in the text, and include Klippel-Feil syndrome, occipitalization of C1, and congenital hemi-atlas. Acquired nonmuscular torticollis that is painful may have a

TABLE 40.1. *Differential Diagnosis*

Congenital
  Congenital muscular
  Vertebral anomalies
  Failure of segmentation
    Klippel-Feil
    Occipitalization of C1
  Failure of formation
    Congenital hemiatlas
  Combined failure of segmentation or formation
  Ocular

Acquired, painful
  Traumatic
    Atlantoaxial rotatory displacement
    Os odontoideum
    C1 fracture
  Inflammatory
    Atlantoaxial rotatory displacement (Grisel)
    Juvenile rheumatoid arthritis
    Discitis or osteomyelitis
    Other infection in neck
  Tumors
    Eosinophilic granuloma
    Osteoid osteoma or osteoblastoma
  Calcified cervical disk
  Sandifer syndrome

Acquired, nonpainful
  Paroxysmal torticollis of infancy
  Tumor of the central nervous system
    Posterior fossa
    Cervical cord
    Acoustic neuroma
  Syringomyelia
  Hysterical
  Oculogyric crisis (phenothiazine toxicity)
  Associated with ligamentous laxity
    Down's syndrome
    Spondyloepiphyseal dysplasia or MPS dysplasia

From, Herring JA, ed. *Tachdjian's pediatric orthopaedics,* 3rd ed. Philadelphia: WB Saunders, 2002, with permission.

traumatic or inflammatory origin, or may be caused by a tumor (eosinophilic granuloma or osteoblastoma). Acquired torticollis that is not painful usually is the result of a central nervous system abnormality. Most of the nonmuscular causes of torticollis are listed in Table 40.1 (29), except for Sandifer syndrome, ocular torticollis, and torticollis caused by posterior fossa tumors, are discussed in other chapters in this text.

Sandifer syndrome is the association of gastroesophageal reflux, often from a hiatal hernia, and torticollis or dystonic body movements. The intermittent occurrence of torticollis with alternating directions, normal sternocleidomastoid muscles, and normal cervical radiographs make Sandifer syndrome a probable diagnosis. Upper gastrointestinal studies are indicated with this clinical picture. Most patients present in infancy. The prevalence of gastroesophageal reflux may be as high as 40% in infants (30). Positioning of the head and neck in a rotated and extended position is believed to provide

relief from the discomfort caused by acid reflux and is a learned movement by the child (31), although Puntis and associates showed that these dystonic movements actually increase the velocity and amplitude of esophageal peristaltic waves (32). A patient with Sandifer syndrome does not have a tight sternocleidomastoid muscle, and the torticollis usually is intermittent. Plain radiographs of the cervical spine eliminate suspicion of congenital anomalies. Contrast studies of the upper gastrointestinal tract usually demonstrate a hiatal hernia and gastroesophageal reflux (33). Esophageal pH studies may be necessary to demonstrate evidence of gastroesophageal reflux (34). Treatment begins with medical therapy; if this fails, a fundoplication can be considered, which usually is curative (10,31).

Ocular torticollis is an abnormal head posture that is adopted by a patient to maintain binocular vision (35). Williams and colleagues found that paralysis of the superior oblique or lateral oblique muscle and nystagmus were causes for ocular torticollis (36). An ocular cause is likely if the head is tilted but not rotated or if the head tilt changes when the child changes positions. Children with ocular torticollis have a full range of cervical motion without any tightness in the sternocleidomastoid muscle. Occlusion of one eye may help to identify ocular torticollis (36). Ophthalmologic evaluation is recommended, and surgical correction of the ocular problem corrects the torticollis.

Posterior fossa tumors or abnormalities also can cause torticollis in infants and children (Fig. 40.5). The contents of the posterior fossa include the cerebellum, brainstem, and most of the cranial nerves (37). Tumors of the posterior fossa account for about 50% of intracranial tumors in infants (38). Children with these tumors tend to maintain a fixed

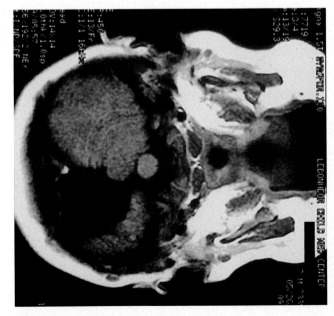

FIG. 40.5. Magnetic resonance image showing posterior fossa abnormality.

posture, with the head tilted and partially externally rotated on one side. Attempts to passively flex the head forward usually are resisted and result in pain (39). Cervical muscle spasm often can be palpated (37). The proposed mechanism of torticollis is stretching and irritation of the dura, innervated by ascending meningeal branches from the upper three cervical nerves (40). The torticollis also can be caused by disruption of normal cerebrospinal fluid flow from the tumor mass. Evaluation should consist of a detailed neurologic examination, plain radiographs, and CT or MRI scans.

Dure and associates reported a child with torticollis caused by a Chiari type I malformation (41). The Chiari I malformation is a downward displacement of the medulla oblongata with extrusion of the cerebellar tonsils through the foramen magnum. The torticollis was associated with headaches and paracervical muscle spasm. MRI is needed to confirm this diagnosis and neurosurgical treatment usually is required.

Natural History

The natural history of congenital muscular torticollis is variable. Infants with a sternocleidomastoid mass and infants with muscular torticollis without a sternocleidomastoid mass have similar outcomes. Resolution of the sternocleidomastoid mass during the first year has been reported in 54% to 70% (17,26,42). Some patients have a degree of residual torticollis that is not an obvious clinical problem and does not require further treatment. Significant torticollis with clinical deformity that requires surgical intervention has been reported to occur in 9% to 21% of patients (7,17,26).

Treatment

Nonoperative treatment recommendations include observation (26,43), application of an orthosis (42,44), an active home program of stimulation exercise and positioning (8,42,44), gentle manual stretching (7,8,26,43,45), and vigorous manual manipulation with rupturing of the tight sternocleidomastoid muscle (27,46). In 90% of patients with congenital muscular torticollis, excellent results can be achieved with gentle manual stretching (26,28,42,43). However, Demirbilek and Atayurt found that the success rate for a stretching program was dependent on the age at which the patient began the stretching program. When stretching was begun in children younger than 3 months of age 100% achieved correction and did not require surgery. The success rate decreased with increasing age. Seventy-five percent of patients between the ages of 3 and 6 months had correction of the deformity, 30% between the age of 6 and 18 months had correction, and none had correction after 18 months of age (47). Initial stretching exercises should be done by a physical therapist, and the parents should be instructed in a home stretching program that consists of rotating the infant's chin to the ipsilateral shoulder and simultaneously tilting the head toward the contralateral shoulder. These should be gentle stretching exercises with the goal of obtaining full passive range of motion in both rotation and tilting (29,44). Other simple measures, such as turning the crib in the opposite direction or placement of toys on one side of the crib, can be used to force the child to look in the opposite direction thereby stretching the sternocleidomastoid muscle.

The use of an orthosis or helmet to correct congenital muscular torticollis and its associated plagiocephaly has not been successful. Emery reported the use of a tubular orthosis to maintain correction after stretching in children older than 4.5 months of age with a residual head tilt of more than 6 degrees (44). Cheng and colleagues have used an orthosis to maintain correction after surgical release of the sternocleidomastoid muscle (48). Except in these situations, the use of an orthosis in the treatment of torticollis is limited.

Nonoperative stretching programs usually are successful in patients up to 1 year of age (43,49), and fewer than 10% eventually require surgery. The indications for surgery include significant head tilt, deficits of passive range of motion of the neck of 10 to 15 degrees in rotation and lateral flexion, and the presence of a tight fibrotic sternocleidomastoid muscle (28). Surgery is only recommended after 1 year of age and after a nonoperative stretching program has failed. The surgical recommendations for congenital muscular torticollis are variable. Some authors recommend surgery any time after 1 year of age, whereas others have found comparable results delaying surgery until around 6 years of age (29). The type of surgery can be a unipolar release (distal) or bipolar release (proximal and distal) (49,50). Surgical techniques vary from a simple tenotomy (50), Z-plasty reconstruction of the sternocleidomastoid muscle (49), endoscopic release (51,52), or partial to almost complete resection of the muscle.

Unipolar release consists of release of the sternocleidomastoid muscle from the mastoid pole at the muscle origin or release of the sternal and clavicular heads of the muscle at its insertion.

Wirth and associates reported excellent long-term results with bipolar release and only had a 2% recurrence rate (50). Ferkel and coworkers reported 92% satisfactory results with bipolar release combined with Z-plasty of the sternal attachment and release of the clavicular attachment (49). The Z-plasty lengthening has the advantage of maintaining the V contour and cosmetic appearance of the neck (Fig. 40.6). Gurpinar and colleagues reported 90% satisfactory results with middle third transection of the sternocleidomastoid muscle (53). Endoscopic release of the fibrotic sternocleidomastoid muscle has been reported in the plastic surgery literature (51,52). This technique does have the advantage of minimal incisions that are easily hidden along the mastoid.

Several technical points need to be emphasized. If a bipolar release is done, the distal incision should be placed in a skin crease above the clavicle. Incisions made directly

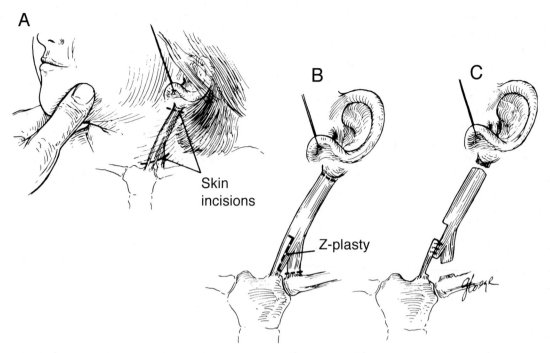

FIG. 40.6. Z-plasty for torticollis. **A:** Location of skin incisions. **B:** Clavicular and mastoid attachments of sternocleidomastoid muscle are cut and z-plasty done on sternal origin. **C:** Completed operation. (From, Ferkel RD, Westin GW, Dawson EG, et al. Muscular torticollis. *J Bone Joint Surg* 1983;65A:894, with permission.)

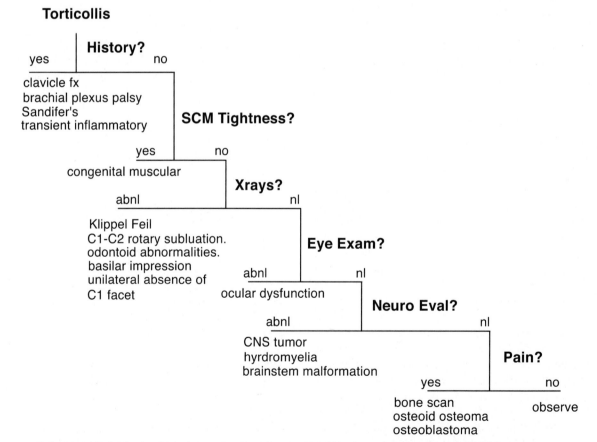

FIG. 40.7. Ballock algorithm for evaluation of torticollis. (From, Ballock RT, Song KM. The prevalence of nonmuscular causes of torticollis in children. *J Pediatr Orthop* 1996;16:500, with permission.)

over the clavicle result in a cosmetically unacceptable scar. The platysma muscle should be separated and repaired at the time of closure to prevent an unsightly depression from resection of the sternocleidomastoid muscle. Structures that can be injured during surgery are the spinal accessory nerve, anterior and external jugular veins, carotid vessels, and facial nerve (10).

SUMMARY

Congenital muscular torticollis is a common disorder in infants and children that has a favorable prognosis with nonoperative treatment. If surgery is required, good results can be expected in about 90% of patients. One of the most important aspects of treatment is to differentiate torticollis resulting from nonmuscular causes from congenital muscular torticollis. Ballock and Song developed an algorithm that may assist in making the correct diagnosis (1) (Fig. 40.7).

REFERENCES

1. Ballock RT, Song KM. The prevalence of nonmuscular causes of torticollis in children. *J Pediatr Orthop* 1996;16:500–504.
2. Wilkins KE. Special problems with the child's shoulder. In: Rockwood CA, ed. *The shoulder.* Philadelphia: WB Saunders, 1990:1055–1071.
3. Davids JR, Wenger DR, Mubarak SJ. Congenital muscular torticollis: sequela of intrauterine or perinatal compartment syndrome. *J Pediatr Orthop* 1993;13:141–147.
4. Von Lackum HL. Torticollis: removal in early life of the fibrous mass from the sternomastoid muscle. *Surg Gynecol Obstet* 1929;48:691–694.
5. Anderson W. Clinical lecture on sternomastoid torticollis. *Lancet* 1893;1:9.
6. Hsu TC, et al. Correlation of clinical and ultrasonographic features in congenital muscular torticollis. *Arch Phys Med Rehabil* 1999. 80:637–641.
7. Ling CM, Low YS. Sternomastoid tumor and muscular torticollis. *Clin Orthop* 1972;86:144–150.
8. Cheng JC, Au AW. Infantile torticollis: a review of 624 cases. *J Pediatr Orthop* 1994;14:802–808.
9. Chandler FA, Altenberg A. Congenital muscular torticollis. *JAMA* 1944;125:476–483.
10. Loder RT. The cervical spine. In: Morrissy RT, Weinstein SL, editors. *Pediatric orthopaedics.* Philadelphia: Lippincott Williams & Wilkins, 2001:799–840.
11. Tang S, et al. Sternocleidomastoid pseudotumor of infants and congenital muscular torticollis: fine-structure research. *J Pediatr Orthop* 1998;18:214–218.
12. Thompson F, McManus S, Colville J. Familial congenital muscular torticollis: case report and review of the literature. *Clin Orthop* 1986;202:193–196.
13. Engin C, Yavuz SS, Sahin FI. Congenital muscular torticollis: is heredity a possible factor in a family with five torticollis patients in three generations? *Plast Reconstr Surg* 1997;99:1147–1150.
14. Sarnat HB, Morrissy RT. Idiopathic torticollis sternocleidomastoid myopathy and accessory neuropathy. *Muscle Nerve* 1981;4:374.
15. Whyte AM, Lufkin RB, Bredenkamp J. Sternocleidomastoid fibrosis in congenital muscular torticollis: MR appearance. *J Comput Assist Tomogr* 1989;13:163.
16. Hosalkar H, et al. Familial torticollis with polydactyly: manifestation in three generations. *Am J Orthop* 2001;30:656–658.
17. Macdonald D. Sternomastoid tumour and muscular torticollis. *J Bone Joint Surg Br* 1969;51:432–443.
18. Morrison DL, MacEwen GD. Congenital muscular torticollis: observations regarding clinical findings, associated conditions, and results of treatment. *J Pediatr Orthop* 1982;2:500–505.
19. Weiner DS. Congenital dislocation of the hip associated with congenital muscular torticollis. *Clin Orthop* 1976;121:163–165.
20. Walsh JJ, Morrissy RT. Torticollis and hip dislocation. *J Pediatr Orthop* 1998;18:219–221.
21. Coventry MB, Harris LE. Congenital muscular torticollis in infancy. *J Bone Joint Surg Am* 1959;41:815.
22. Hollier L, et al. Congenital muscular torticollis and the associated craniofacial changes. *Plast Reconstr Surg* 2000;105:827–835.
23. Tien YC, et al. Ultrasonographic study of the coexistence of muscular torticollis and dysplasia of the hip. *J Pediatr Orthop* 2001;21:343–347.
24. Lin JN, Chou ML. Ultrasonographic study of the sternocleidomastoid muscle in the management of congenital muscular torticollis. *J Pediatr Surg* 1997;32:1648–1651.
25. Chan YL, Cheng JC, Metreweli C. Ultrasonography of congenital muscular torticollis. *Pediatr Radiol* 1992;22:356–360.
26. Cheng JC, et al. Clinical determinants of the outcome of manual stretching in the treatment of congenital muscular torticollis in infants. A prospective study of eight hundred and twenty-one cases. *J Bone Joint Surg Am* 2001;83-A:679–687.
27. Cheng JC, et al. Snapping during manual stretching in congenital muscular torticollis. *Clin Orthop* 2001:237–244.
28. Cheng JC, Tang SP. Outcome of surgical treatment of congenital muscular torticollis. *Clin Orthop* 1999;362:190–200.
29. Herring JA. Disorders of the neck. In: Herring JA, ed. *Tachdjian's pediatric orthopaedics.* Philadelphia: WB Saunders, 2002:172.
30. Darling DB, Fisher JH, Gellis SS. Hiatal hernia and gastroesophageal reflux in infants and children: analysis of the incidence in North American children. *Pediatrics* 1974;54:450.
31. Olguner M, et al. Gastroesophageal reflux associated with dystonic movements: Sandifer's syndrome. *Pediatr Int* 1999;41:321–322.
32. Puntis JWL, et al. Effect of dystonic movements on esophageal peristalsis in Sandifer's syndrome. *Arch Dis Child* 1989;64:1311–1313.
33. Darling DB. Hiatal hernia and gastroesophageal reflux in infancy and childhood: analysis of the radiological findings. *Am J Roentgenol* 1975;123:724.
34. Jolley SG, Johnson DG, Herbst JJ. An assessment of gastroesophageal reflux in children by extended pH monitoring of the distal esophagus. *Surgery* 1978;84:16.
35. Mitchell PR. Ocular torticollis. *Trans Am Ophthal Soc* 1999;XCVII:697–769.
36. Williams CR, et al. Torticollis secondary to ocular pathology. *J Bone Joint Surg Br* 1996;78:620–624.
37. Gupta AK, et al. Torticollis secondary to posterior fossa tumors. *J Pediatr Orthop* 1996;16:505–507.
38. Groover RV. Posterior fossa tumors. In: Swaiman KF, Wright FS, eds. *The practice of pediatric neurology.* St. Louis: CV Mosby, 1982:844–880.
39. Turgut M, et al. Acquired torticollis as the only presenting symptom in children with posterior fossa tumors. *Childs Nerv Syst* 1995;11:86–88.
40. Turgut M. Torticollis secondary to posterior fossa tumors. *J Pediatr Orthop* 1998;18:415.
41. Dure LS, Percy AK, Cheek WR. Chiari type I malformation in children. *J Pediatr* 1989;115:573.
42. Binder H, et al. Congenital muscular torticollis: results of conservative management with long-term follow-up in 85 cases. *Arch Phys Med Rehabil* 1987;68:222–225.
43. Canale ST, Griffin DW, Hubbard CN. Congenital muscular torticollis. A long-term follow-up. *J Bone Joint Surg Am* 1982;64:810–816.
44. Emery C. The determinants of treatment duration for congenital muscular torticollis. *Phys Ther* 1994;74:921–929.
45. Leung YK, Leung PC. The efficacy of manipulative treatment for sternomastoid tumours. *J Bone Joint Surg Br* 1987;69:473–478.
46. Hulbert KE. Congenital torticollis. *J Bone Joint Surg Br* 1950;32:50–59.
47. Demirbilek S, Atayurt HF. Congenital muscular torticollis and sternomastoid tumor: results of nonoperative treatment. *J Pediatr Surg* 1999;34:549–551.
48. Cheng CY, Ho KW, Leung KK. Multi-adjustable post-operative orthosis for congenital muscular torticollis. *Prosthet Orthot Int* 1993;17:115–119.
49. Ferkel RD, Westin GW, Dawson EG. Muscular torticollis: a modified surgical approach. *J Bone Joint Surg Am* 1983;65:894.

50. Wirth CJ, et al. Biterminal tenotomy for the treatment of congenital muscular torticollis. Long-term results. *J Bone Joint Surg Am* 1992; 74:427–434.

51. Burstein FD, Cohen SR. Endoscopic surgical treatment for congenital muscular torticollis. *Plast Reconstr Surg* 1998;101:20–26.

52. Sasaki S, et al. Endoscopic tenotomy of the sternocleidomastoid muscle: new method for surgical correction of muscular torticollis. *Plast Reconstr Surg* 2000;105:1764–1767.

53. Gurpinar A, et al. Surgical correction of muscular torticollis in older children with Peter G. Jones technique. *J Pediatr Orthop* 1998;18:598–601.

Trauma: Fractures and Dislocations

CHAPTER 41

Soft Tissue Neck Injuries

Scott H. Kitchel

Soft tissue injuries of the cervical spine nearly always result from an acceleration injury of the head on the thorax (1). This injury has variously been described as cervical sprain, cervical strain, whiplash, acceleration, deceleration, hyperextension, and soft tissue injury (2). All these descriptive names share the mechanism of tissue stretching and forced range of motion beyond normal restraints.

By far, most cervical soft tissue injuries occur as a result of motor vehicle accidents (3). The incidence of these injuries appears to be increasing due to motor vehicle injuries in both drivers and passengers (4). Sudden oscillation of the head and neck into flexion and extension beyond the individual physiological range may result in painful conditions. Gay and Abbott (5) described the clinical characteristics of the syndrome and divided them into symptoms related to the spinal column, central nervous system, psyche, and others, such as temporomandibular joint or esophagus.

Spinal symptoms include diffuse neck pain with nonradicular radiation, diffuse neck pain with radicular symptoms, cervical radiculopathy, cervical myelopathy, and related lumbar pain syndromes (5). Central nervous system syndromes consist of cerebral concussion, sympathetic dysfunction, cranial nerve dysfunction, chronic headache, and cognitive impairment (5). Psychiatric symptoms include mood and personality change, sleep disturbance, psychoneurotic reaction, depression, and litigation neurosis (5). Any patient with a cervical soft tissue injury may present with combinations of these problems. There is no one specific injury mechanism or threshold of injury (6).

Gay and Abbott (5) described the five most common clinical presentations:

1. *Cervical radiculitis:* Seventy percent of patients experienced cervical pain that radiated to the occiput, jaw, shoulder, upper anterior chest, and arms. Transient reflex and sensory abnormalities were noted in this group.

2. *Cerebral concussion:* Sixty-one percent of patients were initially bewildered, stunned, dazed, or dulled by the accident. Members of this group presented with persistent headaches, vasomotor instability, and vertigo.

3. *Intervertebral disc herniation:* Twenty-six percent of patients presented with radiculopathy, severe neck spasm, and restricted cervical motion.

4. *Persistent psychoneurotic symptoms:* Fifty-two percent of patients developed these problems.

5. *Associated low back injury:* Symptoms of low back pain and lower extremity pain occurred in 30% of patients.

EXPERIMENTAL INJURY PRODUCTION

A great deal of clinical information regarding soft tissue injuries can be learned from the wealth of available experimental data (7). Human subjects as well as anthropomorphic models have been used in many studies. Motion-picture techniques using accelerometers have been able to measure the forces and deflections of the cervical spine in a rear-end collision model (8).

Severy and associates (9) rammed a stationary car equipped with dummy models from the rear with a second car, moving as slowly as 10 miles per hour. The impact accelerated the front car forward. These forces translated to the seated dummy model. The torso and shoulder accelerated with the seat, but because the head was not in contact with the seat, there was a delayed acceleration because of inertia. When the head did accelerate forward, it was propelled from below its center of rotation (starting in extension relative to the body below, which moved with the seat). Therefore, the acceleration of the head was greater than the peak acceleration of the car body. This applied enormous forces to the head and neck complex. Impact at 10 miles per hour produced head acceleration 11 times gravity, with application of distractive forces in excess of 100 pounds to the head and neck. This impact produced initial deflection into hyperextension with rebound into flexion followed by several oscillations of the head back and forth. The maximum hyperextension was 122 degrees, well beyond the normal extension limits of 60 degrees. These data clearly demonstrated how low-speed rear-end collision can apply substantial forces to the cervical soft tissues.

Wickstrom and colleagues (10,11) conducted a series of studies in primates that contributed to our understanding of the chronicity of symptoms. In a rear-end collision model, they found brain injury in 32% of subjects, ligamentous injury between C4 and C7 in 11%, and intervertebral disc damage in 2%. They also noted retropharyngeal hemorrhage beneath the posterior longitudinal ligament and within the paraspinous muscles. The skeletal injuries often involved apophyseal joint damage with capsular tearing, cartilage fissuring, and subchondral bone fracture.

Separately, MacNab (8) performed anatomical dissections on monkeys exposed to hyperextension injuries in a motor vehicle model. He found a number of pathological lesions, including muscle tears of the sternocleidomastoid muscle, rupture of the longus colli muscles with retropharyngeal hematoma, esophageal injury, and disruption of the cervical sympathetic plexus. Several monkeys had disruption of the anterior longitudinal ligament with avulsion of the superior surface of the intervertebral disc from the vertebral body. This avulsion from the bone deprives the disc of one of its normal nutritional pathways and may be an etiology of disc degeneration. These data would be an explanation for why the clinical course of these injuries may be protracted.

Yoganandan and associates (12) replicated soft tissue injuries resulting from a single whiplash acceleration in whole human cadavers. Using cryomicrotomy, they identified stretch and tear of the ligamentum flavum, annulus disruption, and anterior longitudinal ligament rupture and zygapophyseal joint injury with tear of capsular ligaments. In a follow-up study with routine radiography, they could not identify these lesions. They also found computed tomography unable to routinely define these injuries.

CLINICAL PRESENTATION

Soft tissue injuries of the cervical spine most commonly result from motor vehicle accidents (1). Other mechanisms of injury include athletic injuries, blows to the head from falling objects, and direct contact (13). Hyperextension is the most common mechanism, followed by hyperflexion and lateral flexion (13). Generally, injuries produced by hyperflexion and lateral flexion are not as extensive as those produced in hyperextension because of the natural restraints of the chest and shoulders.

The most commonly encountered syndrome is the combination of neck pain, interscapular pain, arm pain, and occipital headache. This syndrome may be combined with features of cranial nerve dysfunction, temporomandibular joint injury, cervical nerve-root trauma, and associated injury to the esophagus, trachea, or vascular structures of the neck (14). Evaluation of patients with a cervical soft tissue injury requires detailed history taking, a careful physical examination, thoughtful review of the diagnostic studies, and often repeat evaluations and examinations. The key points to consider in the history are the mechanism and velocity of the injury (15). Both the severity of the injury and perhaps the prognosis can be suggested from this information. As previously discussed, hyperextension soft tissue injuries are likely to be more severe and more difficult to recover from than hyperflexion or lateral flexion mechanisms. Greater force in the injury generally leads to more extensive injury. Because the force is the product of mass and velocity, increased velocity leads to increased force applied and, presumably, injury (16). Because this injury most commonly involves a motor vehicle accident, the speed at the time of impact should be ascertained, if possible.

Other important information to obtain in the history is the delay between the injury and the onset of symptoms, which may be as much as 2 to 3 days (16). The examiner also should ask specifically about related symptoms, such as may be involved in cranial nerve, esophageal, tracheal, (concussion) brain, and upper extremity injury. Any history of previous neck injury should be noted. Many patients may have associated low back pain (17).

The physical examination of the patient with a cervical soft tissue injury is dictated by the history, but should include evaluation of the head, neck, thorax, and upper extremities. As with any examination, it should begin with inspection and proceed through palpation and functional testing. Symptoms and signs may have a delayed onset and may change greatly over the first few days after the injury.

Inspection of the posture of the patient's neck and the patient's willingness to move the head voluntarily provide information about muscle spasm and may influence treatment decisions. Cranial nerve function can be observed through visual tracking, facial expressions, and speech patterns.

After a general inspection of the head, neck, and upper extremities, palpation for areas of tenderness should be performed, including the occipital pole of the skull, cervical spinous processes, cervical paraspinal muscles, anterior cervical soft tissues, and the temporomandibular joints. As the muscular structures are palpated, the degree of spasm can be judged. Following palpation, the patient should be asked to demonstrate the range of cervical motion within pain tolerance. Flexion, extension, right and left lateral flexion, and right and left rotation should be noted.

The neurologic examination should include assessment of cranial nerves as well as cervical nerve-root function, including motor testing, sensory testing, and reflex evaluation in the extremities. The vascular status of the upper extremity also should be assessed, with palpation of pulses and capillary refill at the fingers.

The typical patient will present with a history of motor vehicle accident and complaints of neck and upper back pain with occipital headache. The patient often holds the head and neck in a stiff posture. Palpation may suggest muscle spasm and focal tenderness in the posterior cervical paraspinal muscles. Range of motion is limited by pain and spasm. The neurologic examination is frequently normal (18).

Radiographic assessment of the patient with soft tissue injuries is negative for evidence of fractures or instability. The most common finding is loss of the normal cervical lordosis on the lateral view (Fig. 41.1) (19). Considerable controversy exists as to whether this finding represents a pathologic finding consistent with muscle spasm or a normal variation (13). Preexisting degenerative disease is often seen and should not be attributed to the accident. Occult fractures, or retropharyngeal soft tissue swelling, should be looked for on the radiographs, but are rarely seen (20).

The loss of cervical lordosis on the lateral radiograph has been evaluated (18,21,22). Mere flattening is not necessarily indicative of any pathology (22); however, a sharply reversed cervical curve may indicate structural damage (21). When a sharp reversal is seen, flexion-extension films usually fail to indicate normal mobility at the involved level (13). Over time, this abnormal curve tends to persist rather than revert to normal (18).

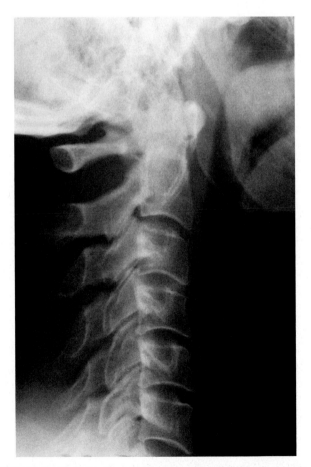

FIG. 41.1. Note the loss of the normal smooth cervical lordosis that occurs secondary to muscle spasm following a musculoligamentous injury in the cervical spine.

Further radiographic diagnostic studies are rarely indicated acutely in the patient with cervical soft tissue injury. The early use of computed tomographic (CT) scanning or magnetic resonance image (MRI) scanning has a limited role. LeBlang (23) and colleagues have found helical CT useful in acute evaluation of cervical injuries; however, this has mostly been for fractures, vascular injuries, and aerodigestive tract lesions. In patients experiencing more lasting symptoms and with findings of persistent restriction of neck movement, repeat plain radiographs with lateral flexion-extension views and special views to show the pillars and articular processes are occasionally useful (13). Bone scans may be useful to screen for occult fractures, which then may be better evaluated and delineated by CT (19). For assessment of ligamentous injuries and annular disc injuries, MRI may be helpful.

Vaccaro and associates (24) have found MRI useful in determining the type and degree of soft tissue disruption in flexion-distraction-type injuries. White and colleagues (25) describe MRI as sensitive in diagnosing acute prevertebral hematoma. Acute MRI scanning for most whiplash injuries has not been successful in correlating pathological findings to symptom development (4). Borchgrevink and coworkers (26) found that an MRI obtained within 48 hours of whiplash neck injury could not detect an abnormality connected to the injury or predict symptom development or outcome.

TREATMENT

Appropriate early intervention and treatment must be tailored to the clinical presentation. Treatment should be based on the pathomechanics and severity of the injury (14). Involving the patient in getting better and more functional, and ensuring that the patient understands the injury and treatment plan are critical (13). The basic treatment for overstretched and injured soft tissues is rest. Depending on the severity of the injury, this may range from avoidance of motion that causes pain to a cervical collar or bed rest.

Use of a soft cervical collar adds comfort to most patients (3). The collar should not be worn regularly for more than 2 to 4 weeks, because this may lead to dependence, muscle atrophy, and reduction of neck motion (27). Rigid collars have not been substantially more effective than soft ones (28). The collar provides support and helps decrease muscle spasms. Application of cold for the first 72 hours following injury may decrease pain and spasm. After that, moist heat may have a similar effect; however, too frequent and prolonged use of heating pads, diathermy, or ultrasound causes irritation and may perpetuate symptoms (13).

A cervical exercise program that includes isometric exercise and gentle range of motion should be instituted as soon as symptoms allow, but usually within 2 weeks (27). Generally, patients tolerate isometric exercises sooner than range of motion or mobilization. Exercises should include neck flexion-extension and lateral flexion and rotation performed several times daily. The assistance of a trained physical therapist is beneficial, as is coordinating the timing for initiating mobilization and range of motion exercises.

Traction in the acute treatment of soft tissue injuries is rarely indicated. It is difficult to rationalize pulling and stretching on tissues that have been injured by a stretching mechanism (13); however, after soft tissue healing has occurred, either manual or mechanical traction may aid in restoring motion (27).

Medications may be helpful in the soft tissue–injured patient, but should be used judiciously (29). Analgesics and sedatives with muscle-relaxing action may be beneficial for a brief period, but should be replaced with active measures and exercise as soon as possible. Dependency on medication in this group of patients develops in a high percentage of cases (5).

The duration of symptoms in cervical soft tissue injuries is variable and does not seem related to severity of injury (14). The role of emotional factors and pending litigation has been evaluated. MacNab (29) had three important observations: (a) patients with chronic symptoms often have sustained more serious injuries, (b) flexion or lateral impact injuries rarely cause prolonged complaints, and (c) 45% of his 266 patients had symptoms persisting 2 years after court settlement. Despite these data and other similar data, most clinicians believe that litigation and emotional factors significantly prolong recovery time.

Studies of patients more than 2 years after injury indicate that from 20% to 90% may have persistent symptoms (21). These symptoms most commonly include neck ache, headache, and stiffness. Follow-up radiographs of patients with no preexisting cervical degenerative disc disease, taken an average of 7 years after injury, show that 39% had developed degenerative disc disease (21), compared with an expected incidence of 6% in age-matched patients. It is interesting to note that the development of degenerative changes had no correlation to persistence of symptoms (21). Many attempts have been made to determine early signs or symptoms that may provide a prognostic index (15). To date, no clear correlations have been developed that are reproduced from one study to the next.

The best outcome can be expected when optimal treatment is undertaken in the acute phase (14). When the symptoms become chronic, the physician must develop a close and trusting relationship with the patient. Attempts to obtain maximum functional recovery within the limits of the disability should be encouraged.

SPINOUS PROCESS FRACTURES

Although spinous process fractures are not isolated soft tissue injuries, they are discussed here because in their most common form, treatment is similar. Spinous process fractures should be thought of in terms of isolated fractures or as part of a more complex pattern (30).

Isolated Injuries

Isolated fractures of the spinous processes may result from hyperextension injuries, hyperflexion injuries, or direct blows (31). The extension injury results in one spinous process abutting the adjacent one and prying it off (31). The flexion injury is actually an avulsion injury termed a *clay-shoveler's fracture*. The spinous process is avulsed by the posterior erector spinal muscles when the head is forced into flexion against their contraction (Fig. 41.2). It can typically be recognized by an oblique fracture line that characterizes this injury. The fracture also may occur without flexion of the head, as a result of forceful contracture of the erector spinal or trapezius muscles (13). Fractures of the spinous process from a direct blow may be caused by a purely external force or by direct penetrating trauma, such as a gunshot wound (30). These fractures may be accompanied by stretching or tearing of the interspinous ligament with minor widening of the adjacent facet joints. As iso-

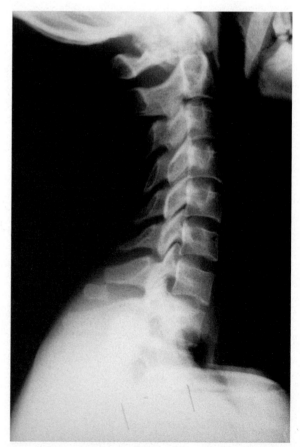

FIG. 41.2. The typical appearance of a bony avulsion fracture secondary to the muscular pull of the trapezius insertion.

lated fractures, all spinous process fractures are considered stable injuries.

The patient with an isolated spinous process fracture most often can provide a history of the event. Occasionally, these injuries occur with accompanying head injuries or multiple trauma, making a history unavailable. When it can be obtained, the history should include an account of the acute event, focusing on the dynamic position of the head and neck, which may provide the examiner a clue as to the etiology of the fracture. The patient usually complains of localized neck pain with muscle spasm and loss of range of motion.

On physical examination, the patient often holds the head and neck quite still and may even support it with his or her hands. Exquisite point tenderness is present at the level of the fracture. The examiner also may palpate protective muscle spasm of the trapezius and erector spinae. The patient is unwilling to allow range of motion testing because of pain and spasm. In cases of penetrating trauma, a wound is found. The neurologic examination is usually normal.

Radiographic examination should include a screening anteroposterior and lateral study. Lateral flexion-extension radiographs confirm the stability of the injury and are mandatory when any evidence of facet joint subluxation or interspinous process widening is seen. No other special radiographic studies are routinely indicated to evaluate these injuries. In the acute phase, motion may be limited because of the pain and spasm.

Once stability of the injury has been determined, management is nonoperative. Supportive care to decrease pain and muscle spasm should be instituted until the fracture heals (31). An external orthosis should be used and the patient given appropriate analgesics and antispasmodics.

Generally, a soft collar or Philadelphia collar is adequate. A sternooccipital mandibular immobilizer (SOMI) type of orthosis may occasionally be used. A halo is not indicated. The duration of collar wear ranges from 3 to 6 weeks, depending on the patient's symptoms and radiographic evidence of fracture healing. At the time of collar removal, repeat flexion-extension radiographs should be obtained to assure stability (31). An active exercise program is then begun to regain strength and cervical motion. When normal motion has been attained and there is evidence of fracture healing, normal activities may be resumed.

Rarely, these fractures may proceed to nonunion, which should not be judged for at least 6 months after injury (28). Should nonunion occur and be symptomatic, the fracture fragment may be surgically excised.

Complex Injuries

Spinous process fractures also may be seen as part of more complex two- and three-column injuries of the cervical spine. In a series of 300 cervical spine fractures requiring hospitalization, 21 fractures included spinous process fractures as part of a more complex injury. Although some of these patients had accompanying paralysis, no neurologic deficit was related to compression of a neurologic structure by the spinous process fracture itself (30). The specific evaluation and treatment of these fractures are discussed in the chapters on fractures and dislocations.

REFERENCES

1. Cailliet R. *Neck and arm pain.* Philadelphia: FA Davis, 1964:60–85.
2. Crowe HD. Whiplash injuries of the cervical spine. In: *Proceedings of the Section of Insurance Negligence and Compensation Law.* Chicago: American Bar Association, 1958:176–184.
3. LaRocca HL. Cervical spine syndrome: diagnosis, treatment and long term outcome. In: Frymoyer JW, Ducker TB, Hadler NM, et al., eds. *The adult spine.* New York: Raven Press, 1991:1051–1062.
4. Petterson K, Hildingsson C, Toolanen G, et al. Disc pathology after whiplash injury. A prospective magnetic resonance imaging and clinical investigation. *Spine* 1997;22:283–287.
5. Gay JR, Abbott KH. Common whiplash injuries of the neck. *JAMA* 1953;152:1968–2704.
6. Davis CG. Injury threshold: whiplash-associated disorders. *Manipulative Physiol Ther* 2000;23:420–427.
7. Panjabi MM, Nibu K, Cholewicki J. Whiplash injuries and the potential for mechanical instability. *Eur Spine J* 1998;7:484–492.
8. MacNab I. Acceleration injuries of the cervical spine. *J Bone Joint Surg Am* 1964;46:1797–1799.
9. Severy DM, Mathewson JH, Bechtol CO. Controlled automobile rear end collisions: an investigation of related engineering and medical phenomenon. *Can Service Med J* 1955;2:727–759.
10. Wickstrom JK, Martinez JL, Rodriguez RPO, et al. Hyperextension and hyperflexion injuries to the head and neck of primates. In: Gurdjian ES, Thomas LM, eds. *Neckache and backache.* Springfield, IL: Thomas, 1970:108–117.
11. Wickstrom JK, Rodriguez RPK, Martinez JL. Experimental production of acceleration-injuries of the head and neck. In: *Accident pathology.* Washington, DC: U.S. Government Printing Office, 185–189.
12. Yoganandan N, Cusick JF, Pintar FA, et al. Whiplash injury determination with conventional spine imaging and cryomicrotomy. *Spine* 2001;26:2443–2448.
13. Hohl M. Soft tissue neck injuries. In: Cervical Spine Research Society, eds. *The cervical spine,* 2nd ed. Philadelphia: JB Lippincott, 1989.
14. Bland JH. *Disorders of the cervical spine.* Philadelphia: WB Saunders, 1987:224–225.
15. Gebhard JS, Donaldson DH, Brown CW. Soft tissue injuries of the cervical spine. *Orthop Rev* 1994(Suppl):9–17.
16. Jolliffe VM. Soft tissue injury of the cervical spine: consider the nature of the accident. *BMJ* 1993;307:439–440.
17. Taylor JRI, Finch PM. Neck sprain. *Austr Fam Physician* 1993;22:1623–1625.
18. Borden AGB, Rechtman AM, Gershon-Cohen J. The normal cervical lordosis. *Radiology* 1960;74:806.
19. Daffner RH. Evaluation of cervical cerebral injuries. *Sem Roentgenol* 1992;27:239–253.
20. Brisner J, Leask WH. Retropharyngeal soft tissue swelling due to soft tissue swelling due to soft tissue injury. *Arch Surg* 1954;68:369.
21. Hohl M. Soft tissue injuries of the neck in automobile accidents: factors influencing prognosis. *J Bone Joint Surg Am* 1974;56:1675–1682.
22. Rechtman AM, Borden AGB, Gersho-Cohen J. The lordotic curve of the cervical spine. *Clin Orthop* 1961;20:208.
23. LeBlang SD, Nunez DB Jr. Helical CT of cervical spine and soft tissue injuries of the neck. *Radiol Clin North Am* 1999;37:515–532.
24. Vaccaro AR, Madigan L, Schweitzer ME, et al. Magnetic resonance imaging analysis of soft tissue disruption after flexion-distraction injuries of the subaxial cervical spine. *Spine* 2001;26:1866–1872.
25. White P, Seymour R, Powell N. MRI assessment of the pre-vertebral soft tissues in acute cervical spine trauma. *Br J Radiol* 1999;72:818–823.

26. Borchgrevink G, Smevik O, Haave I, et al. MRI of cerebrum and cervical columns within two days after whiplash neck sprain injury. *Injury* 1997;28:331–335.

27. Lieberman JS. Cervical soft tissue injuries and cervical disc disease. In: Leek JC, Gershwin ME, Fowler WM Jr, eds. *Principles of physical medicine and rehabilitation in the musculoskeletal diseases.* New York: Grune and Stratton, 1981:263–286.

28. Herowitz HN, Rothman RH. Subacute instability of the cervical spine. *Spine* 19894;9:348–357.

29. MacNab I. Acceleration extension of the cervical spine. In: Rothman RH, Simeone FA, eds. *The spine.* Philadelphia: WB Saunders, 1982:647–660.

30. Bohlman HH. Acute fractures and dislocations of the cervical spine. *J Bone Joint Surg Am* 1979;61:1119–1143.

31. Meyer PR, Heim S. Surgical stabilization of the cervical spine. In: Meyer PR Jr, ed. *Surgery of spine trauma.* New York: Churchill Livingstone, 1989:414.

CHAPTER 42

Cervical Spine Injuries in Athletes

Robert G. Watkins, Lytton Williams, and Robert G. Watkins IV

In many sports, particularly contact sports, the neck is at risk for injury because of an inability to rigidly pad, brace, or protect the cervical spine and allow normal function. The flexibility and motion of the cervical spine must deliver the head and eyes to the right place at the right time. The function of the spine also includes being a conduit for the central nervous system, with the spinal cord and the cervical nerve roots passing through, making injury to the neck a potentially catastrophic event. The incidence of sports-related injuries to the spinal cord in football has been reported by Clark (1) to be 54% of all spinal cord injuries in school and college athletics. Torg (2) has reported on the findings of the National Football Head and Neck Injury Registry, which was established to document the incidence and nature of severe intracranial and cervical spine injuries resulting from tackle football. The criteria for inclusion in the registry are injuries that require hospitalization for at least 72 hours, injuries of the neck involving fracture subluxation or dislocation, injuries involving intracranial hemorrhage, and injuries with associated quadriplegia or death. Between 1971 and 1984, there were 1,412 cervical spine injuries meeting these criteria (2).

The prevention of cervical spine and spinal cord injuries is of paramount importance. The responsibility for educating athletes in methods to prevent neck injury is most important in those sports in which the risk of trauma to the cervical spine is the highest. Contact sports, such as football, rugby, and wrestling, have been identified as being particularly high-risk activities for cervical trauma (2). The use of the head as an offensive weapon to block and tackle makes football a major source of cervical injuries. Even noncontact sports, such as diving, water skiing, surfing, water polo, and body surfing, can be responsible for traumatic spinal injuries (3). The prevention of neck injuries in athletes involves the education of players, trainers, and physicians. Prevention of these injuries must incorporate appropriate rule changes for those sports that are at highest risk. After studies demonstrated the role of head contact in

catastrophic injuries of the head and neck in football players in the mid-1970s, the National Collegiate Athletic Association (NCAA) made rule changes that condemned the use of the head in tackling and effectively outlawed the technique of blocking and tackling known as spearing. These rule changes have had a significant impact on the occurrence of traumatic cervical spine and spinal cord injuries in football players from high school through the professional levels (2). Also, modification of protective gear to incorporate new materials into properly fitting shoulder pads and neck pads has added, it is hoped, to the decreased incidence of neck injuries in athletes.

The treatment of the athlete with neck, cervical spine, or spinal cord trauma remains one of the most medically challenging of all aspects of sports medicine. There have been no miraculous medical breakthroughs that have had a major impact on the catastrophic consequences of a young, active athlete suffering a complete spinal cord injury. Bracken and associates (4) reported that a 24-hour course of high-dose corticosteroids administered within 6 to 8 hours after cervical spinal cord injury may be associated with an improved prognosis for cervical nerve root injuries by recovery of one to two cervical nerve root levels. However, this limited treatment is not enough to allow for complacency in the continual goal of the sports medicine community to decrease the incidence of cervical spine and spinal cord injuries in athletes.

Football players are at greater risk for cervical injury than the average adult in the United States. The nature of the game requires violent contact between the head and shoulders of a player and the body of his opponent or the hard playing field surface. Besides protective equipment and educational techniques to enhance the football player's awareness of the potential for neck injury, several other protective factors can be utilized to decrease the risk of cervical spinal cord injury in these athletes. Neck-strengthening exercises can build muscle bulk and increase the protective capability of the thick sleeve of neck and shoulder muscles that surrounds the cervical spine. The biomechanical advantage afforded by powerful and bulky neck flexors, extensors, and rotators, as well as massive trapezius and shoulder girdle musculature, is evidenced in the modern professional football player. This is particularly true when it is understood that many of the professional football athletes playing today may have narrowed cervical spinal canals secondary to degenerative changes in the cervical discs and cervical facet joints with hypertrophic bony encroachment of the spinal canal. Yet, the prevalence of catastrophic cervical spinal cord injuries in professional football players is exceedingly low. By increasing the level of conditioning of the athlete and improving balance, coordination, and skill, the natural and acquired protective actions of the cervical and shoulder musculature are increased.

The responsibility for teaching and enforcing proper tackling techniques lies with football coaches and referees. Safe tackling techniques must become second nature to the player and must be enforced. Safe blocking and tackling avoid the use of the head in initial contact. Spearing and the use of the head as an offensive weapon increase the risk of cervical spine fractures and quadriplegia. Since the rule changes banning the use of the head as a battering ram, the incidence of quadriplegia in football players has dropped dramatically (2). The biomechanics of cervical spine fractures illustrate that direct head compression, with axial loading and flexion, is a major mechanism of injury (fracture or dislocation) of the cervical spine in football players. To resist the loading impact, attacking players straighten out their cervical spine to a neutral position. The loading on the crown of the athlete's head, coupled with the velocity of body weight, compresses the cervical spine. Just as one would buckle a simple soda straw by squeezing the ends between the fingers, the spine buckles in the middle and produces an axial loading flexion-rotation injury. There is an accordion effect, with bone and ligament failure of the cervical column (2). This is the injury pattern that occurs to the cervical spine when a player uses the head as a battering ram, particularly when that player is fatigued, is wearing inadequate protective equipment, does not have adequate neck strength and muscle bulk, or does not have adequate levels of overall conditioning.

CLINICAL ANATOMY, SIGNS, AND SYMPTOMS

The cervical spinal cord is housed in the neck by the rigid, intercalated spinal motion units. Rigid bony protection against direct blows as well as protection against axial loading, flexion, extension, and torsional injuries is afforded by the laminae, spinous processes, facet joints, and vertebral bodies of the cervical spine. However, with axial loading and bending that surpass the bony or soft tissue element's biomechanical capability and strength, there may be resultant fracture, dislocations, or both. This failure may cause injury to the spinal cord or cervical nerve roots.

Cervical spine or spinal cord injury has a more favorable prognosis when identification of the injury is made prior to any further movement of the injured patient. An unstable fracture or dislocation without neurologic injury can have catastrophic sequelae if improper transportation techniques are utilized, even if performed by well-meaning and concerned individuals. The player with an unstable cervical spine injury may not be aware of the magnitude of the injury because of the minimal amount of pain felt by the player at the time of injury. When in a game situation, it is not unusual for the player to shrug off even the most serious neck injuries as insignificant because of occasional minimal symptomatology noted by the individual. However, once identified as a spinal cord injury, the level of cord injury can be quickly assessed by simple pinprick sensation testing along the cervical dermatomes and by manual muscle strength testing (5).

C3-C4 Level

Injury at the C3-C4 level may result in complete paralysis of the trunk and extremities, with a complete loss of all normal unassisted respirations due to paralysis of the diaphragm as well as of the thoracic musculature. A loss of pain to pinprick to a point just below the clavicle, including the upper extremities, may be evidenced.

C4-C5 Level

With injury at this level, athletes can only shrug their shoulders, via the trapezius, which is innervated by the second and third cervical nerve roots through the spinal accessory nerve. These patients will have only abdominal breathing. Spinal cord swelling or hemorrhage may progress. If only one more segment toward the head is involved, it may mean the cessation of spontaneous respirations. The motor fibers to the diaphragm via the phrenic nerve, from the C3 and C4 nerve cell bodies, exit from the spinal cord with the upper portion of the C5 root. The absence of pain sensation is evident to the level of the outer border of the upper extremity between the shoulder and elbow.

C5-C6 Level

Players with this level injury can flex at the elbows and tend to remain flexed in that position unless they fall prone with gravity. Attempted movements of the hands result in hyperextension at the wrists with inability to close the fingers voluntarily. Extension of the arms is markedly impaired. There may be a loss of sensation over the region of the thumb and index finger of the hand.

C6-C7 Level

With injury at the C6-C7 level, athletes will be able to weakly close their hands and grasp with the fingers. The arms can be flexed and extended weakly at the elbows. They may be unable to spread the fingers because of loss of the intrinsic musculature innervation to the hands. Sensation will be intact over the thumb and index finger, but will usually be lost over the middle and radial half of the ring finger.

C7-T1 Level and Below

Injuries occurring at the C7-T1 junction and below can result in complete sparing of the muscle function of the upper extremities with lower extremity paraplegia. Trunk control, however, including control of the rectus abdominis, internal and external oblique muscles, and the spinal extensor muscles, is affected by the level of the thoracic spinal injury. With a caudal level of thoracic spinal cord injury, there is increased ability of the patient to adapt to activities requiring controlled and coordinated trunk musculature activity. Sensation will be impaired from the dermatomal level corresponding to the level of injury.

Signs and Symptoms

Schneider (6) stressed that gross motor and sensory tests are far from performing a complete neurologic examination and are meant only as a quick method of determining the level of neurologic injury in a player who is, for example, lying on the playing field. A high degree of suspicion must be maintained when examining players injured on the field if there are indications that a neck injury has occurred. When there are questionable findings, or when the examining coach, trainer, or physician believes that a neck injury has occurred, even though the player's complaints include only some vague neck stiffness or neck pain, or when there are minimal objective findings to support concern, these players should be treated as if they have a true injury until this can be proven otherwise.

Much more common than complete or incomplete spinal cord injury are the lesions known as *burners* and *stingers,* which are interchangeable terms. The characteristic motor and sensory manifestations are thought to be quite common among football players. At least 50% of college players have experienced a burner (7). Cervical nerve root or brachial plexus neuropraxia is considered to be the etiology of stingers and burners in younger patients. Older patients are more subject to compression of the dorsal root ganglion in the foramen. Both lesions are identified by intense burning pain accompanied by numbness, paresthesias, and transient weakness in the arm. The symptoms usually last from a few seconds to 15 minutes. The symptoms start immediately after head and shoulder contact, usually with an opponent, but sometimes after striking the playing surface. The pain typically involves the entire arm from the fingertips up to the neck and shoulder. Commonly, the last symptoms to resolve are those of the C5 or C6 roots.

Players may complain of recurrent stingers and burners throughout the season and in the off-season. Almost always, when the symptoms are recurrent, the same motor and sensory deficits are present, and the same biomechanical mechanism of injury is present in the subsequent episodes. However, it is not unusual for a multiroot pattern to be found. Repeated episodes over a season may result in major weakness of the deltoid and biceps (8). A residual neurologic deficit may persist for days to months following more severe episodes. Stingers occur commonly in football and other sports. Understanding the pathomechanics of the stinger and performing comprehensive clinical assessments, along with having a thorough familiarity with rehabilitation techniques, are the keys to properly managing stingers and burners.

The mechanism of injury most often seen in professional football players is an off-center axial load that is applied to the head with the head uncontrollably forced both into extension and lateral flexion. This forces the head toward the ipsilateral side of the resultant burner and stinger. With extension and bending of the cervical spine toward the involved shoulder and arm, the neural foramina are abruptly narrowed, and the bony walls of the neural foramina and the intervertebral disc or osteophytes compress the nerve root and the dorsal root ganglion. The mechanism of injury is equivalent to Spurling's maneuver (9), which is a diagnostic sign that can be elicited in the office setting in the clinical examination of patients with cervical radiculopathy. Spurling's maneuver consists of extension of the head and lateral bending and rotation of the head and neck toward the painful side. When these maneuvers are performed together, a positive Spurling's sign is identified by pain that is reproduced in the patient's shoulder and arm identical to the pain that is the patient's presenting clinical complaint. A positive Spurling's test indicates cervical foraminal stenosis due to either soft disc herniation or osteophyte encroachment of the neural foramina. Foraminal narrowing at one or more levels may be seen on a contrast computed tomographic (CT) scan, or profound central canal and foraminal narrowing may be noted on magnetic resonance imaging (MRI). There are certainly cases, however, when complete diagnostic evaluation, including MRI, CT myelography, and electromyographic (EMG) and nerve conduction studies, fails to reveal the source of the abnormality.

The other possible mechanism of injury in the production of burners and stingers involves an abrupt stretching of the cervical nerve roots or the adjacent brachial plexus. The head is forced away, to the opposite side of the depressed shoulder and symptomatic arm. There is an increased tension on the brachial plexus in this mechanism. Although this mechanism of injury is also associated with transient signs and symptoms, the potential for long-term neurologic deficit is present, as it is with the pinching mechanism previously described. This mechanism is more common in younger patients.

Seddon's classification system of peripheral nerve injuries can be applied to burners and stingers that occur both from dorsal root ganglion compression in the foramen and brachial plexus injury. Seddon (9) classified peripheral nerve injuries into three categories. *Neurapraxia* is the mildest lesion that has identifiable histologic findings and corresponds to demyelinization of the axon sheath without intrinsic axonal disruption. Recovery of neural functioning generally occurs within 3 weeks. *Axonotmesis* includes disruption of the axon and the myelin sheath with preservation of the fibrous epineurium. The epineurium serves as a conduit for the regenerating axon in axonotmesis. In most healthy adults, the rate of recovery in axonotmesis can be expected to be approximately 1 mm per day, with an initial 7-day delay from the time of injury. This expected rate of recovery is measured from the site of injury to the motor end plate to which the nerve supplies motor impulses. *Neurotmesis* corresponds to complete nerve transection. In neurotmesis there is generally no possibility of distal nerve regeneration without surgical repair and reapproximation of the nerve sheath.

Clancy and associates (10) utilized Seddon's classification system for definition of the burner syndrome from brachial plexus injury. Grade I injuries have an initial recovery of motor and sensory function, generally within several minutes of injury, with a complete recovery noticed by 2 weeks. These injuries correspond to Seddon's definition of neurapraxic lesions. Grade II injuries can result in motor loss to the deltoid, biceps, interspinalis, and supraspinalis muscles. Weakness can last from weeks to months and corresponds to axonotmesis. Grade III lesions are quite rare and are more typically seen in trauma patients who have suffered from penetrating injury to the neck or shoulder region from a motor vehicle accident, knife fight, gunshot wound, or shrapnel injury from an explosion. Additionally, falling in this classification of injury is the scapulothoracic dissociation injury that is associated with high-energy trauma and results in evaluation and separation of the shoulder girdle from the thorax. Scapulothoracic dissociation is additionally associated with significant trauma to the traversing major blood vessels and neural and muscular structures. EMG studies demonstrate abnormalities in type II and type III lesions. Generally, type I, grade I neurapraxia does not have EMG or nerve conduction velocity abnormalities.

The long-term EMG findings have been studied in a group of 20 athletes with burners by Bergfeld and colleagues (11). They selected a group of players with clinical findings of severe neurologic involvement after athletic injuries that led to burners or stingers. In this study, the EMG findings generally localized to the upper trunk of the brachial plexus, as well as the cervical nerve root and peripheral nerve root levels. The EMG abnormalities lagged behind the motor recovery of the individual as the injury resolved. They demonstrated that utilizing the EMG as a criterion for return to play after a burner or stinger is an inaccurate and ineffective prognostic measure. The precise history of symptoms, a detailed neurologic examination, and provocative testing such as Spurling's maneuver are

best used to decide on the timing of a player's return to play after a burner or a stinger. An appropriate diagnostic imaging workup should be included in the evaluation of patients with burners or stingers. A severe first-time burner may be the symptom of a cervical disc herniation. Under these circumstances, restricting play until a disc herniation can be ruled out by MRI is an appropriate decision.

Examination of the player on the sidelines will usually reveal the mechanism of injury by careful questioning and head range of motion testing. Spurling's maneuver may reproduce the symptoms. The shoulder abduction test, in which the hand is placed palm down on the top of the head, may decrease the symptoms (7). Davidson and associates (12) reported on a series of patients with cervical myeloradiculopathies due to extradural compressive disease in whom clinical signs included relief of radicular pain with abduction of the shoulder. The mechanism by which shoulder abduction may relieve pain from cervical root impingement at the level of the neural foramen was thought to be due to the shorter distance that the nerve root must traverse; thus, it is under less tension when the shoulder is abducted. In the study by Davidson and colleagues (12), 68% of patients noted relief of pain with abduction of the affected shoulder. On the field, players with burners or stingers classically hold themselves with the head forward and complain of a stiff neck. The arm is too weak to elevate. Attempts to elicit Spurling's sign are generally met with pain. Occasionally, head compression will reproduce the symptoms. This can also be a sign of fracture or disc herniation (13).

PREVENTION OF BURNERS

The primary preventive measure for burners is wearing properly fitting shoulder pads. Shoulder pads should accomplish four basic functions: (a) absorbing shock, (b) protecting the shoulders, (c) fitting the chest, and (d) fixing the midcervical spine to the trunk. The typical shoulder pad (Fig. 42.1) worn by a professional defensive lineman is a soft, thin, padded material that has questionable shock-absorbing properties and fits the chest in a semiarc type of configuration. The fixation to the chest is less than ideal and allows sliding of the shoulder pads on the shoulder during contact. To fit the chest properly, the pads should be more of an A-frame type with rigid, long, anterior and posterior panels. The shoulder pads should fit well to the subxiphoid portion of the chest and fit snugly around the chest. A proper shoulder pad should encompass many of the characteristics of cervicothoracic orthoses. Immobilization of the cervical spine in any type of cervical orthosis requires rigid fixation to the chest. All studies evaluating fixation methods that include only the neck, such as a hard or soft cervical collar, demonstrate poor fixation and limitation of cervical spine motion. It is only when the base is extended and fixed that there is enhanced restriction of cervical spine motion. Although there are limitations on the ability to fix the head to the chest in football players because they must

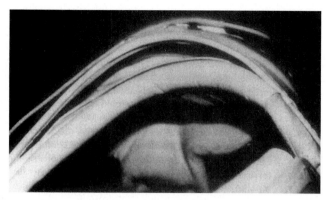

FIG. 42.1. The typical shoulder pad worn by a professional defensive lineman is a soft arc of very thin padded material that has questionable shock-absorbing properties and fits the chest in a semiarc type of configuration.

have full range of motion of the cervical spine, it is possible to fix the chest rigidly to the base of the neck, and the shoulder pads should accomplish this.

The majority of neck rolls that are attached to the top of the shoulder pads rotate away from the neck at the moment of contact (Fig. 42.2). This rolling back of the shoulder pads adds to a lack of protection for the cervical spine in resisting compression. An axial compression mechanism of injury is commonly seen in serious neck injuries and plays a big role in burners. As a shoulder pad rolls back, the head coils into the hole in the shoulder pad. There is no protec-

tion against head compression or from the extension, compression, and rotation mechanism related to burners. It is very difficult to get a collar roll on the back of the shoulder pads that can block extension during contact. One professional veteran used a stiff cervical collar that was tied tightly around his neck posteriorly and attached to the shoulder pads by strings to the laces on the front of the pads. This was an attempt to prevent the failure to block extension seen with collar rolls (Fig. 42.3).

Important characteristics of a proper shoulder pad include a modified A-frame shape to the shoulder pad that fits the chest and prevents shoulder pad roll during contact. Firm circumferential fixation to the chest is important. After fixing the chest, fix the neck to the chest by the fit of the shoulder pad at the base of the neck. Thick, comfortable, stiff pads at the base of the neck are the key. It is this support laterally at the base of the neck that offers fixation to the cervical spine. Some posterior support could be helpful, but is difficult to obtain. Higher, thicker lateral pads inside the shoulder pad that are tighter at the base of the neck can improve fixation of the cervical spine, especially when the pad fits the chest and shoulders well. The lateral pad seen in the Donzis shoulder pad is a good example of a proper pad.

A common method of adapting pads is to add lifters (Fig. 42.4). The lifters provide a pad at the base of the neck that supplements the typical shoulder pad. Often, a combination of lifters, the preexisting pad, and a neck roll improves fit of the pad laterally at the base of the neck. Because approximately 50% of the rotation in the cervical spine occurs at C1-C2, this support should not limit the player's visibility and should provide some added support in the middle and lower portion of the cervical spine.

Regarding the shock-absorbing capability of the shoulder pad, proper fit to the chest is important in distributing shock to the shoulders evenly, over the pad and to the thorax. Better resistive padding and plastics in the outer shell

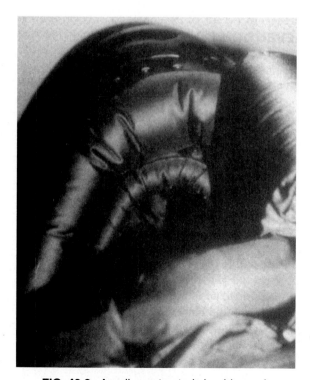

FIG. 42.2. A well-constructed shoulder pad.

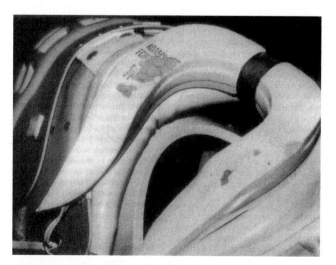

FIG. 42.3. Shoulder pads after they have been modified.

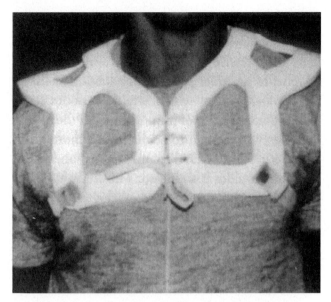

FIG. 42.4. Lifters provide additional neck support.

of the pad will absorb shock and allow the use of the shoulder in proper blocking and tackling techniques. Better shoulder protection should allow one to de-emphasize the use of the head as a blocking and tackling instrument.

Treatment of Burners

In addition to prevention, treatment is critically important. Once symptoms occur, chest-out posturing and thoracic outlet obstruction exercises are helpful. Chest-out posturing produces three effects:

1. It opens the intervertebral foramina to its maximum size. Sticking the chest out brings the head back over the body and produces a strengthening or less extension in the cervical spine. Flexion in the cervical spine, while tightening the nerve roots slightly, does increase the size of the intervertebral foramina. Extension closes the foramina and decreases the central canal's diameter.
2. It reduces the effect of the weight of the head. The lever arm effect of the weight of the head on the cervical spine is eliminated as the head is brought back over the body with the chest-out posturing. This is important in relieving neck strain and decreasing the force exerted on the spine by the weight of the head.
3. It opens the thoracic outlet. By changing the alignment of the scalene muscles and the clavicle relative to the neck, the thoracic outlet is opened with chest-out posturing. A stoop-shoulder, head-forward posture adds to thoracic outlet obstruction and will cause the symptoms of brachial plexus irritation to persist. Many heavily muscled athletes have adopted a round-shoulder, head-forward posture. When they sustain an injury to a nerve root or brachial plexus, symptoms will persist because of an inability to produce proper chest and head alignment.

All strengthening of weak muscles owing to a brachial plexus or nerve root injury should be conducted while emphasizing a chest-out posture.

We frequently use a basic group of preventive and therapeutic exercises designed for neck and shoulder problems. The key to these exercises is emphasizing the chest-out posture. By emphasizing the chest-out posture during upper extremity, shoulder, and neck exercises, proper head and neck alignment is enhanced. A general exercise program could include shoulder and rotator cuff exercises as well as dorsal glides, midline neck isometrics, shoulder shrugs, arm rolls, and a weight program. The athlete should stick the chest out and not attempt to hold the shoulders back or forcefully tuck the chin. The chest, abdomen, and buttock muscles should be used. The important factor is the chest-out posture.

Neck strengthening is also important. Neck and radicular pain will cause muscle weakness and dysfunction in the muscles that support the head. The same emphasis that is used on quadriceps strengthening for knee injuries should be used for neck muscles in neck injuries, but it must be done carefully. Resistive neck exercises are begun very slowly so that the compressive load on the cervical spine does not produce pain. Neck isometrics should be done with the head in the midline only, and resisting forces should be applied perpendicularly to the head from every direction. Very slowly, the head can be taken out of the midline after there is no pain whatsoever with strengthening in the midline, but extremes of head flexion, either anteriorly, posteriorly, or laterally against resistance, are seldom indicated for adequate neck strengthening. Midline isometric strengthening should be emphasized.

Once the symptoms improve, stretching exercises are important to allow for protective flexibility and range of motion of the cervical spine. The reactive stiffness can produce chronic contractures and a loss of range of motion if not corrected. If a contracture exists, sudden motion at a moment of contact through that restricted range of motion can reproduce the injury and severe pain. Use motion into the painless areas initially, then slowly move into the painful areas. Extension is usually the most painful, but it cannot be neglected. Dorsal slides and passive neck stretches are important. Chest-out posturing should also be used during these exercises. Aggressive stretching and motion exercises should be done with extreme caution, as they are the most common cause of flare-ups in therapy.

DECISION MAKING IN NECK INJURIES IN ATHLETES

Decision making in neck injuries to athletes often centers on whether or not a player is cleared to return to play, either on the day of injury or later. The decision that allows a player to resume football play depends on the diagnosis, prognosis, and risk factors for future injury. Crucial to the decision-making process is a physician who is trained in evaluating, diagnosing, and treating neck injuries and who also has a thorough understanding of the game. When dealing with football players, it is important that the physician has an understanding of the mechanics involved in football, as well as the effects of the stress of the game upon the particular injury that the player has received. For the physician to make a reasonable recommendation for return to play, factors such as the mechanism of the player's injury, any prior history of neck injury, the findings on the initial physical examination of the player immediately after injury, and the diagnostic studies that have been obtained must be assessed. Factors to be avoided in this decision-making process are contract provisions, disability contracts, the player's desire to play, and the desires of others (girlfriends, wives, coaches, team owners, parents). Everyone, regardless of what is said, is looking to the team physician for medical advice only. The physician should stick closely to the medical facts of the case and provide the same information to all concerned about the known risk factors.

To help in our decision making, we have developed a system for classifying the risk of continued play or return to play based on the radiographic findings after a specific type of neck injury, the patient's current signs and symptoms, and the patient's detailed prior history of neck injury. The history of prior neck injury must include the frequency of occurrence of such incidents as burners, stingers, transient neuropraxia, and neck stiffness, as well as the length of duration of these episodes of neurologic embarrassment or neck injury. The type of treatments that the player has received and the player's response to these treatments are important in assessing the readiness of the player for return to play. The classification system that has been developed combines the published clinical and scientific information related to specific neck injuries as well as our experience in diagnosing and treating neck injuries in football players. We utilize radiographic component studies and many other factors in the final outcome of the decision-making process. The risk categories are both the risk of permanent injury and the risk of recurrent symptoms.

On-Field Discussion

Decision making begins with a player who has been injured in the game and is down on the field. The only diagnostic capabilities will be the physician's history, physical examination, and knowledge of the mechanics of the injury. The key decision to make is whether to move the player (whether he or she has a spinal cord injury or not). The first issue is whether a player has radiating arm pain and loss of function, such as paresthesias and weakness, or more global paresthesias and weakness indicative of a transient neuropraxia of the cervical spine cord. Radiating arm pain and neurologic deficit can be indicators of a more serious problem, such as spinal instability, that can lead to a permanent neurologic deficit from further cord or nerve root injury. Additionally, some players may be neurologically intact but may have a stiff, painful neck. Neck stiffness and loss of cervical range of motion may indicate a cervical fracture.

Initial muscle spasm that occurs after a cervical spine injury can mask an underlying unstable cervical spine lesion. The patient's pain perception may be altered by the emotion of the game, as well as by the player's dedication to the coach and the team. A controlled head compression test that produces radicular pain may indicate a cervical fracture. Players with new pain, residual loss of neck range of motion, and neck stiffness should not be allowed to return to play until further diagnostic evaluation is performed. No return to play is suggested for players with a significant neck injury until further diagnostic evaluation is performed.

Spinal cord neuropraxia with four-extremity involvement, including, possibly, loss of consciousness, temporary quadriplegia or quadriparesis, or burning dysesthesias of the arms and legs, indicates a significant injury to the spinal cord. Often players who have transient neurapraxia of the spinal cord that lasts for less than 10 to 15 seconds may arise from the playing field and exit the field on their own power; only then, when the player is at the sideline, is the trainer or team physician made aware of the symptoms. Examination of these players on the sideline or on the field involves evaluation for motor weakness, sensory deficits, and signs of myelopathy. It is important that all players with a possible cervical spine injury and acute neurologic deficit be treated with cervical spine immobilization and appropriate transportation and diagnostic studies.

Transportation and Immobilization

Guidelines for transportation and immobilization have been developed by the Inter-Association Task Force for Appropriate Care of the Spine-Injured Athlete (14). The following is an outline of these guidelines.

General Guidelines

- Any athlete suspected of having a spinal injury should not be moved and should be managed as though a spinal injury exists.
- The athlete's airway, breathing and circulation, neurologic status, and level of consciousness should be assessed.
- The athlete should not be moved unless absolutely essential to maintain airway, breathing, and circulation.
- If the athlete must be moved to maintain airway, breathing, and circulation, the athlete should be placed in a supine position while maintaining spinal immobilization.
- When moving a suspected spine-injured athlete, the head and trunk should be moved as a unit. One accepted technique is to manually splint the head to the trunk.
- The Emergency Medical Services system should be activated.

Face Mask Removal

- The face mask should be removed immediately, regardless of current respiratory status.
- Those involved in the prehospital care of injured football players should have the tools for face mask removal readily available.

Helmet and Shoulder Pads

In general, the helmet and shoulder pads should not be removed prior to transport. Indications to remove the helmet and shoulder pads include the following:

- The helmet and shoulder pads do not hold the head securely, such that immobilization of the helmet does not also immobilize the head.
- The design of the helmet and chin strap is such that even after removal of the face mask the airway cannot be controlled or ventilation provided.
- The face mask cannot be removed after a reasonable period of time.
- The helmet prevents immobilization for transportation in an appropriate position.

Spinal immobilization must be maintained while removing the helmet. Helmet removal should be frequently practiced under proper supervision. Specific details for helmet removal have been outlined by the task force (14). In most circumstances, it may be helpful to remove cheek padding and/or deflate air padding prior to helmet removal.

The helmet/shoulder pad unit should be thought of as an all-or-none scenario with regard to spinal immobilization.

- During helmet removal, the shoulder pads must be removed simultaneously.
- Spinal immobilization must be maintained at all times.
- Specific instructions for helmet/shoulder pad removal have been provided by the task force (14).

Transportation

When confronted with an individual on the playing field who complains of symptoms of neck pain or stiffness, or of any upper or lower extremity neurologic manifestations, the initial response of the trainer or team physician should be to ensure prompt and adequate immobilization of the cervical spine and establish an airway. Transportation techniques are vital to avoid increasing neurologic injury in any patient with spinal cord injury. Stabilization of the cervical spine in an injured player does not require routine prehospital removal of the helmet and shoulder pads before transport. No morbidity has been documented because of not removing the helmet and shoulder pads.

In a player with neck injury and respiratory compromise, either the mask must be snapped off the helmet or cut off with large bolt cutters or other tools. The removability of face masks should be continually checked and monitored so that in an emergency easy removal of the face mask will not be a problem. If the provision of an adequate airway is necessary, then the bolt cutters should be utilized to transect the metal stays attaching the face mask to the helmet. If the player is unconscious and having inadequate respiratory effort, then the airway may be opened by grasping the angle of the mandible with both hands and thrusting the jaw forward. Hyperextension of the head to obtain an open airway may not be safe when cervical spine injury is a possibility.

Only after cervical spine immobilization has been provided should the individual be transported to the sidelines, the locker room, or the emergency room. Neck immobilization and transportation of a player with neck injury require proper instruction of the coach and trainer by the team physician as well as practice in the techniques by those involved (Figs. 42.5 and 42.6). The team trainer, as well as rescue personnel in attendance at the game, must be provided with, and be comfortable with the application of, standard cervical immobilization collars. The most common collars in use include the Nec-loc and the Philadelphia collar. When appropriate, these collars can be applied to the player before transportation.

The transport technique should be standardized and practiced by the trainer, coach, and team physician before the start of the playing season. The technique called a six-plus-person lift requires at least six people to move the player safely. Trying to transport the patient with only three people is inappropriate. A frequent error in transport is not having enough people available who know how to transport a player with a potentially unstable cervical spine in-

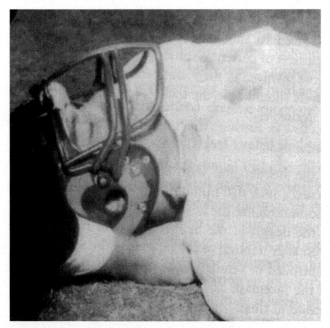

FIG. 42.5. Immobilization of the head to the trunk. The person in charge holds the trapezius-clavicle-scapula area with his or her hands and holds the head between his or her forearms.

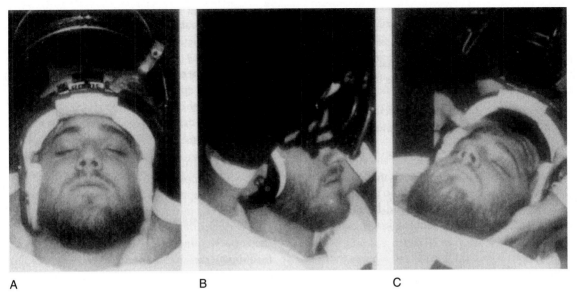

FIG. 42.6. A: Hand position for helmet removal. **B:** Helmet removal, side view. **C:** Helmet removal. The assistant pulls out on the helmet and slips it off.

jury (Fig. 42.7). The most important key to the technique is to have one person controlling the head and shoulders, not just the head. This individual is also in charge of the timing of transportation. This person should grab the trapezial, clavicle, and scapular area with his or her hands while cradling the helmeted head of the player between the forearms. The person in charge should not be responsible for any of the weight of the transfer. The additional members of the transportation team include one individual holding the player's shoulders and upper torso. The third and fourth persons hold the player's trunk and upper thighs on each side of the player. The fifth and sixth members of the turning team are responsible for lifting and turning the legs.

Once all individuals are in place, the team members on each side of the body then join hands in a weaved grip, with the palm placed against the forearm of the individual directly across from them, underneath the player. When the team chief calls the signal, the assistants gently elevate the player off the ground while a rigid backboard is slid directly under the player.

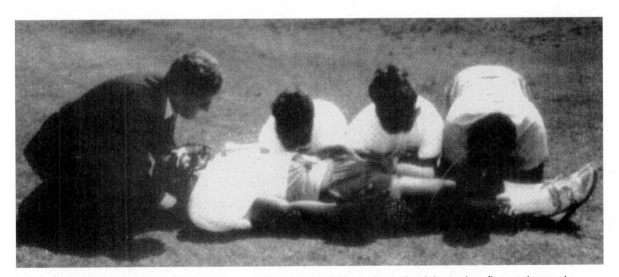

FIG. 42.7. The transport technique should be standardized and practiced; it requires five or six people to move the player safely. This figure illustrates the multiperson carry. The "chief" immobilizes the head, neck, and shoulders and calls the signals. Three people on each side of the body (the three on the near side are not pictured) join hands and lift the player on the chief's command. The spine board is brought underneath the player.

If the player is face down on the field, the chief rotates the player's arms and grasps the player's head and shoulders in a similar fashion. In this situation, it is mandatory that an assistant grasp the chief's arms and squeeze them together to increase the hold on the player's shoulders and head. Safely turning the prone player to the supine position requires multiple assistants to roll the player over gently while the team chief maintains the alignment of the head with the shoulders during the turn. Once the player is turned, the standard transportation protocol is utilized (Fig. 42.8).

Once the player is on the backboard, the player can be safely transported off the field to the appropriate health care facility, while the team chief maintains the grasp on the player's shoulders and head. Once the player is on the backboard, if an appropriate cervical orthosis is available, such as a Philadelphia collar, then the team chief may safely relinquish his or her hold on the neck, at the same time applying the cervical orthosis. If the cervical orthosis cannot be applied because of the helmet or the shoulder pads, then the team chief must maintain his or her grasp on the individual until transportation to the locker room or emergency room is completed. It may be necessary to utilize a backboard that has built-in neck and head supports or utilize sandbags taped into place rather than the original grasp of the person in charge.

Locker Room Decisions

Our decision-making process involves evaluating players for return to play who have had either significant, persistent, or severe enough symptomatology to warrant transportation to a medical facility or to a locker room where radiographs can be obtained.

Radiographic Evaluation

It is mandatory to obtain adequate visualization of the cervicothoracic junction at C7-T1, as well as adequate-

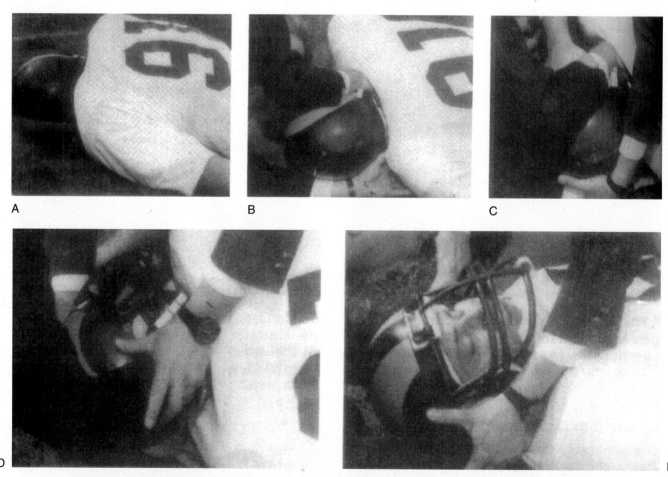

A   B   C

D   E

FIG. 42.8. If the player is facedown on the field (**A**), the chief rotates his or her arms and grasps the player's head and shoulders in a similar fashion (**B**). **C:** In this situation, it is mandatory that an assistant grasp the chief's arms and head. **D:** Safely turning the prone player to the supine position requires multiple assistants to roll the player over gently while the team chief maintains the alignment of the head with the shoulders during the turn. **E:** Once the player is turned, the standard transportation protocol is utilized.

quality films that can be interpreted. Generally, the lateral radiograph is obtained first (Fig. 42.9) and should be interpreted and evaluated before proceeding with the remainder of the radiographic evaluation. The initial sequence of cervical spine films (anteroposterior, lateral, anteroposterior open mouth, and oblique views) (15) should be reviewed and evaluated for any potential instability, fracture, or dislocation before subsequent flexion-extension films are considered. If instability, fracture, or dislocation is identified, then the next appropriate step is to continue cervical spine immobilization and proceed with further diagnostic studies, including CT scan or MRI as indicated by the nature of the lesion.

The radiographs should be evaluated for obvious vertebral body fracture or malalignment; the anterior retropharyngeal space should also be evaluated. At the anterior aspect of the body of C3, there should be no more than 4 mm of space between the posterior pharynx and the anterior vertebral body. Increase in the retropharyngeal space indicates soft tissue swelling and may be indicative of cervical spine injury. The posterior margins of the vertebral bodies and the spinal laminar lines should be evaluated for a symmetric and smooth contour. The facet joints should be evaluated for symmetry and congruity. Changes in the rotational position of the spinal column from one motion segment to the next may be indicative of facet subluxation or dislocation. The criteria of White and Panjabi (16), including subluxation of 3.5 mm or more and kyphotic angulation of the injured level that is 11 degrees or greater than an ad-

jacent level, are generally considered to indicate cervical spine instability. These criteria pertain to any lateral cervical spine view, including flexion view.

The evaluation of C1 through T1 is imperative and can be facilitated by the use of traction on the player's hand in a downward fashion by an assistant during the radiograph or by the use of Boger straps. Boger straps are passive-action Velcro straps that are connected to the wrists and passed around the bottoms of the feet. They are tightened with the knees flexed. As the knees are straightened out by pushing down on the knees, the straps tighten and pull the arms down. A sandbag can be placed on the knees in an unconscious patient, thereby maintaining traction on the arms. We have never had a patient in whom C7 was not visualized using the Boger straps. Occasionally, traction on an arm with cervical radiculopathy produces too much pain to pull for a long time. If Boger straps are not available, then the "swimmer's view" should be employed. This is obtained by centering the beam on the lateral projection at T1; the patient's arm closest to the source of the radiographic beam is kept at the side, while the opposite arm, adjacent to the radiographic plate, is fully abducted over the patient's head. If adequate visualization of the cervicothoracic junction remains a problem after the swimmer's view is obtained, then the next step in radiographic evaluation is a CT scan to include that region. We will not clear a patient's cervical spine film unless the full cervical spine is visualized. Also important on the lateral view is the atlantodens interval. An atlantodens interval of greater than 2 to 3 mm may be considered indicative of cervical spine instability at the atlantoaxial articulation, particularly if it increases on flexion films.

A difficult aspect of the radiographic evaluation is to determine if there is an acute injury, an old injury, or an asymptomatic finding. One complicating factor is the presence of a hypermobile segment over a stiff, arthritic segment. Many athletes have relative osteoarthritic changes in the lower cervical spine. The biomechanical stiffness of these levels may produce a relative increase in mobility through a compensatory mechanism at the levels just above these less mobile lower segments. Although these levels are hypermobile, to find an asymptomatic never-injured level that exceeds the White-Panjabi criteria would be rare (16). Greater than 11 degrees kyphosis relative to an adjacent level usually signifies that the posterior longitudinal ligament is disrupted.

Identification of an area of ligamentous instability may be difficult in acute situations, due to the associated muscle spasm from the injury.

Compression fracture noted in the lateral film must be interpreted with caution. What may be interpreted as a simple compression fracture may, in fact, include an injury with associated cervical spine instability. A review of 27 patients with cervical compression fractures revealed that six of these injuries were later noted to have associated spine instability (17). When doubt continues as to the stability of a

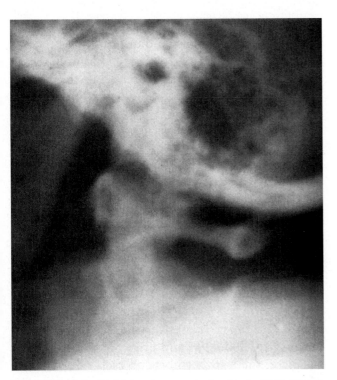

FIG. 42.9. A typical lateral x-ray study of a football player.

cervical spine injury, such as when there is too much spasm to obtain flexion-extension views, continued immobilization with a cervical orthosis is indicated until pain resolves and adequate flexion-extension views can be obtained. Once a fracture has been identified on plain film or CT scan, it should be treated as described in other chapters in this text.

Often important in the radiologic evaluation is the determination of whether a radiographic finding is an acute injury, an old injury, or an asymptomatic degenerative change. Boden and associates (18) have identified the incidence of degenerative changes occurring in the cervical spine in a group of asymptomatic volunteers who underwent MRI of the cervical spine. They were able to identify a 14% to 35% incidence of herniated cervical discs, osteophytes, and degenerative disc disease in these completely asymptomatic individuals. They underscored the importance of clinical correlation with the radiographic findings in individuals being evaluated for cervical injuries.

Once in a controlled environment, removing the player's helmet can be accomplished in a safe fashion. First, remove the face mask. The appropriate hand position of the team chief for helmet removal includes having the team chief grasp the base of the occiput and the base of the neck with open palms and fingers. An assistant may first spread the sides of the helmet, then gently slide the helmet in a cephalad direction and off the player while neck control is maintained by the team chief. Absolutely no cervical flexion should be allowed during this maneuver. If the shoulder pads do not allow for adequate cervical spine examination and radiograph, then they should be removed at this time. They should be removed in a similar fashion, that is, maintaining cervical immobilization and not allowing cervical and head flexion.

When to Do In-Depth Studies

The logical answer to this question is to perform in-depth studies when they are needed to make the diagnosis or when the results would change your treatment. As a practical measure, studies should be obtained on players with severe, persistent, or recurring problems. For a stiff, painful neck due to recent injury, a bone scan may identify an acute fracture. MRI and plain CT scans are helpful, and a contrast CT scan will help identify disc herniations and fractures. An EMG with nerve conduction study is helpful in distinguishing a peripheral nerve problem from a cervical nerve root problem, but not as helpful in following a case for progression. Liberal, repeated use of whatever tests are needed to diagnose the problem properly may be needed.

CONTINUED PLAY DECISIONS: RISK CATEGORIES

In the preseason, the spinal consultant or the team physician is often called upon to examine players and evaluate their risk for play during the upcoming season. Guidelines for participation after injury involve a number of different factors, including age, experience, the individual's level of ability and participation, position played, and the spinal condition itself with its resulting symptoms. Informed consent of all concerned is probably the most important obligation of the physician evaluator. The team physician must be able to give a clear-cut "yes" or "no" answer to the team's management and to the player or the player's parents. It is often the spinal consultant who is asked to make that decision in players who have had documented neck injury and are thought to be at some risk for further play. A comprehensive diagnostic workup involving myelography, contrast CT scan, and MRI is necessary before excluding someone from play after neurologic symptoms resulting from stenosis. The radiographic data will be combined with the history and physical examination of the player to develop a risk category into which a particular player can be placed in regard to his or her chance for permanent damage to the neck, spinal cord injury, permanent nerve root injury with paralysis and pain, or death.

Risks may be categorized in terms of the percentage of the chance of recurrence of symptoms that would hinder future play. Important in this decision is the level of play in which the player participates. In a high school player, of course, the opinion of the parents is important. If there is a suggestion of structural damage and even a minimally increased risk to a high school player, the best choice is often for the athlete to discontinue playing football. In professional football, the players themselves need to be advised of the approximate level of risk, so that they may give informed consent regarding their future play and an appropriate decision can be made by the player and all concerned.

Although no published data can precisely dictate the individual player's risk for return to play, a system that incorporates clinical experience in dealing with football players and the published literature related to cervical spine injuries is utilized. The criteria for return to play has been analyzed by a number of different sources. Each individual injury has its characteristics, which has led investigators to estimate the risks involved in return to play after a player has incurred specific types of injuries or symptoms (5). *Minimal risk* is the term used to suggest that there is very little increased risk, as compared with playing the game as it is normally done. *Moderate risk* means that there is a reasonably high chance that the patient will have recurrence of symptoms and a reasonable chance that the patient will run some risk of permanent damage. *Extreme risk* means that the patient runs a very high risk of permanent damage and recurrence of symptoms. It is critical that all factors related to the player's symptoms, history of injury, radiographic findings, results of any special studies needed, and expectations be included in the ultimate recommendations made to the player in regard to the player's likelihood of injury if he or she returns to the sport of football. When considering other sports that involve bodily contact, similar recommendations can be made.

Congenital Abnormalities

Congenital abnormalities of the cervical spine may or may not place the player at an increased risk for neurologic damage, depending on the precise morphology of the congenital abnormality present. Os odontoideum, which has been documented in the literature as most likely secondary to a traumatic lesion, is a potentially significant unstable situation in which the risk of injury places the player in an extreme-risk category (Fig. 42.10). Not infrequently, os odontoideum will present in the younger player as an asymptomatic and incidental finding and, as such, can be a particularly difficult problem to explain in the otherwise young, healthy, high-caliber athlete.

Multiple levels of failure of segmentation, as found in the Klippel-Feil syndrome, place the adjoining spinal motion units at an increased biomechanical disadvantage secondary to the compensatory increased motion that occurs adjacent to the fused levels. In general, we would list this constellation of segmentation defects as a moderate to extreme risk that would depend somewhat upon the findings on flexion-extension films as well as on the distribution of the fused segments. Sprengel's deformity in association with Klippel-Feil is not unusual and is an extreme risk.

Extreme-Risk Category

Fractures of the first cervical vertebra (Jefferson's fractures) generally represent an axial loading injury, often resulting from head-on collision by the player with an opponent or the ground. The Jefferson's fracture is disruption of the ring of the first cervical vertebra and may be identified on the open-mouth anteroposterior (AP) view as eccentric or excessive overhang of the lateral mass of the first cervical vertebra on the second cervical vertebra. CT scan is excellent for precisely identifying the configuration of a C1 fracture. At the level of the atlas, there is considerable room for the spinal cord secondary to the large central spinal canal at that level. As such, neurologic injury secondary to Jefferson's fracture is unusual. The mechanism of injury involves axial loading that forces the occipital condyles into the lateral mass of the atlas, resulting in failure of the ring of the atlas, often at the thinner region just medial to the trough that lies at the level of the vertebral artery.

Return to play after a recent Jefferson's fracture is contraindicated. It is only after bony healing has occurred and appropriate tests for ligamentous stability can be performed that a recommendation as to return to play can be made. If the bone completely heals; a full, normal range of motion is

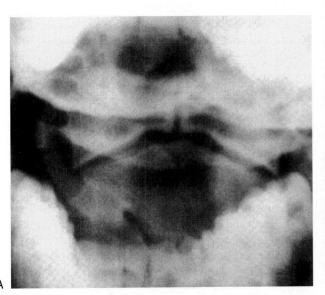

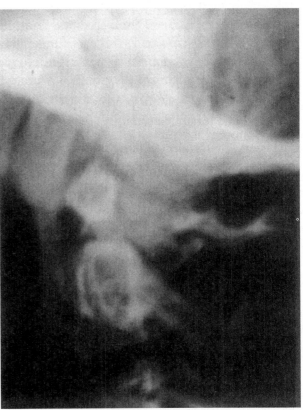

A   B

FIG. 42.10. A: Anteroposterior x-ray study revealing an unstable os odontoideum in a 20-year-old college freshman athlete who suffered pain in his neck for the first time from an automobile accident. **B:** Lateral view.

present; and no residual instability is noted on flexion-extension views, then return to play is possible. If there is any residual instability or if there is residual neck stiffness or discomfort, indicating nonunion or ligamentous injury, then the recommendation for return to play would include placing that player in an extreme-risk category. Occasionally, C1 ring fractures heal with a fibrous union as evidenced on CT scan; in these players with no residual neck stiffness or pain, a moderate risk for return to play would be offered. Figure 42.11 illustrates a Jefferson-type fracture with 7 mm of overhang resulting from head-on collision; the player was a college senior defensive back. The player was projected as a first-round draft choice in the National Football League, so this injury certainly placed the player in a high-risk category.

Transverse ligament ruptures result from high-velocity axial loading injuries. Transverse ligament injuries are quite rare and occur in only 3% of all cervical spine injuries (19). Rupture of the transverse ligament is identified by abnormal motion between the atlas and the odontoid on the flexion-extension views or by an atlantodens interval greater than 5 mm on the neutral lateral film. Partial tears of the transverse ligament may be identified by an atlantodens interval of 2 to 5 mm. We have treated a player who had a partial tear of the transverse ligament; he was a starting professional defensive tackle who had suffered a high-velocity injury with residual stiffness and pain in his neck. This player was thought to be in an extreme-risk category for further play. We have also treated a 17-year-old high school football player who presented after a major neck injury that resulted in upper cervical spine stiffness and pain. He presented with a V-shaped atlantodens interval. The diagnosis for this youngster was a partial transverse ligament tear, even though there have been references made to this entity being an incidental finding. Our recommendation to this boy and his parents was that he would be at an increased risk of neurologic injury from continued participation in football.

The open-mouth and lateral views are utilized to identify odontoid fractures. These are classified according to the system of Anderson and D'Alonzo (20). Odontoid fractures that heal completely, without deformity and with free, unrestricted, pain-free neck motion place that player at a mild risk of secondary injury from continued play. However, any residual deformity or the suggestion of a fibrous union between the odontoid and the body of C2 is a potentially unstable situation. A football player can be expected to place significant biomechanical stress on that fracture and is in an extreme-risk category.

A fracture of the pedicles of C2 ("hangman's fracture") that heals completely, with no fibrous union and with satisfactory reestablishment of the posterior arch of C2, has only a mild risk for subsequent injury. However, any suggestion of fibrous union or significant residual deformity after bony union would increase the chance of injury and would be considered an extreme risk. If the soft tissue injury involves all three columns, it is an extreme-risk injury (21,22).

The hidden flexion injury of McSweeney can be identified as a subtle subluxation presenting on the flexion view that is actually a total ligamentous disruption. This diagno-

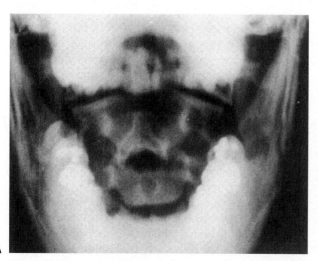

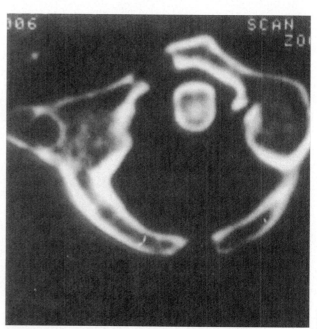

FIG. 42.11. **A:** This flexion fracture results from a head-first tackle. The key measurement is the amount of lateral overhang. An amount over 7 mm may indicate a ruptured transverse ligament. **B:** Computed tomographic scan shows a fracture with separation.

sis is made on the lateral or flexion film (23). The radiographic findings may include a gapping of the spinous processes, a localized end plate deformity, or a subtle avulsion fracture of the anterior edge of the vertebral body. The findings may be quite subtle, and the radiographic findings may take several weeks to become apparent secondary to the residual stiffness and spasm present immediately after the accident. Failure to diagnose this residual ligamentous stability and allowing these players to return to play would be extremely dangerous. This type of residual ligamentous instability places these players at extreme risk. Herkowitz and associates (24) have documented this particular ligamentous and radiographic finding after cervical spine trauma. Delay in the diagnosis and treatment of this injury can also lead to a fixed kyphotic deformity, placing the patient or player permanently in the extreme-risk category.

Fractures of the C3 to C7 vertebral bodies can be associated with compression and flexion forces as well as torsional forces that may leave the player with a significant cervical spine instability. Vertebral burst fractures may include significant spinal cord injury and are occasionally associated with facet dislocations that place the player at significant risk for complete neurologic injury. There is not always good correlation between the degree of spinal cord injury and the amount of bony injury or dislocation on the plain films. The prognosis for return to play after vertebral burst fractures, which may or may not have included subluxation or dislocation in the cervical spine, is dependent on the neurologic injury and the residual deformity present after complete healing. If there is no residual neck pain or stiffness, no residual neurologic deficit, no residual associated cervical instability, and no residual deformity or canal narrowing, then players who have suffered cervical spine compression or burst fractures may be allowed to return to play, but are still at some mild risk.

Both bilateral and unilateral facet injuries can occur with head compression and flexion-rotation injury. The facet dislocation that reduces completely and heals with no residual deformity or instability would place that player in a moderate-risk category because of the damage to ligamentous support for that segment. Facet dislocations that heal with any residual deformity or instability place the player at an extreme risk of further injury.

Other conditions that would qualify as an extreme risk include the following (25,26):

- Clinical history or physical examination findings of cervical myelopathy
- History of a C1-C2 cervical fusion
- C1-C2 rotatory fixation
- Evidence of a spear tackler's spine on radiographic analysis
- A multiple-level Klippel-Feil deformity
- An occipital C1 assimilation
- Radiographic evidence (i.e., MRI) of basilar invagination
- MRI evidence of Arnold-Chiari malformation
- Radiographic evidence of ankylosing spondylitis or diffuse idiopathic skeletal hyperostosis

- More than two previous episodes of a cervical cord neuropraxia
- Status after a cervical laminectomy
- Symptomatic disc herniation
- Clinical or radiographic evidence of rheumatoid arthritis
- Three-level spine fusion

Moderate-Risk Category

Fractures of the cervical facet or pillar fractures through the lateral mass may present like a facet dislocation. For these fractures, the ultimate recommendation regarding return to play depends on any residual deformity that persists after healing has occurred, as well as any residual instability or cervical stiffness that is manifested after treatment.

Herniated cervical discs are reasonably common in adult football players. Most of the herniated cervical discs that we identify in athletes have a lingering, or persistent, radiculopathy in those players with a first-time severe burner at the professional or college level. Because the prevalence of disc bulges and herniations in asymptomatic people and players is significantly high, the finding of a herniated cervical disc in a football player who was completely asymptomatic would not be considered to place that player at an increased risk of injury. However, players who have evidence of radiculopathy are in a moderate-risk category. There is often a great deal of difficulty in determining whether a disc herniation is acute or chronic, hard (as in a cervical osteophyte) or soft, and whether it is a free fragment or simply a contained disc bulge. It is important that any radiographic diagnostic imaging abnormalities in these players be correlated with the physical findings. The physical findings must match the herniation for an accurate prognosis to be made.

The treatment for herniated, extruded cervical discs is an anterior cervical discectomy and fusion. After such treatment, we often place the player in a mild-risk category, secondary to the alterations that occur above and below the fused cervical motion segment. It is for this reason that, given the appropriate clinical indications, we might recommend a microscopic cervical foraminotomy for the treatment of monoradiculopathy secondary to foraminal stenosis in an athlete involved in contact sports. For the athlete with significant intermittent radiculopathy, a positive Spurling's hyperextension test, and foraminal stenosis, a posterolateral foraminotomy is a reasonable approach. The technique of this operation is adopted from Robert Warren Williams (27) and includes a minimal resection of the posterior wall of the foramina only until nerve root pulsations are clearly present. A major facet resection would be a contraindication for return to football.

Other conditions that would qualify as a moderate risk include the following (25,26):

- Previous history of spinal cord neuropraxia. The patient must have full return to baseline strength and cervical range of motion.

- A healed single-level posterior fusion with lateral mass segmental fixation.
- Three or more previous stingers or burners.
- A healed two-level anterior or posterior fusion with or without instrumentation, excluding posterior segmental lateral mass screw fixation.

Minor-Risk Category

Undisplaced fractures that heal without any residual deformity indicate a low risk for return to play. Clay-shoveler fractures are avulsion fractures of the tip of the spinous process of C7 caused by strong muscular contractions of the trapezius and shoulder. They present with point tenderness, otherwise negative studies, and dual rigidity. Lateral mass fractures usually heal, but may have a slight subluxation of one vertebra on another. The degree of risk depends on the degree of subluxation. There is rarely ligamentous damage with this injury. Laminar fractures that heal without deformity are a minor-risk condition. Disc herniations that have become asymptomatic over many months or years are not of significance except if they have left the central canal narrowed. Foraminal stenosis is important when symptomatic, but because of the high incidence of asymptomatic foraminal stenosis, we would not consider a nerve root to be in danger just because radiographic foraminal stenosis was present.

Other conditions that would qualify as minor risks include the following (25,26):

- Single-level Klippel-Feil deformity with no evidence of instability or stenosis
- Spina bifida occulta
- Status after an anterior single-level cervical fusion with or without instrumentation that has healed
- Previous history of a stinger or burner times two
- Status after a single- or multiple-level posterior cervical microforaminotomy

In conclusion, the decision-making process that each team physician uses when approaching the cervical spine–injured football player must rely on the medical facts and current medical knowledge. Attention to detail, structured preplanning, and a practiced on-the-field routine are critical to ensuring that no additional damage is done to the injured player after the accident. Counseling the player and other concerned individuals must be uniform and should only include the medical facts. It is important to remember that the team physician's role is to convey the medical information as well as to instruct and to train the players, coaches, and trainers in techniques that will be useful for preventing player injury and for preventing further injury once a player is down on the field. There are no strict guidelines that have been published that are considered the standard of care. The ultimate recommendation of the team physician must be based on the medical facts as he or she finds them. Familiarity with the game of football or the particular athletic event that the physician is covering, and familiarity with the particular needs and desires of those athletes will help shape a more appropriate decision-making process. An understanding of the relative risk of a spine disorder or a spine injury to an individual player both at the time of injury and for recommending return to play must come from advanced training in sports-related spine injuries or from clinical experience that comes from active participation in the care of athletes on a regular basis.

REHABILITATION OF NECK INJURIES

For the athlete who is expecting to return to contact sports, it is imperative that the individual regains a full, pain-free range of motion of the cervical spine before being allowed to return to the sport. In football, in particular, the interrelationship among the head, neck, and shoulders in the development of a synchronous flow of movement is important to minimize the risk of recurrent injury. The rehabilitative protocol should focus on strength, bulk, and coordination in the rehabilitation of the spinal flexors and extensors, as well as the shoulder girdle musculature. Once the acute phase of the injury has subsided and the player is regaining range of motion of the neck, progressive isometric strengthening of the neck musculature is begun. As symptoms further diminish, the player is progressively allowed to resume a normal weight training schedule to regain lost muscle strength and the muscle bulk that is necessary to protect the underlying skeletal structures. Posture is also important in neck rehabilitation.

We recommend a progressive isometric trunk-strengthening exercise program aimed at placing the neck in a biomechanically sound position with the shoulders, back, and chest in a posturally correct position. This exercise program concentrates on trunk strengthening and trunk mobility. Throughout the program, the patient is instructed in postural modifications emphasizing chest-out posture, which effectively normalizes the lumbar lordosis while bringing the shoulders backward and bringing the head and neck back over the shoulders. This is similar to the military position of attention, in which cervical lordosis is normalized.

Athletes involved in the use of the upper extremities require a rigid cylinder of strength in their torso to transfer torque from their legs to their upper extremities. Trunk and leg strength generate the strength for the upper extremities, while the arms and hands generally provide the fine control. Fatigue in the trunk or legs can reduce the control in the upper extremities available for overhead activities such as required in racquet and throwing sports. With loss of the rigid trunk cylinder strength, there is a resultant loss of synchrony between the arms and legs. There is a similar linkage among the legs, trunk, neck, and head in regard to the control available for blocking and tackling that must be utilized precisely and reproducibly throughout a game. Asymmetrical, asynchronous upper extremity athletic activities can result in neck pain, neck strain, and cervical spine injury.

Interscapular pain can be directly related to bad posture, round shoulder/head forward posture, and asynchronic muscle activity. A weak trunk produces undue arm and shoulder strain because the upper extremity must compensate for the weak trunk, and arm muscles are used for strength instead of fine control (28).

CERVICAL STENOSIS

Cervical spinal stenosis and its associated transient neuropraxia of the cervical spinal cord is a source of great controversy as to recommendations for continued play. Grant (29) first described the clinical entity of cervical spinal cord neuropraxia with transient quadriplegia. Torg and Pavlov (30) described the clinical picture as an acute transient neurologic episode of cervical cord origin with sensory changes that may be associated with motor paresis involving either both arms, both legs, or all four extremities, following forced hyperextension, hyperflexion, or axial loading of the cervical spine. The sensory changes include burning pain, numbness, tingling, and loss of sensation. Congenital cervical spinal stenosis is associated with a decreased anteroposterior diameter of the cervical spinal canal as measured from the posterior vertebral body to the anterior spinal laminar line on the lateral radiograph. Acquired spinal stenosis is more likely to occur in the professional-level football player with multiple levels of degenerative disc disease, multiple levels of osteophyte formation, disc bulging, disc herniation, and hypertrophy of ligamentum flavum as well as hypertrophy of the facet joints.

The absolute sagittal diameter of the cervical spinal canal that can accommodate the spinal cord without cord compression is somewhere between 11 and 13 mm, depending on the relative diameter of the spinal cord. Penning (31) documented that a sagittal diameter less than 11 mm in extension is associated with spinal cord compression. Penning described the "pincer's mechanism," in which the spinal cord is pinched between posterior vertebral osteophytes off of the lip of the vertebral end plate and the posterior lamina. This mechanism of injury is commonly responsible for the production of the central cord syndrome in individuals with preexisting degenerative disc disease and osteophyte formation who suffer a hyperextension injury of the head and neck. However, there is ample clinical experience of professional football players with sagittal cervical spinal canal diameters of less than 11 mm who have no signs or symptoms of spinal cord compression.

Torg has done extensive research on cervical stenosis in football players (26,30,32). Cervical stenosis, defined by a ratio of the diameter of the cervical spinal canal to that of the vertebral body of 0.8 or less, had a high sensitivity with transient neuropraxia. However, its low specificity and low positive predictive value preclude its use as a screening mechanism for determining the suitability of an individual for participation in contact sports. His studies showed no association between developmental narrowing of the cervical canal and quadriplegia. They also showed no association between transient neuropraxia and quadriplegia.

Torg's assessment of the relationship of cervical stenosis to transitory neuropraxia led to the conclusion that developmental narrowing of the cervical canal in a stable spine does not predispose an individual to a permanent catastrophic neurologic injury, and therefore should not preclude an athlete from participating in contact sports. However, he believed that athletes who have developmental spinal stenosis as well as demonstrable cervical spine instability or acute or chronic intervertebral disc disease should not be allowed further participation in contact sports (30).

We believe there are many factors that must be considered prior to making such a determination. As with all radiographic findings, clinical correlation of the radiographic findings with the patient history and physical examination, as well as an understanding of the mechanical considerations of the patient's sport, must be considered before making a judgment as to the individual player's risk category.

Types of Stenosis

There are three basic types of cervical stenosis:

1. *Congenital stenosis:* Typified by short pedicles and a funnel shape to the basic bony structure of the spinal canal, observable on the lateral radiograph.
2. *Developmental stenosis:* Occurs during life and may be the result of thickening of the bone due to increased stress. For example, upper-body weight lifters and people who do upper-body and neck-strengthening exercises produce larger cervical vertebrae, just as they produce larger muscles in the neck and upper extremity; as a result, the spinal canal may narrow as the bone increases in size.
3. *Acquired cervical stenosis:* Due to cervical spondylosis with bone spurs, discs bulging, bulging ligamentum flavum occurring with disc space narrowing, and osteophytes on the facet joints, all contributing to the cervical stenosis.

More than one type of cervical stenosis may be present in any patient.

Measurement of Cervical Stenosis

There are different techniques for measuring the size of the spinal canal in order to assess the presence and degree of cervical stenosis. Torg and Pavlov (30) described a ratio of the central canal sagittal diameter to the vertebral body sagittal diameter measured on the lateral radiograph in order to remove the magnification effect. The determination of what is a normal Pavlov's ratio in certain population groups is still somewhat unclear. The original description of the Torg ratio was a study performed on patients with transient quadriparesis compared with controls. The Torg ratio was not correlated with cervical stenosis based on CT scan or MRI.

In a group of myelopathic and radiculopathic nonfootball patients, Schnebel and associates (33) compared the ratio to central canal diameters as determined by CT scan and found the 0.8 ratio to be an extremely sensitive, but not specific, measurement. Every patient who had 10 mm or less of central canal diameter had a ratio of 0.8 or less. A study by Herzog and colleagues (34) using CT scans and plain radiographs of football players demonstrated that 78% of football players with an abnormal Torg's ratio had a normal-sized spinal canal. The football players had larger vertebral bodies, therefore distorting the ratio and rendering it useless in identifying players with cervical stenosis. The report also showed that standardized-distance lateral radiographs, with calculations done to eliminate magnification, do correctly identify bony spinal stenosis.

Factors in Decision Making in Transient Quadriparesis and Spinal Canal Stenosis

There are numerous decision-making factors in these cases. Among them are the severity of the episode, extent of neurologic deficit, severity of the symptoms, patient age, player position, and neck size. The numerous methods of assessing cervical canal size bear consideration. Regardless of the canal diameter, there is certainly more danger to someone who suffers a greater neurologic injury with the episode.

We have found the rating system shown in Table 42.1 to be helpful in assessing the severity of the episode. However, every factor in a case may be considered in its entirety. In terms of the three major risk factors in Table 42.1, adding in the canal diameter rating to the time and extent of deficit scale, we use a general rating of 6 or below as a mild risk factor, 6 to 10 as a moderate risk, and 10 to 15 as a severe risk. It must be emphasized, however, that each case is individualized. For example, a player with a brief episode with a 4-mm canal or 6 months of myelopathy with a 15-mm canal may be precluded from play forever. The rating scale is only a guideline. To determine return to play, we use the rating scale and extenuating factors such as the level of play and the risk versus the benefit to the patient. The risk versus benefit ratio is often an unquantifiable factor.

An informed consent concerning continued play with cervical stenosis and a prior episode of transient quadriparesis should include an accurate assessment of as many known facts as possible. The prevalence of permanent paralysis in professional football is rare. Permanent paralysis in any football player is primarily related to blocking and tackling techniques. An episode of transient quadriplegia does not necessarily precede an incident of permanent neurologic loss. Cantu (35) reports three cases in which this occurred, but did not have such a case in the Registry.

A good example of a consent would be to inform those concerned that there is no direct predisposition between

TABLE 42.1. *Rating System to Assess Severity[a]*

Rating	Extent of neurologic deficit
1	Unilateral arm numbness or dysesthesia, loss of strength
2	Bilateral upper extremity loss of motor and sensory function
3	Herni arm and leg and trunk loss of motor and sensory function
4	Transitory quadriparesis
5	Transitory quadriplegia

Rating	Time ratings
1	Less than 5 minutes
2	Less than 1 hour
3	Less than 24 hours
4	Less than 1 week
5	Greater than 1 week

Rating of central canal diameter	Canal narrowing
1	Greater than 12 mm
2	Between 10 and 12 mm
3	10 mm
4	10 to 8 mm
5	Less than 8 mm

[a]Any existing neurologic deficit due to a cord neuropraxia should exclude an athlete from play in any case. As a general guideline: less than 4 is a mild episode, 4–7 is a moderate episode, and 8–10 is a severe episode. When combined with canal size, the severity of the episode can lead to some guidelines for recurrence.

having stenosis and getting a fracture dislocation that typically paralyzes football players. Give advice concerning what we do know about nonfootball players. There are several facts known about cervical stenosis in nonfootball players. A report by Eismont and associates (36) demonstrated that the greater the degree of cervical stenosis with a specific cervical spine injury, the greater the neurologic deficit. Matsuura and colleagues (37) found that it is not just the central canal diameter but the shape of the canal that is important. The greater the compression ratio, the greater the degree of neurologic deficit with a spine injury. Edwards and La Rocca (38) demonstrated that an individual with cervical canal stenosis is more likely to require surgery with a cervical disc herniation and less likely to be able to get well nonoperatively (38,39). Radicular pain is more common in smaller canals (40).

Epstein et al. (41) reported that there were 20 patients of 200 admissions to an acute spinal cord injury unit who had no fracture or dislocation, but had complete neurologic deficit. Among these cases were various diagnoses of cervical spondylosis, congenital stenosis, and others. The study indicates that permanent neurologic deficit can occur with spinal stenosis (18). The incidence of permanent tetraplegia in spinal column injury has varied from 4% to 70% of pediatric neck injuries, depending on the sample studied. Others have hypothesized that the etiology of quadriplegia without fracture dislocation is a combination of injury to microvascular blood supply, longitudinal traction on the cord, acute disc prolapse, and/or compromise of the vertebral spinal arterial system (42–46). A common pathology in these cases is a central cord infarct (47). As for recurrence of symptoms, multiple episodes do occur but can potentially be prevented through proper equipment, conditioning, and technique.

OTHER FACTORS IN ANY CONTINUED-PLAY DECISION

Although every position on the football field is subjected to head trauma, the worst are the impact positions of defensive back and linebacker. Blocking and tackling techniques can rarely be changed at the professional level. If the player is a head-hitter, he usually stays a head-hitter. Education for proper blocking and tackling by using the shoulders, not the head, must be aimed at athletes at younger ages, starting with those in grade school and continuing through college.

What are the chances of recurrent injury once a player has been injured? Albright and associates (48) have offered insight into this situation. At the high school level, the reinjury rate after all neck injuries, one-third of which involved extremity or neurologic symptoms, was 17%. The twice-injured players at all levels of play had an 87% chance of future injury. After a time-lost injury, the recurrent injury rate was 42% in the same season, 62% in the next season, and 67% in future seasons (48). Therefore, the recurrent injury rate is substantive regardless of the type of injury received and is higher with the time-lost neck injury.

What can be done to prevent this recurrence? Conditioning can prevent injury. Preconditioned response to predicted head stresses can allow an increased protective muscle reflex response to ward off even relatively unexpected blows (50). Neck strengthening can help protect the player from neck injury (49). Probably the greatest testament to conditioning is the ability of professional football players to deliver or receive high-impact blows without injury.

The most effective method of preventing the high risk of recurrent neck injury is to allow total recovery from pain, relief from tenderness, and restoration of a normal range of motion as well as maximum strength before returning to action.

Responsibility is always a consideration, and it is important to emphasize that the doctor who performs players' physical examinations and clears them to play bears a certain responsibility to the patient. Through proper informed consent, the patient and family are also responsible. The team, as an employer, is responsible for the health of its employees (as in any worker's compensation situation) as well as for fielding an effective team. Earlier, reference was made to risk versus benefit to the patient. The benefit of continued play to the patient is well known to the patient, family, agent, team, and others. The risk to the patient can be very difficult to define as a reality. The physician must present the risks to the patient as clearly as possible. It is hoped that this chapter will provide some guidelines for decision making in situations in which football players have injured their necks and want to return to football. There are many factors to consider in a decision that is of great importance to those involved.

REFERENCES

1. Clark KS. The survey of sports related spinal cord injuries in schools and colleges: 1973–1975. *J Safety Res* 1977;9:140.
2. Torg JS, Vegso JJ, Sennett B, et al. The National Football Head and Neck Injury Registry. 14 year report on cervical quadriplegia, 1971–1984. *JAMA* 1985;254:3439–3443.
3. Burke DC. Spinal cord injuries from water sports. *Med J Austral* 1972;2:1190.
4. Bracken MB, Shepard MJ, et al. A randomized controlled trial of methylprednisolone or naloxone in the treatment of acute spinal cord injury. *N Engl J Med* 1990;322:1405–1411.
5. Schneider RC. The treatment of the athlete with neck, cervical spine and spinal cord trauma. In: Schneider RC, ed. *Sports injuries: mechanisms, prevention and treatment.* Baltimore: Williams & Wilkins, 1985.
6. Schneider RC. Serious and fatal neurosurgical football injuries. *Clin Neurosurg* 1966;12:226.
7. Watkins RG. Neck injuries in football players. *Clin Sports Med* 1986; 5:215–246.
8. Jackson DW, Lohr FP. Cervical spine injuries. *Clin Sports Med* 1986; 5:373–386.
9. Seddon H. *Surgical disorders of the peripheral nerves.* Edinburgh: Churchill Livingstone, 1972.
10. Clancy W, Brand R, Bergfeld J. Upper trunk brachial plexus injuries in contact sports. *Am J Sports Med* 1977;5:209.
11. Bergfeld JA, Hershman EB, Wilbourn AJ. Brachial plexus in sports, a five year followup. *Orthop Transact* 1988;12:743–744.
12. Davidson RI, Dunn EJ, Metzmaker JN. The shoulder abduction test. *Spine* 1981;6:441–446.
13. Garfin SR, Rydevik BL, Brown MD. Compressive neuropathy of spinal nerve roots. *Spine* 1991;16:162–166.
14. Kleiner DM, Almquist JL, Bailes J, et al. *Prehospital care of the spine-injured athlete: a document from the Inter-Association Task Force for the Appropriate Care of the Spine-Injured Athlete.* Dallas, TX: National Athletic Trainers' Association, 2001.
15. Thomas JC. Plain roentgenograms of the spine in the injured athlete. *Clin Sports Med* 1990;5:353–371.
16. White AA III, Johnson RM, Panjabi MM, et al. Biomechanical analysis of clinical stability in the cervical spine. *Clin Orthop Relat Res* 1975;109:89–96.
17. Mazur JW, Stauffer ES. Unrecognized spinal instability associated with seemingly simple cervical compression fractures. *Spine* 1983;8: 687–692.
18. Boden SD, et al. Abnormal magnetic resonance scans of the cervical spine in asymptomatic subjects. A prospective investigation. *J Bone Joint Surg Am* 1990;72:1178–1184.
19. Davis D, Bohlman H, Walker AE, et al. The pathologic findings in fatal craniospinal injuries. *J Neurosurg* 1971;34:603.
20. Anderson LD, D'Alonzo RT. Fractures of the odontoid process of the axis. *J Bone Joint Surg Am* 1974;56:1669.
21. Effendi B, Roy D, Cornish B, et al. Fractures of the rim of the axis. *J Bone Joint Surg Br* 1981;63:319.
22. Levine AM, Edwards CC. The management of traumatic spondylolisthesis of the axis. *J Bone Joint Surg Am* 1985;67:217.
23. Watkins RG. Neck injuries in football players. *Clin Sports Med* 1986; 5:215–246.
24. Herkowitz H, Rothman R. Subacute instability of the cervical spine. *Spine* 1984;9:3348–3357.
25. Vaccaro AR, Watkins B, Albert TJ, et al. Cervical spine injuries in athletes: current return-to-play criteria. *Orthopedics* 2001;24:699–703.
26. Torg JS, Ramsey-Emrhein JA. Suggested management guidelines for participation in collision activities with congenital, developmental, or postinjury lesions involving the cervical spine. *Med Sci Sports Exerc* 1997;29:S256–S272.
27. Williams RW. Microcervical foraminotomy: A surgical alternative for intractable radicular pain. *Spine* 1983;8:708–716.
28. Watkins RG, Buhler W, Loverock P. *Water workout recovery program.* Philadelphia: Contemporary Books, 1988.

29. Grant J, Sears W. Spinal injury and computerized tomography; a review of fracture pathology and a new approach to canal decompression. *Aust NZ J Surg* 1986;56:299–307.
30. Torg JS, Pavlov H. Cervical spinal stenosis with cord neurapraxia and transient quadriplegia. *Clin Sports Med* 1987;6:115–133.
31. Penning L. Some aspects of plain radiography of the cervical spine in chronic myelopathy. *Neurology* 1962;12:513–519.
32. Torg JS. Cervical spinal stenosis with cord neurapraxia in transient quadriplegia. *Clin Sports Med* 1990;9:279–296.
33. Schnebel B, Kingston S, Watkins RG, et al. Comparison of MRI to contrast CT in the diagnosis of spinal stenosis. *Spine* 1989;14:3.
34. Herzog RJ, Weins JJ, Dillingham MF, et al. Normal cervical spine morphometry and cervical spinal stenosis in asymptomatic professional football players. Plain film radiography, multiplanar computer tomography, and magnetic resonance imaging. *Spine* 1991;16(Suppl):178–186.
35. Cantu RC. Head and spine injuries in the young athlete. *Clin Sports Med* 1988;7:459–472.
36. Eismont FJ, Clifford S, et al. Cervical sagittal spinal canal size in spine injuries. *Spine* 1984;9:663–666.
37. Matsuura P, Waters R, Adkins RH, et al. Comparison of computerized tomography parameters of the cervical spine in normal control subjects and spinal cord injured patients. *J Bone Joint Surg Am* 1989;71:183–188.
38. Edwards W, La Rocca H. The developmental segmental sagittal diameter of the cervical spinal canal in patients with cervical spondylosis. *Spine* 1983;8:20.
39. Wolf B, Khulnani M, Malis L. The sagittal diameter of the bony cervical spinal canal and its significance in cervical spondylosis. *J Mt Sinai Hosp* 1976;23:283.
40. Williams JPR, McKibben B. Cervical spine injury in the rugby union football. *Br Med J* 1978;2:17–47.
41. Epstein J, Carras R, Hyman R, et al. Cervical myelopathy caused by developmental stenosis of the spinal canal. *J Neurosurg* 1972;51:362–367.
42. Burke DC. Traumatic spinal paralysis in children. *Paraplegia* 1974;11:268–276.
43. Cheshire DJE. The pediatric syndrome of traumatic myelopathy without demonstrable vertebral injury. *Paraplegia* 1977;15:74–85.
44. Hill SA, Miller CA, et al. Pediatric neck injuries: a clinical study. *J Neurosurg* 1984;60:700–706.
45. Pang D, Wilberger JE Jr. Spinal cord injury without radiographic abnormalities in children. *J Neurosurg* 1982;57:114–129.
46. Scher AT. Vertex impact and cervical dislocation in rugby players. *S Afr Med J* 1981;59:227–228.
47. Ahmann PA, Smith SA, et al. Spinal cord infarction due to minor trauma in children. *Neurology* 1975;25:301–307.
48. Albright JP, Moses JM, Feldick HG, et al. Non-fatal cervical spine injuries in interscholastic football. *JAMA* 1976;236:1243–1245.
49. Reid SE, Reid SE Jr. Advances in sports medicine: prevention of head and neck injuries in football players. *Surg Annu* 1981;13:251–270.
50. Funk FJ, Wells RE. Injuries of the cervical spine in football. *Clin Orthop Relat Res* 1975;109:50–58.

CHAPTER 43

Injuries to the Atlantooccipital Articulation

Paul A. Anderson, Sohail K. Mirza, and Jens R. Chapman

Injuries to the atlantooccipital articulation are being recognized more commonly, and patients surviving with injuries previously thought to be fatal are being increasingly reported. Early trauma care including cardiopulmonary resuscitation at the scene of the accident and proper management of airways has brought patients to emergency rooms who previously would have died. With the increasing sophistication and availability of imaging technology, the likelihood of injury detection has increased (1). The purpose of this chapter is to review the relevant anatomy and biomechanics of the atlantooccipital articulation and to discuss the diagnosis, classification, and treatment of occipital condyle fractures and atlantooccipital dissociation.

ANATOMY

The atlantooccipital articulations form the transition between the cranial vault and the spinal column. The bony elements of the craniocervical junction consist of the occiput, the atlas, and the axis. By the nature of their joint morphology, the five craniocervical articulations provide no inherent stability, but rather rely on ligaments for maintenance of structural integrity. Since these ligaments extend between the occiput to the axis, the craniocervical joints form a close functional unit, which provides approximately half of the range of motion of the cervical spine. Protected within this osseoligamentous unit are the spinal cord, brainstem, and vertebral arteries.

Bony Anatomy

The occipital condyles are paired semilunar-shaped projections from the inferior surface of the occiput. They lie along the anterolateral margins of the foramen magnum and, when viewed from the anterior, are wedge-shaped, extending farther medially than laterally (2,3). The occipital condyles articulate in corresponding concavities of the lat-

eral masses of the atlas. The lateral masses of the atlas are connected to a ring by thin anterior and posterior arches. The cranial surface of the atlantal lateral mass is sloped to match the occipital condyles, which centers the condyles into the atlas (4) (Fig. 43.1). In children, this recess is less well developed. This circumstance may contribute to the higher incidence of atlantooccipital injury in pediatric patients (5).

The transverse atlantal ligament (TAL) attaches to the tubercles emanating from the medial aspect of the lateral masses. Although this arrangement does not significantly increase the load-bearing capacity of the atlas, it contributes to atlantoaxial stability (4). The odontoid closely articulates with the posterior aspect of the anterior arch of the atlas and is secured to the atlas by the TAL and the joint capsules of the atlantoaxial articulations. The corresponding surfaces of the atlantoaxial articulations are bi-convex, which facilitates rotation but provides little intrinsic stability (6).

Ligamentous Anatomy

Ligamentous structures of the neck can be broadly categorized into intrinsic and extrinsic craniocervical ligaments. In humans the intrinsic craniocervical ligaments extend from the occiput to the axis, thereby largely bypassing the atlas. This arrangement allows the atlas to serve as a bushing or washerlike structure and facilitates atlantoaxial rotation (7).

External Craniocervical Ligaments

The ligamentum nucha is a condensation of fibers that spans from the external occipital protuberance and attaches to the posterior tubercle of the atlas and the tips of the spinous processes of the remaining cervical segments. This structure is less well developed in humans than

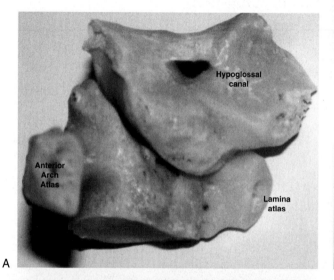

A

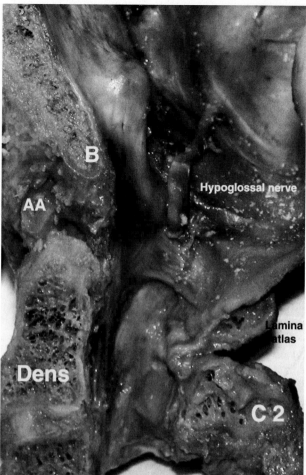

B

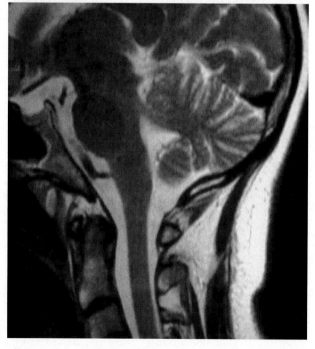

C

FIG. 43.1. The craniocervical articulation offers poor primary bony stability, as demonstrated in this specimen viewed from within the spinal canal **(A)**. Note the proximity of the hypoglossal nerve foramen in the skull base. **B:** A midsagittal cross section of the craniocervical junction. The craniocervical junction with its three bony components and five articulations forms an integrated motion unit. Any injury to any component of the craniocervical junction should be viewed in its potential to impair the integrity of the entire motion unit. AA, anterior atlas arch; B, basion; C2, spinous process of the C2 segment. **C:** A correlating midsagittal T2-weighted magnetic resonance imaging (MRI) scan of the craniocervical junction. This normal MRI scan shows the detail with which the ligamentous support structures of the craniocervical junction can be visualized.

in quadrupeds. The ligamentum flavum and intervertebral discs are absent between the occiput and atlas and between the atlas and axis. Instead, fibroelastic membranes are present posteriorly between the occiput and atlas and between the atlas and axis. Loose joint capsules enclose the atlantooccipital and atlantoaxial articulations. The rostral extension of the anterior longitudinal ligament is referred to as the anterior atlantooccipital and atlantoaxial membranes, which are subdivided into a thinner superficial and a well-developed deep layer. In neutral head position, the anterior atlantooccipital membrane is slightly redundant but serves as an effective check rein against hyperextension. None of the other external ligaments provides a meaningful contribution to the stability of the upper cervical spine (6–8) (Fig. 43.2).

Internal Craniocervical Ligaments

The internal craniocervical ligaments are located within the spinal canal and provide most of the intrinsic stability. These ligaments are arranged in three layers that lie anterior to the dura. From dorsal to ventral, they are the tectorial membrane, the cruciate ligament, and the odontoid ligaments. The tectorial membrane is a broad, flat, ligamentous

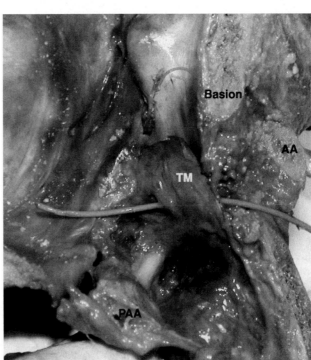

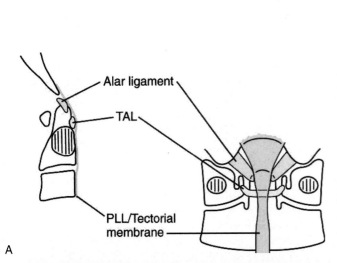

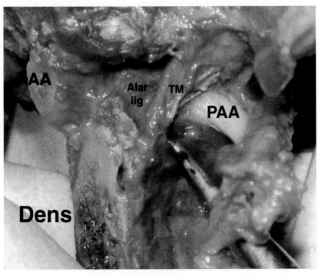

FIG. 43.2. A: The key ligaments of the craniocervical junction. The transverse atlantal ligament (TAL) locks the atlas to the axis and serves as an anchor for the cruciate ligament complex. The alar ligaments connect the medial surface of the occipital condyles to the respective lateral tip of the odontoid. The tectorial membrane can be conceptualized as a rostral continuation of the posterior longitudinal ligament. It originates from the clivus and proceeds caudally along the posterior vertebral body walls of the lower cervical spine. Although the tectorial membrane fulfills a crucial role in resisting vertically oriented cranial displacement, it is a relatively thin ligamentous structure, as represented in the anatomic specimen shown in B. The probe elevates the tectorial membrane. C: The relatively small size of the alar ligaments as pointed out by the surgical probe. AA, anterior atlas arch; PAA, posterior atlas arch; TM, tectorial membrane; Alar lig, alar ligament.

structure that constitutes the rostral continuation of the posterior longitudinal ligament. It attaches to the anterior aspect of the foramen magnum (Fig. 43.2B). Anterior to the tectorial membrane is the cruciate ligament. Its well-developed transverse component is the transverse atlantal ligament, which keys the odontoid process into the atlas with its excursion between the anteromedial aspects of the atlantal condyles. Vertical triangular-shaped bands extend from the transverse ligament and attach to the anterior edge of the foramen magnum and to the axis body.

The most anterior internal craniocervical ligament layer consists of the alar and apical ligaments, which together are referred to as odontoid ligaments. The paired alar ligaments are funnel-shaped, measure 5 to 6 mm in diameter, and consist of a complex multiplanar arrangement of fibers (8,9). They originate from the medial surface of the occipital condyles and converge in a V-shaped fashion on the facies lateralis on either side of the tip of the odontoid process (Fig. 43.2C). The apical ligament is a rudimentary structure that connects the apex of the dens and foramen magnum.

BIOMECHANICS

The five very mobile joints of the upper cervical spine enable a rapid-response, large-scale head movement, whereas the design of the lower cervical spine is more geared toward providing fine adjustment as well as projection of the head. With its unique anatomic arrangement, the upper cervical spine contributes to 60% of rotation and 40% of flexion-extension of overall neck motion by means of coupled, still incompletely understood, joint kinematics. Despite permitting this extensive range of motion, intact craniocervical ligaments with their highly specialized, multilayered configuration restrict distraction or translation of the various bony components to less than 2 mm in any plane (6–10). Complete atlantoaxial rotational excursion from left to right amounts to 80 to 88 degrees. Both the atlantooccipital and atlantoaxial joints are capable of achieving 20 to 30 degrees of motion in the flexion-extension plane. The atlantoaxial joints also permit a total of 20 degrees of left-to-right lateral bending, in addition to 5 to 10 degrees contributed by the atlantooccipital joints (6,11).

The tectorial membrane, the anterior atlantooccipital membrane, and the alar ligaments resist vertical distraction. The alar ligaments, through tightening of the respective contralateral ligament, restrict rotation and lateral bending. Loss of one alar ligament can be expected to increase flexion, rotation, and lateral bending by 30% to 40% in each direction (11). However, unilateral loss of an alar ligament in the absence of functional disruption of the other key ligaments of the craniocervical junction will not result in significant craniocervical instability (9–11). Head extension is initially limited by the anterior atlantooccipital membrane and eventually by impaction of the occiput and posterior elements of the atlas and axis on one another. Flexion is restricted by the tectorial membrane and by impaction of the

basion on the tip of the odontoid. The tectorial membrane limits anteroposterior angulation between the atlas and axis with flexion or extension beyond neutral (7,11). With intact ligaments, anteroposterior translation is further diminished by the occipital condyles being centered in a saddle created by the concavities of the lateral masses of the atlas (4).

While providing a literally vital function, craniocervical ligaments tested in isolation are relatively weak. *In vitro* tensile failure of an alar ligament has been reported to be 210 N, less than half of the load to failure reported for the anterior cruciate ligament of the knee (9). In comparison, the *in vitro* tensile failure of the TAL has been reported to be 350 N. (Intact craniocervical ligaments will usually permit less than 2 mm of distraction or translation between the atlantooccipital or atlantoaxial joints in any plane.)

Forensic Studies

The relative frailty of the human craniocervical ligaments has been used for judicial hangings for centuries. Vehicular trauma has become the leading cause of fatal disruption of the craniocervical junction. Bucholz and Burkhead (12) identified 24 cervical spine injuries in 100 consecutive autopsies of victims of motor vehicular crashes. Eight of the 24 had fatal occipitoatlantal dislocations. Davis and colleagues (13) similarly documented a 10% prevalence of atlantooccipital dislocation in 50 patients who died of vehicular trauma. Jónsson and co-workers (14) examined 22 traffic crash victims with fatal craniocervical trauma using a cryoplaning technique. Fourteen specimens were found to have injuries at the craniocervical junction despite negative radiographs and negative clinical tests for stability as performed by forensic pathologists. Children have been found to be especially at risk for these injuries if subjected to blunt, rapid, deceleration-type trauma such as car crashes or pedestrian versus car trauma. They have shallow or immature concavities of the C1 lateral masses, a relatively large ratio of head to body size, and generalized ligamentous laxity (5,15–18).

EVALUATION OF PATIENTS WITH OCCIPITOCERVICAL INJURIES

Craniocervical injuries have been associated with high-energy injury mechanisms such as road traffic accidents or hanging (12,19–21). Identifying craniocervical injuries in such patients is difficult due to frequent concurrent head trauma and the presence of multiple-system injuries, leading to a primary emphasis on patient resuscitation. All patients with a history of a high-energy injury mechanism should be considered as having a potential craniocervical injury until a complete evaluation has been performed (22,23). Typical clinical complaints associated with craniocervical trauma in an awake patient are headache or pain in the suboccipital region. There are few if any external signs of injury (24).

Physical examination is performed in a methodical, but careful, fashion. Following adequate resuscitation of the patient, the entire posterior aspect of the spine is visually examined and palpated, checking for tenderness, discoloration, and swelling from occiput to coccyx. Removing any external neck immobilization and log rolling the patient with the help of several assistants facilitates this important assessment. An experienced team leader in charge of the turning maneuver holds the patient's head in a neutral position relative to the torso throughout this part of the examination.

The ability to perform a neurologic examination depends on the patient's cognitive status, but should be carried out in every patient and documented according to the guidelines of the American Spinal Injury Association (25). This neurologic examination includes testing of cranial nerve function as well as motor and sensory function in the trunk and extremities. The status of deep tendon reflexes and the presence of pathologic reflexes and sacral sparing are determined. Patients with craniocervical injuries may present with a wide variety of neurologic deficits, ranging from respiratory-dependent quadriplegia to cervicomedullary syndromes such as the cruciate paralysis described by Bell (26). The association of head and brainstem injuries can make a differentiated neurologic assessment very challenging. The examining physician should also be aware of the potential for injuries to cranial nerves VI, VII, IX, XI, and XII in association with craniocervical trauma, which occur in approximately 44% of patients with intact brainstem function (27–30). Neurologic evaluations should be repeated at appropriate intervals to assess for dynamic changes such as secondary deterioration. Some of the causes of secondary neurologic deterioration include thrombosis of vertebral arteries, edema or stroke of the brainstem, and loss of craniocervical alignment (31).

Any patient with craniocervical trauma may require emergent endotracheal airway access and ventilatory support due to secondary respiratory embarrassment. Intubation strategies for patients with an unstable craniocervical junction include nasotracheal intubation under application of manual in-line technique (MILT) or fiberoptic guidance, and tracheostomy if other techniques fail (32).

Radiographic Analysis

Advances in neuroimaging offer unparalleled visualization of the craniocervical junction. Implementation of an effective diagnostic algorithm is essential to minimize missed spinal injuries while maximizing resource utilization. Knowledge of the craniocervical injury entity is an important prerequisite toward the goal of avoiding missed injuries. Because of the closely integrated functional unit that the upper cervical spine forms, any injury to any of its components should prompt further scrutiny to rule out more comprehensive disruption of this structure (Fig. 43.3).

Conventional radiography continues to be the gold standard for spine clearance in trauma patients (33). Of the standard five cervical spine views (lateral, open-mouth odontoid, subaxial anteroposterior, and left as well as right trauma obliques), the lateral and open-mouth views are most relevant for screening and diagnosis of the craniocervical junction anatomy (34). On an anteroposterior open-mouth view the maxilla and teeth frequently override the occipitocervical joints. Because conventional lateral cervical spine projections are centered on the C3 segment, visualization of the craniocervical region can be hampered by obliquity of the atlantooccipital joints relative to the plane of x-ray beams. In case of doubt, a coned-down lateral radiograph of the upper cervical spine or lateral view of the skull can clarify spatial relationships of this region (35).

Indirect warning signs for craniocervical injuries include prevertebral soft tissue swelling, lack of override of the mastoid processes over the odontoid tip, and disruption of the upper cervical spinal laminar line (Fig. 43.3A) (36). If these are found to be out of the ordinary, closer radiographic scrutiny of the upper cervical spine is indicated (37, 38). Multiple screening tests to verify the presence of physiologic craniocervical radiographic alignment have been suggested. Of these tests, Wackenheim's line, Harris' lines, and Powers ratio are effective initial assessment tools (Fig. 43.3B). Wackenheim's line delineates the relationship between the clivus and the odontoid. The clivus is a bony plate that extends from the sella turcica and ends at the basion (anterior ring of the foramen magnum). Normally, a line drawn from the clivus points toward the odontoid and lies within a 5 mm distance from the odontoid tip (39). Powers ratio is the quotient calculated from the distances between the basion and posterior arch of C1 to the distance between the opisthion and anterior arch of C1. Ratios greater than 1.0 imply anterior occipitoatlantal dislocation. This test is not applicable for posterior or rotational atlantooccipital injuries and is of questionable value for vertically distracted injuries (40–43).

Harris et al. (40,44) examined the relationship between the basion and dens in 400 adults and 37 patients with occipital cervical instability. They described the posterior axial line as the rostral extension of the posterior cortex of the axis body. The distance between the basion and posterior axial line is defined as the basion–axis interval (BAI), and the distance between the basion and odontoid tip is the basion–dental interval (BDI). In 98% of normal subjects, the basion–axial and basion–dental intervals were less than 12 mm (Fig. 43.3C). This has been termed the "rule of twelves." In patients with documented occipitocervical instability, the rule of twelves was positive (greater than 12 mm) in 73% of cases. These are important reference lines that should always be verified to determine the status of the occipitoatlantal joints. Although abnormal screening values may not be diagnostic in themselves, they should lead to further neuroimaging tests (33,40).

Computed tomography (CT) is increasingly used for routine assessment of polytraumatized patients (45). It allows

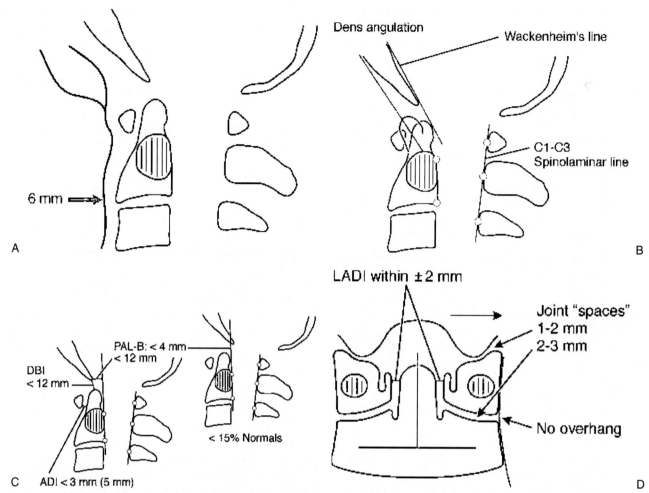

FIG. 43.3. Radiographic reference lines. **A:** *Prevertebral soft tissue shadow.* In a healthy recumbent adult without an endotracheal tube, the prevertebral soft tissue shadow should be less than 6 mm. **B:** Three simple craniocervical radiographic reference lines are depicted. *Dens angulation:* The anterior cortex of the odontoid should parallel the posterior cortex of the anterior ring of the atlas. Any kyphotic or lordotic deviation should be viewed with suspicion for an odontoid fracture or transverse atlantal ligament (TAL) disruption. *Wackenheim's line:* This reference line is drawn as a continuation from the clivus caudally. The tip of the odontoid should be within 1 to 2 mm distance of this line. *C1 to C3 spinolaminar line:* Reference points drawn from the anterior cortex of the laminae of the atlas, axis, and C3 segments should fall within 2 mm of one another. Deviation beyond this should raise suspicion of atlantoaxial translation or disruption of the neural arches of either segment. **C:** Harris lines, which have been shown to have improved sensitivity and specificity compared with other reference systems, such as Powers ratio. *DBI:* The dens–basion interval (DBI) is the distance of the odontoid tip and the distal end of the basion and should measure less than 12 mm in adults. *PAL-B:* The posterior axis line (PAL) should be within 4 mm anterior and 12 mm posterior to the basion. **D:** The lateral atlas–dens interval (LADI) can be measured on open-mouth odontoid views as well as calibrated coronal computed tomographic reformatted views. *LADI:* The left and right lateral atlas–dens intervals should be within 2 mm deviation of one another. The bony components of the occipitocervical joints should be symmetric to one another and not exceed 2 mm distance on open-mouth odontoid films. The C2-C3 facet joints should measure less than 3 mm distance from one another and should be symmetric in appearance as well.

for detailed visualization of the osseous components of the craniocervical junction. Head CT scans have become a routine first-line diagnostic modality for any patient with head injury (46,47). Lowering the caudal window of a routine trauma head CT scan to include the foramen magnum can provide information indicative of craniocervical junction trauma, such as a suboccipital hematoma or an occipital

condyle fracture (48–50). With the emergence of helical CT, comprehensive rapid visualization of the entire cervical spine and its transitional zones can be obtained after a spiral head CT scan has been completed. Definitive osseous craniocervical junction visualization is best achieved with a fine-cut CT of 2 mm or less and sagittal as well as coronal plane reconstructions (50,51). These reconstructed views allow for assessment of congruent fit of the occipital condyles within the concavities of the atlantal lateral masses, with less than 2 mm diastasis or translation in any direction (Fig. 43.3D) (50).

Magnetic resonance imaging (MRI) is indicated to assess neural pathoanatomy and alignment of the craniocervical junction (52). Increased signal intensity on fat suppression techniques, in and around ligamentous structures, reflects probable ligamentous injury (15). Direct imaging of the alar and transverse ligaments by MRI has shown inconsistent results (3).

Occasionally, the aforementioned imaging techniques will fail to answer the basic question of stability of the largely ligamentous craniocervical junction. Cervical traction radiographs under fluoroscopic control are a simple method to conclusively determine stability of this area (53). An experienced surgeon performs this study with the patient placed in a supine position. A true lateral fluoroscopic image of the craniocervical junction is then obtained and printed out for comparison. Cranial traction is then applied with 5 pounds weight with a head halter. Repeat images are then obtained and compared to the initial radiograph. The traction weight is then incrementally increased in 5-pound intervals up to 20 pounds. Any widening of the cranial or atlantoaxial articulations beyond 2 mm is indicative of ligamentous insufficiency (54). Once distractive instability is excluded, passive flexion and extension manipulation can then be performed by the examiner under fluoroscopic imaging to rule out translational instability of the atlanto-occipital and atlantoaxial articulations (53,55).

MECHANISMS OF INJURY

Injury to the craniocervical junction occurs by three primary forces: compression, distraction, and lateral rotation. Axial compression occurs usually from falls from a height or direct blows to the head whereby the cranium compresses downward onto the cervical spine. Occasionally, the skull will fail, resulting in occipital condylar fractures. Distraction injuries are seen more commonly as a result of rapid deceleration, especially in a vehicular crash when the trunk is restrained and the head continues forward, creating tension in the tectorial membrane and alar ligaments (19, 43). Similarly, acceleration injuries occur when a pedestrian is struck by an automobile and can result in similar distractive injuries to the tectorial membrane and alar ligaments. During forced lateral bending or axial rotation, tensile failure of the contralateral alar ligament or bony attachment of the alar ligament may occur. In children younger than 2 years, child abuse in the form of violent shaking ("shaken child syndrome") has been described as a cause of atlantooccipital disruption (56).

Injuries to the occipitocervical junction represent a continuum from mild ligamentous sprains and stable fractures to complete osseoligamentous disruption and instabil-

ity (18,55). Because of the close anatomic relationship of the vertebral arteries, brainstem, cranial nerves, and spinal cord, all injuries should initially be considered life threatening. The remainder of this chapter reviews the diagnosis and treatment of occipital condyle fractures, isolated alar ligament injuries, and occipitoatlantal instabilities.

OCCIPITAL CONDYLE FRACTURES

Outside of the forensic medicine community, occipital condyle fractures historically have remained a relatively obscure injury entity, despite the first case report by Bell dating back to 1817 (57,58). The mechanism of injury is usually either a direct blow to the cranium or rapid deceleration. Many patients are unconscious on admission, and the fracture is incidentally identified on a reformatted head CT. Awake patients may complain of suboccipital pain and occipital headache (58). Tenderness may be difficult to elicit because of the depth of these articulations. Chronic suboccipital pain has been reported in patients with unrecognized occipital condyle fractures (24). Neurologic examination in patients with occipital condyle fractures is most often normal (58). However, fatal brainstem injury, respiratory-dependent quadriplegia, mild degrees of spinal cord injury, and injury to cranial nerves VI, VII, IX, X, XI, and XII have been reported (27–29).

Classification of Occipital Condyle Fractures

Wackenheim, Saternus, and Anderson have proposed classification systems for occipital condyle fractures. Wackenheim (39) gave the first extensive review in 1974, when he reported on six cases. He differentiated avulsion-type injuries, which he found in four cases, and compression injuries, which he found in two cases (39). Saternus (59) differentiated six different injury types based on six different force vectors after autopsy studies on 156 specimens in 1986. Anderson and Montesano (2), in 1988, described a simplified three-part fracture system in which occipital condyle fractures are classified based on CT morphology and the potential for occipitocervical instability. Because the alar ligaments are one of the primary stabilizers of the occipitocervical articulation and attach to the medial surface of the respective occipital condyle, injuries to these structures create the potential for significant instability (10).

Although the system suggested by Saternus (59) is the most comprehensive and is based on a large autopsy series, we prefer the system suggested by Anderson and Montesano (2) for its simplicity and clinical relevance. The following describes this classification (Fig. 43.4).

- Type I injury: A comminuted fracture due to impaction of the occipital condyle into the lateral mass of the atlas. A direct blow to the head causes this most often. In general, it is a stable injury.

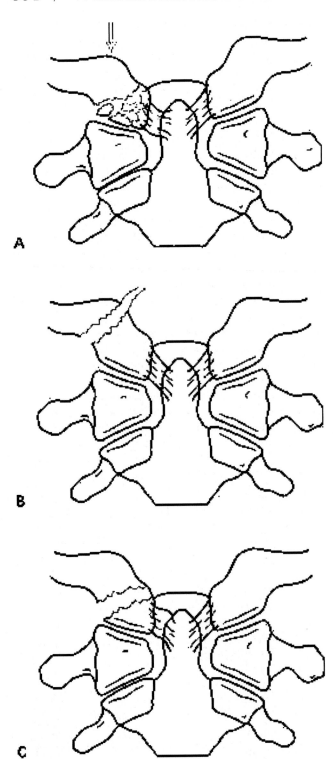

FIG. 43.4. Anderson and Montesano classification of occipital condyle fractures. **A:** Type I injuries are comminuted impaction injuries and are stable. **B:** Type II fractures are impaction fractures extending into the skull base. These injuries are usually stable. **C:** Type III injuries represent avulsion injuries. Type III injuries are likely to be unstable due to their ligamentous nature.

- Type II injury: An occipital condyle fracture associated with a basilar skull fracture. The basilar skull fracture may exit into the foramen magnum through the occipital condyle or the entire condyle may be separated from the skull base by the fracture. These have a similar mechanism as Type I fractures. They are stable, except in the case when the entire condyle has been separated from the occiput.
- Type III injuries: Wedge-shaped avulsion fractures of the attachment of the alar ligaments. The bone fragments are often displaced medially toward the foramen magnum. Frequently they are bilateral and occur in 30% to 50% of cases of atlantooccipital dislocation. A careful assessment of the alignment of the occipitoatlantal and atlantoaxial articulation is required in patients with Type III fractures. This is best determined by high-resolution CT with reformations. Any anteroposterior displacement, joint incongruity, or abnormal diastasis is indicative of occipitocervical instability.

The assessment of occipital condyle fractures should also take into consideration whether the injury is unilateral or bilateral. Presence of bilateral occipital condyle fractures of any subtype in itself is strongly suggestive of a craniocervical disruption (35,55).

Treatment

Treatment options for patients with occipital condyle fractures have to take the overall injury load and constellation of associated trauma into consideration. The presence of displaced skull fractures, chest wall trauma, or noncontiguous spine fractures may necessitate treatment modifications. The treating physician should be aware of any variant of an occipital condyle fracture representing more serious underlying injury to the entire functional unit of the upper cervical spine.

The treatment of stable unilateral Type I and Type II fractures usually consists of cervical immobilization in a hard collar or cervicothoracic brace for 8 to 12 weeks (2). Type II fractures in which the occipital condyle is separated from the occiput may have inadequate lateral column support and therefore should be treated in a halo vest for 8 to 12 weeks. Upright lateral and open-mouth radiographs should be obtained to assure maintenance of satisfactory alignment.

Patients with avulsion injuries of the Type III category should be assessed for potential atlantooccipital instability. In the absence of instability, patients with isolated Type III injury can be treated with external immobilization, such as a hard collar or cervicothoracic brace, for 8 to 12 weeks. Functional radiographs should be obtained to assess stability at the conclusion of immobilization. Type III injuries with minimal displacement can be considered for halo vest treatment after ruling out more comprehensive ligamentous injury. Unstable Type III injuries associated with atlantooccipital instability are best managed with a posterior instrumented occiput-to-C2 arthrodesis. Patients with chronic disabling pain following occipital condyle fracture may be candidates for late occiput-to-C2 arthrodesis (60).

ISOLATED ALAR LIGAMENT INJURIES

Dvorak and Panjabi (9) hypothesized that isolated alar ligament injuries may occur secondary to rapid, forced lateral bending or rotation. Patients may initially present with minimal symptoms, then develop chronic pain as a result of a mild instability due to a lack of a functional alar ligament. A biomechanical study demonstrated an increase of from 4.5 to 9.5 degrees of occipitoatlantal motion and from 31 to 35 degrees of atlantoaxial motion following sectioning of the contralateral alar ligament. Dvorak et al. performed functional CT scans in 43 patients with chronic neck pain following trauma. He found excessive occipitoatlantal rotation or atlantoaxial rotation greater than 10 degrees in 22 of the patients (6,11).

At this time there is no proven efficacious treatment, although external immobilization for 8 to 12 weeks followed by dynamic motion radiographs to assess for craniocervical stability appears to be sufficient for the majority of patients with isolated alar ligament injuries (23). Occipitocervical arthrodesis would be expected to offer pain relief in patients with documented instability or chronic pain (61).

OCCIPITOCERVICAL SUBLUXATION AND DISLOCATION

Craniocervical dissociative injuries were felt to be unsurvivable due to associated neurologic injuries and, therefore, were largely ignored. Until recently, fewer than 20 case reports of survivors had been published. With widespread implementation of the Advanced Trauma Life Support (ATLS) protocols as well as improved pre- and perioperative care, the likelihood for patient survival from these injuries appears to have greatly increased. Newer imaging techniques and the increased vigilance of professionals in charge of trauma health care delivery have resulted in earlier diagnosis of these life-threatening injuries (14,62). Also, patients with less severe instability patterns compared with those with complete dislocations are now being recognized and successfully treated. However, the best treatment choice for patients with these incomplete instability patterns has not been fully elucidated.

Case reports of survivors with occipitocervical dislocation reveal that the majority of patients were subjected to deceleration trauma or pedestrian versus car mechanisms (23,38, 62–65). An alarming prevalence is seen in the pediatric population (5,18,56,66–68). Survivors of craniocervical dislocation commonly had incomplete neurologic deficits such as the Brown-Séquard syndrome, central cord syndrome, or cervicomedullary syndromes (31). Cranial nerve injuries to the sixth, eleventh, and twelfth cranial nerves occurred in over 50% of cases (27,28,62,64).

A missed atlantooccipital dissociation (AOD) remains a formidable problem and is estimated to occur in 50% to 66% of patients (23,55,62,65,69,70). Significant delay in diagnosis of craniocervical dissociation appears to be frequently associated with neurologic deterioration. Chapman and associates (55) reported on complete AODs in nine adult survivors that were missed on initial assessment in six patients, resulting in secondary neurologic deterioration in five of these six patients. Causes for missed diagnoses are multifactorial. Concurrent head trauma, present in over 70% of patients, can disrupt established diagnostic pathways and limit clinical findings (1). Increased awareness of even subtle radiographic findings in the craniocervical region is important due to the potential presence of a spontaneously reduced dislocation. For instance, Type III occipital condyle fractures are concurrent radiographic findings in 30% to 50% of patients with AOD (23,35). An increased atlantodens interval, indicating probable associated injury to the transverse ligament, is present in 36% of patients, although not noted in most published case reports (56,61,71).

Classification of Occipitocervical Instability

Occipitocervical subluxations and dislocations have been classified by Traynelis and associates (30) according to the direction of displacement of the occiput. This is somewhat artificial because these injuries often represent a global craniocervical ligamentous disruption, with displacement often determined by the positioning of the head relative to the thorax for the radiograph. This may explain the high incidence of anterior cranial displacement patterns in children, with their proportionally larger head size (43).

Type I injuries are anterior translocations of the occipital condyle relative to the atlantal lateral masses. These are the most common type and may consist of unilateral or bilateral complete dislocations.

Type II injuries are vertical displacements of the occipital condyles greater than 2 mm of the normal atlantooccipital joint. Such distraction injuries can occur between the occiput and atlas or the atlantoaxial articulation. Because the same ligamentous structures are injured, distractive atlantoaxial injuries are part of the continuum of occipitocervical injuries. Based on a review of case reports, vertically displaced craniocervical dissociations are associated with a higher rate of neurologic deficits than the other types.

Type III injuries are the rarely reported posterior occipital dislocations. The patients in the two case reports both had associated bilateral laminar fractures of the atlas, which probably accounted for the patients' survival.

An alternate approach to classification of atlantocervical dissociations is to differentiate these injuries into three stages of disruption patterns (13,18,55). Injuries are differentiated into incomplete injuries to the craniocervical ligaments (Stage I) and cases of craniocervical dissociation, which in turn are subdivided into occult (Stage II) and overt (Stage III) (Fig. 43.5). In stage I injuries, sufficient residual

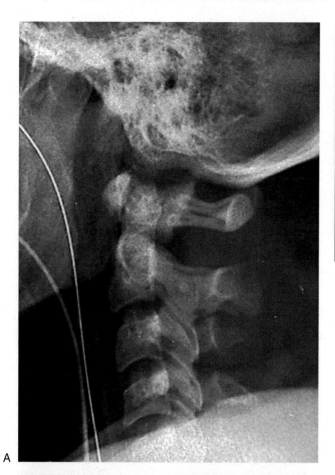

A

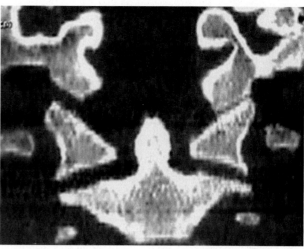

B

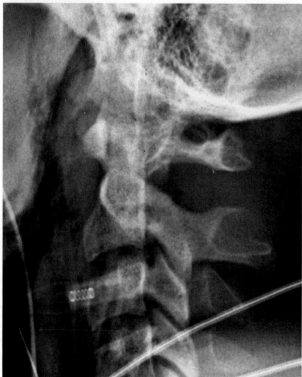

C

FIG. 43.5. Harborview classification of atlantoaxial dissociation (AOD). Stage I atlantooccipital injuries consist of a partial ligamentous disruption without significant displacement. Neurologic injuries are relatively rare. Isolated cranial nerve palsies may be encountered with this condition. The lateral cervical spine radiograph **(A)** shows increased upper cervical soft tissue swelling and a suggestion of widening of the craniocervical junction. A unilateral alar ligament injury was confirmed on computed tomography (CT) and on traction studies **(B)**. The patient was treated nonoperatively with a halo and achieved a satisfactory final healing result. Stage II AOD lesions are essentially joint dislocations, which present in spontaneously reduced state (rebound reduction). The injuries are commonly missed. Devastating secondary neurologic deterioration has been reported with delay in diagnosis and if insufficient stabilization of the craniocervical junction has been provided. **C:** A lateral cervical spine radiograph of a 35-year-old man following a high-speed motor vehicle crash. Traction tests were obtained after CT and MRI scans identified some craniocervical ligamentous trauma. **D:** A normal atlantooccipital articulation (joint lines enhanced by parallel curves). **E:** Atlantooccipital diastasis with 3 mm displacement. Any atlantooccipital diastasis exceeding 1 mm is considered abnormal. The spontaneous reduction is usually induced by residual ligamentous support. These remaining ligamentous structures are, however, unable to withstand physiologic loads without stabilization. Patients with Stage II injuries frequently present with a wide variety of neurologic injuries, ranging from isolated cranial nerve injuries to unusual incomplete spinal cord injuries, such as the cervicomedullary syndrome. **F:** Stage III injuries present with an obvious, complete loss of craniocervical ligamentous support. In the past, Stage III injuries were considered to be incompatible with survival. However, survival of patients with Stage III injuries has been described with increasing frequency. Patients with these injuries are expected to have significant neurologic injuries.

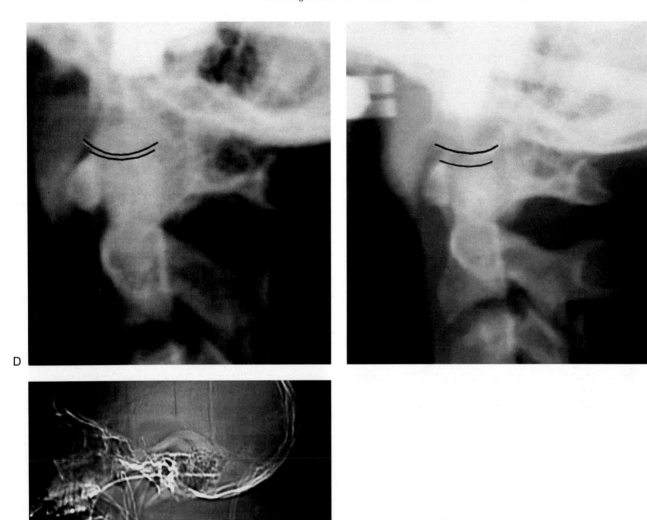

FIG. 43.5. *Continued*

ligamentous support is preserved to restrict atlantooccipital subluxation greater than 2 mm in any direction (Fig. 43.5A,B) (55). Stage I injuries can usually be treated with external immobilization, such as halo vest. Ligamentous disruption of the transverse atlantal ligament, however, has been shown to have poor healing potential if treated nonoperatively (56,71).

Stage II and III injuries represent loss of critical ligamentous support of the craniocervical junction and are invariably unstable. Stage II injuries are less than obvious on initial radiographic survey due to a "rebound phenomenon" caused by residual soft tissue tension, which can lead to a spontaneous partial deformity reduction (Fig. 43.5C–E) (72). Injuries of this severity require dedicated neuroimaging studies and may only become evident on provocative testing, such as traction studies. Patients with this injury subtype may have subtle or no neurologic deficits on initial presentation, but are subject to potentially catastrophic consequences if left undertreated. Posterior instrumented craniocervical arthrodesis is the treatment of choice for this condition.

Stage III injuries present with obvious displacement of the craniocervical junction on the initial lateral cervical spine radiograph. Patients with this injury most often have sustained severe neurologic injuries and have significantly reduced chances of survival or restoration of meaningful vital function (31,64). However, under optimal patient recovery and resuscitation circumstances, patients have survived this injury with recovery of substantial function (Fig. 43.5F) (35,55). Treatment options consist of palliative supportive care for patients with critical and seemingly irreversible central nervous system trauma or early surgical stabilization of the craniocervical junction with rigid internal fixation.

Initial Treatment

The treatment goals for all spine-injured patients are to protect the neural tissues, reduce and stabilize fractures and dislocations, and provide long-term spinal stability. Once recognized, patients with occipitocervical instability must be managed carefully to avoid catastrophic neurologic deterioration. If possible, a spiral CT of the head and neck of the patient is obtained initially (45,50). Following emergent resuscitation and airway management, realignment of the craniocervical junction should be attempted. Obvious dislocations of the craniocervical junction (stage III injuries) can be most effectively reduced under fluoroscopy with a halo ring or halo vest (55). In a multiply injured patient, a halo vest assembly may, however, be contraindicated due to the concurrent presence of a displaced skull fracture or unstable chest wall. If this modality is not applicable, the patient is preferably immobilized on a backboard with the head stabilized by sandbags, tape, and an extraction collar until a spinal injury bed, such as a Roto-Rest bed, becomes available. As is the case with any distractive cervical injury, cranial tong traction has little role in reduction and is potentially harmful (73). If tongs are applied, less than 5 pounds of traction weight should be utilized. Children should have a blanket placed behind the thorax or be placed on a pediatric board to avoid hyperflexion (74). Passive reduction of distractive craniocervical injuries has been observed with a Trendelenburg inclination of the patient's bed, with the patient's head secured by sandbags. Elevation of the head of the bed may lead to worsening of a distractive displacement due to a downward slide of the patient's body (73). Further neuroimaging studies, such as high-resolution CT scanning with reformation or magnetic resonance imaging, should be obtained expediently. This allows for early injury severity assessment and limits potentially precarious patient transfers later on. Repeat lateral radiographs should be checked at intervals to assess for secondary loss of reduction (54).

Due to the evident limitations of both aforementioned immobilization strategies, patients with Stage III dissociative lesions should be considered for early surgical care, if clinically appropriate (Fig. 43.6). Patients with Stage II displacement can usually be maintained reduced in a halo vest at bed rest under full spine precautions until a definitive care plan has been established. To provide long-term stability and to prevent a catastrophic event, a posterior occipitocervical arthrodesis under utilization of rigid instrumentation should be performed in the majority of patients with Stage II injuries. Although substantial cervical motion is sacrificed, an aggressive surgical approach is warranted, considering the potential adverse neurologic consequences.

There are case reports of patients successfully treated for atlantooccipital dissociation in a halo vest without surgery (75). For pediatric patients younger than 2 years, nonoperative management of craniocervical dissociation with closed reduction and recumbent immobilization in a halo vest for 8 weeks followed by 8 weeks of outpatient halo vest management can result in successful restoration of atlantooccipital stability, but may not achieve atlantoaxial translational stability (56,71).

Surgical Treatment

Ideally, the patient is brought to the operating room in a reduced position, immobilized in a halo vest. The patient is then positioned supine on a spinal operating table with turning mechanism, such as the OSI-Jackson table. An awake nasotracheal intubation, aided by fiberoptic endoscopy, is performed. Following intubation, a repeat neurologic check is performed. If available, baseline somatosensory evoked potentials (SSEP) are recorded (32). Control of the patient's head is gained by means of a rigid coupling device to the halo ring or by a triple cranial tong, such as the Mayfield device. With the patient's head thus secured to the operating table, the patient is turned prone while awake and a repeat neurologic exam is performed prior to induction of definitive anesthesia. An image intensifier is then used to recheck spinal alignment and fine-tune craniocervical alignment. Repeat SSEPs are elicited after conclusion of postural manipulation.

Wackenheim's line, with the clivus ridge pointing to the tip of the odontoid, is a simple and reproducible reference line to establish satisfactory reduction (39). Due to the significant contribution of the upper cervical spine motion unit to the overall cervical spine motion, care should also be taken to instrument this region in a neutral craniocervical angle (76). In adults, the most common malalignment consists of a flexed craniocervical position, presumably in order to facilitate exposure (77). This will lead to a compensatory forced hyperextension position of the lower cervical spine and, in turn, may lead to secondary neck pain. In contrast, we have observed secondary neurologic deterioration in a patient instrumented in craniocervical hyperextension. The patient returned to baseline neurologic function after hardware revision. Secondary occipitocervical hyperlordosis due to persistent anterior skeletal growth has also been observed following uninstrumented posterior arthrodesis of the craniocervical junction in pediatric patients (76,78).

Historically, many techniques of occipitocervical arthrodesis have been developed for nontraumatic conditions.

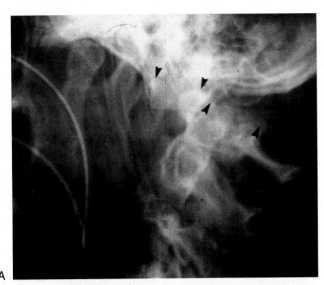

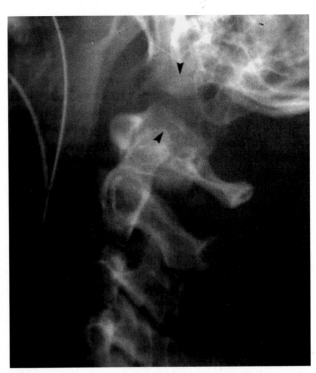

FIG. 43.6. Instability of Stage III atlantoaxial dissociation (AOD) with nonoperable treatment. This patient with a Stage III AOD initially presented with anterior translocation and pentaplegia (high tetraplegia with loss of volitional respiratory impulse), following a pedestrian versus car injury. The injury was missed in initial screening radiographs **(A)**. **B:** The inability to maintain stable reduction with a halo frame. Despite several attempts at maintaining a closed reduction with a halo vest under fluoroscopy, the best reduction result left the patient significantly distracted. The patient was treated with emergent surgical intervention consisting of open reduction and internal fixation. The patient experienced a remarkable recovery over several months following surgery. These image sequences also demonstrate the futility of a directional classification system of atlantooccipital injuries, as suggested by Traynelis. Basically, the head of a patient with a Stage III injury can be placed into any arbitrary position relative to the cervical spine.

Although onlay bone grafts with postoperative halo vest may be appropriate for very young children (5,67, 78–80), the inherent instability of a disrupted craniocervical junction necessitates more rigid fixation strategies and decreases reliance on external immobilization devices such as a halo vest (81). Nonrigid instrumentation techniques, such as precontoured rods affixed to the spine with sublaminar wires and to the occiput with intracranial wire, as suggested by Itoh (82) and Ransford (83) and their respective colleagues, are not routinely recommended, since they offer no discernible advantages over commercially available systems offering rigid segmental fixation.

Roy-Camille (84), Smith (85), and Grob (86,87) and their associates have reported successful utilization of occipital cervical plates. Fixation to the occiput is achieved with bicortical 3.2- or 3.5-mm cortical screws (88). At C2, screws are placed in the pedicles or across the C1-C2 facets utilizing the Magerl technique (86,89). The advantages of the more rigid techniques include maintenance of reduc-

tion, less postoperative bracing, and higher fusion success. More recently, combinations of cervical rod and plating systems have been introduced (89–91) (Fig. 43.7). These systems offer greater flexibility of cervical screw placement and a rigid locking screw–rod interface. As is the case in sublaminar wire placement, disadvantages of screw-based designs are the potential for damage to neural and vascular structures during drilling or screw placement.

Advances in implant design should not obscure the continued importance of achieving a sound arthrodesis by means of a sound bone grafting technique. The technique described by Wertheim and Bohlman (92) using structural autologous iliac crest bone graft affixed to the occiput and cervical spine with cable fixation continues to be the standard for craniocervical arthrodesis. Unless rigid instrumentation techniques are utilized, the patient should be maintained in a halo vest for about 12 weeks. Halo vests continue to be an important adjunctive treatment for patients with metabolically impaired bone structure as well.

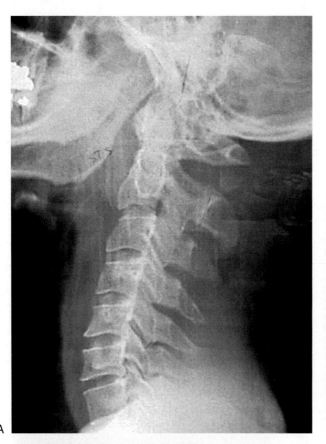

A

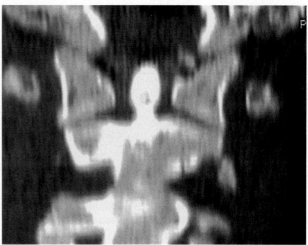

B

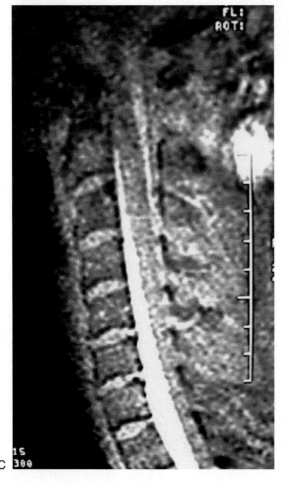

C

FIG. 43.7. Surgical treatment of Stage II atlantoaxial dissociation (AOD). **A:** This 43-year-old man was emergently intubated after a high-speed motor vehicle crash. On arrival the patient was found to be unexaminable due to his head injury. Increased prevertebral soft tissue swelling in the upper cervical spine region led to further radiographic workup of the craniocervical region. **B:** Spiral computed tomography confirmed presence of a Type III occipital condyle avulsion and a 4-mm widening of the atlanto-occipital contralateral articulation. **C:** On magnetic resonance imaging scan, nonspecific findings of soft tissue swelling and bleeding in the posterior atlantoaxial region were identified. **D** and **E:** In order to ascertain craniocervical stability, cervical traction testing under fluoroscopy was performed. The nontraction basion–dens interval (BDI) was 12 mm **(D)**, which increased to 22 mm with 5 pounds of traction **(E)**. Due to absence of any discernible resistive craniocervical ligamentous restraint, the traction test was discontinued at that weight. This test demonstrated an occult Stage II AOD, which if left untreated may result in catastrophic complications. **F** and **G:** Following resuscitation, rigid occipitocervical arthrodesis with a rod-plate instrumentation was performed on postinjury day 3. **F** shows completed rod-plate implantation and cables prepared for implantation of a structural cranioaxial bone graft. The structural femoral allograft is shown locked down with cables in **G. H** and **I:** Flexion-extension radiographs obtained at 6 months' follow-up show solid fusion with satisfactory clinical outcome.

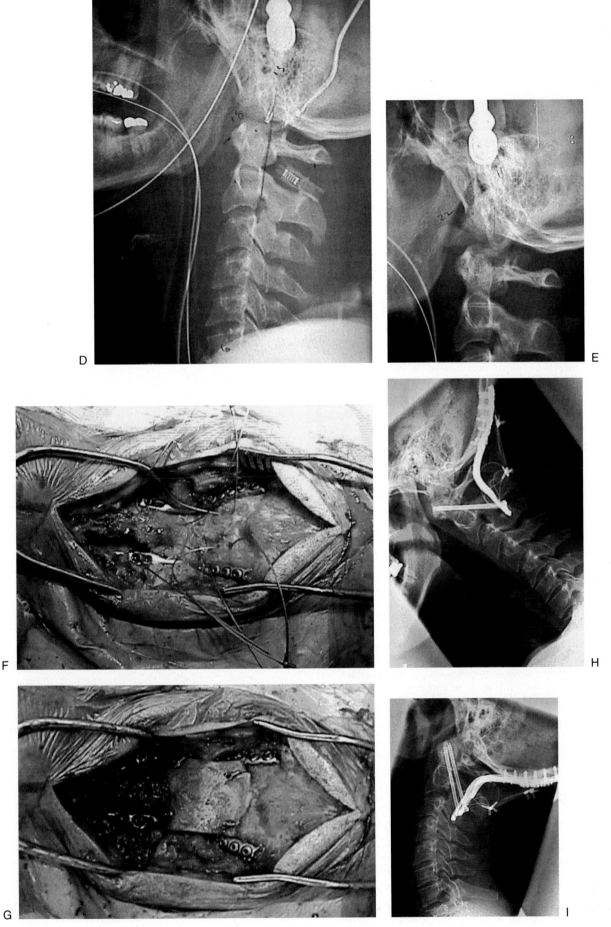

FIG. 43.7. *Continued*

SURGICAL TECHNIQUES OF OCCIPITOCERVICAL FUSION

Because the upper cervical spine forms an integrated motion unit, craniocervical disruption should be treated with an arthrodesis from the occiput to the axis or below. Attempts at limiting an arthrodesis under these circumstances from the occiput to the atlas with techniques such as a transarticular atlantooccipital arthrodesis ignore the likelihood of concurrent atlantoaxial instability and are therefore usually undesirable (86). Conventional occipitocervical arthrodesis techniques, as described by Cone and modified by Bohlman, utilize corticocancellous plates of autogenous iliac grafts affixed with 18- to 20-gauge wires or titanium cables (73, 77,92). The wires or cables are passed through holes drilled into the occiput, through the spinous process of C2, and sublaminarly at C1 (Fig. 43.7F,G). These techniques can be used independently or in conjunction with instrumentation. If performed as a stand-alone procedure, supplemental postoperative halo vest immobilization is required.

Alternative sources of bone graft material have been suggested. Morcellized cancellous iliac crest autograft has been used in conjunction with rigid internal fixation. Various corticocancellous allografts have been recommended as well, but results of long-term follow-up are pending (55). Autologous split-thickness calvarial bone has been suggested for occipitocervical arthrodeses in patients with rheumatoid instability. Limitations of this technique are the limited quantity of structural bone graft obtainable—especially if a C1 laminectomy has to be bridged—and the possibility of compromised screw purchase around the donor site (93).

Bohlman Wire Technique

A midline incision is used, extending from the external occipital protuberance to the spinous process of C2. Wide subperiosteal dissection of the occiput, C1, and C2 is performed. Two parallel 4 × 8-mm troughs are made using an air drill, separated by about 5 to 6 mm of bone located about 2 to 3 centimeters from the foramen magnum. A tunnel is created under the isthmus with angled curettes. A 20-gauge wire is double looped around this bone. Additional wires are looped around the lamina of C1 and through the spinous process of C2. Two corticocancellous bone plates 4 to 5 cm long and approximately 1 cm thick are harvested. The occiput, the lamina of C1, and C2 are decorticated with an air drill. The wires are passed through drill holes placed in the grafts and the wires are tightened. Postoperatively, patients are immobilized in a halo vest for 12 weeks (92).

Posterior Occipitocervical Arthrodesis with Plate or Rod Fixation

The surgeon should be familiar with posterior segmental instrumentation to the cervical spine. Preoperatively, the C2 segment should be closely inspected on CT for ab-normal medial vertebral foramen location, since this may preclude safe posterior screw placement. The patient is positioned and exposure is obtained as described earlier. We recommend performing this procedure under C-arm guidance. The medial edge of the C2 pedicle and the C1-C2 facet joint is exposed by subperiosteal dissection. Identifying the medial edge of the C2 pedicle facilitates safe screw placement. The starting point for screw insertion is 3 to 5 mm above the center of the C2-C3 facet articulation. The screw direction is 20 to 30 degrees cranial and 15 to 20 degrees medial. Using an adjustable drill guide, a 2-mm hole is progressively drilled into the C2 pedicle to a depth of 20 to 22 mm (89,91). If the ring of C1 is intact, this segment can be instrumented with sublaminar wires, which can be passed through a hole in the plate later. Alternatively, C1-C2 screw fixation can be obtained using a C1-C2 transarticular trajectory through which a plate can be affixed. A malleable template is bent to shape and used to determine plate length and contour. This step is crucial in determining the craniocervical angle. Care is taken to place the plate bend above the designated C2 screw hole. If this distance is excessively long, the cranium can be distracted as the plate is seated.

Following plate contouring, the plate is affixed to C2 with a 20- to 24-mm length of 3.5-mm screw. Alternatively, a transarticular screw of 3.5 or 4.0 mm can be placed through the plate hole. If satisfactory bilateral transarticular screw purchase is accomplished, there is no need for further caudal extension of the instrumentation (Fig. 43.7H,I). Should, however, C2 fixation consist of pedicle screw fixation, the instrumentation and arthrodesis is preferably extended to include the C3 segment (55). Bicortical drill holes are placed in the occiput using an adjustable drill guide. The usual occipital screw length is 10 to 12 mm, although if the plates are placed laterally the screw length will be progressively shorter (88). The holes are tapped with a 3.5-mm cortical tap, and two to four screws are placed on each side. Occipital fixation should not extend to the level of the transverse sinus, which extends in perpendicular fashion to the left and right from the inion (88). If wires were passed around the C1 lamina, these can then be tightened over the plate, assuming they are made of similar substances (e.g., titanium, C titanium, or standard steel/stainless steel) (Fig. 43.8). Recently, rod systems have been introduced that allow for adjustable attachment of screws to rods with clamps (90,91). Following decortication of the arthrodesis bed, corticocancellous bone grafts are secured to the occiput and C2 as described previously. Postoperatively, patients are immobilized in a hard collar for 8 to 12 weeks.

Treatment Alternatives

Occipitocervical fixation techniques have been expanded with the emergence of instrumentation of the lateral masses of the atlas with screws and the description of transarticular atlantooccipital screw fixation. The latter technique is

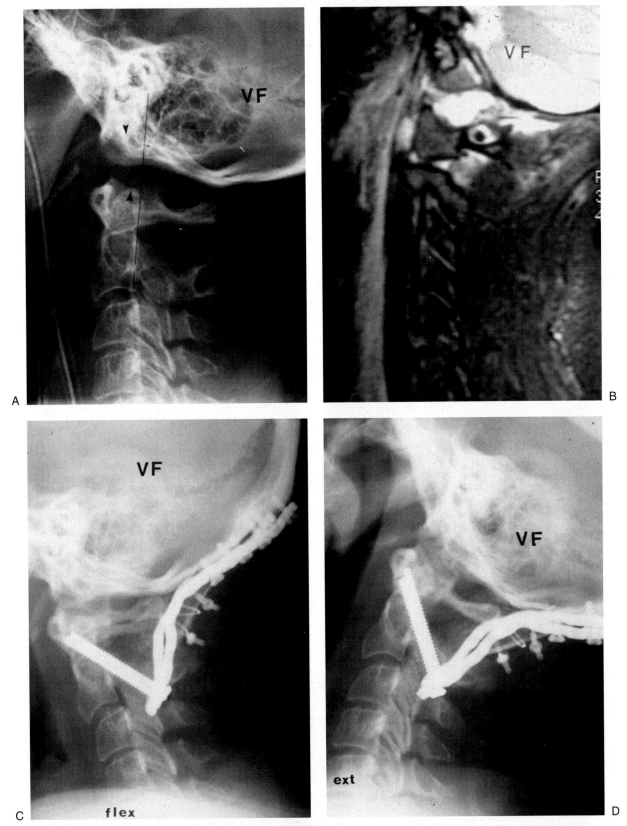

FIG. 43.8. Surgical treatment of Stage III injury. This 54-year-old woman presented after a high-speed motor vehicle crash with pentaplegia. She had received emergent on-scene endotracheal intubation and ventilatory support after having been ejected from her vehicle following a high-speed car crash. **A:** A Stage III distractive atlantooccipital dissociation. **B:** A postreduction magnetic resonance imaging scan showed persistent distraction of the occipitocervical articulation despite attempts at closed reduction with a halo vest. **C:** Open reduction and internal fixation with plates and iliac crest bone graft was performed on a delayed basis on postinjury day 3 due to severe accompanying head injury. **D:** The patient experienced a solid craniocervical fusion with incomplete neurologic recovery.

based on a single patient case report, but generated significant interest (86). This technique presently does not seem appropriate for patients with unstable and displaced craniocervical articulations, but identifies an interesting approach for further study. Moreover, an isolated atlantooccipital arthrodesis in a patient with AOD does not address the con-

currently destabilized atlantoaxial articulation. Screw fixation in the lateral masses of the atlas has been introduced by Harms (91). To date there are no clinical comparison studies of this technique and transarticular screws. Further biomechanical and clinical studies are necessary prior to recommending this technique (Fig. 43.9).

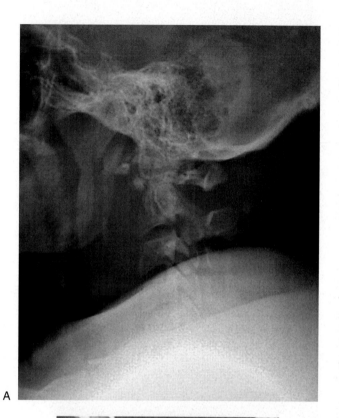

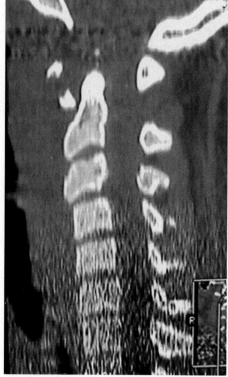

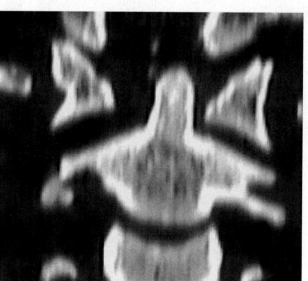

FIG. 43.9. Treatment of atlantoaxial dissociation. **A:** Following a high-speed motor vehicle crash, this 17-year-old morbidly obese girl complained of neck pain and unilateral shoulder weakness. The screening lateral cervical spine radiograph was interpreted to demonstrate prevertebral swelling and a fracture of the atlas. The upper extremity weakness was attributed to a presumed brachial plexopathy secondary to a clavicle fracture. **B** and **C:** Sagittal and coronal computed tomography (CT) reformats confirmed presence of an atlantoaxial dissociation, a variant of AOD. The basion–dens interval as measured on the sagittal reconstruction CT scan was 20 mm (12 mm maximum) with a 7 mm diastasis of the right atlantoaxial articulation (normal maximum 3 mm). **D** and **E:** The patient deteriorated neurologically over the next 24 hours to an American Spinal Injury Association (ASIA) classification B, C3-level incomplete spinal cord injury despite halo immobilization. The magnetic resonance images delineate ligament injury and cord signal changes on the T2-weighted images. In retrospect, the patient had a delayed diagnosis of an incomplete spinal cord injury as described by Wallenberg as a subtype of a cervicomedullary syndrome. **F** and **G:** Due to her fulminant neurologic deterioration, the patient was treated with emergent C1 laminectomy, open reduction of her atlantoaxial dissociation, and occipitocervical fusion with rod-plates and transarticular screws. Fortunately, the patient improved dramatically within days of the surgery and recovered near normal neurologic function (ASIA E) by her 6-month follow-up.

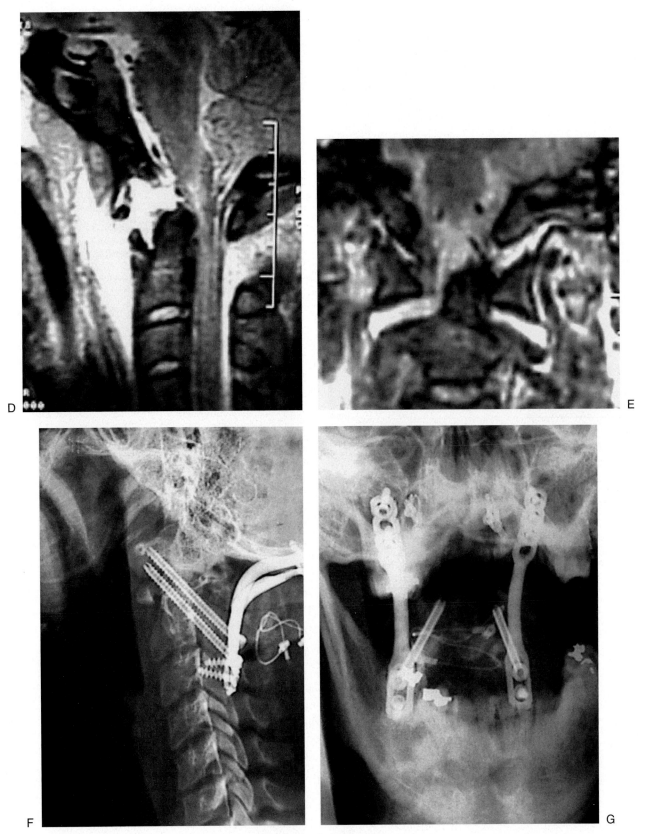

FIG. 43.9. *Continued*

CONCLUSIONS

Occipitocervical injuries are usually highly unstable and frequently result in neurologic injury or death (13). Delays in diagnosis are frequent due to unfamiliarity with the injury entity and difficulty in visualization on plain radiographs. Implementation of a diagnostic algorithm consisting of screening parameters gathered from plain radiographs as well as routine CT scans in high-risk patients should diminish the occurrence of missed injuries. Magnetic resonance imaging and occasional functional assessment tests are important adjuvant diagnostic resources in the management of craniocervical injuries. In cases of ligamentous disruption of the key ligaments of the occipitocervical junction, such as the alar ligaments and tectorial membrane, early instrumented posterior occipitocervical arthrodesis is warranted. Incomplete ligamentous injuries and stable occipital condyle fractures can be treated with external immobilization. In light of technological advances in diagnostic and implant modalities, the main focus should now shift to more timely diagnosis through educational efforts.

REFERENCES

1. Ward WG, Nunley JA. Occult orthopaedic trauma in the multiply injured patient. *J Orthop Trauma* 1991;5:308–312.
2. Anderson PA, Montesano PX. Morphology and treatment of occipital condyle fractures. *Spine* 1988;13:731–736.
3. Pfirrmann CW, Binkert CA, Zanetti M, et al. MR morphology of alar ligaments and occipitoatlantoaxial joints: study in 50 asymptomatic subjects. *Radiology* 2001;218:133–137.
4. Avellino AM, Mann FA, Grady MS, et al. Why acute cervical spine injuries are "missed" in infants and children: 12-year experience from a level 1 pediatric and adult trauma center. In: *Topics Spinal Cord Inj Rehabil* 2000;6(Suppl):203.
5. Gilles FH, Bina M, Sotrel A. Infantile atlantooccipital instability. *Am J Dis Child* 1979;133:30–37.
6. Dvorak J, Schneider E, Saldinger P, et al. Biomechanics of the craniocervical region: the alar and transverse ligaments. *J Orthop Res* 1988;6:452–461.
7. Panjabi MM, Oxland TR, Parks EH. Quantitative anatomy of cervical spine ligaments. Part I. Upper cervical spine. *J Spinal Disord* 1991;4:270–276.
8. Werne S. Studies in spontaneous atlas dislocation. *Acta Orthop Scand Suppl* 1957;32:1–150.
9. Dvorak J, Panjabi MM. Functional anatomy of the alar ligaments. *Spine* 1987;12:183–189.
10. Panjabi M, Dvorak J, Crisco JJ, et al. Effects of alar ligament transection on upper cervical spine rotation. *J Orthop Res* 1991;9:584–593.
11. Crisco JJ, Panjabi MM, Dvorak J. A model of the alar ligaments of the upper cervical spine in axial rotation. *J Biomech* 1991;24:607–614.
12. Bucholz RW, Burkhead WZ. The pathological anatomy of fatal atlanto-occipital dislocations. *J Bone Joint Surg Am* 1979;61:248–250.
13. Davis D, Bohlman HH, Walker AE, et al. The pathological findings in fatal craniospinal injuries. *J Neurosurg* 1971;34:603–613.
14. Jónsson H Jr, Bring G, Rauschning W, et al. Hidden cervical spine injuries in traffic accident victims with skull fractures. *J Spinal Disord* 1991;4:251–263.
15. Grabb BC, Frye TA, Hedlund GL, et al. MRI diagnosis of suspected atlanto-occipital dissociation in childhood. *Pediatr Radiol* 1999;29:275–281.
16. Houle P, McDonnell DE, Vender J. Traumatic atlanto-occipital dislocation in children. *Pediatr Neurosurg* 2001;34:193–197.
17. Kaufman RA, Carroll CD, Buncher CR. Atlantooccipital junction: standards for measurement in normal children. *AJNR Am J Neuroradiol* 1987;8:995–999.
18. Sun PP, Poffenbarger GJ, Durham S, et al. Spectrum of occipito-atlantoaxial injury in young children. *J Neurosurg* 2000;93(Suppl 1):28–39.
19. Alker GJ, Oh YS, Leslie EV, et al. Postmortem radiology of head neck injuries in fatal traffic accidents. *Radiology* 1975;114:611–617.
20. James R, Nasmyth-Jones R. The occurrence of cervical fractures in victims of judicial hanging. *Forensic Sci Int* 1992;54:81–91.
21. Wood-Jones F. The ideal lesion produced by judicial hanging. *Lancet* 1913;23:53.
22. Anderson PA. Occipital cervical instability associated with traumatic tears of the transverse ligament. *Orthop Trans* 1988;12:41.
23. Dickman CA, Papadopoulos SM, Sonntag VK, et al. Traumatic occipitoatlantal dislocation. *J Spinal Disord* 1993;6:300–313.
24. Stroobants J, Fidlers L, Storms JL, et al. High cervical pain and impairment of skull mobility as the only symptoms of an occipital condyle fracture. Case report. *J Neurosurg* 1994;81:137–138.
25. American Spinal Injury Association. *International standards for neurological and functional classification of spinal cord injury*. Chicago, IL: American Spinal Injury Association, 1996.
26. Bell HS. Paralysis of both arms from the injury of the upper portion of the pyramidal decussation: "cruciate paralysis." *J Neurosurg* 1970;33:376–380.
27. Brodke DS, Dailey AT. Upper cervical spine fractures in patients with spinal cord injury. *Spine* 1999;13:70–83.
28. Dickman CA, Hadley MN, Pappas CT, et al. Cruciate paralysis: a clinical and radiographic analysis of injuries to the cervicomedullary junction. *J Neurosurg* 1990;73:850–858.
29. Schliack H, Schaefer P. Hypoglossal and accessory nerve paralysis in a fracture of the occipital condyle. *Nervenarzt* 1965;36:362–364.
30. Traynelis VC, Marano GD, Dunker RO, et al. Traumatic atlanto-occipital dislocation: case report. *J Neurosurg* 1988;65:863–870.
31. Fujimura Y, Nishi Y, Chiba K, et al. Prognosis of neurologic deficits associated with upper cervical spine injuries. *Paraplegia* 1995;33:195–202.
32. Lam AM. Acute spinal cord ischemia: implications for anesthetic management. *Adv Anesth* 1993;10:247–273.
33. Harris, MB, Kronlage SC, Carboni PA, et al. Evaluation of the cervical spine in the polytrauma patient. *Spine* 2000;25:2884–2891.
34. Wholey MH, Bruwer AJ, Hillier LB. The lateral roentgenogram of the neck (with comments on the atlanto-odontoid-basion relationship). *Radiology* 1958;71:350–356.
35. Deliganis AV, Mann FA, Grady MS. Rapid diagnosis and treatment of a traumatic atlantooccipital dissociation. *AJR Am J Roentgenol* 1998;171:986.
36. Monu J, Bohrer SP, Howard G. Some upper cervical spine norms. *Spine* 1987;12:515–519.
37. Ahuja A, Glasauer FE, Alker GJ Jr, et al. Radiology in survivors of traumatic atlantooccipital dislocation. *Surg Neurol* 1994;41:112–118.
38. De Beer JDV, Thomas M, Walters J, et al. Traumatic atlanto-axial subluxation. *J Bone Joint Surg Br* 1998;70:652–655.
39. Wackenheim A. *Roentgen diagnosis of the craniovertebral region*. Berlin: Springer-Verlag, 1974.
40. Harris JH Jr, Carson GC, Wagner LK, et al. Radiologic diagnosis of traumatic occipitovertebral dissociation. 2. Comparison of three methods of detecting occipitovertebral relationships on lateral radiographs of supine subjects. *AJR Am J Roentgenol* 1994;162:887–892.
41. Lee C, Woodring JH, Goldstein SJ, et al. Evaluation of traumatic atlantooccipital dislocations. *AJNR Am J Neuroradiol* 1987;8:19–26.
42. Powers B, Miller MD, Kramer RS, et al. Traumatic anterior atlanto-occipital dislocation. *Neurosurgery* 1979;4:12–17.
43. Weiner BK, Brower RS. Traumatic vertical atlantoaxial instability in a case of atlanto-occipital coalition. *Spine* 1997;22:1033–1035.
44. Harris JH, Carson GC, Wagner LK. Radiologic diagnosis of traumatic occipitovertebral dissociation. 1. Normal occipitovertebral relationships on lateral radiographs of supine subjects. *AJR Am J Roentgenol* 1994;162:881–886.
45. Blackmore CC, Ramsey SD, Mann FA, et al. Cervical spine screening with CT in trauma patients: a cost effectiveness analysis. *Radiology* 1999;212:117–125.
46. Calvy TM, Segall HD, Gilles FH, et al. CT anatomy of the craniovertebral junction in infants and children. *AJNR Am J Neuroradiol* 1987;8:489–494.
47. Kirshenbaum KJ, Nadimpalli SR, Fantus R, et al. Unsuspected upper cervical spine fractures associated with significant head trauma: role of CT. *J Emerg Med* 1990;8:183–198.

48. Gerlock AJ, Mirfakhrace M, Benzel EC. Computed tomography of traumatic atlanto-occipital dislocation. *Neurosurgery* 1983;13:316–319.

49. Przybylski GJ, Clyde BL, Fitz CR. Craniocervical junction subarachnoid hemorrhage associated with atlanto-occipital dislocation. *Spine* 1996;21:1761–1768.

50. Wasserberg J, Bartlett RJ. Occipital condyle fractures diagnosed by high-definition CT and coronal reconstructions. *Neuroradiology* 1995;37(5):370–373.

51. Bloom AI, Neeman Z, Floman Y, et al. Occipital condyle fracture and ligament injury: imaging by CT. *Pediatr Radiol* 1996;26:786–790.

52. Bundschuh CV, Alley JB, Ross M, et al. Magnetic resonance imaging of suspected atlantooccipital dislocation. Two case reports. *Spine* 1992;17:245–248.

53. Davis JW, Parks SN, Detlefs CL, et al. Clearing the cervical spine in obtunded patients: the use of dynamic fluoroscopy. *J Trauma* 1995; 39:435–438.

54. White AA, Panjabi MM. Kinematics of the spine. In: *Clinical biomechanics of the spine,* 2nd ed. Philadelphia: JB Lippincott, 1990:92–97.

55. Chapman JR, Bellabarba C, Newell DW, et al. Craniocervical injuries: atlantooccipital dissociation and occipital condyle fractures. *Semin Spine Surg* 2001;13:90–105.

56. Ghatan S, Newell DW, Grady MS, et al. Traumatic craniocervical instability in the very young: a report of three survivors, their radiological diagnoses, and non-operative management. *J Neurosurg* (in press).

57. Bell C. Surgical observations. *Middlessex Hosp J* 1817;4:469.

58. Clayman D, Sykes C, Vines F. Occipital condyle fractures: clinical presentations and radiologic detection. *Am J Neuroradiol* 1994;15: 1309–1315.

59. Saternus KS. Bruchformen des condylus occipitalis. *Z Rechtsmed* 1987;99:95–108.

60. Lipscomb PR. Cervico-occipital fusion for congenital and post traumatic anomalies of the atlas and axis. *J Bone Joint Surg Am* 1957;39: 1289.

61. Levine AM, Edwards CC. Traumatic lesions of the occipitoatlantoaxial complex. *Clin Orthop* 1989;239:53–68.

62. Matava M, Whitesides T, Davis P. Traumatic atlanto-occipital dislocation with survival. *Spine* 1993;18:1897–1903.

63. Dibenedetto T, Lee CK. Traumatic atlanto-occipital instability: a case report with follow-up and a new diagnostic technique. *Spine* 1990;15: 595–597.

64. Eismont FJ, Bohlman HH. Posterior atlanto-occipital dislocation with fractures of the atlas and odontoid process: report of a case with survival. *J Bone Joint Surg Am* 1978;60:397–399.

65. Montane I, Eismont FJ, Green BA. Traumatic occipitoatlantal dislocation. *Spine* 1991;16:112–116.

66. Birney TJ, Hanley EN Jr. Traumatic cervical spine injuries in childhood and adolescence. *Spine* 1989;14:1277–1282.

67. Eleraky JA, Theodore N, Adams M, et al. Pediatric cervical spine injuries: report of 102 cases and review of the literature. *J Neurosurg (Spine 1)* 2000;92:12–17.

68. Shamoun JM, Riddick L, Powell RW. Atlanto-occipital subluxation/dislocation: a "survivable" injury in children. *Am Surg* 1999;65:317–320.

69. Dublin AB, Marks WM, Weinstock D, et al. Traumatic dislocation of the atlanto-occipital articulation (AOA) with short-term survival: with a radiographic method of measuring the AOA. *J Neurosurg* 1980; 52:541–546.

70. Van Den Bout AH, Commisse GF. Traumatic atlanto-occipital dislocation. *Spine* 1986;11:174–176.

71. Floman Y, Kaplan L, Elidan J, et al. Transverse ligament rupture and atlanto-axial subluxation in children. *J Bone Joint Surg Br* 1991;73: 640–643.

72. Chapman JR, Mirza. Upper cervical spine injuries. In: Rockwood CA Jr, Green DP, Bucholz RW, et al., eds. *Rockwood and Green's fractures in adults,* 4th ed. Philadelphia: Lippincott–Raven Publishers, 1996.

73. Cone W, Nicholson JT. The treatment of fracture dislocations of the cervical vertebra by skeletal traction and fusion. *J Bone Joint Surg Am* 1937;19:584.

74. Herzenberg JE, Hensinger RN, Dedrick DK, et al. Emergency transport and positioning of young children who have an injury of the cervical spine; the standard backboard may be hazardous. *J Bone Joint Surg Am* 1989;71:15–22.

75. Page CP, Story JL, Wissinger JP, et al. Traumatic atlanto-occipital dislocation. Case report. *J Neurosurg* 1973;39:394–397.

76. Rodgers W, Coran D, Kharrazi F, et al. Increasing lordosis of the occipitocervical junction after arthrodesis in young children: the occipitocervical crankshaft phenomenon. *J Pediatr Orthop* 1997;17: 762–765.

77. Newman P, Sweetnam R. Occipito-cervical fusion. *J Bone Joint Surg Br* 1969;51:423–431.

78. Nakagawa T, Kazunori Y, Sakou T, et al. Occipitocervical fusion with C1 laminectomy in children. *Spine* 1997;22:1209–1214.

79. Jevtich V. Traumatic lateral atlanto-occipital dislocation with spontaneous bony fusion: a case report. *Spine* 1989;14:123–127.

80. Schultz KD, Petronio J, Haid RW, et al. Pediatric occipitocervical arthrodesis. *Pediatr Neurosurg* 2000;33:169–181.

81. Anderson PA, Budorick TE, Easton KB, et al. Failure of halo vest to prevent *in vivo* motion in patients with injured cervical spines. *Spine* 1991;16(Suppl 10):S501–505.

82. Itoh T, Tsuji H, Katoh Y, et al. Occipito-cervical fusion reinforced by Luque's segmental spinal instrumentation for rheumatoid diseases. *Spine* 1988;13:1234–1238.

83. Ransford AO, Crockard HA, Pozo JL, et al. Craniocervical instability treated by contoured loop fixation. *J Bone Joint Surg Br* 1986;68: 173–177.

84. Roy-Camille R, Saillant G, Mazel C. Internal fixation of the unstable cervical spine by a posterior osteosynthesis with plates and screws. In: Cervical Spine Research Society, eds. *The cervical spine,* 2nd ed. Philadelphia: JB Lippincott, 1989.

85. Smith SM, Anderson PA, Grady MS. Occipitocervical arthrodesis using contoured plate fixation: an early report on a versatile fixation technique. *Spine* 1993;18:1984–1990.

86. Grob D. Transarticular screw fixation for atlanto-occipital dislocation. *Spine* 2001;26:703–707.

87. Grob D, Dvorak J, Panjabi M, et al. Posterior occipitocervical fusion: a preliminary report of a new technique. *Spine* 1991;12:S17–S24.

88. Haher TR, Yeung AW, Caruso SA, et al. Occipital screw pullout strength. A biomechanical investigation of occipital morphology. *Spine* 1999;24:5–9.

89. Jeanneret B, Magerl F. Primary posterior fusion C1-C2 in odontoid fractures: indications, techniques and results of transarticular screw fixation. *J Spine Disorders* 1992;5:464–475.

90. Abumi K, Takada T, Shono Y, et al. Posterior occipitocervical reconstruction using cervical pedicle screws and plate-rod systems. *Spine* 1999;24:1425–1434.

91. Harms J, Melcher RP. Posterior C1-2 fusion with polyaxial screw and rod fixation. *Spine* 2001;26:2467–2471.

92. Wertheim SB, Bohlman HH. Occipitocervical fusion. Indications, technique, and long-term results in thirteen patients. *J Bone Joint Surg Am* 1987;69:833–836.

93. Robertson SC, Menezes AH. Occipital calvarial bone graft in posterior occipitocervical fusion. *Spine* 1998;23:249–255.

CHAPTER 44

Transverse Ligament Injury

Amir Hasharoni and Thomas J. Errico

Ligamentous injuries to the atlantooccipital region, which range from complete atlantooccipital or atlantoaxial dislocation to an isolated transverse or alar ligament disruption, comprise a hard-to-diagnose and potentially dangerous group of injuries that are relatively rare and often overlooked in the multitrauma patient (1). Transverse ligament complex rupture is now recognized as potentially survivable, although commonly with substantial morbidity. Swift diagnosis is crucial for ensuring prompt, effective treatment and preventing delayed neurologic deficits in patients who survive these injuries.

ANATOMY

The transverse atlantal ligament (TAL) is about 2 to 3 mm thick in its medial portion (2,3). The TAL is separated from the posterior plane of the tectorial membrane by fatty tissues and from the posterior aspect of the odontoid by the cavity of the syndesmoaxoidal joint that lies between the anterior facet of the TAL and the posterior surface of the odontoid process (4–6) (Fig. 44.1).

The TAL is a part of the cruciform ligament, which itself represents only the middle of three layers of the posterior occipitoatlantoaxial ligament complex. The most posterior portion of the cruciform ligament attaches to the anterior edge of the foramen magnum. The descending portion attaches to the body of C2. The most anterior layer of the complex consists of the apical and alar ligaments, which are paired structures attaching to the posterolateral surfaces of the tip of the odontoid and then running obliquely to the medial aspects of the occipital condyles. The apical ligaments connect the tip of the odontoid to the anterior edge of the foramen magnum.

The C1 ring has an anterior–posterior diameter of approximately 3 cm and can be divided according to Steel into thirds, each with separate anatomic components (7). The spinal cord and odontoid process each occupy 1 cm, and the remaining third is "free space" that allows for some anterior displacement without compromising the spinal cord. The spinal cord is not usually endangered unless subluxation exceeds 1 cm. The danger is diminished if the odontoid process is fractured and moves forward with the anterior arch of C1. A hypoplastic or absent odontoid, such as in os odontoideum or in some congenital anomalies, also diminishes the risk of cord compression, presumably because of less space being occupied by rigid structures adjacent to the spinal cord (8).

BIOMECHANICS

The anterior stability of the first cervical vertebra relative to the second is maintained primarily by the transverse and alar ligament complex. The transverse ligament restricts flexion as well as anterior displacement of the atlas, whereas the alar ligaments restrain rotation of the upper cervical spine. A lesion in one or both structures can produce instability that may lead to damage to the neural structures and cause pain.

An intact TAL allows a maximum of 3 mm anterior translation of C1 on C2. Within a range of 3 to 5 mm of anterior translation, failure of the TAL usually occurs. Failure of the TAL is usually a sudden phenomenon at the locus minoris of the TAL, which is the midsubstance. Progressive and slow failure may occur, as well as ligament–bone junction failure, but less often (9).

Jackson (10) used flexion and extension radiographs to study the cervical spine of asymptomatic children and adults. In normal patients, the maximum anterior translation of C1 on C2 was 4 mm in children and 2.5 mm in adults, which correlates well with experimental and clinical data presented by Fielding and others (9,11).

Dickman and associates (12) classified injuries of the transverse ligament as either midsubstance tears (type I) or avulsions at the osseous insertions of the transverse liga-

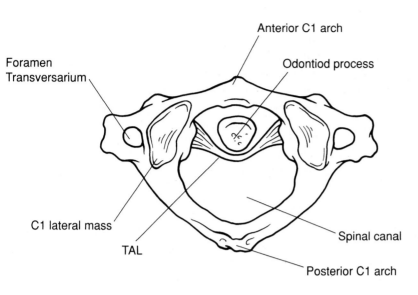

FIG. 44.1. Axial view of the normal C1 vertebra. Both the C1 ring and the transverse ligament are intact.

ment to the lateral masses of C1 (type II). The two types of transverse ligament derangement are usually caused by different injury patterns. Comminuted, or displaced, C1 burst fracture (Jefferson-type fracture) with displacement of the lateral masses of C1 relative to the superior articulating facets of C2 produces disruption of the transverse ligament at its attachments (13), whereas flexion-extension injury tends to produce midsubstance tears (14). The outcome of both injury patterns is the same: C1-C2 instability. According to Dickman and colleagues (12), the healing potential of a midsubstance tear is markedly less than that of the osseous insertion avulsion type of injury.

Transverse ligament disruption without fracture occurs in the elderly and results from a fall with a blow to the occiput. Rupture of the transverse ligaments may occur at the midpoint or may be associated with an avulsion fracture from the lateral mass on either side of the odontoid. These variants are functionally identical clinically, but require different treatment approaches (15,16).

The breaking strength of the transverse ligament complex was found by Dvorak and associates (17), in a mechanical and histologic study of the upper cervical spine, to be 200 N for the alar ligaments and 350 N for the transverse ligaments. Histologic analysis revealed a mainly collagenous nature of these ligaments. The average force required to experimentally rupture the transverse ligament is 84 kg. The remaining ligaments rupture secondarily when the same amount of force is applied (15,18).

The fact that in the clinical setting odontoid fractures often occur, but TAL ruptures rarely occur, suggests that the transverse ligament is strong enough to withstand physiologic loads. The alar ligaments, on the other hand, due to their lower strength and axial direction of loading, might be prone to injury and therefore require stabilization of the occiput-C1-C2 segment more often than normally is assumed (15,17,18). A less severe injury is seen when an isolated rupture of one of the alar ligaments occurs. In this milder injury pattern, a rotatory hypermobility, or instability, of the upper cervical spine appears (19).

CLINICAL PRESENTATION

Traumatic Rupture of the Transverse Atlantal Ligament

Survival after acute traumatic rupture of the TAL is unusual (20–22). This injury has a high incidence of concomitant head trauma. Neurologic symptoms and signs, however, vary and may range from normal function, unilateral numbness or weakness of a single extremity, or delayed neurologic symptoms to a transient quadriparesis. Permanent quadriparesis is almost never seen, basically because at this level the degree of spinal cord injury is usually fatal. Neck muscle spasm usually causes limited range of neck motion. Other clinical signs that may arise include cardiac and respiratory abnormalities, as these control centers are located at this level of the spinal cord. Dizziness, syncope, and blurred vision may also be present, as the vertebral arteries may be injured in their tortuous course between the axis and the atlas while fixed in the foramen transversarium, with excessive C1-C2 displacement compressing these vessels.

The mechanism of injury is probably forward translation (shear) and rotation (9,23). The common mechanism is an anteriorly directed force to the back of the head, frequently with forced flexion, associated with a scalp laceration over the occiput (21,24,25). Acute traumatic rupture of the TAL also may be associated with a burst fracture of C1 (Jefferson's fracture) (26–31) (Fig. 44.2).

Chronic Stress

Congenital bony ankyloses of the cervical spine may impart chronic stresses on the TAL, leading to insufficiency.

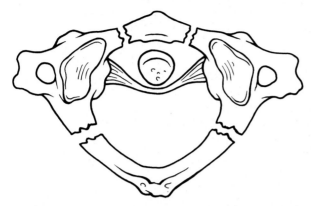

FIG. 44.2. C1 burst fracture. Spreading of the lateral masses of C1 is diagnostic of a burst fracture of the C1 ring. Rupture of the transverse ligament allows further displacement of the lateral masses. In this case the sum of $x + y$ will be greater than 7 mm.

The three most common situations are occipitalization of the atlas, ankylosing spondylitis, and Klippel-Feil syndrome.

Occipitalization or assimilation of the atlas represents partial or complete congenital ankylosis of the bony ring of the atlas to the occiput. Ankylosis usually occurs anteriorly between the anterior arch of the atlas and the rim of the foramen magnum, although posterior together with anterior ankyloses have been reported before (32). Flexion-extension movements are transferred from the occiput-C1 articulation down to the C1-C2 joint, which is not structured for such movement; therefore, laxity of the TAL develops gradually. Anterior atlantoaxial instability is associated with occipitalization of the atlas in 39% to 54% of all cases (25,28,33–42). Forty-seven percent to 68% of patients with occipitalization of the atlas suffer from concomitant congenital ankylosis of C2-C3 (36,43). This association may accelerate the appearance of symptoms and signs of spinal cord compression. About 50% of these patients will develop late-onset atlantoaxial instability and, potentially, cord compromise (44). Occipitalization of the atlas is associated with a high incidence of malpositioned or abnormally long odontoid, which may predispose to earlier compromise of the spinal cord.

Congenital Transverse Atlantal Ligament Insufficiency

Congenital, atraumatic insufficiency of the TAL, either with complete absence or ligamentous laxity, may be seen as an idiopathic insufficiency or in a number of disorders such as Down and Morquio's syndromes.

Atlantoaxial instability may appear in 20% of Down syndrome patients (45,46), due to ligamentous disruption rather than the various bony anomalies frequently seen at the occipitocervical junction in these patients (45). Although most of the patients with TAL insufficiency may be asymptomatic, some may exhibit neurologic deficits with signs of spinal cord compression, torticollis, or neck pain (47,48). Ferguson and associates (49) found no correlation

between C1-C2 subluxation in Down syndrome patients and the neurologic exam. Indications for treatment are controversial and revolve around the need for prophylactic arthrodesis (50). Prophylactic arthrodesis should be performed in those patients with anterior atlantodental interval greater than 7 mm.

Patients with Morquio's syndrome or other congenital disorders associated with anomalies in the occiput to C2 region should be investigated for the presence of TAL insufficiency and treated accordingly.

DIAGNOSIS

To date, the best diagnostic tool for evaluating the function and potency of the transverse ligament is the anterior atlantodental interval (ADI) on flexion-extension radiographs (15). In cases when the odontoid is deficient, the atlantodens interval is measured using a line projected up from the anterior body of the axis to the anterior arch of the atlas. Displacement of 3 to 5 mm in adults is evidence of damage to the transverse ligament. If the displacement exceeds 5 mm, the transverse ligament has ruptured and the alar ligaments are stretched and partially deficient. Displacement of greater than 10 mm indicates that all the ligaments have been disrupted (15).

At the initial emergency room cross-table lateral radiograph, measurement of the distance between the posterior lip of the anterior arch of the atlas to the anterior lip of the dens (ADI) and comparison with normal measurements will help detect injury. In adults, the ADI should not exceed 3 to 3.5 mm. Computed tomography (CT) with sagittal and coronal reformatted images permits optimal detection and evaluation of fracture and subluxation. CT findings that may suggest occipital-C1-C2 injury include joint incongruity, focal hematomas, vertebral artery injury, and capsular swelling. Magnetic resonance imaging (MRI) of the cervical spine with fat-suppressed gradient-echo T2-weighted or short-inversion-time inversion recovery sequences can demonstrate increased signal intensity in the craniocervical ligaments and transverse atlantal ligament (51).

When comparing the diagnostic value of CT and MRI in injuries of the cervical vertebrae, CT can pick up 100% of the fractures but only 33% of the soft tissue lesions, whereas MRI can reveal all the traumatic medullary and paravertebral soft tissue changes but only 50% of the fractures. Based on these results, after primary plain film radiographic imaging, the performance of MRI seems to be recommendable prior to CT in the diagnostic evaluation of traumatic cervical spinal lesions with soft tissue injuries in particular (52).

Gradient-echo MRI pulse sequences provide reliable visualization of the transverse ligament, which exhibits low signal intensity and extends behind the dens between the medial portions of the lateral masses of C1. Dickman and associates (53) studied the transverse ligament for the evaluation of atlantoaxial instability using MRI. The MRI characteristics of the transverse ligament were verified in clinical studies and in postmortem specimens. It is clear now that the treatment of atlantoaxial instability, which was previously based on indirect criteria drawn from CT or plain radiographic studies, can now depend on MRI, which accurately depicts the anatomical integrity of the transverse ligament and serves as a reliable indicator for early treatment (16,53).

TREATMENT

Transverse ligament injuries can be classified into ligamentous injuries (type I) that are incapable of healing without internal fixation, and osseous injuries (type II) that render the transverse ligament physiologically incompetent even though the ligament substance is not torn. These latter can be treated initially with a rigid cervical orthosis. They have a successful healing rate of 74% when treated nonoperatively (12).

Surgery should be reserved for all type I and type II patients who have nonunion with persistent instability after 3 to 4 months of immobilization. Radiographic monitoring of type II injuries is needed to detect patients who will require delayed operative intervention (12).

The purpose of any surgical construct is to reduce and prevent further anterior translation of C1 on C2 (15,54–56). The most secure C1-C2 fixation is a Magerl transarticular screw fixation augmented with a Gallie-type posterior wiring. This provides rigid atlantoaxial stabilization, which has yielded many good clinical results. However, the technique is technically demanding and poses a risk of injury to the nerves and veins around the cord, as well as potential injury to the vertebral arteries. Postoperative stability is excellent, with good stabilization against flexion, extension, lateral bending, and axial rotation (57–59).

Posteriorly, a Gallie-type of wiring, advocated by Fielding (15,54,60), consists of an autogenous bone graft secured under wires passed between the posterior arch of C1 and behind the spinous process of C2. The wire is intended to hold the graft in place, not to effect reduction of the fracture. This construct is effective in stabilizing against flexion.

Another posterior arthrodesis method is the wedge compression technique proposed by Brooks and Jenkins for posterior C1-C2 arthrodesis. This consists of iliac bone grafts compressed under laterally placed wires between the arch of the first vertebra and around the laminae of the second (61). Fixation by posterior wire and graft alone can reduce motion only moderately. To best promote fusion, posterior wire and graft fixation should be used with external immobilization (61).

An intact posterior arch of C1 is a prerequisite for successful surgical stabilization, or postoperative loss of fixation will occur. In cases with comminuted C1 (Jefferson-like) fractures, where neither Magerl screw fixation nor posterior wiring is feasible, patients should be treated in a halo for 6 weeks or until healing of the ring of the atlas can occur

before attempting to fix the C1-C2 instability (23,24). One of the pitfalls in this complex injury is failure to appreciate the transverse ligament tear accompanying the C1 ring fracture (24). The best clue to the existence of such transverse ligament injury is the lateral drift of the lateral masses of the ring of C1 in relation to the lateral masses of C2 as seen on the open-mouth view.

Patients with congenital C1-C2 instability due to TAL insufficiency, and not to aplasia or hypoplasia of the bony elements, should be treated symptomatically. Symptomatic patients with an anterior ADI of more than 5 mm or asymptomatic patients with an anterior ADI of more than 7 mm in flexion should undergo posterior C1-C2 arthrodesis. Although these recommendations are controversial, they at least address the patients with a "cord at risk."

Patients with TAL insufficiency due to congenital bony ankyloses at the occiput-C1 or C2-C3 levels should be treated according to their symptoms because this lesion develops gradually. Asymptomatic patients should have posterior C1-C2 arthrodesis if the anterior ADI is more than 7 mm in flexion. Patients with progressive pain or neurologic symptoms whose anterior ADI in flexion is more than 5 mm should undergo posterior C1-C2 arthrodesis as well. If the C1 ring is fractured or incomplete, then occipital-C2 fusion is necessary.

ATLANTOAXIAL SUBLUXATION IN CHILDREN

Transverse Ligament Disruption

The upper limit of normal C1-C2 translation in children is 4.5 mm (9). Greater values suggest attenuation, or disruption, of the transverse ligament. Only small numbers of cases of acute traumatic rupture of the TAL in children have been reported (27,62,63), with anterior ADIs in flexion ranging from 7 to 15 mm. Any anterior ADI greater than 5 mm in this situation puts the cord at risk. Although this lesion occurs rarely, the only signs and symptoms may be stiffness and pain in the neck after significant head or neck trauma, with neurologic function entirely normal. A CT scan may show a fleck of bone at one of the origins of the transverse ligament, and plain films may show minimal or no thickening of the retropharyngeal space. An active flexion view may be required to demonstrate the instability in a patient with unexplained neck pain or neurologic findings following significant neck trauma (64).

Treatment

Adults and children have different rates of ligament healing with nonoperative treatment. Adults with midsubstance tears of the TAL have low rates of healing and should undergo primary posterior C1-C2 arthrodesis if the anterior ADI is more than 5 mm in flexion. Children have slightly better rates of TAL healing than adults do. Although immediate posterior C1-C2 arthrodesis is the most reliable means of achieving stability, nonoperative treatment in a rigid brace for 2 to 3 months may yield good results in a reasonable number of patients. If pain or an anterior ADI in flexion of more than 5 mm persists after 2 to 3 months of immobilization, posterior C1-C2 arthrodesis should be performed.

In children with posttraumatic C1-C2 instability, the clinical and neurologic presentation may be abnormal, with confusing neurologic signs. Patients should be first treated nonoperatively and operated on secondarily by atlantoaxial arthrodesis using graft and wiring for persistent radiologic instability (65).

SUMMARY

Transverse ligament rupture induced either by burst fracture of the ring of the atlas or by forceful flexion-extension movement that exceeds the ligament's strength can lead to significant C1-C2 instability. The best diagnostic tool for C1-C2 instability is the ADI measurement on the lateral flexion-extension roentgenogram, which may indicate overt instability and the need for emergent MRI. The treatment of choice for isolated midsubstance transverse ligament rupture is a Magerl transarticular screw fixation augmented with a Gallie-type posterior wiring. More conservative treatment can be carried out for children and adults with transverse ligament lateral mass insertion avulsion injuries.

REFERENCES

1. Krantz P. Isolated disruption of the transverse ligament of the atlas: an injury easily overlooked at post-mortem examination. *Injury* 1980;12:168–170.
2. Hecker P. Appareil ligomenteux occipito atloidoaxoidien: etude d'anatomie comparee. *Arch Anat Hist Embryol* 1923.
3. Burguet JL, Sick H, Dirheimer Y, et al. CT of the main ligaments of the cervical occipital hinge. *Neuroradiology* 1985;27:112–118.
4. Willek A. *Munch Med Wschr* 1908;55:1836–1837.
5. Greig DM. *Clinical observations on surgical pathology of bone.* Edinburgh: Oliver and Boyd, 1931.
6. Grisel P. Enucleation de l'atlas et tonicollis Nasopharyngien (French). *Presse Med* 1930;38:50–53.
7. Steel HH. Anatomical and mechanical considerations of the atlanto-axial articulations. *J Bone Joint Surg Am* 1968;50:1481–1482.
8. Fielding JW, Hawkins RJ, Ratzan SA. Spine fusion for atlanto-axial instability. *J Bone Joint Surg Am* 1976;58:400–407.
9. Fielding JW, Cochran GVB, Lawsing JF, et al. Tears of the transverse ligament of the atlas. *J Bone Joint Surg Am* 1974;56:1683–1691.
10. Jackson H. The diagnosis of minimal atlanto-axial subluxation. *Br J Radiol* 1950;23:672.
11. Fielding JW. Normal and selected abnormal motion of the cervical spine from the second cervical vertebra to the seventh cervical vertebra based on cineroentgenography. *J Bone Joint Surg Am* 1964;46:1779.
12. Dickman CA, Greene KA, Sonntag VK. Injuries involving the transverse atlantal ligament: classification and treatment guidelines based upon experience with 39 injuries. *Neurosurgery* 1996;38:44–50.
13. Troyanovich S. C1 burst fracture. *J Manipulative Physiol Ther* 1994; 8:558–561.
14. Oda T, Panjabi MM, Crisco JJ 3rd, et al. Experimental study of atlas injuries. II. Relevance to clinical diagnosis and treatment. *Spine* 1991; 16(Suppl 10):S466–S473.
15. Fielding JW, Hawkins RJ, Ratzan SA. Spine fusion for atlanto-axial instability. *J Bone Joint Surg Am* 1976;58:400–407.
16. Levine AM, Edwards CC. Treatment of injuries in the C1-C2 complex. *Orthop Clin North Am* 1986;17:31–44.
17. Dvorak J, Schneider E, Saldinger P, et al. Biomechanics of the craniocervical region: the alar and transverse ligaments. *J Orthop Res* 1988; 6:452–461.
18. Fielding JW, Cochran GVB, Lansing JF, et al. Tears of the transverse ligaments of the atlas: a clinical and biological study. *J Bone Joint Surg Am* 1974;56:1683–1691.
19. Dvorak J, Panjabi M, Gerber M, et al. CT-functional diagnostics of the rotatory instability of upper cervical spine. 1. An experimental study on cadavers. *Spine* 1987;12:197–205.
20. Dunbar HS, Ray BS. Chronic atlanto-axial dislocations with late neurologic manifestations. *Surg Gynecol Obstet* 1961;113:757.
21. Sherk HH. Lesions of the atlas and axis. *Clin Orthop* 1975;109:33–41.
22. Wigren A, Anici F. Traumatic atlanto-axial dislocation without neurological disorder. *J Bone Joint Surg Am* 1973;55:642.
23. Levine AM, Edwards CC. Traumatic lesions of the occipitoatlanto-axial complex. *Clin Orthop* 1989;239:53–68.
24. Gonzalez TA, Vance M, Helper M, et al. *Legal medicine: pathology and toxicology.* New York: Appleton Century Crofts, 1940:312.
25. Pennecot GF, Leonard P, Des Gachons SP, et al. Traumatic ligamentous instability of the cervical spine in children. *J Pediatr Orthop* 1984;4:339–345.
26. Hamilton AR. Injuries of the atlanto-axial joint. *J Bone Joint Surg Br* 1951;33:434–435.
27. Lipson SJ. Fractures of the atlas associated with fractures of the odontoid process and transverse ligament ruptures. *J Bone Joint Surg Am* 1977;59:940–943.
28. O'Brien JJ, Bullertield WL, Gossling HR. Jefferson fracture with disruption of the transverse ligament. *Clin Orthop* 1977;126:135–138.
29. Spence KF, Decker S, Sell KW. Bursting atlantal fracture associated with rupture of the transverse ligament. *J Bone Joint Surg Am* 1970; 52:543–549.
30. Lippman RK. *J Bone Joint Surg Am* 1953;35:967–979.
31. Greene KA, Dickman CA, Marciano FF, et al. Acute axis fractures. Analysis of management and outcome in 340 consecutive cases. *Spine* 1997;22:1843–1852.
32. Wachenheim A. Occipitalization of the ventral part and vertebralization of the dorsal part of the atlas with insufficiency of the transverse ligament. *Neuroradiology* 1982;24:45–47.
33. Bharucha EP, Dastur HM. Craniovertebral anomalies (a report of 40 cases). *Brain* 1964;87:469–480.
34. McRae DL. Bony abnormalities in the region of the foramen magnum: correlation of the anatomic and neurologic findings. *Acta Radiol* 1953; 40:335–354.
35. McRae DL. The significance of abnormalities of the cervical spine. *AJR Am J Roentgenol* 1960;84:3.
36. McRae DL, Barnum AS. Occipitalization of the atlas. *AJR Am J Roentgenol* 1953;70:23–46.
37. Parke WW, Rothman RH, Brown MD. The pharyngovenebral veins: an anatomical rationale for Grisel's syndrome. *J Bone Joint Surg Am* 1984;66:568–574.
38. Kurt LT, Gartin SR, Fielding JW. The rheumatoid cervical spine. *J Orthop Rheum* 1988;1:71–78.
39. Sullivan AW. Subluxation of the atlanto-axial joint; sequel to inflammatory process of the neck. *J Pediatr* 1949;35:451–464.
40. Watson Jones R. Spontaneous hyperemic dislocation of the atlas. *Proc R Soc Med* 1931–1932;25:586–590.
41. Weisman BNW, Alibadi P, Weinfeld MS, et al. Prognostic features of atlantoaxial subluxation in rheumatoid arthritis patients. *Radiology* 1982;144:745–751.
42. Wilson B, Jarvi BL, Haydon RC. Nontraumatic subluxation of the atlantoaxial joint: Grisel's syndrome. *Ann Otol Rhinol Laryngol* 1987; 96:705–708.
43. Greenberg AD. Atlanto-axial dislocations. *Brain* 1968;91:655–654.
44. Von Torklus D, Gehle W. *The upper cervical spine.* New York: Grune and Stratton, 1972.
45. Manel W, Tishler JM. Observations on the spine in mongoloidism. *AJR Am J Roentgenol* 1966;97:630.
46. Spitzer R, Rabinowitch JY, Wybar KC. A study of the abnormalities of the skull, teeth and lenses in mongolism. *Can Med Assoc J* 1961;84: 567–572.
47. Cunis BH, Blank S, Fisher RL. Atlanto axial dislocation in Down's syndrome. *JAMA* 1968;205:464–465.

48. Dzenitis A. Spontaneous atlanto-axial dislocation in a mongoloid child with spinal cord compression. *J Neurosurg* 1966;25:458–460.

49. Ferguson RL, Putney ME, Allen BL. Comparison of neurologic deficits with atlanto dens intervals in patients with Down syndrome. *J Spinal Disord* 1997;10:246–252.

50. French HG, Burke SW, Whitecloud TS, et al. Chronic atlanto-axial instability in Down's syndrome. *Orthop Trans* 1985;9:135.

51. Deliganis AV, Baxter AB, Hanson JA, et al. Radiologic spectrum of craniocervical distraction injuries. *Radiographics* 2000;20(Suppl): S237–S250.

52. Schroder RJ, Vogl T, Hidajat N, et al. Comparison of the diagnostic value of CT and MRI in injuries of the cervical vertebrae. *Aktuelle Radiol* 1995;5:197–202.

53. Dickman CA, Mamourian A, Sonntag VK, et al. Magnetic resonance imaging of the transverse atlantal ligament for the evaluation of atlanto-axial instability. *Neurosurgery* 1991;75:221–227.

54. Fielding JW. Injuries to the upper cervical spine. In: Griffen PP, ed. *Instructional course lectures*. Chicago: American Academy of Orthopaedic Surgeons, 1987.

55. Griswold DM, Albright JA, Schiffman E, et al. Atlanto-axial fusion for instability. *J Bone Joint Surg Am* 1978;60:285–292.

56. Mazur JM, Stauffer ES. Unrecognized spinal instability associated with seemingly "simple" cervical compression fractures. *Spine* 1983; 8:687–692.

57. King AG. Spinal column trauma. In: Anderson LD, ed. *Instructional course lectures,* vol. 35. St. Louis: CV Mosby, 1986.

58. Tokuhashi Y, Matsuzaki H, Shirasaki Y, et al. C1-C2 intra-articular screw fixation for atlantoaxial posterior stabilization. *Spine* 2000;25: 337–341.

59. Xu R, Ebraheim NA, Misson JR, et al. The reliability of the lateral radiograph in determination of the optimal transarticular C1-C2 screw length. *Spine* 1998;23:2190–2194.

60. White AA, Southwick WO, Panjabi MM. Clinical stability of the lower cervical spine: a review of past and current concepts. *Spine* 1976;1:15–27.

61. Crawford NR, Hurlbert RJ, Choi WG, et al. Differential biomechanical effects of injury and wiring at C1-C2. *Spine* 1999;24:1894–1902.

62. Fielding JW. The cervical spine in the child. *Curr Prac Orthop Surg* 1973;5:31–55.

63. Highland TR, Aron DD. Traumatic rupture of the cervical transverse ligament in a child with a normal odontoid process. *Spine* 1986;11: 73–75.

64. Fielding JW, Hawkins RJ, Hensinger RN, et al. Atlantoaxial rotary deformities. *Orthop Clin N Am* 1978;9:955–967.

65. Filipe G, Berges O, Lebard JP, et al. Post-traumatic instability between the atlas and the axis in children. Apropos of 5 cases. *Rev Chir Orthop Reparatrice Appar Mot* 1982;68:461–469.

CHAPTER 45

Dens Fractures

Ganesh Rao and Ronald I. Apfelbaum

The odontoid process (the dens) of the axis is commonly fractured, accounting for up to 20% of all acute cervical spine fractures (1). Certain types of odontoid process fractures can lead to gross instability of the atlantoaxial complex and present a significant risk for a potentially catastrophic spinal cord injury (2). The treatment of odontoid process fractures remains controversial and ranges from external orthosis to internal fixation techniques that vary significantly. This chapter discusses the development of the odontoid process, types of odontoid fractures, mechanisms of injury, and treatment options.

DEVELOPMENT AND ANATOMY OF THE ODONTOID PROCESS

The complex development of the dens involves two ossification centers, formed during the fifth fetal month, that come together approximately 3 months after birth (3). These centers are separated from the primary ossification center of the vertebral body by the dentocentral synchondrosis, a slow-growing synchondrosis that contributes to the overall heights of both the odontoid process and the body of C2. By 3 to 6 years of age, the dens has fused with the body of C2. Generally, all ossification has occurred by age 7 except for the cartilaginous epiphysis at the tip of the dens, the ossiculum terminale. The ossiculum terminale, a secondary ossification center, forms at the proximal dens epiphysis at 8 to 10 years of age. By 13 years of age, the ossiculum terminale has fused with the rest of the dens.

Discoveries in molecular biology have furthered the understanding of the development of the atlantoaxial complex. Animal models have shown that fusion of the dens to the body of C2 coincides with the decreased expression of the gene *Pax-1* (4). Additionally, mice who have a disruption in the homeobox-containing gene Hoxd-3 will have a deletion of the dens and superior facets of C2, and, in addition, abnormalities of the atlas, including fusion to the oc-

cipital bone. The axis takes on "atlaslike" features, losing the peglike feature of the odontoid process and resembling the ring shape of C1. An appreciation of the embryonic development of the upper cervical spine helps one to understand the complex anatomy of this region.

Vascular Supply of the Dens

The vascular supply of the dens is quite extensive and derives from three main groups of arteries: (a) the paired anterior and posterior ascending arteries arising separately from the vertebral artery at the C2-3 intervertebral level, (b) a pair of transverse arteries in the retropharyngeal cleft arising from the ascending pharyngeal artery, and (c) a branch of the ascending pharyngeal artery that crosses the hypoglossal canal (5–8). These arteries provide the dens with a rich anastomotic network (9–11).

Each anterior ascending artery arises from the anteromedial surface of the respective vertebral artery. The arteries leave the vertebral artery through the neural foramen of C2-C3 and penetrate the longus colli muscle. After coursing through the accessory ligaments to the base of the dens, they anastomose with each other and supply perforators to the anterior surface of the axis and the tip of the dens. The posterior ascending arteries originate from the posteromedial surface of the vertebral arteries. Each artery crosses the junction between the pedicle and the body of C2 and gives off medial branches to the tectorial membrane. Once they cross the posterior border of the alar ligament, only terminal branches remain. One of these branches forms an anastomosis with the rostral-most portion of the anterior ascending artery superior to the alar ligament. The other supplies the tip of the dens and forms an anastomosis with the contralateral artery.

The external carotid artery also contributes via the transverse arteries in the retropharyngeal cleft, which are small vessels that branch from the ascending pharyngeal arteries just before they enter the cranium. These vessels form anastomoses with the anterior ascending arteries lateral to the base of the dens. The ascending pharyngeal arteries provide a minor contribution via the posterior horizontal arteries. These vessels join the apical vasculature after traveling intracranially and emerging through the hypoglossal foramen of the occipital condyle. The ascending pharyngeal artery terminates in two to four branches that enter the base of the skull.

Odontoid fractures, particularly those that occur at the neck of the dens (i.e., the type II odontoid fractures described later in this chapter), are prone to poor healing. It was previously thought that a watershed area existed at the odontoid process, inhibiting bony healing. However, injection studies have shown that there is a rich anastomotic network at the odontoid process (7). Although theoretically a fracture through the neck of the odontoid process may disrupt the ascending arteries, this has not been proven *in vivo*.

Ligaments of the Dens

The ligamentous structures of the atlantoaxial complex are essential for the stability of the upper cervical spine. The main ligaments that provide stability for the atlantoaxial joint are the transverse atlantal, alar, and apical ligaments (Fig. 45.1) (12,13). The transverse atlantal ligament limits flexion and anterior displacement of C1 on C2. The alar ligaments restrain rotation of the occiput-C1-C2 complex, and the tectorial membrane limits extension. The transverse atlantal ligament is the primary stabilizer; this ligament is attached to a tubercle on the anteromedial border of each lateral mass of C1. The ligament passes around the dens at its base and is separated from it by a synovial articulating surface. The transverse ligament is one of the strongest ligaments in the body and, when intact, will not allow the axis to shift on the atlas more than 2 mm in adults, or more than 4 to 5 mm in children (14).

The alar ligaments are attached symmetrically on both sides of the upper dens; the upper portion connects the dens to the occiput, and the remaining, lower portion connects the dens to the atlas (13). The alar ligaments restrict both axial rotation and lateral bending of the occiput-C1-C2 complex. The right alar ligament limits rotation to the left, and the left alar ligament restricts rotation to the right. The apical ligament connects the apex of the dens to the anterior edge of the foramen magnum and is said to make a minor contribution to occiput-C1 stability but no contribution to C1-C2 stability (13).

Anatomic and Biomechanical Considerations

The occipitocervical junction and atlantoaxial complex form the functional components of the upper cervical spine. This region is regarded as a transitional zone that connects the cranium to the spinal column. The weight of the skull is transferred through the occipital condyles and lateral masses of C1 to the lateral masses of C2. From there, most of the weight is transferred anteriorly to the body of C2 and down the spine through the vertebral bodies. The C1-C2 joint is adapted to facilitate rotation and accounts for 50% of the rotation of the head joint. C1 serves as a transitional vertebra. Its superior articulations, which mate with the occipital condyles, are cup shaped. The motion at this level is primarily flexion and extension with virtually no rotation or

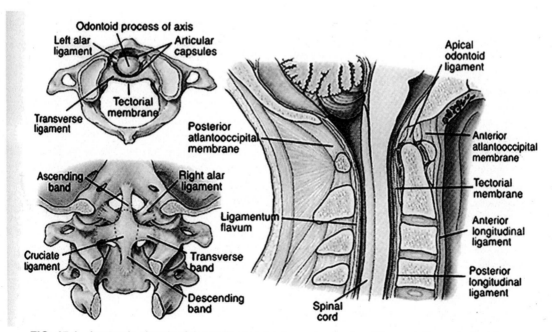

FIG. 45.1. Anatomic sketch of the major ligamentous structures of the occipitocervical region.

translation. There are no intervertebral discs at either the atlantooccipital or atlantoaxial levels. The close apposition of the odontoid process to C1 allows significant rotation of C1 on C2 (13). Both articular surfaces of the C1 and C2 lateral masses have a convex orientation in the sagittal plane that permits significant mobility. Further, the articulating surfaces of C1 and C2 are sloped upward from lateral to medial. As C1 rotates on C2, this sloping allows for a helical motion between C1 and C2. This permits greater excursion before the alar ligament tightens than would be allowed if the surfaces articulated purely horizontally. Unlike the levels inferior to the C1-C2 joint, there is no ligamentum flavum. Instead, a mobile atlantoaxial membrane connects the posterior elements but does not restrict motion. In addition, a generous spinal canal at this level and an axis of rotation in the region of the anterior surface of the spinal cord combine to permit significant rotation without injury to the spinal cord.

A disruption of the C1-C2 complex always leads to atlantoaxial instability. Fractures of the odontoid process or disruption of the transverse ligament permit translation between C1 and C2, compromising the anterior–posterior dimension of the spinal canal and putting the spinal cord at risk for injury. If the instability is due solely to failure of the bony elements, then healing is possible with external immobilization. However, if the transverse ligament is disrupted, surgery is required to achieve bony fusion.

FRACTURES OF THE ODONTOID PROCESS

Odontoid fractures are common cervical spine injuries and account for 10% to 20% of all cervical spine fractures (11,15–20). Anderson and D'Alonzo (21) classified fractures of the odontoid process into three types (Fig. 45.2). Type I is a fracture of the apical portion of the odontoid process. These fractures are rare, and whether they contribute to instability of the atlantoaxial complex is controversial. Type I fractures are typically considered stable, but Scott and associates (22) suggested that they may represent an avulsion of the alar ligaments and thus result in instability. If instability is suspected in a patient with a type I fracture, dynamic imaging may reveal whether there is abnormal motion of the atlantoaxial joint.

Type II fractures involve the neck of the odontoid. These are the most common odontoid fractures and are unstable. A type II fractured odontoid process may be either anterolisthesed or retrolisthesed.

Type III fractures extend into the body of C2. Some type III fractures are comminuted at the base of the dens and are associated with free fracture fragments. This subset of fractures has been termed type IIA (23). Type IIA fractures are less likely to be treated successfully with external immobilization. True type III fractures are typically managed with external immobilization, which is often successful; however, high odontoid process type III fractures are also amenable to surgery (24).

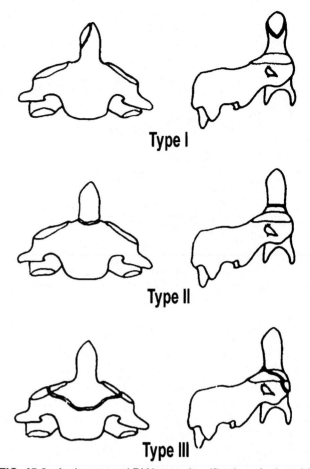

FIG. 45.2. Anderson and D'Alonzo classification of odontoid fractures. (Modified from Anderson LD, D'Alonzo RT. Fractures of the odontoid process of the axis. *J Bone Joint Surg Am* 1974;56:1663–1674, with permission.)

Approximately 90% to 95% of all odontoid fractures are caused by trauma, primarily motor vehicle accidents (15, 25). Althoff (26) performed a definitive study on the mechanisms responsible for the various types of odontoid fractures. In general, the forces that create dens fractures are a combination of horizontal shear and vertical compression. When the forces are applied directly in the sagittal plane, a type III fracture results. At 45 degrees to the sagittal plane, a type II fracture results, and at 90 degrees, a type I fracture results. As the vector producing shear and compression moves out of the sagittal plane more laterally, the fracture of the dens produced is increasingly cephalad (13).

Type II fractures have been further classified, based on the anterior–posterior direction of the fracture line, as anterior oblique, posterior oblique, or horizontal fractures (Fig. 45.3) (15). Anterior oblique fractures slope inferiorly from posterior to anterior, posterior oblique fractures slope superiorly from posterior to anterior, and horizontal fractures slope minimally or not at all. The slope of the fracture line can be an important consideration regarding treatment. For example, an anterior oblique fracture has a lower rate of

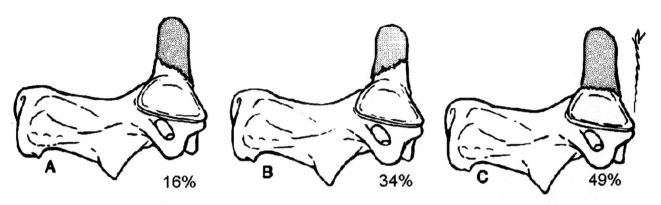

A   16%   B   34%   C   49%

Anterior oblique   Posterior oblique   Horizontal

FIG. 45.3. A classification scheme for type II odontoid fractures describing the slope of the fracture line from its superior to its inferior end. The percentages refer to the incidence in the series reported by Apfelbaum and associates. (From, Apfelbaum RI, Lonser RR, Veres R, et al. Direct anterior screw fixation for recent and remote odontoid fractures. *J Neurosurg* 2000;93(Suppl 2):227–236, with permission).

fusion when treated with a direct anterior odontoid screw (discussed in further detail later in this chapter).

Another entity that should be considered with dens fractures is os odontoideum. Os odontoideum has been defined as a congenital absence of a united odontoid process, which remains as a separate ossicle with smooth circumferential cortical margins that has no connection to the body of C2 (Fig. 45.4) (27,28). The etiology of os odontoideum is con-troversial, although most authors now agree that it most likely results from an unrecognized injury to the odontoid process in childhood. Because os odontoideum is generally not seen in children younger than 5 years of age, it is unlikely that it is congenitally acquired. Regardless of etiology, the presentation of os odontoideum may vary. It can present as occipitocervical pain, myelopathy, and signs or symptoms of vertebrobasilar ischemia (29). There are two anatomic types of os odontoideum: orthoptic and dystopic. The orthoptic type is an ossicle that moves with the anterior arch of C1, whereas the dystopic type is an ossicle that is fused with the basion. The dystopic type of os may sublux anterior to the arch of C1 (14). Most often, anterior instability is identified on imaging, with the os odontoideum subluxing anterior to C2. There are cases, however, when no instability is apparent (14,30).

The evaluation of an odontoid fracture generally begins with plain x-rays (Fig. 45.5), including lateral, anteroposterior, and open-mouth (Fig. 45.6) radiographs of the cervical spine. If an odontoid fracture is suspected, thin-section computed tomography (CT) with reconstructions in the coronal and sagittal planes is recommended for further evaluation (Fig. 45.7) (31,32). Magnetic resonance imaging (MRI) may also be used to assess the integrity of the transverse ligament (31,33).

Because odontoid process fractures render the cervical spine unstable, the patient must be protected from additional neurologic injury during transport to the hospital and during the initial evaluation.

Mortality and Neurologic Injury

Patients with odontoid fractures have varied presentations. Estimates of mortality from dens fractures at the time of the injury range from 25% to 40% (34,35). Survivors of the

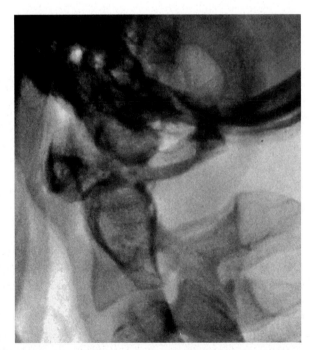

FIG. 45.4. Example of an os odontoideum. Note the rounded, separate ossicle, significant gap between the ossicle and the body of C2, and well-corticated surfaces of both the ossicle and C2.

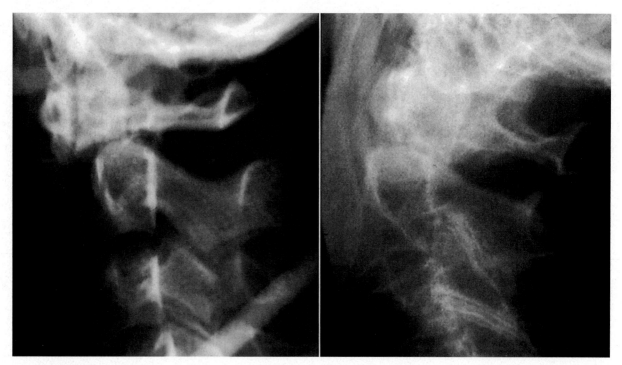

FIG. 45.5. Lateral spine radiograph in two patients with type II odontoid fractures showing the odontoid in an anterolisthesed position on the left and in a retrolisthesed position in the patient on the right.

injury, however, are usually neurologically intact. Anderson and D'Alonzo (21) found that 45 (75%) of the 60 patients in their series had no neurologic deficit initially. The remaining 15 patients (25%) had various neurologic deficits, including Brown-Séquard syndrome, mild upper extremity weakness, hyperreflexia of the lower extremities, and decreased occipi-

tal sensation. Delayed onset of symptoms after the initial injury, which may be catastrophic, has also been reported (2,36). The most common presenting symptom in a patient with an undiagnosed odontoid fracture is neck pain; however, these patients may also complain of hand weakness and lower extremity "stiffness" (2). These fractures must be treated because the potential for ongoing neurologic compromise is well known (36–39).

Over the last few years, the treatment regimen for odontoid fractures has become better delineated. As imaging techniques improve, fractures are being identified earlier, and as surgical techniques become more refined, the indications for their use are becoming more clear. The next section discusses the various treatment options available for odontoid fractures.

TREATMENT OF ODONTOID PROCESS FRACTURES

Type I and type III fractures have been treated with external immobilization with a high degree of success. Julien and associates (40) performed an extensive evidence-based analysis of the literature to evaluate the management of odontoid fractures. Halo/Minerva fixation for 8 to 12 weeks resulted in fusion of all type I odontoid fractures (3 of 3 patients) (40,41). Cervical traction to restore realignment followed by immobilization in a rigid cervical collar also resulted in a successful fusion (3 of 3 patients). For type III odontoid fractures, halo/Minerva immobilization yielded a fusion rate of 84% (67 of 80 patients) (40,41). For type III

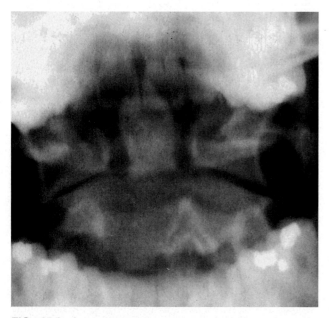

FIG. 45.6. Anteroposterior, open-mouth radiograph showing type II fracture at the base of the odontoid.

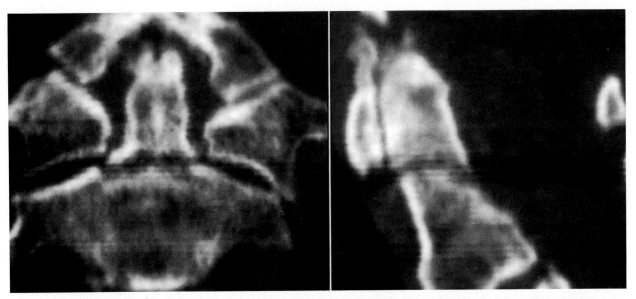

FIG. 45.7. Reconstructed images in the coronal and mid-sagittal planes from thin-section computed tomographic scans allow excellent definition of the fracture. Overlying bone, which can obscure plain film images, is eliminated.

fractures, cervical traction followed by immobilization in a rigid cervical collar for at least 6 weeks resulted in a fusion rate of 88% (57 of 65 patients). Thus, for type I or type III fractures, treatment with cervical traction to restore anatomic alignment followed by at least 6 weeks of immobilization in a cervical collar appears to be effective in most cases.

Cervical traction followed by immobilization is not the most effective treatment of type II odontoid fractures. Cervical traction may be required to alleviate ongoing compression of the neural elements by the C2 body, odontoid process, or C1 posterior ring and to realign the spine and protect the patient from new or additional neural compression. However, Julien and associates (40) reported that treatment of type II odontoid fractures with cervical traction followed by a rigid cervical collar resulted in a fusion rate of only 57% (55 of 97 patients). Management with a halotype orthosis has a variable nonunion rate ranging

from 7% (42) to 100% (43). Nonunion rates have been reported often in the literature, varying from 21% to 45% (17,18,25,44–46). The Cervical Spine Research Society's multicenter survey of dens fractures found a nonunion rate of 32% for odontoid fractures treated nonoperatively (47). Julien and colleagues (40) reported a successful fusion rate of 65% (110 of 168 patients).

Surgery is also an acceptable treatment for odontoid fractures, and several operative options exist. Historically, posterior cervical fusion was the primary operative alternative when external immobilization either failed or was considered unsuitable. Wiring techniques, including those described by Gallie, Brooks, and later Dickman and Sonntag, have been used to achieve posterior cervical fusion (Fig. 45.8). Gallie's technique uses an H-shaped bone graft that is placed between C1 and the spinous process of C2. A superior notch is made in the spinous process of C2 to hold the graft more securely in place, and the graft is secured with a

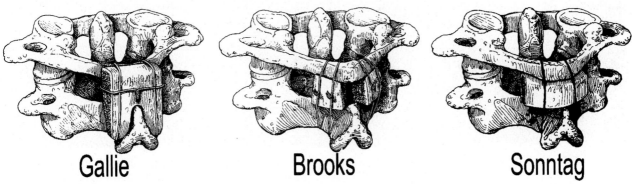

Gallie   Brooks   Sonntag

FIG. 45.8. Artist's drawing of several types of posterior C1-C2 arthrodesis constructs. (Images © BNI 1989. Used with permission.)

wire that is only sublaminar at C1. Brooks's technique involves two wedge bone grafts secured between C1 and C2 with sublaminar wiring. Finally, Dickman and associates described an atlantoaxial arthrodesis secured with a sublaminar wire at C1 and incorporating an iliac crest strut-graft positioned between the posterior arches of C1 and C2. The graft is held in place by a securing wire around the base of the spinous process of the axis (48). Anderson and D'Alonzo (21) and Fielding and colleagues (49) reported excellent results (1 nonunion of 46 Gallie fusions) with posterior fusion for odontoid fractures.

In 1992, Jeanneret and Magerl (50) reported their results with C1-C2 transarticular screw fixation, in addition to posterior fusion, for odontoid fractures. They recommended the use of transarticular screws rather than a Gallie or Brooks arthrodesis alone. They found the technique to be very successful, with a fusion rate of 100%, and reported only one complication of a transient hypoglossal nerve paresis. Dickman and Sonntag (51) compared fusion rates of patients treated with C1-C2 transarticular screws with patients treated with wires and autograft alone for atlantoaxial instability. They reported a 98% fusion rate for patients who received C1-C2 transarticular screw fixation and an 86% fusion rate for patients who received C1-C2 fixation with only wires and arthrodesis.

Important anatomic considerations must be evaluated in patients requiring posterior arthrodesis. Poor bone quality, although not an absolute contraindication, should be of concern. In these cases, rigid external immobilization may be required in addition to internal fixation. For C1-C2 transarticular screw fixation, an adequate pathway for the screw trajectory is essential. The entire pathway for the screw must be inspected carefully on preoperative imaging. We have found that fine-cut CT with reconstructions through the desired screw trajectory is invaluable. The pars interarticularis, the lateral C1-C2 articulation, and the lateral mass of C1 should all be visualized. A dangerous condition that contraindicates screw placement is a vertebral artery that courses into the pars of C2, interfering with potential screw trajectory (Fig. 45.9). Injury to the vertebral artery during screw placement has obvious potentially disastrous neurologic effects.

Successful fusion rates for transarticular screws are almost 100% (51–54). When the anatomy is favorable, this technique is generally preferred because of excellent results. Posterior arthrodesis may be preferred in patients who have a comminuted type II or III fracture, an associated unstable Jefferson's fracture, or who cannot tolerate a halo or other external immobilization. In the review by Julien and associates (40), posterior arthrodesis techniques had a success rate of 100% for type I fractures (1 of 1 patient), 74% for type II fractures (109 of 147 patients), and 97% for type III fractures (28 of 29 patients).

Certain conditions can make C1-C2 transarticular screw placement difficult. These conditions include insufficient space for screw placement in the isthmus of C2 and, as mentioned previously, an anomalous course of the vertebral artery. A new technique has been described by Harms and Melcher (55) for posterior C1-C2 fusion with polyaxial screws placed into the pars or pedicle of C2 and directed into the lateral mass of C1. These are coupled with rods. This construct allows for intraoperative reduction and fixation of the atlantoaxial complex (Fig. 45.10). This technique minimizes the risk of injury to the vertebral artery and is espe-

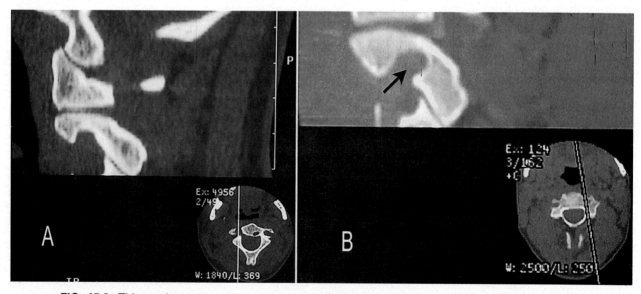

FIG. 45.9. Thin-section computed tomographic reconstructions showing a suitable pathway for transarticular screw placement on the image **(A)**, but insufficient clearance from the vertebral artery foramina (*arrow*) **(B)**. In this patient, only a unilateral transarticular screw was placed.

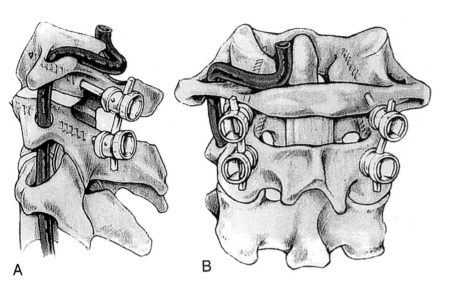

A   B

FIG. 45.10. Harm's technique of C1-C2 posterior fixation. (From, Harms J, Melcher RP. Posterior C1-C2 fusion with polyaxial screw and rod fixation. *Spine* 2001;26:2467–2671, with permission.)

cially valuable when posterior wiring techniques cannot be performed, such as when the posterior elements are deficient. Preliminary data suggest that this technique is safe and effective for managing instability in the atlantoaxial region.

Several other issues must be considered in regard to C1-C2 posterior arthrodesis. The passage of wires or cables into the spinal canal may injure neural elements; this is more likely to occur if C2 sublaminar wires are used. Structural bone grafting should be used to achieve solid fusion and is critical to achieving long-term stability. Any hardware that is placed functions as temporary internal fixation and is unreliable for long-term stability. If an intact posterior arch of C1 is not present, alternative fusion techniques can be applied, such as decortication and bone packing into the C1-C2 joint or the lasso technique (56).

C1-C2 joint fusion eliminates 50% of the rotation of the head, a significant loss of motion. Consequently, an anterior technique for directly treating odontoid fractures has been developed that attempts to preserve the normal motion of the C1-C2 joint. This technique is anterior odontoid screw fixation.

Several authors have described the surgical technique for anterior odontoid screw fixation (16,57–61). Nakanishi first described the technique in 1980 in the Japanese literature (62), and in 1982, Bohler (61) reported his 8-year experience in Europe. Although initial approaches for anterior screw fixation were complex, the technique has gained increased acceptance as instrumentation for the procedure has improved, advances in minimally invasive approaches have been developed, and improvements in fluoroscopic guidance have been made (Figs. 45.11 through 45.16) (63,64). Direct anterior screw fixation is an osteosynthetic technique that provides immediate spinal stabilization. This operation offers the advantages of preservation of rotation of C1 on C2 and a rapid return to normal lifestyle (59,65). Retention of full range of motion has been reported to be as high as 83% (65).

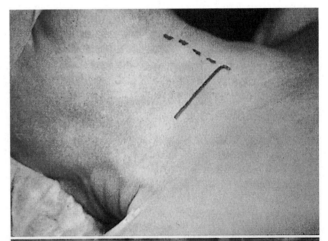

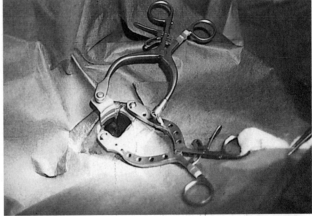

FIG. 45.11. Technique of direct anterior screw fixation, step 1. Skin incision in midcervical region and placement of self-retaining retractor. See reference 63 for full details. (From, Apfelbaum RI. Anterior screw fixation of odontoid fractures. In: Rengachary SS, Wilkins RH, eds. *Neurosurgical operative atlas.* 2nd ed. Baltimore: Williams and Wilkins, 1992:189–199, with permission.)

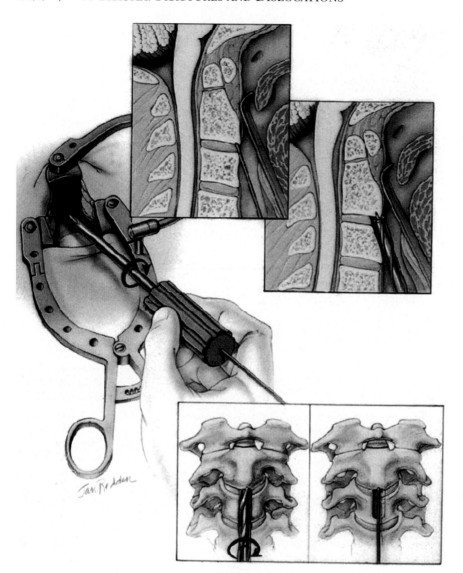

FIG. 45.12. Technique of direct anterior screw fixation, step 2. Placement of K-wire and creation of groove for drill guide in C3. See reference 63 for full details. (From, Apfelbaum RI. Anterior screw fixation of odontoid fractures. In: Rengachary SS, Wilkins RH, eds. *Neurosurgical operative atlas.* 2nd ed. Baltimore: Williams and Wilkins, 1992: 189–199, with permission.)

Various parameters have been identified as predictors of failure to obtain fusion of type II odontoid fractures treated without surgery (23,25,45,66). Higher degrees of displacement of the dens fracture have been associated with increased incidence of nonunion. One series of 229 fractures found that a displacement of greater than 6 mm was associated with a 67% nonunion rate, whereas a displacement of less than 6 mm was associated with a 90% union rate (67). In another retrospective review of 120 patients, Greene and colleagues (1) similarly found that a fracture displacement of 6 mm or greater resulted in a nonunion rate of 86% compared with a nonunion rate of 18% for patients with displacement of 6 mm or less. Another series found that displacement of 4 mm or less was associated with an improved fusion rate (25).

Age is another important factor in the successful healing of odontoid fractures (Fig. 45.17). Children with odontoid process fractures will generally achieve stable fusion with halo immobilization (68–70). Sherk and associates (68)

reported a series of 35 children (age range, 9 months to 7 years) with odontoid fractures in which only 1 failed halo immobilization and required surgical stabilization. Several studies, however, have shown that adult patients have a higher rate of nonunion with external immobilization (71–74). These authors, and others, therefore recommend early surgical stabilization with posterior fusion for the older patient. In a case-control study of 33 patients, Lennarson and associates (75) found that individuals over 50 years old had a nonunion rate 21 times higher than those younger than 50 when treated with halo immobilization. For this reason, they recommend surgical stabilization for patients over age 50. Although Andersson and associates (74) reported only a 20% fusion rate in patients 65 years of age and older who were treated with anterior odontoid screw fixation, Apfelbaum and colleagues (15) performed a multivariate analysis of possible predictors of outcome in patients with odontoid fractures treated with direct anterior odontoid screw fixation and found no correlation between age, sex, number of

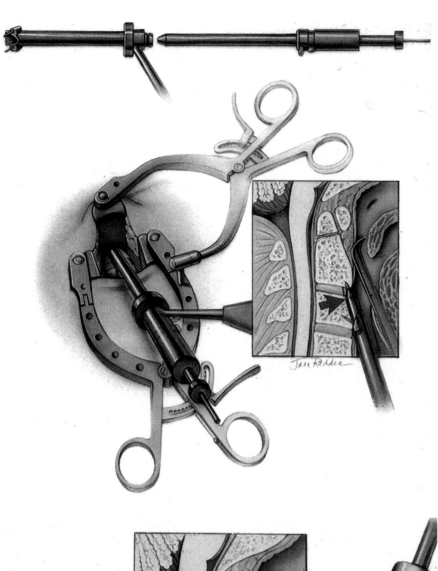

FIG. 45.13. Technique of direct anterior screw fixation, step 3. Drill guide system components mate together and are anchored to C3. See reference 63 for full details. (From, Apfelbaum RI. Anterior screw fixation of odontoid fractures. In: Rengachary SS, Wilkins RH, eds. *Neurosurgical operative atlas.* 2nd ed. Baltimore: Williams and Wilkins, 1992:189–199, with permission.)

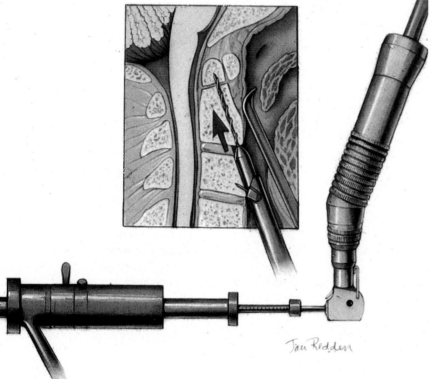

FIG. 45.14. Technique of direct anterior screw fixation, step 4. Drilling screw path through body of C2 into odontoid. This is monitored on biplanar fluoroscopy. See reference 63 for full details. (From, Apfelbaum RI. Anterior screw fixation of odontoid fractures. In: Rengachary SS, Wilkins RH, eds. *Neurosurgical operative atlas.* 2nd ed. Baltimore: Williams and Wilkins, 1992: 189–199, with permission.)

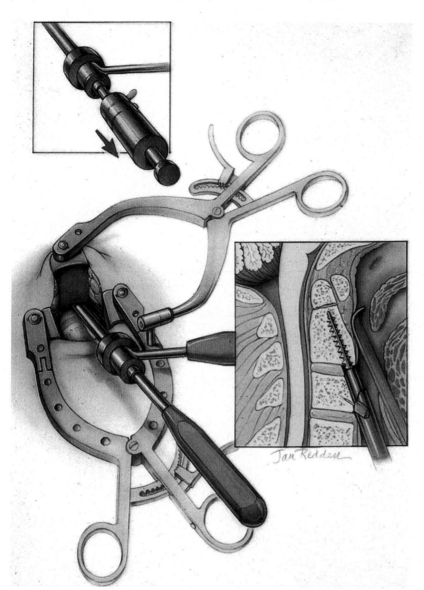

FIG. 45.15. Technique of direct anterior screw fixation, step 5. After drilling the pilot hole, the inner drill guide is removed and the hole is tapped. See reference 63 for full details. (From, Apfelbaum RI. Anterior screw fixation of odontoid fractures. In: Rengachary SS, Wilkins RH, eds. *Neurosurgical operative atlas.* 2nd ed. Baltimore: Williams and Wilkins, 1992:189–199, with permission.)

screws, or degree of odontoid displacement and the fusion rate. The only factors that had a significant impact on the fusion rate were the orientation of the odontoid fragment and the timing of surgery. Both elderly and younger patients had a fusion rate of 88% when treated with direct anterior odontoid screw fixation.

The issue of whether to place one or two odontoid screws is controversial (Fig. 45.18). Some patients do not have an odontoid process large enough to accommodate two screws (76). Two-screw constructs appear to offer the ability to prevent rotation of the dens around a single screw. For this reason, we generally advocate placement of two screws if an odontoid process fracture will accept two screws (Fig. 45.19). There appears to be similar clinical success, however, with both the one- and two-screw constructs (15,77).

For patients who present within the first 6 months of injury and do not have a concomitant transverse ligament rupture, the preferred method of the senior author of this chapter (RIA) is direct anterior screw fixation (15). As noted, the placement of an odontoid screw allows retention of rotation of C1 on C2. The procedure is well tolerated and does not rely on bone graft harvest. Generally, no other postoperative treatment (e.g., a rigid orthosis) is necessary. A fusion rate of 88% has been achieved when the surgery is performed within the first 6 months of injury. However, the bony fusion rate drops to 25% when the operation is performed in patients with remote fractures (i.e., more than 18 months following injury) (15). Therefore, it is clear that the timing of surgery is important. Our results in patients operated upon within 6 months of their injury have not shown a decline in success between those operated on immediately and those operated

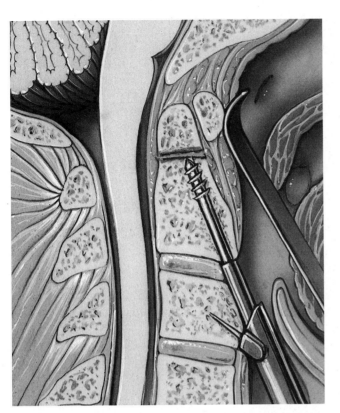

FIG. 45.16. Technique of direct anterior screw fixation, step 6. Screw is placed through the drill guide. See reference 63 for full details. (From, Apfelbaum RI. Anterior screw fixation of odontoid fractures. In: Rengachary SS, Wilkins RH, eds. *Neurosurgical operative atlas.* 2nd ed. Baltimore: Williams and Wilkins, 1992:189–199, with permission.)

on several months later. Thus, if a patient fails external immobilization and is still within 6 months of the injury, anterior odontoid screw placement is an option. We therefore recommend that direct anterior screw fixation be considered in all recent (<6 months' duration) type II odontoid fractures if they have an intact transverse ligament.

Additionally, it is important to consider the orientation of the fracture. Fractures that occur horizontally or in the posterior oblique direction have a higher fusion rate than those that occur in the anterior oblique position (15). Anterior oblique fractures are not an absolute contraindication, but require careful analysis of bone quality and may require supplemental external support. Concomitant C2 body fractures may weaken C2 and prevent screw retention. These, too, are therefore relative contraindications and require careful individual evaluation.

Because remote type II fractures have a higher rate of nonunion, they usually should be treated with posterior C1-C2 fixation and fusion. In addition, when a patient has atlantoaxial instability that is not remediable by placement of an odontoid screw, posterior cervical fusion is indicated. When favorable anatomy exists, placement of C1-C2 transarticular screws may be used for stabilization.

Chronic dens fractures may also result in ventral compression of the spinal cord. Continued ventral compression of the spinal cord, even after fusion to prevent motion, can result in progressive spinal cord damage (2,38,78). For this reason, it is important to realign the spine before posterior fusion. If realignment is not possible, transoral odontoid resection to decompress neural elements before proceeding with the posterior fusion is indicated (2,36,78–80). This procedure has become more common, but remains technically demanding (81).

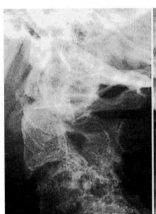
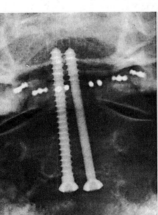
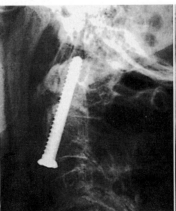
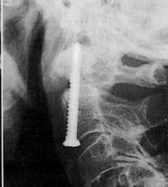

80 y/o; Type II Posterior Oblique Odontoid Fracture

1 month after realignment and screw fixation

3 months post-operation

FIG. 45.17. This 80-year-old osteopenic patient successfully healed her fracture after direct screw fixation. The fracture was reduced from its retrolisthesed position using the drill guide and was fixed with two screws. At 3 months, the fracture appeared healed.

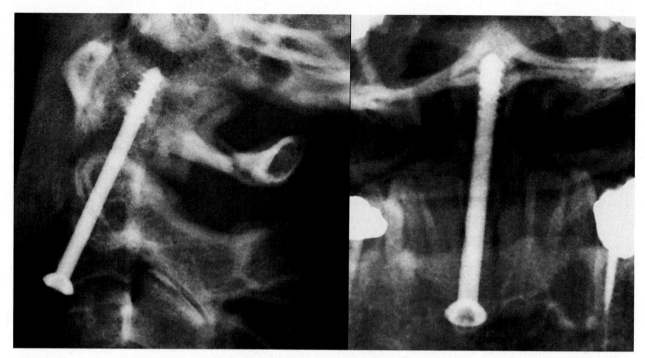

FIG. 45.18. Odontoid screw fixation performed with a single lag screw.

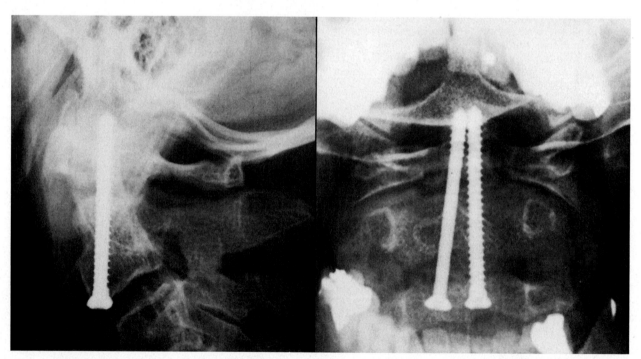

FIG. 45.19. Odontoid screw fixation with two odontoid screws placed to restrict any possible rotation of the odontoid process in relation to C2.

RECOMMENDATIONS FROM THE JOINT SECTION ON DISORDERS OF THE SPINE AND PERIPHERAL NERVES

In 2002, the American Association of Neurological Surgeons/Congress of Neurological Surgeons (AANS/CNS) Joint Section on Disorders of the Spine and Peripheral Nerves published guidelines for the management of acute cervical spinal cord injuries. These guidelines were a result of comprehensive review of all literature specific to injuries of the cervical spine and their treatment modalities. The AANS/CNS were unable to generate treatment standards, citing insufficient evidence in the literature. The guidelines they formulated for the treatment of type II odontoid fractures recommend surgical stabilization and fusion in patients 50 years of age or older. This recommendation is based on one of the better-constructed comparison studies available in the literature (75). For other circumstances, the guidelines state that type I, II, and III fractures may be treated with external immobilization, although type II and III fractures with dens displacement of 5 mm or greater, comminution of the odontoid (type IIA), or inability to maintain fracture alignment with external immobilization should be considered for surgical stabilization.

Controversies Regarding the Guidelines

In general, we agree with the AANS/CNS guidelines. Based on our experience, however, for fractures less than 6 months old and with an intact transverse ligament, we recommend direct anterior screw fixation as the treatment of choice regardless of patient age. This avoids external immobilization and has a very high success rate. Odontoid screw fixation will retain an almost normal rotation of C1 on C2 and results in a rapid return to normal lifestyle.

The AANS/CNS guidelines suggest that patients with os odontoideum, either with or without C1-C2 instability and who have neither symptoms nor neurologic signs, may be managed with clinical and radiographic surveillance. We feel that this suggested treatment ignores the likelihood of future spinal cord injury. Delayed spinal cord injury is a potentially disastrous consequence of an untreated os odontoideum. The biomechanics of the region predict that the absence of an intact odontoid process would create an unstable situation and put the spinal cord at risk in moderate trauma. We are aware of two patients who had been previously diagnosed with os odontoideum and who subsequently sustained additional trauma and became paralyzed. Therefore, the treatment we recommend is posterior fusion, usually using C1-C2 transarticular screws and autologous bone grafting to achieve arthrodesis. This approach has the highest fusion rate and should remove the risk of injury to the spinal cord. Direct anterior screw fixation is usually not an option in os odontoideum because the condition likely results from a remote injury, and there is virtually no chance of achieving a fusion with the direct screw fixation technique.

CONCLUSION

Odontoid fractures are a common injury to the cervical spine. The classification scheme constructed by Anderson and D'Alonzo in 1974 (21) has proven to be useful with minor modifications. In general, type II and shallow type III odontoid fractures are the most common fractures and are often best treated with surgery. Of the surgical techniques available, direct anterior screw fixation appears to be the best option. Retention of the normal rotation of the cervical spine, a rapid return to normal lifestyle, and a high fusion rate are all advantages of this procedure if it is performed when the fracture is reasonably fresh (i.e., less than 6 months old). Remote fractures of the odontoid and os odontoideum should be treated with posterior C1-C2 transarticular screw fixation with arthrodesis. Posterior fixation, preceded by transoral odontoid resection if ventral spinal cord compression is present, may be required for irreducible odontoid fractures. Because delayed neurologic compromise is a well-established danger of dens fractures, physicians should be aware of appropriate treatment measures.

REFERENCES

1. Greene KA, Dickman CA, Marciano FF, et al. Acute axis fractures. Analysis of management and outcome in 340 consecutive cases. *Spine* 1997;22:1843–1852.
2. Crockard HA, Heilman AE, Stevens JM. Progressive myelopathy secondary to odontoid fractures: clinical, radiological, and surgical features. *J Neurosurg* 1993;78:579–586.
3. Ogden JA. Radiology of postnatal skeletal development. XII. The second cervical vertebra. *Skeletal Radiol* 1984;12:169–177.
4. Wilting J, Ebensperger C, Muller TS, et al. Pax-1 in the development of the cervico-occipital transitional zone. *Anat Embryol (Berl)* 1995; 192:221–227.
5. Schiff DC, Parke WW. The arterial supply of the odontoid process. *J Bone Joint Surg Am* 1973;55:1450–1456.
6. Parke WW. The vascular relations of the upper cervical vertebrae. *Orthop Clin North Am* 1978;9:879–889.
7. Haffajee MR. A contribution by the ascending pharyngeal artery to the arterial supply of the odontoid process of the axis vertebra. *Clin Anat* 1997;10:14–18.
8. Althoff B, Goldie IF. The arterial supply of the odontoid process of the axis. *Acta Orthop Scand* 1977;48:622–629.
9. Sherk HH, Dawoud S. Congenital os odontoideum with Klippel-Feil anomaly and fatal atlanto-axial instability. Report of a case. *Spine* 1981;6:42–45.
10. Schatzker J, Rorabeck CH, Waddell JP. Non-union of the odontoid process. An experimental investigation. *Clin Orthop* 1975;108:127–137.
11. Schatzker J, Rorabeck CH, Waddell JP. Fractures of the dens (odontoid process). An analysis of thirty-seven cases. *J Bone Joint Surg Br* 1971;53:392–405.
12. Dvorak J, Schneider E, Saldinger P, et al. Biomechanics of the craniocervical region: the alar and transverse ligaments. *J Orthop Res* 1988; 6:452–461.
13. White AA, Panjabi MM. *Clinical biomechanics of the spine*, 2nd ed. Philadelphia: Lippincott, 1990.
14. Fielding JW, Hensinger RN, Hawkins RJ. Os odontoideum. *J Bone Joint Surg Am* 1980;62:376–383.
15. Apfelbaum RI, Lonser RR, Veres R, et al. Direct anterior screw fixation for recent and remote odontoid fractures. *J Neurosurg* 2000;93(Suppl 2):227–236.
16. Borne GM, Bedou GL, Pinaudeau M, et al. Odontoid process fracture osteosynthesis with a direct screw fixation technique in nine consecutive cases. *J Neurosurg* 1988;68:223–226.

17. Dickson H, Engel S, Blum P, et al. Odontoid fractures, systemic disease and conservative care. *Aust N Z J Surg* 1984;54:243–247.
18. Fujii E, Kobayashi K, Hirabayashi K. Treatment in fractures of the odontoid process. *Spine* 1988;13:604–609.
19. Husby J, Sorensen KH. Fracture of the odontoid process of the axis. *Acta Orthop Scand* 1974;45:182–192.
20. Paradis GR, Janes JM. Posttraumatic atlantoaxial instability: the fate of the odontoid process fracture in 46 cases. *J Trauma* 1973;13:359–367.
21. Anderson LD, D'Alonzo RT. Fractures of the odontoid process of the axis. *J Bone Joint Surg Am* 1974;56:1663–1674.
22. Scott EW, Haid RW Jr, Peace D. Type I fractures of the odontoid process: implications for atlanto-occipital instability. Case report. *J Neurosurg* 1990;72:488–492.
23. Hadley MN, Browner CM, Liu SS, et al. New subtype of acute odontoid fractures (type IIA). *Neurosurgery* 1988;22(1 Pt 1):67–71.
24. Henry AD, Bohly J, Grosse A. Fixation of odontoid fractures by an anterior screw. *J Bone Joint Surg Br* 1999;81:472–477.
25. Apuzzo ML, Heiden JS, Weiss MH, et al. Acute fractures of the odontoid process. An analysis of 45 cases. *J Neurosurg* 1978;48:85–91.
26. Althoff B. Fracture of the odontoid process. An experimental and clinical study. *Acta Orthop Scand Suppl* 1979;177:1–95.
27. Spierings EL, Braakman R. The management of os odontoideum. Analysis of 37 cases. *J Bone Joint Surg Br* 1982;64:422–428.
28. Matsui H, Imada K, Tsuji H. Radiographic classification of os odontoideum and its clinical significance. *Spine* 1997;22:1706–1709.
29. Clements WD, Mezue W, Mathew B. Os odontoideum—congenital or acquired?—that's not the question. *Injury* 1995;26:640–642.
30. Shirasaki N, Okada K, Oka S, et al. Os odontoideum with posterior atlantoaxial instability. *Spine* 1991;16:706–715.
31. Deliganis AV, Baxter AB, Hanson JA, et al. Radiologic spectrum of craniocervical distraction injuries. *Radiographics* 2000;20(Spec No):S237–S250.
32. Nepper-Rasmussen J. CT of dens axis fractures. *Neuroradiology* 1989;31:104–106.
33. Dickman CA, Sonntag VK. Injuries involving the transverse atlantal ligament: classification and treatment guidelines based upon experience with 39 injuries. *Neurosurgery* 1997;40:886–887.
34. Bucholz RW, Burkhead WZ, Graham W, et al. Occult cervical spine injuries in fatal traffic accidents. *J Trauma* 1979;19:768–771.
35. Huelke DF, O'Day J, Mendelsohn RA. Cervical injuries suffered in automobile crashes. *J Neurosurg* 1981;54:316–322.
36. Fairholm D, Lee ST, Lui TN. Fractured odontoid: the management of delayed neurological symptoms. *Neurosurgery* 1996;38:38–43.
37. Sherk HH. Fractures of the atlas and odontoid process. *Orthop Clin North Am* 1978;9:973–984.
38. Moskovich R, Crockard HA. Myelopathy due to hypertrophic nonunion of the dens: case report. *J Trauma* 1990;30:222–225.
39. Bohlman HH. Acute fractures and dislocations of the cervical spine. An analysis of three hundred hospitalized patients and review of the literature. *J Bone Joint Surg Am* 1979;61:1119–1142.
40. Julien TD, Frankel B, Traynelis VC, et al. Evidence-based analysis of odontoid fracture management. *Neurosurg Focus* 2000;8(Article 1).
41. Traynelis VC. Evidence-based management of type II odontoid fractures. *Clin Neurosurg* 1997;44:41–49.
42. Maiman DJ, Larson SJ. Management of odontoid fractures. *Neurosurgery* 1982;11:820.
43. Lind B, Nordwall A, Sihlbom H. Odontoid fractures treated with halovest. *Spine* 1987;12:173–177.
44. Ekong CE, Schwartz ML, Tator CH, et al. Odontoid fracture: management with early mobilization using the halo device. *Neurosurgery* 1981;9:631–637.
45. Hadley MN, Browner C, Sonntag VK. Axis fractures: a comprehensive review of management and treatment in 107 cases. *Neurosurgery* 1985;17:281–290.
46. Wang GJ, Mabie KN, Whitehill R, et al. The nonsurgical management of odontoid fractures in adults. *Spine* 1984;9:229–230.
47. Clark CR, White AA 3rd. Fractures of the dens. A multicenter study. *J Bone Joint Surg Am* 1985;67:1340–1348.
48. Dickman CA, Sonntag VK, Papadopoulos SM, et al. The interspinous method of posterior atlantoaxial arthrodesis. *J Neurosurg* 1991;74:190–198.
49. Fielding JW, Hawkins RJ, Ratzan SA. Spine fusion for atlanto-axial instability. *J Bone Joint Surg Am* 1976;58:400–407.
50. Jeanneret B, Magerl F. Primary posterior fusion C1/2 in odontoid fractures: indications, technique, and results of transarticular screw fixation. *J Spinal Disord* 1992;5:464–475.
51. Dickman CA, Sonntag VK. Posterior C1-C2 transarticular screw fixation for atlantoaxial arthrodesis. *Neurosurgery* 1998;43:275–281.
52. Marcotte P, Dickman CA, Sonntag VK, et al. Posterior atlantoaxial facet screw fixation. *J Neurosurg* 1993;79:234–237.
53. Stillerman CB, Wilson JA. Atlanto-axial stabilization with posterior transarticular screw fixation: technical description and report of 22 cases. *Neurosurgery* 1993;32:948–955.
54. Grob D, Jeanneret B, Aebi M, et al. Atlanto-axial fusion with transarticular screw fixation. *J Bone Joint Surg Br* 1991;73:972–976.
55. Harms J, Melcher RP. Posterior C1-C2 fusion with polyaxial screw and rod fixation. *Spine* 2001;26:2467–2471.
56. Apfelbaum RI. Lasso cabling technique to achieve C1-2 posterior fusion in absence of C1 posterior arch. Presented at the Joint Section on Disorders of the Spine and Peripheral Nerves AANS/CNS Tenth Annual Meeting, 1994.
57. Apfelbaum RI. Anterior screw fixation of odontoid fractures. In: Camins MB, O'Leary PF, eds. *Disorders of the cervical spine*, 2nd ed. Baltimore: Williams and Wilkins, 1992:603–608.
58. Esses SI, Bednar DA. Screw fixation of odontoid fractures and nonunions. *Spine* 1991;16(Suppl 10):S483–S485.
59. Geisler FH, Cheng C, Poka A, et al. Anterior screw fixation of posteriorly displaced type II odontoid fractures. *Neurosurgery* 1989;25:30–38.
60. Lesoin F, Autricque A, Franz K, et al. Transcervical approach and screw fixation for upper cervical spine pathology. *Surg Neurol* 1987;27:459–465.
61. Bohler J. Anterior stabilization for acute fractures and non-unions of the dens. *J Bone Joint Surg Am* 1982;64:18–27.
62. Nakanishi T. Internal fixation of the odontoid fracture. *Cent Jpn J Orthop Traumatic Surg* 1980;23:399–406.
63. Apfelbaum RI. Anterior screw fixation of odontoid fractures. In: Rengachary SS, Wilkins RH, eds. *Neurosurgical operative atlas,* 2nd ed. Baltimore: Williams and Wilkins, 1992:189–199.
64. Aebi M, Etter C, Coscia M. Fractures of the odontoid process. Treatment with anterior screw fixation. *Spine* 1989;14:1065–1070.
65. Montesano PX, Anderson PA, Schlehr F, et al. Odontoid fractures treated by anterior odontoid screw fixation. *Spine* 1991;16(Suppl 3):S33–S37.
66. Dunn ME, Seljeskog EL. Experience in the management of odontoid process injuries: an analysis of 128 cases. *Neurosurgery* 1986;18:306–310.
67. Hadley MN, Dickman CA, Browner CM, et al. Acute axis fractures: a review of 229 cases. *J Neurosurg* 1989;71(5 Pt 1):642–647.
68. Sherk HH, Nicholson JT, Chung SM. Fractures of the odontoid process in young children. *J Bone Joint Surg Am* 1978;60:921–924.
69. Mandabach M, Ruge JR, Hahn YS, et al. Pediatric axis fractures: early halo immobilization, management and outcome. *Pediatr Neurosurg* 1993;19:225–232.
70. Odent T, Langlais J, Glorion C, et al. Fractures of the odontoid process: a report of 15 cases in children younger than 6 years. *J Pediatr Orthop* 1999;19:51–54.
71. Pitzen T, Caspar W, Steudel WI, et al. Dens fracture in elderly patients and surgical management. *Aktuelle Traumatol* 1994;24:56–59.
72. Pepin JW, Bourne RB, Hawkins RJ. Odontoid fractures, with special reference to the elderly patient. *Clin Orthop* 1985;193:178–183.
73. Hanigan WC, Powell FC, Elwood PW, et al. Odontoid fractures in elderly patients. *J Neurosurg* 1993;78:32–35.
74. Andersson S, Rodrigues M, Olerud C. Odontoid fractures: high complication rate associated with anterior screw fixation in the elderly. *Eur Spine J* 2000;9:56–60.
75. Lennarson PJ, Mostafavi H, Traynelis VC, et al. Management of type II dens fractures: a case-control study. *Spine* 2000;25:1234–1237.
76. Schaffler MB, Alson MD, Heller JG, et al. Morphology of the dens. A quantitative study. *Spine* 1992;17:738–743.
77. Jenkins JD, Coric D, Branch CL Jr. A clinical comparison of one- and two-screw odontoid fixation. *J Neurosurg* 1998;89:366–370.
78. Chiba K, Fujimura Y, Toyama Y, et al. Treatment protocol for fractures of the odontoid process. *J Spinal Disord* 1996;9:267–276.
79. Crockard HA, Calder I, Ransford AO. One-stage transoral decompression and posterior fixation in rheumatoid atlanto-axial subluxation. *J Bone Joint Surg Br* 1990;72:682–685.
80. Crockard HA. Anterior approaches to lesions of the upper cervical spine. *Clin Neurosurg* 1988;34:389–416.
81. Crockard HA. Transoral surgery: some lessons learned. *Br J Neurosurg* 1995;9:283–293.

CHAPTER 46

Traumatic Spondylolisthesis of the Axis: "Hangman's Fracture"

Alan M. Levine and Alan Dacre

Death by hanging is an event that has fascinated people for well over a thousand years. Since the introduction of hanging to Western civilization sometime before the tenth century, there has been an effort to produce "the ideal lesion." A variety of methods have been used to perfect the technique so that the victim dies by fracture of the C2 vertebra with transection of the spinal cord and not by either strangulation or decapitation. From early times, the knot was placed in a suboccipital location; but with too short of a drop, asphyxiation might occur by strangulation. When a longer drop became commonplace, occasionally the head was severed from the body.

The first known scientific evidence published in the medical literature of the actual method of injury to the spine was by Reverend S. Houghton in 1866 (1), when he described the fracture dislocation that occurred by execution of criminals. He went so far as to devise a table based on the criminal's weight to calculate the length of the drop necessary to achieve an appropriate execution. It was later demonstrated that a force of 1,260 foot-pounds was necessary to fracture the spine, resulting in death without any extreme trauma to the neck. Based on that, it was decided by the British Commonwealth that the length of the drop could be determined by dividing 1,260 foot-pounds by the weight of the body of the victim in pounds. Marshall (2) in 1888 was the first to propose that hyperextension along with some distraction was in fact the mechanism of injury, resulting in disruption of the spinal cord. He also suggested that a submental placement of the knot was critically important to achieve this hyperextension mechanism.

Frederick Wood-Jones, an anatomist, examined the bony lesions caused by hanging from two different series of specimens. The first were skulls from the Nubian period that had fractures along the base of the skull through the basilar suture lines. He also examined skulls from a series of specimens collected by Captain C. Frasier, who was the one-time superintendent of the Ragoon Central Jail. All these skulls showed a fracture through the second cervical vertebra, and it was known that all were hanged using a submental knot position. He determined that the knot position was critical for determining whether strangulation or fracture of the cervical spine occurred, and that it was necessary to put the knot in a submental position beneath the chin so that in all cases the fracture occurred through the second cervical vertebra. He stated that "it is to be noted the odontoid process plays no part in producing death." The mechanism of death is that the posterior arch of the axis is snapped off and remains fixed to the third cervical vertebra while the dens process and anterior arch of the atlas remain fixed to the skull. This traumatic lesion is caused by the violent hyperextension of the neck causing instantaneous severing of the spinal cord (3–6).

These bipedicular fractures of the second cervical vertebra, sometimes called *periarticular fractures*, have been of extreme interest for more than a century. The term for this particular type of fracture has varied and included *traumatic spondylolisthesis of the axis* (7–14), *fractures of the axis arch* (15), *fractures of the ring of the axis* (16), *fractures of the neural arch* (17), and *hangman's fractures* (13,18–23). In fact, the lesion that is currently seen bears little relationship to that which caused such great fascination, the fracture from judicial hanging. Most current injuries are the direct result of motor vehicle trauma (24,25). It became clear with the increase in vehicular trauma during the twentieth century that this lesion was radiographically similar to those of judicial hanging in terms of the location of the fracture, but the similarity ended there. Early articles (26) attributed the vehicular lesion to the same mechanism, but there were many differences, including the fact that the rate of neurologic deficit was nowhere near similar. The currently accepted term, *traumatic spondylolisthesis of the axis,* was attributed to Garber (27). Subsequently, however, some authors have continued to use the inappropriate term *hangman's fracture* (28).

ANATOMY

The axis (second cervical vertebra) is anatomically extremely different from the five lower cervical vertebrae as well as the atlas above it. The upper cervical unit (occiput-

C1–C2) has been designated the cervicocranium (21) to denote its functioning as a separate unit from the lower cervical spine. Probably the most distinguishing anatomic feature of the axis is the position of the two sets of facet joints. The inferior articular processes are actually posterolateral to the spinal canal and line up with those of the lower cervical spine, whereas the superior articular processes of C2 are anterolateral and line up with those of C1 and the occiput (Fig. 46.1). The pars interarticularis is elongated and func-

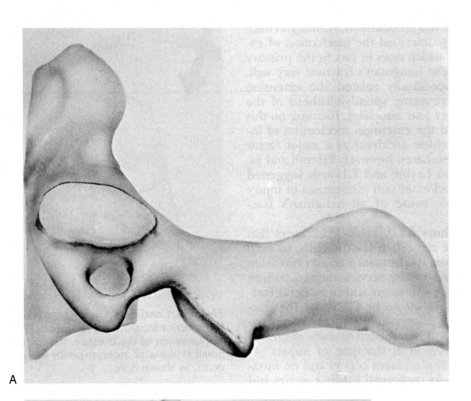

A

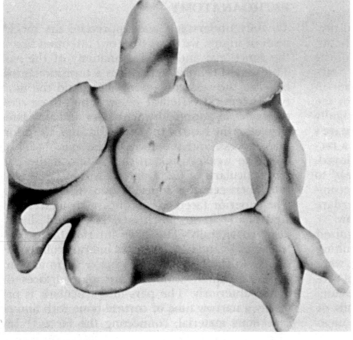

B

FIG. 46.1. A: This lateral view of the C2 vertebra demonstrates the unique relationship of the pars interarticularis to the C1-C2 and C2-C3 articulations. The former are anterior to the spinal canal and biconcave with a slight lateral tilt. The latter are posterolateral to the spinal canal and are oriented similar to the remainder of the joints in the lower cervical spinal. **B:** This oblique view shows the unique relationship of the dens process and the relatively thin anatomic structure of the pars interarticularis.

tions as a junction between the upper and lower cervical spines. The superior articular processes are biconcave and slightly laterally oriented.

The occipitocervical joint allows only flexion and extension (29), whereas the atlantoaxial joints allow flexion, extension, rotation, and vertical approximation as well as lateral gliding. Some of the motions in this complex joint are coupled motions. The predominant motion of the saddle-shaped atlantoaxial joint is rotation, and it contributes about 50% of the total rotation of the cervical spine (29,30). The C2-C3 joint contributes little to the total motion of the cervical spine. The connecting pars interarticularis is primarily a thin tube of cortical bone with only a small amount of cancellous bone and a limited diameter (14).

The axis is both biomechanically and developmentally quite unique. Specifically, the dens process results from the fusion of the axis with the remnant of the body of the atlas. There are strong capsular attachments across the facet joints at the atlantoaxial level as well as some residual components of the anterior longitudinal ligament. In addition, C2 and C1 are directly attached to the skull by the alar, apical, and transverse ligaments. It is this entire complex, with the structure of C2 intimately linked to the base of the skull, that makes this upper area function as a unit, the cervicocranium (21).

The pars is truly a transitional structure, and when marked force is imparted to the skull, it may be directly imparted to this particular transitional area of bone. The weakest part of the entire complex, however, is the area of the posterior arch of C1, which is thinned in the area where the vertebral artery crosses over it. Interestingly, the vertebral artery passes through the body of C2 through the foramen transversarium, which is adjacent to the pars and is another mechanically weak area. The atypical hangman's fracture seems to enter this particular area.

A final important anatomic consideration is that the diameter of the canal at C2 is quite generous. The canal-to-cord ratio is extremely large in the entire upper cervical spine, but the ratio begins to change at about the level of the C2-3 disc. One of the reasons for the minimal incidence of neurologic deficits in vehicular traumatic spondylolisthesis of the axis is the large and forgiving nature of the canal at C2.

CLASSIFICATION AND MECHANISM OF INJURY

Although many attempts have been made at devising a universal classification system for the entire spine, this effort has not been productive. Interestingly, even in those classifications that have attempted to deal with the cervical spine alone, the upper cervical spine has managed to elude classification within those systems. Therefore, classification systems unique to traumatic spondylolisthesis of the axis have been diverse. These have been based on the usual categorizations: (a) anatomic/radiologic, (b) mechanism of injury, and (c) the extent of residual instability. An attempt was made by Francis and associates (31) to translate White

and Panjabi's (32) characteristics for instability of the lower cervical spine into a useful classification for the instability related to traumatic spondylolisthesis, but it has not been widely accepted. The classification used by White and Panjabi in the most recent edition of *Clinical Biomechanics of the Spine* (32) uses a stability/instability classification for treatment along with consideration of the neurologic status and the integrity of the facet joints. Although it is an attempt to categorize by combining neurologic injury with stability, it fails to account for the mechanism of injury and thus omits an important factor in this particular injury; therefore, it is of little help in deciding upon the nature of the treatment for any individual injury.

The classification proposed by Effendi and colleagues (16) and later modified by Levine and Edwards (9) was based on an understanding of the biomechanics of the injury; from that framework, treatment regimens were established (Table 46.1). Because most injuries today occur as a result of motor vehicle accidents, there is little doubt that the basic mechanism of the injury is that of rapid deceleration of the motor vehicle so that the patient's head is thrown forward, usually striking the windshield. This generally subjects the spine to some degree of axial loading, and more importantly in this particular scenario, to hyperextension after impact. Some of the early authors who dealt with this injury seemed to think that this extension mechanism could account for all degrees and types of fractures (7,10,16,21,33); it became apparent, however, that hyperextension and axial load could not be the sole mechanisms for this injury (9–12,16,34).

Some earlier authors believed that continued hyperextension was the cause of increased displacement resulting in rupture of the anterior longitudinal ligament (ALL) (21,32). The hypothesized mechanism was that the hyperextension and axial load caused fracture of the posterior arch. Once that fracture occurred, continuation of this same force on the entire occiput and upper cervical spine caused further extension, with resultant disruption of the ALL and the disc. Occasionally, an avulsion fracture occurred from the anterior superior portion of C3 with the ALL rupture, causing the observed instability. With total disruption of this complex, multidirectional instability could result in subluxation anteriorly and perhaps in some cases posteriorly. It was evident to later authors, however, that a coupling of forces rather than a single extension force was necessary to create the majority of different patterns of injuries. The single force is better related to the mechanism of judicial hanging, whereas the force coupling theory better accounts for the observed pathologic entities (9,10,12,16,20,35).

Although few biomechanical studies have been done to replicate injuries to C2, Teo and associates (36) suggested that the extent of restraint of the posterior elements of C2 could affect the type of fracture produced. A shear force was directed at the odontoid, and either an odontoid fracture or a pars fracture was obtained. When there was less restraint of the C2 posterior elements, a pars fracture occurred; with more restraint, a dens fracture occurred.

TABLE 46.1. *Modified Effendi Classification*

Type	Characteristics	Mechanism
I	Vertical bilateral pars fracture < 3 mm translation No angulation Stable	Hyper-extension, axial load
IA–atypical	Fracture anterior to facets bilateral No angulation < 3 mm translation Fracture line not parallel on x-ray Apparent elongation of pars and body Stable	Hyper-extension, lateral bending
II	Vertical bilateral pars fracture >3 mm translation Compression of anterior C3 Significant angulation of fracture site Potentially unstable	Hyper-extension followed by flexion
IIA	Oblique bilateral pars fracture No compression of anterior C3 Significant angulation Minimal translation Unstable	Flexion distraction, pars fails in tension
III	Type I pars fracture with Unilateral or bilateral facet dislocation Rare disc herniation Unstable	Flexion distraction → hyper-extension

The classification most commonly used today is based on determining the amount of angulation and translation between C2 and C3 (Table 46.1). Angulation is measured by determining the angles between the inferior end plate of the second cervical vertebra and that of the third cervical vertebra. Translation is determined by measuring the distance from the posterior aspect of the third cervical vertebral body and the posterior aspect of the second cervical vertebra at the level of the C2-3 disc. Effendi and colleagues (16) described three major categories of injuries. Levine initially described four patterns (9,10,12), and several authors have described a fifth atypical type (34,37) (Table 46.1).

Type I fracture (Fig. 46.2) is through the neural arch just posterior to the body. Bilateral pars fractures occur at the same portion of the neural arch and are oriented in an almost purely vertical direction in the coronal plane. On lateral roentgenogram, the fracture lines are usually evident. On the initial roentgenogram (Fig. 46.2B), these fractures usually demonstrate less than 3 mm of translation and no angulation. Typically, they are the result of hyperextension and axial load with forces only sufficient to fracture the neural arch. This type of fracture usually does not result in any injuries to the disc or ligamentous structures, nor is it severe enough to lead to significant translation or angulation. To classify a fracture as a type I injury in a neurologically intact patient, a supervised flexion-extension roentgenogram should be done with the patient in the sitting position. In the supine position (the position in which most initial radiographs are taken), the head normally rests in extension, which can cause a type II fracture to reduce and therefore mistakenly be classified as a type I injury. Therefore, inclu-

sion in this category requires the radiologic criteria plus minimal motion on flexion-extension. This relative stability may be accounted for by the fact that the disc and other ligamentous structures remain intact in a type I injury.

Type IA injuries are the most recently recognized and have been denoted as the atypical hangman's fracture. As with other type I fractures, on plain roentgenograms these injuries demonstrate little or no angulation and translation (Fig. 46.3). The fracture lines are generally not parallel (38); therefore, they may not be visible on plain roentgenograms. In fact, there is some controversy about whether this is really a separate fracture type or simply asymmetry in the fracture line of type I or occasionally type II fractures (39). They can be more easily missed than type I fractures because the fractures do not overlap and are not seen on lateral roentgenograms. The most common roentgenographic feature is that of apparent elongation of the C2 body, with perhaps 2 to 3 mm of anterior translation when examining the anterior aspects of the vertebral bodies (Fig. 46.3B).

Type IA fractures are caused by a combination of forces requiring hyperextension associated with lateral bending, creating the asymmetric fracture line. The injury is evaluated most easily with axial images on a computed tomography (CT) scan, where the fracture lines can be better appreciated (Fig. 46.3C). Because the fracture line is oblique, one arm may extend into the vertebral body of C2 (often through the foramen transversarium) (Fig. 46.3C), with the contralateral fracture more posterior in the neural arch. On flexion-extension roentgenograms, these injuries are often demonstrated to be stable. Starr and Eismont (37), however, described two patients with some increased angulation and translation. Samaha and col-

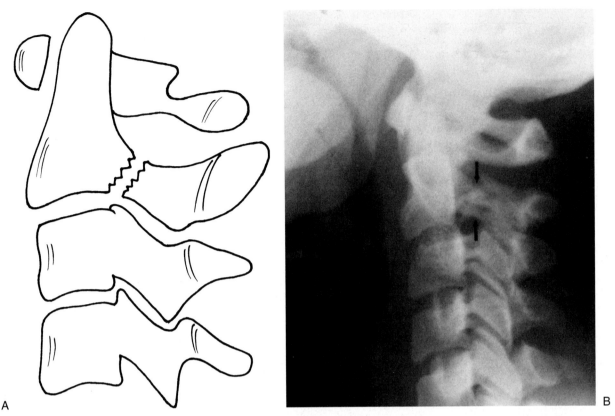

FIG. 46.2. The drawing **(A)** and lateral roentgenogram **(B)** demonstrate the essential features of a type I injury. The fracture line is predominantly vertical in the pars (*arrows*), with minimal separation of the fragments. The hyperextension and axial load mechanism that causes the fracture does not result in any significant angulation or translation.

leagues (39) have also demonstrated that a significant number of pars fractures will be asymmetrical and that this has no relation to stability or whether it is a type I or type II fracture. They felt that the obliquity of the fracture line should not be taken into account when determining treatment.

Type II injuries should be separated into two groups: type II and type IIA. Type II fractures are recognized by the fact that they have more than 3 mm of translation and significant angulation across the fracture site (Fig. 46.4). The amount of angulation and translation depends on two factors. The first is the position in which the roentgenogram is taken. With the patient supine, the cervical spine often falls into slight extension, and the fracture partially reduces. The second factor that determines initial displacement is the amount of force transmitted to the disc during the injury, with the amount of disruption related to the extent of forward translation. The type II injury is a combination injury, with the initial force being hyperextension and axial loading that causes the fracture to the neural arch in a pattern similar to that of a type I injury. Most of these are symmetric vertical fractures through the pars in the coronal plane just posterior to the vertebral body. The second force, flexion, occurs after disruption of the posterior arch and causes disruption of the disc from posterior to anterior. The ALL is generally stripped off the superior aspect of the C3 body (but not disrupted), and a crushing injury occurs to the anterior superior corner of C3 by the inferior aspect of the C2 body (Fig. 46.4B). This combined mechanism is quite compatible with vehicular trauma, during which the patient's neck first extends and then, with deceleration, flexes. The instability of this fracture is related to the combined mechanism, with extension causing only the fracture but the flexion component causing disruption of the disc, often with stripping of the ligament, thus allowing anterior subluxation of C2 over C3.

It was originally suggested that this fracture was the result of continued hyperextension after the original extension injury, but this mechanism cannot be justified on the basis of several clinical features. The continued hyperextension mechanism should result in a rupture of the ALL (21). Therefore, anterior compression of the superior aspect of the C3 body should not occur. In addition, if the ALL were ruptured, longitudinal traction and extension would not cause reduction of type II injuries. If that were so, widening of the disc space should be observed in most patients with this injury. Clinically, that is not the case, and in fact, reduction can be accomplished with 30 pounds of traction and slight extension. In addition, if hyperextension were the primary mechanism, the posterior longitudinal ligament and the posterior aspect of the disc would be spared and thus marked translational instability could not occur.

Type IIA injuries are an important variant (Fig. 46.5). Little or no translation is seen, but significant angulation

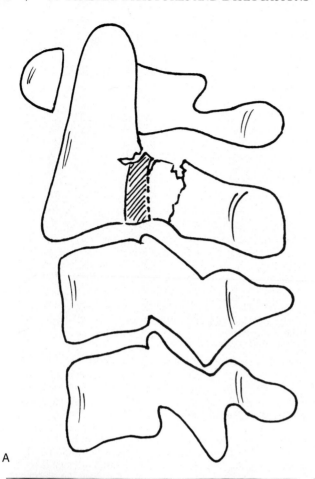

A

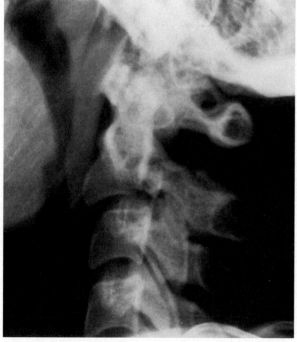

B

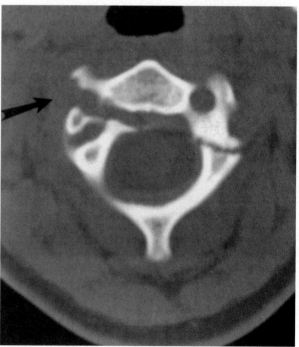

C

FIG. 46.3. A, B: Type IA or atypical traumatic spondylolisthesis of the axis is the result of hyperextension and lateral bending. Similar to standard type I fractures, there is little angulation or translation. The lateral plain roentgenogram **(B)** does not readily demonstrate the fracture line, as it is oblique, but it can be recognized by the irregularity of the superior surface of the pars. In addition, there is apparent elongation of the vertebral body and the pars, often with a 2- to 3-mm step-off at the anterior surface of the bodies between C2 and C3. **C.** Computed tomography scan best reveals the fracture line, which is oblique and may enter the foramen transversarium (*arrow*).

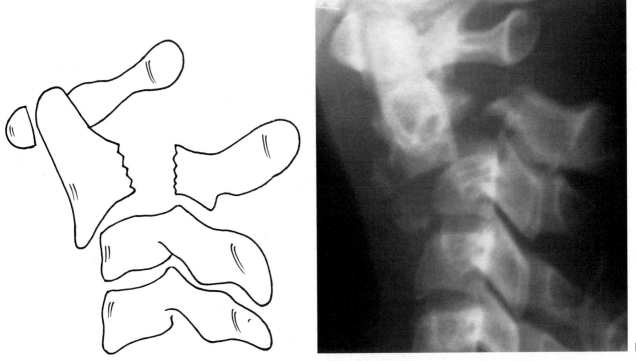

A

B

FIG. 46.4. Type II fractures, as shown in both the drawing **(A)** and the roentgenogram **(B)**, have a relatively vertical fracture line with wide separation of the fragments. The fracture through the pars is created by the same mechanism as a type I fracture (hyperextension and axial load), but the displacement is the result of a secondary flexion force. In most type II fractures, flexion also results in slight compression of the anterior superior corner of the C3 body or, as in this case, avulsion of the corner in continuity with the anterior longitudinal ligament. All type II fractures have both angulation and translation of C2 over C3.

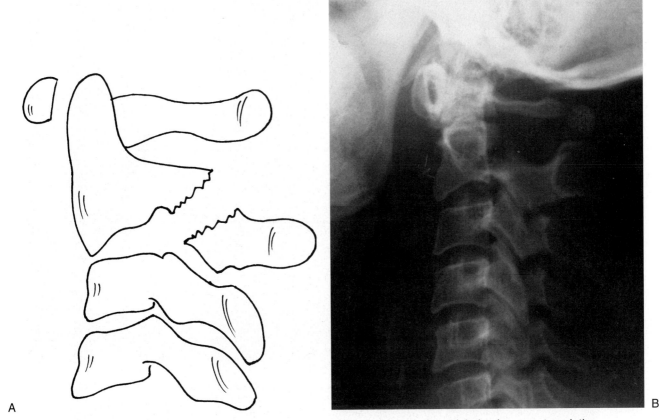

A

B

FIG. 46.5. Type IIA fractures are an important variant. As shown, these injuries have no translation but have significant angulation. In addition, the orientation of the fracture line differs from all the other injuries. This fracture line is oblique, going from anterior-inferior in the pars to posterior-superior. The injury is the result of flexion and distraction, with the pars failing in tension.

often is seen, even with the neck in an extended position. Angulation in this injury can exceed 15 degrees, whereas translation is rarely more than 3 mm. An important distinguishing radiographic feature of type IIA injuries is the direction of the fracture line (Fig. 46.5). Instead of being vertical in the coronal plane at the junction of the pedicle and the posterior aspect of the body, it is most often oblique, running from anterior-inferior to posterior-superior along the length of the pars interarticularis. If interlocking of the fragments occurs related to the direction of the fracture line, the angulation may be maintained. The injury is the direct result of flexion distraction forces. The posterior arch fails in tension, and the disc fails from posterior to anterior, usually leaving the ALL intact. Since there is no axial load or flexion force, there is no crushing of the anterior-superior corner of the C3 body. If patients with these injuries are placed in traction, the angulation will be accentuated because the mechanism is flexion distraction. This injury caused confusion for a number of authors because in those patients who were placed in traction, there was apparent widening of the disc space. This injury is relatively

infrequent, occurring in fewer than 10% of patients with traumatic spondylolisthesis (9,32).

The final type of injury pattern described is a type III fracture (Fig. 46.6), which has been reported to occur in a number of configurations (9–11,16,35); however, the most common form of this injury is a type I pars fracture pattern associated with a bilateral facet dislocation at C2-C3. Other potential patterns include unilateral facet fractures combined with a contralateral neural arch fracture. The critical feature of this injury is that in its classic form the posterior arch of C2 is a free-floating fragment. Because the inferior facets of C2 are dislocated with concomitant posterior ligamentous disruption between C2-C3 combined with fractures across the more proximal portion of the pars, the facet dislocation cannot be reduced closed. This is the only injury that requires operative intervention. The mechanisms of these injuries are unclear. It is conceivable that they result from a flexion distraction injury causing the bilateral facet dislocation, followed sequentially by a hyperextension force causing the traumatic spondylolisthesis. Application of the mechanism in the reverse fashion would not account for the

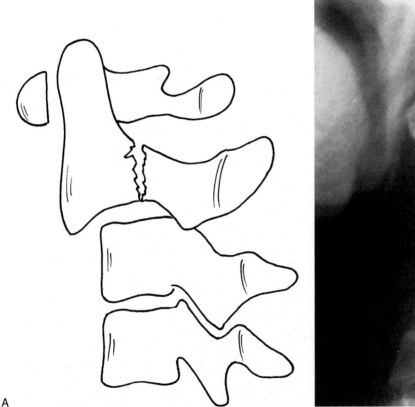

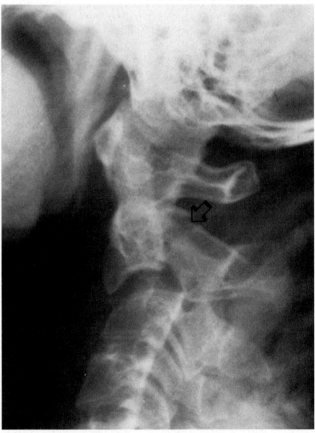

FIG. 46.6. Type III fractures are a combined injury, with a "type I" fracture through the pars but a bilateral or unilateral injury to the facets behind it. In both the drawing **(A)** and the roentgenogram **(B)**, note the fracture through the pars (*arrow*). The mechanism of injury is probably an initial flexion distraction force to create and lock the bilateral facet dislocation, followed by a hyperextension and axial load injury to create the pars fracture. If the pars fracture occurred first, it would be impossible to create the bilateral facet dislocation behind it.

facet dislocation, as there should be no connection between the body of C2 and inferior facets of C2 in that particular combination.

Finally, another group of injuries also can be described as traumatic spondylolisthesis of C2-C3, but these patients do not have bipedicular fractures. These are bilateral laminar fractures of the C2 or bilateral facet fractures of the inferior facets of C2, and may be mistaken for type II traumatic spondylolisthesis (40) but are really "look-alikes." As a result of a flexion or shear mechanism, they are highly unstable and can cause rather dramatic spondylolisthesis. They also may be associated with significant C2-3 discal injury, and like any other facet fracture or dislocation, may be associated with herniation of the C2-3 disc.

RADIOGRAPHIC EVALUATION

Patients presenting to either an emergency department or a trauma unit with traumatic spondylolisthesis of the axis fall into two categories. Because most patients are neurologically intact and usually awake and alert with an isolated cervical spine injury, they can be treated and evaluated like any other patient with a history of spinal trauma. After a general assessment, the most appropriate initial study is a lateral supine cervical spine roentgenogram, which will delineate the injury in most cases.

The second group of patients is those sustaining polytrauma, most commonly with head trauma. They may be uncooperative or totally obtunded, and the cervical spine injury will be evaluated through a routine radiographic trauma series, which will usually include a lateral cervical spine roentgenogram. For traumatic spondylolisthesis, the orientation of the cervical spine on this roentgenogram is the most important factor. The position of the cervical spine in the supine position is commonly lordotic, but the state of reduction of the fracture will depend on the habitus of the patient. The fracture will almost always be visualized, because the C1-C2-C3 complex can usually be visualized radiographically irrespective of the body habitus. If, however, the patient has an extremely large body relative to his or her head or extremely large shoulders, the neck will be in relatively more extension, and therefore the type of traumatic spondylolisthesis may be difficult to determine on a lateral roentgenogram. The patient may have a type II fracture, but because of the relative extension in which the film was taken, it may appear to be a type I fracture (Fig. 46.7). If, on the other hand, the patient is a child and has a relatively large occiput relative to the shoulders or body, the initial roentgenogram may actually be taken in slight flexion, thus accentuating the deformity. Because it is a posterior element injury, rarely is the anterior soft tissue shadow increased. If the soft tissue shadow is in fact increased, some suspicion should be entertained that there is also an injury to the anterior column. The only injury type where the fracture lines are not clearly seen on the lateral roentgenogram is the atypical, or type IA, hangman's fracture, where

because of the obliquity, the fracture lines may not be evident. In this case, the tip-off is that there is an apparent translation, or widening, of the C2 body with reference to the C3 body; in that case, a CT scan should be ordered to define the injury.

In patients who are neurologically intact and who are thought to have a type I traumatic spondylolisthesis of the axis, the next roentgenographic study ordered should be a physician-supervised flexion-extension roentgenogram. If there is compression of the anterior/superior portion of the C3 body, a suspicion should exist that in fact the fracture is a reduced type II injury, and the flexion-extension roentgenograms may show greater instability than suggested by the supine lateral view. If the patient is neurologically compromised or head injured, flexion-extension views should not be obtained. In most type I injuries, flexion-extension roentgenograms will show little motion across the fracture site. Type IA fractures, as previously noted, often need a CT scan to define the injury. It is important that the presence of a fracture through the foramen for the vertebral artery at C2 be identified. If there is any atypical or unaccountable neurologic deficit or stroke-type pattern, a digital subtraction angiogram or magnetic resonance imaging (MRI) angiogram should be done to assess the vertebral flow. In addition, in these injuries, a CT scan is helpful in determining whether there is narrowing of the canal. Type II and type IIA injuries rarely require any additional initial roentgenograms, other than a lateral cervical spine roentgenogram, to make the diagnosis.

Type III injuries, because of their association with facet disruption at C2-C3, may require either a CT scan alone or in combination with an MRI. The CT scan is necessary to help define the nature of the facet disruption. This will define whether it is a simple bilateral facet dislocation at C2-C3 or if there is a facet fracture on one or both sides and whether there is involvement of the lamina. When a bilateral facet dislocation is a component of a type III injury, the reduction of the facet dislocation will need to be done open with the patient under general anesthesia. Therefore, a preoperative MRI is suggested. A small number of patients undergoing open reduction of bilateral facet dislocations at all levels in the cervical spine have been reported to have had subsequent neurologic deficit as a result of a disc herniation. If herniation of the C2-3 disc is noted on preoperative MRI, then an anterior discectomy may be indicated prior to reduction of the facet dislocation.

A critical feature in the evaluation of patients with traumatic spondylolisthesis is to define whether there are other associated spinal injuries; thus, these patients should be carefully evaluated clinically to determine whether there are other areas of tenderness or superficial injuries. If any question exists, appropriate roentgenograms of adjacent areas of the spine should be obtained. A recent study (41) reviewed 784 patients with cervical spine injury and noted that there was a 30% incidence of multiple spinal injury in patients with spondylolisthesis of the axis. This is similar to

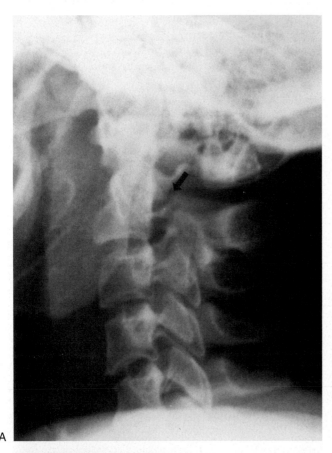

A

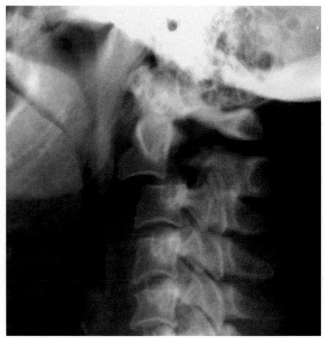

B

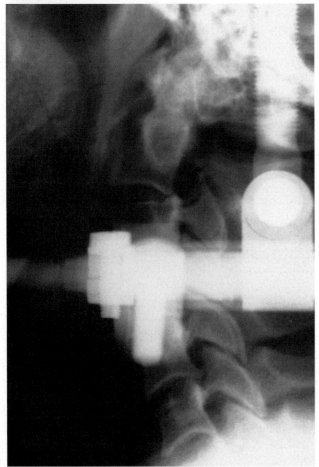

C

FIG. 46.7. This 43-year-old woman sustained this type II traumatic spondylolisthesis of the axis in a motor vehicle accident. She was neurologically intact with an isolated injury. **A:** As a result of her obesity, the initial supine lateral cervical spine roentgenogram fails to demonstrate any displacement or angulation because of the reduction of the fracture due to the extension of her neck in the supine position. **B:** After placement in a collar in the upright position for 2 weeks, significant displacement occurred and was recognized to be a type II fracture. Placement in a halo vest with initial traction resulted in adequate reduction and healing. **C:** Type I fractures in a neurologically intact patient require flexion-extension films for confirmation of stability.

a series of 335 patients who had upper cervical spine fractures, in which Levine and Fischgrund (42) reported a high rate of associated injuries, with 15.2% having two or more fractures in the upper cervical spine and 22.7% having two or more injuries anywhere in the spine. In this group, 131 patients had traumatic spondylolisthesis of the axis, of whom 29 had other cervical spine fractures. Seven had fractures in either the thoracic or the lumbar spine. In most cases, when a patient has two concurrent fractures in the cervical spine, both injuries usually have the same mechanism of injury. Because the mechanism of a type I traumatic spondylolisthesis of the axis is hyperextension and axial load, logically most combined injuries, especially in the upper cervical spine, are of a similar mechanism. Twelve patients in the series (42) had a combination of an atlas fracture (most commonly posterior arch fractures) and traumatic spondylolisthesis of the axis (Fig. 46.8). Six of the 12 patients had a type I traumatic spondylolisthesis of the axis, of whom two of the six had three upper cervical spine injuries, including a type I traumatic spondylolisthesis of the axis, a posterior arch fracture of C1, and a hyperextension teardrop fracture of C2.

Various combinations of the injuries occur, including a hyperextension teardrop fracture of C2 and a traumatic spondylolisthesis of the axis, or a posteriorly displaced dens can be associated with traumatic spondylolisthesis of the axis. Because the other types of traumatic spondylolisthesis have different mechanisms of injury, the associated injuries are also different. Type IA injuries are created by a lateral bending force combined with hyperextension. This is the same mechanism that causes lateral mass fractures in the lower cervical spine, and therefore the two occur in combination. Type II injuries have a flexion mechanism, and type IIA injuries have a flexion distraction mechanism; therefore, the injuries associated with each of these types are generally of the same mechanism.

NEUROLOGIC EVALUATION

Although traumatic spondylolisthesis of the axis frequently results from a vehicular injury, it is rarely associated with a neurologic deficit. This is one of the features that differentiates it from a judicial hanging injury, which is always associated with either death by strangulation or by severing of the spinal cord. In a study reported by Francis and associates (31) in which neurologic deficit was assessed for a large group of mixed injury types, the total prevalence of neurologic deficit was only 6.5% of patients.

When broken down according to types of injuries (9), rarely does neurologic deficit occur in type I or type II injuries except when associated with closed head injuries. Type III injuries are most commonly associated with neurologic deficit, although it has been reported (37) that the asymmetric canal narrowing associated with atypical hangman's fractures (type IA) also can result in neurologic deficit. Two patients in this series had incomplete quadriplegia, believed to be caused by cord impingement. In addition, with a type IA injury, an ischemic insult could potentially occur (34) because the lesion may, with some frequency, extend through the foramen for the vertebral artery and cause vertebral artery disruption.

TREATMENT

The treatment of traumatic spondylolisthesis of the axis has evolved over time. Perhaps one of the most common errors made in treatment of traumatic spondylolisthesis has been overestimation of the instability of these fractures and thus overimmobilization during treatment. As a general principle, treatment of traumatic spondylolisthesis of the axis is based on an understanding of the mechanism of the injury and the resultant instability. Correct assessment of the degree of instability associated with these injuries is the key to management of the patient. For traumatic spondylolisthesis of the axis, the major purpose of the classification schema (9) is to divide the injuries into groups related to mechanism and stability and therefore treatment. Separating type I and type II injuries by the anatomic patterns of the fracture, and when necessary by flexion-extension roentgenograms in the neurologically intact patient, defines the degree of instability for most patients with this injury. Type III injuries by definition are unstable and also irreducible and thus require surgical intervention as a general rule.

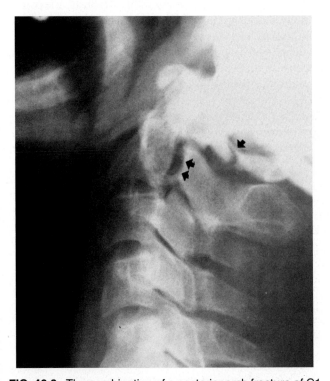

FIG. 46.8. The combination of a posterior arch fracture of C1 (*single arrow*) and a type I traumatic spondylolisthesis of the axis (*two arrows*) is relatively common. Both injuries have the same injury mechanism: hyperextension and axial load. Individually, these are stable injuries that can simply be treated in a collar; the combination can be treated likewise.

The components of treatment of these injuries should be divided into acute and definitive treatment. Upon establishing that a patient has been admitted with a traumatic spondylolisthesis of the axis, the type of injury should be defined as accurately as possible on the initial lateral roentgenogram. Irrespective of the degree of displacement, the transporting backboard can be removed and collar immobilization used if the patient is neurologically intact, which will allow adequate mobility for the workup. The only absolute indication for immediate application of the halo traction might be an accompanying associated displaced injury, such as a severely displaced dens fracture, or the presence of neurologic deficit. Thus, acute treatment consists initially of preliminary assessment of the nature of the injury, examination of the patient for neurologic injury, and application of external immobilization, which can be a collar in most cases and skeletal traction in the minority.

The range of definitive treatment is from cervical orthotic immobilization to halo traction/halo vest immobilization and finally surgery. Early studies on the treatment of this injury advocated a variety of methods of treating this fracture in its acute phase. Schneider and colleagues (21) treated seven of eight patients with prolonged skeletal traction followed by immobilization in a cast or a vest. One patient failed to unite and had a late anterior C2-C3 fusion. At the same time, however, Cornish (7) condemned the use of traction and suggested that an anterior C2-C3 arthrodesis was the treatment of choice for all patients with a hangman's fracture. He treated 11 patients with an anterior C2-C3 arthrodesis and obtained a 100% fusion rate but with a high complication rate, including 3 patients with Horner's syndrome and other complications. Others have advocated this method of treatment (43); more recently (28), anterior C2-C3 plating has been advocated for treatment of this fracture. Nonoperative treatment, however, has been the predominant modality utilized in most studies, ranging from collar mobilization to traction and halo immobilization. Brashear and colleagues (17) suggested cervical traction for 6 weeks followed by halo immobilization. Francis and associates (31) reported on a large multicenter study using either immediate mobilization in a halo vest or short-term traction (8 days) and then mobilization in a halo vest. Overall, for a mixture of injury types in most series, the union rate approaches 95% after 3 months of immobilization.

Treatment based on the type of injury is a much more predictable and reliable method (9,16). In some series, patients with minimal instability were treated in a halo vest, which is excessive. Therefore, based on the currently accepted classification schema (38), treatment can be assigned based on an understanding of the mechanism of the injury and the resultant instability (Table 46.2). Type I injuries, defined as having less than 3 mm of translation and minimal angulation confirmed by flexion-extension roentgenograms, are stable injuries. The disc is mechanically intact, and there is little or no ligamentous instability. Because the two fracture fragments are in close association and primary healing occurs with predictability, final stability is accomplished by fracture union. A halo vest does not restrict all toggle and does not provide any more substantial immobilization at the C2-C3 level for this injury than a cervical collar (32,44,45). Therefore, the most reasonable alternative for treatment of these injuries is collar mobilization. This should be a semirigid-type collar, such as a Philadelphia or Miami J collar, which should be left in position for approximately 3 months, as this is the usual time to fracture healing.

In a review of 64 patients, 39 of whom had less than 6 mm of displacement, treated with nonrigid immobilization, all showed stable healing (46). Failures of this type of treatment most often manifest by increasing displacement with immobilization in the collar, suggesting that the fracture was perhaps originally a type II injury. These were believed to be type I based on a supine roentgenogram, and were not verified to be type I injuries based on flexion-extension roentgenograms. One contraindication to cervical immobilization in an orthosis for a type I injury is body

TABLE 46.2. *Treatment Algorithm*

Evaluation and Classification ↓							
Type I or atypical ↓		Type II ↓		Type IIA ↓		Type III ↓	
Collar immobilization × 3 months	↓ <5 mm displacement ↓	↓ >5 mm displacement ↓	Reduction in halo ↓		C-spine MRI ↓	↓
	Flexion-extension radiographs ↓	reduction in traction	↓ Maintain in halo	↓ Osteosynthesis (operative fixation)	↓ Disc herniation ↓	↓ No disc herniation ↓
	<2 mm motion ↓	>2 mm motion ↓	Osteosynthesis			Anterior/posterior discectomy fusion	Posterior reduction and fixation
	Collar immobilization × 3 months	Halo or operative fixation					

habitus, as patients who are obese and have short necks may have difficulty wearing a semirigid collar.

It should also be noted that if combination injuries occur, treatment is directed at the most unstable of the injuries. In addition, treatment is based on assessment of individual injuries, not a subjective compilation of the injuries. Therefore, for a patient with a type I traumatic spondylolisthesis of the axis, which can be treated in collar immobilization, the addition of a posterior arch fracture, which if occurring alone would be treated in collar immobilization, need not necessarily change the treatment plan. The two injuries together do not make the cervical spine more unstable and warrant treatment in a halo vest. On the other hand, a patient with a posteriorly displaced type II dens fracture should be treated appropriately for the type II dens fracture with either surgery or halo immobilization. If the latter is the recommended treatment, the addition of a traumatic spondylolisthesis of the axis does not alter that treatment. Should the patient need stabilization of the dens fracture, postoperative immobilization in a collar is generally sufficient to achieve both goals.

Atypical or type IA traumatic spondylolisthesis of the axis is again a predominantly stable injury. In the patient without a neurologic deficit, flexion-extension roentgenograms should be done after completion of the CT scan, and then external immobilization can be applied. Because the fractures are in close apposition, primary healing will occur even in a slightly displaced position (Fig. 46.9).

Type II fractures should be divided into type II and type IIA. Both are unstable injuries (9,28), although the nature of the instability is different, and the two groups of injuries require different treatment. Type II fractures result from a hyperextension axial load, causing a vertical fracture of the arch, followed by a subsequent flexion force that disrupts the disc and leads to the deformity (Fig. 46.10A). Thus, with this injury type (II), the resultant instability is a flexion type, related to the mechanism that caused the soft tissue disruption and not related to the extension/axial load portion of the force that caused the bony fractures. In addition, generally there is disruption of the anterior-superior corner of C3, often with some stripping of the ALL, although the ALL in this type of fracture is intact.

These fractures can be reduced by a maneuver to counteract the forces that have caused the deformity. Because the deformity was caused by flexion and some compression, reduction can be achieved in traction with extension. Traction is best applied either through Gardner-Wells tongs or a halo. Most commonly, a halo ring should be applied, as this will allow easy conversion from the traction modality to halo vest immobilization (Fig. 46.10B). Patients who have halo traction (usually 25 to 30 pounds of traction in addition to extension over a roll) may lose their reduction if mobilized immediately in a halo vest because the halo vest does not maintain axial traction. A certain degree of toggling and slight axial loading of the cervical spine occur with position change (supine to erect), and the fracture may redisplace, generally to its original degree of deformity.

The decision about the definitive type of treatment for these patients with displaced unstable type II injuries is based on the necessity of achieving a union to reestablish stability at C2-C3, which can be achieved either through primary bony healing across the fracture site or anterior ankylosis at C2-C3 as a result of the bone healing generated by stripping of the ALL and disc. The goals of treatment should include anatomic alignment so that there is minimal angular deformity remaining at this level. Angulation at the fracture site is not acceptable, because it will generally cause extreme hyperextension at the level above and below and may lead to early degenerative disease and late pain, requiring an arthrodesis. In general, patients who have between 3 and 5 mm of displacement with less than 10 degrees of angulation can be reduced in halo traction and immediately immobilized in a halo vest. Vaccaro and colleagues (47) demonstrated that those patients with 11 degrees or less of angulation could be reduced in short-term traction and placed in a halo vest with a satisfactory result. Those with 11.5 degrees of angulation or more required long-term traction to maintain reduction. The expectation is that the patient with a minimally displaced fracture, once mobilized in the halo vest, will lose most of the reduction achieved in traction, but the fracture fragments should be in close enough proximity to heal. The relative alignment of the spine is acceptable enough that healing in that position should give a satisfactory clinical result.

For type II fractures that have more than 5 mm of translation or 10 degrees of angulation, placing the patient immediately in a halo vest may lead to the fracture fragments settling into the position of maximal displacement, which may result in an unacceptable result for one of two reasons. The first is that the fracture fragments may be so separated that there is not close enough approximation to allow primary healing of the fracture, and nonunion may occur with resultant instability. The second is that with significant angulation, the sagittal alignment may be unacceptable and lead to long-term pain complaints. Therefore, for patients with significant initial displacement, two methods of treatment are possible. Both methods rely on anatomic reduction of the fracture, which can be achieved in the following fashion: A halo is placed on the patient and traction is applied, in most cases on a Stryker frame, beginning with 10 pounds and slowly increasing the weight in 5-pound increments until the fracture is reduced (Fig. 46.10B). If the height of the C2-3 interspace seems to be restored but the angulation is not improving and there is no pathologic widening of the C2 disc space, the weight can be increased to as much as 40 pounds. A towel roll, approximately 4 inches in diameter, centered at the C6 level should also be placed to help achieve extension along with distraction. Because this reduction maneuver takes both axial distraction and extension, it is critical that the fractures be appropriately classified. If a type IIA injury is mistakenly placed in axial traction and extension, the deformity will be markedly accentuated.

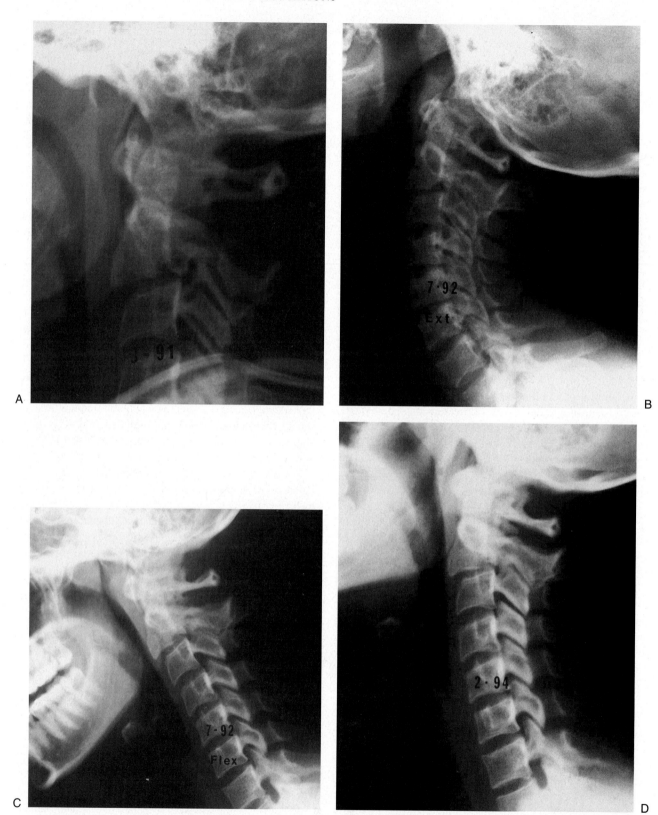

FIG. 46.9. A: This 23-year-old woman sustained a type IA (atypical) traumatic spondylolisthesis of the axis in a motor vehicle accident. She had slight translation and was treated in external immobilization for 3 months. **B, C:** One year after completing treatment, flexion-extension roentgenograms were done and showed restoration of stability. **D:** Three years after injury, she was asymptomatic.

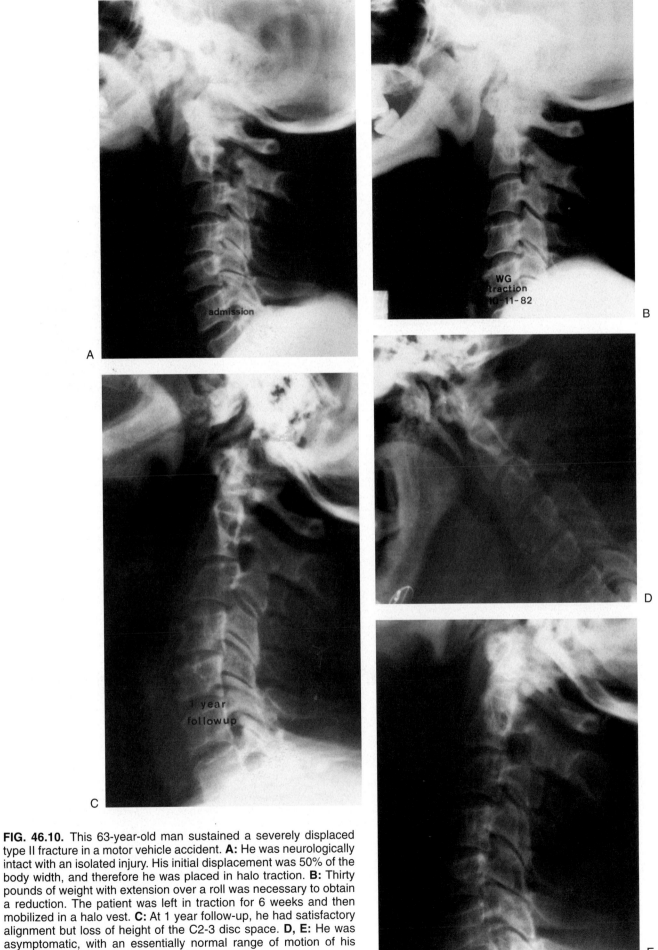

FIG. 46.10. This 63-year-old man sustained a severely displaced type II fracture in a motor vehicle accident. **A:** He was neurologically intact with an isolated injury. His initial displacement was 50% of the body width, and therefore he was placed in halo traction. **B:** Thirty pounds of weight with extension over a roll was necessary to obtain a reduction. The patient was left in traction for 6 weeks and then mobilized in a halo vest. **C:** At 1 year follow-up, he had satisfactory alignment but loss of height of the C2-3 disc space. **D, E:** He was asymptomatic, with an essentially normal range of motion of his neck and stable flexion-extension views.

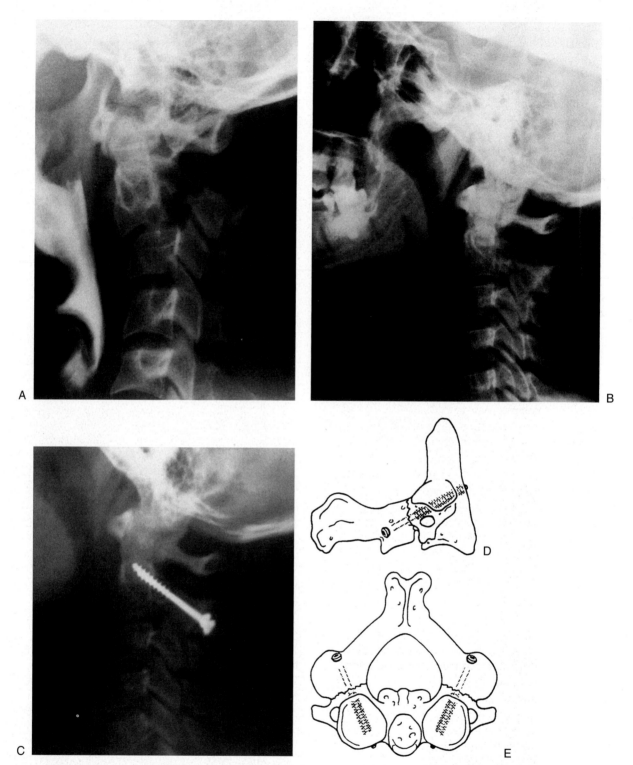

FIG. 46.11. A: The patient sustained multiple injuries, including a significantly displaced type II traumatic spondylolisthesis of the axis. **B:** Reduction was achieved using halo traction. **C:** Transpedicular fixation was achieved, allowing immediate mobilization in a collar. **D, E:** Orientation of the screws in the pedicles is achieved using biplanar image intensification.

Once the anatomic reduction is achieved, either of two treatment modalities can be undertaken. A patient can be left in traction, allowing primary union of the fracture fragments to occur. With close approximation, a callus will form and preliminary stability may be seen as early as 4 weeks. This stability should be tested at the end of 4 weeks by removing all traction weight from the head and leaving the patient on the Stryker frame for an hour. If displacement does not recur, the patient may be mobilized in a halo vest. After 24 hours of ambulation in the halo vest, the reduction should again be checked by a lateral roentgenogram. If it remains stable, the patient can be discharged in the halo vest for the remaining portion of his or her 12-week treatment (Fig. 46.10C–E). If the patient is not stable at the end of 4 weeks in the supine or in the erect position, or if position is lost because of the plasticity of the fracture callus, the patient should be placed back in traction for an additional week or taken to surgery. The entire cycle is repeated at that point, again if unsuccessful at 5 weeks, and again at 6 weeks. No patient should be maintained in traction longer than 6 weeks. Many adolescents will have enough fracture callus at the end of 4 weeks to achieve mobilization. Older persons may require longer, and this treatment is not appropriate for them.

In the patient in whom there is significant risk or who does not desire prolonged bedrest, or if reduction cannot be maintained, surgical treatment can be undertaken. Once the fracture is reduced in traction (Fig. 46.11A,B), surgical stabilization by osteosynthesis along the pedicle can be achieved (Fig. 46.11C) (48), which can be done with screws placed through the C2 pedicle. The patient is placed in a prone position in traction, with biplanar image intensification used to localize the pedicles. An alternative method has been described using CT guidance within the operating suite (49), with recent evidence suggesting that this may be performed with computer-aided navigational devices (50). Dissection of the lamina of C2 is undertaken. A small no. 4 Penfield elevator then can be placed along the medial side of the pedicle to identify its direction. A 2-mm burr is used to make an opening in the midportion of the lamina just medial to the C2-C3 facet joint. The starting hole is placed somewhat more proximal than for a Magerl-type C1-C2 arthrodesis, because this screw is directed into the pedicle (Fig. 46.11D,E). After localizing the direction of the pedicle on a lateral view and establishing the medial-most aspect of the pedicle by visual inspection and palpation, a 3.5-mm drill bit can be used to overdrill the posterior fragment of the fracture composed of the lamina and generally the pedicle of C2. This step is done under image intensification to verify that the drill is being advanced in the correct anterior-posterior as well as the medial-lateral positions. After overdrilling the pedicle with a 3.5-mm drill hole, a 2.7-mm drill is used to drill the vertebral body. The anterior aspect of the body does not need to be penetrated, because the reduction is usually almost complete and the additional purchase is not necessary. Either a 3.5-mm screw can be used to lag the fracture, or a partially threaded screw can be used. For most average-sized persons, a 30- to 35-mm screw length with 20 mm of unthreaded portion and 15 mm of thread is adequate. The 20 mm will generally traverse the fracture site nicely. With symmetric lagging of the two sides, a no. 4 Penfield elevator can be used to palpate the closure of the fracture site, which can be visualized on anteroposterior and lateral image intensification. Postoperatively, the patient can be mobilized in a semirigid collar. For patients in whom at least a partial reduction cannot be achieved or, most appropriately, in whom a displaced nonunion exists, an anterior C2-C3 arthrodesis can be undertaken.

Although both are unstable, type IIA fractures must be differentiated from type II fractures, because the former are flexion distraction injuries (Fig. 46.12A) and application of axial traction will widen the disc space and cause inadvertent displacement of the fracture (Fig. 46.12B). The criteria for differentiating a type II from a type IIA fracture have been identified previously, but most critically, the features are angulation without significant translation and an oblique fracture line rather than a vertical fracture one (Fig. 46.12A). The mechanism of injury is flexion distraction; thus, to counteract that instability and deformity, opposing forces of extension and axial load should be applied. Type IIA fractures are unstable injuries but should be reduced by applying slight extension and axial compression to the neck. Again, for definitive treatment, a halo vest is applied immediately without any traction. The halo vest then can be used to extend and compress the neck, which should reduce the fracture (Fig. 46.12C). Occasionally, there is interdigitation of the fracture fragments, as they have somewhat jagged edges, and complete reduction of the fracture cannot be achieved. If the degree of angulation is less than 10 degrees and there is good apposition of the fracture fragments, however, this should still yield a good clinical result. The patient should be mobilized in the vest and alignment checked at 24 hours. Maintenance for 3 months in a halo vest is associated with a better than 95% union rate, although due to the small incidence of this fracture, comparison to other treatment methods has not been done.

Type III fractures are a combination of essentially a type I traumatic spondylolisthesis of the axis and a facet injury at C2-C3. The most common entity is a bilateral facet dislocation at C2-C3 with a "type I fracture pattern," and can comprise bilateral facet fractures or even a unilateral facet fracture in association with a type I traumatic spondylolisthesis of the axis. The type III fracture that is associated with a C2-C3 bilateral facet dislocation is the only absolute surgical indication in all of the hangman's fractures. The inferior articular processes of C2, which are dislocated with reference to the superior articular processes of C3, are not connected to any other bony structure because of the bipedicular fracture lying just anterior to them and are irreducible by closed traction. This type of injury requires open reduction and internal fixation using bipedicular screws in C2 with a plate to the lateral mass of C3, depending on the nature of the fracture (9). Because such a patient will require reduction of the facet

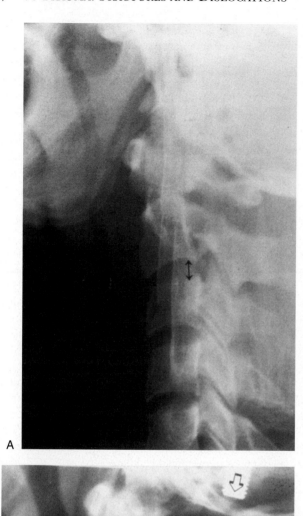

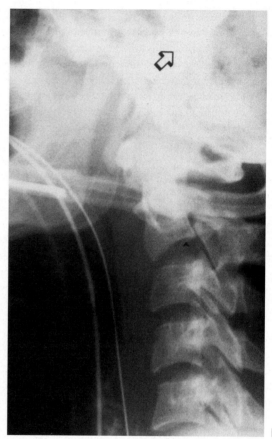

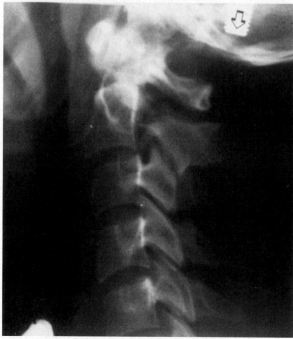

FIG. 46.12. A: This 24-year-old man sustained a type IIA injury, with the initial lateral supine roentgenogram demonstrating angulation (*double-headed arrow*) without translation and an oblique fracture line. **B:** This pattern was not recognized by the treating physician, who immediately placed the patient in traction (*arrow*) Gardner-Wells tongs and displaced the fracture. **C:** On recognizing the nature of the injury, the patient was converted to a halo vest and compression was applied (*arrow*), achieving complete reduction of the deformity.

dislocation component of the injury under general anesthesia, we suggest that an MRI be done preoperatively to assess the degree of disruption or herniation of the C2-3 disc. Although the theoretic possibility of herniation exists, it is exceedingly rare to have a clinically significant disc disruption at this level. If no disc herniation is found on an MRI, the technique for reduction of the facet dislocation component of the type III injury is similar to other bilateral facet dislocations.

After complete dissection of the posterior elements at C2 and C3, the articular cartilage is removed from the exposed

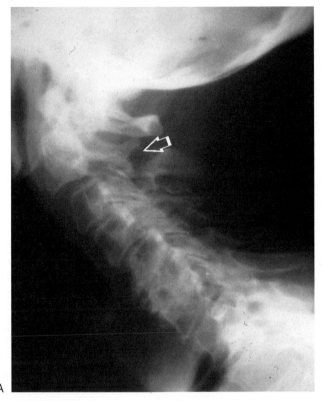

A

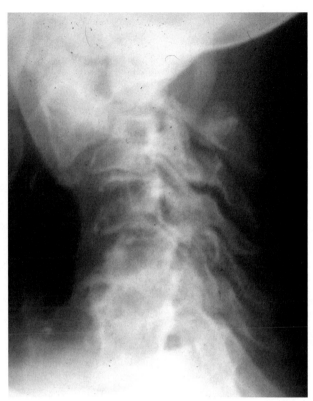

B

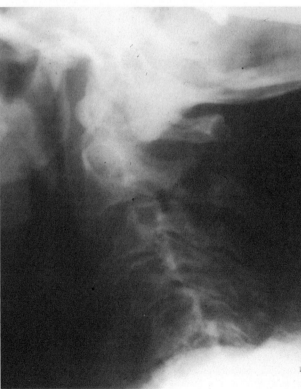

C

FIG. 46.13. A: This elderly gentleman was involved in a motor vehicle accident and had neck pain immediately without neurologic deficit. A lateral roentgenogram taken in the emergency room demonstrated a laminar fracture (*arrow*), which was missed initially. **B:** Two weeks later the patient was seen because he had neck pain and was unable to get his chin off his chest. He still was neurologically intact but had complete spondylolisthesis of C2 over C3 secondary to bilateral fact fractures. **C:** He was reduced in traction and taken to the operating room for stabilization. The patient tolerated the procedure and was discharged 4 days later.

superior facets of C3. Gentle distraction should be applied via towel clips on the spinous processes and, if necessary, slight leverage on the facets using a Penfield elevator to achieve reduction, maintaining the facet architecture for maximal stability after reduction. Theoretically, if there are no laminar or facet fractures, an interspinous wire can be used to stabilize the injury. Plate fixation is necessary if there are facet or laminar fractures. In that instance, it is necessary to use pedicle screws in the C2 pedicle because there is no lateral mass at C2 in which to place the screws at that level. The screws placed through the plate at the C3 level are directed in a standard fashion into the lateral mass. The screws at the C2 level also may be used to stabilize the accompanying pedicular fracture. The technique is the same as for displaced type II fractures (that is, reduction of the traumatic spondylolisthesis and a lag screw placed across the fracture), but this time the screw is placed through the plate and used to stabilize the C2-C3 facet injury. Alternatively, the screws in the C2 pedicle can be placed short (less than 20 mm), simply down the direction of the pedicle, but not across the fracture so that they do not distract the fracture.

Although neither the use of pedicle screws in C2 nor the use of posterior cervical plates are currently approved by the U.S. Food and Drug Administration (FDA), they are certainly preferable to other alternatives that require extension of the construct to the next more proximal level (occiput). If fractures exist at the C2 level that preclude fixation at that level, inclusion of the C1 ring would be necessary. That technique, however, includes a normal C1-C2 joint and significantly increases the morbidity (increased loss of range of motion) and also the risk of nonunion.

Finally, in the event the preoperative MRI showed a large herniated disc fragment within the canal, the surgical technique would differ significantly. The initial approach would be anterior, with removal of the disc fragment. Because the posterior elements are not connected to the vertebral bodies, however, reduction of the facet dislocation could not be achieved from an anterior approach as is sometimes done with lower cervical spine facet dislocations. For the type III injury, after disc evacuation is complete from an anterior approach, a posterior approach is necessary to reduce and stabilize the facet dislocation components.

Other combinations of injuries may specifically resemble a type III spondylolisthesis, including unilateral pars fractures with laminar fractures and facet dislocation (40). Therefore, careful evaluation is very important. It is also important not to confuse a bilateral facet fracture with spondyloptosis of C2 over C3 (Fig. 46.13) with traumatic spondylolisthesis; both, however, are extremely rare. There can be a spondylolisthesis of C2 over C3 without any pedicular fractures simply by massive disruption of the injured space with a standard bilateral facet fracture with a significant shear component. These injuries are treated like other bilateral facet fractures, with reduction in traction (Fig. 46.13) followed by plate fixation with screws directed down the C2 pedicle (because of the lack of a sufficient lateral mass at the C2 level) into the lateral mass of C3.

RESULTS AND COMPLICATIONS

The treatment of type I traumatic spondylolisthesis involves few complications and even fewer long-term problems. Probably because of the lack of neurologic deficit as well as the lack of difficulty in treating these fractures, no long-term follow-up series are available confirming these good results. However, there are long-term unpublished data from Levine's series of traumatic spondylolisthesis (9), originally published in 1985. The union rate of type I fractures, because of the close approximation of the fracture fragments, approaches 100%. In our experience, there have only been two nonunions of type I fractures (9,12). Nonunions of this injury can be treated either by osteosynthesis using a pedicle screw (48) across the fracture or by an anterior C2-C3 arthrodesis (28,51). About 10% of patients with type I traumatic spondylolisthesis will end up with symptomatic degenerative changes at C1-C2 as a result of the original injury (unpublished data). Because the mechanism of injury is hyperextension, considerable crushing of the C2-C3 facet cartilage may occur as well as resultant traumatic arthritis with loss of the facet cartilage space with specific localized pain at that particular area. These patients often have pain with palpation over C2, and their symptoms may be exacerbated by weather-related phenomena. This problem occurs more frequently than in type II fractures because these patients rarely develop spontaneous ankylosis between C2 and C3, which is seen more frequently in type II traumatic spondylolisthesis.

Type IA fractures unite with the same relative frequency as type I fractures and maintain fracture position during treatment in most cases and have no specific long-term problems. Few patients present with neurologic deficit (5, 42,52); however, because this type of injury has been reported only recently, follow-up in terms of neurologic recovery is short and cannot be determined from the available literature.

Patients with type II traumatic spondylolisthesis constitute a large spectrum of individual considerations based on the amount of displacement. About 70% of patients develop an anterior C2-C3 ankylosis either as a primary response in stabilizing the injury (9,12,53) or related to the degree of the stripping of the ALL at C2-C3 (Fig. 46.14). If this does not occur and there is a wide separation between the fracture fragments because of lack of reduction, nonunion is a possibility with type II fractures. Treatment criteria are similar to those described for type I fractures. When a nonunion develops in a type II fracture, it does not have the same degree of instability as the original injury. Although many type II injuries can initially have in excess of 5 mm of translation (and therefore instability on flexion-extension), the segment usually becomes stiffer and less mobile as the nonunion develops. Therefore, a nonunion that may have more than 5 mm of

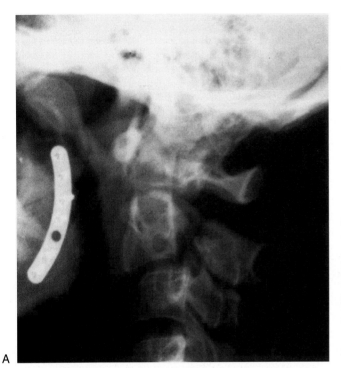
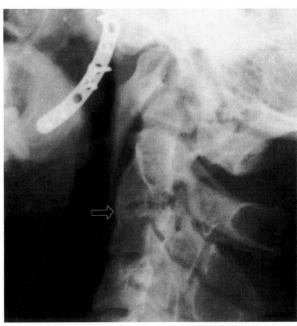

A   B

FIG. 46.14. A, B: This patient sustained multiple injuries in a motor vehicle accident, including a moderately displaced type II fracture and facial fractures. As a result of the limited degree of displacement, the patient was treated primarily in a halo vest, and the degree of displacement was accepted. Nine months later, a spontaneous C2-C3 arthrodesis had occurred as a result of the severe disruption of the disc space.

residual translation may now have only 1 to 2 mm of motion on flexion-extension roentgenograms. Thus, the decision to correct a nonunion surgically can be delayed and should not be considered before 6 months of treatment. Occasionally, these fractures unite late in the clinical course. When surgical intervention is needed, the approach can be by posterior osteosynthesis if the fracture can be reduced; if it cannot be reduced, the approach can be an anterior C2-C3 arthrodesis, either with or without a plate fixation in the symptomatic patient. Patients may have long-term pain complaints if they are left in more than 10 degrees of kyphosis, leading to hyperextension of the level above and below to maintain the normal sagittal alignment of the head over the trunk. They will have normal flexion but markedly decreased extension on physical examination.

Although patients may have a normal flexion, a study demonstrated that at 18 months' follow-up, patients who underwent screw fixation of the fracture with preservation of the C2-3 disc space will still have reduced motion at that segment. Nearly 70% of patients had 4 degrees of motion or less (mean 3.5 degrees of motion) (53). Thus, the injury causes disruption of the disc, with either spontaneous ankylosis or decreased motion.

Patients with type III injuries constitute a small group, many of whom have neurologic deficit because of the bilateral facet dislocation. Patients with high levels of quadriplegia generally have a poor long-term prognosis; however,

the number of patients is few and the follow-up short. Thus, no long-term data are currently available.

CONCLUSION

Traumatic spondylolisthesis of the axis, as currently understood, must be separated from the injury associated with judicial hangings. Over the last 25 years, significant progress has been made in delineating the mechanisms of the injury and the resultant instabilities. The most commonly used classification system consists of five major subtypes and defines both the mechanism and the instability. Most patients with these injuries can be treated nonoperatively and heal readily. It is uncommon for these patients to have neurologic deficits, and the only absolute indication for operative treatment is the type III traumatic spondylolisthesis associated with a bilateral facet dislocation. Perhaps the most exciting aspect of these injuries is the morbid fascination we have with its namesake, the hangman's fracture.

REFERENCES

1. Haughton S. On hanging, considered from a mechanical and physiological point of view. *Philos Mag J Sci* 1866;32:23–34.
2. Marshall JJD. Judicial executions. *BMJ* 1888:779–782.
3. Annotation: judicial hanging. *Lancet* March 1, 1913:629.
4. Marshall JJD. Letter to the Editor. *Lancet* January 18, 1913:194.

5. Marshall JJD. The executioner surgeon. Letters, notes and answers. *BMJ* November 13, 1913:1340.

6. Wood-Jones F. The ideal lesion produced by judicial hanging. *Lancet* January 4, 1913:53.

7. Cornish BL. Traumatic spondylolisthesis of the axis. *J Bone Joint Surg Br* 1968;50:31–43.

8. Gerlock AJ, Mirfakhraee M. Computed tomography and hangman's fractures. *South Med J* 1983;76:727–728.

9. Levine AM, Edwards CC. The management of traumatic spondylolisthesis of the axis. *J Bone Joint Surg Am* 1985;67:217–226.

10. Levine AM, Edwards CC. Treatment of injuries in the C1-C2 complex. *Orthop Clin North Am* 1986;17:31–44.

11. Levine AM, Edwards CC. Traumatic lesions of the occipitoatlanto-axial complex. *Clin Orthop* 1989;239:53–68.

12. Levine AM, Rhyne AL. Traumatic spondylolisthesis of the axis. *Semin Spine Surg* 1991;3:47–60.

13. Pepin JW, Hawkins RJ. Traumatic spondylolisthesis of the axis: hangman's fracture. *Clin Orthop* 1981;157:133–138.

14. Sherk HH, Howard T. Clinical and pathologic correlations in traumatic spondylolisthesis of the axis. *Clin Orthop* 1983;174:122–126.

15. Marar BC. Fracture of the axis arch. "Hangman's fracture" of the cervical spine. *Clin Orthop* 1975;106:155–165.

16. Effendi B, Roy D, Cornish B, et al. Fractures of the ring of the axis: a classification based on the analysis of 131 cases. *J Bone Joint Surg Br* 1981;63:319–327.

17. Brashear HR Jr, Venters GC, Preston ET. Fractures of the neural arch of the axis. *J Bone Joint Surg Am* 1975;57:879–887.

18. Bucholz RW. Unstable hangman's fractures. *Clin Orthop* 1981;154:119–124.

19. Mollan RAB. Hangman's fracture: injury. *Br J Accident Surg* 1982;14:265–267.

20. Roda JM, Castro A, Blazquez MG. Hangman's fracture with complete dislocation of C-2 on C-3. *J Neurosurg* 1984;60:633–635.

21. Schneider RC, Livingston KE, Cave AJE, et al. "Hangman's fracture" of the cervical spine. *J Neurosurg* 1965;22:141–154.

22. Seljeskog EL, Chou SN. Spectrum of the hangman's fracture. *J Neurosurg* 1976;45:3–8.

23. Termansen NB. Hangman's fracture. *Acta Orthop Scand* 1974;45:529–539.

24. Hadley MN, Sonntag VKH, Graham, et al. Axis fractures resulting from motor vehicle accidents: the need for occupant restraints. *Spine* 1986;11:861–864.

25. Hadley MN, Browner C, Sonntag VKH. Axis fractures: a comprehensive review of management and treatment in 107 cases. *Neurosurgery* 1985;17:281–290.

26. Grogono BJS. Injuries of the atlas and axis. *J Bone Joint Surg Br* 1954;36:397–410.

27. Garber JN. Abnormalities of the atlas and axis vertebrae—congenital and traumatic. *J Bone Joint Surg Am* 1964;46:1782–1791.

28. Tuite GF, Papadopoulos MD, Sonntag VK. Caspar plate fixation for the treatment of complex hangman's fractures. *Neurosurgery* 1992;30:761–765.

29. Hohl M. Normal motions in the upper portion of the cervical spine. *J Bone Joint Surg Am* 1964;46:1777.

30. Fielding JW. Normal and selected abnormal motion of the cervical spine from the second cervical vertebra to the seventh cervical vertebra based on cineroentgenography. *J Bone Joint Surg Am* 1964;46:1779–1781.

31. Francis WR, Fielding JW, Hawkins RJ, et al. Traumatic spondylolisthesis of the axis. *J Bone Joint Surg Br* 1981;63:313–318.

32. White AA, Panjabi MM. *Clinical biomechanics of the spine*, 2nd ed. Philadelphia: J.B. Lippincott, 1990:208–215.

33. Williams TG. Hangman's fracture. *J Bone Joint Surg Br* 1975;57:82–88.

34. Levine AM, Kleeman J, Crain E. Atypical hangman's fracture (in preparation).

35. Dussault RG, Effendi B, Roy D, et al. Locked facets with fracture of the neural arch of the axis. *Spine* 1983;8:365–367.

36. Teo EC, Paul JP, Evans JH, et al. Biomechanical study of C2 axis fracture: effect of restraint. *Ann Acad Med Singapore* 2001;30:582–587.

37. Starr JK, Eismont FJ. Atypical hangman's fractures. *Spine* 1993;18:1954–1957.

38. Hadley MN, Dickman CA, Browner CM, et al. Acute axis fractures: a review of 229 cases. *J Neurosurg* 1989;71:642–647.

39. Samaha C, Lazennec JY, Laporte C, et al. Hangman's fracture: the relationship between asymmetry and instability. *J Bone Joint Surg Br* 2000;82:1046–1052.

40. Choi WG, Vishteh AG, Baskin JJ, et al. Completely dislocated hangman's fracture with a locked C2-3 facet. Case report. *J Neurosurgery* 1997;87:7557–7560.

41. Gleizes V, Jacquot FP, Signoret F, et al. Combined injuries in the upper cervical spine: clinical and epidemiological data over a 14-year period. *Eur Spine J* 2000;9:386–392.

42. Levine AM, Fischgrund J. Fractures of the C1-C2 complex. *Concurrent Spinal Injuries* (in press).

43. Norrell H, Wilson CB. Early anterior fusion for injuries of the cervical portion of the spine. *JAMA* 1970;214:525–530.

44. Johnson RM, Hart DL, Simmons EF, et al. Cervical orthoses: a study comparing their effectiveness in restricting cervical motion in normal subjects. *J Bone Joint Surg Am* 1977;59:332–339.

45. Whitehill R, Richman JA, Glaser JA. Failure of immobilization of the cervical spine by the halo vest. *J Bone Joint Surg Am* 1986;68:326–332.

46. Coric D, Wilson JA, Kelly DL Jr. Treatment of traumatic spondylolisthesis of the axis with nonrigid immobilization: a review of 64 cases. *J Neurosurg* 1996;85:550–554.

47. Vaccaro AR, Madigan L, Bauerle WB, et al. Early halo immobilization of displaced traumatic spondylolisthesis of the axis. *Spine* 2002;27:2229–2233.

48. Roy-Camille R, Saillant G, Bouchet T. Technique du vissage des pedicules de C2 (French). In: Roy-Camille R, ed. *5emes Journees d'Orthopedie de la Pitie, Rachis Cervical Superieur*. Paris: Masson, 1986:41–43.

49. Taller S, Suchomel P, Lukas R, et al. CT-guided internal fixation of a hangman's fracture. *Eur Spine J* 2000;9:393–397.

50. Arand M, Hartwig E, Kinzl L, et al. Spinal navigation in cervical fractures—a preliminary clinical study on judet-osteosynthesis of the axis. *Comp Aid Surg* 2001;6:170–175.

51. Vieweg U, Meyer B, Scramm J. Differential treatment in acute upper cervical spine injuries: a critical review of a single-institution series. *Surg Neurol* 2000;54:203–210; discussion 210–211.

52. Moon MS, Moon JL, Moon YW, et al. Traumatic spondylolisthesis of the axis: 42 cases. *Bull Hosp Jt Dis* 2001–2002;60:61–66.

53. Verheggen R, Jansen J. Hangman's fracture: arguments in favor of surgical therapy for type II and III according to Edwards and Levine. *Surg Neurol* 1998;49:253–262.

CHAPTER 47

Classification of Lower Cervical Spine Injuries

D. Greg Anderson and Alexander R. Vaccaro

The classification of cervical spine injuries is important for several reasons. First, classification facilitates accurate communication regarding an injury. Second, classification may be used to determine the most appropriate treatment of an injury. Third, classification may be the best way to determine accurate injury prognosis. Fourth, classification allows valid and reliable research to be performed and is especially crucial when research is performed at multiple centers. In addition, some classification systems aid in understanding the injury mechanism and pathomechanics.

A myriad of classification systems have been proposed to describe injuries of the cervical spine. Classification systems have traditionally been based on a variety of factors, including mechanisms of injury, radiographic descriptions, injury biomechanics, and neurologic status. All of these systems have their individual strengths and weaknesses. To use a system appropriately, one must understand the rationale of the classification so that an injury can be viewed in the appropriate context.

Injuries to the cervical spine are often referred to by their radiographic descriptions, such as "compression fracture," "burst fracture," "teardrop fracture," or "bilateral facet dislocation." Although these names will continue to be used, it is our belief that a more exact description of the injury mechanism and severity is useful. Mechanistic classifications enhance an understanding of the injury pathomechanics and assist in establishing appropriate treatment based on spinal biomechanics. A thorough understanding of the injury mechanism is especially crucial in the operative treatment of spinal injuries, where the methods of reduction and instrumentation chosen must address the specific compromised anatomy.

The ideal classification system would allow all injuries to be placed into a specific category. The system would have a perfect degree of inter- and intraobserver reliability. The system should allow the clinician to better understand the injury, dictate the best treatment, and predict the outcome. Finally, the system should be simple enough to use

clinically, while specific enough to allow research to be performed. Needless to say, this "ideal" classification system is not yet available.

This chapter focuses on the most useful classification systems that are currently available for lower cervical spine trauma. We find it useful to consider a given injury by first classifying the mechanism of injury. This provides a good understanding of specific anatomical disruption. Next, we consider the stability of the injury based on biomechanical principles. Finally, we provide an accurate classification of the neurologic status of the patient. On the basis of these considerations, we are then able to develop a logical treatment plan for the patient.

ANATOMY

The unique anatomy of the lower cervical spine is worthy of review because a thorough understanding of the anatomy will assist in understanding the injury patterns seen in the lower cervical spine. The anatomy of the lower cervical spine has been described by various authors using either a two-column (1,2) or three-column system (3,4). Although both systems have merits, the two-column system probably provides the best understanding of the common injury patterns seen in the lower cervical spine and will be used in our description. The two-column spine consists of an anterior column and posterior column. The anterior column contains the anterior longitudinal ligament (ALL), intervertebral disc, vertebral body, and the posterior longitudinal ligament (PLL). The posterior column is made up of the posterior bony elements, facet capsules, interspinous and supraspinous ligaments, and the ligamentum flavum (LF). The most important stabilizer of the anterior column is the annulus fibrosus, whereas the facet joints are the most important stabilizers of the posterior column (2).

The facet joints are unique in the lower cervical spine. They overlap one another in the coronal plane and are oriented approximately 45 degrees to the horizontal in the sagittal plane. The inclination of the facets gradually increases as one progresses cranially from C7 toward C2. The facets joints allow relatively large ranges of motion to occur in flexion, extension, and lateral bending. Due to the orientation of the facets, the motions of lateral bending and rotation are coupled, causing the spinous processes to rotate toward the convexity of the lateral curve. The facet joints serve as the major structure resisting forward subluxation of the vertebrae during flexion. Zdeblick and associates (5, 6) studied the facet joints and facet capsules and concluded that there is a statistically significant increase in posterior flexion strain and decreased torsional stiffness of the vertebral segment when greater than 50% of the facet joint or facet capsule is removed.

The functional spinal unit consists of two vertebrae, the intervening intervertebral disc, and associated ligamentous and capsular structures. It is important to understand which structures resist hypermobility during segmental motion. For instance, the ALL and anterior annulus act as a tension band during extension of the motion segment, whereas the posterior ligamentous structures act as a tension band during flexion. Compressive loads are resisted by the vertebral bodies, intervertebral discs, and facet joints. Pure tensile loads are resisted by the annulus, interspinous ligament, LF, and facet capsule. Flexion is resisted by the interspinous ligaments, facet capsules and facet joints, PLL, and posterior annulus. Extension is resisted by the ALL and anterior annulus, as well as by compression of the facet joints. The maximal sagittal plane translation occurring under physiologic loads is 2 to 2.7 mm (2). Lower cervical spine injuries can be understood as failure of the structures designed to resist the forces and moments occurring at the time of the injury.

Finally, it is important to recognize that in lower cervical spine injuries, it is often the soft tissue disruption that is the most critical aspect of the injury when determining the degree of instability present. When reviewing plain radiographs, the obvious bony injury should be used as a clue to understanding the degree of soft tissue disruption present. The treating physician may then gain an understanding of the "personality" of the injury and thus the tendency for displacement under physiologic loads.

MECHANISTIC CLASSIFICATION SYSTEMS

Whitley and Forsyth (7) described an early mechanistic classification of cervical spine injuries in 1960. The classification system was based on a review of 159 patients with cervical fractures. The authors described the injury mechanism of many common cervical spine fractures. The injury mechanisms discussed included flexion injuries, extension injuries, combined flexion-extension injuries, burst-type injuries, and direct trauma. The authors further divided flexion and extension injuries into those occurring with and without compression. This classification system retains historical importance because it promoted thinking about cervical spine injuries in terms of the mechanism of injury.

In 1982, Allen and associates (8) published a classification system based on the clinical review of 165 patients with indirect lower cervical spine trauma. This system continues to be the most comprehensive and useful mechanistic classification available. Lower cervical injuries are divided into "phylogenies" based on a common mechanism of injury, emphasizing the orderly sequence of injury progression. Within each phylogeny, a series of injuries are described, ranging from mild to severe. Six categories of injury—compressive flexion, vertical compression, distractive flexion, compressive extension, distractive extension, and lateral flexion—are included. The names of each category describe the attitude of the cervical spine at the time of injury and the dominant force vector. The authors also acknowledge minor injury vectors, which may cause separate or combined injuries. Rotation in this system is not treated as a major vector but is thought to localize the injury more to one side, creating the asymmetry often seen on radiographs. In general, the risk and severity of neurologic injury were found to increase in relation to the injury stage.

Compressive Flexion

Compressive flexion (CF) injuries comprised 36% of the injuries in the series by Allen and associates (8). CF injuries (Fig. 47.1) were divided into five stages: CF stage 1 (CFS1) injuries result in a rounded shape to the anterior superior vertebral body without any posterior ligamentous disruption; CF stage 2 (CFS2) injuries demonstrate a "beaked" appearance of the anterior vertebral body with loss of anterior height due to compression failure; CF stage 3 (CFS3) injuries contain an oblique fracture line traversing from the anterior superior vertebral body to the inferior end plate or a fracture of the "beak" of the CFS2 injury; CF stage 4 (CFS4) injuries demonstrate up to 3 mm of posterior translation of the posterior vertebral body into the neural canal; and CF stage 5 (CFS5) lesions have gross (>3 mm) displacement of the posterior aspect of the vertebral body into the neural canal. In addition, some CFS4 and most CFS5 injuries demonstrate subluxation of the facets and widening of the space between the spinous processes at the injured motion segment due to disruption of the posterior annulus and posterior ligamentous complex. Sagittal body fractures and posterior lamina fractures are frequently associated with CF injuries.

Vertical Compression

Vertical compression (VC) injuries accounted for 14% of all cervical injuries in the series of Allen and associates (8). These injuries demonstrate compression failure

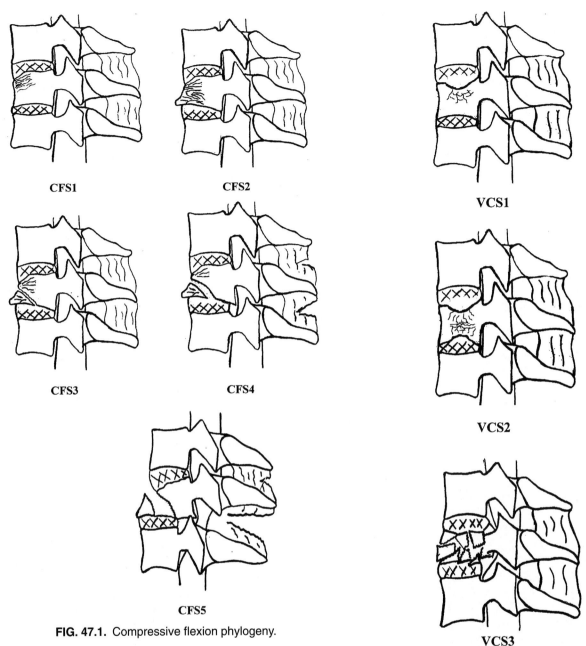

CFS1

CFS2

CFS3

CFS4

CFS5

FIG. 47.1. Compressive flexion phylogeny.

VCS1

VCS2

VCS3

FIG. 47.2. Vertical compression phylogeny.

of the vertebral body (Fig. 47.2), which is divided into three stages: VC stage 1 (VCS1) demonstrates failure or "cupping" of either the superior or inferior end plates; VC stage 2 (VCS2) injuries have failure of both end plates with the "cupping" deformity. There may also be fracture lines through the centrum with minimal displacement; and in VC stage 3 (VCS3), there is comminution of the vertebral body with a radial displacement of the fragments. Often, fragments of bone are displaced into the spinal canal. The posterior ligamentous complex may be intact or disrupted, which can be determined by looking for widening between the spinous processes and subluxation of the facet joint. In some cases, the posterior elements may be fractured. The associated posterior column dis-

ruptions are important in determining injury stability and are thought to be caused by the head going into flexion or extension late in the injury after the vertical crush to the centrum.

Distractive Flexion

Distractive flexion (DF) injuries accounted for 61% of the injuries in the series (8). DF injuries (Fig. 47.3) demonstrate progressive failure of the posterior ligamentous complex and annulus fibrosus in tension. DF stage 1 (DFS1) demonstrates forward subluxation of the upper

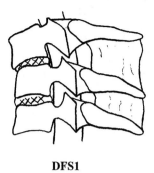

DFS1

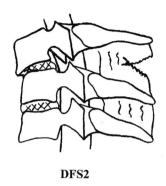

DFS2

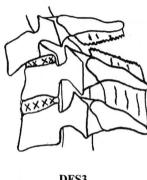

DFS3

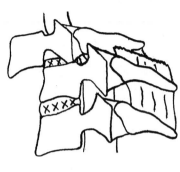

DFS4

FIG. 47.3. Distractive flexion phylogeny.

facet in the motion segment with widening of the space between the spinous processes. This results from a stretch injury to the posterior ligamentous complex. In DF stage 2 (DFS2), there is a unilateral facet dislocation demonstrating up to 25% forward subluxation of the vertebral body in the motion segment. In DF stage 3 (DFS3), there is a bilateral facet dislocation with approximately 50% anterior subluxation of the upper vertebra in the motion segment. DF stage 4 (DFS4) demonstrates gross anterior displacement of the upper vertebra on the lower vertebra in the motion segment, creating the "floating vertebra." Disruption of the posterior ligamentous complex is variable in DFS2 injuries but is always seen in DFS3 and DFS4 injuries.

Compressive Extension

Compressive extension (CE) injuries made up 40% of the series of Allen and associates (8). CE injuries (Fig. 47.4) occur with compressive failure of the posterior bony elements and variable shear forces to the motion segment. CE stage 1 (CES1) demonstrates a unilateral vertebral arch fracture (pedicle, facet, and/or lamina) with or without rotational displacement of the vertebral body. CES1 injuries were noted to be the most prevalent injury in the series. CE stage 2 (CES2) injuries demonstrate bilateral laminar frac-

tures, often at multiple contiguous levels but without evidence of other soft tissue failure.

CE stages 3 and 4 (CES3 and CES4) injuries were not seen in the series but were described on a theoretical basis as the logical progression of the primary force vector and as links to the stage 5 CE (CES5) injury. CES3 consists of bilateral disruption of the articular pillars (pedicle, facet, and/or lamina) without displacement, whereas CES4 is a similar injury with partial forward subluxation of the fractured vertebra on the vertebra below.

CES5 consists of bilateral vertebral arch fracture with full vertebral body width displacement of the fractured vertebra on the vertebra below. The posterior bony elements of the fractured vertebra are left behind. The posterior soft tissue disruption occurs between the fractured vertebra and the one above, while anterior soft tissue disruption occurs between the fractured vertebra and the one below. Because of the separation of the anterior and posterior elements in the CES5 injury, there is a high incidence of partial or complete spinal cord sparing with this injury, which is surprising given the gross displacement.

Distractive Extension

Distractive extension (DE) injuries accounted for 9% of the series (8). DE injuries (Fig. 47.5) are characterized

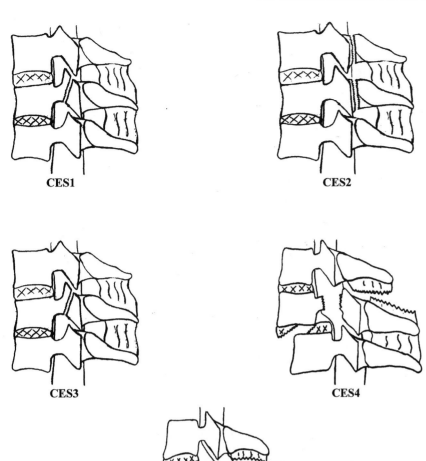

CES1

CES2

CES3

CES4

CES5

FIG. 47.4. Compressive extension (CE) phylogeny. Note that a CE stage 3 injury has bilateral fractures of the pars or articular facets. CE stages 3 and 4 were not seen in the series but were described on a theoretical basis.

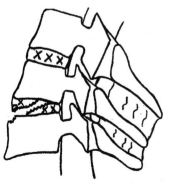

DES1

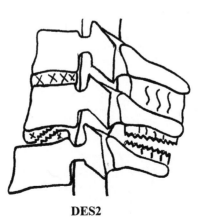

DES2

FIG. 47.5. Distractive extension phylogeny.

by progressive failure of the motion segment in an anterior to posterior direction. DE stage 1 (DES1) injuries consist of failure of the ALL and annulus fibrosus with widening of the disc space anteriorly seen on x-ray. There may be a small avulsion fracture at the anterior margin of the disc space, but no posterior subluxation is seen. DE stage 2 (DES2) injuries have the same findings as DFS1 but also demonstrate posterior displacement of the upper vertebra in the motion segment. The magnitude of posterior displacement is often minimized by neutral positioning of the head at the time of the radiograph. DES2 injuries have disruption of the posterior annulus and posterior ligamentous complex sufficient to allow the posterior subluxation. DE injuries in the series were shown to occur more commonly in older patients and often were the result of a fall on the face.

Lateral Compression

Lateral compression (LC) injuries accounted for 5% of the series (8). LC injuries (Fig. 47.6) demonstrate an asymmetric compression of the vertebral motion segment, with one side sustaining more collapse, resulting in a lateral deviation of the spine on the anteroposterior x-ray. LC stage 1 (LCS1) demonstrates asymmetric compression failure of the vertebral body with an ipsilateral, undisplaced vertebral arch fracture. LC stage 2 (LCS2) is similar to the LCS1 injuries but demonstrates displacement of the vertebral arch fracture or widening of the contralateral articular processes, demonstrating tension failure opposite the compression injury. The forced lateral flexion of the neck causing this injury pattern has been associated with injuries to the brachial plexus by other authors (9), but no plexus injuries were noted in the series of Allen and associates (8).

Biomechanical Assessment of Stability

The concept of spinal stability is important, but the exact criteria for instability remain elusive. Stability has been defined by White and Panjabi (2) as "the ability of the spine under physiologic loads to limit patterns of displacement so as not to damage or irritate the spinal cord or nerve roots and, in addition, to prevent incapacitating deformity or pain due to structural changes." Allen and associates (8) defined instability as "greater than normal range of motion within a motion segment." Allen viewed instability as a spectrum ranging from slight, benign increase in motion to a dangerous, gross loss of segmental integrity. From a clinical prospective, it is important to be able to determine which lower cervical spine injuries have enough loss of stability that a specific treatment intervention is warranted to prevent further injury.

Holdsworth (1) and others (9,10) have emphasized the importance of the posterior ligamentous complex in conferring stability to the spine. In their descriptions, the disruption of the posterior ligamentous complex is the primary determinant of instability.

White and Panjabi (2) have emphasized that similar injury mechanisms can produce different injury patterns due to the complexity of the specific forces, moments, and positions of the affected joints at the time of force application. They have described a point-based system for assessing stability in lower cervical spine injury, which is summarized in Table 47.1. Clinical data and *in vitro* biomechanical testing of cervical spine injury patterns are the basis for this system. To use the system, radiographic criteria, physical examination, and a stretch test are required. Five or more points in this system predict spinal instability (11).

The stretch test is performed by placing a patient in halter or tong traction with a roller beneath the head to reduce

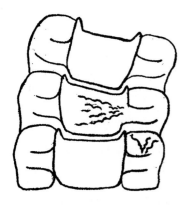

LFS1

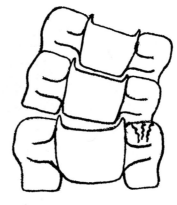

LFS2

FIG. 47.6. Lateral flexion phylogeny.

TABLE 47.1. *The Diagnosis of Clinical Instability in the Middle and Lower Cervical Spine*

Element	Point value
Anterior elements destroyed or unable to function	2
Posterior elements destroyed or unable to function	2
Positive stretch test	2
Radiographic criteria	
A. Flexion-extension radiographs	
1. Sagittal plane translation > 3.5 mm or 20°	2
2. Sagittal plane rotation > 20°	2
or	
B. Resting radiographs	
1. Sagittal plane displacement > 3.5 mm	2
2. Relative sagittal plane angulation > 11°	2
Developmental narrow spinal canal	1
1. Sagittal diameter < 13°	
2. Pavlov ratio < 0.8	
Abnormal disc narrowing	1
Spinal cord damage	2
Nerve root damage	1
Dangerous loading anticipated	1

Total of 5 or more points = unstable.

friction. Initial lateral radiographs of the cervical spine with 10 pounds of traction are carefully analyzed to rule out a disruption of the occipitocervical junction. Serial weight is sequentially added in 10-pound increments, performing neurologic testing with each addition of weight. The end point of the test is reached when "instability" is noted on x-rays, there is a change in neurologic exam, or the weight limit (65 pounds or one-third body weight) is reached. Instability on the stretch test is defined as distraction of a vertebral interspace by 1.7 mm greater than the resting film or a change in segmental alignment of 7.5 degrees (11).

From a practical standpoint, performance of the stretch test is rarely required because most significant injuries can be classified as stable or unstable by understanding the specific tissue disruptions present. This is facilitated by use of a mechanistic classification as described previously. The criteria of the point-based system of White and Panjabi are valuable to consider when evaluating stability, particularly in equivocal cases. Finally, it is important to realize that "subacute instability" may exist even when injury radiographs are normal. Herkowitz and Rothman (12) presented a series of patients with normal initial radiographs and neurologic examination who were noted to have an unstable cervical injury on follow-up radiographs at an average of 14.3 days postinjury. Five of the six patients demonstrated an objective neurologic deficit at follow-up. The authors recommended immobilization of cervical trauma for 3 weeks until the initial pain and muscle spasm subsided. Repeat examination and radiographs (including flexion and extension films) should then be performed to rule out subacute instability.

NEUROLOGIC ASSESSMENT AND CLASSIFICATION

Classification of associated neurologic injuries is important to consider. Neurologic classification is paramount for determining the appropriate timing and intervention to be rendered. The neurologic examination and classification should be repeated frequently in the early course following a spinal cord injury because the examination will often change and will potentially alter management. Accurate neurologic classification is crucial to the study of therapeutic interventions such as the second National Acute Spinal Cord Injury Study, which demonstrated the usefulness of early high-dose steroids for incomplete spinal cord injury (13).

Numerous authors have noted a poor correlation between the severity of the spinal injury and the severity of the neurologic injury (14–17). Total quadriplegia may occur without an apparent spinal column disruption; conversely, a widely displaced cervical dislocation may sometimes be seen in a neurologically intact patient. Allen and associates (8) noted a correlation between the severity of spinal column injury and the risk and degree of neurologic injury using their classification system. However, even with this system the neurologic status is only moderately related to the injury, and many exceptions exist. Therefore, the neurologic status should be considered as a separate and equally important consideration along with the spinal column injury in determining the appropriate treatment of the patient.

The American Spinal Injury Association (ASIA) developed its standard neurologic classification of spinal cord injury in 1992 (18,19). The ASIA clinical format for recording neurologic examination is shown in Figure 47.7. Sensory and motor testing is done separately for each side of the body over 28 standardized dermatomes and 10 standardized myotomes. Sensation is tested for pinprick and light touch modalities. The neurologic level is recorded as the most distal level with normal function. In cases where there is a discrepancy between sides of the body or between sensory and motor testing, it is recommended that each modality be individually recorded. Because many key muscles have neurologic input from more than one nerve root level, mild weakness may be present when a portion of the normal nerve supply is absent due to a neurologic injury. In this case, the most distal muscle with a motor function of 3 or greater is designated as the motor level when more proximal muscles show normal strength. Testing of the most distal sacral levels (S4-S5) for sensation and testing the motor function of the anal sphincter are important to determine if some sacral sparing is present, which improves injury prognosis. Functional impairment can be categorized using the ASIA Impairment Scale (Table 47.2), which is a modification of the original Frankel grading system.

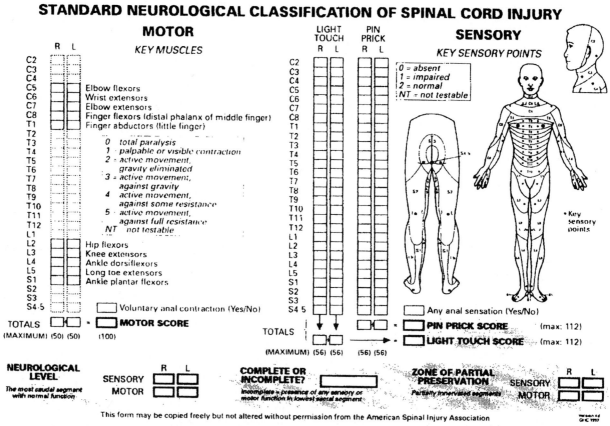

FIG. 47.7. American Spinal Injury Association (ASIA) standard neurological examination form. ASIA impairment scale.

SUMMARY

Careful classification is important to our understanding and communication of lower cervical spine injuries. We have found it useful to categorize the skeletal injury and its severity using the mechanistic classification system of Allen and associates (8). With an understanding of the specific tissue disruptions present, we then seek to categorize the stability of the injury. The biomechanical principles of White and Panjabi (2) are helpful in this regard. Finally, we accurately classify the neurologic status using the ASIA

committee system (18). With a complete understanding of the injury, stability, and neurologic status, a logical treatment plan may then be organized and executed.

REFERENCES

1. Holdsworth F. Fractures, dislocations and fracture-dislocations of the spine. *J Bone Joint Surg Br* 1963;45:6–20.
2. White AA, Panjabi MM. *Clinical biomechanics of the spine.* Philadelphia: JB Lippincott, 1978:102–107.
3. Denis F. The three-column spine and its significance in classification of acute thoracolumbar spine injuries. *Spine* 1989;8:817–831.
4. Stauffer ES. Management of spine fractures C3-C7. *Orthop Clin North Am* 1977;17:45–53.
5. Zdeblick TA, Abitbol JJ, Kunz DN. Cervical stability after sequential capsule resection. *Spine* 1993;18:2005–2008.
6. Zdeblick TA, Zou D, Warden KE. Cervical stability after foraminotomy. *J Bone Joint Surg Am* 1992;74:22–27.
7. Whitley JE, Forsyth HF. The classification of cervical spine injuries. *Am J Roentgenogr Radiat Ther Nucl Med* 1960;83:633–644.
8. Allen BL, Ferguson RL, Lehmann TR, et al. A mechanistic classification of closed indirect fractures and dislocations of the lower cervical spine. *Spine* 1982;7:1–27.
9. Roaf RR. A study of the mechanics of spinal injuries. *J Bone Joint Surg Br* 1960;42:810–823.
10. Beatson TR. Fractures and dislocations of the cervical spine. *J Bone Joint Surg Br* 1963;45:21–35.
11. Bernhardt M, White AA, Panjabi MM. Biomechanical considerations of spinal stability. In: Herkowitz HN, et al., eds. *The spine.* Philadelphia: WB Saunders, 1999:1071–1096.

TABLE 47.2. *ASIA Impairment Scale*

A. Complete. No sensory of motor function is preserved in the sacral segments S4-S5.
B. Incomplete. Sensory but not motor function is preserved below the neurologic level and extends through the sacral segments S4-S5.
C. Incomplete. Motor function is preserved below the neurologic level, and the majority of key muscles below the neurologic level have a muscle grade of less than 3.
D. Incomplete. Motor function is preserved below the neurologic level, and the majority of key muscles below the neurologic level have a muscle grade of greater than or equal to 3.
E. Normal. Sensory and motor function is normal.

12. Herkowitz HN, Rothman RH. Subacute instability of the cervical spine. *Spine* 1984;9:348–357.
13. Bracken MB, Shepard MJ, Collins WF Jr, et al. Methylprednisolone or naloxone treatment after acute spinal cord injury: 1-year follow-up data. Results of the second National Acute Spinal Cord Injury Study. *J Neurosurg* 1992;76:23–31.
14. Barnes RW. Fractures and dislocations of the cervical spine. *Postgrad Med* 1964;35:588–599.
15. Durbin FC. Fractures-dislocations of the cervical spine. *J Bone Joint Surg Br* 1957;39:23–38.
16. White AA, Johnson RM, Panjabi MM. Biomechanical analysis of clinical stability in the cervical spine. *Clin Orthop* 1975;109:85–95.
17. White AA, Panjabi MM, Saja S. Biomechanics of the axially loaded cervical spine: development of a clinical test for ruptured ligaments. *J Bone Joint Surg Am* 1978;57:582–587.
18. American Spinal Injury Association, ed. *Standards for neurologic and functional classification of spinal cord injury,* rev. ed. Chicago: American Spinal Injury Association, 1992.
19. Ditunno JF, Young W, Donovan WH, et al. The International Standards Booklet for Neurological and Functional Classification of Spinal Cord Injury. *Paraplegia* 1994;32:10–80.

CHAPTER 48

Flexion Injuries

Michael J. Vives and Steven R. Garfin

Traumatic injuries to the subaxial cervical spine are a common cause of morbidity and mortality in both developed and undeveloped nations. Most patients with closed spinal column injury are young adult males, whose injury often results from motor vehicle accidents, falls, or sports injuries. A second peak in prevalence also exists in people aged 50 years and older. Injuries in this age group are predominantly related to falls. Categorizing these injuries by their mechanism has allowed the spine care practitioner to more adeptly evaluate and treat the patients who experience them. This chapter focuses on acute injuries of the cervical spine due to flexion.

ANATOMY AND PATHOMECHANICS

Although the atlantoaxial joint and subaxial spine contribute equally to rotation, most of the flexion and extension in the cervical spine occurs from C3 to C7. Up to 17 degrees of sagittal plane motion occurs at individual motion segments of the subaxial spine. Coronal plane motion ranges from 4 to 11 degrees per motion segment in this region (1). The anterior two-thirds of the vertebral body, in concert with the anterior longitudinal ligament and annulus fibrosis, acts as a tension band limiting extension. Posteriorly, the supraspinous and interspinous ligaments, the ligamentum flavum, and the facet capsules resist flexion (2).

Motor vehicle accidents and shallow dives are the most common scenarios leading to flexion injuries of the cervical spine. Experiments in human cadavers loaded axially to the posterior skull vertex demonstrated cervical motion segment failure in extension, while those loaded anterior to the skull vertex failed in flexion (3). Porcine models have demonstrated great variations in resultant fracture patterns with small variations in distance of load application anteriorly or posteriorly from neutral to the point of axial loading (4–6). The initial head-neck-thorax position and loading conditions determine cervical spine response to impact, as shown

in studies of both human cadaveric and calf spines (7–10). When the cervical spine is straight and colinear with an axial force, the spine buckles after a sudden "give," or deformation, in structure. In human cadaveric studies, prepositioning the head in a mildly flexed position, eliminating the normal cervical lordosis (that is, straightening the spine), results in the least amount of axial deformation per given axial load. Large amounts of energy are absorbed by the spinal column until it buckles, rapidly dissipating stored energy to the surrounding soft tissues. In theory, the relatively straight position of the spine at initial loading may lessen the ability of the surrounding muscles and ligaments to dissipate the applied energy to surrounding structures. Specimens prepositioned in more flexion and then axially loaded failed in flexion at substantially lower loads than did the neutral-positioned specimens (3). These studies, along with mathematical models, have suggested that the straightened (rather than the kyphotic) cervical spine will withstand the highest external axial load (11,12).

Even in the absence of an external axial load, excessive flexion or combined flexion-rotation may result in injury to the cervical spinal column. Pure flexion injuries generally produce a compression fracture of the vertebral body. More substantial flexion moments can result in associated disruption of the posterior ligaments. The resultant injury often manifests radiographically as angulation of the compressed anterior vertebral body with widening of the interspinous space. There may be associated perching of the facets with minimal vertebral body translation. Large amounts of translation, however, generally indicate a more substantial rotatory force with facet dislocation (13).

When the major injury vector is a flexion bending moment near, but anterior to, the sagittal plane, posterior distraction forces disrupt the posterior ligaments and facet capsules, often without compressive force transmitted to the vertebral bodies. With lower magnitudes of force, subluxation of the facets may occur. With higher levels of force, bilateral perching or even dislocation of the facets may occur, with more extensive injury to the ligamentum flavum and intervertebral disc occurring concomitantly (14). The addition of a rotational force to the flexion distraction mechanism can result in a unilateral facet dislocation. The failure of the interspinous ligament combined with the unilateral disruption of the facet capsule and posterolateral annulus allows a rotational deformity to result.

CLASSIFICATION

Although a universally accepted classification system for fractures and dislocations of the lower cervical spine does not exist, those based on mechanism of injury have generally been found useful. The classification by Allen and associates (15) is one of the most widely quoted today. This system is based on a retrospective evaluation of 165 cases of cervical spine trauma. The authors proposed six categories, each named for the presumed position of the cervical spine at the moment of injury and the initial principal mechanism of load to failure. The categories proposed by those authors were vertical compression, compressive flexion, distractive flexion, lateral flexion, compressive extension, and distractive extension (Fig. 48.1). They demonstrated that the probability of related neurologic injury could be predicted based on the type and severity of the spinal column injury.

The classification describes a continuum of injury severity related to the force dissipated to the spine at the time of trauma. This chapter focuses on the compressive flexion (CF) and distractive flexion (DF) phylogenies.

Compressive Flexion Injuries

- Compressive flexion stage 1 (CFS1): The CFS1 lesion is produced by a compressive force oriented obliquely downward and posterior in the sagittal plane causing deformation of the centrum. This manifests as blunting of the anterior-superior margin of the vertebral body, producing a rounded contour. The posterior ligamentous complex remains intact (Fig. 48.2A).
- Compressive flexion stage 2 (CFS2): The CFS2 lesion involves the same predominant injury vector as the stage 1 lesion, with presumed greater force transmitted. The resultant injury consists of the changes seen in CFS1 along with obliquity of the anterior vertebral body and loss of some anterior height, resulting in a "beaked" appearance of the anterior-inferior vertebral body. Increased concavity of the inferior end plate may be noted on plain radiographs, but a vertical fracture line through the centrum is often missed (Fig. 48.2B).
- Compressive flexion stage 3 (CFS3): In the stage 3 lesion, the same obliquely oriented compressive forces are involved with the addition of shear stress generated by the bending moment. The resulting injury includes the features of the CFS2 lesion as well as an oblique fracture extending from the anterior surface of the vertebral body

to the inferior subchondral plate with a fracture of the beak (Fig. 48.2C).
- Compressive flexion stage 4 (CFS4): The CFS4 injury is produced by the same predominant injury vector, presumably with more force. Allen and associates (15) proposed that the production of the oblique fracture, as seen in the CFS3 lesion, resolves the compressive stress. As a result, the CFS4 and CFS5 lesions demonstrate no greater deformation of the centrum. A tension/shear component, however, is transmitted through the posterior part of the anterior elements. As a result, along with the findings of a CFS3 injury, CFS4 lesions demonstrate mild displacement (less than 3 mm) of the inferior-posterior vertebral margin into the neural canal at the involved motion segment (Fig. 48.2D).
- Compressive flexion stage 5 (CFS5): The CFS5 lesion has the injury features of a CFS3 lesion and more pronounced displacement of the posterior vertebral body fragment into the neural canal. The posteroinferior margin of the upper vertebra may approximate the lamina of the subjacent vertebra. This degree of displacement indicates disruption of the posterior ligamentous complex. The facets are separated or perched, with associated widening of the distance between spinous processes (Fig. 48.2E).

In the authors' series of 36 cases with the CF phylogeny, complete spinal cord injury was present in 25% of CFS3 injuries, 38% of CFS4, and 91% of CFS5 injuries. Thus, the higher stages of the CF phylogeny are felt to be caused by greater force and reflect a greater degree of spinal instability.

Although radiographic descriptive classifications can be useful for unique injuries, they can often be confusing due to their ambiguity and the lack of mechanistic information inferred by their labeling. Two radiographic patterns, however, have been described that are frequently referred to in the spine literature: the teardrop and quadrangular fractures. The flexion teardrop fracture was described by Harris (16,17), who characterized it as complete ligamentous and disc disruption at the level of the injury, including disruption of the facet joints. Additionally, a large triangular anterior bone fragment was thought to be "squeezed off" by the vertebral bodies above and below. The spine proximal to the injury level is usually flexed. Whereas Harris felt these injuries were produced by flexion moments, Allen and associates (15) felt they were produced by combined injury mechanisms of compressive flexion and vertical compression.

The quadrangular fragment fracture was described by Favero and Van Petegham (18) as a variant of a CFS5 injury. The four characteristics of this fracture are an oblique fracture of the vertebral body extending from the anterior-superior margin of the vertebral cortex to the inferior end plate, posterior subluxation of the upper vertebral body on the lower vertebral body, variable degree of angular kyphosis, and disruption of the disc and ligaments anteriorly and posteriorly. The authors felt this pattern implied a greater

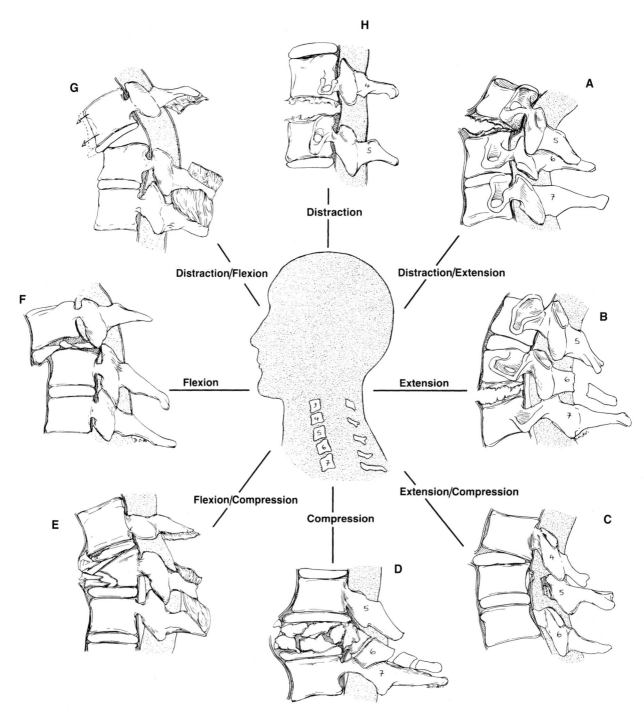

FIG. 48.1. Lower cervical spine injuries. Allen and Ferguson's classification grouped injuries into patterns named for the presumed position of the cervical spine at the moment of injury and the initial principal mechanism of load to failure. **A:** Distractive extension injury. **B:** Extension injury with associated spinous process fracture. **C:** Compressive extension injury. **D:** Axial compression injury. **E:** Compressive flexion injury. **F:** Flexion injury. **G:** Distractive-flexion injury. **H:** Distraction injury. (From, Frymoyer JW, ed. *The adult spine: principles and practice.* New York: Raven, 1991, with permission.)

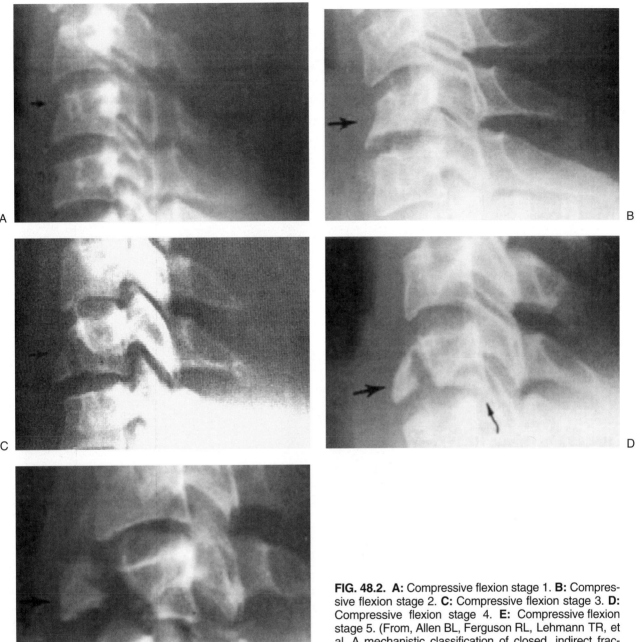

FIG. 48.2. A: Compressive flexion stage 1. **B:** Compressive flexion stage 2. **C:** Compressive flexion stage 3. **D:** Compressive flexion stage 4. **E:** Compressive flexion stage 5. (From, Allen BL, Ferguson RL, Lehmann TR, et al. A mechanistic classification of closed, indirect fractures and dislocations of the lower cervical spine. *Spine* 1982;7:1–27, with permission.)

degree of instability, requiring both anterior and posterior stabilization.

Distractive Flexion Injuries

- Distractive flexion stage 1 (DFS1): The DFS1 lesion is commonly referred to as a "flexion sprain." The stage 1 lesion probably involves a variable degree of disruption of the posterior ligaments and facet capsules, while leaving the intervertebral disc uninjured. The injury is manifest as facet subluxation in flexion, with increased divergence of the spinous processes spanning the injury level (Fig. 48.3A).
- Distractive flexion stage 2 (DFS2): The injury typically catalogued as DFS2 is the unilateral facet dislocation (Fig. 48.3B). Rotary listhesis may be detected by widening of the uncovertebral joint on the side of the dislocation and displacement of the tip of the spinous process toward the dislocated facet. When the forces causing the dislocation cease, subsequent muscle contractions lock

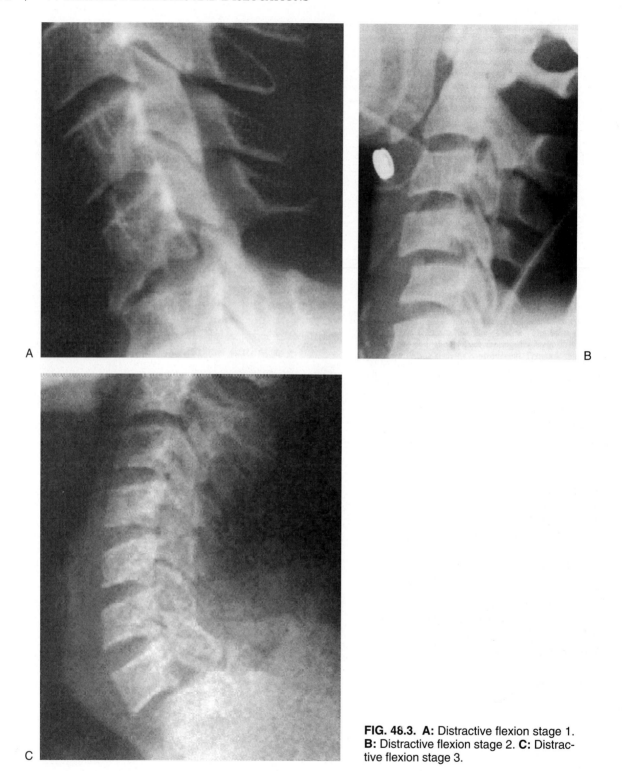

FIG. 48.3. A: Distractive flexion stage 1. **B:** Distractive flexion stage 2. **C:** Distractive flexion stage 3.

the dislocated facet in a position with the inferior articular process of the superior vertebra anterior to the superior articular process of the inferior vertebra (19).

- Distractive flexion stage 3 (DFS3): The DFS3 lesion consists of bilateral facet dislocation (Fig. 48.3C). There is generally at least 50% anterior displacement of the superior vertebral body with respect to the inferior vertebra. The anterior superior margin of the inferior vertebra may be blunted into a rounded contour.

- Distractive flexion stage 4 (DFS4): The final category in this phylogeny, DFS4, consists of bilateral facet dislocation with displacement full body width anteriorly.

Although grouped together as a general injury category, it is recognized that these "stages" do not necessarily represent elements in a spectrum of one injury mechanism. Unilateral facet dislocations (DFS2) may involve a rotational moment combined with flexion and distraction forces. Bilateral facet dislocations (DFS3), in contrast, can be produced by pure flexion or distraction forces.

The contribution to stability by the surrounding soft tissue structures must be assessed and better understood. In an anatomical model using cadaveric spines, Sim and associates (20) implicated the ipsilateral articular capsule, anulus fibrosis, and ligamentum flavum as the soft tissue restraints that must be disrupted to produce a unilateral facet dislocation (DFS2). Disruption of the anterior and posterior longitudinal ligaments and the interspinous ligaments was not necessary to produce a unilateral dislocation. Although many authors feel that an extrinsic rotational vector is necessary to produce such a unilateral dislocation (21–23), the experimental model used in the study by Sims and colleagues (20) demonstrated that unilateral distraction with the physiologic coupled rotation (due to facet geometry) was sufficient to result in a DFS2 lesion. The DFS3 lesion appears to be associated with greater soft tissue disruption. In a retrospective study using magnetic resonance analysis of flexion distraction injuries, Vaccaro and associates (24) reported that disruption of the anterior and posterior longitudinal ligaments was consistently seen in bilateral facet dislocations, compared with unilateral facet dislocations.

Ebraheim and colleagues (25) investigated the effect of different degrees of anterior translation on the spinal canal in a cadaveric simulation of distractive flexion injuries. After 3 mm of anterior translation, the average area of the spinal canal at the level of the inferior vertebra was 75% for C6, 77% for C7, and 79% for T1. After 6 mm of anterior translation (approximately 50% translation), the average spinal canal area decreased to 59% at C6, 51% at C7, and 56% at T1 (25). The rate of spinal cord injury for unilateral facet dislocation is on the order of 25%, whereas for bilateral facet dislocations the rate is close to 50%. Kang and colleagues (26) reported an association between the space available for the cord at the injury level and the risk for spinal cord injury. A sagittal canal diameter of less than 13 mm was associated with injury to the spinal cord.

Distractive flexion injuries have recently been shown to be associated with a substantial rate of injury to the vertebral artery. One recent study demonstrated that the static deformity associated with advanced injuries (DFS2 or higher) results in considerable deformation of the vertebral vasculature (27). Vaccaro and associates (28) demonstrated in a follow-up study that the majority of these injuries do not recannulate, indicating significant disruption of the vessel anatomy. Fortunately, the majority of these injuries are asymptomatic, requiring only observation.

ASSESSMENT

All patients with head injury, high-energy trauma, complaints of neck pain, or neurologic deficit should be assumed to have a cervical spine injury following a traumatic event. In the field, immediate stabilization and focus on protection of the cervical spine is mandatory. With coordinated movements, the neck should be palpated for tenderness and any evidence of step-off. A thorough sensorimotor examination should be documented at initial presentation, along with documentation of perianal sensory sparing and the presence or absence of a bulbocavernosus reflex.

The initial radiographic evaluation should include an anteroposterior and lateral cervical view (including the cervicothoracic junction) and an open-mouth odontoid view. This radiographic protocol detects the majority of cervical spinal injuries (29–31). Up to 16% of patients will have noncontiguous spine fractures, with fractures at the C1-C2 level along with a remote subaxial fracture being one of the most common patterns (32). The radiographic criteria for spinal stability continue to evolve. Angulation greater than 11 degrees compared with adjacent normal segments or translation greater than 3.5 mm were guidelines developed by serial sectioning studies in cadavers (1).

If the plain radiographs reveal osseous abnormalities, computed tomography (CT) may help define the extent of bony damage (Fig. 48.4). CT is also helpful when the lower cervical spine cannot be adequately visualized on plain radiographs. Magnetic resonance imaging (MRI) may be indicated in the following: patients with neurologic deficits (to localize and quantify the degree of cord compression),

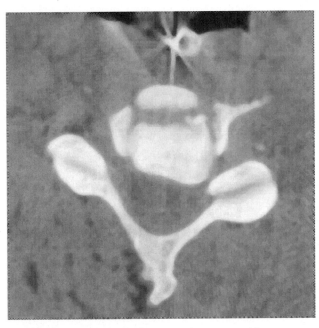

FIG. 48.4. A transaxial computed tomographic scan revealing multiple fracture planes involving the centrum of the vertebral body.

particularly when CT does not demonstrate a reason for the deficit; patients with deteriorating neurologic status; and cases of suspected posterior ligamentous injury not evident by plain radiographs or on CT reconstructions (33). Controversy exists regarding the timing of obtaining these modalities in the acute trauma setting. The authors favor early restoration of cervical alignment and protection, with traction, in the alert and cooperative patient prior to pursuit of an advanced imaging work-up, which may require delay or repeated transfers.

Lateral flexion-extension radiographs are rarely indicated in the acute trauma setting. The patient should be able to position his or her neck voluntarily. These views should not be obtained with physical or radiographic findings of bony, ligamentous, or neurologic injury. The information gained on flexion-extension films in the acute setting is also limited because of pain. A negative study does not preclude significant soft tissue disruption (34) because muscle spasm can mask instability for up to 2 weeks. Follow-up films in that time frame are therefore necessary.

TREATMENT

Compressive Flexion Injuries

In CFS1 and CFS2 injuries, the structural integrity of the anterior column retains partial competence. The posterior annulus and posterior ligamentous structures remain intact. Most patients can be managed with a rigid cervical orthosis or, in cases of questionable compliance, a halo vest, until bony healing. Ten to 12 weeks of immobilization is often necessary. Patients should be monitored for improvement of symptoms and radiographic signs of healing. Flexion-extension lateral radiographs should be obtained prior to cessation of immobilization. Abnormal motion in this circumstance may be an indication for a posterior arthrodesis (13).

Stage 3 injuries (teardrop fragment without subluxation) are potentially unstable. Evaluation by MRI should be performed to assess possible injury to the disc and posterior ligamentous complex. In the absence of injury to these soft tissues, the fracture may be managed in a halo brace until healing. For those injuries with associated posterior ligamentous injury, anterior or posterior arthrodesis may be indicated due to the risk of late kyphotic deformity. The authors prefer the anterior approach in the management of this fracture pattern, although a posterior arthrodesis with triple wiring (35) or lateral mass plating is often adequate (33,36). In the setting of a neurologic deficit, especially with evidence of significant anterior thecal sac compression from retropulsed bone or an extruded disc fragment, an anterior decompressive and reconstructive procedure is indicated. These injuries may progress into kyphosis if treated in an orthosis, even in a halo. If this method is selected, frequent radiographs should be obtained in the brace.

Subluxation of the inferior body fragment posteriorly into the neural canal (CFS4) suggests a more unstable lesion.

Traction with Gardner-Wells tongs and an extension roll placed beneath the scapula lengthwise is useful, but often results in incomplete realignment. Definitive halo vest immobilization without surgical stabilization is often unsuccessful due to progressive loss of cervical alignment over time. In a neurologically intact patient, posterior stabilization may suffice. However, in the presence of an incomplete neurologic injury with objective anterior thecal sac compression, an anterior decompression, strut graft placement, and plating is often indicated (37–39). Supplemental posterior arthrodesis may be indicated with extensive posterior ligamentous injury. Fixation posteriorly can be achieved through interspinous wiring or lateral mass plating.

More extensive subluxation (greater than 3 mm) with retropulsion of the posteroinferior vertebral body into the spinal canal defines a CFS5 injury (Fig. 48.5). An isolated posterior arthrodesis in this circumstance is inadequate due to the extensive degree of anterior and posterior osteoligamentous instability present. There is disruption of the anterior longitudinal ligament, the entire annulus fibrosus including the disc, the posterior longitudinal ligament, and often the posterior bony elements. Thus, all three columns are significantly involved, usually over the course of two motion segments (40). This pattern is best addressed through an anterior approach. Again, in the presence of a neurologic deficit with bony encroachment of the neural canal, this facilitates complete decompression of the spinal canal. Strut grafting and anterior plating provide stabilization. More secure stabilization can be achieved through a combined anterior and posterior stabilization approach. If such a combined approach is felt to be necessary, the authors favor performing the anterior procedure first, followed by the posterior procedure under the same anesthesia.

The surgical procedure of choice in these advanced-stage compressive flexion injuries remains controversial. Biomechanical studies in models depicting anterior injuries with posterior ligamentous disruption have cited anterior plating techniques as inadequate fixation. In a bovine model, Sutterlin's group (41) found inadequate restoration of flexural or axial stability using anterior Caspar instrumentation. They therefore recommended additional posterior stabilization (41). The same group reached similar conclusions in a human cadaver model of distractive flexion injuries treated with anterior plating (but without structural bone graft) (42).

In contrast, clinical reports of anterior plating and structural grafting without supplemental posterior fixation have been more favorable. Several authors have reported success with varied anterior plating systems in lower cervical spine injuries with and without postoperative halo use (37,38,43–45). Garvey and colleagues (46) reported their clinical experience using stand-alone anterior Caspar plating and structural bone grafting. This study focused on a narrow population of 14 patients with mechanically unstable cervical spine injuries (CFS4 or CFS5 and DFS2 or DFS3). At an average follow-up of 30 months, no patient had loss of fixation, and all had radiographically solid anterior fusions. Eleven of the 14 patients wore a rigid plastic

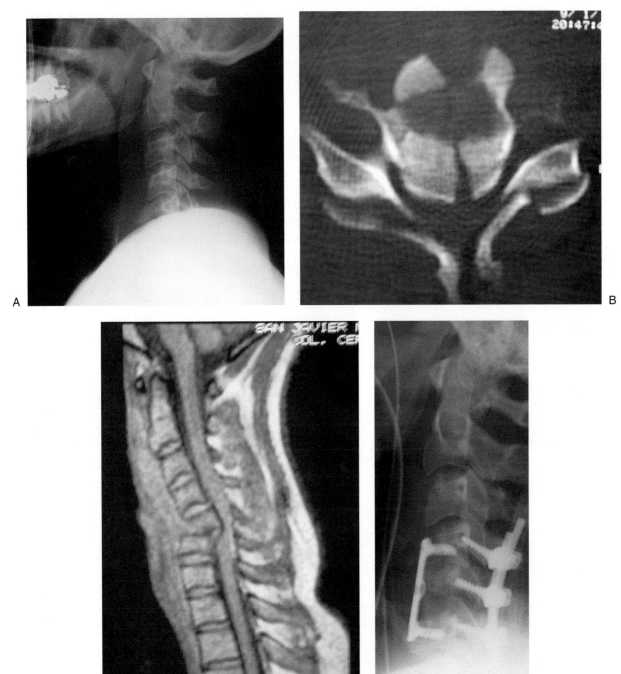

FIG. 48.5. A: A lateral cervical radiograph revealing a stage V flexion compression cervical spine injury. **B:** Axial computed tomographic scan showing posterior displacement of the posterior vertebral margin into the spinal canal. **C:** Sagittal magnetic resonance imaging demonstrating the pronounced posterior displacement of the vertebral body into the canal with spinal cord compression. **D:** An anterior-posterior approach was used to decompress the cervical canal and stabilize the subaxial cervical spine. This is seen on the lateral radiograph following anterior iliac crest strut graft placement, anterior cervical plate instrumentation, and posterior lateral mass fixation.

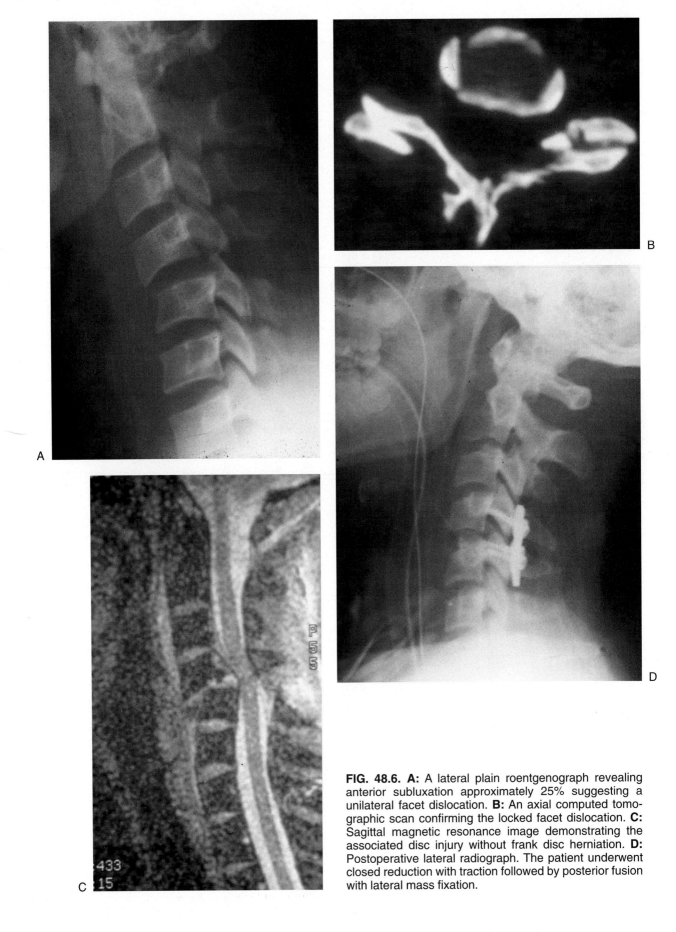

FIG. 48.6. A: A lateral plain roentgenograph revealing anterior subluxation approximately 25% suggesting a unilateral facet dislocation. **B:** An axial computed tomographic scan confirming the locked facet dislocation. **C:** Sagittal magnetic resonance image demonstrating the associated disc injury without frank disc herniation. **D:** Postoperative lateral radiograph. The patient underwent closed reduction with traction followed by posterior fusion with lateral mass fixation.

collar postoperatively, with only 3 immobilized in halo vests. Based on the results, the authors suggested that the addition of anterior plating to anterior structural grafting could obviate the need for additional posterior plating.

Distractive Flexion Injuries

Low-grade injuries of the "flexion sprain" variety (DFS1) can generally be treated with immobilization in a rigid cervical orthosis. Six weeks of immobilization is generally recommended, although the exact length of such treatment can be modified based on symptoms and radiographic signs of stability on flexion-extension views.

Unilateral facet dislocations (DFS2) should be promptly reduced, when possible, with traction. Skeletal traction is best applied through Gardner-Wells tongs. A lateral radiograph should be obtained after the initial 10 to 15 pounds to rule out overdistraction and occult occipitocervical injury. Serial neurologic exams and lateral radiographs should be performed after each weight increment. A manipulative reduction may be required once perching of the facets is achieved with traction. Distraction away from the dislocated facet is followed by rotation of the head toward the side of the dislocation (47). This can be performed manually through the tongs, or gradually by altering the pull of the traction. These dislocations often reduce over time, in traction, without excessive weights (60 lb) or manual manipulation techniques. Some surgeons favor obtaining a prereduction MRI to rule out a disc herniation at the injured segment, which may be displaced into the canal with the reduction maneuver (48). Although some surgeons treat successfully reduced unilateral facet dislocations with halo or rigid orthotic immobilization, many favor immediate operative stabilization (Fig. 48.6). Traditional interspinous wiring techniques have demonstrated consistently good results if the facet is not fractured (49,50). Lateral mass fixation is another alternative that has been associated with good clinical outcomes (51). A variety of plate and screw systems, as well as rod and screw systems, are currently available.

Bilateral facet dislocations (DFS3 and DFS4) should also be treated with prompt reduction. Neurologic injury in this setting is common, and administration of methylprednisolone following the guidelines of the third National Acute Spinal Cord Injury Study is often considered (52). Final reduction of the facets sometimes requires an anteriorly directed force followed by extension once the facets are distracted (47). Disc herniation can be present prior to reduction in up to 55% of bilateral facet dislocations. As in DFS2 injuries, controversy exists over the practicality of obtaining an MRI before reduction in an alert and neurologically intact patient. Most of the cases of reported neurologic deficit occurred during surgical reduction under general anesthesia. It has been demonstrated that immediate traction and reduction can be performed safely when the patient is awake and alert (53). Such an approach allows for the most expedited reduction, which may promote the best chance for recovery in cases with incomplete spinal cord injury. If this technique is chosen and the patient deteriorates or does not improve, an MRI can be obtained at that time.

Immobilization of this unstable lesion in a halo vest often results in recurrent subluxation or dislocation. Reduction is therefore usually followed by a posterior stabilization procedure, such as a conventional wiring technique or lateral mass plating. Some surgeons prefer an anterior approach with discectomy and structural grafting accompanied by rigid plating. Again, biomechanical studies of anterior plating (without structural bone graft) had led to concerns regarding the adequacy of this type of fixation for this injury pattern (41,42,54). Clinical data on anterior structural grafting with a rigid plate, however, have demonstrated good results, even without postoperative halo immobilization (46,55).

In situations in which attempts at closed reduction of unilateral or bilateral facet dislocations fail, open reduction and fusion is indicated. Prior to open reduction, an MRI should be performed to exclude a disc herniation, since serial neurologic examinations during the operative reduction are impractical. Also, one reason for failure of closed reduction is the presence of a large disc herniation. In the setting of a frank disc herniation at the dislocated segment, anterior discectomy and arthrodesis should be considered. In some cases the facets cannot be reduced during the anterior procedure. This may necessitate an intermediate stage involving open posterior reduction and instrumented arthrodesis followed by reopening the anterior wound for anterior interbody arthrodesis and plating. An alternate technique has been reported (56) in which the interbody graft is placed after end plate preparation and a buttress plate is fixed to the superior vertebral body. The anterior wound is then closed and the reduction and arthrodesis performed posteriorly, pulling the graft into the interspace as the superior body is reduced onto the inferior one (56).

SUMMARY

Flexion injuries of the lower cervical spine are relatively common. These injuries can be mechanistically classified, with higher stages representing more unstable lesions. More severe lesions are associated with high rates of neurologic injury. Cervical orthoses may suffice for benign compression fractures with little deformity or for flexion sprains without frank facet incongruity. Higher-grade lesions, however, may require single or combined stabilization procedures. Although the classification system presented may help outline treatment recommendations, more unstable injuries warrant individualized strategies.

REFERENCES

1. White AA III, Southwick WO, Panjabi MM. Clinical instability in the lower cervical spine—a review of past and current concepts. *Spine* 1976;1:15–27.
2. White AA III, Panjabi MM, Saha S, et al. Biomechanics of the axially loaded cervical spine: development of a clinical test for ruptured ligaments. *J Bone Joint Surg Am* 1975;57:582.

3. Maiman DJ, Sances A, Myklebust JB, et al. Compression injuries of the cervical spine: a biomechanical analysis. *Neurosurgery* 1983;13:254–260.

4. Oxland TR, Panjabi MM, Southern EP, et al. An anatomic basis for spinal instability: a porcine trauma model. *J Orthop Res* 1991;9:452–462.

5. Panjabi MM, Durancea JS, Oxland TR, et al. Multidirectional instabilities of traumatic cervical spine injuries in a porcine model. *Spine* 1989;14:1111–1115.

6. Southern EP, Oxland TR, Panjabi MM, et al. Cervical spine injury patterns in three modes of high-speed trauma: a biomechanical porcine model. *J Spinal Disord* 1990;3:316–328.

7. Alem NM, Nusholtz GS, Melvin JW. Head and neck response to axial impacts. In: *Proceedings of the 28th STAPP Car Crash Conference.* Warrendale, PA: Society of Automotive Engineers, 1984.

8. Hodgson VR, Thomas LM. Mechanisms of cervical spine injury during impact to the protected head. In: *Proceedings of the 24th STAPP Car Crash Conference.* Warrendale, PA: Society of Automotive Engineers, 1980:17.

9. Nusholtz GS, Huelke DE, Lux P, et al. Cervical spine injury mechanisms. In: *Proceedings of the 27th STAPP Car Crash Conference.* Warrendale, PA: Society of Automotive Engineers, 1983:179–197.

10. Shono Y, McAffe PC, Cunningham BW. The pathomechanics of compression injuries of the cervical spine. *Spine* 1993;18:2009–2019.

11. Helleur C, Gracovetsky S, Farfan H. Tolerance of the human cervical spine to high acceleration: a modeling approach. *Aviat Space Environ Med* 1984;55:903–909.

12. Yoganandan N, Sances A, Maiman DJ, et al. Experimental spinal injuries with vertical impact. *Spine* 1986;11:855–860.

13. Abitbol JJ, Kostuik JP. Flexion injuries to the lower cervical spine. In: Clarke CR, Ducker TB, Dvorak J, et al., eds. *The cervical spine,* 3rd ed. Philadelphia: Lippincott–Raven, 1998:457–464.

14. Vaccaro AR, Falatyn SP, Flanders AE, et al. Magnetic resonance evaluation of the intervertebral disc, spinal ligaments, and spinal cord before and after closed traction reduction of cervical spine dislocations. *Spine* 1999;24:1210–1217.

15. Allen BL, Ferguson RL, Lehmann TR, et al. A mechanistic classification of closed, indirect fractures and dislocations of the lower cervical spine. *Spine* 1982;7:1–27.

16. Harris JH, Edeiken-Monroe B, Kopaniky DR. A practical classification of acute cervical spine injuries. *Orthop Clin North Am* 1986;17:15–30.

17. Harris JH. Radiographic evaluation of spinal trauma. *Orthop Clin North Am* 1986;17:75–86.

18. Favero KJ, Van Petegham PK. The quadrangular fragment fracture: roentgenographic features and treatment protocol. *Clin Orthop* 1989;239:40–46.

19. Braakman R, Vinken PJ. Unilateral facet locking in the lower cervical spine. *J Bone Joint Surg Br* 1967;49:249–257.

20. Sim E, Vaccaro AR, Berzlanovich A, et al. *In vitro* genesis of subaxial cervical unilateral facet dislocations through sequential soft tissue ablation. *Spine* 2001;26:1317–1323.

21. Argenson C, Lovet J, Sansouiller JL, et al. Traumatic rotatory displacement of the lower cervical spine. *Spine* 1988;13:767–773.

22. Burke CD, Berryman D. The place of closed manipulation in the management of flexion-rotation dislocations of the cervical spine. *J Bone Joint Surg Br* 1971;53:165–182.

23. Young JWR, Resnik CS, DeCandido P, et al. The laminar space in the diagnosis of rotational flexion injuries of the cervical spine. *AJR Am J Roentgenol* 1989;152:103–107.

24. Vaccaro AR, Madigan L, Schweitzer ME, et al. Magnetic resonance imaging analysis of soft tissue disruption after flexion-distraction injuries of the subaxial cervical spine. *Spine* 2001;26:1866–1872.

25. Ebraheim NA, Xu R, Ahmad M, et al. The effect of anterior translation of the vertebra on the canal size in the lower cervical spine: a computer-assisted anatomic study. *J Spinal Disord* 1997;10:162–166.

26. Kang JD, Figgie MP, Bohlman HH. Sagittal measurements of the cervical spine in subaxial fractures and dislocations: an analysis of two hundred and eighty-eight patients with and without neurological deficits. *J Bone Joint Surg Am* 1994;76:1617–1628.

27. Sim E, Vaccaro AR, Berzlanovich A. The effects of staged cervical flexion-distraction deformities on the patency of the vertebral arterial vasculature. *Spine* 2000;25:2180–2186.

28. Vaccaro AR, Klein G, Flanders AE, et al. Long term evaluation of vertebral artery injuries following cervical spine trauma using magnetic resonance angiography. *Spine* 1998;23:789–795.

29. Streitweiser DR, Knopp R, Wales LR, et al. Accuracy of standard radiographic views in detecting cervical spine fractures. *Ann Emerg Med* 1983;12:538–542.

30. Clark CR, Ingram CM, El-Khoury GY, et al. Radiographic evaluation of cervical spine injuries. *Spine* 1988;13:742–747.

31. Freemyer B, Knopp R, Piche J, et al. Comparison of five-view and three-view cervical spine series in the evaluation of patients with cervical trauma. *Ann Emerg Med* 1989;18:818–821.

32. Vaccaro AR, An HS, Lin SS, et al. Noncontiguous injuries of the spine. *J Spinal Disord* 1992;5:320–329.

33. Rizzolo SJ, Cotler JM. Unstable cervical spine injuries: specific treatment approaches. *J Am Acad Orthop Surg* 1993;1:57–63.

34. Wang JC, Hatch JD, Sandu HS. Cervical flexion and extension radiographs in acutely injured patients. *Clin Orthop* 1999;365:111–116.

35. Stauffer ES. Wiring techniques of the posterior cervical spine for the treatment of trauma. *Orthopedics* 1988;11:1543–1548.

36. Anderson PA, Henley MB, Grady MS, et al. Posterior cervical arthrodesis with AO reconstruction plates and bone graft. *Spine* 1991;16:72–79.

37. Bohler J, Gaudernak T. Anterior plate stabilization for fracture-dislocations of the lower cervical spine. *J Trauma* 1980;20:203–205.

38. Cabenela ME, Ebersold MJ. Anterior plate stabilization for bursting teardrop fractures of the cervical spine. *Spine* 1988;13:888–891.

39. Ripa DR, Kowall MG, Meyer PR, et al. Series of ninety-two traumatic cervical spine injuries stabilized with anterior ASIF plate fusion technique. *Spine* 1991;16:46–55.

40. Meyer PR. Cervical spine fractures: changing management concepts. In: Bridwell KH, DeWald RL, eds. *The textbook of spinal surgery.* Philadelphia: Lippincott–Raven, 1997:1679–1742.

41. Sutterlin CE III, McAfee PC, Warden KE, et al. A biomechanical evaluation of cervical spine stabilization methods in a bovine model. Static and cyclic loading. *Spine* 1988;13:795–802.

42. Coe JD, Warden KE, Sutterlin CE III, et al. Biomechanical evaluation of cervical spine stabilization methods in a human cadaveric model. *Spine* 1989;14:1122–1131.

43. Aebi M, Mohler J, Zach GA, et al. Indications, surgical technique, and results of 100 surgically treated fractures and fracture-dislocations of the cervical spine. *Clin Orthop* 1986;203:244–256.

44. Caspar W, Barbier DD, Klara PM. Anterior cervical fusion and Caspar plate stabilization for cervical trauma. *Neurosurgery* 1989;25:491–502.

45. Suh PB, Kostuik JP, Esses SI. Anterior cervical plate fixation with the titanium hollow screw plate system. A preliminary report. *Spine* 1990;15:1079–1080.

46. Garvey TA, Eismont FJ, Roberti LJ. Anterior decompression, structural bone grafting, and Caspar stabilization for unstable cervical spine fractures and/or dislocations. *Spine* 1992;17(Suppl 10):S431–S435.

47. Cotler HB, Miller LS, DeLucia FA, et al. Closed reduction of cervical spine dislocations. *Clin Orthop* 1987;214:185–194.

48. Eismont FJ, Arena MJ, Green BA. Extrusion of an intervertebral disc associated with traumatic subluxation or dislocation of cervical facets. *J Bone Joint Surg Am* 1991;73:1555–1560.

49. Rogers WA. Fracture and dislocations of the cervical spine: an end-result study. *J Bone Joint Surg Am* 1957;39:341–376.

50. Weiland DJ, McAfee PC. Posterior cervical fusion with triple-wire strut graft technique: one hundred consecutive patients. *J Spinal Disord* 1991;4:15–21.

51. Fehlings MG, Cooper PR, Errico TJ. Posterior plates in the management of cervical instability: long term results in 44 patients. *J Neurosurg* 1994;81:341–349.

52. Bracken MB, Shepard MJ, Holfors TR, et al. Administration of methylprednisolone for 24 or 48 hours or tirilazad mesylate for 48 hours in the treatment of acute spinal cord injury: results of the third National Acute Spinal Cord Injury randomized controlled trial. *JAMA* 1997;277:1597–1604.

53. Star AM, Jones AA, Cotler JM, et al. Immediate closed reduction of cervical spine dislocations using traction. *Spine* 1990;15:1068–1072.

54. Ulrich C, Woersdoefer O, Kalff R. Biomechanics of fixation systems to the cervical spine. *Spine* 1991;16(Suppl 3):S4–S9.

55. Razack N, Green BA, Levi AD. The management of traumatic cervical bilateral facet fracture-dislocations with unicortical anterior plates. *J Spinal Disord* 2000;13:374–381.

56. Allred CD, Sledge JB. Irreducible dislocations of the cervical spine with a prolapsed disc: preliminary results from a treatment technique. *Spine* 2001;26:1927–1930.

CHAPTER 49

Extension Injuries

Michael J. Vives and Steven R. Garfin

Cervical spine injuries are a major cause of morbidity in today's society. Injuries to the subaxial cervical spine are commonly caused by extension forces in association with compression, distraction, or rotation. These injuries are the focus of this chapter. Soft tissue injuries about the cervical spine from acceleration of the head on the thorax (whiplash) are discussed elsewhere.

INCIDENCE

Extension injuries frequently lack demonstrable radiographic abnormalities. As a result, there is no agreement about the rate of occurrence of these injuries. Whitley and Forsyth (1) reported a frequency nearly equal to flexion injuries. Kiwerski (2) estimated that 26% of his large series of cervical spinal injuries were a result of a hyperextension mechanism. In detailing the experiences of a large tertiary spinal injury center over a 27-year period, Meyer (3) reported that approximately one-third of injuries were due to hyperextension.

ANATOMY AND PATHOMECHANICS

Extension injuries are often the result of falls or trauma in which the point of force application involves the patient's head or face. The anterior longitudinal ligament and the anterior annulus are the structures that resist extension. In an immature calf spine model, Shono and associates (4) demonstrated predictable anterior avulsion fractures, anterior longitudinal ligament disruptions, and disc injuries. In severe injuries, muscular avulsions of the sternocleidomastoid, strap muscles, longus colli, or end plate have been reported (5,6). With forced hyperextension or application of compressive forces with a posterior eccentricity, there is impaction of the posterior arches and compression of the facet joints (7). With sufficient force, fractures of the posterior elements occur. Fractures of the spinous processes,

laminae, articular pillars, and pedicles can occur alone or in combination. With more substantial force, the extension moment can cause failure of the posterior longitudinal ligament with posterior displacement of the vertebral body into the spinal canal. In these cases, the spinal cord may be pinched between the posterior portion of the cephalad vertebral body and the next caudal lamina.

White and Panjabi (8) developed a cadaveric testing model in which soft tissue constraints were sectioned from anterior to posterior with concurrent application of a hyperextension load. They noted small increments of change in both angular and translational displacement until the posterior longitudinal ligament was sectioned, with ensuing catastrophic failure. Several postmortem studies in patients who had sustained hyperextension injuries have corroborated these experimental findings (9–11).

CLASSIFICATION

Although a universally accepted classification system for fractures and dislocations of the lower cervical spine does not exist, those based on mechanism of injury have generally been found useful. The classification by Allen and associates (12) is one of the most widely used today. This system is based on a retrospective evaluation of 165 cases of cervical spine trauma. The authors proposed six categories, each named for the presumed position of the cervical spine at the moment of injury and the initial principal mechanism of load to failure. The categories proposed by the authors were vertical compression, compressive flexion, distractive flexion, lateral flexion, compressive extension, and distractive extension (Fig. 49.1). The authors demonstrated that the probability of related neurologic injury could be predicted based on the type and severity of the spinal injury (12).

The classification discusses a continuum of injury severity related to the force dissipated to the spine at the time of

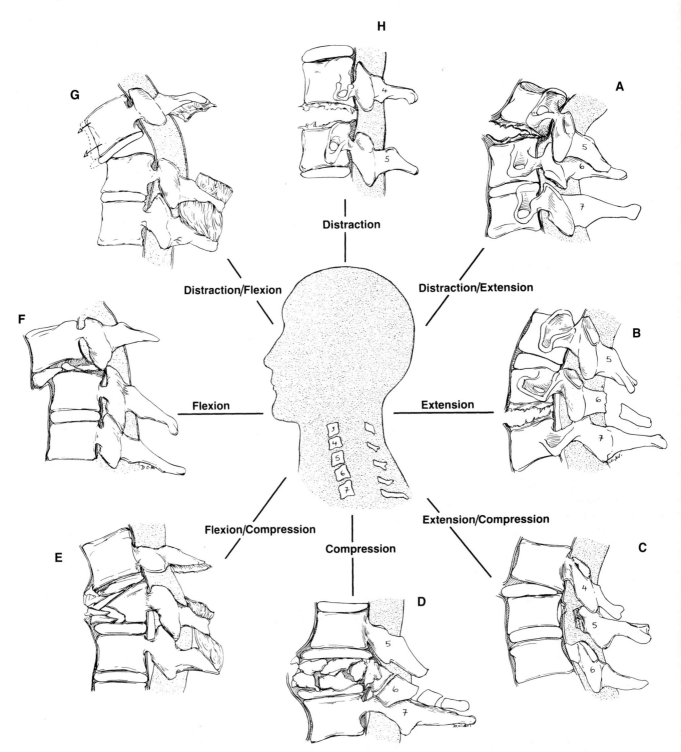

FIG. 49.1. Lower cervical spine injuries. Allen and Ferguson's classification grouped injuries into patterns named for the presumed position of the cervical spine at the moment of injury and the initial principal mechanism of load to failure. **A:** Distractive extension injury. **B:** Extension injury with associated spinous process fracture. **C:** Compressive extension injury. **D:** Axial compression injury. **E:** Compressive flexion injury. **F:** Flexion injury. **G:** Distractive flexion injury. **H:** Distraction injury. (From, Frymoyer JW, ed. *The adult spine: principles and practice*. New York: Raven, 1991, with permission.)

trauma. This chapter focuses on the compressive extension (CE) and distractive extension (DE) phylogenies.

Compressive Extension Injuries

- Compressive extension stage 1 (CES1): The stage 1 lesion involves a unilateral posterior arch fracture. Anterorotary displacement of the vertebral centrum may or may not be present. The posterior element fracture may consist of a linear fracture through the articular pillar, an ipsilateral pedicle and laminar fracture resulting in the "horizontal facet" appearance, or a combination of ipsilateral articular process and pedicular fracture (Fig. 49.2A).
- Compressive extension stage 2 (CES2): The stage 2 lesion involves bilaminar fractures without evidence of failure of anterior constraints. Multiple contiguous levels are often involved (Fig. 49.2B).
- Compressive extension stages 3 and 4 (CES3, CES4): The CES3 lesion involves bilateral vertebral arch "cor-

ner" fractures—laminae, pedicles, or articular processes (or some bilateral combination)—without displacement of the vertebral body. The stage 4 lesion involves bilateral posterior arch fractures with partial vertebral body displacement anteriorly. These two stages were not encountered in Allen and colleagues' study group (12), but were hypothesized to be the link between the mild and advanced lesions of the CE phylogeny.

- Compressive extension stage 5 (CES5): The stage 5 lesion consists of bilateral posterior arch fractures with vertebral body displacement anteriorly the full width of the centrum. The posterior fragment of the arch does not displace, while the anterior portion of the fractured arch remains with the vertebral body. Shear forces result in ligamentous failure at two different levels. Posteriorly, failure occurs between the suprajacent and the fractured vertebrae, while anteriorly failure ensues between the fractured vertebra and the next caudal vertebra. Typically, the anterior-superior portion of the subjacent vertebral body is sheared off as displacement occurs (Fig. 49.2C).

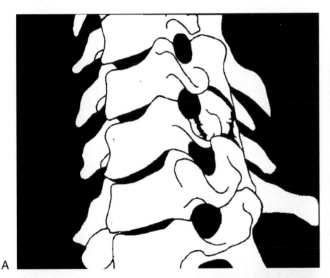

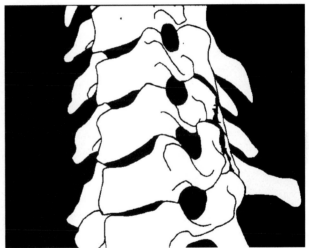

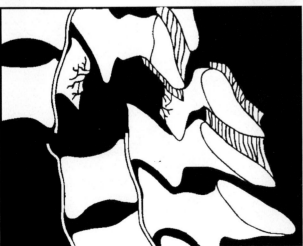

FIG. 49.2. A: Compressive extension stage 1. **B:** Compressive extension stage 2. **C:** Compressive extension stage 5. (From, Cotler JM, ed. *Surgery of spinal trauma.* Philadelphia: Lippincott, 1999, with permission.)

In the series by Allen and associates (12), 32 of the 40 cases they cataloged as CE in nature were CES1. They attributed this high frequency to lateralization of the compressive stress by associated rotational forces. Twenty-five percent of the patients with a CES1 lesion had root level involvement, 12.5% a central cord lesion, and 1 patient (of 32) had a complete cord lesion. Two of the five patients with CES2 lesions had complete spinal cord injuries. The authors noted that none of the three patients with CES5 injuries had complete cord lesions (one radicular, one partial, and one central cord injury). Therefore, for this particular phylogeny, the severity of anatomic damage did not correlate with the severity of the neurologic deficit.

The CES1 lesion with horizontalization of a unilateral facet has also been described by various other authors (1,13,14). This injury may be associated with disruption of the anterior longitudinal ligament and fissure of the disc above and below. The plain radiographic appearance of this injury pattern may be confused with distractive flexion stage 2 (DFS2) injuries involving unilateral facet dislocations. Both may show evidence of anterior subluxation. The appearances on computed tomographic (CT) scanning, however, are fairly distinct. Fractures seen in the DFS2 category are generally of the marginal avulsion nature. In CE mechanisms, the articular pillars experience an impacting-type fracture with alteration of the shape or production of a linear fracture through the body of the articular process, pedicle, or some combination of these (14).

The CES5 lesion resembles what other authors have called the "extension teardrop fracture." This fracture is characterized by a bilateral fracture of the posterior arch between the superior and the inferior articular processes and anterolisthesis of the cephalad vertebra with a postero-inferior marginal fracture. This fracture line runs obliquely from the midpoint of the posterior margin of the vertebra through the intervertebral disc to the anterosuperior margin of the underlying vertebra. The posterior arch is separated from the anteriorly displaced centrum, as in spondylolisthesis (15). Due to the anterolisthesis, Burke termed this a hyperextension injury masquerading as a flexion injury. Forsyth (9) described the mechanism as the head moving through an arc. The hyperextension force is first directed backward and then downward, fracturing the articular processes or pedicles. If allowed to continue, it will finally rebound in a forward direction, with the force pushing the vertebral body anteriorly (9).

Distractive Extension Injuries

- Distractive extension stage 1 (DES1): The stage 1 lesion is caused by a hyperextension vector, with failure of the anterior ligamentous complex (anterior longitudinal ligament and intervertebral disc) or a transverse failure through the bony centrum. In the stage 1 lesion there is no translation or posterior displacement. In injuries that are primarily through the soft tissues, disc space widening may be the only feature on plain radiographs (Fig. 49.3A). Alternatively, there may be a fracture through the margin of an adjacent vertebral body.
- Distractive extension stage 2 (DES2): In addition to the features seen in DES1, the stage 2 lesion involves failure of the posterior ligamentous complex. The resultant instability may allow displacement of the upper vertebral body posteriorly into the spinal canal (Fig. 49.3B). Such displacement may reduce spontaneously when the head is neutrally positioned.

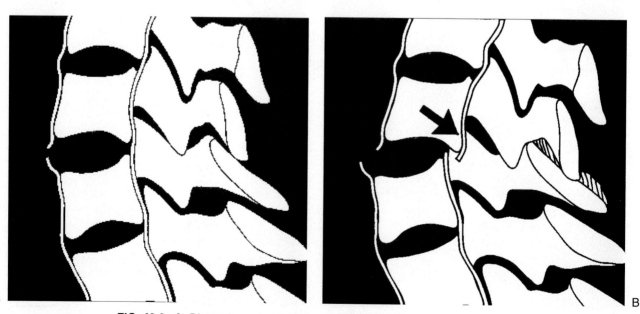

FIG. 49.3. A: Distractive extension stage 1. **B:** Distractive extension stage 2.

Distractive extension injuries account for 8% to 22% of subaxial cervical injuries (16–19). The initial tensile failure of the anterior ligamentous complex implies a major injury vector directed in hyperextension, away from the trunk. In the stage 2 lesion the stress is also transmitted to the posterior elements, resulting in tension/shear failure. Forsyth (9) described the mechanism for the same injury pattern in 1964. He postulated that when the head and neck are hyperextended without compression, the spinous and articular processes are forced together and act as a fulcrum. After rupture of the anterior longitudinal ligament, separation may occur between the end plate and disc. The remainder of the cervical spine cephalad to the separation continues posteriorly, stripping the longitudinal ligament away from the vertebral body below. The data accumulated in the series of Allen and associates (12) suggested that in this phylogeny the neck is in a position of extension and a force is applied over the face or anterior calvaria.

Neurologic injuries in the setting of DES1 lesions are rarely reported. The stage 2 lesion, however, often results in neurologic impairment. Six of the seven patients with this injury pattern in the series of Allen and colleagues (12) had some degree of spinal cord injury. Taylor and Blackwood (19) had previously described an extension dislocation with spontaneous reduction causing the syndrome of a paraplegic patient with normally aligned cervical vertebrae. The pathoanatomy of the neural injury presumably involves compression of the cord between the stable lamina and ligamentum flavum below and the mobile posteroinferior edge of the cephalad vertebral body (20).

Extension Injuries in Patients with Cervical Spondylosis and Ankylosing Spondylitis

In addition to the categories presented previously, hyperextension may produce neural injury in patients with spondylosis and cervical stenosis. Disc degeneration and posterior end plate osteophyte formation along with hypertrophied, infolded ligamentum flavum may result in significant reduction in the space available for the cord. Taylor (20) performed experiments demonstrating the forward bulging of the ligamentum flavum produced by hyperextension. Schneider and associates (21) described the syndrome of acute central cervical spinal cord injury characterized by motor impairment that was greater in the upper than in the lower extremities, bladder dysfunction, and varying degrees of sensory loss, often minimal, below the level of the lesion. These authors postulated that the structural distortion of the cord, greatest in the central portion, damages predominantly the inner portion of the lateral pyramidal tract, corresponding to fibers destined to the upper extremities.

Ankylosing spondylitis represents the extreme end of the spectrum of arthritic involvement of the cervical spine.

Cervical ankylosis develops in 75% of patients whose disease duration is greater than 16 years (22). This results in a rigid, yet brittle, cylinder of bone surrounding the spinal cord, which has diminished capacity to accommodate extension force vectors. The most common presentation is a fracture through a calcified lower cervical intervertebral disc (Fig. 49.4) or through the upper portion of the vertebral body (23,24). Falls that result in a blow to the head, motor vehicle accidents, or apparently trivial injuries can be the source of these fractures. If the trauma is minor, the initial injury may go unrecognized and present later as an advancing flexion deformity (25).

ASSESSMENT

All patients with head injury, high-energy trauma, complaints of neck pain, and/or neurologic deficit should be assumed to have a cervical spine injury. In the field, immediate stabilization and focus on protection of the cervical spine is mandatory. Extension injuries most commonly occur as a result of direct trauma to the forehead or face, so complaints of a painful cervical spine with evidence of facial or forehead trauma should raise suspicion of extension injury. Motor vehicle accidents with violent hyperextension of the head are also commonly associated with these injury patterns (2,14,26). As previously stated, aged patients with advanced spondylosis or ankylosing spondylitis may sustain substantial injuries with minimal trauma. With coordinated movements, the neck should be palpated for tenderness and any evidence of step-off. A motor and sensory root/cord specific examination should be documented at initial presentation, along with assessment of perianal sensory sparing and the presence or absence of a bulbocavernosus reflex, in patients who otherwise appear to have complete injuries.

The initial radiographic evaluation should include an anteroposterior and lateral cervical view (including the cervicothoracic junction) and an open-mouth odontoid view. This radiographic protocol detects the majority of cervical spinal injuries (27–29). Up to 16% of patients will have noncontiguous spine fractures, with fractures at the C1-C2 level along with a remote subaxial fracture being one of the most common patterns (26). The radiographic criteria for spinal stability continue to evolve. Angulation greater than 11 degrees compared with adjacent normal segments and translation greater than 3.5 mm were flexion injury guidelines developed by serial sectioning studies in cadavers (30). The plain radiographic findings in extension injuries, however, may be subtle. Anterior disc space widening or an increase in the retropharyngeal space may be the only features in some injuries.

If the plain radiographs reveal osseous abnormalities, computed tomography (CT) may help define the extent of bony damage. CT is particularly helpful in delineating fractures of the posterior elements in the compressive extension phylogeny. CT is also commonly employed when the lower

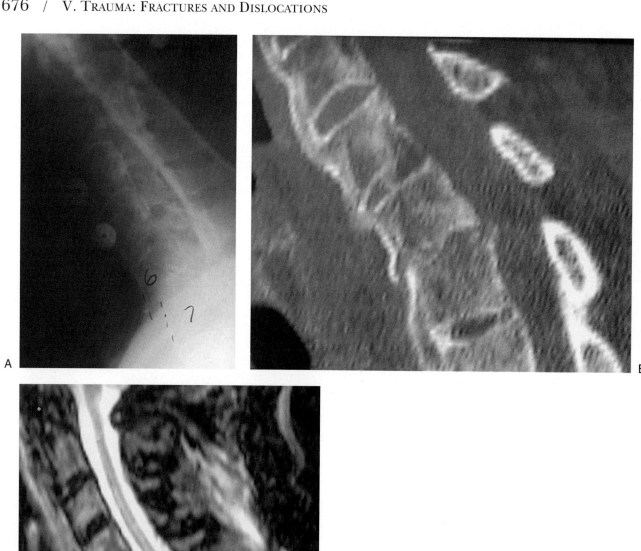

FIG. 49.4. A: Extension injury through a lower cervical disc in a patient with ankylosing spondylitis. **B:** Sagittal reconstruction computed tomography of same patient demonstrating diffuse calcification of the cervical intervertebral discs. **C:** Sagittal magnetic resonance image demonstrating the disruption of the C6-7 disc.

cervical spine cannot be adequately visualized on plain radiographs. Magnetic resonance imaging (MRI) is particularly helpful in the evaluation of patients with suspected extension injuries due to its ability to detect soft tissue injury (31). Davis and associates (32) demonstrated the effectiveness of MRI in evaluating patients without abnormality

on plain radiographs. Fifty of 130 patients with normal radiographs were found to have discal or soft tissue injuries (32). MRI is also helpful in the evaluation of patients with neurologic deficits because of its ability to demonstrate cord injury and spinal stenosis. Schaefer and colleagues (33) demonstrated the usefulness of MRI in differentiating intramedullary cord hematoma from localized or multisegmental edema. The median motor recovery for those with intramedullary hematoma was 9%; for those with edema involving multiple motion segments, 41%; and for those with edema involving only one motion segment, 72% (33).

In most extension injuries, initial immobilization with lateral sandbags or a plastic collar is appropriate. Accurate recognition of the injury pattern prior to application of tong traction is necessary to avoid excessive widening of a fissured disc in extension. If cervical traction is desired to maintain alignment, a flexed position should be utilized. As discussed previously, spinal cord injury is common in this setting, and administration of methylprednisolone following the guidelines of the third National Acute Spinal Cord Injury trial is often instituted (34). In spinal cord–injured patients, early attention to prevention of pressure ulcers should be instituted, either by use of a Roto-Rest bed (if the patient is in traction) or by alternating inclination on cushions if the patient is in a collar.

TREATMENT

The definitive treatment of an extension injury is dependent on the degree of instability and/or neurologic impairment. Although stability continues to be imprecisely defined, it can be simplistically thought of as a condition that allows greater than physiological motion across a motion segment. This excess motion may or may not pose a threat to neural function, either immediately due to frank static malalignment or as a late sequela. Alternatively, this excess motion may predispose to increasing deformity or chronic pain.

Compressive Extension Injuries

The stage 1 lesion involves anterior annular disruption under tension and a unilateral pedicle or lateral mass fracture due to compression. This results in rotational instability around the intact lateral mass. Retrospective data (14) on patients treated in either a hard collar or halo brace demonstrated that such management was universally unsuccessful. Neither method was able to achieve or maintain adequate reduction of the rotary subluxation. Persistence of the presenting neurologic deficit was also common.

Posterior approaches for such fracture separations of the lateral mass have been employed. Because the lateral mass is freely floating, two consecutive facet joints are disrupted, resulting in two levels of instability. Because the injury is rotationally unstable, most midline wiring techniques are not ideal. The Bohlman triple-wire technique may be considered if the adjacent spinous processes are intact. This technique, however, generally cannot achieve or maintain reduction of the lateral masses, so patients with radiculopathy do not experience the benefit of decompression of the involved root (35). Jeanneret and associates (36) have described a technique utilizing a transpedicular screw for direct osteosynthesis of the fracture. This technique, however, has not become widely used due to the small size of the subaxial pedicles (except C7). The emergence of new image guidance systems (incorporating downloaded CT data) may lead to a renewed interest in this method. Lateral mass screw fixation utilizing plates or rods must involve three levels (Fig. 49.5). Instrumenting the uninjured side first may facilitate reduction and stabilization of the injured side. On the injured side, standard screw trajectories can be utilized, although stabilizing the floating lateral mass with a Penfield 4 may be necessary. Alternatively, the screw in the fractured level can be directed 15 degrees lateral and 10 degrees inferior, with the intention of crossing the inferior facet joint to stabilize the fragment (35).

Conceptually, treating this injury with an anterior discectomy, interbody graft, and plating seems ideal, because this is the site of soft tissue disruption. Lifeso and Colucci (14) performed a prospective study involving 18 patients with CES1 injuries treated in this manner. All went on to successful arthrodesis without residual deformity. All patients that had root involvement or incomplete cord injury demonstrated improvement compared with their presenting deficit. The same authors reported retrospective data on 11 patients with CES1 injuries treated through a posterior approach. They reported 5 of the 11 failed due to development of late kyphosis from disc degeneration (n = 3), malreduction of the fracture (n = 2), or persistent neural deficits (n = 2).

The isolated laminar fractures seen in CES2 lesions rarely are associated with neurologic injuries. Bohlman, in his report on cervical injuries (37), found that all laminar fractures associated with paralysis also had associated vertebral body or articular process fractures. Hahnle and Nainkin (38) reported a case of Brown-Séquard syndrome in an 18 year old after a head-on collision in which the patient's head struck the dashboard. The patient was noted to have a nondisplaced hangman's fracture and fourth and fifth laminae fractures that were invaginated unilaterally into the spinal canal. In the more common setting of the neurologically intact patient, immobilization in a rigid cervical orthosis or halo vest is usually sufficient (39).

Although not always associated with severe neurologic deficit, the higher-grade lesion in this phylogeny (CES5) always involves circumferential instability. If neurologic injury exists, preoperative MRI may be considered. Given the extreme disruption of both columns, combined anterior and posterior fusion with instrumentation may be the best approach to management. Anterior discectomy and interbody arthrodesis of the discs above and below the translated centrum should be followed by anterior plating. The addition of posterior lateral mass fixation may enhance the overall stability in these complex injuries. Currently, more data on these specific lesions are necessary to make meaningful

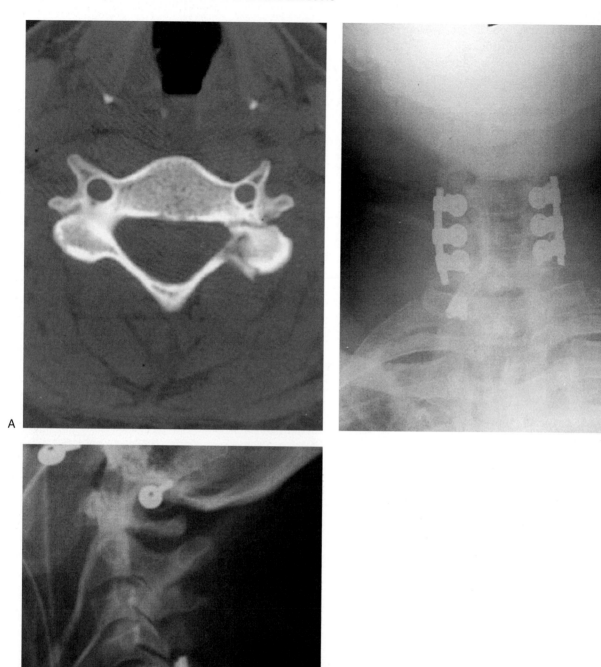

FIG. 49.5. A: Axial computed tomographic scan demonstrating "floating facet." **B, C:** Postoperative radiographs after posterior lateral mass stabilization.

predictions of success with either one-column or combined approaches.

Distractive Extension Injuries

The type 1 DES injury may occur exclusively through the intervertebral disc or involve the bony centrum. Those that involve largely bony injury may be managed in a halo vest (40). The definitive management of DES1 lesions that are purely through the anterior longitudinal ligament and disc, or those that are associated with a small "teardrop" avulsion fracture, is less clear. Levine and Lutz (41) reported on 24 patients with the latter injury who were treated nonoperatively in a cervical orthosis. Twenty-one of 24 achieved stability uneventfully at mean follow-up of 2.5 years.

Conversely, both operative (40) and nonoperative treatment (35) has been recommended for DES1 lesions that involve purely soft tissue disruption. This category actually represents a spectrum of injuries that involve disruption of the anterior restraints from the anterior annulus and longitudinal ligament to the posterior annulus and posterior longitudinal ligament. It is unclear whether MRI or early, supervised flexion-extension films can accurately demonstrate the extent of instability produced by this spectrum of anterior soft tissue injuries. If an initial nonsurgical route is chosen, immobilization in either a rigid orthosis or halo should be accompanied by serial radiographic follow-up. Immobilization for 10 to 12 weeks should be followed by flexion-extension films to determine stability. Continued instability may warrant surgical intervention. If surgical treatment is selected, either primarily or after failed nonoperative treatment, then anterior reconstruction with a plate acting as a tension band seems the ideal treatment (Fig. 49.6). Vaccaro and associates (40) reported signs of neurologic dysfunction (two electrophysiologically and one clinically) due to presumed overdistraction at the time of graft placement. They postulated that this was the result of cord lengthening and vascular ischemia from overdistraction at the disc space in the setting of an already lengthened and edematous cord (from the injury vector). They therefore recommended meticulous contouring of the graft to fit the anterior column defect with minimal distraction. Because ligaments often do not heal, the authors of the current chapter prefer early surgical stabilization.

Patients with DES2 lesions demonstrate translation (>3 mm) in addition to widening of the disc space. These injuries involve disruption of both the anterior and posterior columns. Combined anterior and posterior stabilization procedures may ensure better long-term stability (Fig. 49.7). Consideration may be given to initially approaching

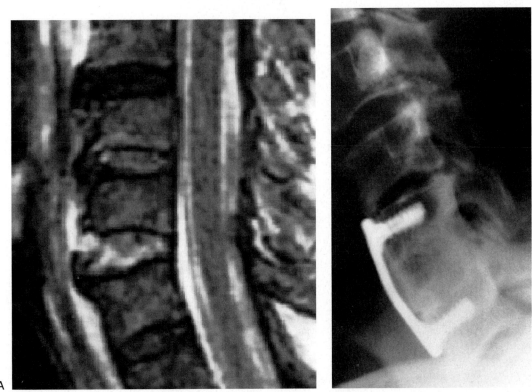

FIG. 49.6. A: Sagittal magnetic resonance image of a patient with a DES1 injury. **B:** Postoperative radiograph after anterior cervical discectomy and fusion with an anterior plate acting as a tension band. (Courtesy of Alexander R. Vaccaro, M.D., with permission.)

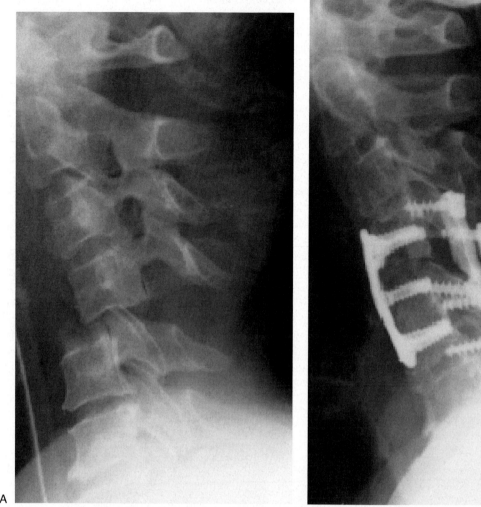

FIG. 49.7. A: Lateral radiograph of a patient with a DES2 injury, with marked vertebral retrolisthesis at C4-5. **B:** Postoperative radiograph after treatment of the same patient with anterior-posterior decompression and reconstruction with instrumentation. (From, Vaccaro AR, Klein GR, Thaller JB, et al. Distraction extension injuries of the cervical spine. *J Spinal Disorders* 2001;14(3):193–200, with permission.)

the spine posteriorly to adequately align the spine in the sagittal plane prior to anterior column reconstruction (40). In the series by Vaccaro and associates (40) of 24 patients with DE injuries, 46% were noted to have radiographic evidence of ankylosing spondylitis or diffuse idiopathic skeletal hyperostosis. The authors suggested that the reduced capacity of the brittle spine to accommodate substantial distractive extension force vectors was responsible for the strong association. They reported that with prompt recognition of the associated pathology and careful management, no differences in radiographic or neurologic outcomes were noted in this subset of patients (40).

In cases where multilevel cervical stenosis coexists with the destabilizing lesion, an adjunctive decompressive procedure may be warranted. Again, reestablishing sagittal alignment with posterior fixation may be helpful

as the initial stage. The decision to perform the decompressive procedure through a laminectomy/laminoplasty versus multilevel discectomies or corpectomies should be individualized, considering the nature of the compressive pathology (by the preoperative advanced imaging studies) and the overall alignment reestablished at the time of the posterior reduction and stabilization or with traction. Extending the posterior instrumentation to include all levels decompressed may help avoid the development of late deformity.

Treatment of patients with cervical spondylosis and central cord syndrome after a destabilizing extension injury can be managed in accordance with the guidelines presented earlier. Management of traumatic central cord injuries in the absence of demonstrated instability is more controversial. Advocates for nonsurgical treatment have cited substantial recovery of function in patients treated nonoperatively. Tow and Kong (42) reported on the results of 73 patients with central cord syndrome who were treated nonoperatively. They noted significant improvements in the admission/discharge American Spinal Injury Association (ASIA) motor scores and Modified Barthel Index (MBI) scores. In their series, 92% of patients were continent of bladder on discharge, compared with 64% on admission. Newey and associates (43) presented the long-term outcome in patients with central cord syndrome treated nonoperatively. At a mean follow-up of 8.6 years, all six patients younger than 50 years could walk independently and had bladder control. In patients aged 50 to 70 years, 77% could walk independently and 69% had bladder control at final follow-up. Of the ten patients older than 70 years in this study, only three were alive at final follow-up; one patient could ambulate independently, and none had bladder control.

Other studies have suggested that in selected patients, operative intervention may improve the rate and degree of motor recovery. Chen and colleagues (44) presented a retrospective study of 114 patients who sustained traumatic central cord injuries between 1988 and 1994. Better results in terms of motor and sensory improvement were noted in patients with clinically correlated encroaching cord lesions who received surgical decompression in the early subacute period. Bose and associates (45) performed a retrospective analysis of 28 patients treated at the Delaware Valley Regional Spinal Cord Injury Center. They reported benefit both in rate and degree of motor recovery in patients treated operatively who had failed to improve progressively after an initial period of improvement, with persistent compression of neural tissue visualized on myelography. Therefore, consideration can be given to treating such injuries nonoperatively for a 6-week period with monitoring of patients' neurologic function. Those patients whose recoveries plateau may benefit from surgical decompression. Again, because multilevel stenosis may be involved, the route and extent of the decompressive procedure should be individualized based on the number of levels involved and the overall alignment. Currently, there are no prospective, randomized studies we are aware of that can definitively guide the decision to operate, the timing, or the surgical approach in these patients.

SUMMARY

Extension injuries to the cervical spine are common both in young adults and the elderly. A high index of suspicion is necessary because plain radiographic findings may be subtle. Advanced imaging studies may be indicated to accurately delineate bony and soft tissue disruption, as well as to define associated neurologic injuries. Mechanistic classifications may help determine appropriate interventions to treat instability. Surgical intervention should be considered in cases with neurologic injury and in those with primarily soft tissue (ligament and disc) disruption, although more data are needed to clarify the timing and method.

REFERENCES

1. Whitley JF, Forsyth HF. Classification of cervical spine injuries. *AJR Am J Roentgenol* 1960;83:633–644.
2. Kiwerski J. Hyperextension-dislocation injuries of the cervical spine. *Injury* 1993;24:674–677.
3. Meyer P Jr. Cervical spine fractures, changing management concepts. In: Bridwell KJ, DeWald RL, eds. *The textbook of spinal surgery.* Philadelphia: JB Lippincott, 1991:1004.
4. Shono Y, McAfee PC, Cunningham BW. The pathomechanics of compression injuries in the cervical spine. Nondestructive and destructive investigative methods. *Spine* 1993;18:2009–2019.
5. Hohl M. Soft tissue injuries of the neck in automobile accidents. *J Bone Joint Surg Am* 1974;56:1675–1682.
6. Jonsson H Jr, Bring G, Rauschning W, et al. Hidden cervical spine injuries in traffic accident victims with skull fractures. *J Spinal Disord* 1991;4:251–263.
7. White AA, Panjabi MM. The problem of clinical instability in the human spine: a systematic approach. In: White AA, Panjabi MM, eds. *Clinical biomechanics of the spine,* 2nd ed. Philadelphia: JB Lippincott, 1990:277–378.
8. White AA III, Johnson RM, Panjabi MM, et al. Biomechanical analysis of clinical stability in the cervical spine. *Clin Orthop* 1975;109:85–96.
9. Forsyth HF. Extension injuries of the cervical spine. *J Bone Joint Surg Am* 1964;46:1792–1797.
10. Marar BC. Hyperextension injuries of the cervical spine. *J Bone Joint Surg Am* 1974;56:1655–1662.
11. Kinoshita H, Hirakawa H. Pathological studies and pathological principles on the management of extension injuries of the cervical spine. *Paraplegia* 1989;27:172–181.
12. Allen BL, Ferguson RL, Lehmann TR, et al. A mechanistic classification of closed, indirect fractures and dislocations of the lower cervical spine. *Spine* 1982;7:1–27.
13. Sears W, Fazi M. Prediction of stability of cervical spine fracture managed in the halo vest and indications for surgical intervention. *J Neurosurg* 1990;72:426–432.
14. Lifeso RM, Colucci MA. Anterior fusion for rotationally unstable cervical spine fractures. *Spine* 2000;25:2028–2034.
15. Louis R, Louis CA, Aswad R. Extension injuries of the lower cervical spine. In: Clark CR, ed. *The cervical spine.* Philadelphia: Lippincott, 1998.
16. Nazarian SM, Louis RP. Posterior internal fixation with screw plates in traumatic lesions of the cervical spine. *Spine* 1991;16:S64–S71.
17. Slucky AV, Eismont FJ. Treatment of acute injury of the cervical spine. *J Bone Joint Surg Am* 1994;76:1882–1896.
18. Reich SM, Cotler JM. Mechanism and patterns of spine and spinal cord injuries. *Trauma Q* 1993;9:7–28.
19. Taylor AR, Blackwood W. Paraplegia in hyperextension cervical injuries with normal radiographic appearances. *J Bone Joint Surg Br* 1948;33:245–248.
20. Taylor AR. The mechanism of injury to the spinal cord in the neck without damage to the vertebral column. *J Bone Joint Surg Br* 1951;33:543–547.
21. Schneider RC, Thompson JM, Rebin J. The syndrome of acute central cervical spinal cord injury. *J Neurol Neurosurg Psychiatry* 1958;21:216–227.
22. Wilkenson M, Bywaters EGL. Clinical features and course of ankylosing spondylitis. *Ann Rheum Dis* 1958;17:209–228.
23. Harding JR, McCall IW, Park WM, et al. Fracture of the cervical spine in ankylosing spondylitis. *Br J Radiol* 1985;58:3–7.
24. Murray GC, Persellin RH. Cervical fracture complicating ankylosing spondylitis: a report of eight cases and review of the literature. *Am J Med* 1981;70:1033–1041.
25. Simmons EH. The surgical correction of flexion deformity of the cervical spine in ankylosing spondylitis. *Clin Orthop* 1972;86:132.
26. Vaccaro AR, An HS, Lin SS, et al. Noncontiguous injuries of the spine. *J Spinal Disord* 1992;5:320–329.
27. Streitweiser DR, Knopp R, Wales LR, et al. Accuracy of standard radiographic views in detecting cervical spine fractures. *Ann Emerg Med* 1983;12:538–542.
28. Clark CR, Ingram CM, El-Khoury GY, et al. Radiographic evaluation of cervical spine injuries. *Spine* 1988;13:742–747.
29. Freemyer B, Knopp R, Piche J, et al. Comparison of five-view and three-view cervical spine series in the evaluation of patients with cervical trauma. *Ann Emerg Med* 1989;18:818–821.

30. White AA III, Southwick WO, Panjabi MM. Clinical instability in the lower spine—a review of past and current concepts. *Spine* 1976;1:15–27.

31. Halliday AL, Henderson BR, Hart BL, et al. The management of unilateral lateral mass/facet fractures of the subaxial cervical spine; the use of magnetic resonance imaging to predict instability. *Spine* 1997;22:2614–2621.

32. Davis SJ, Teresi LM, Bradley WG Jr, et al. Cervical spine hyperextension injuries: MR findings. *Radiology* 1991;180:245–251.

33. Schaefer DM, Flanders AE, Osterholm J, et al. Prognostic significance of magnetic resonance imaging in the acute phase of cervical spine injury. *J Neurosurg* 1992;76:218–223.

34. Bracken MB, Shepard MJ, Holfors TR, et al. Administration of methylprednisolone for 24 or 48 hours or tirilazad mesylate for 48 hours in the treatment of acute spinal cord injury: results of the third National Acute Spinal Cord Injury randomized controlled trial. *JAMA* 1997;277:1597–1604.

35. Levine AM. Facet fractures and dislocations. In: Levine AM, Eismont FJ, Garfin SR, et al., eds. *Spinal trauma*. Philadelphia: WB Saunders, 1998.

36. Jeanneret B, Gebhard JS, Magerl F. Transpedicular screw fixation of articular mass fracture-separation: results of an anatomical study and operative technique. *J Spinal Disord* 1994;7:222–229.

37. Bohlman HH. Acute fractures and dislocations of the cervical spine—an analysis of three-hundred hospitalized patients and review of the literature. *J Bone Joint Surg Am* 1979;61:1119–1142.

38. Hahnle UR, Nainkin L. Traumatic invagination of the fourth and fifth cervical laminae with acute hemiparesis. *J Bone Joint Surg Br* 2000;82:1148–1150.

39. Brodke DS, Harris M. Subaxial cervical trauma; evaluation and management options. *Semin Spine Surg* 2001;13:128–141.

40. Vaccaro AR, Klein GR, Thaller JB, et al. Distraction extension injuries of the cervical spine. *J Spinal Disord* 2001;14:193–200.

41. Levine AM, Lutz B. Extension teardrop fractures of the cervical spine. Presented at the 20th annual meeting of the Cervical Spine Research Society, Palm Desert, CA, December 3–5, 1992. Abstract 49.

42. Tow AM, Kong KH. Central cord syndrome: functional outcome after rehabilitation. *Spinal Cord* 1998;36:156–160.

43. Newey ML, Sen PK, Fraser RD. The long-term outcome after central cord syndrome: a study of the natural history. *J Bone Joint Surg Br* 2000;82:851–855.

44. Chen TY, Lee ST, Lui TN, et al. Efficacy of surgical treatment in traumatic central cord syndrome. *Surg Neurol* 1997;48:435–440.

45. Bose B, Northrup BE, Osterholm JL, et al. Reanalysis of central cervical cord injury management. *Neurosurgery* 1984;15:367–372.

CHAPTER 50

Subaxial Cervical Spine Burst Fractures

Anis O. Mekhail, Michael P. Steinmetz, and Edward C. Benzel

DEFINITION, PATHOMECHANICS, AND CLASSIFICATION

Definition

A burst fracture is characterized by an incomplete or complete fragmentation of the vertebral body, widening of the interpedicular distance, loss of the vertebral body height, retropulsion of one or several posterior wall fragments, and involvement of one or both adjacent discs (Fig. 50.1). True burst fractures, although common in the thoracolumbar spine (70% to 80%), are rare in the cervical spine (1).

Pathomechanics of Injury

A burst fracture results from an axial load leading to failure of the vertebral body. An associated injury can occur, depending on the relation of the axial load to the instantaneous axis of rotation, as well as the position of the cervical spine at the time of impact. A true axial load applied to a lordotic subaxial spine is likely to result in an isolated burst fracture. If the force is ventral to the instantaneous axis of rotation, an associated dorsal distraction injury will occur (Fig. 50.2). Most traumatic cervical spine lesions are associated with compression damage to the dorsal elements (the application of compressive forces dorsal to the instantaneous axis of rotation) because of the normal cervical lordosis (2). If a burst component is present, it is usually combined with a dorsal lesion. Therefore, the burst element is only the expression of a more severe lesion. Exposing cervical burst fractures to extension or further compression can worsen spinal canal compromise (3).

The amount of canal involvement at the time of injury—and therefore, perhaps, spinal cord injury—is not always seen on the first radiographs. Zhu and colleagues (4), in a biomechanical study, demonstrated that cervical spine instability occurred after high-speed axial compression of young male cadaver cervical spines using 30 J of impact energy. However,

only after 50 J of impact energy was applied was a bony injury observed. Chang and associates (5) and Carter and colleagues (6), in two separate biomechanical studies using ligament-intact human cadaveric cervical spines subjected to a fast loading rate to produce a burst fracture, demonstrated that the transient spinal canal narrowing was significantly greater than the postinjury canal narrowing. There was, however, no significant correlation between the transient and the postinjury values. Chang and associates (5) found that there was significant recovery of axial height after impact. They also showed that the transient midsagittal diameter at impact was significantly less than the postinjury midsagittal diameter and found a weak, but significant, correlation between the transient and the postinjury values. Carter and colleagues (6) demonstrated that slow loading produced wedge compression fractures. In conclusion, both studies demonstrated that the postinjury radiographic measurements significantly underestimate the actual transient injury.

Retropulsion of a bony fragment into the spinal canal by itself does not imply that the lesion should be termed a burst fracture. The teardrop fracture of the cervical spine is not truly a burst fracture (7,8). Instead, it is a lesion with significant focal dorsal element disruption. Torg and associates (9) reported on 55 patients with teardrop fractures obtained from the National Football Head and Neck Injury Registry. They described two fracture patterns associated with a ventral caudal corner (teardrop) fracture fragment: (a) the isolated fracture, which is usually not associated with permanent neurologic sequelae; and (b) a three-part, two-plane fracture in which there is an associated sagittal vertebral body fracture and a fracture of the posterior neural arch. The latter fracture was nearly always associated with permanent neurologic sequelae, specifically quadriplegia. Their conclusion was that axial loading of the cervical spine is the mechanism of injury in both fracture patterns.

Korres and colleagues (10) classified the teardrop fracture of the lower cervical spine into four types. They em-

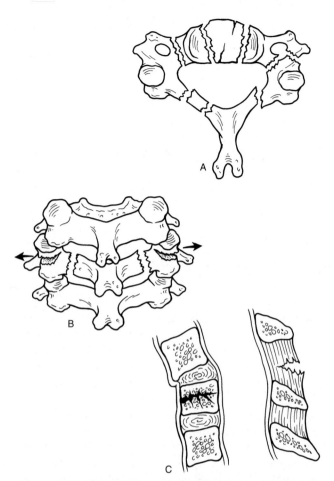

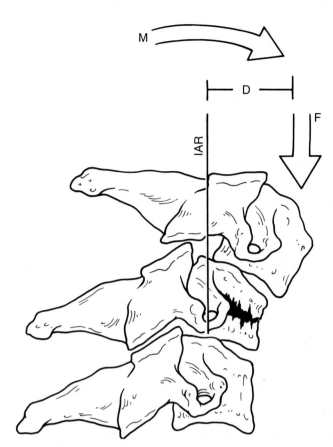

FIG. 50.1. A burst fracture is characterized by an incomplete or complete fragmentation of the vertebral body **(A)**, secondary widening of the interpeduncular distance **(B)**, and a loss of vertebral body height and the involvement of one or both adjacent discs **(C)**. (Adapted from Aebi M, Benzel E. Cervical spine burst fractures. In: Cervical Spine Research Society, eds. *The cervical spine*, 3rd ed. Philadelphia: Lippincott–Raven Publishers, 1998:465–473.)

FIG. 50.2. If a force vector (F) passes in a plane that is adjacent to the instantaneous axis of rotation (IAR), a bending (and failure) of the spine toward the side of the force application (M) is applied and is defined by the product of F and D (the distance from the IAR), as depicted. (Adapted from Aebi M, Benzel E. Cervical spine burst fractures. In: Cervical Spine Research Society, eds. *The cervical spine*, 3rd ed. Philadelphia: Lippincott–Raven Publishers, 1998:465–473.)

phasized the association of a ligamentous lesion with this injury and its contribution to the degree of instability. They believe that the mechanism of injury for the teardrop fracture is a combination of flexion and compression applied simultaneously. The main difference between the pattern of teardrop fractures and that of burst fractures is that the coronal fracture line typically begins in the ventral wall of the vertebral body and proceeds inferiorly in the former injury and not in the upper end plate, as in the latter.

Classification

There are few universally discussed, or accepted, classification systems for cervical spine injuries. One of the most complete is the mechanistic classification by Allen and associates (7) (Table 50.1). Knowing the mechanism of injury can help treatment by reversing (or resisting) the forces producing the injury. In their classification, the posterior

longitudinal ligament and the structures anterior to it are considered the ventral column of the spine, and the structures posterior to the posterior longitudinal ligament are considered the posterior column. Vertical compression injuries are most common following motor vehicle accidents, diving accidents, and direct blows to the top of the skull

TABLE 50.1. *Allen and Associate's Mechanistic Classification of Closed, Indirect Fracture and Dislocation of the Lower Cervical Spine*

Compression flexion	CF1–5
Vertical compression	CV1–3
Distractive flexion	DF1–4
Compressive extension	CE1–5
Distractive extension	DE1–2
Lateral flexion	LF1–2

From, Allen BL, Ferguson RL, Lehmann TR, et al. A mechanistic classification of closed, indirect fractures and dislocations of the lower cervical spine. *Spine* 1982;7:1–27, with permission.

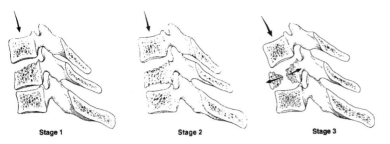

Stage 1 **Stage 2** **Stage 3**

FIG. 50.3. The stages of vertical compression injury. Stage 1: Central cupping fracture of superior or inferior end plate. Stage 2: Similar to stage 1, but fracture of both end plates; any fracture of the centrum is minimal. Stage 3: Fragmentation and displacement of vertebral body. (Adapted from Rizzolo SJ, Cotler JM. Unstable cervical spine injuries: specific treatment approaches. *J Am Acad Orthop Surg* 1993;1:57–66.)

(Fig. 50.3). The most common level of injury is at C6-C7 (11). Stage 3 vertical compression injuries are referred to as *burst fractures*. Similarly, the AO (Arbeitsgemeinschaft für Osteosynthesefragen) comprehensive classification scheme of the thoracic and lumbar injuries employs the two-column concept (12).

Denis described several fracture types, and accompanying modes of failure, of the thoracolumbar spine (13). His classification depends on his three-column concept of spinal stability. According to this classification, burst fractures result from failure of the anterior and middle columns in compression.

A recent mechanistic classification of cervical spine injuries based on plain radiographs and computed tomographic (CT) scans included burst fractures under compressive hyperflexion injuries (14).

According to the classification of Magerl and associates (1), which is a pathomorphologic classification combined with functional motions (Tables 50.2 and 50.3), most cervical spine fractures are B or C lesions, whereas most thoracolumbar lesions are A lesions.

The load-sharing classification is a radiographic classification, based on plain radiographs as well as CT axial and sagittal reconstruction images, that grades the amount of damaged vertebral body (extent of comminution), the spread of the fragments, and the amount of corrected traumatic kyphosis (Fig. 50.4) (15). It can be useful in estimating the degree of instability of the injured spine and thus can aid in planning the length of the construct and the need for a combined ventral and dorsal surgical stabilization.

DIAGNOSIS

Clinical Evaluation

Initially, priority is directed to maintenance of airway, breathing, and circulation. If the patient has a spinal cord

TABLE 50.3. *Definition of the Three Major Lower Cervical Spine Fracture Types*

Posterior element injury?

No	Yes
↓	Distraction ↙ ↘ Torsion
Type A	Type B Type C

If no posterior element injury is present, a burst fracture is classified as type A. If posterior element distraction is present, it is classified as type B, whereas if a rotational component is superimposed, it is classified as type C.

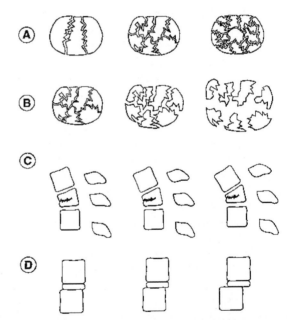

FIG. 50.4. Thoracic and lumbar fracture assessment. The extent of comminution fracture **(A)** (Adapted from Benzel E. Trauma, tumor, and infection. In: Benzel E, ed. *Biomechanics of spine stabilization.* Rolling Meadows, IL: American Association of Neurological Surgeons, 2001:61–82.). The extent of dispersion of the fragments **(B)** (Modified from McCormack T, Karaikovic E, Gaines RW. The load sharing classification of spine fractures. *Spine* 1994;19:1741–1744.). The extent of angular deformation **(C)**. The extent of translation (in any plane) **(D)**. These factors are used to determine axial load-bearing capacity **(A, B, and C)** and the angular and translational deformation resistance ability **(C and D)**.

TABLE 50.2. *Classification of Lower Cervical Spine Injuries*

Type	Description
A	Vertebral body fractures (compressive lesions)
B	Posterior disruptions (distractive lesions)
C	Rotational dislocation combined with type A, B, or both (special lesions)

injury, hypotension and bradycardia are often present due to neurogenic shock. After initial hemodynamic stabilization with fluids and possibly vasopressors, the neurologic status of the patient should be carefully assessed. The history should include the mechanism of injury (direction and magnitude). It is to be noted, however, that the patient's account of the injury is not always consistent with the mechanism of injury inferred from the radiographic studies. The complex buckling of the cervical spine that results from vertical impact of the head may cause concomitant flexion and extension in different regions of the cervical spine (16).

The physical examination should include inspection and palpation of the entire spine and the head searching for ecchymoses, swelling, and tenderness, and for gaps between the cervical spinous processes. The neurologic status should be recorded, employing assessment tools such as the Frankel or the American Spinal Injury Association (ASIA) classification scheme (17). Subsequent neurologic evaluation should be undertaken to detect any neurologic deterioration.

Radiographic Studies

Plain Radiographs

A three-film cervical spine series consisting of a cross-table lateral view, an anteroposterior view, and an odontoid view reveals 83% to 99% of cervical spine injuries (18). Plain radiography is useful for the determination of subluxation. Width of the prevertebral soft tissue of more than 10 mm at C1, more than 4 to 5 mm at C3-C4, and more than 15 to 20 mm at C6 is suggestive of soft tissue swelling, indicating disruptive acute trauma (19). On the lateral radiograph, four lordotic lines can be drawn: along the ventral margins of the vertebral bodies, the dorsal vertebral margins, the ventral cortical margins of the spinous processes, and the tips of the spinous processes. Disruption of these lines suggests significant injury. In a review of the lateral radiographs and CT scans of cervical spine injuries, the dorsal vertebral body line seen on the lateral radiograph was found to be disrupted in all 36 pure cervical spine burst fractures (20). It is important to be able to visualize C7-T1 on the lateral radiograph in order to avoid missing caudal lesions. A swimmer's view may be necessary if the lateral radiograph with caudal traction of the shoulders fails to visualize the C7-T1 level.

As long as the dorsal tension band system is intact, burst fractures may be biomechanically stable. However, if a coexistent flexion component occurs, resulting in distraction failure of the dorsal elements, the lesion should be considered to be unstable and have poor healing potential (7, 8,21,22). When there is a wedge-shaped deformity of the vertebral body, there is a high probability of a coexisting lesion of the dorsal complex. An association between the space available for the spinal cord and the severity of neurologic injury in trauma patients has been demonstrated (23,24). If dorsally displaced bone fragments compromise more than 50% of the spinal canal, significant spinal cord injury may occur (25).

Computed Tomography

CT is most useful for the visualization of bony injury. It is invaluable in the assessment of burst fractures and bony fragment retropulsion. CT, used as a primary screening tool, has a sensitivity of 90% and a specificity of 100% in detecting cervical injury.

Magnetic Resonance Imaging

Magnetic resonance imaging (MRI) is most useful for the evaluation of neural element distortion, compression, and injury. It is also the study of choice for determining the extent of soft tissue injury and the presence of an associated disc herniation.

MRI has also been shown to provide information that allows, to some extent, prognosis of the spinal cord injury. Hemorrhage in the spinal cord is associated with a poor prognosis for neurologic recovery, whereas cord edema has a better prognosis (26,27). Magnetic resonance angiograms can be useful in detecting vertebral artery injuries (28).

TREATMENT

The goals of treatment of spinal injury are to provide spinal stability, restore anatomic alignment, preserve and improve neurologic function, and prevent late deformity (29). To minimize the progression of the primary injury, the following steps should be undertaken:

1. Spinal immobilization
2. Hemodynamic and medical resuscitation
3. Early reduction and maintenance of spinal alignment
4. Neurodiagnostic studies
5. Decompression of the injured neural elements (if necessary)
6. Spinal stabilization

Surgery is indicated when nonoperative management fails to achieve these treatment goals. The theoretical benefit of early neural decompression is that it limits the secondary injury cascade created by edema, regional hematoma, neural membrane destabilization, and mechanical compression by the fractured fragments.

Initial Management

Methylprednisolone is the most widely used pharmacotherapeutic agent for the prevention or treatment of the secondary biochemical injury cascade. It exerts its protective effects by decreasing lipid oxidation, stabilizing the cell membranes, enhancing spinal cord blood flow, and decreasing vascular permeability and edema (30). Its effectiveness beyond root injury recovery, however, has been questioned. Although its routine use is controversial, at this time it appears to be a standard component in the early treatment of patients with spinal cord injuries.

The unstable cervical spine in the acute setting should be stabilized in a rigid cervical collar, a spine board, and sandbags (or equivalent strategies). Depending on the pathology, the cervical spine can be initially reduced and stabilized by skull tong traction. Harrington and associates (31), in a biomechanical study, showed that regardless of the relative sagittal plane angulation of the vertebrae, distraction was the main factor in generating force in the posterior longitudinal ligament. However, it was not possible to produce a ventrally directed force in the posterior longitudinal ligament at less than 35% canal narrowing. Also, because lordosis slackens the posterior longitudinal ligament, they recommend that distraction be applied before angular positioning of the vertebrae.

Nonoperative Treatment

Burst fractures without neurologic abnormalities and without significant posterior column involvement may be treated nonoperatively with bracing. Acute fractures are easier to reduce with traction than chronic fractures. A C-arm image intensifier or repeat lateral radiographs are essential to tell whether ligamentous structures are disrupted during the application of traction. Adequacy of reduction can usually be verified by diagnostic studies. Ducker and colleagues (32) continued traction for 4 weeks, followed by a halo vest for 8 weeks. Flexion deformity should be prevented. A collar was then used for an additional 4 weeks. Using this protocol, they reported that fewer than 10% of pure burst fractures required delayed spinal fusion. Most surgeons would apply a halo vest or a hard cervicothoracic orthosis for 2 to 3 months for stable fractures. After that, flexion-extension films are obtained to detect any residual instability. Physical therapy, in the form of active neck strengthening exercises, can be instituted after complete healing is obtained.

Surgical Indications and Timing

In a retrospective review of cervical burst and flexion teardrop fractures by Koivikko and associates (33), 34 patients were treated nonoperatively with skull traction or halo vest, and 35 patients with ventral decompression, bone grafting, and fixation by a Caspar plate. Operatively treated patients recovered more often, with at least one Frankel grade improvement, and presented less narrowing of the spinal canal and less kyphotic deformity. Kiewerski (34) discussed 273 patients with burst fractures of the cervical spine: Nonoperative treatment in the form of skull traction and long periods of bed care was used in 70 patients, and the remainder were treated by ventral decompression and fusion. Neurologic improvement was obtained in 14%

of the nonoperative and 44% of the operative groups. Hospital stays were shorter in the operative group.

Factors that influence management decisions include the presence or absence of neurologic deficit (radiculopathy or myelopathy), the extent of spinal canal compromise, the extent of disruption of spinal integrity, and the potential for deformity of the cervical spine.

Neurologic Deficit

Neurologic involvement can be grouped into one or a combination of four categories: (a) normal, (b) incomplete myelopathy, (c) complete myelopathy, or (d) isolated nerve root dysfunction—radiculopathy. Spinal cord decompression is mainly indicated in patients with incomplete spinal cord injury and concomitant spinal cord compression. The extent of their neurologic deficit can be diminished by decompression (35). Nerve root decompression may be beneficial in patients with complete myelopathy in whom nerve root dysfunction occurs in relation to compression at or near the segmental level of injury. In this case the surgical goals are related more to nerve root salvage than to spinal cord function (36). Decompression is not generally indicated in the neurologically intact patient unless significant spinal canal compromise is present.

Extent of Spinal Canal Compromise

According to Bedbrook (25), there is a correlation between neurologic deficit and the extent of spinal canal encroachment when canal narrowing of 50% or more is present. In a patient with spinal canal narrowing and a normal neurologic examination, decompressive surgery is controversial. Spontaneous remodeling of the retropulsed bone fragments may occur over time, leading to an increase in spinal canal diameter, if anatomic alignment can be maintained.

Instability

White and Panjabi (37) have developed criteria for the diagnosis of clinical instability (Table 50.4). In the presence of failure of the dorsal elements (dorsal osteoligamentous complex), management is different from that of only a vertebral body burst fracture due to the poorer healing potential of the former (38). Signs of an associated distractive injury of the dorsal osteoligamentous elements (type B lesions) or a rotational injury (type C lesions) indicate a significant potential for deformity and/or instability that may endanger neural integrity or cause chronic pain (1). The radiographic signs of complex burst fractures (B and C injuries) include the following:

- Sagittal or frontal plane translation or dislocation that is only possible with a disruption of the dorsal osteoligamentous complex.

TABLE 50.4. *Quantification of Acute Instability for Subaxial Cervical, Thoracic, and Lumbar Injuries*

Condition	Points assigned
Loss of integrity of anterior (and middle) column[a]	2
Loss of integrity of posterior column(s)[a]	2
Acute resting translational deformity[b]	2
Acute dynamic translation deformity exaggeration[c]	2
Acute dynamic angulation deformity exaggeration[c]	2
Neural element injury[d]	3
Acute disc narrowing at level of suspected pathology	1
Dangerous loading anticipated	1

A score of 5 points or more implies the presence of overt instability. A score of 2 to 4 points implies the presence of limited instability.

[a]By clinical examination, magnetic resonance imaging (MRI), computed tomography, or radiography. A single point may be allotted if incomplete evidence exists; for example, only MRI evidence of dorsal ligamentous injury (i.e., evidence of only interspinous ligament injury on T2-weighted images). Columns are defined as per Bailey, Denis (13), and Louis.

[b]From static resting anteroposterior and lateral spine radiographs. Must be the result of an acute clinical process. Tolerance for this criterion is variable with respect to surgeon and clinical circumstances. Guidelines as per White and Panjabi (37).

[c]From dynamic (flexion and extension) spine radiographs. Recommended only after other mechanisms of instability assessment have been exhausted, and then only by an experienced clinician. Usually indicated only in cervical region. Must be the result of an acute clinical process. Tolerance for this criterion is variable with respect to surgeon's opinion and clinical circumstances. Guidelines as per White and Panjabi (37).

[d]Three points for cauda equina, 2 points for spinal cord, or 1 point for isolated nerve root neurologic deficit. The presence of neural element injury indicates that a significant spinal deformation occurred at the time of impact, implying that structural integrity may well have been disturbed.

Adapted from White and Panjabi (37) as modified in Benzel E. Stability and instability of the spine. In: Benzel E, ed., *Biomechanics of spine stabilization*. Rolling Meadows, IL: American Association of Neurological Surgeons, 2001: 29–43.

- Incongruity of the facet joints, either by joint capsule disruption or by a combination of disruption and fracture. Visualization is optimized with oblique radiographs and/or CT (1-mm cuts in a plane that is perpendicular to the joint orientation).
- Rotational deformity, as identified on an anteroposterior (AP) radiograph, with a laterally offset spinous process.
- Asymmetric widening of the disc space on the AP radiograph at the level of the uncinate process. This is evidence to support a rotational dislocation.

Timing of Surgery

Some studies of early surgical intervention (within 3 to 5 days) have shown increased morbidity and mortality in patients with acute spinal cord injury (39). However, others have demonstrated that early decompression and stabilization of cervical spine injuries allows early patient mobilization and rehabilitation, as well as decreasing overall morbidity, hospital stay, and cost of treatment (40–42). Vaccaro and colleagues (42) noted no significant neurologic benefit in patients who underwent surgery within 72 hours of injury. Results in animal studies seem to favor surgical decompression within 8 to 12 hours (43). The evidence available to date is not sufficient to unequivocally support either early or delayed surgery.

Selection of Surgical Procedures and Implants

The following issues should be addressed when deciding on the type of surgery to perform:

1. Determine whether the burst fracture requires ventral surgery, including decompression, bone grafting, and possibly instrumentation, or whether a dorsal approach can be used.
2. Determine the indication for combined ventral and dorsal surgery.
3. Determine the number of segments that should be included in the fusion or fixation construct.
4. Determine the type of instrumentation that should be used.

Ventral Surgery

Ventral surgery for cervical burst fractures is in general superior to dorsal surgery (44–48). Ventral surgery is a relatively atraumatic approach to the spine that directly addresses the pathologic anatomy. Blood loss may be less than in the dorsal approach because of the relatively easily dissected planes in the ventral approach. Fragments of the burst fracture can be removed under direct vision, and spinal cord and nerve root decompression can be effectively accomplished. Through the ventral approach, a disc fragment that may displace into the spinal canal during a reduction maneuver can be removed before reduction. In addition, it is not necessary to position the patient in the arguably unfavorable prone position.

Load distribution and anatomic nuances are factors that favor a ventral arthrodesis, because the bone graft can be incorporated under axial compression in a well-vascularized bony bed. The bone healing process (i.e., fusion) and rehabilitation can be improved by applying a plate under axial compression (44,49). After performing a C5 corpectomy with transection of ligamentous and capsular structures, Grubb and associates (49) found that ventrally plated specimens had flexural and lateral bending and torsional stiffness values that were similar to or greater than those of intact control specimens. In a retrospective study of ventral decompression, interbody fusion, and plating of 26 patients with three-column cervical spine injuries, Böhler and Gaudernak (51) reported that all patients achieved solid fusion without recurrence of the deformity. None of the patients was placed in an orthotic device since the surgeon felt the internal fixation was rigid enough. Controversy exists, however, as to the adequacy of ventral cervical plating alone without a dorsal stabilization procedure in advanced-stage axial compression and in cases of osteopenic bone. Aebi and associates (44) reported a 1% nonunion rate with ventral plating (range of 0% to 3%). A summary of the results from various reports indicates that the true nonunion rate is approximately 3% (49).

For burst fractures with an intact inferior one-third of the vertebral body and inferior end plate, fixation may be limited to the injured segment. In these cases, the caudal screws of a ventral plating system should be inserted into the intact lower third of the vertebral body, in the subchondral bone, if possible (Fig. 50.5).

Unicortical screws have been shown to be as efficacious as bicortical screws in long-term follow-up studies, without the potential complications related to spinal canal penetration. In most systems the screws should converge in the transverse plane for better holding power. Intermediate screws placed within the graft are to be avoided because of the potential weakening of the graft related to the hole created for the screw (52). Ventral plating with locked fixation screws provides better stability than ventral plating with no screw-plate lock mechanism (50,53).

Dorsal Surgery

Dorsal spinal wiring has been the standard method of dorsal cervical stabilization in patients with competent dorsal elements. This technique provides stability mainly in flexion, but lacks significant stability in extension and rotation (54–56). The most common complication associated with wiring techniques is loss of fixation and subsequent bony nonunion.

Lateral mass plating with optional C2 and/or C7 pedicle screw placement for dorsal cervical fixation is a more rigid construct than wiring techniques. It is also beneficial in cases with dorsal element deficiency. Dorsal screws, however, carry the risk of neural injury as well as vertebral artery injury. For this reason, a preoperative CT scan may be useful in selected cases to identify the morphology of the lateral masses and the pedicles and their relationship with the vertebral artery and the neural foramina. A relative contraindication for this technique is osteopenic bone. Despite the high success rate with this technique (57,58), careful patient selection is required because of the relatively high risk of radiculopathy. Unicortical purchase of the lateral mass decreases the risk of nerve root injury while sacrificing only 28% of the screws' pull-out strength. Cervical instability patterns that may benefit from lateral mass plating include multilevel fusions, especially following a long-segment cervical corpectomy and strut fusion or in cases of dorsal element deficiency. Plate-rod devices allow for hook stabilization in the thoracic spine along with cervical lateral mass fixation, avoiding canal penetration by hooks in the cervical spine.

Fehlings and associates (59) reported 44 patients with cervical spine instability who were treated by lateral mass plating. The patients were kept in a Philadelphia collar postoperatively. Solid arthrodesis was achieved in 93% of cases. Three patients required revision of the cervical plating. Screw loosening was noted in 5 patients. The authors concluded that lateral mass plating is highly effective in the management of cervical spine instability and that supplemental bone grafting was generally not required for recent trauma.

Most of the experimental work comparing the stability and strength of dorsal with ventral constructs demonstrated superior characteristics of the dorsal fixation approaches. For the most part, these studies have been conducted with spines from predominantly aged cadavers or calf spines. These experiments poorly represent the *in vivo* situation and do not entirely respect the proper combination of the implant, bone graft, and type of lesion (54,55,60). In a biomechanical study, Koh and colleagues (61) demonstrated that dorsal plating with interbody grafting was biomechanically superior to ventral plating with locked fixation screws for stabilizing burst-type injuries. The authors concluded that combined ventral and dorsal fixation might not improve the stability significantly as compared with dorsal grafting with lateral mass screws and interbody grafting.

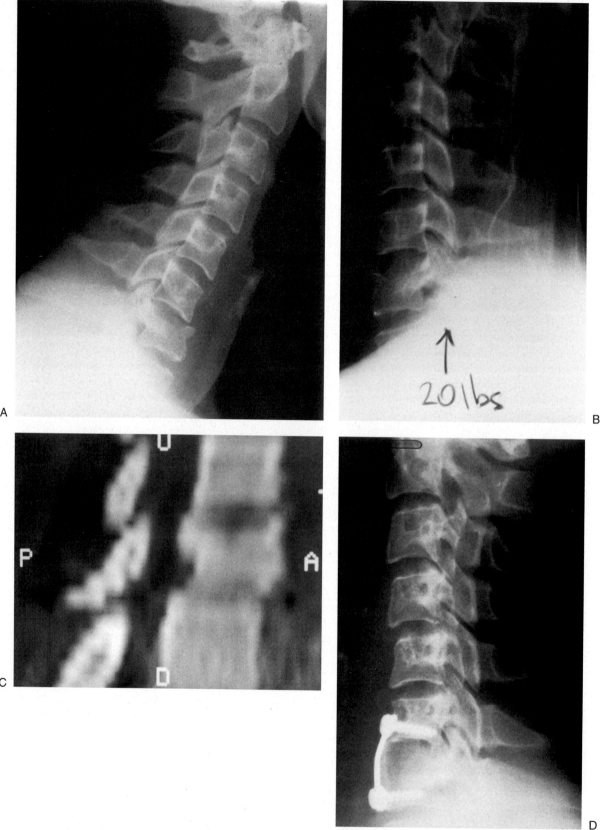

FIG. 50.5. A burst fracture of C7. **A:** Lateral burst with kyphosis deformity. **B:** After axial traction with 20 pounds, satisfactory reduction was achieved. **C:** Sagittal computed tomographic reconstruction demonstrating the fractured posterior wall of C7. **D:** Following anterior decompression, a monosegmental anterior fusion of C6-C7 using a simple Orozco plate with titanium plasma cover and 3.5-mm screws that did not protrude through the posterior wall was performed. Note that the distal screws are placed in the subchondral bone of the C7 distal end plate. (Adapted from Aebi M, Benzel E. Cervical spine burst fractures. In: Cervical Spine Research Society, eds. *The cervical spine*, 3rd ed. Philadelphia: Lippincott–Raven Publishers, 1998:465–473.)

They recommended that rigid postoperative external orthoses be considered if the ventral plating is used alone for the treatment of unstable cervical injuries.

In 1977, Stauffer and Kelly (22) stated that ventral surgery was contraindicated in lesions with dorsal element disruption. This is no longer always applicable, because surgically induced or traumatic instability in most cases can be controlled effectively with ventral plating.

Combined Surgery

With associated dislocation and disruption of the dorsal elements, reduction by axial traction alone leads to appropriate alignment of the injured segment or segments in the majority of cases. However, the more easily a dislocation or a malalignment is reduced, the greater the associated instability (21,45,46). If significant dorsal osteoligamentous injury exists, the primary emphasis should be directed ventrally to decompress the spinal cord and to establish ventral column integrity. An additional dorsal stabilization procedure can then be performed, especially if a ligamentous injury is present (Fig. 50.6). Dorsal stabilization alone for a three-column injury is likely to result in persistent instability (62). An alternative approach in the presence of an associated dorsal bony injury is ventral fusion with instrumentation and rigid bracing (with a cervical brace or cervicothoracic orthosis or a halo). In cases of a complete myelopathy, the stabilization procedure may be performed in conjunction with foraminotomies in the hope that local nerve root function may be improved (7,25,36).

McNamara and colleagues (63) recommend a single-stage ventral and dorsal approach in cases with both ventral and dorsal column instability. They perform the dorsal wiring procedure first in order to restore dorsal ligamentous integrity and act as a tension band. They believe that this technique minimizes the risk of graft dislodgement and anterior overdistraction. They obtained solid fusion in their six patients. The postoperative care included halo immobilization for 12 weeks followed by a Philadelphia collar for another 4 weeks. In the elderly or debilitated patient, a

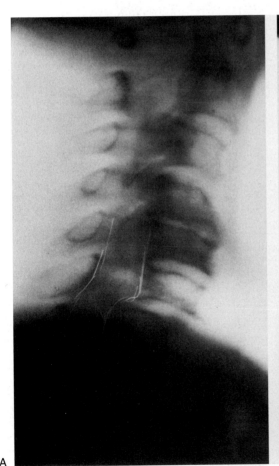
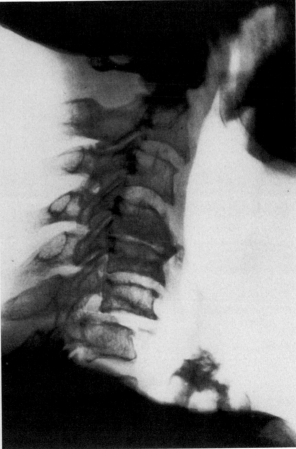

A

FIG. 50.6. A: An 80-year-old man with significant degenerative stiff cervical spine who sustained a fracture dislocation of C6-C7 and incomplete tetraplegia. **B:** Posterior reduction and wire stabilization was inadequate. **C:** An anterior plate fixation was added and provided sufficient stability for rehabilitation without external bracing. The patient became an independent walker. (Adapted from Aebi M, Benzel E. Cervical spine burst fractures. In: Cervical Spine Research Society, eds. *The cervical spine*, 3rd ed. Philadelphia: Lippincott–Raven Publishers, 1998:465–473.)

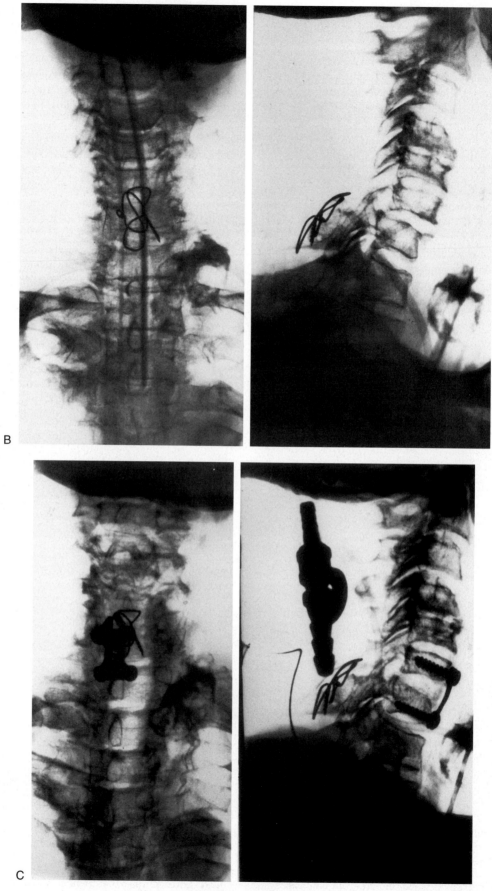

FIG. 50.6. *Continued*

staged approach with ventral decompression and fusion, followed in 7 to 10 days by dorsal instrumentation and fusion, may be considered.

McAfee and Bohlman (64) reported on 10 unstable cervical spine injuries that were treated by one-stage ventral cervical decompression and fusion followed by posterior triple wiring and fusion. The indication for surgery was a fixed kyphosis and an incomplete neurologic deficit or cervical instability. They concluded that although the operation took an average of 7 hours, its use was justified in patients with the appropriate indication.

In a biomechanical study evaluating different ventral constructs after corpectomy combined with a dorsal construct, Shono and associates (65) showed that a carbon fiber composite cage packed with cancellous bone graft was more rigid than conventional iliac crest strut graft or polymethylmethacrylate in flexion and extension (65). They concluded that after anterior decompression and strut fusions, supplemental dorsal wiring should be considered.

Special Considerations in the Pediatric and Geriatric Populations

Cervical Spine Injuries in Children

Cervical spine injuries in children are rare, with estimates ranging from 2% to 12% of all spine fractures (66, 67). Nonoperative treatment is successful in most patients (68); however, it is associated with a high risk of kyphotic deformation. Herzenberg and associates (69) have shown that younger children were forced into kyphosis when placed on a standard backboard in the acute setting. This kyphosis was attributed to the disproportionate head-to-body-size ratio in children younger than 8 years. They recommended either a modified backboard with a dropout for the occiput or padding under the thorax. Surgical stabilization is usually recommended for burst fractures associated with neurologic injuries (68). Cervical laminectomy is to be avoided because it increases instability with the development of subsequent kyphosis (70,71) and subjects the spinal cord to dorsal migration and increased neurologic deficit.

Cervical Spine Injuries in Elderly

Cervical spine injuries in the elderly are usually due to a minor trauma or a fall. Burst fractures from that common mechanism of injury are rare in this age group. Older people poorly tolerate bed rest and traction; however, most injuries can be treated nonoperatively (72). When surgery is considered, it is important to note that tenuous fixation may be achieved with ventral plating because of the weak pull-out strength of screws placed in osteopenic bone. Possible solutions include bicortical fixation, supplemental dorsal fixation, or the addition of a halo vest or Minerva jacket, especially in patients who cannot tolerate long surgery. Similarly, cages are

relatively contraindicated in the face of osteopenic vertebrae because of the risk of axial subsidence.

Complications

Cervical spine injuries can involve the following complications.

- Neurologic: Early identification and proper management of cervical spine injuries are essential in order to avoid the occurrence or deterioration of neurologic injuries. Ascending paralysis is rare, but can be seen any time after injury. It is usually secondary to ascending central necrosis of the gray matter, with an enlarging central syrinx. MRI is usually diagnostic.
- Spinal deformity: Unrecognized instability, either due to the injury itself or surgically induced, can result in late deformity, especially kyphosis. Hardware failure and nonunion can eventually lead to instability and deformity. Scoliosis can also occur caudal to the level of injury due to paralysis of the back muscles, especially in children.
- Operative: Operative complications include infection, esophageal perforation, dysphagia, vascular injury, neurologic injury, dural injury, and bone graft complications.
- Gastrointestinal bleeding: Gastrointestinal bleeding occurs in up to 40% of patients. It is most common 10 to 14 days following injury (56,73). The risk of ulceration may be aggravated by corticosteroid administration. To decrease the risk of ulceration, H2 blockers and early enteral feeding are recommended.
- Deep venous thrombosis (DVT): The incidence of DVT in spinal cord injury patients has been reported to be as high as 95%. It is clinically relevant in 25% to 35% of patients. This is predominantly due to the loss of vasomotor tone and prolonged immobility. For this reason, DVT prophylaxis (mechanical and pharmacologic) should be considered and instituted, if medically appropriate, in spinal cord injury patients.
- Pulmonary: Hypoventilation can result from paralysis of the intercostal muscles and the diaphragm. Atelectasis and pneumonia are common complications and should be treated aggressively. Pulmonary embolism is another significant problem that can be minimized by DVT prophylaxis.
- Skin complications: Skin care is crucial in spinal cord–injured patients. Vigilant nursing care, rotating beds, and pressure-relieving mattresses should be used as soon as possible. Ulcers should be aggressively treated with debridement, local wound care, and pressure relief. Pin-site care is also important in patients in a halo vest.

SUMMARY

True isolated burst fractures of the cervical spine are relatively uncommon. They result from axial compression of the vertebral body. Treatment of isolated burst fractures with relative preservation of body height and without significant spinal canal compromise or neurologic manifestation is usually accomplished with bracing.

In cases of significant vertebral body collapse, neurologic compromise, or dorsal element injury, ventral decompression and fusion (and possibly dorsal instrumentation) can be performed with the goal of attaining healing of the fracture in a stable, well-aligned position, preserving or regaining neurologic function, and preventing late deformity. Dorsal instrumentation is indicated in unstable three-column injuries. However, it carries the risks of added surgery, including increasing the operative time. An alternative approach in these injuries is to employ a halo or cervicothoracic orthosis after ventral interbody fusion and instrumentation.

REFERENCES

1. Magerl F, Aebi M, Gertzbein SD, et al. A comprehensive classification of thoracic and lumbar injuries. *Eur Spine J* 1994;3:184–201.
2. Aebi M, Nazarian S. Klassification der Halswirbelsaulenverletzungen (German). *Orthopade* 1987;16:27–36.
3. Ching RP, Watson NA, et al. The effect of post-injury spinal position on canal occlusion in a cervical spine burst fracture model. *Spine* 1997;22:1710–1715.
4. Zhu Q, Ouyang J, Lu W, et al. Traumatic instabilities of the cervical spine caused by high-speed axial compression in a human model. *Spine* 1999;24:440–444.
5. Chang DG, Tencer AF, Ching RP, et al. Geometric changes in the cervical spinal canal during impact. *Spine* 1994;19:973–980.
6. Carter JW, Mirza SK, Tencer AF, et al. Canal geometry changes associated with axial compressive cervical spine fracture. *Spine* 2000;25:46–54.
7. Allen BL, Ferguson RL, Lehmann TR, et al. A mechanistic classification of closed, indirect fractures and dislocations of the lower cervical spine. *Spine* 1982;7:1–27.
8. Schneider RC, Kahn EA. Chronic neurological sequelae of acute trauma to the spine and spinal cord. I: The significance of the acute flexion or "tear-drop" fracture dislocation of the cervical spine. *J Bone Joint Surg Am* 1956;38:985–997.
9. Torg JS, Pavlov H, O'Neill MJ, et al. The axial load teardrop fracture: a biomechanical, clinical, and roentgenographic analysis. *Am J Sports Med* 1991;19:355–364.
10. Korres DS, Stamos K, Andreakos A, et al. The anterior inferior angle fracture of a lower cervical vertebra. *Eur Spine J* 1994;3:202–205.
11. Rizzolo SJ, Cotler JM. Unstable cervical spine injuries: specific treatment approaches. *J Am Acad Orthop Surg* 1993;1:57–66.
12. Aebi M, Thalgott JS, et al., eds. *AO ASIF principles in spine surgery.* Berlin: Springer-Verlag, 1988:1–143.
13. Denis F. The three-column spine and its significance in the classification of acute thoracolumbar spine injuries. *Spine* 1983;8:817–831.
14. Daffner RH, Brown RR, Goldberg AL. A new classification for cervical vertebral injuries: influence of CT. *Skeletal Radiol* 2000;29:125–132.
15. McCormack T, Karaikovic E, Gaines RW. The load sharing classification of spine fractures. *Spine* 1994;19:1741–1744.
16. Nightingale RW, McElhaney JH, Richardson WJ, et al. Experimental impact injury to the cervical spine: relating motion of the head and the mechanism of injury. *J Bone Joint Surg Am* 1996;78:412–421.
17. American Spinal Injury Association. *Standards for neurologic and functional classification of spinal cord injury, revised.* Chicago, IL: American Spinal Injury Association, 1992.
18. MacDonald RL, Schwartz ML, Mirich D, et al. Diagnosis of cervical spine injury in motor vehicle crash victims: how many x-rays are enough? *J Trauma* 1990;30:392–397.
19. Meyer PR Jr. *Surgery of spine trauma.* New York: Churchill Livingstone, 1989:210.
20. Daffner RH, Deeb ZL, Rothfus WE. The posterior vertebral body line: importance in the detection of burst fractures. *AJR Am J Roentgenol* 1987;148:93–96.
21. Raynor RB, Kingman AF. Cervical spine injuries. *J Trauma* 1968;8:597–604.
22. Stauffer ES, Kelly EG. Fracture dislocations of the cervical spine. *J Bone Joint Surg Am* 1977;59:45–48.
23. Eismont FJ, Clifford S, Goldberg M, et al. Cervical sagittal spinal canal size in spine injury. *Spine* 1984;9:663–666.
24. Kang JD, Figgie MP, Bohlman HH. Sagittal measurements of the cervical spine in subaxial fractures and dislocations. An analysis of two hundred and eighty-eight patients with and without neurologic deficits. *J Bone Joint Surg Am* 1994;76:1617–1628.
25. Bedbrook GM. Spinal injuries with tetraplegia and paraplegia. *J Bone Joint Surg Br* 1979;61:267–284.
26. Cotler HB, Kulkarni MV, Bondurant FJ. Magnetic resonance imaging of acute spinal cord trauma. *J Orthop Trauma* 1988;2:1–4.
27. Flanders AE, Spettell CM, Tartaglino LM, et al. Forecasting motor recovery after cervical spinal cord injury: value of MR imaging. *Radiology* 1996;201:649–655.
28. Willis BK, Greiner F, Orrison WW, et al. The incidence of vertebral artery injury after midcervical spine fracture or subluxation. *Neurosurgery* 1994;34:435–441.
29. Aebi M, Mohler J, Zach GA, et al. Indication, surgical technique, and results of 100 surgically-treated fractures and fracture-dislocations of the cervical spine. *Clin Orthop Rel Res* 1986;203:244–257.
30. Bracken MB, Shepard MJ, Holford TR, et al. Administration of methylprednisolone for 24 or 48 hours or tirilazad mesylate for 48 hours in the treatment of acute spinal cord injury: results of the third National Acute Spinal Cord Injury randomized controlled trial. *JAMA* 1997;277:1597–1604.
31. Harrington RM, Budorick MS, Hoyt J, et al. Biomechanics of indirect reduction of bone retropulsed into the spinal canal in vertebral fracture. *Spine* 1993;18:692–699.
32. Ducker TB, Bellegarrigue R, Salcman M, et al. Timing of operative care in cervical spinal cord injury. *Spine* 1984;9:525–531.
33. Koivikko MP, Myllynen P, Kajalainen M, et al. Conservative and operative treatment in cervical burst fractures. *Arch Orthop Trauma Surg* 2000;120:448–451.
34. Kiewerski JE. Early anterior decompression and fusion for crush fractures of cervical vertebrae. *Int Orthop* 1993;17:166–168.
35. Benzel EC, Larson SJ. Functional recovery after decompressive spine operation for cervical spine fractures. *Neurosurgery* 1987;30:742–746.
36. Benzel EC, Larson SJ. Recovery of nerve root function after complete quadriplegia from cervical spine fractures. *Neurosurgery* 1986;19:809–812.
37. White AA III, Panjabi MM. The problem of clinical instability in the human spine: a systematic approach. In: White AA, Panjabi MM, eds. *Clinical biomechanics of the spine*, 2nd ed. Philadelphia: JB Lippincott, 1990:277–378.
38. Holdsworth FW. Fractures, dislocations, and fracture dislocations of the spine. *J Bone Joint Surg Am* 1970;52:1534–1551.
39. Marshall LF, Knowlton S, Garfin SR. Deterioration following spinal cord injury: a multicenter study. *J Neurosurg* 1987;66:400–404.
40. Duh MS, Shepard MJ, Wilberger JE, et al. The effectiveness of surgery on the treatment of acute spinal cord injury and its relation to pharmacological treatment. *Neurosurgery* 1994;35:240–249.
41. Schlegel J, Bayley J, Yuan H, et al. Timing of surgical decompression and fixation of acute spinal fractures. *J Orthop Trauma* 1996;10:323–330.
42. Vaccaro AR, Daugherty RJ, Sheehan TP, et al. Neurologic outcome of early versus later surgery for cervical spinal cord injury. *Spine* 1997;22:2609–2613.
43. Ducker TB, Salcman M, Daniel HB. Experimental spinal cord trauma. III: Therapeutic effect of immobilization and pharmacologic agents. *Surg Neurol* 1978;10:71–76.
44. Aebi M, Zuber K, Marchesi D. The treatment of cervical spine injuries by anterior plating. *Spine* 1991;16:38–45.
45. Bohler J, Gaudernak T. Anterior plate stabilization for fracture-dislocation of the lower cervical spine. *J Trauma* 1980;20:203–205.
46. Bombart M, Canevet D, Deckard J. Comparison sur l'ensemble de la serie des resultants de la chirurgie par voie anterieure et par voie posterieure. *Rev Chir Orthop* 1984;70:533–536.
47. Cabanel ME, Ebersold MJ. Anterior plate stabilization for bursting teardrop fractures of the cervical spine. *Spine* 1988;13:888–891.

48. Gassman J, Seligson D. The anterior cervical plate. *Spine* 1983;8:700–707.
49. Aebi M, Webb J. The spine. In: Muller ME, Allgower M, Schneider R, et al., eds. *Manual of internal fixation*, 3rd ed. Berlin: Springer, 1991.
50. Grubb MR, Currier BL, Shih JS, et al. Biomechanical evaluation of anterior cervical spine. *Spine* 1998;23:886–892.
51. Böhler J, Gaudernak T. Anterior plate stabilization for fracture-dislocations of the lower cervical spine. *J Trauma* 1980;20:203–205.
52. Vaccaro AR, Singh K. Principles of spinal instrumentation for cervical spinal trauma. In: An HS, Cotler JM, eds. *Spinal instrumentation*, 2nd ed. Philadelphia: Lippincott Williams & Wilkins, 1999:85–97.
53. Spivak JM, Chen D, Kummer FJ. The effect of locking fixation screws on the stability of anterior cervical plating. *Spine* 1999;24:334–338.
54. Coe JD, Warden KE, Sutterlin CE, et al. Biomechanical evaluation of cervical spine stabilization methods in a human cadaveric model. *Spine* 1989;14:1122–1131.
55. Sutterlin CE, McAfee PC, Warden JE, et al. A biomechanical evaluation of cervical spine stabilization methods in a bovine model: static and cyclical loading. *Spine* 1988;13:795–802.
56. Bohlman HL. Acute fractures and dislocations of the cervical spine: an analysis of three hundred hospitalized patients and review of the literature. *J Bone Joint Surg Am* 1979;61:1119–1142.
57. Graham A, Swank M, Kinard R, et al. Posterior cervical arthrodesis and stabilization with a lateral mass plate. *Spine* 1996;21:323–329.
58. Swank M, Sutterlin C, Bossons C, et al. Rigid internal fixation with lateral mass plates in multilevel anterior and posterior reconstruction of the cervical spine. *Spine* 1997;22:274–282.
59. Fehlings MG, Cooper PR, Errico TJ. Posterior plates in the management of cervical instability: long-term results in 44 patients. *J Neurosurg* 1994;81:341–349.
60. Ulrich C, Worsdorfer O, Claes L, et al. Comparative study of the stability of anterior and posterior cervical spine fixation procedures. *Arch Orthop Trauma Surg* 1987;106:226–231.
61. Koh YD, Lim T, You JW, et al. A biomechanical comparison of modern anterior and posterior plate fixation of the cervical spine. *Spine* 2001;26:15–21.
62. Cybulski GR, Douglas RA, Meyer PR, et al. Complications in three-column cervical spine injuries requiring anterior-posterior stabilization. *Spine* 1992;17:253–256.
63. McNamara MJ, Devito DP, Spengler DM. Circumferential fusion for the management of acute cervical spine trauma. *J Spinal Disord* 1991;4:467–471.
64. McAfee PC, Bohlman HH. One-stage anterior cervical decompression and posterior stabilization with circumferential arthrodesis. *J Bone Joint Surg Am* 1989;71:78–88.
65. Shono Y, McAfee PC, Cunningham BW, et al. A biomechanical analysis of decompression and reconstruction methods in the cervical spine. *J Bone Joint Surg Am* 1993;75:1674–1684.
66. Aufdermaur M. Spinal injuries in juveniles: necropsy findings in twelve cases. *J Bone Joint Surg Br* 1974;56:513–519.
67. Hause M, Hoshiro R, Omato S, et al. Cervical spine injuries in children. *Fukushima J Med Sci* 1974;20:114.
68. Evans DL, Bethem D. Cervical spine injuries in children. *J Pediatr Orthop* 1989;9:563–568.
69. Herzenberg JE, Hensiger RN, Dedrick DK, et al. Emergency transport and positioning of young children who have an injury of the cervical spine: The standard backboard may be dangerous. *J Bone Joint Surg Am* 1989;71:15–22.
70. Sim F, Svien H, Bickel W, et al. Swan-neck deformity following extensive cervical laminectomy. *J Bone Joint Surg Am* 1974;56:564–580.
71. Yasuoko S, Peterson H, MacCarty C. Incidence of spinal column deformity after multilevel laminectomy in children and adults. *J Neurosurg* 1982;57:441–445.
72. Lieberman IH, Webb JK. Cervical spine injuries in the elderly. *J Bone Joint Surg Br* 1994;76:877–881.
73. Albert TJ, Levine MJ, Balderston RA, et al. Gastrointestinal complications in spinal cord injury. *Spine* 1991;16(Suppl 10):S522–S525.
74. Bailey RW. Fractures and dislocations of the cervical spine: Orthopedic and neurological aspects. *Postgrad Med* 1964;35:588–599.
75. Louis R. Stability as defined by the three-column spone concept. *Anat Clin* 1985;7:33–42.

CHAPTER 51

Cervical Instrumentation for Traumatic Injuries

Mark A. Prévost and Robert A. McGuire, Jr.

Spinal instability can result from fracture of the bony elements of the cervical spine as well as disruption of the soft tissue restraints of the vertebral segment. This instability can lead to bony malalignment or displacement with resulting neural compromise. The use of instrumentation provides a method to stabilize the spine, protect the neural elements, and enhance bone healing following trauma.

Because of anatomical and biomechanical considerations, cervical spine fixation should be divided into three separate regions: (a) occipitocervical junction, (b) C1-C2 fixation, and (c) C2 to C7 stabilization. Occipitocervical stabilization can be attained using onlay bone graft wired into position, contoured rods wired to the spine, or contoured plates or rods attached to the skull and posterior spinal elements by screws. C1-C2 stabilization can be achieved with odontoid screws, transarticular screw stabilization posteriorly, various posterior wiring techniques, or clamp fixation, depending on the pathology. C2 to C7 stabilization can be obtained by using anterior struts of bone or cement, anterior plating techniques, posterior spinous process wiring, or posterior plate/rod and screw combinations. Techniques involving instrumentation and the clinical outcomes obtained with their use are the subject of this chapter.

OCCIPITOCERVICAL BIOMECHANICS

Stability of the occipitocervical junction is maintained by a combination of bony and ligamentous constraints. The bony constraints are limited to the occipital condyles, which are wedge-shaped structures on the inferior aspect of the occipital bone just lateral and anterior to the foramen magnum. They have a convex semilunar shape and articulate with the concave lateral masses of C1. The main ligamentous constraints include the paired alar ligaments and the tectorial membrane as a continuation of the posterior longitudinal ligament. Other ligamentous constraints include the apical ligaments, the atlantooccipital joint capsules, and the anterior and posterior atlantooccipital membranes. Panjabi and associates (1) have studied the three-dimensional movements of the occiput to C1 junction and have reported the following range of motion: flexion, 3.5 degrees; extension, 21 degrees; lateral bending, 5.5 degrees; and axial rotation, 7.2 degrees.

Occipitocervical dislocation occurs generally as a result of hyperextension and distraction; the patient rarely survives the injury (2,3). If the patient does survive, external immobilization of the occipitocervical junction is often difficult. Because most of these injuries involve soft tissues rather than bone, the potential for instability with perhaps catastrophic neurologic compromise can exist following nonoperative treatment; therefore, operative stabilization should be considered early in the treatment plan.

Treatment Techniques for Occipitocervical Fusions

Operative treatment of C0-C1 instability is generally performed with a fusion from C0 to C2 or lower, depending on the injury, to obtain adequate stability. A fusion from the occiput to the atlas may not be biomechanically solid enough to support this type of instability. Many techniques for posterior occipitocervical fusion with good results have been described. Most of these are a modification of three basic techniques: occipitocervical wiring of onlay bone graft, contoured rods wired into position, or some combination of rods and plates with screw fixation.

Robinson and Southwick (4) originally described a method of onlay bone graft wiring in 1960. Fixation to the skull was accomplished by making two burr holes adjacent to the foramen magnum, about one-quarter inch from its margin and about three-eighths inch lateral to the midline. Wire was then passed through the foramen from the burr hole on each side. This wire is sutured to the graft through a drill hole in the graft. The graft was also wired to the first,

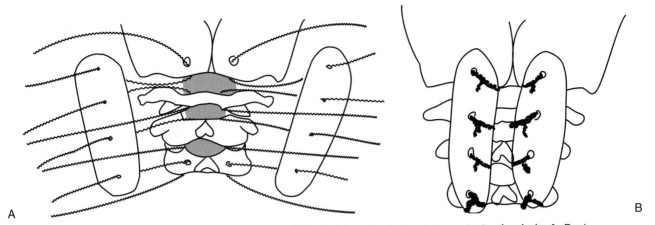

FIG. 51.1. An adaptation of the Robinson and Southwick method of occipitocervical arthrodesis. **A:** Position of drill holes and wires in relationship to graft. **B:** Position of the iliac bone graft after wire fixation.

second, and third cervical vertebrae, either to the spinous process or passed under the lamina (Fig. 51.1).

Wertheim and Bohlman (5) described a modification of the Robinson and Southwick technique that avoids intracranial placement of the wire in stabilizing onlay bone to the skull. The bone at the external occipital protuberance is very thick, allowing passage of wires without going through both tables of the skull. A burr is used to create a trough on either side of the protuberance; these are then connected with a towel clip. A 20-gauge wire is looped through the hole and around the ridge. A second wire is looped around the arch of the atlas, and a third is passed through a drill hole in the base of the spinous process of the axis. These are then used to tie down the bone grafts. Postoperatively, the patient should be immobilized in a halo vest until bony fusion has occurred.

Ransford and associates (6) reported on the ability to stabilize the occipitocervical junction using a contoured Luque rod wired to the skull and cervical spine. Wires are passed through burr holes and withdrawn through the foramen magnum, and additional sublaminar wires are placed at the levels to be fused. The sublaminar and occipital wires are then secured to an anatomically conforming occipitocervical loop fashioned from a Luque rod. Iliac cancellous bone graft is then applied generously to the decorticated posterior elements and occiput.

More recently, several methods of occipitoatlantoaxial fixation have been presented using either C2 pedicle screws or C1-C2 transarticular screws to improve postoperative stability. Techniques using posterior wiring usually require longer fusions or external rigid immobilization. These newer instrumentation methods allow for immobilization in a hard cervical collar if good fixation is achieved. In a biomechanical study of five different occipitoatlantoaxial fixation techniques, Oda and associates (7) demonstrated that C2 transpedicular and C1-C2 transarticular screws significantly increased the stabilizing effect compared with sublaminar

wiring and lamina hooks. The reader is referred to the latter parts of this chapter for techniques of transpedicular or C1-C2 transarticular screw placement. If plates are to be used, these screws are generally placed first. If a screw-rod system is used, the surgeon has more flexibility in the sequence of screw placement. Fixation of C1 can be augmented with wire or cable around the lamina and attached to the plate or rod (Fig. 51.2). For fixation below C2, lateral mass screws are used for stabilization.

Haher and colleagues (8) performed a biomechanical study on occipital screw pull-out strength. The greatest pull-out strength was at the occipital protuberance, with bicortical pull-out strength 50% greater than unicortical. Wire pull-out strength was similar to the unicortical screw. Unicortical pull-out strength at the occipital protuberance was comparable with bicortical screws at other locations. Two bicortical screws on each side are usually placed below the superior nuchal line to avoid the confluence of sinuses. Unicortical screws at or above this line can also be used. Possible penetration of the sinuses could cause thrombosis (9).

Occipitocervical Clinical Evaluation and Results

Wertheim and Bohlman (5) reported 13 patients treated with their technique that avoids intracranial placement of the wire in stabilizing onlay bone to the skull, all of whom achieved successful fusion. Elia and associates (10) reported 28 occipitocervical fusions using the onlay technique, with a primary fusion rate of 89%; postoperatively, a halo was used. Ranford and colleagues (6) reported on the ability to stabilize the occipitocervical junction using a contoured Luque rod wired to the skull and cervical spine in three cases. Sasso and associates (11) reported on 23 patients with occipitocervical fusions with posterior plate and screw instrumentation. All 23 patients attained solid fusions with only simple orthosis wear for an average of 11 weeks. Smith and co-workers (12) described a technique using

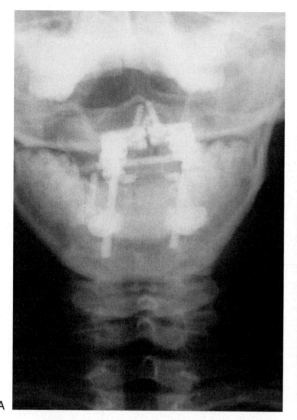
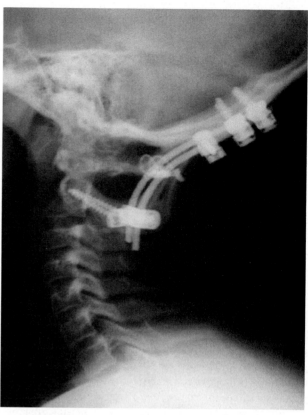

A

B

FIG. 51.2. A: This 13-year-old boy presented with an occipitocervical dislocation and complete T11 lower cord injury. The patient was treated with an occipitocervical arthrodesis using a rod, wire, and polyaxial screws. **B:** Lateral radiograph showing C2 pedicle screws, sublaminar wire around the arch of C1, and bicortical screws in the skull.

contoured plate fixation on 14 patients with excellent fusion results, minimal complications, and the ability to use a collar rather than a halo postoperatively. Abumi and associates (13) reported the results in 26 patients treated with occipitocervical reconstruction using pedicle screws in the cervical spine and occipitocervical rod systems. Solid fusion was achieved in all patients except two who had metastatic vertebral tumors.

C1-C2 BIOMECHANICS

The atlantoaxial joint consists of four separate joints: two intervertebral and two odontoid joints. The two intervertebral joints are between the lateral masses of C1 and C2. Both surfaces are convex, providing little inherent bony stability. In addition, the joint capsules are loose, permitting the wide range of motion seen at this articulation. The two odontoid "joints" are between the dens and the arch of the atlas anteriorly and the strong transverse ligament posteriorly.

The orientation of the C1-C2 facet complex does not provide adequate mechanical support to prevent instability should damage to the dens or transverse ligament occur. Stability of this unique segment relies on the ligamentous components. These structures include the anterior longitudinal ligament, alar ligaments, ligamentum flavum, and most importantly the transverse ligament, which prevents anterior dislocation of C1 on C2. Approximately 50% of axial rotation of the cervical spine occurs at the C1-C2 articulation (14). Three-dimensional movement studies by Panjabi and associates (1) showed the following range of motions for C1-C2: flexion, 11.5 degrees; extension, 10.9 degrees; lateral bending, 6.7 degrees; and axial rotation to each side, 38.9 degrees.

Anterior Techniques

Anterior screw stabilization of the odontoid allows preservation of axial rotation. Sasso and colleagues (15) compared the use of one or two screws for stabilization of the odontoid. Mechanically produced type II odontoid fractures in ten C2 vertebral specimens were stabilized with either one or two 3.5-mm screws. The stabilized specimen construct was then tested to failure. Data obtained after internal fixation demonstrated that the stability of the segment was restored to half that of the unfractured odontoid. The use of two screws did not significantly enhance stability in testing to refailure, as there was no significant difference between the failure load of the one-screw construct versus the two-screw technique. In an anatomic study, Heller and associates (16) found that the odontoid was often too small to accept two screws and cautioned that attempts to place these could lead to complications. In another anatomic study using computed tomography (CT) for evaluation, Nucci and co-workers (17) found that the critical diameter for the placement of two 3.5-mm cortical screws with tapping over a guide wire was 9.0 mm. This dimension was present in 95% of the 92 CT scans of C2 studied. Without tapping, only 33% of patients had odontoids capable of housing two 3.5-mm. screws.

Graziano and associates (18) performed a comparative study of anterior odontoid screws using either one or two 3.5-mm bone screws or a posterior C1-C2 Brooks sublaminar wiring construct using 18-gauge wire. There were no significant differences between bending and torsional stiffness for the one-screw or two-screw specimens, nor was there significant difference between one- or two-screw fixation and posterior C1-C2 wiring in the torsional mode. Bending stiffness was significantly greater with either one or two screws than with the posterior wire fixation technique. This study is in agreement with that of Sasso and colleagues (15), who reported no difference using either one or two screws to enhance the stability of the fractured dens.

The posterior approaches for C1-C2 fusions are by far the most frequently used approaches due to their ease and familiarity. However, when the posterior approach is not a viable option or is undesirable, anterior approaches can be useful. The anterior approaches include transmucosal, lateral retropharyngeal, and anterior retropharyngeal. Vaccaro and associates (19) described an anterior retropharyngeal approach to place left (or left and right) anterior C1-C2 transarticular screws.

Anterior Clinical Evaluation and Results

Odontoid fractures are classified using the criteria of Anderson and D'Alonzo (20). A type I fracture is an oblique fracture through the apex of the dens and probably represents an avulsion of the alar ligaments. Type II fractures occur at the junction of the dens with the body of the axis, which is below the level of the transverse ligament. This fracture is the most common, as well as the most controversial regarding treatment. Type III fractures extend in an oblique manner caudally from the base of the dens to the anterior body of the axis.

Indications for anterior stabilization include a type II or shallow type III displaced odontoid fracture; a type II fracture with an intact transverse ligament and posterior C1 arch fracture, which would preclude an initial posterior wiring procedure and require prolonged halo immobilization to allow healing of C1 before operative stabilization; and patients who wish to retain C1-C2 mobility. Contraindications include dens fractures with oblique configurations

that prevent adequate stability when compressed following internal fixation and fractures resulting from a pathologic process (21).

Bohler (22) reported on a series of 15 patients in whom a 100% fusion was achieved after anterior screw fixation. Montesano and colleagues (23) treated 14 patients with odontoid fractures with odontoid screws. The rate of union was 86% (12 of 14). All of the six fractures treated with a single screw achieved a solid fusion, as did six of eight fractures when two screws were employed. ElSaghir and Bohm (24) reported their results in 30 patients treated with two 2.7-mm cortical titanium screws. They reported no cases of nonunion and no major complications. In a report on 81 patients, Henry and associates (25) noted a union rate of 92%. There was one major complication in an 83-year-old woman who was tetraparetic after the procedure. All patients were treated with a single 3.5-mm screw.

Conclusion

Anterior fixation of odontoid fractures provides excellent stability to facilitate fracture union while maintaining normal C1-C2 motion. The technique is demanding and requires meticulous attention to detail—from positioning to the surgical technique—to minimize the risks of intraoperative and postoperative complications.

C1-C2 Posterior Biomechanics

In evaluating posterior wiring techniques, Hanley and Harvell (26) compared a simple midline wiring to the Gallie and Brooks techniques. The Brooks stabilization achieved twice the stiffness of the simple midline wiring and Gallie technique in resisting flexion and extension movements. In evaluation of torsional stability, the Brooks technique was found to be five times the stiffness of the others. All three methods reestablished the prefracture stability of the C1-C2 segment.

Grob and colleagues (27) compared the Gallie and Brooks wiring techniques, Magerl transarticular screw method, and a Halifax clamp in reestablishing stability to the C1-C2 segment. All specimens were loaded using pure moments in flexion-extension, axial rotation, and lateral bending. Although all the procedures decreased motion across this segment, the Gallie technique was least effective, and the Magerl transarticular screw technique was the most effective in limiting motion. The Gallie system allowed significantly more rotation in flexion-extension, axial rotation, and lateral bending than the other fixation techniques. Although there were no statistically significant differences between the Brooks, Magerl, or the Halifax clamp techniques, the Magerl technique tended to allow the least rotation.

Crisco and associates (28) evaluated graft translation using the same fixation techniques as Grob and colleagues. They reported no significant difference between any of the fixations and the average axial translation. The Magerl technique, however, significantly decreased motion in the shear mode compared with the other techniques. Montesano and co-workers (29) found greater stiffness in rotation and no translation with the screw fixation technique compared with wiring alone. Naderi and associates (30) studied four combinations of cable-graft-screw fixation at C1-C2. They reported that the transarticular screws prevented lateral bending and axial rotation better than the posterior cable-graft. The cable-graft prevented flexion and extension better than screw fixation. They concluded that it was mechanically advantageous to include as many fixation points as possible when treating C1-C2 instability. Three-point fixation may be the treatment of choice for C1-C2 fixation when instability is a concern.

Mandel and co-workers (31) examined the C2 isthmus dimensions for the placement of transarticular screws. They concluded that placing a 3.5-mm screw in a narrow C2 isthmus (smaller than 5 mm in height or width) would be technically difficult. Based on the 205 specimens examined, approximately 10% of patients may be at risk for a vertebral artery injury with the placement of C1-C2 transarticular screws. Paramore and associates (32) reported that 18% of 94 patients on CT reconstructions had a high-riding transverse foramen for the C2 vertebral artery on at least one side that would prevent safe passage of a screw. Because of the concern regarding vertebral artery and neurologic injury, several image-guided surgery systems have evolved. Weidner and colleagues (33) used CT data to plan optimal screw trajectory before surgery and then used that data during surgery to guide screw placement in 37 patients. These were compared with a historic control group of 78 patients. Their results showed that image-guided surgery reduced, but did not eliminate, screw misplacements.

Tokuhashi and associates (34) reported a posterior stabilization technique using the Halifax interlaminar clamp in combination with an intraarticular screw. Bony fusion was obtained with no vascular or neural complications in the 11 patients treated with this technique.

Clinical Evaluation of Posterior Results

Jeanneret and Magerl (35) reported on C1-C2 posterior fixation in which 13 patients stabilized with the transarticular screw technique achieved a solid arthrodesis (Fig. 51.3). In a similar study by McGuire and Harkey (36), eight patients in whom the transfacet screw technique was used achieved solid arthrodesis. Fielding and associates (37) reported a series of 46 patients whose fractures were treated using the Gallie technique; 45 attained a solid arthrodesis. Brooks and Jenkins (38) used a sublaminar C1-C2 wiring technique in 15 patients, of whom 14 achieved a solid arthrodesis. Griswold and colleagues (39) reported an arthrodesis rate of 100% in 30 patients treated with the Brooks technique. Statham and associates (40) showed the Halifax clamp to be less effective than the other methods; the complication rate was 31%.

Conclusion

It is evident from the biomechanical and clinical data that the stability of the C1-C2 articulation can be reestablished using a variety of techniques. Biomechanically, the Magerl transarticular screw technique provides better fixation in all studies performed, but clinical results are good regardless of the procedure chosen.

C2 TO C7 STABILIZATION

Anterior Construct Biomechanics

For stabilization of the C2 to C7 segment in patients with spinal instability, the use of an anterior strut alone is not recommended. In 1977, Stauffer and Kelly (41) reported 16 patients with fracture-dislocations and significant cervical instability, all of whom failed to regain stability when an anterior strut alone, without significant external restraint or secondary internal fixation, was employed.

Anterior cervical plating can be used to provide stability to the fractured cervical spine. Montesano and associates (29) compared Rogers wiring versus an anterior plate using bicortical screws in a distraction flexion injury model with no interposition graft. These investigators found the posterior wiring construct to be stiffer than the anterior plate and suggested that a combined anterior-posterior reconstruction be used simultaneously.

Abitbol and colleagues (42) compared anterior plates with posterior cervical stabilization. A distraction flexion type III injury was created in the spines of human cadavers at the C4-C5 level. Five posterior stabilization systems were tested in a random sequence: Rogers wiring, cervical modular fixation with screws and rods, 3.5 Synthes reconstruction plates, Haid plates, and Harms plates. The specimens then were retested after fixation with an anterior Caspar or Morsher plate. In torsion, the Synthes reconstruction plate, Harms, and modular fixation systems were the stiffest constructs, with no statistically significant difference between them. The anterior plates allowed significantly greater motion than the posterior devices. In flexion testing, the Rogers wiring, the Synthes plate, and the modular system provided significantly greater flexural stiffness compared with the Caspar plate, the Morsher plate, and the Haid and Harms devices. The anterior plates provided the most rigid stabilization compared with the posterior devices in spinal extension testing. With axial loading, the posterior Synthes reconstruction plate supplied the stiffest construct, with the Morsher and Caspar anterior plates the least. The investigators concluded that anterior plating alone may not restore complete stability to the spine and that additional posterior stabilization may be necessary to enhance spinal stiffness.

Grubb and associates (43) evaluated anterior plates using a flexion compression injury model in a porcine spine. Three constructs were tested: a cervical spine locking plate, the Caspar plate with unicortical screws, and the Caspar plate with bicortical screws. Interposition grafts were used

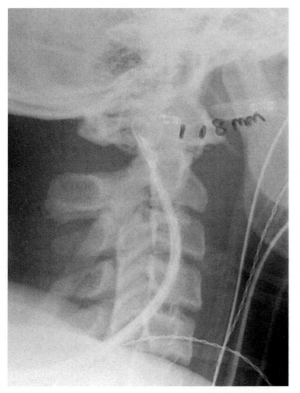

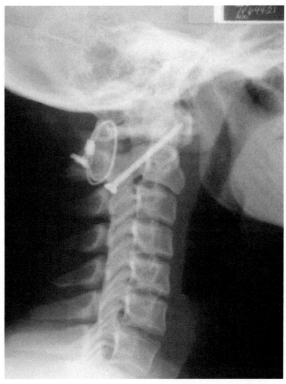

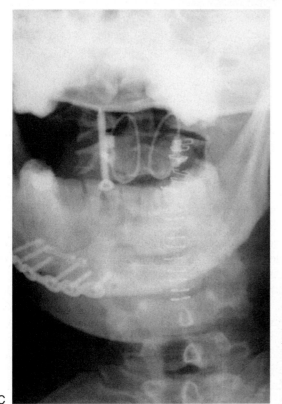

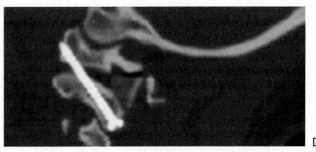

FIG. 51.3. A: Lateral radiograph taken after a motor vehicle accident revealing an increased atlanto-dens interval in a patient who presented with upper cervical pain. **B, C:** Anteroposterior and lateral radiograph after C1-C2 fusion with unilateral Magerl transarticular screw technique and posterior Brooks fusion. After studying preoperative computed tomographic (CT) scans it was felt only one side was safe for the transarticular screw. **D:** CT reconstruction showing placement of transarticular screw.

in testing these constructs to failure. Unlike the results in previous studies, the instrumented constructs were comparable to intact specimens in flexural stiffness, lateral bending, and torsional stiffness. The cervical spine locking plate had a significantly higher failure moment, in which the mode of failure was the screws pulling out of the bone. No screw–plate interface loosening was noted with this system. On the other hand, the mode of failure with the Caspar system using a unicortical screw fixation was screw pull-out combined with loosening of the plate–screw interface. The failure mode for the Caspar plate with bicortical screw purchase was plate deformation and screw–plate interface loosening, but no significant screw pull-out from bone. Kotani and associates (44) showed that front and back approaches using anterior plate and posterior stabilization with the triple-wire technique and pedicle screw fixation provided distinct biomechanical advantages *in vitro* when spinal instability involved three-column injury or multi-level constructs.

Clinical Outcome of Anterior Constructs

Although *in vitro* biomechanical testing procedures do not appear to indicate that use of an anterior plate alone would be sufficient, Garvey and associates (45) reported a series of 14 patients with significant fracture dislocation and posterior instability who were treated with bone grafting and anterior plating alone. Fusion was achieved in all of the patients, with no loss of fixation or development of kyphosis (Fig. 51.4). Similarly, Aebi and colleagues (46) reported a series of 86 patients with 22 fractures and 64 posterior ligamentous disruptions who were treated with anterior interposition grafting and plating. Only one reoperation was necessary for replacement of the graft; all fractures healed, and no evidence of plate breakage or loss of spinal alignment was seen.

More recently, Razack and associates (47) reported on single-level anterior cervical discectomy and stabilization for bilateral facet fracture dislocations using bone graft and anterior titanium plates with unicortical screws in 22 patients. They reported one instrumentation failure, but all 22 patients had evidence of stability at the instrumented level on final follow-up. Lifeso and Colucci (48) reported on 32 rotationally unstable cervical fractures treated with either brace or posterior surgical constructs and fusion, and compared these with a second group of 18 patients treated with early anterior discectomy, fusion, and plating. Their results showed that nonoperative treatment was uniformly unsuccessful. Posterior stabilization and fusion had unsuccessful results in 45% due to late kyphosis or inability to control rotational instability. Anterior fusion resulted in solid union without residual deformity in all cases. They concluded that although posterior bony injury is the usual radiographic finding, disruption of the anterior disc and longitudinal ligament is the more significant injury and leads to late collapse and deformity.

Conclusion

Analysis of these clinical studies, although biomechanically unsupported by experimental biomechanical data, indicates that anterior plating alone provides excellent clinical outcome in flexion distraction injuries of the cervical spine.

Posterior Construct Biomechanics

Coe and colleagues (49) tested eight posterior techniques using a distraction flexion stage 3 injury model. Eight constructs were tested using cyclic loads to simulate cervical compression, flexion, extension, and rotation with measurements of axial load, axial displacement, torque, rotation, and anterior and posterior strains. They tested: (a) an intact spinal segment, (b) a sublaminar wire fixation technique, (c) Rogers' wiring technique, (d) Bohlman's triple-wire technique, (e) Roy-Camille posterior plate fixation, (f) AO posterior hook-plate fixation, (g) Caspar anterior plate with bicortical fixation, and (h) the AO posterior hook plate with Caspar anterior plate fixation. No significant differences in flexural or torsional stiffness were noted. There was a significant difference noted in the posterior strain during flexion and axial loading when the Caspar anterior plate construct was compared with all the posterior stabilization methods. The differences between the anterior Caspar plating system and the posterior constructs were significant. If the bony posterior elements are intact, this study supports the use of the interspinous wiring techniques of Rogers and Bohlman in providing as much rigidity as the other posterior fixation constructs. Conversely, Ulrich and colleagues (50) found that posterior wiring was not as effective in preventing translational displacement as the posterior hook plate or anterior plate and that fatigue of the wire could occur with complete discoligamentous injuries. With this type of instability, internal fixation with external immobilization is recommended if either posterior wiring or anterior plating is used exclusively.

Posterior stabilization also can be provided by posterior plating techniques (Fig. 51.5). These methods become important when there is compromise of the laminae or spinous processes resulting from previous surgery, fractures, or tumors. These techniques also can be used when the anterior column is incapable of weight bearing. Screw direction into the lateral mass is important in imparting stability to the posterior construct. Errico and associates (51) evaluated the pull-out strength of screws inserted by the Magerl technique, in which the screw is placed into the lateral mass in an anterior lateral and cranial direction, compared with the Roy-Camille technique, in which the screw is placed in a parasagittal plane in the lateral mass. There were significant differences in the pull-out strength between these two techniques: The Magerl was stronger than the Roy-Camille technique. Montesano and colleagues (52) compared the two screw-insertion techniques placed into C4-C5

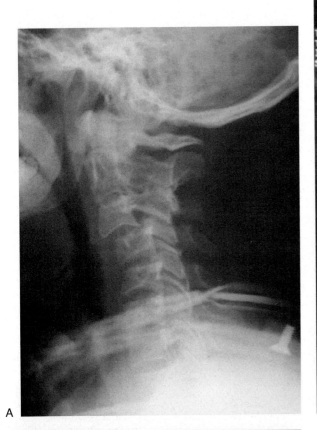

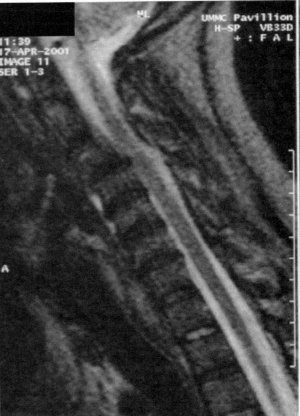

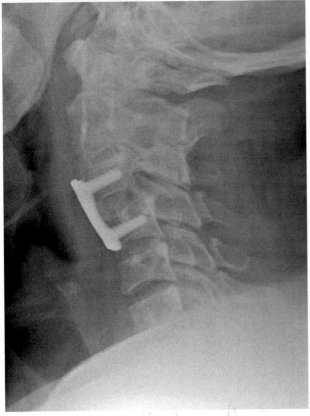

FIG. 51.4. A: This 31-year-old man was involved in a motor vehicle collision and suffered a fracture of the C3 left facet and lateral mass with good initial alignment. He was initially treated with halo fixation; this lateral radiograph at his first follow-up shows subluxation at C3-C4 measuring 5 to 6 mm. **B:** Magnetic resonance imaging shows a herniated disc at this level. **C:** Lateral radiograph shows stabilization with anterior cervical plate and autograph bone graft.

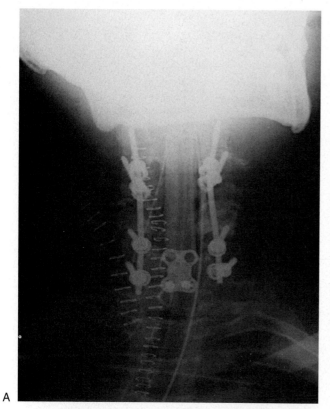
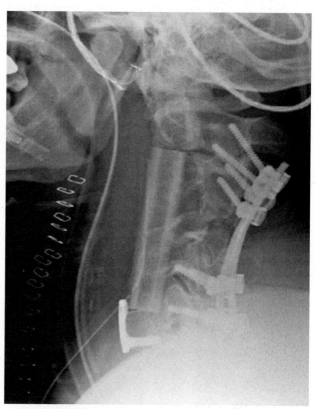

A   B

FIG. 51.5. A: This 32-year-old man had a previous history of a C3-C4 fracture dislocation and subsequent arthrodesis at C3-C4. He was then involved in a repeat motor vehicle collision with ligamentous disruption at C2-C3 and a fracture dislocation at C5-C6 producing an incomplete spinal cord injury. From his previous injury, he had a severe kyphotic deformity at C3 to C5 with block arthrodesis of the anterior and posterior elements. The patient underwent a 540-degree procedure with corpectomies at C3 to C5, posterior osteotomies at C3 to C5 and arthrodesis from C2 to C6. **B:** Lateral radiograph showing fibular strut graft with antikickout plate and posterior instrumentation.

and C5-C6 segments (Fig. 51.6). Both methods employed stainless steel reconstruction plates and 3.5-mm cancellous screws. Significant differences in the mean failure load were noted: The Magerl technique failed at 885 N, compared with 152 N for the Roy-Camille technique. The mechanisms of failure were also significantly different. The failure of the Magerl technique was caused by the plate bending, whereas the Roy-Camille technique failed by caudal screw pull-out. Screw placement with the Magerl technique has several advantages, notably that the neurovascular structures and intact motion segments are relatively protected. It also provides stability in a spine in which the anterior column is not totally functional; however, it involves a steeper angle of insertion, which clinically may be difficult in the lower cervical spine.

Other methods of posterior screw fixation have been described and can provide stable fixation in cases of unusual anatomy or stripped screws. Transfacet screws were first described by Roy-Camille and associates and offer an alternative to lateral mass screws. In a biomechanical study by Klekamp and colleagues (53), pull-out strength for the screws placed across the facets was 467 N, compared with

360 N for the lateral mass screws. Cervical pedicle screws have also been reported as an alternative fixation technique for posterior cervical plating. Jones and co-workers (54) studied the biomechanical pull-out properties of pedicle screws compared with lateral mass screws. The mean load to failure was 677 N for the cervical pedicle screws and 355 N for the lateral mass screws. They observed minor pedicle wall violations in 13% of cases.

In their evaluation of posterior plating constructs, Gill and associates (55) found no significant biomechanical differences between wiring techniques and plating techniques in the stability afforded the spine, which would again reinforce the conclusion of Coe and colleagues (49) that interspinous wiring techniques impart minimal risks to the patient and supply excellent stability to the spine provided the posterior elements are intact.

Clinical Outcome of Posterior Technique

In a clinical evaluation of posterior cervical fusions with the Bohlman triple-wire technique, Weiland and

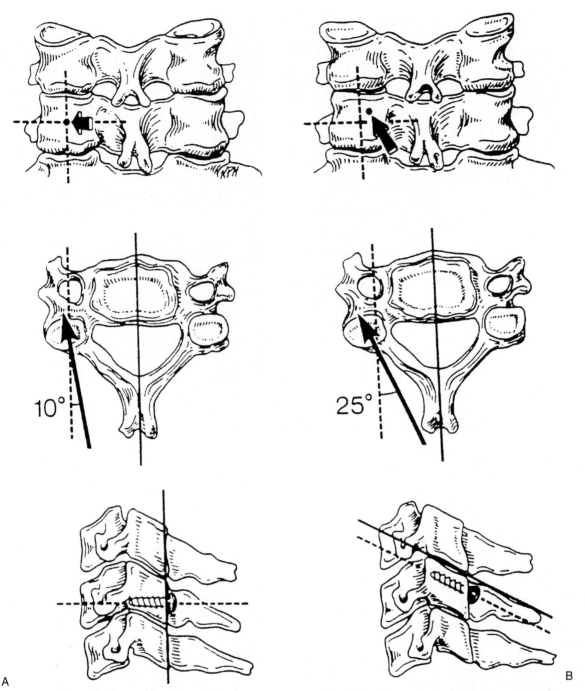

FIG. 51.6. A: The Roy-Camille technique can potentially jeopardize the neurovascular structures and unaffected facet joints. The failure mode of the construct is screw pullout. **B:** The Magerl technique provides excellent fixation. It provides relative protection for the neurovascular structures, but care must be exercised to avoid damage to the root above during the drilling and screw insertion maneuvers. The mode of failure in this construct is usually through plate bending rather than screw pullout.

McAfee (56) reported on 60 patients who underwent subaxial fusions. Of this total, only 2 were placed in a halo vest; the remaining patients were managed postoperatively in cervical or cervicothoracic orthoses. The fusion rate was 100%, with no infections or iatrogenic neuro-logic injuries (Fig. 51.7). Anderson and associates (57) reported on a series of 30 patients treated with posterior plating, all of whom healed with no vascular or neuro-logic injury. No failure of the constructs or increased kyphosis occurred.

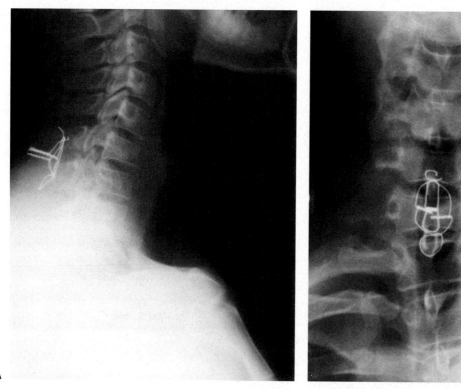

A   B

FIG. 51.7. A, B: This lateral and anteroposterior radiograph demonstrates the Bohlman triple-wire technique, which is useful when spinous processes are available. This technique does not jeopardize the neural elements, because the wire passage is dorsal to the spinolaminar line.

Conclusion

Posterior wiring techniques provide enhanced stability to the spine as long as the anterior weight-bearing column and posterior elements are present. If the anterior column is significantly damaged, or compromise of the laminae or spinous processes occurs, techniques using lateral mass screws with posterior plates or rods provide excellent stability to the spine with successful clinical outcomes.

REFERENCES

1. Panjabi M, Dvorak J, Duranceau J, et al. Three-dimensional movements of the upper cervical spine. *Spine* 1988;13:726–730.
2. Davis D, Bohlman H, Walker E, et al. The pathologic findings in fatal cranio-spinal injuries. *J Neurosurg* 1971;34:603–615.
3. Bucholz RW, Burkhead WZ. The pathologic anatomy of fatal atlanto-occipital dislocations. *J Bone Joint Surg Am* 1979;61:248–250.
4. Robinson RA, Southwick WO. Surgical approaches to the cervical spine. In: American Academy of Orthopedic Surgeons, eds., *Instructional course lectures,* vol. 17. St. Louis, MO: CV Mosby, 1960:299–330.
5. Wertheim SB, Bohlman HH. Occipitocervical fusion: indications, techniques, and long-term results in 13 patients. *J Bone Joint Surg Am* 1987;69:833–836.
6. Ransford AO, Crockard HA, Pozo JL, et al. Craniocervical instability treated by contoured loop fixation. *J Bone Joint Surg Br* 1986;68:173–177.
7. Oda I, Abumi K, Sell L, et al. Biomechanical evaluation of five different occcipito-atlanto-axial fixation techniques. *Spine* 1999;24:2377–2382.
8. Haher T, Yeung A, Caruso S, et al. Occipital screw pullout strength: a biomechanical investigation of occipital morphology. *Spine* 1999;24:5–9.
9. Heywood A, Learmonth I, Thomas M. Internal fixation for occipito-cervical fusion. *J Bone Joint Surg Br* 1988;70:708–711.
10. Elia M, Mazzara J, Fielding J. Onlay technique for occipitocervical fusion. *Clin Orthop* 1992;280:170–174.
11. Sasso R, Jeanneret B, Fischer K, et al. Occipitocervical fusion with posterior plate and screw instrumentation: a long-term follow-up study. *Spine* 1994;19:2364–2368.
12. Smith MD, Anderson P, Grady MS. Occipitocervical arthrodesis using contoured plate fixation. *Spine* 1993;18:1984–1990.
13. Abumi K, Takada T, Shono Y, et al. Posterior occipitocervical reconstruction using cervical pedicle screws and plate-rod systems. *Spine* 1999;24:1425–1434.
14. Penning L. Normal movements of the cervical spine. *AJR Am J Roentgenol* 1979;130:317–319.
15. Sasso RC, Heggeness MH, Dohrety BJ. Biomechanics of odontoid fracture fixation: comparison of one and two screw techniques. *Spine* 1993;18:1950–1953.
16. Heller JG, Also MD, Schaffler MB, et al. Quantitative dens morphology. *Orthop Trans* 1990;14:693.
17. Nucci R, Seigal S, Merola A, et al. Computed tomographic evaluation of the normal adult odontoid: implications for internal fixation. *Spine* 1995;20:264–270.
18. Grazino G, Jaggers C, Lee M, et al. A comparative study of fixation techniques for type II fractures of odontoid process. *Spine* 1993;18:2383–2387.
19. Vaccaro A, Lehman A, Ahlgren B, et al. Anterior C1-C2 screw fixation and bony fusion through an anterior retropharyngeal approach. *Orthopedics* 1999;22:1165–1170.
20. Anderson LD, D'Alonzo RT. Fractures of the odontoid process of the axis. *J Bone Joint Surg Am* 1974;56:1663–1664.
21. Etter C, Coscia M, Jaberg H, et al. Direct anterior fixation of dens fracture with a cannulated screw system. *Spine* 1991;16:525–532.

22. Bohler J. Anterior stabilization for acute fracture and nonunions of the dens. *J Bone Joint Surg Am* 1982;64:18–27.
23. Montesano PX, Anderson PA, Schehr F, et al. Odontoid fractures treated by anterior odontoid screw fixation. *Spine* 1991;16:533–537.
24. ElSaghir H, Bohm H. Anderson type II fracture of the odontoid process: results of anterior screw fixation. *J Spinal Disord* 2000;13:527–530.
25. Henry A, Bohly J, Grosse A. Fixation of odontoid fractures by an anterior screw. *J Bone Joint Surg Br* 1999;81:472–477.
26. Hanley EN, Harvell JC. Immediate postoperative stability of the atlanto-axial articulation: a biomechanical study comparing simple midline wiring, and the Gallie and Brook's procedures. *J Spinal Disord* 1992;5:306–310.
27. Grob D, Crisco JJ, Panjabi MM, et al. Biomechanical evaluation of four different posterior atlantoaxial fixation techniques. *Spine* 1992;17:480–490.
28. Crisco JJ, Panjabi MM, Oda T, et al. Bone graft translation of four upper cervical spine fixation techniques in a cadaveric model. *J Orthop Res* 1991;9:835–846.
29. Montesano PX, Juach EC, Andersen PA, et al. Biomechanics of cervical fixation. *Spine* 1991;16(Suppl):S10–S16.
30. Naderi S, Crawford N, Song G, et al. Biomechanical comparison of C1-C2 posterior fixations cable, graft and screw combinations. *Spine* 1998;23:1946–1956.
31. Mandel I, Kambach B, Petersilge C, et al. Morphologic considerations of C2 isthmus dimensions for the placement of transarticular screws. *Spine* 2000;25:1542–1547.
32. Paramore CG, Dickman CA, Sonntag VH. The anatomic suitability of the C1-C2 complex for transarticular screw fixation. *J Neurosurg* 1996;85:221–224.
33. Weidner A, Wahler M, Chiu S, et al. Modification of C1-C2 transarticular screw fixation by image-guided surgery. *Spine* 2000;25:2668–2673.
34. Tokuhashi Y, Matsuzaki H, Shirasaki Y, et al. C1-C2 intra-articular screw fixation for atlantoaxial posterior stabilization. *Spine* 2000;25:337–341.
35. Jeanneret B, Magerl F. Primary posterior fusion of C1-2 in odontoid fractures: indications, techniques, and results of transarticular screw fixation. *J Spinal Disord* 1992;5:464–475.
36. McGuire RA, Harkey HL. Modification of technique and results of atlantoaxial transfacet stabilization. *Orthopedics* 1995;18:1029–1032.
37. Fielding JW, Hawkins RJ, Ratzan SA. Spine fusion for atlanto-axial instability. *J Bone Joint Surg Am* 1976;58:400–407.
38. Brooks AL, Jenkins EW. Atlanto-axial arthrodesis by the wedge compression method. *J Bone Joint Surg Am* 1978;60:279–284.
39. Griswold DM, Albright JA, Schiffman E, et al. Atlantoaxial fusion of instability. *J Bone Joint Surg Am* 1978;60:285–292.
40. Statham P, O'Sullivan M, Russell T. The Halifax interlaminar clamp for posterior cervical fusion: initial experience in the United Kingdom. *Neurosurgery* 1993;32:396–399.
41. Stauffer ES, Kelly EG. Fracture-dislocations of the cervical spine. *J Bone Joint Surg Am* 1977;59:45–48.
42. Abitbol JJ, Zdeblick T, Kunz D, et al. A biomechanical analysis of modern anterior and posterior cervical stabilization techniques. Presented at the Cervical Spine Research Society, 1992.
43. Grubb MR, Currier BL, Bonin V, et al. Biomechanical evaluation of the anterior cervical spine stabilization in a porcine model. *Orthop Trans* 1993;17:617.
44. Kotani Y, Cunningham B, Abumi K, et al. Biomechanical analysis of cervical stabilization systems. *Spine* 1994;19:2529–2539.
45. Garvey TA, Eismont FJ, Roberti U. Anterior decompression, structural bone grafting, and cast bar plate stabilization for unstable spine fractures and dislocations. *Spine* 1992;17(Suppl):S431–S435.
46. Aebi M, Zuber K, Marchesi D. Treatment of cervical spine injuries with anterior plating: indications, techniques, and results. *Spine* 1991;16:538–545.
47. Razack N, Green B, Levi A. The management of traumatic cervical bilateral facet fracture-dislocations with unicortical anterior plates. *J Spinal Disorders* 2000;13:374–381.
48. Lifeso R, Colucci MA. Anterior fusion for rotationally unstable cervical spine fractures. *Spine* 2000;25:2028–2034.
49. Coe JD, Warden KE, Sutterlin CE, et al. Biomechanical evaluation of cervical spinal stabilization methods in a human cadaveric model. *Spine* 1989;14:1122–1130.
50. Ulrich C, Woersdoerfer O, Kalff R, et al. Biomechanics of fixation systems to the cervical spine. *Spine* 1991;16:54–59.
51. Errico T, Uhl R, Cooper P, et al. Pull out strength comparison of two methods of orienting screw insertion in the lateral masses of the bovine cervical spine. *J Spinal Disord* 1992;5:459–469.
52. Montesano PX, Jauch EC, Jonsson H. Anatomic and biomechanical study of posterior cervical spine plate arthrodesis and evaluation of two different techniques of screw pull out. *J Spinal Disord* 1992;5:303–305.
53. Klekamp JW, Ugbo J, Heller J, et al. Cervical transfacet versus lateral mass screws: a biomechanical comparison. *J Spinal Disord* 2000;13:515–518.
54. Jones E, Heller J, Silcox H, et al. Cervical pedicle screws versus lateral mass screws: anatomic feasibility and biomechanical comparison. *Spine* 1997;22:977–982.
55. Gill K, Paschal S, Corin J, et al. Posterior plating of the cervical spine, a biomechanical comparison of different posterior fusion techniques. *Spine* 1988;13:813–816.
56. Weiland DJ, McAfee PC. Posterior cervical fusion with triple wire strut graft technique: one hundred consecutive patients. *J Spinal Disord* 1991;4:15–21.
57. Anderson PA, Henley MB, Grady MS, et al. Posterior cervical arthrodesis with AO reconstruction plates and bone graft. *Spine* 1991;16:572–579.

SECTION VI

Spinal Cord Injury

CHAPTER 52

Acute Spinal Cord Injuries

Pathophysiologic Mechanisms and Experimental Therapy

Andrew V. Slucky

Acute spinal cord injury (SCI) continues to remain a problem of substantial patient morbidity and socioeconomic expense. Each year, an estimated 12,000 new cases of paraplegia and quadriplegia occur in the United States (1–4). Of those injured, 4000 die before reaching the hospital and 1,000 die during the course of hospitalization. In reflection on the improved methods of initial injury management, the incidence rate of those patients reaching the hospital alive increased from 17 per million (1935 to 1944) to 50 per million in the 1975 to 1981 period (5).

Conversely, because the initial injury incidence has not appeared to decrease over time, initial injury survival has increased along with the consequent socioeconomic cost. The average initial hospitalization costs for a patient with high-level quadriplegia and respirator dependency can be in excess of $250,000 (6,7), with an additional $1.5 million expended in lifetime medical costs and lost earnings (8). In 1990, an estimated $4 billion was spent in the management of all SCI in the United States (9).

Over several decades, major gains have been made in the understanding of SCI, including the development of reproducible SCI models and identification of biochemical pathways leading to SCI. An evolution of proposed injury mechanisms has developed sequentially from an initial understanding of neurocellular function, to the activation of pathologic injury pathways, and ultimately, to an understanding of the neurocellular injury response and a reversal of SCI pathophysiology.

Despite these advancements, substantial hurdles remain in the understanding and treatment of acute SCI. Although numerous elements have been identified as factors involved

in SCI, to date, no *unified* theory of spinal cord pathomechanics has been defined. Ambiguity remains concerning causal relationships of suspect elements, whether they are the promoters of SCI or the end results of injury-induced cellular necrosis. Finally, difficulties in logistics and expense severely limit development of large-scale clinical trials of potential therapeutic agents. Compounding these difficulties is the ethical issue of withholding agents of known benefit in comparative trials against agents of theoretic benefit, given the devastating consequences of SCI. The following section reviews the known pathologic mechanisms of SCI and discusses the status of current experimental therapies.

PATHOPHYSIOLOGY

Injury Mechanism

The spinal cord is particularly susceptible to injury in the cervical region because of the coupling of a large mass, the head, to a lever arm of great flexibility, the cervical spine. The spinal cord is injured when the ligaments, muscles, and bony structures between the skin and spinal cord fail to dissipate the energy of impact (10,11). Transmission of the energy of impact to the cervical spinal cord results in microhemorrhage in the central gray matter and, typically, loss of neuroconduction in the adjacent white matter.

The spinal cord can be traumatically injured by excessive flexion, extension, rotation or axial loading with resultant: (a) impact plus compression; (b) impact alone with transient compression; (c) distraction; and (d) laceration/transection (12). Fracture-dislocation is the most common cause of cervical SCI; however, the spinal cord also can be injured without radiographic evidence of injury to the vertebral column. This latter condition is termed spinal cord injury without radiographic abnormality (SCIWORA), and typically occurs in very young or in older patients with cervical spondylosis (13).

The risk of SCI with damage to cervical vertebrae is increased in persons with narrow spinal canal diameters (14,15). Patients with a narrow midsagittal spinal canal diameter have an increased chance of developing a severe neurologic injury with a given spinal fracture, dislocation, or both compared with patients with a larger midsagittal canal diameter (14).

Injury Models

Design of clinically relevant animal models of SCI has been difficult because of the multifactoral nature of human injuries (16). The numerous variables include age, sex, and preexisting clinical conditions. Logistical variables include the type of force applied (compression or distraction), velocity, duration, point of impact (ventral or dorsal), and quantification of energy imparted. Additional limitations of animal modeling of SCI include the necessity of preinjury anesthesia in the animal, the necessity to violate a major body cavity to impart the experimental load (e.g., a laminectomy or corpectomy for application of a load), and the fact that human injuries typically occur in a closed vertebral system, whereas most animal models use an open approach for lesioning.

Currently, most laboratory research on SCI uses the classic weight-drop contusion model first developed by Allen (17,18) in 1911. The method consists of dropping a known weight through a tube placed on the exposed *thoracic* cord. The severity of the SCI is graded by varying either the weight or the height of the drop; injury magnitude is recorded as the force product in gram-centimeters (g-cm). Disadvantages of the system are that quantification of g-cm is not a true representation of the energy imparted to the cord; a 20-g mass dropped 5 cm transfers more than 100 times greater energy to the cord compared with a 2-g mass dropped 50 cm, even though both are equivalent injury products (100 g-cm) (19). Furthermore, the cord is compressed dorsally, which differs from the more common ventral or circumferential compression seen in human injuries. Despite these drawbacks, the weight-drop technique has been modified by numerous investigators and has successfully created spinal cord lesions in several animal models.

In 1978 Rivlin and Tator (20) described the use of a modified aneurysm clip for application of circumferential compression to the spinal cord in a rat model. This model was adopted by several other investigators and found to be reliable and inexpensive (8). Advantages of the model include precise delivery of a known force of finite duration. Disadvantages of this method are that it requires more manipulation of the exposed cord because the clip must be placed under its ventral as well as over its dorsal aspect. Additionally, the biomechanics of the injury does not mimic the human condition.

Alternative models include the use of balloon or cuff compression techniques. In 1953 Tarlov and associates (21) described insertion of a balloon in the spinal extradural space of dogs to produce paralysis. The technique was later modified and applied in monkey (22) and rat (23) models. Disadvantages of the model include technical difficulty in positioning the balloon; the inability to quantify cord pressure; the difficulty of performing this technique in the small animal model; and that the model biomechanics do not closely imitate human injury. Other investigators also have described a laser-lesion model of SCI with some experimental success (24).

Primary Versus Secondary Injury

Animal-modeling studies of acute SCI suggest that spinal cord lesions produced by physical contusion progress over a period of several hours to days (17,18,25–28). Current concepts suggest that two separate components, a *primary* and *secondary* injury, contribute to the final neurologic damage of acute SCI. The primary injury typically results in acute paralysis and is accompanied by membrane shifts in electrolytes, a decrease in membrane bound Na^+-K^+-adenosine triphosphatase (ATPase), a loss of energy stores, and early morphologic changes (28–31). The secondary injury appears to consist of a series of autodestructive processes characterized by a biochemical cascade and cellular response, variably lasting for hours or days, which destabilize the neurologic membrane of surviving axons with a resultant progressive and heretofore irreversible pattern of spinal cord cystic degeneration and neurolysis (28,29). The important distinction between primary and secondary injury is that although the primary process occurs passively, subsequent to the initial mechanical disruption of the axons, the secondary injury cascade is actively mediated by cellular and molecular processes (32–35).

Primary Mediators of Spinal Cord Injury

Mechanical disruption of the spinal cord results in a loss of neurophysiologic conduction across the lesion site (36–40). In addition, initial injury results in hemorrhage, abnormal intracellular electrolyte flux, loss of energy stores, and the release of normal metabolites and lysozymes from injured cells (Table 1) (41).

Mechanical Compression

Traumatic SCI occurs with direct force transduction to the spinal cord and initiation of the injury cascade. Subsequent to impact injury, the persistence of compression has been implied as a primary mediator of SCI. Conversely, the reversal of such mechanism (i.e., decompression) has been

TABLE 52.1. *Pathomechanisms of Traumatic Spinal Cord Injury*

Primary injury mechanisms
Mechanical disruption
Electrolyte flux
  Increased intracellular sodium
  Increased extracellular potassium
  Increased intracellular calcium
    Neurogenic shock, hypotension
    Hemorrhage

Secondary injury mechanisms
Posttraumatic ischemia
  Loss of microcirculation
  Reduced spinal cord blood flow
  Endogenous opiod release
  Decreased adenosine triphosphate production
Ionic disequilibrium
  Accelerated calcium influx
  Altered sodium and magnesium homeostsis
  Activation of ionotropic-Ca^{2+} channels
  Glutamate-mediated excitotoxicity
Free radical formation
  Phospholipase A_2-arachidonic acid release
  Hemorrhage [Fe^{2+}] free radical formation
  Lipid membrane peroxidation
Inflammation
  Nuclear factor, _B activation
Eicosanoid production
  Leukotriene production
  Kininogen-kinin cascade

Terminal mechanisms
Necrosis
  Apoptosis

a point of significant surgical contoversy regarding application and timing (42). Numerous animal models have demonstrated that decompression of the spinal cord improves recovery after SCI with recovery substantially dependent on time of decompression (36,43–50). Presumably, relief of compressive forces returns the injured spinal section to its native cellular environment and homeostasis, albeit the effects of the consequent injury cascade. However, as a viscoelastic substance, the spinal cord tissues demonstrate significant relaxation properties implying an injury mechanism supplement to persistent compression. In a SCI canine model, using a mechanical plunger for compression to 50% of cord diameter, Carlson et al. (51) reported a reduction in initial piston–cord interface pressures to 49% at 5 minutes postcompression and 13% at 90 minutes postcompression. Recovery of evoked potentials occurred with decompression at the 5- and 60-minute groups, but not with later groups. Delamarte et al. (46) in a canine model, and Dimar et al. (47) in a rat model, reported a significant dependence of functional recovery to time of decompression, with the greatest recovery of evoked potentials occurring in animals decompressed within 60 to 120 minutes. These studies suggest that despite intrinsic pressure gradient relaxation, residual spinal cord displacement remains a factor in the promotion of acute

SCI. Specific to the deformational forces of spinal cord compression, Blight and DeCristo (52) noted that axial compression of the spinal cord matrix resulted in an increased longitudinal cord shear stress with microvascular insult as a possible compressive injury mechanism.

Electrolytes

Numerous experiments demonstrated altered intracellular electrolyte flux after contusive acute SCI. The initial cellular disruption and consequent equilibration of intracellular contents with extracellular fluids suggest strongly that contusion of the spinal cord disrupts most cells at the injury site (53); however, the mechanisms of cellular injury appear to differ substantially between gray and white matter (54–56). Compared with gray-matter neurons, axons in the spinal cord white matter demonstrate voltage-gated sodium channels and several ion exchangers yet lack receptor-coupled and voltage-sensitive calcium channels (55–58), suggesting that the mechanisms for posttraumatic fluxes in ion gradients appear to differ in neurons and axons (59).

Sodium

Total tissue sodium concentration ($[Na]_t$) is normally 55 mM in the cat spinal cord with a measured extracellular sodium concentration ($[Na^+]_e$) of approximately 150 mM and a calculated intracellular sodium concentration ($[Na^+]_i$) of 31 mM (60–63). Cellular disruption of the axonal membrane allows equilibration of the intracellular and extracellular space, resulting in a *decrease* in $[Na^+]_e$. Some investigators hypothesize that this initial leakage of Na^+ results in the early conduction block of acute SCI (64). Rises in $[Na^+]_i$ can lead to intracellular acidosis, cytotoxic cell edema, and stimulation of intracellular phospholipase activity (54–56,65–67). In studies of cats using a weight-drop contusive model, Young and DeCriscito (62) demonstrated that postinjury $[Na^+]_e$ levels fall from normal levels of 150 mM to below 70 mM and remain below 100 mM more than 5 hours after injury. Within 1 hour postinjury, $[Na^+]_i$ had increased at the lesion site by 40% and was 100% greater than normal within 3 hours (68). Such ionic shifts are believed to result in substantial osmotic gradients at the lesion site, with resultant tissue swelling and pressures high enough to account for the observations of reduced spinal cord blood flow.

Beyond its role as a primary mediator, Fehlings and Agrawal (59) reported on potential mechanisms of sodium-induced cell injury as an element in the secondary injury cascade. Replacement of $[Na^+]_e$ with the impermeable cation, *N*-methyl-D-glutamine (NMDG+), blockade of voltage-gated Na^+ channels with procaine, or inhibition of the Na^+-H^+ exchanger with amiloride provided significant neuroprotection after traumatic axonal injury. Subsequent blockage of the Na^+-Ca^{2+} exchanger with benzamil did not produce any significant neuroprotection, suggesting that the mechanism of Na+-associated cytotoxicity does not involve reverse gating of the Na+-Ca2+ exchanger.

Potassium

Mechanical disruption of the axon results in a substantial flux of intracellar potassium ($[K^+]_i$). Total tissue potassium concentration ($[K^+]_t$) is normally 89 mM in the cat spinal cord with a measured extracellular ionic activity ($[K^+]_e$) of approximately 3 to 4 mM and a calculated intracellular potassium concentration $[K^+]_i$ of 110 (60–63,69,70). Cellular disruption of the axonal membrane allows equilibration of the intracellular and extracellular space, resulting in an *increase* in $[K^+]_e$.

Disruption of sodium and potassium extracellular gradients profoundly affects spinal cord function. Vyklicky and Sykova (71) reported that a $[K^+]_e$ greater than 10 mM can block axonal conduction. This finding suggests that the initial paralysis resulting from contusive injury is probably caused by the rise in $[K^+]_e$. In 1975, Eidelberg and associates (38) reported large increases of potassium in superfusants obtained from spinal cords subject to prolonged compression. Later, using ion-selective microelectrodes, Young and colleagues (70) showed that $[K^+]_e$ rises from a preinjury level of 4 mM to a mean of 54 mM and as high as 87 mM within seconds after contusion. The potassium ions cleared, with an exponential half-time of 31 to 38 minutes, depending on blood flow; evoked potentials, which disappeared immediately after injury, returned as the $[K^+]_e$ fell below 15 mM. In further studies, Young and associates (70) noted that after $[K^+]_e$ returned toward normal, there were no further increases in $[K^+]_e$ despite significantly decreased white matter blood flow. The absence of secondary increase in $[K^+]_e$ in the face of hypoperfusion was attributed to the magnitude of the total tissue potassium loss that occurred within the first hour of injury (63).

Calcium

Postinjury axonal calcium flux has been implicated in acute SCI as both a primary and secondary injury mediator. Normal extracellular calcium concentrations ($[Ca^{2+}]_t$) are a thousandfold greater than intracellular concentrations, and active maintenance of the membrane gradient is necessary for normal neuronal function (72). Contusive injury to the spinal cord results in profound decrease in $[Ca^{2+}]_t$ levels within minutes from levels of 1.2 mM (73) to levels of about 0.01 mM (309,358). Extracellular calcium in white matter at the lesion site recovers during the first hour but declines between 1 to 3 hours to below 0.01 mM; $[Ca^{2+}]_t$ in the surrounding cord returns close to preinjury values by 3 hours (74). This substantial fall in $[Ca^{2+}]_t$ is on an order of one magnitude or greater than that expected with the equilibration of intracellular and extracellular fluid (53). Several researchers (28,75,76) report that $[Ca^{2+}]_t$ at the injury site increases by four to eight times normal, suggesting that a large amount of calcium enters and precipitates in injured tissues.

Calcium plays an important role in modulating the neuronal cytoskeleton and enzyme function, the regulation of sodium and potassium conductance during neuronal excitation, and the storage and release of synaptic neurotransmitters (77–81). Neurons normally regulate intracellular calcium activity by binding Ca^{2+} ions with mitochondria (82–86) or cytoplasmic substance (72,86–90), or by transmembrane transport (91). Calcium entry into cells activates phospholipases and phosphatases (92), leading to the release of as much as 80% of tissue phosphates for binding calcium ions (53). Young (93) and Altman and Dittmer (94) noted that phosphates are present at extraordinarily high levels in the mammalian (especially the human) spinal cord and may play an important protective role in the postinjury precipitation of calcium ions. Conversely, it is believed that these precipitant reactions and other calcium-based actions lead to further progression of secondary injury.

Metabolites

In the acute phase of experimental SCI, marked metabolic alterations have been noted, including changes in glucose use, decreased tissue pO_2 levels and a depletion of high-energy phosphates. Rawe and associates (95) described an initial increase in both gray and white matter glucose use after acute injury for up to 1 hour in the canine model. Subsequently, gray matter glucose use decreased and remained below baseline for 3 to 8 hours, whereas white matter glucose use returned to baseline or with more severe injury decreased below baseline over the same observation period. The transient increase in glucose use is hypothesized to be secondary to the continued delivery of glucose substrate in the face of ischemia and an enhancement of anaerobic glycolysis (16,95).

Several investigators reported a rapid decline in gray and white matter tissue oxygen tension beginning as early as 15 minutes after trauma and lasting for several hours, suggesting that tissue hypoxia is a major factor in SCI (96–101). Concurrently, other studies have shown that a depletion of high-energy phosphates (ATP and phosphocreatinine) occurs after injury (102,103) and is associated with a lactic acid buildup and oxidative shifts in the NAD+-NADH of injured spinal cord tissues (102–106). A decrease in energy stores is believed to affect critical membrane enzyme function necessary for the maintenance of ionic gradients. Clendenon and associates (107) reported a marked reduction in the specific activity of the membrane-bound Na+-K+ ATPase pump within 5 minutes of acute injury, which is necessary for the maintenance of membrane ionic gradients.

Injury Site Morphology

The contusive impact of SCI results in initial microscopic tissue injury. As first described by Allen (17) in

1911, within 15 minutes of acute injury, petechial hemorrhages occurred in the gray matter and edema in the white matter. Hemorrhage increased during the first 2 hours, and by 4 hours there occurred "numerous swollen axis cylinders," that is, axonal edema. Using electron microscopy, Dohrmann and colleagues (108) noted ruptures in the walls of the muscular venules of the gray matter as early as 5 minutes after injury; at 15 and 30 minutes postinjury, perivascular extravasation of erythrocytes and axonal edema occurred. By 4 hours, there were visible disruption of myelin sheaths, some axonal degeneration, and ischemic endothelial injury. Other investigators (25,30,109) report that by 4 hours after injury the hemorrhagic changes had coalesced at the injury site into an area of hemorrhagic necrosis that extended in a fusiform shape along the longitudinal axis of the cord. The acute damage appears initially central in the gray matter. White matter changes begin in areas adjacent to hemorrhagic gray matter and spread radially to involve more peripheral regions (30,31,110,111). In electron microscopic studies of axons, Balentine (26) noted granular dissolution of the axoplasm and vesicular disruption of the white matter myelin. Bresnahan (111,112) observed axonal and periaxonal enlargments containing numerous cytoplasmic organelles, which he attributed to axoplasmic stasis. Frank demyelination of the dorsal column was observed within 24 hours, as well as diffuse tissue edema and necrosis of the initial central zone of hemorrhage (113,114). By the end of 1 week, cystic degeneration and cavitation were evident at the injury site and in adjacent areas (30).

Secondary Mediators of Spinal Cord Injury

A large body of experimental data has been collected suggesting the involvement of secondary injury mechanisms in the progression of SCI. Notable are the phenomenon of transient return of evoked potentials, which later permanently abolish hours to days after injury (68,115,116), the delay of substantial decreases in white matter blood flow until 1 to 4 hours after severe SCI (96,97,117–119), and, most compelling, the reported beneficial effects of various agents in minimizing acute SCI, suggesting blockade of a secondary injury pathway (119–126). Numerous secondary mechanisms have been implicated in the progression of primary SCI, including ischemia (8,32,119,127–131), calcium influx (29,75,76,132–135), edema (28,136,137), free-radical generation (138–142), release of vasoactive or neurotoxic substances (25,143–149), inflammation and immunogenic response (86,147,150–155), and finally, concepts of programmed cell death, *apoptosis* (156–158). However, the role of secondary tissue damage needs to be critically assessed in that many phenomena attributed to secondary tissue damage may be manifestations, rather than causes, of tissue death (53). Verification of a causal relationship is most strongly supported by experiments that demonstrate

that elimination of a specific mechanism also produces a notable functional recovery.

Posttraumatic Ischemia

A substantial body of evidence implicates posttraumatic changes in spinal cord blood flow (SCBF) as a principal element of the secondary SCI cascade (8,41). Subsequent to acute injury, both systemic and local changes appear to contribute to a progressive altered cellular environment and consequent SCI.

Neurogenic shock, defined as inadequate tissue perfusion caused by serious paralysis of vasomotor input and characterized by bradycardia and hypotension with decreased peripheral resistance and depressed cardiac output, can occur in acute SCI (12,159,160). Left uncorrected, these systemic perturbations can lead to global systemic ischemia as well as local exacerbation of neural tissue damage. Implicated mechanisms include uncompensated decreased sympathetic tone, depressed myocardial function from increased vagal tone, and consequent decreased cardiac output and peak organ perfusion pressure (159,160).

Compounding a global systemic dysfunction is the loss of protective regional autoregulation in acute SCI neural tissues. Autoregulation of blood flow in the normal spinal cord occurs within the same range as the brain (~50 to ~130 mm Hg) (161–163). Several investigators showed impairment of spinal cord autoregulation after experimental SCI (130,164–166). Experimentally, it appears that autoregulation is intact during the initial 60 to 90 minutes after SCI but is lost coincident with the onset of ischemia (167). Furthermore, several studies noted that restoration of normotension or induced hypertension does not necessarily reverse the injury ischemia, but instead caused marked hyperemia at adjacent sites (167–170).

At the local injury site, relative differences in spinal cord tissue vascularity affect injury response. In the normal condition, gray matter to white matter blood flow is maintained at a 3:1 ratio (26,171). Initial white matter injury response is variably one of brief decreased perfusion with early return to a normal or hyperemic state before onset of necrotic lesioning (150,167,172,173). Kobrine (64) reported that posttraumatic white matter SCBF doubled within 4 hours after injury, returned to normal after 8 hours, and remained in the normal range for 24 hours. In contradistinction, central gray matter hemorrhages occur as early as 5 minutes postinjury with marked decreased SCBF, if not vascular standstill, within 1 hour after injury and persisting up to 24 hours postinjury (8,167,128,131,162,168,174,175).

Futher evidence suggestive of a role of ischemia in the progression of SCI includes reports of lactate increases in lesioned area (104); reports of a significant decrease in tissue oxygen content after trauma (96–99,176); reports of spinal cord ischemia models producing changes comparable with those produced by spinal trauma (177); and, most compelling, reports of posttraumatic hypoperfusion demonstrating a linear relationship among white matter SCBF, severity of injury, and neurophysiologic function (89), including evoked motor and sensory potentials. In an animal model study using dextran to counteract systemic hypotension and nimodipine, a calcium channel blocker known for its selective vasodilation of cerebral vasculature, Fehlings and colleagues (168) reported significant elevation of posttraumatic SCBF and improved axonal function as measured by evoked potentials. Improvement in axonal function was highly correlated with the improvement in blood flow, suggesting that reversal of ischemia minimizes its role as a secondary injury mechanism. The causes of posttraumatic ischemia are unknown. Osterholm (149,178) initially reported increased norepinephrine at the lesion site and its possible role in promoting posttraumatic ischemia; however, similar results could not be reproduced by others (179). Tator and Koyanagi studied the spinal cord arterial microstructure, noting that the centrifugal sulcal arterial system supplies the anterior half of the posterior gray matter and posterior white columns, and the inner half of the anterior and lateral white columns (180–182). Modeling studies of mechanical stress in the traumatized spinal cord have demonstrated that anteroposterior compressive forces produce longitudinal stress most significant in the cord centrum (52). As such, large surface vessels of the cord adjacent to the pia matter are less subject to damaging shear stress than smaller vessels of the intermedullary plane. In comparing microangiography of injured versus uninjured human spinal cord tissue, Koyanagi and Tator (180–182) noted no occulusion of the major spinal vessels. Principal damage appeared to occur at the anterior sulcal artery within a short distance from its origin at the anterior spinal artery, resulting in a large region of gray matter hypoperfusion. Further experimental evidence suggests that venous congestion plays a secondary injury role, predominantly in the posterior columns (181,183–186). Additional proposed ischemic mechanisms include endothelial swelling and edema (29,108,176,187–190), thrombosis or platelet aggregation (191), thromboxane A activation (92,151), or the action of excitatory amino acids (120,192–197). Arguably, posttraumatic decreases in SCBF may be simply manifestations of injury as opposed to being the cause of tissue damage (28). Young (198) postulated that posttraumatic ischemia indeed may have a protective effect by limiting the diffusion of calcium ions into the intracellular space, and thus minimizing further metabolic derangement. Arguing against this are the findings of Fehlings and associates (168,199) demonstrating that treatment of ischemia restores cord function.

Calcium Disequilibrium and Excitatory Amino Acids

As discussed in the primary mechanisms section, acute SCI results in a significant intracellular Ca^{2+} influx with precipitation and prolonged suppression of extracellular Ca^{2+} levels. Calcium itself plays a critical intracellular role in the regulation of normal neuronal function. Conversely, calcium disequilibrium plays a significant role in the pro-

pogation of secondary SCI mechanisms (196). Uncontrolled Ca^{2+} influx alters intracellular transport (69) and membrane ionic permeability (200–202). In addition, Ca^{2+} binds to mitochondria (72,82,83,87–90,203,204), resulting in an uncoupling of oxidative phosphorylation (205,206), depletion of energy stores (207,208), and a release of hydrogen ions (84,85). Influx of calcium ions is believed to promote the activation of phospholipase A_2, lipoxygenase, and cyclooxygenase, as well as other calcium-dependent proteases (calpains), with resultant liberation of membrane phospholipid arachidonic acid, generation of free radicals, peroxidation of membrane lipids, and degradation of structural central nervous system proteins, including the axon-myelin unit (16,132,196,209–213).

Calcium mediated activation of phospholipases and liberation of arachoidonic acid is associated with inhibition of Na^+-K^+ ATPase and tissue edema (214), upregulation of cyclooxygenase-1 (COX-1) expression (215), and reduction of blood flow by causing platelet aggregation and vasoconstriction (12). Cyclooxygenase-2 (COX-2) expression has been induced after experimental SCI and may represent a common substrate linking membrane damage and Ca^{2+}-mediated neuronal damage (216). Selective inhibition of COX-2 appears to improve outcome of SCI in experimental animal models (216,217).

Beyond its apparent direct role as a mediator of cellular injury or death, uncontrolled calcium infusion at initial SCI appears to trigger adjunct pathways sustaining intracellular calcium excess (196). Recent research has implicated the excitatory amino acid, glutamate, as an important component in the promotion of postinjury calcium influx (120, 218–222). In brief, glutamate appears to stimulate neurons and glia via a series of receptors, subdivided as ionotropic and metabothropic. Start Glutamate ionotropic receptors are further subdivided as N-methyl-D-aspartate (NMDA) and non–NMDA kainate (KA) receptors. Activation of ionotropic receptors results in the opening of their ionic channels typified by their respective cation permeabilities (e.g., Na^+, K^+, Ca^{2+}) (192). Current views are that uncontrolled NMDA receptor activation appears most associated with the rapid gray matter neurodegeneration similar to that seen in focal ischemic injuries (223,224). Conversely, KA receptor-mediated injury has been associated with a more delayed form of gray matter neurodegeneration such as that seen with global cerebral ischemia (196,225,226). Glutamate receptor expression in axonal white tracts appears more variable, with both NMDA- and KA-glutamate receptor mechanisms reportedly active in promoting postinjury Ca^{2+} influx (192,196,227).

Postinjury breakdown of neural membrane potential and subsequent cellular energy failure results in a reversal of energy-dependent ionic pumps. Consequent membrane depolarization appears to cause the opening of voltage-gated Ca^{2+} channels allowing for further calcium influx (228). Unregulated depolarization also acts to dislodge positively charged magnesium cations from NMDA channel pores, where they normally act to prevent ion fluxes (229). Depolarization increases synaptic terminal release of glutamate that, coupled with a decline in energy-dependent glutamate reuptake, results in an accelerated calcium influx promoting further neural membrane destabilization and injury extension, hence the term *excitotoxicity* (39). The mechanism of this neurotoxicity appears to involve an early intracellular accumulation of sodium cytotoxic-producing edema and delayed destruction of neurons associated with an elevated concentration of intracellular calcium and activation of calcium-dependent cyteine proteases, the calpains (8,227, 230). Because of their apparent high Ca^{2+} permeability as compared with other receptors, glutamate-evoked Ca^{2+} influx through NMDA receptor channels appears more neurotoxic than equivalent KA or voltage-gated calcium channels (224).

Current research has demonstrated a benefit from specific glutamate NMDA and KA receptor blockade; however, given the multitude of calcium influx pathways, it is apparent that blocking a single pathway of Ca^{2+} influx may not provide complete neural protections against Ca^{2+}-mediated neurotoxicity (196).

Edema

Several investigators theorized that the development of posttraumatic edema contributes to secondary injury in the spinal cord (29,53). In 1911, Allen (17), and later others (7,136,188,210,231,232), reported histologic evidence of edema in acute SCI. Using fluorescent tracers, several investigators (31,188,233) detailed the development of posttraumatic edema. Posttraumatic edema appears initially in the central gray matter of the cord and progressively spreads into the adjacent white matter (31,188,233). Histologic and ultrastructural changes characteristic of edema were most severe 2 to 3 days after injury, with some normalization by 7 days (212), although one study (234) reported continued changes in spinal cord tissue water content 3 to 5 days after injury. Nemecek and colleagues (233) described the existence of a secondary edema in distinction to the vasogenic type, the former of which appeared more gradually and had the characteristics of a plasma ultrafiltrate. The severity of injury was correlated with the longitudinal extension of the edema within the spinal cord (235).

The pathogenesis of posttraumatic edema is not yet defined, although some investigators (53,236) suggest that initial ionic shifts could generate substantial tissue swelling, possibly enough to reduce blood flow by the observed amounts. Additional processes could include capillary leakage at endothelial tight cell junctions (237) or an increase in vesicular transport across the endothelium (112,238).

Free-Radical Formation and Oxidative Stress

Oxygen-radical–induced lipid peroxidation appears active as a secondary injury mechanism in acute SCI (129,138). *Free radicals* are molecules that lack an electron in the outer orbit; this characteristic makes them highly reactive, particularly in their ability to propagate through chain reactions (239). Reactive species include: superoxide anion (O_2^-), hydroxyl (HO) and nitric oxide (NO) radicals. Lipid peroxidation involves the reaction of fatty acids in oxygen-based free-radical chain reactions. Membrane phospholipid and cholesterol components appear to be biologically most susceptible to free-radical damage. In the normal condition, cellular metabolism involving oxygen reduction produces oxygen free radicals. In postinjury states, additional sources of free radicals include the oxidation of arachidonic acid by prostaglandin-forming enzymes (240); hemorrhage products, which release ferrous ions to catalyze oxygen-based free radical and lipid peroxidation reaction (241–243); and the "respiratory burst" of invading neutrophils (244,245). Cells normally control the deleterious effects of free radicals through endogenous agents, including superoxide dismutases, catalases, ascorbic acid, alpha-tocopherol (vitamin E), glutathione peroxidase reduction of glutathione (GSH), and steroids. Cellular *oxidative stress* refers to the cellular inability to control aberrant free radical formation. The spinal cord is particularly vulnerable to oxidative stress because of a very high proportion of polyunsaturated fatty acids and comparative low content of GSH in neuronal tissues (244).

Numerous investigators have implied a role for free radicals in the progression of acute SCI. Suggestive factors include the measured increases in peroxidized polyunsaturated fatty acid and cholesterol metabolites (139,142, 246,247), the decreases in endogenous tissue antioxidants (α-tocopherol and ascorbic acid) (248,249), and the inhibition of phospholipid-dependent membrane-bound Na+-K+-ATPase (107). However, the most compelling evidence has been the efficacy of antioxidants in the treatment of experimental SCI (125,143,246,250,251).

Inflammation Cascade and Immunologic Response

The cardinal features of acute inflammatory processes have been shown in several animal models of SCI (252). Several studies (25,253) showed an early lesional platelet deposition after acute SCI. Morphologic and enzymatic studies demonstrated early infiltration of polymorphonuclear leukocytes and their role in neurophagia acutely after SCI (25,254–256). Primary activation of arachidonic acid metabolism results in an accumulation of proinflammatory mediators, including prostaglandin and the eicosanoids, thromboxane, and leukotriene (147,151,153,155). Chao and colleagues (86) demonstrated an increased accumulation of kininogen and its conversion to proinflammatory kinins in the injured spinal cord. Concordant activation of the kininogen-kinin cascade possibly acts to mediate inflammation further and sustain the activation of phospholipases and their end-product metabolites (prostaglandins and eicosanoids) (257,258).

The role of inflammation as an agent versus a product of secondary injury mechanisms remains unclear (259). Resnick et al. (216) demonstrated increased cyclooxygenase

(COX-2) mRNA and protein expression after acute SCI. Furthermore, there appears to be a biphasic leukocyte response after SCI. Initially, an infiltration by neutrophils predominates followed by a second phase involving recruitment of macrophages with phagocytosis of damaged tissues (260). Macrophages and microglia have been regarded as integral components of neural regeneration (244). Conversely, numerous studies report macrophage activation associated with tumor necrosis factor (__X-TNF)_ and nitric oxide production, neuronal death, and demyelination (229, 260,261). Recruitment of leukocytes to the site of injury is dependent on a series of adhesive proteins (chemokimes), including intercellular adhesion molecule 1 (ICAM-1), P-selectin, and cytokines interleukin-1 and −6, and TNF (152,154). In an experiment using ICAM-knockout mice subject to SCI, Farooque (152) demonstrated reduced neutrophil recruitment and enhanced motor recovery function.

The most compelling evidence of inflammation as an active mediator of the secondary injury process are the recent reports of nuclear factor-kappa B (NF-κB) activation after traumatic SCI. The NF-κB family of transcription factors is required for the activation of a variety of genes regulating the inflammatory, proliferative, and cell death responses of cells. Using electrophoretic and histologic assay techniques, Bethea and colleagues (262) have demonstrated direct evidence for the activation of NF-κB after SCI trauma.

Apoptosis

Intuitively, the entropic consequence resultant from loss of cellular energy stores, actively maintained ionic gradients, and membrane structural integrity is cellular demise and necrosis. Presumably, such terminal events are limited to the corresponding magnitude of overall cellular injury. Recent research has identified an alternative cellular death pathway, *apoptosis*, which appears to play a significant role in the process of delayed neuronal death after traumatic injury. Pathologically, apoptosis involves a compaction of the cellular body with nuclear fragmentation and formation of surface blebs as compared to the typical structural dissolution associated with necrosis. Physiologically, apoptotic function appears to be a programmed process whereby nonfunctional neurons are removed during development or regeneration.

There appear to be two main pathways of apoptosis in SCI: extrinsic or receptor-*dependent* and intrinsic or receptor-*independent* (12). Receptor-dependent apoptosis appears activated by extracellular signaling complexes, the most important being TNF. Interactively, a family of cysteine proteins, the caspases, is thought to play an important role in apopotosis (157,158,167,263). Eldadah and Faden (264) report early accumulation of TNF in experimental SCI with resultant activation of *Fas* receptors in neurons, oligodendrocyte, and microglia with subsequent activation of caspase-8 as the inducer caspase and caspase-3 and -6 as effector caspases. Consequent activation of effector caspases results

in cellular demise (12,157,158). As an adjunct mediator, nitric oxide synthase (NOS) induction reportedly results in caspase-3 activation and programmed cell death (265).

Activation of the receptor-independent pathway reportedly occurs in SCI neurons subject to high intraneuronal calcium concentrations with induction of mitochondrial damage and cytochrome *c* release (264). Cytochrome c couples with apoptosis activating factor-1 to activate the inducer caspase-9, which in turn activates effector caspases-3 and -6 with resultant cellular demise (266).

Recent clinical reports have demonstrated apoptosis activity within 3 hours of human acute SCI at the lesion epicenter, as well as within areas of wallerian degeneration in both ascending and descending white matter tracts (156, 157). Increasing evidence suggests an excitotoxic mechanism in the initiation of apoptosis, although other reports suggest that ultimately the form of cell death may depend on the concentration of glutamate to which cells are exposed, with high levels resulting in necrosis and lower levels leading to apoptosis (267). As an inducible mechanism, current efforts are being directed at inhibition of postinjury apoptotic pathways that may limit neural tissue death in the zone of SCI.

EXPERIMENTAL THERAPIES

Animal modeling of acute SCI provides a better understanding of injury mechanisms and allows opportunities for the development of interventional therapies. Simpson and associates (252) stated that "... confirmation of the animal studies in a human trial using a rigorously designed protocol has significant laboratory and clinical implications. It establishes the precedent that the therapeutic success of SCI models in animals can be duplicated in patients with a similar disorder." Interpretation of therapeutic treatments in animal models requires critical evaluation of the methodology, however, including the animal species used, injury method, severity of injury, anesthetic, drug regimen, and methods used to measure functional outcome. Measures of physical outcome in animals must have some practical application to the human condition. Unfortunately, many studies lack morphologic correlation of the anatomic and physiologic basis for recovery and therefore limit our understanding of the anatomy required for the preservation of locomotive capacity. Likewise, clinical studies need standardized outcome measurements to allow rational comparisons among treatment regimens. Only recently have major organizations in the field taken steps toward application of a standard injury scoring (Fig. 1) (268).

Steroids

Numerous animal studies document the beneficial effect of steroids in treating experimental SCI (32,123,242,269–271). The presumed mechanism of action is multifactorial, including reversal of intracellular potassium loss and intracellular calcium accumulation (136,271); reversal of

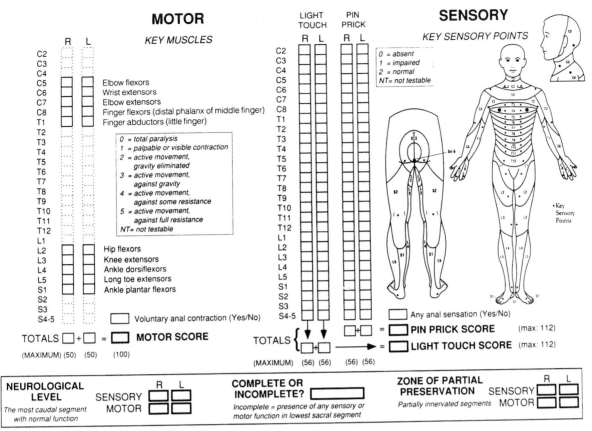

FIG. 52.1. The 1992 Standard Neurological Classification of Spinal Cord Injury. Copies of the standard can be obtained by contacting: American Spinal Injury Association, c/o Lesley M. Hudson, MA, 2020 Peachtree Road, NW, Atlanta, GA 30309. (From: American Spinal Injury Association. *Standards for neurological classification of spinal cord injury, revised 1992.* Chicago: American Spinal Injury Association, 1992, with permission.)

SCI hypoperfusion (271–273); enhancement of postinjury Na^+-K^+-ATPase activity (240) inhibition of vasoactive prostaglandin E_2 and thromboxane A_2 formation (274,275) and most importantly, an inhibition of lipid peroxidation resultant from postinjury free-radical formation (124,240). Despite variability of study methods, a significant body of evidence was collected to warrant a series of large clinical trials based on the results of experimental steroid treatments.

Methylprednisolone

Consequent to experimental modeling, methylprednisolone (MP) has become the clinical corticosteroid of choice in the treatment of SCI (276). In comparison with dexamethasone and hydrocortisone, MP appears to possess superior antioxidant properties, passes through cell membranes more rapidly, and appears more effective in inhibiting activated complement components (276–278).

To date, three large clinical trials termed the National Acute SCI Study (NASCIS) have been completed using MP and other agents in treating acute SCI. In 1984, the initial NASCIS 1 clinical trial enrolled 330 patients and compared the efficacy of high-dose (1,000-mg IV bolus followed by 250 mg every 6 hours for 10 days) versus low-dose (100-mg IV bolus then 25 mg every 6 hours for 10 days) MP protocols (277). At 6 month follow-up, there were no significant differences in neurologic outcome found between groups attributable to treatment. A higher incidence of infection was observed in the high-dose group (9.3%) versus the low-dose group (2.6%). The study did not incorporate a placebo group on the basis of ethical issues in withholding a presumed effective treatment.

In the ensuing interval until the next trial, experimental animal studies reported a biphasic dose-response curve to the beneficial antioxidant effects of MP with inhibition of lipid peroxidation at intravenous dosing of 30 mg/kg, but not at 60 mg/kg. Additionally, MP distribution in tissues was found to decrease rapidly after insult and that the beneficial antioxidant effects paralleled tissue distribution and elimination of MP (274). Design considerations for MP in future studies were to include bolus dosing at 30 mg/kg with early initial dosing and frequent maintenance dosing.

In 1990, the NASCIS 2 trial was implemented as a multicenter, randomized double-blinded, placebo-controlled study for acute SCI comparing MP (30 mg/kg IV bolus followed by a 5.4 mg/kg per hour continuous infusion for 23 hours) and the opioid antagonist naloxone (5.4 mg/kg bolus followed by a 4 mg/kg per hour continuous infusion for 23 hours) versus placebo infusion (279). Initial release of study results at 6-month follow-up reported improvement in the motor scores of 47 patients who had an incomplete motor lesion and had been managed *within 8 hours* after the injury with MP compared with those of similar patients managed with naloxone (37 patients) or placebo (46 patients) treatments. No significant difference was noted between treatment groups, comprising 337 patients, managed 8 hours *after the injury*. Complications after treatment with steroids included an increased, although not statistically significant prevalence of wound infection [8%, 3%; and 4% for patients given methylprednisolone, naloxone, and placebo, respectively ($p = 0.21$)] and gastrointestinal hemorrhage [5%, 2%, and 3% for patients given methylprednisolone, naloxone, and placebo, respectively ($p = 0.44$)]. Criticisms of the study include the lack of control over subsequent operative intervention in the long-term follow-up period, stratification of the patient population, use of summed motor scores, and absence of functional assessment with respect to improvement in motor score (280,281). Initial evaluation criteria of the NASCIS 2 trial did not allow for investigators to determine if MP improved neurologic function via recovery of segmental function at the level of injury or via recovery of function below the level of injury because of recovery of long spinal tract function (276). In *post hoc* analysis by the primary investigators, separate analysis of the lumbosacral segments revealed significantly improved motor scores for patients who had received methylprednisolone within 8 hours compared with those who had received a placebo (282). These results suggest that the beneficial effects of MP were not limited to segments close to the injury lesion. At 1 year after injury, the probability of improved motor function was reportedly greater in patients managed with MP than in patients who had received placebo (283).

In 1997, the NASCIS 3 trial was performed as a double-blinded, randomized, non–placebo-controlled study with the objective of determining whether extending the NASCIS 2 MP protocol to 48 hours would be beneficial (284,285). Additional objectives included a subgroup analysis of early (<3 hours from time of injury) versus late (3 to 8 hours after injury) administration of MP within the first 8 hours after injury, as well as inclusion of a tirilazad mesylate (TM) trial arm, a potent nonglucocorticoid inhibitor of lipid peroxidation. Revision of recovery criteria include addition of Functional Independence Measure (FIM) to determine improvements in everyday function including self-care, sphincter control, mobility, locomotion, communication, and social cognition. At 1 year follow-up, there was no significant difference in motor function between the two MP groups (285). Most benefit from the 48-hour regime occurred in patients whose initial MP administration was delayed from 3 to 8 hours after injury. Greater gains were seen in FIM scores in patients whose treatment could not be started until after 3 hours of injury, but none of the comparisons reached

nominal levels of statistical significance at last follow-up (285). Overall mortality rates were comparable between groups; however, there was a 2× higher incidence of severe pneumonia and a 4× higher incidence of severe sepsis in the 48-hour group compared with the 24-hour group (281, 284,285). The investigators concluded that the NASCIS 3 findings supported the continued clinical use of MP in acute SCI.

The current recommendations for MP use in acute SCI are: (a) the 24-hour regimen for treatment at less than 3 hours from time of injury; (b) the 48-hour regimen for treatment at 3 to 8 hours after time of injury; and (c) no MP treatment at greater than 8 hours after time of injury. The use of MP in acute *penetrating* SCI is not indicated (285). Although recommended, there remains notable controversy and variable consensus regarding the statistical significance of MP treatment results and safety concerns (281,286).

21-Aminosteroids (Lazaroids)

The 21-aminosteroid compounds are a group of nonglucocorticoid MP analogs without the 11-β-hydroxyl function that is known to be essential for glucocorticoid-receptor binding (287). These drugs appear to lack the drawbacks of the glucocorticoid-modulated systemic effects associated with the 11-β-hydroxyl moiety (288). Their mechanism of action appears to be the scavenging of lipid peroxyl radicals, facilitation of endogenous vitamin E prevention of lipid peroxidation, and apparent membrane stabilization resulting from a decrease in membrane fluidity (274,288). The principal agent developed for clinical trials is TM. Numerous animal models of experimental SCI showed a substantial neuroprotective effect with TM, with a greater antioxidant efficacy than achieved with high-dose methylprednisolone (287–290). Its inclusion in the NASCIS 3 protocol was to define the role of lipid peroxidation in the secondary injury cascade associated with acute SCI (291) and conversely, the role of inflammation as both a cellular and humoral mediator in the secondary injury cascade, given the lack of glucocorticoid effects with TM (252).

Results of the TM treatment arm in NASCIS 3 were equivocal. Forty-eight hour treatment with TM appeared as efficacious as 24-hour treatment with MP, but not as effective as 48-hour treatment with MP. TM treatment did not result in any higher complications than other treatment groups. Because no placebo arm was included in the study, the presumption of treatment effectiveness is relative to the conclusions of the NASCIS 2 study regarding MP effectiveness in acute SCI (276). At current status, the clinical use of TM is deferred in the treatment of acute SCI pending further study with alternative dosing regimes.

GM-1 Ganglioside

Gangliosides are complex acidic glycolipids present in high concentration in cells of the central nervous system;

they form a major component of the cell membrane, predominantly in the outer leaflet of the cell membrane's lipid bilayer (292–294). In a small, prospective, randomized, placebo-controlled clinical trial, the administration GM-1 ganglioside (Sygen) was shown to markedly enhance neurologic motor function at 1 year of follow-up (294). Thirty-four patients were given either 100 mg of GM-1 intravenously or a placebo each day for 18 to 32 doses, with the first dose taken within 72 hours after the injury. All patients also received a 250-mg MP bolus followed by intravenous administration of 125 mg of MP every 6 hours for up to 72 hours. Patient improvement was attributed to the return of useful motor strength in initially paralyzed muscles rather than to the strengthening of paretic muscles. This finding correlates with experimental injury studies in which an increase in axonal survival, from less than 3% to more than 6% at the site of injury allowed neurologic function to return caudal to the injury (i.e., paralyzed muscles regained motor function) (295,296). It has been postulated that the mechanism of GM-1 ganglioside is facilitation of neurite growth, attenuation of retrograde neural degeneration, modulation of glutamate-mediated endotoxicity and protein-kinase activity, or a combination of these actions (293,294,297).

In 2001, results of a large clinical trial, the Sygen Multicenter SCI Study were released (298). Seven hundred and sixty patients with nonpenetrating acute SCI completed the randomized, double-blind, sequential, placebo-controlled trial receiving one of three interventions: (a) placebo; (b) low-dose GM-1 (300 mg IV loading dose followed by 100 mg/d × 56 days); or (c) high-dose GM-1 (600 mg IV loading dose followed by 200 mg/d × 56 days). All patients received the NASCIS 2 protocol dosage of MP. At final evaluation, utilizing the initial study criteria, the neurologic outcomes at 26 weeks between GM-1 and placebo were similar, despite a more rapid time course of neurologic recovery in the Sygen group ($p = 0.01$) (298,299). There were no significant differences in mortality between the placebo and Sygen groups. *Post hoc* analysis showed mild neuroprotective effects favoring Sygen respective to: (a) an improvement in sensory (but not motor) scores at 26 and 52 weeks; (b) significantly enhanced neurologic function at 8 weeks; and (c) some improvement in bladder function ($p = 0.06$) (298). The described effects were most evident in the motor-incomplete patients. The less than promising outcome of the recent clinical trial comparted to the early clinical trial could possibly result from patient variability in the initial clinical trail, the effects of MP–GM-1 interaction, or the scheduled delay in GM-1 administration consequent to completion of the NASCIS 2 MP regimen in the study SCI patients (299). Constantini and Young (297) have demonstrated that GM-1 induces a blockade of the lipocortin-mediated antiinflammatory effects of high-dose MP. Given the issues and outcome, current clinical use of GM-1 in acute SCI remains subject to formal evidence-based guideline review or limited to further clinical studies in selected patients with SCI.

Opiate Antagonists

Both naloxone and thyrotropin-releasing hormone are opiate receptor antagonists. The theoretic benefit of these compounds is their blockade of endogenous spinal cord opioid release with a reversal of injury-induced systemic hypotension and its coupled decrease in SCBF.

Naloxone

Despite controversial success in some animal studies (116,119,300,301) and failure in others (302,303), the inclusion of naloxone in NASCIS 2 demonstrated no apparent clinical benefit (279,283,291,304); however, experimental work with other opiate receptors suggested that κ-receptor (the receptor for dynorphin A) antagonists may be protective after an acute SCI (305–308). Other researchers reported additional naloxone effects at alternative cellular sites, including a reversal of posttraumatic calcium and ascorbic acid derangements (100,248), inhibition of proteolysis (309), and neutrophil superoxide release (310,311), and stabilization of lysosomal membranes (309). Ildan and associates (312) demonstrated a posttraumatic attenuation by naloxone of Na^+-K^+/Mg^{2+}-ATPase activity, lipid peroxidation, and early ultrastructural changes caused by experimental SCI.

Thyrotropin-Releasing Hormone

Thyrotropin-releasing hormone (TRH) is a pituitary tripeptide that has many physiologic effects, including the ability to act *in vivo* as a partial physiologic opiate antagonist. Pharmacologically, TRH differs from naloxone in that it does not act as an opiate receptor and reverses opioid autonomic and behavioral effects while maintaining opioid analgesic effects (300,313). The major limitation of this peptide is its short half-life. In animal models, TRH and associated analogs improved neurologic recovery from experimental SCI, suggesting that it has therapeutic potential (314,315). In a small clinical trial, Pitts et al. (316) demonstrated that intravenous TRH (0.2 mg/kg IV bolus followed by 0.2 mg/kg/h × 6 hours; administered within 1 hour of injury) resulted in significant sensory and motor function improvement at 4 months after injury. Other investigators (16) reported TRH to be of no benefit in experimental SCI. Similar to naloxone, TRH has demonstrated nonopioid neurologic effects, including a potentiation of spinal reflexes and trophic effects on cholinergic spinal neurons (317,318). Such findings suggest a possible role for TRH in the recovery phase, versus the acute phase, of SCI (16).

Excitatory Amino Acid Antagonists

Under certain pathologic conditions (e.g., cerebral ischemia, brain, or spinal cord trauma), the overactivation of excitatory amino acid antagonists (EAAs), most specifically, the NMDA and KA receptors, has been postulated to contribute to neuronal death through a process of excitotoxicity. Receptor overactivation is thought to initiate this damage through uncontrolled influx of Na^+, Cl^-, and Ca^{2+} ions through EAA-receptor channels with resultant toxic effects of edema, osmotic damage, and activation of calcium-dependent degradative enzymes (218–220). Wada (319) demonstrated NMDA-receptor activation promoting delayed neuronal and glial death resulting from apoptosis both 24 hours and 7 days after experimental acute SCI.

Characterization of the NMDA receptor has defined a transmitter binding site, a modulatory site that binds glycine, and an ion channel that is permeable to Na^+, K^+, and Ca^{2+} ions (220,320,321). The NMDA receptor can be blocked by competitive antagonists (AP5, AP7, CPP) at the transmitter site or by noncompetitive agonists (Mg^{2+}, phencyclidine, ketamine, memantine, MK-801) at the receptor ion channel (220,319,321,322). Presently, only the noncompetitive NMDA receptor antagonists have been shown to be protective in models of SCI and ischemia (192,194,323). Faden and colleagues (122) and others (323,324) demonstrated a significant postinjury protective effect with the noncompetitive antagonist MK-801 in experimental injury models. Wrathall and colleagues (325,326) studied the effects of NBQX, a highly selective KA-receptor antagonist, and noted reduced lesion volumes in both gray and white matter and improved distal neurologic function. Other ion-channel antagonists studied include phencyclidine and ketamine, both of which can demonstrate significant psychotomimetic side effects (16). Alternatively, the dextrarotary opioid compounds, dextrophan and dextromethorphan, inhibit NMDA receptor channel function (327,328) without the disadvantages of phencyclidine-like compounds.

Unfortunately, many EAA antagonist agents appear toxic at therapeutic doses, whereas agents of lesser toxicity appear to lack sufficient receptor affinity (276). The use of EAA antagonists remains experimental at this time.

Membrane Ion-Channel Modulation

Calcium-Channel Blockers

The benefit of calcium-channel blockers with regard to posttraumatic spinal cord ischemia is controversial. The presumed mechanism of action is through stabilization of postinjury calcium influx and enhancement of SCBF (8). Several calcium-channel blockers (nifedipine, nimodipine, and flunarizine) have decreased posttraumatic spinal cord ischemia in some models (127,329) and not in others (330–333). The role of calcium-channel blockers in acute injury is unclear given their pronounced induction of systemic hypotension in most models. In dose-response studies using intravenous nimodipine, Guha (334) defined an optimal dose of 0.05 mg/kg as producing a 40% increase in SCBF, with only a 25% reduction in mean arterial pressure.

Subsequent studies combining nimodipine and vasopressive agents resulted in improved posttraumatic SCBF (169,170) and improved axonal function (168) as measured by evoked potentials. However, difficulties in treatment include restoration of mean systemic arterial pressure to normotensive levels only, given reports of enhanced intramedullary hemorrhage in injured tissues from hypertension and hyperemia (335–337). Furthermore, postinjury increases in intracellular calcium ion have been reported to occur by alternative pathways not affected by calcium-channel blockade, including NMDA-receptor channels and calcium released from injured intracellular organelles into the axon cytosol.

Sodium-Channel Blockers

Reversal of postinjury intracellular sodium accumulation has been postulated as a therapeutic treatment in acute SCI (59,338–340). Tetrodotoxin, although excessively toxic, demonstrated significant long-term tissue sparing and reduced functional deficit in experimental SCI (340). QX-314, a potent sodium-channel blocker, demonstrated some tissue sparing but no significant improvement in postinjury neurologic function (338). Schwartz and Fehlings (339) reported significant neuroprotection with sparing of gray and white matter and improvement in behavioral recovery using the compound riluzole in acute rodent SCI. The current clinical application of such agents remains investigational.

Magnesium

Magnesium [Mg^{2+}] homeostasis has recently gained some attention in acute SCI relative to results in experimental brain injury (276). Normally, Mg^{2+} acts to block NMDA channel pores and prevent Ca^{2+} influx. Membrane depolarization acts to dislodge Mg^{2+} with resultant activation of NMDA currents and Ca^{2+} influx by EEAs (341). Experimental rat models of brain injury have shown improved neurologic outcome with Mg^{2+} pretreatment (342). Suzer (343) demonstrated significant improvement in axonal function and decrease lipid peroxidation with use of high-dose Mg^{2+} (600 mg/kg $MgSO_4$) in acute rat SCI.

Modulation of Inflammation and Apoptosis

A growing body of evidence supports modulation of the inflammatory and apoptotic cascades as a therapeutic treatment for acute SCI. Specific therapies directed at inhibition of enzymatic conversion of arachadonic acid have demonstrated some success in experimental SCI (216,217,344, 345). Resnick (216) reported an unregulation of COX-2 with experimental acute SCI and that treatment with the selective COX-2 inhibitor, SC58125, improved functional outcome after experimental SCI. Similar results were reproduced in an experimental model of reversible spinal cord ischemia with the selective COX-2 inhibitor, SC-236 (217).

Gabexate mesylate, a protease inhibitor with both antiinflammatory and anticoagulant activity, also has demonstrated some neuroprotective effect with reduction of motor disturbances and leukocyte inflammation in SCI rats (346).

The delineation of apoptotic mechanisms in acute SCI lends itself to future therapeutic treatments. Recent studies have demonstrated neuroprotective benefit with inhibition of caspase-3 with intraperitoneal zDEVD-fmk (347). The antiapoptotic protein, Bcl-2, has demonstrated similar neuroprotective properties in experimental SCI (348), further confirmed by experiments that transgenic mice overexpressing this protein are resistant to ischemic injury (349). Prospectively, inhibition of postinjury inflammation and apoptosis remain as viable treatment pathways of significant clinical interest in acute SCI.

Other Pharmacologic Agents

Vitamin E

Pretreatment with vitamin E (α-tocopherol) reduces morbidity after experimental SCI (250). The presumed mechanism of action is through an antioxidation effect and phospholipid membrane stabilization. Clinical shortcomings include the need for injury pretreatment, thus limiting the benefit of this agent in the treatment of acute injuries. Conversely, possible aggressive nutritional support with such agents following acute SCI can contribute to maximizing intrinsic antioxidant defenses (244).

Osmotic Diuretics

Despite experimental success with edema-reducing agents, including mannitol, glycerol, and low-molecular-weight dextran, there has been no compelling evidence of clinical effectiveness of these agents with regard to posttraumatic SCI (151,212). As a combined therapy, Legos et al. (350) reports that concurrent adminstration of hypertonic saline with MP may enhance their combined neuroprotective effect in experimental SCI.

Physical Approaches

Hypothermia

Cooling of posttraumatic spinal cord segments is of some benefit (212,351,352). A combined review of 11 clinical trails demonstrated that 28 (45%) of 62 patients who had a SCI with no motor or sensory sparing had neurologic improvement and 10 (16%) regained the ability to walk (353). These results can be compared with the historically poor results of conventional treatment in which only 2% to 10% of patients who had a complete injury on presentation exhibited substantial distal motor function after the period of spinal shock (354–356); however, the clinical results of cord cooling have been clouded by the concurrent use of steroids in many studies. The theoretical mechanism of action of cord cooling is a local decrease in spinal cord metabolism and oxygen consumption, with a resultant reduction of edema and the blockade of the secondary injury biochemical cascade. Mathematical modeling studies suggest that additional benefit is derived from cerebrospinal fluid convection within injured spinal levels (357).

Controversy exists with regard to the degree and duration of cooling required for benefit. Recent experimental studies demonstrated moderate temperature decreases of 1 to 3°C to be of value (352).

Cooling has serious disadvantages: the acute operative intervention in a traumatized patient, the need for a wide multilevel laminectomy and prolonged operative exposure, and the technical difficulties inherent in the currently available cooling devices (151,352,353). At this time, the clinical role of spinal cord cooling is experimental.

FUTURE DIRECTIONS

As discussed, acute, contusive spinal cord trauma results in primary tissue disruption with propagation of the injury through secondary injury–mediated mechanisms. Morphologic studies showed a remarkably consistent histological appearance of spinal cord injured tissues with progression of initial gray matter petechiae over several hours to central hemorrhagic necrosis over several days to injury site cavitation over several weeks.

Despite such overt damage, the gross histologic appearance of the spinal cord does not correlate absolutely with the degree of function or predict the functional recovery (52). Remyelination of injured axons can improve conduction in the surviving axons (358). Young and colleagues (296,358) compared total postinjury axonal count in an animal injury model with remaining neurologic function and noted surprisingly that the mean axon count was only 60,000 in animals that recovered locomotion compared with 20,000 in those that remained paralyzed. This difference of 40,000 axons is less than 10% of the normal axonal population and suggests that only relatively moderate levels of improvement in the number of functioning axons could lead to substantial improvement in physiologic function. Future directions include continued treatment efforts at minimization of the acute SCI cascade and maximization of surviving axons, including possible repair or regeneration.

Given the growing identification of acute SCI pathways and their subsequent complex interaction, future treatment protocols will be forced to address issues of combined versus sequential therapies. Clearly, no one dominant injury pathway, or for that matter, clinically significant treatment therapy, has been identified. Implementation of combined therapies may overcome single agent therapy weakness by summative effect, yet is subject to the complex, and possible inhibitory, action of combined elements (359,297). Sequential therapies would appear to more appropriately act upon the various stages of the induced acute SCI event, however, their determined order of treatment and possible competitive effects remain indeterminate at our current level of understanding in acute SCI.

REFERENCES

1. Albin MS, White RJ. Epidemiology, pathophysiology, and experimental therapeutics of acute spinal cord injury. *Crit Care Clin* 1987; 3:441–452.
2. Garfin SR, Shackford SR, Marshall LF, et al. Care of the multiply injured patient with cervical spine injury. *Clin Orthop Res Res* 1989; 239:19–29.
3. Kalsbeek WD, McLaurin RL, Harris BSH III, et al. The National Head and Spinal Cord Injury Survey: major findings. *J Neurosurg* 1980;53(Suppl):S19–31.
4. Kraus JF, Franti CE, Riggins RS, et al. Incidence of traumatic spinal cord lesions. *J Chron Dis* 1975;28:471–492.
5. Griffin MR, Opitz JL, Kurland LT, et al. Traumatic spinal cord injury in Olmstead County, Minnesota, 1935–1981. *Am J Epidemiol* 1985; 121:884–895.
6. De Vivo MJ, Kartus PL, Stover SL, et al. Benefits of early admission to an organized spinal cord injury care system. *Paraplegia* 1990;28: 545–555.
7. Whiteneck GG, Menter RR, Charlifue SW, et al. Short- and long-term costs of spinal cord injury. *Paraplegia* 1987;15:113.
8. Tator CH, Fehlings MG. Review of the secondary injury theory of acute spinal cord trauma with emphasis on vascular mechanisms. *J Neurosurg* 1991;75:15–26.
9. Stripling TE. The cost of economic consequences of traumatic spinal cord injury. *Paraplegia* 1987;25:225–228.
10. Bunegin L, Hung TH, Chang GL. Biomechanics of spinal cord injury. *Crit Care Clin* 1987;3:453–470.
11. Sonntag VKH, Douglas RA. Management of cervical spinal cord trauma. *J Neurotrauma* 1992;9(Suppl 1):S385–396.
12. Dumont RJ, Verma S, Okonkwo DO, et al. Acute spinal cord injury., Part I: Pathophysiologic mechanisms. *Clin Neuropharm* 2001;24:254–264.
13. Tator CH. Spine-spinal cord relationships in spinal canal trauma. *Clin Neurosurg* 1983;30:479–494.
14. Eismont FJ, Clifford S, Goldberg M, et al. Cervical sagittal spinal canal size in spine injury. *Spine* 1984;7:663–666.
15. Torg JS, Pavlov H, Genuario SE, et al. Neuropraxia of the cervical spinal cord with transient quadriplegia. *J Bone Joint Surg Am* 1986; 68:1354–1370.
16. Martinez-Arizala A, Green BA, Bunge RP. Experimental spinal cord injury: pathophysiology and treatment. In: Rothman RH, Simione FA, eds. *The Spine*. Philadelphia: WB Saunders, 1992:1247–1276.
17. Allen AR. Surgery of experimental lesion of spinal cord equivalent to crush injury of fracture dislocation. *JAMA* 1911;50:941–952.
18. Allen AR. Remarks on histopathological changes in spinal cord due to impact: an experimental study. *J Nerv Ment Dis* 1914;41:141–147.
19. Dohrmann GJ, Panjabi MM, Banks D. Biomechanics of experimental spinal cord trauma. *J Neurosurg* 1978;48:993–1001.
20. Rivlin AS, Tator CH. Effect of duration of acute spinal cord compression in a new acute cord injury model in the rat. *Surg Neurol* 1978;939–943.
21. Tarlov IM, Klinger H, Vitale S. Spinal cord compression studies: I. Experimental techniques to produce acute and gradual compression in dogs. *Arch Neurol Psychiat* 1953;70:813–819.
22. Tator CH. Acute spinal cord injury in primates produced by an inflatable extradural cuff. *Can J Surg* 1972;16:222–231.
23. Kahn M, Gabriel R. Acute spinal cord injury in the rat: comparison of three experimental techniques. *Can J Neurosci* 1983;10:161–165.
24. Watson BD, Prado R, Dietrich WD, et al. Photochemically induced spinal cord injury in the rat. *Brain Res* 1986;367:296–300.
25. Balentine JD. Pathology of experimental spinal cord trauma. I. The necrotic lesion as a function of vascular injury. *Lab Invest* 1978;39: 236–253.
26. Balentine JD. Pathology of experimental spinal cord trauma: II. Ultrastructure of axons and myelin. *Clin Invest* 1978;39:254–266.
27. Goodkin R, Campbell JB. Sequential pathological changes in spinal cord injury. *Surg Forum* 1969;20:430–432.
28. Young W. Blood flow, metabolic and neurophysiological mechanisms in spinal cord injury. In: Becker PB, Povlishock JT (eds.). *Central Nervous System Trama Report.* Bethesda: National Institute of Neurological and Communicative Disorder and Stroke, National Institutes of Health, 1985:463–473.
29. Balentine JD. Hypotheses in spinal cord trauma research. In: Becker DP, Povlishock JT, eds. *Central nervous system trauma status report.* Bethesda, MD: National Institute of Neurological and Communicative Disorders and Stroke, National Institutes of Health, 1985:455–461.
30. Ducker TB, Kindt GW, Kempe LG. Pathological findings in acute experimental spinal cord trauma. *J Neurosurg* 1971;35:700–708.
31. Green BA, Wagner FC Jr. Evolution of edema in the acutely injury spinal cord: a fluorescence microscopic study. *Surg Neurol* 1973;1: 98–101.
32. Ducker TB, Hamit HF. Experimental treatments of acute spinal cord injury. *J Neurosurg* 1969;30:693–697.
33. Koenig C, Dohrman GJ. Histopathological variability in "standardized" spinal cord trauma. *J Neurol Neurosurg Psychiatr* 1977;40:1203.
34. Molt JT, Nelson LR, Poulos DA, et al. Analysis and measurement of some sources of variability in spinal cord trauma. *J Neurosurg* 1979;50:784–791.
35. O'Brien MF, Lenke LG, Lou J, et al. Astrocyte response and transforming growth factor-β_ localization in acute spinal cord injury. *Spine* 1994;19:2321–2330.
36. Martin SH, Bloedel JR. Evaluation of experimental spinal cord injury using cortical evoked potentials. *J Neurosurg* 1973;39:75–81.
37. D'Angelo CM, Vangilder JC, Taub A. Evoked clinical potentials in experimental spinal cord trauma. *J Neurosurg* 1973;38:332–336.
38. Eidelberg E, Sullivan J, Bringham A. Immediate consequences of spinal cord injury: possible role of potassium in axonal conduction block. *Surg Neurol* 1975;3:317–321.
39. Olney JW. Neurotocity of excitatory amino acids. In: McGeer EG, Olney JW, McGeer PI, eds. *Kainic acid as a tool in neurobiology.* New York: Raven Press, 1978:95–121.
40. Singer JM, Russel GV, Coe JE. Changes in evoked potentials after experimental cervical spinal cord injury in the monkey. *Exp Neurol* 1970;29:449–461.
41. Tator CH. Review of experimental spinal cord injury with emphasis on local and systemic circulatory effects. *Neurochirurgie* 1991;37: 291–302.
42. Fehlings MH, Sekhon LHS, Tator CH. The role of timing and decompression in acute spinal cord injury. What do we know? What should we do? *Spine* 2001;26(Suppl):101–110.
43. Bohlman HH, Bahniuk E, Raskulinecz G, et al. Mechanical factors affecting recovery from incomplete cervical spinal cord injury: preliminary report. *John Hopkins Med J* 1979;145:115–125.
44. Brodkey JS, Richards DE, Blasingame, et al. Reversible spinal cord trauma in cats: additive effects of direct pressure and ischemia. *J Neurosurg* 1972;37:591–593.
45. Carlson GD, Minato Y, Okada A, et al. Early time-dependent decompression for spinal cord injury: vascular mechanisms of recovery. *J Neurotrauma* 1997;14:951–962.
46. Delamarter RB, Sherman J, Carr JB. Pathophysiology of spinal cord injury: recovery after immediate and delayed decompression. *J Bone Joint Surg Am* 1995;77:1042–1049.
47. Dimar JR, Glassman SD, Raque GH, et al. The influence of spnal canal narrowing and timing of decompression on neurologic recovery after spinal cord contusion in a rat model. *Spine* 1999;24:1623–1632.
48. Kobrine AI, Evans DE, Rizzoli H. Correlation of spinal cord blood flow and function in experimental compression. *Surg Neurol* 1978; 10:54–59.
49. Nystrom B, Berglund JE. Spinal cord restitution following compression injuries in rats. *Acta Neurol Scand* 1988;78:467–472.
50. Zhang Y, Hillered L. Olsson Y, et al. Time course of energy perturbation after compression trauma to the spinal cord: an experimental study in the rat using microdialysis. *Surg Neurol* 1993;39:297–304.
51. Carlson GD, Warden KE, Barbeau JM, et al. Viscoelastic relaxation and regional blodd flow response to spinal cord compression and decompression. *Spine* 1997;22:1285–1291.
52. Blight AR, DeCristo V. Morphometric analysis of experimental spinal cord injury in the cat: the relation of injury intensity to survival of myelinated axons. *Neuroscience* 1986;19:321–341.
53. Young W, Ransohoff J. Acute spinal cord injuries: experimental therapy, pathophysiologic mechanisms, and recovery of function. In:

Sherk HH, ed. *The cervical spine*, 2nd ed. Philadelphia: JB Lippincott, 1989:464–495.

54. Regan RF, Choi DW. Glutamate neurotoxicity in spinal cord culture. *Neuroscience* 1991;43:585–591.

55. Stys PK, Waxman SG, Ransom BR. Na$^+$-Ca^{2+} exchanger mediates Ca^{2+} influx during anoxia in mammalian central nervous system white matter. *Ann Neurol* 1991;30:375–380.

56. Stys PK, Waxman SG, Ransom Br. Ionic mechanisms of anoxic injury in mammalian CNS white matter: role of Na$^+$ channels and the Na$^+$-Ca^{++} exchanger. *J Neurosci* 1992;12:430–439.

57. Mullins LJ, Requena J, Whittembury J. Ca^{2+} entry in squid axons during voltage-clamp pulses is mainly Na$^+$/Ca^{2+} exchange. *Proc Natl Acad Sci USA* 1985;82:1847–1851.

58. Reithmeier RAF. Mammalian exchangers and co-transporters. *Curr Opin Cell Biol* 1994;6:583–594.

59. Fehlings MG, Agrawal S. Role of sodium in the pathophysiology of secondary spinal cord injury. *Spine* 1995;20:2187–2191.

60. Nicholson C. Measurements of extracellular ions in the brain. *Trends Neurosci* 1980;3:216–218.

61. Nicholson C, Phillips KJM. Ion diffusion modified by tortuosity and volume fraction in the extracellular microenvironment of the rat cerebellum. *J Physiol Lond* 1981;321:225–257.

62. Young W, DeCrescito V. Sodium ionic changes in injured spinal cords: mechanisms of edema. *Proc Soc Neurosci* 1986;16(A):267.

63. Young W, Koreh I. Potassium and calcium changes in injured spinal cords. *Brain Res* 1986;365:42–53.

64. Kobrine AI. The neuronal theory of experimental traumatic spinal cord dysfunction. *Surg Neurol* 1975;3:261.

65. Friedman JE, Haddad GG. Removal of extracellular sodium prevents anoxia-induced injury in freshly dissociated rat CA1 hippocampal neurons. *Brain Res* 1994;641:57–64.

66. Gusovskky F, Hollingsworth EB, Daly JW. Regulation of phosphatidylinositol turnover in brain synaptosomes: stimulatory effects of agents that enhance influx of sodium ions. *Proc Natl Acad Sci USA* 1986;83:3003–3007.

67. Haigney MCP, Lakatta EG, Stern MD, Silverman HSet al. Sodium channel blockade reduces hypoxic sodium loading and sodium-dependent calcium loading. *Circulation* 1994;90:391–399.

68. Young W, Tomasula JJ, DeCrescito V, et al. Vestibulospinal monitoring in experimental spinal trauma. *J Neurosurg* 1980;52:64–72.

69. Nicholson C. Dynamics of the brain cell microenvironment. *Neurosci Res Prog Bull* 1980;18:177–322.

70. Young W, Koreh I, Yen V, et al. Effect of sympathectomy on extracellular potassium activity and blood flow in experimental spinal cord contusion. *Brain Res* 1982;253:115–124.

71. Vyklicky L, Sykova E. The effects of increased extracellular potassium in the isolated spinal cord on the flexor reflex of the frog. *Neurosci Lett* 1975;19:203–207.

72. Baker PF. The regulation of intracellular calcium. *Symp Soc Exp Biol* 1976;30:67–88.

73. Nicholson C. Modulation of extracellular calcium and its functional implications. *Fed Proc* 1980;39:1519–1523.

74. Stokes BT, Fox P, Hallinden G. Extracellular calcium activity in the injured spinal cord. *Exp Neurol* 1983;80:561–572.

75. Hapel RD, Banik NL, Balentine JD, et al. Tissue calcium levels in CaCl$_2$-induced myelopathy. *Neurosci Lett* 1984;49:279–283.

76. Hapel RD, Smith K, Powers JM, et al. Ca^{+2} accumulation in experimental spinal cord trauma. *Brain Res* 1983;211:476–479.

77. Abood LG, Hoss W. Excitation and conduction in the neuron. In: Siegel GJ, Albers RW, Katzman R, et al, eds. *Basic Neurochemistry*. Boston: Little, Brown, 1976:103–124.

78. Forscher P. Calcium and phosphoinositide control of cytoskeletal dynamics. *Trends Neurol Sci* 1989;12:468–474.

79. Huang KP. The mechanism of protein kinase C activation. *Trends Neurol Sci* 1989;12:425–432.

80. Kennedy MB. Regulation of neuronal function by calcium. *Trends Neurosci* 1989;12:417–420.

81. Malenka RC, Kauer JA, Perkel DJ, et al. The impact of post-synaptic calcium on synaptic transmission—its role in long-term potentiation. *Trends Neurol Sci* 1989;12:444–450.

82. Brinley FJ. Calcium buffering in squid axons. *Ann Rev Biophys Bioeng* 1978;7:363–392.

83. Brinley FJ, Tiffert T, Scarpa A. Mitochondria and other calcium buffers of squid axon studied in situ. *J Gen Physiol* 1978;72:101–127.

84. Carafoli E, Lehninger AL. A survey of the interaction of calcium ions with mitochondria from different tissues and species. *Biochem J* 1971;122:681–690.

85. Carafoli E, Crompton M. The regulation of intracellular calcium by mitochondria. *Ann NY Acad Sci* 1978;307:269–284.

86. Chao J, Xu J, Hsu CY. Kinonogen and kinins in experimental spinal cord injury. *FASEB J* 1988;2:145.

87. Baker PF. Transport and metabolism of calcium ions in nerve. *Prog Biophys Mol Biol* 1972;24:177–223.

88. Baker PF. The regulation of intracellular calcium in giant axons of Loligo and Myxicola. *Ann NY Acad Sci* 1978;207:250–268.

89. Baker PF, Hodgkin AL, Ridgeway EB. Depolarization and calcium entry into squid giant axons. *J Physiol (Lond)* 1971;218:709–755.

90. Baker PF, Umbach JA. Calcium buffering in axons and axoplasm of Loligo. *J Physiol Lond* 1987;383:369–394.

91. Hodgkins AL, Keynes RD. Active transport of cations in giant axons from Sepia and Loligo. *J Physiol Lond* 1957;128:28–60.

92. Feder J. The phosphatases. In: Griffith EJ, Beeton A, Spencer JM, et al, eds. *Environment phosphorus handbook*. New York: Wiley, 1972:475–508.

93. Young W. Cellular defenses against excessive calcium entry in trauma and ischemia. In: Cerra FB, Shoemaker WC, eds. *Critical care: state of the art*. Fullerton, CA: The Society of Critical Care Medicine 1987:71–98.

94. Altman PL, Dittmer DS. *Biology data book*, 2nd ed. Washington, DC: Federation of American Society for Experimental Biology, 1973:1206–1229.

95. Rawe SE, Lee WA, Perot PL. Spinal cord glucose utilizationuse after experimental spinal cord injury. *Neurosur* 1981;9:40–47.

96. Hayashi N, de la Torre JC, Green BA. Regional spinal cord blood flow and tissue oxygen content after spinal cord trauma. *Surg Forum* 1980;31:461–463.

97. Hayashi N, de la Torre JC, Green Ba, et al. Rat spinal cord laminar blood flows of gray and white matter using multiple micro-electrode hydrogen clearance. *Neurology* 1980;30:406.

98. Kelly DL, Lassiter RRL, Calogero JA, et al. Effects of local hypothermia and tissue oxygen studies in experimental paraplegia. *J Neurosurg* 1970;33:554–563.

99. Kelly DL, Lassiter RRL, Vongsvivut A, et al. Effects of hyperbaric oxygenation and tissue oxygen studies in experimental paraplegia. *J Neurosurg* 1972;36:425–429.

100. Stokes BT, Fox P, Hollinden G. Extracellular metabolites: their measurement and role in the acute phase of spinal cord injury. In: Dacey RG Jr, Winn HR, Rimmel RW, et al, eds. *Trauma of the central nervous system*. New York: Raven Press, 1985:309–323.

101. Stokes BT, Garwood M. Traumatically induced alterations in the oxygen fields in the canine spinal cord. *Exp Neurol* 1982;75:665–677.

102. Anderson DK, Means ED, Waters TR, et al. Spinal cord energy metabolism following compression trauma to the feline spinal cord. *J Neurosurg* 1980;53:375–380.

103. Kahn T, Green B, Raimondi AJ. Energy metabolism of acutely injured spinal cord of cat. *J Neuropathol Exp Neurol* 1975;34:84–85.

104. Locke GE, Yashon D, Feldman RA. Ischemia in primate spinal cord injury. *J Neurosurg* 1971;84:614–617.

105. Rosental M, Lamanna J, Yamada S, et al. Oxidative metabolism, extracellular potassium, and sustained potential shift in cat spinal cord in situ. *Brain Res* 1979;162:113–127.

106. Yammada S, Sanders D, Maeda G. Oxidative metabolism during the following spinal cord ischemia. *Neurol Res* 1981;3:1–16.

107. Clendenon NR, Allen N, Gordon WA, et al. Inhibition of Na$^+$-K$^+$-activated ATPase activity following experimental spinal cord trauma. *J Neurosurg* 1978;49:563–568.

108. Dohrmann GJ, Wagner FC Jr, Bucy PC. The microvasculature in transitory traumatic paraplegia. An electron microscopic study in the monkey. *J Neurosurg* 1971;35:263–271.

109. McVeigh JF. Experimental cord crushes with special references to the mechanical factors involved and subsequent changes in the areas affected. *Arch Surg* 1923;7:573–600.

110. Bresnahan JO. An electron-microscopic analysis of axonal alterations following blunt contusion of the spinal cord of the rhesus monkey (*Macaca mulatta*). *J Neurol Sci* 1978;37:59–82.

111. Bresnahan JC, King JS, Martin GF, et al. A neuroanatomical analysis of spinal cord injury in the rhesus monkey. *J Neurol Sci* 1976;28:521–542.

112. Beggs JL, Waggener JD. Transendothelial vesicular transport of protein following compression injury to the spinal cord. *Lab Invest* 1976;34:428–439.

113. Gledhill RF, Harrison BM, McDonald WI. Demyelination and remyelination after acute spinal cord compression. *Exp Neurol* 1973; 38:472–487.

114. Tator CH, Rowed DW. Current concepts in the immediate management of acute spinal cord injuries. *Can Med Assoc* 1979;121:1453–1464.

115. Ducker TB, Saleman M, Lucas JT, et al. Experimental spinal cord trauma, II: Blood flow, tissue oxygen, evoked potentials in both paretic and plegic monkeys. *Surg Neurol* 1987b;10:64–70.

116. Flamm ES, Young W, Demophoulus HB, et al. Experimental spinal cord injury: treatment with naloxone. *Neurosurgery* 1982;10:227–231.

117. Hall ED, Wolf DL. Post-traumatic spinal cord ischemia: relationship to injury severity and physiological parameters. *CNS Trauma* 1987; 4:15–25.

118. Lohse DC, Senter HJ, Kauer JS, et al. Spinal cord blood flow in experimental transient paraplegia. *J Neurosurg* 1980;52:335–345.

119. Young W, Flamm ES, Demopoulos HB, et al. Effect of naloxone on posttraumatic ischemia in experimental spinal contusion. *J Neurosurg*. 1981;55:209–219.

120. Choi DW. Glutamate neurotoxicity in cortical cell culture is calcium dependent. *Neurosci Lett* 1985;58:2931–2937.

121. Faden AI, Jacobs PT, Holaday JW. Opiate antagonist improves neurologic recovery after spinal injury. *Science* 1981;211:493–494.

122. Faden AI, Lemke M, Simon RP, et al. *N*-methyl-*D*-aspartate antagonist MK801 improves outcome following traumatic spinal cord injury in rats: behavioral, anatomic, and neurochemical studies. *J Neurotrauma* 1988;5:33–45.

123. Green Ba, Kahn T, Klose KI. A comparative study of steroid therapy in acute experimental spinal injury. *Surg Neurol* 1980;13:91–97.

124. Hall ED, Braughler JM. Acute effects of intravenous glucocorticoid pre-treatment on the in vitro peroxidation of spinal cord tissue. *Expl Neurol* 1981;72:321–324.

125. Hall ED, Braughler JM. Glucocorticoid mechanisms in acute spinal injury: a review and therapeutic rationale. *Surg Neurol* 1982;18: 320–331.

126. Means Ed, Anderson DK, Waters TR, et al. Effect of methylprednisolone in compression trauma to the feline spinal cord. *J Neurosurg* 1981;55:200–208.

127. De Ley G, Leybaert L. Effect of flunarizine and methylprednisolone on functional recovery after experimental spinal cord injury. *J Neurotrauma* 1993;10:25–35.

128. Griffiths IR. Spinal cord blood flow after acute experimental cord injury in dogs. *J Neurol Sci* 1976;27:247–259.

129. Hall ED, Braughler JM, McCall JM. New pharmacological treatment of acute spinal cord trauma. *J Neurotrauma* 1988;5:81–89.

130. Kobrine AI, Doyle TF, Rizzoli HV. Spinal cord blood flow as affected by changes in systemic arterial blood pressure. *J Neurosurg* 1976;44: 12–15.

131. Senter HJ, Venes JL. Altered blood flow and secondary injury in experimental spinal cord trauma. *J Neurosurg* 1978;49:569–578.

132. Balentine JD, Green W. Ultrastructural pathology of axons and myelin in calcium induced myelopathy. *J Neuropathol Exp Neurol* 1984;43:500–510.

133. Balentine JD, Spector M. Calcification of axons in experimental spinal cord trauma. *Ann Neurol* 1977;2:520–523.

134. Young W. The role of calcium in spinal cord injury. *CNS Trauma* 1985;2:109–114.

135. Young W, Yen V, Blight A. Extracellular calcium ionic activity in experimental spinal cord contusion. *Brain Res* 1982;253:105–113.

136. Lewin MG, Hansebout RR, Pappius HM. Chemical characteristics of traumatic spinal cord edema in cats: effects of steroids on potassium depletion. *J Neurosurg* 1974;40:65–75.

137. Young W. Correlation of somatosensory evoked potentials and neurological findings in clinical spinal cord injury. In: Tator CH, ed. *Early management of cervical spinal injury*. New York: Raven Press, 1981: 153–166.

138. Demopoulos HB, Flamm ES, Pietronigro DD, et al. The free radical pathology and the microcirculation in the major central nervous system disorders. *Acta Physiol Scand* 1980;492(Suppl):91–119.

139. Demopolulus HB, Flamm ES, Seligman MC, et al. Further studies on free radical pathology in the major central nervous system disorders: effects of very high doses of methylprenisolone on the functional

140. Flamm ES, Demopoulos HB, Seligman ML, et al. Ethanol potentiation of central nervous system trauma. *J Neurosurg* 1977;46:328.

141. Flamm ES, Demopoulus HB, Seligman ML, et al. Free radicals in cerebral ischemia. *Stroke* 1978;9:445.

142. Milvy P, Kakari S, Campbell JB, et al. Paramagnetic species and radical products in cat spinal cord. *Ann NY Acad Sci* 1973;222: 1102–1111.

143. Anderson DK, Means ED. Iron-induced lipid peroxidation in spinal cord: protection with mannitol and methyleprednisolone. *J Free Radiol Biol Med* 1985;1:59–64.

144. Braughler JM, Hall ED. Correlation of methylprednisolone pharmacokinetics in cat spinal cord with its effect on (Na^+-K^+)-ATPase, lipid peroxidation and motor neuron function. *J Neurosurg* 1981;56: 838–844.

145. Demediuk P, Saunders RD, Anderson DK, et al. Membrane lipid changes in laminectomized and traumatized cat spinal cord. *Proc Natl Acad Sci USA* 1985;82:7071–7075.

146. Hall ED, Braughler JM. Role of lipid peroxidation in post-traumatic spinal cord degeneration—a review. *CNS Trauma* 1986;3:281–294.

147. Hsu CY, Halushka PV, Hogan EL, et al. Alteration of thromboxane and prostacyclin levels in experimental spinal cord injury. *Neurology* 1985;35:1003–1009.

148. Jonsson HT, Daniell HB. Altered levels of PCF in cat spinal cord tissue following traumatic injury. *Prostaglandins* 1976;11:51–61.

149. Osterholm JL. Noradrenergic mediation of traumatic spinal cord autodestruction. *Life Sci* 1974;14:1363.

150. Bingham WG, Goldman H, Friedman SJ, et al. Blood flow in normal and injured monkey spinal cord. *J Neurosurg* 1975;43:162–171.

151. de la Torre JC. Spinal cord injury: review of basic and applied research. *Spine* 1981;6:315–335.

152. Farooque M, Isaksson J, Olsson Y. Improved recovery after spinal cord trauma in ICAM-1 and P-selectin knockout mice. *Neuroreport* 1999;10:131–134.

153. Hsu CY, Liu TH, Hogan EL. Lipid inflammatory mediators in ischemic brain edema, and injury. In: Bazan ND, ed. *New trends in lipid mediators*, vol 4. Basel: Karger, 1990:85–112.

154. Klusman I, Schwab ME. Effects of pro-inflammatory cytokines in experimental spinal cord injury. *Brain Res* 1997;762:173–184.

155. Matteo MR, Smith RS. Neurophil-dependent tissue damage. *Agents Actions* 1988;25:61–62.

156. Emery E, Aldana P, Bunge MB, et al. Apoptosis after traumatic human spinal cord injury. *J Neurosurg* 1998;89:911–920.

157. Lou J, Lenke LG, Ludwig FJ, et al. Apoptosis as a mechanism of neuronal cell death following acute experimental spinal cord injury. *Spinal Cord* 1998;36:683–690.

158. Lu J, Ashwell KWS, Waite P. Advances in secondary spinal cord injury. Role of apoptosis. *Spine* 2000;25:1859–1866.

159. Guha A, Tator CH. Acute cardiovascular effects of experimental spinal cord injury. *J Trauma* 1988;28:481–490.

160. Kiss ZHT, Tator CH. Neurogenic shock. In: Geller ER, ed. *Shock and resuscitation*. New York: McGraw-Hill, 1993:421–440.

161. Hickey R, Allen MS, Bunegin L, et al. Autoregulation of spinal cord blood flow: is the cord a microcosm of the brain *Stroke* 1986;17: 118–119.

162. Kobrine AI, Doyle TF, Martins AN. Autoregulation of spinal cord blood flow. *Clin Neurosurg* 1975;22:573–581.

163. Marcus ML, Heistad DD, Ehrhardt J, et al. Regulation of total and regional spinal cord blood flow. *Circ Res* 1977;41:128–134.

164. Senter HJ, Venes JI. Loss of autoregulation and posttraumatic ischemia following experimental spinal cord trauma. *J Neurosurg* 1979; 50:198–206.

165. Smith AJK, McCreery DB, Bloedel JR, et al. Hyperemia, CO_2 responsiveness, and autoregulation in the white matter following experimental spinal cord injury. *J Neurosurg* 1978;48:239–251.

166. Young W, DeCrescito V, Tomasula JJ. Effect of sympathectomy on spinal blood flow autoregulation and posttraumatic ischemia. *J Neurosurg* 1982;56:706–710.

167. Sekhon LHS, Fehlings MG. Epidemiology, demographics, and pathophysiology of acute spinal cord injury. *Spine* 2001;26(Suppl):2–12.

168. Fehlings MG, Tator CH, Linden RD. The effect of nimodipine and dextran on axonal function and blood flow following experimental spinal cord injury. *J Neursurg* 1989;71:403–416.

169. Guha A, Tator CH, Piper I. Effect of a calcium channel blocker on posttraumatic spinal cord blood flow. *J Neurosurg* 1987;66:423–430.

170. Guha A, Tator CH, Smith CR, et al. Improvement in posttraumatic spinal cord blood flow with a combination of a calcium channel blocker and a vasopressor. *J Trauma* 1989;29:1440–1447.

171. Hayashi N, Green B, Gonzalez-Carvajal M, et al. Local blood flow, oxygen tension, and oxygen consumption in the rat spinal cord. *J Neurosurg* 1983;58:516–525.

172. Chehrazi BB, Scremin O, Decima EE. Effect of regional spinal cord blood flow and central control in recovery from spinal cord injury. *J Neurosurg* 1989;71:747–753.

173. Kobrine AI, Doyle TF, Martins AN. Local spinal cord blood flow in experimental traumatic myelopathy. *J Neurosurg* 1975;42:144–149.

174. Dohrmann GJ, Allen WE. Microcirculation of traumatized spinal cord: correlation of microangiography and blood flow patterns in transitional and permanent paraplegia. *J Trauma* 1975;15:1003–1013.

175. Freid LC, Goodkin R. Microangiographic observations of the experimentally traumatized spinal cord. *J Neurosurg* 1971;35:709–714.

176. Ames A III, Wright RL, Kowada M, et al. Cerebral ischemia II. The no-reflow phenomenon. *Am J Pathol* 1968;52:437–453.

177. Zivin JA, Degirolami V. Spinal cord infarction: a highly reproducible stroke model. *Stroke* 1980;11:200–204.

178. Osterholm JL. The pathophysiological response in spinal cord injury. *J Neurosurg* 1974;40:5–33.

179. Schultz TW, DeLuca DC, Reding DL. Norepinephrine levels in traumatized spinal cord of catecholamine depleted cats. *Brain Res* 1976;109:367–374.

180. Koyanagi I, Tator CH, Lea PJ. Three-dimensional analysis of the vascular system in the rat spinal cord with scanning electron microscopy of vascular corrosion cast: 1. Normal spinal cord. *Neurosurgery* 1993;33:277–284.

181. Koyanagi I, Tator CH, Lea PJ. Three-dimensional analysis of the vascular system in the rat spinal cord with scanning electron microscopy of vascular corrosion cast: 2. Acute spinal cord injury. *Neurosurgery* 1993;33:285–292.

182. Tator CH, Koyanagi I. Vascular mechanisms in the pathophysiology of human spinal cord injury. *J Neurosurg* 1997;86:483–492.

183. Kim RC, Smith HR, Henbest ML, et al. Nonhemorrhagic venous infarction of the spinal cord. *Ann Neurol* 1984;15:379–385.

184. Koyanagi I, Tator CH, Theriault E. Silicone rubber microangiography of acute spinal cord injury in rats. *Neurosurgery* 1993;32:260–268.

185. Rao KR, Donnenfeld H, Chisud JG, et al. Acute myelopathy secondary to spinal venous thrombosis. *J Neurol* 1982;56:107–113.

186. Shingu H, Kimura I, Nasu Y, et al. Microangiographic study of spinal cord injury and myelopathy. *Paraplegia* 1989;27:182–189.

187. Fisher EG, Ames AIII, Hedley-Whyte ET, et al. Reassessment of cerebral capillary changes in acute global ischemia and their relationship to the "no-reflow phenomenon." *Stroke* 1977;8:36–39.

188. Griffiths IR, Miller R. Vascular permeability to protein and vasogenic oedema in experimental concussive injuries to the canine spinal cord. *J Neurol Sci* 1974;22:291–304.

189. Hsu CY, Hogan EL, Gadsden RHS, et al. Vascular permeability in experimental spinal cord injury. *J Neurol Sci* 1985;70:275–282.

190. Stewart WB, Wagner FC. Vascular permeability changes in the contused feline spinal cord. *Brain Res* 1979;169:163–167.

191. Nemecek S. Morphological evidence of microcirculatory disturbances in experimental spinal cord trauma. *Adv Neurol* 1978;20:395–405.

192. Faden AI, Simon RP. A potential role for excitotoxins in the pathophysiology of spinal cord injury. *Annl Neurol* 1988;23:623–626.

193. Jorgensen MB, Diemer NH. Selective neuron loss after cerebral ischemia in the rat: possible role of transmitter glutamate. *Acta Neurol Scand* 1982;66:536–546.

194. Martinez-Arizala A, Rigamonti DD, Long JB, et al. Effects of NMDA receptor antagonists following spinal ischemia in the rabbit. *Exp Neurol* 1990;108:232–240.

195. Panter SS, Yum SW, Faden AI. Alteration in extracellular amino acids after traumatic spinal cord injury. *Ann Neurol* 1990;24:96–99.

196. Tymianski M, Tator CH. Normal and abnormal calcium homeostasis in neurons: a basis for the pathophysiology of traumatic and ischemic central nervous system injury. *Neurosurgery* 1996;38:1176–1195.

197. Wieloch T. Neurochemical correlates to selective neuronal vulnerability. *Prog Brain Res* 1985;63:69–85.

198. Young W. The post-injury response in trauma and ischemia: secondary injury or protective mechanisms *CNS Trauma* 1987;4:27–51.

199. Fehlings MG, Tator CH, Linden TD. The relationships among the severity of spinal cord injury, motor and somatosensory evoked potentials and spinal cord blood flow. *Electroencephalogr Clin Neurophysiol* 1989;74:241–259.

200. Krnjevic K, Lisiewicz A. Injection of calcium ions in spinal motoneurones. *J Physiol Lond* 1972;225:363–390.

201. Maury JF. Effect of Ca on membranes. *Fed Proc* 1966;25:1804–1810.

202. Meech RW. Intracellular calcium and the control of membrane permeability. *Symp Soc Exp Biol* 1976;30:161–191.

203. Brinley FJ, Tiffert T, Scarpa A, et al. Intracellular calcium buffering capacity in isolated squid axon. *J Gen Physiol* 1977;70:355–384.

204. Nicholls D, Akenman K. Mitchondrial calcium transport. *Biochim Biophys Acta* 1982;805:393–404.

205. Cittadini A, Boss D, Wolf F, et al. The role of intracellular $Ca^{2+}Ca^{2+}/Mg^{2+}$ ratio in bioenergetic reactions. In: Anghileri LJ, Tuffet-Anghileri AM, eds. *The role of calcium in biological systems.* Boca Raton, FL: CRC Press, 1982:189–200.

206. Kretsinger RH. Calcium in neurobiology: a general theory of its function and evolution. In: Schmitt FO, Worden FG, eds. *The neurosciences: fourth study program.* Cambridge, MA: MIT Press, 1979:617–622.

207. Chance B. The energy-linked reaction of calcium with mitochondria. *J Biol Chem* 1965;240:2729–2748.

208. Lehninger AL. Mitochondria and calcium in transport. *Biochem J* 1970;119:129–138.

209. Balentine JD, Dean D. Calcium-induced spongiform and necrotizing myelopathy. *Lab Invest* 1992;47:286–295.

210. Balentine JD, Hilton CW. Ultrastructural pathology of axons and myelin in calcium-induced myelopathy. *J Neuropathol Exp Neurol* 1980;139:339.

211. Banik NL, Hogan EL, Whetstine LJ, et al. Changes in myelin and axonal proteins in $CaCl_2$-induced myelopathy in rat spinal cord. *CNS Trauma* 1984;1:131–138.

212. Janssen L, Hansebout RR. Pathogenesis of spinal cord injury and newer treatments. *Spine* 1989;14:23–32.

213. Shields DC, Schaecher KE, Hogan EL, et al. Calpain activity and expression increased in activated glial and inflammatory cells in penumbra of spinal cord injury lesion. *J Neurol Sci Res* 2000;61:146–150.

214. Faden AI, Chan PH, Longar S. Alterations in lipid metabolism, Na,K-ATPase activity and tissue water content of spinal cord after experimental traumatic injury. *J Neurochem* 1987;48:1809–1816.

215. Schwab JM, Brechtel K, Nguyen TD, et al. Persistent accumulation of cyclooxygenase-1 (COX-1) expressing microglial/macrophages and upregulation of endothelium following spinal cord injury. *J Neuroimmunol* 2000;111:122–130.

216. Resnick DK, Graham SH, Dixon CE, et al. Role of cyclooxygenase-2 in acute spinal cord injury. *J Neurotrauma* 1998;15:1005–1013.

217. Lapchak PA, Araujo DM, Song D, et al. Neuroprotection by the selective cyclooxygenase-2 inhibitor SC-236 results in improvements inbehavioral deficits induced by reversible spinal cord ischemia. *Stroke* 2001;32:1220–1225.

218. Choi DW. Ionic dependence of glutamate neurotoxicity. *J Neurosci* 1987;7:369–379.

219. Choi DW. Glutamate neurotoxicity and diseases of the nervous system. *Neuron* 1988;1:623–634.

220. Cotman CW, Bridges RJ, Taube JS, et al. The role of the NMDA receptor in central nervous system plasticity and pathology. *J NIH Res* 1989;1:65–74.

221. Lipton Sa, Rosenberg PA. Excitatory amino acids as a final common pathway for neurologic disorders. *N Engl J Med* 1994;330:613–622.

222. Rothman SM, Olney JW. Excitotoxicity and the NMDA receptor. *Trends Neurol Sci* 1987;10:299–302.

223. Ozawa K, Seta K, Araki H, et al. The effects of ischemia on mitochondrial metabolism. *J Biol Chem* 1967;61:512–514.

224. Tymianski M, Charlton MP, Carlen PL, et al. Source specificity of early calcium neurotoxicity in cultured embryonic spinal neurons. *J Neurosci* 1993;13:2085–2104.

225. Koh JY, Goldberg MP, Hartley DM, et al. Non-NMDA receptor-mediated neurotoxicity in cortical culture. *J Neurosci* 1990;10:696–705.

226. Rothman SM, Thurston JH, Hauart RE. Delayed neurotoxicity of excitatory amino acids in vitro. *Neuroscience* 1987;22:471–480.

227. Agrawal SK, Fehlings MG. Role of NMDA and non-NMDA ionotropic glutamate receptors in traumatic spinal cord axonal injury. *J Neurosurg* 1997;17:1055–1063.

228. Imaizumi T, Kocsis JD, Waxman SG. The role of voltage-gated Ca^{2+} channels in axonic injury of spinal cord white matter. *Brain Res* 1999;817:84–92.

229. Rhoney DH, Luer MS, Hughes M, et al. New pharmacologic approaches to acute spinal cord injury. *Pharmacotherapy* 1996;16:382–392.

230. Saido TC, Sorimachi H, Suzuki K. Calpain: new perspectives in molecular diversity and physiological-pathological involvement. *FASEB J* 1994;8:814–822.

231. Kapadia SE. Ultrastructural alterations in blood vessels of the white matter after experimental spinal cord trauma. *J Neurosurg* 1984;61:539–544.

232. Richardson HD, Nakamaura S. An electron microscopic study of spinal cord edema and the effect of treatment with steroids, mannitol, and hypothermia. In: *Proceedings of the Virginia Spinal Cord Injury Conference* 1971:10–16.

233. Nemecek S, Petr R, Suba P, et al. Longitudinal extension of oedema in experimental spinal cord injury: evidence for two types of posttraumatic oedema. *Acta Neurochir (Wright)* 1977;37:7–16.

234. Yashon D, Bingham WG Jr, Faddoul EM, et al. Edema the spinal cord following experimental impact trauma. *J Neuros* 1973;38:693–697.

235. Wagner FC Jr, Stewart WB. Effect of trauma dose on spinal cord edema. *J Neurosurg* 1981;54:802–806.

236. Balentine JD, Hogan EL, Banik NL, et al. Calcium and the pathogenesis of spinal cord injury. In: Dacey RG Jr, Winn HR, Rimmel RW, et al, eds. *Trauma of the central nervous system.* New York: Raven Press, 1985:285–295.

237. Struder RK, Welch DM, Siegel BA. Transient alteration of the blood-brain barrier: effect of hypertonic solutions administered via carotid artery injection. *Exp Neurol* 1974;44:266–273.

238. Hirano A, Becker NH, Zimmerman HM. Pathological alterations in the cerebral endothelial cell barrier to peroxidase. *Arch Neurol* 1969;20:300–308.

239. del Maestro R. An approach to free radicals in medicine and biology. *Acta Physiol Scand* 1980;492(Suppl):153–168.

240. Braughler JM, Hall ED. Correlation of methylprednisolone levels in cat spinal cord with its effects on $(Na^+\text{-}K^+)$-ATPase, lipid peroxidation, and alpha motor neuron function. *J Neurosurg* 1982;56:838–844.

241. Aust SD, Morehouse LA, Thomas CE. Role of metals in oxygen radical reactions. *J Free Rad Biol Med* 1985;1:3–23.

242. Black P, Markowitz RS. Experimental spinal cord injury in monkeys: comparison of steroids and local hypothermia. *Surg Forum* 1971;22:409–411.

243. Sadrzadeh SM, Graft E, Panter SS, et al. Hemoglobin, a biological Fenton reagent. *J Biol Chem* 1984;259:14354–14356.

244. Juurlink BHJ, Paterson PG. Review of oxidative stress in brain and spinal cord injury: suggestions for pharmacologic and nutritional management strategies. *J Spinal Cord Med* 1998;21:309–334.

245. McCord JM. Oxygen-derived radicals: a link between reperfusion injury and inflammation. *Fed Proc* 1987;46:2402–2406.

246. Anderson DK, Saunders RD, Demediuk P, et al. Lipid hydrolysis and peroxidation in injured spinal cord: partial protection with methylprednisolone or vitamin E and selenium. *CNS Trauma* 1985;2:256–267.

247. Kurihara M. Role of monoamines in experimental spinal cord injury: relationship between $Na^+\text{-}K^+$-ATPase and lipid peroxidation. *J Neurosurg* 1985;62:743–749.

248. Pietronigro RD, Hovsepian M, Demophoulus HB, et al. Loss of ascorbic acid from injured feline spinal cord. *J Neurochem* 1983;41:1072–1076.

249. Saunders RD, Dungan LL, Demediuk P, et al. Effects of methylprednisolone and the combination of alpha tocopherol and selenium on arachidonic acid metabolism and lipid peroxidation in traumatized spinal cord tissue. *J Neurochem* 1987;49:24–31.

250. Anderson DK, Waters TR, Means ED. Pretreatment with alpha tocopherol enhances neurologic recovery after experimental spinal cord injury compression. *J Neutrauma* 1988;5:61–67.

251. Hall ED, Braughler JM, McCall JM. Antioxidant effects in brain and spinal cord injury. *J Neurotrauma* 1992;9(Suppl 1):S165–172.

252. Simpson RK, Hsu CY, Dimitrijevic MR. The experimental basis for early pharmacologic intervention in spinal cord injury. *Paraplegia* 1991;29:364–372.

253. Goodman JG, Bingham WG, Hunt WE. Platelet aggregation in experimental spinal cord injury. *Arch Neurol* 1979;30:197–201.

254. Faden AI. Neuropeptides and central nervous system injury. *Arch Neurol* 1986;43:501–504.

255. Means ED, Anderson DK. Neuronophagia by leukocytes in experimental spinal cord injury. *J Neurophathol Exp Neurol* 1983;43:707–719.

256. Xu J, Hsu CY, Liu TH, et al. Leukotriene B, release and polymorphonuclear cell infiltration in spinal cord injury. *J Neurochem* 1990;55:907–912.

257. Kontos HS, Wei EP, Ellis EF, et al. Appearance of superoxide anion radical in cerebral extracellular space during increased prostaglandin synthesis in cats. *Circ Res* 1985;57:142–151.

258. Kontos HS, Wei EP, Povlishock JT, et al. Oxygen radicals mediate the cerebral arteriolar dilation from arachidonate and bradykinin in cats. *Circ Res* 1984;55:295–303.

259. Popovich PG, Stokes BT, Whitacre CC. Concepts of autoimmunity following spinal cord injury: possible roles of T lymphocytes in the traumatized central nervous system. *J Neurosci Res* 1996;45:349–363.

260. Schwab ME, Bartholdi D. Degeneration and regeneration of axons in the lesion spinal cord. *Physiol Rev* 1996;76:319–370.

261. Merrill JE, Ignarro LJ, Sherman MP, et al. Microglial cell cytotoxicity of oligodendrocytes is mediated through nitric oxide. *J Immunol* 1993;151:2132–2140.

262. Bethea JR, Castro M, Keanne RW, et al. Traumatic spinal cord injury induces nuclear factor-_B activation. *J Neurosci* 1998;18:3251–260.

263. Springer JE, Azbill RD, Knapp PE. Activation of the caspase-3 apoptotic cascade in traumatic spinal cord injury. *Nat Med* 1999;5:943–946.

264. Eldadah BA, Faden AI. Caspase pathways, neuronal apoptosis, and CNS injury. *J Neurotrauma* 2000;17:811–829.

265. Satake K, Matsuyama Y, Kamiya M, et al. Nitric oxide via macrophage iNOS induces apoptosis following traumatic spinal cord injury. *Brain Res Mol Brain Res* 2000;85:114–122.

266. Budd SL, Tenneti L, Lishnal T, et al. Mitochondrial and extrachondrial apoptotic signaling pathways in cerebrocortical neurons. *Proc Nat Acad Sci USA* 2000;97:6161–6166.

267. Bonfoco E, Kraine D, Ankarcrona M, et al. Apoptosis and necrosis: two distinct events induced, respectively, by mild and intense insults with *N*-methyl-*D*-aspartate or nitric oxide/superoxide in cortical cell cultures. *Proc Natl Acad Sci USA* 1995;92:7162–166.

268. American Spinal Injury Association. *Standards for neurological classification of spinal cord injury revised 1992.* Chicago: American Spinal Injury Association, 1992.

269. de la Torre JC, Johnson CM, Goode DJ, et al. Pharmacologic treatment and evaluation of permanent experimental spinal cord trauma. *Neurology* 1975;25:508–514.

270. Faden AI, Jacobs TP, Patrick DH, et al. Megadose corticosteroid therapy following experimental spinal injury. *J Neurosurg* 1984a;60:712–717.

271. Young W, Flamm ES. Effect of high dose corticosteroid therapy on blood flow, evoked potentials, and extracellular calcium in experimental spinal injury. *J Neurosurg* 1982;57:667–673.

272. Anderson DK, Means ED, Waters TR, et al. Microvascular perfusion and metabolism in injured spinal cord after methylprednisolone treatment. *J Neurosurg* 1982;56:106–113.

273. Hall ED, Wolf DJ, Braughler JM. Effects of a single large dose of methylprednisolone sodium succinate on experimental posttraumatic spinal cord ischemia. *J Neurosurg* 1984;61:124–130.

274. Hall ED. Neuroprotective actions of glucocorticoid and nonglucocorticoid steroids in acute neuronal injury. *Cell Mol Neurobiol* 1993;13:415–432.

275. Hall ED. The neuroprotective pharmacology of methylprednisolone. *J Neurosurg* 1993;76:13–22.

276. Dumont RJ, Verma S, Okonkwo DO, et al. Acute spinal cord injury, Part II: Contemporary pharmacology. *Clin Neuropharm* 2001;24:265–279.

277. Bracken MB, Collins WF, Freeman DF, et al. Efficacy of methylprednisolone in acute spinal cord injury. *JAMA* 1984;251:45–52.

278. Braughler JM. Lipid peroxidation-induced inhibition of gammabutyric acid uptake in rat brain synaptosomes: protection by glucocorticoids. *J Neurochem* 1985;44:1282–1288.

279. Bracken MD, Shepard MJ, Collins WF, et al. A randomized controlled trial of methylprednisolone or naloxone in the treatment of acute spinal cord injury. N Engl J Med 1990;332:1405–1411.

280. Ducker TB, Zeidman SM. Spinal cord injury: role of steroid therapy. Spine 1994;19:2281–2287.

281. Hulbert RJ. The role of steroids in acute spinal cord injury. An evidence-based analysis. Spine 2001;26(Suppl):39–46.

282. Bracken MB, Holford TR. Effects of timing of methylprednisolone or naloxone administration on recovery of segmental and long-tract neurological function in NASCIS 2. J Neurosurg 1993;79:500–507.

283. Young W, Bracken MB. The Second National Acute Spinal Cord Injury Study. J Neurotrauma 1992;9(Suppl 1):S397–405.

284. Bracken MB, Shepard MJ, Holford TR, et al. Administration of methylprednisolone for 24 or 48 hours or tirilazad mesylate for 48 hours in the treatment of acute spinal cord injury. Results of the third National Acute Spinal Cord Injury Randomized Controlled Trial. JAMA 1997;227:1597–1604.

285. Bracken MB, Shepard MJ, Holford TR, et al. Methylprednisolone or tirilazad mesylate administration after acute spinal cord injury: 1-year follow-up. Results of the third National Acute Spinal Cord Injury Randomized Controlled Trial. J Neurosurg 1998;89:699–706.

286. Fehlings MG. Summary statement: the use of methylprednisolone in acute spinal cord injury. Spine 2001;26(Suppl):55.

287. Hall ED, Yonkers PA, Andrus PK, et al. Biochemistry and pharmacology of lipid antioxidants in acute brain and spinal cord injury. J Neurotrauma 1992;9(Suppl 2):S425–442.

288. Hall ED. Effects of the 21-aminosteroid U74006F on posttraumatic spinal cord ischemia in cats. J Neursurg 1988;68:462–465.

289. Anderson DK, Braughler JM, Hal ED, et al. Effects of treatment with U-74006F on neurological outcome following experimental spinal cord injury. J Neurosurg 1988;69:562–567.

290. Francel PC, Long BA, Malik JM, et al. Limiting ischemic spinal cord injury using a free radical scavenger 21-aminosteroid and/or cerebrospinal fluid drainage. J Neurotrauma 1993;79:742–751.

291. Bracken MB. Pharmacologic treatment of acute spinal cord injury: current status and future projects. J Emerg Med 1993;11:43–48.

292. Geisler FH. GM-1 ganglioside and motor recovery following human spinal cord injury. J Emerg Med 1993;11:49–55.

293. Geisler FH, Dorsey FC, Coleman WP. Recovery of motor function after spinal cord injury: a randomized placebo-controlled trial with GM-1 ganglioside. N Engl J Med 1991;324:1829–1838.

294. Geisler FH, Dorsey FC, Coleman WP. GM-1 ganglioside in human spinal cord injury. J Neurotrauma 1992;(Suppl 1):S407–416.

295. Young W. Recovery mechanisms in spinal cord injury: implications for regenerative therapy. In: Seil FJ, ed. Neural regeneration and transplantation frontiers of clinical neurosciences. New York: Liss, 1989:157–169.

296. Young W. Secondary injury mechanisms in acute spinal cord injury. J Emerg Med 1993;11:13–22.

297. Constantini S, Young W. The effects of methylprednisolone and the ganglioside GM-1 on acute spinal cord injury in rats. J Neurosurg 1994;80:97–111.

298. Geisler FH, Coleman WP, Grieco G, et al. The Sygen multicenter acute spinal cord injury study. Spine 2001;26(Suppl):87–98.

299. Fehlings MG, Bracken MB. Summary statement: the Sygen (GM-1 Ganglioside) clinical trail in acute spinal cord injury. Spine 2001;26(Suppl):99–100.

300. Faden AI, Jacobs TP, Holaday JW. Thyrotropin-releasing hormone improves neurologic recovery after spinal trauma in cats. N Engl J Med 1981;305:1063–1067.

301. Faden AI, Jacobs TP, Mougey E, et al. Endorphins in experimental spinal injury. Ann Neurol 1981;10:326–332.

302. Black P, Markowitz RS, Cooper V, et al. Models of spinal cord injury. Part 1, static load technique. Neurosurgery 1986;19:752–762.

303. Wallace MC, Tator CH. Failure of naloxone to improve spinal cord blood flow and cardiac output after spinal cord injury. Neurosurgery 1986;18:428–432.

304. Bracken MB, Shepard MJ, Collins WF, et al. Methylprednisolone or naloxone treatment after acute spinal cord injury: 1 year follow-up data: results of the second NASCIS. J Neurosurg 1992;76:23–31.

305. Faden AI. Opioid and nonopioid actions mechanisms may contribute to dynophin's pathophysiological actions in spinal cord injury. Ann Neurol 1990;24:67–74.

306. Faden AI, Sacksen I, Noblle LJ. Opiate receptor antagonist nalmefene improves neurological recovery after traumatic spinal cord injury in rats through a central mechanism. J Pharmacol Exp Ther 1988;245:742–748.

307. Faden AI, Takemori AE, Portoghese TS. Kappa-Selective opiate antagonist nor-binaltorphimine improves outcome after traumatic spinal cord injury in rats. CNS Trauma 1987;4:227–237.

308. Hall ED, Wolf DL, Althaus JS, et al. Beneficial effects of the kappa opioid receptor agonist U-50488H in experimental acute brain and spinal cord injury. Brain Res 1987;435:174–180.

309. Curtis MT, Lefer AM. Protective actions of naloxone in hemorrhagic shock. Am J Physiol 1980;239H416–H421.

310. Koreh K, Seligamn ML, Flamm ES, et al. Lipid antioxidant properties of naloxone in vitro. Biochem Biophys Res Commun 1984;102:1317–1322.

311. Simpkins CO, Alailima ST, Tate EA. Inhibition by naloxone of neutrophil superoxide release: a potentially useful anti-inflammatory effect. Circ Shock 1986;20:181–191.

312. Ildan F, Polat S, Oner A, et al. Effects of naloxone on sodium- and potassium-activated and magnesium-dependent adenosine-5±-triphosphate activity and lipid peroxidation and early ultrastructural findings after experimental spinal cord injury. Neurosurgery 1995;36:797–805.

313. Holaday JW, D'Amato RJ, Faden AI. Thyrotropin-releasing-hormone improves cardiovascular function in experimental endotoxic and hemorrhagic shock. Science 1981;213:216–218.

314. Faden AI. TRH analog YM-14673 Improves outcome following traumatic brain and spinal cord injury in rats: dose-response studies. Brain Res 1989;486:228–235.

315. Faden AI, Jacobs TP, Smith MT. Thyrotropin-releasing hormone in experimental spinal injury: dose response and late treatment. Neurology 1984;34:1280–1284.

316. Pitts LH, Ross A, Chase GA, et al. Treatment with thyrotropin-releasing hormone (TRH) in patients with traumatic spinal cord injuries. J Neurotrauma 1995;12:235–243.

317. Fukuda H, Ono H. Ventral root depolarization and spinal reflex augmentation by a TRH analog in spinal cord. Neuropharmacology 1982;21:739–744.

318. Schmidt-Achert KM, Askansas V, Engel WK. Thyrotropin-releasing hormone enhances choline acetyl transferase and creatine kinase in culture spinal ventral horn neurons. J Neurochem 1984;43:586–589.

319. Wada S, Yone K, Ishidou Y, et al. Apoptosis following spinal cord injury in rats and preventative effect of N-methyl-D-aspartate receptor antagonist. J Neurosurg 1999;91(Suppl):98–104.

320. Kemp JA, Foster AC, Wong EH. Noncompetitive antagonists of excitatory amino acid receptors. Trends Neurosci 1987;10:294–298.

321. Monaghan DT, Bridges RJ, Cotman CW. The excitatory amino acid receptors: their classes, pharmacology, and distinct properties in the function of the central nervous system. Ann Rev Pharmacol Toxicol 1989;29:365–402.

322. Von Euler M, Li-Li M, Whitemore S, et al. No protective effect of the NMDAS antagonist memantine in experimental spinal cord injuries. J Neurotrauma 1997;14:53–61.

323. Kochlar A, Zivin JA, Lyde PD, et al. Glutamate antagonist therapy reduces neurologic deficits produced by focal central nervous system ischemia. Arch Neurol 1988;45:148–153.

324. Yanase M, Sakou T, Fukuda T. Role of N-methly-D-aspartate receptor in acute spinal cord injury. J Neurosurg 1995;83:884–888.

325. Rosenberg LJ, Teng YD, Wrathall JR. 2,3-dihydroxy-6-nitro-7-sulfamoyl-benzo(f)quinoxaline reduces glial loss and acute white matter pathology after experimental spinal cord contusion. J Neurosci 1998;19:464–475.

326. Wrathall JR, Teng YD, Marriott R. Delayed antagonism of AMPA/kainate receptors reduces long-term functional deficits resulting from spinal cord trauma. Exp Neurol 1997;145:565–573.

327. Lehmann J, Sills MA, Tsai C, et al. Dextromethophan modulates the NMDA-type receptor-associated ion channel by binding to its closed state. In: Cavalheiro EA, et al, eds. Frontiers in excitatory amino acid research. New York: Allan R. Liss, 1988:571–578.

328. Steinberg, GK, Saleh J, Kunis D. Delayed treatment with dextromethorphan and dextrophan reduces cerebral damage after transient focal ischemia. Neurosci Lett 1988;89:193–197.

329. Pointillart V, Gense D, Gross C, et al. Effects of nimodipine on post-traumatic spinal cord ischemia in baboons. *J Neurotrauma* 1993;10:201–213.

330. Faden AI, Jacobs TP, Smith MT. Evaluation of the calcium channel antagonist nimodipine in experimental spinal cord ischemia. *J Neurosurg* 1984;60:796–799.

331. Ford RW, Malm DN. Failure of nimodipine to reverse acute experimental spinal cord injury. *CNS Trauma* 1985;2:9–17.

332. Holtz A, Nystrom B, Gerdin B. Spinal cord injury in rats: inability of nimodipine or antineutrophil serum to improve spinal cord blood flow neurologic status. *Acta Neurol Scand* 1989;79:460–467.

333. Shi RY, Lucas JH, Wolf A, et al. Calcium antagonists fail to protect mammalian spinal neurons after physical injury. *J Neurotrauma* 1989;6:261–276.

334. Guha A, Tator CH, Piper I. Increase in rat spinal cord blood flow with the calcium channel blocker, nimodipine. *J Neurosurg* 1985;63:250–259.

335. Alderman JL, Osterholm JL, D'Amore BR, et al. Influence of arterial blood pressure upon central hemorrhagic necrosis after severe spinal cord injury. *Neurosurgery* 1979;4:53–55.

336. Croft TJ, Brodkey JS, Nulsen FE. Reversible spinal cord trauma: a model for electrical monitoring of spinal cord function. *J Neurosurg* 1972;36:402–406.

337. Rawe SE, Roth RH, Collins WF. Norepinephrine levels in experimental spinal cord trauma. Part 2. Histopathological study of hemorrhagic necrosis. *J Neurosurg* 1977;46:350–357.

338. Agrawal SK, Fehlings MG. The effect of the sodium channel blocker QX-314 on recovery after acute spinal cord injury. *J Neurotrauma* 1997;14:81–88.

339. Schwartz G, Fehlings MG. Evaluation of the neuroprotective effects of sodium channel blockers after spinal cord injury: improved behavioral and neuroanatomical recovery with riluzole. *J Neurosurg* 2001;94(Suppl 2):245–256.

340. Teng YD, Wrathall JR. Local blockade of sodium channels by tetrodotoxin ameliorates tissue loss and long-term functional deficits resulting from experimental spinal cord injury. *J Neurosci* 1997;17:4359–4366.

341. Cox JA, Lysko PG, Henneberry RC. Excitatory amino acid neurotoxicity at the *N*-methyl-*D*-aspartate receptor in cultured neurons: role of voltage-dependent magnesium block. *Brain Res* 1989;499:267–272.

342. McIntosh TK, Vink R, Yamakami I, et al. Magnesium protects against neurologic deficit after brain injury. *Brain Res* 1989;482:252–260.

343. Suzer T, Coskun E, Islekel H, et al. Neuroprotective effect of magnesium on lipid pereoxidation and axonal function after experimental spinal cord injury. *Spinal Cord* 1999;37:480–484.

344. Hall ED, Wolf DL. A pharmacological analysis of the pathophysiologic mechanisms of posttraumatic spinal cord ischemia. *J Neurosurg* 1986;65:951–961.

345. Hallenback JM, Jacobs TP, Faden AI. Combined PGI$_2$, indomethicin, and heparin improved neurologic recovery after spinal cord injury in cats. *J Neurosurg* 1983;58:749–754.

346. Taoka Y, Okajima K, Uchiba M, et al. Activated protein C reduces the severity of compression-induced spinal cord injury in rats by inhibiting activation of leukocytes. *J Neurosci* 1998;38:1393–1398.

347. Arnold PM, Citron BA, Ameenuddin S, et al. Caspase-3 inhibition is neuroprotective after spinal cord injury [abstract]. *J Neurochem* 2000;74:S73B.

348. Takahashi K, Schwartz E, Ljubetic C, et al. DNA plasmid that codes for human Bcl-2 gene preserves axotomized Clarke's nucleus neurons and reduces atrophy after spinal cord hemitransection in adult rats. *J Comp Neurol* 1999;404:159–171.

349. Martinou JC, Dubois-Dauphin M, Staple JK, et al. Overesxposure of Bcl-2 in transgenic mice protects neurons from naturally occurring death and experimental ischemia. *Neuron* 1994;33:1017–1030.

350. Legos JJ, Gritman KR, Tuma RF, et al. Coadministration of methylprednisolone with hypertonic saline solution improves overall neurologic function and survival rates in a chronic model of spinal cord injury. *Neurosurgery* 2001;49:1427–1433.

351. Hansebout RR, Kuchner EF, Romero-Sierra C. Effects of local hypothermia and of steroids upon recovery from experimental spinal cord compression injury. *Surg Neurol* 1975;4:531–535.

352. Martinez-Arizala A, Green BA. Hypothermia in spinal cord cooling. *J Neurotrauma* 1992;9(Suppl 2):S497–505.

353. Hansebout RR, Tanner JA, Romero-Sierra C. Current status of spinal cord cooling in the treatment of acute spinal cord injury. *Spine* 1984;9:508–511.

354. Bosch A, Stauffer ES, Nickel VS. Incomplete traumatic paraplegia: a ten-year review. *JAMA* 1971;216:473–478.

355. Ducker TB, Russo GL, Bellegarrique R. Complete sensorimotor paralysis after cord injury: mortality, recovery, and therapeutic implications. *J Trauma* 1979;19:837–840.

356. Hansebout RR. A comprehensive review of methods of improving cord recovery after acute spinal cord injury. In: Tator CH, ed. *Early management of acute spinal cord injury: seminars in neurologic surgery*. New York: Raven Press, 1982:181–190.

357. Goetz T, Romero-Sierra C, Ethier R, et al. Modeling of therapeutic dialysis of cerebrospinal fluid by epidural cooling in spinal cord injuries. *J Neurotrauma* 1988;5:139–150.

358. Blight AR, Young W. Central axons in injured cat spinal cord recover electrophysiologic function following remyelination by Schwann cells. *J Neurosci* 1989;91:15–34.

359. Bracken MB. Methylprednisolone and acute spinal cord injury. An update of the randomized evidence. *Spine* 2001;26(Suppl):47–54.

CHAPTER 53

Acute Injuries to the Spine and Spinal Cord: Evaluation and Early Treatment

Bruce E. Northrup

Acute injury of the cervical spine and spinal cord often presents a difficult therapeutic problem; excellent reviews have been written by Chestnut (1), Garfin and associates (2), Rizzolo and co-workers (3), Slucky and Eismont (4), Kilburn and Hadley (5), and Fehlings and Louw (6). Knowledge of the best treatment of neural injury is limited. Exacerbation of the spinal cord injury is an ever-present concern.

TREATMENT GOALS AND STEPS

The goals of treatment of the injured spinal cord are to prevent worsening of the injury and to maximize the inherent reparative processes. There are five key steps to obtaining these goals: early recognition, prompt resuscitation, stabilization of the injury, prevention of additional injuries, and avoidance of complications.

Recognition has two aspects: clinical and radiologic. Early recognition is aided in large part by the patient's complaints of pain and neurologic deficit. Clearly, the patient who is obtunded because of drugs, alcohol, or associated central nervous system injury is unable to cooperate (7). Some patients, although alert, will not complain of notable neck pain and yet may have unstable cervical spine fractures. Because of associated neural injury, a patient with one spine injury can have a second spine injury that is asymptomatic. The spine surgeon treating a trauma patient must be vigilant to identify the patient with a second spinal injury (8). The American Spinal Injury Association (ASIA) has developed new standards that aid in the neurologic examination (9), and in this way have improved our ability to define the injury.

The radiologic part of spinal injury recognition is enhanced greatly by the appreciation of injury patterns such as those described by Allen and associates (10), who devised the most widely accepted classification of cervical fractures based on the mechanism of injury. They divided the fractures into distraction or compression in the sagittal plane related to the pathological anatomy of the fracture fragments. One should become familiar with these categories to better recognize radiographic patterns and to treat spinal injuries more systematically. In younger patients, radiographs may be misleading, because a number of patients may have completely normal radiographs (11).

Prompt resuscitation involves the recognition of other soft tissue injuries in the abdomen, chest, or extremities that may be hidden by the sensory deficit of the spinal cord injury. Just as we always assume that a patient with a head injury has a cervical spine fracture, we should proceed as if every patient with a cervical spine fracture, cervical spinal cord injury, or clouded consciousness due to injury or drugs has an occult thoracic or abdominal injury. General surgeons specializing in trauma and spine surgeons have developed more cooperative relationships in recent times. Attention to rapid restoration of physiological homeostasis helps to prevent worsening of the neurologic deficit, and Vale and colleagues (12) have shown that neurologic recovery is substantially improved in those patients whose hemodynamic deficits are quickly corrected.

Stabilization of the injury begins in the field and is directly related to the goal of prevention of additional injuries. Increased care at the accident site and improved methods of immobilization during extraction and transportation to the treating facility have resulted in fewer patients with complete injuries and more patients with incomplete spinal cord injuries (13). Stabilization of the injury can be accomplished in the field with adhesive tape, a spine board, and a cervical collar; improved immobilization can be achieved in the hospital using skeletal traction or a halo vest or both. In spite of this, approximately 3% of patients with spinal injuries worsen neurologically before reaching the hospital (14–16).

In some cases this may be related to poor stabilization of the injury.

The final goal is to avoid complications. Many complications that occur in patients with cervical spine injury are related to sepsis and occur days after the patient has reached the hospital. The source of the sepsis is often related to paralysis and immobilization, especially involving the bladder and lungs. Venous thrombosis and potential embolization are other examples of complications secondary to immobilization. These and other related topics are covered in Chapter 54, "Medical Rehabilitation of Patients After Spinal Cord Injury."

Over the past 20 years, early mortality for cord injury has declined substantially (17–20). In most spinal cord injury centers, mortality is currently about 7%. Therefore, 93% of patients survive the initial hospitalization (21). This substantial reduction in mortality is due to improvements in many areas, including emergency medical procedures in the field and in the emergency room, improved imaging of the injury, and the development of technology to minimize certain complications such as deep venous thrombosis and to better treat other complications such as respiratory insufficiency (22,23). Additionally, the development of improved techniques of stabilization and aggressive, enthusiastic rehabilitation programs has done much to speed the mobilization of patients with spinal cord injury. These improvements have not occurred without substantial increases in the cost of care.

EPIDEMIOLOGY

Approximately 14,000 spinal cord injuries occur each year; of these instances, 10,000 patients survive to reach a treatment facility (that is, 3.2 to 5.3 spinal cord injuries per 100,000 population) (2,24–26). The incidence of cord injuries peaks during the summer months. The injury affects both the old and the young, with most cord injuries occurring in the 15-to-24 age group. Spinal cord injury occurs substantially more often in males and is distributed bimodally among two age groups. In the group of patients aged 15 to 24 years, motor vehicle accidents or sports-related injuries are most commonly responsible for the injury. In the second group of patients, aged 55 years and older, falls are most frequently the cause. The mortality in the latter group is high, likely related to the patients' age and associated medical problems.

The more frequent use of seat belts and the addition of shoulder harnesses has reduced the prevalence of injuries related to motor vehicle accidents. The seat belt may, however, still produce either an extension injury (if the individual slides under the belt) or a flexion-distraction injury with a cervical spine fracture/dislocation (27,28). The exact importance of air bags is unknown, but clearly they reduce injury to the head and spine in the event of a motor vehicle collision (29). New patterns of injury affecting smaller individuals traveling in the front seat have emerged as a result of air bag use. These injuries often occur in low-speed collisions (30).

PREVENTION

A variety of educational approaches have been taken to teach youth, who are most at risk for spinal cord injury, the effects of trauma. One of the most widespread of these programs is Think First, a joint effort of the American Association of Neurologic Surgeons and the Congress of Neurologic Surgeons, which endorses one or two injured persons to speak to youths about trauma and cord injury. Although the effects of these programs are difficult to assess, similar programs have been effective in industry.

PREHOSPITAL CARE

Initial responders in the field assess the patient for airway patency, ventilation, pulse, and level of consciousness. The patient's inability to move his or her extremities may identify potential spinal injuries.

Airway patency is always the first priority in prehospital stabilization of the trauma patient. Neck motion can be minimized with the chin-lift maneuver, as opposed to the jaw-thrust maneuver when establishing an open airway (1). In an unconscious patient, an oropharyngeal or nasopharyngeal airway may be necessary to maintain a patent airway (31,32). In a conscious patient, an oral airway suffices, although it may occasionally serve as an irritant and jeopardize immobilization in an uncooperative patient (33).

If oropharyngeal or nasopharyngeal placement does not improve breath sounds, endotracheal intubation should be performed. Blind nasotracheal intubation does not extend the neck and a priori might seem safer than orotracheal intubation; however, a comparison of the two methods showed them to be equivalent (34,35). A tracheostomy may be used to establish a patent airway and does not increase the risk of infection should an anterior-approach spinal operation be needed at a later date (36). Supplemental oxygen should be provided once an airway is established.

Extrication without additional injury is possible only when cervical spine immobilization is achieved with a collar that adds stability to the neck in extension (37). Although a neutral position of the head is desirable, attempts to achieve a neutral position should cease if resistance is met. Following extrication, a spine board to which the head, torso, and extremities are taped provides the safest means of immobilization (37). Sandbags placed on each side of the head and attached to the board with tape aid in cervical spine immobilization. The so-called log-rolling maneuver for placing the patient on the spine board, although usually regarded as a safe maneuver, may increase the opportunity for movement of any fracture fragments (38). The posture of a child's neck will be relatively flexed if the posterior skull is flattened against the spine board due to children having a relatively large head in comparison to the thorax.

In children, the hollow of the neck must be supported to maintain the neutral position, or a board with a recess for the occiput should be utilized. The patient should be transported to the hospital in the Trendelenburg position to avoid blood pooling in the lower extremities.

Prevention of aspiration and delivery of an adequate volume of air for respiration are essential to prehospital care. Aspiration of gastric contents occurs frequently and is common in patients who do not survive spinal cord injury (39). In the event of emesis, the hypopharynx should be suctioned. If no suction is available, patients should be log-rolled to their sides to prevent aspiration. An esophageal obturator also may be helpful. The mechanism of gastric contraction alone is sufficient to produce vomiting in a patient following spinal cord injury because striated muscular contractions below the lesion cannot take place in a quadriplegic patient. The chronic effect of quadriplegia is to delay gastric emptying. The acute effects may be similar (40,41), further increasing the likelihood of aspiration.

IN-HOSPITAL CARE

Any trauma patient with cutaneous evidence of an injury above the clavicle, disturbed consciousness, a complaint of spine pain, or pain elicited by palpation of the spine should arouse suspicion of concomitant spine or spinal cord injury. The neck must be immobilized, either in a semirigid collar or secured to a spine board, and this immobilization must not be removed until the neck has been judged radiographically to be free of cervical injury, including the C7-T1 junction (42). Patients should not be allowed to sit up if a spinal cord injury is suspected.

A number of clues suggest concomitant spinal cord injury in an obtunded patient. When the injury is at the mid-cervical level, the patient often exhibits a characteristic posture of the forearms flexed on the chest because the injury has produced paralysis of extensor muscles and spared flexor muscles. This is often the first clue that the patient has a cord injury. Other characteristic signs of spinal cord injury include diaphragmatic breathing due to paralyzed intercostal muscles, flaccid areflexia related to spinal shock, absent motor responsiveness when stimulation is applied to the portion of the body below the sensory level, priapism, warm distal extremities due to vasoparalysis (in a warm patient), and a slow pulse in the presence of a low blood pressure. A patient presenting with warm feet and dilated superficial veins along with a low blood pressure may also have a spinal cord injury.

Before the American College of Surgeons organized trauma services, approximately one-third of diagnosed spinal cord injuries were initially missed (17). In many patients, multiple injuries may mask the spinal injury, and vice versa. The loss of sensation experienced from a spinal cord injury may mask an acute abdominal injury.

External evidence of injury (ecchymosis, abrasion, or laceration of various parts of the face or head) often reveals the mechanism of injury. The posterior aspect of the spine may be evaluated by carefully log-rolling the patient to the side. Gentle palpation of the supine patient is a safer practice when possible. The presence of a muffled voice with reduced resonance (due to the reduction in volume of the column of resonating air) is a sign in upper cervical spinal cord injury, suggesting a retropharyngeal hematoma related to the soft tissue injury associated with a cervical fracture. The voice sounds as if the patient were trying to speak with a large mouthful of hot food. When present, this sign should arouse suspicion that the patient may develop acute respiratory collapse.

Fluid Resuscitation

Spinal cord injury produces a loss of sympathetic tone and widespread vasodilatation below the level of the lesion. Thus, the peripheral vascular volume is relatively expanded compared with the circulation blood volume. In this situation, the blood pressure is reduced by a relative oligemia. Patients with spinal cord injury also experience a relatively increased effect of the vagus nerve on the heart. The resultant bradycardia and pooling of blood peripherally reduce cardiac output and diminish systemic blood pressure (43,44). Hypoxia worsens the effects of the oligemia produced by the cardiac effects of spinal cord injury (39,45). The use of supplemental oxygen is important to minimize the hypoxia.

Following an isolated spinal cord injury, the patient may have a blood pressure as low as 70 mm Hg and a pulse rate below 60 beats per minute (bpm). In sharp contrast to this are patients in hemorrhagic shock, who are more likely to demonstrate a blood pressure of 70 mm Hg and a pulse rate of 120 bpm. Atropine (0.04 mg) may be given to combat the bradycardia resulting from spinal cord injury (46). Fluid infusion alone should not be used to correct the hypotension associated with neurogenic shock because the volumes required are usually large and will usually aggravate any associated pulmonary compromise. Such attempts usually result in fluid overload since vasomotor tone, not fluid, needs restoration. Normal vasomotor tone, and subsequently blood pressure, may be restored by the careful administration of pressor agents, such as dopamine (47).

Fluid resuscitation is aided by raising the patient's legs, which minimizes pooling of blood in the lower portion of the body. Patients who require resuscitation should have a Swan-Ganz catheter or a central venous catheter placed. Vasoparalysis alters the relationships among circulation, blood volume, and intravascular pressure, making it impossible in many patients, particularly the elderly, to determine precisely the patient's volume status without the information provided by these catheters. Hypotension, however, should not be attributed to a neurogenic cause unless occult bleeding has been ruled out.

A substantial number of patients with a spinal cord injury will have additional serious injuries, including blunt abdominal trauma (for example, a lacerated liver, spleen, or disrupted hollow viscus) (45,48) as well as extremity or rib fractures. These injuries may have a much greater impact on the survival of the patient than the primary spinal cord injury and must not be overlooked. It is ideal for a team of physicians that includes general surgeons specializing in trauma to evaluate the patient with spinal injuries. Trauma surgeons are routinely in charge of initially examining the patient for extraspinal injuries and the general resuscitation of the patient that may be necessary on arrival in the emergency department. They often supplement the abdominal examination with diagnostic peritoneal lavage, computed tomography (CT) of the abdomen, or abdominal ultrasound (45).

Neurologic Examination

In 1992, under the leadership of John Ditunno, ASIA, which consists of orthopedists, neurosurgeons, physiatrists, and statisticians (9), revised the functional and neurologic standards by which spinal cord injury is classified. These international standards defining neurologic impairment have restructured the neurologic examination and the quantification of neurologic impairment and functional disability. This essential revision permits accurate communication between clinicians. The key points are summarized here.

The ASIA committee provided a standardized classification of spinal cord injury in terms of spinal level (right and left, motor and sensory) and functional grade. The standards define level of injury as the most caudal segment of the cord with normal function. The classification system identifies ten muscles and 28 key sensory points to be graded. The sensory points are stimulated with pinpricks (pain) and light touch and scored on a three-point scale using 0 for absent sensation, 1 for impaired or partial sensation, 2 for normal sensation, and NT for areas rendered inaccessible. The level of spinal injury should be marked on the patient's skin for subsequent examiners. All dermatomes should be methodically tested (Table 53.1). Failure to test the dermatomes of the upper extremities is a common error.

The key muscles are graded on a six-point scale developed by the Medical Research Council:

5: Normal muscle strength
4: Just noticeable weakness against moderate resistance
3: Muscles that overcome gravity but not additional resistance
2: Muscles that cannot overcome gravity but can flex and extend with gravity eliminated
1: Contractions cause only visible or palpable change in muscle shape or tension but no movement
0: Total muscle paralysis

A change in neurologic function can be delineated accurately by using the six-point scale in each examination.

TABLE 53.1. *The Twenty-Eight Dermatomes and Key Points for Examination[a]*

C2	Occipital protuberance
C3	Supraclavicular fossa
C4	Top of the acromioclavicular joint
C5	Lateral side of the antecubital fossa
C6	Thumb—dorsal surface
C7	Middle finger—dorsal surface
C8	Little finger—dorsal surface
T1	Medial (ulnar) side of the antecubital fossa
T2	Apex of the axilla
T3	Third intercostal space
T4	Fourth intercostal space
T5	Fifth intercostal space (midway between T4 and T6)
T6	Sixth intercostal space (level of xiphisternum)
T7	Seventh intercostal space (midway between T6 and T8)
T8	Eighth intercostal space (midway between T6 and T10)
T9	Ninth intercostal space (midway between T8 and T10)
T10	Umbilicus
T11	Eleventh intercostal space (midway between T10 and T12)
T12	Inguinal ligament at midpoint
L1	Half the distance between T12 and L2
L2	Mid-anterior thigh
L3	Medial femoral condyle
L4	Medial malleolus
L5	Dorsum of the foot at the third metatarsal phalangeal joint
S1	Lateral heel
S2	Popliteal fossa in the midline
S3	Ischial tuberosity
S4–S5	Perianal area (taken as one level)

[a]Dermatomal key points to be tested bilaterally with both pinprick and touch.

Modified from Ditunno JF, Young W, Creasey G. International standards for neurological and functional classification of spinal cord injury: revised 1992. *Paraplegia* 1994;32:70–80.

The spinal levels and the muscle groups innervated by them are as follows:

C5: Elbow flexors (biceps, brachialis)
C6: Wrist extensors (extensors carpi radialis longus and brevis)
C7: Elbow extensors (triceps)
C8: Finger flexors (flexor digitorum profundus to the middle finger)
T1: Small finger abductors (abductor digiti minimi)
L2: Hip flexors (iliopsoas)
L3: Knee extensors (quadriceps)
L4: Ankle dorsiflexors (tibialis anterior)
L5: Long toe extensors (extensor hallucis longus)
S1: Ankle plantar flexors (gastrocnemius, soleus)

These muscles were chosen to be graded in the case of spinal injury because of consistent and reliable innervation and ease of testing in the recumbent position. The deltoid, for example, was not chosen because it is difficult to test in the recumbent position without compromising spine immobilization.

The ASIA impairment scale describes the degree of functional disability:

A: Patients with no motor function and no sensory function preserved in the sacral segments S4 and S5
B: Patients with preservation of sensation but no motor function below the neurologic level of spinal cord injury extending through the sacral segments
C: Patients with motor preservation and key muscles with a grade greater than 3
D: Patients with motor preservation and key muscles with a grade greater than 3
E: Patients without spinal cord injury

In addition to determining neurologic deficit, ASIA recommends assessing functional impairment using the functional independence measure (FIM). This standard measure of daily life activity performance includes six areas of function: self-care, sphincter control, mobility, locomotion, communication, and social cognition.

SPINAL CORD INJURY SYNDROMES

Spinal cord injuries may be complete or partial. A patient with a complete spinal cord injury has no evidence of neurologic function below the spine level of the lesion. If the spinal cord injury is complete for more than 48 hours, neurologic recovery will not occur. Partial spinal cord injuries show a variable degree of neurologic recovery and usually plateau at 2 years after injury. Immediately after sustaining a complete spinal cord injury, the patient may experience a poorly understood condition called *spinal shock* in which deep tendon reflexes and many cutaneous reflexes (including withdrawal reflexes and the bulbocavernosus reflex) are absent. The reappearance of these reflexes indicates the end of the spinal shock period. If there is not motor or sensory sparing after the end of spinal shock, then the person is judged to have sustained a complete spinal cord injury. Many patients with a complete spinal cord lesion do not experience spinal shock.

Partial spinal cord injuries are divided into a number of spinal cord syndromes and have a variety of symptoms and signs that characterize the anatomy of the lesion.

Anterior Cord Syndrome

Characteristically, the spinal cord injury resulting in anterior cord syndrome involves the anterior two-thirds of the spinal cord. The posterior regions of the spinal cord are intact, and patients appreciate touch or vibration in these areas. Pain and temperature sensations are carried in nerve fibers traversing the anterior portions of the lateral funiculus and are generally more severely affected in anterior cord syndrome. Most often, these sensations are not present caudal to the spinal cord injury. A rectal examination is a vital component of the physical examination of a patient with a spinal cord injury because sensation may be restricted to the perineal region alone.

There is a subset of patients with a sustained mild anterior spinal cord injury who clearly perceive pain elicited by a pinprick in the lower extremities. Approximately 70% of these patients will regain the ability to walk (49,50). For the remainder of patients experiencing incomplete sensory loss, the likelihood of neurologic and functional recovery is poor. Magnetic resonance imaging (MRI) has demonstrated a high incidence of cervical disc herniation in response to all traumatic spinal injuries (51), but the anterior spinal cord syndrome is associated with a particularly high prevalence of such disc herniations. Prompt imaging in this variety of partial spinal cord injury is therefore advised. Patients with anterior cord syndrome correspond to group B of the ASIA impairment scale.

Central Cord Syndrome

Central cord syndrome is characterized by a disproportionate impairment of the upper extremities rather than the lower extremities. Dr. Richard Schneider, who originally reported a number of central cord syndrome cases, identified some patients in this group with a hematoma in the central portion of the spinal cord. The mechanism of the hematoma was believed to be due to lamination of the spinothalamic tracts. Recent work, however, has cast doubt on the existence of such laminae in humans, and the presence of a hematoma is not essential to the lesion (52). The prognosis for functional recovery from central cord syndrome is fair. In a study by Penrod and associates (53), 23 of 59 patients with central cord syndrome regained functional walking ability. When the patients were divided into ASIA impairment scale groups C and D, all of the group D patients walked, regardless of age. In group C, 70% of patients younger than 50 years walked, and 40% of the patients over the age of 50 walked.

The bony lesion associated with the central cord syndrome is variable. Although the characteristic paralysis may be seen with any bony injury, it is most commonly seen in elderly patients with spondylosis and spinal stenosis and no fracture. A substantial number of these older patients have sustained a hyperextension injury, either pinching the spinal cord between a posteriorly subluxed vertebral body and the lamina of the inferior vertebra or impinging the spinal cord by a hypertrophic ligamentum flavum bulging posteriorly into the spinal canal.

Brown-Séquard Syndrome

Brown-Séquard syndrome results from an injury involving predominantly one-half of the spinal cord. The spinothalamic fibers represent contralateral pain and temperature sensations, whereas the posterior columns and corticospinal tracts mediate ipsilateral touch and motor movements. Therefore, patients with Brown-Séquard syndrome have an ipsilateral loss of touch and motor function and a contralateral loss of pain and temperature sensation. Penetrating spinal cord injury as well as a variety of spine fractures may produce this lesion. The potential for recovery is generally good, with approximately 90% recovering the ability to walk. This pattern of neurologic deficit is often superimposed on the central cord syndrome (54).

Posterior Cord Syndrome

Posterior cord syndrome is an uncommon manifestation of spinal cord injury characterized by loss of dorsal column function. Although motor function is preserved, walking becomes quite difficult because proprioception is markedly impaired.

RADIOGRAPHIC IMAGING

Although the type and degree of neurologic deficit ultimately prove to be the most important determinants of eventual functional outcome, the bony and ligamentous abnormalities dictate the practical treatment of the patient with a spinal injury. Imaging of bony and ligamentous abnormalities characterizes the spinal injury and indicates how to best achieve and maintain reduction and decompression of the neural tissue.

Radiographic imaging will usually be performed while the patient is still restrained on a spine board. Plain x-ray film imaging remains the standard of care because supplementary studies generally are not required to recognize a bony abnormality. Lateral radiographs usually demonstrate the pathology and suggest the proper treatment. In a review of a group of patients examined in 17 hospital emergency departments, Shaffer and Doris (55) reported that the crosstable lateral image was effective in diagnosing three-fourths of the bony abnormalities; the remaining bony abnormalities were diagnosed correctly with open-mouth and anteroposterior (AP) views. This study suggests that the radiographic examination should begin with a lateral radiograph of the cervical spine. A so-called swimmer's view is utilized if the top of T1 cannot be seen on the lateral radiograph. After visualizing all cervical vertebrae, the base of the skull, and the top of the T1 vertebra, the other radiographs, such as right and left oblique views, may be taken to further elucidate any bony abnormality. Supine oblique projection of the cervical spine can be accomplished without moving the patient by aligning the x-ray beam 45 degrees medially and 15 degrees cephalad (56).

Often, computed tomography (CT) scans reformatted into coronal and sagittal views best demonstrate the odontoid or the junction of the cervical and thoracic spine. Cervical fractures are identified in a higher percentage of cases when CT is used as the imaging modality as opposed to plain x-rays.

The decision as to when a patient should have spine radiographs taken is an important one. Davis and colleagues

(57) suggest that the head and neck be considered as one unit in trauma cases. Similarly, the American College of Surgeons Committee on Trauma (31) approaches the issue conservatively, suggesting that all patients with a high probability of cervical spine trauma (patients with supraclavicular trauma, obtundation, or high-velocity injuries) receive a lateral spine radiograph early during resuscitation efforts. An alert, asymptomatic patient rarely has a cervical spine fracture. Kreipke and associates (58) found no fractures in alert asymptomatic patients and recommended that no cervical spine radiographs be taken in this group. A prospective study of alert, asymptomatic patients performed by Roberge and co-workers (59) also found no fractures among patients with a negative examination. McKee and associates (7), however, reported one patient with an asymptomatic cervical fracture; this case report led them to urge caution in withholding radiographic evaluation of the cervical spine in complex medical situations in which multiple injuries, excitement, and age might serve to mask the symptoms of spine fracture.

I suggest that a full set of cervical spine radiographs that includes lateral, AP, and open-mouth views be taken for the following patients: all alert patients with neck pain or tenderness on careful physical examination; all patients with neurologic deficit, polytrauma, or craniofacial injuries; all intoxicated or unconscious patients; and all older patients who are at increased risk of spine fracture.

Fractures may be hidden and difficult to diagnose at either end of the cervical spine, specifically at the occiput–C2 complex and at the junction of the lower cervical spine and upper thoracic spine where overlying shoulders obscure the vertebrae. Other common causes of missed spine fractures are multiple trauma, altered consciousness due to either coma or intoxication, and the presence of noncontiguous fractures (8). All patients with a known cervical spine fracture should have a complete set of spine radiographs taken, because approximately 14% of patients with cervical spine fractures have additional fractures.

To confirm a fracture in a difficult-to-diagnose area and to delineate nondisplaced fractures of the posterior elements, CT may be helpful. Reconstructed CT sagittal and coronal images may be the only way to visualize some fractures of the odontoid process and cervicothoracic junction. When CT and polytomography were compared for diagnostic value, CT better displayed laminar fractures, posterior element fractures, and C1 fractures, whereas polytomography better demonstrated facet fractures (60). CT myelography will show areas of neural compression.

MRI supplements rather than substitutes for the information provided by plain films, CT, and polytomography. Epidural hematoma, herniated disc, spinal cord compression, and spinal cord displacement from osteophytes or stenosis are conditions better recognized with MRI than with other imaging modalities. In addition, MRI demonstrates abnormalities within the spinal cord (hemorrhage, edema) and in the extraspinal soft tissues and ligaments (33,61). It also offers prognostic ability in terms of neurologic recovery (51,61,62).

Magnetic resonance angiography yields detailed information regarding the vertebral arteries, which supply the spinal cord and brainstem. These arteries frequently are affected in cases of spine and spinal cord injury, although the clinical importance of vertebral artery injury remains unclear (63). In fatal instances of spinal cord injury, the vertebral artery is often intact, only showing signs of occlusion in 4% of cases (57).

Although an MRI provides useful information, it also has drawbacks. Access to the patient is limited while an MRI is performed. This type of imaging procedure cannot be used for patients who have pacemakers, aneurysm clips, metallic fragments (for example, gunshot wounds), or who are receiving intravenous pressors via pumps as part of pressure support during MRI scanning.

The Eastern Association for the Surgery of Trauma (EAST) developed a prospectively tested imaging protocol (64,65) that proved helpful in the examination of obtunded patients. The protocol included a CT of the upper cervical spine, including coronal and sagittal reformats. Although lower cervical spine imaging was not included in the EAST protocol, the evaluation of its usefulness is planned for future study.

MECHANICAL PATHOPHYSIOLOGY

During the instantaneous development of a spinal injury, soft tissues (including muscles, discs, and ligaments) and bony tissues (including facet joints and vertebral bodies) may fail to absorb the full energy of impact. Tissues are often displaced from their anatomic position, and the mechanical energy of the deforming force may be transmitted to the spinal cord (4). Mechanical failure is commonly evidenced radiographically. In many patients after injury, loads incurred in the course of performing normal daily activities produce additional bony tissue displacement and perhaps progressive neural injury. Following trauma, both pediatric and elderly patients can experience spinal cord injury without a fracture or dislocation. Excessive spine flexibility in the young and spondylosis causing a reduction of space between the spinal cord and the bony and soft tissue elements in the elderly can impart a direct force to the spinal cord. In children, this condition has been termed SCIWORA (spinal cord injury without radiographic abnormality).

REDUCTION OF DISLOCATIONS

The timing of reducing a dislocation remains controversial. A number of authors believe that early decompression of the spinal cord immediately follows early reduction of a dislocation. This group of surgeons advocates aggressive reduction as soon as a dislocation is imaged on plain films. Cotler and associates (66) reviewed the rationale for early reduction of cervical spine dislocations in patients with neurologic deficit and suggested that early resolution of neural compression resulted in improved recovery. The study concluded that weights up to 140 pounds were safe for reduction of cervical spine dislocations, and that reduction could be accomplished in 187 minutes. These authors emphasized that reduction and decompression were accomplished in awake patients capable of cooperating with neurologic monitoring. Blumberg and colleagues (67) noted the necessity of using ferromagnetic skull pins with increased weight, because MRI-compatible pins failed above 50 pounds of traction.

Cotler and associates (66) avoided the delay that would be imposed by performing imaging studies before reduction by proceeding with traction immediately following the demonstration of a cervical spine dislocation on plain lateral radiographs. The authors rapidly added weights until the dislocation was reduced. Some case reports indicate that urgent reduction of the dislocated spine may provide rapid neurologic improvement (20). Patients who are uncooperative because of head injury, drugs, or mental illness are not candidates for closed reduction without prior imaging to determine whether the patient has a concomitant disc herniation. Such patients cannot be properly monitored. Disc herniations, if present, are best removed anteriorly prior to reduction. Patients with a spine dislocation most often worsen neurologically when under general anesthesia, when a spontaneous reduction occurs, or when undergoing rapid-sequence reduction while awake. Similarly, the use of sedative or paralytic drugs should be avoided because of the reduced ability of patients to cooperate in serial neurologic examinations. Complete interference with muscular contraction also theoretically could permit overdistraction of the dislocated spine.

Although some authors advocate early reduction of a spine dislocation, others support a more conservative approach to dislocation management. A number of authors worldwide have reported cases in which rapid reduction of spinal dislocations resulted in catastrophic neurologic worsening with rapid onset of quadriplegia (68–75). Many, but not all, of these reductions occurred during surgery or were spontaneous and not physician controlled. In some cases, there was considerable delay between reduction of the spine dislocation and the onset of quadriplegia (71,72). A few of the reductions resulting in poor outcomes, however, occurred in awake patients reduced with careful monitoring. These reports emphasize the possibility of herniated disc tissue located behind the dislocated superior vertebra, such that disc fragments reside in the spinal canal and become more prominent following reduction. This finding prompted Eismont and associates (70) and others to delay reduction until an MRI (or CT myelography) had been obtained, and to remove any demonstrated disc herniation prior to reduction. Pratt and colleagues (76) also emphasized the importance of an MRI prior to surgery to identify disc herniations behind the cephalad vertebrae to avoid posing a risk of neurologic injury. In a case analysis (75) of a patient with a spine dislocation and a known disc herniation, seven of nine spine surgeons agreed that the disc fragments should be removed anteriorly prior to the reduction of the dislocation. The prevalence of serious neurologic worsening following reduction is unknown, but is assumed to be low because large numbers of patients have undergone reduction of spine dislocations without neurologic loss (4,34,66,77–81).

It may be possible to identify patients at greater risk for postreduction neurologic injury. Berrington and associates (68) concluded that patients with smaller intervertebral disc height between the dislocated vertebral bodies tend to have larger disc fragments in the canal, therefore increasing their risk for neurologic worsening. Also, patients with anterior cord syndromes are commonly found to have disc herniations, which could serve as a clinical element in identifying patients at greater risk for neurologic worsening.

The risk of spinal cord injury is related to the amount of room available for the spinal cord. Patients with a spinal cord injury generally have a narrower spinal canal (82) than the population at large. Lintner and associates (83), however, found that the spinal canal diameter of patients with facet injuries did not allow prediction of neurologic impairment, which emphasizes the importance of injury force and radiolucent anatomic structures (for example, discs and ligaments). Therefore, intervertebral space height, canal size, and anterior cord involvement are often factors that may predict which patients will be more severely affected by a herniated disc fragment.

TIMING OF SURGERY

Controversy still exists regarding the proper timing of surgery for patients with spinal cord injuries. Patient outcomes supporting the proponents for both early and late surgery can be cited. Some reports suggest that early surgery worsens the neurologic deficit. Lawrence Marshall (15,16) convened a number of neurosurgeons and orthopedists from various centers in the United States. The panel reviewed nearly 300 patients with spinal cord injuries and found that in the small percentage of patients who worsened following spinal cord injury surgery, all of the operations occurred within 5 days of sustaining the injury. They concluded that surgery should be delayed for 5 days postinjury. Heiden and associates (84), in a separate review, indicated that surgery prior to 1 week after sustaining the spinal cord injury was associated with neurologic worsening.

A spontaneous rate of neurologic worsening following a spinal cord injury exists. Frankel and co-workers (14) reported a 2% prevalence of spontaneous neurologic worsening. This percentage agrees well with that reported by Marshall (15,16) and suggests that the neurologic worsening that occurs following spinal cord surgery in some patients

may be unrelated to mechanical factors. In a prospective study, Vaccaro and associates (85) compared patients randomly assigned to early- or late-surgery groups. The early-surgery group was operated upon prior to 72 hours postinjury, and the late-surgery group was operated on more than 5 days after injury. Both groups fared equally well in terms of neurologic recovery, suggesting that early surgery caused no harm.

One argument supporting early surgery for spinal cord injury is that recovery can occur more effectively if compression of the spinal cord is relieved earlier. Benzel and Larson (86) discounted this logical argument after evaluating the functional recovery achieved by patients in whom surgery was performed after neurologic recovery had plateaued. They found that substantial functional recovery could occur even when surgery was delayed up to 173 days postinjury. Similar results were found by Anderson and Bohlman (87) for delayed surgery in patients with incomplete traumatic myelopathies.

The modern trend supports earlier surgical intervention in patients with nonspinal multiple trauma, such as abdominal trauma. The rationale for earlier surgical intervention is that the first few minutes to several hours after a traumatic injury serve as a window of opportunity during which the patient is free of complications involving yet additional organ systems. The patient is a better candidate for surgery immediately postinjury and is likely to improve more with earlier correction of systemic abnormalities. Thus, the "golden period" refers to the first few hours after sustaining a severe injury.

The same rapid deterioration of multiple organ systems may occur in patients with spinal cord injury. Commonly, one-fourth of patients with cervical spinal cord injuries develop atelectasis, and one-third develop pneumonia. Although the systemic complication rate is not increased by early surgery (88), often these complications begin to occur at postinjury day 3 to 5, and they interfere with the scheduling of "delayed" surgery.

Glucocorticoids given more than 8 hours postinjury have proved ineffective for treating patients with spinal cord injuries. Young and Bracken (89) suggested that the 8-hour therapeutic window seen in the pharmacologic treatment of spinal cord injury may be the same for surgical treatment of spinal cord injury. Rapid progression of neuropathologic changes occurs during the first 24 hours postinjury. Despite this fact, a review of surgical results with regard to timing in the second National Acute Spinal Cord Injury Study (NASCIS II) found no substantial advantage to early surgery (<24 hours postinjury) in terms of neurologic recovery (82).

There are two reasons to advocate early surgery for spinal cord injury. The first is avoidance of systemic complications, and the second is rapid decompression of the partially injured spinal cord to preserve neurologic function. Wilberger (90) showed an increased incidence of systemic complications in patients operated on more than 24 hours postinjury. Krengel and associates (91) indicated that systemic complications were reduced greatly in patients operated on acutely following injury. Levi and colleagues (92) suggested that early surgery provided greater ease of patient care, earlier rehabilitation, and improved recovery in patients with cervical spinal cord injuries. There remains no agreement on the optimal time to operate; however, most would agree that prompt surgery is necessary in patients who exhibit progressive neurologic worsening.

EARLY STEROIDS

NASCIS II (17) demonstrated the beneficial use of steroids within 8 hours of spinal cord injury in all groups except patients with a penetrating spinal cord injury (93). In the latter group, steroids increased the number of infectious complications. The dosage of methylprednisolone is 30 mg/kg given as a bolus, followed by 5.4 mg/kg given as a continuous infusion over the next 24 hours. (This and other treatments for spinal cord injury are detailed in Chapter 52.)

REFERENCES

1. Chestnut RM. Emergency management of spinal cord injury. In: Narayan RK, Wilberger JE, Povlishock JT, eds. *Neurotrauma*. New York: McGraw Hill, 1995:1113–1121.
2. Garfin SR, Shackford SR, Marshall LF, et al. Care of the multiply injured patient with cervical spine injury. *Clin Orthop* 1989;239:19–29.
3. Rizzolo SJ, Vaccaro AR, Cotler JM. Cervical spine trauma. *Spine* 1994;19:2288–2298.
4. Slucky AV, Eismont FJ. Treatment of acute injury of the cervical spine. *J Bone Joint Surg Am* 1994;76:1882–1986.
5. Kilburn MBP, Hadley MN. Contemporary treatment paradigms in spinal injuries. *Clin Neurosurg* 1998;46:153–169.
6. Fehlings MG, Louw D. Initial stabilization and medical management of acute spinal cord injury. *Am Fam Physician* 1996;54:155–161.
7. McKee TR, Tinkoff G, Rhodes M. Asymptomatic occult cervical spine fracture: case report and review of the literature. *J Trauma* 1990;30: 623–626.
8. Vaccaro AR, An HS, Lin S, et al. Noncontiguous injuries of the spine. *J Spinal Disord* 1992;5:320–329.
9. Ditunno JF, Young W, Creasey G. International standards for neurological and functional classification of spinal cord injury: revised 1992. *Paraplegia* 1994;32:70–80.
10. Allen BL, Ferguson RL, Lehmann TR, et al. A mechanistic classification of closed, indirect fractures and dislocations of the lower cervical spine. *Spine* 1982;7:1–27.
11. Pang D, Pollack IF. Spinal cord injury without radiographic abnormality in children—the SCIWORA syndrome. *J Trauma* 1989;29:654–664.
12. Vale FL, Burns J, Jackson AB, et al. Combined medical and surgical treatment after acute spinal cord injury: results of a prospective pilot study to assess the merits of aggressive medical resuscitation and blood pressure management. *J Neurosurg* 1997;87:239–246.
13. Tator CH, Duncan EG, Edmonds VE, et al. Changes in epidemiology of acute spinal cord injury from 1947 to 1981. *Surg Neurol* 1993;40: 207–215.
14. Frankel HL, Hancock DO, Hyslop G, et al. The value of postural reduction in the initial management of closed injuries of the spine with paraplegia and tetraplegia. Part I. *Paraplegia* 1969;7:179–192.
15. Marshall LF, Garfin S. Incidence and causes of neurological deterioration following spinal cord injury. In: Piepmeier JM, ed. *The outcome following traumatic spinal cord injury*. Mount Kisco, NY: Futura Publishing, 1992:13–30.
16. Marshall LF, Knowlton S, Garfin SR, et al. Deterioration following spinal cord injury. *J Neurosurg* 1987;66:400–404.
17. Bohlman HH. Acute fractures and dislocations of the cervical spine. *J Bone Joint Surg Am* 1979;61:1119–1141.
18. DeVivo MJ, Black EJ, Stover SL. Causes of death in the first 12 years after spinal cord injury. *Arch Phys Med Rehabil* 1993;74:248–254.
19. DeVivo MJ, Rutt RD, Black KJ, et al. Trends in spinal cord injury demographics and treatment outcomes between 1973 and 1986. *Arch Phys Med Rehabil* 1992;73:424–430.
20. Ducker TB, Russo GL, Bellegarrique R, et al. Complete sensorimotor paralysis after cord injury: mortality, recovery and therapeutic implications. *J Trauma* 1979;19:837–840.
21. DeVivo MJ, Richards JS, Stover SL, et al. Spinal cord injury—rehabilitation adds life to years. *West J Med* 1991;154:602–606.
22. Lanig IS, Lammertse DP. The respiratory system in spinal cord injury. *Phys Med Rehabil Clin North Am* 1992;3:725–740.
23. Park PK, Ziring BS, Merli GJ. Prophylaxis of deep venous thrombosis in patients with acute spinal cord injury. *Trauma Quarterly* 1993;9: 93–99.
24. Kalsbeek WD, McLaurin RL, Harris BS, et al. The national head and spinal cord injury survey: major findings. *J Neurosurg* 1980;53:5–19.
25. Kraus JF, Franti CE, Riggins RS, et al. Incidence of traumatic spinal cord lesions. *J Chron Dis* 1975;28:471–492.
26. Stover SL, Delisa JA, Whiteneck GC. *Spinal cord injury: clinical outcomes from the model systems*. Gaithersburg, MD: Aspen Publishers, 1995.
27. Saldeen T. Fatal neck injuries caused by use of diagonal safety belts. *J Trauma* 1967;7:856.
28. Taylor TKF, Nade S, Banister JH. Seat belt fractures of the cervical spine. *J Bone Joint Surg Br* 1976;58:328.
29. Kuner EH, Schlickewer W, Oltmanns D. Protective airbags in traffic accidents: change in injury patterns and reduction in the severity of injuries. *Unfallchirurgie* 1995;21:92–99.
30. Maxeiner H, Hahn M. Airbag induced lethal cervical trauma. *J Trauma* 1997;42:1148–1151.
31. Alexander RH, Proctor HI. Spine and spinal cord trauma. In: *Advanced trauma life support program for physicians*. Chicago: American College of Surgeons, 1993:191–203.
32. Bivins HG, Ford S, Bezmalinovic Z, et al. The effect of axial traction during orotracheal intubation of the trauma victim with an unstable cervical spine. *Ann Emerg Med* 1988;17:25–29.
33. Beers GJ, Raque GH, Wagner GG, et al. MR imaging in acute cervical spine trauma. *J Comput Assist Tomogr* 1988;12:755–761.
34. Beyer CA, Cabanela ME, Berquist TH. Unilateral facet dislocations and fracture-dislocations of the cervical spine. *J Bone Joint Surg Br* 1991;73:977–981.
35. Suderman VS, Crosby ET, Lui A. Elective oral tracheal intubation in cervical spine-injured adults. *Can J Anaesth* 1992;38:785–789.
36. Northrup BE, Vaccaro A, Rosen J. The occurrence of infection in anterior cervical fusion for spinal cord injury following tracheostomy. *Spine* 1995;20:2449–2453.
37. Podolsky S, Baraff LJ, Simon RR, et al. Efficacy of cervical spine immobilization methods. *J Trauma* 1983;23:461–465.
38. McGuire RA, Neville S, Green BA, et al. Spinal instability and the log-rolling maneuver. *J Trauma* 1987;27:525–531.
39. Green BA, Eismont FJ, O'Heir JT. Prehospital management of spinal cord injuries. *Paraplegia* 1987;25:229–238.
40. Fealey RD, Szurszewski JH, Merrit JL, et al. Effect of traumatic spinal cord transection on human upper gastrointestinal motility and gastric emptying. *Gastroenterology* 1984;87:69–75.
41. Segal JL, Milne N, Brunnemann SR, et al. Metoclopramide-induced normalization of impaired gastric emptying in spinal cord injury. *Am J Gastroenterol* 1987;82:1143–1148.
42. MacDonald RL, Schwartz ML, Mirich D, et al. Diagnosis of cervical spine injury in motor vehicle crash victims: how many x-rays are enough? *Trauma* 1990;30:392–397.
43. Lehman KG, Lane JG, Piepmeier JM, et al. Cardiovascular abnormalities accompanying acute spinal cord injury in humans: incidence, time course and severity. *J Am Coll Cardiol* 1987;10:46–52.
44. Levi L, Wolf A, Belzberg H. Hemodynamic parameters in patients with acute cervical cord trauma: description, intervention and prediction of outcome. *Neurosurgery* 1993;33:1016–1017.
45. Soderstrom CA, McArdle DQ, Ducker TB, et al. The diagnosis of intraabdominal injury in patients with cervical cord trauma. *J Trauma* 1983;23:1061–1065.

46. Cohen M. Initial resuscitation of the patient with spinal cord injury. *Trauma Quarterly* 1993;9:38–43.

47. Rosner M. Medical management of spinal cord injury. In: Pitts LH, Wagner FC, eds. *Craniospinal trauma.* New York: Thieme Medical Publishers, 1990:213–225.

48. Saboe LA, et al. Spine trauma and associated injuries. *J Trauma* 1991; 31:43–48.

49. Crozier KS, Graziani V, Ditunno JF, et al. Spinal cord injury: prognosis for ambulation based on sensory examination in patients who are initially motor complete. *Arch Phys Med Rehabil* 1991;72:119–121.

50. Northrup BE, Ball D, Osterholm JL. Initial sensory examination as a predictor of neurologic recovery following anterior spinal cord injury. In: Kehr P, Weidner A, eds. *Cervical spine,* vol. I. New York: Springer Verlag, 1987:81–84.

51. Schaeffer DM, Flanders AE, Osterholm JL, et al. Prognostic significance of magnetic resonance imaging in the acute phase of cervical spine injury. *J Neurosurg* 1992;76:218–230.

52. Quencer RM, Bunge RP, Egnor M, et al. Acute traumatic central cord syndrome MRI: pathological correlations. *Neuroradiology* 1992;34:85–94.

53. Penrod LE, Hegde SK, Ditunno JF. Age effect on prognosis for functional recovery in acute, traumatic central cord syndrome. *Arch Phys Med Rehab* 1990;71:963–968.

54. Little JW, Halar E. Temporal course of motor recovery after Brown-Sequard spinal cord injuries. *Paraplegia* 1985;23:39–46.

55. Shaffer MA, Doris PE. Limitation of the cross table lateral view in detecting cervical spine injuries: a retrospective analysis. *Ann Emerg Med* 1981;10:508–513.

56. McCall IW, Park WM, McSweeney T. The radiological demonstration of acute lower cervical injury. *Clin Radiol* 1973;24:235–240.

57. Davis D, Bohlman H, Walker AE, et al. The pathological findings in fatal craniospinal injuries. *J Neurosurg* 1971;34:603–613.

58. Kreipke DL, Gillespie KR, McCarthy MC, et al. Reliability of indications for cervical spine films in trauma patients. *J Trauma* 1989;29:1438–1439.

59. Roberge RJ, Wears RC, Kelly M, et al. Selective application of cervical spine radiography in alert victims of blunt trauma: a prospective study. *J Trauma* 1988;28:784–788.

60. Clark CR, Igram CM, El-Khoury GY, et al. Radiographic evaluation of cervical spine injuries. *Spine* 1988;13:742–747.

61. Flanders AE, Tartaglino LM, Friedman DP, et al. Magnetic resonance imaging in acute spinal cord injury. *Semin Roentgenol* 1992;27:271–298.

62. Marciello MA, Flanders AE, Herbison GJ, et al. Magnetic resonance imaging related to neurologic outcome in cervical spinal cord injury. *Arch Phys Med Rehabil* 1993;74:940–946.

63. Friedman DP, Flanders AE. Unusual dissection of the proximal vertebral artery: a description of three cases. *AJNR Am J Neuroradiol* 1992; 13:283–286.

64. Pasquale M, Fabian TC. Practice management guidelines for trauma from the Eastern Association for the Surgery of Trauma. *J Trauma* 1998;44:941–956.

65. Schenarts PJ, Diaz J, Kaiser C, et al. Prospective comparison of admission computed tomographic scan and plain films of the upper cervical spine in trauma patients with altered mental status. *J Trauma* 2001;51:663–668.

66. Cotler JM, Herbison GJ, Nasuti JF, et al. Closed reduction of traumatic cervical spine dislocation using traction weights up to 140 pounds. *Spine* 1993;18:386–890.

67. Blumberg KD, Catalano JB, Cotler JM, et al. The pullout strength of titanium alloy MRI-compatible and stainless steel MRI-incompatible Gardner-Wells tongs. *Spine* 1993;18:1895–1896.

68. Berrington NR, vanStaden JF, Willers JG, et al. Cervical intervertebral disc prolapse associated with traumatic facet dislocations. *Surg Neurol* 1993;40:395–399.

69. Burke DC, Berryman D. The place of closed manipulation in the management of flexion-rotation dislocations of the cervical spine. *J Bone Joint Surg Br* 1971;53:165–182.

70. Eismont FJ, Arena MJ, Green BA. Extrusion of an intervertebral disc associated with traumatic subluxation or dislocation of cervical facets. *J Bone Joint Surg Am* 1991;73:1555–1560.

71. Mahale YJ, Silver JR, Henderson NJ. Neurological complications of the reduction of cervical spine dislocations. *J Bone Joint Surg Br* 1993;75:402–409.

72. Mahale YJ. Progressive paralysis after bilateral facet dislocation of the cervical spine. *J Bone Joint Surg Br* 1992;74:219–223.

73. Olerud C, Jonsson H. Compression of the cervical spine cord after reduction of fracture dislocations. *Acta Orthop Scand* 1991;62:599–601.

74. Robertson PA, Ryan MD. Neurological deterioration after reduction of cervical subluxation. *J Bone Joint Surg Br* 1992;74:224–227.

75. Zeidman S. Traumatic quadriplegia with dislocation and central disc herniation. *J Spinal Disord* 1991;4:490–491.

76. Pratt ES, Green DA, Spengler DM. Herniated intervertebral discs associated with unstable spinal injuries. *Spine* 1990;15:662–666.

77. Hadley MN, Fitzpatrick BC, Sonntag VKH, et al. Facet fracture-dislocation injuries of the cervical spine. *Neurosurgery* 1992;30:661–666.

78. Harrington JF, Likavec MJ, Smith AS. Disc herniation in cervical fracture subluxation. *Neurosurgery* 1991;29:374–379.

79. Sabiston CP, Wing PC, Schweigel JF, et al. Closed reduction of dislocations of the lower cervical spine. *J Trauma* 1988;28:832–835.

80. Shapiro SA. Management of unilateral locked facet of the cervical spine. *Neurosurgery* 1993;33:832–837.

81. Wolf A, Levi L, Mirvis S, et al. Operative management of bilateral facet dislocation. *J Neurosurg* 1991;75:883–890.

82. Duh MS, Shepard MJ, Wilberger JE, et al. The effectiveness of surgery for the treatment of acute spinal cord injury and its relationship to pharmacologic treatment. *Neurosurgery* 1994;35:240–248.

83. Lintner DM, Knight RQ, Cullen JP. The neurologic sequelae of cervical spine facet injuries. *Spine* 1993;18:725–729.

84. Heiden JS, Weiss MH, Rosenberg AW, et al. Management of cervical spinal cord trauma in southern California. *J Neurosurg* 1975;43:732–736.

85. Vaccaro AR, Dougherty RJ, Sheehan TP, et al. Neurologic outcome of early vs. late surgery for cervical spinal cord injury. *Spine* 1997;22:2609–2613.

86. Benzel EC, Larson SJ. Functional recovery after decompressive spine operation for cervical spine fractures. *Neurosurgery* 1987;20:742–746.

87. Anderson PA, Bohlman HH. Anterior decompression and arthrodesis of the cervical spine: long-term motor improvement. Part I: Improvement in incomplete traumatic quadriparesis. *J Bone Joint Surg Am* 1992;74:671–682.

88. Wolf A, Wilberger JE. Timing of surgical intervention after spinal cord injury. In: Narayan RK, Wilberger JE, Povilshock JT, eds. *Neurotrauma.* New York: McGraw-Hill, 1996:1193–1199.

89. Young W, Bracken MB. The second National Acute Spinal Cord Injury Study. *J Neurotrauma* 1992;9:S397–S404.

90. Wilberger JE. Diagnosis and management of spinal cord trauma. *J Neurotrauma* 1991;8:S21–S28.

91. Krengel WF, Anderson PA, Yuan H, et al. Early versus delayed stabilization after cervical spinal cord injury. Presented at the Cervical Spine Research Society annual meeting, Philadelphia, December 1991.

92. Levi L, Wolf A, Rigamonti D, et al. Anterior decompression in cervical spine trauma: does timing of surgery affect the outcome? *Neurosurgery* 1991;29:216–221.

93. Heary RF, Vaccaro AR, Northrup BE, et al. Long-term outcome of victims of cervical gunshot wounds. Presented at the Congress of Neurological Surgeons annual meeting, San Francisco, 1995.

SUGGESTED READING

Anglen J, Meltzer M, Bunn P, et al. Flexion and extension views are not cost effective in a cervical spine clearance protocol for obtunded trauma patients. *J Trauma* 2002;52:54–59.

Benzel EC, Doezema D. Prehospital management of spinally injured patient. In: Narayan RK, Wilberger JE, Povlishock JT, eds. *Neurotrauma.* New York: McGraw-Hill, 1995:1113–1121.

Bracken MB, Shepard MJ, Collins WF, et al. A randomized, controlled trial of methylprednisolone or naloxone in the treatment of acute spinal cord injury. *N Engl J Med* 1990;322:1405–1411.

Eismont FJ, Clifford S, Goldberg M, et al. Cervical sagittal spinal canal size in spine injury. *Spine* 1984;9:663–666.

Schenants PJ, Diaj J, Kaiser C, et al. Prospective comparison of admission computed tomographic scan and plain films of the upper cervical spine in trauma patients with altered mental status. *J Trauma* 2001;51:663–668.

CHAPTER 54

Medical Rehabilitation of Patients After Spinal Cord Injury

Jack E. Zigler

Spinal cord injury (SCI) is a catastrophic event that, in an instant, can irrevocably change the course of an otherwise healthy young person's life. The individual, typically a young male, is suddenly immersed into a new world of emergency medical care, spinal immobilization, emergency room assessment, possible surgical intervention, and initial total dependency on strangers to provide all the basic aspects of self-care that were previously taken completely for granted. Additionally, social, emotional, physical, and economic concerns are quickly factored into the new equation of life for this individual.

The acute care hospital offers the first steps in medical and surgical stabilization, but it is in the rehabilitation facility that the patient is helped to regain the emotional stability, the physical strength, and the daily life skills he or she must learn in order to reintegrate into society at the maximal level attainable for his or her level of injury. Spinal cord injury rehabilitation centers make use of the multidisciplinary team approach, so that specialized workers can use their unique expertise to address the complex problems of these patients in a complementary fashion. This system has been honed in the last 50 years and has shown measurable and important results in improving quality of care.

Since 1973, the National Spinal Injury Database has captured data from an estimated 13% of new SCI cases in the United States. As of May 2001, this database contained information on nearly 21,000 patients with acute spinal cord injuries. In 1979, the federal Model Systems grant empowered institutions that had acute care neurotrauma facilities, inpatient rehabilitation units, and outpatient care systems to receive monies for operations and participation in data sharing through a centralized database. Twenty-nine Model Systems facilities were funded in 2000 and are providing care today as regional SCI centers. Their goal is to oversee the patient's care from the emergency facility through inpatient rehabilitation and on to outpatient and community services.

Sharing data and clinical information in providing care has resulted in significant cost savings and improved patient outcomes (1). For those entered into Model Systems management immediately following injury, the average number of days hospitalized in the acute care facility has declined from 26 days in 1974 to 16 days in 1999. Days in the rehabilitation unit during the same interval have decreased from 115 days to 44 days. After his Chicago unit joined the Model Systems, Meyer reported in 1980 that cases of complete SCI at the unit decreased from 50% to 39% of new injuries, reflecting improved care in handling the newly traumatized individual (1). Similarly, Tator reported in 1993 a decrease in complete injuries from 65% to 46% in his Toronto spinal injury unit, and noted a decrease in overall morbidity from 20% to 9% (1).

Rehabilitation efforts are patient-centered. The goal of the health care team is to educate patients so that they may make appropriate care decisions in their lives. Patients are instructed in the self-care skills they will need to maintain their health. Family members are encouraged to participate in the rehabilitation process. Short- and long-term goals are established for the patient and the family, tailored to maximize each individual's potential. Strengthening a wrist extensor muscle in a patient with poor C6 function may allow that patient, with an appropriate orthosis, to independently grasp a utensil and feed himself or herself. This small act may reaffirm some measure of independence in an individual who feels that he or she has lost much control over life. Strengthening a triceps muscle by therapy or muscle transfer surgery may allow a C7 tetraplegic patient to transfer independently from wheelchair to bed, and may obviate the need for a full-time attendant. This results in cost savings as well as increased self-esteem.

The long-term results of this organized system of care are encouraging. By postinjury year 10, 32% of paraplegics and 24% of tetraplegics are employed. Of all persons discharged from the system, 88.7% are sent to a private, non-institutional residence (in most cases, their homes before injury). Only 4.8% are discharged to nursing homes. Life expectancies for persons with SCI continue to increase, but remain 10% to 20% below their age-matched able-bodied cohorts. Mortality rates are higher during the first year postinjury, especially for the severely injured. The most common causes of death for the individuals followed in the database since 1973 have been pneumonia, pulmonary emboli, and septicemia (2).

TEAM APPROACH

In no other aspect of medical care is a team approach as necessary as in spinal cord injury. Vernon Nickel used the multidisciplinary approach that had worked well for polio rehabilitation at Rancho Los Amigos when he developed Rancho's spinal injury rehabilitation center. Nursing, physical and occupational therapy, catheter care, psychology, sexual counseling, recreational therapy, speech therapy, and social services are all key components of the team giving input to each patient's care plan. Team rounds allow the various disciplines involved in the patient's care to have concurrent input into the care plan, and different services enjoy goal-oriented interaction. Mutually acceptable decisions are made at these team meetings, so that patients are presented with a unified care plan that all services have helped establish.

Spine surgeons, who were instrumental in establishing spinal injury rehabilitation centers and traditionally played key roles in the multidisciplinary team, have stepped back to allow other members of the team to assume more prominent roles. Most units are now directed by nonsurgeons.

Rehabilitation Nursing

Understanding coexisting medical diseases and the accurate delivery of care for patients with diabetes or cardiopulmonary disease is the daily responsibility of the nursing team. Similarly, adequate nutrition needs to be monitored so the patient can maximize the benefits of the full program. Most patients lose 10% of their body weight in the first 4 weeks after injury, paralleled by nitrogen excretion. Calcium excretion usually plateaus at 150% above baseline (3,4). Bowel programs are instituted upon admission after the neurologic lesion is diagnosed. Bladder protocols are designed by a urology consultant, but are typically implemented by a catheter care team and the nursing service.

Poor nursing care can significantly impair the achievement of rehabilitation goals. Complications of poor skin care can be very costly in both dollars and time. Skin breakdown usually reflects suboptimal early postinjury management, and may occur in 28% to 85% of patients (5,6). A full-thickness sacral decubitus may prolong hospitalization and cost up to $70,000 in additional health care costs. Prevention requires nursing vigilance, proper patient positioning, and strongly interactive patient education. As with many preventable problems, prophylaxis begins with the nursing staff education program.

Nurses provide the first line of awareness for several potentially life-threatening problems that can affect this specific patient population. Acute pulmonary obstruction in a tetraplegic patient who cannot clear secretions requires close nursing observation as well as frequent position changes and suctioning. Early and aggressive pulmonary toilet and early patient mobilization are recommended, but up to 62% of SCI patients still encounter serious respiratory morbidity (7).

Vital signs may be altered following acute SCI, and normal sympathetic adjustments may not occur, resulting in exaggerated orthostatic changes. The average tetraplegic patient has a resting heart rate of 60 and a blood pressure of 100/60 mm Hg. Patients with SCI may have been fluid overloaded in the field as a result of these vital signs, and may be at risk for acute respiratory distress syndrome (ARDS) within the first few days of injury.

Autonomic dysreflexia, caused by stimulation of the sympathetic and parasympathetic systems, results in a reflex rise in blood pressure that cannot be relieved by the normal compensatory mechanisms. Symptoms of headache, sweating above the injury level, facial flushing, urticaria, or nasal congestion may occur with bladder distention, kidney stones, bladder infection, spasms, blocked catheter tubing, or too-rapid bladder emptying. Other common causes are colonic distention, skin irritation, or even a tight leg bag. Treatment demands early recognition by the nursing service, sitting the patient up, close monitoring of vital signs, loosening clothing, checking catheter tubing, and carefully monitoring bladder drainage.

Consulting Services

Orthopaedic surgery, neurosurgery, urology, internal medicine, plastic surgery, general surgery, otolaryngology, and dental services are all required on a consulting basis to the spinal cord injury rehabilitation team. If appropriate specialty services are not available in the rehabilitation facility, patients may need to spend more time in the acute care hospital, which delays their program completion. Urologic intervention may be needed for urinary tract infections and calculi, as well as for drainage procedures. Surgical treatment of contractures and pressure sores may be required despite the best active preventive care.

Psychological intervention helps the patient deal with the many changes that are occurring in the individual's life as a result of the spinal cord injury. The adjustment to a major neurologic injury is similar to the stages of grieving: denial, anger, bargaining, depression, and acceptance. Another theory proposes five phases of adjustment in which the patient passes through shock, panic, defensive retreat, acknowledgment, and ultimately adaptation. The rehabilitation team uses its regular meetings as a forum to help ensure that the patient's adaptive behaviors do not interfere with the overall progress toward his or her individually developed goals. The patient's family often needs to be involved in these meetings and in dealing with the phases of the acceptance process.

Sexual counseling and education is of prime concern to young patients. Neurologic education, alternative behaviors, and precautions are all discussed with the patient and his or her significant other.

Physical Therapy

A comprehensive evaluation of the patient's neurologic status and the condition of the musculoskeletal system is performed prior to treatment. This evaluation provides the functional level, which serves as the basis for development of a treatment plan to achieve long-term goals specific for each patient. The American Spinal Injury Association (ASIA) standards are universally accepted for evaluation, which allows consistent data for communication between clinicians and centers regarding SCI. The comprehensive evaluation consists of eight major areas of emphasis: sensory testing, motor control, respiratory function, joint range of motion (ROM), muscle tone, skin integrity, functional level, and bulbar function.

Muscle testing utilizing the ASIA standards identifies key muscles in the upper and lower extremities that correspond to each neurologic level. ASIA defines a functional muscle as having a grade of 3 on a five-point scale (ability to move a joint through a full ROM against gravity, but not against resistance). However, many clinicians use 3+ as a minimal functional grade, requiring the ability to work against some resistance. A manual muscle grade below the "functional level" implies that the patient will not have the endurance to perform functional tasks and will not have enough strength to move objects against gravity (Table 54.1).

Spinal cord–injured patients are generally described by whether their injury is complete or incomplete and by their level of injury. In most spinal injury rehabilitation centers, the level of injury, or the functional level, is defined by the motor level that is 3+ or better and has bilaterally intact sensation. This level is used by the entire team in establishing a diagnosis and prognosis, as well as for anticipated functional outcome.

Defining complete versus incomplete spinal cord injury requires that the patient be out of spinal shock during the evaluation, and that the presence or absence of sacral sparing be ascertained (Table 54.2). If there is any communication between the cerebral cortex and the conus medullaris, the injury is incomplete and the possibility of potential return of neurologic function is improved.

Occupational Therapy

The occupational therapist's goal is to help the patient attain the greatest possible degree of self-sufficiency and independence in activities of daily living (ADLs). Equipment is prescribed by the therapist to enhance the functioning of patients, particularly tetraplegics. From a practical standpoint, occupational therapists tend to work with upper extremity function, whereas physical therapists tend to work with lower extremity and trunk function, as well as ambulation and wheelchair skills.

The occupational therapist's evaluation is similar to that of the physical therapist, but typically also includes a home and community evaluation, a prevocational evaluation, and a driving evaluation. Long-term ADL goals are set for discharge from the rehabilitation hospital. Age, height, weight, physical endurance, and lifestyle may all influence the optimal level of function, so it is not merely a reflection of the patient's neurologic level.

TABLE 54.1. *Spinal Level of Injury and Key Muscle Groups*

Level	Muscle group(s)
C5	Elbow flexors (biceps, brachialis)
C6	Wrist extensors (extensors carpi radialis longus and brevis)
C7	Elbow extensors (triceps)
C8	Finger flexors (flexor digitorum profundus) to middle finger
T1	Small finger abductor (abductor digiti minimi)
L2	Hip flexors (iliopsoas)
L3	Knee extensors (quadriceps)
L4	Ankle dorsiflexors (tibialis anterior)
L5	Long toe extensors (extensor hallucis longus)
S1	Ankle plantar flexors (gastrocnemius, soleus)

TABLE 54.2. *American Spinal Injury Association Impairment Scale*

Grade	Category	Description
A	Complete	No sensory or motor function is preserved in the sacral segments S4–S5.
B	Incomplete	Sensory but not motor function is preserved below the neurologic level and extends through the sacral segments S4–S5.
C	Incomplete	Motor function is preserved below the neurologic level, and the majority of key muscles below the neurologic level have a muscle grade below 3.
D	Incomplete	Motor function is preserved below the neurologic level, and the majority of key muscles below the neurologic level have a muscle grade of 3 or higher.
E	Normal	Sensory and motor function are normal.

FUNCTIONAL SKILLS

In tetraplegic patients, each spinal nerve level that can be spared is of critical importance for the patient's ultimate function. A patient with a C5 injury can flex and abduct the shoulders and flex the elbows. Although these patients may be able to propel a manual wheelchair with adapted hand rims over short distances, muscle weakness and limited endurance will necessitate a power wheelchair with hand controls. Such a patient will require assistance for all transfers and bed mobility activities.

When the C6 level is functional, normal shoulder girdle muscle strength allows better wheelchair propulsion endurance, may allow looping sliding board transfers, and provides the capacity for independent pressure relief by leaning forward in the wheelchair. When C7 is intact, the patient has full innervation to the clavicular portion of the pectoralis major, the serratus anterior, and all the wrist extensor muscles. Additionally, the sternal pectoralis major, the triceps, and the latissimus dorsi muscles are all partially innervated. The presence of the serratus and latissimus provides the essential components of the force couple for shoulder girdle stability, allowing depression-type raises for pressure relief, independent transfers, and the ability to propel a manual wheelchair over a variety of surfaces and inclines.

Wheelchair skills are an integral part of the reintegration process by which the individual with SCI rejoins society. Higher-level wheelchair skills include the ability to propel the chair on uneven surfaces such as grass, gravel, and dirt; to safely propel up and down a 10-degree slope; to handle curb cut-outs; and to perform wheelies over small obstacles or curbs. Most paraplegics are able to acquire these skills. Lower cervical level tetraplegic patients may eventually acquire these skills, but the lack of trunk balance musculature makes these tasks more difficult. The most difficult advanced skills are transferring from ground to wheelchair (e.g., after falling out of the chair) and wheelies.

SPECIAL CONSIDERATIONS

Deep venous thrombosis has been reported historically to occur after SCI in 14% to 16% of patients based on clinical parameters, but in 47% to 100% using more sophisticated diagnostic tools (e.g., Doppler ultrasonography, iodine-125 fibrinogen scans, contrast dye venography). The severity of the motor deficit and injury at a thoracic level both increase the risk of thromboembolic complications (8–10). The major factors predisposing persons with acute SCI to venous thromboembolism include venous stasis secondary to failure of the venous muscle pump (a consequence of the paralysis) and a transient hypercoagulable state. Various management modalities (exercise and early mobilization, intermittent compression boots, and anticoagulant prophylaxis within 72 hours of injury) have resulted in a lower incidence of deep venous thrombosis, reported by some centers to be as low as 5%.

Heterotopic ossification occurs following both adult brain injury and spinal cord injury. Early diagnosis based on clinical findings of warmth and swelling (often in an insensate joint area) and corroboration on bone scan should alert the team to initiate treatment. Antiinflammatory medication has been used in the past, but disodium etidronate, which works by inhibiting the formation and growth of hydroxyapatite crystals, has been successfully used in combination with aggressive physical therapy (11,12). Surgical resection is sometimes necessary when joint malalignments interfere with skin care or cause pressure ulcerations. Surgery is associated with a high morbidity, including hemorrhage, sepsis, and reankylosis (13).

Osteoporosis results from marked calcium resorption following SCI. Bone loss following SCI appears to follow a selective pattern, with the most significant loss involving the hips, relatively sparing the lumbar spine. Using dual-energy x-ray absorptiometry (DEXA) scans, Garland demonstrated mean bone mineral density in patients with SCI and fractures to be significantly lower than in those with SCI and no fractures, although both groups were below the fracture threshold of 1 g/cm^2. The fracture group's bone mineral density was 49% of able-bodied controls. Pharmacologic agents (calcitonin, bisphosphonates) are generally utilized but have not yet been shown to be effective in reducing osteoporosis in patients with SCI.

Spasticity is defined as a velocity-dependent increase in stretch reflexes. Patients with incomplete lesions usually exhibit greater spasticity than those with complete lesions. A physical therapy stretching program is the first line of treatment. Muscle relaxers, such as baclofen, potentiate the inhibitory effect of gamma aminobutyric acid (GABA). Other medications that are occasionally useful are benzodiazepams, dantrolene, and clonidine.

Contractures may occur despite ROM stretching programs and splinting. Surgery is sometimes required, and tendon lengthenings, tenotomies, and neurectomies are occasionally necessary. Hip adductors, the Achilles tendon, and the obturator nerve are the most common sites of surgical intervention.

Spinal cord pain may be manifested as a constant burning, numbness, or tingling below the level of injury. Gunshot wounds to the spine are notoriously associated with spinal pain syndromes. Various medications such as antidepressants, anticonvulsants, sodium channel blockers, opioids, clonidine, potassium channel blockers, and specific receptor agonists have been prescribed with somewhat uneven success. Electrical stimulation and nerve blocks may be tried, but are rarely helpful. Surgical intervention is sometimes attempted as a last resort, but it, too, has a generally poor success rate (14).

PROGNOSIS AND OUTCOMES

Initially, the medical care of the patient with a spinal cord injury is shared between the surgical team and the rehabilitation team. The surgical team's goals are prevention of progression of the neurologic deficit. These goals are addressed through temporary mechanical stabilization, medical stabilization, and surgical stabilization with possible decompression of the spine. The focus of the rehabilitation team is to assess and maintain the multiple organ systems potentially affected by the injury and to prepare the patient for a return to the community by restoring, substituting, and modifying function.

Neurologic exams performed soon after injury are often used for diagnostic labeling as well as to help formulate expected functional outcomes for each injured patient. This information is important to the patient and family, the health care team, and to third-party payers to justify the appropriateness of medical intervention and rehabilitation expenses. The 72-hour examination and the 1-month postinjury examination are the most useful as predictors of recovery and outcome.

In complete tetraplegia, there is little chance of functional motor recovery after 1 month postinjury. Weak muscles in the upper extremity, however, may continue to strengthen to functionally significant levels, and root escape to the next level may occur in 70% to 80% of patients. The majority of neurologic recovery in patients with complete injuries occurs during the first 6 to 9 months, with a rapid plateau occurring thereafter at 12 to 18 months.

Incomplete injuries show greater recovery potential. In incomplete paraplegia, 85% of muscles that were grades 1 or 2 at 1 month recovered to at least grade 3 by 1 year postinjury. In comparison, only 26% regained "motor useful" function if they were graded 0/5 at 1 month. In both incomplete tetraplegia and paraplegia, the most improvement was noted within the first 6 to 9 months, and a plateau was reached at 1 year (15).

SUMMARY

A spinal cord injury has a profound impact on the life of an individual, and demands multidisciplinary care that can best be delivered in a rehabilitation facility equipped with the appropriate personnel and services. Historical data support the advantages of regionalized care in the rehabilitation of SCI. Specialized skills are required for initial stabilization and assessment, as well as for aggressive goal-directed treatment programs. Early examinations can provide important information regarding recovery potential and anticipated outcomes. Day-to-day care by allied health personnel is essential to maximize the patient's potentials for functional recovery and reintegration into society.

REFERENCES

1. Stover SL, DeLisa JA, Whiteneck GG. *Spinal cord injury: clinical outcomes from the Model Systems.* Gaithersburg, MD: Aspen, 1995.
2. Stover SL, Fine PR. *Spinal cord injury: the facts and figures.* Birmingham: University of Alabama at Birmingham, 1986.
3. Halm MA. Elimination concerns with acute spinal trauma: assessment and nursing interventions. *Crit Care Nurs Clin North Am* 1990;2:385–398.
4. Rodriguez DJ, Benzel EC, Clevenger FW. The metabolic response to spinal cord injury. *Spinal Cord* 1997;35:599–604.
5. Mawson AR, Biundo JJ Jr, Neville P, et al. Risk factors for early occurring pressure ulcers following spinal cord injury. *Am J Phys Med Rehabil* 1988;67:123–127.
6. Mawson AR, Siddiqui FH, Biundo JJ. Enhancing host resistance to pressure ulcers: a new approach to prevention. *Prev Med* 1993;22:433–450.
7. Lam AM. Acute spinal cord injury: monitoring and anesthetic implications. *Can J Anaesth* 1991;38(4 Pt 2):60–73.
8. Green D. Prevention of thromboembolism after spinal cord injury. *Semin Thromb Hemost* 1991;17:347–350.
9. Kulkarni JR, Burt AA, Tromans AT, et al. Prophylactic low dose heparin anticoagulant therapy in patients with spinal cord injuries: a retrospective study. *Paraplegia* 1992;30:169–172.
10. Merli GJ. Management of deep venous thrombosis in spinal cord injury. *Chest* 1992;102(Suppl 6):652–657.
11. Garland DE. Clinical observations on fractures and heterotopic ossification in the spinal cord and traumatic brain injured populations. *Clin Orthop* 1988;233:86–101.
12. Garland DE, Alday B, Venos KG, et al. Diphosphonate treatment for heterotopic ossification in spinal cord injury patients. *Clin Orthop* 1983;176:197–200.
13. Garland DE, Orwin JF. Resection of heterotopic ossification in patients with spinal cord injuries. *Clin Orthop* 1989;242:169–176.
14. Burchiel KJ, Hsu FPK. Pain and spasticity after spinal cord injury: mechanisms and treatment. *Spine* 2001;26(24S):S146–S160.
15. Burns AS, DiTunno JF. Establishing prognosis and maximizing functional outcomes after spinal cord injury. *Spine* 2001;26(24S):S137–S145.

CHAPTER 55

Nontraumatic Syringomyelia

Andrew R. Brodbelt, Marcus A. Stoodley, and Nigel R. Jones

HISTORY

Syringomyelia remains one of the most enigmatic conditions affecting the nervous system. Descriptions of cystic cord cavitation were made by Estienne (1) in 1546, Brunner in 1688, and Morgagni in 1761 (2). Ollivier d'Angers (3) described pathological dilatation of the central canal, which he believed was a developmental anomaly, in 1824. The first clinical correlation was made by Portal (4), who in 1804 recognized that progressive sensory loss and paralysis of the limbs of a servant was associated with cystic spinal cord cavitation. Further observations were made by Gull in 1862 and Clarke in 1865 (5); in 1882, Schultze (6) described the classic clinical syndrome, including reduced sensation of pain and temperature. The presentation of the disease was well recognized by Gowers (7) in his *Manual of Diseases of the Nervous System* in 1886. Since the first operative decompression of a spinal cord cyst by Abbe and Coley (8) in 1892, the treatment of syringomyelia has been essentially surgical.

The association between syringomyelia and other nervous system abnormalities was made by Langhans, who described a case associated with cerebellar deformity (5). Chiari described three types of cerebellar malformation in 1891, two of which (types I and II) were associated with "hydromyelia" (5). Syringomyelia is now known to be associated with many abnormalities of the nervous system, but despite being the subject of extensive speculation, its pathogenesis remains unknown.

DEFINITIONS

Ollivier (3) introduced the term *syringomyelia* in 1827 to describe pathological dilatation of the central canal, after the Greek *syrinx,* meaning pipe, tube, or channel, and *myelus,* meaning marrow. In Greek lore, the nymph Syrinx, while being chased by Pan, prayed to be turned into a clump of weeds. On embracing her, Pan found he was clutching a handful of reeds. Sighing, he elicited a pleasant sound from the reeds. *Syrinx* or *syringe* thus came to mean a shepherd's pipe or tube (9).

After publication of Stillings's work in 1856 (10), *hydromyelia* was used to describe a dilatation of the central canal, and *syringomyelia* to refer to a cystic cavity separate from the central canal (11,12). In attempts to avoid confusion, *syringohydromyelia, hydrosyringomyelia,* and *progressive posttraumatic cystic myelopathy* have been used as encompassing terms for both types of cavity (13–16). Pseudosyringomyelia was introduced to differentiate cysts occurring in association with tumors, hemorrhage, or necrosis, in the belief that these cysts are not formed as a result of altered cerebrospinal fluid (CSF) dynamics (17).

In the current text, syringomyelia will be used to describe all abnormal fluid-filled cavities within the spinal cord except small nonenlarging cavities secondary to trauma or necrosis occurring at the site of injury (18). Qualifying terms, such as *posttraumatic,* are used when necessary to differentiate various types of syringomyelia.

EPIDEMIOLOGY

Syringomyelia affects mainly children and young adults, with an average age of presentation before 29 years (15, 19,20). Although it was once regarded as rare, magnetic resonance imaging (MRI) studies now show that 57% to 65% of patients with a Chiari malformation and up to 28% of all spinal injury patients have syringomyelia (19,21–24). Reported demographic data relied on limited population studies performed prior to the development of MRI and almost certainly underestimated the true frequency of the diagnosis. These reports suggested a prevalence of 5.6 to 9 per 100,000 population, an incidence of 0.09 to 0.44 cases per year per 100,000 population, and approximately 22,000 people affected in the United States (25–28). A prevalence of 130 per 100,000 has been reported for some regions of the Russian Federation (29).

There have been several reports of familial syringomyelia and of syringomyelia occurring in siblings with healthy parents (19,30–34). There is no clinical difference between these familial and the vastly more common sporadic cases (33). Human leukocyte antigen (HLA) A9 appears to be more frequent in patients with syringomyelia (34,35). Both autosomal recessive and dominant inheritance have been implicated, but case numbers are too few to be conclusive (19,34). Inheritance of associated predisposing conditions does lead to a higher frequency of syringomyelia (34).

ASSOCIATED CONDITIONS

Syringomyelia occurs in association with a wide array of congenital and acquired conditions. Most cases are associated with an abnormality at the craniocervical junction, a localized spinal abnormality, or trauma (Fig. 55.1). Other common associations include occult spinal dysraphism, intramedullary and extramedullary tumors, and arachnoiditis. Idiopathic cases are rare and may represent missed pathology. Focal areas of arachnoiditis or arachnoid webs are easily overlooked with standard imaging studies (36,37).

Malformations at the Craniocervical Junction

Most, if not all, abnormalities occurring at the craniocervical junction causing compression of the medulla or spinal cord have been reported in association with syringomyelia. Such syrinxes are often immediately caudal to the level of compression, but there may be an intervening segment of normal spinal cord.

In the Chiari type I malformation, there is overcrowding of the hindbrain by mesenchymal underdevelopment of the posterior cranial fossa, and caudal displacement of the cerebellar tonsils of usually more than 5 mm (19,38,39). The Chiari II malformation is a neuroectodermal defect associated with myelomeningocele, consisting of downward displacement of the caudal cerebellum and medulla in association with myelodysplasia and complex brain anomalies (19). Both types are seen commonly in association with syringomyelia, although not all patients with Chiari malformations develop syrinxes (19,40). Syrinxes are found in 65% of symptomatic patients with Chiari I malformations (19). There is disagreement concerning the relationship of syringomyelia to the extent of tonsillar herniation (41,42).

Syrinxes may be seen with chronic tonsillar herniation associated with other congenital abnormalities or with herniation secondary to lumbar CSF shunting, cerebellar tumors, or supratentorial lesions (Table 55.1). The Dandy-Walker malformation (cystic dilatation of the fourth ventricle and dysgenesis of the vermis) usually is associated with hydrocephalus and occasionally with a syrinx (43).

Syringomyelia also may accompany virtually any other congenital or acquired chronic compression at the craniocervical junction.

Congenital Spinal Malformations

Syringomyelia may be seen with congenital spinal malformations. Syrinxes have been reported to develop in 35% of patients with occult spinal dysraphism, 37% to 53% of patients with diastematomyelia, and 24% of patients with a tethered spinal cord (44–46). Syrinxes associated with occult spinal dysraphism occur predominantly in the caudal third of the spinal cord and may form rostral or caudal to the lesion but are usually in close proximity and rostral (45).

Spinal Intramedullary Tumors

Syringomyelia may be seen with virtually any intramedullary tumor (Fig. 55.2) (47–49). Two thirds of patients with hemangioblastomas and half of those with spinal ependymomas had an associated syrinx (50–53). Intramedullary spinal cord tumors were found at postmortem in 10% to 16% of patients with syringomyelia (54,55). Conversely, syrinxes were seen in 31% to 58% of autopsied cases of spinal cord tumor (49,55,56). In a series of 100 patients with intramedullary tumors, 45 had a syrinx (49). Of these syrinxes, 49% were rostral to the tumor, 11% were caudal, and 40% were both above and below the tumor (49). Syrinxes were seen in 50% of adult patients and 21% of pediatric patients. There appears to be a higher incidence of syringomyelia with tumors of the more rostral spinal cord (49).

Chronic Extramedullary Spinal Cord Compression

Syringomyelia in association with an extramedullary mass is not common but may be seen with neoplasms, cysts, lipomas, cervical disc disease, or spondylosis (52,57–59). The syrinx may be caudal or rostral to the lesion, but is usually caudal (60–62). We have seen syrinxes caudal to cervical disc protrusions, tumors, spinal deformity, and arachnoid cysts. In a series of 51 cases of syringomyelia reported by Milhorat and colleagues (59), 25 were associated with extramedullary lesions causing chronic cord compression, although the authors included 14 cases of Chiari malformation in this group. Cervical disc protrusions, tumors, and craniospinal deformity accounted for the other cases. In each case, the syrinx arose immediately caudal to the lesion and did not extend rostrally. Longer lesions were found in younger patients (59). In two of three cases of cervical disc protrusion, the syrinx resolved following discectomy, and excision of other extramedullary masses resulted in resolution of the syrinxes (59).

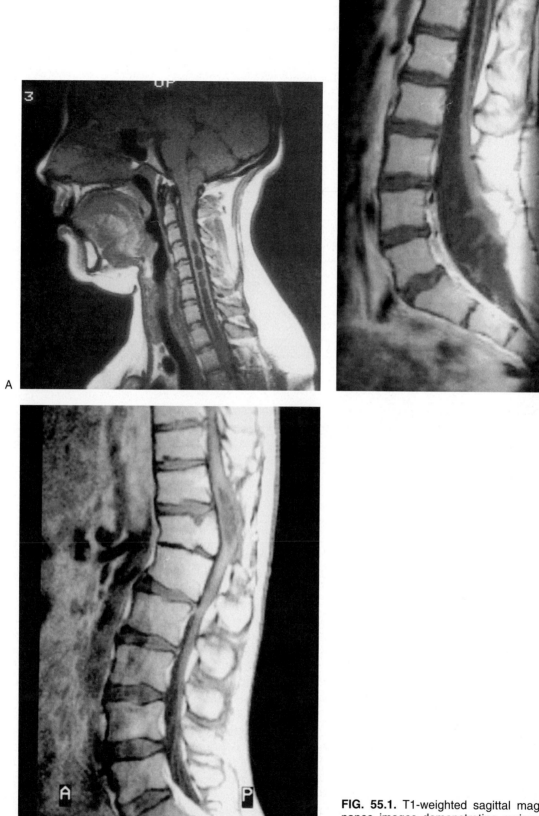

FIG. 55.1. T1-weighted sagittal magnetic resonance images demonstrating syringomyelia associated with Chiari malformation **(A)**, lipomyelomeningocele **(B)**, and spinal trauma **(C)**.

TABLE 55.1. *Conditions Associated with Syringomyelia*

Craniocervical junction	Spine
Congenital	
Chiari malformation type I (19)	Myelomeningocele
Chiari malformation type II	Tethered spinal cord (44,225)
Dandy-Walker malformation (43)	Diastematomyelia (45,226)
Posterior fossa arachnoid cysts (43,227)	Lipomyelomeningocele (228,229)
Apert's syndrome with tonsillar herniation (230,231)	Spinal dermoid (45)
Crouzon's syndrome (230)	Neurenteric cyst (232)
Noonan's syndrome (233,234)	Sacral agenesis (235)
Achondroplasia (236)	Anorectal anomalies (237)
	Familial spinal arachnoiditis (238)
Acquired	
Tonsillar herniation secondary to	*Intramedullary*
Posterior fossa tumor (239)	Neoplastic
Supratentorial tumors (240)	Primary: Ependymoma, hemangioblastoma, astrocytoma, lymphoma (48–51)
Lumboperitoneal shunts (91,241)	Metastases (47)
Chronic subdural hematoma (242)	Nonneoplastic
Lhermitte-Duclos disease (243)	Spinal trauma
Nocardia brain abscess (244)	Demyelination, multiple sclerosis (245)
Basilar impression (61)	Spinal sarcoidosis (246); tuberculosis (247)
Pannus deformity of the odontoid (61)	*Extramedullary*
Arachnoiditis	Neoplastic: Meningioma (62,248), schwannoma (249), lymphoma (250), myeloma (251,252), lipomatosis (251,253)
Idiopathic (58)	Nonneoplastic
	Intervertebral disc protrusion (59)
	Cervical spinal stenosis (57,59)
	Arachnoiditis (58,68)
	Arachnoid telangiectasia inducing arachnoiditis (254)
	Intraventricular hemorrhage, subarachnoid hemorrhage, meningitis (58)
	Arachnoid web (37)
	Arachnoid ossification (255)
	Sarcoidosis (246)
	Spinal lipomas (256)
	Multiple sclerosis (257)
	Idiopathic (58)

Adapted from Stoodley MA, Jones NR. Syringomyelia. In: Cervical Spine Research Society, eds. *The cervical spine.* Philadelphia: Lippincott–Raven Publishers, 1998.

Arachnoiditis

Arachnoiditis of the posterior fossa or spine may be associated with syringomyelia (60,63–65). The arachnoiditis may follow bacterial meningitis, subarachnoid hemorrhage, tuberculosis, syphilitic pachymeningitis, trauma (including birth-related trauma), injected radiopaque dyes, surgery, or spinal anesthetics, or it may be idiopathic (33,37,58,63–68). The syrinx usually forms caudal to the area of arachnoiditis (33). Arachnoiditis is common in patients with noncommunicating syringomyelia, usually in association with trauma, previous meningitis, or subarachnoid hemorrhage (15,64,69–72).

Spinal Trauma

Until recently, posttraumatic syringomyelia was considered a rarity (53,73,74). Symptomatic syringomyelia develops in 1% to 9% of spinal injury patients (14,22,24,33,72, 75–77). Of patients who suffered a spinal injury and were imaged between 1 and 30 years after injury, 21% to 28% had a syrinx, and 30% to 50% had some sort of spinal cord cystic change (21,22,24,78–80). Syringomyelia does not appear to be more common after tetraplegia than after paraplegia, but does occur more frequently after a complete cord lesion than after a partial lesion (15,27,33,72,76,78). Whether the development of syringomyelia in this context is associated with the degree of spinal canal stenosis remains unclear (21,22,24).

Symptoms may occur as early as 2 months or as long as 35 years after the injury, with a mean of 7 to 13 years (27,33,72–74,76,81,82). Neurologic symptoms and signs usually begin unilaterally and progress cephalad in almost all patients, although a caudal progression may be seen (33,73). The cysts are usually juxtaposed to the injury site: rostral in 81%, caudal in 4%, and in both directions in 15% of cases (15,78). For more details, readers are referred to Chapter 56, "Posttraumatic Syringomyelia."

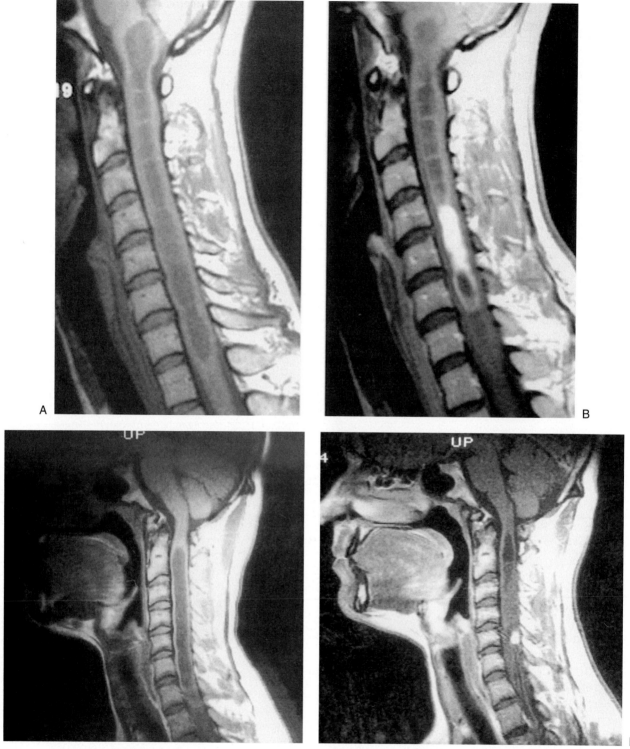

FIG. 55.2. Syringomyelia associated with intramedullary tumors. T1-weighted magnetic resonance imaging (MRI) before **(A)** and after **(B)** administration of intravenous paramagnetic contrast in a case of spinal cord fibrillary astrocytoma. The syrinx is seen on the precontrast scan as a low-signal area within the cord, but the tumor is not discernible. After contrast administration, the tumor becomes apparent as a high-signal lesion at the caudal end of the syrinx. Intramedullary hemangioblastoma is seen on a precontrast T1-weighted MRI **(D)** as a high-signal nodule that was not seen on the precontrast scan **(C)**.

PATHOLOGY

Syrinxes most commonly occur in the low cervical and upper thoracic spinal cord (15,18,33,43,58). A patient may have single or multiple, uni- or multiloculated cysts involving separate portions of the spinal cord (83,84). In one pathological study of 105 cases, the syrinx extended 2 to 5 levels in 32%, 6 to 10 levels in 37%, and 11 to 20 levels in 9%, and 24% had a holocord cavity (58). This distribution is somewhat different from that encountered in clinical practice, due to the inclusion of large numbers of extensive communicating syrinxes associated with severe congenital defects in the pathological series. Three percent to 17% of posttraumatic syrinxes extend more than 10 levels (15,58). Syrinxes can extend into the brainstem or even supratentorially (85). Syrinx enlargement often affects the crossing spinothalamic tracts (Fig. 55.3).

The histologic changes in the parenchyma surrounding syrinxes are similar regardless of the associated condition and represent the nonspecific results of a distensile force (18,58,86). Syrinx walls are generally formed of compressed glial tissue and flattened ependyma surrounded by gliosis (58,87,88). There is evidence of wallerian degeneration, macrophage infiltration, and demyelination in the surrounding white matter and of central chromatolysis and neuronophagia in the gray matter (58). Vascular changes may be seen around the cyst, including hyalinized and thickened vessels, edema, and hemorrhages. Aberrant nerve fibers may be seen in the wall of the cavity; these may arise from spinal ganglia and enter through the dorsal horns (33). Enlargement of the perivascular spaces may be observed (87).

Milhorat and associates (54,58,89) have classified syrinxes according to pathological and MRI findings as follows: (a) communicating central canal syrinxes, (b) noncommunicating central canal syrinxes, (c) extracanalicular syrinxes, (d) atrophic cavitations, and (e) neoplastic cavities (Fig. 55.4). The clinical findings with each type correlate with parenchymal damage, such as dissection, caused by the syrinx rather than with syrinx size alone.

Communicating Central Canal Syrinxes

Communicating central canal syrinxes consist of a dilated central canal in continuity with the fourth ventricle and are often associated with hydrocephalus. They occur in children and young adults with conditions such as the Chiari II malformation or Dandy-Walker cyst that obstruct CSF outflow from the fourth ventricle (58). In patients with an obstructed aqueduct of Sylvius, the fourth ventricle is isolated from the cerebral ventricles and its outlets are occluded. In these cases, the dilated upper central canal communicates with the isolated fourth ventricle. The cavities are lined wholly or in part by ependyma and are defined at their caudal end by central canal

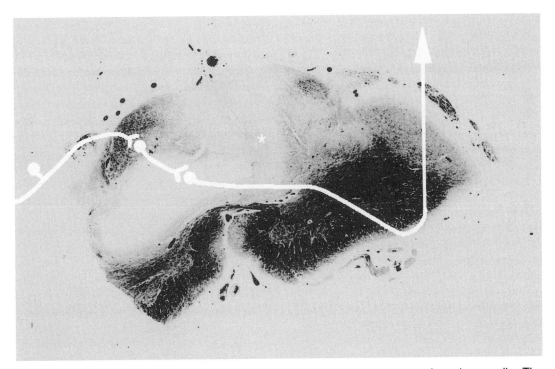

FIG. 55.3. Cross section of cervical spinal cord of a patient with posttraumatic syringomyelia. The crossing fibers of the lateral spinothalamic tract are preferentially affected by the enlarging syrinx as compared with relative preservation of the dorsal columns, producing the classic dissociated sensory loss. Enlargement of the central canal (*) and paracentral dissection, as occurs with canalicular syringomyelia, would also selectively damage the crossing spinothalamic fibers. (Pathological specimen courtesy of Dr. P. Blumbergs, with permission.)

I. Communicating

II. Noncommunicating
Canalicular

Extracanalicular

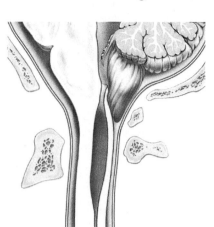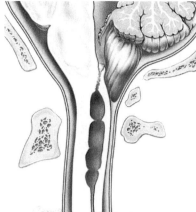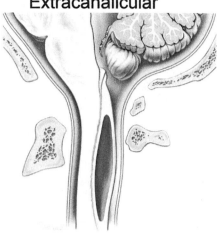

Other
III. Atrophic cavitiations (Syringomelia ex vacuo)
IV. Neoplastic cavitations

FIG. 55.4. Anatomical classification of syrinx cavities. Communicating syrinxes are associated with obstruction of the outlets of the fourth ventricle and often hydrocephalus. The syrinx communicates directly with the fourth ventricle via the central canal. Noncommunicating canalicular syrinxes start as dilatations of the central canal that do not communicate with the fourth ventricle, but may then rupture into the spinal cord. These are more common with chronic posterior fossa compression such as the Chiari type I malformation. Noncommunicating extracanalicular syrinxes form as a cavity separate to the central canal, and may occur after spinal cord trauma (From, Milhorat TH. Classification of syringomyelia. *Neurosurg Focus* 2000;8:1–6.).

stenosis. Because rupture or dissection of the enlarged central canal rarely occurs, this type of syrinx is asymptomatic or associated with nonspecific clinical findings (54,58,89).

Noncommunicating Central Canal Syrinxes

Noncommunicating central canal syrinxes are dilatations of the central canal found at a variable distance caudal to the fourth ventricle and are associated with conditions such as Chiari I malformation, cervical spinal stenosis, spinal arachnoiditis, and basilar impression. Most cavities are closed at their rostral end by canal stenosis, but some have an apparent communication with the fourth ventricle through a patent, although not enlarged, central canal. The cavities are complex, with extensive ependymal denudation and intracanalicular septations of spongy glial tissue (58,86). Paracentral dissection has been reported to occur in over 40% of cases, and therefore patients with this type of syrinx are more likely to have segmental neurologic deficits (54,58,89).

Extracanalicular Syrinxes

Noncommunicating extracanalicular syrinxes are associated with spinal trauma, infarction, hemorrhage, or transverse myelitis. The cavities are usually in the central gray matter, dorsal and lateral to the central canal. Most extra-

canalicular syrinxes are found in the central and dorsolateral gray matter, a vascular watershed, while 9% have been reported to occur in the white matter alone (33,58). Extracanalicular syrinxes are irregular in shape and commonly have hemosiderin-containing macrophages and microglia in the wall (58,88). In contrast to canalicular syrinxes, ependymal cells are not seen. In both noncommunicating canalicular and noncommunicating extracanalicular syrinxes, there may be direct communication with the subarachnoid space at the dorsal nerve root entry zones or ventromedian fissure (33, 58,86). Segmental neurologic deficits correlating with the extent of cord damage are common (54,58,89).

PATHOGENESIS

Early pathogenic theories included incomplete neural tube fusion, central cord necrosis, chronic inflammation, and neoplasia (2,11,65,90). The first suggestion of a role for CSF hydrodynamics in the formation of syrinxes came in 1908, although Morgagni had previously suggested that oversecretion of CSF distended the central nervous system, causing a dilated central canal and spina bifida (91, 92). Recent theories have centered on hydrodynamic factors, which can be divided into (a) the initiating factor or factors, (b) the source and fluid route into a syrinx, and (c) the driving force behind syrinx enlargement (Fig. 55.5).

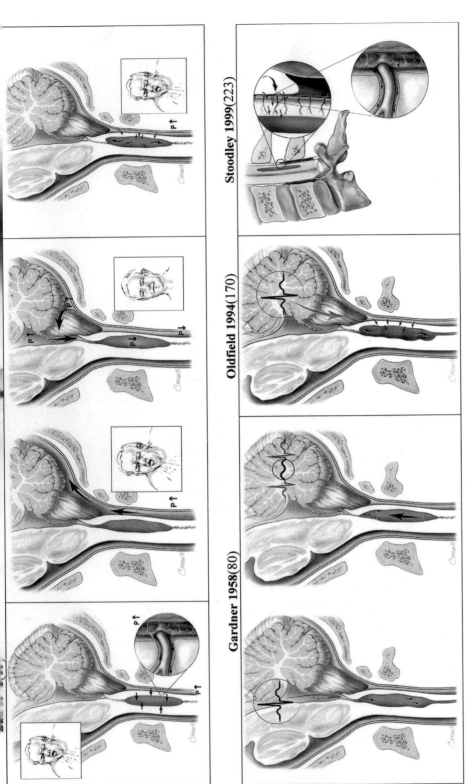

FIG. 55.5. Etiological theories of syringomyelia. Ball and Dayan (118) proposed that Valsalva maneuvers produce pressure waves within the subarachnoid space (SAS) that force fluid down perivascular spaces into the cord and syrinx. The syrinx was initiated by the coalescence of small pools of extracellular water. Williams and Fahy (215) suggested that the Valsalva maneuver forces fluid from the SAS of the spinal canal into the cranial cavity. After relaxation, cerebellar tonsils obstruct return flow into the spinal SAS, so fluid is "sucked" into the fourth ventricle and central canal. The syrinx is initiated by these pressure waves along the central canal, which also maintains it. Williams (80) later reasoned that, in some patients, the dilated central canal, once formed, becomes isolated. Valsalva-induced pressure waves on the surface of the cord compress the cavity, forcing fluid to "slosh" to the poles, dissecting normal spinal cord tissue and enlarging the syrinx. Gardner and Angel (121) contended that systole produces pressure waves in cerebrospinal fluid in the fourth ventricle, forcing fluid down the central canal because of congenital obstruction of the outlets of the fourth ventricle. In diastole the rostral central canal acts as a valve reducing fluid return. Oldfield and associates (146) suggested that during systole the cerebellar tonsils enlarge, causing a pressure wave down the SAS and forcing fluid across the spinal cord to form and enlarge a syrinx. Systolic-induced pressure waves on the surface of the cord could also compress the cavity, forcing fluid to move to the poles, dissecting normal spinal cord tissue and enlarging the syrinx, similar to Williams's slush theory. Finally, Stoodley and colleagues (139) believe that the penetrating arteries within the perivascular space act as a fluid pump continually forcing fluid into the spinal cord. An isolated cavity—either an isolated segment of spinal canal or previous hematoma cavity—aids syrinx initiation, and perturbations of subarachnoid space compliance alter inflow or outflow of the pump, producing a syrinx.

Cerebrospinal Fluid Hydrodynamic Factors

Syrinx Initiation

There is evidence to suggest that the initial formation of a spinal cord cavity in some circumstances may involve different mechanisms than those that lead to subsequent enlargement of such a cyst to form a syrinx. Loculated portions of the central spinal cord canal, as well as intraparenchymal inflammation, ischemia, excitotoxic amino acid release, hematoma formation, neoplasia, and arachnoiditis have all been implicated in the formation of isolated cavities.

Loculated segments of the central spinal cord canal are common. Central canal stenosis or occlusion has been reported to be present in 75% to 97% of autopsy cases after the third decade, and isolated segments occur between stenotic regions (93–95). Small incidental dilatations of these segments are occasionally seen at autopsy (58). It should be noted that cyst formation and edema are standard responses to injury in the central nervous system, and occur after parenchymal injury in the spinal cord (96–100). Arachnoiditis has been suggested to cause cord ischemia and repeated microtrauma with subsequent cyst formation (15,101). Compression at the foramen magnum is claimed to interfere with venous drainage, causing necrosis and cavities (102,103). However, widespread venous anastomoses and alternative venous channels in this area make this mechanism unlikely (104).

Pencil-shaped infarcts of the spinal cord, with a shape and location similar to syringomyelic cysts, are seen in compression myelopathy secondary to extradural tumor and also are observed in cases of spinal trauma, arachnoiditis, intramedullary tumors, and metastases (105,106). Further evidence for an ischemic role in syrinx initiation is that the common site of extracanalicular syrinxes is the vascular watershed within the cord (58). Experimental animal work also suggests that cysts formed by focal parenchymal injury precede syrinx development (107). After both spinal cord injury and ischemia, selective motor neuronal cell death occurs by glutamate receptor activation and calcium influx (108,109). Intraspinal injection of an excitatory amino acid produces extracanalicular syrinxes (110). The presence of an intraparenchymal hematoma after spinal trauma increases the likelihood of developing a syrinx and affects the size and speed of formation of the syrinx (15).

Some noncommunicating or extracanalicular syrinxes may form without an initial isolated cavity. Spinal cord edema has been noted prior to syrinx formation, and coalescence into larger fluid-filled cavities has been suggested (96,111).

Fluid Source and Route

Syrinx fluid almost certainly arises from CSF in the subarachnoid and interstitial spaces. Supporting evidence for this theory includes the similar chemical composition of CSF and syrinx fluid, the lack of an anatomical barrier to fluid flow across ependymal and pial surfaces, and tracer studies that show rapid flow between the subarachnoid and interstitial spaces via perivascular spaces (112–117). Although theoretical alternative sources also include intracellular and intravascular fluid, there are substantial differences in fluid composition as well as anatomical barriers limiting flow, such as cell membranes and the blood–brain barrier.

The possible routes of flow from the subarachnoid space to a syrinx cavity are from the fourth ventricle and central canal, transparenchymal flow, or along perivascular spaces (15,80,93,118–120). The original hydrodynamic theories of syrinx formation relied on fluid flow from the fourth ventricle into the central canal (Table 55.2). Gardner and Angel (121) suggested that congenital atresia of the outlets of the fourth ventricle channels choroid plexus systolic pulses of CSF (the waterhammer) down the narrow cervical central canal, which then acts as a one-way valve limiting return flow and causes progressive central canal enlargement (Fig. 55.5). Williams (122) suggested that CSF flowed from the spinal subarachnoid space into the cranial compartment during a Valsalva maneuver, and then flowed preferentially down the central canal during relaxation because the cerebellar tonsils obstructed return flow into the spinal subarachnoid space (the so-called suck mechanism, Fig. 55.5). According to this theory, noncommunicating syrinxes had either lost their original communication with the fourth ventricle or developed from an isolated cavity, with fluid derived from damaged cells and capillaries (122). Furthermore, external pressure on the cord could compress the cord and propel the syrinx contents longitudinally, dissecting the cord and enlarging the syrinx (the so-called slush mechanism) (122).

There is overwhelming evidence against these mechanisms in noncommunicating types of syringomyelia. Embryologic studies suggest that the outlets of the fourth ventricle do not rupture due to pressure but involute (123, 124). Extracanalicular noncommunicating syrinxes and intrasyrinx septations are difficult to explain by these theories, because there is no direct continuity with the central canal (58,125). In patients with syringomyelia, pathological data, myelography, and magnetic resonance imaging studies show little evidence of communication between the fourth ventricle and syrinx, and the incidence of canal stenosis in syrinx patients is similar to the normal population (27,58,126). The exception is in children with hydrocephalus and a Chiari II malformation—the enlarged central canal in these cases does communicate with the fourth ventricle (58).

In some human studies there is a substantial delay between intrathecal contrast injection and its appearance within the syrinx, and this has been used to suggest transmedullary penetration as opposed to direct flow (Fig. 55.6) (93–95,119). Recent animal work suggests that in extracanalicular syrinxes, transparenchymal flow occurs

TABLE 55.2. *Current Hypotheses for Syrinx Formation and Associated Difficulties*

Author and year (ref.)	Associated abnormality	Fluid source and route	Driving force	Comments and critique
Gardner and Angel, 1958 (121)	Atresia of fourth ventricle outlets; Chiari malformation	CSF, central canal	Arterial: Pulse in ventricular CSF	**Pathological and MRI studies** provide findings that are difficult to reconcile. Intrasyrinx septations exist, fourth ventricular outlet obstruction is uncommon, few fourth ventricles communicate with the central canal, and syrinx cavities can be completely extracanicular and noncommunicating (27,54,137,164,244). **Embryology** of fourth ventricle outlets suggests they do not rupture due to pressure, but involute (57,123).
Ball and Dayan, 1972 (118)	Chiari, acquired Chiari, and arachnoiditis	CSF, perivascular	Valsalva movement	**Physiology:** A calculated pulse pressure down the aqueduct is only on the order of 4×10^{-5} mm Hg and unlikely to drive fluid down the central canal (118). **Physiology:** Arterial pulsations are probably more important than venous transmitted pressure waves (3,27,99,139,141,142,177).
Williams and Fahy, 1980 (215)	Chiari	Central canal	Valsalva: Suck and slosh	**Pathological and MRI studies** show few fourth ventricles communicate with the central canal (27,54,137,164,181). A syrinx cavity can be completely extracanalicular and noncommunicating (137,244). **Physiology:** Arterial pulsations are probably more important than venous transmitted pressure waves (3,27,99,139,141,142,177). In a child with Chiari II, lumbar spinal pressures were always greater than intracranial pressures (181). Calculated pulse pressures down the aqueduct are only on the order of 4×10^{-5} mm Hg and unlikely to drive fluid down the central canal (118).
Williams, 1992 (80)	Adhesions	Cervical central canal before closure, perivascular	Valsalva: Slosh	**Physiology:** Arterial pulsations are probably more important than venous transmitted pressure waves (3,27,99,139,141,142,177). There is no experiment to indicate that fluid movement within the syrinx is large enough to dissect the cord.
Oldfield et al., 1994 (146)	Chiari I	CSF, perivascular, transparenchymal	Arterial: Tonsillar pulse in spinal CSF	**Pathology:** Explains only noncommunicating canalicular syrinxes. **Physiology:** The biomechanics of how CSF is forced across the spinal parenchyma and preferentially into the syrinx is not explained. **Treatment:** Syringosubarachnoid shunts should not work.
Stoodley et al., 1999 (139)	Isolation + CSF block	CSF, perivascular	Arterial	**Pathology:** 31% (18 of 58) of noncommunicating syrinxes (NCC and NCE) communicate with the subarachnoid space (137,146, 201,248). **Physiology:** Local spinal cord blood flow improves after syrinx decompression, suggesting an increase in perivascular fluid flow (19).

CSF, cerebral spinal fluid; NCC, noncommunicating canalicular; NCE, noncommunicating extracanalicular.

along the dorsal horn, and may indicate syrinx outflow (127).

Perivascular Fluid Flow

There is an anatomical pathway from the subarachnoid space to a syrinx cavity via the perivascular space. As arteries penetrate the central nervous system, they lose their pial coat (128–130). Some investigators argue that a pial coat distinctive from the adventitia is discernible around arterioles as they enter the spinal cord and becomes fragmented at its deeper aspect (131,132). In either case, the space between the blood vessel and the spinal cord is the Virchow-Robin space and is continuous with the subpial space and the interstitial

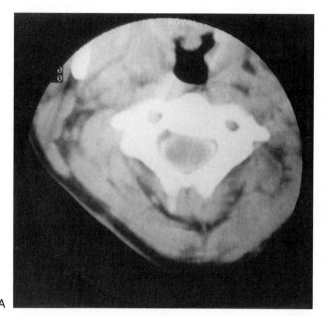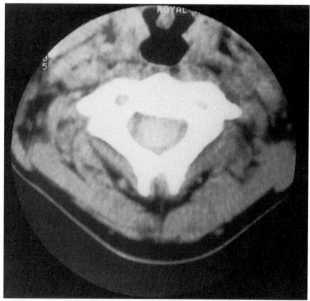

A   B

FIG. 55.6. Computed tomography myelogram immediately after intrathecal contrast injection **(A)**, and 48 hours later **(B)**. In the delayed scan, contrast is seen filling the syrinx cavity.

space (128–132). In all syrinxes, the discontinuous ependymal wall, if present, provides little barrier to fluid movement between the syrinx and the interstitial space.

Tracers placed in the cisterna magna rapidly appear in the perivascular space and migrate into the central canal (118,133–135). Ink injected into a syrinx at necropsy rapidly moves to the perivascular space (118). The pia mater is fully permeable, at least to solutes and horseradish peroxidase (HRP), although it appears to prevent the passage of larger objects such as erythrocytes (113,129,132,135). In animal models of noncommunicating canalicular and extracanalicular syringomyelia, the CSF tracer HRP rapidly flows from the subarachnoid space along the perivascular space and into the syrinx (Fig. 55.7) (120,127). Further evidence of perivascular flow into syrinxes is the dilated perivascular spaces that have been observed in some cases of syringomyelia (118,120).

Because there is evidence for rapid flow into syrinxes, there must be a route for fluid outflow. The role of perivenular spaces and transparenchymal routes in fluid outflow has not yet been investigated.

The Driving Force for Syrinx Enlargement

Syrinx enlargement must result from an imbalance of inflow and outflow. It is also reasonable to assume that the pressure within an enlarging syrinx must exceed the surrounding parenchymal pressure, and even the subarachnoid pressure. Intrasyrinx pressures of 0.5 to 22 cm of water have been measured, albeit in prone ventilated patients, often with the dura open and the arachnoid CSF drained (27,73,136,137). Syrinx pressures increase during respira-

tion (mean, 1.1 cm) and cardiac systole (mean, 0.7 cm) (27, 73,137). Histologic tissue changes surrounding syrinxes are consistent with the results of a nonspecific distensile force (18,58,86).

Theoretical mechanisms able to produce a high-pressure syrinx and rapid fluid flow include intraabdominal or intrathoracic pressure changes transmitted via the venous system, an arterial pulsation–driven system, a diffusion gradient, or active transport at the cellular level. Most evidence supports an arterial or venous mechanism. Tracer studies in animals have suggested a rapid perivascular flow (10 minutes from foramen magnum to perivascular space) that is arterial pulsation dependent (133,134,138,139). Other researchers have suggested that substantial flow takes much longer, and that larger particles and edema delay the process (133,140). This evidence is not absolute, and specific mechanisms of action are not proven.

CSF flow is influenced by respiratory function (27,122, 141–143). Williams (122) measured CSF flow in patients during a cough or Valsalva maneuver and found cranial flow, which he attributed to epidural venous engorgement, followed by caudal flow. Pressure waves in the subarachnoid space attributable to respiratory function have been demonstrated in humans and dogs (122,144). In recent canine investigations and human MRI studies, lumbar CSF pulse waves consisted of spinal arterial pulsations (39.4%), venous pulsations in the lumbar canal (37.6%), and intracranial pulsations (23%) (142,145). Studies using magnetic resonance phase imaging have raised doubts about the importance of respiratory pressures on the subarachnoid space pressure in patients with a Chiari malformation (27, 122).

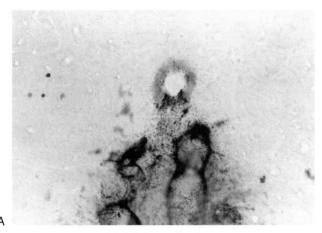

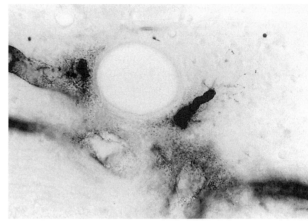

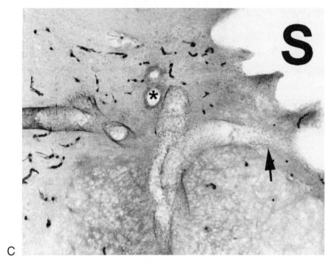

FIG. 55.7. Evidence for fluid flow from perivascular space into the central canal in canalicular and extracanalicular syrinxes. Horse radish peroxidase (HRP) injected into the subarachnoid space of a normal rat **(A)** rapidly outlines the perivascular spaces (*arrow*) and flows into the central canal (***). Six weeks after intraepenchymal kaolin injection, the central canal has become dilated **(B)**, but rapid flow of cerebrospinal fluid into the central canal continues. In a separate experimental group, intraspinal quisqualic acid combined with subarachnoid kaolin induces an extracanalicular syrinx at 6 weeks **(C)**. Fluid in this group also flows from perivascular spaces (*arrow*) into the syrinx cavity (*S*). (Sections of rat cervical spinal cord, HRP/tetramethylbenzidine, 20×)

Local or cranial arterial pulsation has been suggested as the driving force behind CSF flow across the cord and into the syrinx (27,120,146). Magnetic resonance phase imaging, intraoperative ultrasound, and animal experimental work support a dominant role of cardiac pulsation in relation to CSF flow (27,138,141–143,146,147). The mechanism of cardiac-to-CSF pulse transference is debated. Observed peak CSF velocities within the lower fourth ventricle, followed by the aqueduct and the foramen of Monroe, have implicated movement of the cerebellum, tonsils, and choroid plexus in the initiation of CSF flow (27,121,142,146–148). In patients with Chiari I and symptomatic syringomyelia, CSF flow was reduced and prolonged, although CSF velocity was increased at the foramen magnum (27,146). This information is used to support the theory that cerebellar tonsils are forced down with systole to act as a piston on the isolated spinal CSF, imparting a pressure wave on the surface of the spinal cord, which could cause progression of syringomyelia by compressing the cord and propelling the syrinx contents longitudinally (Fig. 55.5) (27,146). According to this theory, a syrinx could therefore originate and be extended by the pressure wave forcing fluid along perivascular and inter-

stitial spaces. No evidence has been produced to suggest that this theory applies to extracanalicular or communicating syringomyelia, or to demonstrate the route of fluid flow into the cord in any type of syrinx (149). CSF flow in posttraumatic syringomyelia patients may be turbulent and influenced by a locally tethered cord and blockage of the subarachnoid space (70,150). Spinal cord movement and cord systolic expansion also produce substantial local CSF flow, which is more important beyond the caudal cervical spine and may be important in syrinx pathogenesis (142).

In an animal model, perivascular flow into the spinal cord does not occur if arterial pulsations are damped (138). This suggests that a possible mechanism of noncommunicating canalicular and extracanalicular syrinx formation is arterial pulsation–driven CSF flow into an isolated segment of central canal or a central gray matter cyst. A cyst forming in the central gray matter after hemorrhage or infarction will enlarge by the continued arterial pulsation–driven flow of CSF. Presumably, CSF flowing into the central canal normally reaches the subarachnoid space via the fourth ventricle or the caudal opening of the central canal. If a segment of central canal becomes isolated by two levels of occlusion, the continuing arterial pulsation–driven flow of CSF into the canal will enlarge it to form a syrinx.

Communicating canalicular syringomyelia probably results from occlusion of the outlets of the fourth ventricle, with subsequent enlargement of all ventricles and the central canal (54). Experimental evidence for syrinxes forming in this way has been provided by numerous studies using cisternal kaolin injections to occlude the outlets of the fourth ventricle, causing hydrocephalus and syringomyelia (151,152).

Tumor-Associated Syringomyelia

Tumor-associated syrinxes can be formed adjacent to intramedullary tumors such as astrocytomas and ependymomas (54). These cysts contain proteinaceous fluid and are lined by tumor or tightly packed glial cells around a mural nodule (54). The mechanism of cyst formation may be direct fluid secretion, ischemia, hemorrhage, interference with tissue fluid drainage, secretion of an edema-generating factor, or production of conditions conducive to syrinx formation by alteration of subarachnoid space compliance (49, 122,153–155).

CLINICAL FEATURES

The mean age at the onset of symptoms is approximately 30 years, regardless of whether a Chiari malformation is present, although symptoms may occur from infancy to 70 years (15,33,156,157). The onset of symptoms in patients with syringomyelia is earlier than in patients who have a Chiari malformation without a syrinx (19,158). The spinal cord damage caused by a syrinx dictates the clinical features. Usually, there is an insidious onset of motor and sensory symptoms, but there is considerable variation (27,159–161). There may be a rapid onset spontaneously or after mild cervical trauma, coughing, straining, or sneezing (29,157,160–164). The classic dissociated sensory loss affects the ulnar border of the forearm, extending into the arm and the chest in a cape or half-cape distribution, but this is in fact uncommon (161). The most common presenting symptoms are lower limb stiffness and pain and numbness of the hands (15,16,72,75,76). Other presenting features include oscillopsia, diplopia, stridor, urinary incontinence, dysesthesia, ataxia, dyshydrosis, and respiratory paralysis (33,92,163,165,166).

Pain is often restricted to the suboccipital and neck area, associated with coughing (probably due to cervicomedullary compression) or a burning, aching pain on the side of the sensory loss (72,158,167). If the dorsal root entry zone is affected, all sensation may be lost unilaterally (167). Sensory disturbance may extend to the face if the syrinx extends into the upper cervical cord or brainstem. The first motor signs are often seen in the upper limbs, with wasting and weakness of the hands (33,158). Wasting of the hypothenar eminence with lower cervical lesions is a notable feature. Hypotonia, areflexia, and fasciculations may

be seen (33,92,158). Spastic paraparesis and brisk reflexes may be due to cervicomedullary compression or from syrinx involvement of descending motor tracts (167). Upper limb girdle joints may be affected by arthropathy, spontaneous fractures, and calcification of the soft tissues in the late stages of the disease (33,168,169).

The presenting features differ in children. The first manifestation is often scoliosis, and focal neurologic deficits may not follow for many years (92,168,170,171). Scoliosis may be present in up to half of the cases of hindbrain-related syringomyelia, and it may improve after treatment of the syrinx (169,172–174). Conversely, only 4% of children with scoliosis will have a syrinx as the underlying cause (175).

Syringobulbia usually occurs as an extension of syringomyelia, but it may occur separately (33). Nystagmus, the most common sign, may be due to either compression by a hindbrain malformation or to parenchymal damage by the syrinx. Facial sensory loss in an onion-skin pattern, pharyngeal and laryngeal dysfunction, and other bulbar signs may be seen (33). Damage to the chemosensitive regions and the nucleus tractus solitarius may cause carbon dioxide insensitivity and respiratory failure (176,177). Syringobulbia may be more common in non-hindbrain-related cases, perhaps because compression of the upper end of the cord prevents upward extension of a cyst (169).

NATURAL HISTORY

The natural history of syringomyelia is not well established (159). Symptoms may progress for a few years and then remain static, or there may be a slow and intermittent or continuous deterioration (29,52). The majority of patients seem to have a slow progression of symptoms and signs over many years (29,52,157,172,178). A few progress more rapidly, sometimes associated with myelography or as a result of hemorrhage into the syrinx from vessels in the wall of the cavity (33,76,179). In small observational series, 17% to 50% of patients remained static without treatment for over 10 years or more (157,172,180,181). In one study of 10 patients with posttraumatic syringomyelia, those patients undergoing rehabilitation without surgery did better than those with surgical treatment (182). There are a number of reports of spontaneous resolution in adults and children, which may be due to decompression of the syrinx into the subarachnoid space (183–185).

INVESTIGATIONS

Before the introduction of modern neuroimaging techniques, the diagnosis of syringomyelia was difficult to make (52,159,171,173). Plain radiographs may reveal associated skeletal abnormalities such as basilar impression, platybasia, scoliosis, segmentation abnormalities of the cervical spine, associated cervical spine instability, or an enlarged spinal canal if the syrinx has been present since childhood (33,36,168,169,171,186–188). Myelography may reveal an enlarged cord, but the demonstration of syringomyelia or the

Chiari malformation is unreliable (33,159,189). In air myelography, the so-called collapsing cord sign indicates syrinx presence: The upper part of the cord collapses, with concomitant dilation of the dependent cord, when the patient is vertical (33,173).

Plain computed tomography (CT) is not reliable for the diagnosis of syringomyelia, primarily because of image degradation by surrounding bone, but will demonstrate posterior fossa size and bony anatomy, which may be useful for planning surgery (33,36). Combined with contrast myelography, CT is capable of demonstrating Chiari malformations and subarachnoid adhesions, but 10% to 50% of syrinxes will be missed if the CT scan is done immediately after myelography (37,73,92,188). Three hours following myelography, CT imaging demonstrates loss of the sharp margins of the cord, whereas after 6 to 24 hours, the cavity is filled with contrast medium and the subarachnoid space may be clear of contrast (Fig. 55.6) (33,173,119,188). Acute neurologic deterioration may follow myelography, presumably due to dissection of the syrinx into cord parenchyma.

Currently, magnetic resonance imaging (MRI) is the imaging modality of choice for the diagnosis and monitoring of syringomyelia (36,150,188). MRI is more sensitive in detecting syrinxes than myelography, is noninvasive, can demonstrate fluid movement, and clearly demonstrates most—some authors suggest all—associated abnormalities (19,33,36,70). MRI demonstrates that syrinxes are often asymmetrical, loculated, or multiple, which may aid in operative planning (23,73,188). Intramedullary tumors associated with syringomyelia may be shown with MRI after administration of intravenous paramagnetic contrast agents such as gadolinium (Fig. 55.2). Due to partial volume effects, MRI may not adequately demonstrate cavities within small spinal cords or in patients with scoliosis (33,169,190). One assessment of the severity of syringomyelia is by measuring the cross-sectional area of syrinxes and calculating the percentage of spinal cord area occupied by the cyst (29,45). The thinner the neural tissue around the cyst, the more severe or rapidly progressive the syrinx is suggested to be. Regions of edematous signal change within the cord (low signal on T1-weighted and high signal on T2-weighted images), with or without a syrinx, may precede the development or active advancement of a syrinx (96,111,191).

In addition to standard T1, T2, and T1 with gadolinium axial and sagittal views, MRI can provide information on fluid flow. Phase-contrast cine MRI may be used to determine which patients with "borderline" tonsillar herniation might benefit from decompression, and demonstrate normalization of CSF flow following surgery (27,36,188,192). Cine MRI may also be used to help confirm spinal cord tethering and communication of spinal cord cysts with the subarachnoid space (150).

Intraoperative ultrasonography and electrophysiology have a role. Ultrasonography can be useful to localize the syrinx, to reveal dural and subarachnoid adhesions and webs, to define septations within the cyst, and to aid in optimal shunt placement (Fig. 55.8) (27,36,146,150,188). Intraoperative somatosensory evoked potentials of median or tibial nerves may help alert the surgeon to developing neuronal damage, especially during initial positioning and tonsillar manipulation (70). We have not found preoperative electrophysiology useful in the diagnostic workup of patients with a syrinx (36).

TREATMENT

There is no entirely satisfactory treatment for syringomyelia. Surgery has included posterior fossa decompres-

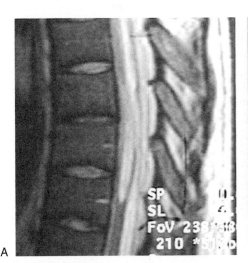
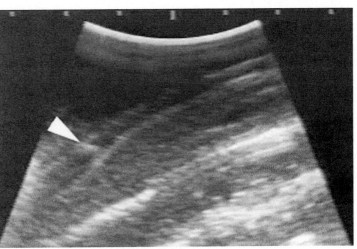

A   B

FIG. 55.8. A patient diagnosed with transverse myelitis who deteriorated following revision of a baclofen pump had a syrinx visible on preoperative T2-weighted images **(A)**. Intraoperative ultrasound **(B)** demonstrated a highly localized band of arachnoid adhesions (*arrow*) visible at operation but not in preoperative imaging.

sion, various shunting procedures, and opening the cyst directly into the subarachnoid space. There is often short-term improvement; however, the variable and long course of the disease makes it difficult to determine the effectiveness of treatment based on small studies with short follow-up periods (157,159,193). No symptomatic improvement occurs in up to 50% of cases regardless of the method of treatment or presence of radiologic improvement (36,157,182,194–198). Surgical intervention appears to be most effective at alleviating cough headache and stabilizing the sensory loss and weakness, and least effective in improving spasticity or burning dysesthetic pain (36,199).

The appropriate timing of surgical treatment has been controversial. Many authors advocate surgical treatment only in cases with progression of signs and symptoms; however, it seems that results are better in patients with a short duration of symptoms (36,92,181,200–202). Other than medically infirm and pregnant patients, we prefer to treat patients as soon as the disease is diagnosed because of the tendency for rapid advancement of deficits in some cases and the likelihood that established neurologic deficits are irreversible (104,169). Pregnant patients with syringomyelia usually have an elective cesarian section under general anesthesia before any syrinx surgery (203,204).

Posterior Fossa Decompression

First advocated by Gardner and Goodall (205), posterior fossa decompression is used in an attempt to correct presumed abnormalities in craniospinal CSF flow. The mechanism by which decompression results in resolution of syrinxes is not clear (169). Improvement may occur even when there is no change in craniospinal pressure relationships, which may be due to alteration of the capacitance of the neuraxis and change in the pulsation characteristics (104). Decompression can increase subarachnoid space compliance and reduce intraspinal pressure (27). It may be that alterations of these factors affect the pulsation-driven perivascular flow of CSF (139).

There are several variations in surgical technique. These include the size of the craniectomy or craniotomy, leaving dura intact or dissecting only the external layer of dura, preserving or opening the arachnoid, subpial resection or suturing back the cerebellar tonsils, leaving the dura open, or inserting a dural graft (36,206–209). Transoral decompression is sometimes used in cases of anterior compression (210). Often there is a combination of anterior and posterior compression; in these cases, we perform a posterior decompression first unless the anterior compression is particularly severe. Plugging the opening of the central canal was originally advocated to prevent CSF flow into the syrinx from the fourth ventricle (121). It does not improve the success rate and leads to a higher rate of complications (36,159, 167,211).

Posterior fossa decompression has been used with some success for nonhindbrain-related syrinxes, where no patho-

logical abnormality could be found (212). Posterior fossa decompression is our initial preference for cases of chronic compression at the craniocervical junction (Fig. 55.9). We perform a wide posterior bony decompression, removing as many posterior vertebral arches as necessary to expose the entire compressive lesion (Fig. 55.10). The dura is opened in a Y shape over the cerebellar hemispheres and inferiorly to expose the tips of the cerebellar tonsils in the case of a Chiari malformation. We attempt to leave the arachnoid intact unless arachnoid bands or adhesions are present. We use artificial dura to close the dural defect, avoiding autologous tissue such as fascia lata, which we believe is more likely to promote scarring and fibrosis.

Complication rates of up to 28% are reported; these include infection, aseptic meningitis, CSF fistula, hematoma, hydrocephalus, cerebellar slump, cerebellar or cerebral infarction, transient brainstem or cranial nerve dysfunction, syrinx recurrence, and death in 1% (36,213,214).

Shunting

The simplest approach to syrinx drainage is percutaneous aspiration, but improvements tend to be short-lived (181). Similarly, open myelotomy may produce temporary benefit, but long-term results are plagued by postoperative adhesive arachnoiditis and refilling of the syrinx cavity (33,202, 215). Terminal ventriculostomy is an option in paraplegic patients; improvement is seen in some cases, but most patients continue to deteriorate (33,181,193,215).

Shunt insertion as a primary treatment method is indicated only when no presumptive causative condition can be treated. Conditions requiring a shunt include posttraumatic syrinxes with extensive arachnoiditis, some intramedullary tumors, and other causes of extensive arachnoiditis. Patients who deteriorate, or fail to improve, after posterior fossa decompression despite imaging evidence of satisfactory fluid flow are treated with shunts as a second line of therapy (Fig. 55.11).

When syrinx drainage is required, some form of Silastic shunting device is usually used, with the specific type dictated largely by personal preference. Patients with a Chiari malformation and hydrocephalus can sometimes be treated successfully with a ventriculoperitoneal shunt (36,89). Syringosubarachnoid shunts are frequently used for posttraumatic syrinxes, but some authors believe this may result in poor absorption of fluid (73,74,216). The distal end of the shunt tubing must be proximal to the site of obstruction to CSF flow. Syringoperitoneal shunts allow ready absorption of CSF, but syringopleural shunts are easier to perform and are our preferred method of treatment when a shunt is required, provided pulmonary reserve is adequate (73,197, 217).

All implantable devices have potential complications, and shunts for syringomyelia are no exception. Catheters may dislodge or become blocked. Complication rates of between 10% and 100% are reported, with most series having around

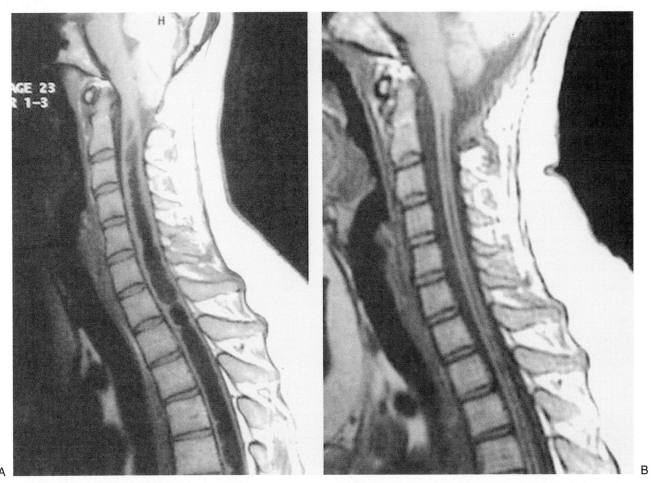

FIG. 55.9. Syringomyelia associated with the Chiari type I malformation **(A)** treated with posterior fossa decompression. The cerebellar hernia resolved, and there was a marked reduction in the size of the syrinx **(B)**.

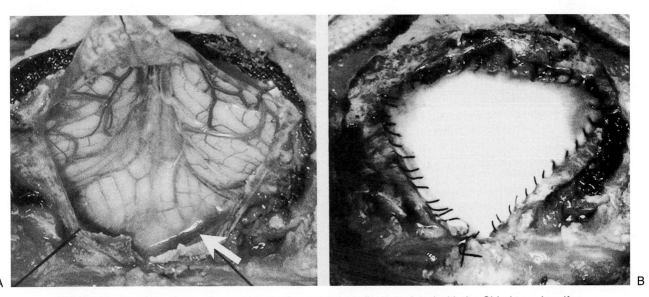

FIG. 55.10. Posterior fossa decompression for syringomyelia associated with the Chiari type I malformation. A wide suboccipital craniectomy is performed, the posterior arch of C1 is removed to expose the tips of the cerebellar tonsils (*arrow*), and the arachnoid is left intact if possible **(A)**. Artificial dura is used to close the dural defect **(B)**.

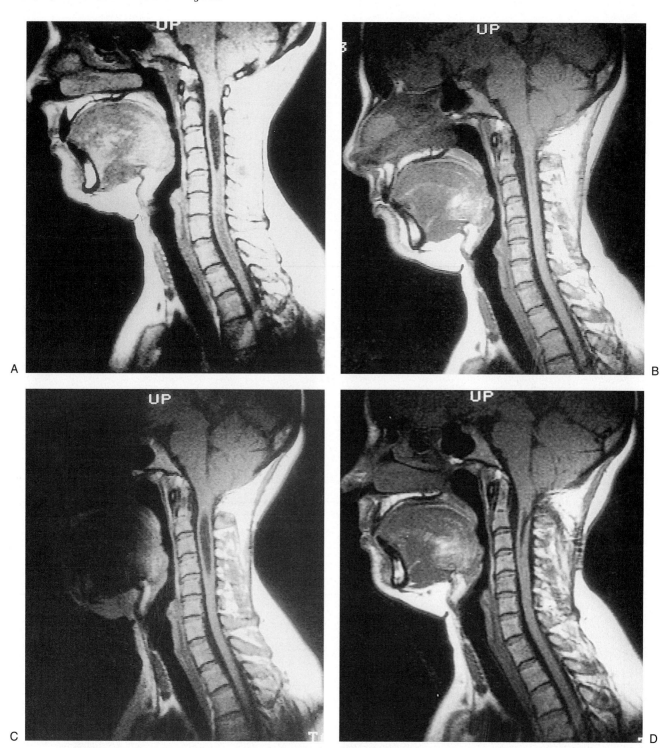

FIG. 55.11. Syringomyelia associated with the Chiari type I malformation **(A)**. The syrinx resolved after posterior fossa decompression **(B)** but recurred 12 months later **(C)**. The syrinx collapsed again after syringopleural shunting **(D)**. The shunt tubing is seen on the magnetic resonance scan (*arrow*).

50% (15,36,71,196,197,218). There are reports of 97% success with shunt insertion as a primary treatment for Chiari-associated syringomyelia with 5-year follow-up (219). We find catheter-related complications to be less common when ventricular catheters in the syrinx are used instead of fine-caliber T tubes, when it is technically feasible to use the larger catheter. The larger-diameter catheters also have the advantage of being detectable on MRI, confirming their position within the syrinx. Septated syrinxes have been reported to collapse after simple syringosubarachnoid shunting procedures, but if the syrinx is truly multiloculated, endoscopic catheter placement may address this problem

(220). Intraoperative ultrasound can aid in selecting the best site for catheter insertion and confirm suitable placement (33,221). The addition of a chamber into the shunt system allows for shunt function studies in the case of suspected blockage, although we have not found this very useful. Even with a catheter inside the syrinx, CSF overdrainage may occur, producing low-pressure headaches, and in these circumstances the addition of a programmable valve may help. Other complications of shunting procedures include spinal cord damage, spinal instability (after extensive laminectomy), deafferentation pain, CSF fistula, and infection, including pyosyrinx (36).

Although debate still reigns, shunting procedures now appear inferior to procedures that deal directly with the underlying problem (36,69,146,197). Dramatic short-term improvement after shunting is common, but long-term results are not very good (222,223).

In patients with localized areas of spinal arachnoid adhesions and syringomyelia, reports of primary lysis have suggested good results with low complication rates (36, 37,71,81,224). Extensive arachnoidal adhesions may be impossible to divide adequately, and shunting is required in these cases. Pseudomeningocele formation may have better results than shunting in posttraumatic syringomyelia (80,223).

SUMMARY

Syringomyelia is predominantly a disease of children and young adults, with a long course of pain and progressive neurologic deficits. It is associated with a wide array of conditions, notably craniocervical junction abnormalities and spinal trauma. Syrinxes may be classified into three types: (a) communicating central canal syrinxes, (b) noncommunicating central canal syrinxes, and (c) extracanalicular syrinxes. The mechanism of cyst formation in each of these types is unknown, but may involve a combination of hydrodynamic factors, local or distal arterial pulsations, isolated cavities, and altered subarachnoid space compliance. The wide variety of treatment options is testament to the fallibility of treatment and the high incidence of symptom progression after treatment. Our preference is to treat the underlying abnormality whenever possible and to use syringopleural shunting only for those patients with extensive arachnoiditis or failure of other treatments.

Greater understanding of the pathophysiology of syringomyelia is needed to improve the treatment and prognosis of this enigmatic condition.

REFERENCES

1. Estienne C. *La Dissection des Parties du corps humain divisee en trois livres.* Paris: Simon de Collines, 1546.
2. Lotbinière ACJd. Historical considerations. In: Anson JA, Benzel EC, Awad IA, eds. *Syringomyelia and the Chiari malformations.* Park Ridge, IL: American Association of Neurological Surgeons, 1997:1–26.
3. Ollivier CP. *Traité des maladies de la Moelle Épinié, contenant l'histoire anatomique, physiologique et pathologique de ce centre nerveux chez l'homme.* Paris: Méquignon-Marvis père et fils, 1827:178–183.
4. Portal A. De la Moelle épinière. In: *Cours D'Anatomie Médicale, ou élémens de l'anatomie de l'homme, avec des remarques physiologiques et pathologiques, et les resultants de l'observation sur le siege et la nature des maladies, d'après l'ouverture des corps.* Paris: Baldouin, 1805:61–120.
5. Foster JB, Hudgson P. Historical introduction. In: Barnett HJM, Foster JB, Hudgson P. *Syringomyelia.* London: WB Saunders, 1973:3–10.
6. Schultze F. Über Spalt, Höhlen und Ghombildung im Rückenmark und in der Medullar oblongata. *Virchows Arch* 1882;87:510–540.
7. Gowers WR. *A manual of diseases of the nervous system.* London: Churchill, 1886.
8. Abbe R, Coley WB. Syringomyelia, operation, exploration of cord, withdrawal of fluid. *J Nerv Ment Dis* 1892;19:512–520.
9. Haubrich WS. *Medical meanings: a glossary of word origins.* San Diego: Harcourt Brace Jovanovich, 1984.
10. Stilling B. Neue Untersuchungen uber den au des Ruckenmarks. In: Cassel, Verlag von Heinrich Hotop, 1856:4–27.
11. Hallopeau FH. Contributions à l'étude de la sclerose diffuse peri-épendymaire. *Gaz Med Paris* 1870;25:394.
12. Simon T. Über syringomyelia und Geschwulstbildung in Rückenmark. *Arch Psychiatr Nervenkrankh* 1875;5:120–163.
13. Ballentine HT, Ojemann RG, Drew JH. Syringohydromyelia. In: *Progress in neurological surgery.* Basel: Karger, 1971:227–245.
14. Barnett HJM, Botterell EH, Jousse AT, et al. Progressive myelopathy as a sequel to traumatic paraplegia. *Brain* 1966;89:159–174.
15. Edgar R, Quail P. Progressive post-traumatic cystic and non-cystic myelopathy. *Br J Neurosurg* 1994;8:7–22.
16. Hoffman HJ, Neill J, Crone KR, et al. Hydrosyringomyelia and its management in childhood. *Neurosurgery* 1987;21:347–351.
17. Escourolle R, Poirier J. *Manual of basic neuropathology.* Philadelphia: WB Saunders, 1978.
18. Stoodley MA, Jones NR. Syringomyelia. In: Cervical Spine Research Society, eds. *The cervical spine.* Philadelphia: Lippincott–Raven Publishers, 1998:565–583.
19. Milhorat TH, Chou MW, Trinidad EM, et al. Chiari I malformation redefined: clinical and radiographic findings for 364 symptomatic patients [see comments]. *Neurosurgery* 1999;44:1005–1017.
20. Moriwaka F, Tashiro K, Tachibana S, et al. Epidemiology of syringomyelia in Japan—the nationwide survey. *Rinsho Shinkeigaku* 1995; 35:1395–1397.
21. Abel R, Gerner HJ, Smit C, et al. Residual deformity of the spinal canal in patients with traumatic paraplegia and secondary changes of the spinal cord. *Spinal Cord* 1999;37:14–19.
22. Perrouin-Verbe B, Lenne-Aurier K, Robert R, et al. Post-traumatic syringomyelia and post-traumatic spinal canal stenosis: a direct relationship. Review of 75 patients with a spinal cord injury. *Spinal Cord* 1998;36:137–143.
23. Pillay PK, Awad IA, Little JR, et al. Symptomatic Chiari malformation in adults: a new classification based on magnetic resonance imaging with clinical and prognostic significance. *Neurosurgery* 1991;28:639–645.
24. Wang D, Bodley R, Sett P, et al. A clinical magnetic resonance imaging study of the traumatised spinal cord more than 20 years following injury. *Paraplegia* 1996;34:65–81.
25. Brewis M, Poskanzer DC, Rolland C, et al. Neurological disease in an English city. *Acta Neurol Scand* 1966;42:1–89.
26. Ferrero Arias J, Pilo Martin I. Prevalence of several neurological diseases in the central provinces of the Iberian Peninsula in eighteen-year-old males. *Neurologia* 1991;6:89–94.
27. Heiss JD, Patronas N, DeVroom HL, et al. Elucidating the pathophysiology of syringomyelia. *J Neurosurg* 1999;91:553–562.
28. Hertel G, Ricker K. A geometrical study on the distribution of syringomyelia in Germany. In: *Neurology: proceedings of the 11th World Congress of Neurology.* Amsterdam: Excerpta Medica, 1978:353–365.
29. Bogdanov EI, Mendelevich EG. Syrinx size and duration of symptoms predict the pace of progressive myelopathy: retrospective analysis of 103 unoperated cases with craniocervical junction malformations and syringomyelia. *Clin Neurol Neurosurg* 2002;104:90–97.
30. Bentley SJ, Campbell MJ, Kaufman P. Familial syringomyelia. *J Neurol Neurosurg Psychiatry* 1975;38:346–349.
31. Cavender RK, Schmidt JH 3rd. Tonsillar ectopia and Chiari malformations: monozygotic triplets. Case report. *J Neurosurg* 1995;82:497–500.

32. Myrianthopoulos NC. Epidemiology of central nervous system malformations. *Handbook of Clinical Neurology* 1987;6:49–69.
33. Nogues MA. Syringomyelia and syringobulbia. *Handbook of Clinical Neurology* 1987;6:443–464.
34. Zakeri A, Glasauer FE, Egnatchik JG. Familial syringomyelia: case report and review of the literature. *Surg Neurol* 1995;44:48–53.
35. Newman PK, Wentzel J, Foster JB. HLA and syringomyelia. *J Neuroimmunol* 1982;3:23–26.
36. Klekamp J, Samii M. *Syringomyelia: diagnosis and management.* Berlin: Springer, 2002.
37. Mallucci CL, Stacey RJ, Miles JB, et al. Idiopathic syringomyelia and the importance of occult arachnoid webs, pouches and cysts. *Br J Neurosurg* 1997;11:306–309.
38. Badie B, Mendoza D, Batzdorf U. Posterior fossa volume and response to suboccipital decompression in patients with Chiari I malformation. *Neurosurgery* 1995;37:214–218.
39. Nishikawa M, Sakamoto H, Hakuba A, et al. Pathogenesis of Chiari malformation: a morphometric study of the posterior cranial fossa. *J Neurosurg* 1997;86:40–47.
40. Batzdorf U. Chiari I malformation with syringomyelia. Evaluation of surgical therapy by magnetic resonance imaging. *J Neurosurg* 1988;68:726–730.
41. Masur H, Oberwittler C. Syringomyelia in Chiari malformation: relation to extent of cerebellar tissue herniation. *Neurosurgery* 1993;33:948–949.
42. Stovner LJ, Rinck P. Syringomyelia in Chiari malformation: relation to extent of cerebellar tissue herniation. *Neurosurgery* 1992;31:913–917.
43. Banna M. Syringomyelia in association with posterior fossa cysts. *AJNR Am J Neuroradiol* 1988;9:867–873.
44. Erkan K, Unal F, Kiris T. Terminal syringomyelia in association with the tethered cord syndrome. *Neurosurgery* 1999;45:1351–1360.
45. Iskandar BJ, Oakes WJ, McLaughlin C, et al. Terminal syringohydromyelia and occult spinal dysraphism. *J Neurosurg* 1994;81:513–519.
46. Koyanagi I, Iwasaki Y, Hida K, et al. Surgical treatment of syringomyelia associated with spinal dysraphism. *Childs Nerv Syst* 1997;13:194–200.
47. Foster O, Crockard HA, Powell MP. Syrinx associated with intramedullary metastasis. *J Neurol Neurosurg Psychiatry* 1987;50:1067–1070.
48. Landan I, Gilroy J, Wolfe DE. Syringomyelia affecting the entire spinal cord secondary to primary spinal intramedullary central nervous system lymphoma. *J Neurol Neurosurg Psychiatry* 1987;50:1533–1535.
49. Samii M, Klekamp J. Surgical results of 100 intramedullary tumors in relation to accompanying syringomyelia. *Neurosurgery* 1994;35:865–873.
50. Fox JL, Bashir R, Jinkins JR, et al. Syrinx of the conus medullaris and filum terminale in association with multiple hemangioblastomas. *Surg Neurol* 1985;24:265–271.
51. Nagahiro S, Matsukado Y, Kuratsu J, et al. Syringomyelia and syringobulbia associated with an ependymoma of the cauda equina involving the conus medullaris: case report. *Neurosurgery* 1986;18:357–360.
52. Netsky MG. Syringomyelia, a clinicopathological study. *Arch Neurol Psychiat* 1953;70:741–777.
53. Nyland H, Krogness KG. Size of posterior fossa in Chiari type 1 malformation in adults. *Acta Neurochir* 1978;40:233–242.
54. Milhorat TH. Classification of syringomyelia. *Neurosurg Focus* 2000;8:1–6.
55. Poser CM. *The relationship between syringomyelia and neoplasm.* Springfield, IL: Charles C Thomas, 1956.
56. Sloof JL, Kernohan TW, MacCarthy CS. *Primary intramedullary tumor of the spinal cord and filum terminale.* Philadelphia: WB Saunders, 1964:155–164.
57. Kaar GF, N'Dow JM, Bashir SH. Cervical spondylotic myelopathy with syringomyelia. *Br J Neurosurg* 1996;10:413–415.
58. Milhorat TH, Capocelli AL Jr, Anzil AP, et al. Pathological basis of spinal cord cavitation in syringomyelia: analysis of 105 autopsy cases. *J Neurosurg* 1995;82:802–812.
59. Milhorat TH, Johnson RW, Johnson WD. Pathogenesis of syringomyelia with description of non-communication type that arises immediately caudal to obstructive lesions. In: Matsumoto S, Tamaki N, eds. *Hydrocephalus: pathogenesis and treatment.* Tokyo: Springer-Verlag, 1992:218–228.
60. Barnett HJM. Syringomyelia associated with spinal arachnoiditis. In: Barnett HJM, Foster JB, Hudgson P. *Syringomyelia.* London: WB Saunders, 1973:220–244.
61. Milhorat TH, Miller JI, Johnson WD, et al. Anatomical basis of syringomyelia occurring with hindbrain lesions. *Neurosurgery* 1993;32:748–754.
62. Wasserberg J, Marks P, Hardy D. Syringomyelia of the thoracic spinal cord associated with spinal meningiomas. *Br J Neurosurg* 1987;1:485–488.
63. Brammah TB, Jayson MI. Syringomyelia as a complication of spinal arachnoiditis. *Spine* 1994;19:2603–2605.
64. Caplan LR, Norohna AB, Amico LL. Syringomyelia and arachnoiditis. *J Neurol Neurosurg Psychiatry* 1990;53:106–113.
65. Charcot JM, Joffroy A. Deux cas d'atrophie musculaire progressive avec lésions de la substance grise et des faisceaux antérolatéraux de la moelle épinière (French). *Arch Physiol Norm Pathol* 1869;2:354–367, 629–649, 744–760.
66. Falcone S, Quencer RM, Green BA, et al. Progressive posttraumatic myelomalacic myelopathy: imaging and clinical features. *AJNR Am J Neuroradiol* 1994;15:747–754.
67. Foster JB, Hudgson P. Basal arachnoiditis. In: Barnett HJM, Foster JB, Hudgson P. *Syringomyelia.* London: WB Saunders, 1973:30–49.
68. Parker F, Aghakhani N, Tadie M. Non-traumatic arachnoiditis and syringomyelia. A series of 32 cases [in French]. *Neurochirurgie* 1999;45(Suppl 1):67–83.
69. Batzdorf U, Klekamp J, Johnson JP. A critical appraisal of syrinx cavity shunting procedures. *J Neurosurg* 1998;89:382–388.
70. Klekamp J, Batzdorf U, Samii M, et al. Treatment of syringomyelia associated with arachnoid scarring caused by arachnoiditis or trauma. *J Neurosurg* 1997;86:233–240.
71. Lee TT, Alameda GJ, Gromelski EB, et al. Outcome after surgical treatment of progressive posttraumatic cystic myelopathy. *J Neurosurgery (Spine)* 2000;92:149–154.
72. Schurch B, Wichmann W, Rossier AB. Post-traumatic syringomyelia (cystic myelopathy): a prospective study of 449 patients with spinal cord injury. *J Neurol Neurosurg Psychiatry* 1996;60:61–67.
73. Davis CH, Symon L. Mechanisms and treatment in post-traumatic syringomyelia. *Br J Neurosurg* 1989;3:669–674.
74. Hida K, Iwasaki Y, Imamura H, et al. Posttraumatic syringomyelia: its characteristic magnetic resonance imaging findings and surgical management. *Neurosurgery* 1994;35:886–891.
75. El Masry WS, Biyani A. Incidence, management, and outcome of post-traumatic syringomyelia. In memory of Mr Bernard Williams. *J Neurol Neurosurg Psychiatry* 1996;60:141–146.
76. Rossier AB, Foo D, Shillito J, et al. Posttraumatic cervical syringomyelia. Incidence, clinical presentation, electrophysiological studies, syrinx protein and results of conservative and operative treatment. *Brain* 1985;108:439–461.
77. Tobimatsu Y, Nihei R, Kimura T, et al. A quantitative analysis of cerebrospinal fluid flow in post-traumatic syringomyelia. *Paraplegia* 1995;33:203–207.
78. Backe HA, Betz RR, Mesgarzadeh M, et al. Post-traumatic spinal cord cysts evaluated by magnetic resonance imaging. *Paraplegia* 1991;29:607–612.
79. Squier MV, Lehr RP. Post-traumatic syringomyelia. *J Neurol Neurosurg Psychiatry* 1994;57:1095–1098.
80. Williams B. Pathogenesis of post-traumatic syringomyelia. *Br J Neurosurg* 1992;6:517–520.
81. Levi AD, Sonntag VK. Management of posttraumatic syringomyelia using an expansile duraplasty. A case report. *Spine* 1998;23:128–132.
82. Rossier AB, Foo D, Shillito J, et al. Progressive late post-traumatic syringomyelia. *Paraplegia* 1981;19:96–97.
83. Gardner WJ, McMurray FG. "Non-communicating" syringomyelia: a non-existent entity. *Surg Neurol* 1976;6:251–256.
84. Gower DJ, Pollay M, Leech R. Pediatric syringomyelia. *J Child Neurol* 1994;9:14–21.
85. Berry RG, Chambers RA, Lublin FD. Syringoencephalomyelia (syringocephalus). *J Neuropathol Exp Neurol* 1981;40:633–644.
86. Reddy KK, Del Bigio MR, Sutherland GR. Ultrastructure of the human posttraumatic syrinx. *J Neurosurg* 1989;71:239–243.
87. Durward QJ, Rice GP, Ball MJ, et al. Selective spinal cordectomy: clinicopathological correlation. *J Neurosurg* 1982;56:359–367.
88. Foo D, Bignami A, Rossier AB. A case of post-traumatic syringomyelia. Neuropathological findings after 1 year of cystic drainage. *Paraplegia* 1989;27:63–69.
89. Milhorat TH, Johnson RW, Milhorat RH, et al. Clinicopathological correlations in syringomyelia using axial magnetic resonance imaging. *Neurosurgery* 1995;37:206–213.

90. Joffroy A, Archard. De la myélite cavitaire (French). *Arch Physiol Norm Pathol* 1887;10:435–472.

91. Chumas PD, Armstrong DC, Drake JM, et al. Tonsillar herniation: the rule rather than the exception after lumboperitoneal shunting in the pediatric population [see comments]. *J Neurosurg* 1993;78:568–573.

92. Foster JB. Hydromyelia. *Handbook of Clinical Neurology* 1987;6: 425–433.

93. Aboulker J. La syringomyelie et les liquides intra-rachidiens (French). *Neurochirurgie* 1979;25(Suppl 1):1–44.

94. Milhorat TH, Kotzen RM, Anzil AP. Stenosis of central canal of spinal cord in man: incidence and pathological findings in 232 autopsy cases. *J Neurosurg* 1994;80:716–722.

95. Yasui K, Hashizume Y, Yoshida M, et al. Age-related morphologic changes of the central canal of the human spinal cord. *Acta Neuropathol* 1999;97:253–259.

96. Fischbein NJ, Dillon WP, Cobbs C, et al. The "presyrinx" state: a reversible myelopathic condition that may precede syringomyelia. *AJNR Am J Neuroradiol* 1999;20:7–20.

97. Guizar-Sahagun G, Grijalva I, Madrazo I, et al. Development of posttraumatic cysts in the spinal cord of rats subjected to severe spinal cord contusion. *Surg Neurol* 1994;41:241–249.

98. Kakulas BA. A review of the neuropathology of human spinal cord injury with emphasis on special features. *J Spinal Cord Med* 1999; 22:119–124.

99. Levy LM. Toward an understanding of syringomyelia: MR imaging of CSF flow and neuroaxis motion. *AJNR Am J Neuroradiol* 2000; 21:45–46.

100. Tator CH, Fehlings MG. Review of the secondary injury theory of acute spinal cord trauma with emphasis on vascular mechanisms [see comments]. *J Neurosurg* 1991;75:15–26.

101. Klekamp J, Volkel K, Bartels CJ, et al. Disturbances of cerebrospinal fluid flow attributable to arachnoid scarring cause interstitial edema of the cat spinal cord. *Neurosurgery* 2001;48:174–186.

102. Sherk HH, Charney E, Pasquariello PD, et al. Hydrocephalus, cervical cord lesions, and spinal deformity. *Spine* 1986;11:340–342.

103. Taylor AR. Another theory of the aetiology of the syringomyelic cavity. *J Neurol Neurosurg Psychiatry* 1975;38:825.

104. Williams B. A critical appraisal of posterior fossa surgery for communicating syringomyelia. *Brain* 1978;101:223–250.

105. Hashizume Y, Iljima S, Kishimoto H, et al. Pencil-shaped softening of the spinal cord. Pathologic study in 12 autopsy cases. *Acta Neuropathol* 1983;61:219–224.

106. Hirose G, Shimazaki K, Takado M, et al. Intramedullary spinal cord metastasis associated with pencil-shaped softening of the spinal cord: case report. *J Neurosurg* 1980;52:718–721.

107. Brodbelt AR, Stoodley MA, Brown CJ, et al. Time and dose profiles of experimental excitotoxic post-traumatic syringomyelia. *ANZ J Surgery* 2001;71:A66.

108. Liu D, Thangnipon W, McAdoo DJ. Excitatory amino acids rise to toxic levels upon impact injury to the rat spinal cord. *Brain Res* 1991; 547:344–348.

109. Simpson RK Jr, Robertson CS, Goodman JC. Spinal cord ischemia-induced elevation of amino acids: extracellular measurement with microdialysis. *Neurochem Res* 1990;15:635–639.

110. Yezierski RP, Sanata M, Park SH, et al. Neuronal degeneration and spinal cavitation following intraspinal injections of quisqualic acid in the rat. *J Neurotrauma* 1993;10:445–456.

111. Levy EI, Heiss JD, Kent MS, et al. Spinal cord swelling preceding syrinx development. Case report. *J Neurosurg* 2000;92:93–97.

112. Cserr HF, Knopf PM. Cervical lymphatics, the blood-brain barrier and the immunoreactivity of the brain: a new view. *Immunol Today* 1992;13:507–512.

113. Davson H, Segal MB. *Physiology of the CSF and blood brain barriers*. Boca Raton, FL: CRC Press, 1996.

114. Foldi M. The brain and the lymphatic system revisited. *Lymphology* 1999;32:40–44.

115. Kida S, Weller RO, Zhang ET, et al. Anatomical pathways for lymphatic drainage of the brain and their pathological significance. *Neuropathol Appl Neurobiol* 1995;21:181–184.

116. Rosenberg GA. *Brain fluids and metabolism*. Oxford, UK: Oxford University Press, 1990.

117. Weller RO. Pathology of cerebrospinal fluid and interstitial fluid of the CNS: significance for Alzheimer disease, prion disorders and multiple sclerosis. *J Neuropathol Exp Neurol* 1998;57:885–894.

118. Ball MJ, Dayan AD. Pathogenesis of syringomyelia. *Lancet* 1972; 799–801.

119. Ikata T, Masaki K, Kashiwaguchi S. Clinical and experimental studies on permeability of tracers in normal spinal cord and syringomyelia. *Spine* 1988;13:737–741.

120. Stoodley MA, Gutschmidt B, Jones NR. Cerebrospinal fluid flow in an animal model of noncommunicating syringomyelia. *Neurosurgery* 1999;44:1065–1075.

121. Gardner WJ, Angel J. The cause of syringomyelia and its surgical treatment. *Cleve Clin Q* 1958;25:4–8.

122. Williams B. On the pathogenesis of syringomyelia: a review. *J R Soc Med* 1980;73:798–806.

123. Brocklehurst G. The development of the human cerebrospinal fluid pathway with particular reference to the roof of the fourth ventricle. *J Anat* 1969;105:467–475.

124. Jones HC, Sellars RA. The movement of cerebrospinal fluid through the rhombencephalic roof in fetal and neonatal rats. *J Physiol* 1982; 2P.

125. Yamada H, Yokota A, Haratake J, et al. Morphological study of experimental syringomyelia with kaolin-induced hydrocephalus in a canine model. *J Neurosurg* 1996;84:999–1005.

126. Milhorat AT, Johnson MD, Miller JI, et al. Surgical treatment of syringomyelia based on magnetic resonance imaging criteria. *Neurosurgery* 1992;31:231–244.

127. Brodbelt AR, Stoodley MA, Watling A, et al. Cerebrospinal fluid flow in the excitotoxic model of post-traumatic syringomyelia. *ANZ J Surg* 2002;72(Suppl):A64.

128. Esiri MM, Gay D. Immunological and neuropathological significance of the Virchow-Robin space. *J Neurol Sci* 1990;100:3–8.

129. Hutchings M, Weller RO. Anatomical relationships of the pia mater to cerebral blood vessels in man. *J Neurosurg* 1986;65:316–325.

130. Nicholas DS, Weller RO. The fine anatomy of the human spinal meninges. A light and scanning electron microscopy study. *J Neurosurg* 1988;69:276–282.

131. Adachi M, Hosoya T, Haku T, et al. Dilated Virchow-Robin spaces: MRI pathological study. *Neuroradiology* 1998;40:27–31.

132. Zhang ET, Inman CB, Weller RO. Interrelationships of the pia mater and the perivascular (Virchow-Robin) spaces in the human cerebrum. *J Anat* 1990;170:111–123.

133. Ichimura T, Fraser PA, Cserr HF. Distribution of extracellular tracers in perivascular spaces of the rat brain. *Brain Res* 1991;545:103–113.

134. Rennels ML, Blaumanis OR, Grady PA. Rapid solute transport throughout the brain via paravascular fluid pathways. *Adv Neurol* 1990;52:431–439.

135. Rennels ML, Gregory TF, Blaumanis OR, et al. Evidence for a "paravascular" fluid circulation in the mammalian central nervous system, provided by the rapid distribution of tracer protein throughout the brain from the subarachnoid space. *Brain Res* 1985;326:47–63.

136. Asano M, Fujiwara K, Yonenobu K, et al. Post-traumatic syringomyelia. *Spine* 1996;21:1446–1453.

137. Milhorat TH, Capocelli AL Jr, Kotzen RM, et al. Intramedullary pressure in syringomyelia: clinical and pathophysiological correlates of syrinx distension [see comments]. *Neurosurgery* 1997;41:1102–1110.

138. Stoodley MA, Brown SA, Brown CJ, et al. Arterial pulsation-dependent perivascular cerebrospinal fluid flow into the central canal in the sheep spinal cord. *J Neurosurg* 1997;86:686–693.

139. Stoodley MA, Jones NR, Brown CJ. Evidence for rapid fluid flow from the subarachnoid space into the spinal cord central canal in the rat. *Brain Res* 1996;707:155–164.

140. Blaumanis OR, Rennels ML, Grady PA. Focal cerebral edema impedes convective fluid/tracer movement through paravascular pathways in cat brain. *Adv Neurol* 1990;52:385–389.

141. Greitz D, Greitz T, Hindmarsh T. A new view on the CSF-circulation with the potential for pharmacological treatment of childhood hydrocephalus. *Acta Paediatr* 1997;86:125–132.

142. Henry-Feugeas MC, Idy-Peretti I, Baledent O, et al. Origin of subarachnoid cerebrospinal fluid pulsations: a phase-contrast MR analysis. *Magn Reson Imaging* 2000;18:387–395.

143. Levy LM. MR imaging of cerebrospinal fluid flow and spinal cord motion in neurologic disorders of the spine. *MRI Clin North Am* 1999;7:573–587.

144. Hall P, Turner M, Aichinger S, et al. Experimental syringomyelia: the relationship between intraventricular and intrasyrinx pressures. *J Neurosurg* 1980;52:812–817.

145. Urayama K. Origin of lumbar cerebrospinal fluid pulse wave. *Spine* 1994;19:441–445.

146. Oldfield EH, Muraszko K, Shawker TH, et al. Pathophysiology of syringomyelia associated with Chiari I malformation of the cerebellar tonsils. Implications for diagnosis and treatment. *J Neurosurg* 1994;80:3–15.

147. Nitz WR, Bradley WG Jr, Watanabe AS, et al. Flow dynamics of cerebrospinal fluid: assessment with phase-contrast velocity MR imaging performed with retrospective cardiac gating. *Radiology* 1992;183:395–405.

148. Bering EA. Circulation of the cerebrospinal fluid: demonstration of the choroid plexus as the generator of the force for flow of fluid and ventricular enlargement. *J Neurosurg* 1962;19:405–413.

149. Atkinson LD, Lane JI. Communicating syringomyelia. *J Neurosurg* 1994;81:500–502.

150. Schwartz ED, Falcone SF, Quencer RM, et al. Posttraumatic syringomyelia: pathogenesis, imaging, and treatment. *Am J Roentgenol* 1999;173:487–492.

151. Chakrabortty S, Tamaki N, Ehara K, et al. Experimental syringomyelia in the rabbit: an ultrastructural study of the spinal cord tissue. *Neurosurgery* 1994;35:1112–1120.

152. McLaurin RL, Bailey OT, Schurr PH, et al. Myelomalacia and multiple cavitations of spinal cord secondary to adhesive arachnoiditis. *Arch Pathol* 1954;57:138–146.

153. Gardner WJ. Hydrodynamic mechanism of syringomyelia: its relationship to myelocele. *J Neurol Neurosurg Psychiatry* 1965;28:247–259.

154. Pillay PK, Awad IA, Hahn JF. Gardner's hydrodynamic theory of syringomyelia revisited. *Cleve Clin J Med* 1992;59:373–380.

155. Solomon RA, Stein BM. Unusual spinal cord enlargement related to intramedullary hemangioblastoma. *J Neurosurg* 1988;68:550–553.

156. Jacob RP, Rhoton AL Jr. The Chiari I malformation. In: Anson JA, Benzel EC, Awad IA, eds. *Syringomyelia and the Chiari malformations.* Park Ridge, IL: American Association of Neurological Surgeons, 1997:57–68.

157. Mariani C, Cislaghi MG, Barbieri S, et al. The natural history and results of surgery in 50 cases of syringomyelia. *J Neurol* 1991;238:433–438.

158. Banerji NK, Millar JH. Chiari malformation presenting in adult life. Its relationship to syringomyelia. *Brain* 1974;97:157–168.

159. Levy WJ, Mason L, Hahn JF. Chiari malformation presenting in adults: a surgical experience in 127 cases. *Neurosurgery* 1983;12:377–390.

160. Schlesinger EB, Antunes JL, Michelsen WJ, et al. Hydromyelia: clinical presentation and comparison of modalities of treatment. *Neurosurgery* 1981;9:356–365.

161. Tashiro K, Fukazawa T, Moriwaka F, et al. Syringomyelic syndrome: clinical features in 31 cases confirmed by CT myelography or magnetic resonance imaging. *J Neurol* 1987;235:26–30.

162. Barnett HJM. Syringomyelia consequent on minor to moderate trauma. In: Barnett HJM, Foster JB, Hudgson P. *Syringomyelia.* London: WB Saunders, 1973:174–178.

163. Foster JB, Hudgson P. The clinical features of communicating syringomyelia. In: Barnett HJM, Foster JB, Hudgson P. *Syringomyelia.* London: WB Saunders, 1973:11–15.

164. Zager EL, Ojemann RG, Poletti CE. Acute presentations of syringomyelia. Report of three cases. *J Neurosurg* 1990;72:133–138.

165. Fuller R, Stanners A. A cough, then respiratory failure. *Lancet* 2000;355:284.

166. Sudo K, Fujiki N, Tsuji S, et al. Focal (segmental) dyshidrosis in syringomyelia. *J Neurol Neurosurg Psychiatry* 1999;67:106–108.

167. Logue V, Edwards MR. Syringomyelia and its surgical treatment—an analysis of 75 patients. *J Neurol Neurosurg Psychiatry* 1981;44:273–284.

168. Williams B. Orthopaedic features in the presentation of syringomyelia. *J Bone Joint Surg Br* 1979;61:314–323.

169. Williams B. Surgery for hindbrain related syringomyelia. *Adv Tech Stand Neurosurg* 1993;20:107–164.

170. Isu T, Iwasaki Y, Akino M, et al. Hydrosyringomyelia associated with a Chiari I malformation in children and adolescents. *Neurosurgery* 1990;26:591–597.

171. Wisoff JH, Epstein F. Management of hydromyelia. *Neurosurgery* 1989;25:562–571.

172. Boman K, Iivanainen M. Prognosis of syringomyelia. *Acta Neurol Scand* 1967;43:61–68.

173. Cahan LD, Bentson JR. Considerations in the diagnosis and treatment of syringomyelia and the Chiari malformation. *J Neurosurg* 1982;57:24–31.

174. Sengupta DK, Dorgan J, Findlay GF. Can hindbrain decompression for syringomyelia lead to regression of scoliosis? *Eur Spine J* 2000;9:198–201.

175. Arai S, Ohtsuka Y, Moriya H, et al. Scoliosis associated with syringomyelia. *Spine* 1993;18:1591–1592.

176. Haponik EF, Givens D, Angelo J. Syringobulbia-myelia with obstructive sleep apnea. *Neurology* 1983;33:1046–1049.

177. Nogues M, Gene R, Benarroch E, et al. Respiratory disturbances during sleep in syringomyelia and syringobulbia. *Neurology* 1999;52:1777–1783.

178. Tator CH. Acute spinal cord injury: a review of recent studies of treatment and pathophysiology. *Can Med Assoc J* 1972;107:143–145.

179. Perot P, Feindel W, Lloyd-Smith D. Hematomyelia as a complication of syringomyelia: Gowers' syringeal hemorrhage. Case report. *J Neurosurg* 1966;25:447–451.

180. Anderson NE, Willoughby EW, Wrightson P. The natural history and the influence of surgical treatment in syringomyelia. *Acta Neurol Scand* 1985;71:472–479.

181. Peerless SJ, Durward QJ. Management of syringomyelia: a pathophysiological approach. *Clin Neurosurg* 1983;30:531–576.

182. Ronen J, Catz A, Spasser R, et al. The treatment dilemma in posttraumatic syringomyelia. *Disabil Rehabil* 1999;21:455–457.

183. Avellino AM, Britz GW, McDowell JR, et al. Spontaneous resolution of a cervicothoracic syrinx in a child. Case report and review of the literature. *Pediatr Neurosurg* 1999;30:43–46.

184. Olivero WC, Dinh DH. Chiari I malformation with traumatic syringomyelia and spontaneous resolution: case report and literature review. *Neurosurgery* 1992;30:758–760.

185. Sun PP, Harrop J, Sutton LN, et al. Complete spontaneous resolution of childhood Chiari I malformation and associated syringomyelia. *Pediatrics* 2001;107:182–184.

186. Appleby A, Foster JB, Hankinson J, et al. The diagnosis and management of the Chiari anomalies in adult life. *Brain* 1968;91:131–140.

187. Foster JB, Hudgson P, Pearce GW. The association of syringomyelia and congenital cervico-medullary anomalies: pathological evidence. *Brain* 1969;92:25–34.

188. Schenk M, Ruggieri PM. Imaging of syringomyelia and the Chiari malformations. In: Anson JA, Benzel EC, Awad IA, eds. *Syringomyelia and the Chiari malformations.* Park Ridge, IL: American Association of Neurological Surgeons, 1997:41–56.

189. Bidzinski J. Pathological findings in suboccipital decompression in 63 patients with syringomyelia. *Acta Neurochir Suppl* 1988;43:26–28.

190. Samuelsson L, Saaf J, Wahlund LO, et al. Evaluation of syringomyelia and Chiari malformations using ultra-low magnetic resonance imaging. *Magn Reson Imaging* 1990;8:123–129.

191. Jinkins JR, Reddy S, Leite CC, et al. MR of parenchymal spinal cord signal change as a sign of active advancement in clinically progressive posttraumatic syringomyelia. *AJNR Am J Neuroradiol* 1998;19:177–182.

192. Menick BJ. Phase-contrast magnetic resonance imaging of cerebrospinal fluid flow in the evaluation of patients with Chiari I malformation. *Neurosurg Focus* 2001;11:1–4.

193. Bidzinski J. Late results of the surgical treatment of syringomyelia. *Acta Neurochir Suppl* 1988;43:29–31.

194. Aschoff A, Kunze S. 100 years syrinx surgery—a review. *Acta Neurochir (Wien)* 1993;123:157–159.

195. Faulhauer K, Loew K. The surgical treatment of syringomyelia. Long-term results. *Acta Neurochir* 1978;44:215–222.

196. Schaller B, Mindermann T, Gratzl O. Treatment of syringomyelia after posttraumatic paraparesis or tetraparesis. *J Spinal Disorders* 1999;12:485–488.

197. Sgouros S, Williams B. A critical appraisal of drainage in syringomyelia. *J Neurosurg* 1995;82:1–10.

198. Umbach I, Heilporn A. Post-spinal cord injury syringomyelia. *Paraplegia* 1991;29:219–221.

199. Barbaro NM, Wilson CB, Gutin PH, et al. Surgical treatment of syringomyelia. Favorable results with syringoperitoneal shunting. *J Neurosurg* 1984;61:531–538.

200. Nishizawa S, Yokoyama T, Yokota N, et al. Incidentally identified syringomyelia associated with Chiari I malformations: is early interventional surgery necessary? *Neurosurgery* 2001;49:637–641.

201. Rhoton AL Jr. Microsurgery of Arnold-Chiari malformation in adults with and without hydromyelia. *J Neurosurg* 1976;45:473–483.

202. Tator CH, Meguro K, Rowed DW. Favorable results with syringosubarachnoid shunts for treatment of syringomyelia. *J Neurosurg* 1982;56:517–523.

203. Daskalakis GJ, Katsetos CN, Papageorgiou IS, et al. Syringomyelia and pregnancy—case report. *Eur J Obstet Gynecol Reprod Biol* 2001;97:98–100.

204. Murayama K, Mamiya K, Nozaki K, et al. Cesarean section in a patient with syringomyelia. *Can J Anaesth* 2001;48:474–477.

205. Gardner WJ, Goodall Robert J. The surgical treatment of Arnold-Chiari malformation in adults. *J Neurosurgery* 1950;7:199–206.

206. Genitori L, Peretta P, Nurisso C, et al. Chiari type I anomalies in children and adolescents: minimally invasive management in a series of 53 cases. *Childs Nerv Syst* 2000;16:707–718.

207. Isu T, Sasaki H, Takamura H, et al. Foramen magnum decompression with removal of the outer layer of the dura as treatment for syringomyelia occurring with Chiari I malformation. *Neurosurgery* 1993;33:844–850.

208. Munshi I, Frim D, Stine-Reyes R, et al. Effects of posterior fossa decompression with and without duraplasty on Chiari malformation-associated hydromyelia. *Neurosurgery* 2000;46:1384–1390.

209. Sahuquillo J, Rubio E, Poca MA, et al. Posterior fossa reconstruction: a surgical technique for the treatment of Chiari I malformation and Chiari I/syringomyelia complex—preliminary results and magnetic resonance imaging quantitative assessment of hindbrain migration. *Neurosurgery* 1994;35:874–884.

210. Kohno K, Sakaki S, Shiraishi T, et al. Successful treatment of adult Arnold-Chiari malformation associated with basilar impression and syringomyelia by the transoral anterior approach. *Surg Neurol* 1990;33:284–287.

211. Halliday AL. Suboccipital and cervical decompression. In: Anson JA, Benzel EC, Awad IA, eds. *Syringomyelia and the Chiari malformation*. Park Ridge, IL: American Association of Neurological Surgeons, 1997:145–150.

212. Iskandar BJ, Hedlund GL, Grabb PA, et al. The resolution of syringohydromyelia without hindbrain herniation after posterior fossa decompression. *J Neurosurg* 1998;89:212–216.

213. Menezes AH. Chiari I malformations and hydromyelia—complications. *Pediatr Neurosurg* 1991;17:146–154.

214. Paul KS, Lye RH, Strang FA, et al. Arnold-Chiari malformation. Review of 71 cases. *J Neurosurg* 1983;58:183–187.

215. Williams B, Fahy G. A critical appraisal of "terminal ventriculostomy" for the treatment of syringomyelia. *J Neurosurg* 1983;58:188–197.

216. Suzuki M, Davis CH, Symon L, et al. Syringoperitoneal shunt for treatment of cord cavitation. *J Neurol Neurosurg Psychiatry* 1985;48:620–627.

217. Phillips TW, Kindt GW. Syringoperitoneal shunt for syringomyelia: a preliminary report. *Surg Neurol* 1981;16:462–466.

218. Iwasaki Y, Hida K, Koyanagi I, et al. Reevaluation of syringosubarachnoid shunt for syringomyelia with Chiari malformation. *Neurosurgery* 2000;46:407–412.

219. Hida K, Iwasaki Y, Koyanagi I, et al. Surgical indication and results of foramen magnum decompression versus syringosubarachnoid shunting for syringomyelia associated with Chiari I malformation. *Neurosurgery* 1995;37:673–678.

220. Vaquero J, Martinez R, Arias A. Syringomyelia-Chiari complex: magnetic resonance imaging and clinical evaluation of surgical treatment. *J Neurosurg* 1990;73:64–68.

221. Dohrmann GJ, Rubin JM. Intraoperative ultrasound imaging of the spinal cord: syringomyelia, cysts, and tumors—a preliminary report. *Surg Neurol* 1982;18:395–399.

222. Foster JB, Hudgson P. The surgical treatment of communicating syringomyelia. In: Barnett HJM, Foster JB, Hudgson P. *Syringomyelia*. London: WB Saunders, 1973:64–78.

223. Schaan M, Jaksche H. Comparison of different operative modalities in post-traumatic syringomyelia: preliminary report. *Eur Spine J* 2001;10:135–140.

224. Ohata K, Gotoh T, Matsusaka Y, et al. Surgical management of syringomyelia associated with spinal adhesive arachnoiditis. *J Clin Neurosci* 2001;8:40–42.

225. Tripathi RP, Sharma A, Jena A, et al. Magnetic resonance imaging in occult spinal dysraphism. *Australas Radiol* 1992;36:8–14.

226. Schlesinger AE, Naidich TP, Quencer RM. Concurrent hydromyelia and diastematomyelia. *AJNR Am J Neuroradiol* 1986;7:473–477.

227. Arunkumar MJ, Korah I, Chandy MJ. Dynamic CSF flow study in the pathophysiology of syringomyelia associated with arachnoid cysts of the posterior fossa. *Br J Neurosurg* 1998;12:33–36.

228. Brophy JD, Sutton LN, Zimmerman RA, et al. Magnetic resonance imaging of lipomyelomeningocele and tethered cord. *Neurosurgery* 1989;25:336–340.

229. Chapman PH, Frim DM. Symptomatic syringomyelia following surgery to treat retethering of lipomyelomeningoceles. *J Neurosurg* 1995;82:752–755.

230. Cinalli G, Renier D, Sebag G, et al. Chronic tonsillar herniation in Crouzon's and Apert's syndromes: the role of premature synostosis of the lambdoid suture. *J Neurosurg* 1995;83:575–582.

231. Vollmer DG, Park TS, Cail WS, et al. Hydromyelia complicating Apert's syndrome: a case report. *Neurosurgery* 1985;17:70–74.

232. Puca A, Cioni B, Colosimo C, et al. Spinal neurenteric cyst in association with syringomyelia: case report. *Surg Neurol* 1992;37:202–207.

233. Finsterer J. Holocord syringomyelia as the dominant feature in Noonan's syndrome. *Eur Neurol* 2000;44:181–182.

234. Peiris A, Ball MJ. Chiari (type 1) malformation and syringomyelia in a patient with Noonan's syndrome. *J Neurol Neurosurg Psychiatry* 1982;45:753–754.

235. O'Neill OR, Roman-Goldstein S, Piatt JH Jr. Sacral agenesis associated with spinal cord syrinx. *Pediatr Neurosurg* 1994;20:217–220.

236. Uematsu S, Wang H, Kopits SE, et al. Total craniospinal decompression in achondroplastic stenosis. *Neurosurgery* 1994;35:250–257; discussion 257–258.

237. Rivosecchi M, Lucchetti MC, Zaccara A, et al. Spinal dysraphism detected by magnetic resonance imaging in patients with anorectal anomalies: incidence and clinical significance. *J Pediatr Surg* 1995;30:488–490.

238. Nagai M, Sakuma R, Aoki M, et al. Familial spinal arachnoiditis with secondary syringomyelia: clinical studies and MRI findings. *J Neurol Sci* 2000;177:60–64.

239. Klekamp J, Samii M, Tatagiba M, et al. Syringomyelia in association with tumours of the posterior fossa. Pathophysiological considerations, based on observations on three related cases. *Acta Neurochir (Wien)* 1995;137:38–43.

240. Sheehan JM, Jane JA Sr. Resolution of tonsillar herniation and syringomyelia after supratentorial tumor resection: case report and review of the literature. *Neurosurgery* 2000;47:233–235.

241. Welch K, Shillito J, Strand R, et al. Chiari I "malformations"—an acquired disorder? *J Neurosurg* 1981;55:604–609.

242. Morioka T, Shono T, Nishio S, et al. Acquired Chiari I malformation and syringomyelia associated with bilateral chronic subdural hematoma. Case report. *J Neurosurg* 1995;83:556–558.

243. Siddiqi SN, Fehlings MG. Lhermitte-Duclos disease mimicking adult-onset aqueductal stenosis. Case report. *J Neurosurg* 1994;80:1095–1098.

244. Young WF. Syringomyelia presenting as a delayed complication of treatment for nocardia brain abscess. *Spinal Cord* 2000;38:265–269.

245. Iwasaki Y, Ikeda K, Ichikawa Y, et al. Multiple sclerosis and syrinx formation. *Acta Neurol Scand* 2000;101:346.

246. Vinas FC, Rengachary S. Diagnosis and management of neurosarcoidosis. *J Clin Neurosci* 2001;8:505–513.

247. Kobayashi R, Togashi S, Nagasaka T, et al. Intramedullary tuberculoma with syringomyelia. *J Spinal Disord* 2002;15:88–90.

248. Hirata Y, Matsukado Y, Kaku M. Syringomyelia associated with a foramen magnum meningioma. *Surg Neurol* 1985;23:291–294.

249. Jamjoom AB, Davies KG. Syringomyelia associated with a spinal schwannoma: a case report. *J Neurol Neurosurg Psychiatry* 1990;53:438–439.

250. Hormigo A, Lobo-Antunes J, Bravo-Marques JM, et al. Syringomyelia secondary to compression of the cervical spinal cord by an extramedullary lymphoma. *Neurosurgery* 1990;27:834–836.

251. Quencer RM, el Gammal T, Cohen G. Syringomyelia associated with intradural extramedullary masses of the spinal canal. *AJNR Am J Neuroradiol* 1986;7:143–148.

252. Rhyner PA, Hudgins RJ, Edwards MS, et al. Magnetic resonance imaging of syringomyelia associated with an extramedullary spinal cord tumor: case report. *Neurosurgery* 1987;21:233–235.

253. Citow JS, Kranzler L. Thoracic epidural lipomatosis with associated syrinx: case report. *Surg Neurol* 2000;53:589–591.

254. Buxton N, Jaspan T, White B. Arachnoid telangiectasia causing meningeal fibrosis and secondary syringomyelia. *Br J Neurosurg* 2001;15:54–57.

255. Slavin KV, Nixon RR, Nesbit GM, et al. Extensive arachnoid ossification with associated syringomyelia presenting as thoracic myelopathy. Case report and review of the literature. *J Neurosurg* 1999;91:223–229.

256. Xenos C, Sgouros S, Walsh R, et al. Spinal lipomas in children. *Pediatr Neurosurg* 2000;32:295–307.

257. Solaro C, Uccelli A, Gentile R, et al. Multiple sclerosis and noncommunicating syringomyelia: a casual association or linked diseases? *Acta Neurol Scand* 1999;100:270–273.

CHAPTER 56

Posttraumatic Syringomyelia

Michael Y. Wang and Barth A. Green

HISTORICAL REVIEW

The earliest reports describing spinal cord cavitation date back to Etienne in the mid-1500s (1). Numerous authors, including Brunner (1688), Morgagni (1740), and Santorini subsequently contributed to the description of this entity (2). Portal (1804) was the first to recognize the neurologic finding of motor weakness as a clinical manifestation of syringomyelia (3), and Shultze (1887) and Kahler (1888) went on to describe the characteristic constellation of clinical symptoms and signs associated with syringomyelia that are recognized today (2).

Early case reports proposing a connection between cystic degeneration of the spinal cord and traumatic injury date back to the writings of Bastian and Strumpell in the late 19th century (4). Although their trauma patients were recognized as having spinal syrinxes, the lack of imaging technology precluded correlations between cyst development and neurologic deterioration. In 1890, Schmasus was able to link spinal cord trauma to cystic cavitation in a rabbit animal model. Further recognition of the connection between trauma and syringomyelia came after Charcot (1892) and Cushing (1898) reported patients who developed the clinical symptoms of syringomyelia soon after spinal cord injury (2,5,6). In 1935 Tauber and Langworthy (7) reported the first case of delayed syringomyelia of which we are aware, in which a patient became symptomatic 8 years after trauma.

With improvements in the acute and long-term management of spinal injury, the survival of these patients has greatly improved. Posttraumatic spinal cord cavitation became more prevalent, as reflected by the larger case series of Barnett (1965), Seibert (1981), and Lyons (1987) and their associates (8–10). They delineated the syndrome of delayed neurologic deterioration due to spinal cord cysts. In the past three decades, more sophisticated imaging modalities such as computed tomography (CT), CT myelography, magnetic resonance imaging (MRI), and cine MRI have facilitated making the correct diagnosis, following the pathology, and appropriately treating patients with posttraumatic syrinxes (Fig. 56.1).

EPIDEMIOLOGY

Symptomatic posttraumatic cystic myelopathy, syrinxes, or cystic cavitation of the spinal cord occurs in up to 3.2% of spinal cord injury patients (11). Some authors have reported a higher prevalence of cysts based on MRI studies that include asymptomatic patients (12,13). The time span between injury and the onset of symptoms has been reported to range from 2 months to 30 years (11). The severity of injury has been hypothesized to influence the likelihood of cyst formation (14–16). Up to 8% of patients with complete injuries develop the clinical signs and symptoms of syringomyelia (16), a rate that is two to three times higher than with incomplete lesions (17). Injury severity has also been shown to accelerate the rapidity with which patients become symptomatic after injury. In the series by Lyons and associates (10,17), the mean time to presentation was 101 months in patients with incomplete injury as compared with 39 months in patients with complete lesions.

Penetrating missile injuries are more likely than blunt injuries to cause cyst formation, presumably because of the increased prevalence of posttraumatic intradural adhesions. Similarly, intracanalicular bone fragments and dural tears promote extensive scarring between the spinal cord and dura. The resulting myelomalacia, arachnoiditis, and cord tethering all contribute to abnormal flow patterns in the spinal fluid, promoting cyst formation. Prolonged immobility after injury may also play a role in the development of posttraumatic cysts. With the patient in a dependent position, neural edema and posttraumatic intradural blood clots promote adhesions between the spinal cord and dura.

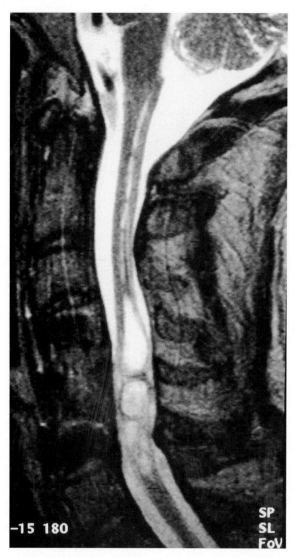

-15 180

SP
SL
FoV

FIG. 56.1. Midcervical multiloculated syrinx in a patient who fell from a tree and was suffering incomplete quadriplegia. Ascending myelopathy prompted magnetic resonance imaging evaluation.

PATHOGENESIS

The pathophysiological mechanism that results in the formation of a posttraumatic cyst is poorly understood and remains a topic of considerable controversy. Gardner and McMurray (18) originally proposed that an obstruction to cerebrospinal fluid (CSF) flow at the craniocervical junction causes pulse waves to be transmitted caudally through the spinal cord. Fluid is forced into the Virchow-Robin space or central canal of the spinal cord. These theories were supported by case reports of patients with syringomyelia in which a connection was demonstrated between the syrinx and the ventricular system (19–21). Although this original theory was based on studies of nontraumatic lesions, it became accepted as a pathophysiological explanation for all syrinxes.

Other theories later emerged to explain the development of posttraumatic syringomyelia (22,23). Milhorat and associates (24) showed that the histopathology and clinical findings seen in posttraumatic syringomyelia were different from lesions of nontraumatic origin (2). A two-step process was proposed to explain posttraumatic cysts: cyst formation followed by cyst expansion. Cyst formation is a direct result of the initial injury, which causes tissue edema, hemorrhage, and cell loss. Macroscopically, this results in degenerated spinal cord parenchyma and myelomalacia. Local microcystic cavitation also occurs, and these lesions may become contiguous to form a larger cyst. Cavitation may be aggravated by additional factors, such as hematoma liquefaction, cord ischemia, release of intracellular lysosomal enzymes, and mechanical crush injury (11,17). The gray matter adjacent to the central canal between the dorsal horns is especially prone to cyst cavity formation due to its poor vascularity and lack of connective tissue support.

After initial cyst formation, cyst expansion may occur due to derangements in CSF flow. Cord tethering occurs due to the arachnoiditis that results from intradural blood and inflammatory mediators. Tethering of the spinal cord to the surrounding meninges sets up abnormal flow dynamics, which forces fluid into existing cavities via transmural migration (17,25). Experimental animal models of arachnoiditis in rabbits treated with intrathecal kaolin injection support these theories (26). Spinal cord tethering also creates areas of CSF turbulence, further promoting cavity expansion. The fixed spinal cord is also unable to accommodate the mechanical forces associated with flexion and extension and changes in intrathoracic pressure.

Spinal cord tethering remains central to most theories of cyst expansion. Tethering and the resultant perturbations in CSF flow are central to the "slosh" and "suck" theories proposed by Williams (27). The "slosh" hypothesis theorizes that Valsalva maneuvers such as coughing and sneezing create a rise in epidural venous pressure that cannot by dissipated when there is interference with CSF flow. These forces are transmitted to the spinal cord, which compresses the cystic cavity, distorting areas of structural weakness within the cord parenchyma (3,11,17). The "suck" hypothesis proposes that increases in epidural venous pressure create a pressure gradient around a partial subarachnoid block. This causes CSF to be rapidly forced upward and then sucked back down slowly around the block. Positive pressure proximal to the block leads to cephalad cyst extension. Hughes (28) theorized that a valvelike connection between the subarachnoid space and the cyst allows CSF to enter but not exit from the syrinx (2,11). Mechanical compression from a large disk herniation, subluxation, gibbus, kyphoscoliosis, or canal instability may also cause tethering and result in syringomyelic cavities.

CLINICAL PRESENTATION

The most common initial complaint of a patient with a posttraumatic syringomyelia is pain (11,17,29,30), the quality of which can be dull, aching, sharp, or stabbing. Milhorat and associates (31) reported that painful dysesthesias occur in up to 40% of patients. Hyperesthesias in a dermatomal distribution are also frequently observed. Pain commonly occurs at or above the original site of injury, and cyst expansion with an ascending pain syndrome is a characteristic finding. The pain may be worsened with a Valsalva maneuver.

Sensory loss is the second most common complaint and often occurs in a dissociated pattern. The usual location of syrinx cavities results in the preferential impairment of pain and temperature sensation, with proprioception being spared. Sensory loss may be patchy in some cases, whereas other patients manifest an ascending sensory level. Decreased sensation can be bilateral, unilateral, or can alternate sides depending on the patient's position.

Progressive motor weakness is the third most common symptom and rarely occurs as an isolated phenomenon. It is commonly associated with an ascending sensory level or the loss of deep tendon reflexes (4,17,32). Loss of deep tendon reflexes in the upper limbs can be an early clinical sign of syringomyelia, particularly with descending lesions (17,33,34). Other symptoms include changes in tone (either increased spasticity or decreased tone), hyperhidrosis, autonomic dysreflexia, an alternating Horner's syndrome, sphincter dysfunction, and respiratory insufficiency. These signs may be unilateral, bilateral, or posturally dependent.

IMAGING

The earliest cases of syringomyelia were diagnosed solely on clinical findings. Definitive diagnosis relied on exploratory laminectomy or postmortem studies. Air myelography allowed the preoperative confirmation and localization of syrinx cavities (17,35), but the invasive nature and morbidity associated with this technique was a great limitation. The advent of CT myelography after water-soluble contrast injection greatly advanced the preoperative diagnosis of posttraumatic syringomyelia (36). Delayed views were particularly helpful in delineating cystic fluid collections. However, difficulty distinguishing cysts from intramedullary tumors remained a problem with this imaging modality.

MRI is currently the most sensitive diagnostic tool for evaluating cases of possible posttraumatic cystic myelopathy (2,11,29). MRI is noninvasive, and gadolinium contrast is well tolerated. Because of the excellent soft tissue definition, MRI is superior for detecting tumors and intramedullary scarring (11). Myelomalacic cavities can also be distinguished from true syrinxes by their irregularly demarcated borders, moderate hypointensity on T1-weighted images, and nonCSF signal intensity on proton-density-weighted images (11,29,30,37). In cases with instrumentation, fast spin echo T2-weighted images are optimal for minimizing metal artifact.

The noninvasive assessment of CSF flow dynamics has more recently been made possible with cine MRI. Spinal cord tethering can be assessed in detail by this technique, because an interruption in normal CSF flow is evident around areas where the spinal cord is adherent to the surrounding dura. Cyst pulsatility, which occurs when the syrinx communicates with the subarachnoid space, can also be seen with cine MRI (11). This finding may be predictive of future cyst expansion. MRI is also the study of choice for following cyst progression.

Intraoperative ultrasound is highly useful in the surgical management of syringomyelia. Following laminectomy, ultrasound can be used for cyst localization. The excellent visualization of adhesions, points of tethering, and septations offered by ultrasound can be used to guide intraoperative treatment. Ultrasound can also be used to assess shunt placement and document collapse of the cyst cavity.

SURGICAL MANAGEMENT

Radiographic or clinical evidence of cyst expansion is an indication for surgical intervention. Because neurologic deterioration can only be halted with collapse of the syrinx, this is the most compelling indication for surgery. Expanding cysts produce neurologic deficits locally. Cyst expansion in rostral and/or caudal directions leads to characteristic ascending and descending deficits. Sudden, permanent neurologic impairment as a result of trivial trauma has also been described as a consequence of syringomyelia. This has prompted some authors to recommend surgery in an attempt to forestall these disastrous incidents (2,16).

Advances in noninvasive imaging techniques have increased the frequency with which asymptomatic spinal cord cysts are detected. Surgical intervention in these cases is more controversial. Small cysts less than 1 centimeter in rostrocaudal extent that are not causing substantial displacement of the surrounding spinal cord are managed conservatively. Narrow, asymptomatic cysts spanning several spinal segments that do not expand the spinal cord can also be followed with serial imaging studies every 3 to 6 months. Large cysts that expand the spinal cord and obliterate the surrounding subarachnoid space usually produce neurologic symptoms and signs and should prompt a detailed physical examination to search for missed findings. In cases followed conservatively, documentation of a detailed history and physical examination of the sensory system are essential to detect any evidence of cyst enlargement. Pain drawings may be a useful adjunct for assessing changes in symptomatology. In some cases the loss of spinal cord function is heralded only by the conversion of upper motor neuron findings (for example, spasticity) to lower motor neuron findings (for example, loss of tone). Although this may appear to be a benign phenomenon, it is associated with increased risks of decubitus ulcers and difficulty with bowel and bladder care.

Contemporary sophisticated imaging techniques have led to the evolution of radiographic predictors of cyst enlargement. It is our experience that cysts having pulsatile CSF flow on cine MRI are more frequently symptomatic and will require surgical intervention. Asano and co-workers (38) used the flow-void sign on T2-weighted MRI to distinguish between cases of high-pressure and low-pressure cysts in their series. In that series, cysts with high pressure showed more clinical and radiographic improvement after surgery than low-pressure cysts.

Presurgical evaluation should determine the exact location and extent of the syrinx, along with any associated pathology such as cord tethering, subarachnoid cysts, and fissures. Surgery should be carried out with continuous monitoring of somatosensory and motor evoked potentials and with the aid of the operating microscope. After laminectomy with exposure of the dura, intraoperative ultrasonography is employed to localize the cyst and to visualize any areas of cord tethering. Because cysts and tethering frequently occur at sites of previous intradural surgery, special care must be taken in exposing the dura to free it from extradural adhesions so that ultrasound can be used and good planes are available for duraplasty. Frequently, a plane can be found using a sharp curette. If this is not possible, soft tissue may be left on the dura and opened along with it in the midline. Before the dura is tacked away from the midline, care must be taken to free it from any neural tissue to prevent inadvertent traction on the spinal cord. In the event of midline dorsal dural adhesions that cannot be separated from the spinal cord with microdissection, it is safer to leave the adherent dura attached to the spinal cord surface.

A key component of the operative intervention is spinal cord untethering with careful sharp dissection of adhesions (39). In our experience, proper lysis of adhesions alone will lead to immediate collapse of the syrinx in greater than 50% of cases (Fig. 56.2). This is accomplished primarily with sharp dissection using a no. 11 blade, round knife, or microscissors. Attention must always be directed to the lateral gutters to ensure free CSF communication. Tethering to

the ventral dura may be difficult to lyse and should be done only with the strictest caution to avoid neurovascular injury. It is our practice to repeat intraoperative ultrasonography after untethering to assess cyst size (Fig. 56.3). If the cyst has not collapsed, shunting of the syrinx is necessary. We attempt to avoid shunts, especially pleural and peritoneal shunts, because of their associated complications. Shunt failure rates have been reported to be as high as 50% in some long-term studies (40–43).

In the event that a shunt is needed, we prefer cyst-to-subarachnoid shunts or shunt stents. Shunts that drain into the pleural or peritoneal cavities are reserved for cases with diffuse arachnoiditis or extensive levels of tethering. The shunt entry point should be chosen at an area where the overlying neural tissue is thinnest and pial arteries are absent. In most cases the caudal end of the cyst is chosen. At this point a 2-millimeter section of pia is cauterized with bipolar current. A vertical myelotomy is then made using a no. 11 blade. The myelotomy can be made at the dorsal root entry zone for eccentrically located cysts. A Silastic microcatheter is then directed into the cyst in a cephalad direction. Preoperative measurement of the length of the syrinx will allow an appropriate length of tubing to be used. In the rare event that one tube will not traverse a multiloculated or double-barreled cyst, additional myelotomies and shunt catheter placements may be necessary.

After catheter placement, an x-ray is taken to ensure that the catheter has not kinked or folded over on itself. Intraoperative ultrasound is performed to confirm that the tube is in the syrinx cavity and to evaluate the degree of cyst collapse. One or two centimeters of tubing should extend from the myelotomy into the dorsal expanded subarachnoid space created by the duraplasty. Once catheter placement has been confirmed, a 6–0 Prolene suture is used to secure it to the pia, preventing dislodgement. If substantial dorsal adhesions are present, the risk of distal shunt occlusion is significant; the tube may be directed between the nerve

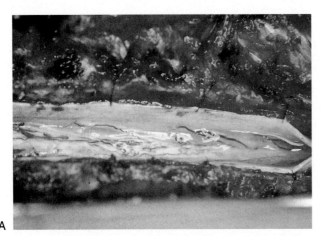

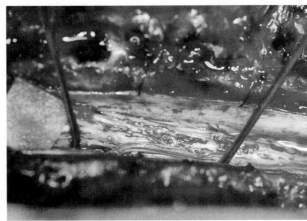

A

B

FIG. 56.2. Intraoperative views. **A:** The thoracic spinal cord, showing subarachnoid adhesions to the surrounding dura. **B:** After adhesions have been sharply dissected, the spinal cord is untethered from the surrounding dura.

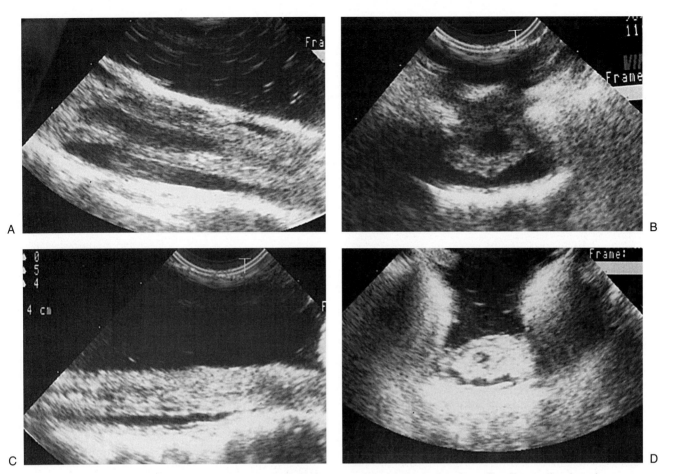

FIG. 56.3. Intraoperative ultrasounds. **A, B:** Before opening the dura, showing adhesions to the dorsal surface and the intramedullary cyst. **C, D:** After untethering, showing cyst collapse.

roots into the ventral subarachnoid space. Hemostasis is essential to prevent scarring and retethering; this is achieved using thrombin-soaked Gelfoam and careful microbipolar coagulation. All Gelfoam is removed prior to closure.

The prevention of retethering is critical to ensure the long-term success of the surgery. We regularly perform a duraplasty using a freeze-dried dural allograft to expand the dorsal subarachnoid space (Fig. 56.4). The dural graft must be circumferentially sewn in a watertight fashion using a 6–0 Prolene running suture with the stitches spaced closely together. In regions with irregular, thin, or disrupted dura, a fat or muscle graft can be sewn over any remaining defects.

Postoperatively, patients are carefully positioned in a semiprone position to keep the spinal cord from resting in a dependent position upon the graft and suture line. Log rolling is performed religiously from semiprone to semiprone every 2 hours for the next 48 hours while the patient is on strict bedrest. The patient is then mobilized to a wheelchair or walking, avoiding the supine position for more than 30 minutes at a time for the next 30 days. Valsalva maneuvers are also discouraged during this time period. By 30 days any initial scar formation will have already occurred. Patients who are doing well are followed with cine MRI scans, annually at first and then less frequently as time goes on.

In summary, posttraumatic syringomyelia is now recognized as a major issue following spinal cord injury and spinal cord surgery. Our current management protocol includes early mobilization in a Roto-Rest bed after injury and early surgery for decompression and stabilization. These measures

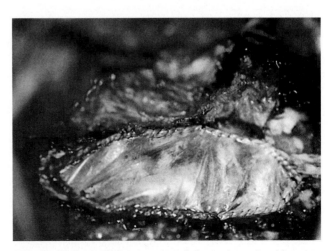

FIG. 56.4. Duraplasty to expand the subarachnoid space and prevent retethering.

are intended to decrease the likelihood of delayed spinal cord tethering and associated syrinx formation. We apply similar management principles postoperatively after intradural surgery for neoplasms. This includes untethering of any adhesions found during surgery, expansile duraplasty in select cases, and postural therapy postoperatively.

REFERENCES

1. Finlayson AI. Syringomyelia and related conditions. In: Joynt RJ, ed. *Clinical neurology,* vol. 3. Philadelphia: JB Lippincott, 1989:1–17.
2. Madsen PW, Falcone SF, Bowen BC, et al. Posttraumatic syringomyelia. In: Levine A, Eismont F, Garfin S, et al., eds. *Spine trauma.* Philadelphia: WB Saunders, 1998:608–629.
3. Wilson SAK. Syringomyelia: syringobulbia. In: Bruce AN, ed. *Neurology,* vol. 3. Baltimore: Williams and Wilkins, 1955:1187–1202.
4. Vernon JD, Silver JR, Ohry A. Posttraumatic syringomyelia. *Paraplegia* 1982;20:339–364.
5. Barnett HJM, Jousse AT. Posttraumatic syringomyelia. In: Vinken PJ, Bruyn GW, eds. *Injuries of the spine and spinal cord, part II. Handbook of clinical neurology,* vol. 26. Amsterdam: North-Holland, 1976: 113–157.
6. Cushing HM. Haematomyelia from gunshot wounds of the spine. A report of two cases with recovery following symptoms of hemilesion of the cord. *Am J Med Sci* 1898;115:654–683.
7. Tauber ES, Langworthy OR. A study of syringomyelia and the formation of cavities in the spinal cord. *J Nervous Mental Dis* 1935;81:245–264.
8. Barnett HJM, Botterell EH, Jousse AT, et al. Progressive myelopathy as a sequel to traumatic paraplegia. *Brain* 1965;89:159–178.
9. Seibert CE, Dreisbach JN, Swanson WB, et al. Progressive posttraumatic cystic myelopathy: neuroradiologic evaluation. *AJR Am J Roentgenol* 1981;136:1161–1165.
10. Lyons BM, Brown DJ, Calvert JM, et al. The diagnosis and management of posttraumatic syringomyelia. *Paraplegia* 1987;25:340–350.
11. Schwartz ED, Falcone SF, Quencer RM, et al. Posttraumatic syringomyelia: pathogenesis, imaging and treatment. *AJR Am J Roentgenol* 1999;173:487–492.
12. Backe HA, Betz RR, Mesgarzadeh M, et al. Posttraumatic spinal cord cysts evaluated by magnetic resonance imaging. *Paraplegia* 1991;29: 607–612.
13. Hussey RW, Ha CY, Vijay M, et al. Prospective study of the occurrence rate of posttraumatic cystic degeneration of the spinal cord utilizing magnetic resonance imaging. *J Am Paraplegia Soc* 1990;13:16.
14. Edgar R, Quail P. Progressive posttraumatic cystic and non-cystic myelopathy. *Br J Neurosurg* 1994;8:7–22.
15. Levi AD, Sonntag VK. Management of posttraumatic syringomyelia using an expansile duraplasty: a case report. *Spine* 1998;23:128–132.
16. Rossier AB, Foo D, Shillito J, et al. Posttraumatic cervical syringomyelia: incidence, clinical presentation, electrophysiological studies, syrinx protein and results of conservative and operative treatment. *Brain* 1985;108:439–461.
17. Biyani A, El Masry WS. Posttraumatic syringomyelia: a review of the literature. *Paraplegia* 1994;32:723–731.
18. Gardner WJ, McMurray FG. "Non-communicating" syringomyelia: a non-existent entity. *Surg Neurol* 1976;6:251–256.
19. Ellertsson AB, Greitz T. Myelocystographic and fluorescein studies to demonstrate communication between intramedullary cysts and the cerebrospinal fluid space. *Acta Neurol Scand* 1969;45:418–430.
20. McLean DR, Miller JDR, Allen PBR, et al. Posttraumatic syringomyelia. *J Neurosurg* 1973;39:485–492.
21. Oakley JC, Ojemann GA, Alvord EC. Posttraumatic syringomyelia: case report. *J Neurosurg* 1981;55:276–281.
22. Nurick S, Russell JA, Deck MDF. Cystic degeneration of the spinal cord following spinal cord injury. *Brain* 1970;93:211–222.
23. Williams B, Terry AF, Jones HWF, et al. Syringomyelia as a sequel to traumatic paraplegia. *Paraplegia* 1981;19:67–80.
24. Milhorat TH, Capoceli AL, Anzil AP, et al. Pathological basis of spinal cord cavitation in syringomyelia: analysis of 105 autopsy cases. *J Neurosurg* 1995;82:802–812.
25. Williams B. Pathogenesis of posttraumatic syringomyelia [Editorial]. *Br J Neurosurg* 1992;6:517–520.
26. Cho KH, Iwasaki Y, Imamura H, et al. Experimental model of posttraumatic syringomyelia: the role of adhesive arachnoiditis in syrinx formation. *J Neurosurg* 1994;80:133–139.
27. Williams B. The distending force in the production of "communicating syringomyelia." *Lancet* 1969;2:189–193.
28. Hughes JT. Pathologic changes after spinal cord injury. In: Illis LS, ed. *Spinal cord dysfunction: assessment.* Oxford: Oxford University Press, 1988:34–40.
29. Green BA, Lee TT, Madsen PW, et al. Management of posttraumatic cystic myelopathy. *Topics Spinal Cord Inj Rehab* 1997;2:36–46.
30. Lee TT, Arias JM, Andrus HL, et al. Progressive posttraumatic myelomalacic myelopathy: treatment with untethering and expansile duraplasty. *J Neurosurg* 1997;86:624–628.
31. Milhorat TH, Kotzen RM, Mu HT, et al. Dysesthetic pain in patients with syringomyelia. *Neurosurgery* 1996;38:940–947.
32. Anton HA, Schweigel JF. Posttraumatic syringomyelia: the British Columbia experience. *Spine* 1986;11:865–868.
33. Dworkin GE, Stass WE. Posttraumatic syringomyelia. *Arch Phys Med Rehab* 1981;66:329–331.
34. Watson N. Ascending cystic degeneration of the cord after spinal cord injury. *Paraplegia* 1981;19:89–95.
35. Rossier AB, Foo D, Naheedy MH, et al. Radiography of posttraumatic syringomyelia. *AJNR Am J Neuroradiol* 1983;4:637–640.
36. Li KC, Chui MC. Conventional and CT metrizamide myelography in Arnold-Chiari I malformation and syringomyelia. *AJNR Am J Neuroradiol* 1987;8:11–17.
37. Falcone S, Quencer RM, Green BA, et al. Progressive posttraumatic myelomalacic myelopathy: imaging and clinical features. *AJNR Am J Neuroradiol* 1994;15:747–754.
38. Asano M, Fujiwara K, Yonenobu K, et al. Posttraumatic syringomyelia. *Spine* 1996;21:1446–1453.
39. Williams B. Posttraumatic syringomyelia: an update. *Paraplegia* 1990; 28:296–313.
40. Batzdorf U, Klekamp J, Johnson JP. A critical appraisal of syrinx cavity shunting procedures. *J Neurosurg* 1998;89:382–388.
41. Lee TT, Alameda GJ, Gromelski EB, et al. Outcome after surgical treatment of progressive posttraumatic cystic myelopathy. *J Neurosurg (Spine 2)* 2000;92:149–154.
42. Sgouros S, Williams B. A critical appraisal of drainage of syringomyelia . *J Neurosurg* 1995;82:1–10.
43. Sgouros S, Williams B. Management and outcome of posttraumatic syringomyelia. *J Neurosurg* 1996;85:197–205.

CHAPTER 57

Spinal Cord and Nerve Regeneration

M. Darryl Antonacci and Marion Murray

Peripherally directed axons can regenerate to form functional connections, but central nervous system (CNS) axons do not. Aguayo and his colleagues (1–3), in the 1980s, demonstrated, however, that many CNS neurons could indeed regenerate their axons for long distances if a favorable environment was provided. In those studies, transplants of peripheral nerves were used to provide the more favorable physical and chemical environment needed for axonal regeneration. This important finding implicated an intrinsically nonpermissive adult CNS environment as a major reason for the failure of axonal regeneration.

REPAIR STRATEGY

After initial injury to the spinal cord, a secondary cascade of events occurs that creates a hostile environment for surviving neurons and those not directly injured. This hostile environment is in part a consequence of the loss of neurotrophic and other growth-promoting factors. Additionally, release of toxic molecules from dying cells, deleterious effects of the immune response, programmed cell death (apoptosis), and the development of an astrocyte barrier at the site of the lesion contribute to a nonpermissive environment and inhibit axonal regeneration. CNS neurons are also intrinsically poor regenerators and do not respond to injury with the robust upregulation of gene expression necessary for axonal regeneration. Over the last two decades, as details of the injury cascade and the inhibitors of the regenerative process have become better elucidated, strategies have emerged to counter these effects. Axonal regeneration can now be enhanced by providing specific neurotrophic factors, cell adhesion molecules, and extracellular matrix molecules that stimulate and modulate growth, as well as by blocking growth-inhibitory molecules. Components of the immune response can be suppressed pharmacologically, and modern gene therapy techniques can introduce the necessary genes required to stimulate and provide growth-related protein

synthesis. It is now evident that although there are substantial obstacles to regeneration in the CNS, each of these obstacles also has potential solutions.

The first step in promoting repair is to support neuron survival (neuroprotection). At the time of an acute injury, whether from causes such as gunshot wounds, stab wounds, penetration by bony shards, or through injuries that lead to contusion of the spinal cord, some neurons are directly destroyed, but many injured neurons survive, often in an atrophic and probably compromised state. For instance, corticospinal tract neurons do not typically die after axonal injury, although they may atrophy. Other axotomized neurons may die through retrograde degeneration, or undergo such severe atrophy they are no longer recognized. Of the neurons that survive, some sprout new axons. Because some recovery and restoration of functional neuronal circuits is potentially possible when neurons survive, neuroprotection is an important first step in repair strategies (4–6).

A second step is to modulate the typically inhibitory CNS. This includes blocking growth-inhibitory proteins normally present in the adult CNS as well as countering toxic effects of the injury, including the astrocytic response, proteoglycan upregulation, and scar formation.

A third step is to support axonal growth and promote regeneration by providing a favorable molecular environment for surviving neurons. Delivering appropriate trophic and tropic factors is a powerful strategy that stimulates axonal outgrowth. Although there are various delivery methods, the repair process is likely to combine delivery with provision of a "bridge" by using cellular and noncellular transplants. This would allow regenerating axons to cross the site of injury and reach target neurons from which they have been separated. Cellular transplants can also be modified using gene therapy to allow for controlled patterns of gene expression at the site of repair and thereby provide neuroprotection, promote regeneration, and counter the nonpermissive CNS environment. Gene therapy, therefore, has emerged as a very powerful component of modern repair strategy in spinal cord injury.

Increase Neuronal Survival

Interventions that target the prevention of apoptotic cell death or provide neurotrophic factors are promising neuroprotective strategies (7–13). One method to inhibit neuronal death would be to block the caspase-induced execution phase of apoptosis (14,15). For example, YVAD and DEVD-CHO are inhibitors of specific caspases and have been shown to arrest the programmed cell death of motor neurons (16–18). Another important family of peptides that may be strategically useful in the prevention of apoptosis is related to the protooncogene Bcl-2. These peptides function prior to caspase activation (16,19). Some of these peptides, namely Bcl-2 and Bcl-xL, are potent inhibitors of apoptosis. Bcl-2 is localized to mitochondria, endoplasmic reticulum, and nuclear membranes. It inhibits the release of cytochrome c. Cytochrome c in combination with ATP participates in activating the autocatalysis of procaspase 9 into caspase 9, and thereby triggers the execution phase of apoptosis (16,20,21). Bcl-2, therefore, blocks the apoptotic cascade. It has also been shown that axotomized neurons have increased survival when Bcl-2 is overexpressed (22–28). Bcl-2 also serves to protect cells in other ways, by inhibiting the release of calcium from mitochondria and by suppressing lipid peroxidation (29–32). Consequently, inhibitors of apoptosis such as members of the Bcl-2 family may serve as powerful adjuncts to other neuroprotective strategies such as the provision of neurotrophic factors (16).

Although endogenous levels are not sufficient, exogenous administration of neurotrophic factors has been shown to rescue axotomized neurons from retrograde cell death (33–37). Neurotrophic factors have been supplied via various routes (see "Delivering Neurotrophic Factors," later in this chapter) and have been shown to effectively rescue neurons after exogenous administration and after transplantation of fetal tissue or cells genetically modified to secrete specific neurotrophic factors. The neuroprotective effect of trophic factors may be limited to within 1 week of injury, however, because delayed administration at 2 or more weeks demonstrates no protective effects (38). Moreover, some neuronal populations respond to provision of one trophic factor, whereas others require more than one factor (35). Because most spinal cord injuries involve mixed populations of injured neurons, provision of a cocktail of trophic factors is probably necessary to optimize their rescue. Although providing neurotrophic factors may prevent retrograde cell death, surviving neurons are atrophic and most likely compromised in function to some degree. Nonetheless, neuroprotective strategies directed at inhibiting apoptotic cell death and providing the required levels of neurotrophic factors will maximize the number of surviving neurons available for regeneration.

Overcome Inhibitory Central Nervous System Environment

The CNS environment is inhibitory to axonal growth and becomes more so after injury. The mechanical barrier formed by the astrocytic glial scar poses a physical and chemical obstacle to regenerating axons. In addition, cavitation and cyst formation eliminates a terrain through which axons can grow. The astrocytic response to CNS injury is limited in the first 10 days. At that time there is a change in astrocyte morphology and an upregulation in the expression of proteoglycans (39). These molecules (for example, phosphacan, brevican, neurocan, and NG2) are inhibitory to axonal regeneration (40,41). Their inhibitory effects vary depending on the size of the associated glycosaminoglycan side chain and degree of sulfation. They likely block the growth-promoting effects of cell adhesion molecules such as laminin through direct interaction with their protein cores. They also variably inhibit other growth-promoting extracellular matrix molecules depending on their side chains. *In vitro,* proteases can degrade the proteoglycans and have been shown to diminish their inhibitory effects (28,42). Administering enzymes to lesioned rat dorsal columns that attenuate the inhibitory activity resulted in growth of both corticospinal axons and ascending sensory axons (43). Provision of neurotrophic factors may also enable regenerating axons to overcome these growth-inhibitory effects (40,44).

The scar and extracellular matrix contain many other inhibitory molecules, which negatively modulate axon growth. In 1988, Caroni and Schwab (45) purified two membrane proteins found on the surface of differentiated rat oligodendrocytes and in CNS myelin that inhibited neurite growth. The axon growth-inhibitory properties of these myelin molecules, NI-35 and NI-250, as well as the subsequently cloned Nogo-A, were neutralized by a monoclonal antibody (IN-1). When antibodies to block the growth-inhibitory molecules were administered, axonal regeneration occurred into optic nerve explants (45,46). In another study, regrowth of brainstem spinal and corticospinal axons following a spinal cord lesion in adult rats was described after application of IN-1 antibodies (47). Specific reflex and locomotor functions (contact-placing responses) recovered but were abolished after removal of the sensorimotor cortex. The authors suggested that the recovery was dependent on the growth of these axons after effective neutralization of the growth-inhibitory molecules of CNS myelin.

Other neurite inhibitory molecules have also been discovered in CNS myelin. In 1994, two groups of investigators using different experimental approaches described the strong growth-inhibiting effects of myelin-associated glycoprotein (MAG) (48,49). *In vivo,* MAG contributes to axonal growth inhibition after injury. Priming neurons with neurotrophins or increasing cAMP levels has been shown to successfully block MAG- and myelin-derived inhibition of neurite growth (50). However, overcoming the inhibitory effects of MAG depends on the selection of the neurotrophic factor. Brain- or glial-derived neurotrophic factors (BDNF or GDNF) blocked the effect of MAG, whereas nerve growth factor (NGF) did not. Countering the growth-inhibiting molecular components of the myelin sheath using specific blocking agents has thus become an important part of the repair strategy.

Promote Regeneration

Using Peripheral Nerve Grafts

In the years preceding their 1928 publication, Ramon y Cajal and his student, Tello, suggested that central nervous system neurons could regenerate in the right milieu; Aguayo and his colleagues later showed the effectiveness of using peripheral nerve grafts in CNS axonal regeneration. Peripheral nerve transplantation provides a source of trophic factors (1,2,3,51–53), and the grafts lack CNS myelin inhibitory factors. Although axons could enter and grow for long distances within the peripheral nerve graft, they were not successful in penetrating the host spinal cord, presumably because they could not overcome the CNS inhibitory environment. In 1996, Cheng and associates (54) used multiple peripheral nerve transplants to study axonal regeneration across a completely transected spinal cord in the adult rat. They placed 18 small-diameter peripheral nerves into a 3- to 5-mm spinal cord defect, directing these grafts from white matter to gray matter. The grafted area was stabilized with fibrin glue containing acidic fibroblast growth factor (FGF-1), a factor shown to support neurite outgrowth (55). They described successful regeneration of corticospinal tract axons and several bulbospinal pathways through the peripheral nerve graft and also into host tissue. Hind limb function improved progressively during the first 6 months. This study did not show, however, whether the use of multiple peripheral nerve grafts alone allows growth of regenerating axons into host CNS tissue.

Regardless, the amount of peripheral nerve that would be needed and the graft lengths likely to be necessary in human spinal cord injuries limit the use of peripheral nerve grafts. In some cases of spinal cord injuries, or in cases of syringomyelia, these lesions can be quite large. Peripheral nerve grafts also tend to have reduced viability after storage (56–58). One approach to overcome these limitations has been the isolation from the peripheral nerves of Schwann cells, the peripheral myelin-forming cell (59,60). Once isolated, Schwann cells do not lose their ability to express crucial trophic factors (61–64). Another major advantage of using Schwann cells over peripheral nerve grafts is that, once isolated, the number of Schwann cells can be expanded greatly *in vitro*.

Using Schwann Cell Grafts

Enhanced axonal regeneration using peripheral nerve grafts has been largely attributed to Schwann cell expression of trophic factors (51). The basement membranes of Schwann cell tubes also contain many adhesion molecules, such as L1, J1, integrins, and laminin. These molecules have been shown to enhance axonal growth and provide guidance cues to regenerating axons (65–71). In 1997, Xu and colleagues (72) substantially improved upon earlier techniques in the isolation and expansion of Schwann cells in culture. Their study obtained an increase in the yield of Schwann cells by approximately 17,000-fold. Such high cell numbers would be necessary for transplantation into spinal cord defects (60).

Several techniques have been used to transplant Schwann cells into the spinal cord. Schwann cells have been injected not only by a comparatively nontraumatic air pressure microtransplantation system but also nontraumatically by glass micropipette (73,74). In these studies, high Schwann cell survival after transplantation was documented. Other investigators injected a suspension of 10,000 Schwann cells into an upper cervical lesion of the corticospinal tract. As early as 4 days after transplantation, Schwann cells were documented along the perivascular space, and at 6 weeks, they not only remained viable but also had myelinated several segments of the host's corticospinal tract (75). These investigators concluded that Schwann cells integrated into the cytoarchitecture of the myelinated adult host corticospinal tract in a nonrandom manner, resulting in the formation of organized central and peripheral tissue.

The effectiveness of Schwann cell transplantation is affected by the time of transplantation after injury. Schwann cells injected immediately or 10 days after low thoracic injury in adult female rats survived better than when the Schwann cells were injected 3 days after injury secondary to reduced posttraumatic micro- and macrocavitation (76). It is likely that graft survival is affected by the presence or buildup of toxic metabolites, or the absence of necessary neurotrophins (60,76). Although increased neuronal survival occurred with immediate transplantation, the time for optimal axonal regeneration remains to be determined.

To maximize the effectiveness of Schwann cell transplantations, Schwann cells have been transplanted with different matrix carriers, for example, collagen, Matrigel, and carbon filaments. Matrigel contains extracellular matrix molecules such as laminin, collagen 4, entactin, and proteoglycans (60). After a complete spinal cord transection, a Matrigel bridge containing Schwann cells had eight times more nonmyelinated axons within the transplanted graft than a pure Schwann cell graft. In addition, nearly 2,000 myelinated axons were found within the combined Matrigel and Schwann cell graft (72). In this study, the transplanted Schwann cells supported regrowth of both ascending and descending axons, but not corticospinal fibers. Limited regrowth of serotonergic and noradrenergic fibers from the rostral stump also occurred.

In a thoracic hemisection model, Schwann cell transplants in a Matrigel carrier supported the regeneration of some axons from propriospinal, sensory, and as many as 19 different brainstem areas that projected not only into the graft but also into distal spinal cord tissue for distances up to 3.5 mm (77). These axons coursed into the gray matter and formed terminal boutonlike structures. A similar study was performed using fibrin glue instead of Matrigel. Although axons penetrated the graft, the grafts were not as stable as those using a Matrigel carrier (60,78).

Interestingly, Schwann cells harvested from adult human donors have also survived transplantation into a spinal cord injury in an immunodeficient rat, which does not generate a strong immune response (55,79). Several neuronal populations, including propriospinal, sensory, motoneuronal, and brainstem neurons, regenerated into these human Schwann cell grafts. As many as 1,500 myelinated axons were found within the graft. Using anterograde and retrograde tracers, regeneration of propriospinal neurons, but not motoneuronal axons, up to 2.6 mm beyond grafts into host tissue was noted. Schwann cells are therefore effective in filling the defect and attracting many types of axons but may not be able to provide for long-distance growth within the host.

Combining additional strategies with Schwann cell bridges appears to improve transgraft regeneration of brainstem neurons. Chen and associates (80) administered methylprednisolone along with the Schwann cell transplantation into a thoracic cord lesion. Over 3,000 myelinated axons were subsequently demonstrated within the graft. Brainstem serotonergic and adrenergic axons were found up to 2.5 mm into the graft and some in the distal spinal cord tissue. Immunosuppression improved the regeneration in this model (60). The addition of neurotrophic factors to Schwann cell grafts also improved regeneration. Xu and colleagues (81) delivered BDNF and NT-3 in conjunction with a Schwann cell graft. The neurotrophins were delivered for 14 days, and the rats were sacrificed 2 weeks later. Approximately 1,500 myelinated axons were found within the grafts, and retrograde labeling demonstrated that 67% of these were from brainstem vestibular nuclei. Thus, the combination of neurotrophins with Schwann cell/Matrigel grafts increased propriospinal axon regeneration and, more important, supported growth from distant brainstem neuron populations (60,81). Insulin-like derived growth factor 1 (IGF-1) and platelet-derived growth factor (PDGF) have also been shown to support regeneration into Schwann cell/Matrigel grafts (82). Although there was an increase in the ratio of myelinated to unmyelinated axons and in the thickness of the myelination, fewer

axons regenerated into the graft. Thus, choice of growth factors for axonal regeneration is important.

Using Olfactory Ensheathing Glia

In recent years, increasing interest has been paid to olfactory ensheathing glia (OEG) cells. Olfactory axons are able to regenerate and reestablish synaptic contacts with their targets, even in adults. In the olfactory bulb, olfactory ensheathing glia support the growing neurites, possibly isolating them from the nonpermissive environment of the CNS (60,83–85). The OEG cells are present at the junction where the axons leave the peripheral environment to enter the central nervous system, and produce several trophic factors, including PDGF, NGF, BDNF, NT-3, and neurotrophin-4 (60). OEG cells also express many cell adhesion molecules (for example, L1, N-CAM, laminin, fibronectin, and glia-derived nexin) that may enhance axonal elongation (60,71,83,86–96). They are now obtainable through various culture techniques from either embryonic, neonatal, or adult rat olfactory bulbs (84–86,97,98), making them more readily available for further investigation.

Early studies suggest that OEG cells may support axonal regeneration. In one study, rhizotomies were performed (98). The root stump was then microsurgically anastomosed to the cord, and a suspension of ensheathing cells was transplanted in the spinal cord at the dorsal root entry zone. Three weeks after the transplantation, dorsal root ganglion axons had crossed the root–cord transition zone, entered the spinal cord, and elongated through spinal cord gray matter to innervate laminae 1 through 5 ipsilaterally, reaching the dorsal gray commissure and lamina 4 of the contralateral side. Neither the OEG cells nor the regenerating axons they accompanied entered laminae not normally innervated by dorsal roots. Li and associates (75) created stereotaxic corticospinal lesions and injected a suspension of OEG cells into the site. Corticospinal axons regenerated through the lesion/transplant site, and OEG cells were found associated with these axons.

Investigators have also shown that OEG cells are capable of remyelinating dorsal column axons. In addition, the remyelinated axons improved conductive velocities and frequency–response properties (99,100). Although much more research needs to be done, OEG cells may contribute to combined repair strategies in the future and potentially play a role in the treatment of demyelinating diseases.

Delivering Neurotrophic Factors

Exogenous administration of trophic factors, such as BDNF, NT-3, NGF, and aFGF, into the spinal cord has been successful in promoting some regeneration by all descending pathways and, where it has been studied, in promoting neuroprotection (34). Specific neuronal cell populations have specific receptors and specific requirements for neurotrophic factors. Studies with NT-3 and BDNF have shown preferential effects on the corticospinal tract and rubrospinal tract, respectively (101,102). Other axons, such as the vestibulospinal, reticulospinal, propriospinal, and dorsal roots, also have receptors for one or more of these trophic factors. Because most spinal cord injuries involve mixed populations of neurons, identifying the optimal combinations of neurotrophins and the best method of delivery will be necessary to optimize regeneration.

Systemic administration of trophic factors is limited by variable pharmacokinetics, development of antibodies, and the need to pass the blood–brain barrier (16). There can also be systemic side effects at therapeutic concentrations of neurotrophic factors, even if minimized by intrathecal delivery (103). Intrathecal effectiveness is variable depending on the neurotrophic factor involved. Brain-derived neurotrophic factor, for instance, is bound by ependymal cell receptors (Trk B receptors) and is therefore ineffective by this route (16,104). Bradbury and colleagues (105) showed the intrathecal effectiveness of NT-3 over BDNF following crush injury of the ascending sensory tracts of the dorsal columns. After NT-3 but not BDNF administration, abundant sprouting of axons occurred at the lesion site. An additional problem for a local delivery is presented by the upregulation of Trk B receptors by astrocytes. These receptors have a high affinity for brain-derived neurotrophic factor as well as other neurotrophic factors such as NT-4 and NT-5 (106). Such receptors thus compete with the axotomized axons for the availability of neurotrophic factors and diminish their effectiveness (16). Transplants of cells that provide neurotrophic factors, and of other cells modified to do so by gene therapy, potentially overcome some of the limitations posed by other local delivery mechanisms.

GENE THERAPY TO DELIVER GENE PRODUCTS AND PROMOTE REGENERATION

It is now clear that regeneration of CNS axons can be elicited by exogenous administration of neurotrophic factors. Over the last decade, substantial advances have been made in techniques that allow more precise delivery of substances at physiological doses. More specifically, gene therapy has developed as a very powerful strategy. The principle behind gene therapy is that genetic sequences coding for specific proteins can be incorporated into the genetic sequence of cells such that the desired protein can be produced in a controlled fashion. The process of introducing the genetic sequence into the cell is known as *gene transfer*. *Ex vivo* gene therapy is a technique in which cultured cells are genetically modified *in vitro* using recombinant vectors and subsequently transplanted into a host. *In vivo* gene therapy is a technique in which genes are introduced into the host directly through special vectors such as viruses. As the genetic sequences of more proteins become known, these techniques become more powerful. For instance, with respect to spinal cord injury repair, substances for which genetic sequences are known include molecules such as neurotrophins, neurotransmitters, antiapoptotic factors, structural proteins, extracellular matrix molecules, and many others (107). Gene therapy therefore has the potential to provide gene products required for neuroprotection, regeneration, and for establishing a more permissive environment.

Gene therapy has three components: the cell that needs to be modified, the vector for the gene that introduces the genetic sequence into the cell, and the protein that has been genetically coded for (that is, the gene product). The delivery mechanism used for gene transfer typically is either a viral or nonviral vector. The transgene, or the gene of interest, which is transferred to the donor cell, might also include genetic sequences for promoter or reporter genes. The ability to include additional sequences in the gene of interest plays a powerful role in controlling the expression of the therapeutic gene. For instance, specific promoters can be included that allow for overexpression in order to deliver a high dose of the gene product. Conversely, inhibitory sequences can be included that allow for time-specific or dose-specific expression of the target gene product. One can also include sequences that allow tracing of the cells that express the gene. For example, the genetic sequence for green fluorescent protein can be introduced with the gene of interest and allow identification of gene product expression (107).

Vectors

The use of a viral vector is based on the ability of viruses to infect host cells and thereby introduce virally encoded sequences into the host DNA and protein manufacturing process (107). Typically, when viral vectors are used, they have been made replication deficient and therefore are no longer infectious. The choice of a particular viral vector depends on the size of the transgene of interest, because different viruses are able to incorporate different-sized genes. Another consideration is the type of genetic material one is trying to incorporate, either DNA or RNA. The primary viruses that have been evaluated and used in studies include the herpes simplex virus, retroviral viruses, adenoviruses, adeno-associated viruses, and lentiviruses (107). The herpes simplex virus, retroviruses, and adenoviruses have been the most thoroughly studied, but continued development of other vectors can be expected.

The herpes simplex virus is a large DNA virus with a carrying capacity of up to 35 kb of additional DNA. These viruses are capable of infecting a broad range of host cell types, including neurons and glial cells. They have typically been used for *in vivo* gene delivery in the CNS. The expression of the desired gene product, however, is usually transient, lasting only about 2 weeks (107). Disadvantages of the virus include a low viral titer and a requirement for a helper virus. Long-term safety is unknown (108,109).

Retroviral RNA viruses have a carrying capacity of less than 7 kb. These viruses utilize an enzyme called *reverse transcriptase,* which converts the RNA into a proviral DNA, or cDNA. The transgene is then randomly incorporated into the host cell genetic sequence, unlike the herpes simplex virus, which remains in an epichromosomal stage. Retroviral viruses therefore cause a permanent modification of the host cell, and transgene dilution does not occur with cell division. This may also be a disadvantage because overexpression of the transgene may lead to an accumulation of the gene product, which may be toxic (107). Additionally, there is greater potential for insertional mutagenesis using retroviruses (110,111). These limitations make retroviruses more useful for *ex vivo* applications (102, 112).

Adenoviral vectors infect a broad range of cells, including neurons and glia. They modify both dividing and postmitotic cells and are therefore useful in both *in vivo* and *ex vivo* gene therapy (102,107,112–114). Adenoviruses, however, generate a strong host immune reaction (115,116).

Nonviral vector systems such as plasmids, liposomes, and receptor-mediated endocytosis are easy to synthesize and modify and have no limitations on the size of the transgene (107). Their limitations include less efficient gene transfer and some cytotoxicity as well as limited target cell populations (109,110,117,118).

Donor Cells

One advantage of *ex vivo* gene therapy is that there are virtually unlimited numbers of potential donor cells. The use of transplants of specific donor cells to allow for expression of specific proteins in spinal cord injury will permit the formation of a controlled environment that is more amenable to regeneration. The transplanted cells can also fill the injury site, providing a terrain that is potentially permissive to growing axons. Cells to be used in transplantation should optimally be nontumorigenic, nonimmunogenic, and allow optimal expression of the gene product for a desired length of time. The categories of potential donor cell candidates include nonneuronal cells and neural precursor cells. Nonneuronal cells include fibroblasts, astrocytes, Schwann cells, and marrow stromal cells. Neural precursor cells include neural stem cells and immortalized stem cell lines (107).

Nonneuronal Cells

Primary fibroblasts are easily obtained from skin biopsy, easily cultured to expand their numbers, and easily stored. Both autografts and allografts have been transplanted into spinal cord injury models in adult rats (114,119,120). Allograft transplants of fibroblasts combined with immunosuppressants such as cyclosporin A have demonstrated fibroblast survival and favorable expression of the desired gene products (107,114). Several gene products have been introduced

into the fibroblast, including neurotrophins. Most of the studies of genetically modified fibroblasts have noted high protein expression within approximately 2 weeks after transplantation, but decreased expression at approximately 8 weeks after transplantation (107,114,121). Several mechanisms, including promoter downregulation, aggressive host immune response, and transgene dilution secondary to cell division, are probable reasons for the diminished expression at 8 weeks after transplantation (107,114,121). It is possible, however, that the effects on neuroprotection and regeneration may be most important during the first few weeks and that downregulation after this time may in fact be beneficial.

In addition to primary nonneuronal cells such as fibroblasts or Schwann cells (see "Using Schwann Cell Grafts," earlier in this chapter), established cell lines derived from chromocytomas, neuroblastomas, gliomas, and schwannomas have been used in gene therapy experiments (122–127). These are less desirable than primary cells, however, because they have the continued risk of tumorigenesis (107).

Certain cells found in bone marrow are similar to stem cells and are referred to as *marrow stromal cells* (MSCs). These cells are easily harvested from bone marrow. Harvested marrow stromal cells can differentiate into a variety of different types of cells. They are also easily modifiable through *ex vivo* gene therapy to deliver several different therapeutic gene products, including neurotrophins (107, 128,129). Human marrow stromal cells have been grafted into the rat CNS and have been found to generate a minimal immune response and to survive for several months (128). The combination of easy isolation from human donors as well as easy genetic modifiability makes marrow stromal cells a very attractive candidate for *ex vivo* gene therapy in spinal cord injuries (107). They may also be advantageous as allografts.

Neural Precursor Cells

Using gene transfer techniques that allow for the immortalization of cell lines, including the transfer of oncogenes, a large number of neural progenitor cell lines have been created (107). Such cell lines have been developed from oligodendrocytes, astrocytes, and neuroblasts (130–132). Similar to true stem cell lines, immortalized progenitor cell lines are self-renewing, can be genetically modified, and, like stem cells, can differentiate into a variety of different types of cells (133). These cells have been grafted into adult mammalian CNS and have been demonstrated to differentiate into neurons and glial cells in response to CNS signals (134–136).

True neural stem cells offer even greater potential than neural progenitor cell lines because stem cells inherently have the ability for unlimited self-renewal and differentiate into a much greater range of types of cells. They are, therefore, more readily prepared and stored. Progenitor cells are one step closer to terminal differentiation and therefore have a relatively more limited capacity for further differentiation (107,137–140).

REGENERATION STUDIES USING *EX VIVO* GENE THERAPY

Fibroblasts

Expression of substances by genetically modified cells has been the focus of much research in recent years, and modified fibroblasts are perhaps the best studied and most successful method. Transgene expression of neurotrophic factors (NGF, NT-3, and BDNF) has been a primary focus (102,120,124,141–143). Genetically modified fibroblasts have been shown to be neuroprotective in spinal cord injury models (107). Fibroblasts genetically modified to secrete the neurotrophin NT-3 rescued approximately 30% of Clarke's nucleus neurons (corticospinal tract) from cell death, although the cells remained somewhat atrophic. Those modified to secrete BDNF rescued many of the red nucleus neurons (rubrospinal tract) that would have died and also prevented much of the atrophy (144,145).

Use of genetically modified fibroblasts has also induced axonal regeneration into transplanted grafts and distal spinal cord tissue. Primary fibroblasts genetically modified to secrete BDNF were grafted into a cervical hemisection in adult rats. The lesion destroys the ipsilateral rubrospinal tract. After sacrifice, retrograde and anterograde labeling demonstrated that up to 10% of the rubrospinal tract axons had regenerated up to ten segments distal to the lesion (102). In this study, the animals were tested for functional recovery of forelimb usage. After the BDNF/fibroblast transplant, the animals partially recovered forelimb function, but this recovery was abolished by a second lesion just rostral to the transplant. This indicated a significant functional recovery that was dependent on the presence of the transplanted tissue.

Fibroblasts have also been genetically engineered to express other substances, such as the neural cell adhesion molecule L1 (107,146). These L1-secreting fibroblasts were also transplanted into a hemisection spinal cord injury model and elicited enhanced axon ingrowth into the transplanted grafts. Other preliminary data from our laboratory using fibroblasts modified to secrete BDNF and NT-3 have shown long-distance regeneration of serotonergic axons transplanted after a complete thoracic transection. Regenerating axons enter and traverse the grafted site into distal host tissue for up to 6 to 12 mm. Whether these traversing axons reestablish a functional neuronal connection in the distal host tissue is under investigation.

Schwann Cells

Schwann cells have also been genetically modified to produce specific gene products. The inherent ability of Schwann cells to express cell adhesion type molecules (for example, L1, integrin) and extracellular matrix molecules (for example, collagen and laminin), as well as neurotrophic factors such as NGF and BDNF, is well documented and known to promote regeneration in the CNS (2,3,55,58,75,121). Regeneration completely through the Schwann cell grafts into host spinal cord tissue remains limited, however. *Ex vivo* gene therapy may improve penetration of distal spinal cord tissue by delivery of specific neurotrophic factors.

In recent years, attempts have been made to genetically alter Schwann cells to deliver specific neurotrophic factors directly. Menei and associates (147) in 1998 altered Schwann cells via viral factors to deliver brain-derived neurotrophic factor. In this study, Schwann cells were also injected into caudal spinal cord tissue distal to the transection for a distance of 5 mm to serve as a guidance tract. One month after grafting, axons were documented to traverse the transection and were found within the Schwann cell trails. Unlike earlier studies in which Schwann cells were used without BDNF, Schwann cells modified to secrete BDNF enhanced brainstem axonal growth across the spinal cord transection and also into distal spinal cord tissue, mostly from reticular and raphe nuclear sites (81).

SUMMARY

The studies performed in the last 15 years have provided important data suggesting that spinal cord injury is treatable and the obstacles are solvable. After the primary injury, whether from a contusion, ischemic event, or axotomy, many of the pathophysiological mechanisms that subsequently ensue in the secondary cascade of injury are similar and respond to similar interventions. The primary objective after initial spinal cord injury should be to minimize further injury, enhance neuronal survival, and modify the microenvironment to be conducive to axonal regeneration. Much of the data obtained in the last decade suggests that neuronal survival after injury can be enhanced through the provision of exogenous neurotrophic factors or antiapoptotic molecules. The precise timing and sequence for the provision of such factors remains to be clearly delineated; however, there is good evidence that suggests increased neuronal survival is currently possible through these various means.

Effective mechanisms of delivery for exogenous trophic factors as well as other substances such as antiapototic factors, cell adhesion molecules, cytoskeletal proteins, and extracellular matrix molecules are currently available and will continue to be greatly improved as data are derived from studies on gene therapy using various donor cells and delivery vectors. In conjunction with the delivery of exogenous trophic factors through *ex vivo* gene therapy, the provision of a substrate for axonal growth is likely to greatly enhance regeneration after transplantation. Some studies have been performed comparing different matrices and polymer guidance channels, which enhance axonal regeneration in combination with cellular transplantation. The optimal carrier matrix has not yet been defined.

Future directions for research and transfer into the clinical setting will no doubt also involve aggressive patient rehabilitation and training for patterned locomotion. Ambulation in humans, as in animals, is likely to be organized by a central pattern generator (CPG), which is a local neuronal circuit allowing for reflex patterned gait. Data suggest that not only can the CPG be trained to elicit a primitive reflex walking pattern, but also that provision of pharmacologic agonists and antagonists of the CPG circuit, or exogenous delivery of neurotransmitters by regenerating axons after transplant of genetically modified cells, may enhance this intrinsic reflex gait. When combined with other strategies such as functional electrical stimulation, early impact in the clinical setting should be possible. Although much research remains to be done, the future is now bright for individuals with spinal cord injuries, and the tempo has changed. We now know we can induce axons in the spinal cord to regrow. We know these regenerating axons can make connections with remaining neuronal circuits. And we know that these connections can be made to work.

REFERENCES

1. David S, Aguayo AJ. Axonal elongation into peripheral nervous system "bridges" after central nervous system injury in adult rats. *Science* 1981;214:931–933.
2. Richardson PM, Issa VMK, Aguayo AJ. Regeneration of long spinal axons in the rat. *J Neurocytol* 1984;13:165–182.
3. Richardson PM, McGuinness UM, Aguayo AJ. Axons from CNS neurons regenerate into PNS grafts. *Nature* 1980;284:264–265.
4. Bracken MB, Shepard MJ, Collins WF, et al. Methylprednisolone or naloxone treatment after acute spinal cord injury; one year follow-up data. Results of the second National Acute Spinal Cord Injury Study. *J Neurosurg* 1992;76:23–31.
5. Hall ED. The neuroprotective pharmacology of methylprednisolone. *J Neurosurg* 1992;76:13–22.
6. Stuart EG. Tissue reactions and possible mechanisms of piromen and desoxycorticosterone acetate in central nervous system regeneration. In: Windle WF, ed. *Regeneration in the central nervous system.* Springfield, IL: Thomas, 1955:162–170.
7. Davis JN, Antonawich FJ. Role of apoptotic proteins in ischemic hippocampal damage. *Ann N Y Acad Sci* 1997;835:309–320.
8. Garcia-Valenzuela E, Gorczyca W, Darzynkiewicz Z, et al. Apoptosis in adult retinal ganglion cells after axotomy. *J Neurobiol* 1993;25:431–438.
9. Grafstein B. Axonal transport: function and mechanisms. In: Waxman SG, Kocsis JD, Stys PK, eds. *The axon.* New York: Oxford University Press, 1995:185–191.
10. Grafstein B. Forward: half a century of regeneration research. In: Ingoglia NA, Murray M, eds. *Axonal regeneration in the central nervous system.* New York: Marcel Dekker, 2001:1–17.
11. Groves MJ, Christopherson T, Giometto B, et al. Axotomy-induced apoptosis in adult rat primary sensory neurons. *J Neurocytol* 1997;26:615–624.
12. Levi-Montalcini R. Neuronal regeneration *in vitro*. In: Windle WF, ed. *Regeneration in the central nervous system.* Springfield, IL: Thomas, 1955:54–65.
13. Lindholm D. Role of neurotrophins in preventing glutamate-induced neuronal cell death. *J Neurol* 1994;242:S16–S18.
14. Hayashi T, Sakurai M, Abe K, et al. Apoptosis of motor neurons with induction of caspases in the spinal cord after ischemia. *Stroke* 1998;29:1007–1012.
15. Villa T, Kaufmann SH, Earnshaw WC. Caspases and caspase inhibitors. *Trends Biochem Sci* 1997;22:388–393.
16. Himes TB, Tessler A. Neuroprotection from cell death following axotomy. In: Ingoglia NA, Murray M, eds. *Axonal regeneration in the central nervous system.* New York: Marcel Dekker, 2001:477–503.
17. Li L, Prevette D, Oppenheim RW, et al. Involvement of specific caspases in motoneuron cell death *in vivo* and *in vitro* following trophic factor deprivation. *Mol Cell Neurosci* 1998;12:157–167.
18. Milligan CE, Prevette D, Yaginuma H, et al. Peptide inhibitors of the ICE protease family arrest programmed cell death of motoneurons *in vivo* and *in vitro*. *Neuron* 1995;15:385–393.
19. Holtzman DM, Deshmukh M. Caspases: a treatment target for neurodegenerative disease? *Nature Med* 1997;3:954–955.
20. Stout AK, Raphael HM, Kanterewicz BI, et al. Glutamate-induced neuron death requires mitochondrial calcium uptake. *Nature Neurosci* 1998;1:366–373.
21. Thornberry NA, Lazebnik Y. Caspases: enemies within. *Science* 1998;281:1312–1316.
22. Alberi S, Raggenbass M, Debilbao F, et al. Axotomized neonatal motoneurons overexpressing the Bcl-2 proto-oncogene retain functional electrophysiological properties. *Proc Natl Acad Sci USA* 1996;93:3978–3983.
23. Antonawich FJ, Federoff HJ, Davis JN. Bcl-2 transduction, using a herpes simplex virus amplicon, protects hippocampal neurons from transient global ischemia. *Exp Neurol* 1999;156:130–137.
24. Antonawich FJ, Krajewski S, Reed JC, et al. Bcl-x(1) Bax interaction after transient global ischemia. *J Cereb Blood Flow Metab* 1998;18:882–886.
25. Cenni MC, Bonfanti L, Martinou JC, et al. For long-term survival of retinal ganglion cells following optic nerve section in adult Bcl-2 transgenic mice. *Eur J Neurosci* 1996;8:1735–1745.
26. Coulpier M, Junier MP, Peschanski M, et al. Bcl-2 sensitivity differentiates two pathways for motoneuronal death in the wobbler mutant mouse. *J Neurosci* 1996;16:5897–5904.
27. Farlie PG, Dringen R, Rees SM, et al. Bcl-2 transgene expression can protect neurons against developmental and induced cell death. *Proc Natl Acad Sci USA* 1995;92:4397–4401.
28. Zuo J, Ferguson TA, Hernandez VJ, et al. Neuronal matrix metalloproteinase-2 degraded and inactivated a neurite inhibiting chondroitin sulfate proteoglycan. *J Neurosci* 1998;18:5203–5211.
29. Davies AM. Bcl-2 family of proteins, and the regulation of neuronal survival. *Trends Neurosci* 1995;18:355–358.
30. Green DR, Reed JC. Mitochondria and apoptosis. *Science* 1998;281:1309–1312.
31. Hockenbery DM, Oltvai ZN, Yin XM, et al. Bcl-2 functions in an antioxidant pathway to prevent apoptosis. *Cell* 1993;75:241–251.
32. Krajewski S, Mai JK, Krajewska M, et al. Upregulation of Bax protein levels in neuron following cerebral ischemia. *J Neurosci* 1995;15:6364–6376.
33. Giehl KM, Tetzlaff W. BDNF and NT-3, but not NGF, prevent axotomy-induced death of rat corticospinal neurons *in vivo*. *Eur J Neurosci* 1996;8:1167–1175.
34. Murray M. Therapies to promote CNS repair. In: Ingoglia NA, Murray M, eds. *Axonal regeneration in the central nervous system.* New York: Marcel Dekker, 2001:649–673.
35. Shibayama M, Hattori S, Himes BT, et al. Neurotrophin-3 prevents death of axotomized Clarke's nucleus neurons in adult rat. *J Comp Neurol* 1998;390:102–111.
36. Sperry RW. Functional regeneration in the optic system. In: Windle WF, ed. *Regeneration in the central nervous system.* Springfield, IL: Thomas, 1955:66–76.
37. Tuszynski MH, Gage FH. Bridging grafts and transient nerve growth factor infusions promote long-term central nervous system neuronal rescue and partial functional recovery. *Proc Natl Acad Sci USA* 1995;92:4621–4625.
38. Shibayama M, Matsui N, Himes BT, et al. Critical interval for rescue of axotomized neurons by transplants. *Neuroreport* 1998;9:11–14.
39. Fawcett JW. Intrinsic control of regeneration. In: Ingoglia NA, Murray M, eds. *Axonal regeneration in the central nervous system.* New York: Marcel Dekker, 2001:161–184.
40. Plant GW, Dimitropoulou A, Bates ML, et al. The expression of inhibitory proteoglycans following transplantation of Schwann cell grafts into a completely transected adult rat spinal cord. *Soc Neurosci Abstr* 1998;33:8.

41. Snyder SE, Li J, Schauwecker PE, et al. Comparison of RPTP zeta/beta, phosphacan, and Trkb mRNA expression in the developing and adult rat nervous system and induction of RPTP zeta/beta and phosphacan mRNA following brain injury. *Brain Res Mol Brain Res* 1996; 40:79–96.

42. Muir E, Du J-S, Fok-Seang J, et al. Increased axon growth through astrocyte lines transfected with urokinase. *Glia* 1998;23:24–34.

43. Bradbury EJ, Moon LDF, Popat RJ, et al. Chondroitinase ABC promotes functional recovery after spinal cord injury. *Nature* 2002;416: 636–640.

44. McEwen BS, Grafstein B. Fast and slow components in axonal transport of protein. *J Cell Biol* 1968;38:494–508.

45. Caroni P, Schwab ME. Two membrane protein fractions from rat central myelin with inhibitory properties for neurite growth and fibroblast spreading. *J Cell Biol* 1988;106:1281–1288.

46. Caroni P, Schwab ME. Antibody against myelin-associated inhibitor of neurite growth neutralizes nonpermissive substrate properties of CNS white matter. *Neuron* 1988;1:85–96.

47. Bregman BS, Kunkel-Bagden E, Schnell L, et al. Recovery from spinal cord injury mediated by antibodies to neurite growth inhibitors. *Nature* 1995;378:498–501.

48. McKerracher L, David S, Jackson DL, et al. Identification of myelin-associated glycoprotein as a major myelin-derived inhibitor of neurite growth. *Neuron* 1994;13:805–811.

49. Mukhopadhyay G, Doherty P, Walsh FS, et al. A novel role for myelin-associated glycoprotein as an inhibitor of axonal regeneration. *Neuron* 1994;13:757–767.

50. Cai D, Shen Y, DeBellard ME, et al. Prior exposure to neurotrophins blocks inhibition of axonal regeneration by MAG and myelin via a cAMP-dependent mechanism. *Neuron* 1999;1:85–96.

51. Fawcett JW, Keynes RJ. Peripheral nerve regeneration. *Annu Rev Neurosci* 1990;13:43–60.

52. Son YJ, Thompson WJ. Nerve sprouting in muscle is induced and guided by processes extended by Schwann cells. *Neuron* 1996;14: 133–141.

53. Son YJ, Thompson WJ. Schwann cell processes guide regeneration of peripheral axons. *Neuron* 1996;14:125–132.

54. Cheng H, Cao Y, Olson L. Spinal cord repair in adult paraplegic rats: partial restoration of hind limb function. *Science* 1996;273:510–513.

55. Guest JD, Hesse D, Schnell L, et al. Influence of IN-1 antibody and acidic FGF-fibrin glue on the response of injured corticospinal tract axons to human Schwann cell grafts. *J Neurosci Res* 1997;50:888–905.

56. Berry M, Hall SM, Rees L, et al. Response of axons and glia at the site of anastomosis between the optic nerve and cellular or acellular sciatic nerve grafts. *J Neurocytol* 1988;17:727–744.

57. Hall SM. Regeneration in the peripheral nervous system. *Neuropathol Appl Neurobiol* 1989;15:513–529.

58. Levi AVO, Bunge RP. Studies of myelin formation after transplantation of human Schwann cells into the severe combined immunodeficient mouse. *Exp Neurol* 1994;130:41–52.

59. Bunge RP. Changing usage of nerve tissue culture 1950–1975. In: Tower DB, ed. *The nervous system, vol. 1: The basic neurosciences*. Raven Press: New York, 1975:31–42.

60. Plant GW, Ramon-Cueto A, Bunge MB. Transplantation of Schwann cells and ensheathing glia to improve regeneration in adult spinal cord. In: Ingoglia NA, Murray M, eds. *Axonal regeneration in the central nervous system*. New York: Marcel Dekker, 2001:529–561.

61. Casella GTB, Bunge RP, Wood TM. Improved method for harvesting human Schwann cells from mature peripheral nerve and expansion in vitro. *Glia* 1996;17:327–338.

62. Levi ADO. Characterization of the technique involved in isolating Schwann cells from adult human peripheral nerve. *J Neurosci Methods* 1996;68:21–26.

63. Li RH, Chen J, Hammonds G, et al. Identification of GAS six as a growth factor for human Schwann cells. *J Neurosci* 1996;16:2012–2019.

64. Morrissey TK, Kleitman N, Bunge RP. Isolation and characterization of Schwann cells derived from adult peripheral nerve. *J Neurosci* 1991;11:2433–2442.

65. Bunge MP. Schwann cell regulation of extra cellular matrix biosynthesis and assembly. In: Dyck PJ, Thomas PK, Griffin JW, eds. *Peripheral neuropathy*, 3rd ed. Philadelphia: WB Saunders, 1993:299–316.

66. Daniloff JK, Levi G, Grumet M, et al. Altered expression of neuronal cell adhesion molecules induced by nerve injury and repairs. *J Cell Biol* 1986;103:929–945.

67. Guenard V, Xu X, Bunge M. The use of Schwann cell transplantation for faster central nervous system repair. *Semin Neurosci* 1993;5:401–411.

68. Kuffler DP. Isolated satellite cells of a peripheral nerve direct the growth of regenerating frog axons. *J Comp Neurol* 1986;249:57–64.

69. Martini R, Schachner M, Fassner A. Enhanced expression of extracellular matrix molecules J1/tenascin in the regenerating adult mouse sciatic nerve. *J Neurocytol* 1990;19:601–616.

70. Mirsky R, Jessen KR. Schwann cell development and regulation of myelination. *Semin Neurol* 1990;2:423–435.

71. Schachner M. Functional implications of glial cell recognition molecules. *Semin Neurosci* 1990;2:497–507.

72. Xu XM, Chen A, Guenard V, et al. Bridging Schwann cell transplants promote axonal regeneration from both the rostral and caudal stumps of transected adult rat spinal cord. *J Neurocytol* 1997;26:1–16.

73. Brook GA, Lawrence JM, Raisman G. Morphology and migration of cultured Schwann cells transplanted into the fimbria and hippocampus in adult rats. *Glia* 1993;9:292–304.

74. Emmet CJ, Jaques-Berg W, Seeley PJ. Microtransplantation of neural cells into adult rat brain. *Neuroscience* 1990;38:213–222.

75. Li Y, Raisman G. Integration of transplanted cultured Schwann cells into the long myelinated fiber tracts of the adult spinal cord. *Exp Neurol* 1997;145:397–411.

76. Martin LJ, Al-Abdulla NA, Bram Brink AM, et al. Neurodegeneration in excitotoxicity, global cerebral ischemia, and target deprivation: a prospective on the contributions of apoptosis and necrosis. *Brain Res Bull* 1998;46:281–309.

77. Xu XM, Zhang SX, Li H, et al. Regrowth of axons into the distal spinal cord through a Schwann cell-seeded mini-channel implanted into hemisected adult rat spinal cord. *Eur J Neurosci* 1999;11:1723–1740.

78. Bamber NI, Li H, Lu X, et al. Fibrin "glue" as an alternative matrix for implanting Schwann cells into partially injured adult rat spinal cords. *Soc Neurosci Abstr* 1998;24:69.

79. Guest JD, Rao A, Olson L, et al. The ability of human Schwann cell grafts to promote regeneration in the transected nude rat spinal cord. *Exp Neurol* 1997;48:502–522.

80. Chen A, Xu XM, Kleitman N, et al. Methylprednisolone administration improves axonal regeneration into Schwann cell grafts in transected adult rat thoracic spinal cord. *Exp Neurol* 1996;138:261–276.

81. Xu XM, Guenard V, Kleitman N, et al. A combination of BDNF and NT-3 promotes supraspinal axonal regeneration into Schwann cell grafts in adult rat thoracic spinal cord. *Exp Neurol* 1995;134:261–272.

82. Oudega M, Xu XM, Guenard V, et al. A combination of insulin-like growth factor-1 and platelet derived growth factor enhances myelination but diminishes axonal regeneration into Schwann cell grafts in the adult rat spinal cord. *Glia* 1997;19:247–258.

83. Doucette JR. Glial influences on axonal growth in the primary olfactory system. *Glia* 1990;3:433–449.

84. Ramon-Cueto A, Avila J. Olfactory ensheathing glia: properties and function. *Brain Res Bull* 1998;46:175–187.

85. Ramon-Cueto A, Plant GW, Avila J, et al. Long distance axonal regeneration in the transected adult rat spinal cord is promoted by olfactory ensheathing glia transplants. *J Neurosci* 1998;18:3803–3815.

86. Barnett SC, Hutchins AM, Noble M. Purification of olfactory nerve ensheathing cells from the olfactory bulb. *Dev Biol* 1993;155:337–350.

87. Franceschini IA, Barnett SC. Low-affinity NGF-receptor and E-N-CAM expression define two types of olfactory nerve ensheathing cells that share a common lineage. *Dev Biol* 1996;173:327–343.

88. Goodman MN, Silver J, Jacobberger JW. Establishment and neurite outgrowth properties of neonatal and adult rat olfactory bulb glial cell lines. *Brain Res* 1993;619:199–213.

89. Kafitz KW, Greer CA. Role of laminin in axonal extension from olfactory receptor cells. *J Neurobiol* 1997;32:298–310.

90. Key B, Akeson RA. Olfactory neurons expressed a unique glycosylated form of neural cell adhesion molecule (N-CAM). *J Cell Biol* 1990;110: 1729–1743.

91. Liesi P. Laminin immunoreactive glia distinguish regenerative adult CNS systems from non-regenerative ones. *EMBO J* 1985;4:2505–2511.

92. Miragell F, Kadmon G, Husmann M, et al. Expression of cell adhesion molecules in the olfactory system of the adult mouse: presence of the embryonic form of N-CAM. *Dev Biol* 1988;129:516–531.

93. Pixley SK. The olfactory nerve contains two populations of glia, identified both *in vivo* and *in vitro*. *Glia* 1992;5:269–284.

94. Pixley SK. Characteristics of olfactory receptor neurons and other cell types in the associated rat olfactory cell cultures. *Int J Dev Neurosci* 1996;14:823–839.

95. Ramon-Cueto A, Nieto-Sampedro M. Glial cells from the adult rat olfactory bulb: immunocytochemical properties of pure cultures of ensheathing cells. *Neuroscience* 1992;47:213–220.

96. Reinhardt E, Meier R, Halfter W, et al. Detection of glia-derived nexin in the olfactory system of the rat. *Neuron* 1988;1:387–394.

97. Doucette JR. Glial progenitor cells of the nerve fiber layer of the olfactory bulb. Effect of astrocyte growth media. *J Neurosci Res* 1993;35:274–287.

98. Ramon-Cueto A, Nieto-Sampedro M. Regeneration into the spinal cord of transected dorsal root axons is promoted by ensheathing glia transplants. *Exp Neurol* 1994;127:232–244.

99. Franklin RJM, Gilson JM, Franceschini IA, et al. Schwann cell-like myelination following transplantation of an olfactory bulb-ensheathing cell line in two areas of demyelination in the adult CNS. *Glia* 1996;17:217–224.

100. Imaizumi T, Lankford KL, Waxman SG, et al. Transplanted olfactory ensheathing cells remyelinate and enhanced axonal conduction in the demyelinated dorsal columns of the rat spinal cord. *J Neurosci* 1998;18:6176–6185.

101. Grill R, Murai K, Blesch A, et al. Cellular delivery of neurotrophin-3 promotes corticospinal axonal growth and partial functional recovery after spinal cord injury. *J Neurosci* 1997;17:5560–5572.

102. Liu Y, Kim D, Himes BT, et al. Transplants of fibroblasts genetically modified to express BDNF to promote regeneration of adult rat rubrospinal axons. *J Neurosci* 1999;19:4370–4387.

103. Penn RD, Kroin JS, York MM, et al. Intrathecal ciliary neurotrophic factor delivery for treatment of amyotrophic lateral sclerosis (phase 1 trial). *Neurosurgery* 1997;40:94–100.

104. Yan Q, Matheson C, Sun J, et al. Distribution of intracerebral ventricularly-administered neurotrophins in rat brain and its correlation with Trk receptor expression. *Exp Neurol* 1994;127:23–36.

105. Bradbury EJ, Khemani S, Von R, et al. NT-3 promotes growth of lesioned adult rat sensory axons ascending in the dorsal columns of the spinal cord. *Eur J Neurosci* 1999;11:3873–3883.

106. Frisen J, Verge VM, Fried K, et al. Characterization of glial Trk B receptors: differential response to injury in the central and peripheral nervous systems. *Proc Natl Acad Sci USA* 1993;90:4971–4975.

107. Fischer I, Liu Y. Gene therapy strategies. In: Ingoglia NA, Murray M, eds. *Axonal regeneration in the central nervous system.* New York: Marcel Dekker, 2001:563–601.

108. Hermens WT, Verhaagen J. Viral vectors, tools for gene transfer in the nervous system. *Prog Neurobiol* 1998;55:399–432.

109. Neve RL. Adenovirus factors enter the brain. *Trends Neurosci* 1993;16:251–253.

110. Crystal RG. Transfer of genes to humans: early lessons and obstacles to success. *Science* 1995;270:404–410.

111. Miller AD. Human gene therapy comes of age. *Nature* 1992;357:455–460.

112. Blomer U, Naldini L, Verma IM, et al. Applications of gene therapy to the CNS. *Hum Molec Genet* 1996;5:1397–1404.

113. Davidson BL, Bohn MC. Recombinant adenovirus: a gene transfer vector for study and treatment of CNS diseases. *Exp Neurol* 1997;144:125–130.

114. Liu Y, Himes BT, Tryon B, et al. Intraspinal grafting of fibroblasts genetically modified by recombinant adenoviruses. *Neuroreport* 1998;9:1075–1079.

115. Byrnes AP, Rusby JE, Wood MJ, et al. Adenovirus gene transfer causes inflammation in the brain. *Neuroscience* 1995;66:1015–1024.

116. Yang Y, Nunes FA, Berencsi K, et al. Cellular immunity to viral antigens limits E1-deleted adenoviruses for gene therapy. *Proc Natl Acad Sci USA* 1994;91:4407–4411.

117. Miller N, Vile R. Targeted vectors for gene therapy. *FASEB J* 1995;9:190–199.

118. Scherman D, Bessodes M, Cameron B, et al. Application of lipids and plasmid design for gene delivery to mammalian cells. *Curr Opin Biotechnol* 1998;9:480–485.

119. Kawaja MD, Fagan AM, Firestein BL, et al. Intracerebral grafting of cultured autologous skin fibroblasts into the rat striatum and assessment of graft size and ultrastructure. *J Comp Neurol* 1991;307:695–706.

120. Tuszynski MH, Peterson DA, Ray J, et al. Fibroblasts genetically modified to produce nerve growth factor induced robust neuritic ingrowth after grafting to the spinal cord. *Exp Neurol* 1994;126:1–14.

121. Snyder EY, Senut MC. The use of nonneuronal cells for gene delivery. *Neurobiol Dis* 1997;4:69–102.

122. Cunningham LA, Short MP, Vielkind U, et al. Survival and differentiation within the adult mouse striatum of grafted rat pheochromocytoma cells (PC 12) genetically modified to express recombinant beta-NGF. *Exp Neurol* 1991;11:174–182.

123. Gage FH, Wolff JA, Rosenberg MB, et al. Grafting genetically modified cells to the brain: possibilities for the future. *Neuroscience* 1987;23:795–807.

124. Rosenberg MB, Friedman T, Robertson RC, et al. Grafting genetically modified cells to the damaged brain: restorative effects of NGF expression. *Science* 1988;242:1575–1578.

125. Schinstine M, Fiore VM, Winn SR, et al. Polymer-encapsulated schwannoma cells expressing human nerve growth factor to promote the survival of cholinergic neurons after a fimbria-fornix transection. *Cell Transplant* 1995;4:93–102.

126. Tornatore C, Baker-Cairns B, Yadid G, et al. Expression of tyrosine hydroxylase in an immortalized human fetal astrocyte cell line, *in vitro* characterization and engraftment into the rodent striatum. *Cell Transplant* 1996;5:145–163.

127. Whittemore SR, Holet VR, Keane RW, et al. Transplantation of a temperature-sensitive, nerve growth factor-secreting, neuroblastoma cell line into adult rats with fimbria-fornix lesions rescues cholinergic septal neurons. *J Neurosci Res* 1991;28:156–170.

128. Azizi SA, Stokes D, Augelli BJ, et al. Engraftment and migration of human bone marrow stromal cells implanted in the brains of albino rats—similarities to astrocyte grafts. *Proc Natl Acad Sci USA* 1998;95:3908–3913.

129. Himes BT, Chow S, Jin H, et al. Grafting human bone marrow stromal cells into injured spinal cord of adult rats. *Soc Neurosci Abstr* 1999;25:213.

130. Almazan G, Mckay R. An oligodendrocyte precursor cell line from rat optic nerve. *Brain Res* 1992;579:234–245.

131. Giordano M, Takashima H, Herranz A, et al. Immortalized GABAergic cell lines derived from rat striatum using a temperature-sensitive allele of the SV 40 large T antigen. *Exp Neurol* 1993;124:395–400.

132. Radany EH, Brenner M, Besnard F, et al. Directed establishment of rat brain cell lines with the phenotypic characteristics of type I astrocytes. *Proc Natl Acad Sci USA* 1992;89:6467–6471.

133. Martinez-Serrano A, Bjorklund A. Immortalized neural progenitor cells for CNS gene transfer and repair. *Trends Neurosci* 1997;20:530–538.

134. Onifer SM, Whittemore SR, Holets VR. Variable morphological differentiation of a raphe-derived neuronal cell line following transplantation into the adult rat CNS. *Exp Neurol* 1993;122:130–142.

135. Shihabuddin LS, Hertz JA, Holets VR, et al. The adult CNS retains the potential to direct region-specific differentiation of a transplanted neuronal precursor cell line. *J Neurosci* 1995;15:6666–6678.

136. Snyder EY, Deitcher DL, Walsh C, et al. Multipotent neural cell lines can engraft and participate in development of mouse cerebellum. *Cell* 1992;68:33–51.

137. Gage FH, Ray J, Fisher LJ. Isolation, characterization, and use of stem cells from the CNS. *Annu Rev Neurosci* 1995;18:159–192.

138. McKay R. Stem cells in the central nervous system. *Science* 1997;276:66–71.

139. Weiss S, Dunne C, Hewson J, et al. Multipotent CNS stem cells are present in the adult mammalian spinal cord and ventricular neuroaxis. *J Neurosci* 1996;16:7599–7709.

140. Weiss S, Reynolds BA, Vescovi AL, et al. Is there a neural stem cell in the mammalian forebrain? *Trends Neurosci* 1996;19:387–393.

141. Chen KS, Gage FH. Somatic gene transfer of NGF to the aged brain: behavior and morphological amelioration. *J Neurosci* 1995;15:2819–2825.

142. Kawaja MD, Rosenberg MB, Yoshida K, et al. Somatic gene transfer of nerve growth factor promotes the survival of axotomized septal neurons and the regeneration of their axons in adult rats. *J Neurosci* 1992;12:2849–2864.

143. Tuszynski MH, Gabriel K, Gage FH, et al. Nerve growth factor delivery by gene transfer induces differential outgrowth of sensory, motor, and noradrenergic neurites after spinal cord injury. *Exp Neurol* 1996;137:157–173.

144. Himes BT, Solowska-Baird J, Boyne L, et al. Grafting of genetically modified cells that produce neurotrophins in order to rescue axotomized neurons in rats spinal cord. *Soc Neuro Sci Abstr* 1995;21:537.

145. Tessler A, Fischer I, Giszter S, et al. Embryonic spinal cord transplants enhance locomotor performance in spinalized new born rats. In: Seil FJ, ed. *Neuronal regeneration, reorganization and repair.* New York: Raven Press, 1997.
146. Kobayashi S, Miura M, Asou H, et al. Grafts of genetically modified fibroblasts expressing neural cell adhesion molecule L1 into transected spinal cord of adult rats. *Neurosci Lett* 1995;188:191–194.
147. Menei P, Montero-Menei C, Whittemore SR, et al. Schwann cells genetically modified to secrete BDNS promote enhanced axonal regrowth across transected adult rat spinal cord. *Eur J Neurosci* 1998;10:607–621.

SUGGESTED READING

Acheson A, Barker PA, Alderson RS, et al. Detection of brain-derived neurotrophic factor-like activity in fibroblasts and Schwann cells: inhibition by antibodies to NGF. *Neuron* 1991;7:265–275.

Anderson JK, Garber DA, Meaney CA, et al. Gene transfer into a mammalian central nervous system using herpes virus vectors: extended expression of bacterial Lac Z in neurons using the neuron-specific enolase promoter. *Hum Gene Ther* 1992;3:487–499.

Chen DF, Schneider GE, Martinou JC, et al. Bcl-2 promotes regeneration of severed axons in mammalian CNS. *Nature* 1997;385:434–439.

Chiocca EA, Choi BB, Cai WZ, et al. Transfer and expression of the Lac Z gene in rat brain neurons mediated by herpes simplex virus mutants. *New Biologist* 1990;2:739–746.

Doucette JR. Immunocytochemical localization of laminin, fibronectin, and collagen type I and V in the nerve fiber layer of the olfactory bulb. *Int J Dev Neurosci* 1996;14:945–959.

Fournier AE, McKerracher L. Expression of specific tubulin isotypes increases during regeneration of injured CNS neurons, but not after application of brain-derived neurotrophic factor (BDNF). *J Neurosci* 1997;8:1167–1175.

Martin D, Robe P, Franzen R, et al. Effects of Schwann cell transplantation in a contusion model of rat spinal cord injury. *J Neurosci Res* 1996;45:588–597.

Mikucki SA, Oblinger MM. Corticospinal neurons exhibit a novel pattern of cytoskeletal gene expression after injury. *J Neurosci Res* 1991;30:213–225.

Navarro X, Valero A, Gudino G, et al. Ensheathing glia transplants promote dorsal root regeneration and spinal reflex restitution after multiple lumbar rhizotomy. *Ann Neurol* 1999;45:207–215.

Pandtlow CE, Heumann R, Schwab ME, et al. Cellular localization of nerve growth factor synthesis by *in situ* hybridization. *EMBO J* 1987;6:891–899.

Ramon-Cueto A, Valverde F. Olfactory bulb ensheathing glia: a unique cell type with axonal growth-promoting properties. *Glia* 1995;14:163–173.

Rende M, Muir D, Ruoslahdi E, et al. Immunolocalization of ciliary neurotrophic factor in adult rate sciatic nerve. *Glia* 1992;5:25–32.

Rossiter JP, Riopelle RJ, Bisby MA. Axotomy-induced apoptotic cell death of neonatal rat facial motoneurons: time course analysis in relation to NADPH-diaphorase activity. *Exp Neurol* 1996;138:33–44.

Ryder EF, Snyder EY, Cepko CL. Establishment and characterization of multipotent neural cell lines using retrovirus vector-mediated oncogene transfer. *J Neurobiol* 1990;21:356–375.

So KF, Yip HK. The use of peripheral nerve transplants to enhance axonal regeneration in CNS neurons. In: Ingoglia NA, Murray M, eds. *Axonal regeneration in the central nervous system.* New York: Marcel Dekker, 2001:505–528.

Tuszynski MH, Weidner N, McCormack M, et al. Grafts of genetically modified Schwann cells to the spinal cord: survival, axon growth and myelination. *Cell Transplant* 1998;7:187–196.

Zhou L, Connors T, Chen DF, et al. Red nucleus neurons of Bcl-2 overexpressing mice are protected from cell death induced by axotomy. *Neuroreport* 1999;10:3417–3421.

SECTION VII

Tumors and Spinal Infection

CHAPTER 58

Intradural Intramedullary and Extramedullary Tumors

Seth M. Zeidman

Spinal cord tumors account for about 15% of central nervous system neoplasms and arise from the spinal cord parenchyma, nerve roots, meningeal coverings, intraspinal vascular network, sympathetic chain, or vertebral column (1). Metastatic involvement of the spinal intradural compartment occurs rarely. Intradural spinal tumors are broadly categorized by their relationship to the spinal cord.

Discussion of spinal cord tumors is usually organized according to location in the spinal canal: (a) extradural; (b) intradural extramedullary; or (c) intramedullary. Intradural tumors are classically divided into extramedullary and intramedullary lesions. Intramedullary tumors arise within the spinal cord, whereas extramedullary tumors are extrinsic to the cord. Signs and symptoms, the radiologic features, and surgical approach are more a function of the involved anatomic compartment than distinct tumor histology.

Extradural tumors (55%). These lesions are the most common spine tumors and arise outside the dura in vertebral bodies or epidural tissues. Metastatic lesions constitute most extradural tumors.

Intradural extramedullary tumors (40%). These lesions arise from leptomeninges or roots. Only 4% of metastases occur here (Fig. 58.1).

Intramedullary spinal cord tumors (5%). These lesions arise within the substance of the spinal cord and displace or invade white-matter tracts and neuron bodies. Only 2% of metastases occur in this compartment (Fig. 58.2).

INTRADURAL EXTRAMEDULLARY TUMORS

Included within this group are meningiomas and nerve sheath tumors, which constitute about 85% of all intradural extramedullary tumors. Sarcoma and lipoma account for an additional 10%. Less common entities include dermoid, epidermoid, angioma, and lymphoma.

Meningioma

Meningiomas arise from arachnoid villi cells embedded in the dura at the nerve root sleeve, thus explaining their propensity for lateral or ventrolateral locations (Fig. 58.3). They can typically be dissected free from the nerve roots. Upper cervical tumors are more commonly found in an anterolateral location. Lower cervical meningiomas are unusual.

The typical patient with a spinal meningioma is female (female-to-male ratio, 10:1), older (most in the fifth and seventh decade), with a solitary (multiple tumors occur only 2% of the time), entirely intradural (10% of lesions involve both intradural and extradural compartments) lesion.

Nerve Sheath Tumors

The classification of nerve sheath tumors is complicated by the use of the terms neurofibroma and schwannoma, and the persistence of the inaccurate terms neuroma, neurinoma, and neurolemmoma. In patients with neurofibromatosis, nerve sheath tumors are usually asymptomatic and multiple, with histology consistent with neurofibromas. In patients with neurofibromatosis, these tumors are multiple and occur at numerous levels of the spinal canal. In the absence of neurofibromatosis, the tumors are nearly always schwannomas.

Nerve sheath tumors typically arise from the dorsal nerve roots. These tumors are relatively avascular, globoid, and without calcification. The dorsal root is intimately involved in the tumor and can rarely be preserved during surgical resection.

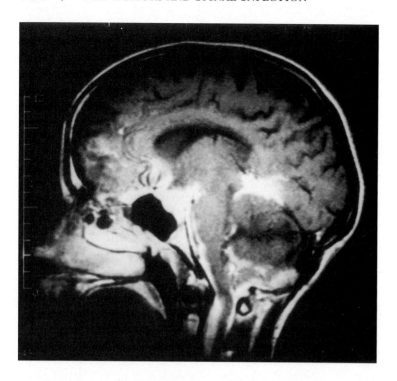

FIG. 58.1. Intradural extramedullary metastasis. Sagittal magnetic resonance imaging shows leptomeningeal spread of melanoma.

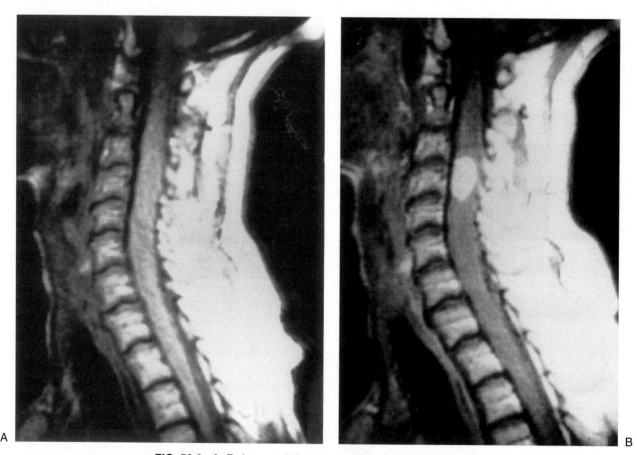

A   B

FIG. 58.2. A, B: Intramedullary metastasis: an unusual lesion.

Schwannomas originate from Schwann cells, but the origin of neurofibromas is uncertain. It has been postulated that neurofibromas arise from mesenchymal cells (fibroblasts). Neurofibromas produce a fusiform dilation of the involved sensory nerve root, with no apparent plane between nerve and tumor. Occasionally, they straddle the neural foramen and enlarge in the paraspinal tissues, resulting in a so-called dumbbell tumor with the narrowest portion within the foramen. When these tumors have a dumbbell configuration, the size of the extradural component may greatly exceed that of the intradural component. Multiple neurofibromas contribute to establishing the diagnosis of neurofibromatosis, but the entity should be considered in any patient with even a solitary tumor (Fig. 58.3).

Most intraspinal nerve sheath tumors are schwannomas. They occur with about the same frequency as meningiomas, but in a more even distribution along the spine. They are slightly more common in men, with a peak incidence in the third and fifth decades. Like neurofibromas, schwannomas originate from sensory roots. In distinction to neurofibromas, schwannomas can often be separated from the nerve root. They are generally connected to a few fascicles without fusiform root enlargement.

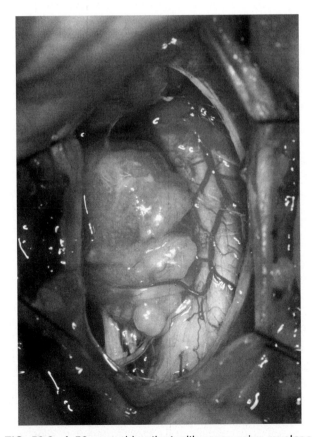

FIG. 58.3. A 56-year-old patient with progressive myelopathy. Cervical intradural extramedullary lesion. The tumor was a meningioma. Tumors that are inside the dura but outside the spinal cord such as this meningioma can be totally resected. The cerebellum can be identified at the superior end of the picture.

Clinical Features

The clinical manifestations of extramedullary intradural tumors are neither unique nor distinct. Classically, these tumors present with radicular symptoms that often evolve into myelopathy as the tumor enlarges and compresses the spinal cord. Preoperative symptom duration is variable but generally extended, often exceeding 2 years. By the time of diagnosis, most patients have objective neurologic deficits. The symptoms may be difficult to differentiate from those of intramedullary and extradural tumors or nonneoplastic conditions such as syringomyelia, spondylotic myelopathy, multiple sclerosis (MS), or spinal arteriovenous malformation.

Pain, either local or radicular, is the most common symptom. Unilateral radicular pain is common with nerve sheath tumors because of their dorsal root origin. Occipital headaches may accompany high cervical or foramen magnum tumors. Local pain is more typical of dural irritation from meningiomas. Nocturnal pain (pain when laying flat in bed) should alert the examiner to a potential spinal cord tumor.

Segmental sensory or motor root deficits generally appear after pain and before myelopathy. The earliest and most common sign of cord compression is corticospinal tract dysfunction. The symptoms may be unilateral or bilateral and include stiffness, gait disturbance, and incoordination of fine hand movement. Sphincter dysfunction is an unusual sign and tends to occur late. In general, the clinical progression is most closely related to tumor location and speed of growth.

Radiographic Diagnosis

Except for occasionally demonstrating foraminal enlargement, bony erosion, or occult instability, plain roentgenograms and plain computed tomography (CT) scans contribute little to the diagnostic evaluation of a patient with an intradural extramedullary lesion. MRI remains the procedure of choice for localizing and identifying intradural tumors. MRI will generally identify the pathology and define the relationship to the spinal cord and related structures, such as the vertebral artery, and it may provide clues to the histology of the lesion. It may be particularly helpful in dumbbell lesions, by better delineating the extradural component. Meningiomas appear isointense on both T1-weighted and T2-weighted sequences and intensely enhance with the administration of gadolinium contrast. Nerve sheath tumors usually have a higher signal intensity than meningiomas on T2-weighted images. These tumors likewise enhance intensely with the administration of gadolinium.

Myelography, postmyelographic CT scanning, and MRI with gadolinium enhancement are among the most informative diagnostic studies. Myelography is as sensitive as MRI in identifying intradural pathology and may be more sensitive in the lower lumbar region. CT with intrathecal contrast provides excellent delineation of the interface between tumor and spinal cord as well as superior imaging of bone detail. For suspected meningeal carcinomatosis not apparent on radiographic studies, cytologic examination of cerebrospinal fluid obtained by lumbar puncture is essential.

Surgical Therapy

Because most intradural extramedullary tumors are benign, the goal of surgery is complete and total resection. The treatment of intraspinal meningiomas, neurofibromas, and schwannomas is surgical excision (2). This may include excision of the involved portion of the dura mater (meningioma) or the involved nerve rootlets or entire root (schwannoma, neurofibroma). In nerve sheath tumors arising from the dorsal roots, the nerve root is intimately involved in the tumor and can rarely be separated. Dorsal roots may be sacrificed over a few segments in the thoracic region; however, very few dorsal rootlets can be safely sacrificed in the cervical or lumbar region. These tumors are rarely adherent to the spinal cord and can easily be separated away from it (3).

At the level of involvement, neurofibromas and schwannomas typically grow on the dorsal (sensory) root in preference to the ventral (motor) root, and it is generally possible to spare motor function during tumor removal. In neurofibromas, such tumors are part of a more widespread process (neurofibromatosis), in which there are similar tumors on multiple other nerve roots and nerves. Although follow-up surveillance may be needed, most patients with solitary intraspinal lesions (meningioma, neurofibroma, or schwannoma) can be cured with gross total removal of the lesion.

The critical element to successful excision is adequate initial exposure. The posterior midline approach with laminectomy allows adequate access for most of these tumors. Even ventrally located lesions can be safely excised using this approach because the enlarging tumor slowly displaces the spinal cord. The laminectomy must be performed in a nontraumatic fashion to avoid canal compromise. To minimize injury, the dura should be widely opened. The arachnoid is initially preserved to prevent spinal cord herniation and to minimize bleeding into the subarachnoid space. Dentate ligament section allows gentle mobilization of the spinal cord. If a posterior root has been sacrificed, this can also be used to rotate the cord. Both anterior and posterior roots from C2 to C4, as well as in the thoracic spine, can be sectioned safely. From C5 to T1, there is minimal deficit if one posterior root is sectioned. Even anterior root section, often required for dumbbell tumor removal, often results in surprisingly minimal deficit. Dense attachments may only allow a piecemeal removal of the tumor to minimize the risk for producing a significant neurologic deficit.

Small tumors may be removed en bloc, but larger tumors necessitate intracapsular decompression. This can be performed safely with the ultrasonic aspirator. Once the tumor size is reduced, development of the dissection plane can proceed, using the reflected arachnoid or the tumor capsule. After the tumor has been removed, it is important to disrupt the arachnoid trabeculae and irrigate out any residual blood products. This will minimize postoperative arachnoid adhesions and intramedullary cyst development from impaired cerebrospinal fluid flow. The dura must be closed in a watertight fashion. Sometimes with meningiomas, this may require a patch graft and fibrin glue or other sealant.

There are two ways of dealing with the dural attachment of an isolated intradural spinal meningioma. One is complete resection of the involved dura together with the tumor, and the other is coagulation only of the tumor base of the dura. A third option is separation of the inner and outer dural layers and resection of the inner layer with the tumor and preservation of the outer, uninvolved layer (4).

With dumbbell neurofibromas, there is usually significant extradural extension out the neural foramina. Single, staged, or simultaneous approaches should be based on the size and location of the tumor. The intradural portion should be resected first to minimize spinal cord manipulation during removal of the extradural component. If the patient is elderly, medically unstable, and not symptomatic from the extradural portion, it may not be crucial to remove the extradural tumor. It is important, when the nerve root is sectioned laterally, to section it proximal to the ganglion to minimize painful neuralgias postoperatively.

Surgery for metastases within the subarachnoid space is generally not required unless the diagnosis is in question or functional improvement with good life expectancy is felt likely. These are ordinarily managed with radiotherapy, hormonal therapy, or chemotherapy (5).

Results

Surgical results for most intradural benign lesions are quite good, often with rapid improvement of neurologic deficits. Final clinical outcome is dependent on the severity of initial deficits, age, and duration of symptoms. Excision of solitary nerve sheath tumors is generally considered curative. For meningiomas and ependymomas, recurrence rates differ depending on the histology of the tumor. Similarly, angiomas and dermoids are not expected to recur if completely resected.

INTRAMEDULLARY NEOPLASMS

Intramedullary spinal cord tumors account for 3% of all central nervous system tumors and for about 25% of spinal neoplasms. Astrocytomas and ependymomas are the most common tumors, constituting 45% and 35%, respectively, of intramedullary lesions. The remaining 20% are divided among several different tumor types, including hemangioblastomas (10%), lipomas (2%), dermoids (1%), epidermoids (1%), teratomas (1%), neuroblastomas, and mixed tumors. Primary lymphoma, oligodendroglioma, cholesteatoma, subependymoma, PNETs, and intramedullary metastases are extremely rare (Fig. 58.4).

Intramedullary spinal cord tumors occur at all ages, predominantly in young or middle-aged adults and less com-

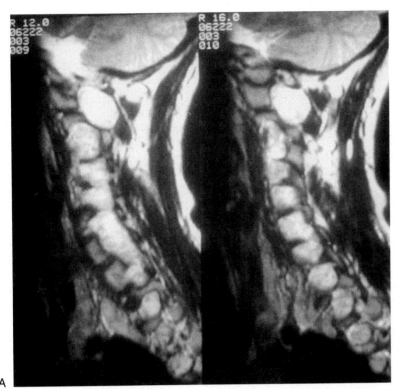
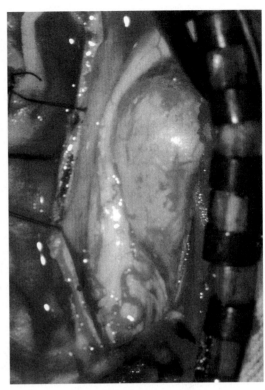

FIG. 58.4. Neurofibromatosis with multiple lateral enhancing lesions. Tumors extend laterally out through and expanding the foramina. **A:** Sagittal magnetic resonance imaging delineates the multiple lesions in this patient. **B:** Intraoperative photograph demonstrates a clear plane between the lesion and spinal cord.

monly in children and in elderly (>60 years old) patients. In children, astrocytomas predominate, but in adults, ependymomas and astrocytomas occur more equally. An equal distribution between males and females has been reported.

Clinical Features

The clinical manifestations of intramedullary spinal cord tumors are not pathognomonic and are identical with many other conditions affecting the spinal cord. The clinical course is variable and dependent on tumor histology. Patients with malignant tumors typically progress from symptom onset to surgery within 10 months. Intramedullary tumors occur most commonly in adults; however, children can also present with these neoplasms. The symptoms in these two groups are similar. However, most intramedullary spinal cord tumors are subtle in symptomatology and only present over a period of years. Patients note slowly developing clumsiness, weakness, or sensory symptoms. Presentation as the initial manifestation of scoliosis is common.

The most common manifestation of intramedullary spinal cord tumors is neck pain. Persistent diffuse pain in a dermatomal origin is often a clue to an intramedullary neoplasm. Sensory symptoms typically precede motor dysfunc-

tion. Posterior column dysfunction may occur in a slow but progressive fashion. The classic central cord syndrome is a rare presentation for these neoplasms. These symptoms are generally progressive with few remissions or exacerbations. A suspended sensory loss involving the upper extremities or trunk, indistinguishable from that seen with syringomyelia, can be seen. Motor symptoms are less subtle. Patients may have progressive unilateral or bilateral weakness. Children may not complain of weakness, but parents may notice a new gait ataxia or disuse of the involved extremity. Cervical lesions produce paresthesias, dysesthesias, and areas of sensory loss involving one or both upper extremities.

Many patients experience progressive myelopathy. Children may present with abdominal pain as a nonspecific symptom that makes accurate diagnosis particularly difficult. It is not uncommon for these children to undergo an extensive gastrointestinal evaluation before diagnosis of an intraspinal neoplasm.

Imaging

Plain X-Rays

Fewer than 20% of patients with intramedullary spinal cord tumors have abnormal plain x-rays of the spine. Plain radiographs may reveal some degree of bony erosion but otherwise are of limited value once the diagnosis of an intramedullary spinal cord tumor has been established. Widening of the pedicles on the frontal projection may suggest an intraspinal mass, but intramedullary location and a focused differential diagnosis cannot be determined. The use of plain radiographs is otherwise limited in the diagnosis of intramedullary tumors. CT myelography can reveal swelling of the spinal cord but does not delineate the pathology within the cord (6).

Magnetic Resonance Imaging

Magnetic resonance imaging (MRI) is the preferred diagnostic modality for the evaluation of intramedullary spinal cord tumors and is generally the only examination necessary for diagnosis. Unlike CT myelography, which visualizes the external configuration of the spinal cord, MRI can image the spinal cord itself with minimal artifact from surrounding osseous structures. It also can define the relationship of the spinal cord to surrounding bone and soft tissue structures. Intramedullary tumors produce fusiform spinal cord expansion with variable signal change on T1-weighted imaging depending on the histology. Most intramedullary tumors are isointense or slightly hypointense with respect to the surrounding spinal cord on T1-weighted images. There is variability in signal intensity due to tumor cellularity, cysts, edema, calcification, and hemorrhage. However, gadolinium eliminates the confusion of the variable signal intensities. The borders of the tumor may be more clearly identified on T1-weighted images with the administration of gadolinium.

MRI has become increasingly accurate in predicting the histologic tumor type. Sagittal T1-weighted images with gadolinium enhancement are also useful for demonstrating the presence of associated peritumoral cysts, syringomyelia, or edema. MRI provides a triplanar view of the neoplasm, which allows accurate differentiation between intramedullary and extramedullary tumors. Although this imaging study is very accurate, occasionally it is difficult to differentiate an inflammatory process such as sarcoidosis, MS, or amyloid angiopathy from neoplasm.

MRI evaluation of the spinal cord should start with imaging of the spinal cord in the sagittal plane with T1- and T2-weighted images. Axial views then should be obtained at the levels of suspected pathology. Gadolinium-enhanced images define the configuration and extent of the lesion. Intramedullary tumors are often associated with syringomyelia, and any cystic process in the spinal cord must be proved unrelated to a tumor process. Tumor-associated cysts often have a high protein content and may be indistinguishable from the adjacent tumor on nonenhanced studies. These cysts do not enhance with gadolinium and can thus be distinguished from spinal cord widening by tumor.

Imaging patterns, specifically T2 signal characteristics and gadolinium uptake, can help narrow the differential diagnosis by suggesting tumor histology. Most astrocytomas have an eccentric location within the cord. The MRI appearance of astrocytomas is variable. T1-weighted images show diffuse spinal cord enlargement with irregular margins and heterogeneous enhancement due to hemorrhage or cystic changes. T2-weighted images demonstrate areas of high signal intensity. T1-weighted sequences following contrast administration help delineate tumor from surrounding edema. Often, a cyst can be differentiated from the solid part of the neoplasm. MRI cannot differentiate high-grade from low-grade neoplasms. Although the MRI appearance of astrocytomas and ependymomas can be nearly identical, ependymomas are generally bright on gadolinium-enhanced T1-weighted images, with sharp borders and moderate uptake of gadolinium. Despite these patterns, there is enough overlap in appearance that pathologic analysis is required for diagnosis. Postoperatively, MRI allows sensitive follow-up for tumor recurrence. This is important because most patients develop radiologic recurrence before they manifest symptoms. In addition to preoperative assessment, a postoperative MRI study can define the extent of resection, hematomas, cyst drainage, and cerebrospinal fluid collections.

Intense gadolinium enhancement with flow voids suggests hemangioblastoma. MRI is invaluable in localizing small hemangioblastomas, particularly when associated with a large cyst. Lipomas have a characteristic high signal intensity on T1-weighted images and do not enhance with gadolinium. MRI can be quite helpful in identifying vascular malformations.

Spinal Cord Angiography

Spinal cord angiography is indicated in the evaluation of intramedullary spinal cord tumors only when the clinical history or MRI suggests an arteriovenous malformation or a hemangioblastoma. In both of these entities, spinal angiography clarifies the diagnosis and lesion anatomy.

Differential Diagnosis

Several nonneoplastic lesions may mimic intramedullary spinal cord neoplasm in their radiographic and clinical presentation. These can be classified as either infectious (tuberculosis; fungal, bacterial, or parasitic infection; syphilis; cytomegalovirus, herpes simplex virus) and noninfectious (sarcoid, MS, myelitis, acute disseminating encephalomyelitis, systemic lupus erythematosus) inflammatory lesions, idiopathic necrotizing myelopathy, unusual vascular lesions (amyloid, infarct, isolated intramedullary vascular lesions), and radiation myelopathy. Although biopsy may be indicated in many cases, the mistaken diagnosis of intramedullary neoplasm can often be eliminated preoperatively. MRI facilitates differentiation of intramedullary spinal cord tumors from other entities. Nevertheless, the clinical presentation of two nonneoplastic entities, MS and syringomyelia, can be strikingly similar to that seen with these tumors. Because the MRI may also be misleading in these conditions, MS and syringomyelia warrant particular attention.

Multiple Sclerosis

MS involving the spinal cord can precisely replicate the signs and symptoms of an intramedullary spinal cord tumor. Onset of the neurologic deficit is typically more rapid in patients with MS, and remissions and exacerbations are an essential aspect of diagnosis. In contrast, the clinical course of a patient with an intramedullary spinal cord neoplasm is one of relentless progression, although the rapidity of progression can vary from patient to patient.

Evaluation of the cerebrospinal fluid is often positive for oligoclonal bands, and triple evoked responses may be abnormal. MRI of the brain often identifies lesions consistent with plaques. The MRI appearance of spinal cord lesions caused by MS may bear a superficial resemblance to that of intramedullary spinal cord tumors. The spinal cord lesions of MS are almost always limited in their rostral-caudal extent to one or two spinal segments. Although the signal intensity of the acute MS lesion may be similar to that seen with intramedullary spinal cord tumors and may enhance after administration of gadolinium, spinal cord widening is generally minimal, a sharp contrast to the pattern seen with intramedullary spinal cord tumors. Demyelinating disease can mimic a spinal cord tumor, even on MRI, and must be considered in the differential diagnosis of a symptomatic spinal cord mass.

Syringomyelia

The clinical course of syringomyelia tends to be more indolent than that of intramedullary spinal cord tumors, but in many other respects, the two entities are indistinguishable. Administration of gadolinium is essential to exclude enhancement from a small tumor. Visualization of the cervicomedullary junction in the sagittal plane can be evaluated for a Chiari-associated syrinx in the absence of enhancement.

Management Decisions

The presence of an intramedullary spinal cord tumor does not necessarily mandate operative removal. The decision to operate on patients with advanced neurologic deficits must be made in concert with the patient and the family with realistic expectations. These include a desire to preserve residual sphincter function or to preserve sensation in bedridden patients who are at risk for skin breakdown. Although patients who cannot stand are unlikely to regain enough motor function to ambulate as a result of tumor resection, surgery may maintain the quality of a patient's life by preserving the ability to transfer or to turn in bed. Patients with complete motor and sensory deficits will not improve with surgery and are not operative candidates except when the diagnosis is in doubt.

Ambulatory patients with progressive neurologic deficits are ideal operative candidates. Surgical intervention can halt or slow neurologic deterioration and improve motor and sensory function. Although surgery risks increasing neurologic deficits, once a motor deficit appears, neurologic dysfunction tends to progress relentlessly. Patients with intramedullary spinal cord tumors who forego surgery will inevitably progress to a complete neurologic deficit. Thus, the risks of operation are more than outweighed by the natural history of the disease.

Surgery for anaplastic spinal cord astrocytomas does not appear to have lasting benefits except in obtaining an accurate diagnosis. Although a rapid clinical course may strongly suggest the presence of a malignant astrocytoma, only histologic examination of tissue obtained at operation can establish a diagnosis definitively.

Making a decision regarding the patient presenting only with neck or back pain, mild sensory symptoms, and a paucity of objective deficits is more difficult. Many patients with minor symptoms and no significant functional impairment are unwilling to risk neurologic deterioration as a result of an operation. In this situation, the patient should be closely followed for the appearance of additional symptoms or an objective deficit. After symptoms progress, patients frequently are more prepared psychologically to face the risks of surgery.

Surgical Technique

The patient should be positioned prone. When the tumor is at or above T2, the patient should be placed in a three-pin headholder with the neck in a neutral, unrotated position. The horseshoe-shaped headrest should be avoided because skin breakdown of the face or forehead can occur following extended procedures. Antibiotics and steroids, using the spinal cord injury dosing with a gradual taper, are given during the perioperative period. I routinely use somatosensory evoked potential (SSEP) monitoring during spinal cord surgery. Many centers also use motor evoked potentials (MEPs). Whereas SSEPs are mediated principally by the dorsal columns, MEPs monitor the integrity of the descending motor pathways. Although continuous evoked response monitoring during spinal surgery is of unproven efficacy, I use it on every case to avoid excessive retraction.

A standard midline approach with a careful, wide laminectomy is performed to expose completely the rostral-caudal extent of the lesion. Tumor-associated cysts are frequently more extensive than the tumor itself. It is unnecessary to extend the laminectomy to include areas of cystic enlargement. The cyst fluid disappears with total tumor removal, and the cyst walls are composed of nonneoplastic tissue, which does not need to be resected. One must remain cognizant of the fact that the underlying spinal cord may be compromised.

Placement of instruments under the lamina is contraindicated. A high-speed drill or a double-action rongeur is preferable.

Because of the high incidence of postlaminectomy kyphosis in children, block removal of the laminae is performed to allow for laminoplasty reconstruction. I do not recommend this in the adult population because the incidence of postlaminectomy kyphosis is quite low.

Meticulous hemostasis is essential. Bone wax should be applied to the bone edges. Strips of thrombin-soaked Gelfoam are placed along the lateral gutters of the laminectomy site, and moist cotton strips are draped over the adjoining muscle edges. After the laminectomy is performed, ultrasound should be used to confirm the location of solid tumor and any adjacent cysts. I recommend introducing the operating microscope at this point. The dura is opened, and tacking sutures are placed. Sharp dissection of arachnoid from adherent vessels by microsurgical technique is undertaken to avoid vessel avulsion.

Although hemangioblastomas will typically have a pial presentation, most intramedullary tumors do not present on the surface. Hemangioblastoma nearly always reaches the pia at some aspect. It is helpful to search for this site because it will facilitate dissection and isolation of these vascular tumors from the circulation.

Intraoperative ultrasound is very useful for localizing tumor, identifying associated cysts, as well as delineating the extent of resection. The myelotomy should be performed at or near the posterior median septum, preferably at a point where the normal neurologic tissue appears most thinned. When an extensive myelotomy is planned, it is preferable to make a midline myelotomy even when this is not the most attenuated portion of the cord. Sometimes, being certain of the exact midline is difficult because the spinal cord anatomy may be distorted by the tumor. Therefore, because normally the midline is midway between the left and right dorsal roots, both the left and right dorsal roots should be identified before initiating the myelotomy. Extension of a myelotomy situated in the area of the dorsal root entry zone can be disastrous. The most common technical error associated with this surgery is inadequate exposure of the tumor poles.

During pial incision, all attempts should be made to preserve any large, longitudinally oriented veins. If necessary, midline veins or arteries should be cauterized along with the pia-arachnoid by using the bipolar cautery at a low setting. The pia-arachnoid and dorsal surface of the spinal cord then should be incised sharply to a depth of 2 to 3 mm over the length of the spinal cord occupied by the solid tumor. Pial and arachnoid sutures can be placed and tacked to the dura. The pia-arachnoid and dorsal surface of the spinal cord should be held apart by placing gentle traction on 6–0 sutures placed through the pia-arachnoid on either side of the midline. If the tumor is not immediately visible, dissection within the spinal cord should be continued in a ventral direction until the tumor is encountered. As the myelotomy is performed, the normal spinal tissue will retract laterally with the pia, and the tumor–spinal cord interface will appear with minimal manipulation.

In the case of large nonvascular tumors, internal debulking using the ultrasonic surgical aspirator allows for simpler dissection of tumor margins. Gentle traction on the surface of the tumor serves to expose bridging vessels at the tumor margin that can be cauterized safely. The tumor bed should be carefully inspected under high magnification because many of these tumors are friable and unencapsulated and small fragments can be left behind inadvertently. When gross total excision is the goal, I believe the first surgical intervention offers the best chance for cure. Delayed reoperation can be difficult, especially in the setting of previous irradiation. The dura is invariably adherent to the underlying cord, and the tumor–spinal cord interface tends to be obscured by scar.

After the tumor resection is completed, the pial sutures should be removed, but closure of the myelotomy is not performed. The dura must be closed in a watertight fashion with interrupted or running sutures. If the dura cannot be closed without undue tension, a dural patch should be used. Additionally, if residual tumor is present or the spinal cord remains swollen, a dural graft should be placed to avoid spinal cord constriction. Late neurologic deterioration from arachnoidal adhesions has been observed, and this can be lessened by placement of an adequate dural patch, thereby establishing normal CSF pathways circumferentially. The remainder of the closure should be standard.

Specific Tumor Types

Astrocytoma

Intramedullary spinal cord astrocytomas are usually located several millimeters beneath the dorsal surface of the spinal cord, and although they may be distinguished from the surrounding spinal cord, they blend imperceptibly with the spinal cord at their margins, rendering complete lesion extirpation impossible. Morphologically, astrocytomas typically have a gray or whitish-yellow, stringy tough edematous stroma. The lower-grade lesions are relatively avascular and lend themselves to resection with the ultrasonic aspirator (Fig. 58.5). Resection of these infiltrating lesions should be continued until the interface with the spinal cord becomes indistinguishable or until resection produces changes in the evoked potentials. These tumors may infiltrate viable functioning spinal cord pathways at the periphery of the tumor and result in postoperative exacerbation of neurologic deficits, even when the surgeon is confident that resection is confined strictly to grossly apparent tumor. An intramedullary astrocytoma ordinarily cannot be completely removed surgically. However, in some cases, especially at the cervicomedullary junction, cleavage planes can be defined and gross total resection achieved. Gross total resection can result in extended clinical (neurologic) stabilization and effective cure.

Tumor cysts may be located rostral or caudal to the tumor. Lack of cyst enhancement in cavities adjacent to tumor suggests the presence of a benign reactive syrinx rather than a frankly neoplastic cyst.

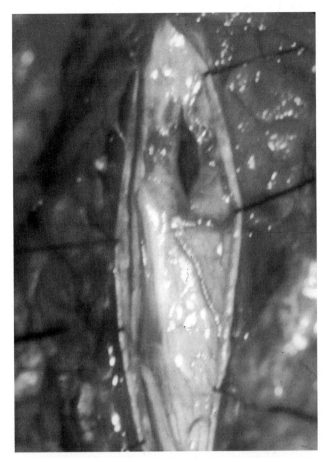

FIG. 58.5. Astrocytoma, low grade. This low-grade localized glioma can be removed partly. Adjuvant radiation may be helpful for some of these lesions.

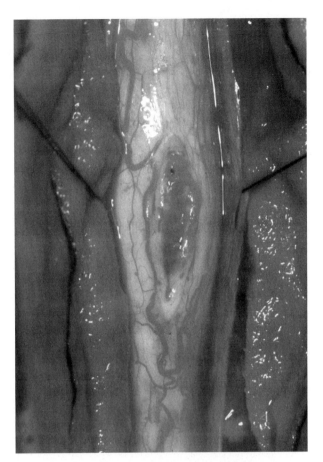

FIG. 58.6. Astrocytoma, intraoperative.

Histologically, compared with the more benign astrocytomas, malignant astrocytomas tend to be more vascular and exhibit a less distinct interface with the spinal cord, making it more difficult to identify a surgical plane between the tumor and normal spinal cord (7) (Fig. 58.6). If biopsy confirms a malignant astrocytoma, further tumor removal is generally unwarranted. There is no evidence that surgical debulking of a malignant astrocytoma is beneficial.

Factors positively influencing the prognosis are low histologic grade of the tumor and good preoperative and postoperative general conditions. Among the grade II astrocytomas, the fibrillary and protoplasmatic types presented longer survival times regardless of the type of removal performed. In anaplastic astrocytomas, the simultaneous presence of certain morphologic features indicative of higher malignancy negatively influenced survival. The degree of resection did not influence average survival within each histologic grade.

Because ependymomas cannot be reliably distinguished from astrocytomas by clinical presentation or currently available imaging techniques, all intramedullary spinal cord tumors should be aggressively explored so that curable lesions are not overlooked.

Ependymoma

Ependymomas are the most common intramedullary neoplasm in adults, whereas in children, they account for only 12% of all intramedullary tumors. They occur throughout the spinal axis, originating from ependymal rests along the central canal. As they grow from their point of origin, they push the adjacent spinal cord aside and are distinct from the surrounding spinal cord. They are histologically benign and typically have a central location in the spinal cord. Intraoperatively, they are firm and have a shaggy reddish-purple, gray, or yellow appearance with variable blood supply, which always comes from the anterior spinal artery. At surgery, ependymomas appear reddish gray. Ependymomas are well delineated from the surrounding parenchyma and usually can be totally excised. Cysts are frequently found at either or both ends of the tumor and aid in dissection. Ependymomas typically have a clear plane of dissection, and surgical cure is usually possible with preservation of the surrounding spinal cord.

Although smaller lesions often may be removed en bloc, generally, the bulk of the tumor should be reduced first in piecemeal fashion to avoid excessive manipulation of adjacent neural structures. If the tumor is highly vascular, tumor reduction can be accomplished by shrinking the surface with the bipolar cautery on a low setting. If the lesion is relatively avascular, the center of the tumor may be debulked with the ultrasonic aspirator. A cleavage plane between tumor and adjacent tissue can be developed by retracting tumor into the residual cavity. As the tumor is lifted out of the spinal cord, its vascular supply can be cauterized and cut and the tumor removed from its bed.

In most patients, total resection is possible (8,9) (Fig. 58.7). Unfortunately, ependymomas may blend imperceptibly with the spinal cord at their point of origin, and in these cases, total resection is impossible without injuring the cord. Resection should be stopped when the interface between the tumor and normal spinal cord is indiscernible. Intraoperative findings of arachnoid scarring and cord atrophy are ominous for surgical morbidity. There is typically a portion of the tumor adherent to the anterior median raphe that should be removed sharply to avoid traction injury to the anterior spinal artery. If only a partial resection can be achieved, postoperative irradiation may be required.

Complete removal can be achieved in almost all cases of intramedullary spinal cord ependymomas in children, and the long survival rates justify avoiding postoperative radiation therapy.

Hemangioblastoma

Hemangioblastomas account for 3% to 7% of intramedullary spinal cord tumors and are particularly rare in children (10). They occur throughout the spinal canal and are most commonly located on the dorsal or dorsolateral surface of the spinal cord. On MRI, hemangioblastomas are typically cystic lesions with a strongly enhancing mural nodule. T1-weighted images reveal a well-circumscribed tumor with decreased signal intensity, whereas T2-weighted images reveal hyperintense lesion. Flow voids from a feeding vessel are often discernible.

Hemangioblastomas are typically red and nodular with a clear plane of dissection, and surgical cure is usually possi-

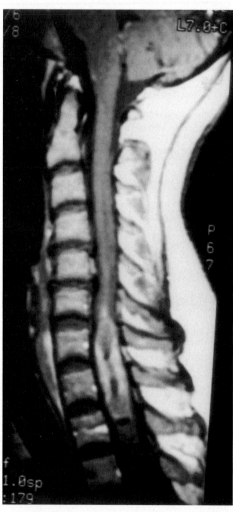
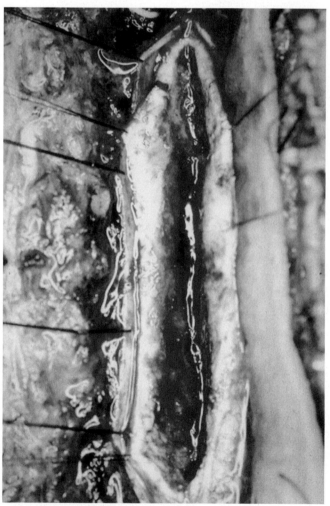

FIG. 58.7. A, B: A 43-year-old patient with complaints of numbness and clumsiness in the hands with mechanical neck pain. Magnetic resonance imaging showed enhancing intramedullary spinal cord tumor. Final pathology report was ependymoma. Patient is functional in computer work 3 years later with minimal deficit.

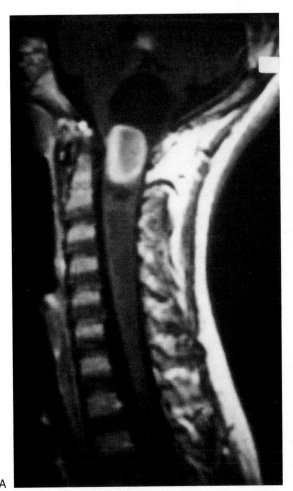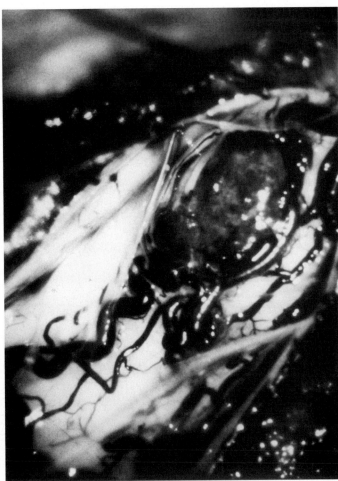

A   B

FIG. 58.8. Hemangioblastoma. **A:** Sagittal magnetic resonance imaging with gadolinium enhancement that reveals an adjacent tumor associated cyst. **B:** Intraoperative photograph of hemangioblastoma showing dilated, tortuous vessels around a prominent nidus.

ble with maintenance of the surrounding spinal cord (Fig. 58.8). They are immediately apparent on the surface of the spinal cord, along with a collection of vessels that supply and drain the lesion. They range in size from a few millimeters in diameter to the size of a large grape and are well-defined from the surrounding spinal cord (11).

These lesions are highly vascular, and no attempt should be made to enter these tumors until the vascular supply is interrupted totally because consequent bleeding may be difficult to control. The arterial supply, part of which is visible on the dorsal surface of the spinal cord, should be coagulated and cut, and the tumor very slowly reduced in size with bipolar cautery of the feeding vessels and tumor capsule. After this is done, the tumor may be dissected more easily from the adjacent spinal cord. This dissection exposes additional vascular supply, which should be interrupted sequentially, allowing total removal. It is generally advisable to preserve at least one venous pedicle until all feeding arteries are divided.

Hemangioblastomas are curable tumors but may recur as a result of the growth of residual tumor or, as is more commonly the case, growth of additional lesions that were clinically or radiographically inapparent at the time of the first surgery. Hemangioblastomas are relatively benign in their clinical and histologic behavior and can be meaningfully resected by careful microsurgical technique.

Ganglioglioma

Gangliogliomas are benign neoplasms, common in children and young adults. They consist of a mixture of well-differentiated neoplastic neurons and glial elements. The glial elements are usually astrocytes, and the neoplastic neurons are characteristically large and relatively mature. The neurons are readily recognized by their characteristic nuclear and nucleolar features, abundance of cytoplasm, content of Nissl substance, and presence of argyrophilic neuritic processes. Their expression of neuronal markers like synaptophysin and neurofilament proteins also serves to identify these abnormal neurons. Most gangliogliomas grow slowly and have an indolent course. Like astrocytomas, these tumors do not have a well-demarcated cleavage plane.

Lipoma

Lipomas of the spinal cord are rare congenital tumors. Intramedullary (subpial) lipomas not associated with spinal dysraphism are very unusual. These tumors are not neoplasms; they are histologically identical to normal adipose tissue and are located on the dorsal surface of the spinal cord covered by little or no neural tissue. They increase in size and in relation to fatty tissue elsewhere in the body.

Myelopathic signs and symptoms evolve slowly and generally are first manifest during rapid growth spurts or after excessive weight gain. Preoperative diagnosis is usually possible with MRI. Although distinct from adjacent spinal cord and noninvasive, these lesions adhere densely to normal spinal cord, so that total removal is impossible without creating unacceptable neurologic deficits.

The most effective operative strategy consists of subtotal removal, with a rim of tumor left at the interface with the spinal cord. The laser is ideal for removal of lipomas because the fibrous interstices of the lesion make removal with the ultrasonic aspirator difficult. The laser does an excellent job with many of these tumors. Lipomas simply melt away with minimal manipulation of the nerves. These lesions grow slowly, but they may recur as a result of continued growth of residual tumor.

Patients with intramedullary spinal cord lipoma who present with significant neurologic compromise have a very poor prognosis with regard to neurologic function and generally show no improvement with surgical resection.

Intramedullary Metastatic Tumors

Metastases to the spinal cord are rare and represent fewer than 8% of all intramedullary spinal cord tumors. Tumors that metastasize to the spinal cord include lung and breast carcinoma. Less commonly, lymphoma, colon adenocarcinoma, head and neck carcinoma, and renal cell carcinoma may produce spinal cord metastases. With the availability of more sensitive imaging techniques, these tumors are being diagnosed with increasing frequency. MRI is sensitive, but nonspecific, in distinguishing intramedullary spinal cord metastases from primary cord tumors. Urgent biopsy is often necessary before definitive treatment. Radiation with chemotherapy significantly prolongs survival.

These lesions tend to be vascular and well defined from the adjacent spinal cord. The most effective operative strategy consists of slow bipolar coagulation of the tumor to reduce the bulk of the lesion, followed by visualization and section of the vascular supply and total removal. Radical subtotal resection may offer additional quality survival, especially in cases of metastatic melanoma with an occult primary.

Intramedullary spinal cord metastasis is a devastating condition, but with appropriate diagnosis and aggressive treatment, selected patients may have substantially increased survival. Regardless of treatment, many patients survive less than 1 year.

Technical Adjuncts to Intramedullary Spinal Cord Tumor Removal

Intraoperative Spinal Sonography (Ultrasound)

High-frequency sector scanning allows excellent visualization of the spinal canal during surgery on spinal cord tumors. Intraoperative spinal sonography (IOSS) is performed by filling the operative field with saline solution to maintain an acceptable distance from the probe to the spinal cord. Tumors within the cervical spinal canal are ideal for localization and characterization with IOSS (12). I have had the opportunity to image a large variety of cervical tumors and have rarely failed to identify readily the neoplasms. The only significant exception to this has been with spinal hemangioblastomas, which are often isoechogenic with normal spinal cord. These can be identified with use of intraoperative color-flow Doppler ultrasound. With vascular tumors, color-flow Doppler studies demonstrate the position of high-flow vessels in the region of tumor dissection. IOSS images the tumors, the relationships of the lesions to the spinal cord, and the normal internal structures of the cord itself at the margins. In cases of intramedullary tumors, IOSS defines the extent of the required myelotomy, the presence of syringomyelic cavities caudal and cranial to the tumor, and the relationship of tumor depth to the anterior cord surface. Before the dura is opened, the overall extent of the tumor is visualized, and specific areas of interest such as cysts or calcified regions are defined and localized. This imaging guides the dural opening and often directs the surgeon to a particular location to initiate the myelotomy and exploration. If rostral or caudal cysts are present, the myelotomy is initiated at the cyst–tumor junction. If no cysts are present, the myelotomy is performed over the most voluminous portion of the tumor, where the possibility of damaging functional neural tissue is much less.

In cystic tumors such as astrocytomas or hemangioblastomas, ultrasound identifies the specific mural nodule of tumor. With intramedullary tumors, the "central canal" virtually always is absent to ultrasound imaging. This is helpful in determining the longitudinal extent of tumors. Edema proximal or distal to the tumor also causes spinal cord widening and loss of the central canal, thus creating some confusion in determining the absolute limits of the tumor. In most cases, the tumor border is quite well defined, and the edema is less echogenic. The routine use of IOSS during surgery for spinal tumors facilitates determination of the precise locations for biopsy of intramedullary lesions and directs the optimum surgical progression.

Occasionally, intraoperative ultrasound is less helpful, only demonstrating widening of the spinal cord with an imaging pattern similar to that of adjacent cord. In this situation, the major neoplastic differential diagnostic considerations include astrocytoma and ependymoma.

The diagnosis and intraoperative management of intramedullary spinal cord tumors has been significantly influenced by new diagnostic and surgical tools such as IOSS.

With the help of these tools, most intramedullary spinal cord tumors may be diagnosed and treated surgically with significantly decreased risk.

Finally, ultrasound can be extremely useful in monitoring ongoing tumor resection. A persistent abnormal signal or persistent uncollapsed intratumoral cyst encourages continued tumor removal. Thus, ultrasound facilitates a radical resection of intramedullary tumors.

Intraoperative ultrasonography should be used routinely during surgery for spinal tumors to reduce the extent of the laminectomy, dural opening, and myelotomy. A good correlation exists between signal intensity on T1-weighted MRI, the echographic aspect of the tumor, and the pathologic findings at operation.

Ultrasonic Aspirator

The ultrasonic aspirator combines tissue fragmentation, irrigation, and aspiration capability in procedures requiring precise, selective tissue removal with minimal trauma to surrounding tissue. The ultrasonic aspirator emits a variable ultrasonic energy field that emulsifies tissue immediately in front of the unit's tip. A small amount of water is injected into the field to liquefy further the emulsification, and the slurry is then aspirated by the unit. This allows for removal of tissue, with little energy being imparted to surrounding tissue (as would happen with simple aspiration, during which a pulling force can be exerted).

Placing the aspirator tip in contact with the tumor permits relatively atraumatic tumor resection while avoiding manipulation of adjacent spinal cord. The ultrasonic aspirator allows preservation of blood flow in adjacent white matter within 0.5 to 1 mm of the resection bed. The end result is less injury to surrounding structures. This is particularly helpful with tumors resistant to regular suction. Without the ultrasonic aspirator, tumor removal requires sharp dissection and increased spinal cord manipulation, often resulting in permanent loss of function. The force of the unit can be adjusted so that it is unlikely to injure blood vessels adjacent to the tissue being removed.

Laser

The laser is sometimes useful for resecting intramedullary spinal cord tumors. The surgeon can target using the microscope and activate the laser by the microscope. The laser beam is directed through the lens of the operating microscope using a series of mirrors to vaporize tumor. The CO_2 laser is favored for its ability to deliver variable amounts of energy that is highly focused. It is one of the most precise tools for removal of small amounts of tissue and can be used with high precision. The CO_2 laser cauterizes vessels the size of capillaries but will cut through larger vessels with resultant hemorrhage. Its two major drawbacks are the very slow speed at which it works and its poor cauterization ability (blood vessels are cut but not sealed and thus bleed). It is helpful in resecting tumors that cannot be removed with the ultrasonic aspirator.

The neodymium:yttrium-aluminum-garnet (Nd:YAG) laser delivers more diffuse energy to a larger area of tissue around the target point. Tissues surrounding the target are injured, and there is less associated bleeding because it is more effective at cauterizing blood vessels. The beam is transmitted down a fiberoptic strand to a hand-held wand.

Evoked Potential Recordings

Continuous evoked response monitoring is a potentially useful adjunct to surgical therapy (13). However, the true efficacy of evoked potential monitoring in improving outcome after operation for intramedullary spinal cord lesions remains unclear. Intraoperative evoked potential monitoring has been demonstrated to provide critical information during spinal surgery. However, evoked potentials may not be as useful for patients with spinal cord tumors because the functional integrity of the sensory and motor pathways may already be disrupted. Nevertheless, intraoperative monitoring of SSEPs during intramedullary spinal cord surgery is commonly employed. Intraoperative monitoring of the functional integrity of the spinal cord during removal of intramedullary spinal cord lesions is an aid in intraoperative decision making and a primary tool for the prediction of neurologic outcome.

Dorsal column and spinothalamic tract injury is reflected in amplitude or latency changes of the recorded waveforms. Patients with profound sensory deficits have evoked responses that are either absent or of such low amplitude that meaningful recordings cannot be obtained. Currently available SSEP monitoring techniques do not provide real-time intraoperative guidance. A delay of up to 60 seconds occurs from the time of injury until changes in the evoked potential waveform are observed. Irreversible damage may occur from operative maneuvers performed before the injury is reflected by changes in the potentials.

Monitoring sensory pathways provides no direct information regarding the integrity of the corticospinal tract. Injury may occur to the motor pathways without any change in the SSEPs. In practice, the corticospinal and the spinothalamic tracts are in such close proximity that injury to motor pathways is usually reflected in changes of the sensory evoked potentials. However, false-negative study results do occur.

Several new approaches have been used recently in an attempt to obviate some of the disadvantages of standard evoked potential monitoring techniques. MEPs allow assessment of descending fiber tracts. Morota reported that the presence of monitorable MEPs in adults before myelotomy was a better predictor of surgical outcome than is the patient's preoperative motor status.

MEP monitoring has become the neurophysiologic monitoring technique of choice for that purpose. MEPs, elicited with a short train of transcranial electrical stimuli and recorded from limb muscles, reflect the functional integrity of the corticospinal tract. Both epidural and muscle MEPs correlate closely with postoperative neurologic function. Over time, the technique's reliable power of predicting clinical outcome and its practical versatility have altered the surgical approach in that gross total resections are more readily attempted as long as MEP data indicate the intact functional integrity of the corticospinal tract.

Stimulation and recording of both sensory and motor pathways permit a more complete assessment of spinal cord function. However, it must be recognized that no study has conclusively demonstrated that use of intraoperative evoked potentials, sensory or motor, results in an improved clinical outcome.

Management

Before recent advances, the mainstay of therapy for spinal cord tumors was biopsy followed by radiation therapy. Currently, standard treatment for intradural spinal cord tumors remains microsurgical resection. Attempts at surgical resection should be performed before significant neurologic deterioration. Preoperative neurologic status is the best predictor of functional status postoperatively.

Neurologic outcome in the immediate postoperative period is related most closely to the patient's immediate preoperative neurologic state. Rarely, patients who have no motor function may regain a small amount of function after operation, but most likely they will not be able to walk or stand as a result of tumor resection. Similarly, patients who cannot stand are unlikely to be able to walk in the postoperative period.

Complications

Exacerbation of Neurologic Deficit

Neurologic deterioration is less a function of tumor histology or the extent of surgical resection than preoperative status. Patients with severe preoperative motor deficits have the highest likelihood of sustaining a permanent neurologic deficit postoperatively. Nearly 20% of patients experience a permanent increase in their deficits.

Dorsal column injury will cause loss of proprioception and may occur as a result of the myelotomy. Lateral dissection can injure the spinothalamic tracts and produce sensory dysfunction. Diminution of SSEPs may indicate disturbance or injury to these pathways.

Dysesthesias, hyperesthesias, and hyperpathia are terrible postoperative complications. These entities may render an otherwise functional extremity useless and prevent a patient with minimal or no motor deficit from returning to a former occupation or resuming a normal social life. Frequently, these symptoms are present preoperatively from tumor invasion of sensory pathways and persist or are exacerbated as a result of tumor removal.

Neurologic deterioration can occur several days after surgery and has been attributed to too rapid steroid taper. Subsequent increase in corticosteroid dosage does not always restore neurologic function. Potentially reversible etiologies such as postoperative hematoma and vascular insults must be considered and treat as appropriate.

Operative Wound Breakdown

Wound breakdown is unusual in patients who have not been previously operated on. However, in the setting of a previous operation and irradiation, wound dehiscence, cerebrospinal fluid fistulae, and meningitis occur commonly, regardless of how meticulously the closure is performed. For this reason, the operative incision in the patient who previously underwent operation and irradiation should be closed with rotational flaps of the trapezius or latissimus dorsi muscles from beyond the irradiated field.

Spinal Deformities

Postlaminectomy kyphosis and the swan-neck deformity are well-recognized complications of surgery for intramedullary spinal cord tumors. Children with intramedullary spinal cord tumors are at risk for the development of these deformities after surgery. Children under 3 years of age, those with preoperative spinal deformity, and those with preoperative neurologic deficits are at greatest risk. In the absence of preoperative kyphosis, development of postlaminectomy kyphosis in adults is extremely rare. Osteoplastic laminotomy is performed to forestall the development of progressive spinal deformity.

In the cervical spine, laminectomy and denervation of the paraspinous muscles likely lead to flexion deformity. Severe, untreated flexion deformity may result in spinal cord compression and progressive neurologic deficit, which may be mistaken for tumor recurrence. Because postoperative spinal deformities commonly occur in children, frequent follow-up is essential. In the cervical spine, early fusion at the first sign of flexion deformity is indicated.

Adjunctive Treatment

Radiation Therapy

No study has demonstrated a beneficial effect of radiation therapy on neurologic function or survival in patients with glial spinal cord tumors. Guidetti and associates did not find any consistent benefit from radiation therapy (14). Other investigators reported improvement or disappearance of deficits after irradiation, but none of these studies was controlled and no proof exists that the radiation treatment itself resulted in improvement. Although surgery is the treatment of choice for both intramedullary and extramedullary tumors, some authors recommend biopsy and radiation for astrocytomas and ependymomas. The beneficial results of these studies may be related to the effects of the decompressive laminectomy rather than the adjuvant treatment of intradural extramedullary tumors other than metastatic disease.

The efficacy of radiation therapy is difficult to determine because the natural history of low-grade astrocytomas is unpredictable and long-term survival without radiation may occur (15,16). It appears to be reasonable to irradiate all adult patients with spinal cord astrocytomas, regardless of the surgeon's impression of the completeness of removal or the histologic grade of the tumor. Treatment consists of 4,500 Gy given in divided doses to the region of the tumor. Garcia noted improved outcomes in patients treated with 4,000 Gy compared with those treated with smaller doses (17). Marsa and co-workers used doses of more than 5,000 Gy, but such treatment is not recommended because of the risk for radiation myelopathy (18).

Because of the detrimental effect of radiation therapy on development in children, most pediatric patients who are believed to have had a gross total resection of their tumors are not irradiated. However, radiation therapy has been proposed for recurrent low-grade tumors in children or as an initial treatment postoperatively, particularly in patients who have had rapid neurologic deterioration. These patients must be followed with serial MRI scans to detect tumor recurrence.

Patients with ependymomas who are believed to have had complete removal should not be irradiated. Instead, they should be followed closely with frequent MRI and treated with reoperation or radiation if recurrence becomes apparent. When removal of an ependymoma is incomplete, local radiation may be given to the area of residual tumor.

Chemotherapy

Adjuvant treatment for intramedullary tumors is based on radiotherapy. The place of chemotherapy in this setting has yet to be determined. For the past decade, chemotherapeutic agents such as carmustine (BCNU) have been a standard part of the management protocol for treating patients with brain astrocytomas. However, the efficacy of this and similar agents in managing spinal cord astrocytomas is unknown. As a large proportion of intramedullary malignancies occur in children, who are more sensitive to the deleterious effects of irradiation, chemotherapy assumes an important role. The efficacy of chemotherapy in patients with intramedullary glial tumors calls for further trials in this setting, especially in young children and patients with metastases. Systemic chemotherapy is reserved for treatment of malignant spinal cord tumors such as glioblastoma multiforme as an adjunct to surgical resection.

Long-Term Outcomes

Long-term survival and postoperative neurologic function are related to tumor histology, the patient's preoperative neurologic status, and the extent of tumor resection. Most intramedullary spinal cord tumors grow slowly, and long-term survival is the rule. Epstein has noted that gross total removal of low-grade spinal cord astrocytomas is associated with no evidence of tumor progression clinically or radiologically for many months (19). However, higher-grade astrocytomas (anaplastic) often cannot be radically resected owing to the infiltrative nature of the tumor. Although the outlook for patients with low-grade astrocytomas is better, slow progression of tumors in the cervical region can result in death from respiratory paralysis. Degeneration of low-grade tumors into malignant ones may occur and further affects the outcome adversely. Patients with malignant astrocytomas have a particularly dismal outcome (20).

Fortunately, the long-term survival of patients with ependymomas is less bleak than is the case for patients with astrocytomas. Gross total removal of spinal cord ependymomas is associated with extended disease-free survival. Unlike the outcome associated with astrocytomas, the outcome in patients with ependymomas does not appear to be related to histologic grade. Although ependymomas may seed the subarachnoid space, this method of dissemination appears to be the exception rather than the rule.

Hemangioblastomas are benign tumors that are curable if they are removed totally. In practice, hemangioblastomas are found frequently in multiple locations, and the patient's outcome is determined by the behavior of tumors located elsewhere in the nervous system or systemically.

Extent of Tumor Resection

Spinal cord tumors usually grow slowly, so that the relationship between outcome and the extent of tumor resection must be examined at an extended interval from surgery. Estimates of the completeness of tumor resection by the operating surgeon are prone to overestimation. Because astrocytomas are infiltrating, complete resection is achieved less frequently than previously believed. Patients with astrocytomas who underwent gross total resection have a high incidence of recurrence and neurologic progression. This finding suggests that complete or nearly complete removal is rarely achieved. The incidence of tumor recurrence is less a function of whether total removal has been achieved than of the length of follow-up. The extent of resection of astrocytomas correlates poorly with the risk for recurrence, patient survival, and neurologic outcome. Unfortunately, systematic follow-up has been lacking from most clinical studies.

CONCLUSION

Development of new technologies for the diagnosis and treatment of intramedullary tumors, including MRI, the operating microscope, ultrasound, laser, and ultrasonic tissue aspirator have radically changed the results of surgery, perioperative management and long-term outcome results. Unsatisfactory outcomes with standard operative therapies before the introduction of these new technologies led many surgeons to conclude that the least harmful strategy was limited biopsy with adjuvant postoperative irradiation. These developments have allowed more accurate preoperative diagnosis and safer, more effective operative interventions.

REFERENCES

1. Stein BM. Intramedullary spinal cord tumors. *Clin Neurosurg* 1983; 30:717–741.
2. Klekamp J, Samii M, Surgical results for spinal meningiomas. *Surg Neurol* 1999;52(6):552–562.
3. McCormick PC. Anatomic principles of intradural spinal surgery. *Clin Neurosurg* 1994;41:204–223.
4. Saito T, Arizono T, Maeda T, et al. A novel technique for surgical resection of spinal meningioma. *Spine* 2001;26(16):1805–1808.
5. Schick U, Marquardt G, Lorenz R. Intradural and extradural spinal metastases. *Neurosurg Rev* 2001;24(1):1–5; discussion, 6–7.
6. Wang TC, Huang KM, Liu HM, et al. CT myelography for differential diagnosis between intramedullary and intradural-extramedullary spinal tumors in the region of the conus medullaris. *J Formos Med Assoc* 1991;90(1):66–71.
7. Maira G, Amante P, Denaro L, et al. Surgical treatment of cervical intramedullary spinal cord tumors. *Neurol Res* 2001;23(8):835–842.
8. Brotchi J. Intrinsic spinal cord tumor resection. *Neurosurgery* 2002; 50(5):1059–1063.
9. Chang UK, Choe WJ, Chung SK, et al. Surgical outcome and prognostic factors of spinal intramedullary ependymomas in adults. *J Neurooncol* 2002;57(2):133–139.
10. Wanebo JE, Lonser RR, Glenn GM, et al. The natural history of hemangioblastomas of the central nervous system in patients with von Hippel-Lindau disease. *J Neurosurg* 2003;98(1):82–94.
11. Pluta RM, Iuliano B, DeVroom HL, et al. Comparison of anterior and posterior surgical approaches in the treatment of ventral spinal hemangioblastomas in patients with von Hippel-Lindau disease. *J Neurosurg* 2003;98(1):117–124.
12. Mimatsu K, Kawakami N, Kato F, et al. Intraoperative ultrasonography of extramedullary spinal tumours. *Neuroradiology* 1992;34(5): 440–443.
13. Wagner W, Peghini-Halbig L, Maurer JC, et al. Intraoperative SEP monitoring in neurosurgery around the brain stem and cervical spinal cord: differential recording of subcortical components. *J Neurosurg* 1994;81(2):213–220.
14. Guidetti B, Mercuri S, Vagnozzi R. Long-term results of the surgical treatment of 129 intramedullary spinal gliomas. *J Neurosurg* 1981;54 (3):323–330.
15. Isaacson SR. Radiation therapy and the management of intramedullary spinal cord tumors. *J Neurooncol* 2000;47(3):231–238.
16. Przybylski GJ, Albright AL, Martinez AJ. Spinal cord astrocytomas: long-term results comparing treatments in children. *Childs Nerv Syst* 1997;13(7):375–382.
17. Garcia DM. Primary spinal cord tumors treated with surgery and postoperative irradiation. *Int J Radiat Oncol Biol Phys* 1985;11(11):1933–1939.
18. Marsa GW, Goffinet DR, Rubinstein LJ, et al. Megavoltage irradiation in the treatment of gliomas of the brain and spinal cord. *Cancer* 1975; 36(5):1681–1689.
19. Epstein FJ, Farmer JP, Freed D. Adult intramedullary astrocytomas of the spinal cord. *J Neurosurg* 1992;77(3):355–359.
20. Santi M, Mena H, Wong K, et al. Spinal cord malignant astrocytomas. Clinicopathologic features in 36 cases. *Cancer* 2003;98(3):554–561.

CHAPTER 59

Cervical Spine Metastases

Louis G. Jenis and Howard S. An

The most common site of spread of skeletal metastases occurs within the vertebral column. The propensity for tumor deposits to invade the spine varies by location, with the lumbar and thoracic areas being the most common and the cervical region being the least common (1,2). The presentation and management of metastatic disease of the cervical spine differs from the other spinal locations and also depending on whether the atlantoaxial or subaxial regions are involved.

The annual rate of spinal metastases is estimated to occur in 5% of cancer patients or 18,000 patients in the United States (3,4). The cervical spine is the least frequent site of spread of spinal metastatic deposits. Brihaye and associates reviewed the literature on the distribution of spinal metastases from 1959 to 1985 and reported on 1,585 cases of symptomatic epidural deposits, with 70.3% localized to the thoracic and thoracolumbar spine, 21.6% in the lumbar and sacral spine, and 8.1% in the cervical spine (5). Recent studies suggest that cervical involvement may be more prevalent, occurring in up to 20% of all spinal metastases (6–9). The wide range of quoted incidence of tumor spread is likely related to whether the symptomatic or asymptomatic involvement is reported.

Each primary tumor varies in its propensity to metastasize to the skeleton, with breast, lung, prostate, renal, and thyroid neoplasms accounting for nearly 40% of reported cases in 1988 (10). The overall incidence of metastatic spread to the vertebral column from breast tumors ranges from 16.5% to 37% (5–7,11). In women, spinal metastases from breast tumors account for nearly 54% of all secondary site neoplasms (6). Primary lung tumors have been reported to spread to the spine in 12% to 15% of cases and to be more prevalent in males (5,6,12). Prostate tumors have been reported to spread to the spine in 9.2% to 15% of cases, whereas estimates for renal tumors are 3% to 6.5%, and for thyroid tumors, nearly 4% (5,6). Other, less common primary tumors reported to metastasize to the spinal column include gastrointestinal tumors (4.7%), gyneco-

logic tumors (9.4% in women), and melanoma (1% to 2%) (6). In addition, tumors of unknown origin may be identified in 10% to 12% of spinal metastases (3,13). In the cervical spine, tumors from breast, lung, prostate and myeloma are the most prevalent. Multiple myeloma is a primary neoplasm with some propensity for the spine.

PATHOPHYSIOLOGY AND PATHOANATOMY

The exact mechanism of metastatic spread of tumors to the spine remains incompletely understood. The mechanical hypothesis of Ewing suggests that the bony trabeculae of the vertebral bodies present an ideal site for lodging of metastatic emboli secondary to the low-flow state within the venous sinusoids (13). However, other low venous flow sites throughout the body also exist and provide an area for seeding. Paget's theory suggests that there are unique anatomic and biologic factors allowing selective tumor adherence in certain tissues (14). The specific host tissue site provides a suitable environment for establishment of metastatic deposits. The most reasonable explanation for metastatic deposits in the spine is likely multifactorial, including mechanistic aspects of both theories.

The route of spread is most commonly through the venous system, although direct spread from adjacent tumors into the vertebral bodies or into the spinal canal through the neuroforamina may occur. In addition, arterial and lymphatic spread may contribute to tumor deposits within the spine. The perivertebral venous plexus, as described by Batson (15), is a series of valveless channels allowing bidirectional flow and may be a potential source of metastatic spread. Increased intraabdominal or intrathoracic pressure diverts venous flow into the epidural space from the pelvic or azygous system and subsequently into the vertebral trabecular system. Seeding of the axial skeleton or epidural space and rarely intradural structures is possible with this shunting of venous flow. Constans and co-workers have classified four principal types of metastatic lesions based on the actual site of seeding and the relationship to the vertebral body or posterior elements and spinal cord or thecal sac (6). The types include complex or associated lesions (83.5%) responsible for both bony and neural compression, primarily bony lesions (10.3%), epidural lesions (5.0%), and intradural lesions (1% to 2%).

The vertebral body is the primary site of seeding of metastatic deposits in the cervical spine. The posterior half of the vertebral body is initially involved when the venous system is responsible for tumor spread. The anterior vertebral body, laminae, pedicles, and lateral masses are usually involved later in the disease process as cortical bone destruction proceeds (16). The establishment of tumor deposits within the vertebrae allow for cancellous bone destruction through multiple mechanisms, including direct tumor cell bony lysis or osteoclastic activation. Trabecular erosion ensues, causing biomechanical weakening of the vertebra and increases the risk for pathologic collapse. Asdourian and associates have described the pathogenesis of vertebral body collapse and etiology of spinal canal compromise in a series of patients with metastatic breast cancer and related this to the development of spinal deformity (11,17).

The manifestations of collapse vary within the cervical spine and differ in the upper cervical and subaxial regions. In the subaxial spine, vertebral body collapse may lead to an angular kyphotic deformity with or without posterior cortical wall retropulsion. Neurologic dysfunction may transpire from tumor or bone advancing into the epidural space with compression of the spinal cord or anterior spinal artery system or with tenting of the dural sac over an acute angular deformity. Pathologic fracture may also develop without significant angular deformity if the preexisting cervical lordotic sagittal alignment has been maintained. In this situation, as the line of weight-bearing passes posterior to the vertebral body, collapse occurs symmetrically in an axial direction with or without epidural space involvement (11). Although the intervertebral disc is usually resistant to tumor encroachment, the weakened vertebral end plates may allow for disc collapse into the vertebral bodies. The presence of disc space collapse associated with vertebral body destruction may lead to confusion in the diagnosis of cervical metastatic disease (i.e., discitis) and require advanced imaging studies for differentiation from other disease processes (18).

The occipitoatlantoaxial complex is an anatomically and biomechanically unique area. Metastatic involvement in this area is rare and may involve the lateral masses of C1 and the body or posterior elements of C2 (19). The spinal canal area at the C1-C2 level is the largest in the spine, and therefore neurologic signs generally develop from mechanical instability rather than from slow, direct tumor spread. Biomechanical stability of the upper cervical spine is primarily dependent on the intact lateral articular masses and transverse ligament. Destruction of the lateral masses may lead to a painful rotatory instability unlike the angular kyphosis and flexion instability of subaxial vertebral body involvement. A kyphotic deformity may develop from destruction of the C2 spinous process with subsequent detachment of the paraspinal musculature from its insertion (19).

CLINICAL PRESENTATION

The syndrome of cervical spine metastatic disease may present with varied clinical signs and symptoms. Rao and co-workers identified 11% of patients presenting with cervical lesions that were asymptomatic and were recognized only through routine screening studies (8). Symptoms may range from local nonmechanical and referred pain to mechanical pain of pathologic fracture or instability to neurologic manifestations of nerve root and spinal cord compression (20,21). The average age range of patients diagnosed with cervical spine metastases is 58 to 61 years, without male or female predominance (7,16,22).

Pain is the predominant symptom in most patients with metastatic disease of the cervical spine, with localized, unremitting discomfort reported in 89% to 93% (8,22). The nonmechanical pain due to tumor infiltration is often described as a progressively worsening symptom not related to activities and present at night, when sleep interruption is common. Pain may be unilateral or bilateral, with referred pain to the upper trapezial and shoulder area. In a patient with a previous history of known carcinoma, a new onset of nonmechanical neck pain should encourage evaluation for metastatic disease rather than the typical pain of cervical spondylosis. Studies have suggested that cervical metastases may appear up to 29 months after the initial diagnosis of the primary neoplasm (8,22). Local mechanical pain present with discomfort exacerbated by motion and relieved with rest or relative immobilization may indicate pathologic instability.

A sudden onset of pain with minimal trauma or applied force to the neck may indicate a pathologic fracture, although deformity associated with an acute fracture is rare. Deformity in the lower cervical spine is usually a slowly developing angulation from anterior and middle vertebral body collapse. Destruction of the C2 spinous process with detachment of the insertion of the paraspinal musculature may lead to a progressive feeling of head "heaviness" and an inability to hold the head upright without assistance (19).

Neurologic dysfunction is estimated to occur in 5% to 10% of patients with metastatic spine disease and may present with variable intensity and rapidity of onset. Although uncommon, cervical radiculopathy may result from tumor metastasis into the epidural space in the foramen or from retropulsion of weakened bony fragments from invasion of tumor tissue. Patients describe a burning, dysesthetic-type pain radiating in a specific dermatomal pattern suggestive of nerve root involvement. Weakness and sensory and reflex deficits may also accompany the primary symptom of pain. Spinal cord compression with symptoms and signs of myelopathy may also develop and become a presenting feature of cervical metastatic disease. Spinal cord compression is more common in the subaxial cervical area as opposed to the atlantoaxial region secondary to the differential size of the spinal canal at these levels. Motor deficits are often initial presenting features, most likely from the anterior epidural space being invaded by tumor from the vertebral body. Long tract signs, including lower extremity spasticity, weakness and difficulty with ambulation, myelopathic hand syndrome (23), and intrinsic hand muscle atrophy, may be seen. Sphincter disturbance is usually a late finding of spinal cord compression and portends a poor prognosis for eventual recovery of function (24).

DIAGNOSTIC EVALUATION

The initial evaluation of patients with persistent or nonmechanical neck pain, which is concerning for a pathologic process, includes plain radiographic examination. This is especially important in a patient with a previous history of known cancer in whom the possibility of metastasis must be considered (16). Plain radiographs require 30% to 50% demineralization before detecting a destructive process within the vertebral body and their sensitivity as a screening tool is limited (25). This may leave up to 60% of patients with metastatic spinal disease without evidence of involvement on plain radiographs (26). When destructive changes are present, they may include loss of visualization of the pedicle on the anteroposterior radiograph ("winking owl sign"), osteolysis of the vertebral body with or without collapse, spinous process erosion, and elevation of soft tissue shadows (16). Osteoblastic lesions may present with metastatic deposits arising from prostate and less commonly lung and breast cancers.

Plain radiographs allow for the determination of the location and extent of spinal metastases and the presence or absence of spinal stability. Although subjective, findings consistent with progressive deformity, significant angulation or translation, or vertebral end plate fracture may be considered signs of instability (16).

In addition to evaluation of the cervical spine, a skeletal screen should be obtained to identify nonspinal bony metastases because reports suggest that nearly 95% of lesions are present in the appendicular skeleton in the presence of spinal lesions (8). A complete thoracic-lumbar-sacral series may also confirm the presence of other spinal deposits.

For patients with known primary cancer, bone scintigraphy is an excellent screening test for identifying metastatic lesions. However, the use of bone scanning to detect metastatic lesions in the spine has limitations, including the lack of specificity, inability to provide detailed description of the anatomy of the area being investigated, and inability to provide evidence of neurocompression. Although bone scans are sensitive in determining the presence of a high bone turnover state, they cannot differentiate whether the process is from spondylosis, infection, healing fracture, or

tumor. In addition, bone scanning may not reveal a high turnover state, such as in myeloma, in which osteoclastic activity far outweighs osteoblastic bone production. The main indications for this test in a patient with known cervical metastatic disease are to identify skip lesions within the spine and to evaluate the appendicular skeleton for possible impending fractures.

The use of more advanced neurodiagnostic studies such as computed tomography (CT), either alone or combined with water-soluble myelography (CT myelography), and magnetic resonance imaging (MRI) has become commonplace in the evaluation of spinal metastases. Often, there is a role for the use of both of these studies in determining the degree of bony and soft tissue involvement and spinal cord compression. CT permits direct visualization of the bony anatomy and spinal canal and osseous compressive structures. CT myelography infers neural compression by deformity of the dural sac or exiting nerve roots in the cervical spine and is not a direct detector of actual spinal cord impingement.

The use of MRI has several advantages over CT myelography in determining the actual site of cord compression, identification of intramedullary cord signal changes, and direct evaluation of bone marrow changes that are consistent with pathologic processes. In addition, MRI can provide information at multiple spinal levels and can be used as a screening study with sagittal plane evaluation of the entire spinal column. MRI provides direct evidence of cord compression and the degree of canal compromise present based on the intrinsic "contrast" effect of the high signal intensity cerebrospinal fluid on T2-weighted imaging.

Metastatic lesions to the vertebral bodies replace normal marrow fat with tumor tissue that can be detected on MRI scanning. The use of gadolinium (gadopentetate dimeglumine) on T1-weighted images may further enhance the tumor tissue and improve on the delineation of normal and abnormal processes. The characteristics of marrow replacement allow MRI to differentiate metastases from infectious processes (2). Bone marrow signal in tumor and infection show diminished intensity on T1-weighted views and increased intensity on T2-weighted views. In tumor replacement, the signal changes often show multiple focal defects with involvement of the posterior elements, whereas, in infection, the marrow alterations were located adjacent to the vertebral end plates and are usually absent from the posterior bony column.

MANAGEMENT

General Principles

The management of patients with metastatic disease of the cervical spine or any region of the skeleton requires an aggressive multidisciplinary approach including input from the treating family practitioner, medical and radiation oncologists, and spine surgeon. Several factors must be considered when recommending the type of treatment, whether nonoperative or operative; these include patient characteristics such as age, medical condition, and overall life expectancy and tumor characteristics such as location, type, radiosensitivity, degree of instability, and presence of neurologic compromise.

Although age itself is not a contraindication to spinal surgery, the medical status of the patient can present problems with the management of systemic cancer disease. The risks of surgery must be balanced against the benefits of improving the patient's quality of life and must be dealt with on an individualized basis. In addition, life expectancy must be considered before embarking on surgical intervention. Patients with less than 8 to 12 weeks remaining are possibly more appropriate candidates for nonoperative measures. This magnifies the importance of identification of the primary neoplasm because different prognoses are likely. The survival of patients with bony lung metastases is near 7 to 9 months, as compared with that of patients with breast carcinoma with skeletal lesions, which is closer to 30 months (16). In one study, the average survival time following diagnosis of cervical spine metastases of all tumor types was 14.7 months (8).

In an attempt to provide prognosis or determination of the type of treatment that should be rendered to each patient, classification systems have been described. Harrington has proposed a five-level classification scheme, including (a) no significant neurologic involvement, (b) bony involvement without collapse or instability, (c) neurologic involvement without spinal instability or collapse, (d) painful bony collapse without significant neurologic compromise, and (e) bony collapse associated with significant neurologic compromise (26). It was suggested that categories 1, 2, and 3 be treated with a nonoperative protocol, whereas patients with manifestations of category 4 or 5 disease are more likely candidates for surgery.

The Kostuik classification system attempts to identify which lesions will cause mechanical instability and are suitable for surgical intervention (27). This system divides the cross-sectional image of the vertebral body into quartiles and the posterior elements into left and right halves to create six zones. Tumor involvement of three or more zones may result in spinal instability from mechanical causes, and severe instability is suggested when five or six columns are replaced with metastasis (13,27).

DeWald and co-workers developed a classification system to determine treatment, including bony and neurologic involvement but also the immunocompetency of each patient (28). The presence of marked bony deformity along with neurologic compromise in the setting of an immunosuppressed patient may be best treated by nonoperative measures, as suggested by this classification scheme. In addition, this classification attempts to identify those findings of impending spinal instability, including more than 50% destruction of the vertebral body or destruction of both pedicles, to determine whether surgical intervention is needed.

Raycroft and colleagues have proposed a specific classification system applied to the management of cervical metastatic tumors (29). Their classification scheme is based on location and extent of the lesion along with neurologic status. Three categories are described, including (a) localized painful tumor involvement without neurologic compromise confined to the anterior column only, (b) bony and neurologic involvement with spinal cord compression, and (c) diffuse bony involvement including both the anterior and posterior columns without significant neurologic compromise. The main purpose of this classification is to determine the type of surgical treatment appropriate for each category following a failure of conservative treatment.

Tokuhashi and associates have devised a scoring system that may assist in differentiating which patients are appropriate for surgical versus nonoperative treatment (30). Preoperative parameters that were considered include the patient's overall condition, presence of extraspinal skeletal metastases, other vertebral metastases, extraskeletal metastases, primary origin of the tumor, and neurologic status.

There is currently no specific classification system available that can address all issues and direct the management of the patient with metastatic cervical disease. It remains that each patient must be evaluated on an individual basis and that each lesion must be "personalized" to determine the most effective treatment of the disease.

Nonoperative Treatment

The treatment goals of cervical spinal metastases are to provide pain control, relieve or prevent neural deficit, and establish and maintain a quality of life that is consistent with the patient's desires. Various nonoperative treatment methods are available, including radiotherapy, hormonal therapy, chemotherapy, and high-dose steroid therapy.

The presence of epidural or bony metastatic deposits producing pain or neural deficit without evidence of instability or bony collapse is an ideal situation for the use of radiotherapy (Fig. 59.1). Minimally displaced odontoid fracture, diffuse involvement of the C2 vertebral body, or isolated posterior element involvement at C2 without evidence of instability may be treated with collar immobilization and radiation therapy (19,31). Careful monitoring of these patients during their radiation protocol is imperative to identify early signs of instability such as acute pain exacerbation or development of neurologic symptoms. Immobilization should be continued until there is radiographic evidence of consolidation or healing of the lesions. Whether immobilization is achieved with a rigid orthosis such as a sternal-occipital-mandibular immobilization (SOMI) or halo brace is based on the discretion of the treating physician. A stable neurologic deficit, multiple noncontiguous areas of spinal cord compression, or a long-term prognosis of less than several weeks would also be considered an indication for initial treatment with radiation (17). The goal

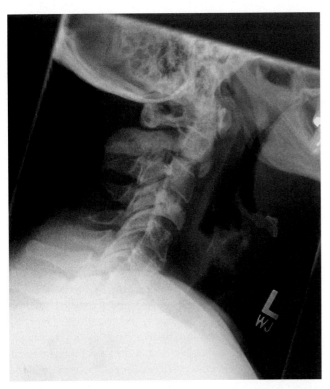

FIG. 59.1. This 42-year-old woman presented with gradual onset of upper neck pain. Plain lateral radiograph depicts osteoblastic lesion of C2 without significant angulation or translation. Neurologic examination was normal. Treatment included immobilization and radiation and hormonal therapy for metastatic breast cancer.

of radiation therapy is to deliver enough energy to an area where the tumor cells are killed and remaining normal cells may still survive. This can be performed with external-beam delivery systems such as cobalt-60 or linear accelerators (teletherapy) or by insertion of the energy source within the tumor tissue itself (brachytherapy) (32). The response to radiation therapy differs among tumor types, with breast cancer, prostate cancer, myeloma, and lymphoma being more radiosensitive than lung or renal tumors (12). If a tumor is to respond to radiation, it generally will do so very early in the course of treatment, manifested as diminished local pain and tumor size (33).

Whether to apply radiation or chemotherapy in the preoperative or postoperative period remains controversial. Patients who present with significant deformity, progression of neurologic deficit, radioresistant or chemoresistant tumors, spinal instability, or previous maximum-dose radiation treatments are candidates for initial surgical management followed by treatment to prevent tumor regrowth. Perioperative radiation therapy may compromise incorporation of the fusion. Studies have examined the role of postoperative radiation in animal models of fusion in both anterior and posterior constructs (34,35). These studies suggest that preoperative radiation most likely does not affect

strut graft incorporation. However, immediate postoperative radiation did have significant detrimental effects on the biomechanical and histologic properties of bone grafts, and it is currently recommended that radiation treatments, if indicated, be delayed for at least 3 to 6 weeks after surgery (34). Similar recommendations exist for the role of chemotherapeutic agents (13).

Numerous radiation dosage protocols have been proposed for the treatment of painful bony metastases. Manipulation of the dosage and fractionation of the delivered radiation has resulted in different institutions applying varied protocols (36). There have been no randomized controlled studies to confirm the most optimum schedule for the treatment of cervical metastatic disease.

The use of radiation therapy to treat neurologic deficits from spinal cord compression has become popular. The use of this modality to treat spinal cord compression from epidural metastases requires a prompt diagnosis and early intervention (37–40). The factors that have been identified as having prognostic significance include the ability to ambulate, rate of development of neurologic compromise, and duration of symptoms (24,32). There is also a different response to radiation therapy in treating cord compression from soft tissue metastases as opposed to bony fragments, with clinical improvement noted more likely with the former (24,41).

The role of steroids in the treatment of spinal cord compression from metastatic disease is to diminish localized intramedullary spinal cord edema (42). Steroids are indicated in the initial treatment of acute neurologic compromise from cord compression before definitive treatment such as surgical decompression is applied. A high-dose protocol followed by a gradual taper over several days is often used and may be combined with radiation therapy in the treatment of a gradually evolving neurologic deficit.

Chemical hormone–sensitive tumors may also be treated with chemotherapy or hormonal therapy. Several chemotherapeutic agents are currently used to combat sensitive tumor types, including breast, thyroid, and small cell lung carcinomas (13). Differential effects on the growth of cancer cells within bone can be achieved despite the significant side effects of many of these agents. Chemotherapy is not a treatment option for spinal instability or fracture causing neurologic dysfunction or for the treatment of generally resistant tumors such as adenocarcinoma of the lung or gastrointestinal tract, squamous cell carcinoma of the lung, renal cell carcinoma, or metastatic melanoma (13). More recent research has focused on the role of immunoglobulins in the treatment of metastatic renal cell carcinoma; however, these protocols are still being tested (43,44). Hormonal therapy for sensitive tumors such as breast or prostate carcinoma may improve the overall prognosis when treatment is combined with other regimens. Tumor cell growth may be limited with the use of tamoxifen or antiandrogen agents, respectively, in these instances (13,45).

SURGICAL INTERVENTION

The general indications for the surgical treatment of cervical metastatic disease include spinal instability or progressive deformity from bone destruction or fracture, progressive neurologic deficit unresponsive to nonoperative treatment, neurologic deficit associated with significant spinal cord compression from bony structures, requirement for a tissue diagnosis by biopsy, and intractable neck pain recalcitrant to nonoperative means of therapy. However, it is necessary to consider other factors when deciding on surgery, including the location within the cervical spine and other specific characteristics of the tumor itself along with patient life expectancy. Issues regarding surgical indications and management differ for upper and lower cervical lesions and certainly by tumor type, number of sites involved, location within the vertebra, and presence or absence of other spinal or extraspinal sites of involvement.

Occipitocervical Spine

Involvement of the upper cervical spine by metastatic disease is uncommon, and few reports have been published to direct treatment specifically (19,31). Presenting symptoms are generally severe pain because neurologic compromise is unlikely secondary to the large canal size at this level. When neurologic findings do appear, they are often created by malalignment such as lateral mass collapse or an odontoid fracture with displacement rather than pure epidural metastasis (19).

The indications for surgical intervention of upper cervical lesions include evidence of gross instability due to fracture or bony destruction, gross malalignment such as a kyphotic deformity from muscle detachment of the C2 spinous process, or neurologic compromise from malalignment or tumor compression. The basic goals of surgery are to realign, stabilize, and decompress the spinal column.

Many techniques exist to stabilize the upper cervical spine (46). The posterior approach allows for indirect reduction of the spinal canal compromise through realignment and stabilization. Anterior approaches may be indicated when residual neurologic compromise remains after posterior stabilization. Before embarking on a complex surgery, a full evaluation of the cervical spine is necessary to identify any skip lesions in the lower vertebrae that may alter the operative plan. Often, the C1 and C2 lateral masses are destroyed in the metastatic process, causing rotatory instability and requiring fusion from the occiput to C2 or lower, depending on the presence of other lesions. Preoperative evaluation of the base of the skull for lesions that may limit fixation is imperative in these situations.

Intraoperative considerations require careful patient positioning to minimize the risk for neurologic injury or further deterioration. Awake fiberoptic intubation may be required in situations in which significant instability is present. The head is stabilized with Mayfield tongs to the operating table, and all bony prominences are well padded when in the prone position. An alternative is preoperative placement of halo external fixation along with gentle, awake realignment of the upper cervical deformity with attention to neurologic status for acute changes. The halo may then be used to maintain stability intraoperatively. A midline posterior approach is performed to the upper cervical spine. Careful dissection through the ligamentum nuchae is followed by subperiosteal dissection on the spinous processes and laminae. Metastatic involvement of the spinous processes and laminae should be noted preoperatively because weakened bone may allow penetration into the spinal canal with an iatrogenic fracture of the posterior elements.

Posterior atlantoaxial stabilization is indicated when there is no involvement of the C1 lateral masses or posterior elements allowing adequate wire fixation techniques. Numerous techniques for stabilization are available, including Brooks or Gallie-type arthrodesis or transarticular screw fixation. Fixation may be extended into the lower cervical spine as needed.

Extension of the fusion to the occiput should be considered when extensive involvement of the atlas is encountered. Posterior occipitocervical arthrodesis can be accomplished by several techniques, including wire or plate stabilization. The Wertheim and Bohlman technique involves passage of wires through the outer table of the occiput, sublaminar at C1, and through the spinous process at C2 (47). The wires are then tightened around corticocancellous grafts. Further fixation into the lower cervical spine may be required as well as external halo immobilization. Occipitocervical plate fixation may be used as a means of stabilizing the upper cervical spine. Bone quality allowing adequate screw purchase may be the limiting factor, especially with more widespread disease. Consideration must be given to postoperative external halo immobilization when fixation is not ideal. Luque rods or rectangles attached to the spine with sublaminar cables or wires are another alternative form of fixation when incorporation of the skull is necessary.

The use of autogenous bone graft is recommended to achieve fusion, especially in patients with a relatively slow-growing tumor and a prolonged life expectancy. Preoperative evaluation of the iliac crest with a screening bone scan may be the best available study to determine the presence of metastatic deposits in the iliac crest. The role of polymethylmethacrylate (PMMA) cement in the treatment of posterior cervical stabilization is limited (48). McAfee and associates reported a retrospective review of nine patients treated with adjunctive PMMA for instability from neoplastic disease and identified eight failures (49). Loss of fixation at the bone–cement junction was the most common mechanism of failure in the posterior constructs. The authors recommend using PMMA as a salvage procedure only, or in patients with a very limited lifespan, and always combined with autogenous bone graft.

Although unlikely, recurrent neurologic compromise following posterior stabilization or the presence of a radioresistant tumor within the body of C2 may require an anterior decompression of the upper cervical spine. The approach to this area may be accomplished by an anterior retropharyngeal dissection, as described by McAfee and colleagues (50), or a transoral-transpharyngeal approach (51). Anterior decompression should be accompanied by a posterior stabilization procedure performed concomitantly or as a staged procedure.

Subaxial Cervical Spine

Preoperative and intraoperative considerations applied to the upper cervical region are similar to those in the subaxial spine. As opposed to C1 and C2 deposits, metastatic involvement of the lower cervical spine is more likely to cause neurologic compression based on the smaller canal size in this region and also the greater volume of cancellous bone in the subaxial vertebral bodies (22). Anterior column involvement is nearly universal in this area and may be accompanied by additional posterior disease (16). The goals of surgery are to decompress the spinal cord and prevent worsening of neurologic status and to achieve or maintain stability with rigid fixation.

The approach to the anterior cervical spine for metastatic disease is the same as for the treatment of degenerative disc disease or trauma. If realignment of the spine is necessary, either preoperative awake halo traction may be applied or intraoperative application of skeletal traction may be undertaking using Gardner-Wells tongs. Awake fiberoptic intubation should be considered for evidence of instability or the presence of preoperative neurologic symptoms. In addition, spinal cord monitoring is advised to decrease the risk for neurologic deterioration. The anterior Smith-Robinson approach is used for access to the anterior cervical spine, whereas a modified approach has been described for lesions at the cervicothoracic junction (52). Decompression is completed with corpectomy of as many vertebral bodies as necessary to accomplish the goals of treatment based on preoperative evaluation. Performance of a corpectomy, especially in tumor tissue, may lead to excessive bleeding. This may be controlled with thrombin-soaked gelatin sponges or bone wax. Massive intraoperative hemorrhage has been noted in metastatic thyroid and renal cell carcinoma, and consideration should be given to preoperative embolization in these tumors (53). Preoperative angiography and embolization should be followed by surgical intervention within 24 hours to avoid untimely revascularization from collateral circulation (54,55).

Stabilization may be completed with autograft or allograft struts either from iliac crest or fibular origin depending on the length of the construct needed. In this group of patients with a limited life expectancy, in whom it is important to diminish operative and perioperative morbidity, allografts are generally a better choice for anterior bone constructs when feasible. Bone graft may be used alone with rigid external fixation such as a halo device; however, this may add to morbidity and a delay in postoperative mobilization. Titanium

mesh implants packed with bone graft or PMMA may also be considered (Fig. 59.2). In an attempt to improve on the postoperative quality of life of the patient, consideration should be given to the addition of internal rigid fixation with less reliance on external immobilization. This can be accomplished with internal fixation such as anterior plating, PMMA, vertebral body ceramic replacement, or combinations thereof.

The role of anterior cervical plating in traumatic conditions has been well documented (56–58). The use of adjunctive plate fixation in improving stability in metastatic cervical disease is not well established. Hall and Webb reported on five patients with neoplastic involvement of the cervical spine treated with decompression and vertebral body replacement with a strut graft or PMMA followed by AO plating (59). Concerns of adequate fixation in adjacent vertebral bodies for screw purchase are prevalent along with loss of fixation from postoperative irradiation of the surgical field that may lead to compromised fixation and resultant spinal instability. If plates are used, the screws at the upper and lower levels should be placed in tumor-free vertebrae.

Others have recommended the use of PMMA combined with instrumentation as a means of achieving stability (48, 60). This should be considered only in those individuals with a relatively poor life expectancy in whom the role of PMMA is immediate stability only. Clark and co-workers (61) and Sundaresan and colleagues (62) reported on the use of Steinmann pins inserted into the vertebral bodies incorporated into PMMA as a means of vertebral body replacement. Others have reported modifications of such techniques combined with PMMA in anterior spinal fixation, including K wires driven into the vertebral bodies (16) and Harrington and Knodt rods (26,63).

The use of a ceramic prosthesis for vertebral body replacement has been described (64,65). Hosono and associates reported on 90 patients with metastatic cervical disease treated with an alumina ceramic prosthesis and noted pain relief in 94% of patients with recovery of ambulation in 81% (66). Matsui and associates evaluated 10 patients with cervical metastases treated with this technique of vertebral body replacement and noted satisfactory pain relief and stability at follow-up of 22.3 months (67). No interference with local radiation therapy was noted.

The decision to perform a combined anterior and posterior approach to the cervical spine depends on the type, degree, and location of spinal cord compression. In instances in which a napkin-ring type of circumferential encroachment on the spinal canal is noted, consideration should be given to a combined decompressive and stabilization procedure. Other factors that must be taken into consideration include the patient's overall medical condition, ability to withstand a same-day or staged procedure and life expectancy and the tumor being treated. Patients with a long life expectancy from a relatively slow-growing tumor may be treated anteriorly with decompression and strut grafting without PMMA augmentation, followed by an additional posterior stabilization procedure (Fig. 59.3) to avoid rigid

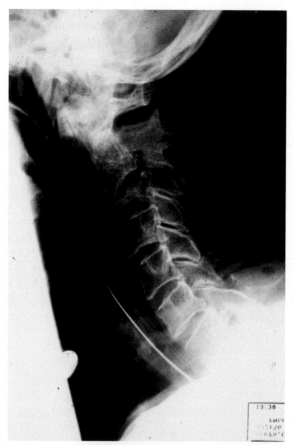

A

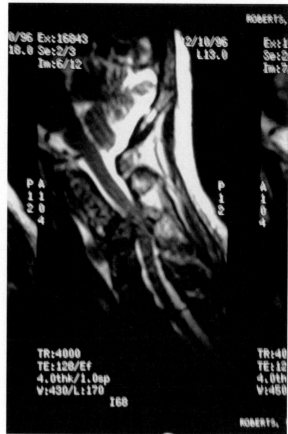

B

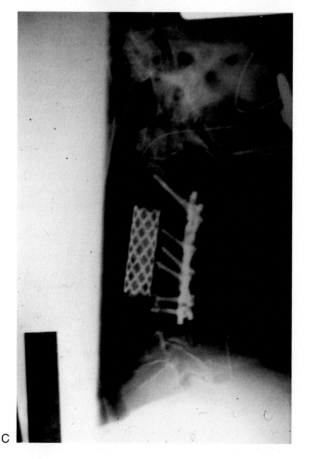

C

FIG. 59.2. This 54-year-old man presented with acute onset of neck pain and inability to maintain his head on a level position (relative kyphosis). Neurologic examination was normal. **A:** Lateral plain radiograph depicts a lytic lesion at C3 with collapse. **B:** Magnetic resonance imaging shows bony destruction and tumor infiltration with canal compromise. Evaluation confirmed multiple myeloma with numerous other sites of bony involvement. **C:** The patient was treated surgically for progressive kyphosis, including an anterior cervical corpectomy at C3 and C4 and strut reconstruction with a polymethylmethacrylate-packed titanium mesh cage. A posterior instrumented spinal fusion from C2 to C5 was also performed as a same-day combined stabilization procedure. The patient was treated postoperatively with soft collar immobilization and radiation therapy to the other bony lesions. The patient succumbed to his disease about 4 months later.

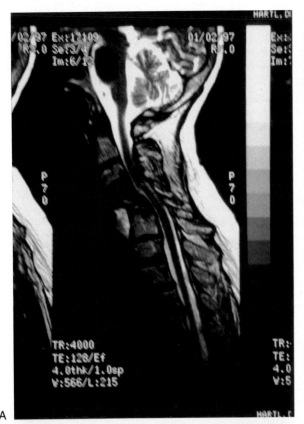

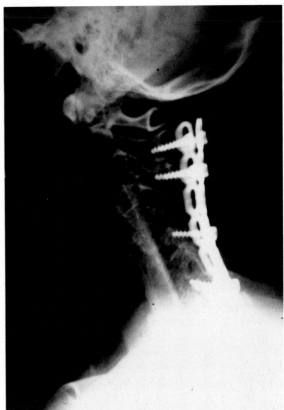

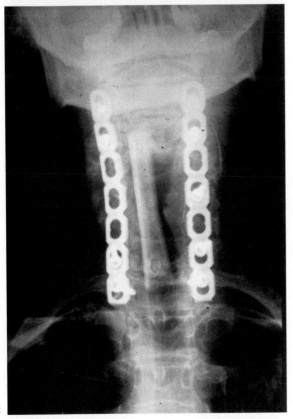

FIG. 59.3. This 55-year-old woman presented with gradual onset of neck pain and severe myelopathy, including urinary incontinence. **A:** Magnetic resonance imaging sagittal view shows a translatory deformity to the spine with kinking of the spinal cord at the C5 level. **B, C:** The patient was treated with anterior cervical corpectomy from C4 to C6, followed by realignment and strut grafting with allograft fibula. Tissue diagnosis was consistent with breast carcinoma. A combined same-day posterior instrumented fusion from C2 to C7 was performed. The lateral view (**B**) shows the hardware in position and restoration of sagittal alignment. (Note some loss of posterior fixation at C2 screws, which was asymptomatic.) The anteroposterior view (**C**) shows the instrumentation and cage in position. The patient was treated on a delayed basis with radiation and chemotherapy.

external immobilization. The anterior approach and decompression along with realignment and stabilization is the initial procedure. This can then be followed by posterior stabilization with or without decompression including laminectomy. Posterior decompression alone for circumferential compression has not been shown to be more effective than radiation therapy alone and should not be considered as a sole means of treatment (68).

SUMMARY

The treatment of cervical metastatic disease requires a multidisciplinary team approach to evaluation and management and demands consideration of multiple factors before accepting a regimen. The patient's overall functioning and medical status and life expectancy, history of previous treatment, tumor type, and location within the cervical spine and individual vertebrae must all be carefully evaluated. Most lesions are amenable to nonoperative aggressive modalities aimed at shrinking tumor size and halting growth. Surgical intervention is limited to specific indications, including spinal instability, progressive neurologic deterioration from bony collapse and compression, intractable pain, and failure of conservative means of treatment. Several options exist for the types of procedure available to the spinal surgeon, including realignment, decompression, and stabilization. Each case must be dealt with on an individual basis to determine the most appropriate technique in terms of accomplishing the goals of improving quality of life and preserving or improving neurologic function.

REFERENCES

1. Kleinman W, Kiernan H, Michelsen W. Metastatic cancer of the spinal column. *Clin Orthop Relat Res* 1978;136:166–173.
2. Perrin R, McBroom, R, Perrin R. Metastatic tumors of the cervical spine. *Clin Neurosurg* 1991;37:740–755.
3. Black P. Spinal metastasis: current status and recommended guidelines for treatment. *Neurosurgery* 1979;5:726–746.
4. O'Connor M, Currier B. Metastatic disease of the spine. *Orthopedics* 1992;15:611–620.
5. Brihaye J, Ectors P, Lemort M, et al. The management of spinal epidural metastases. *Adv Tech Stand Neurosurg* 1988;16:121–176.
6. Constans J, de Divitiis E, Donzelli R, et al. Spinal metastases with neurological manifestations: review of 600 cases. *J Neurosurg* 1983; 59:111–118.
7. Hammerberg K. Surgical treatment of metastatic spine disease. *Spine* 1992;17:1148–1153.
8. Rao S, Badini K, Schildhauer T, et al. Metastatic malignancy of the cervical spine. A nonoperative history. *Spine* 1992;17S:407–412.
9. Schaberg J, Gainor B. A profile of metastatic carcinoma of the spine. *Spine* 1985;10:19–20.
10. Silverberg E, Lubera J. Cancer statistics, 1988. *Cancer* 1988;381:5–22.
11. Asdourian P, Mardjetko S, Rauschning W, et al. An evaluation of spinal deformity in metastatic breast cancer. *J Spinal Disord* 1990;3: 119–134.
12. Tolli T, Cammisa F, Lane J, et al. Metastatic disease of the spine. In: Wiesel S, ed. *Seminars in spine surgery*, Vol 7. Philadelphia: WB Saunders, 1995:277–287.
13. Mardjetko S, DeWald C. Management of metastatic spinal disease. In: *Spine: state of the art reviews*, Vol 10. Philadelphia: Hanley & Belfus, 1996:89–95.
14. Poste G, Fidler I. Pathogenesis of cancer metastasis. *Nature* 1980;283: 139–146.
15. Batson O. The role of the vertebral veins in metastatic processes. *Ann Intern Med* 1942;16:38–45.
16. Rao S, Davis R. Cervical spine metastases. In: Clark C, ed. *The cervical spine*, 3rd ed. The Cervical Spine Research Society. Philadelphia: Lippincott-Raven, 1998:603–619.
17. Asdourian P. Metastatic disease of the spine. In: Bridwell K, ed. *Textbook of spinal surgery*, 2nd ed. Philadelphia: Lippincott-Raven, 1997:2007:2050.
18. An H, Vaccaro, A, Dolinskas C, et al. Differentiation between spinal tumors and infections with magnetic resonance imaging. *Spine* 1991; 16S:334–338.
19. Phillips E, Levine A. Metastatic lesions of the upper cervical spine. *Spine* 1989;14:1071–1077.
20. Boland P, Lane J, Sundaresan N. Metastatic disease of the spine. *Clin Orthop* 1982;169:95–102.
21. Frank C, Brantigan J, McGuire M. Evaluation of patients with spinal column tumors. In: *Spine: state of the art reviews*, Vol 10. Philadelphia: Hanley & Belfus, 1996:13–22.
22. Atanasiu J, Badatcgeff F, Pidhorz L. Metastatic lesions of the cervical spine. *Spine* 1993;18:1279–1284.
23. Ono K, Ebara T, Fuji K, et al. Myelopathy hand: new signs of cervical cord damage. *J Bone Joint Surg Br* 1987;69:215–219.
24. Siegal T, Siegal T. Current considerations in the management of neoplastic spinal cord compression. *Spine* 1989;14:223–228.
25. Chabot M, Herkowitz H. Spine tumors: patient evaluation. In: Weisel S, ed. *Seminars in spine surgery*, Vol 7, No 4. Philadelphia: WB Saunders; 1995:260–268.
26. Harrington K. The use of methylmethacrylate for vertebral-body replacement and anterior stabilization of pathological fracture-dislocations of the spine due to metastatic malignant disease. *J Bone Joint Surg Am* 1981;63:36–46.
27. Kostuik J, Weinstein J. Differential diagnosis and surgical treatment of metastatic spine tumors. In: Frymoyer J, ed. *The adult spine: principles and practice*. New York: Raven, 1991:861–888.
28. DeWald R, Bridwell K, Prodromas C, et al. Reconstructive spinal surgery as palliation for metastatic malignancies of the spine. *Spine* 1985; 10:21–26.
29. Raycroft J, Hockmann R, Southwick W. Metastatic tumors involving the cervical vertebrae: surgical palliation. *J Bone Joint Surg Am* 1978; 60:763–768.
30. Tokuhashi Y, Matsuzaki H, Teviyama S, et al. Scoring system for the preoperative evaluation of metastatic spine tumor prognosis. *Spine* 1990;15:1110–1113.
31. Sundaresan N, Galicich J, Lane J, et al. Treatment of odontoid fractures in cancer patients. *J Neurosurg* 1981;54:187–192.
32. Kagan AR. Radiation therapy for metastases and myeloma. In: *Spine: state of the art reviews*, Vol 10. Philadelphia: Hanley & Belfus, 1996: 183–190.
33. Orcutt F, Wong G. Radiation therapy for metastatic disease of the spine. In: Bridwell K, ed. *Textbook of spinal surgery*, 2nd ed. Philadelphia: Lippincott-Raven, 1997:2051–2055.
34. Bouchard J, Koka A, Bensauan M, et al. Effect of irradiation on posterior spinal fusions. A rabbit model. *Spine* 1994;19:1836–1841.
35. Emery S, Brazinski M, Koka, A, et al. The biological and biomechanical effects of irradiation on anterior spinal bone grafts in a canine model. *J Bone Joint Surg Am* 1994;76:540–548.
36. Tombolini V, Zurlo A, Montagna A, et al. Radiation therapy of spinal metastases: results with different fractionations. *Tumori* 1994;80:353–356.
37. Bruckman J, Bloomer W. Management of spinal cord compression. *Semin Oncol* 1978;5:135–140.
38. Maranzano E, Latini P, Checcaglini F, et al. Radiation therapy in metastatic spinal cord compression. A prospective analysis of 105 consecutive patients. *Cancer* 1991;67:1311–1317.
39. Maranzano E, Latini P. Effectiveness of radiation therapy without surgery in metastatic spinal cord compression: final results from a prospective trial. *Int J Radiat Oncol Biol* 1995;32:959–967.
40. Patterson R. Metastatic disease of the spine: surgical risk versus radiation therapy. *Clin Neurosurg* 1980;27:641–644.
41. Tomita T, Galicich J, Sundaresan N. Radiation therapy for spinal epidural metastases with complete block. *Acta Radiol Oncol* 1983;22: 135–143.

42. Weissman D. Glucocorticoid treatment for brain metastases and epidural spinal cord compression. A review. *J Clin Oncol* 1988;3:543–551.

43. Gleave M, Elhilali M, Fradet Y, et al. Interferon gamma-1b compared with placebo in metastatic renal cell carcinoma. *N Engl J Med* 1998;338:1265–1271.

44. Negrier S, Escudier B, Lasset C, et al. Recombinant human interleukin-2 recombinant, human interferon alfa-2a, or both in metastatic renal-cell carcinoma. *N Engl J Med* 1998;338:1272–1278.

45. Smalley R, Sconga D, Malmud L. Advanced breast cancer with bone only metastases: a chemotherapeutically responsive pattern of metastases. *Am J Clin Oncol* 1988;5:161–166.

46. Sherk H, Synder B. Posterior fusions of the upper cervical spine: indications, techniques and prognosis. *Orthop Clin North Am* 1978;9:1091–1099.

47. Wertheim S, Bohlman H. Occipitocervical fusion. Indications, technique, and long-term results in thirteen patients. *J Bone Joint Surg Am* 1988;70:658–667.

48. Dunn E. The role of methyl methacrylate in the stabilization and replacement of tumors of the cervical Spine. *Spine* 1977;2:15–24.

49. McAfee P, Bohlman H, Ducker T, et al. Failure of stabilization of the spine with methylmethacrylate. A retrospective analysis of twenty-four cases. *J Bone Joint Surg Am* 1986;65:1145–1157.

50. McAfee P, Bohlman H, Riley L Jr, et al. The anterior retropharyngeal approach to the upper part of the cervical spine. *J Bone Joint Surg Am* 1987;69:1371–1383.

51. Fang H, Ong G. Direct anterior approach to the upper cervical spine. *J Bone Joint Surg Br* 1962;44:1588–1604.

52. Kurz L, Pursel S, Herkowitz H. Modified anterior approach to the cervicothoracic junction. *Spine* 1991;16:542–547.

53. King G, Kostuik J, McBroom R, et al. Surgical management of metastatic renal cell carcinoma of the spine. *Spine* 1991;16:265–271.

54. Gellad F, Sadato N, Numaguchi Y, et al. Vascular metastatic lesions of the spine: preoperative embolization. *Radiology* 1990;176:683–686.

55. Roscoe M, McBroom R, St. Louis E, et al. Preoperative embolization in the treatment of osseous metastases from renal cell carcinoma. *Clin Orthop* 1989;238:302–307.

56. Aebi M, Zuber K, Marchesi D. Treatment of cervical spine injuries with anterior plating. Indications, techniques and results. *Spine* 1991;16S:38–45.

57. Jonsson H, Cesarini K, Petren-Mallmin M, et al. Locking screw-plate fixation of cervical spine fractures with and without ancillary posterior plating. *Arch Orthop Trauma Surg* 1991;111:1–12.

58. Mann D, Bruner C, Keen, J, et al. Anterior plating of unstable cervical spine fractures. *Paraplegia* 1990;28:564–572.

59. Hall D, Webb J. Anterior plate fixation in spine tumor surgery. *Spine* 1991;16S:80–83.

60. Sherk H, Nolan J, Mooar P. Treatment of tumors of the cervical spine. *Clin Orthop* 1988;233:163–167.

61. Clark C, Keggi K, Panjabi M. Methylmethacrylate stabilization of the cervical spine. *J Bone Joint Surg Am* 1984;66:40–46.

62. Sundaresan N, Galicich J, Lane J, et al. Treatment of neoplastic epidural cord compression by vertebral body resection and stabilization. *J Neurosurg* 1985;63:676–684.

63. Siegal T, Tiqva P, Siegal T. Vertebral body resection for epidural compression by malignant tumors. Results of forty-seven consecutive operative procedures. *J Bone Joint Surg Am* 1985;67:375–382.

64. Ono K, Tada K. Metal prosthesis of the cervical vertebra. *J Neurosurg* 1975;42:562–566.

65. Solini A, Orsini G, Broggi S. Metal cementless prosthesis for vertebral body replacement of metastatic malignant disease of the cervical spine. *J Spinal Disord* 1989;2:254–262.

66. Hosono N, Yonenobu K, Fuji T. Vertebral body replacement with a ceramic prosthesis for metastatic spinal tumors. *Spine* 1995;20:2454–2462.

67. Matsui H, Tatezaki S, Tsuji H. Ceramic vertebral body replacement for metastatic spine tumors. *J Spinal Disord* 1994;7:248–254.

68. Nicholls P, Jarecky T. The value of posterior decompression by laminectomy for malignant tumors of the spine. *Clin Orthop* 1985;201:210–213.

CHAPTER 60

Benign Tumors of the Cervical Spine

Alan M. Levine and Stefano Boriani

Most patients who present with cervical spine pain are older than 40 years of age and eventually are found to have a diagnosis of cervical spondylosis. However, a small number of predominantly younger patients are found to have a neoplasm in their cervical region. These neoplasms can be either paraspinal soft tissue lesions, intraosseous bony lesions, or intradural and extradural neoplasms involving the neural elements. Whereas the paraspinal lesions are most commonly paraspinal soft tissue sarcomas, occasionally benign soft tissue lesions such as lipomas do occur. The most common subset of intraosseous bony lesions of the cervical spine in patients older than 40 years of age are metastatic lesions to the vertebral bodies with or without soft tissue extension into the paraspinal region or extradurally into the spinal canal. If radiographs are not obtained initially, the symptoms may easily be confused with those of cervical spondylosis even in the patient with a history of cancer. Of the primary bone tumors, benign lesions of the cervical spine are less frequent than malignant lesions (1–7), in contrast to the remainder of the spine, where benign tumors are more frequent than malignant lesions (7). As with other benign bony spinal lesions, however, these tumors occur predominantly in young persons. The final group of benign tumors of the cervical spine includes those involving the neural elements, which can either be intradural (meningiomas) or extradural (neurofibromas, schwannomas and paragangliomas) (8).

Within this subset of benign spinal lesions, a number of different histologic types can be found with widely different pathologic behaviors ranging from minimally destructive and relatively avascular (osteoid osteoma) to highly destructive and extremely vascular (osteoblastoma or aneurysmal bone cyst). Likewise, these tumors can range from small lesions occurring predominantly in the posterior elements (2, 5,9–12) to larger expansile lesions occurring in the vertebral body with or without expansion into the pedicles and the posterior elements (12–15). Despite the pathologic and size differences, they have many common features and pre-

sent similar treatment problems as a result of the association with both neural and vascular structures in close proximity in the neck. They also occur predominantly in patients in the second and third decades of life; thus, a unique set of surgical problems is associated with even limited resections of the cervical spine in this age group.

The diagnosis of these lesions has changed dramatically in the past 15 years, first with the advent of computed tomography (CT) but more importantly with the development of magnetic resonance imaging (MRI) (16). In most series describing these lesions before 1980, major delays in diagnosis and treatment of benign tumors of the cervical spine were common because the only effective radiographic studies were plain films and bone scans (2,9,10,13,17,18). For small lesions hidden in the complex anatomy of the cervical spine, plain radiographs even with multiple views were often insufficient to allow visualization of the lesion. The advent of plain film tomography enhanced visualization to some degree; however, the rapid expansion of imaging modalities with CT scan, MRI (42), and finally single-photon emission CT (SPECT) bone scans have made even the smallest lesions visible. More accurate definition of neural, vascular, and soft tissue involvement with noninvasive modalities resulted in much earlier diagnosis and treatment for patients of the past decade. Similarly, CT-guided biopsy frequently made it possible to achieve a definitive histologic diagnosis to plan surgery without the morbidity or risk associated with open biopsy (1,20–23). Definitive imaging patterns, such as the CT appearance of an osteoid osteoma or the fluid-fluid levels on the MRI of an aneurysmal bone cyst (19), made it feasible to plan surgery without biopsy, with the definitive diagnosis made intraoperatively by frozen section. Embolization both as a definitive modality and as a preoperative adjunct decreased the morbidity of dealing with highly vascular lesions (11,24,25). Advances in anesthesiology and intraoperative monitoring of motor- and sensory-evoked potentials now have made it possible to perform surgical excisions of complex benign lesions more safely. Finally, although it may seem incongruous to consider treating a benign lesion with either radiation or chemotherapy, selective indications have appeared in the literature. Improvements in delivery techniques have made use of adjuvant treatments possible in the most complex or recurrent cases (26,27). New technologies such as stereotactic radiosurgery are emerging and may in the future provide alternative methods for treatment of patients whose tumors have either not responded to more conventional treatment or in whom the risks associated with surgical resection appear to be excessive (8).

Therefore, to care effectively for patients with benign tumors of the cervical spine, it is important to understand the patterns of presentation as well as the natural history and potential for progression of the various tumor types. Especially in the pediatric population, it is necessary to be able to inform the parents fully of the expected response to treatment and the likelihood of recurrence requiring secondary procedures.

PATIENT POPULATION

Although each tumor type has a slightly different age range and gender predilection, generally men are affected twice as often as women (6,7,9,25). For patients with aneurysmal bone cysts, the male and female incidences are about equal (25,28). Both giant cell tumors and hemangiomas, on the other hand, show a slight female predominance and a peak incidence in the third decade (4,29,30). This finding is compatible with the occurrence of giant cell tumors throughout the remainder of the skeleton. Most other primary cervical tumors occur in a population younger than 20 years of age (Fig. 60.1), as in one series of patients with a mean age of 16 years and an age range of 2 to 40 years (7). Interestingly, this demo-

graphic profile fits patients with osteoid osteomas, osteoblastomas, aneurysmal bone cysts, and osteochondromas most closely. Eosinophilic granuloma may occur in a somewhat younger population (31–33) but still with a male predominance.

With each of the various histologic types of tumors, there seems to be a relatively random occurrence of lesions within the various segments of the cervical spine. Few lesions occur in C1 (18), but the distribution from C2 to C7 shows slight variation from series to series (Fig. 60.2). Predilection for location within the vertebral elements is relatively specific for each tumor, as is the relative occurrence in the cervical spine versus the thoracic, lumbar, and sacral regions. Osteoid osteomas and osteoblastomas occur predominantly in the posterior elements of the spine, especially in the areas of the facet joints and pedicles (3,13). Osteoblastomas and occasionally osteoid osteomas (34) can arise in the anterior elements of the spine. About 25% of all spinal osteoid osteomas and osteoblastomas occur in the cervical region, with predominance in the lumbar region (13,34,35). Aneurysmal bone cysts occur frequently in the posterior elements, especially the spinous processes, lamina, and pedicles, and when the vertebral body is involved, the tumor is usually circumferential (5,24,25,28,36). Again, as in osteoid osteomas and osteoblastomas, lumbar involvement is most common, with cervical involvement about half as common. Osteochondromas were thought to be reasonably rare lesions, although two recent reports (37,38) have suggested that they are slightly more common than previously assumed. They can occur anywhere in the cervical spine and are more common in males, occurring usually around the third decade of life.

Langerhans cell histiocytosis (LCH) (previous referred to as *eosinophilic granuloma*) typically involves the vertebral body and only rarely the pedicles and posterior elements even in multifocal and advanced cases. The lumbar

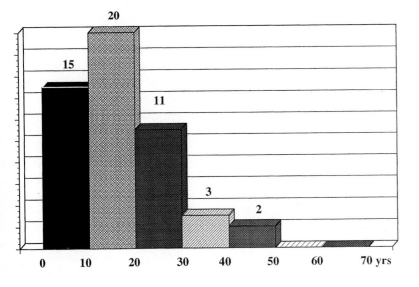

FIG. 60.1. Age distribution of 51 cases of benign tumors of the cervical spine observed at the Rizzoli Institute.

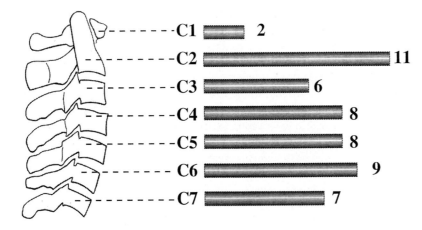

FIG. 60.2. Occurrence in the cervical spine of 51 cases of benign tumors observed at the Rizzoli Institute.

and thoracic spines are much more commonly affected than the cervical spine. The nomenclature for this tumor has been changed by the World Health Organization. The eponymic terms, *Hand-Schüller-Christian disease* and *Letterer-Siwe disease*, have been dropped in favor of the term *multicentric bone and systemic involvement*. The patterns of vertebral involvement are similar in all forms of the tumor. Giant cell tumors were the fourth most common benign tumor in the spine in Dahlin and Unni's series (39), but more than half of those tumors occurred in the sacrum. About 5% of all giant cell tumors occur in the spine; the predominant involvement is in the vertebral body. Within the mobile spine, a cervical location is as common as a thoracic or lumbar location. Other tumors can occur in the cervical spine, such as chondromyxoid fibroma (40) or fibrous dysplasia (41), but so infrequently that characterization of the patterns of vertebral involvement are not relevant.

DIAGNOSIS

Signs and Symptoms

The clinical onset of primary benign tumors of the cervical spine is usually nonspecific (6,7,42–44) and typically consists of either diffuse or localized neck pain. The pain in some cases is constant and in other cases episodic, but usually it is localized in asymmetric lesions to the involved side of the neck. In osteoid osteomas, the pain is nocturnal in about 50% of the patients but is relieved by the use of salicylates in only 30% of patients (45–51). When any tumor, especially an osteoid osteoma or osteoblastoma, encroaches on a neuroforamen, radicular symptoms and signs may be present. Myelopathy from encroachment on the dural sac is extremely infrequent, although it can occur with the more aggressive tumor types such as giant cell tumor, aneurysmal bone cyst, or osteoblastoma (52, 53). On the other hand, most hemangiomas of the spine are asymptomatic. However, when they are symptomatic, the presentation is highly variable and usually associated with muscle spasm (46,54–56). Tumors that preferentially in-

volve the vertebral body as opposed to the posterior elements (giant cell tumor, eosinophilic granuloma, circumferential aneurysmal bone cyst) often present with a more constant type of pain or even neural injury, especially when associated with pathologic fracture and collapse of the vertebral body (57). Exophytic tumors occasionally may cause dysphagia because they intrude on the esophagus. As previously mentioned, in a large series of cervical benign tumors (7), the duration of symptoms averaged 19 months but ranged from 1 to 60 months, including tumors presenting over several decades, and thus patients did not benefit from current methods of evaluation. Even so, those patients with LCH and those with aneurysmal bone cyst had relatively short symptomatic periods as a result of the severity of the pain. More current series suggest that the average duration of symptoms in the adolescent population with neck pain averages less than 2 months. In a series of 41 patients (7), 39 presented with neck pain. Persistent cervical pain and muscular spasm occur in most of these patients. Torticollis (the equivalent of scoliosis in the thoracic and lumbar spine) was present in 12 of 41 patients. Presentation with a mass is relatively rare, but patients with osteochondromas and aneurysmal bone cysts involving the posterior elements may exhibit that finding.

Neurologic signs and symptoms should be considered as either radicular (relatively frequent) or myelopathic, related to cord compression (relatively infrequent). Radicular pain has been reported to occur in 20% to 50% of all patients; however, demonstrable radicular findings, such as changes in reflexes, sensation, muscle strength, muscle atrophy, or paresis, occur in fewer than 20% of all patients. In more aggressive tumors, cord compression from the tumor or from pathologic fracture of the vertebral body has been reported to occur (41,53,57,58), but it is more frequent in the thoracic spine (4,13,43). Circumferential vertebral involvement as occurs in hemangiomas (54–56) and aneurysmal bone cysts (5,12,59) may cause gradual constriction of the neural canal and myelopathy. Likewise, in the patient with multifocal hemangiomas (about one third of all patients) or in the pregnant patient, the prevalence of neurologic deficit is higher.

Imaging Studies

The radiographic evaluation of any spinal lesion and most especially the cervical spine always begins with plain radiographs in the patient with localizing symptoms. At least two orthogonal views are necessary [anteroposterior (AP) and lateral]. Although plain radiographs may identify the location of the lesion, often bone scan, CT scan, or MRI will allow definitive identification in patients suspected of having a tumor (60). Symptoms that should suggest further studies after a negative plain roentgenogram are dysphagia, persistent night cervical pain, muscular spasm not relieved by medication, painful torticollis, sudden occurrence of neurologic symptoms, and extremity pain, which may or may not fit a dermatomal distribution. Because most patients are children or teenagers, any patient with persistent neck pain unresponsive to conservative measures after 1 month with negative plain radiographs should be subjected to a bone scan or MRI, depending on the clinical circumstance.

Plain Radiographs

A standard radiographic series to evaluate the cervical spine for the presence of a tumor should consist of an AP and lateral view. If the physical examination suggests symptoms in the craniocervical area, an open-mouth view should be added. Likewise, pillar or oblique views will help define a lesion in the pedicles or facets. Because of the complex anatomy of the cervical spine and multiple overlapping structures, the plain radiograph may appear normal in some smaller lesions, but specific tumors may have a typical appearance. For example, exostoses are ossified and lobulated masses. Hemangioma has a striated or honeycomb pattern. Osteoblastoma produces enlargement of the vertebral borders and is often associated with granular ossifications, whereas osteoid osteoma (when visible) has a radiolucent nidus with variable ossified reaction. Fibrous dysplasia causes gross deformation of the outline with architectural derangement of cancellous bone and frosted-glass pattern. The later stages of LCH (eosinophilic granuloma or histiocytosis X) may have the distinctive appearance of a vertebra plana.

Conversely, aneurysmal bone cyst and giant cell tumor appear mostly as radiolucent areas with variable definitions of their margins and are often difficult to distinguish on plain radiographs. The specific radiographic appearance of each lesion is discussed later.

Bone Scan

Technetium-99m (^{99m}Tc) isotope labeling is of great value in detecting many tumors not visible on standard radiographs. Most benign cervical lesions are evident on bone scan. The only lesion that in its early stages may not exhibit intense activity is an LCH, which will become more evident after collapse of the vertebral body. Activity on ^{99m}Tc may be faint and visible only on a SPECT scan until pathologic fracture has occurred and the lesion is visible as a vertebra plana on plain radiograph. The most common benign lesion that might be symptomatic but not readily visible on plain roentgenogram is the osteoid osteoma; however, osteoid osteomas are easily detected as a typical "hot spot" and osteoblastomas as larger hyperactive areas. Aneurysmal bone cyst may present as negative area with positive border. On the other hand, the specificity of bone scan is minimal: fractures, infections, and osteoarthrosis can provoke increased uptake as well.

Computed Tomography

The CT scan is highly sensitive to early bone destruction and remains unsurpassed for both evaluation of and planning for surgical intervention for a benign lesion of the cervical spine. For bony lesions of the cervical spine initially detected on either plain radiograph or bone scan, the next step for accurate definition of the lesion is axial CT scan images because cross-sectional imaging helps to enhance the understanding of the inherently complex anatomy of the cervical spine. It best evaluates cortical lesions and matrix calcification. For small lesions in the cervical spine or for accurate two- or three-dimensional reconstructions, 2-mm cuts are necessary through the area of interest. Use of both bone and soft tissue windows allows definition of not only the extent of vertebral involvement but also the presence or absence of a soft tissue mass and a suggestion of either vertebral artery, nerve root, or cord compression. Contrast enhancement can be used for careful evaluation of the tumor margins and intrinsic vascularity. Some CT scan images are considered pathognomonic, such as the nidus in osteoid osteoma. Highly suggestive are "polka dot" or "corduroy" patterns typical of hemangioma or the granular ossifications within a lytic area in the osteoblastomas (16).

Magnetic Resonance Imaging

For detecting occult lesions not visualized on standard radiographs, MRI has greater sensitivity than bone scan. Compared with normal bone marrow, most tumors demonstrate decreased signal intensity on T1-weighted images and increased signal on T2-weighted images (16,61). MRI is rarely necessary in the primary evaluation of benign lesions of the cervical spine because other studies more often initially reveal their presence. The MRI is a useful tool for completing the evaluation of tumors that may have a major soft tissue mass (giant cell tumor), involvement of the vertebral artery (giant cell tumor, aneurysmal bone cyst), or compression of the nerve roots or dural sac (any lesion). The MRI allows noninvasive evaluation, which once required either angiography or myelography. Interpreting the MRI, however, requires a greater competence than CT and must be considered together with other imaging techniques to avoid incorrect diagnosis. On MRI, the nidus of a small osteoid osteoma, for example, may remain undetected, whereas the surrounding reactive area can be interpreted as a permeative infiltration into the cancellous bone.

Angiography

Angiography alone is rarely used as a primary tool to evaluate the vascularity of a lesion to aid in diagnosis (62) because magnetic resonance angiography (MRA) is less invasive and easier to do. Today, angiography is used primarily for selective vascular studies before embolization. Embolization can then be used either as a primary therapeutic modality (aneurysmal bone cyst, giant cell tumor, hemangioma) or as a preoperative adjunct to decrease the vascularity and thus the morbidity of resecting lesions such as hemangiomas, giant cell tumor, osteoblastomas, or aneurysmal bone cyst. The shared branches to the tumor and spinal cord make embolization technically more difficult in the cervical spine than in the thoracic or lumbar regions. For the purpose of angiographic studies, the cervical spine should be divided into the upper cervical spine (C1 to C3) and the lower cervical spine. A variety of arteries are evaluated, including the vertebral, occipital, ascending pharyngeal, thyrocervical, and costocervical arteries. Each of the benign lesions has a different radiologic appearance, but none has the arteriovenous (A-V) shunting characteristic of malignant tumors. Embolization of these tumors is generally not curative but may be palliative in the sense that symptoms, especially pain, may be reduced and tumor growth retarded. The type of embolization is based on the flow characteristics and the size of the lesion. Gelfoam, polyvinyl alcohol foam, stainless steel coils, and cyanoacrylate are the most commonly used substances. Embolization preoperatively must be done within 24 hours of surgery to achieve maximal effect and prevent revascularization of the tumor.

Biopsy Techniques

The problems and complications of biopsy of bone and soft tissue lesions are myriad but are also well documented (21,43). Clearly, the hazards are more substantial in malignant tumors than in benign ones irrespective of the location; however, even biopsy of benign lesions can be complicated by such events as implantation and recurrence of the tumor in the biopsy tract (giant cell tumor) or excessive bleeding (aneurysmal bone cyst). Therefore, the basic principles of tumor biopsy should be followed strictly and include (a) placing the biopsy tract in line with the incision for definitive treatment, (b) achieving minimal tissue contamination by avoiding dissection of tissue planes and going directly to the tumor, (c) obtaining adequate tissue for diagnosis (and confirming, if possible, by frozen section that the tissue is viable and satisfactory for diagnosis), (d) obtaining adequate hemostasis to prevent contamination by hematoma,

and (e) draining all open biopsy wounds. The basic criteria for correct biopsy technique are important for all musculoskeletal biopsies (3,63) but may be more difficult to adhere to in the spine than in other areas as a result of the limited number of approaches and the proximity to critical vascular structures that can be easily contaminated. Fortunately, benign cervical lesions are for the most part more forgiving to violations of standard technique than malignant ones.

Biopsies of benign lesions of the cervical spine vary with the location, size, nature, and definitive therapy of the spinal tumor. Biopsies can be needle biopsy, incisional, or excisional. Needle biopsies can be either fine-needle aspiration or a core biopsy. In lesions in which the radiographic picture is quite characteristic and the lesion is relatively small, an excisional biopsy is safe and efficacious. In a larger lesion that has a soft tissue component with either anterior or posterior involvement for which surgery is considered, the treatment of choice, an incisional biopsy followed by a frozen section, is recommended. In lesions that have a soft tissue component and may not require surgical treatment or may be part of a larger differential diagnosis, a needle aspiration may provide sufficient pathologic material. This is often true of an LCH or when trying to differentiate an infection from a tumor, which most appropriately is done under CT guidance (1).

The approach to anterior lesions in the cervical spine is from lateral with a metal maker placed on the skin and a trajectory constructed to the lesion (Fig. 60.3). If a larger-bore needle is needed, alternatively, an anterior approach is possible in the upper cervical spine, traversing the thyroid gland. In the lower cervical spine, the needle is introduced just posterior to the border of the sternocleidomastoid manually, displacing the carotid sheath anteriorly. For lesions in the posterior aspect of the cervical spine, biopsy is relatively easy with CT control. Depth of biopsy and avoidance of both the spinal canal and the vertebral artery can be accomplished. Control by CT scan will reduce morbidity and frequently make it possible to reach even small tumors. Even in suspected benign cervical tumors, the preoperative biopsy allows adequate staging of the tumor and thus planning of the reconstruction of difficult tumors (giant cell tumor, aneurysmal bone cysts, osteoblastomas, and others) with confidence before beginning the definitive procedure. The only contraindications are thrombocytopenia and extremely vascular lesions in which obtaining hemostasis after biopsy may be difficult. In the literature, the success rate of needle biopsies of the spine has varied considerably from 50% to 90%. This rate depends somewhat on whether the series has reported biopsies of all regions of the spine as well as the nature of the lesions. Ottolenghi (23), in 1964, was the first to report a series of cervical aspiration biopsies with a 79% success rate; later series have reported higher success rates (20). The most common adverse outcome of needle biopsy of the spine is obtaining nondiagnostic tissue or nonrepresentative tissue in the more complex lesions.

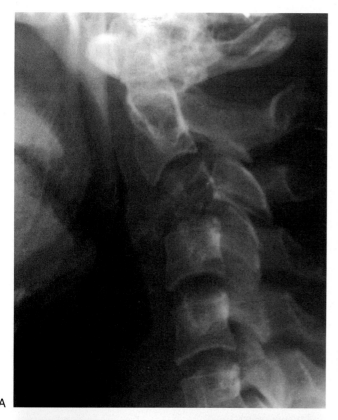

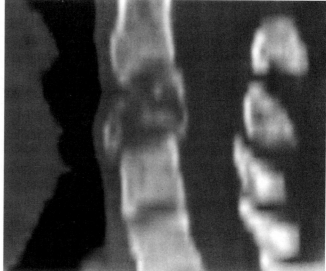

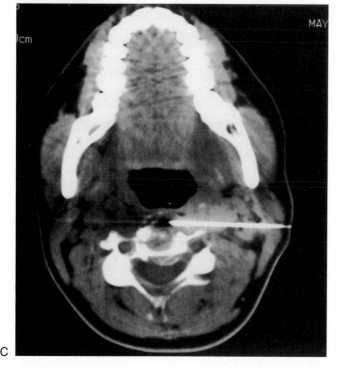

FIG. 60.3. A: This 27-year-old woman presented with the gradual onset of neck pain. She had a sudden onset of increased pain as a result of the pathologic fracture of C3. **B:** Computed tomography scan shows destruction of the C3 body without matrix calcification and with periosteal new bone formation. Magnetic resonance imaging demonstrates cord impingement but with no soft tissue mass outside the confines of the vertebral body. **C:** Before surgical planning, a needle biopsy was done to confirm the histologic diagnosis of giant cell tumor. The patient had a two-stage resection consisting of anterior resection with methylmethacrylate body replacement both as reconstruction and as adjuvant therapy. The second stage was a posterior stabilization with plating and autologous bone graft for fusion.

STAGING AND TREATMENT PLANNING

Oncologic Staging

Oncologic and surgical staging is of the utmost importance to perform appropriate treatment. Oncologic staging (3,45,64) is based on the histology and the local aggressive-ness of the tumor and defines its biologic behavior. The WBB (Weinstein, Boriani, Biagini) surgical staging (42) describes the extension of the tumor and provides a tool for planning surgery, exchanging information, and evaluating the relationship between treatment and outcome. The Enneking staging system (45), which divides benign tumors into three stages and localized primary malignant tumors into four stages, is based on clinical features, radiographic pattern, CT scan, MRI data, and histologic findings. It was formerly described for long bone tumors (45) and adapted to spinal tumors (3,4,7,13,42,64).

The first stage of a benign tumor (S1, latent, inactive) includes asymptomatic lesions bordered by a true capsule (Fig. 60.4). A well-defined margin around the circumference of the lesion is seen even on plain radiographs. These tumors are latent and do not require treatment unless pathologic fracture occurs.

Benign stage 2 tumors (S2, active) grow slowly, causing mild symptoms. The tumor usually remains within the confines of the bone border of the vertebra but may expand it and be bordered by a thin capsule and by a layer of reactive tissue (Fig. 60.4B), which may be defined on plain radiograph as enlargement of the tumor's boundaries or more clearly identified by MRI. A radioisotope scan is often positive. There is some neovascularity as part of the tumor expansion.

The third stage of benign tumors (S3, aggressive) includes rapidly growing benign tumors, which often are associated with symptoms due to cord compression or pathologic fracture. The capsule is very thin, discontinuous, or absent. The tumor invades the neighboring compartments, and a reactive hypervascularized tissue (pseudocapsule) is found, sometimes permeated by neoplastic interdigitations (Fig. 60.4C). Bone scan is highly positive, and fuzzy limits are seen on plain radiographs. The CT scan shows compartmental extension, and MRI defines a pseudocapsule and the apparent relationship with the neurologic structures. En bloc resection, even if marginal, is the treatment of choice.

During the surgical planning, reconstruction of the spine must be taken into consideration (65). Most resections of the posterior elements of the cervical spine destabilize the spine to some degree. The degree of destabilization is dependent on the patient's age and the extent of the posterior element resection. In the adult, a one- or two-level midline laminectomy, which does not involve the facets or pedicles, is well tolerated without fusion. In skeletally immature children, however, certainly anything in excess of a midline one-level laminectomy in the cervical spine frequently leads to secondary kyphosis. The resultant kyphosis is more difficult to correct after it occurs as opposed to prophylactic fixation and fusion at the time of resection. Therefore, skeletally immature children should have a posterior arthrodesis traversing the extent of the laminectomy (7) (Fig. 60.5).

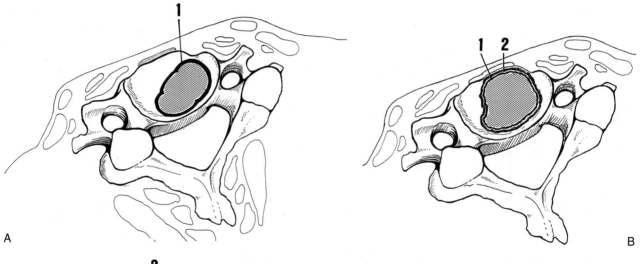

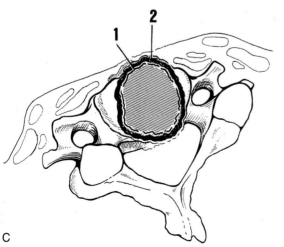

FIG. 60.4. Oncologic staging of benign bone tumors by Enneking (64,91). The capsule is indicated with 1, the reactive pseudocapsule with 2. **A:** Stage 1. Benign latent inactive lesions: these asymptomatic lesions are bordered by a true capsule, which is shown even on plain radiographs by well-defined margins. **B:** Stage 2. Benign active lesions grow slowly and cause mild symptoms. The tumor usually remains within the confines of the bone border of the vertebra but may expand it and may be bordered by a thin capsule and by a layer of reactive tissue, which may be defined on plain radiograph as enlargement of the tumor's boundaries or more clearly identified by magnetic resonance imaging. **C:** Stage 3. Benign aggressive lesion includes rapidly growing benign tumors, often associated with symptoms resulting from cord compression or pathologic fracture. The capsule is quite thin, discontinuous, or absent. The tumor can invade the neighboring compartments. A reactive hypervascularized tissue (pseudocapsule) is found, sometimes permeated by neoplastic digitations.

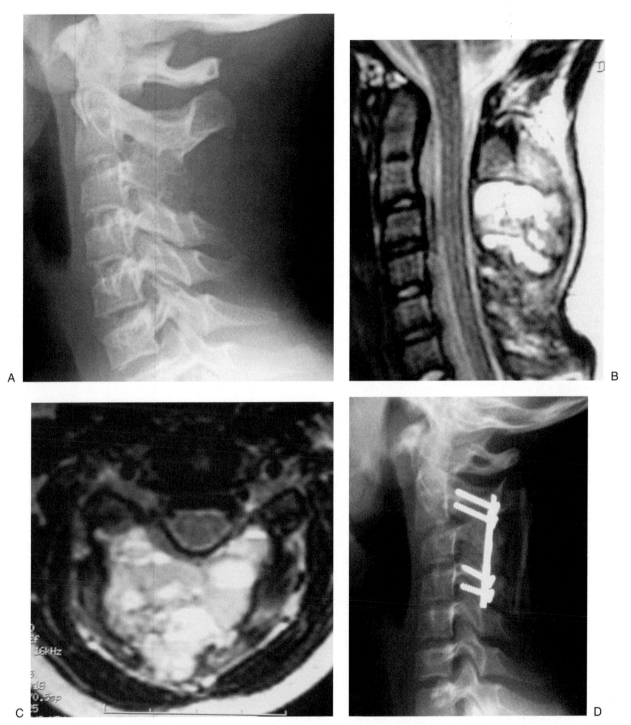

FIG. 60.5. An 8-year-old girl presented with pain in her neck and a palpable mass. **A:** Plain lateral radiograph demonstrates absence of the C3 spinous process with suggestion of a large soft tissue mass. **B:** Sagittal magnetic resonance imaging (MRI) shows the aneurysmal bone cyst expansion of the spinous process. **C:** On the axial MRI, the fluid-fluid levels are well visualized. **D:** The patient underwent resection of the spinous process, lamina, and lateral masses, which were all involved, and arthrodesis from C2 to C4.

In the adult, resection of any component of the lateral mass or pedicle on one side will destabilize that segment of the spine (66). Generally, instrumentation and arthrodesis should be done simultaneously using the remaining posterior spinal elements and confining the fusion and instrumentation to the affected levels. For example, if an entire lateral mass is removed on one side with a portion of the lamina, the posterior cervical plate on the contralateral side will span the level above to the level below with screws in all three levels but with screws in only the level above and below on the resected side. If only one articular process is removed, that fixation can be restricted to one level. Arthrodesis should be done with autologous graft taken from the iliac crest with a separate surgical setup.

In the anterior cervical spine, after corpectomy, replacement of the vertebral segment or segments can be done in several ways. For giant cell tumor and most stage 3 lesions, replacement with methylmethacrylate anteriorly gives immediate stability when combined with and augmented by posterior autologous arthrodesis and plating. This mode of reconstruction has the advantage of allowing rapid recognition of early recurrence and immediate stability to limit the degree of postoperative immobilization. In the case of giant cell tumor, the heat of polymerization can contribute to the local control as it does with extremity lesions. For most stage II benign tumors, autologous strut graft with anterior plating is sufficient to achieve stability and fusion. Alternatively, use of a titanium or carbon fiber cage filled with autologous bone graft is a reasonable option. In patients undergoing an anterior and posterior resection, both anterior and posterior instrumentation should be used to regain stability. Instrumentation preferably should be titanium to allow adequate follow-up

using either MRI or CT scan as dictated by the case. Autologous graft should be used posteriorly at a minimum, and some type of structural replacement should be used anteriorly.

Surgical Approach

The extent and difficulty of the surgical approach are based primarily on the location and size of the tumor (67) (Fig. 60.6). More benign tumors of the cervical spine involve the posterior elements (2,6,42,68), especially the more common lesions, osteoid osteoma and osteoblastoma (13,14,44–46,48,50,51,69). Benign posteriorly based tumors, whether completely intraosseous or with a soft tissue component, can most often be treated through a midline posterior approach (Fig. 60.5). In most lesions, the paraspinal musculature is retained; therefore, the most physiologic method is a midline approach. Although beyond the purview of this review, aggressive soft tissue lesions involving the spine indeed may require an incision and approach over the posterolateral aspect of the neck. However, a midline approach provides exposure from the base of the occiput to the thoracic spine and laterally to the edges of the lateral masses in the lower cervical spine and the vertebral artery and joints of the craniocervicum. The only major pitfalls to this approach are potential for injury to the greater occipital nerve in the proximal end of the incision and destabilization of the paraspinal musculature when the laminectomy extends proximal to C2. The posterior arch of C2 is critical for stable attachment of the muscles, and if resection of the C2 arch is necessary, adequate restabilization of the musculature is necessary. Not attending to this element of the reconstruction may result in gap-

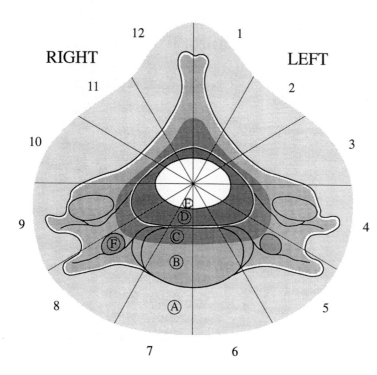

FIG. 60.6. Surgical staging of cervical tumors by the Weinstein-Boriani-Biagini system (42). The transverse section is divided into 12 sectors (in a clockwise order) and into 6 concentric layers. **A:** Expansion in the surrounding soft tissues. **B:** Intraosseous. **C:** Involvement of the canal wall. **D:** Extrusion into the epidural space. **E:** Involvement of the dura. **F:** Involvement of the vertebral artery canal. The combination of these figures identifies each tumor and allows correct planning of the surgical treatment.

ping of the paraspinous muscles, anterior subluxation, and neck pain.

Anteriorly, the surgical approach is limited by many vascular structures (common carotid artery and its terminal branches, the deep jugular veins, and vertebral arteries), by nerves (vagus, hypoglossal, facial, lingual), and by the trachea and esophagus (70). A circumferential approach for en bloc resection is limited by both the position of the vertebral artery and, more importantly, the exiting nerve roots. Unilateral sacrifice of nerve roots is more debilitating than in either the thoracic spine or sacrum and thus harder to accept for treatment of benign tumors. The vertebral arteries lie within the bone structure, compelling the surgeon to perform difficult dissections, which sometimes necessitate ligation or bypass of one vertebral artery. Generally, two surgical approaches are possible to the lower cervical spine—the posterior midline and the anterolateral prevascular, expanded inferiorly by sternotomy (71), sternal window, or third-rib thoracotomy. Most lower cervical spine tumors can be handled through a standard anterior approach. The only modification necessary is use of a longitudinal skin incision rather than a transverse incision. The longitudinal incision is placed on the anterior edge of the sternocleidomastoid and allows visualization from T1 to C4. In the lower cervical spine, anterolateral lesions (such as osteochondromas) may present a more difficult technical problem with involvement of the vertebral artery and the thoracic duct. Alternatively, Verbeist (72,73) described a more lateral approach to the cervical spine originally used for cervical spondylosis. Again, the oblique incision along the anterior border of the sternocleidomastoid is used, and the muscle is either retracted laterally or detached at its superior insertion. The trachea and esophagus are retracted medially and the carotid sheath laterally to expose the lateral aspect of the anterior tubercle of the transverse process. The anterior attachments of the longus colli are detached from the tubercles protecting the sympathetic chain. Both the nerve root and the vertebral artery can be visualized directly when removing the tumor from this approach.

The upper cervical spine can be approached by one of three methods, depending on the location of the tumor and the extent of dissection necessary to remove it. The most extensile approach is the high retropharyngeal approach, technically an extension of the approach to the lower cervical spine (74). This approach allows exposure in the relatively normal or thin patient from the anterior arch of C1 continuously to the lower cervical spine. The skin incision is made along the inferior edge of the mandible back to the anterior edge of the sternocleidomastoid and then along the anterior border of that muscle. After dividing the platysma along the incision lines, flaps are made in that plane. The marginal mandibular branch of the facial nerve is identified and preserved. The submandibular salivary gland is resected, and the digastric tendon is divided and tagged. The hyoid and pharynx can then be mobilized medially. Superior exposure is obtained in the retropharyngeal space by sequentially dividing the vascular leashes, including the superior thyroidal, lingual, superior pharyngeal, and fascial artery and vein. The prevertebral fascia is transected longitudinally in the standard fashion, giving extensile exposure. This can be augmented when necessary by the use of a mandibular splitting approach yielding more direct access to the upper portion of C2 and the C1 arch. Alternatively, the transoral approach for C1 and C2 can be used, depending on the anatomy of the mandible; this can be enlarged by the extensile transmandibular approach (75,76). The transoral approach is most useful for resection of small, anteriorly based tumors. A separate posterior approach can then be used for occiptocervical or C1-C2 arthrodesis. An additional approach popularized by Whitesides and Kelly (77) allowed a lateral approach to the upper cervical spine. It is extremely limited but allows direct exposure of one side or the other at the level of the C1-C2 articulation.

Adjuvant Treatments

Adjuvant treatments for benign spinal tumors are becoming more commonly used either to make surgery safer or in lieu of surgery in large unresectable or recurrent tumors. As modalities such as embolization, radiofrequency ablation, and stereotactic radiosurgery become safer and more often used, they may have increasing applications in benign tumors of the cervical spine. Most adjuvant modalities are used in stage 3 tumors, especially those occurring in the sacrum (26,78–80).

Although chemotherapy is rarely used for benign or even aggressive tumors, agents such as bisphosphonates (81) or interferon may have a role in the future. Chemotherapy is commonly used in the treatment of the disseminated bony systemic forms of LCH (vinblastine plus or minus prednisone), and some have suggested that local injection of prednisone in solitary lesions may be effective.

The most commonly used adjuvant is embolization. Although the cervical spine represents a more difficult region to apply this technique because of the potential for flow of the agent into the cerebral circulation or because of the potential for vascular insult to the cord, it is an effective preoperative and palliative modality. Preoperative embolization of vascular tumors such as giant cell tumor or aneurysmal bone cyst can diminish blood loss substantially. However, it has also been shown to be adequate definitive treatment in recurrent or unresectable tumors (24,25,79,80).

Another commonly used adjuvant treatment is radiation therapy, which has been reported for a number of different benign but locally aggressive tumors, including giant cell tumor (82,83), osteoblastoma, LCH, and aneurysmal bone cyst (24–26). Treatment is reasonably well established in LCH, requiring only 800 cGy to achieve a predictable response, but is less commonly used now than previously. Giant cell tumors have been treated for many years with radiation, but early studies showed a 10% rate of malignant transformation especially in the sacral lesions. New techniques reported in more current studies seem to have a lower incidence of malignant transformation and thus may in the future have greater applicability (82,83). Current recommendations are for 5,000 cGy to be used only in recurrent unresectable lesions. Aneurysmal bone cyst may be either primary or secondary, associated with giant cell tumor, osteoblastoma, and so forth. Although surgery remains the primary treatment modality for both initial and recurrent tumors, radiation has been shown to be effective (24–26). There is limited literature (13) on the use of radiation for the treatment of recurrent stage 3 osteoblastomas of the spine. It does appear, however, to have some effect on tumor regrowth. The use of brachytherapy or stereotactic radiosurgery may be considered after excision in the recurrent osteoblastoma.

For more than 20 years, topical adjuvants have been used for the treatment of giant cell tumors of bone and include phenol, liquid nitrogen, and methylmethacrylate. All can be considered for use in the cervical spine, depending on the local toxicity and the ability to control the agent based on the size and distribution of the tumor. Methylmethacrylate has a particular advantage in the spine because it is reasonably controllable, it can be used easily to substitute for the destroyed vertebral body structurally, and it does not interfere with repeat imaging to evaluate for recurrence. Liquid nitrogen probes also allow controllable freezing as an adjuvant technique, and their success in the cervical spine has been reported.

SPECIFIC TUMORS

Hemangioma

Hemangiomas of the spine are the most common benign tumor and occur in about 10% of the population but are usually asymptomatic. When they do become symptomatic, they are usually the result of either pathologic fracture or expansion of the bony architecture. Expansion of the neural arch may result in compression of the epidural space and thus pain (55). Women are affected more commonly than men, and the cervical spine is a relatively rare location compared with the thoracic spine. This benign condition is almost always diagnosed as stage 1 and is usually an incidental radiographic finding. In a review of 148 cases of symptomatic hemangioma of the literature, Nguyen and colleagues (84) found 10 in the cervical spine. Of the 18 symptomatic hemangiomas registered at the Rizzoli Institute, only 1 case was observed in the cervical spine.

The radiographic appearance is that of striated or honeycomb texture, expression of hamartomatous growth of vascular tissue within the vertebral body, and rare involvement of the posterior arch. A wedge-shaped collapse of the vertebral body is rarely observed and obscures the preexisting honeycomb or striated pattern. More commonly, minor fractures of the expanded trabeculae occur, causing the pain. On CT scan, small round ossifications are found (the

typical polka-dot appearance), which represents transverse images of thickened trabeculae. The cortices become somewhat fuzzy and ill defined; the outer border is not always intact. Paravertebral soft tissue masses can occur. On T1-weighted MRI, the intraosseous portions appear mottled, with increased signal intensity due to adipose tissue interspersed within the bony trabeculae. On MRI, an extraosseous extension of a hemangioma displays a lower signal intensity. On T2-weighted images, hemangiomas demonstrate increased signal intensity. Focal fat deposition may mimic vertebral hemangiomas on T1-weighted images but does not present the same increased signal intensity on T2-weighted images (61). Pathologically, capillary, venous, and cavernous types occur in the spine. All vascular spaces are lined by endothelial cells, which may differentiate the cavernous type from aneurysmal bone cysts. No treatment is required in asymptomatic lesions. Surgery is considered only rarely in these benign tumors; however, when necessary, an angiogram is an important part of the preoperative evaluation because it helps to diminish blood loss and blood flow and can be a treatment itself. The common vascularity of the spinal cord and affected vertebrae may preclude angiographic treatment, however. Vertebroplasty with methylmethacrylate has been used predominantly in the thoracic spine, but the results to date have very short follow-up. Radiation therapy has been used with relative success in symptomatic hemangiomas and has been used for the treatment of pain as well as the neurologic deficit. Use of radiation therapy remains controversial because the long-term effects of 4,000 cGy in a young population are not well documented (54). Stereotactic radiosurgery may provide another alternative because it has been shown to be effective in the treatment of other benign tumors of the spine (8) and can markedly limit the dose to surrounding tissues. Surgical intervention is indicated in the patient with unremitting pain, especially with neural compression. Embolization is a necessary precursor of surgical intervention and has been documented to reduce neural compression. Surgical decompression should be directed to the area of the mass lesion. Because most patients have a predominance of disease in the vertebral body, corpectomy followed by strut grafting should give both adequate stabilization and decompression. Too few patients are reported in the literature to evaluate the relative merits of this approach. If the compression appears to be posterior, laminectomy may be reasonable, although the patient with posterior arch involvement will more than likely have body involvement as well.

Gorham Disease

Gorham disease is extremely rare, and its origin and pathogenesis are unknown. A massive regional osteolysis with proliferation of capillaries occurs and progresses slowly, generally arresting spontaneously (7,85). One case

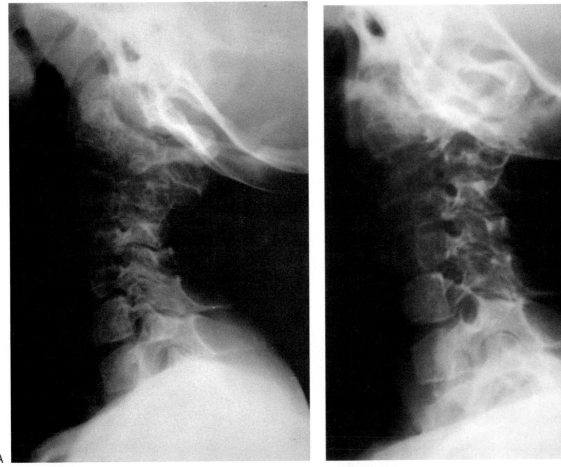

FIG. 60.7. A: Gorham disease in a child aged 4 years involving C1 to C4: massive lytic erosion. **B:** Same case, 2 years later (no surgical treatment performed). Spontaneous evolution toward ossification of the involved segments.

of cervical localization of this disease was observed in our series (Fig. 60.7). In a 4-year-old child, three vertebrae were involved by massive lytic osseous destruction, with consequent stiffness and torticollis. This child was treated by halo cast after histologic confirmation. The destruction progressed slowly but arrested itself 2 years later with partial reconstitution and incomplete fusion (Fig. 60.7B).

Aneurysmal Bone Cyst

Aneurysmal bone cyst of the spine accounts for about 10% of all such lesions seen in the body (5). This lesion generally occurs in the first two decades of life without male or female predilection (24–26,28). Isolated disease more commonly occurs in the posterior arch, but many patients have circumferential involvement (12). Aneurysmal bone cyst is a pseudotumoral, hyperplastic, and hemorrhagic lesion whose pathogenesis is unknown. It occurs frequently in the spine, arising mostly in the posterior elements, frequently involving one side of the vertebral body (Fig. 60.8A). It is more commonly located in the thoracic

or lumbar spine (28). Twenty-five percent of aneurysmal bone cysts of the spine observed at the Rizzoli Institute arose in the cervical spine (5,7). Plain radiographs show progressive bone destruction and ballooning out of the cortex and periosteum to form a poorly demarcated soft tissue mass (Fig. 60.8B and C). A surrounding bony shell is sometimes detectable (Figs. 60.3 and 60.4). The CT scan and MRI show multiple fluid-filled cavities. On MRI, the numerous cystic cavities are surrounded by a rim of low signal intensity; however, a wide range of signal intensities are seen depending on the various blood products present within the tumor.

Enormous size can sometimes be reached before diagnosis is made (Fig. 60.2). In the stage of stabilization, when expansion ceases, a multilocular appearance with osseous septa is found. Healing seldom occurs spontaneously (5, 7,12,23,30). Although radiation therapy has been given as definitive treatment, it is rarely used today as the primary treatment (5,26). In addition, there is concern about the effect of growth retardation by radiation therapy in the growing spine. However, with modern techniques and use

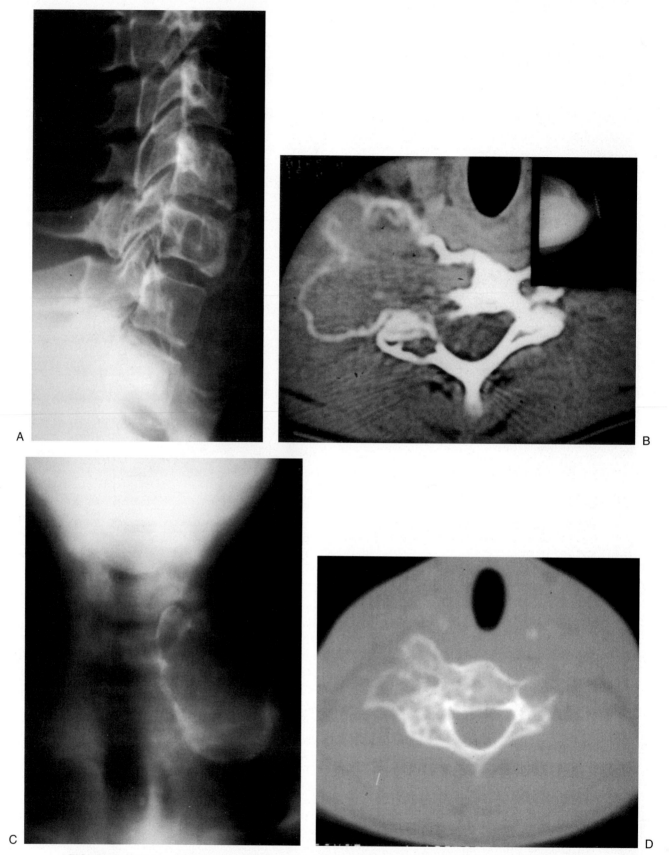

FIG. 60.8. Aneurysmal bone cyst arising from the C5 body invading the left mass and producing a huge mass in the prevertebral region. **A:** Standard radiograph. **B:** Computed tomography (CT) scan showing the prevertebral mass bordered by a thin ossified margin. **C:** Conventional tomogram demonstrating vertical extension of the mass with its thin ossified margin. **D:** CT scan 4 years later. The patient had been submitted to radiation therapy (32 Gy). The mass is dramatically reduced and ossified.

of 26 to 30 Gy, the treatment has been reported to be both safe and effective (26). The risk for spinal cord damage with higher doses and induced sarcomas also must be considered, as should the difficulties in irradiating large masses. The healed appearance is a thick, domelike, peripheral bony shell, with actual transformation into a solid mass of bone (Fig. 60.8D).

The course of symptoms is generally slow, with spinal cord compression possible as the circumferential cystic growth constricts the canal. Embolization may be quite effective in decreasing the vascularity of aneurysmal bone cyst, making surgical resection and decompression less morbid. There is the possibility of communications between the afferents of the cyst and the blood supply to the spinal cord, which must be carefully watched during embolization. The most effective treatment is curettage or marginal resection followed by reconstructive surgery with autologous graft and stabilization. Circumferential vertebral involvement is best approached by a posterior resection and stabilization followed by a piecemeal corpectomy and strut grafting or cage (24,25,28). The recurrence rate, however, has been reported to be at least 25% after curettage and grafting. Recurrence is a less frequent complication in older patients (12).

Langerhans Cell Histiocytosis

Previously called *eosinophilic granuloma* and *histiocytosis X*, LCH is a reticuloendotheliosis of unknown origin, probably viral, which may involve the bone marrow, internal organs, skin, and mucosae. It is more common in the first two decades of life and in males. Spinal localization may be solitary or multiple and usually involves only the body. Rarely is there involvement of the pedicle. A common radiographic manifestation of this systemic condition is *vertebra plana*, which is actually a late radiographic pattern and may occur almost insidiously without significant symptoms (Fig. 60.9). It is collapsed bony trabeculae following the erosive activity of the LCH and is more common in younger children than adolescents. It is sometimes asymptomatic and discovered only on a casual radiograph. In the cervical spine, a less frequent site than thoracolumbar, the usual clinical finding is neck pain and torticollis in a preadolescent patient. Discovered by standard radiographs (Fig. 60.9A) or CT scan, a purely lytic lesion necessitates the differential diagnosis with Ewing sarcoma or lymphoma. Small amounts of tumor tissue are typical of LCH (Fig. 60.9B) and explain the difficulties in finding adequate specimen for histologic diagnosis during biopsy. Frequently, the diagnosis can be made by needle aspiration and smear, thus obviating the need for any open procedure.

LCH can be a self-limited disease and may heal spontaneously. After collapse, during the healing phase, especially in younger patients, the body may in fact regain some of its original height (Fig. 60.9C and D). A report of six cases demonstrated spontaneous regression and healing without injection, radiation, or surgery (32). When the diagnosis could be obtained by aspiration smear or frozen section, local steroid injection has been done as a form of treatment; however, its effectiveness is unproven. Radiation therapy of only 8 Gy also has been effective for both extremity and spinal lesions and has not been shown to have detrimental effects on spinal growth. The most effective part of the treatment is external immobilization to prevent occurrence of kyphosis during the acute stage. Surgical débridement and stabilization followed by immobilization by halo cast (Fig. 60.9C) is extremely rare in the treatment of this condition and should be reserved for the child with multilevel disease and severe kyphosis. A bone scan is necessary both as a baseline and as follow-up for at least 2 years from the time of occurrence. Chemotherapy is indicated for disseminated disease.

Fibrous Dysplasia

Vertebral location is extremely rare for this otherwise frequent hamartomatous condition, which sometimes occurs with polyostotic distribution. Asymptomatic and usually discovered incidentally, it is a typical stage 1 lesion. Weakening of trabecular structures and vertebral collapse are responsible for neck pain, muscle spasm, and associate torticollis (Fig. 60.10). The radiographic picture shows an expanded vertebral outline with faded radiolucency of the vertebral body. When the lytic processes are more intense, especially in the adolescent, collapse may occur with a pattern quite similar to vertebra plana. No treatment is indicated in latent lesions. Stabilization is needed when mechanical failure occurs or is impending (86). In active lesions, radiotherapy is to be avoided. It is not effective and has been responsible for radiation-induced sarcoma. Curettage and bone grafting are advised only in rare cases in the adults. The lesion does recur in children, and the grafts are often absorbed (63).

Osteoid Osteoma

Osteoid osteomas and osteoblastomas are histologically similar lesions that are differentiated predominantly by the size of the lesions; however, as recently demonstrated (7, 13), osteoblastomas and osteoid osteomas have distinctly different rates of spinal occurrence, rates of recurrence, biologic aggressiveness, and certainly size. Osteoid osteoma is an osteoblastic benign tumor that most frequently arises in the posterior arch and, as demonstrated (7), is the most frequent benign tumor in the cervical spine (Table 60.1). There is a clear male predominance with a ratio of 2:1 (45,48, 50,51,69). Most cases present before the age of 25 years. About 10% of all reported osteoid osteomas occur in the spine. About 50% of all lesions occur in the lumbar spine, 30% in the cervical spine, and the remainder in the thoracic and sacral regions.

Persistent neck pain in an adolescent or young adult, frequently associated with radiation to the upper limb without specific dermatomal distribution, interfering with sleep, relieved by salicylates, and sometimes concomitant with muscle spasm, is consistent with the suspicion of osteoid

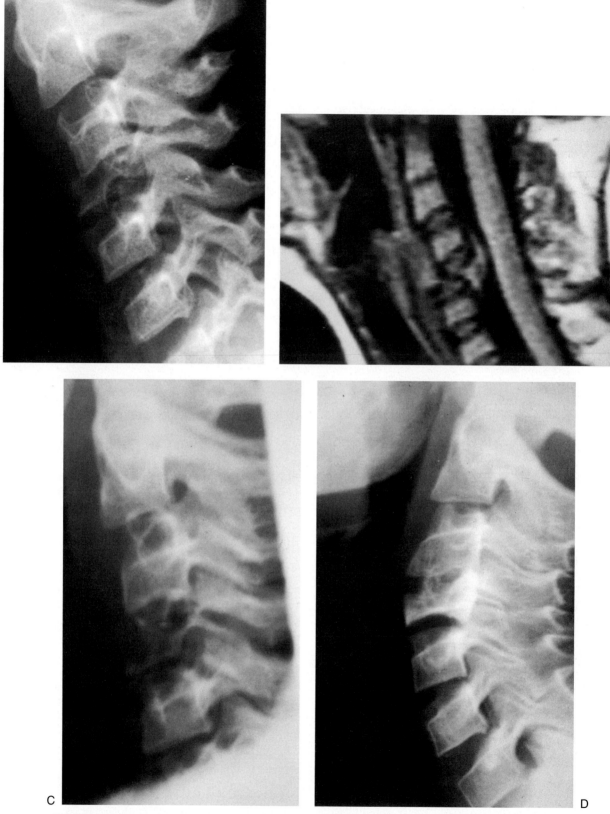

FIG. 60.9. Eosinophilic granuloma occurring in a child aged 7 years who complained of mild pain and muscular spasm. **A:** Lytic erosion of C4 vertebral body with collapse and subluxation. **B:** T1-weighted magnetic resonance imaging shows a small amount of pathologic tissue with initial invasion of the canal. **C:** Reduction in halo cast after corticosteroid injection during open biopsy procedure with frozen-section histology. **D:** Plain radiograph 2 years later shows partial reconstruction of the affected vertebra.

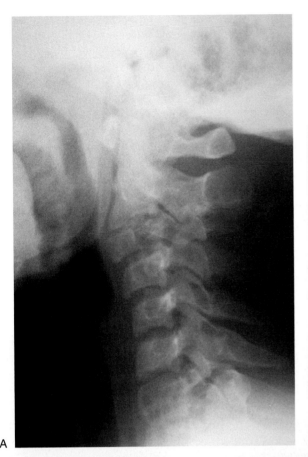

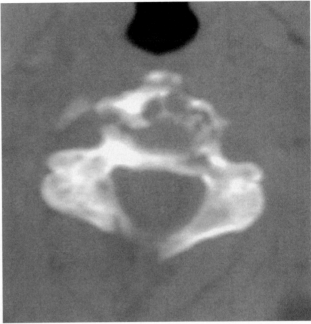

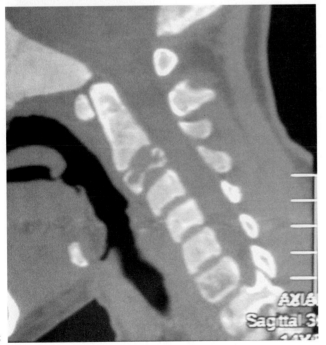

FIG. 60.10. This 14-year-old girl with know Albright syndrome presented with pain in her cervical spine. The lateral radiograph (**A**) demonstrated a pathologic fracture of C3. Immobilization did not improved the pain, and computed tomography scan with reconstruction (**B, C**) showed involvement of the body of C3 with fibrous dysplasia.

TABLE 60.1. *Histologic Diagnoses of 51 Cases of Benign Tumors of the Cervical Spine at Rizzoli Institute, Bologna, Italy*

Diagnosis	No. of cases
Eosinophilic granuloma	7
Exostosis	2
Osteoid osteoma	15
Osteoblastoma	7
Giant cell tumor	3
Fibrous dysplasia	1
Gorham disease	1
Aneurysmal bone cyst	15

osteoma. About one third of patients respond to aspirin. Torticollis may be present but is notably less frequent than associated scoliosis in the thoracolumbar spine (50). The lesions most commonly occur in the lamina or pedicle (50%) and less frequently in the facet, transverse spinous process, or body. The tumor itself is a small lucent area and is more commonly visualized by the zone of reactive sclerosis around it. A bone scan (Fig. 60.11A) usually must be performed because standard radiographs, even the best quality, may be negative as a result of other superimposing anatomic structures. When visible, the radiolucent nidus is surrounded

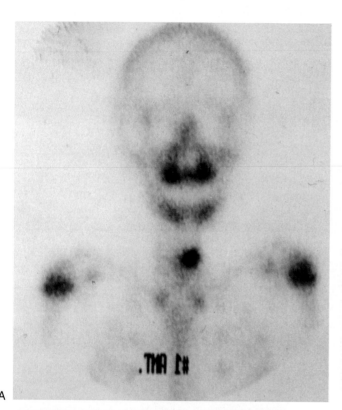

A

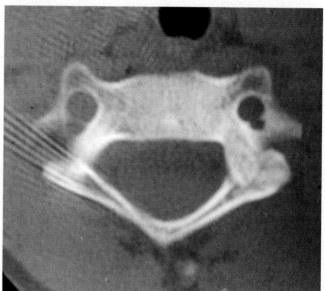

B

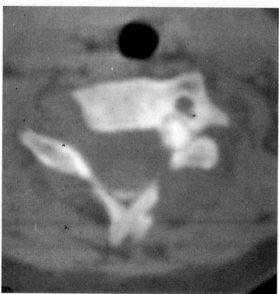

C

FIG. 60.11. A: A 14-year-old boy with nocturnal cervical pain. The isotope scan shows a "hot spot" image in the lower cervical spine. **B:** Computed tomogram shows a dense lesion in the left lateral mass of C6 with the typical pattern of osteoid osteoma. **C:** Recurrence after incomplete excision.

by a variable amount of sclerosis, which sometimes obscures the nidus and is an obstacle to diagnosis. An enlargement of the profile may result when the osteoid osteoma arises from the posterior element neural arch. The typical hot spot on bone scan associated with osteoid osteoma helps to focus the examination of standard radiographs and localizes the CT scan to the suspected lesion. Two different CT scan pictures are consistent with the diagnosis of an osteoid osteoma; the most common is a small, rounded radiolucent area, frequently but not always surrounded by a sclerotic reaction. When arising on the surface of the bone, it appears as a rounded, ovoid, small mass that is dense (Fig. 60.11B) or sclerotic. Sometimes MRI is deceiving because the surrounding reactive zone enhances (Fig. 60.12). If the nidus is not included in the slice, the surgeon can be deceived into performing a biopsy on the reactive tissue because of suspecting either an osteomyelitis or a lymphoma.

Although some cases of spontaneous regression of osteoid osteomas have been reported, treatment is usually surgical. Intralesional excision (*curettage*) has been the treatment of choice. However, for nonspinal lesions, percutaneous radiofrequency ablation as been shown to be equally effective (87), although at this point there is limited experience in the spine and even less experience in the cervical spine. Even so, this is a developing technology with potential. Currently, curettage of the nidus remains the effective treatment, and it is not necessary to remove the reactive bone because it usually regresses spontaneously, as does the torticollis. "Recurrence" of this lesion usually results from incomplete excision of the nidus (35) or missing the nidus completely (Fig. 60.11C). Although a variety of techniques have been reported to enhance the capability of delineating and excising the nidus at surgery,

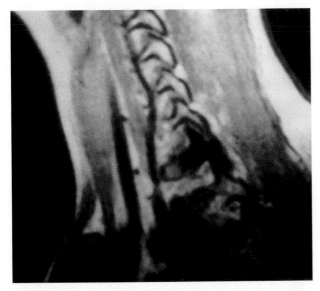

FIG. 60.12. T1-weighted magnetic resonance imaging of an osteoid osteoma of the area on the posterior arch. A wide hyperdense image prevents localizing the source of the pain and could suggest a biopsy in a reactive area.

good preoperative planning using a high-resolution CT scan most likely will lead to a successful result. The nidus is also most often easily recognized by its reddish berry-like appearance.

Osteoblastoma

Although histologically similar to the osteoid osteoma, these lesions are much larger (>2 cm) and less common. Forty percent of cases have been reported in the spine (39, 63,88,89). There is a predominance in males, and the main occurrence is before the age of 25 years (mean age, about 18 years) (13,14). About 50% of osteoblastomas occur in the lumbar spine; the remainder are split evenly between the thoracic and cervical spine (2). The prevalence of scoliosis or torticollis depends on the duration of symptoms. This tumor has a much higher incidence of neurologic involvement than osteoid osteoma. It most commonly arises from the posterior elements, sometimes invading the body, rarely occurring within the body (Fig. 60.13A and B).

Osteoblastomas tend to involve more than one element of the spine, commonly as a result of their larger size. Neurologic signs and symptoms in the form of radiculopathy may be present up to 50% of the time, with myelopathy occurring in 25%, most frequently in the thoracic spine. In the cervical spine, symptoms may range from nocturnal pain similar to that of osteoid osteoma to severe neck pain with muscular spasm (59). Osteoblastoma can be identified by plain radiographs. Its pattern varies from that of a giant osteoid osteoma, a rounded radiolucent mass larger than 2 cm with variable amount of scanty ossifications (Fig. 60.13B), to that of a highly aggressive purely lytic lesion, to be distinguished from low-grade osteosarcoma (39,63,85,90). About two thirds of lesions are stage 2, and one third are stage 3 (13). The "active" lesions (S2) (64) are positive on bone scan (Fig. 60.13B) and present on CT scan, with well-marginated sclerotic borders (Fig. 60.13C) and a thin reactive shell that thickens the cortical outline. These lesions can be treated by curettage, including the pseudocapsule (13) (Fig. 60.13D and E), and have a relatively low local recurrence rate of 5% to 10%. The "aggressive" lesions (S3) (64) are surrounded by a large pseudocapsular hypervascularized reaction, observed by contrast-enhanced CT scan, and quickly expanding to the epidural space (13). In S3 lesions, intralesional curettage is associated with a high rate of local recurrence of about 20%, especially when associated with areas of aneurysmal bone cyst. Profuse bleeding can be associated with these tumors from their reactive tissue and from the associated epidural veins; the morbidity of surgery can be decreased significantly by preoperative embolization. For this reason, the treatment of choice is en bloc excision (64,91,92); a "marginal" margin may be adequate (13). If it is feasible, selective arterial embolization is mandatory to reduce bleeding before curettage and may serve as a treatment option or adjuvant. Further adjuvants like cryotherapy or postoperative radiotherapy have been considered for better local control, but these treatments are

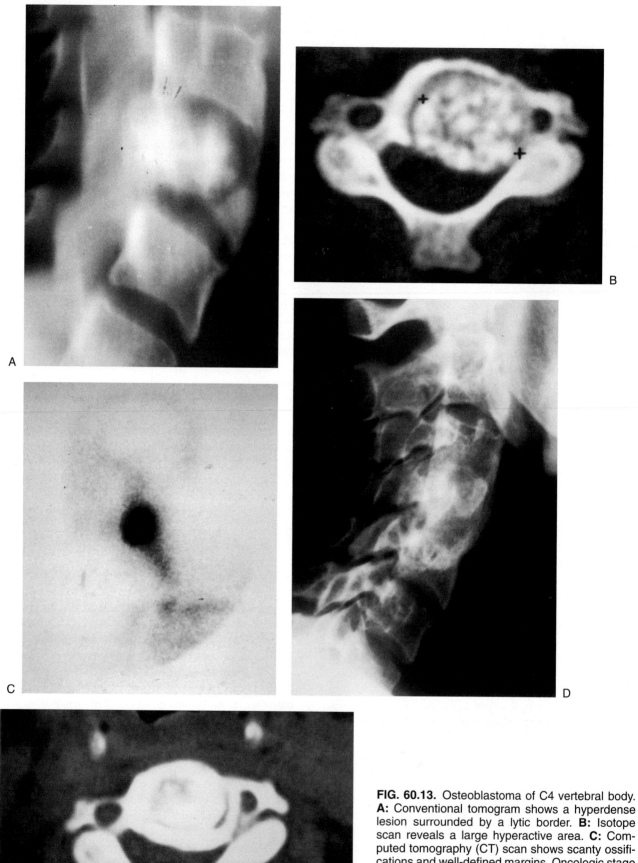

FIG. 60.13. Osteoblastoma of C4 vertebral body. **A:** Conventional tomogram shows a hyperdense lesion surrounded by a lytic border. **B:** Isotope scan reveals a large hyperactive area. **C:** Computed tomography (CT) scan shows scanty ossifications and well-defined margins. Oncologic stage S2. Suggested surgery: intralesional excision. **D:** Standard radiograph at 5 years' follow-up after curettage of the lesion and autogenous grafting. No recurrence, fusion of the graft. **E:** CT scan at the last follow-up.

not benign. In the patient with multiple recurrences, radiation therapy in the form of brachytherapy could be combined with marginal resection.

Giant Cell Tumor

Giant cell tumors are indeed a contradiction in terms, considered by some to be benign but having a significant recurrence rate after curettage of 50%, a small occurrence of "benign" pulmonary metastases, and up to a reported 10% rate of malignant transformation after radiation treatment to these tumors in the sacrum. Thus, the term *conventional* (rather than *benign*) is used by some for this locally aggressive, sometimes unpredictable tumor originating from histiofibroblastic elements. The prevalence in the spine is low (2% to 10%), and the frequency is much lower in the cervical spine than in the sacrum. The age and gender distribution differs slightly from other tumors in that occurrence in females is more common, and the peak incidence is in the third decade. Giant cell tumor often manifests as purely lytic lesions (Fig. 60.14A) arising mostly in the vertebral body. It is frequently visible on plain radiographs, especially in the cervical spine (Fig. 60.4A). Staging of this tumor is usually done by a combination of plain films, bone scan, CT scan, and MRI. As a result of the sometimes aggressive-looking appearance in the spine, staging requires biopsy to be complete (Fig. 60.4C). The extent of the lesion is usually visible on CT scan; the bony destruction and the cortical expansion (Fig. 60.14B) with periosteal new bone formation are seen on CT scan. On the other hand, the soft tissue involvement and the neural compression are best seen on MRI.

The decision about the nature of the surgical procedure is based on the staging of the tumor and the degree of involvement of critical vascular and neural structures. Stage 2 lesions may be treated using intralesional excision (curettage) plus adjuvant therapy (phenol, liquid nitrogen, or methylmethacrylate), whereas stage 3 lesions may require marginal en bloc resection. The clinical onset is not specific: slow in S2 lesions (appearing as well-defined lytic areas without ossification or reactive bone formation), and quite rapid in S3, involving most of the vertebra, with frequent pathologic fracture and nerve root or cord compression (4). The biologic behavior of giant cell tumor is sometimes unpredictable; evolution from S2 to S3 and (rare) progression to malignancy can be seen. Tumors that demonstrate malignant transformation most often are treated by radiation therapy with doses of at least 5,000 cGy and are located in the sacrum.

Curettage is the treatment of choice and must include the pseudocapsule. Curettage is often followed by adjuvant radiotherapy in S3 lesions. A potential hazard is the extreme vascularity of some giant cell tumors. For any type of surgical procedure, intralesional or excisional, preoperative embolization should be considered to reduce blood loss and morbidity, especially if there is a component of aneurysmal bone cyst associated with the giant cell tumor. Additionally, to reduce this risk, a marginal en bloc excision can be planned (4,29). This procedure in the cervical spine often requires a multistaged approach, including in some instances ligature or bypass of the vertebral artery and significant risk for cranial nerve or spinal cord injury. En bloc resections with this degree of risk clearly should be reserved for the aggressive stage 3 lesion or the recurrent tumor. Frequently, the extent of the tumor and its location prevent performance of en bloc surgery and require staged procedures of intralesional excision (68) (Fig. 60.14B to D). Although these procedures may be considered radical for what some consider a benign lesion, the locally aggressive nature of the tumor can lead to both severe neurologic deficit and death. Radiation therapy has not been reported to be as morbid in the mobile spine as in the sacrum (82, 83). A number of different alternatives exist for the recurrent tumor that has no re-resection possibility. Repeated embolization has been shown to be able to control or perhaps even cure (79,80) the very large lesion. In addition, cryosurgery (78), bisphosphonates (81), and interferon may hold some potential for control of the lesion. Finally, radiotherapy may be delivered with modern techniques in doses ranging from 25 to 45 Gy. Pathologically, multinucleated giant cells are the peculiarity of this condition; however, giant cells are present as occasional reactive elements in a number of other tumoral and pseudotumoral conditions (aneurysmal bone cyst, histiocytic fibroma, chondroblastoma, hyperparathyroidism, and others).

Osteochondroma

Osteochondroma is a hamartoma that develops from an aberrant germ cell of fetal cartilage. It is the second most frequent bone tumor but rarely occurs in the spine, accounting for about 1% to 3% of cases. Dahlin and Unni (39) reported eight cases in the cervical spine of 615 exostoses. In our series, two cases were located in the cervical spine. Frequently asymptomatic (S1), an exostosis may become symptomatic if and when it grows toward the spinal canal (Fig. 60.15) or if it develops a large subcutaneous protuberance. Exostosis is to be differentiated from enchondral osteophytes protruding into the vertebral canal. Rose and Fekete (93) described an osteochondroma of the odontoid that caused sudden death by partial transection of the cervical cord. Tully and colleagues (94) described a case of progressively increasing spasticity in a child that resulted from an exostosis arising from the body of C5. In most cases, a palpable painless mass arising from the anterior or anterolateral surface of the vertebral body is found by the patient during skeletal maturation. The tumor forms dense conglomerate masses (Fig. 60.15) containing radiolucent areas with clusters of calcifications; typically, the cortex of the host is evaginated, with the cancellous bone continuing directly into the vertebral cancellous bone (85). Radiopaque calcifications within the mass are not consistent with malignant

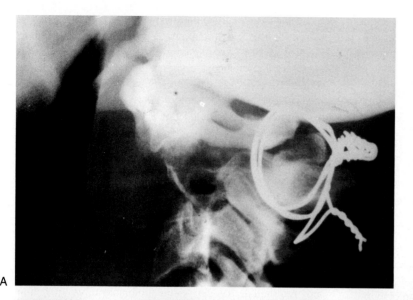

A

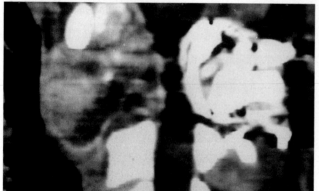

B

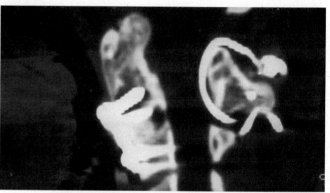

C

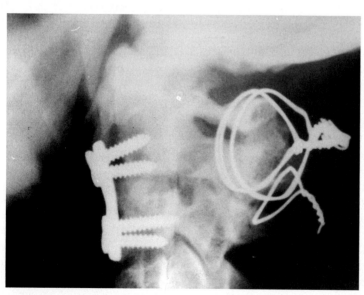

D

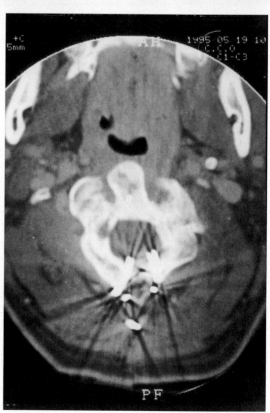

E

FIG. 60.14. Giant cell tumor arising from the body of C2 in a 21-year-old man. **A:** Lateral radiograph at referral to the Rizzoli Institute shows complete destruction of the C2 body and indirect signs of a huge anterior mass. The patient had been submitted elsewhere to posterior wiring and fusion. **B:** Preoperative sagittal reconstruction showing the large anterior tumor mass. **C:** Two-year follow-up midsagittal reconstruction now shows fusion with satisfactory alignment and absence of recurrence. **D:** Intralesional excision and grafting; standard radiogram 2 years later. **E:** Computed tomography (CT) scan at last follow-up. No recurrence, fusion of the graft. (From Laus M, Pignatti G, Malaguti MC, et al. Anterior extraoral surgery to the upper cervical spine. *Spine* 1996;21:1687–1693, with permission.)

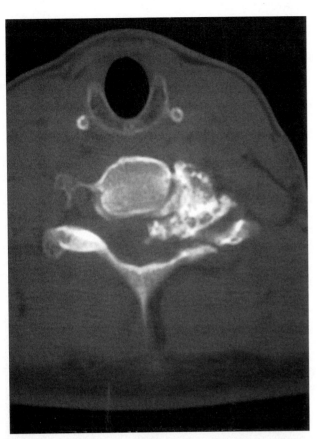

FIG. 60.15. Osteochondroma (exostosis) of left C6 mass protruding into the canal. Asymptomatic. Oncologic stage S1.

lesions and of the surgical anatomy of the region. Oncologic staging and surgical staging are mandatory to decide on treatment. Even in benign tumors, adjuvant therapies such as radiation, embolization, cryotherapy, and chemotherapy all must be considered by the treatment team. For the more aggressive lesions such as giant cell tumor, aneurysmal bone cyst, and osteoblastoma, adequate treatment for the particular lesion is mandatory the first time. Incomplete or unnecessary treatments that expose the patient to the unnecessary risk for recurrence or, even worse, an adverse survival outcome, must be avoided. On the other hand, overaggressive treatments may put a patient at unnecessary risk (a vertebrectomy for an aneurysmal bone cyst), thus submitting the patient to the risk for a major surgical procedure without an appropriate oncologic indication.

In summary, primary tumors of the spine are uncommon and those of the cervical spine even more uncommon. Few centers evaluate enough spine tumors to have sufficient experience and knowledge in the management of such cases. In a recent study of primary giant cell tumors of the spine, recurrence rates were three to four times higher when patients were initially treated at centers with limited experience (7). Thus, understanding the nature and correctly staging even the benign tumors of the cervical spine significantly affect patient outcome. The regional anatomy makes it even more difficult to adhere to the principles of oncologic surgery, which are known to improve patient outcome.

degeneration; the depth of the cartilaginous cap is directly correlated and is the most reliable indicator of malignancy when the cap is larger than 2 cm.

CONCLUSION

Primary bone tumors are quite rare in the cervical spine; they affect mainly children or young adults, with a 2:1 male-to-female ratio. The most common symptoms are often persistent neck pain and stiffness; neurologic involvement is infrequent. Malignant tumors seem to arise in older patients, always from the vertebral body, and they frequently are associated with major neurologic problems at the onset (11 of 18 cases). The most frequently affected vertebra is C2. Plain roentgenograms may not delineate the lesion clearly because of the small size and the complex anatomy of the cervical vertebra. Bone scan, CT scan, and MRI are commonly used. The location of the tumor is often helpful in defining the nature of the lesion. Osteoid osteoma and osteoblastomas most often arise from the pedicle and facet region; aneurysmal bone cysts arise from the neural arch, sometimes expanding asymmetrically from the vertebral body. All other histologic types usually arise from the vertebral body.

Surgical treatment of primary bone tumors of the cervical spine requires knowledge of the biologic behavior of these

REFERENCES

1. Babu NV, Titus VTK, Chittaranjan S, et al. Computed tomographically guided biopsy of the spine. *Spine* 1994;19:2436–2442.
2. Bohlman HH, Sachs BL, Carter JR, et al. Primary neoplasms of the cervical spine. *J Bone Joint Surg Am* 1986;68:483–494.
3. Campanacci M, Boriani S, Savini R. Staging, biopsy, surgical planning of primary spine tumors. *Chir Organi Mov* 1983;75[Suppl 1]:99–103.
4. Campanacci M, Boriani S, Giunti A. Giant cell tumors of the spine. In: Sundaresan SN, Schmidek HH, Schiller AL, et al., eds. *Tumors of the spine: diagnosis and clinical management.* Philadelphia: WB Saunders, 1990:163–172.
5. Capanna R, Albisinni U, Picci P, et al. Aneurysmal bone cyst of the spine. *J Bone Joint Surg Am* 1985;67:527–531.
6. Dreghorn CR, Newman RJ, Hardy GJ, et al. Primary tumors of the axial skeleton experience of the Leeds Regional Bone Tumor Registry. *Spine* 1990;15:137–139.
7. Levine AM, Boriani S, Donati D, et al. Benign tumors of the cervical spine. *Spine* 1992;17:S399–406.
8. Gerszten PC, Ozhasoglu C, Burton SA, et al. CyberKnife frameless single-fraction stereotactic radiosurgery for benign tumors of the spine. *Neurosurg Focus* 2003;14:1–5.
9. Fraser RD, Paterson DC, Simpson DA. Orthopaedic aspects of spine tumours in children. *J Bone Joint Surg Br* 1977;59:143–151.
10. Gabrielsen TO, Seeger JF. Vertebral angiography in the diagnosis of intraspinal masses in upper cervical region. *Neuroradiology* 1973;5:7–12.
11. Gellad FE, Sadato N, Numaguchi Y, et al. Vascular metastatic lesions of the spine: pre-operative embolization. *Radiology* 1990;176:683–686.
12. Hay MC, Paterson D, Taylor TKF. Aneurysmal bone cysts of the spine. *J Bone Joint Surg Br* 1978;60:406–411.
13. Boriani S, Capanna Donati D, Levine A. Osteoblastoma of the spine. *Clin Orthop* 1992;278:37–45.

14. De Souza Dias, L, Frost HM. Osteoblastoma of the spine: a review and report of eight new cases. *Clin Orthop* 1973;91:141–151.

15. Fielding JW, Ratzan S. Osteochondroma of the cervical spine. *J Bone Joint Surg Am* 1973;55:640–641.

16. Flemming DJ, Murphey MD, Carmichael BB, et al. Primary tumors of the spine. *Semin Muskuloskelet Radiol* 2000;4:299–320.

17. Fielding JW, Pyle RN Jr, Fietti VG. Anterior cervical vertebral body resection and bone-grafting for benign and malignant tumors. *J Bone Joint Surg Am* 1979;61:251–253.

18. Hastings DE, MacNab I, Lawson, V. Neoplasms of the atlas and axis. *Can J Surg* 1968;11:290–296.

19. Keogh C, Bergin D, Brennan D, et al. MR imaging of bone tumors of the cervical spine. *MRI Clin North Am* 2000;8:513–527.

20. Kattapuram SV, Rosenthal DI. Percutaneous biopsy of the cervical spine using CT guidance. *Am J Roentgenol* 1987;149:539–541.

21. Mankin HJ, Lange TA, Spanier S. The hazards of biopsy in patients with malignant primary bone and soft tissue tumors. *J Bone Joint Surg Am* 1982;64:1121.

22. Mankin HJ, Mankin CJ, Simon MA. The hazards of biopsy revisited for the members of the musculoskeletal tumor society. *J Bone Joint Surg Am* 1996;78:656.

23. Ottolenghi CE, Schajowicz F, DeSchant FA. Aspiration biopsy of the cervical spine: technique and result in thirty-four cases. *J Bone Joint Surg Am* 1964;46:715–733.

24. Boriani S, De Lure F, Campanacci L, et al. Aneurysmal bone cyst of the mobile spine: report on 41 cases. *Spine* 2001;26:27–35.

25. Papagelopoulos PJ, Currier BL, Shaughnessy WJ, et al. Aneurysmal bone cyst of the spine: management and outcome. *Spine* 1998;23:621–628.

26. Feigenberg SJ, Marcus RB Jr, Zlotecki RA, et al. Megavoltage radiotherapy for aneurysmal bone cysts. *Int J Radiat Oncol Biol Phys* 2001;49:1243–1247.

27. Suit HD, Goiten M, Munzenreider J, et al. Definitive radiation therapy for chordoma and chondrosarcoma of base of skull and cervical spine. *J Neurosurg* 1982;56:377–385.

28. de Kleuver M, van der Heul RO, Veraart BEEMJ. Aneurysmal bone cyst of the spine: 31 cases and the importance of the surgical approach. *J Pediatr Orthop* 1998;7:286–292.

29. Sanjay BK, Sim FH, Unni KK, et al. Giant cell tumors of the spine. *J Bone Joint Surg Br* 1993;78:148–154.

30. Verbiest H. Giant cell tumours and aneurysmal bone cysts of the spine. *J Bone Joint Surg Br* 1965;47:699–713.

31. Fowles JV, Bobechko WP. Solitary eosinophilic granuloma in bone. *J Bone Joint Surg Br* 1970;52:238–243.

32. Seimon LP. Eosinophilic granuloma of the spine. *J Pediatr Orthop* 1981;1:371–336.

33. Siberstein MJ, Sundaram M, Akbarnia B, et al. Eosinophilic granuloma of the spine. *Orthopedics* 1985;8:267–274.

34. Suttner NJ, Chandy KJ, Kellerman AJ. Osteoid osteomas of the body of the cervical spine. Case report and review of the literature. *Br J Neurosurg* 2002;16:69–71.

35. Ozaki T, Liljenqvist U, Hillmann S, et al. Osteoid osteoma and osteoblastoma of the spine: experiences with 22 patients. *Clin Orthop* 2002;397:394–402.

36. Khoshyomn S, Lew SM, Wilson JT. Aneurysmal bone cyst of the cervical spine. *Pediatr Neurosurg* 2002;37:48–49.

37. Khosla A, Martin DS, Awwad EE. The solitary intraspinal vertebral osteochondroma. An unusual cause of compressive myelopathy: features and literature review. *Spine* 1999;24:77–81.

38. Sharma MC, Arora R, Deol PS, et al. Osteochondroma of the spine: an enigmatic tumor of the spinal cord—a series of 10 cases. *J Neurosurg Sci* 2002;46:66–70.

39. Dahlin DC, Unni KK. *Bone tumors: general aspects and data on 8,542 Cases*, 4th ed. Springfield, IL: Charles C Thomas, 1986.

40. Lopez-Ben R, Siegal GP, Hadley MN. Chondromyxoid fibroma of the cervical spine: case report. *Neurosurgery* 2002;50:409–411.

41. Lomasney LM, Basu A, Demos TC, et al. Fibrous dysplasia complicated by aneurysmal bone cyst formation affecting multiple cervical vertebrae. *Skeletal Radiol* 2003;32:533–536.

42. Boriani S, Weinstein JN. Differential diagnosis and surgical treatment of primary benign an malignant neoplasm. In: Frymoyer JW, ed. *The adult spine: principles and practice,* 2nd edition. Philadelphia: Lippincott-Raven, 1996.

43. Macdonald DR. Clinical manifestations. In: Sundaresan SN, Schmidek HH, Schiller AL, et al., eds. *Tumors of the spine: diagnosis and clinical management.* Philadelphia: WB Saunders, 1990:6–21.

44. Marsh BW, Bonfiglio M, Brady LP, et al. Benign osteoblastoma: range of manifestations *J Bone Joint Surg Am* 1975;57:1–9.

45. Fielding J, Keim HA, Hawkins RJ, et al. Osteoid osteoma of the cervical spine. *Clin Orthop* 1977;128:163–164.

46. Glasauer FE. Benign lesions of the cervical spine. *Acta Neurochir (Wien)* 1978;42:161–175.

47. Janin Y, Epstein JA, Carras R, et al. Osteoid osteoma and osteoblastomas of the spine. *Neurosurgery* 1981;8:31–38.

48. Maclellan DJ, Wilson FC Jr. Osteoid osteoma of the spine. *J Bone Joint Surg Am* 1967;49:111–121.

49. Maiuri F, Signorelli C, Lavano A, et al. Osteoid osteomas of the spine. *Surg Neurol* 1986;25:375–380.

50. Pettine KA, Klassen RA. Osteoid-osteoma and osteoblastoma of the spine. *J Bone Joint Surg Am* 1986;68:354–361.

51. Raskas DS, Graziano GP, Herzenberg JE, et al. Osteoid osteoma of the spine. *J Spinal Disord* 1992;5:204–211.

52. Garcia-Bravo A, Sanchez-Enriquez J, Mendez-Suarez JJ, et al. Secondary tetraplegia due to giant-cell tumors of the cervical spine. *Neurochirurgie* 2002;48:527–532.

53. Schneider M, Sabo D, Gerner HJ, et al. Destructive osteoblastoma of the cervical spine with complete neurologic recovery. *Spinal Cord* 2002;40:248–252.

54. Einstein S, Spiro F, Browde S, et al. The treatment of symptomatic vertebral hemangioma by radiotherapy. *Spine* 1986;11:640–642.

55. McAllister VL, Kendall BE, Bull JWD. Symptomatic vertebral haemangiomas. *Brain* 1975;98:71–79.

56. Mohan V, Gupta SK, Tuli SM, et al. Symptomatic vertebral haemangiomas. *Clin Radiol* 1980;31:575–579.

57. Kanamiya T, Asakawa Y, Naito M, et al. Pathological fracture through a C-6 aneurysmal bone cyst—Case report. *J Neurosurg* 2001;94[2 Suppl]; 302–304.

58. Michalowski MB, Pagnier-Clemence A, Chirossel JP, et al. Giant cell tumor of cervical spine in an adolescent. *Med Pediatr Oncol* 2003;41: 58–62.

59. Parrish FF, Pevey JK. Surgical management of aneurysmal bone cyst of the vertebral column. *J Bone Joint Surg Am* 1967;49:1597–1604.

60. Giunti A, Laus M. *Radicolapatie spinali.* Bologna: A. Gaggi, 1992: 216–220.

61. Masaryk TJ. Spine tumors. In: Modic MT, Masaryk TJ, Ross JS, eds. *Magnetic resonance imaging of the spine.* Chicago: Year Book Medical Publishers, 1989:183–213.

62. Spiegel PK, Koch-Weser PT. Angiography of high cervical extramedullary tumours. *Clin Radiol* 1975;26:385–338.

63. Campanacci M. *Tumors of bone and soft tissues.* Bologna: Aulo Gaggi; Berlin: Springer Verlag, 1990.

64. Enneking WF, Spainer SS, Goodman MA. A system for the surgical staging of musculoskeletal sarcomas. *Clin Orthop* 1980;153:106–120.

65. Weinstein JN. Differential diagnosis and surgical treatment of primary benign and malignant neoplasms. In: Frymoyer JW, ed. *The adult spine: principles and practice.* New York: Raven Press, 1991.

66. Kostuik JP, Errico TJ, Gleason TF, et al. Spinal stabilization of vertebral column tumors. *Spine* 1988;13:250–256.

67. Lassale B, Guigui P, Delecourt C. Voies d'abord du rachis. In: *Encycl Med Chir Techniques Chir Ort Traum* (Paris) 1995:44–150.

68. Laus M, Pignatti G, Malaguti MC, et al. Anterior extraoral surgery to the upper cervical spine. *Spine* 1996;21:1687–1693.

69. Kirwan E O'G, Hutton N, Pozo JL, et al. Osteoid osteoma and benign osteoblastoma of the spine. *J Bone Joint Surg Br* 1984;66:21–26.

70. Standefer M, Hardy RW Jr, Marks K, et al. Chondromyxoid fibroma of the cervical spine—a case report with a review of the literature and a description of an operative approach to the lower anterior cervical spine. *Neurosurgery* 1982;11:288–292.

71. Sunderesan N, DiGiacinto GV. Surgical approaches to the cervicothoracic junction. In: Sundaresan SN, Schmidek HH, Schiller AL, et al. *Tumors of the spine: diagnosis and clinical management.* Philadelphia: WB Saunders, 1990:358–368.

72. Verbiest H. Anterolateral operation for fractures and dislocations in the middle and lower parts of the cervical spine. *J Bone Joint Surg Am* 1969;51:1489–1530.

73. Verbiest H. Tumors involving the cervical spine: benign tumors. In: *The cervical spine.* Philadelphia: JB Lippincott, 1990:430–476.

74. McAfee PC, Bohlman HH, Riley LH, et al. Anterior retropharyngeal approach to the upper part of the cervical spine. *J Bone Joint Surg Am* 1987;69:1371–1383.

75. Honma G, Murota K, Shiba R, et al. Mandible and tongue-splitting approach for giant cell tumor of axis. *Spine* 1989;14:1204–1210.

76. Shah JP, Shaha AR. Transmandibular approaches to the upper cervical spine. In: Sundaresan SN, Schmidek HH, Schiller AL, et al., eds. *Tumors of the spine: diagnosis and clinical management.* Philadelphia: WB Saunders, 1990:329–335.

77. Whitesides TE Jr, Kelly RP. Lateral approach to the upper cervical spine for anterior fusion. *South Med J* 1966;59:879–883.

78. Kollender Y, Meller I, Bickels J, et al. Role of adjuvant cryosurgery in intralesional treatment of sacral tumors: results of a 3–11 year follow-up. *Cancer* 2003;97:2830–2838.

79. Lackman RD, Khoury LD, Esmail A, et al. The treatment of sacral giant-cell tumours by serial arterial embolisation. *J Bone Joint Surg Br* 2002;84:873–877.

80. Lin PP, Guzel VB, Moura MF, et al. Long-term follow-up of patients with giant cell tumor of the sacrum treated with selective arterial embolization. *Cancer* 2002;95:1317–1325.

81. Fujimoto N, Nakagawa K, Seichi A, et al. A new bisphosphonate treatment option for giant cell tumors. *Oncol Reports* 2001;8:643–647.

82. Caudell JJ, Ballo, MT, Zagars GK, et al. Radiotherapy in the management of giant cell tumor of bone. *Int J Radiat Oncol Biol Phys* 2003; 57:158–165.

83. Khan DC, Malhotra S, Stevens RE, et al. Radiotherapy for the treatment of giant cell tumor of the spine: a report of six cases and review of the literature. *Cancer Invest* 1999;17:110–113.

84. Nguyen JP, Djindjian M, Badiane S. Hemangiomes vertebraux avec signes neurologiques. *Neurochirurgie* 1989;35:270–274.

85. Wilner D. *Radiology of bone tumors and allied disorders.* Philadelphia: WB Saunders, 1990.{REF}

86. Hu SS, Healey JH, Huvos AG. Fibrous dysplasia of the second cervical vertebra: a case report. *J Bone Joint Surg Am* 1990;72:781–783.

87. Rosenthal DI, Hornicek, FJ, Wolfe MW, et al. Percutaneous radiofrequency coagulation of osteoid osteoma compared with operative treatment. *J Bone Joint Surg Am* 1998;80:815–821.

88. Mirra JM, Picci P, Gold RM. *Bone tumors: clinical radiologic and pathologic correlation.* Philadelphia/London: Lea & Febiger, 1989.

89. Schajowicz F. *Tumors and tumorlike lesions of bone and joints.* Berlin: Springer Verlag, 1981.

90. Marsh HO, Choi CB. Primary osteogenic sarcoma of the cervical spine originally mistaken for benign osteoblastoma *J Bone Joint Surg Am* 1970;52:1467–1471.

91. Enneking WF. Spine. In: *musculoskeletal tumor surgery.* New York: Churchill Livingstone, 1983:303–329.

92. Weatherley CR, Jaffray D, O'Brien JP. Radical excision of an osteoblastoma of the cervical spine. *J Bone Joint Surg Br* 1986;68:325–328.

93. Rose EF, Fekete A. Odontoid osteochondroma causing sudden death. *Am J Clin Pathol* 1964;42:606–668.

94. Tully RJ, Pickens J, Oro J, et al. Hereditary multiple exostoses and cervical cord compression: CT and MR studies. *J Comput Assist Tomogr* 1989;13:330–333.

CHAPTER 61

Primary Malignant Tumors of the Cervical Spine

Stefano Boriani, Stefano Bandiera, and James N. Weinstein

Rarity of occurrence and proximity to vital structures make it difficult to diagnose and treat primary malignant bone tumors in the cervical spine. Excluding metastases and plasmacytomas, most bone tumors of the cervical spine are benign (1–5). Slow evolution and nonspecific symptoms frequently result in late diagnosis. Computed tomography (CT) scan and magnetic resonance imaging (MRI) could allow early detection of these lesions, but it is uncommon to order such expensive diagnostic studies in the face of neck pain unaccompanied by neurologic deficit. Therefore, these conditions are discovered when pain becomes intractable or when neurologic symptoms or anatomically related symptoms (like dysphagia) occur.

The high-grade malignancies (osteosarcoma, malignant fibrous histiocytoma) often are discovered earlier because of their more rapidly evolving clinical picture. In most cases, malignant tumors of the cervical spine are expansive and involve more anatomic "compartments" at the first detection (6). Their proximity to anatomic structures that cannot be sacrificed makes it difficult to treat these lesions according to commonly accepted oncologic criteria. In some cases, these lesions can be impossible to treat surgically and such treatment would be ill advised once they have recurred.

Malignant hemoglobinopathies are more common in the cervical spine than are primary malignant bone tumors, but the role of surgery in these conditions remains controversial. Surgical treatment of primary malignant bone tumors of the cervical spine, when indicated, is always difficult and frequently requires multiple approaches. Institutions without significant experience in the diagnosis, staging, and treatment options in these cases should refer them to a center where such experience exists. As with most tumors, the coordinated effort of an experienced unit is important to the management of such cases.

Advances in anesthesiology have made it possible to perform these often long and bloody procedures more safely. Performing a posterior approach in the sitting position is an example (7,8). Unlike benign lesions of the cervical spine, malignant lesions are seen more often in elderly patients (i.e., those with chordoma or plasmacytoma), adding further anesthesiologic risk and associated morbidity.

Often, the rapid evolution or the late discovery of such lesions makes it difficult to identify the site of origin within the vertebra of primary malignant tumors of the cervical spine. These primary malignancies often involve the whole vertebra (or most of it) and the surrounding tissues at the time of discovery. In this chapter, we discuss the role of imaging techniques, oncologic surgical planning, and the expected outcome of different histologic tumor types by using the published literature and our institutional experience.

A word of caution is in order. These tumors in and of themselves provide even the most skilled clinician with a diagnostic and therapeutic challenge that is in many ways the most difficult in medicine. One should seek all the available help necessary for the patient to have the best possible opportunity for success. Finally, it is often difficult to make definitive treatment suggestions because each tumor in each patient is different, and generalities or algorithmic approaches to such cases do not have evidenced-based support. Cancer, in and of itself, is difficult for patients and their families to deal with, but "shared decision making" with our patients in such cases is essential. All options must be considered and the patient's values entered into the treatment equation.

POPULATION

Of 613 cases of primary bone tumors of the spine treated at C. A. Pizzardi and Rizzoli Institutes in Bologna, Italy,

TABLE 61.1. *Histologic Diagnoses of 31 Cases of Primary Malignant Tumors of the Cervical Spine Treated at C. A. Pizzardi and Rizzoli Institute, Bologna, Italy*

Diagnosis	No. of cases
Chordoma	12
Chondrosarcoma	3
Ewing sarcoma	4
Osteosarcoma	4
Malignant fibrous histiocytoma	1
Rabdomiosarcoma	1
Fusated cells sarcoma	1
Non-Hodgkin lymphoma	4
Solitary plasmocytoma	16
Total	**46**

125 cases (20%) occurred in the cervical spine, and 46 of these were primary malignant (Table 61.1). Males were affected three times more than females (35 versus 11 cases), 65% of the cases occurred in patients older than 50 years, and 50% were in patients older than 60 years. Eleven cases arose from C2, five from C3, seven from C4, nine from C5, eight from C6, and six from C7.

Most chordomas occurred at either C2 or C3; the osteosarcomas, malignant fibrous histiocytomas, and chondrosarcomas were located at the lower cervical segments. As an initial presentation, multisegmental involvement was seen in six cases (chordoma, chondrosarcoma, Ewing sarcoma). Although all malignant histologic types, except for chondrosarcomas, originated from the vertebral body, extension to include the whole vertebra was often the case at the time of diagnosis.

DIAGNOSIS

Signs and Symptoms

The clinical onset of primary tumors of the cervical spine is usually nonspecific (1,9). Persistent cervical pain, mostly night pain, and muscular spasm occur in most patients. Dysphagia is associated with large lesions arising from C2 that extend anteriorly (chordoma, Ewing sarcoma, plasmacytoma) and was observed in 8 of 46 cases (17.4%).

Pathologic fracture is the result of neoplastic erosion of the cortex or the collapse of the vertebral body after massive destruction of the cancellous bone and substitution with neoplastic tissue. Before 1980, 10 of 12 cases of primary tumor of the cervical spine presented with symptoms related to a pathologic fracture (83%). In more recent times, with a high index of suspicion, early detection of these tumors is possible with bone scan, CT scan, or MRI. Thus, the rate of pathologic fractures at the onset of symptoms in primary malignant bone tumors of the cervical spine has fallen (20.6%; 7 of 34 observed since 1980).

Major neurologic symptoms occurred in 14 patients (30%). Five chordomas and one Ewing sarcoma presented with signs of cord compression and slow development of incomplete quadriplegia; in two other cases (plasmacytoma and osteosarcoma), root compression with mild cord involvement was present at baseline.

Diagnostic Imaging Studies

In the past, primary tumors of the cervical spine were discovered only by standard radiographs when associated with significant bone loss. Today, although plain radiographs remain the first imaging study, bone scan, CT scan, and MRI help to make definitive identification in patients suspected of having a tumor (10). Symptoms that should suggest performing further studies after a negative plain radiograph are dysphagia, persistent night pain, sudden occurrence of neurologic symptoms, and extremity pain, which may or may not fit a dermatomal distribution.

Standard Radiographs

Because of the superposition of lines typical of the cervical spine standard radiographic picture, the plain radiograph may be normal in some smaller lesions and in some myxoid tumors with expansion outside the vertebral body without evidence of bone involvement (Fig. 61.1). Specific tumors have a more typical appearance; for example, chondrosarcomas are frequently calcified and lobulated (Fig. 61.2), and plasmacytomas and chordomas appear mostly as pure radiolucent lesions with variable definitions of their margins and are often difficult to distinguish from one another on plain

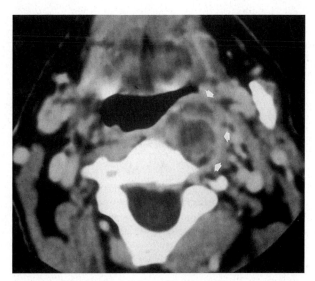

FIG. 61.1. Chordoma of C3: a wide myxoid mass (*white arrows*) expanding from the vertebral body causing dysphagia, the only symptom complained of by the patient. Standard radiographs were negative.

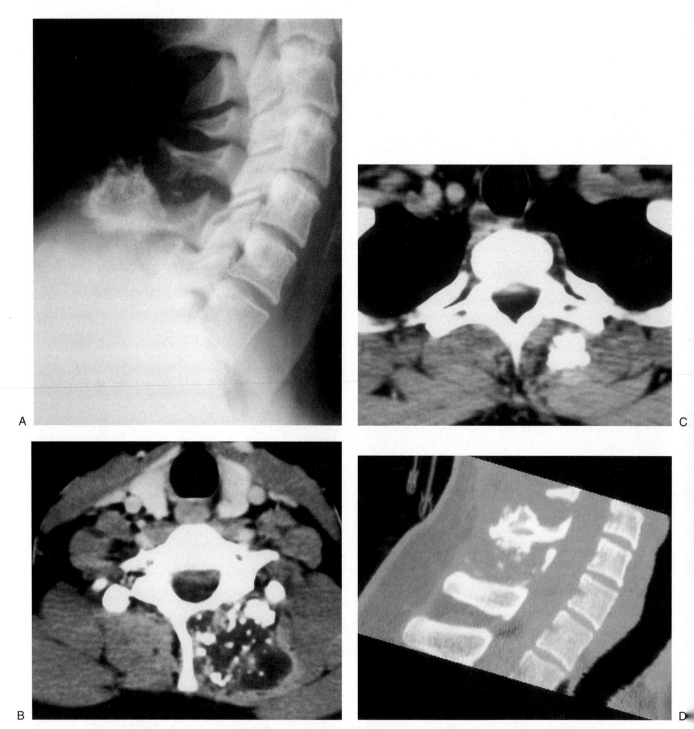

FIG. 61.2. Peripheral chondrosarcoma in a 31-year-old man. **A:** On standard radiograph, a soft tissue mass containing granular ossifications is seen arising from the C6 spinous process and extending proximally to C4 and distally to the T1 lamina. **B:** Computed tomography (CT) scan shows a cartilaginous growth including granules (**C**) completely ossified distally. **D, E:** The full extension of the tumoral mass is confirmed on the sagittal CT scan view. A low-grade malignant extracompartmental tumor (Enneking IB) is supposed and en bloc excision performed. **F:** Radiograph of the specimen in lateral view: the spinous processes of C5 to T1 are recognized. **G:** Radiograph of the specimen in transverse view. The spinous processes (*small arrows*) and the laminae can be recognized (*large arrow* indicates the inner surface of the lamina). The histologic diagnosis was grade 2 peripheral chondrosarcoma. Wide tumor-free margins are histologically demonstrated all around the tumor. **H:** Isola posterior stabilization and posterior bone grafting are performed.

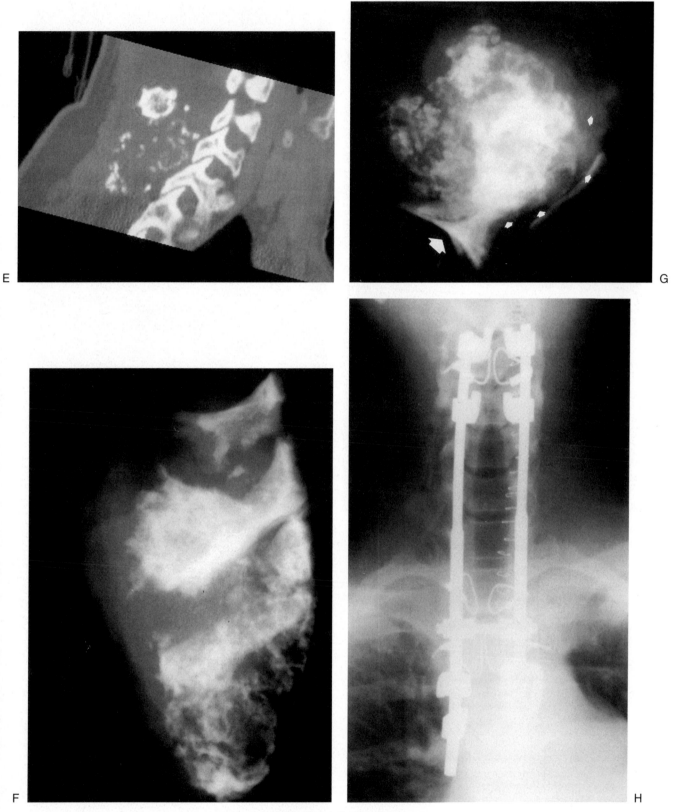

FIG. 61.2. *Continued.*

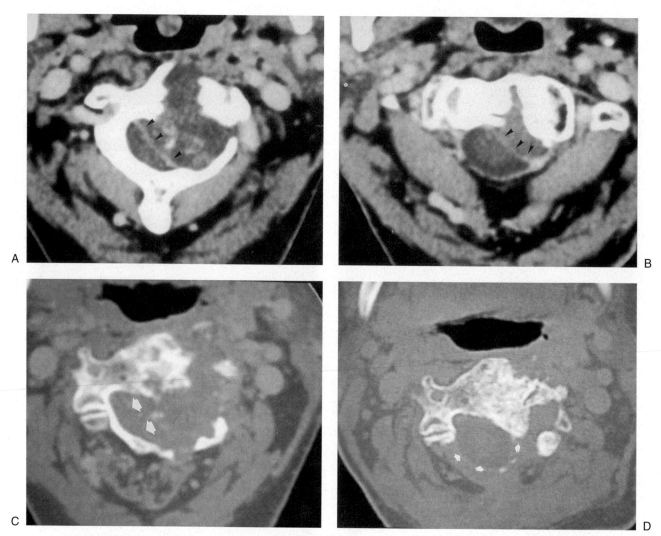

FIG. 61.3. Chordoma in a woman aged 67 years. **A:** Huge myxoid mass arising from C2 and expanding to C1–C2. **B:** Compressing the dural sac (*arrowheads*). The patient was referred to our institution with severe motor weakness in all four limbs. Computed tomography (CT) scan through the C2 vertebral body performed at admission (**C**) and at 4-year follow-up (**D**) shows the dural sac (*white arrows*) and the reconstruction of the vertebra after intralesional excision and radiation therapy. There was no sign of local disease or distant spread at 4-year follow-up. This figure was not included.

radiographs (Figs. 61.3 to 61.6). High-grade malignancy, such as an osteosarcoma, typically presents as an aggressive, osteolytic destructive process accompanied by variable amounts of ossification. Round cell tumors (i.e., Ewing sarcoma and lymphomas) present with a typical permeative pattern and an associated soft tissue mass before there is any bone destruction (Fig. 61.7). The discs are involved only rarely but sometimes are surrounded by the tumor. This factor is important in distinguishing tumors from pyogenic and tuberculous spinal infections.

Bone Scan

The technetium 99m (^{99m}Tc) scan in the workup of a malignant tumor is rarely necessary to find the lesion, which is almost always evident on standard radiographs. More frequently, the bone scan is used for detection of possible distant metastases. Only in cases of tumors like chordoma, which are difficult to see on plain radiographs because of infiltrative pattern of growth, are isotope scans helpful in guiding the use of a CT scan or MRI. Plasmacytomas are not always detectable by bone scan. Tomographic bone scan technology, however, can improve the sensitivity but not necessarily the specificity.

Computed Tomography

The CT scan is highly sensitive to early bone destruction and in some clinicians' minds remains unique for planning definitive surgical treatment. Contrast enhancement is often

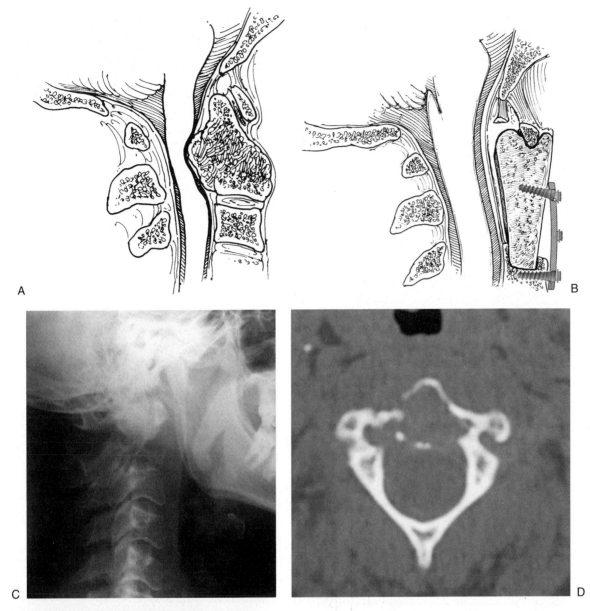

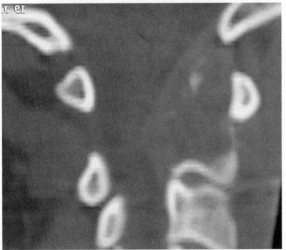

FIG. 61.4. **A:** Typical lateral view of a malignant tumor of C2 in our artist's interpretation. Huge myxoid mass arising from C2 and expanding to C1–C2. **B:** Reconstruction after C2 corpectomy by a shaped tricortical iliac autogenous graft. Posterior approach for extracapsular excision and additional stabilization and fusion are sometimes required. **C:** C2 chordoma in a man 55 years of age. Standard radiogram showing complete bone, soft tissue swelling, erosion, and instability. **D:** Computed tomography (CT) scan of the same case: the tumor eroded the anterior cortex and expanded in the anterior retropharyngeal region. **E:** The sagittal CT reconstruction shows the epidural extension of the tumor. **F:** After corpectomy, a tricortical autogenous graft is prepared with a high-speed drill. **G:** At 2-year follow-up, sagittal CT reconstruction shows the graft fusion and its relationship with the anterior C1 arch. The patient underwent adjuvant radiation therapy. **H:** At 2-year follow-up, CT scan confirms the good relationship of the graft with the anterior C1 arch. There is no sign of local disease or distant metastases.

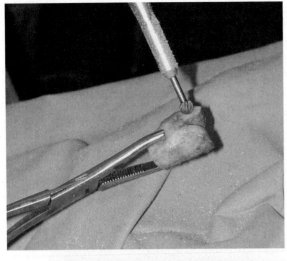

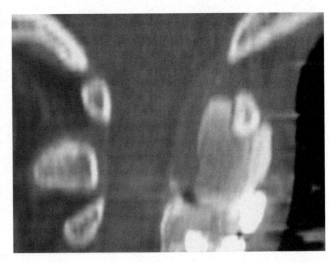

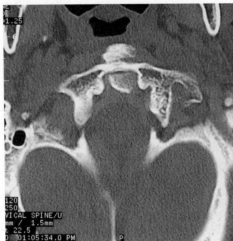

FIG. 61.4. *Continued*

requisite to the careful evaluation of tumor margins and the tumor's intrinsic vascularity.

Magnetic Resonance Imaging

The MRI has greater sensitivity than the bone scan in detecting occult lesions not visualized on standard radiographs. The advantages are particularly evident for plasmacytomas. Furthermore, it is usually well tolerated, noninvasive, and safe. Compared with normal bone marrow, most tumors demonstrate decreased signal intensity on T1-weighted images and increased signal on T2-weighted images (11). Also, MRI is extremely sensitive to alterations in the vertebral body marrow, but it lacks specificity as to the etiology of the various pathologic processes. Any disorder or therapeutic procedure resulting in loss of myeloid elements, such as radiation therapy, may demonstrate increased signal intensity in the marrow secondary to fatty replacement of hematopoietic tissue (12). Soft tissue extension of a tumor and its particular relationship with the dura are better visualized by MRI than by CT scan.

Myelography

In most countries, myelography has now been replaced by MRI to assess spinal cord or nerve root compression, but it still can be useful in concert with CT when a stainless steel device, which is known to cause metal artifacts, is present.

Angiography

Angiography allows visualization of the vascularity of the tumor and the relationships of the tumor mass with the vertebral arteries. Preoperative embolization of the tumor is helpful in reducing intraoperative bleeding when an intralesional procedure is planned, but it can be performed only rarely because of common vascularity with

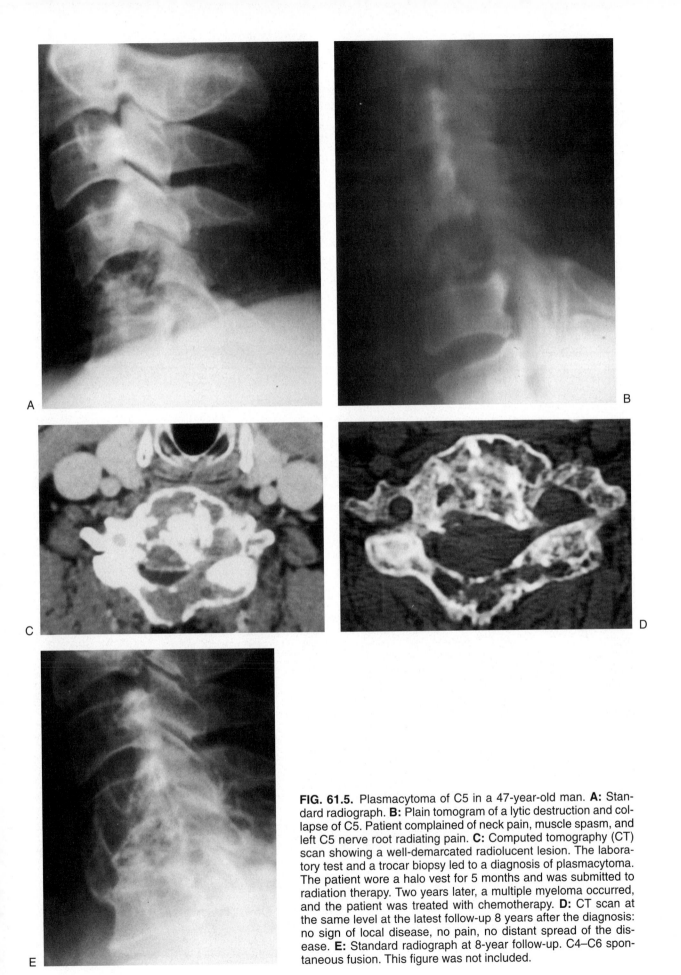

FIG. 61.5. Plasmacytoma of C5 in a 47-year-old man. **A:** Standard radiograph. **B:** Plain tomogram of a lytic destruction and collapse of C5. Patient complained of neck pain, muscle spasm, and left C5 nerve root radiating pain. **C:** Computed tomography (CT) scan showing a well-demarcated radiolucent lesion. The laboratory test and a trocar biopsy led to a diagnosis of plasmacytoma. The patient wore a halo vest for 5 months and was submitted to radiation therapy. Two years later, a multiple myeloma occurred, and the patient was treated with chemotherapy. **D:** CT scan at the same level at the latest follow-up 8 years after the diagnosis: no sign of local disease, no pain, no distant spread of the disease. **E:** Standard radiograph at 8-year follow-up. C4–C6 spontaneous fusion. This figure was not included.

847

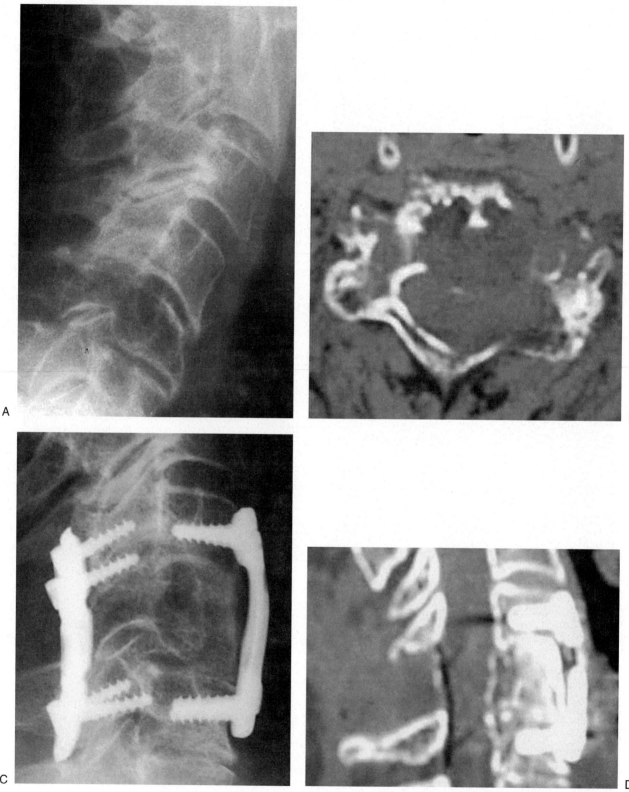

FIG. 61.6. Plasmacytoma of C5 in a 52-year-old man. **A:** Standard radiograph: it is possible to detect the disappearance of the posterior wall of the C5 body. **B:** Computed tomography (CT) scan showing a radiolucent lesion occupying almost the whole vertebra (sectors 4 to 12, layers A to F), severely compromising the stability. The laboratory test and a trocar biopsy led to a diagnosis of plasmacytoma. The patient required urgent surgery. Complete intralesional excision was planned, requiring double approach, followed by chemotherapy. **C:** Standard radiograph at 2-year follow-up. Graft incorporation and C4 to C6 fusion. Restoration of lordosis. **D:** CT scan at 2-year follow-up. Full recovery, no sign of local disease, no pain, no distant spread of the disease.

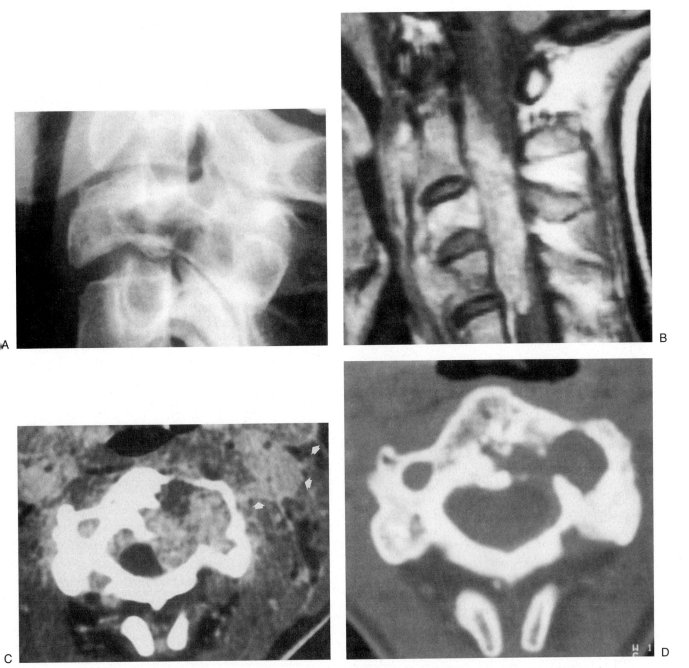

FIG. 61.7. Ewing sarcoma in an 18-year-old woman. **A:** Standard radiogram: reduction of the height of C3 vertebral body; lytic permeative aspect, well appreciated on T2-weighted magnetic resonance imaging section. **B:** A hyperlucent tumoral tissue invading the canal. **C:** Computed tomography (CT) scan shows the tumoral mass arising from the C3 vertebral body and expanding both in the canal and in the prevertebral soft tissues (*arrows*). Open biopsy allowed a diagnosis of Ewing sarcoma. The patient underwent radiation therapy and polychemotherapy. **D:** CT scan at latest follow-up (58 months after treatment): no sign of local disease. The patient has been continuously disease free with no pain and no distant spread of the disease.

the cervical cord and should be performed only in experienced institutions.

Biopsy Techniques

Histologic confirmation of the diagnosis is mandatory to distinguish between primary and secondary malignan-cies and to differentiate malignancies that require varied treatments (e.g., chordoma versus plasmacytoma). Trocar-needle biopsy under CT scan control (Fig. 61.8) is theoreti-cally a good way to achieve a diagnosis and usually does not require general anesthesia. Often, CT scanning helps in reaching even the smallest of lesions. Correct use of this technique (13) minimizes tumor contamination. The trocar-

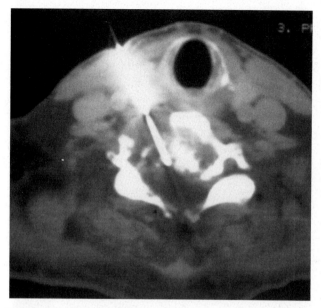

FIG. 61.8. Trocar biopsy under computed tomography scan control of a C4 chordoma.

needle should be introduced at a point within the incision line, and the direction should pass through a muscle to resect the complete scar and needle track together with the tumor; pressure should be applied to reduce bleeding as the trocar is removed. In the cervical spine, this procedure is technically demanding and frequently not well tolerated by the patient. Knowing that these malignant primary tumors of the cervical spine are often extracompartmental at the time of discovery, it is generally not feasible to perform an en bloc resection. However, perioperative frozen sections should be examined before submitting the patient to an intralesional excision. The extent of surgical extirpation, together with the necessity of adjuvant therapies, is decided by this important information obtained for histologic diagnosis. In rare cases of resectable tumors (small and often posteriorly located), particular attention should be given to the imaging studies. In fact, the peculiar pattern of chondrosarcoma or chordoma must make the surgeon vigilant. In these cases, the risk for contamination by the myxoid tissue is extremely high and at times justifies performing primary en bloc resection without histologic confirmation (Fig. 61.2).

STAGING

Oncologic Staging

Oncologic and surgical staging is of the utmost importance to provide appropriate treatment. The oncologic staging (14) is based on the histology and the local aggressiveness of the tumor and defines its biologic behavior. The WBB surgical staging system (15–17) describes the extension of the tumor and provides a tool for planning surgery, exchanging information, and evaluating the relationship between treatment and outcome. The Enneking staging system (6) divides benign tumors into three stages and localized primary malignant tumors into four stages. This system is based on clinical features, radiographic patterns, CT scan, MRI data, and histologic findings. It was formerly described for long bone tumors (6) and later applied to spinal tumors (1,4,9,15,17–25). With regard to malignant tumors, histologically low-grade malignant tumors are included in stage I, subdivided into IA (the tumor remains inside the vertebra) and IB (the tumor invades perivertebral compartments). No capsule is found, but a thick pseudocapsule of reactive tissue is permeated by small microscopic islands of tumor. High-grade malignancies are defined as IIA and IIB. The neoplastic growth is so rapid that the host has no time to form a continuous reactive tissue layer. These rapidly growing tumors are known to seed locally with satellite lesions or to have skip metastases at a distance from the main tumor mass. These malignancies are usually seen on plain radiographs as radiolucent and destructive and may be associated with a pathologic fracture. The CT scan and MRI define the transverse and longitudinal extent of tumor and may confirm the absence of a reactive tissue layer.

Surgical Planning

The experience collected with primary tumors of the limbs shows that performing the surgical procedure according to well-established oncologic criteria (6,13) leads to significant control of local recurrences. Unfortunately, en bloc excisions are seldom feasible in the cervical spine; in most cases, only intralesional excision is possible (22,26). This situation obviously worsens prognosis and requires the use of local adjuvants or polychemotherapy (27).

A new system of surgical staging is now under clinical trial to correlate the extension of the spine tumor, surgical procedure, and outcome. This system (WBB) was proposed by Weinstein (16) and subsequently modified (15, 17) to identify each lesion in a consistent manner. On the transverse plane, the vertebra is divided into 12 radiating zones (numbered 1 to 12 in a clockwise order) and into five layers (A to E from the perivertebral to intradural involvement, F indicating the involvement of the foramen transversarium). This system is based on the need (anatomically based) to approach the cervical spine considering the cord as an unresectable structure, the vertebral arteries as a special additional layer, whose invasion must be separately considered in the surgical planning. The validity of this attitude is confirmed by Lassale (28), presenting the surgical approaches in the spine with a similar sectorialization. In our opinion, this system allows a rational approach to surgical planning, provided that all efforts are made to perform surgery along the required margins. Appropriate attention to such detail can affect not only the margins of excision but also local recurrences and distal spread, which in these malignant tumors obviously can affect survival.

TREATMENT

Surgery

Surgical Approaches

The surgical approach is often limited by the many vascular and neural structures (common carotid artery and its terminal branches, the deep jugular veins, and vertebral arteries; and the vagus, hypoglossal, facial, lingual, laryngeal, and recurrent nerves) (29–33) as well as the trachea and esophagus. With this in mind, the classic surgical routes may provide the only alternative for intralesional surgery. In some cases, combined anterior and posterior approaches are warranted. Two surgical approaches are generally acceptable for the lower cervical spine (28,32): the posterior midline and the anterolateral prevascular. This approach can be expanded inferiorly by a sternotomy (34) or third-rib thoracotomy (35). The posterior approach can be performed with minimal bleeding with the patient in sitting position (6,8). The upper cervical spine can be reached by extrapharyngeal approaches (32,36,37) or by transoral approach (38). The retropharyngeal approach (39) requires a careful dissection of the spinal accessory nerve and detachment of the sternocleidomastoid muscle. The submandibular approach (37) requires resection of the submaxillary gland, extensive dissection of the regional structures, and risk for glossopharyngeal nerve palsy. Alternatively, the transoral approach can be used and can be enlarged by the extensile transmandibular approach (26,40). A circumferential approach for vertebrectomy is also limited by the brachial plexus. Sacrifice of cervical nerve roots is more difficult to accept than in other regions of the spine; the vertebral arteries (26,31,41,42) lying within the bone structure compel the surgeon to perform difficult dissections that sometimes necessitate ligature or bypass of one vertebral artery.

Surgical Procedures

Surgery in the cervical spine is associated with high rate of complications (43–46). The aforementioned anatomic constraints make it difficult to perform complete excision of tumor, even intralesional. The oncologically appropriate surgical technique for malignant tumors is en bloc excision, but the classic techniques of en bloc excision of the vertebral body described for the thoracic and lumbar spine (25, 47–49) cannot be performed in the cervical spine. Only with some smaller lesions of the body is en bloc excision a viable option (50). Appropriate evaluation and discussion of the risk-to-benefit ratio should take place before the operation. En bloc removal of tumors located in sectors 5 to 7 (C3 to C7) can be performed by a triple approach: first posterior to remove sectors 2 to 4, then anterior presternocleidomastoid to perform discectomies and to remove sectors 7 or 8 to visualize the dura, isolating and saving the vertebral artery. Finally, an anterior contralateral approach is performed to ligate the vertebral artery if enclosed in the tumor (it has been recently pointed out that unilateral verte-

bral artery ligation is safe) (51), to complete the discectomies and finally to remove tumor sectors 4 to 7 en bloc. Fujita and associates (50) recently described the en bloc excision of a chordoma located in sectors 6 to 8 according to the Tomita technique (25). These authors report intralesional margin in layer D (epidural), making doubtful the risk-to-benefit ratio of such a difficult and risky technique versus complete extracapsular intralesional excision. Conversely, en bloc resection of the posterior arch (sectors 10 to 3) (Fig. 61.9) does not present specific difficulties (47) but requires careful fixation of the head to modify the patient's position during resection and reconstruction. A long posterior midline approach with lateral dissection on the articular masses must be followed by long arthrodesis in a physiologic position (Fig. 61.2).

In most cases, primary malignant tumor excision requires 360-degree surgery to perform a complete excision, even intralesionally, because this procedure must remove also the pseudocapsule of the tumor ("extracapsular" excision)

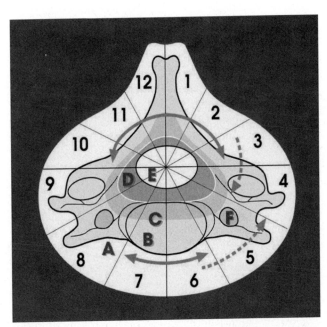

FIG. 61.9. The WBB system (14,87,88) applied to the cervical spine. On the transverse plane, the vertebra is divided into 12 radiating zones (numbered 1 to 12 in a clockwise order) and into five layers. When the tumor erodes the peripheral cortex and expands into the soft tissues, it occupies layer A. Layer B defines a tumor expanding within the bone without eroding the cortex. When the tumor involves the posterior wall of the body, it occupies layer C, and if it expands into the canal, it occupies layer D. Layer E denotes intradural involvement, and layer F indicates involvement of the foramen transversarium. The *arrows* indicate the possibility of performing en bloc resection. En bloc resection of the posterior arch (sectors 10 to 3) does not present specific difficulties, whereas the anterior resection is very technically demanding (30). *Dotted arrows* indicate a theoretical extension of the excision. The staging system can also be useful to plan intralesional surgery and to exchange information among institutions.

to reduce the risk for recurrence. In the lower cervical spine (Fig. 61.6), this procedure is technically demanding only with respect to the vertebral artery and with reference to the biomechanical requirement of the reconstruction. Angiographic study is needed to confirm that the other vertebral artery is large enough and that simultaneous occlusion testing of the involved vertebral artery is uneventful (51).

When the tumor occurs from C1 and C2, circumferential excision is much more technically demanding (26), and reconstruction requires special combinations of plate and shaped graft (Fig. 61.4).

Reconstruction

Anterior (52–54) and posterior devices for stabilization are commonly used in most countries. Most of the recent papers refer to fixation in the higher levels (29,55–57); to the use of navigation, especially in the higher levels (58–61); and to the proposal of implanting the screw in the small cervical pedicle (55,62,63) instead of the most popular technique of fixation in the articular masses (64,65).

Fibular vascularized graft has been shown to have increased compressive strength compared with rib or iliac crest grafting and is particularly indicated when immediate radiation therapy must be delivered (66). Conversely, owing to the common fear of interfering with leg functioning (67,68) and to the demanding microsurgical technique, tricortical graft is more popular, even if associated with high rate of patient discomfort because of persistent pain (69,70). Titanium, ceramic, and carbon fiber spacers are frequently used to replace vertebral bodies. Contemporary anterior and posterior plating minimizes fusion extension and enhances immediate stability (53,71) (Figs. 61.4 and 61.6).

Adjunctive Techniques

Radiation: Indications and Timing

Advances in anesthesiologic and surgical techniques have reduced the indications for radiation therapy. The risk for radiation-induced sarcomas and radiation-related myelopathy must be considered when thinking about radiation therapy as an isolated treatment for a primary spine tumor. Well-collimated megavoltage radiation or proton-beam therapy can provide an effective and safe adjuvant to surgery or can be used as an independent but acceptable palliation treatment. Ewing sarcoma and plasmacytomas are the most radiation-sensitive conditions, but timing of treatment is quite different. Ewing sarcoma (Fig. 61.5) is often submitted to radiation therapy (40 to 44 Gy) after short courses of chemotherapy and as an alternative to surgery when the tumor in question does not allow for an appropriate surgical margin resection (as a result of extension of the tumor mass). In cases of Ewing sarcoma responsive to chemotherapy, surgical extirpation following chemotherapy of the extensively necrotic tumor can be

considered. Conversely, radiation therapy is the treatment of choice for plasmacytoma (Fig. 61.5) and is combined with chemotherapy in multiple myeloma. Only in cases of severe tumor destruction with vertebral collapse or neurologic compromise is surgery (corpectomy) suggested, followed by adjuvant radiation therapy.

In the extremities, surgical resection must be performed with the aim of achieving a wide margin. It is still debatable whether in the cervical spine, when wide resection is not feasible or requires a significant functional sacrifice, it is better to perform an intralesional procedure or to reject surgery in favor of radiation and chemotherapy. The latter may be best in cases of plasmacytoma (Fig. 61.5), Ewing sarcoma (Fig. 61.7), and lymphomas. A correctly planned extracapsular excision combined with careful radiation probably results in better function with the least risk for local recurrence. Unresectable chondrosarcomas and chordomas of the occipitocervical junction have been treated successfully by high-energy radiotherapy and 160-MV proton-beam radiation therapy (72).

Chemotherapy: Indications and Timing

Ewing sarcoma and osteosarcoma require a combination of therapies in which chemotherapy is the cornerstone. The actual protocols of chemotherapy for both conditions require preoperative intravenous or intraarterial administration of combinations of drugs like adriamycin, methotrexate, cisplatin, and hypophamine. Two difficulties are often encountered in cervical spine Ewing sarcomas and osteosarcomas. First, it is impossible to perform intraarterial administration; second, there is the risk of the tumor growing during the courses of therapy, thus preventing appropriate surgery or provoking unacceptable neurologic damages. Furthermore, it is often risky or even impossible to perform such major surgery on a patient who has only recently been subjected to polychemotherapy. On the other hand, if the tumor is sensitive, chemotherapy helps to shrink the tumor, makes surgery somewhat easier, reduces the volume of the tumor mass, and makes it easier to dissect the tumor from neighboring structures. Decisions regarding the timing of intravenous chemotherapy must be made by the team on a case-by-case basis.

Embolization: Indications, Timing, Results

Embolization has therapeutic importance in the treatment of aneurysmal bone cyst, especially in surgically inaccessible sites, like the pelvis. Its role in treatment as an adjuvant for malignant tumors of the cervical spine is well known. Reducing the amount of bleeding in and of itself is a good indication, but a selective angiogram is necessary to exclude common branches with the cord vascularity.

SPECIFIC TUMORS

Chondrosarcoma

Chondrosarcoma is a malignant bone tumor whose cells tend to differentiate into cartilage. The reported prevalence of chondrosarcoma in the spine is more than 6% (19,24) without significant prevalence among the spinal regions. It is frequently evident even on plain radiographs. A peripheral chondrosarcoma is in some cases thought to originate from a preexisting exostosis. On the other hand, it is almost impossible to state the same for central chondrosarcomas arising from enchondroma. A slowly growing mass is the only presenting symptom, possibly combined with the symptoms associated with adjacent compressed neural or vascular structures. On plain radiographs, an extraosseous mass is found arising from the posterior elements of the involved vertebra, irregularly ossified, lobulated, bumpy like a cauliflower, with fuzzy limits extending out toward the soft tissues. On CT scan, the cartilaginous cap can be carefully examined (Fig. 61.2).

The most appropriate treatment is en bloc excision with wide margins (6,13,19,24,73). The feasibility criteria for such resections were previously described for the lower cervical spine: small lesions located in the anterior part of the cervical spine (sectors 4 to 8 or 5 to 9) and even huge posterior lesions (Fig. 61.2), if confined to sectors 11 to 2 (no pedicle involvement), are amenable to en bloc resections. When chondrosarcoma occurs at C1 or C2, piecemeal excision is the only possible surgical procedure (26,74).

Conventional radiation therapy and chemotherapy are not effective. Some relatively good results have been reported from high-energy x-rays and 160-MV proton-beam radiation therapy (72) for chondrosarcoma of the clivus.

Histologic grading is of utmost prognostic importance. Recurrences after intralesional surgery for histologic grade 1 chondrosarcoma are not as frequent, occur late, and can be reexcised because they rarely metastasize. Local recurrences and metastases are more frequent in histologic grade 2 and 3 lesions but generally occur late. In these tumors, when resection is not feasible, prognosis is not good: most patients die after many surgeries and multiple recurrences (19,24) (mean survival of 20% at 5 years). Because of the late occurrence of metastases, a 5-year minimum follow-up is required for treatment evaluation of chondrosarcomas.

In the series from the C. A. Pizzardi and Rizzoli Institutes, cervical chondrosarcoma is quite rare (3 cases of 29 spinal chondrosarcomas). One was a grade 1 peripheral chondrosarcoma arising from the lateral mass of C6 and developing posteriorly submitted to en bloc resection on the basis of the preexisting exostosis. The patient was disease free 14 years later. The second case was a histologic grade 2 peripheral chondrosarcoma arising from the posterior arch of C6 and C7 that was submitted to intralesional excision and recurred 8 years later with a huge mass expanding to the posterior arches of T1 to T3. The neoplastic mass extended into the pleural cavity. Using a double approach, a marginal en bloc resection was performed. No recurrence

was found at 8-year follow-up. The patient complained of the residual cervicothoracic kyphoscoliosis because no stabilization was performed.

The third case was a huge grade 2 peripheral chondrosarcoma arising from the C6 spinous process. It spanned four vertebral segments (C4 to T1). An en bloc excision was performed, achieving a wide margin (Fig. 61.2). Posterior C2 to T4 stabilization and grafting were performed. There has been no recurrence at 6 years follow-up.

Chordoma

Chordoma has an estimated incidence of 0.5% per million population; fewer than 15% of chordomas arise in the spine above the sacrum, and fewer than 5% occur before patients are 20 years old (75). This malignant tumor is a neoplastic transformation of ectopic notochordal remnants and typically is seen in the sphenooccipital region (including the first cervical vertebra) and sacrum. It represents 1% to 4% of all primary malignant bone tumors (13,73). Chordomas grow slowly (76), manifesting clinically after the fifth decade in most cases. Chordomas of the cervical spine occur almost exclusively from the vertebral body. A long history of mild neck pain is the common complaint, together with symptoms related to an anterior slow-growing mass (76–78): dysphagia, upper respiratory obstruction, Claude-Bernard-Horner syndrome, or slow cord and nerve root compression (2,18,79) in expansile chordomas within the spinal canal. A palpable mass in rare cases may be appreciated; cranial nerve compression can be provoked by craniocervical chordomas (22). Radiographically, this tumor often appears totally radiolucent. In some instances, calcifications are found within the tumor mass (78) and are difficult to appreciate at early stages by plain radiographs (80). CT scans offer better detail of semifluid-like masses (Figs. 61.1 and 61.3), sometimes to be differentiated from a tuberculous abscess. Invasion of the layers A and D is commonly found at the clinical onset of the disease (80). A variable amount of gelatinous substance is contained within these lobular structures of chordomas, divided by fibrous septa (81). On MRI, chordomas appear isointense or, less frequently, hypointense on T1-weighted images. On T2-weighted images, increased signal intensity is appreciated with low signal septa. The relationship of this tumor with adjacent neurovascular structures is detailed well by MRI (78,82).

Histologically, these tumors are arranged in lobules containing vacuolated cells (*physaliferous cells*), sometimes assuming a signet-ring appearance and surrounded by mucin. Some chordomas contain cartilage and therefore must be distinguished from chondrosarcomas (75,79,83).

The treatment of choice of chordoma is wide en bloc excision; however, this margin is frequently impossible to achieve in cervical chordomas (Figs. 61.1, 61.3, 61.4, and 61.6) because en bloc resection is rarely feasible owing to the tumoral expansion through unresectable anatomic structures. Radiation therapy of chordomas has long been a matter of discussion (72,84–86), most of which concludes by stressing the importance of CT-guided therapy plans, hyperfractionation, and particle-beam therapy. These refinements in treatment techniques allow radiation to be effective in achieving prolonged remission of the disease, especially when piecemeal surgical excision of the tumoral mass (Figs. 61.3, 61.4, and 61.6) can be performed (18, 83), including the pseudocapsule of the tumor (double approach mostly required). Metastases are rare and late (18, 85); local progression of the disease is the most frequent cause of death.

Twelve cases were observed and treated at C. A. Pizzardi and Rizzoli Institutes, located mainly at C2 (6 cases), from a total of 42 chordomas of the mobile spine. Two cases expanded to the adjacent vertebra. Average patient age was 52 years; two patients were older than 70 years. Two patients were submitted to radiation therapy only, and they died after 1 and 11 months from the treatment. Three patients died at average 56 months after palliative surgery combined with adjuvant therapy. In two cases, an intralesional excision only was performed, but both patients died in the postoperative period from interstitial pneumonia. Five cases were submitted to an intralesional excision combined with adjuvant therapy. At the final follow-up, 3 patients are continuously disease free (9 to 55 months; average, 28 months). One is alive with disease at 112 months after the treatment; this patient was submitted to a second intralesional excision plus radiation therapy for a local recurrence observed after 89 months. One patient died after 12 months from tumor progression.

Malignant Fibrous Histiocytoma

Malignant fibrous histiocytoma is a sarcoma of histiocytic origin that consists generally of histiocytes and fibroblasts and is quite rare in the cervical spine (13,73). It appears as a pure osteolytic lesion with fuzzy borders. In the cervical spine, pathologic fracture (and associated neurologic symptoms) may occur at onset as a result of the rapid collapse of the bone. These cases can be confused in the second and third decades of life with eosinophilic granuloma, but the rapid evolution and the associated large soft tissue mass in a short period suggest malignancy. The appropriate treatment is en bloc excision (wide margin) and chemotherapy (6). In the cervical spine, because of tumor mass extension among unresectable anatomic structures at diagnosis, a palliative curettage, macroscopically complete, is the only realistic surgical treatment and generally should be combined with radiation and chemotherapy.

Only one case of malignant fibrous histiocytoma of the cervical spine has been observed at the Rizzoli Institute, in 1970. Surgery was considered impractical, and no chemotherapy was available at that time. Radiation therapy was not effective, and the patient died 5 months later with local progression and pulmonary metastases.

Osteosarcoma

The most frequent malignant bone tumor (characterized by cells that tend to differentiate into osteoblasts and to produce neoplastic bone) is extremely rare in the spine. In their review of 1,122 cases of osteosarcoma, Shives and colleagues (23) found 30 cases in the spine, 4 of which were cervical. In a review of 1,000 osteosarcomas, 10 occurred in the spine above the sacrum and none in the cervical spine (87).

Spinal osteosarcoma arises from the vertebral body (69,88,89) or from the posterior elements, but frequently it involves the whole vertebra at the time of diagnosis (90,91). The radiographic picture may present different patterns: from a totally radiolucent vertebra with collapse and kyphosis to so-called ivory vertebra with variable amounts of neoplastic tissue around.

Some reported cases of osteosarcoma of the spine are secondary, arising from Paget disease (87) or after radiation therapy (87–89); therefore, compared with the population of osteosarcoma in the limbs, older persons are affected more often.

The course of the disease is rapid, with early lung metastases. The prognosis of osteosarcoma of the limb is improved (60% to 70% without evidence of disease after 5 years) thanks to protocols of neoadjuvant chemotherapy and to surgical criteria that cannot be applied to the cervical spine (27). At best, an intralesional extracapsular excision of the whole mass can be performed (6), sometimes requiring a procedure that is very technically demanding and complex (38), but a poor prognosis must be expected (23,87). Bielack ad co-workers (27) reported 5.7% local control in osteosarcoma of the trunk versus 60% in the limbs. Chemotherapy is mandatory before or after surgery, and radiotherapy can be used as an adjuvant even in the face of finding no evidence of radiosensitivity of these tumors.

Four cervical cases were observed at C. A. Pizzardi and Rizzoli Institutes from a series of 18 osteosarcomas of the spine. These cases were located at C6 and at C7 in three young adults (aged 17 to 24 years) and in a 56-year-old man. In all cases, an intralesional excision was performed combined with chemotherapy and radiation therapy. One patient died after 24 months. Three patients were alive without evidence of the disease after an average of 58 months (13 to 146 months).

Ewing Sarcoma

Ewing sarcoma, a high-grade sarcoma uniformly formed by small round cells, is rarely observed in the spine and is exceptionally rare in the cervical spine. Grubb and colleagues (92) reported no cases in the cervical spine in 19 cases observed in the mobile spine. Differential diagnosis can be difficult (not only on imaging, but also on the histologic picture) with metastases from neuroblastoma or lymphoma. The course of symptoms in the cervical sites is very rapid, and cord compression may be the only associated symptom. The plain radiograph shows a totally lytic process collapsing the vertebra and expanding into the neighboring soft tissues. Differential diagnosis should include eosinophilic granuloma, which usually does not produce the wide shadow of the extraosseous mass; the fast-growing Ewing sarcoma can inundate the disc and therefore can be confused with tuberculous spondylitis. Both CT scan and MRI detail the neoplastic mass and its expansion toward the vital structures. Treatment must be based on combined radiation and chemotherapy protocols. Surgery should be regarded as palliative because it is impossible to resect Ewing sarcoma in the cervical spine with adequate margin because of the early extracompartmental extension of the tumor mass, typically semifluid and infiltrating. The goals should be to remove or prevent any cord compression and to stabilize the spine.

Four cervical cases were observed at the Rizzoli Institute of a series of 28 primary Ewing sarcomas of the spine. Two cases were multisegmental at diagnosis. One patient was submitted only to partial surgical excision (in the 1970s) and died 10 months later. Another was submitted to megavoltage radiation and chemotherapy (in the 1980s) and died 1 year after diagnosis. Two more recent cases were submitted to palliative surgery (decompressive laminectomy) in one case and to external immobilization (halo cast) in the other, both combined with polychemotherapy and megavoltage radiotherapy (up to 51 Gy). These patients are alive without signs of disease at 24 and 130 months (Fig. 61.5), respectively, after diagnosis. A postlaminectomy kyphosis developed in the 9-year-old child submitted to posterior decompression.

Solitary Plasmacytoma

Plasmacytoma is a primary systemic malignant neoplasm of the bone marrow originating from B-lymphoid cells in plasmacellular differentiation. Existence of a true solitary plasmacytoma of the bone is therefore doubtful (93). Slow-growing lesions associated with neck pain and muscle spasm were the common complaint in all cases; one case had associated bilateral root compression. A radiolucent area, central in the vertebral body with early collapse, without ossifications, and with fuzzy limits is the typical radiographic pattern, mostly evolving toward a complete disappearing of the vertebral outline. This picture in an individual older than 60 years suggests the diagnosis of plasmacytoma and the need to perform appropriate laboratory tests: serum proteins electrophoresis, urinary Bence Jones protein, complete blood count (anemia), and bone marrow smear, to rule out multiple myeloma. Bone scan is not consistently sensitive, but MRI is able to show radiographically undetected foci of the disease (94) and to determine the relationship of the tumor mass to the spinal cord, nerve roots, and other vital structures.

If biochemical tests are positive, indicating the existence of gammopathy (i.e., myeloma), and no neurologic injury or instability is present, the treatment of choice is radiotherapy (Fig. 61.5) combined with chemotherapy.

A CT-guided trocar-needle biopsy is indicated to achieve a definitive histologic diagnosis, unless the diagnosis of multiple myeloma has been established.

Surgery may be indicated in cases of neurologic compromise or when stabilization of the spine is thought to be necessary. The role of surgery for "solitary plasmacytoma" without neurologic compromise or instability is at best controversial. We favor intralesional excision, stabilization, and adjuvant treatment to improve the long-term outcome. En bloc spondylectomy is considered overaggressive treatment because plasmacytomas are believed to be systemic lesions and generally are responsive to radiation, even if the initial laboratory studies are negative.

When indicated (rarely), surgery should be planned in advance of radiotherapy, avoiding associated complications of infection and serious wound problems. An anterior presternocleidomastoid approach for corpectomy and prosthetic replacement (or autogenous graft and adjuvant fixation) is the procedure suggested for C3 to C7 plasmacytomas, and lateral retrovascular for C1 to C2 plasmacytomas. If a direct approach to this region is necessary, it can be associated with significant morbidity. In such cases, a posterior occipitocervical fusion might be appropriate to consider when secondary radiation therapy is to follow and stability may be at issue.

Sixteen cervical tumors of 98 spinal plasmacytomas fulfilling the inclusive criteria of Bacci and associates (95) were included in the series from C. A. Pizzardi and Rizzoli Institutes. Most patients were male (81 cases), and the youngest patient was 38 years of age. All the cervical vertebrae except C1 were involved. A complete intralesional surgical excision (corpectomy), combined with radiation therapy, was performed in 10 cases. A combination of chemotherapy and radiation was given in the other 6 cases. Eight of the 16 patients developed systemic disease within 2 years, 5 of whom died 11 to 89 months after diagnosis. The 11 survivors have had follow-up of 2 to 12 years (average, 43 months). Of the 10 patients who underwent corpectomy, 2 died 65 and 89 months after treatment, 6 are continuously disease free 2 years after treatment, and 2 are alive after sequential treatment of myeloma. Of the 6 patients treated by chemotherapy and radiation only, 3 died 1, 2, and 5 years after treatment, 2 are alive after sequential treatment of myeloma 8 and 12 years after treatment, and 1 one is alive with disease after 32 months.

CONCLUSION

Primary bone tumors are quite rare in the cervical spine. They affect mainly children or young adults with a 3.2:1 ratio of male prevalence. Malignant tumors seem to arise in the older patients, more frequently from the vertebral body, and frequently are associated with major neurologic problems at the onset (14 of 46 cases in our series). The more frequently affected vertebrae are C2 and C5.

Surgical treatment of primary bone tumors of the cervical spine requires a comprehensive knowledge of the biologic behavior of these lesions and of the surgical anatomy of the region. Oncologic and surgical staging are mandatory to decide on treatment. Adjuvant therapies like radiation, embolization, and chemotherapy all must be considered by the oncologic team. Adequate treatment for a particular lesion is mandatory the first time. Incomplete or unnecessary treatments that expose the patient to unnecessary risk for recurrence or, even worse, an adverse survival outcome, must be avoided. On the other hand, overaggressive treatments may put a patient at unnecessary risk without an appropriate oncologic indication. Primary malignant tumors of the spine are uncommon and those of the cervical spine even more uncommon; diagnosis, staging, and treatment should be centralized in a referral center where all necessary information should be obtained before any invasive intervention is performed, including biopsy.

ACKNOWLEDGMENTS

This work is dedicated to the memories of Mario Campanacci and Bertil Stener.

We extend special thanks to Carlo Piovani for his invaluable help preparing the drawings and images used in this chapter.

REFERENCES

1. Abdu WA, Provencher M. Primary bone and metastatic tumors of the cervical spine. *Spine* 1998;23:2767–2776.
2. Bohlman HH, Sachs BL, Carter JR, et al. Primary neoplasms of the cervical spine. *J Bone Joint Surg Am* 1986;68:483–494.
3. Boriani S, Capanna R, Donati D, et al. Osteoblastoma of the spine. *Clin Orthop* 1992;278:37–45.
4. Levine AM, Boriani S, Donati D, et al. Benign tumors of the cervical spine. *Spine* 1992;17:S399–406.
5. Touboul E, Khelif A, Guerin RA. Les tumeurs primitives du rachis. *Neurochirurgie* 1989;35:312–316.
6. Enneking WF. *Musculoskeletal tumor surgery.* New York: Churchill Livingstone, 1983:69–122.
7. De Iure F, Boriani S, Biagini R, et al. Tecnica chirurgica. La posizione seduta nell'accesso posteriore al rachide cervicale per neoplasia ossea. *Chir Organi Mov* 1995;80:77–84.
8. Matjasko J, Petrozza P, Cohen M, et al. Anesthesia and surgery in the seated position: analysis of 554 cases. *Neurosurgery* 1985;17:695–699.
9. Boriani S, Weinstein JN. Differential diagnosis and surgical treatment of primary benign and malignant neoplasms. In: Frymoyer JW, ed. *The adult spine: principles and practice,* 2nd ed. Philadelphia: Lippincott-Raven, 1997:951–987.
10. Wilner D. *Radiology of bone tumors and allied disorders.* Philadelphia: WB Saunders, 1990.
11. Masaryk TJ. Spine tumors. In: Modid MT, Masaryk TJ, Ross JS, eds. *Magnetic resonance imaging of the spine.* Chicago: Year Book Medical Publishers, 1989:183–213.
12. Boden SD, Lee RR, Herzog RJ. Magnetic resonance imaging of the spine. In: Frymoyer JW, ed. *The adult spine: principles and practice,* 2nd ed. Philadelphia: Lippincott-Raven, 1997:563–630.
13. Campanacci M. *Tumors of bone and soft tissues.* Bologna: Aulo Gaggi; Berlin: Springer Verlag, 1990.
14. Ebraheim NA, Lu J, Yang H, et al. Vulnerability of the sympathetic trunk during the anterior approach to the lower cervical spine. *Spine* 2000;25:1603–1606.
15. Boriani S, Weinstein JN, Biagini R. Spine update: a surgical staging system for therapeutic planning of primary bone tumors of the spine. A contribution to a common terminology. *Spine* 1997;22:1036–1044.
16. Weinstein JN. Spine neoplasms. In: Weinstein S, ed. *The pediatric spine.* New York: Raven Press, 1994:887–916.
17. Weinstein J, Hart R, Boriani S, et al. Spine tumors: surgical staging and clinical outcome. Application to giant cell tumors of the spine. 21st Meeting of the ISSLS Proceedings, Seattle, Washington, June 21–25, 1994.
18. Boriani S, Chevalley E, Weinstein JN, et al. Chordoma of the spine above sacrum—treatment and outcome in 21 cases. *Spine* 1996;21:1569–1571.
19. Camins MB, Duncan AW, Smith J, et al. Chondrosarcoma of the spine. *Spine* 1978;3:202–209.
20. Campanacci M, Boriani S, Savini R. Staging, biopsy, surgical planning of primary spine tumors. *Chir Organi Mov* 1983;75:95–103.
21. Campanacci M, Boriani S, Giunti A. Giant cell tumors of the spine. In: Sundaresan SN, Schmidek HH, Schiller AL, et al., eds. *Tumors of the spine: diagnosis and clinical management.* Philadelphia: WB Saunders, 1990:163–172.
22. Giunti A, Laus M. *Radicolopatie spinali.* Bologna: A. Gaggi Ed., 1992:216–220.
23. Shives TC, Dahlin DC, Sim FH, et al. Osteosarcoma of the spine. *J Bone Joint Surg Am* 1986;68:660–668.
24. Shives TC, McLeod RA, Unni KK, et al. Chondrosarcoma of the spine. *J Bone Joint Surg Am* 1989;71:1159–1165.
25. Tomita K, Kawahara N, Baba H, et al. Total en bloc spondylectomy for solitary spinal metastases. *Int Orthop* 1994;18:291–298.
26. Harms J. 360 Degree surgery for high cervical vertebral tumours. Proceedings of 18th Annual Meeting of CSRS, Paris 2002:114.
27. Bielack SS, Wulff B, Delling G, et al. Osteosarcoma of the trunk treated by multimodal therapy: experience of the Cooperative Osteosarcoma Study Group (COSS). *Med Pediatr Oncol* 1995;24:6–12.
28. Lassale B, Guigui P, Delecourt C. Voies d'abord du rachis. *Encycl Méd Chir Techniques Chir Orth Traum* 1995;8:44–150.
29. Ebraheim NA, Rollins JR Jr, Xu R, et al. Anatomic consideration of C2 pedicle screw placement. *Spine* 1996;21:691–694.
30. Ebraheim NA, Xu R, Yeasting RA. The location of the vertebral artery foramen and its relation to posterior lateral mass screw fixation. *Spine* 1996;21(11):1291.
31. Heary RF, Albert TJ, Ludwig SC, et al. Surgical anatomy of the vertebral arteries. *Spine* 1996;21:2074–2080.
32. Lu J, Ebraheim NA, Nadim Y, et al. Anterior approach to the cervical spine: surgical anatomy. *Orthopedics* 2000;23:841–845.
33. Sengupta DK, Grevitt MP, Mehdian SM. Hypoglossal nerve injury as a complication of anterior surgery to the upper cervical spine. *Eur Spine J* 1999;8:78–80.
34. Sundaresan N, DiGiacinto GV. Surgical approaches to the cervicothoracic junction. In: Sundaresan SN, Schmidek HH, Schiller AL, et al., eds. *Tumors of the spine: diagnosis and clinical management.* Philadelphia: WB Saunders, 1990:358–368.
35. Kurz LT, Brower RS, Herokwitz HN, et al. Surgical approaches to the cervico-thoracic junction. In: Sherk HH, ed. *The cervical spine: an atlas of surgical procedures.* Philadelphia: JB Lippincott, 1994.
36. Laus M, Pignatti G, Malaguti MC, et al. Anterior extraoral surgery to the upper cervical spine. *Spine* 1996;21:1687–1693.
37. McAfee PC. Anterior surgical approaches to the lower and upper cervical spine. In: Sherk HH, ed. *The cervical spine: an atlas of surgical procedures.* Philadelphia: JB Lippincott, 1994:37–70.
38. Sar C, Eralp L. Transoral resection and reconstruction for primary osteogenic sarcoma of the second cervical vertebra. *Spine* 2001;26:1936–1941.
39. Whitesides TE. Lateral retropharyngeal approach to the upper cervical spine. In: Sherk HH, ed. *The cervical spine: an atlas of surgical procedures.* Philadelphia: JB Lippincott, 1994:71–78.
40. Shah JP, Shaha AR. Transmandibular approaches to the upper cervical spine. In: Sundaresan SN, Schmidek HH, Schiller AL, et al., eds. *Tumors of the spine: diagnosis and clinical management.* Philadelphia: WB Saunders, 1990:329–335.
41. Curylo LJ, Mason HC, Bohlman HH, et al.: Tortuous course of the vertebral artery and anterior cervical decompression: a cadaveric and clinical case study. *Spine* 2000;25:2860–2864.
42. Golfinos JG, Dickman CA, Zabramski JM, et al. Repair of vertebral artery injury during anterior cervical decompression. *Spine* 1994;9:2552–2556.

43. Apfelbaum RI, Kriskovich MD, Haller JR. On the incidence, cause, and prevention of recurrent laryngeal nerve palsies during anterior cervical spine surgery. *Spine* 2000;25:2906–2912.

44. Gaundinez RF, English GM, Gebhard JS, et al. Esophageal perforation after anterior cervical surgery. *J Spinal Disord* 2000;13:77–84.

45. Smith MD, Emery SE, Dudley A, et al. Vertebral artery injury during anterior decompression of the cervical spine. *J Bone Joint Surg Br* 1993,75:410–415.

46. Winslow CP, Meyers AD. Otolaryngologic complications of the anterior approach to the cervical spine. Am J Otolaryngol 1999,20:16–27.

47. Boriani S. Subtotal and total vertebrectomy for tumors. Editions Scientifique at Medicales Elsevier SAS (Paris). *Surg Tech Orthop Traumatol* 2000;55–070-A-10.

48. Roy-Camille R, Mazel C, Saillant G, et al. Treatment of malignant tumors of the spine with posterior instrumentation. In: Sundaresan N, Schmidek HH, Schiller AL, et al., eds. *Tumors of the spine: diagnosis and clinical management.* Philadelphia: WB Saunders, 1990:473–487.

49. Stener B. Surgical treatment of giant cell tumors, chondrosarcomas, and chordomas of the spine. In: Uhthoff HK, ed. *Current concepts of diagnosis and treatment of bone and soft tissue tumors.* Berlin: Springer-Verlag, 1984:233–242.

50. Fujita T, Kawahara N, Matsumoto T, et al. Chordoma in the cervical spine managed with en bloc excision. *Spine* 1999;24:1848–1859.

51. Hoshino Y, Kurokawa T, Nakamura K, et al. A report on the safety of unilateral vertebral artery ligation during cervical spine surgery. *Spine* 21(12):1454–1457.

52. Caspar W, Pitzen T, Papavero L, et al. Anterior cervical plating for the treatment of neoplasm in the cervical vertebrae. *J Neurosur (Spine)* 1999;90:27–34.

53. Epstein NE. The value of anterior cervical plating in preventing vertebral fracture and graft extrusion after multilevel anterior cervical corpectomy with posterior wiring and fusion: indications, results, and complications. *J Spinal Disord* 2000;13:9–15.

54. Heidecke V, Rainov NG, Burkert W. Anterior cervical fusion with the Orion locking plate system. *Spine* 1998;23:1796–1803.

55. Abumi K, Shono Y, Ito M, et al. Complications of pedicle screw fixation in reconstructive surgery of the cervical spine. *Spine* 25(8):962–969.

56. Harms J, Melcher RP. Posterior C1-C2 fusion with polyaxial screw and rod fixation. *Spine* 2001;26:2467–2471.

57. Henriques T, Cunningham BW, Olerud C, et al. Biomechanical comparison of five different atlantoaxial posterior fixation techniques. *Spine* 2000;25:2877–2883.

58. Gebhard JS, Schimmer RC, Jeanneret B. Safety and accuracy of transarticular screw fixation C1-C2 using an aiming device: an anatomic study. *Spine* 1998;23:2185–2189.

59. Goffin J, Van Brussel K, Martens K, et al. Three-dimensional computed tomography-based, personalized drill guide for posterior cervical stabilization at C1-C2. *Spine* 2001;26:1343–1347.

60. Todd JA, Gregg R. Klein, et al. Image-guided anterior cervical corpectomy: a feasibility study. *Spine* 1999;24:826.

61. Weidner A, Wähler M, Chiu ST, et al. Tumor surgery of the upper cervical spine: a retrospective study of 13 cases. *Acta Neurochir* (Wien) 2001;143:217–225.

62. Ludwig SC, Kramer DL, Balderston RA, et al. Placement of pedicle screws in the human cadaveric cervical spine: comparative accuracy of three techniques. *Spine* 2000;25:1655–1667.

63. Karaikovic EE, Daubs MD, Madsen RW, et al. Morphologic characteristics of human cervical pedicles. *Spine* 1997;22:493–500.

64. Graham AW, Swank ML, Kinard RE, et al. Posterior cervical arthrodesis and stabilization with a lateral mass plate: clinical and computed tomographic evaluation of lateral mass screw placement and associated complications. *Spine* 1996;21:323–328.

65. Seybold EA, Baker JA, Criscitiello AA, et al. Characteristics of unicortical and bicortical lateral mass screws in the cervical spine. *Spine* 1999;24:2397.

66. Wright NM, Kaufman BA, Haughey BH, et al. Complex cervical spine neoplastic disease: reconstruction after surgery by using a vascularized fibular strut graft. Case report. *J Neurosurg* (Spine) 1999;90:133–137.

67. Lang CJ, Frederick RW, Hutton WC. A biomechanical study of the ankle syndesmosis after fibular graft harvest. *J Spinal Disord* 1998;11: 508–513.

68. Vail TP, Urbaniak JR. Donor-site morbidity with the use of vascularized autogenous fibular grafts. *J Bone Joint Surg Am* 1996;78:204–211.

69. Fielding W, Pyle RN, Fietti VG. Anterior cervical body resection and bone grafting for benign and malignant tumors: a survey under the auspices of the cervical Spine Research Society. *J Bone Joint Surg Am* 1979;61:251–253.

70. Kurz LT, Garfin SR, Booth RE. Harvesting autogenous iliac bone grafts: a review of complications and techniques. *Spine* 1989;14:1324–1331.

71. Schultz KD, McLaughlin MR, Haid RW, et al. Single-stage anterior-posterior decompression and stabilization for complex cervical spine disorders. *J Neurosurg* 2000;93:214–221.

72. Suit HD, Goiten M, Munzenreider J, et al. Definitive radiation therapy for chordoma and chondrosarcoma of base of skull and cervical spine. *J Neurosurg* 1982;56:377–385.

73. Dahlin DC. Bone tumors. *General aspects and data on 6221 cases.* Springfield, IL: Charles C. Thomas, 1978.

74. Blaylock RL, Kempe LG. Chondrosarcoma of the cervical spine. *J Neurosurg* 1976;44:500–553.

75. Wojne KJ, Hruban RH, Garin-Chesa P, et al. Chondroid chordomas and low-grade chondrosarcomas of the craniospinal axis: an immunohistochemical analysis of 17 cases. *Am J Surg Pathol* 1992;16:1144–1152.

76. Shallat RF, Taekman MS, Nagle RC. Unusual presentation of cervical chordoma with long term survival. *J Neurosurg* 1982;57:716–718.

77. Laurent P, Linarte R, Noblia B, et al. Chordomes vertebraux: problemes diagnostiques at therapeutiques. *Rev Chir Orthop Reparatrue Appar Mot* 1981;67:137–140.

78. Winants D, Bertal A, Hennequin L, et al. Imagerie des Chordomes cervicaux et thoraciques. *J Radiol* 1992;73:169–174.

79. Mindell ER. Chordoma: current concepts review. *J Bone Joint Surg Am* 1981;63A:501–555.

80. Wippol FJ, Koeller KK, Smirniotopoulos JG. Clinical and imaging features of cervical chordoma. *Am J Roentgenol* 1999;172:1423–1426.

81. Rodde A, Becker S, Stines J, et al. Chordomes du rachis cervical aspects radiologiques caracteristiques: a propos de 2 observations. *J Radiol* 1987;68:587–591.

82. Sze G, Vichanco LS, Brant-Zawadzki MN, et al. Chordomas: MR imaging. *Radiology* 1988;166:187–191.

83. Reddy EK, Mansfield CM, Hartman GV. Chordoma. *Int J Radiat Oncol Biol Phys* 1981;7:1709–1711.

84. Amendola BE, Amendola MA, Oliver E, et al. Chordoma: role of radiation therapy. *Radiology* 1986;158:839–843.

85. Sundaresan N, Galicich JH, Chu FC, et al. Spinal chordomas. *J Neurosurg* 1979;50:312–319.

86. Tewfik HH, McGinnis WL, Nordstrom DG, et al. Chordoma: evaluation of clinical behavior and treatment modalities *Int J Radiat Oncol Biol Phys* 1977;2:959–962.

87. Barwick KW, Huvos AH, Smith J. Primary osteogenic sarcoma of the vertebral column: clinicopathologic correlation of ten patients. *Cancer* 1980;46:595–604.

88. Lang G, Kher P, Paternotte H, et al. Osteosarcome post-radiotherapique de la 6eme vertebre cervicale: a propos d'un cas. *Rev Chir Orthop* 1981;67:691–693.

89. Roy-Camille R, Saillant G, Chiras J, et al. Osteosarcome de C4-C5 radio-induit. Interet des exploration preoperatoires et da la resection chirurgicale *Rev Chir Orthop* 1984;70[Suppl 1]:90–100.

90. Mnaymneh W, Brown M, Tejada F, et al. Primary osteogenic sarcoma of the second cervical vertebra: case report. *J Bone Joint Surg Am* 1979;61:460–442.

91. Yoshino MT, Carmody RF. Osteosarcoma of the cervical spine. *Am J Roentgenol* 1991;157:1357.

92. Grubb MR, Currier BL, Pritchard DJ, et al. Primary Ewing's sarcoma of the spine. *Spine* 1994;19:309–313.

93. McLain RE, Weinstein JN. Solitary plasmacytomas of the spine: a review of 84 cases. *J Spinal Disord* 1989;2:69–74.

94. Moulopoulos LA, Dimopoulos MA, Weber D, et al. Magnetic resonance imaging in the staging of solitary plasmacytoma of bone. *J Clin Oncol* 1993;11:1311–1115.

95. Bacci G, Savini R, Calderoni P, et al. Solitary plasmacytoma of the vertebral column: a report of 15 cases. *Tumori* 1982;68:271–275.

96. Poulsen JJO, Jensen JT, Thommesen P. Ewing's sarcoma simulating vertebra plana. *Acta Orthop Scand* 1975;46:211–215.

CHAPTER 62

Cervical Spinal Infections

Bradford L. Currier, Choll W. Kim, John G. Heller, and Frank J. Eismont

Advances in the diagnosis and treatment of infectious disease have dramatically improved the prognosis for patients with spinal infections. Before antibiotics were available, 60% of patients with neurologic compromise subsequent to tuberculous spondylitis died (1). Today, less than 5% of patients similarly affected die of the disease (2,3). Despite this encouraging statistic, spinal infections still can have devastating consequences.

Infections do not involve the cervical region as frequently as they do the thoracic or lumbar spine. However, cervical infections have the highest rate of neurologic compromise and the greatest potential for causing disability. Prompt evaluation and treatment are essential when a cervical spinal infection is suspected. Spinal infections may be classified by the cause or anatomic site of the infection. This chapter covers these variations and highlights the differences in evaluation, management, and prognosis.

PYOGENIC INFECTIONS

Iatrogenic Wound and Disc Space Infections

Epidemiology and Etiology

The prevalence of infection varies with the approach and the magnitude of the procedure. Transoral procedures once were associated with a high infection rate (4). Later series (5–7) proved that infection rates were low when the oral approach was used for decompression only and antibiotics were given prophylactically. Hadley and associates (6) reported only one infection in 53 transoral decompressions. Bone grafting through the transoral approach may increase the infection rate and has caused at least one fatality (6). Several successful cases of transoral arthrodesis have been reported (6,8), but McAfee and others (9) prefer the anterior retropharyngeal approach. They reported no infections in 15 patients who had arthrodesis performed through the retropharyngeal approach. The prevalence of infection after an extrapharyngeal approach to the subaxial cervical spine ranges between 0% and 2% (9–11).

In patients undergoing lumbar procedures the infection rate increases from 0.7% for a simple discectomy, to 2% for an uninstrumented fusion, and to up to 6% for an instrumented fusion (12). Arthrodesis and instrumentation increase only minimally the risk for infection in the cervical spine. Lundsford and colleagues (13) found an infection rate of 0.6% after anterior cervical discectomy without fusion and a rate of 1.4% after anterior cervical discectomy with arthrodesis. An infection in the bone graft donor site occurred in another 2 of the 140 patients who underwent arthrodesis (1.4%). Espersen and associates (14) reported that infections developed in 1.8% of 1,106 patients treated with the Cloward technique by various graft types. A superficial infection occurred in 1% of patients, a deep infection in 0.27%, and a donor-site infection in 0.5%. The infection rate following anterior cervical decompression and arthrodesis with a plate is low. No infections were encountered in one series of 261 patients who underwent corpectomy and reconstruction with allograft fibula and anterior plating for spinal stenosis (15). Longer follow-up may reveal a higher infection rate for instrumentation procedures because delayed implant failure may lead to esophageal rupture and infection (16–18). Late infections caused by hematogenous seeding also have been reported after thoracic and lumbar instrumentation procedures (19,20). The rate of infection after laminectomy was 1.2% in one large series (21) and 1.5% in another report (22).

The infection rate after a posterior cervical arthrodesis ranges from 0% to 18% (23–26). Several factors are responsible for the high rate reported in some series. Weiland and McAfee (25) observed no infections in a series of 100 patients. Twenty-seven of their patients had rheumatoid arthritis. Most other large series of patients with rheumatoid arthritis have high infection rates ranging from 5% to

18% (23,24,26,27). Patients with Down syndrome also have a higher rate of infection (28).

Arthrodesis to the occiput does not appear to increase the infection rate. McAfee and associates (9) described 37 patients who had an occipitocervical fusion without instrumentation. The only infections involved the donor site in two patients and halo pin sites in two. Instrumentation used to augment an occipitocervical fusion did not increase the risk for infection (29,30). Itoh and co-workers (31) reported one infection in 17 cases (6%) of occipitocervical arthrodesis with Luque segmental instrumentation, but all the patients in that series had rheumatoid arthritis.

The infection rates have varied widely after posterior cervical lateral mass plating in the subaxial spine. Heller and colleagues (32) reported that one in a series of 78 consecutive patients developed a superficial infection after treatment that included lateral mass plating. Three other groups described infections occurring in 1 of 30 patients (3.3%) (33), 2 of 44 patients (4.5%) (34), and 3 of 24 patients (12.5%) (35).

Use of methylmethacrylate cement compromises local immune mechanisms and increases the risk for infection (36,37). Several studies (38–40) reported infection rates of less than 3% after insertion of methylmethacrylate. One group (41) reported a rate of 7.1% and another group (23) reported an infection rate of 18% when methyl methacrylate was used. The highest rate (23) occurred in patients with rheumatoid arthritis. When patients with rheumatoid arthritis were excluded and methylmethacrylate was used for traumatic patients, the infection rate was still slightly higher than the rate without the use of cement: 2.5% (40) and 3% (38). Eismont and Bohlman (42) and McAfee and colleagues (43) advised against the use of methylmethacrylate because of the increased infection rate and poor mechanical properties of cement.

Infections may occur after percutaneous diagnostic and therapeutic procedures (44). Connor and Darden (45) reported that cervical discography caused an infection in two of 31 patients (6.5%). In one patient, an epidural abscess developed that led to myelopathy and eventual quadriplegia. However, most large series show that the rate of infection as a result of cervical discography is low. Guyer and co-workers (46) showed that 2 of 269 cervical discograms (0.74%) led to discitis. Similarly, Grubb and Kelly (47) showed that only 3 of 807 cervical injections (0.37%) led to an infection. Finally, Zeidman and associates (48), in a large series of 4,400 diagnostic cervical injections, showed that only 8 resulted in an infection.

Esophageal perforation can lead to a life-threatening infection. The perforation may occur during exposure of the spine (49), from blunt cervical spinal traumas (50), from the sharp edge of a bone graft (51), or from erosion of the wall of the esophagus from anterior hardware (17,18).

The risk factors for a postoperative spinal infection can be classified as *controllable* or *uncontrollable*. Factors be-

yond the control of the surgeon include older patient age (52), use of corticosteroid therapy (53), and immunosuppression (54). Controllable risk factors include malnutrition (55,56), a concurrent remote infection (57,58), cigarette smoking (59), poorly controlled diabetes mellitus (54,60), and preoperative hospitalization (60). Cruse and Foord (60) found that the infection rate doubles for each additional week that patients are hospitalized preoperatively. Measures that help decrease infection intraoperatively include double gloving, limiting traffic and conversation in the operating room (55), handling tissues carefully, and periodically releasing self-retaining retractors to allow reperfusion of muscle (61).

Antibiotics administered prophylactically have proved effective in decreasing the rate of infection after thoracolumbar spinal procedures (62). Antibiotics are most effective when administered before bacteria infect the wound (63,64). The appropriate duration of prophylaxis is controversial. Use of drugs probably could be stopped after the first dose or two, but many surgeons prefer to continue antibiotic therapy until all drains have been removed. Antibiotic therapy should not be continued for more than 24 to 48 hours postoperatively (58,65,66). The choice of antibiotic depends on many factors, including spectrum of activity, adverse effects, cost, and pharmacokinetics (54,67,68). Host factors must also be considered, such as preoperative hospitalization, exposure to antibiotics, compromise of the immune system, and remote infections.

Clinical Presentation

Superficial Infections

Wound infections may be classified as superficial or deep. A superficial infection is characterized by pain, tenderness, and the typical signs of infection: erythema, swelling, fluctuation, drainage, and fever. By definition, the infection is located superficial to the deep fascia. Superficial infections may extend below the deep fascia, and therefore all wound infections must be treated aggressively.

Deep Infections

Infections that occur below the deep fascia are more insidious than superficial infections. The only symptoms may be fever and progressive neck pain out of proportion to the expected postoperative course. The wound may appear completely benign (69).

Discitis

A patient with a postoperative disc space infection may present with axial or radicular pain, fever, chills, and night sweats. Neurologic signs and symptoms suggest that the disc space infection has been complicated by an epidural abscess (53,70).

Diagnostic Evaluation

The erythrocyte sedimentation rate (ESR) and C-reactive protein (CRP) value are usually increased in the early postoperative period after uncomplicated procedures (71) (Fig. 62.1). After lumbar procedures, the CRP level peaked after 2 to 3 days and returned to normal 5 to 14 days after surgery. The ESR peaked 5 days after surgery and declined slowly and irregularly. Similar data for cervical spinal procedures are not available. An ESR or CRP level that is higher than expected and increasing after 3 to 5 days suggests infection. The white blood cell count is generally unremarkable but may be increased, especially if a deep wound infection or epidural abscess has occurred (69).

The presence of bacteria confirmed by Gram stain or culture is diagnostic of infection. It is not necessary to culture a draining wound preoperatively if antibiotics can be withheld until after surgery. Exploration and débridement of the wound should be performed urgently, and tissue samples for cultures can be obtained at surgery. If the wound appears benign but a deep infection is suspected, the contents of the wound can be aspirated to obtain a specimen for Gram stain and culture. After surgical preparation of the wound, a spinal needle can be advanced down to bone, and the contents of the wound can be aspirated. If the tap is nonproductive, a new needle can be inserted in another quadrant of the wound and the procedure repeated until fluid is obtained for analysis. If all four quadrants of the wound produce no aspirate, the examination is considered to have a negative result. The sensitivity and specificity of percutaneous aspirations of the cervical spine are not known. If signs of superficial infection are present, the deep aspiration is not performed until the superficial space is clean because the needle may contaminate the deep space. Patients with presumed disc space infections should undergo an open or closed (needle) biopsy (discussed later).

Imaging studies are generally not helpful in the diagnosis of wound infections, and treatment should not be delayed for these studies to be performed. Plain radiography, computed tomography (CT), magnetic resonance imaging (MRI), and radionuclide studies all have a role in the diagnosis of postoperative discitis and are discussed in the following section on hematogenous osteomyelitis.

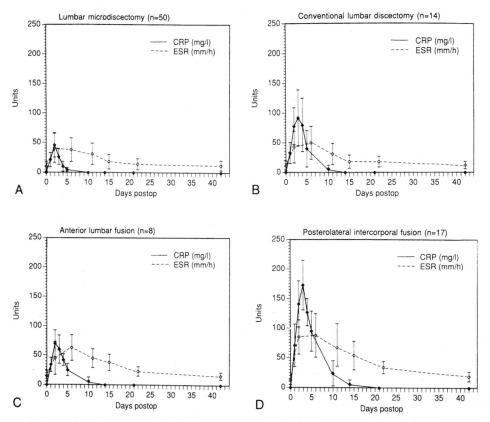

FIG. 62.1. A–D: Serial mean values of C-reactive protein (CRP) and erythrocyte sedimentation rate (ESR) before and after four types of uncomplicated spinal operations. (From Thelander U, Larsson S. Quantitation of C-reactive protein levels and erythrocyte sedimentation rate after spinal surgery. *Spine* 1992;17:400–404, with permission.)

Management

The principles of treatment of postoperative wound infections include (a) thorough irrigation and débridement, (b) appropriate antibiotic therapy, (c) proper nutrition and medical management, and (d) appropriate wound care. The management of postoperative discitis is the same as the treatment for hematogenous disc space infection and is discussed in a later section.

Treatment of a wound infection must be expeditious. The wound should be opened and explored without delay. If the infection is superficial, the deep fascia should be left intact. Samples of the subcutaneous tissues should be cultured, and the tissues should be copiously irrigated and débrided. The fascia then is inspected for any signs of communication between the layers. If the fascia is intact and the patient does not have signs of septicemia, some surgeons recommend leaving the fascia closed and draining the superficial space only. The subfascial plane can be aspirated and left undisturbed if results of the aspirate are negative (69). Others (72) believe it is necessary to open and débride the wound (one layer at a time) down to the bone in all cases. All devitalized tissue should be removed from the wound. Bone graft that becomes loosened by irrigation or grossly infected should be removed. It is not necessary or desirable to remove all the bone graft because it is needed to achieve a solid fusion and its presence may help to resolve the infection (62,68,69,70, 73,74). If hardware is present, it should be left in place unless it has failed (59,62,69,70,73,74). Methylmethacrylate, if present, should be removed from the wound (42,43) (Fig. 62.2). Multiple débridements may be required to control the infection.

The technique and timing of wound closure are based on the nature of the infection, the appearance of the wound, the clinical response, and patient risk factors. The options include wound closure over drains in each layer, open packing with delayed closure, and open packing with healing by second intention.

Prognosis

The prognosis for a patient treated for postoperative infection is based on the nature of the infection, the health of the patient, and the adequacy of treatment. Information on cervical infections is limited, and guidelines must be extrapolated from the literature on thoracolumbar infections. Massie and colleagues (72) described 22 patients with postoperative spinal infections. Five patients required reoperation, and 10 were allowed to heal by second intention, but all wounds eventually healed, and chronic drainage, osteomyelitis, or death did not occur. Stambough and Beringer (56) described 11 patients with deep infections, 4 with superficial infections, and 4 with iliac crest donor-site infections. The hardware was removed in 3 of the 11 patients with deep infections but retained in all others. Solid fusion occurred in 17 of 18 patients, and all but one infection eventually resolved.

Hematogenous Vertebral Osteomyelitis and Disc Space Infection

Epidemiology and Etiology

The incidence of vertebral osteomyelitis is increasing, which may be an effect of the increasing numbers of elderly and immunocompromised persons in the population. The cervical spine is involved in about 6% of cases of vertebral osteomyelitis (75,76). The incidence of cervical infection is higher in series comprising intravenous drug users (77–79). In the series reported by Sapico and Montgomerie (78), 27% of the infections occurred in the cervical spine. Use of the jugular vein for injection may explain this association (77). Immunocompromised hosts, especially patients who are diabetic or are human immunodeficiency virus (HIV) positive, are particularly susceptible to the development of vertebral osteomyelitis (79,80).

Hematogenous vertebral osteomyelitis may be caused by any condition that results in bacteremia. Infections of the urinary tract, soft tissues, or respiratory tract and intravenous drug use are all common causes (79).

Microbiology

In the preantibiotic era, *Staphylococcus aureus* was the causative organism in almost every case of vertebral osteomyelitis and is still the most common pathogen, accounting for 50% of all spinal infections (76). The most frequent gram-negative pathogens are *Pseudomonas* species organisms, *Escherichia coli,* and *Proteus* species, which are common causes of urinary tract infections (81–84). *Pseudomonas aeruginosa* is identified frequently as the organism responsible for vertebral osteomyelitis in heroin users (79,85,86). Anaerobic infections are uncommon and generally are associated with open fractures, infected wounds, human bites, foreign bodies, or diabetes mellitus (76,87). *Salmonella* species osteomyelitis is encountered rarely and has a tendency to infect sites of preexisting disease (88,89).

Pathogenesis

The nucleus pulposus is an avascular tissue that is metabolically active (90). The nucleus pulposus receives nutrients from diffusion across the end plates and from the blood vessels in the annulus fibrosis (90,91). In the developing spine, the end plate has an orderly arrangement of cartilage canals that contain vascular organs resembling glomeruli (91,92) (Fig. 62.3). After birth, the cartilage end plates become progressively thinner, and by adulthood, most of the vessels of the cartilage canals are obliterated (93,94). In children, microorganisms have nearly direct access to the nucleus pulposus through the cartilage canals, allowing infection to begin spontaneously in the disc and then spread to adjacent bone. Pediatric discitis is relatively common in the lumbar spine but exceedingly rare in the cervical spine. In adults, hematogenous infection begins in the metaphysis

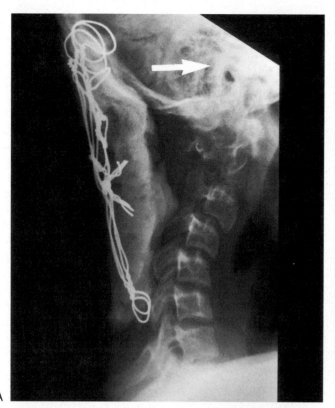

A

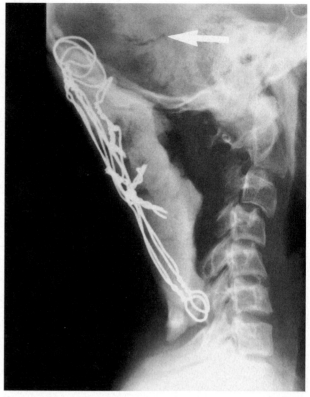

B

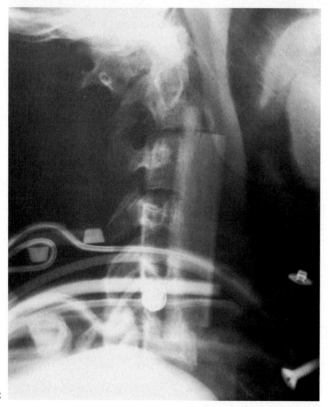

C

FIG. 62.2. Postoperative wound infection. In this 16-year-old boy, Gorham disease of the cervical spine developed and was treated elsewhere by laminectomies of C1 through C5, methyl methacrylate stabilization, and radiation therapy. Progressive pain and swan neck developed 4 months after operation. On presentation, the patient had an unstable cervical spine and a deep wound infection. He was treated by débridement of the posterior wound, application of a halo vest, intravenously administered antibiotics, and anterior fusion of C2 through C6 with a fibular strut graft. Deep culture specimens from the posterior wound grew *Staphylococcus aureus*. The wound healed uneventfully, but the upper end of the graft dislodged from the C2 body, and progressive kyphosis and instability developed. He was treated by posterior arthrodesis from the occiput through C6 and postoperative halo immobilization. At final follow-up 1 year after the last procedure, his fusion was solid, the cervical spine infection was resolved, and he had no notable neck pain or neurologic deficit. Lateral cervical spine radiographs in flexion (**A**) and extension (**B**) demonstrate stabilization of the occiput through C6 with methyl methacrylate and wires and swan neck with instability. **C:** Lateral cervical radiograph taken after removal of posterior construct and anterior arthrodesis of C2 through C6 with fibular strut graft. **D:** Lateral cervical radiograph demonstrates extrusion of upper end of bone graft and progression of deformity. **E:** One year after posterior arthrodesis of the occiput through C6, solid anterior and posterior fusion is seen.

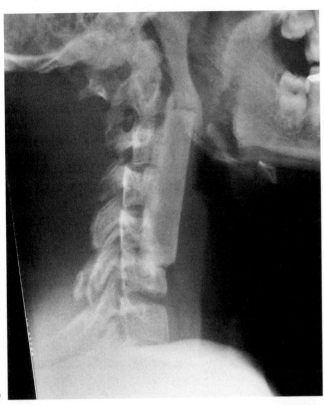

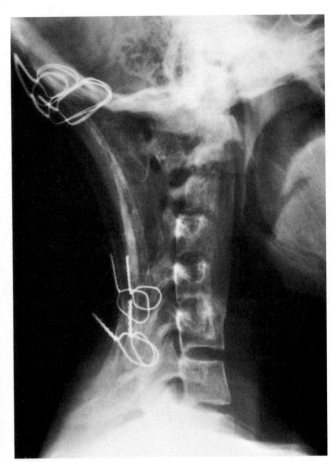

D   E

FIG. 62.2. *Continued*

and spreads across the disc by lysosomal destruction of the nucleus pulposus or through the annular vessels. Segmentation of sclerotomes during development leads to the vascular arrangement of a single artery supplying adjacent vertebral bodies. Wiley and Trueta (95) demonstrated that bacteria could gain access to the metaphyseal region of adjacent vertebrae through these arteries and cause infection.

Disc space infection and vertebral osteomyelitis once were thought to be distinct clinical entities (96). Because the clinical manifestations and treatment of septic discitis and vertebral osteomyelitis are similar, it is best to consider them as related conditions in a spectrum of disease (97,98).

The pathogenesis of neurocompromise associated with vertebral osteomyelitis may be related to direct compression by bone or disc, from spinal instability and deformity, or by epidural pus and granulation tissue. The neural tissue may also sustain ischemic damage from septic thrombosis or be impaired by inflammatory infiltration of the dura (76,96,99).

Clinical Presentation

The presentation may be acute, subacute, or chronic, depending on the host's resistance and the organism's viru-

lence. A literature review published in 1979 (76) indicated that 50% of the patients had symptoms for more than 3 months before seeking help, and only 20% had symptoms for less than 3 weeks before presentation. Infants and intravenous drug users generally have a more acute presentation than other subgroups of patients (76,79,100,101).

Neck pain is present in more than 90% of patients with a cervical spinal infection (78). The pain frequently radiates to the trapezius region and the shoulder. About 50% of patients have a fever (76); fever is a common symptom in patients with acute infections. Patients occasionally complain of radicular pain and may have signs of radiculopathy or myelopathy when the infection is complicated by an epidural abscess. Atypical symptoms, such as headache, chest pain, dysphasia, meningeal irritation, or respiratory problems, occur in about 15% of patients (76,80,102). Rarely, patients present with signs of septicemia (103). Unilateral neck pain with radiculopathy may indicate an infection of the cervical facet. Although rare, facet infections are often found together with an epidural abscess (104).

The most common findings on physical examination are tenderness, spasm, and limited motion. Torticollis also may be present (105,106). Neurologic deficits occur in about

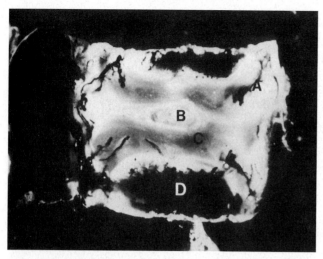

FIG. 62.3. Sagittally sectioned human fetal specimen (26 weeks' gestation) injected, cleared, and transilluminated shows cartilage canals and absence of vessels in nucleus pulposus. **A:** Cartilage canal. **B:** Nucleus pulposus. **C:** Hyaline cartilage end plate. **D:** Ossified vertebral body (original magnification × 10). (From Whalen JL, Parke WW, Mazur JM, et al. The intrinsic vasculature of developing vertebral end plates and its nutritive significance to the intervertebral disks. *J Pediatr Orthop* 1985;5:403–410, with permission.)

17% of all patients with vertebral osteomyelitis (76). The rate of neurologic deficits is higher with cervical lesions. Stone and colleagues (107) found that more than half their patients with cervical infection had neurologic deficits. In a series described by Eismont and associates (44) 82% of the patients with cervical lesions were paralyzed. Predisposing factors for paralysis include diabetes mellitus, rheumatoid arthritis, older age, systemic corticosteroid therapy, and a more cephalad level of infection (44,76,108). Abscess formation is more common in cervical infections than in lumbar infections, but since the start of the antibiotic era, severe abscesses occur infrequently in any region of the spine (82). Abscesses may occur in the retropharyngeal region, the lateral region of the neck, the epidural space, or the posterior mediastinum (99).

Diagnostic Evaluation

The differential diagnosis of pyogenic disc space infection and vertebral osteomyelitis includes granulomatous infections, metastatic carcinoma, multiple myeloma, degenerative disease, trauma, fractures associated with osteoporosis, destructive spondyloarthropathy, gout, and Scheuermann disease (76, 109–112).

The white blood cell count is increased in only 42% of patients overall and is usually normal in patients with chronic infections (76,82). ESR is increased in more than 90% of patients (76). An increased ESR is not specific for infection, but it is a good indicator test and is also useful for following the response to treatment (76,81,96,110,113).

The CRP value is a more recent method of evaluating a systemic inflammatory response. It has advantages over the ESR in the evaluation and follow-up of patients with vertebral osteomyelitis because the level increases more rapidly and has a much shorter half-life (114). Blood cultures have positive results in 24% of patients with pyogenic spinal infections (76).

Plain radiographic findings are characteristic but are not evident until 2 to 4 weeks after the onset of the disease (75, 82,115–117). The earliest sign of infection is narrowing of the disc space and abnormal prevertebral soft tissue contours. Paraspinal soft tissue swelling is found in one third of patients with pyogenic infections compared with two thirds of patients infected with tuberculosis (118). Destructive changes in the end plates and the anterior aspect of the vertebral body are present after 3 to 6 weeks (Fig. 62.4). The late changes seen on plain radiographs include reactive bone formation, fracture, collapse, kyphosis, and enlarging abscesses (76). The process may extend to adjacent levels; 79% of cases involve at least two vertebrae (75). The overall accuracy of plain radiographs is 74% (119). Tomograms often show abnormalities earlier than plain radiographs.

Radionuclide studies allow detection of spinal infections earlier than plain radiography (96,119,120,121). These studies provide a survey of the entire body and may detect multiple sites of infection, which occur in 4% of patients (119). Gallium scans show evidence of infection earlier in the course of the disease than technetium scans (120,122). Gallium scans are more useful for following the response to treatment because they appear normal during resolution of the infection; technetium scans remain positive for many months after the disease has resolved (120). Gallium scans have slightly higher specificity than technetium scans (85% versus 78%). Both studies have about 90% sensitivity and 85% accuracy (119,120). Single-photon emission CT (SPECT) is more sensitive and has better contrast resolution than planar scintigraphy; it also allows three-dimensional localization (123). Feiglan and associates (124) found the sensitivity of technetium planar scintigraphy to be 74% compared with 92% for SPECT scans. Gallium planar scintigraphy had a sensitivity of 69% compared with 92% for SPECT scans. Indium scans are not particularly helpful in the evaluation of spinal infections because of low sensitivity. The specificity is 100%, but the sensitivity is only 17% and the accuracy 31% (125).

Use of CT may be helpful in distinguishing infection from malignancy and in demonstrating clearly the extent of bony destruction and the formation of soft tissue abscesses (126–128). The soft tissue mass, frequently seen in the prevertebral area in infections, usually surrounds the spine anteriorly, in contrast to neoplasms, which are more likely to have a partial paravertebral soft tissue mass or no extension beyond the vertebrae. Neoplasms are more likely than infections to involve the posterior elements and may be osteoblastic compared with the osteolytic appearance of infections (128).

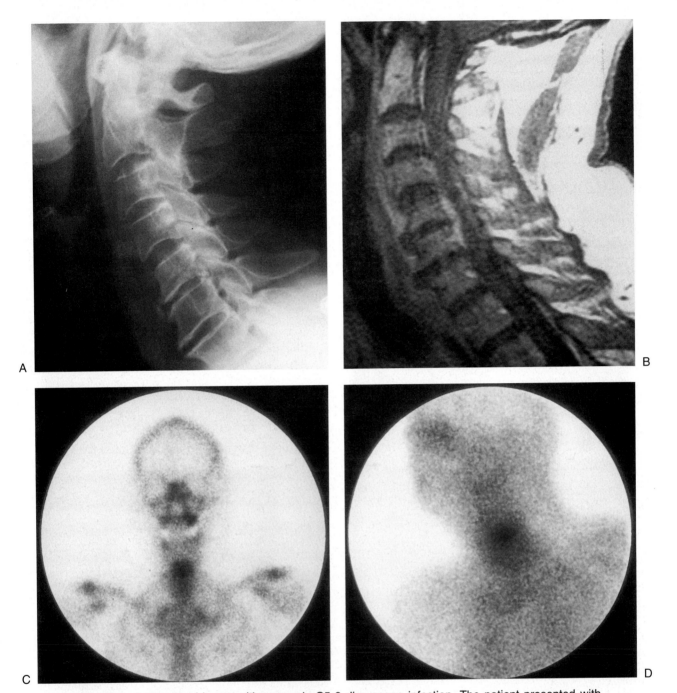

FIG. 62.4. A 72-year-old man with pyogenic C5-6 disc space infection. The patient presented with neck pain and arm pain, greater on the right than the left, 1 week after a stellate ganglion block for postherpetic neuralgia. He had mild hyperreflexia and an up-going toe on the right. Sedimentation rate was 30 mm/1 h. Magnetic resonance imaging (MRI) suggested infection, and a computed tomography (CT) myelogram demonstrated a complete block. A CT-guided biopsy initially had negative results, and the patient was placed in a Philadelphia collar and observed. *Propionibacterium acnes* grew on culture after 7 days, but the treating physician considered the organism to be a contaminant. At $2\frac{1}{2}$ weeks after the biopsy, plain radiographs demonstrated progressive collapse and led to an anterior discectomy and iliac crest arthrodesis. Intraoperative cultures were positive for coagulase-negative staphylococci. After operation, a halo vest was applied for 3 months, and antibiotics were administered intravenously for 6 weeks. One year after operation, the patient was completely asymptomatic and had a normal neurologic examination. **A:** Lateral cervical spine radiograph demonstrates narrowing of C5-6 disc space with degenerative changes. **B:** T1-weighted sagittal MRI with gadolinium shows enhancement in the epidural space at C5-6. **C:** Technetium bone scan demonstrates increased uptake at the C5-C6 level. **D:** Gallium scan demonstrates increased uptake at the C5-C6 level. **E:** Anteroposterior myelogram shows complete block to flow of contrast material at C5-C6. **F:** Postmyelographic CT shows epidural compression at C5-C6. **G:** Lateral cervical spine radiograph 3 weeks after presentation demonstrates collapse of C5-6 disc space with kyphotic deformity. **H:** Lateral cervical spine radiograph demonstrates solid fusion 1 year after operation.

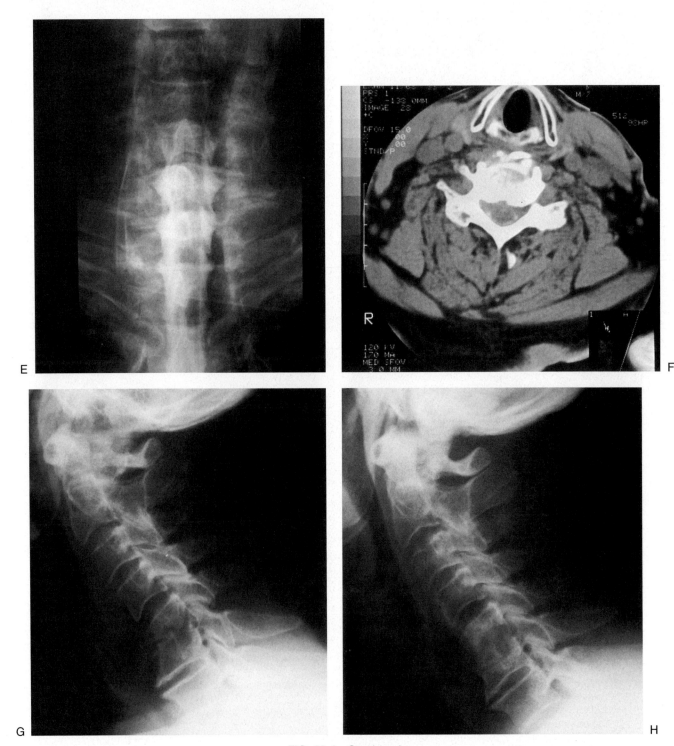

FIG. 62.4. *Continued*

Postmyelography CT or MRI is indicated in the presence of neurologic signs or symptoms to eliminate the possibility of epidural and subdural abscesses (Fig. 62.4). Spinal fluid should be examined during myelography to eliminate the possibility of meningitis.

Use of MRI allows early diagnosis of infection and recognition of abscess formation without the risk for in-

trathecal injection (129,130) (Fig. 62.4). This study provides much more anatomic information than radionuclide studies, and results become positive at about the same time as a gallium scan (119). MRI has 96% sensitivity, 93% specificity, and 94% accuracy in detecting vertebral osteomyelitis and is considered the diagnostic modality of choice (119).

On T1-weighted sequences, the signal intensity in the peridiscal area is decreased, and the junction between the disc and the vertebral body is indistinct. On T2-weighted sequences, the signal intensity is higher than normal in the disc. Gadolinium, a paramagnetic contrast material, causes enhancement of the disc space and allows better delineation of epidural abscesses (131). The enhanced images allow localization of optimal sites for percutaneous biopsy and may distinguish active infections from those responding to treatment (131). Over time, the T1-weighted sequences revert from a hypointense signal in the vertebral body to a hyperintense fat signal, and the hyperintense signal on the T2-weighted sequence gradually diminishes. In the healed stage, the disc space is narrowed or obliterated, and spontaneous fusion is common (132,133).

In almost all cases, MRI distinguishes tumor from infection. Tumors rarely involve the disc spaces and do not have the typical T1- and T2-weighted changes described for infection. Contiguous vertebral involvement is seen more frequently in infections than in tumors. Fat planes often are obscured diffusely as a result of edema with infection, whereas they are often intact or only focally altered with tumors (134).

Despite the accuracy of MRI, an absolute diagnosis must be based on bacteriologic or histologic examination of the pathologic tissue (99,135,136). The only circumstances in which the diagnosis may be made without a tissue biopsy include pediatric discitis (rare in the cervical spine) and signs and symptoms of spinal infection in a patient with a positive blood culture.

Needle biopsies can be performed safely throughout all regions of the spine (137,138). A definite diagnosis is possible with a percutaneous needle biopsy in 68% to 86% of patients (76,82,137,139,140,141). A false-negative result of a needle biopsy occurs often in patients being treated with antibiotics at the time of the biopsy. Open biopsies have lower false-negative rates because the surgeon can select grossly abnormal tissue and provide the pathologist with a larger tissue sample (76). In the cervical spine, open biopsy is often performed as part of the definitive surgical procedure.

During evaluation of a patient with suspected cervical spinal infection, the spine must be protected, and the patient's neurologic status must be examined frequently. Infections in the cervical spine are more likely to lead to instability and neurologic compromise than involvement of the thoracolumbar region (Fig. 62.4). A severe or progressive neurologic deficit is a surgical and medical emergency. If the spine is unstable, MRI-compatible Gardener-Wells tongs and cervical traction should be applied, and MRI or CT should be performed urgently.

Management

The goals of treatment are to establish the diagnosis, to prevent or reverse neurologic deficits, to relieve pain, to establish spinal stability, to eradicate the infection, and to prevent relapses. Antibiotic therapy and surgery play major roles in the treatment of spinal infections, but attention to good general medical care remains a vital part of the treatment. Associated conditions that compromise wound healing or immune response should be managed aggressively. Proper nutrition and the reversal of metabolic deficits and hypoxia are essential. Diabetes mellitus and other systemic illnesses, including coexistent infections, should be brought under control (44). Most infections in the thoracic and lumbar spine can be managed effectively with antibiotics and immobilization. Infections in the cervical spine have a higher risk for complications, and surgical treatment is often required in addition to antibiotic therapy.

When possible, the choice of antibiotic agent should be determined by the culture and sensitivity results so that the most specific and least toxic agent can be used. Antibiotic treatment should be withheld until an organism is identified on culture of a biopsy specimen because, in some cases, a second biopsy is required for additional culture material. Patients who have systemic toxicity or neurologic deficit, however, should be treated with maximal doses of broad-spectrum antibiotics as soon as the biopsy has been completed before culture results are available. Antibiotics should be administered parenterally for 6 weeks, followed by an oral course of antibiotics until the disease is resolved. Parenteral therapy for less than 4 weeks results in a higher rate of failure (44,75,76,81).

The ESR is a reasonable guide to assess the therapeutic response and can be expected to decrease to one half to two thirds of pretreatment levels by the completion of successful treatment (76,81,96,110,115). Repeat biopsy is indicated if the ESR does not decrease with treatment or if the patient does not respond clinically as expected. The CRP level provides another method of following treatment response. Preliminary data suggest that it is as good as the ESR for monitoring the effectiveness of treatment (142).

Patients should be immobilized to control pain and to prevent deformity or neurologic deterioration. The requirements for bracing patients in the postoperative period or in selected individuals not undergoing surgery depend on the severity of the infection, the quality of host bone, and, if surgery is performed, the stability of the bone graft. In general, upper cervical spinal infections require a halo vest. Lesions in the lower cervical spine can be managed in a cervicothoracic orthosis or hard collar if resection and grafting have involved one or two levels. For more extensive infections, a halo vest is recommended.

Surgical treatment is indicated in the following circumstances: (a) to obtain a bacteriologic diagnosis; (b) to drain a severe abscess (spiking fevers and septic course); (c) to treat infections refractory to nonoperative treatment (persistently increased ESR or CRP or persistent pain); (d) to decompress neural elements in the presence of a neurologic deficit; and (e) to prevent or correct spinal deformity or instability (44,75,143,144).

The timing of surgery must be individualized. A progressive neurologic deficit or a severe abscess is a surgical emergency, but most spinal infections can be managed less urgently. Preoperative traction is recommended for spinal realignment and indirect spinal cord decompression in patients with extensive bony collapse and deformity.

In nearly all patients, the spine should be approached anteriorly to provide direct access to the infected tissues and to allow adequate débridement. In patients with epidural extension, the posterior longitudinal ligament should be excised to ensure that the neural elements are decompressed and the infected tissue is removed. Infections in the cervical spine may lead to extensive bone destruction extending laterally to the foramen transversarium and placing the vertebral artery at risk during débridement (145). The risk can be higher if the vertebral artery is tortuous, which has been shown in cadaver studies to occur in 2.7% of cases (146). Anterior exposure allows stabilization of the spine by bone grafting, which promotes rapid healing without collapse and facilitates rehabilitation (44,147–150). Laminectomy is contraindicated in most cases because it may lead to neurologic deterioration and increased instability (44,151, 152) (Fig. 62.5).

After débridement of the infected focus, autogenous iliac crest grafting can be performed during the same procedure. The graft should extend from healthy bone above to healthy bone below (44,143,148,149,153,154). Autogenous bone grafting after vertebral body resection in the presence of active infection is safe and effective (155,156). The mean number of vertebrae involved is two (75). When débridement requires more than a two-level corpectomy, a fibular graft may be used (157). In cases of severe kyphotic deformity, anterior débridement and reconstruction with autogenous bone grafts should be the first procedure (147,148, 149,157,158). Posterior stabilization and arthrodesis are indicated in cases of severe kyphosis or spinal instability or when postoperative bracing is not possible (148,151,157). Posterior instrumentation in the setting of active disease is controversial, and no series has been reported showing acceptable results in the cervical spine, although a recent report by Przybylski and Sharan (159) included two patients with cervical discitis and osteomyelitis treated successfully by single-stage autogenous bone grafting and internal fixation. Posterior instrumentation of the thoracolumbar spine has been effective in tuberculous infections (160,161) and pyogenic infections (157,162–169) and may prove to be acceptable in the cervical spine.

Zigler and others (106) described five patients with pyogenic osteomyelitis of the upper cervical spine and occiput treated by antibiotics and surgery. Two were treated by anterior débridement and occipitocervical arthrodesis, one by transoral drainage, one by posterior occipitocervical arthrodesis, and one by posterior arthrodesis of C1 and C2; all five patients recovered. Loembe (170) described three patients treated in a delayed fashion with anterior plate fixation. The procedure was performed after 3 weeks of intravenously administered antibiotics and cervical traction. More recently, Rezai and associates (168) reported on

the treatment of spinal infections by one-stage surgical débridement and stabilization. Their series included 26 cervical infections, of which 19 were treated with anterior instrumentation at the time of initial deébridement. They found that use of cervical instrumentation did not preclude the successful eradication of infection.

Prognosis

Relapse of infection occurs in up to 25% of patients but is much less common if antibiotics are administered for more than 28 days (44,76). The mortality rate is less than 5%, and death is much more likely in elderly patients and those with an underlying disease (44,76). Factors that predispose a patient to paralysis include older age, a more cephalad level of infection, and a history of diabetes mellitus or rheumatoid arthritis (44). Fewer than 7% of patients overall have residual neurologic deficits (44,76). Diabetic patients are more likely to have neurologic deficits, and patients with thoracic involvement are the least likely to recover (44,76).

Eismont and associates (44) described the results of operation on 14 patients with spinal cord paralysis. The condition of the 7 patients who underwent laminectomy deteriorated, and the condition of 4 remained unchanged. In contrast, half the patients treated by an anterior procedure recovered normal or nearly normal function, and no patient's condition was made worse by the procedure. They found that the prognosis of the patients with paralysis from cervical spinal infection is better with surgical treatment. The results of anterior débridement and primary bone grafting in conjunction with the full course of antibiotics are favorable (44,75,107,143,147,154,171,172). Stone and colleagues (107) described 18 patients treated surgically for osteomyelitis of the cervical spine. Nine patients had myelopathy, and four had radiculopathy. Solid fusion was achieved in all patients, and at the final follow-up, all were ambulatory and neurologically intact.

Spontaneous fusion occurs in about 50% of patients treated nonoperatively for vertebral osteomyelitis (76,118,173). The more cephalad the level of infection is the higher the rate of spontaneous fusion. Almost all patients with cervical infection experience spontaneous fusion (110,174).

Infants with vertebral osteomyelitis have a poor prognosis and a high recurrence rate (100,101). Intravenous drug users have a surprisingly good prognosis; in 67 patients (18 with cervical infection) reported in the literature (79), no deaths or permanent neurologic sequelae occurred. HIV status does not appear to affect the neurologic outcome of patients with spinal infections (175).

Spinal Infection from Traumatic Injuries

Penetrating Trauma

High-velocity combat injuries require aggressive débridement of the missile tract to prevent infection. Low-velocity

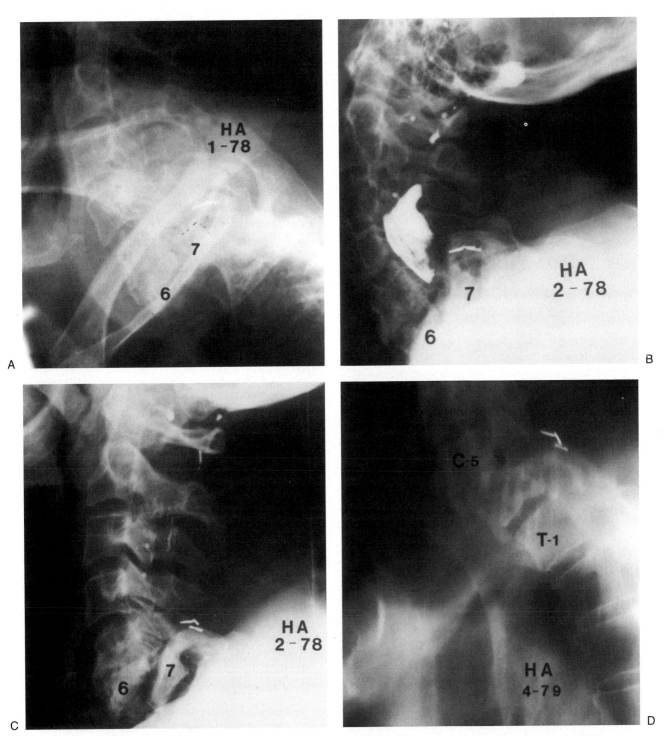

FIG. 62.5. Cervical instability secondary to laminectomy for treatment of an epidural abscess. This patient presented with progressive quadriplegia from an epidural abscess. The extent of anterior involvement was not recognized, and he was treated with laminectomies of C5 through C7. Shortly after surgery, he dislocated C6 on C7, and his neurologic status deteriorated. He was placed in skeletal traction to reduce the dislocation and to decompress the spinal cord and subsequently underwent anterior decompression and fusion. He recovered to normal neurologic function. **A:** Lateral radiograph shows C6-C7 dislocation after laminectomies of C5 through C7. **B:** Lateral myelogram shows complete block at C6 and C7. **C:** Lateral radiograph taken with skeletal traction applied shows partial reduction of C6-C7 dislocation. **D:** Lateral tomogram taken 1 year after anterior decompression and fusion shows solid anterior fusion and good spinal alignment. (Courtesy of H. H. Bohlman.)

gunshot wounds and stab wounds, on the other hand, generally can be treated nonoperatively. Low-velocity gunshot wounds to the spine do not require débridement so long as the bullet does not traverse the esophagus or pharynx (68,176–183). Treatment of gunshot wounds that traverse contaminated viscus is controversial.

Schaefer and co-workers (184,185) recommend aggressive management for transpharyngeal gunshot wounds. If a pharyngeal wound is identified by endoscopy, they recommend intravenous administration of broad-spectrum antibiotics, neck wound exploration to repair soft tissue and to débride the cervical spine, and external immobilization for about 6 weeks.

Kupcha and colleagues (178) described 28 patients with low-velocity gunshot wounds to the cervical spine and found that routine exploration without specific indications was not beneficial. They recommended panendoscopy and arteriography for all patients and a short course (<7 days) of antibiotics given intravenously. If the bullet traverses the pharynx, they recommended following the guidelines from Schaefer and colleagues (185). The group at the Thomas Jefferson Medical Center subsequently concluded that débridement of the spinal wound is not necessary and recommend endoscopy with individualized management of the esophageal wound, 48 hours of antibiotics given intravenously, and no spinal débridement (Alex Vaccaro, M.D., personal communication, November 1995).

Blunt Trauma

Two groups (112,186) reported a total of eight cases of vertebral osteomyelitis at the site of a spine fracture. Osteomyelitis may develop as a complication of the fracture because the fracture creates a favorable environment for hematogenous infection. Alternatively, osteomyelitis may develop within the central portion of an osteoporotic vertebral body, perhaps because the bone is more hyperemic or because of vascular stasis. Infection may lead to a pathologic fracture of the vertebrae without the usual involvement of the disc space (112). This is an infrequent occurrence but should be considered in certain clinical settings.

Vertebral osteomyelitis has been reported to occur in the cervical and upper thoracic spine after blunt traumatic esophageal rupture (50,187). The esophageal injury may be due to direct trauma from bone fragments or vertebral osteophytes, from breakdown of contused esophageal tissue anterior to a fracture site, or from a rapid increase in intraluminal pressure (112,186). Patients may present with pain, fever, neck swelling, dysphagia, or odynophagia. Failure to make the diagnosis may lead to mediastinitis, airway compromise, and septicemia. Treatment requires surgical repair of the rupture, nasogastric drainage, and antibiotic therapy (50).

INFECTIONS OF THE SPINAL CANAL

Epidural Abscess

Epidemiology and Etiology

The incidence of pyogenic infections in the epidural space appears to be increasing (53,188,189). Nussbaum and co-workers (53) described 40 patients seen at one institution between 1979 and 1991. A substantial increase in infections was noted after 1988. They attributed the change to several factors, including an increase in the use of illicit drugs, increasing rates of spinal surgery and spinal anesthesia, and a heightened awareness of the disorder. Hlavin and associates (189) also documented an increasing incidence of epidural abscess, up to 1.96 patients per 10,000 admissions per year. Most patients are in the sixth decade of life (53,188,190). In a referral setting, an epidural abscess can be expected to occur in about 7% of the spinal infections encountered (191). The male-to-female ratio is about 1::1 (188,190). The cervical spine is involved in 6% to 18% of patients in most series (188, 191–195). Fifty-eight percent of cases occurred in the cervical spine in the series reported by Nussbaum and colleagues (53) and by Rigamonti and associates (196). They attributed the disproportionate number of cervical cases to the large number (40%) of intravenous drug users in their series. Redekop and co-workers (197) also reported a higher than expected percentage of cases occurring in the cervical spine (52%). Alcohol or drug use was a factor in only 4 of their 25 patients.

The primary source of infection can be identified in about 60% of cases (188). Infection may occur by hematogenous spread from a remote infection (53,188,190,192–194,198), by spread from a contiguous focus of vertebral osteomyelitis or a disc space infection, or by direct inoculation at the time of surgery, epidural corticosteroid injection, lumbar puncture, or epidural catheterization (53,188,190,192–194,198–200). Factors associated with a higher incidence of infection include diabetes mellitus, intravenous drug use, previous back trauma, and pregnancy (188,191,192,196,201).

Microbiology

In the preantibiotic era, S. aureus was the pathogen in almost all cases in which the organism was known (194). In later series (188,192–194,198), S. aureus accounted for about 60% of cases. From the results in 166 patients from five series, S. aureus accounted for 62%, aerobic streptococci for 8%, Staphylococcus epidermidis for 2%, gramnegative rods for 18%, anaerobes for 2%, and other bacteria for 1%; 6% of the organisms were unidentified (188,192–194,198). Intravenous drug users are frequently infected with gram-negative organisms, especially Pseudomonas species (53,198), although one series (202) documented a high percentage of drug users infected with S. aureus.

Pathogenesis and Pathology

Most epidural abscesses occur in the regions of the spinal canal where the epidural space is largest. Dandy's (203) cadaver dissections demonstrated that the epidural space is filled with fat and loose areolar tissue containing numerous veins. The size and shape of this space are determined by variations in the size of the spinal cord. The cervical spine has almost no fat between bone and dura. Except for a space dorsal to the origin of the spinal nerves, the epidural space is mostly a potential space. Ventrally, the dura is closely applied to the spinal canal from C1 through S2. Posteriorly, the space begins to appear at C7 and gradually deepens along the thoracic vertebrae to a depth of 0.5 to 0.75 cm between T4 and T8. The epidural space communicates with the posterior mediastinal spaces through the intervertebral foramina (204). The abscesses are more common anteriorly in the cervical spine, whereas most abscesses in the thoracolumbar spine occur posteriorly (3:1) (188,190,192–194,197,205,206,207). A higher prevalence of vertebral osteomyelitis, or discitis, in association with cervical epidural abscesses may be responsible for this observation (193,205).

The pathogenesis of the neurologic manifestations is related to either direct compression from epidural pus or granulation tissue or to embarrassment to the intrinsic circulation of the cord (192,194,201,208). A microangiographic study (209) in rabbits demonstrated that the initial neurologic deficit is related to compression rather than to ischemia.

Several authors have identified a correlation between the duration of infection and the gross appearance at surgery or postmortem examination. Corradini and associates (210) described an early presuppurative phase in which the inflammatory lesion was characterized by an epidural mass of swollen, red, friable fat without any gross pus. In patients who have had symptoms for less than 2 weeks, gross pus with varying amounts of red granulation tissue has been identified (188,192,201,210,211). In patients with symptoms of longer duration, granulation tissue is often identified on the dura (188,192,210,211). In delayed cases when symptoms have been present for 150 days or more, grayish white granulation tissue or fibrous tissue has been found (211). Some authors (193,194,198) argue that it is not always possible to predict whether pus or granulation tissue is likely to be found at surgery.

Clinical Presentation

Patients with an epidural abscess have varied presentations, which causes initial misdiagnosis in about 50% of cases (188). Long delays between presentation and definitive treatment are common.

Most authors attempt to distinguish between acute and chronic disease, but this distinction is somewhat arbitrary.

Most patients with an acute epidural abscess present with fever, axial pain, and spinal tenderness. These signs and symptoms may be lacking in patients with chronic disease (191–194,201,211). Several authors have claimed that the distinction between acute and chronic disease is not clinically relevant (53,189,197,212).

Without treatment, the disease frequently progresses through four stages: local spinal pain, radicular pain, weakness, and paralysis (194,201,210). The transition from one stage to another is highly variable; weakness and paralysis may not develop for many months, or they may occur suddenly and unpredictably in a matter of hours (188,191). Nuchal rigidity may occur in patients with an epidural abscess; therefore, this sign is not helpful in distinguishing an epidural abscess from meningitis or spinal cord abscess (192).

Diagnostic Evaluation

Patients with an acute epidural abscess generally appear sicker than those with vertebral osteomyelitis. The white blood cell count and the ESR generally are increased (191). Patients with chronic disease often appear to have fewer toxic responses, and the white blood cell count is normal (192). The definitive diagnosis is based on identification of the organism. Culture specimens taken directly from the abscess are positive in about 90% of cases. Blood cultures have positive results in 60% of cases, and cultures of cerebrospinal fluid (CSF) yield the organism in about 11% of cases (188,192–194,198). Plain radiographs frequently are normal unless an established disc space infection or focus of vertebral osteomyelitis is present (Fig. 62.3). Radionuclide studies may be helpful, but they are nonspecific. Results may be falsely negative (202) and may result in a delay in treatment. A gallium scan may be slightly more sensitive than a technetium scan (202).

In the past, myelography was the standard imaging modality. It was often necessary to perform injections at sites above and below the abscess to demonstrate the extent of the epidural compression. A high-grade block is commonly seen. The lateral myelogram demonstrates whether the abscess is located anteriorly or posteriorly and is helpful for surgical planning (192,198,211). If pus is encountered during needle insertion, a specimen should be taken for a culture, but the thecal sac should not be entered. A second puncture for myelography should be performed at a different level. The CSF should be sampled at the time of myelography for cell count, glucose measurement, protein measurement, and culture. Bacteria may be present in the CSF in the 7% to 13% of cases in which the epidural abscess is complicated by meningitis or, more rarely, a subdural abscess (192,188,198,211). The CSF generally reflects a parameningeal infection with increased protein content.

Plain CT has a high false-negative rate, and in one study, it was diagnostic in only four of nine cases. Contrast-enhanced CT has been advocated by some authors (213). Unfortunately, it may miss the area of interest unless a myelogram is performed in conjunction with the study.

MRI is considered the imaging modality of choice (53,214–217). It is noninvasive and safe and can visualize the degree of cord compression and extent of the abscess in all directions. The MRI also permits diagnosis of disc space infection or vertebral osteomyelitis. Areas of infection appear as high signal intensity on T2-weighted images. False-negative results may occur with nonenhanced MRI, especially with extensive abscesses that do not have discrete cephalad and caudad borders (191). MRI also may be falsely negative in patients with concomitant meningitis because the signal changes in the abscess may be similar to those in the infected CSF (130). When the result of MRI is negative, myelography and postmyelographic CT should be performed if an epidural abscess is suspected. Some authors (214) claim that pus has a much higher signal intensity on T2-weighted sequences than granulation tissue and surrounding inflammatory edema. Other investigators (130) believe it is not possible to make such a distinction even with gadolinium-enhanced images.

Contrast enhancement is valuable for the detection of an epidural abscess as well as other spinal infections, especially if the infection spans multiple segments (89,130,131). Follow-up studies (218) on treated infection demonstrated a decrease in abscess size, but enhancement may persist in the disc or epidural space despite clinical improvement. This persistent enhancement may represent chronic granulation tissue or scar formation (218).

The differential diagnosis of an epidural abscess includes acute transverse myelitis (219), osteomyelitis, discitis, meningitis, subdural or intramedullary abscesses, vascular lesions, disc herniation, epidural hematoma, and tumors.

Management

An epidural abscess is a medical and surgical emergency. The goals of treatment are to eradicate the infection to preserve or improve the patient's neurologic status, to relieve pain, and to preserve spinal stability. A review of the literature from 1970 to 1990 (220) revealed 37 reported cases of epidural abscess that had been treated conservatively. These patients represented 6.6% of all published cases of patients with epidural abscess. During that time, 63% of the cases were managed successfully; although outcomes were disastrous in some. Baker and colleagues (192) noted that all five patients managed without surgery in their series died. Danner and Hartman (188) described six patients, and Hlavin and colleagues (189) reported eight patients, who required emergent laminectomy for neurologic deterioration while being treated with appropriate antibiotics for epidural abscesses. Piccolo and associates (221) reported on five patients treated surgically for cervical epidural ab-

scesses. They noted that patients did poorly if they had diabetes mellitus, if the epidural lesion was higher than C4, or if more than three levels were involved. Occipitocervical infections may fare better with nonoperative treatment (222).

Even the most ardent proponents (213,223) of nonoperative management of epidural abscesses recommend a nonsurgical approach only in selected cases: in poor surgical candidates, when the abscess involves a considerable length of the vertebral canal, when no severe neurologic deficit is present, or when complete paralysis has lasted more than 3 days. These authors think that patients whose condition is deteriorating neurologically should undergo operation.

Most authors consider surgical decompression in combination with antibiotic therapy to be the treatment of choice in all patients except those who could not tolerate an operation. The surgical approach depends on the location of the abscess. When the abscess is located posteriorly, laminectomy is the preferred treatment and is the most common procedure for thoracolumbar epidural abscesses (192,194). If a laminectomy is performed, the facet joints should be left intact to preserve spinal stability. Intraoperative ultrasonography after laminectomy allows the epidural mass to be localized (130). After a laminectomy, the wound may be closed over drains or packed open (188,192,194). Instrumentation and fusion may be necessary in patients in whom spinal stability has been compromised by decompression. In these patients, long-term follow-up is essential because of the risk for pseudarthrosis and persistent infection. Most cervical spinal epidural abscesses occur anteriorly; therefore, most abscesses in this region are débrided through an anterior approach (196,207).

As soon as the diagnosis is made, specimens should be obtained, and antibiotic therapy should be started immediately based on the results of the Gram stain and the known bacteriologic basis of the disease. Initial therapy should include a first-line antistaphylococcic agent. Gram-negative organisms should be suspected if the patient has a history of a spinal procedure or intravenous drug use. S. epidermidis should also be considered after spinal procedures (188). The definitive antibiotic therapy should be based on the culture and sensitivity results. Antibiotics should be given in maximum dosages for at least 2 weeks, and most authors recommend 3 to 4 weeks of parenteral therapy (188,192). Antibiotics must be administered parenterally for at least 6 to 8 weeks for coexistent vertebral osteomyelitis or disc space infection (188,192).

Prognosis

The natural history of an untreated epidural abscess is relentless progression of symptoms and possible death. In the preantibiotic era, the overall mortality rate was between 55% and 70% (201,208,224). The outcomes of patients with epidural abscess treated with surgical decompression and antibiotics appear to have improved in recent years as a result of improved diagnostic imaging, antibiotic therapy, and surgical techniques. A review (188) of early studies indicated that 39% of patients recovered fully, 26% had residual weakness but were able to ambulate, 22% were paralyzed, and 13% died. A combination of five later series (53,189,197,212, 225,226) indicated that 78% of patients treated surgically recover fully or with minimal weakness.

The prognosis for neurologic recovery depends on the duration and severity of the neurologic deficit (188,191, 194,198,227). Heusner (194) found that most patients with paresis for less than 36 hours had a complete recovery. No patient with a complete paralysis for longer than 36 to 48 hours recovered adequate neurologic function (194,228). Complete sensory loss is also considered a poor prognostic factor (228). Patients who have an acute progressive syndrome with complete paraplegia occurring within the first 12 hours have a poor prognosis, presumably because of spinal cord infarction rather than mechanical compression (202).

The prognosis for patients who have a cervical epidural abscess is not as favorable as that for patients who have infections in the thoracic and lumbar spine. The mortality rate is higher, and the neurologic deficits are more severe and refractory to treatment. The mortality rate in one recent series was 38% despite aggressive treatment (191). In another study of 23 patients treated in the past decade, only 4 of 10 patients who initially had less than antigravity strength improved enough to be ambulatory and continent of bowel and bladder despite surgical intervention within 36 hours of presentation (196). Other associated conditions thought to be poor prognostic factors are diabetes mellitus, advanced stage, female sex (191), HIV infection (202), and vertebral osteomyelitis (194).

Several authors have claimed that the distinction between acute and chronic disease has no prognostic importance. They found no difference in terms of clinical grade on presentation or functional recovery when patients were classified by duration of illness (53,212,189,197).

Subdural Abscess

Epidemiology and Etiology

Since Sittig first described spinal subdural empyema in 1927 (229), 44 cases have been described in the literature (230). Only 10 cases occurred in the cervical spine. The condition involves intrathecal infection of the spinal meninges. Similar to other infections of the spinal canal, a subdural abscess may occur by hematogenous spread from a distant focus of infection, by spread from a contiguous infection, or by direct inoculation (230,231). There is no apparent predilection for any age group, and the female-to-male ratio is about 2:1. Pregnant women and diabetic patients are two groups at risk for infection.

Pathogenesis, Pathology, and Microbiology

The paucity of reported cases prohibits definitive statements about the pathogenesis of this disorder. Autopsy results have been reported in only six cases. In their review of the literature, Levy and colleagues (230) identified five authors who stated specifically that spinal cord inflammation was not present. Most reports described local liquefaction necrosis with wallerian degeneration without evidence for microemboli or inflammation. Levy and colleagues (230) favored ischemia occurring after spinal cord compression as the pathogenesis of the neurologic sequelae that result from subdural abscesses. Most infections are caused by *S. aureus*, although other organisms, including streptococci, *E. coli,* and *Pseudomonas* species, have been reported (230).

Clinical Presentation

Fraser and associates (232) suggested that a patient with a subdural abscess presents similarly to one with an epidural abscess, except often there is no spinal percussion tenderness. In the review of the literature by Levy and colleagues (230), only one third of patients complained of spinal tenderness. In addition, not all patients with an epidural abscess have spinal tenderness, making that feature unreliable for distinguishing the two disorders (193,228). The clinical triad of fever, spinal pain, and spinal cord compression was present in about 40% of all cases reported in the literature (230).

Diagnostic Evaluation

The findings on laboratory analysis are similar to those in patients with epidural abscess. The white blood cell count and ESR are generally increased. CSF findings generally are consistent with a parameningeal process with increased protein level, a moderate pleocytosis, and a low to normal glucose level (230,232).

Myelography reveals an intradural extramedullary filling defect, usually with a complete spinal block, and may demonstrate defects at several levels (230–233). Fraser and associates (232) noted that there is no major anatomic barrier in the subdural space; therefore, an abscess in this location could extend more easily than an epidural abscess. They believed that the myelographic finding of multiple defects favors a diagnosis of a subdural abscess over an epidural abscess. Fraser and colleagues (232) also suggested that the radiographic finding of osteomyelitis in association with a myelographic block favors a diagnosis of epidural abscess because an infection in the subdural space is unlikely in association with vertebral osteomyelitis.

In the diagnosis of subdural abscess, MRI has been reported to be effective. The findings are similar to those of an epidural abscess (230). Similar to the arguments Fraser and colleagues (232) made for myelography, the findings of adjacent osteomyelitis suggest an epidural abscess, and multilevel or multiply loculated collections favor a diagnosis of subdural abscess (230).

Management

The appropriate treatment for subdural abscess is urgent decompressive laminectomy with irrigation and drainage in conjunction with appropriate antibiotic therapy. Because most subdural abscesses are caused by *S. aureus*, the initial antibiotic regimen must treat gram-positive cocci until culture and sensitivity results are available (230). Only one documented case was reported of a patient's condition improving after antibiotic therapy alone (234).

The prognosis for patients treated surgically and with antibiotics is reasonably good overall but guarded when the infection involves the cervical spine. Levy and colleagues (230) collected all cases reported in the literature through 1993. Thirty-two patients were treated with surgery and antibiotics after 1948, and documentation was adequate to assess the response to treatment: 12 patients made a full recovery, 11 had a marked recovery, 4 showed moderate recovery, 1 had mild recovery, and 4 died. Ten of the 32 patients had isolated cervical spinal involvement: 2 made a full recovery, 3 had a marked recovery, 1 showed moderate improvement, and all 4 deaths in the overall series occurred in patients with a subdural abscess in the cervical spine.

Intramedullary Spinal Abscess

Epidemiology and Etiology

Intramedullary spinal abscesses are rare infections. Bartels and colleagues found fewer than 100 cases reported since Hart first described the condition in 1830 (235,236). The thoracic cord was involved in 30 cases, the cervical spine in 16, and the lumbar cord in 12. Nineteen cases occurred in the thoracolumbar region, 6 occurred in the cervicothoracic area, and 10 involved the entire spine (235). The male-to-female ratio is about 3:1. The average age of affected females is younger than male patients.

Spinal cord abscesses generally occur by hematogenous spread from a distant focus of infection and, like abscesses in the epidural space, may be caused by a contiguous infection or by direct inoculation. In contrast to epidural abscesses, most patients are healthy before the onset of infection. A review of the literature revealed that only 3 of 93 infections occurred in diabetic patients, and only two reported patients were intravenous drug users (235).

Microbiology

The agents responsible for abscesses in the spinal cord are similar to the pathogens causing epidural abscesses. In 56 reported cases in which the organism was identified, *Staphylococcus* was the causative agent in 22, and *Strepto-*

coccus was found in 15. The remaining cases were caused by various organisms, including gram-negative bacteria. In 10 patients, multiple organisms were cultured (235).

Clinical Presentation

Initial symptoms of an intramedullary spinal abscess include weakness (38.6% of patients), spinal pain (36.1%), fever (27.7%), and radicular pain (26.5%). At presentation, most patients have weakness (88.9%), and many have sensory loss (47.7%), sphincter disturbance (40%), and fever (25.6%) (235). The rarity of the condition and the unusual constellation of symptoms may lead to a considerable delay in diagnosis. The progressive clinical stages described for epidural abscess are usually not encountered in patients with spinal cord abscess, and the rate of progression of the disease is unpredictable.

Diagnostic Evaluation

Surprisingly, analysis of CSF often yields normal findings or shows nonspecific increase in protein. Occasionally, inflammation or pus is encountered. Plain CT scans may show a widened cord and possibly demonstrate the intramedullary abscess. Myelography and postmyelographic CT scans usually show a block and a widening of the cord. Although MRI has been described (235) in only eight cases, it is now the diagnostic method of choice. In addition to a widened cord, the lesion may have signal characteristics typical for infection. The lesion is usually isointense or hypointense on T1-weighted sequences. In three of five cases, signal intensities were increased on T2-weighted sequences. The lesions enhanced with gadolinium administration in two of three cases (235). Definitive diagnosis is made from culture results of a biopsy specimen taken during surgery.

Management and Prognosis

Treatment of a spinal cord abscess is urgent surgical drainage and antibiotic therapy. The disease was universally fatal in the preantibiotic era, and several patients treated later with antibiotics but not surgically also died. Only 8 of the 59 patients reported in the literature who have been treated surgically have died, 6 of whom did not receive antibiotics postoperatively. With appropriate treatment, the prognosis is favorable: 22% of patients made a complete recovery, 55.9% had improvement, 6.8% had no change, 1 patient's condition deteriorated, and 2 patients died (235).

GRANULOMATOUS INFECTIONS (TUBERCULOSIS)

Granulomatous infections may be caused by fungi, certain bacteria, and spirochetes. These disorders have similarities in clinical presentation and in histologic features. Most bacteria cause pyogenic infections, but bacteria in the order Actinomycetales cause chronic granulomatous infections. This order includes the following families of pathogens: Mycobacteriaceae (genus: *Mycobacterium*), Actinomycetaceae (genera: *Actinomyces, Arachnia*), and Nocardiaceae (genus: *Nocardia*). Tuberculosis is the most common granulomatous spinal infection worldwide. The clinical features of the other granulomatous infections are similar to tuberculous spondylitis, and the surgical principles are the same (97,217). The chemotherapeutic management of these infections is highly variable and is beyond the scope of this discussion. The help of an infectious disease specialist is often required when treating these conditions.

Epidemiology and Etiology

The incidence of tuberculous spondylitis (Pott disease) varies considerably throughout the world and is generally proportional to the quality of the public health services available. In affluent countries, the incidence has decreased dramatically in the past 30 years, and until recently, the disease was quite uncommon. In 1986, the number of new cases of tuberculosis increased 2.6% for the first time in several decades (237). The growing number of patients immunocompromised by the acquired immunodeficiency syndrome (AIDS) or other conditions is thought to be responsible for the resurgence of tuberculosis.

Spinal involvement develops in about 50% of patients with tuberculosis (238). Hsu and Leong (239) reviewed the Hong Kong experience with cervical Pott disease. Of 1,100 patients with spinal tuberculosis, 40 (3.69) had disease localized between C2 and C7. In a larger series (240) of 5,393 cases of spinal tuberculosis, the atlantoaxial level was involved in only 15 cases (0.3%). Fang and co-workers (241) noted that, between 1957 and 1959, a total of 587 cases of spinal tuberculosis were seen, and 42 of the cases (7.2%) occurred in the cervical spine. The total number of involved cervical vertebrae was 99, of which 18 involved either C1 or C2. Lifeso and associates (3) had a disproportionately large number of patients with C1 and C2 involvement in their series of 107 patients from Saudi Arabia. Six patients had atlantoaxial involvement, and 9 patients had disease localized from C3 through C7.

Spinal tuberculosis generally occurs by hematogenous spread from a distant focus of infection. The pulmonary and genitourinary systems are the most frequent sources, but tuberculosis also may spread from other skeletal lesions (242,243). The spine also may become infected by direct extension from visceral lesions (242).

Pathogenesis and Pathology

The three major types of spinal involvement are peridiscal, central, and anterior, listed in decreasing order of prevalence (244). Atypical forms of spinal tuberculosis include those with neural arch involvement only and rare cases of epidural or intradural tuberculomas without bony involvement (245–247).

With peridiscal disease, the infection begins in the metaphyseal area and spreads under the anterior longitudinal ligament to involve the adjacent bodies. In contrast to pyogenic infections, the disc is relatively resistant to infection and may be preserved, even with extensive bone loss.

In patients with primarily anterior involvement, the infection spreads beneath the anterior longitudinal ligament and may extend over several segments. The scalloping erosion of the anterior aspect of the vertebral body may be from changes in local vertebral body blood supply (248).

With central involvement, the disease begins within the middle of the vertebral body and remains isolated to one vertebra. Central lesions tend to lead to vertebral collapse and therefore are the most likely type to produce severe spinal deformity (242).

Several pathogenic findings distinguish tuberculous spondylitis from pyogenic infections. In tuberculous infections, large paraspinal abscesses are more common, and the disc is more resistant. The pathologic changes generally take longer to develop and frequently are associated with greater deformity in tuberculosis (115,117,242,249). In 13 of the patients described by Hsu and Leong (239), cord compression was caused by an abscess; in 4 patients, the cause was a kyphotic deformity. Fang and colleagues (241) noted that the upper cervical cord can be damaged from tuberculosis by atlantoaxial subluxation (Fig. 62.6), upward translocation of the dens, compression from an abscess, or tuberculous invasion of the cord.

An epidural granuloma is analogous to a pyogenic epidural abscess. Most frequently, the granuloma arises by spread from the adjacent bone, but it occurs rarely by hematogenous seeding without any bony involvement (3,173, 245,247). Other lesions that may cause a neurologic deficit without bony involvement are tuberculous arachnoiditis, meningitis, and intradural extramedullary and intramedullary tuberculomas (3,173,250,251). Paraplegia from extraosseous disease occurs in about 5% of cases (3). The pathologic features of tuberculous spondylitis may be altered by secondary pyogenic infection that may occur through sinus tracts or after débridement (242).

Clinical Presentation

The classic presentation of a patient with tuberculous spondylitis includes spinal pain with manifestations of chronic illness, such as weight loss, malaise, and intermittent fever. The physical findings include local tenderness, muscle spasm, and restricted motion. Retropharyngeal abscesses may lead to swallowing problems or airway obstruction (239–241,252) (Fig. 62.6). The patient also may have a spinal deformity and neurologic deficit. In developing countries, the complications of neglected disease, such as paraplegia, kyphosis, and draining sinuses, may be the

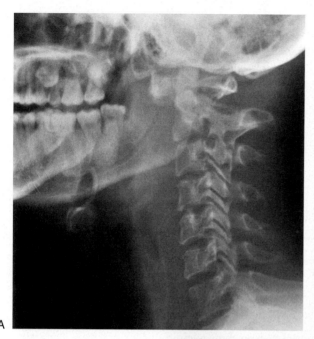

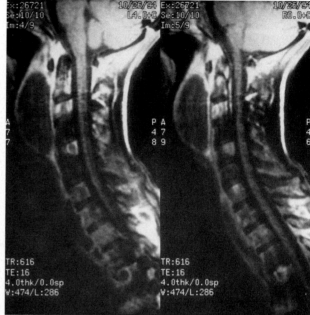

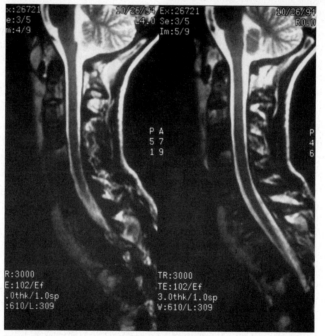

FIG. 62.6. A 25-year-old man presented with dysphagia and respiratory distress. He had a 5-month history of pain in the left wrist, left ankle, and right thigh and intermittent fever. Emergency studies revealed a large retropharyngeal abscess, involvement of multiple cervical and thoracic vertebrae, and C1-C2 instability. The patient was placed in traction immediately, and a tracheostomy was performed, followed by anterior cervical incision and drainage. The wound was closed over a drain. Posterior C1-C2 fusion was performed 5 days after incision and drainage, and the patient was maintained in a halo vest for 3 months. Multiple-extremity soft tissue abscesses and sinus tracts were present, and all resolved with antibiotic therapy. The left distal radius also required incision and drainage. *Mycobacterium tuberculosis* grew on cultures, and the patient was treated with isoniazid, rifampin, pyroxamine, and ethambutol. **A:** Lateral radiograph shows C1-C2 subluxation and large retropharyngeal abscess. **B:** T1-weighted magnetic resonance imaging (MRI) with gadolinium shows large retropharyngeal abscess with peripheral enhancement extending from the skull base to the inferior aspect of T9. There is bony involvement of all cervical and upper thoracic vertebral bodies, with sparing of the disc spaces. **C:** T2-weighted sagittal sequences show similar findings, but the retropharyngeal mass is not as well seen. **D:** Axial T1-weighted sequences show a large retropharyngeal abscess with extension into the epidural space and involvement of the atlantoaxial joints. The airway is narrowed and displaced anteriorly. **E:** The wall of the abscess cavity was opened, and 275 mL of purulent material was drained. **F:** Lateral cervical spine radiograph shows solid C1-C2 fusion 3 months after operation.

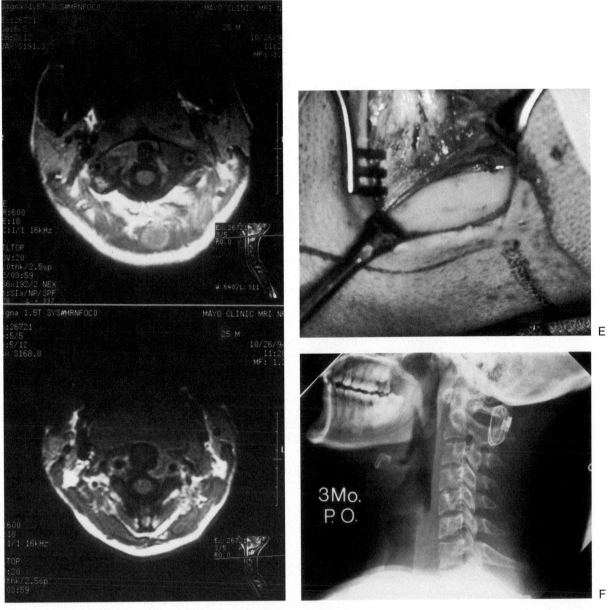

FIG. 62.6. *Continued*

presenting complaints (253–256). In the two series from Hong Kong, torticollis was present in 45% of patients with subaxial involvement (239), and five of six patients with atlantoaxial disease (241). One of the patients had rotatory fixation of the C1 and C2 joints. Eleven of the 40 patients with subaxial involvement (239) presented with deformity. Kyphosis averaged 26 degrees.

Retropharyngeal abscesses are common, especially in young children (239,241). Two of six patients with atlanto-axial involvement had a discharging sinus in the neck (241). Five of 40 patients with subaxial involvement had discharging sinuses, but none communicated with the spine (239). The authors noted that the thick cervical prevertebral fascia contained the abscess preventing sinus formation.

In 10% to 47% of patients, neurologic deficits develop during the course of the disease (1,243,248,249,257–259). The incidence of paralysis is highest with spondylitis in the thoracic and cervical spine (239,241,246,259). Spinal cord involvement was present in the Hong Kong series in 43% of the patients with subaxial disease (239) and in four of six patients with atlantoaxial involvement (241). Hsu and Leong (239) noted that the clinical findings of subaxial tuberculosis are influenced by age. Children younger than 10 years had extensive involvement with large abscesses. Patients older than 10 years had more localized disease with less pus but a higher incidence of paralysis (17% compared with 81%).

A distinct syndrome has been reported in heroin users with tuberculous spondylitis. All five patients in one series

(257) had an acute toxic reaction with fever, back pain, weight loss, night sweats, and rapidly evolving neurologic deficits. All patients had disseminated tuberculosis with involvement of extravertebral sites.

Diagnostic Evaluation

The diagnosis of cervical tuberculosis is frequently delayed as a result of the rarity of the condition and the nonspecific initial symptoms (239,252,260). The differential diagnosis of cervical Pott disease includes pyogenic vertebral osteomyelitis or other granulomatous spine infections, retropharyngeal abscesses, primary bone tumors or metastatic disease, trauma, and degenerative disease.

The ESR generally is increased with tuberculous spondylitis. The tuberculin purified protein derivative skin test result is usually positive and indicates past or present exposure to Mycobacterium (3). Cultures of early-morning urine samples may be helpful in patients with renal involvement, and sputum specimens and bronchial washings may be positive with active pulmonary disease. These laboratory findings are helpful, but an absolute diagnosis can be made only by biopsy of the spinal lesion or associated soft tissue mass (149). Because the vertebral lesions frequently are lytic and may be associated with a paraspinal abscess, CT-directed fine-needle biopsies have proved effective in confirming the diagnosis (261). Because most patients with cervical involvement undergo surgery, the biopsy can be performed in an open fashion. Culture of the aspirate from a subcutaneous abscess may reveal the organism and obviate the need for a spinal biopsy.

The earliest finding on plain radiographs is bone rarefaction. With peridiscal involvement, disc space narrowing is followed by bone destruction similar to pyogenic infections. With anterior multilevel spinal involvement, the anterior aspect of several adjacent vertebrae may be eroded in a scalloped fashion. Central body involvement generally resembles a tumor with central rarefaction and bone destruction followed by collapse (244).

Radionuclide scanning with technetium or gallium may help define the extent of disease (262). Unfortunately, radionuclide scans are not sensitive for tuberculous infection. Technetium bone scans are negative in 35% of cases, and gallium scans are negative in 70% (3). SPECT scans may prove to have better sensitivity than planar scans (124). CT is useful to delineate soft tissue changes around the spine and in the canal and clearly demonstrates the extent of bony involvement. Postmyelographic CT is helpful in cases with neurologic involvement but is performed less commonly now because of the availability of MRI.

MRI is the imaging modality of choice because it demonstrates the bony and soft tissue involvement and is capable of direct imaging in multiple planes. The intervertebral disc may have a normal signal on MRI, reflecting the resistance of the disc to tuberculous infection. The MRI findings are different from those in pyogenic infection and reflect the

pathologic types described earlier (263,264). The signal changes on T1- and T2-weighted sequences are similar to those described for pyogenic infections (133), except the disc may not have an increased signal on T2-weighted images (264) (Fig. 62.6). Gadolinium-enhanced scans are helpful in demonstrating abscesses as well as the extent of osseous involvement (118,131,133). Enhanced MRI can distinguish abscesses from granulation tissue. A mass with enhancement at the periphery but not the center is generally an abscess, whereas a mass with near-total enhancement is generally granulation tissue (265).

Management

The goals of management are to eradicate the infection and to prevent or treat neurologic deficits and spinal deformity or instability. Chemotherapy is an integral part of the management of spinal tuberculosis. The only cases in which chemotherapy is not indicated are those in which late-onset paraplegia from progressive deformity occurred in a patient with healed inactive disease. Drug therapy usually is started preoperatively but may be started postoperatively if a biopsy is necessary. The first-line drugs currently in use include isoniazid, rifampin, pyrazinamide, streptomycin, and ethambutol. The second-line agents used occasionally in special circumstances include ethionamide, cycloserine, kanamycin, capreomycin, and p-aminosalicylic acid. The choice of agents, dosages, and duration of therapy should be directed by an infectious disease expert. Multiple drugs are used because of the potential for resistance to a single agent. Selection of rational combinations of drugs is based on the mechanism of action and toxicity of the agents (266).

In 1963, the Medical Research Council Committee for Research on Tuberculosis in the Tropics began to investigate the widely divergent forms of treatment available at that time. A subcommittee, the Working Party on Tuberculosis of the Spine, initiated several large-scale, controlled prospective trials of treatment methods. The design of each study was based on the available resources in areas where tuberculosis was endemic. The Research Council concluded that the treatment of choice for spinal tuberculosis in developing countries is ambulatory chemotherapy with 6- or 9-month regimens of isoniazid and rifampin. Surgery was recommended only for biopsy or the management of myelopathy, abscesses, or sinuses (267,268). The latest 15-year follow-up supports these initial recommendations (269). Furthermore, the Council showed that bed rest, cast immobilization, and long-term antibiotic therapy (18-month regimen) were no better than out-patient short-course antibiotic therapy (269). Surgery, however, was better when patients were younger than 15 years old or a kyphotic deformity was greater than 30 degrees (270).

Unlike thoracolumbar Pott disease, however, surgery plays a primary role in the treatment of cervical tuberculous spondylitis. Disease in the cervical spine is frequently associated with neurologic compromise (241), and the prognosis of patients treated surgically is better than that of patients managed nonoperatively (3,248,257,258). Surgery is also indicated for biopsy, the management of severe abscesses, failed medical therapy, and deformity. The surgical approaches to the cervical spine are simple and have low morbidity.

Before surgery, patients with pathologic fractures, kyphotic deformity, or spinal instability should be immobilized in skeletal traction. Realignment of the spine decompresses and protects the cord. Surgical treatment is best performed soon after diagnosis because the procedure is technically easier and the prognosis of neurologic recovery is better. Abscesses tend to dissect along tissue planes. If surgery is delayed, fibrosis makes the procedure more difficult. The duration of neurologic symptoms before operation and the time for recovery of neurologic deficits correlate directly (257,271). Surgery also may be performed for late-onset paralysis associated with cord compression by a hard bony ridge in association with kyphosis.

When surgical treatment is necessary, radical débridement and anterior strut graft fusion in association with chemotherapy (the Hong Kong operation) are recommended (148,165,248,249,253,256,272,273). The spine is approached anteriorly so that the affected area may be treated most directly. Upper cervical spinal infections may be débrided through a transoral approach (3,4,240,241) or through the anterior retropharyngeal approach (274). Lesions between C3 and C7 may be approached through the anterior triangle or the posterior triangle. The latter may be preferable in some cases because abscess cavities often extend into the posterior triangle, making dissection easier (275).

The sequestered bone and caseous material must be débrided to bleeding bone above and below and to the posterior longitudinal ligament. The decompression should expose the dura in patients with neurologic deficit when spinal cord decompression is necessary (276). The angular deformity is corrected by insertion of a strut graft. Autogenous bone grafting at the time of the primary débridement is reliable in adults and children (36,148,149,248,249, 253,257,277,278). The choice of graft material is based on considerations of graft incorporation and structural support. In general, autograft is preferred over allograft bone, although no series have compared the two types of grafts. Iliac crest graft is usually preferred when the defect involves one or two levels. Fibular grafts are useful to span larger defects. In children, allograft struts may be sufficient to achieve solid fusion with no recurrence of infection (279,280).

Because of the potential for wound dehiscence in patients who may be immunocompromised and have poor wound-healing potential, the wounds should be closed in layers with interrupted nonabsorbable sutures.

The only indication for a laminectomy in the treatment of spinal tuberculosis is atypical disease involving the neural arch and causing posterior spinal cord compression (151, 152,247,281). It is also reasonable in rare circumstances with posterior epidural or intradural tuberculomas without bony involvement (245,250); in all other cases, laminectomy is contraindicated because the procedure destabilizes the spine and may lead to further deformity and neurologic damage (152). If laminectomy is indicated, a fusion should be performed if any of the facets are removed or if a kyphotic deformity is already present (151).

In the series by Fang and colleagues (241) of six patients with upper cervical tuberculous infections, a supplementary arthrodesis of C1 and C2 was performed in one patient, and a posterior arthrodesis of C1 through C3 was used as the sole procedure in another patient. Hsu and Leong (239) described four patients with subaxial cervical involvement who underwent primary posterior arthrodesis. All four patients subsequently required an anterior débridement and arthrodesis, two for progressive kyphosis and two for suspected persistence of disease. Others (241,272) found that posterior arthrodeses alone were inadequate to maintain spinal alignment or to prevent late kyphosis and neurologic compromise. Güven and colleagues (282) recommended a single-stage posterior approach with rigid internal fixation without any anterior procedure for thoracolumbar tuberculosis. They described 10 patients who underwent that procedure. In all patients, stable fusion was achieved with resolution of the tuberculosis: the mean loss of correction was only 3.4 degrees. The authors did not recommend a single-stage posterior approach in patients with paraplegia, in the presence of a huge abscess requiring drainage, or in multisegmental involvement (more than two vertebral bodies).

Some authors recommend a two-stage procedure with an instrumented posterior fusion followed by anterior débridement and fusion for thoracolumbar tuberculosis. The rationale for a two-stage procedure is that, after anterior débridement and arthrodesis alone, an extensive portion of the correction is lost in the first 6 months to 2 years postoperatively (283,284). Anterior grafts do not always provide stable fixation, especially in cases in which the graft spans more than two disc spaces (285). Moon and others (160) reported on 39 adults undergoing a two-stage procedure for thoracolumbar tuberculosis. The instrumented posterior arthrodesis was followed by anterior débridement and fusion either in the same operative session or in a delayed fashion. They achieved excellent deformity correction without prior anterior release, and the loss of correction did not exceed 3 degrees. The tuberculosis resolved completely in all patients.

Yau and associates (286) performed two-stage procedures for severe kyphotic deformities of the spine. Only 1 of the 30 patients had deformity involving the cervical spine (C7 through T6). Halo pelvic traction was used for 40 weeks between the two stages, and the patient eventually had resolution of disease and 50% reduction in the deformity. Treatment was associated with substantial morbidity and mortality in the other 29 patients, including three deaths.

The traction caused posterior cervical joint degeneration in 18 patients, and severe neck stiffness developed in 8 of them. Avascular necrosis of the odontoid also developed in 9 patients. Aside from the morbidity of traction, extended periods of traction are not feasible in the current health care environment. Severe deformities are now managed in a single operative session or in closely staged procedures.

The risk of using spinal instrumentation despite active tuberculosis infection was studied by Oga and others (161), who evaluated 11 patients undergoing combined posterior instrumented arthrodesis and anterior débridement and arthrodesis. In none of the patients did infection persist or recur; no kyphotic deformities occurred postoperatively. The authors also evaluated the adherence properties of *Mycobacterium tuberculosis* and *S. epidermidis* to stainless steel. Scanning electron microscopy showed that the surface of the stainless steel was heavily colonized by *Staphylococcus* species and covered with a thick adherent biofilm. In contrast, only a few biofilm-covered microcolonies of *M. tuberculosis* were observed. They concluded that posterior instrumentation is not associated with persistence or recurrence of spinal tuberculosis infection.

Rare case reports (287) documented success in treating spinal infection in the thoracolumbar spine with anterior decompression and fusion with anterior instrumentation. Recently, Yilmaz and associates (288) described 38 patients treated with anterior débridement, strut grafting, and anterior instrumentation in those with kyphosis. All patients had thoracic or thoracolumbar involvement. In their series, 37 of 38 patients had less than 3 degrees loss of correction; 1 patient died. None had recurrence of disease. However, use of anterior instrumentation in the setting of infection must be done with caution. In one unreported case seen by one of the authors (JGH), anterior instrumentation failed because of the poor bone quality of the vertebral bodies adjacent to the infection. Further study may produce a definitive treatment algorithm, particularly for the cervical spine (289).

With the advent of posterior cervical lateral mass rods and plates, a single-stage posterior approach or two-stage procedure with posterior instrumentation may prove effective in selected cases of cervical spine involvement, but no series we are aware of have been reported to support that concept. Postoperative immobilization is generally accomplished with a halo vest or cervicothoracic orthosis. Posterior cervical instrumentation may obviate the need for such external support in the future, but the risks of the procedure have to be weighed against the standard approach of anterior radical débridement, arthrodesis, and postoperative external immobilization.

Many complications have been reported after surgery to treat spinal tuberculosis. Operative risk is greatest in elderly patients with extensive disease. In one series (273), the operative mortality was 2.9%, and an additional 1% of the patients died of the disease later. Early complications include wound sepsis, pleural effusion, pulmonary embolism, CSF fistula into the pleural cavity, progressive neurologic deficit, loss of graft fixation or graft fracture, atelectasis, pneumonia, air leak, Horner syndrome, and injury to one of the great vessels (290). Late complications include graft resorption, graft fracture, nonunion, and progressive kyphosis (158,285). The complication rates in the two Hong Kong series (239,241) of cervical spinal tuberculosis described earlier were minimal. Two of four anterior facet joint grafts of C1 and C2 became dislodged, and one of these patients had resubluxation of the atlantoaxial joint. A supplementary posterior arthrodesis after anterior débridement without fusion prevents that problem (Fig. 62.5).

Prognosis

The prognosis of patients treated for tuberculous spondylitis depends on the age and general health of the patient, the severity and duration of the neurologic deficit, and the treatment selected. Before the advent of chemotherapy, the mortality rate for patients treated nonoperatively was 12% to 43% (246,291). The rate for patients with a neurologic deficit was close to 60% (1). With the chemotherapeutic regimens now available, the mortality rate is generally less than 5% if the disease is diagnosed early, the patient complies with the regimen, and follow-up is frequent (2,3). The relapse rate approaches zero (3).

The risk factors for neural deficit include older age, more cephalad level of infection, increased loss of vertebral body height, and absence of paraspinal abscesses (259). These risk factors seem self-evident except for the absence of extensive paravertebral abscess. Drainage of pus and debris from the spinal canal releases pressure on the cord (259). Patients with neurologic deficit may improve spontaneously without operation or chemotherapy (281) or with chemotherapy alone (243,292), but in general, the prognosis is better with early operation (3,248, 258).

In the study of subaxial disease by Hsu and Leong (239), the results of anterior débridement and fusion were excellent. All patients were relieved of their neck pain within a few days after surgery, and at 9 months, all patients were clinically free of disease. Kyphosis was corrected from an average of 25.5 degrees before operation to 5.4 degrees at follow-up. All 12 patients with cord compression had complete neurologic recovery: eight patients recovered by 2 weeks, three within 3 months, and one after 4 months. Three of the four patients with neurologic symptoms from atlantoaxial involvement (241) were completely relieved of symptoms immediately after transoral decompression. The fourth patient had undergone a posterior fusion of C1 through C3 after a prolonged course of halo traction. This patient's condition deteriorated postoperatively but gradually improved during the ensuing 9 months. Solid fusion was achieved in all patients, and five of six patients had no neck symptoms other than mild torticollis in two.

GRISEL SYNDROME

Epidemiology and Etiology

Grisel syndrome refers to atlantoaxial subluxation as a result of ligamentous laxity induced by parapharyngeal inflammation. Sir Charles Bell (293) described the first case in 1830. His patient suffered a dislocation of the atlas as a result of a deep ulcer involving the posterior pharynx that "destroyed the transverse ligament." Other physicians (294) described similar cases in the 100 years between Bell's report and Grisel's article (295) in 1930. Desfosses (296) published a case report in the same year and called the condition *maladie de Grisel*. The eponym *Grisel syndrome* has been in common use since. Lopes and Li recently reported on two cases of midcervical instability in infants caused by upper respiratory tract infections (297). These may represent a variant of Grisel disease in the subaxial spine. Both patients were successfully treated nonoperatively.

In two large reviews (298,299) of the literature from the 1940s, more than three fourths of patients with Grisel syndrome were younger than 13 years. In 1969, Keuter (300) noted that the incidence of the condition in adults was increasing relative to that in children. Between 1981 and 1989, 11 patients with Grisel syndrome were described in the North American literature; their average age was 17.5 years (301). The widespread use of antibiotics for childhood infections may be responsible for the shift in age distribution (301). The disease still primarily affects persons younger than 30 years, in contrast to vertebral osteomyelitis, which is much more common in elderly persons (97).

Watson Jones (302) noted that the infection causing atlantoaxial subluxation did not need to be in the nasopharyngeal region "as suggested by Grisel." That fact has been confirmed by many authors (294,298,299,301,303–306), who have reported cases resulting from a wide variety of conditions, including upper respiratory tract infection, sinusitis, tonsillitis, otitis media, parotiditis, mastoiditis, acute rheumatic fever, and others.

Pathophysiology and Pathology

The pathophysiology of Grisel syndrome is not well defined; pathologic information is scant because most patients survive the condition. Parke and colleagues (307) performed injection studies of the valveless epidural sinuses of human perinatal cadavers. They demonstrated retrograde filling of a series of veins that had numerous lymphatic anastomoses and appeared to drain the posterosuperior pharyngeal region. They called these the pharyngovertebral veins (Fig. 62.7) and thought they could serve as a pathway for the spread of inflammatory processes to the atlantoaxial complex. Parke and colleagues (307) postulated that the age distribution of patients who have Grisel syndrome may be explained partly by the fact that the peripharyngeal lymphoid tissue is hypertrophic in childhood. The adenoids are

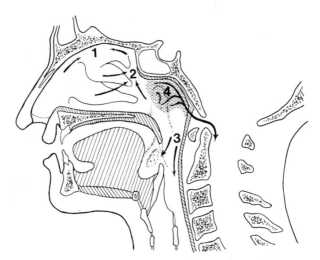

FIG. 62.7. Venous drainage of nasal cavity, nasopharynx, and oral pharynx. The upper lateral wall of the nasal cavity drains through the ethmoidal veins (1). The lower lateral wall of the nasal cavity drains into the pterygoid plexus (2). The oropharynx drains into the maxillary veins and posterior pharyngeal plexus (3). The posterior nasopharyngeal region (*cross-hatched area*, 4) drains by way of the pharyngovertebral veins through the pharyngobasilar fascia and anterior atlantooccipital membrane to communicate with the periodontoidal plexus and epidural veins. (From Parke WW, Rothman RH, Brown MD. The pharyngovertebral veins: an anatomical rationale for Grisel's syndrome. *J Bone Joint Surg Am* 1984;66:568–574, with permission.)

especially susceptible to inflammation in children and are located in the area drained by the pharyngovertebral venous plexus. This venous system provides an anatomic rationale for Grisel syndrome because it allows a hematogenous route for peripharyngeal septic exudates to enter the periodontoidal venous plexus and suboccipital epidural sinuses.

Parke and colleagues (307) suggested that surgical trauma may enhance the transport of inflammatory products into the pharyngeal vertebral plexus. This possibility would explain the cases of Grisel syndrome that occur after procedures such as tonsillectomy, adenoidectomy, or mastoidectomy. Positioning of the patient for these procedures also may be a factor (298,306,308,309). Because upper respiratory tract infections are so much more common than Grisel syndrome, Parke and colleagues (307) theorized that affected children must have an anatomic predisposition to instability.

The upper cervical spinal joints are much more mobile in children than in adults, and this trait is manifested by a greater atlantodental interval (310–312) and subaxial pseudosubluxation (313). Kawabe and associates (314) found that the facets of the axis in children are more steeply inclined in the coronal plane and more curved in the sagittal plane than in those of adults. Children with the greatest mobility presumably would be at higher risk for Grisel syndrome.

There are many theories concerning the pathologic changes that occur as a result of periodontoidal inflammation and lead to the development of atlantoaxial subluxation and rotatory deformities. Wittek (315) suggested that an effusion develops in the C1-C2 joints that stretches the facet capsules, and this stretching leads to excessive laxity. Coutts (316) implicated infolded inflammatory synovial fringes as the mechanism preventing reduction of the displaced joints. Grisel (295) believed that muscle spasm was primarily responsible for the displacement. Watson Jones (302) theorized that decalcification of the bone adjacent to the ligamentous attachments occurs as a result of inflammatory hyperemia and leads to ligamentous laxity. Hess and colleagues (308) suggested that reduction in the early stages of the disease is prevented by a combination of factors, including muscle spasms. Fielding and co-workers (317) concluded that a combination of swollen capsular and synovial tissues and muscle spasm is responsible for blocking reduction in the early stages. If the deformity is not reduced, ligament and capsular contractures can occur, leading to atlantoaxial rotatory fixation. Wortzman and Dewar (318) proved that muscle spasm alone is not the mechanism that prevents reduction of rotatory displacement. They described four patients who underwent infiltration of local anesthetic into the C1 and C2 joints. The patients experienced pain relief with decreased muscle spasm, allowing improvement in range of motion, but radiographs showed persistent rotatory deformity of C1 and C2.

Kawabe and colleagues (314) provided more information on the synovial fringes described by Coutts (316). They identified meniscus-like synovial folds at the occipitoatlantal and lateral atlantoaxial joints in infant cadavers but not in adults (Fig. 62.5). Inflammation, infolding, or rupture of the folds into the joints were cited as the explanation for rotatory fixation. Atrophy of the synovial folds with advancing age may be another explanation for the age distribution of atlantoaxial rotatory deformities.

Clinical Presentation

Patients with Grisel syndrome present with increasing pain in the neck region, spasm, and restricted motion. Fever may be present as well as the sign of the underlying infectious process. Rest and support of the head and neck may provide relief of pain, and patients may present supporting their heads in their hands.

If atlantoaxial rotatory deformity has occurred, torticollis is evident. The patient's head is rotated away from the anteriorly displaced C1 and C2 joints and tilted toward the involved side "like a bird with his head cocked listening for a worm" (318). The patient may be able to increase the deformity actively but cannot overcome the torticollis beyond the neutral position. Attempts to correct the deformity are painful (206,295,303,319,320). The sternocleidomastoid muscle on the side opposite the tilt may be in spasm as if

attempting to correct the deformity (295,320,321). On palpation, the C2 spinous process may be prominent and deviated to the side to which the chin is pointed, secondary to the lateral tilt of the head (319,320) or possibly from counterrotation of C2 in an attempt to realign the head (298). This phenomenon is known as the *Sudeck sign* (319,309), although it was described in 1907 by Corner (319), who also pointed out that the prominence of the C2 spinous process is caused by flexion and forward displacement of the head. Before the advent of radiography, examination of the pharynx was an important part of the assessment. Corner (319) noted that two prominences in the pharynx could be identified. The transverse process of the anteriorly rotated atlas would be palpated on one side, and the lateral mass of the axis would be prominent on the other side if the corresponding lateral mass of the atlas was rotated posteriorly.

Neurologic complications are uncommon (298,299,302–305,308,322). Only a few cases of neurologic involvement have been reported, ranging from hyperreflexia to quadriplegia (299,305,306,323,324). The neurologic deficit in one patient described by Wilson and co-workers (306) may well have been secondary to the patient's underlying meningitis.

Occipital neuralgia may occur because the greater occipital nerve is in close proximity to the facet capsule of C1 and C2 (303,320,325). In patients with long-standing atlantoaxial rotatory fixation, facial flattening may occur. This feature was noted on presentation in 7 of 17 patients in the series by Fielding and Hawkins (320).

With time, the torticollis may eventually resolve despite the persistence of the rotatory deformity of C1 and C2. This phenomenon was first described by Wortzman and Dewar (318), who noted that the abnormality returned to normal in only 1 of 23 cases. They thought that the improvement in head position was the result of compensation in the lower cervical spine. More recently, the compensatory rotation has been shown to occur primarily at the occipitoatlantal joint (320,326,327). Adults have less capacity for counterrotation of the occiput through C1 and therefore may have persistent deformity (327).

Diagnostic Evaluation

The ESR and white blood cell count may be increased, depending on the severity of the underlying infectious process. A spinal tap may be required to exclude the diagnosis of meningitis. In the absence of torticollis, static plain radiographs may be unremarkable, or they may show prevertebral soft tissue swelling, locally destructive processes, or subluxation of C1 and C2. Lateral flexion and extension radiographic views may demonstrate atlantoaxial instability. When torticollis is present, plain radiographs are difficult to interpret because of the rotation and tilt of the occiput through C2 complex (328). The lateral masses of the atlas may obscure the odontoid because of the forward location of one relative to the other (319). The two sides of the posterior arch of C1 may not be superimposed on a lateral radiograph because of the tilt of C1 (303,319). The transverse ligament may be incompetent, leading to a widened atlantodental interval. It is difficult to measure the atlantodental interval on plain radiographs. Lateral tomograms or CT scans (329) are often necessary to assess this critical factor. The atlantodental interval normally measures up to 3 mm in adults (312) and 4 mm (311,312,330,331) or 4.5 mm (310) in children.

On the anteroposterior, open-mouth projection, the lateral mass of the atlas that is rotated anteriorly appears wider and closer to the midline than its counterpart on the opposite side (318,319). The joint spaces of C1 and C2 appear asymmetric, often leading to a narrow joint space on one side and a widened space on the opposite side (303,318, 319). The spinous process of the axis may be rotated away from the side of the anteriorly displaced facet joint of C1 and C2 (Sudeck sign) (309,319).

Ironically, lateral flexion of the head causes more rotation of C2 than pure rotation of the head. Because of coupled motion, the spinous process of the axis is rotated to the side opposite the direction of head tilt and tilted in the same direction. Torticollis from any cause generally involves both rotation and head tilt, and therefore the axis often is rotated in one direction and tilted in the other (319).

In patients with Grisel syndrome, CT may be helpful for distinguishing cellulitis from an abscess (303). The alar and transverse ligaments can be visualized by CT, and thus it provides some information on the integrity of these structures (332,333). Plain CT is an excellent means of demonstrating abnormal relationships of C1 and C2 (99,303,321, 327,329,333,334). However, unless the facet joints of C1 and C2 are dislocated, the rotational deformities seen on a static CT scan may represent simple head rotation in a normal person because the joints are held within the physiologic range in most cases of atlantoaxial rotatory deformity.

Rinaldi and associates (334) were the first to recommend dynamic CT for the diagnosis of atlantoaxial rotatory fixation. Many authors have confirmed that obtaining a CT scan in maximal head rotation to the left and maximal rotation to the right is the best means of demonstrating the condition (99,321,326,327,333). It may be necessary to use MRI to exclude abscess formation (Fig. 62.6), cord compression, vertebral osteomyelitis or discitis, intraspinal abscess, and tumors suggested by the clinical findings.

Management

The goals of management are to treat the underlying infectious process, to restore normal pain-free range of motion, to prevent or reverse neurologic compromise, and to restore spinal stability. Antibiotic therapy and occasionally incision and drainage may be required to treat the infection. The spine should be immobilized and activities restricted until the process has resolved. Radiographs in flexion and extension can be taken after complete resolution of symptoms to determine whether the spine is stable. Attentive follow-up is essential because recurrence of deformity (321), ligamentous laxity (319), or potentially unstable counterrotation of the occiput (326,327,329) may occur.

The management of patients with atlantoaxial rotatory deformity caused by Grisel syndrome is based on the time from the onset of symptoms to presentation. If the deformity has been present for less than 1 week, Phillips and Hensinger (321) advise immobilization in a soft collar and bed rest for 1 week. If the deformity does not reduce, they advise hospitalization and the institution of traction. If the deformity has been present for more than 1 week but less than 1 month, they advise in-hospital traction followed by immobilization. If the patient presents more than 1 month after the onset of symptoms, they recommended attempting traction for up to 3 weeks, but if no reduction is achieved, arthrodesis should be considered for symptomatic patients. After reduction, they advise immobilization to allow the stretched and edematous ligaments to heal (321).

Fielding and Hawkins (320) advise immobilization for 3 months after reduction. Other authors recommended a period of 6 to 8 weeks (294) or until the patient has full pain-free range of motion (321). After immobilization, radiographs in flexion and extension should be obtained to exclude instability. Surgical management is advised for patients with atlantoaxial rotatory deformity with spinal instability (manifested by an atlantodental interval of more than 4 mm after adequate conservative management), for patients with neural involvement, or when conservative measures fail to achieve or maintain reduction (319).

When operation is indicated, a posterior arthrodesis of C1 and C2 is the procedure of choice. Preoperative traction should be attempted to reduce the deformity. If traction is not successful, however, in situ arthrodesis of C1 and C2 may be performed (319,321,335). Alternatively, the deformity can be reduced at surgery and the alignment maintained using minipolyaxial screws and rods, as described by Harms and Melcher (336). Three factors should be considered when performing in situ arthrodesis. First, the passage of wires may be more dangerous because the canal is narrowed with fixed atlantoaxial subluxation or rotation (303). Second, the final clinical result, although acceptable, may not be as good as fusion following reduction (335). Third, the improvement in torticollis is a consequence of compensatory occiput to C1 rotation (327). Conceivably, the abnormal position of the occiput and C1 joints may place the patient at some increased risk during future traumatic episodes, and the long-term effects of occiput and C1 hypermobility are unknown.

Prognosis

The prognosis for patients with Grisel syndrome is related to the duration of symptoms before institution of treatment and the degree of laxity of the transverse ligament. In the report by Phillips and Hensinger (321) of rotatory atlantoaxial subluxation, 16 children were examined less than

1 month after the onset of symptoms, and all had reduction of the deformity either spontaneously or after a short period of traction. Three of the seven children who were seen more than 1 month after the onset of symptoms eventually required fusion.

Recurrence of deformity in the series by Phillips and Hensinger (321) was much more common in the group with a longer delay before diagnosis or a more severe lesion. Recurrence developed in five patients with type II deformities (mild laxity of the transverse ligament), whereas none of the children with type I deformities (intact transverse ligament) had recurrence. The recurrences were within 2 weeks in two children, within 2 months in two, and within 4 months in one. No specific cause for the recurrences was identified. The cause of the initial subluxation was trauma in two and unknown in one; none of the nine children with Grisel syndrome had a recurrent deformity. The children with recurrences were rehospitalized and placed in traction. Reduction was achieved and maintained in three children, but the deformity in the other two could not be reduced, and they underwent arthrodeses.

Neurologic deficits, vertebral artery compromise, and fatalities are uncommon, but all have been reported with atlantoaxial rotatory deformity, especially in cases associated with transverse ligament laxity (303,319). Most cases of neurologic compromise secondary to Grisel syndrome resolved with appropriate treatment (299,305,306,323,324).

Facial asymmetry was found in 41% of the patients with atlantoaxial rotatory fixation described by Fielding and Hawkins (320). Only one of five patients who underwent arthrodesis had postoperative facial asymmetry. Two patients refused surgery and were treated conservatively; 8 years later, the symmetry of one patient's face remained unchanged, and the other had no clinical deformity or facial asymmetry (320).

Because 50% of cervical rotation occurs at the atlantoaxial joint, some loss of rotation occurs after fusion of C1 and C2. Fielding and colleagues (317) found that the motion was less restricted than expected and was age dependent. The average rotation lost was 13% in patients aged 20 years or younger, 25% in those aged 20 to 40 years, and 28% in those older than 40 years. Compensatory hypermobility of the occiput-C1 articulation may be responsible for the minimal loss of motion after fusion of C1 and C2. Persistent radiographic rotatory deformity of C1 and C2 occurs in a considerable number of patients and is often associated with compensatory counterrotation of C0 and C1 (327).

REFERENCES

1. Bosworth DM, Pietra AD, Rahilly G. Paraplegia resulting from tuberculosis of the spine. *J Bone Joint Surg Am* 1953;35:735–740.
2. Adendorff JJ, Boeke EJ, Lazarus C. Tuberculosis of the spine: results of management of 300 patients. *J R Coll Surg Edinb* 1987;32:152–155.
3. Lifeso RM, Weaver P, Harder EH. Tuberculous spondylitis in adults. *J Bone Joint Surg Am* 1985;67:1405–1413.
4. Fang SY, Ong GB. Direct anterior approach to the upper cervical spine. *J Bone Joint Surg Am* 1962;44:1588–1604.
5. Alonso WA, Black P, Connor GH, et al. Transoral transpalatal approach for resection of clival chordoma. *Laryngoscope* 1971;81:1626–1631.
6. Hadley MN, Spetzler RF, Sonntag VKH. The transoral approach to the superior cervical spine: a review of 53 cases of extradural cervicomedullary compression. *J Neurosurg* 1989;71:16–23.
7. Spetzler RF, Selman WR, Nash CL, et al. Transoral microsurgical odontoid resection and spinal cord monitoring. *Spine* 1979;4:506–510.
8. Ashraf J, Crockard HA. Transoral fusion for high cervical fractures. *J Bone Joint Surg Br* 1990;72:76–79.
9. McAfee PC, Cassidy JR, Davis RF, et al. Fusion of the occiput to the upper cervical spine. *Spine* 1991;16:S490.
10. Bertalanffy H, Eggert HR. Complications of anterior cervical diskectomy without fusion in 450 consecutive patients. *Acta Neurochir (Wien)* 1989;99:41–50.
11. Cuatico W. Anterior cervical diskectomy without interbody fusion: an analysis of 81 cases. *Acta Neurochir (Wien)* 1981;57:269–274.
12. Heller JG. Postoperative infections of the spine. In: Rothman RH, Simeone FA, eds. *The spine*, 3rd ed. Philadelphia: WB Saunders, 1992:817.
13. Lunsford LD, Bissonette DJ, Jannetta PJ, et al. Anterior surgery for cervical disk disease. I. Treatment of lateral cervical disk herniation in 253 cases. *J Neurosurg* 1980;53:1–11.
14. Espersen JO, Buhl M, Eriksen EF, et al. Treatment of cervical disk disease using Cloward's technique. I. General results, effect of different operative methods and complications in 1,106 patients. *Acta Neurochir (Wien)* 1984;70:97–114.
15. Mayr MT, Subach BR, Comey CH, et al. Cervical spinal stenosis: outcome after anterior corpectomy, allograft reconstruction, and instrumentation. *J Neurosurgery* 2002;96[Suppl 1]:10–16.
16. Kuriloff DB, Blaugrund S, Ryan J, et al. Delayed neck infection following anterior spine surgery. *Laryngoscope* 1987;97:1094–1098.
17. Newhouse KE, Lindsey RW, Clark CR, et al. Esophageal perforation following anterior cervical spine surgery. *Spine* 1989;14:1051–1053.
18. Smith MD, Bolesta MI. Esophageal perforation after anterior cervical plate fixation: a report of two cases. *J Spinal Disord* 1992;5:357–362.
19. Heggeness MH, Esses SI, Errico T, et al. Late infection of spinal instrumentation by hematogenous seeding. *Spine* 1993;18:492.
20. Richards BS. Delayed infections following posterior spinal instrumentation for the treatment of idiopathic scoliosis. *J Bone Joint Surg Am* 1995;77:524–529.
21. Henderson CM, Hennessy RG, Shuey HM, et al. Posterior-lateral foraminotomy as an exclusive operative technique for cervical radiculopathy: a review of 846 consecutively operated cases. *Neurosurgery* 1983.
22. Raaf JE. Surgical treatment of patients with cervical disk lesions. *J Trauma* 1969;9:327–338.
23. Bryan WJ, Inglis AE, Sculco TP, et al. Methylmethacrylate stabilization for enhancement of posterior cervical arthrodesis in rheumatoid arthritis. *J Bone Joint Surg* 1982;64:1045–1050.
24. Santavirta S, Slatis P, Kankaapaa U, et al. Treatment of the cervical spine in rheumatoid arthritis. *J Bone Joint Surg Am* 1988;70:658–667.
25. Weiland DJ, McAfee PC. Posterior cervical fusion with triple-wire strut graft technique: one hundred consecutive patients. *J Spinal Disord* 1991;4:15–21.
26. Wertheim SB, Bohlman HH. Occipitocervical fusion: indications, technique, and long-term results in thirteen patients. *J Bone Joint Surg Am* 1987;69:833–836.
27. Clark CR, Goetz DD, Menezes AH. Arthrodesis of the cervical spine in rheumatoid arthritis. *J Bone Joint Surg Am* 1989;71:381–392.
28. Segal LS, Drummond DS, Zanotti RM, et al. Complications of posterior arthrodesis of the cervical spine in patients who have Down syndrome. *J Bone Joint Surg Am* 1991;73:1547–1554.
29. Fehlings MG, Errico T, Cooper P, et al. Occipitocervical fusion with a five-millimeter malleable rod and segmental fixation. *Neurosurgery* 1993;32:198–207.
30. Sasso RC, Jeanneret B, Fischer K, et al. Occipitocervical fusion with posterior plate and screw instrumentation-a long-term follow-up study. *Spine* 1994;19:2364.
31. Itoh TI, Tsuji H, Katoh Y, et al. Occipito-cervical fusion reinforced by Luque's segmental spinal instrumentation for rheumatoid arthritis. *Spine* 1988;13:1234–1238.

32. Heller JG, Silcox DH 3rd, Sutterlin CE 3rd. Complications of posterior cervical plating. *Spine* 1995;20:2442–2448.

33. Anderson PA, Henley MB, Grady MS, et al. Posterior cervical arthrodesis with AO reconstruction plates and bone graft. *Spine* 1991;16[3 Suppl]:S72–S79.

34. Fehlings MG, Cooper PR, Errico TJ. Posterior plates in the management of cervical instability: long-term results in 44 patients. *J Neurosurg* 1994;81:341–349.

35. Levine AM, Mazel C, Roy-Camille R. Management of fracture separations of the articular mass using posterior cervical plating. Spine 1992;17[Suppl]:5445.

36. Petty W. The effect of methylmethacrylate on bacterial phagocytosis and killing by human polymorphonuclear leukocytes. *J Bone Joint Surg Am* 1978;60:752–757.

37. Petty W. The effect of methylmethacrylate on chemotaxis of polymorphonuclear leukocytes. *J Bone Joint Surg Am* 1978;60:492–498.

38. Branch CL, Kelly DL, Davis CH, et al. Fixation of fractures of the lower cervical spine using methylmethacrylate and wire: technique and results in 99 patients. *Neurosurgery* 1989;25:503–513.

39. Clark CR, Keggi KJ, Panjabi MM. Methylmethacrylate stabilization of the cervical spine. *J Bone Joint Surg Am* 1984;66:40–46.

40. Duff TA, Khan A, Corbett JE. Surgical stabilization of cervical spine fractures using methyl methacrylate. *J Neurosurg* 1992;76:440–443.

41. Wilde GP, Hopkins JS. The use of acrylic bone cement for cervical fusion in patients with rheumatoid arthritis. *J R Soc Med* 1988;81:523–525.

42. Eismont FJ, Bohlman HH. Posterior methylmethacrylate fixation for cervical trauma. *Spine* 1981;6:347–353.

43. McAfee PC, Bohlman HH, Ducker T. Failure of stabilization of the spine with methylmethacrylate: a retrospective analysis of twenty four cases. *J Bone Joint Surg Am* 1986;68:1145–1157.

44. Eismont FJ, Bohlman HH, Soni PL, et al. Pyogenic and fungal vertebral osteomyelitis with paralysis. *J Bone Joint Surg Am* 1983;65:19–29.

45. Connor PM, Darden BV 2nd. Cervical discography complications and clinical efficacy. *Spine* 1993;18:2035–2038.

46. Guyer RD, Ohnmeiss DD, Mason SL, et al. Complications of cervical discography: findings in a large series. *J Spinal Disord* 1997;10:95–101.

47. Grubb SA, Kelly CK. Cervical discography: clinical implications from 12 years of experience. *Spine* 2000;25:1382–1389.

48. Zeidman SM, Thompson K, Ducker TB. Complications of cervical discography: analysis of 4400 diagnostic disc injections. *Neurosurgery* 1995;37:414–417.

49. van Berge Henegouwen DP, Roukema JA, de Nile JC, et al. Esophageal perforation during surgery on the cervical spine. *Neurosurgery* 1991;29:766–768.

50. Pollock RA, Purvis JM, Apple DF, et al. Esophageal and hypopharyngeal perforation injuries in patients with cervical spine trauma. *Ann Otol* 1981;90:323–327.

51. Whitehill R, Sirna EC, Young DC, et al. Late esophageal perforation from an autogenous bone graft. *J Bone Joint Surg Am* 1985;67:644–645.

52. National Academy of Sciences-National Research Council. Postoperative wound infections and the influence of ultraviolet irradiation of the operating room of various other factors. *Ann Surg* 1964;160[Suppl]:1–192.

53. Nussbaum ES, Rigamonti D, Standiford H, et al. Spinal epidural abscess: a report of 40 cases and review. *Surg Neurol* 1992;38:225–231.

54. Polk Jr HC. Principles of preoperative preparation of the surgical patient, In: Sabiston, ed. *Textbook of surgery: the biological basis of modern surgical practice*, 13th ed. Philadelphia: WB Saunders, 1986:87–98.

55. Polk Jr HC, Simpson CJ, Simmons BP, et al. Guidelines for prevention of surgical wound infection. *Arch Surg* 1983;118:1213.

56. Stambough JL, Beringer D. Postoperative wound infections complicating adult spine surgery. *J Spinal Disord* 1992;5:277–285.

57. Monson TP, Nelson CL. Microbiology for orthopaedic surgeons: selected aspects. *Clin Orthop* 1984;190:14–22.

58. Nelson CL, Green TG, Porter RA. One day versus seven days of preventive antibiotic therapy in orthopaedic surgery. *Clin Orthop* 1983;176:258–263.

59. Thalgott JS, Cotler HB, Sasso RC, et al. Postoperative infections in spinal implants: classification and analysis: a multicenter study. *Spine* 1991;16:981.

60. Cruse PJE, Foord R. A five-year prospective study of 23,649 surgical wounds. *Arch Surg* 1973;107:206–210.

61. Whitecloud TS, Butler JC, Cohen JL. Complications with the variable spinal plating system. *Spine* 1989;14:472.

62. Keller RB, Pappas AM. Infections after spinal fusion using internal fixation instrumentation. *Orthop Clin N Am* 1972;3:99.

63. Burke JF. The effective period of preventive antibiotic action in experimental incisions and dermal lesions. *Surgery* 1961;50:161–168.

64. Horwitz NH, Curtin JA. Prophylactic antibiotics and wound infections following laminectomy for lumbar disk herniation: a retrospective study. *J Neurosurg* 1975;43:727–731.

65. Fitzgerald RH, Thompson RL. Current concepts review: cephalosporin antibiotics in the prevention and treatment of musculoskeletal sepsis. *J Bone Joint Surg Am* 1983;65:1201–1205.

66. Mader JT, Cierny G. The principles of the use of preventive antibiotics. *Clin Orthop* 1984;190:72–82.

67. Scuderi GJ, Greenberg SS, Banovak K, et al. Penetration of glycopeptide antibiotics in nucleus pulposus. *Spine* 1994;18:2039.

68. Velmahos G, Demetriads D. Gunshot wounds of the spine: should retained bullets be removed to prevent infection. *Ann R Coll Surg Engl* 1994;76:85–87.

69. Gepstein R, Eismont F. Postoperative spine infections, In: SR, ed. *Complications of spine surgery*. Baltimore: Williams & Wilkins, 1989:302–322.

70. Gaines DL, Moe JH, Bocklage J. Management of wound infections following Harrington instrumentation and spine fusion. *J Bone Joint Surg Am* 1970;42:404–405.

71. Thelander U, Larsson S. Quantitation of C-reactive protein levels and erythrocyte sedimentation rate after spinal surgery. *Spine* 1992;17:400–404.

72. Massie JB, Heller JG, Abitbol JJ, et al. Postoperative posterior spinal wound infections. *Clin Orthop* 1992;284:99–108.

73. Lonstein J, Winter R, Moe J. Wound infection with Harrington instrumentation and spine fusion for scoliosis. *Clin Orthop* 1973;96:222.

74. Moe JH. Complications of scoliosis treatment. *Clin Orthop* 1967;53:21.

75. Malawski SK, Lukawski S. Pyogenic infection of the spine. *Clin Orthop* 1991;272:58–66.

76. Sapico FL, Montgomerie JZ. Pyogenic vertebral osteomyelitis: report of nine cases and review of the literature. *Rev Infect Dis* 1979;1:754–776.

77. Endress C GD, Fata J, Salciccioli G. Cervical osteomyelitis due to IV heroin use: radiologic findings in 14 patients. *AJR Am J Roentgenol* 1990;155:333–335.

78. Sapico FL, Montgomerie JZ. Vertebral osteomyelitis. *Infect Dis Clin North Am* 1990;4:539–550.

79. Sapico FL, Montgomerie JZ. Vertebral osteomyelitis in intravenous drug abusers: report of three cases and review of the literature. *Rev Infect Dis* 1980;2:196–206.

80. Stone DB, Bonfiglio M. Pyogenic vertebral osteomyelitis: a diagnostic pitfall for the internist. *Arch Intern Med* 1963;112:491–500.

81. Frederickson B, Yuan H, Orlans R. Management and outcome of pyogenic vertebral osteomyelitis. *Clin Orthop* 1978;131:160–167.

82. Garcia A Jr, Grantham SA. Hematogenous pyogenic vertebral osteomyelitis. *J Bone Joint Surg Am* 1960;42:429–436.

83. Genster HG, Andersen MJF. Spinal osteomyelitis complicating urinary tract infection. *J Urol* 1972;107:109–111.

84. Redfern RM, Cottam SN, Phillipson AP. Proteus infection of the spine. *Spine* 1988;13:439–441.

85. Lewis R, Gorbach S, Altner P. Spinal *Pseudomonas* chondroosteomyelitis in heroin users. *N Engl J Med* 1972;286:1303.

86. Wiesseman GJ, Wood VE, Kroll LL. Pseudomonas vertebral osteomyelitis in heroin addicts: report of five cases. *J Bone Joint Surg Am* 1973;55:1416–1424.

87. Incavo SJ, Muller DL, Krag MH, et al. Vertebral osteomyelitis caused by *Clostridium difficile*: a case report and review of the literature. *Spine* 1988;13:111–113.

88. Carvell JE, Maclarnon JC. Chronic osteomyelitis of the thoracic spine due to salmonella typhi: a case report. *Spine* 1981;6:527–530.

89. Sandiford JA, Higgins GA, Blair W. Remote salmonellosis: surgical masquerader. *Am Surg* 1982;48:54–58.

90. Brown MD, Tsaltas TT. Studies on the permeability of the intervertebral disk during skeletal maturation. *Spine* 1976;1:240–244.

91. Hassler O. The human intervertebral disk: a microangiographical study on its vascular supply at various ages. *Acta Orthop Scand* 1970;40:765–772.

92. Whalen JL, Parke WW, Mazur JM, et al. The intrinsic vasculature of developing vertebral end plates and its nutritive significance to the intervertebral disks. *J Pediatr Orthop* 1985;5:403–410.

93. Coventry MB, Ghormley RK, Kernohan JW. The intervertebral disk: its microscopic anatomy and pathology. I. Anatomy, development and physiology. *J Bone Joint Surg* 1945;27:105–112.

94. Rudert M, Tillman B. Lymph and blood supply of the human intervertebral disk. *Acta Orthop Scand* 1993;64:37–40.

95. Wiley AM, Trueta J. The vascular anatomy of the spine and its relationship to pyogenic vertebral osteomyelitis. *J Bone Joint Surg Br* 1959;41:796–809.

96. Kemp HBS, Jackson JW, Jeremiah JD, et al. Pyogenic infections occurring primarily in intervertebral disks. *J Bone Joint Surg Br* 1973;55:698–714.

97. Currier BL, Eismont FJ. Infection of the spine, In: Herkowitz H, Garfin S, Balderston R, et al., eds. *The spine*, 4th ed. Philadelphia: WB Saunders, 1992:1207–58.

98. Wenger DR, Bobechko WP, Gilday DL. The spectrum of intervertebral disk-space infection in children. *J Bone Joint Surg Am* 1978; 60:100.

99. Kowalski HM, Cohen WA, Cooper P, et al. Pitfalls in the CT diagnosis of atlantoaxial rotary subluxation. *AJR Am J Roentgenol* 1987; 149:595–600.

100. Eismont FJ, Bohlman HH, Soni PL, et al. Vertebral osteomyelitis in infants. *J Bone Joint Surg Br* 1982;64:32–35.

101. Pritchard AE, Thompson WAL. Acute pyogenic infections of the spine in children. *J Bone Joint Surg Br* 1960;42:86–89.

102. Puig Guri J. Pyogenic osteomyelitis of the spine: differential diagnosis through clinical and roentgenographic observations. *J Bone Joint Surg* 1946;28:29–39.

103. Barron MM. Cervical spine injury masquerading as a medical emergency. *Am J Emerg Med* 1989;7:54–56.

104. Muffolerro AJ, Nader R, Westmark RM, et al. Hematogenous pyogenic facet joint infection of the subaxial cervical spine. A report of two cases and review of the literature. *J Neurosurg* 2001;95:135–138.

105. Visudhiphan P, Chiemchanya S, Somburanasin R, et al. Torticollis as the presenting sign in cervical spine infection and tumor. *Clin Pediatr* 1982;21:71–76.

106. Zigler JE, Bohlman HH, Robinson RA, et al. Pyogenic osteomyelitis of the occiput, the atlas, and the axis: a report of five cases. *J Bone Joint Surg Am* 1987;69:1069–1073.

107. Stone JL, Cybulski GR, Rodriguez J, et al. Anterior cervical débridement and strut-grafting for osteomyelitis of the cervical spine. *J Neurosurg* 1989;70:879–883.

108. Kulowski J. Pyogenic osteomyelitis of the spine: an analysis and discussion of 102 cases. *J Bone Joint Surg* 1936;18:343–363.

109. Cohn SL, Akbarnia BA, Luisiri A, et al. Disk-space infection versus lumbar Scheuermann's disease. *Orthopedics* 1988;11:330–335.

110. Collert S. Osteomyelitis of the spine. *Acta Orthop Scand* 1977;48:283–290.

111. Duprez TP, Malghem J, Vande Berg BC, et al. Gout in the cervical spine: MR pattern mimicking diskovertebral infection. *AJNR Am J Neuroradiol* 1996;17:151–153.

112. McHenry MC, Duchesneau PM, Keys TF. Vertebral osteomyelitis presenting as spinal compression fracture: six patients with underlying osteoporosis. *Arch Intern Med* 1988;148:417–423.

113. Schofferman L, Schofferman J, Zucherman J, et al. Occult infections causing persistent low-back pain. *Spine* 1989;14:417–419.

114. Fouquet B, Goupille P, Jattiot F, et al. Diskitis after lumbar disk surgery: features of "aseptic" and "septic" forms. *Spine* 1992;17:356–358.

115. Digby JM, Kersley JB. Pyogenic nontuberculous spinal infection: an analysis of 30 cases. *J Bone Joint Surg Br* 1979;61:47–55.

116. Onofrio BM. Intervertebral diskitis: incidence, diagnosis and management. *Clin Neurosurg* 1980;27:481–516.

117. Ross PM, Fleming JL. Vertebral body osteomyelitis: spectrum and natural history: a retrospective analysis of 37 cases. *Clin Orthop Res* 1976;118:190–198.

118. King DM, Mayo KM. Infective lesions of the vertebral column. *Clin Orthop* 1973;96:248.

119. Modic MT, Feiglin DH, Piraino DW. Vertebral osteomyelitis: assessment using MR. *Radiology* 1985;157:157–166.

120. Bruschwein DA, Brown ML, McLeod RA. Gallium scintigraphy in the evaluation of the disk-space infections: concise communication. *J Nucl Med* 1980;21:925–927.

121. Staab EV, McCartney WH. Role of gallium 67 in inflammatory disease. *Semin Nucl Med* 1978;8:219–234.

122. Norris S, Ehrlich MG, McKusick K. Early diagnosis of disk-space infection with 67 Ga in an experimental model. *Clin Orthop* 1979; 144:293–298.

123. Swayne LC, Dorsky S, Caruana V, et al. Septic arthritis of a lumbar facet joint: detection with bone SPECT imaging. *J Nucl Med* 1989; 30:1408–1411.

124. Feiglan D, Modic M, Piraino D, et al. Evaluation of MRI and nuclear medicine in spinal infection: a reappraisal. *J Nucl Med* 1985;26:672.

125. Whalen JL, Brown ML, McLeod R, et al. Limitations of indium leukocyte imaging for diagnosis of spine infections. *Spine* 1991;16:193.

126. Golimbu C, Firooznia H, Rafii M. CT of osteomyelitis of the spine. *AJR Am J Roentgenol* 1984;142:159–163.

127. Kattapuram SV, Phillips WC, Boyd R. CT in pyogenic osteomyelitis of the spine. *Am J Radiol* 1983;140:1199–1201.

128. Van Lom KJ, Kellerhouse LE, Pathria MN, et al. Infection versus tumor in the spine: criteria for distinction with CT. *Radiology* 1988; 166:851–855.

129. Bruns J, Maas R. Advantages of diagnosing bacterial spondylitis with magnetic resonance imaging. *Arch Orthop Trauma Surg* 1989; 108:30–35.

130. Post MJD, Quencer RM, Montalvo BM, et al. Spinal infection: evaluation with MR imaging and intraoperative US. *Radiology* 1988; 169:765–771.

131. Post MJD, Sze G, Quencer RM, et al. Gadolinium enhancing MR in spinal infection. *J Comput Assist Tomogr* 1990;14:721–729.

132. Sharif HS. Role of MR imaging in the management of spinal infections. *AJR Am J Roentgenol* 1992;158:1333.

133. Van Tassel P. Magnetic resonance imaging of spinal infections. *Top Magn Reson Imaging* 1994;6:69–81.

134. An HS, Vaccaro AR, Dolinskas CA, et al. Differentiation between spinal tumors and infections with magnetic resonance imaging. *Spine* 1991;16[Suppl]:S334–S338.

135. Eismont FJ, Green BA, Brown MD, et al. Coexistent infection and tumor of the spine: a report of three cases. *J Bone Joint Surg Am* 1987;69:452–458.

136. Nagel DA, Albright JA, Keggi KJ, et al. Closer look at spinal lesions: open biopsy of vertebral lesions. *JAMA* 1965;191:103–106.

137. Ottolenghi CE. Aspiration biopsy of the spine: technique for the thoracic spine and results of twenty-eight biopsies in this region and overall results of 1050 biopsies of other spinal segments. *J Bone Joint Surg Am* 1969;51:1531–1544.

138. Ottolenghi CE, Schajowicz F, De Schant FA. Aspiration biopsy of the cervical spine: technique and results in thirty-four cases. *J Bone Joint Surg Am* 1964;46:715–733.

139. Armstrong P, Green G, Irving JD. Needle aspiration/biopsy of the spine in suspected disk-space infection. *Br J Radiol* 1978;51:333–337.

140. Brugieres P, Revel MP, Dumas JL, et al. CT-guided vertebral biopsy: a report of 89 cases. *JNR* 1991;18:351–359.

141. Ghelman B, Lospinuso MF, Levine DB, et al. Percutaneous CT-guided biopsy of the thoracic and lumbar spine. *Orthop Trans* 1991; 16:736–739.

142. Brown EM. Infections in neurosurgery: using laboratory data to plan optimal treatment strategies. *Drugs* 2002;62:909–913.

143. Emery SE, Chan DPK, Woodward HR. Treatment of hematogenous pyogenic vertebral osteomyelitis with anterior débridement and primary bone grafting. *Spine* 1989;14:284–291.

144. Forsythe M, Rothman RH. New concepts in the diagnosis and treatment of infections of the cervical spine. *Orthop Clin North Am* 1978;9:1039–1051.

145. Smith MD, Emery SE, Dudley A, et al. Vertebral artery injury during anterior decompression of the cervical spine. A retrospective review of ten patients. *J Bone Joint Surg Br* 1993;75:410–415.

146. Curylo LJ, Mason HC, Bohlman HH, et al. Tortuous course of the vertebral artery and anterior cervical decompression: a cadaveric and clinical case study. *Spine* 2000;25:2860–2864.

147. Fang D, Cheung KMC, Dos Remedios IDM, et al. Pyogenic vertebral osteomyelitis: treatment by anterior spinal débridement and fusion. *J Spinal Disord* 1994;7:173–180.

148. Kemp HBS, Jackson JW, Jeremiah JD, et al. Anterior fusion of the spine for infective lesions in adults. *J Bone Joint Surg Br* 1973;55:715–734.

149. Kirkaldy-Willis WH, Thomas TG. Anterior approaches in the diagnosis and treatment of infections of the vertebral bodies. *J Bone Joint Surg Am* 1965;47:87–110.

150. Southwick WO, Robinson RA. Surgical approaches to the vertebral bodies in the cervical and lumbar regions. *J Bone Joint Surg Am* 1957;39:631–644.

151. Kemp HBS, Jackson JW, Shaw NC. Laminectomy in paraplegia due to infective spondylosis. *Br J Surg* 1974;61:66–72.

152. Seddon HJ. Pott's paraplegia: prognosis and treatment. *Br J Surg* 1934–35;22:769–799.

153. Cahill DW, Love LC, Rechtine GR. Pyogenic osteomyelitis of the spine in the elderly. *J Neurosurg* 1991;74:878–886.

154. Liebergall M, Chaimsky G, Lowe J, et al. Pyogenic vertebral osteomyelitis with paralysis: prognosis and treatment. *Clin Orthop* 1991;269:142.

155. McGuire RA, Eismont FJ. The fate of autogenous bone graft in surgically treated pyogenic vertebral osteomyelitis. *J Spinal Disord* 1994;7:206–215.

156. Wiltberger BR. Resection of vertebral bodies and bone grafting for chronic osteomyelitis of the spine. *J Bone Joint Surg Am* 1952;34:215–218.

157. Graziano GP, Sidhu KS. Salvage reconstruction in acute and late sequelae from pyogenic thoracolumbar infection. *J Spinal Disord* 1993;6:199–207.

158. Rajasekaran S, Soundarapandian S. Progression of kyphosis in tuberculosis of the spine treated by anterior arthrodesis. *J Bone Joint Surg Am* 1989;71:1314–1323.

159. Przybylski GJ, Sharan AD. Single-stage autogenous bone grafting and internal fixation in the surgical management of pyogenic discitis and vertebral osteomyelitis. *J Neurosurg* 2001;94:1–7.

160. Moon MS, Woo YK, Lee KS, et al. Posterior instrumentation and anterior interbody fusion for tuberculous kyphosis of dorsal and lumbar spines. *Spine* 1995;20:1910.

161. Oga M, Arizono T, Takasita M, et al. Evaluation of the risk of instrumentation as a foreign body in spinal tuberculosis. *Spine* 1993;18:1890–1894.

162. Abramovitz JN, Batson RA, Yablon JS. Vertebral osteomyelitis. The surgical management of neurologic complications. *Spine* 1986;11:418–420.

163. Carragee EJ. Instrumentation of the infected and unstable spine: a review of 17 cases from the thoracic and lumbar spine with pyogenic infections. *J Spinal Disord* 1997;10:317–324.

164. Dietze DD Jr, Fessler RG, Jacob RP. Primary reconstruction for spinal infections. *J Neurosurg* 1997;86:981–989.

165. Fountain SS. A single-stage combined surgical approach for vertebral resections. *J Bone Joint Surg Am* 1979;61:1011–1017.

166. Rath SA, Neff U, Schneider O, et al. Neurosurgical management of thoracic and lumbar vertebral osteomyelitis and discitis in adults: a review of 43 consecutive surgically treated patients. *Neurosurgery* 1996;38:926–933.

167. Redfern RM, Miles J, Banks AJ, et al. Stabilisation of the infected spine. *J Neurol Neurosurg Psychiatry* 1988;51:803–807.

168. Rezai AR, Woo HH, Errico TJ, et al. Contemporary management of spinal osteomyelitis. *Neurosurgery* 1999;44:1018–1025; discussion, 25–26.

169. Safran O, Rand N, Kaplan L, et al. Sequential or simultaneous, same-day anterior decompression and posterior stabilization in the management of vertebral osteomyelitis of the lumbar spine. *Spine* 1998;23:1885–1890.

170. Loembe PM. Tuberculosis of the lower cervical spine (C3-C7) in adults: diagnostic and surgical aspects. *Acta Neurochir (Wien)* 1994;131:125.

171. Felländer M. Paraplegia in spondylitis: results of operative treatment. *Paraplegia* 1975;13:75–88.

172. Lifeso RM. Pyogenic spinal sepsis in adults. *Spine* 1990;15:1265.

173. Freilich D, Swash M. Diagnosis and management of tuberculous paraplegia with special reference to tuberculous radiculomyelitis. *J Neurol Neurosurg Psychiatry* 1979;42:12–18.

174. Messer HD, Litvinoff J. Pyogenic cervical osteomyelitis. Chondroosteomyelitis of the cervical spine frequently associated with parenteral drug use. *Arch Neurol* 1976;33:571–576.

175. Heary RF, Hunt CD, Krieger AJ, et al. HIV status does not affect microbiologic spectrum or neurologic outcome in spinal infections. *Surg Neurol* 1994;42:417–423.

176. Heary R, Vaccaro A, Mesa JJ, et al. Thoracolumbar infections in penetrating injuries to the spine. *Orthop Clin North Am* 1996;27:69–81.

177. Kihtir T, Ivatury RR, Simon R, et al. Management of transperitoneal gunshot wounds of the spine. *J Trauma* 1991;31:1579.

178. Kupcha PC, An HS, Cotler JM. Gunshot wounds to the cervical spine. *Spine* 1990;15:1058–1063.

179. Lin SS, Vaccaro AR, Reisch S, et al. Low velocity gunshot wounds to the spine with an associated transperitoneal injury. *J Spinal Disord* 1995;8:136–144.

180. Maier RV, Carrico CJ, Heinbach DM. Pyogenic osteomyelitis of axial bones following civilian gunshot wounds. *Am J Surg* 1979;137:378.

181. Roffi RP, Waters RL, Adkins RH. Gunshot wounds to the spine associated with a perforated viscus. *Spine* 1989;14:808–811.

182. Romanick PC, Smith TK, Kopaniky DR, et al. Infection about the spine associated with low-velocity-missile injury to the abdomen. *J Bone Joint Surg Am* 1985;67:1195.

183. Yoshida GM, Garland D, Waters RL. Gunshot wounds to the spine. *Orthop Clin North Am* 1995;26:109–116.

184. Jones RE, Bucholz RW, Schaefer SD. Cervical osteomyelitis complicating transpharyngeal gunshot wounds to the neck. *J Trauma* 1979;19:630–634.

185. Schaefer SD, Bucholz RW, Jones RE, et al. The management of transpharyngeal gunshot wounds to the cervical spine. *Surg Gynecol Obstet* 1981;152:27–29.

186. Lowe J, Kaplan L, Liebergall M, et al. *Serratia* osteomyelitis causing neurological deterioration after spine fracture: a report of two cases. *J Bone Joint Surg Br* 1989;71:256–258.

187. Ring D, Vaccaro AR, Scuderi G, et al. Vertebral osteomyelitis after blunt traumatic esophageal rupture. *Spine* 1995;20:98–101.

188. Danner RL, Hartman BJ. Update of spinal epidural abscess: 35 cases and review of the literature. *Rev Infect Dis* 1987;9:265–274.

189. Hlavin ML, Kaminski HJ, Ross JS, et al. Spinal epidural abscess: a 10-year perspective. *Neurosurgery* 1990;27:177–184.

190. Darouiche RO, Hamill RJ, Greenberg SB, et al. Bacterial spinal epidural abscess: review of 43 cases and literature survey. *Medicine* 1992;71:369–385.

191. Gardner RD, Cammisa FP, Eismont FJ, et al. Nongranulomatous spinal epidural abscesses. *Orthop Trans* 1989;13:562–563.

192. Baker AS, Ojemann RG, Swartz MN, et al. Spinal epidural abscess. *N Engl J Med* 1975;293:463–468.

193. Hancock DO. A study of 49 patients with acute spinal extradural abscess. *Paraplegia* 1973;10:285–288.

194. Heusner AP. Nontuberculosis spinal epidural infections. *N Engl J Med* 1958;239:845–854.

195. Lasker BR, Harter DH. Cervical epidural abscess. *Neurology* 1987;37:1747–1753.

196. Rigamonti D, Liem L, Wolf AL, et al. Epidural abscess in the cervical spine. *Mt Sinai J Med* 1994;61:357.

197. Redekop GJ, Del Maestro RF. Diagnosis and management of spinal epidural abscess. *Can J Neurol Sci* 1992;19:180–187.

198. Kaufman DM, Kaplan JG, Litman N. Infectious agents in spinal epidural abscesses. *Neurology* 1980;30:844–850.

199. Bergman I, Wald ER, Meyer JD, et al. Epidural abscess and vertebral osteomyelitis following serial lumbar punctures. *Pediatrics* 1983;72:476–480.

200. Fine PG, Hare BD, Zahniser JC. Epidural abscess following epidural catheterization in a chronic pain patient: a diagnostic dilemma. *Anesthesiology* 1988;69:422–424.

201. Browder J, Meyers R. Infection of the spinal epidural space: an aspect of vertebral osteomyelitis. *Am J Surg* 1937;37:4–26.

202. Koppel BS, Tuchman AJ, Mangiardi JR. Epidural spinal infection in intravenous drug abusers. *Arch Neurol* 1988;45:1331–1337.

203. Dandy WE. Abscesses and inflammatory tumors in the spinal epidural space (so-called pachymeningitis externa). *Arch Surg* 1926;13:477–494.

204. de Villiers JC, de Clüver PF. Spinal epidural abscess in children. *Afr J Surg* 1978;16:149–155.

205. Kricun R, Shoemaker EI, Chovanes GI, et al. Epidural abscess of the cervical spine: MR findings in five cases. *AJR Am J Roentgenol* 1992;158:1145.

206. North JB, Brophy BP. Epidural abscess: a hazard of spinal epidural anaesthesia. *Aust N Z J* 1979;49:484–485.
207. Williams JW, Powell T. Epidural abscess of the cervical spine: case report and literature review. *Br J Radiol* 1990;63:576–578.
208. Browder J, Meyers R. Pyogenic infections of the spinal epidural space: a consideration of the anatomic and physiologic pathology. *Surgery* 1941;10:296–308.
209. Feldenzer JA, McKeever PE, Schaberg DR. The pathogenesis of spinal epidural abscess: microangiographic studies in an experimental model. *J Neurosurg* 1988;69:110–114.
210. Corradini EW, Turney MF, Browder EJ. Spinal epidural infection. *NY State J Med* 1948;48:2367–2370.
211. Russell NA, Vaughan R, Morley TP. Spinal epidural infection. *Can J Neurol Sci* 1979;6:325–328.
212. Curling OD, Gower DJ, McWhorter JM. Changing concepts in spinal epidural abscess: a report of 29 cases. *Neurosurgery* 1990;27:185–192.
213. Leys D, Lesoin F, Viaud C. Decreased morbidity from acute bacterial spinal epidural abscesses using computed tomography and nonsurgical treatment in selected patients. *Ann Neurol* 1985;17:350–355.
214. Angtuaco EJ, McConnell JR, Chadduck WM, et al. Mr imaging of spinal epidural sepsis. *AJR Am J Roentgenol* 1987;149:1249–1253.
215. Bertino RE, Porter BA, Stimac GK, et al. Imaging spinal osteomyelitis and epidural abscess with short t1 inversion recovery (stir). *AJNR Am J Neuroradiol* 1988;9:563–564.
216. Erntell M, Holtas S, Norlin K. Magnetic resonance imaging in the diagnosis of spinal epidural abscess. *Scand J Infect Dis* 1988;20:323–327.
217. Garvey TA, Eismont FJ. Tuberculosis and fungal osteomyelitis of the spine. *Semin Spine Surg* 1990;2:295–2308.
218. Sadato N, Numaguchi Y, Rigamonti D, et al. Spinal epidural abscess with gadolinium-enhanced MRI: serial follow-up studies with clinical correlations. *Neuroradiology* 1994;36:44–48.
219. Altrocchi PH. Acute spinal epidural abscess vs. Acute transverse myelopathy: a plea for neurosurgical caution. *Arch Neurol* 1963;9:17–25.
220. Wheeler D, Keiser P, Rigamonte D. Medical management of spinal epidural abscesses: case report and review. *Clin Infect Dis* 1992;15:22–27.
221. Piccolo R, Passanisi M, Chiaramonte I, et al. Cervical spinal epidural abscesses. A report on five cases. *J Neurosurg Sci* 1999;43:63–67.
222. Spies EH, Stucker R, Reichelt A. Conservative management of pyogenic osteomyelitis of the occipitocervical junction. *Spine* 1999;24:818–822.
223. Mampalam TJ, Rosegay H, Andrews BT. Nonoperative treatment of spinal epidural infections. *J Neurosurg* 1989;71:208–210.
224. Mixter WJ, Smithwick RH. Acute intraspinal epidural abscess. *N Engl J Med* 1932;207:126–131.
225. Corboy JR, Price RW. Myelitis and toxic, inflammatory, and infectious disorders. *Curr Opin Neurol Neurosurg* 1993;6:564–570.
226. McGee-Collett M, Johnston IH. Spinal epidural abscess: presentation and treatment. *Med J Aust* 1991;155:14.
227. Hulme A, Dott NM. Spinal epidural abscess. *BMJ* 1954;1:64–68.
228. Hakin RN, Burt AA, Cook JB. Acute spinal epidural abscess. *Paraplegia* 1979;17:330–336.
229. Sittig O. Metastatischer ruckenmarksabscess bei sepischem abortus. *Z Gesamte Neurol Psychiatr* 1927;107:146–151.
230. Levy ML, Wieder BH, Schneider J, et al. Subdural empyema of the cervical spine: clinical pathologic correlates and magnetic resonance imaging. *J Neurosurg* 1993;79:929–935.
231. Lownie SP, Ferguson GG. Spinal subdural empyema complicating cervical diskography. *Spine* 1989;14:1415–1417.
232. Fraser RAR, Ratzan K, Wolpert SM, et al. Spinal subdural empyema. *Arch Neurol* 1973;28:235–238.
233. Butler EG, Dohrmann PJ, Stark RJ. Spinal subdural abscess. *Clin Exp Neurol* 1988;25:67–70.
234. Kurokowa Y, Hashi K, Fujishige M, et al. Spinal subdural empyema diagnosed by MRI and recovered by conservative treatment. *No To Shinkei* 1989;41:513.
235. Bartels RHMA, Gonera EG, van der Spek JAN, et al. Intramedullary spinal cord abscess. *Spine* 1995;20:1199–1204.
236. Hart J. Case of encysted abscess in the centre of spinal cord. *Dublin Hosp Rep* 1830;5:522.
237. Fertel D, Pitchenik AE. Tuberculosis in acquired immune deficiency syndrome. *Semin Respir Infect* 1989;4:198–205.
238. Tuli SM, Srivastava TP, Varma BP, et al. Tuberculosis of spine. *Acta Orthop Scand* 1967;38:445–458.
239. Hsu LCS, Leong JCY. Tuberculosis of the lower cervical spine (C2 to C7): a report on 40 cases. *J Bone Joint Surg Br* 1984;66:1–5.
240. Wang LX. Peroral focal débridement for treatment of tuberculosis of the atlas and axis. *Chin J Orthop* 1981;1:207.
241. Fang D, Leong JCY, Fang HSY. Tuberculosis of the upper cervical spine. *J Bone Joint Surg Br* 1983;65:47–50.
242. Compere EL, Garrison M. Correlation of pathologic and roentgenologic findings in tuberculosis and pyogenic infections of the vertebra: the fate of the intervertebral disk. *Ann Surg* 1936;104:1038–1067.
243. Friedman B. Chemotherapy of tuberculosis of the spine. *J Bone Joint Surg Am* 1966;48:451–474.
244. Doub HP, Badgley CE. The roentgen signs of tuberculosis of the vertebral body. *AJR Am J Roentgenol* 1932;27:827–837.
245. Babhulkar SS, Tayade WB, Babhulkar SK. Atypical spinal tuberculosis. *J Bone Joint Surg Br* 1984;66:239–242.
246. Dobson J. Tuberculosis of the spine: an analysis of the results of conservative treatment and of the factors influencing the prognosis. *J Bone Joint Surg Br* 1951;33:517–531.
247. Naim UR, Al Arabi K, Khan F. A typical form of spinal tuberculosis. *Acta Neurochir (Wein)* 1987;88:26–33.
248. Bailey HL, Gabriel SM, Hodgson AR, et al. Tuberculosis of the spine in children: operative findings and results in 100 consecutive patients treated by removal of the lesion and anterior grafting. *J Bone Joint Surg Am* 1972;54:1633–1657.
249. Hodgson AR, Yau A, Kwon JS, et al. A clinical study of 100 consecutive cases of Pott's paraplegia. *Clin Orthop* 1964;36:128–150.
250. Lin SK, Wu T, Wai YY. Intramedullary spinal tuberculomas during treatment of tuberculous meningitis. *Clin Neurol Neurosurg* 1994;96:71–78.
251. Mathuriya SN, Khosla VK, Banerjee AK. Intradural extramedullary tuberculous spinal granulomas. *Clin Neurol Neurosurg* 1988;90:155–158.
252. Neal SL, Kearns MJ, Seelig JM, et al. Manifestations of Pott's disease in the head and neck. *Laryngoscope* 1986;96:494.
253. Hodgson AR. Report on the findings and results in 300 cases of Pott's disease treated by anterior fusion of the spine. *J West Pacific Orthop Assoc* 1964;1:3.
254. Medical Research Council Working Party on Tuberculosis of the Spine. A controlled trial of anterior spinal fusion and débridement in the surgical management of tuberculosis of the spine in patients on standard chemotherapy: a study in two centers in South Africa. *Tubercle* 1978;59:79–105.
255. Medical Research Council Working Party on Tuberculosis of the Spine. A controlled trial of débridement and ambulatory treatment in the management of tuberculosis of the spine in patients on standard chemotherapy: a study in Bulawayo, Rhodesia. *J Trop Med Hyg* 1974;77:72–92.
256. Medical Research Council Working Party on Tuberculosis of the Spine. A controlled trial of six month and nine month regimens of chemotherapy in patients undergoing radical surgery for tuberculosis of the spine in Hong Kong. *Tubercle* 1986;67:243–259.
257. Forlenza SW, Axelrod JL, Grieco MH. Pott's disease in heroin addicts. *J Am Med Assoc* 1979;241:379–380.
258. Martin NS. Pott's paraplegia: a report of 120 cases. *J Bone Joint Surg Br* 1971;53:596–608.
259. Subhadrabandhu T, Laohacharoensombat W, Keorochana S. Risk factors for neural deficit in spinal tuberculosis. *J Med Assoc Thai* 1992;75:453–460.
260. Walker GF. Failure of early recognition of skeletal tuberculosis. *Br Med J* 1968;1:682–683.
261. Mondal A. Cytological diagnosis of vertebral tuberculosis with fine-needle aspiration biopsy. *J Bone Joint Surg Am* 1994;76:181–184.
262. Sarkar SD, Ravikrishnan KP, Woodbury DH, et al. Gallium 67-citrate scanning-a new adjunct in the detection and follow-up of extrapulmonary tuberculosis: concise communication. *J Nucl Med* 1979;20:833–836.
263. Sharif HS, Aideyan OA, Clark DC, et al. Brucellar and tuberculous spondylitis. Comparative imaging features. *Radiology* 1989;171:419–425.
264. Smith AS, Weinstein MA, Mizushima A, et al. Mr imaging characteristics of tuberculous spondylitis vs vertebral osteomyelitis. *AJR Am J Roentgenol* 1989;153:399–405.
265. Kim NH, Lee HM, Suh JS. Magnetic resonance imaging for the diagnosis of tuberculous spondylitis. *Spine* 1994;19:2451–2455.

266. Haas DW, Des Prez RM. Mycobacterium tuberculosis, In: Mandell, Bennett, R, eds. *Principles and practice of infectious diseases*, 4th ed. New York: Churchill Livingstone, 1995:2213–2242.

267. Medical Research Council Working Party on Tuberculosis of the Spine. A comparison of 6 or 9 month course regime of chemotherapy in patients receiving ambulatory treatment or undergoing radical surgery for tuberculosis of the spine. *Ind J Tuberculosis* 1989;36[Suppl]:1.

268. Medical Research Council Working Party on Tuberculosis of the Spine. A controlled trial of ambulant out-patient treatment and in-patient rest in bed in the management of tuberculosis of the spine in young Korean patients on standard chemotherapy: a study in Masan, Korea. *J Bone Joint Surg Br* 1973;55:678–697.

269. Medical Research Council Working Party on Tuberculosis of the Spine. A 15-year assessment of controlled trials of the management of tuberculosis of the spine in Korea and Hong Kong. Thirteenth report of the medical research council working party on tuberculosis of the spine. *J Bone Joint Surg Br* 1998;80:456–462.

270. Parthasarathy R, Sriram K, Santha T, et al. Short-course chemotherapy for tuberculosis of the spine. A comparison between ambulant treatment and radical surgery—ten-year report. *J Bone Joint Surg Br* 1999;81:464–471.

271. Hodgson AR, Stock FE. Anterior spine fusion for the treatment of tuberculosis of the spine: the operative findings and results of treatment in the first 100 cases. *J Bone Joint Surg Am* 1960;42:295–310.

272. Hodgson AR, Stock FE. Anterior spinal fusion: a preliminary communication on the radical treatment of Pott's disease and Pott's paraplegia. *Br J Surg* 1956;44:266–275.

273. Hodgson AR, Stock FE, Fang HSY, et al. Anterior spinal fusion: the operative approach and pathological findings in 412 patients with Pott's disease of the spine. *Br J Surg* 1960;48:172–178.

274. McAfee PC, Bohlman HH, Riley LH, et al. The anterior retropharyngeal approach to the upper part of the cervical spine. *J Bone Joint Surg Am* 1987;69:1371–1383.

275. Hodgson AR. An approach to the cervical spine (C3-C7). *Clin Orthop* 1965;39:129–134.

276. Medical Research Council Working Party on Tuberculosis of the Spine. Five year assessments of controlled trials of ambulatory treatment, débridement and anterior spinal fusion in the management of tuberculosis of the spine: studies in Vulawayo (Rhodesia) and in Hong Kong. *J Bone Joint Surg Br* 1978;60:163–177.

277. Allen AR, Stevenson AW. Follow-up notes on articles previously published in the journal: a 10-year follow-up of combined drug therapy and early fusion in bone tuberculosis. *J Bone Joint Surg Am* 1967;49:1001–1003.

278. Medical Research Council Working Party on Tuberculosis of the Spine. A 10-year assessment of a controlled trial comparing débridement and anterior spinal fusion in the management of tuberculosis of the spine in patients on standard chemotherapy in Hong Kong. *J Bone Joint Surg Br* 1982;64:393–398.

279. Govender S, Parbhoo AH. Support of the anterior column with allografts in tuberculosis of the spine. *J Bone Joint Surg Br* 1999;81:106–109.

280. Govender S, Parbhoo AH, Kumar KP. Tuberculosis of the cervicodorsal junction. *J Pediatr Orthop* 2001;21:285–287.

281. Garceau GJ, Brady TA. Pott's paraplegia. *J Bone Joint Surg Am* 1950;32:87–96.

282. Güven O, Kumano K, Yalçin S, et al. A single-stage posterior approach and rigid fixation for preventing kyphosis in the treatment of spinal tuberculosis. *Spine* 1994;19:1039–1043.

283. Kim BJ, Koh S, Lim Y, et al. The clinical study of the tuberculous spondylitis. *J Korean Orthop Assoc* 1993;28:2221.

284. Lee EY, Hahn MS. A study of influences of the anterior intervertebral fusion upon the correct ability of kyphosis in tuberculous spondylitis. *J Korean Orthop Assoc* 1968;3:31.

285. Rajasekaran S, Shanmugasundaram TK. Prediction of the angle of gibbus deformity in tuberculosis of the spine. *J Bone Joint Surg Am* 1987;69:503–509.

286. Yau ACMC, Hsu LCS, O'Brien JP, et al. Tuberculous kyphosis. *J Bone Joint Surg Am* 1974;56:1419–1434.

287. Kostuik JP. Anterior spinal cord decompression for lesions of the thoracic and lumbar spine, techniques, new methods of internal fixation, results. *Spine* 1983;8:512.

288. Yilmaz C, Selek HY, Gurkan I, et al. Anterior instrumentation for the treatment of spinal tuberculosis. *J Bone Joint Surg Am* 1999;81:1261–1267.

289. Faraj AA. Anterior instrumentation for the treatment of spinal tuberculosis. *J Bone Joint Surg Am* 2001;83:463–464.

290. Hodgson AR, Yau ACMC. Anterior surgical approaches to the spinal column. *Recent Adv Orthop* 1969;1:289–323.

291. Adams ZB. Tuberculosis of the spine in children: a review of 63 cases from the Lakeville State Sanatorium. *J Bone Joint Surg* 1940;22:860–861.

292. Tuli SM. Results of treatment of spinal tuberculosis by "middle-path" regime. *J Bone Joint Surg Br* 1975;57:13–23.

293. Bell C. *The nervous system of the human body*. London: Longman, 1830.

294. Wetzel FT, LaRocca H. Grisel's syndrome. *Clin Orthop* 1989;240:141.

295. Grisel P. Enucleation de l'atlas torticolis naso-pharyngyngien. *Presse Med* 1930;38(4):50–54.

296. Desfosses P. Un cas de maladie de Grisel. Torticollis nasopharyngien par subluxation de l'atlas. *Presse Med* 1930;138:1179–1180.

297. Lopes DK, Li V. Midcervical postinfectious ligamentous instability: a variant of Grisel's syndrome. *Pediatr Neurosurg* 1998;29:133–137.

298. Sullivan AW. Subluxation of the atlanto-axial joint: sequel to inflammatory processes of the neck. *J Pediatr* 1949;354:451–464.

299. Wilson MJ, Michele AA, Jacobson EW. Spontaneous dislocation of the atlanto-axial articulation including a report of a case with quadriplegia. *J Bone Joint Surg* 1940;22:698.

300. Keuter EJW. Non-traumatic atlanto-axial dislocations associated with nasopharyngeal infections (Grisel's disease). *Acta Neurochir (Wien)* 1969;21:11.

301. Mathern GW, Batzdorf U. Grisel's syndrome. *Clin Orthop* 1989;244:131.

302. Watson Jones R. Spontaneous hyperaemic dislocation of the atlas. *Proc R Soc Med* 1932;25:586–590.

303. Berkheiser EJ, Seidler F. Nontraumatic dislocations of the atlanto-axial joint. *J Am Med Assoc* 1931;96:517–523.

304. Bredenkamp JK, Maceri DR. Inflammatory torticollis in children. *Arch Otolaryngol Head Neck Surg* 1990;116:310–313.

305. Marar BC, Balachandran N. Non-traumatic atlanto-axial dislocation in children. *Clin Orthop* 1973;92:220.

306. Wilson BC, Jarvis BL, Haydon RC. Nontraumatic subluxation of the atlantoaxial joint: Grisel's syndrome. *Ann Otol Rhinol Laryngol* 1987;96:705–708.

307. Parke WW, Rothman RH, Brown MD. The pharyngovertebral veins: an anatomical rationale for Grisel's syndrome. *J Bone Joint Surg Am* 1984;66:568–574.

308. Hess JH, Bronstein IP, Abelson SM. Atlantoaxial dislocations unassociated with trauma and secondary to inflammatory foci in the neck. *Am J Dis Child* 1935;49:1137–1147.

309. Sudek P. Ueber drehungsverrenkung des atlas. *Dtsch Zeitschrift Chir* 1923;183:289–303.

310. Jackson H. The diagnosis of minimal atlanto-axial subluxation. *Br J Radiol* 1950;23(275):672–674.

311. Locke GR, Gardner JI, van Epps EF. Atlas-dens interval (ADI) in children: a survey based on 200 normal cervical spines. *AJR Am J Roentgenol* 1966;97:135.

312. Steel HH. Anatomical and mechanical considerations of the atlanto-axial articulations. *J Bone Joint Surg Am* 1968;50:1481–1482.

313. Cattell HS, Filtzer DL. Pseudosubluxation and other normal variations in the cervical spine in children. *J Bone Joint Surg Am* 1965;47:1295–1309.

314. Kawabe N, Hirotani H, Tanaka O. Pathomechanism of atlantoaxial rotatory fixation in children. *J Pediatr Orthop* 1989;9:569–574.

315. Wittek A. Ein fall von distensions luxation in atlanto-epistropheal-gelenke. *Müncherer Medizinische Wochenschrift* 1836;55:1836–1837.

316. Coutts MB. Atlanto-epistropheal subluxations. *Arch Surg* 1934;29:297.

317. Fielding JW, Hawkins RJ, Ratzan SA. Spine fusion for atlanto-axial instability. *J Bone Joint Surg Am* 1976;58:400–407.

318. Wortzman G, Dewar FP. Rotary fixation of the atlantoaxial joint. *Radiology* 1968;90:479–487.

319. Corner EM. Rotary dislocations of the atlas. *Ann Surg* 1907;45:9–26.

320. Fielding JW, Hawkins RJ. Atlantoaxial rotatory fixation. *J Bone Joint Surg Am* 1977;59:37–44.

321. Phillips WA, Hensinger RN. The management of rotatory atlanto-axial subluxation in children. *J Bone Joint Surg Am* 1989;71:664.

322. Washington ER. Non-traumatic atlanto-occipital and atlanto-axial dislocation: a case report. *J Bone Joint Surg Am* 1959;41:341–344.

323. Hunter GA. Non-traumatic displacement of the atlanto-axial joint: a report of 7 cases. *J Bone Joint Surg Br* 1968;50:44.

324. Woltman HW, Meyerding HW. Spontaneous hyperemic dislocation of the atlanto-axial joint. *Surg Clin North Am* 1934;14:581–588.

325. Crisco III JJ, Oda T, Panjabi MM, et al. Transections of the C1-C2 joint capsular ligaments in the cadaveric spine. *Spine* 1991;16[10 Suppl]:S474–S479.

326. Clark CR, Kathol MH, Walsh T, et al. Atlantoaxial rotatory fixation with compensatory counter occipito-atlantal subluxation. *Spine* 1986; 11:1048–1050.

327. Ono K, Yonenobu K, Fuji T, et al. Atlantoaxial rotatory fixation. Radiographic study of its mechanism. *Spine* 1985;10:602.

328. Fielding JW. Cineroentgenography of the normal cervical spine. *J Bone Joint Surg Am* 1957;69:1280–1288.

329. Fielding JW, Stillwell WT, Chynn KY, et al. Use of computed tomography for the diagnosis of atlanto-axial rotatory fixation. *J Bone Joint Surg Am* 1978;60:1102–1104.

330. Fielding JW. Selected observations of the cervical spine in the child. *Curr Pract Orthop Surg* 1973;5:31–55.

331. Fielding JW, Cochran GV, Lawsing JF, et al. Tears of the transverse ligament of the atlas. *J Bone Joint Surg Am* 1974;56:1683–1691.

332. Daniels DL, Williams AL, Haughton VM. Computed tomography of the articulations and ligaments at the occipito-atlantoaxial region. *Radiology* 1983;146:709–716.

333. Dvorak J, Panjabi MM, Gerber M, et al. CT functional diagnostics of the rotatory instability of the upper cervical spine: 1. An experimental study on cadavers. *Spine* 1987;12:197–205.

334. Rinaldi I, Mullins WJ, Delaney WF, et al. Computerized tomographic demonstration of rotational atlantoaxial fixation. *J Neurosurg* 1979; 50:115.

335. Goddard NJ, Stabler J, Albert JS. Atlantoaxial rotatory fixation and fracture of the clavicle. *J Bone Joint Surg Br* 1990;72:72.

336. Harms J, Melcher RP. Posterior C1-C2 fusion with polyaxial screw and rod fixation. *Spine* 2001;26:2467–2471.

CHAPTER 63

Syringomyelia

Geoffrey P. Zubay, Shahram Partovi, and Curtis A. Dickman

The term *syringomyelia* was coined by Charles Prosper Ollivier D'Angers in 1827 (1). Ollivier used the term to describe the abnormal dilation of the central canal of the spinal cord and hypothesized that it was the result of arrested development in the intrauterine period. In time it would be realized that the cystic dilation of the spinal cord involved the central canal in some cases (2). This realization led to the adoption of the terms *hydromyelia* and *syringomyelia* to differentiate the two processes. Hydromyelia was used to describe the abnormal dilation of the central canal. Work by subsequent investigators focused on elucidating the congenital and acquired origin of these abnormalities.

Early work searching for the etiology of congenital syringomyelia focused on the histopathologic abnormalities noted in autopsy specimens (3,4). Derangements of normal cell layers in the central canal were thought to result from abnormal migration of cells during embryologic development. It was not until 1883 when John Cleland described a case of hydrocephalus associated with spina bifida that syringomyelia and hindbrain abnormalities were recognized as associated with each other (1). Cleland hypothesized that closure of the canal between the fourth ventricle and spinal canal led to distention of the canal and its subsequent rupture into open spina bifida.

In the following years, researchers were unable to identify a common origin for syringomyelia, which was associated with tumors, infection, embryonic maldevelopment, Chiari malformations, and trauma. The numerous theories of its pathogenesis failed to provide a comprehensive theory of how the syrinx evolved. It became apparent that syrinxes of the spinal cord could form from a variety of conditions and causes, each with a different pathogenetic mechanism and each potentially deserving separate consideration when choosing a therapeutic treatment.

Advances in magnetic resonance imaging (MRI) led to the greatest advances in the understanding of syringomyelia.

The increased resolution of imaging and the development of imaging techniques able to evaluate cerebrospinal fluid (CSF) flow in the spinal canal qualitatively and quantitatively improved the pathogenetic understanding of different forms of syringomyelia.

When syringomyelia is considered from clinical and pathologic perspectives, using a classification system based on the anatomic nature of the syrinx provides the most useful working framework. Based on his review of 927 patients with cavitary lesions of the spinal cord, Milhorat developed such a classification system (5). This chapter considers syringomyelia as a clinical problem and uses this classification system to provide a reasonable and logical framework for the clinical management of this disease process.

CLINICAL MANIFESTATIONS

The clinical manifestations of syringomyelia depend on the underlying pathologic process causing the dilation of the spinal cord. Typically, a syrinx declares itself over a protracted clinical course; an acute presentation is unusual (6). Some authors have speculated that patients may present acutely from acute extension of a syrinx, hemorrhage into a syrinx, or clinical events related to dysfunction acquired from the presence of the syrinx (i.e., involvement of the intermediolateral cell column may cause postural imbalance).

The classic clinical description of syringomyelia is a constellation of symptoms related to the location of a syrinx in the cervical spinal cord. The constellation of symptoms relates to the loss of lower motoneurons at the level of the syrinx, the loss of descending upper motoneurons passing below the syrinx, and the loss of spinothalamic fibers crossing in the anterior commissure at the level of the syrinx. The result is weakness or wasting with hyporeflexia in the arms, spasticity in the legs, and a capelike distribution of lost pain and temperature sensation at the levels of the syrinx. However, the clinical picture is rarely this simple.

Typically, patients exhibit a constellation of symptoms related to the precise location of the syrinx and the underlying pathologic process.

CLASSIFICATION

Traditionally, the term *syringomyelia* has been used to describe a fluid-filled cavity within the spinal cord, whereas *hydromyelia* has been used to describe a dilation of the central canal of the spinal cord. Unfortunately, today, syringomyelia tends to be used to describe all cases of cystic dilation of the spinal cord. By being merely descriptive, older classification schemes bear the same handicap. Descriptive classification schemes often lack utility because they fail to distinguish between cases with similar anatomic morphology but different pathologic etiologies. Consequently, they do not facilitate decision making in terms of surgical therapy.

Barnett is credited with the first English monograph on syringomyelia (1). His work was remarkable for distinguishing types of syringomyelia based on etiology. This system classified syringomyelia into five categories. In the first category, communicating syringomyelia (syringohydromyelia), the term *communicating* was used to indicate communication with the CSF space and not with the fourth ventricle. This type of syringomyelia is associated with developmental anomalies at the foramen magnum and in the posterior fossa. It is also associated with acquired abnormalities at the base of the brain (basal arachnoiditis, posterior fossa tumors, and cysts). In the second category, syringomyelia is a late sequel to trauma. In the third, syringomyelia is a sequel to spinal arachnoiditis. In the fourth, syringomyelia is associated with spinal cord tumors. The final category is idiopathic syringomyelia.

Milhorat's classification is based on more sophisticated information obtained from contemporary MRI techniques (5). His system was based on his review of 927 cases of cavitary lesions of the spinal cord evaluated with MRI techniques. In contrast to Barnett's classification system, Milhorat's scheme incorporated a more sophisticated compendium of information regarding the pathophysiologic disturbance of normal CSF flow at the foramen magnum, in the spinal central canal, and in the spinal arachnoid space.

Milhorat classified tubular enlargements of the spinal canal based on their anatomic location and communication (4,5,7). He excluded two separate conditions that also cause tubular enlargements of the spinal cord because of their discretely different pathogenesis: atrophic cysts related to myelomalacic changes in the spinal cord and cysts related to neoplasms. His three general categories are (a) dilations of the central canal that communicate with the fourth ventricle (communicating syringomyelia), (b) dilations of the central canal that do not communicate with the fourth ventricle (noncommunicating syringomyelia), and (c) extracanalicular syrinxes that originate in the spinal cord parenchyma and that do not communicate with the central canal or fourth ventricle (primary parenchymal cavitations).

Communicating Syringomyelia

Dilations of the central canal that communicate with the fourth ventricle are caused by obstruction of CSF outflow at the level of the fourth ventricle. Because CSF outflow to the subarachnoid space is obstructed, CSF flow is diverted to the central canal. Dilations of the cerebral ventricles and a central canal syrinx may extend caudally variable distances. The earlier the inciting process occurs in life, the more caudally the syrinx extends, presumably because central canal stenosis, which occurs as an age-related phenomenon, limits its extension in adults and the elderly. Initially, the cavity is lined by ependymal cells, which become discontinuous as the cavity enlarges. For unknown reasons, these syrinxes are less likely to rupture into the surrounding spinal subarachnoid space than noncommunicating syringes.

Communicating syringomyelia can result from posthemorrhagic hydrocephalus, postmeningitic hydrocephalus, and complex hindbrain herniated malformations such as Chiari II malformations and Dandy-Walker malformations (8–10).

Noncommunicating Syringomyelia

Dilations of the central canal that do not communicate with the fourth ventricle are associated with disturbances of normal CSF flow patterns below the foramen magnum. Unlike syrinxes that communicate with the fourth ventricle, the noncommunicating syrinxes tend to be complex lesions frequently associated with intracanalicular septae and paracentral dissection into the spinal subarachnoid space. The dorsolateral paracentral location of parenchymal dissections may be related to the location of the arterial watershed zone between the anterior and posterior spinal arteries (Fig. 63.1). Patients often exhibit discrete neurologic symptoms that correlate with the location of the paracentral dissection.

Noncommunicating syrinxes tend to be associated with Chiari I malformations, basilar invagination, tethered cord, and acquired tonsillar herniation. Gardner and Angel originally proposed that the central canal dilation occurred in Chiari I malformations as a result of obstruction of the foramen of the fourth ventricle, which herniates through the foramen magnum (11). However, this theory required the syrinx to communicate with the fourth ventricle. Recent investigations have shown that such communication seldom exists (12). Using phase-contrast MRI techniques to evaluate CSF flow patterns, Pinna and colleagues found that CSF did not pass from the fourth ventricle to the central spinal canal in any of their 32 patients with syringomyelia associated with a Chiari I malformation (13).

During the cardiac cycle in normal patients, there is pulsatile expansion and contraction of the brain parenchyma.

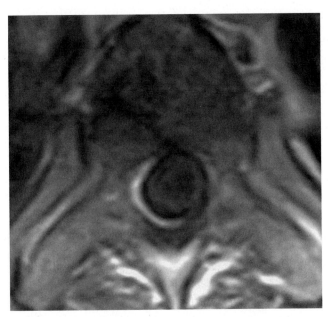

FIG. 63.1. Axial T1-weighted magnetic resonance image of a Chiari I malformation shows a central orientation of the syrinx within the spinal cord.

Because the cranial vault is an incompressible space, systolic expansion of the brain parenchyma leads to its downward herniation into the foramen magnum. In normal patients, this downward herniation of the brain does not prevent the normal bidirectional flow of CSF across the foramen magnum.

In 1994, Heiss and associates proposed a unique explanation for the etiology of the noncommunicating syrinx observed in some cases of Chiari I malformations (12). Pulsatile expansion during systole leads to downward herniation of the tonsils through the foramen magnum, obstructing the normally observed bidirectional CSF flow at the level of the foramen magnum. Because the spinal subarachnoid space is poorly compliant to pressure changes, such obstruction generates abnormal pulsatile pressure waves in the spinal subarachnoid space associated with the systolic phase of the cardiac cycle. Further investigation supports that this abnormal pulsatile waveform may have three effects: (a) it may force CSF along the periarterial Virchow-Robin spaces into the central canal, leading to formation of a syrinx; (b) it may force CSF through the interstitial fluid spaces into the central canal, leading to formation of a syrinx; and (c) it may subject the central canal dilation to pressure disturbances facilitating upward or downward expansion of the syrinx (13). This hypothesis has led to a new theory that a presyrinx state may exist, during which the spinal cord has not yet developed a frank cavitation. Instead, it shows signs of CSF accumulation characterized by spinal cord edema and fattening on T2-weighted MRI and by a clinically reversible myelopathic state (14).

Primary Parenchymal Cavitations

Tubular cavitations of the spinal cord that do not arise from the central canal and that do not communicate with the fourth ventricle are called *primary parenchymal cavitations* (5). They arise after injury to the spinal cord (e.g., trauma, ischemia, infarction, and intramedullary hemorrhage).

Typically, these cavitations form in the watershed zone of the spinal cord in the dorsolateral quadrant. Because the inciting cause is usually related to an injury, the cavity is characterized by a lining of fibroglial tissue with various degrees of necrosis, neuronophagia, and wallerian degeneration.

Similar to that of noncommunicating syringomyelia, the genesis of the cavitation is thought to be related to disturbances in spinal subarachnoid CSF flow. Local arachnoiditis or stenosis may lead to local perturbation of spinal subarachnoid CSF flow, which may be susceptible to pulsatile wave disturbances as observed in noncommunicating syringomyelia. CSF may be forced from the subarachnoid space though the interstitial spaces and perivascular spaces into the substance of the spinal cord, leading to the genesis of the cavity.

Atrophic Cavitations

Local disturbances in CSF flow lead to the distention and propagation of primary parenchymal cavitations; atrophic cavitations are associated with no local or regional disturbances in CSF flow (5). Atrophic cavitations may result from many of the same causes that underlie primary parenchymal cavitations. However, the absence of disturbances in CSF flow results in a regional atrophy of the spinal cord unaccompanied by fluid accumulation. The result is a collection of microcysts, clefts, and dilations of the central canal in the background of regional spinal cord atrophy. Atrophic cavitations are nonpathologic. They do not propagate or cause symptoms related to intralesional pressure or distention. Some authors refer to this condition as syringomyelia *ex vacuo*.

Many investigators have alluded to the notion that the event or condition that leads to regional disturbances in CSF flow may be arachnoid scarring or local spinal canal stenosis. The presence or absence of these conditions in the setting of an infarct, trauma, or degenerative changes may result in the genesis of primary parenchymal cavitations or atrophic cavitations, respectively.

IMAGING

Advances in imaging technology have led to many advances in the understanding of the pathophysiologic basis of syringomyelia. Most of these advances have occurred in static and dynamic MRI techniques. When patients are unable to undergo MRI, computed tomography (CT) can be used.

Computed Tomography Myelography

CT alone is unable to identify syringomyelia or related abnormalities consistently. The administration of intrathecal contrast allows the consistent identification of cavitations of the spinal cord. Typically, the contrast agent requires 4 hours to migrate into the spinal cord. Sometimes migration of the contrast agent may require as long as 12 to 24 hours. Therefore, when a syrinx is not identified on initial delayed scanning, a CT scan should be repeated 12 to 24 hours after contrast administration.

The major limitation of CT myelography is its lack of specificity and sensitivity. Contrast uptake by the spinal cord may occur in regions of myelomalacia; subsequent CT imaging may produce an image that mimics the appearance of a spinal cord syrinx (i.e., false-positive result). Furthermore, reports comparing CT to MRI have documented a false-negative rate as high as 27% (7,13,15). Consequently, CT myelography should be the imaging modality of choice only when MRI is contraindicated or when artifact from metal implants precludes an adequate MRI study from being obtained.

Magnetic Resonance Imaging

MRI techniques are the superior imaging modality for defining syringomyelic changes in the spinal cord. Because high-contrast resolution and multiplanar imaging are available, syringomyelic alterations of the spinal cord can be defined accurately.

Many parameters can be modified during MRI. Therefore, physicians must understand which parameters are important for defining a syrinx to optimize the amount of useful information that can be obtained from an MRI study and to avoid misinterpretation of images.

Slices in the sagittal and axial planes should be obtained in 3-mm and 5-mm cuts to limit partial-volume effects and to ensure that small cavitations can be visualized. Attention should also be paid to the field of view and the matrix size of the scan. If the field of view is too large and the matrix size is too small, truncation artifacts can arise. Truncation artifact occurs at high-contrast signal interfaces. On T1-weighted MRI, the signal interface between CSF and the spinal cord is less pronounced. Therefore, T1-weighted MRI

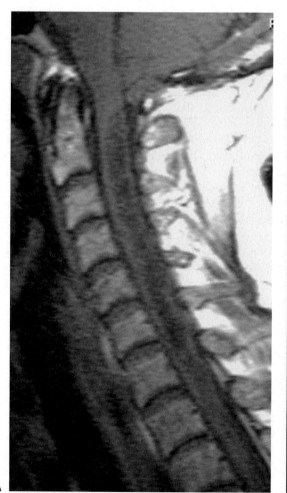
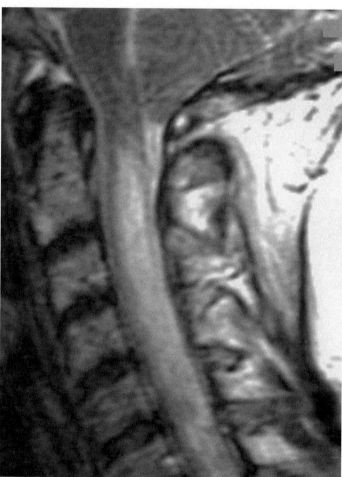

A   B

FIG. 63.2. Sagittal T1-weighted (**A**) and T2-weighted (**B**) magnetic resonance imaging studies of a Chiari I malformation show the margins and morphology of the syrinx associated with the Chiari malformation (**A**) and the complex internal architecture of the syrinx with associated septations (**B**).

is less susceptible to these artifacts. In contrast, there is a significant signal interface between CSF and the spinal cord on T2-weighted imaging. When too large of a field of view is used with too small of a matrix, the signal of the CSF in the spinal cord is magnified, creating the false appearance of a holocord syrinx.

T1-weighted images are best for defining the morphology of the syrinx. Axial images are useful in delineating an eccentric morphology, the presence of septations, and the degree of adjacent spinal cord thinning (Fig. 63.1). T2-weighted images best define actual changes in the spinal cord substance, for example, the presence of gliosis, myelomalacia, or tumor (Fig. 63.2). Intermediate-weighted images help differentiate between myelomalacia and CSF, both of which frequently appear bright on T2-weighted images.

MRI also allows accurate assessment of the anatomy at the craniovertebral junction. MRI techniques accurately depict Chiari malformations. When no obvious etiology for a syrinx can be ascribed, the administration of gadolinium can help to identify or rule out the presence of an associated tumor.

Newer MRI techniques obtain discrete information based on the flow patterns and velocity of CSF within the spinal cord. On routine spin-echo images, artifact is produced by fluid motion. For example, on T2-weighted images without flow compensation, regions of pulsatile flow appear as signal voids, as routinely demonstrated in blood vessels and large CSF reservoirs. In the spinal canal, these signal voids in the CSF surrounding the spinal cord can be misinterpreted as the signal voids from large draining veins associated with an arteriovenous malformation.

MRI phase studies take advantage of bipolar gradients to encode velocity along a preselected direction and can quantify slow flow. Molecules acquire a magnetic spin from the pulse. When they move along the direction of the bipolar gradient, they acquire a phase shift proportional to their velocity. This phase shift is then interpreted for velocity and direction. Cine formats are obtained by formatting the pulses generated to the cardiac cycle (i.e., peripheral pulse gating or cardiac gating).

These imaging techniques capture detailed information about the motion of the brain and CSF during the cardiac cycle. During systole, blood flows into the brain parenchyma. The expansion of the brain causes CSF to flow out of the ventricles and compress the subarachnoid space surrounding the brain. Compression of the subarachnoid space causes CSF to flow downward toward the basal cisterns and into the spinal canal. During diastole, the direction of CSF flow reverses.

TREATMENT

In the past, numerous treatment modalities focused on the syringomyelic cavitations of the spinal cord. The principal reason for the failure of this treatment paradigm is that syringomyelia is not a disease process. Rather, it is a secondary manifestation of one of many pathophysiologic disturbances of normal CSF physiology in the spinal cord. Therefore, treatment should be targeted at the inciting process. In individual cases, the difficulty lies in determining the underlying disease process.

Atrophic cavitations of the spinal cord deserve no surgical treatment. Cystic cavitations related to intramedullary or extramedullary tumors should resolve with appropriate tumor resection (16). Persistence of spinal cord cysts after tumor resection should alert physicians to the possibility of tumor regrowth, spinal cord tethering at the site of tumor resection, arachnoid scarring at the site of tumor resection, or acquired stenosis of the spinal canal at the site of dural closure. Most of these conditions can be prevented with meticulous dural closure and the liberal use of dural patches to prevent unwanted intrathecal stenosis.

Communicating Syringomyelia

In communicating syringomyelia, the pathogenesis of the spinal cord syrinx is related to the obstruction of CSF outflow at the level of the fourth ventricle (9,17,18). Therefore, therapy should be targeted at this underlying pathologic process. In cases of posthemorrhagic hydrocephalus or postmeningitic hydrocephalus, ventriculoperitoneal shunting is typically adequate. In cases of congenital syndromes associated with complex hindbrain herniation, therapy may require posterior fossa decompression, ventriculoperitoneal shunting, or both, depending of the patient's individual needs.

Noncommunicating Syringomyelia

In noncommunicating syringomyelia, the pathogenesis of the spinal cord syrinx is obstruction of CSF flow between the fourth ventricle and central spinal canal. Classically, this abnormality is associated with the Chiari I malformation (17–19). Although numerous hypotheses have been proposed, they agree on the following premise. Hindbrain herniation compresses the cervicomedullary junction and alters normal CSF flow dynamics in the spinal cord (12,13,20). The most compelling theory has been proposed by Oldfield (21). Abnormal pulsations in the spinal canal lead to paracentral cavitation of the spinal cord when CSF migrates into the spinal cord because abnormal pulsatile waveforms are transmitted to the intrathecal space during the cardiac cycle (12,13). Septations are common because the cavitation is paracentral and unrelated to direct dilation of the central canal as in communicating syringomyelia.

Therapy is therefore directed at treatment of the Chiari I malformation (22–26). Although some physicians advocate bony decompression at the cervicomedullary junction alone, most advocate enlargement of the potential space surrounding the cervicomedullary junction at the level of the foramen magnum either by opening the dura alone or by using a dural patch. Authors tend to disagree about what else is needed. Gardner's original hydrodynamic theory attributed the genesis of the syrinx to CSF pulsations transmitted from the fourth ventricle into the spinal canal (11).

Based on his conclusions, numerous investigators have advocated microsurgical lysis of adhesions around the outlet of the fourth ventricle and plugging the obex with muscle to prevent transmission of the CSF pulsations into the central canal of the spinal cord. Based on contemporary data primarily obtained from phase-contrasted MRI, the lack of communication between the fourth ventricle and the central canal in syrinxes associated with Chiari I malformations suggests that these maneuvers probably do not alter surgical outcomes. Because skull base surgery is associated with serious consequences, it is becoming less common.

If, however, obstruction of the foramen magnum by the descended tonsils is the inciting pathologic process, then shrinking the tonsils by using microsurgical techniques can be beneficial if the craniovertebral junction cannot be decompressed adequately with the above techniques. The author (CAD) advocates making small microsurgical incisions only at the posterior border of the tonsils and performing a modest subpial tonsillar resection. The authors (CAD, GPZ) suggest that this approach reduces complications related to delayed arachnoid scarring from bipolar electrocauterization of the pial-arachnoid surface of the tonsils.

Primary Parenchymal Cavitations

In primary parenchymal cavitations, an acquired cavitation of the spinal cord pathologically fills and distends because regional CSF flow has been disturbed by local arachnoid scarring or stenosis of the spinal canal (5). Treatment is required because these cavitations tend to propagate or progress. In contrast, simple atrophic cavitations seldom enlarge, presumably because there are no regional disturbances in CSF flow.

The original cavitation typically results from local trauma, an infarct, or hemorrhage (8,27,28). Pathologic distention of the cavitation results from the local disturbance in CSF flow. Therefore, resolution of the local disturbance in CSF flow is the appropriate surgical therapy. Surgery may consist of spinal canal decompression or local detethering of the spinal cord with placement of a non-scar-promoting dural patch.

Shunting Procedures for Syrinx Cavitation

The historical use of shunting to treat syringomyelia underscores the lack of understanding of the underlying pathogenetic process. Numerous procedures have been advocated for the treatment of syringomyelia: terminal ventriculostomy, syringocisternostomy, lumboperitoneal shunting, thecoperitoneal shunting, syringoperitoneal shunting, and syringosubarachnoid shunting (1,10,23–25).

Terminal ventriculostomy used to be the treatment for syrinxes. This procedure involves excision of the filum terminale and the tip of the conus medullaris to provide an outlet for CSF flow from the syrinx. Williams critically reviewed this procedure and concluded that it typically resulted in poor outcomes (1,29). Of his 31 patients, 29 either deteriorated or showed no improvement.

Milhorat and colleagues advocated syringocisternostomy as an alternative to syringosubarachnoid shunting (4,5,7). This group argued that when CSF flow is obstructed above a syrinx, shunting to the subarachnoid space below the level of obstruction will provide no clinical benefit. By extending the shunt to the posterior fossa, they obtained clinical and radiographic improvement in four patients with Chiari-related syringomyelia.

Lumboperitoneal shunting has also been suggested as a possible therapy. Theoretically, shunting fluid from the subarachnoid space could reduce the transmural gradient favoring the movement of CSF into a syrinx. Park and colleagues reported that four of six patients improved after being treated with lumboperitoneal shunts, myelotomy, and placement of a syringopleural shunt 1 month after the myelotomy (30).

Thecoperitoneal shunting works on the same principles as lumboperitoneal shunting. The proximal catheter of the shunt is placed in the subarachnoid space adjacent to the syrinx instead of within the syrinx. Vengsarkar and co-workers (31) used this modality to treat three patients. Each had a Chiari I malformation associated with the syrinx, and two had undergone a prior Chiari decompression. The three patients improved both radiographically and clinically.

In contrast to thecoperitoneal shunting, the proximal catheter on syringoperitoneal shunts is placed directly in the syrinx. Syringoperitoneal shunting has been documented extensively. Some authors (32,33) report good outcomes in patients bearing syrinxes associated with and without Chiari malformations. If drainage of fluid into the peritoneum is complicated, CSF may be diverted to the pleural cavity.

Finally, syringosubarachnoid shunting is the simplest of the above procedures. It involves placing a tube to connect the syrinx with the subarachnoid space. Hida and associates (20) treated 70 patients with either foramen magnum decompression or syringosubarachnoid shunting. Patients with symptoms referable to foramen magnum compression underwent foramen magnum decompression, whereas patients with large syrinxes and symptoms related to spinal cord cavitation underwent syringosubarachnoid shunting. Patients who received a syringosubarachnoid shunt uniformly did well, suggesting that syringosubarachnoid shunting may be a reasonable first-line treatment for syrinxes associated with Chiari I malformations. However, Tator and Briceno (34) obtained less convincing results with 20 patients who received syringosubarachnoid shunts. In their series, only 2 of the 4 patients with cerebellar tonsillar ectopia did well with shunting.

The use of shunting procedures for syrinxes is compelling. However, numerous other authors have reported adverse outcomes after shunting procedures. Based purely on pathophysiologic information, if the inciting cause for the syrinx can be identified and treated, it makes more sense to consider this approach as the first-line therapy.

The use of shunts in communicating syringomyelia makes sense. Because the syrinx communicates with the fourth ventricle, shunting of the ventricular system is adequate, and direct shunting of the syrinx is neither necessary nor desirable.

The use of shunts in noncommunicating syringomyelia is less well founded based on anatomic and physiologic data. The frequent presence of septations within the syrinx precludes adequate shunting of the syrinx alone. The absence of communication between the syrinx and the fourth ventricle precludes the use of a regular ventriculoperitoneal shunting procedure. Furthermore, in the absence of treatment directed at the primary abnormality, there is little rationale to suggest why the syrinx will not recur.

In primary parenchymal cavitations, initial therapy should be directed at treating any local cause of disturbance in CSF flow. Failure of this therapy should prompt reexamination of the adequacy of the surgical procedure. The regional CSF flow disturbance should be resolved before local syrinx shunting or fenestration is considered.

If this first line of therapy fails, shunting may be a good second line of intervention. The results of subarachnoid, syrinx, and regional CSF shunting are unclear, and the rate of shunt failure is high. Comparing the different techniques, no clear winner emerges. Therefore, choosing the simplest procedure may afford the patient the least risk. By applying this rationale when conventional treatment modalities fail, syringosubarachnoid shunting would be the preferred modality.

SURGICAL TECHNIQUE

Of the techniques described earlier, the surgical treatment of the Chiari I malformation is the procedure most commonly performed. It has been described with numerous variations. No studies support the appropriateness of one particular technique compared with another. We describe the nuances of the technique used at our institution to treat Chiari I malformations.

The patient is positioned prone with the head fixated in the Mayfield headholder in a bicoronal orientation (Fig. 63.3). The head is flexed in a military fashion to open the occipitocervical joint. Somatosensory evoked potentials are typically recorded before and after positioning.

The neck is shaved just rostral to the inion. The opening incision proceeds from the inion to just below the C2 spinous process. The soft tissue is dissected in the relatively avascular nuchal midline (Fig. 63.4). Care is taken to prevent the detachment of any muscles from the C2 spinous process. If a C2 laminectomy is unnecessary, this maneuver avoids complications with postoperative pain management. A C1 laminectomy is performed using Kerrison rongeurs. A suboccipital craniectomy is performed below the level of the transverse sinus. At the foramen magnum, the craniectomy is extended laterally until the occipital condyle is identified. This maneuver affords a wide bony decompression at the foramen magnum.

The tonsils are freed of any arachnoid tethering until the obex of the fourth ventricle is identified. If the tonsils are

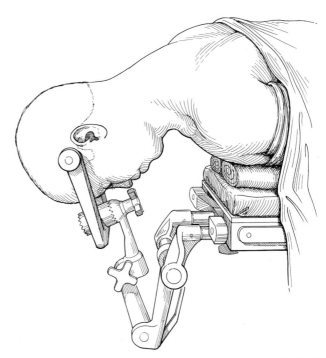

FIG. 63.3. The patient is positioned prone with the Mayfield head holder affixed to the operating room table. The military orientation of the neck facilitates exposure of the occipitocervical junction. (Courtesy of Barrow Neurological Institute, St. Joseph's Hospital and Medical Center, Phoenix, Arizona.)

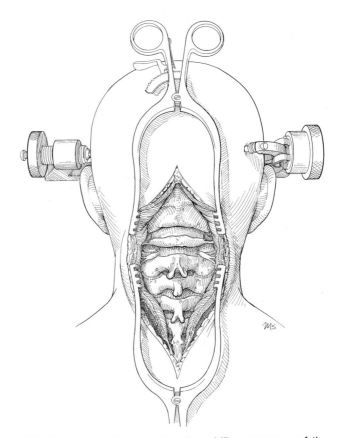

FIG. 63.4. Illustration showing the midline exposure of the occipitocervical junction. (Courtesy of Barrow Neurological Institute, St. Joseph's Hospital and Medical Center, Phoenix, Arizona.)

abnormally large or significantly descended, they are surgically shrunk in the following fashion. Using bipolar electrocauterization, a longitudinal opening in the pial plane of the tonsil is made to permit a subpial resection of the tonsil. The pial plane of the tonsil abutting the fourth ventricle must not be violated to prevent unnecessary scarring.

A triangular bovine pericardial patch is fashioned and sewn to the surrounding dural margins to create a patulous subarachnoid space at the foramen magnum. A watertight closure is obtained using a 6–0 Prolene suture.

To prevent any complications related to cerebellar sag, a portion of the craniotomy is reattached to the inferior margin of the craniectomy. Before the bone is reaffixed, it is modified so that it does not crowd the foramen magnum and does not compress the contents of the posterior fossa.

CONCLUSION

Syringomyelia is a complex disorder, and its clinical manifestations can be devastating. Appropriate surgical treatment of a syrinx begins with accurate identification of the underlying pathologic process that led its genesis. Many failures in syrinx treatment may be avoidable by improving diagnosis of the underlying pathologic process. Although numerous classification schemes exist for syringomyelia, Milhorat's system offers a rational treatment paradigm because it is based on the pathologic origin of the syrinx. Advances in noninvasive imaging are helping to improve our understanding of the underlying pathologic processes that lead to the formation of a syrinx. The use of sophisticated pulse sequences with higher-strength MRI may help identify the pathologic process underlying the formation of a syrinx and may help make surgical decision making a more straightforward process.

REFERENCES

1. Williams B. Syringomyelia. Neurosurg Clin N Am 1990;1(3):653–685.
2. Wisoff JH. Hydromyelia: a critical review. Childs Nerv Syst 1988;4(1):1–8.
3. Batzdorf U. Primary spinal syringomyelia: a personal perspective. Neurosurg Focus 2000;8(3):Article 7.
4. Milhorat TH, Capocelli AL Jr, Anzil AP, et al. Pathological basis of spinal cord cavitation in syringomyelia: analysis of 105 autopsy cases. J Neurosurg 1995;82:802–812.
5. Milhorat TH. Classification of syringomyelia. Neurosurg Focus 2000; 8(3):Article 1.
6. Zager EL, Ojemann RG, Poletti CE. Acute presentations of syringomyelia. Report of three cases. J Neurosurg 1990;72:133–138.
7. Milhorat TH, Chou MW, Trinidad EM, et al. Chiari I malformation redefined: clinical and radiographic findings for 364 symptomatic patients. Neurosurgery 1999;44(5):1005–1017.
8. Schurch B, Wichmann W, Rossier AB. Post-traumatic syringomyelia (cystic myelopathy): a prospective study of 449 patients with spinal cord injury. J Neurol Neurosurg Psychiatry 1996;60(1):61–67.
9. Rauzzino M, Oakes WJ. Chiari II malformation and syringomyelia. Neurosurg Clin N Am 1995;6(2):293–309.
10. Stoodley MA, Jones NR. Syringomyelia. In: The Cervical Spine Research Society Editorial Committee, ed. The cervical spine, 3rd ed. Philadelphia: Lippincott-Raven, 1998:565–582.
11. Gardner WJ, Angel J. The mechanism of syringomyelia and it surgical correction. Clin Neurosurg 1958;6:131–140.
12. Heiss JD, Patronas N, DeVroom HL, et al. Elucidating the pathophysiology of syringomyelia. J Neurosurg 1999;91:553–562.
13. Pinna G, Alessandrini F, Alfieri A, et al. Cerebrospinal fluid flow dynamics study in Chiari I malformation: implications for syrinx formation. Neurosurg Focus 2000;8(3):Article 3.
14. Fishbein NJ, Dillon WP, Cobbs C, et al. The "presyrinx" state: is there a reversible myelopathic condition that may precede syringomyelia? Neurosurg Focus 2000;8(3):Article 4.
15. Tanghe HL. Magnetic resonance imaging (MRI) in syringomyelia. Acta Neurochir (Wien) 1995;134(1–2):93–99.
16. Keung YK, Cobos E, Whitehead RP, et al. Secondary syringomyelia due to intramedullary spinal cord metastasis. Case report and review of literature. Am J Clin Oncol 1997;20(6):577–579.
17. Cai C, Oakes WJ. Hindbrain herniation syndromes: the Chiari malformations (I and II). Semin Pediatr Neurol 1997;4(3):179–191.
18. Nishikawa M, Sakamoto H, Hakuba A, et al. Pathogenesis of Chiari malformations: a morphometric study of the posterior cranial fossa. J Neurosurg 1997;86:40–47.
19. Bindal AK, Dunsker SB, Tew JM Jr. Chiari I malformation: classification and management. Neurosurgery 1995;37(6):1069–1074.
20. Stoodley MA, Jones NR, Yang L, Brown CJ. Mechanisms underlying the formation and enlargement of noncommunicating syringomyelia: experimental studies. Neurosurg Focus 2000;8(3):Article 2.
21. Oldfield EH. Cerebellar tonsils and syringomyelia. J Neurosurg 2002; 97(5):1009–1010.
22. Hida K, Iwasaki Y, Koyangi I, et al. Surgical indication and results of foramen magnum decompression versus syringosubarachnoid shunting for syringomyelia associated with Chiari I malformation. Neurosurgery 1995;37(4):673–679.
23. Mariani C, Cislaghi MG, Barbieri S, et al. The natural history and results of surgery in 50 cases of syringomyelia. J Neurol 1991;238(8):433–438.
24. Goel A, Desai K. Surgery for syringomyelia: an analysis based on 163 surgical cases. Acta Neurochir 2000;142:293–302.
25. Ellenbogen RG, Armonda RA, Shaw DWW, et al. Toward a rational treatment of Chiari I malformation and syringomyelia. Neurosurg Focus 2000;8(3):Article 6.
26. Grabb PA, Mapstone TB, Oakes WJ. Ventral brain stem compression in pediatric and young adult patients with Chiari I malformations. Neurosurgery 1999;44(3):520–528.
27. Yang L, Jones NR, Stoodley MA, et al. Excitotoxic model of post-traumatic syringomyelia in the rat. Spine 2001;26(17):1842–1849.
28. Lee TT, Almeda GJ, Camilo E, et al. Surgical treatment of post-traumatic myelopathy associated with syringomyelia. Spine 2001;26(24S):S119–S127.
29. Williams B. Surgical treatment of syringobulbia. Neurosurg Clin N Am 1993;4(3):553–571.
30. Park TS, Cail WS, Broaddus WC, et al. Lumboperitoneal shunt combined with myelotomy for treatment of syringohydromyelia. J Neurosurg 1989;70(5):721–727.
31. Vengsarkar US, Panchal VG, Tripathi PD, et al. Percutaneous thecoperitoneal shunt for syringomyelia. Report of three cases. J Neurosurg 1991;74(5):827–831.
32. Lesoin F, Petit H, Thomas CE 3rd, et al. Use of the syringoperitoneal shunt in the treatment of syringomyelia. Surg Neurol 1986;25(2):131–136.
33. Suzuki M, Davis C, Symon L, et al. Syringoperitoneal shunt for treatment of cord cavitation. J Neurol Neurosurg Psychiatry 1985;48(7):620–627.
34. Tator CH, Briceno C. Treatment of syringomyelia with a syringosubarachnoid shunt. Can J Neurol Sci 1988;15(1):48–57.

SECTION VIII

Inflammatory Conditions

CHAPTER 64

Rheumatoid Arthritis in the Cervical Spine

Charles W. Cha, Scott D. Boden, and Charles R. Clark

Rheumatoid arthritis in the cervical spine results in anatomic abnormalities as a consequence of the destruction of synovial joints, ligaments, and bone. Inflammatory synovitis can produce erosion of both bone and ligament, resulting in pain, instability, bony subluxations, and ultimately spinal cord or brainstem compression. Compression of the cervical spinal cord or brainstem or both may result either from direct compression by synovial pannus or from indirect compression due to cervical subluxations. Atlantoaxial subluxation is attributed to erosive synovitis in the atlantoaxial, atlantoodontoid, and atlantooccipital joints, as well as the synovium-lined bursa between the odontoid and the transverse ligament. Atlantoaxial impaction (cranial settling, upward translocation of the odontoid, pseudobasilar invagination, vertical subluxation) describes the settling of the skull on the atlas, and the atlas on the axis, resulting from erosion and bone loss in the occipitoatlantal and atlantoaxial joints. Subaxial subluxations occur through destruction of the facets, interspinous ligaments, and intervertebral discs (spondylodiscitis).

Although much is known about the natural history, pathophysiology, pharmacologic management, and operative stabilization of patients with rheumatoid disease in the cervical spine, the clinically relevant question of when to undertake operative intervention in the cervical spine remains somewhat unclear. Operative stabilization or arthrodesis has traditionally been reserved for patients with severe progressive neurologic deficit or intractable pain (1). The early experience with many of these patients demonstrated a high operative morbidity as well as variable neurologic recovery once notable paralysis had occurred. Complicating the operative decision further is the fact that although many patients have radiographic evidence of cervical spine involvement, not all have progression of their cervical disease and develop paralysis. Therefore, a difficult clinical issue remains as to how to identify patients before they develop irreversible neurologic deficit and when

one should proceed with operative stabilization in this select group.

Although the answer to this question is still not completely clear, we can shed some light on it by examining what is known about the predictors of paralysis as well as the predictors of the potential for neurologic recovery after operations in patients with rheumatoid disease in the cervical spine. After such an analysis is undertaken, a rational scheme can then be devised to monitor patients safely and cost effectively, to decide when secondary neurodiagnostic imaging studies should be performed, and finally, to offer recommendations for the timing of operative stabilization. Because the techniques of operative stabilization are covered in the chapters that follow, this chapter focuses primarily on developing a strategy for timely and cost-effective evaluation and management of these challenging patients.

PREDICTORS OF PARALYSIS

Natural History

Defining the natural history of a particular disease is important because it serves as a baseline from which one can gauge the potential of certain therapeutic modalities to alter or affect the natural course of a disease process. Unfortunately, with chronic diseases such as rheumatoid arthritis, establishing the natural history of the disease can be problematic for several reasons. First, gauging the natural progression of a disease requires long-term prospective studies that follow untreated patients. In situations where effective therapies are known to exist, it is unethical to withhold those beneficial therapies for the sake of research. Second, the logistics of completing these long-term studies can be complicated. As a result, knowledge of the natural history of cervical spine involvement in the rheumatoid patient is limited. Only a few studies address this topic, and current knowledge is based on smaller, retrospective evaluations.

Reports documenting the prevalence of cervical subluxations in the rheumatoid population vary widely. Between 43% to 86% of rheumatoid patients have radiographic evidence of cervical instability (2). The most common type of cervical subluxation in rheumatoid patients is atlantoaxial subluxation, which represents approximately 65% of all cervical subluxations (Fig. 64.1). Of patients with atlantoaxial subluxation, most have anterior subluxation, although approximately 20% may have lateral subluxations and less than 10% have posterior subluxation. Rotatory subluxations have been reported, but are rare (3). Approximately 20% of rheumatoid subluxations involve basilar invagination (cranial settling), alone or in combination with atlantoaxial subluxation. About 15% of rheumatoid patients with cervical subluxations may also have subaxial subluxation, which frequently occurs at multiple levels. Rheumatoid patients may present with any combination of these three main types of cervical instability.

Despite the high prevalence of radiographic changes seen in the rheumatoid cervical spine, associated neurologic deficits are reported to occur in only 7% to 58% of patients (4,5). The wide variation in the reported prevalence of neurologic deficits can be attributed to the variability in the neurologic classification systems as well as to the difficulty in detecting subtle neurologic changes in this group of patients. Regardless, it is clear that many patients with pain and radiographic changes do not display a neurologic deficit.

To better characterize the natural history of cervical disease in the rheumatoid population, studies have evaluated the rate of progression for both radiographic as well as neurologic changes. Rana (6) followed the radiographs of 41 patients with atlantoaxial instability for a period of 10 years. Twenty-seven percent of these patients were noted to have radiographic subluxations that progressed, whereas 61% showed no radiographic changes and 12% actually improved radiographically. In 1981, Pellicci and colleagues (2) noted that although 80% of their patients with rheumatoid arthritis who had cervical involvement showed radiographic progression, only 36% had neurologic progression. Boden and associates (7) evaluated the clinical course of 73 patients for an average of 7.1 years. Of the 73 patients, 42 (58%) developed paralysis. The majority of these patients were treated operatively; however, 7 were treated nonoperatively because they either refused surgery or had medical contraindications to sur-

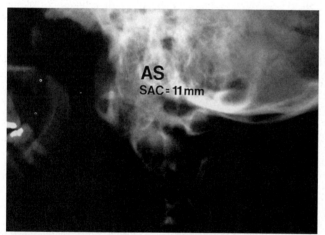

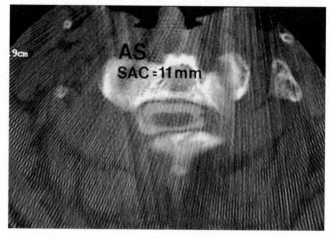

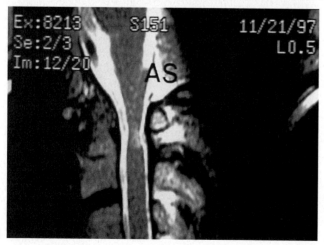

FIG. 64.1. Lateral radiograph of the upper cervical spine shows atlantoaxial instability **(A)**, computed tomographic myelogram shows spinal cord deformation **(B)**, and magnetic resonance imaging reveals the myelomalacia that has developed from the chronic compression **(C)**.

gery. Six of 7 patients had a deterioration of neurologic function, and all were dead within 4 years of onset of paralysis; 5 of the 7 deaths could be directly attributed to the cord compression.

These studies indicate that although rheumatoid patients are likely to have radiologic progression of their cervical disease, the majority will not go on to develop a neurologic deficit. However, once paralysis develops, the natural history seems to be one of progressive neurologic deterioration, which ultimately can lead to death. In fact, sudden death in the rheumatoid patient with cervical involvement is a substantial concern and occurs secondary to medullary compression caused by upper cervical instability. Postmortem analyses indicate that sudden death from medullary compression can occur in as many as 10% of patients (8).

Our knowledge of the natural history of rheumatoid cervical disease indicates that a wide variation exists in radiographic measurements. There is also a substantial amount of overlap between symptomatic and asymptomatic patients. These factors combine to make the radiographic definition of instability elusive in this patient population. Furthermore, the poor correlation of neurologic symptoms with radiographic evidence of instability makes the identification of an impending neurologic deficit, and therefore of the ideal candidate for surgical treatment, difficult.

To better identify the rheumatoid patient with an impending neurologic deficit, investigators have evaluated certain clinical and radiographic parameters for predicting which patients are at a higher risk for neurologic compromise.

Clinical Presentation

The findings that accompany cervical involvement with rheumatoid arthritis can be very subtle. A careful history and physical examination are crucial in the spinal evaluation of the rheumatoid patient. Typically, these patients manifest with pain, frequently at the craniocervical junction. Patients may also complain of occipital headaches, which may be secondary to an occipital neuralgia precipitated by compression of the greater occipital branch of C2. If the greater auricular branch is involved, then the patients may develop ear pain. Compression of the trigeminal nucleus with vertical settling can present as facial pain. Neurologic symptoms are multiple and can be vague, ranging from paresthesias in the hand to Lhermitte phenomena, which are electrical sensations traveling through the body. Vertebrobasilar insufficiency, which is associated with basilar invagination, may cause tinnitus, vertigo, loss of equilibrium, and visual disturbances. Diplopia, dysphagia, and urinary dysfunction, frequency, or retention are important warning signs that are caused by bulbar involvement. Vertical nystagmus and Cheyne-Stokes respirations can be associated with brainstem compression. Joint crepitation and instability may be palpated in the upper cervical spine and noted with range of motion, sometimes in the form of a "clunk."

Physical examinations are difficult to interpret in this population because subtle neurologic changes may be masked for a variety of reasons and are often confused or misattributed to other musculoskeletal manifestations of this disease. For example, motor strength testing may be difficult in the patient with multiple joint deformities and tendon subluxations or ruptures. These patients typically have a baseline weakness due to muscular atrophy. Peripheral nerve entrapment may also confuse the neurologic examination. Detection of long tract signs, which herald the onset of early myopathy, can be very difficult given all of the peripheral involvement that can occur with this disease. Therefore, the clinician must be astute in detecting the subtle changes that accompany neurologic compression of the cervical spine.

Studies have evaluated the use of certain clinical parameters to help predict which patients are at risk of developing progressive cervical disease and neurologic deficit. The clinical risk factors that have been identified include male gender, severe peripheral disease, the use of corticosteroids, and age of onset of disease (9–11). It is difficult to determine whether the use of corticosteroids is truly an independent risk factor or just an association with patients with severe peripheral disease. A study of 149 patients attempted to correlate laboratory values with the development of cervical spine subluxations in the rheumatoid population. Subluxation in the cervical spine was associated with the presence of HLA-DW2 and HLA-B7 cross-reacting group. Using these laboratory values along with the age of onset of disease, the researchers were able to successfully predict radiologic outcome in 82% of the patients (12). Unfortunately, these clinical parameters that include history, physical examination, and laboratory evaluation are only a moderate help at predicting which of these patients are at risk for developing a neurologic deficit.

Radiographic Predictors of Paralysis

Clinicians must often rely heavily on expensive, often invasive, and less than perfect imaging studies to identify the patient who is at risk of developing a neurologic deficit. Prediction of the timing of onset of myelopathy in any given patient is difficult—not unlike predicting an earthquake before it occurs. Studies of large populations of rheumatoid patients have enabled the establishment of parameters for predicting patients at higher risk for neurologic compromise.

Plain Radiography

Plain radiographs are the basis of radiographic evaluation of the rheumatoid cervical spine. Although magnetic resonance imaging (MRI) is the superior imaging modality for demonstrating cord compression from subluxation or synovial pannus, it is expensive and somewhat time-consuming, and therefore not practical to use on a routine or ongoing basis to screen all patients with rheumatoid arthritis. Therefore, it is important to review plain radiographs and to assess what can and cannot be learned from such studies.

Anterior atlantoaxial subluxation may be assessed on a lateral cervical spine radiograph by measuring the anterior atlantodental interval (AADI) from the midposterior margin of the anterior ring of C1 to the anterior surface of the odontoid. If this interval measures more than 3 mm in an adult or 4 mm in a child, it is considered abnormal and spinal cord function may be in jeopardy. The interval is generally accentuated on a flexion view if instability or excessive motion is present. In fact, the amount of dynamic motion present at the atlantodental interval, measured as the change between flexion and extension, may be more clinically relevant than the maximal interval on a single flexion view.

Anterior atlantoaxial subluxation may also be assessed by measurement of the posterior atlantodental interval, which is measured from the posterior aspect of the odontoid to the anterior margin of the C1 lamina. This interval does not represent the space available for the cord in patients with rheumatoid arthritis because the retroodontoid synovial pannus may occupy 1 to 3 mm or more of that space.

Vertical migration of the odontoid can be assessed radiographically in a variety of ways (Fig. 64.2). McRae's line connects the front of the foramen magnum to the back, and the odontoid should not project above this line. The upper tip of the odontoid process normally lies 1 cm below the anterior margin of the foramen magnum. Chamberlain's line is drawn from the posterior margin of the hard palate to the posterior margin of the foramen magnum. The tip of the odontoid should not project more than 3 mm above this line; projection 6 mm above this line is considered pathologic. Commonly, however, the margins of the foramen magnum are difficult to define without a tomogram. McGregor's line is easier to use because it connects the posterior margin of the hard palate to the most caudal point of the occiput. The tip of the odontoid should not project more than 4.5 mm above this line.

Because the odontoid tip may be difficult to identify, particularly with rheumatoid-related osteopenia or destruction, another measurement was described by Redlund-Johnell and Pettersson (13). The McGregor line is drawn on a lateral cervical radiograph with the head in neutral position. The distance to the lower end plate of the C2 vertebral body is then measured. Less than 34 mm in men and less than 29 mm in women is defined as vertical migration of the odontoid. Clark and associates (14) have described the so-called station of the atlas, which notes the relationship between the anterior arch of the atlas and the axis. Normally, the atlas lies adjacent to the upper portion of the dens. If the arch lies adjacent to the base of the dens or body of the axis, moderate to severe cranial settling may be present. All these measurements, as well as others (15,16), attempt to identify and quantitate the degree of odontoid encroachment on space normally occupied by the brainstem and spinal cord.

Subaxial subluxations tend to occur at multiple levels in a given patient, producing a "staircase" or "stepladder" deformity (Fig. 64.3). Lack of osteophyte formation is typical of rheumatoid arthritis, as is involvement of C2-C3 and C3-C4, which are not commonly involved in degenerative disease. Subaxial subluxation may be quantitated on lateral cervical radiographs as relative translation, with the distance of the forward slip (in millimeters) expressed as a percentage of the total anteroposterior diameter of the inferior vertebral body. Alternatively, this deformity may be described by measuring the minimum spinal canal diameter behind the slipped vertebra. The latter measurement may more closely reflect potential spinal cord compression. Ascertaining whether the subluxations are fixed or mobile on flexion-extension radiographs is also important.

An increasing number of studies assessing the measurements made from plain lateral cervical radiographs have shown that the AADI is unreliable at discriminating patients with rheumatoid arthritis from those without neurologic deficit. One example is a study by Collins and co-workers (17), which showed that 61% of rheumatoid patients undergoing total joint replacement operations had radiographic

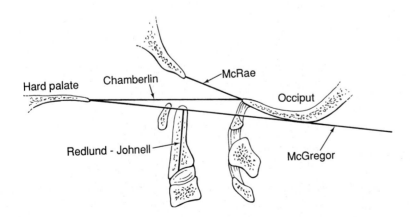

FIG. 64.2. Schematic (lateral view) of upper cervical spine showing some of the reference lines for measuring basilar invagination.

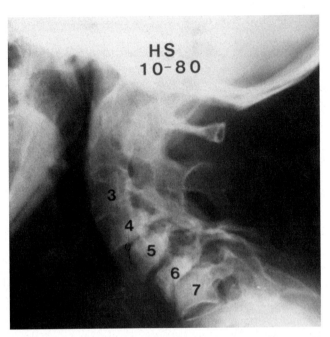

FIG. 64.3. Lateral radiograph of a patient with rheumatoid arthritis with progressive multiple-level subaxial subluxations from the third through seventh cervical vertebrae. The patient developed slowly progressive cervical myelopathy and required surgery. (From Boden SD, Dodge LD, Bohlman HH, et al. Rheumatoid arthritis of the cervical spine. *J Bone Joint Surg Am* 1993;75:1282–1297, with permission.)

10 mm, depending on the series, has been recommended (6,11,14). Other investigators (19) have suggested that it is not the absolute amount of subluxation present but the degree of mobility that is most important. In addition, neurologic progression is generally considered inevitable once any degree of cord compromise is present. Unfortunately, there is poor correlation between vertebral subluxation on plain radiographs (measured by the AADI) and cord compression as shown by MRI (20).

Traditionally, the AADI as measured on lateral cervical radiographs has been used clinically to follow patients with rheumatoid arthritis affecting the cervical spine. However, the ability of this measurement to identify patients with paralysis prior to its onset is unreliable, as demonstrated by calculations made in a recent large series of rheumatoid patients (7). This can be more clearly documented by examining the sensitivity, specificity, accuracy, positive predictive value, and negative predictive value calculated for the AADI in predicting paralysis depending on where the cutoff value for the interval is set. For example, if the critical AADI is set at greater than or equal to 8 mm, the sensitivity, or ability to detect patients with paralysis, is 59%; however, the specificity, or the ability to remain normal in the absence of clinical disease, is only 58% (Table 64.1). Although increasing the cutoff of the AADI to greater than or equal to 10 mm raises the specificity of the test to 90%, it decreases the sensitivity and ability to detect patients with paralysis to 35%. More important, the negative predictive value (which represents the percentage of patients below that interval who would not have paralysis) is only 56%.

The posterior atlantodental interval (PADI) is measured from the posterior aspect of the dens to the anterior aspect of the C1 lamina (Fig. 64.4). This measurement was extensively evaluated and compared with the traditional anterior interval in a long-term series (7). Use of a PADI with a cutoff of less than or equal to 14 mm yielded a sensitivity (ability to detect patients with paralysis) of 97%, far superior to that of the anterior interval (Table 64.1). The specificity using the posterior interval was only 52% and was

evidence of atlantoaxial instability, yet only 50% of patients had any signs or symptoms of their cervical disease. In some studies, investigators attempted to use the AADI as a potential criterion for recommending operative intervention in patients with rheumatoid arthritis affecting the cervical spine. Although the normal atlantodental interval is 3 mm, more than 5 mm of subluxation is considered to represent atlantoaxial instability (18). In studies of patients with rheumatoid arthritis, operative intervention for an atlantodental interval greater than 8 mm, greater than 9 mm, or greater than

TABLE 64.1. *Reliability of Anterior and Posterior Atlantodental Intervals in Predicting Paralysis in Patients with Rheumatoid Arthritis of the Cervical Spine*

Test and cutoff interval	Sensitivity (%)	Specificity (%)	Accuracy (%)	Positive predictive value (%)	Negative predictive value (%)
AADI					
≥8 mm	59	58	58	61	56
≥9 mm	41	77	58	67	55
≥10 mm	35	90	62	80	56
≥11 mm	18	97	55	86	52
PADI					
≥12 mm	76	90	83	90	78
≥13 mm	91	71	82	78	88
≥14 mm	97	52	75	69	94

AADI, anterior atlantodental interval; PADI, posterior atlantodental interval.
Data calculated from a series of 73 patients. (From Allmann K-H, Uhl M, Uhrmeister P, et al. Functional MR imaging of the cervical spine in patients with rheumatoid arthritis. *Acta Radiologica* 1998;39:543–546, with permission.)

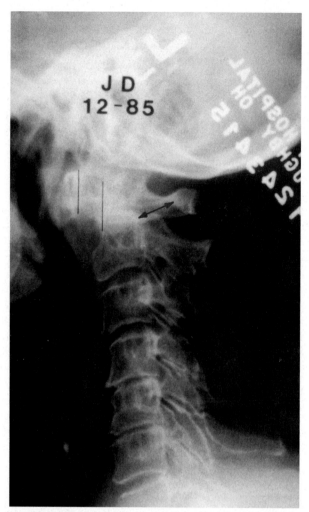

FIG. 64.4. Lateral cervical radiograph of a rheumatoid patient with atlantoaxial subluxation. Both the anterior atlantodental interval (*vertical lines*) and the posterior atlantodental interval (*arrowheads*) are marked.

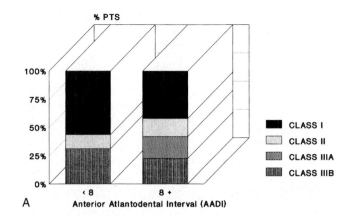

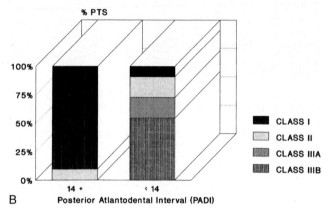

FIG. 64.5. Prediction of the development of paralysis in 73 patients who had rheumatoid arthritis of the cervical spine. **A:** Paralysis in rheumatoids predicted by the anterior atlantodental interval (AADI). **B:** Paralysis in rheumatoids predicted by the posterior atlantodental interval (PADI). Although the AADI did not correlate well with paralysis ($p > 0.10$), a PADI of 14 mm clearly demarcated neurologically intact patients (Ranawat class I) from those in whom paralysis developed (classes II and III) ($p = 0.000001$). (From Boden SD, Dodge LD, Bohlman HH, et al. Rheumatoid arthritis of the cervical spine. *J Bone Joint Surg Am* 1993;75: 1282–1297, with permission.)

comparable to the anterior interval. More important, the negative predictive value using the PADI increased to 94%. The importance of this latter phenomenon is that if the PADI is greater than 14 mm, the chance that the patient will not have paralysis is 94%. Indeed, the negative predictive value is probably the most important value to examine for a diagnostic test used as a screening tool to indicate patients who require further study or even the potential for operative intervention. The primary goal of such a screening test is to avoid missing patients with disease or paralysis; a secondary goal is to minimize the number of false-positive results. The PADI is clearly superior in this regard (Fig. 64.5).

For similar reasons, in patients with subaxial subluxations, the residual posterior canal diameter is a more useful measurement than the percentage of anterior vertebral slippage. As with the AADI, these measurements from plain lateral radiographs are not equal to the space available for the cord, due to the unknown thickness of the synovial pan-

nus not visible on plain films. Therefore, although a PADI greater than 14 mm is generally safe, a patient with a PADI of 13 mm could have as much as 12 mm to as little as 8 or 9 mm available for the cord, depending on the thickness of pannus (7).

Polytomography

Although often replaced by more modern techniques, tomograms are particularly useful for quantitating the amount of basilar invagination present in the cervical spine and may be obtained if there is any suggestion of such deformity on plain radiographs. Protrusion of the tip of the dens above the opening of the foramen magnum defines basilar

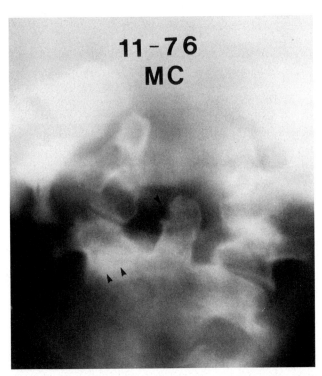

FIG. 64.6. Anteroposterior tomogram demonstrating erosions of the odontoid process (*arrowhead*) and atlantoaxial joint (*arrowheads*). (From Boden SD, Dodge LD, Bohlman HH, et al. Rheumatoid arthritis of the cervical spine. *J Bone Joint Surg Am* 1993;75:1282–1297, with permission.)

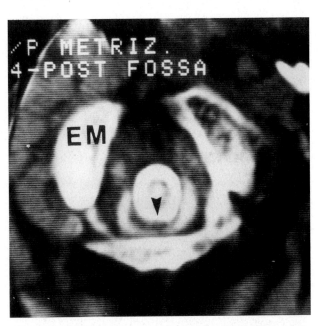

FIG. 64.7. Computed tomographic scan, made after myelogram, shows posterior displacement of the odontoid resulting in severe spinal cord compression (*arrowhead*). (From Boden SD, Dodge LD, Bohlman HH, et al. Rheumatoid arthritis of the cervical spine. *J Bone Joint Surg Am* 1993;75: 1282–1297, with permission.)

invagination (Fig. 64.6). Protrusion of more than 4.5 mm above McGregor's line (drawn from the top of the hard palate to the base of the occiput) is another definition. Several other lines and measurements can be made, as already described, to quantitate the extent of settling; however, the most important factor is simply to recognize any degree of basilar invagination when present and to determine whether it is a fixed or mobile deformity.

Computed Tomography

Computed tomography (CT), particularly when used after performing a myelogram with intrathecal contrast, can be useful for demonstrating spinal cord compression in patients with upper cervical rheumatoid disease (Fig. 64.7). CT has a much higher correlation with neurologic status and development of paralysis than does measurement of the traditional AADI from lateral cervical radiographs (21). In one study of 19 patients identified with a widened anterior atlantodental interval, CT demonstrated spinal cord compression in 11 and absence of any neurologic compression in the remaining 8 subjects (22). In other studies, multiplanar CT demonstrated unsuspected areas of compromise in 9 of 14 patients with rheumatoid arthritis, frequently resulting in altered operative plans (15).

Magnetic Resonance Imaging

The chief limitation of the use of plain radiographs is that the presence or absence of neural compromise must be indirectly inferred from the bony landmarks that outline the spinal canal. MRI has afforded the ability to directly visualize neural compression not only from bone, but also from the soft tissue pannus that develops with rheumatoid arthritis (Fig. 64.8). Dvorak and colleagues (23) showed that two-thirds of rheumatoid patients with atlantoaxial subluxation had a pannus greater than 3 mm in diameter. The implication of this finding is that the space available for the spinal cord can frequently be considerably less than the bony canal diameter demonstrated on plain radiographs. In a comparison of plain radiographs to MRI scans, Kawaida and associates (24) noted that spinal cord compression was found only variably in patients who had an AADI greater than or equal to 8 mm as measured on plain radiographs. The explanation for this phenomenon lies in the variability of the soft tissue pannus behind the dens as well as the variability in the width of the dens and the anterior and posterior interval in different patients.

Because MRI defines the space available for the cord more accurately than plain radiographs, some authors have attempted to set parameters for the minimal acceptable space available for the cord as visualized on MRI. For example, Kawaida and associates (24) showed that all patients with rheumatoid arthritis had spinal cord compres-

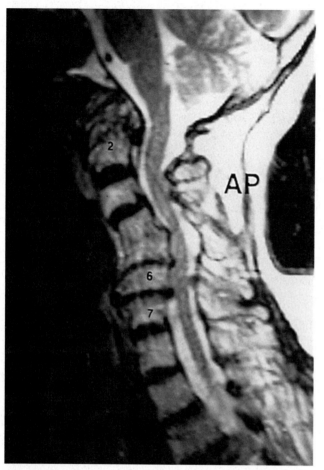

FIG. 64.8. Sagittal magnetic resonance scan of the cervical spine demonstrating a large soft tissue pannus involving the atlantoaxial joint.

sion when the space available for the cord, as shown on MRI scan, was less than or equal to 13 mm. Dvorak and colleagues (23) recommended operative intervention if the spinal cord diameter was less than 6 mm in flexion. Regardless of these arbitrary thresholds, an advantage to the use of MRI is the capacity to directly visualize spinal cord compression, and it is the presence or absence of cord compression that should guide decision making in the treatment of these patients.

In contrast with plain radiography, the presence of spinal cord compression as seen on the MRI correlates well with neurologic function in the rheumatoid patient. In a prospective analysis by Reijnierse and colleagues (25) of 63 consecutive patients with rheumatoid arthritis, subarachnoid space encroachment anywhere along the cervical spine was found to significantly correlate with neurologic classification. Hamilton and associates (26) found that evidence of cord compromise at the atlantoaxial level on the MRI was associated with neurologic deterioration that ultimately led

to either surgical intervention or death within a 12-month period.

Some controversy exists as to whether provocative dynamic MRI is necessary to elicit spinal cord compression that may be missed with static MRI. Detractors from the use of dynamic MRI suggest that the technique is unnecessary and adds the theoretical risk of precipitating a neurologic event. Flexion MRI has been documented to cause narrowing of the subarachnoid space in 12% to 20% of patients (27,28) and has been shown to change the cervicomedullary angle. In a prospective analysis of 42 rheumatoid patients who underwent flexion MRI, the technique was safe and did not cause a neurologic change (28). Narrowing was observed in the subarachnoid space with flexion; however, the clinical management was not changed by the additional findings seen with the flexion MRI views. No patient with a normal subarachnoid space in the neutral position had significant compression in the flexed position. Those who did show cord compromise on flexion views already had a compromised subarachnoid space on neutral views. Another important finding available with MRI is the cervicomedullary angle, which normally is 135 degrees to 175 degrees. In patients with rheumatoid arthritis, a cervicomedullary angle of less than 135 degrees correlated highly with the presence of clinical myelopathy and paralysis (29).

PREDICTORS OF NEUROLOGIC RECOVERY

Far less has been studied about the predictors of the potential for neurologic recovery after operation in patients with rheumatoid arthritis than is available regarding the natural history. Several factors appear not to be strongly correlated with recovery after operation. These include age, sex, duration of paralysis before operation, preoperative AADI (in patients with atlantoaxial subluxation), and preoperative percent slippage of vertebral body (in patients with subaxial subluxation).

Several factors have been shown to correlate with the potential for neurologic recovery after operative stabilization. The Ranawat classification (16) is an approximate gauge of the presence and severity of neurologic deficit (Table 64.2). It appears to be correlated with recovery after operation, in that patients with more severe deficits tend to have poorer neurologic recovery and a higher perioperative morbidity (Fig. 64.9). The location of rheumatoid pathology in the cervical spine also apparently had some prognostic value for recovery, in that patients with any notable degree of basilar invagination appeared to have a poorer prognosis for motor recovery following operation. Pseudarthrosis after an attempted fusion was also correlated with poor recovery.

More recently, available data suggest that the preoperative posterior atlantodental interval (in patients with atlan-

TABLE 64.2. *Ranawat Classification of Neurologic Deficit*

Class I	Pain, no neurologic deficit
Class II	Subjective weakness, hyperreflexia, dysesthesias
Class III	Objective weakness, long tract signs
Class IIIA	Class III, ambulatory
Class IIIB	Class III, nonambulatory

From Ranawat CS, O'Leary P, Pellicci P, et al. Cervical fusion in rheumatoid arthritis. *J Bone Joint Surg Am* 1979;61: 1003–1010, with permission.

toaxial subluxation) and the postoperative subaxial canal diameter (in patients with subaxial subluxation) may be predictors of potential for neurologic recovery after operation (7). Patients whose PADI is less than 10 mm prior to surgery have a poor prognosis for neurologic recovery. In contrast, patients with a PADI of 14 mm or greater tend to experience significant motor recovery after appropriate surgery (Fig. 64.10). Patients with a residual postoperative subaxial canal diameter less than 14 mm also may achieve less recovery.

A SCHEME FOR SERIAL EVALUATION AND TIMING OF OPERATIVE INTERVENTION

With an understanding of the predictors of paralysis and the predictors of the potential for neurologic recovery after operative stabilization, we can begin to establish a rational scheme both for serial evaluation of patients who undergo nonoperative management and for key check points at which operation should be considered. The goals of management of such patients are threefold: to avoid development of an irreversible neurologic deficit, to avoid onset of sudden death due to unrecognized spinal cord compression, and to avoid unnecessary operations. Ideally, these three

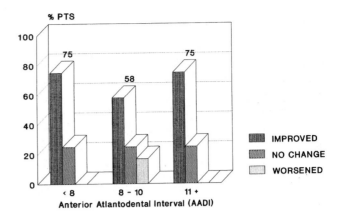

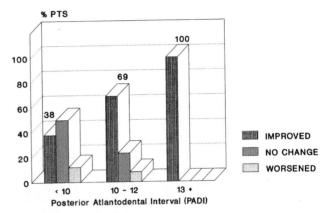

PREDICTED BY PADI

FIG. 64.10. Postoperative neurologic recovery in 35 patients with rheumatoid arthritis of the cervical spine grouped by radiographic measurements. **Top:** Neurologic recovery predicted by anterior atlantodental interval (AADI). **Bottom:** Neurologic recovery predicted by posterior atlantodental interval (PADI). Although the AADI did not correlate with neurologic recovery ($p > 0.10$), the PADI showed a strong correlation with recovery ($p = 0.0001$). (From Boden SD, Dodge LD, Bohlman HH, et al. Rheumatoid arthritis of the cervical spine. *J Bone Joint Surg Am* 1993;75:1282–1297, with permission.)

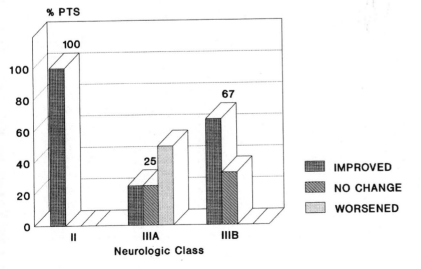

FIG. 64.9. Postoperative neurologic recovery in 35 rheumatoid patients with arthritis of the cervical spine grouped by original Ranawat class. (From Boden SD, Dodge LD, Bohlman HH, et al. Rheumatoid arthritis of the cervical spine. *J Bone Joint Surg Am* 1993;75:1282–1297, with permission.)

goals should be accomplished with a scheme that is cost-effective and easy to follow.

The basis for such a management scheme must embrace three important concepts. First, because of the seemingly increased morbidity in patients with more severe neurologic deficits who undergo operation, investigators believe that earlier operative intervention yields a better outcome (30). Second, about 10% of all patients with rheumatoid arthritis may die suddenly owing to unrecognized cord compression; this must be prevented. Finally, because 50% of patients with rheumatoid arthritis and radiographic evidence of instability as measured by the AADI do not develop neurologic symptoms (2), it is also important that any scheme avoid operation in such patients. With these concepts in mind, we can now focus on a rational scheme for serial patient evaluation and indications for surgery in patients with rheumatoid arthritis of the cervical spine. Because no algorithm will cover 100% of the patients, clinical judgment must always prevail.

Patients with intractable pain, a clear-cut neurologic deficit, or both, are generally candidates for operative management. Therefore, the remainder of our discussion focuses on the more controversial group of patients with rheumatoid arthritis with radiographic evidence of instability with some pain or no pain, but no neurologic deficit. The most cost-effective method of screening patients in the cervical spine for rheumatoid involvement is plain radiographs followed with tomograms if there is any suggestion of basilar invagination. On the basis of these two studies, patients can be separated into those with atlantoaxial subluxation, basilar invagination, subaxial subluxation, or some combination of the three (Fig. 64.11).

Atlantoaxial Subluxation

In patients with atlantoaxial subluxation and without neurologic deficit, if the posterior atlantodental interval measures more than 14 mm on the plain radiographs, continued observation is generally safe treatment. If, however, the PADI is 14 mm or less, performing an MRI to evaluate the true space available for the cord, accounting for the amount of space occupied by the synovial pannus, is advisable. If the MRI scan demonstrates a cervicomedullary angle less than 135 degrees, or any evidence of cord impingement, then a posterior atlantoaxial fusion should be strongly considered.

Atlantoaxial Subluxation with Basilar Invagination

In patients with atlantoaxial subluxation and any notable degree of basilar invagination but with no neurologic deficit, an MRI scan in flexion is still advisable to evaluate specifically the amount of spinal cord compression present (Fig. 64.12). The high morbidity of operation in patients with progressive basilar invagination and their poor potential for recovery warrant a more aggressive approach in such patients. Therefore, if there is any evidence of cord compression, cervical traction is appropriate; if reduction is achieved, occipitocervical fusion should be performed. If cord compression is not relieved with traction, then either a C1 laminectomy or an anterior resection of the odontoid should be performed in addition to the occipitocervical fusion (31). For patients who have isolated and fixed basilar invagination with no symptoms and no evidence of notable cord compression, observation may be continued.

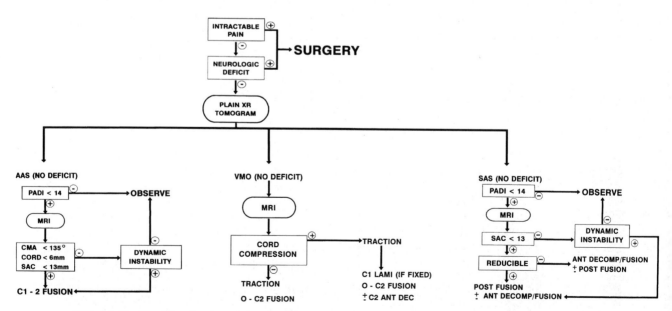

FIG. 64.11. Algorithm for the evaluation and management of rheumatoid patients with cervical spine involvement.

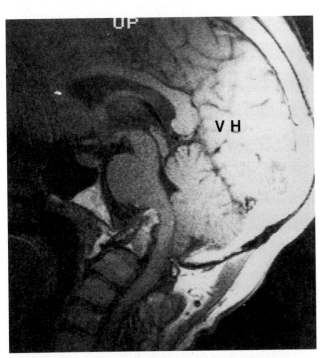

FIG. 64.12. Sagittal magnetic resonance scan demonstrating severe compression of the brainstem resulting from basilar invagination of the odontoid process. Note the relationship of the body of the axis to the clivus anteriorly. (From Boden SD, Dodge LD, Bohlman HH, et al. Rheumatoid arthritis of the cervical spine. *J Bone Joint Surg Am* 1993;75:1282–1297, with permission.)

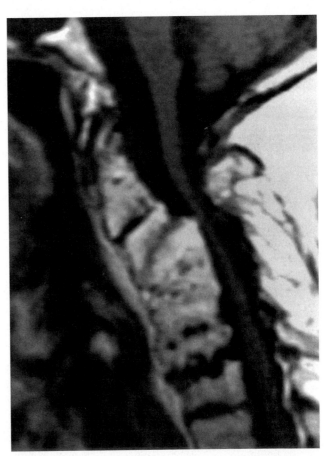

FIG. 64.13. Sagittal magnetic resonance scan of the cervical spine demonstrating subaxial subluxation and cord impingement.

Subaxial Subluxation

Patients with subaxial subluxation and no neurologic deficit should be followed with plain cervical radiographs (Fig. 64.13). If the residual subaxial canal diameter is more than 14 mm in the area of interest, it is generally safe to continue observation. If, however, the posterior subaxial canal diameter is less than 14 mm, an MRI scan should be obtained to evaluate the true space available for the cord. If any cord impingement is observed or a notable degree of mobility is present at that segment, operative arthrodesis is recommended. In most cases, a posterior cervical fusion is the procedure of choice. However, if a notable neurologic deficit is present and the subluxation is not readily reduced, an anterior decompression and fusion in lieu of or in addition to the posterior stabilization may be advisable. Instability may result from an anterior decompression and fusion alone, and such patients should be carefully monitored with plain radiographs postoperatively. If any further subluxation is noted, a posterior arthrodesis may be necessary.

Combined Subluxations

In patients with combinations of upper cervical and lower cervical subluxations, the processes must be addressed to-

gether; frequently, an occipitocervical arthrodesis will have to be carried down into the subaxial cervical spine to avoid deterioration below an upper fusion. Although some researchers have suggested that progression of subaxial disease accelerates after atlantoaxial fusion, this possibility is difficult to confirm from the available data.

Clinical Outcomes and Operative Complications

Certainly some investigators may consider it overly aggressive to perform a prophylactic arthrodesis on the basis of radiographic instability in patients who are not yet experiencing clinical symptoms or neurologic deficit. However, it is also clear that many patients present with an initial deficit so severe that it is potentially irreversible. Outcome after operative arthrodesis is good when patients have not yet developed severe myelopathy. In addition, operative morbidity and anesthetic complications are less common when the operation is performed earlier in the course of the disease. Some evidence suggests that early atlantoaxial arthrodesis may prevent cranial settling (32).

Monitoring a patient's disease progression by following the AADI on plain lateral radiographs is an unreliable method at best. Plain radiographs can be more useful if the PADI and subaxial canal diameters are measured instead. These radiographs can be used as the screening tool and should be followed up with MRI scans only when indicated based on the criteria already outlined. As more work is done using somatosensory and motor evoked potentials, these electrophysiologic diagnostic studies may also be useful in predicting the potential for postoperative neurologic recovery. Once any notable demyelination occurs, it cannot be reversed.

The clinical success rate for cervical fusions in patients with rheumatoid arthritis of the cervical spine ranges from 60% to 90%. This variance is explained in part by variable disease severity at the time of operation and the precise definition of clinical success in a patient with a progressive systemic disease. The most common complications of cervical spine operation in rheumatoid arthritis include death (5% to 10%), infection, wound dehiscence, wire breakage and loss of reduction, nonunion (5% to 20%), and late subaxial subluxation below a fused segment (4). Thus, anatomically involved levels should be incorporated into a fusion even if distal to the site of the primary pathology. In addition, because previously asymptomatic levels can develop subluxation below rigid segments, continued clinical monitoring is imperative. Not all nonunions are symptomatic, and their management must be individualized.

SUMMARY

The primary goal in management of patients with rheumatoid arthritis of the cervical spine is to prevent onset of irreversible neurologic deficit. Patients should be followed and evaluated by careful physical examination to avoid masking of subtle changes of myelopathy by severe peripheral joint disease. Use of the PADI and subaxial canal diameters measured on plain lateral cervical radiographs is a reliable screening tool to identify high-risk patients who require further evaluation with MRI or CT myelography. The primary technical objective of operation is stabilization of diseased spinal segments and relief of spinal cord compression through reduction of subluxation or decompression. Complications are not uncommon, but tend to occur less frequently in patients who have operative intervention before onset of severe myelopathy. Pain relief is generally good when a solid arthrodesis is achieved, and neurologic recovery is most favorable when severe cord compression is not present preoperatively.

REFERENCES

1. Ferlic D, Clayton ML, Leidholt JD, et al. Surgical treatment of the symptomatic unstable cervical spine in rheumatoid arthritis. *J Bone Joint Surg Am* 1975;57:349–354.

2. Pellicci PM, Ranawat CS, Tsairis P, et al. A prospective study of the progression of rheumatoid arthritis of the cervical spine. *J Bone Joint Surg Am* 1981;68:342–350.
3. Bogduk N, Major GA, Carter J. Lateral subluxation of the atlas in rheumatoid arthritis: a case report and post-mortem study. *Ann Rheum Dis* 1984;43:341–346.
4. Conaty JP, Mongan ES. Cervical fusion in rheumatoid arthritis. *J Bone Joint Surg Am* 1981;63:1218–1227.
5. Sherk HH. Atlantoaxial instability and acquired basilar invagination in rheumatoid arthritis. *Orthop Clin North Am* 1978;9:1053–1063.
6. Rana NA. Natural history of atlanto-axial subluxation in rheumatoid arthritis. *Spine* 1989;14:1054–1056.
7. Boden SD, Dodge LD, Bohlman HH, et al. Rheumatoid arthritis of the cervical spine: a twenty year analysis with predictors of paralysis and recovery. *J Bone Joint Surg Am* 1993;75:1282–1297.
8. Mikulowski P, Wollheim FA, Rotmil P, et al. Sudden death in rheumatoid arthritis with atlanto-axial dislocation. *Acta Med Scand* 1975;198:445–451.
9. Lipson SJ. Rheumatoid arthritis in the cervical spine. *Clin Orthop* 1989;239:121–127.
10. Rasker JJ, Cosh JA. Radiological study of cervical spine and hand in patients with rheumatoid arthritis of 15 years duration: an assessment of the effects of corticosteroid treatment. *Ann Rheum Dis* 1978;37:529–535.
11. Weissman BNW, Aliabadi P, Weinfeld MS, et al. Prognostic features of atlantoaxial subluxation in rheumatoid arthritis patients. *Radiology* 1982;144:745–751.
12. Cabane J, Michon A, Ziza JM, et al. Comparison of long term evolution of adult onset and juvenile onset Still's disease, both followed up for more than 10 years. *Ann Rheum Dis* 1990;45:283–285.
13. Redlund-Johnell I, Petterson H. Radiographic measurements of the cranio-vertebral region. *Acta Radiol Diagn* 1984;25:23–28.
14. Clark CR, Goetz DD, Menezes AH. Arthrodesis of the cervical spine in rheumatoid arthritis. *J Bone Joint Surg Am* 1989;71:381–392.
15. Fischgold H, Metzger J. Etude radiographic de l'impression basilaire (French). *Rev Rheum* 1952;19:161.
16. Ranawat CS, O'Leary P, Pellicci P, et al. Cervical fusion in rheumatoid arthritis. *J Bone Joint Surg Am* 1979;61:1003–1010.
17. Collins DN, Barnes CL, FitzRandolph RL. Cervical spine instability in rheumatoid patients having total hip or knee arthroplasty. *Clin Orthop* 1991;272:127–135.
18. Fielding JW, Hawkins RJ, Ratzan SA. Spine fusion for atlanto-axial instability. *J Bone Joint Surg Am* 1976;58:400–407.
19. Heywood AWB, Learmonth ID, Thomas M. Cervical spine instability in rheumatoid arthritis. *J Bone Joint Surg Br* 1988;70:702–707.
20. Breedveld FC, Algra PR, Vielvoye CJ, et al. Magnetic resonance imaging in the evaluation of patients with rheumatoid arthritis and subluxations of the cervical spine. *Arthritis Rheum* 1987;30:624–629.
21. Braunstein EM, Weissman BN, Seltzer SE, et al. Computed tomography and conventional radiographs of the craniocervical region in rheumatoid arthritis: a comparison. *Arthritis Rheum* 1984;27:26–31.
22. Raskin RJ, Schnapf DJ, Wolf CR, et al. Computerized tomography in evaluation of atlantoaxial subluxation in rheumatoid arthritis. *J Rheum* 1983;10:33–41.
23. Dvorak J, Grob D, Baumgartner H, et al. Functional evaluation of the spinal cord by magnetic resonance imaging in patients with rheumatoid arthritis and instability of upper cervical spine. *Spine* 1989;14:1057–1064.
24. Kawaida H, Sakou T, Morizono Y, et al. Magnetic resonance imaging of upper cervical disorders in rheumatoid arthritis. *Spine* 1989;14:1144–1148.
25. Reijnierse M, Bloem JL, Dijkmans BAC, et al. The cervical spine in rheumatoid arthritis: relationship between neurologic signs and morphology on MR imaging and radiographs. *Skeletal Radiol* 1996;25:113–118.
26. Hamilton JD, Johnston RA, Madhok R, et al. Factors predictive of subsequent deterioration in rheumatoid cervical myelopathy. *Rheumatology* 2001;40:811–815.
27. Allmann K-H, Uhl M, Uhrmeister P, et al. Functional MR imaging of the cervical spine in patients with rheumatoid arthritis. *Acta Radiologica* 1998;39:543–546.

28. Reijnierse M, Breedveld FC, Kroon HM, et al. Are magnetic resonance flexion views useful in evaluating the cervical spine of patients with rheumatoid arthritis? *Skeletal Radiol* 2000;29:85–89.
29. Bundschuh C, Modic MT, Kearney F, et al. Rheumatoid arthritis of the cervical spine. *AJR Am J Roentgenol* 1988;151:181–187.
30. Zoma A, Sturrock RD, Fisher WD, et al. Surgical stabilization of the rheumatoid cervical spine: a review of indications and results. *J Bone Joint Surg Br* 1987;69:8–12.
31. Crockard HA, Calder I, Ransford AO. One-stage transoral decompression and posterior fixation in rheumatoid atlanto-axial subluxation. *J Bone Joint Surg Br* 1990;72:682–685.
32. Kraus DR, Peppelman WC, Agarwal AK, et al. Incidence of subaxial subluxation in patients with generalized rheumatoid arthritis who have had previous occipital cervical fusions. *Spine* 1991;16:S486–S489.

CHAPTER 65

Rheumatoid Arthritis

Upper Cervical Involvement

Alan Crockard and Dieter Grob

From 1969 to 1984, 1,294 clinical cases of patients with rheumatoid arthritis (RA) presented to the Schulthess Klinik for treatment by orthopaedic surgery. Of these patients, 248 (19.2%) had reported pain related to their cervical spine at least once, and underwent clinical and radiographic examination. To date, 46 (18.5%) of these selected patients have undergone operation on their cervical spine. Within 5 years of serologic confirmation of the diagnosis of RA, one-third to one-half of the patients will have some degree of atlantoaxial subluxation (1,2). Only a few of these (2% to 3%) will become myelopathic approximately 10 years later (12 to 15 years); of these myelopathic patients, half will be dead in a year.

The challenge, then, is obvious: to identify those who are at risk and to prevent whatever factor leads to neuraxial damage. But who is at risk? Is the symptomatic patient with a reducible 5-mm anterior atlantodental interval (AADI) less at risk than a patient with an AADI of 7 mm? Does an inflammatory mass (pannus) associated with significant odontoid translocation alter the surgical decisions? Can the neurologic deficit be reversed? Will operative stabilization cause further subaxial problems? Although much is known about RA of the cervical spine, questions remain; it is likely that some of these questions will be answered within the next decade.

This chapter outlines the pathologic changes that occur at the craniocervical joint in order to correlate them with symptoms and signs and to outline the indications for and the types of operative intervention. It also reviews outcome criteria and the complications of treatment.

PATHOLOGY

The pathologic process begins as an inflammatory synovitis, which in turn causes articular cartilage and sub-

chondral damage, with disorganization of the joint, damage to the capsule, and resultant strain on the associated ligaments. The inflammatory process also affects the ligaments, and the combined stresses result in tears and ruptures. Drugs, age, and disability combine to produce osteopenia, but no evidence indicates that avascular necrosis or vasculitis is a factor in the process; rather, there is ample evidence of ongoing remodeling throughout the degenerative process.

Atlantoaxial subluxation may be caused by damage to the ligamentous apparatus, to the odontoid process (dens), or both. Damage to the transverse atlantal ligament alone will allow as much as 3 or 4 mm of subluxation; a greater AADI implies damage to the alar–apical ligament complex or an incomplete odontoid peg or resorbed dens. Translocation (cranial settling) results from progressive destruction of the lateral mass joints (atlantoaxial and occipitoatlantal) and the lateral masses themselves; unequal destruction on one side will result in torticollis. If the translocation continues, the atlantoaxial joint may lock and the impacted odontoid will appear to be "fixed" in position, giving rise to the mistaken clinical impression that the joint that once had an increasing AADI is now safe because the bones no longer appear to move. Translocation of more than 1 cm can occur only if the ring of atlas is disrupted. Coupled with these changes is translation, with the atlas moving forward and further compromising the subarachnoid space and compressing the posterior aspect of the spinal cord. Posterior dislocation occurs in cases with bony destruction of the dens (Fig. 65.1). Its prevalence is reported to be not more than 6.7% of all atlantoaxial subluxations (3). Every flare-up of the inflammatory process will cause an acute synovitis, and the pannus will further compromise the neuraxis;

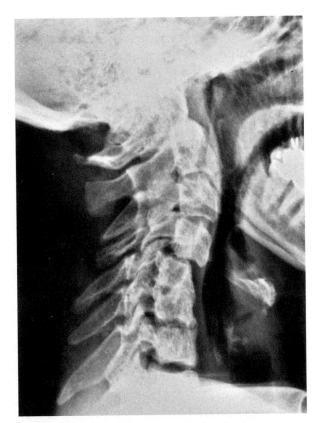

FIG. 65.1. A patient with rheumatoid arthritis with posterior dislocation of the atlantoaxial segment due to bony destruction of the dens. The patient also has subaxial subluxation at C4-C5 and ankylosis of C5 to C7.

immobilization of the joint by rest, external orthosis, or operative fixation of the joint will cause its resolution. The compression may be so great and so acute that fixation alone may be dangerous and some form of operative decompression should be considered.

Neuropathologic (4) and neuroradiologic studies (5) by one of us (AC) have indicated the possible mechanisms causing the myelopathy. Again, as in the histology of bone, there is no evidence of vasculitis or endarteritis. The spinal cord is thin and atrophic and the anterior spinal artery is usually patent. In the white matter tracts, there are axonal retraction balls, the end result of torn axons, whereas in the anterior horn cells chromatolysis is evident. These findings are characteristic of repetitive trauma as the cord is impacted during head movements against the osteophytes or the subluxations of the cervical vertebrae.

CLINICAL FINDINGS

Most patients with RA of the cervical spine have some neck pain, but C2 root pain should alert the clinician to atlantoaxial instability. Often misinterpreted as mastoid pain, earache, or migraine, this pain radiates in the distribution of

the posterior primary ramus. Cranial nerve palsies have been reported to be common, but detailed studies have suggested that they are extremely uncommon (6). Clinical examination of a patient with RA with a painful cervical spine often discloses tenderness over the neck and shoulder muscles. In some instances, the atlantoaxial instability and joint crepitation may be felt on palpation of the atlantoaxial segment. Lhermitte's sign can sometimes be provoked by flexing the head, which may be associated with a palpable subluxation ("clunk test").

Specific signs of brainstem compression have been very rare, although respiratory inadequacies have been noted (7) but may be due to central and peripheral causes. Specific neurologic signs such as nystagmus may be due to a coincidental Chiari malformation. Loss of joint position sense is evident when the cord is compressed posteriorly, and that or nystagmus, or both, should alert the clinician to potential dangers with a posterior fixation procedure.

Typical signs of cord compression are rarely evident. Instead, patients report decreasing ambulation and dexterity, stiffness and, occasionally, altered sensation. Stiff, "frozen" shoulders are almost always neurogenic rather than due to capsulitis. Very rarely, the patient presents with spinal myoclonus, a condition characterized by involuntary semirhythmic contractions of skeletal muscle groups (8). Histologically, cord compression is characterized by vacuolar degeneration of the anterior horn cells (9), which is the end stage of the repetitive trauma and possibly the effect of medication used in treatment of RA. It is extremely responsive to clonazepam. Because of joint deformity, previous surgery, and long-term medication causing some peripheral neuropathy, formal reflex changes in patients with RA are not as reliable a sign as in patients without RA.

Gross deformities of the large joints often require surgical replacement or correction. As a result of the procedures, the normal neural reflex pathways will be disturbed, making accurate neurologic assessment difficult in patients with numerous joint replacements.

CLINICAL ASSESSMENT

As in any progressive multisystem disease, characterization of the extent of the condition and the effects of treatment must be standardized if there is to be any objective assessment of one center's treatment as compared with that of another. For the reasons already given, a formal neurologic examination will not be useful; however, functional grading is a useful crude guide. Currently, the Ranawat classification (10) is the one most widely used, but there is little in this classification to distinguish a severely affected (myelopathic ambulatory) patient from a myelopathic but bed-bound patient. At present, attempts are being made to digitize certain aspects of the Stanford Health Activity Questionnaire (HAQ) (11,12).

RADIOLOGY

Conventional anteroposterior and lateral radiographs are the basis of radiologic investigations. The transoral view to visualize the atlantoaxial joints often cannot be taken because patients cannot be positioned correctly. Bone structure, posture and alignment, calcification, and structure should be examined. The degree of horizontal atlantoaxial subluxation and upward migration of the dens can be measured in the lateral view of the craniocervical junction (13,14). The Redlund-Johnell method, which measures from the base of C2 to the foramen magnum, proved to be the most accurate technique in a comparative study (15).

Measurement of the posterior atlantodental interval (PADI) appears to be more accurate than the conventional AADI (16), since it indicates the real space available for the cord, but even this does not provide information about the soft tissue that might cause compression (17). Functional radiographs in flexion and extension not only allow detection of instabilities in the atlantoaxial segment and the subaxial cervical spine but also provide information about the reducibility of the subluxation (Fig. 65.2).

Computed Tomography and Magnetic Resonance Imaging

Computed tomography (CT) and magnetic resonance imaging (MRI) have become indispensable imaging modalities in the surgical evaluation process. They can accurately locate bony (CT more than MRI) or soft tissue (MRI more than CT) compression or obstruction and allow precise operative planning of decompression. MRI in flexion and extension (Fig. 65.3) identifies by direct visualization the extent of compression of the retrodental inflammatory tissue in both positions and can provide information concerning the indications for anterior decompression (17,18). An absolute cord diameter less than 6 mm will leave the patient susceptible to myelopathy.

For follow-up, lateral cervical radiographs are usually sufficient; however, patients with deteriorating neurologic function should undergo MRI, and fixation with an implant composed of titanium or another nonferrous compound should be considered.

MANAGEMENT DECISIONS

Operative management decisions are always difficult when the disease is ongoing because bone quality is likely to deteriorate, and acceleration of subaxial changes due to the fusion itself is possible. Until recently, long-term outcome has not been known, and operative preferences have been based on an individual's experience. Some broad principles are emerging (Tables 65.1 and 65.2).

Although most researchers advocate operative intervention for patients with myelopathy, much evidence shows that patients who are bed-bound for more than 3 months fare badly after operation. The overall operative mortality for Ranawat class IIIB patients is 12.5%, but assessment of survivors at 1 year after surgery shows a mortality rate of 61% in the first year. Whether such patients should be subjected to cervical surgery at all is quite debatable (10,16,19,20). Nevertheless, no clear guidelines exist for operation on patients with asymptomatic reducible atlantoaxial

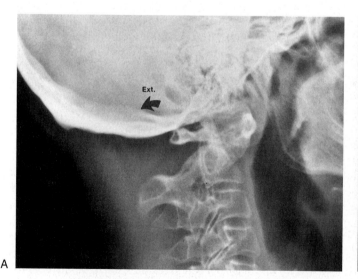
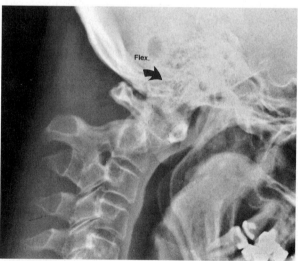

FIG. 65.2. A patient with rheumatoid arthritis with severe atlantoaxial subluxation and anterior shifting of the atlas. The radiographs in extension **(A)** and flexion **(B)** demonstrate the limited reduction of the subluxation. No decompression of the neural structures will be achieved by simple posterior fixation of the dislocated segment, and sublaminar wires at C1 would be dangerous.

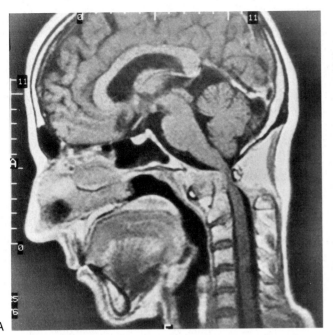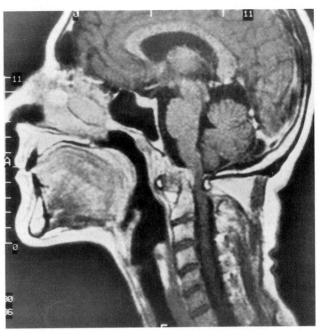

A   B

FIG. 65.3. Functional MRI scan shows subluxation of C1 on C2. MRI provides information about the degree of the displacement and the changes in neural compression in flexion **(A)** and extension **(B)**.

subluxation. A multicenter controlled trial would be of value.

Painless isolated atlantoaxial instability is considered common, but some researchers believe that there are no clear indications for operation (21–23). However, this view does not take into consideration the possibility that repeat trauma-tization of the medulla due to the instability may cause permanent damage and that an unstable atlantoaxial segment represents a potential risk of severe cord lesion with minor trauma (24). For these symptomless patients, we advocate a careful clinical evaluation that includes neurophysiologic evaluation with electromyography (EMG) to identify peripheral problems such as carpal tunnel syndrome and motor and sensory evoked potentials (MEP, SSEP) to study spinal cord function. In the absence of pathologic findings, an anticipatory attitude seems to be justified. Regular annual checkups with thorough investigations are necessary to allow rapid intervention in case of radiologic progression or clinical deterioration.

We consider radiologically verified progression of atlantoaxial subluxation without neurologic deficit to represent an indication for arthrodesis (Table 65.2). Because better

TABLE 65.1. *Indications for Posterior Fusion*

Atlantoaxial segment
   Clinically relevant cervical myelopathy
   Pathologic neurophysiologic changes (MEP and SSEP)
   Spinal cord less than 6 mm in flexion (MRI)
   Spinal canal less than 10 mm in flexion (radiographs)
   Retrodental pannus more than 10 mm (MRI)
   Increasing AADI or cranial settling
   Intractable neck pain
   Incapable of wearing an external support
   Instability due to decompressive laminectomy
Inclusion of the occiput
   Vertical instability (cranial settling)
   Pathologic changes in the atlantooccital joints
      (radiographs, CT, MRI)
   Instability of the ring of the atlas in RA (decompressive
      procedures)

MEP, motor evoked potentials; SSEP, somatosensory evoked potentials; MRI, magnetic resonance imaging; CT, computed tomography; AADI, anterior atlantodental interval; RA, rheumatoid arthritis.
From, Dvorak J, Grob D, Baumgartner H, et al. Functional evaluation of the spinal cord by magnetic resonance imaging in patients with rheumatoid arthritis and instability of upper cervical spine. *Spine* 1989;14:1057, with permission.

TABLE 65.2. *Rationale for Surgery*

To justify surgical intervention of the cervical spine in patients with rheumatoid arthritis, the following items should be achieved:
1. Relief of pain
2. Reduction of dislocation and maintenance of anatomic position
3. Decompression of neurologic tissue
4. Prevention of neurologic deterioration
5. Adequate postoperative management
6. Low mortality/complication rate
7. Reasonable amount of surgery

results are obtained when operation is performed before myelopathy occurs (25), waiting for deterioration does not appear to be justifiable. In addition, the clinical outcome and pain reduction is better if arthrodesis is performed earlier. In a series of 70 patients with RA and atlantoaxial instability, the outcome after fusion was directly correlated with the stage of the disease at which operation was performed (26).

Treatment of compressive inflammatory pannus is another difficult problem. Transoral decompression is advocated but requires special instrumentation and skills. Posterior fixation in the presence of compression may cause neurologic deterioration. Immobilization in an external orthosis for weeks or months will allow resorption of the inflammatory tissue, but the inconvenience and time required are factors for both the patient and clinician to consider. External bracing itself can produce problems in patients deformed by RA.

Skull traction for reduction of translocation or atlantoaxial subluxation is another management problem. Although a short period of traction may be useful, prolonged traction (more than 7 to 10 days) causes problems such as pressure sores and hypostatic pneumonia. Again we emphasize the importance of a policy that documents the overall morbidity and mortality of clinical management of the patient rather than only operative decisions and discussions based on operative mortality or morbidity that may mask the true seriousness of RA of the cervical spine.

Because morbidity is associated with harvesting of bone graft and there is a high rate of nonunion in patients with RA, some researchers consider that in this condition bone graft may not always be required (27). Although use of bone graft in young fit patients is practicable, its use in elderly patients with end-stage RA has been questioned, and in one 10-year series there was little evidence of instrumentation failure or pull-out without graft (18).

WHICH OPERATION?

The type and extent of operation for patients with RA varies with the individual surgeon's practice as well as with the patient's condition; there are many methods of stabilization, and we clearly have our own preferences.

Anterior decompression is recommended for patients with neuraxial compression and a significant anterior pannus and/or irreducible odontoid, or marked (5 mm) vertical translocation.

We do not recommend anterior fixation. Posterior stabilization is always required after anterior decompression in rheumatoid disease.

In young, fit (Ranawat class I and II) patients, atlantoaxial fixation is all that is required even in the presence of some irreducible subluxation or mild translocation (25). In end-stage conditions, in which profound translocation may exist, transoral surgery may be required. If there is a "staircase" subaxial slip combined with atlantoaxial subluxation,

a long fixation from the occiput that includes most of the cervical spine may be used (Table 65.1).

OPERATIVE PROCEDURES

We do not describe full preoperative preparation for surgical techniques; this has been well described previously (28).

Transoral Odontoidectomy

The minimal requirement for transoral odontoidectomy is that the patient's mouth open more than 25 mm for the routine procedure. Temporomandibular arthritis or a subaxial kyphos may prevent the lower jaw from opening. In such a patient requiring decompression, access may be gained by a midline mandibular split with lateral traction, which allows the tongue to be retracted downward to gain access. We have found that there is nothing to gain from midline division of the tongue (it is the mandible that prevents access) or a subglottic suprahyoid approach, which still places considerable limitations on visibility. In our extensive experience with transoral procedures, such techniques have been necessary in fewer than 1% of cases.

The risk of sepsis should always be considered. Poor dentition or sepsis must be treated preoperatively. Other fears such as the risk of meningitis have perhaps been exaggerated, although great care is required during the procedure. Provided that the pharyngeal mucosa is protected from operative trauma and there are clean incisions that are carefully resutured, there is little risk of sepsis. In our practice, the mucosa is protected by instrumentation as much as possible; retraction with temporary stitches causes trauma, particularly if the high-speed drill catches the stitches.

Dural penetration increases the risks of intradural sepsis, since it is extremely difficult to provide a watertight closure by dural sutures; if a leak occurs, a multilayer closure, oxidized cellulose, thrombin/fibrin glue, and a lumbar cerebrospinal fluid drain should be used.

We do not use anterior bone grafting in patients with RA; we concentrate instead on posterior fixation and arthrodesis.

Postoperative intraoral swelling can be a great problem. Prolonged vigorous retraction with no relaxation is the usual cause. Tongue swelling may be caused by retracting the tongue against the teeth; great care should be taken to prevent this. In our own experience, the use of 1% hydrocortisone ointment applied to the tongue and buccal mucous membranes before and 4 hours after operation has significantly reduced this complication.

Division of the palate is usually not required for operations below the foramen magnum; the palate may be adequately retracted. In cases of extensive translocation or when the head cannot be extended to gain exposure, division of the soft palate is necessary. Careful two-layer closure of this sphincter of the nasal passages is essential to allow normal postoperative function.

In terms of operative exposure, the anterior tubercle on the arch of the atlas is the key to the area. A 4-cm midline incision of the pharynx will provide adequate access above and below the arch. The vertebral artery is at least 20 mm to each side in adults, and there is little danger in removing 10 mm of the arch to atlas to expose the odontoid and inflammatory tissue. At the foramen magnum and at the base of the axis, the vertebral artery is much closer to the midline.

Decompression of the dural sac is the object of the anterior procedure. This involves use of a high-speed air drill to remove the odontoid process; long bayoneted instruments are useful to remove the soft tissue. The inflammatory tissue should be removed to the greatest degree possible, as well as the thickened cruciate ligament and remnants of the transverse and alar apical complex. Until the dural pulsations can be seen, the decompression is inadequate.

When there is marked translocation of the odontoid, the peg may be extracted without removal of any of the anterior rim of the foramen magnum by disconnecting the peg from the axis and pulling the tip of the peg down with long forceps to allow division of the apical alar complex.

Posterior Cervical Arthrodesis

Historical Background

Painful instabilities of the atlantoaxial joint and the suboccipital area in patients with RA have been well known since the last century and were probably first described in 1890 by Garrod (29). Mixter and Osgood (30) published a technique for posterior atlantoaxial arthrodesis with silk suture, forming a loop between the posterior arch of the atlas and the spinous process of C2, and referred to an earlier publication by Lane in 1892 (31); however, grafting was not mentioned. In 1891, Hadra (32) used a wire loop for the same procedure, but all of the patients in his series had instability secondary to Pott's disease.

In 1939, Gallie (33) published his well-known paper on posterior atlantoaxial arthrodesis for different etiologies. This technique, with a median bone graft fixed to the atlas and the axis with wires, underwent several modifications in subsequent years, mainly in the wiring technique. Brooks (34) obtained improved stability (35,36) by using two wedge-shaped bone grafts placed between the arch of the atlas and the lamina of C2. However, this increased stability required instrumentation with wire loops in the spinal canal. Guyotat (37) and Holness (38) and their colleagues replaced the wires with posterior clamps, fixing the atlas and the axis posteriorly. Direct transarticular fixation of the atlantoaxial joint was first described by Barbour in 1971 (39). His technique required a bilateral approach to the C1-C2 joints from the lateral sides. A direct atlantoaxial transarticular screw fixation by a posterior approach was first performed by Magerl in 1979 (40–42). As an innovation, this method offered true three-point fixation of the atlantoaxial segment by adding a posterior bone graft.

Reports on occipitocervical arthrodesis are fewer. In 1927, Foerster (43) described a technique with a fibular strut graft between occiput and lower cervical spine in a patient with progressive atlantoaxial instability after a fracture of the dens. The difficulties involved in fixing graft bone or internal fixation devices on the convexity of the surface of the occiput led to numerous attempts to solve this problem. Wires (44,45), screws (46,47), rods (27,48–50), bone cement (44,51–53), and plates (54–56) were advocated for internal fixation. Despite the original problems, the new implants, even without bone graft, have increased postoperative stability and have provided good long-term results (18).

Atlantoaxial Arthrodesis

The most common technique for posterior atlantoaxial arthrodesis is one of the Gallie-type procedures (33). Several modifications have been reported (57–59). The essence of this arthrodesis procedure consists of an autologous bone graft fixed with a wire loop to the posterior part of the atlas and the spinous process of the axis. Its advantage lies in the simplicity of the operation. Its major disadvantages result from the inferior stability afforded and the lack of resistance to translational displacement in cases of atlantoaxial subluxation (35). Improved rotational stability is provided by bilateral fixation-type procedures such as the Brooks procedure (34), in which two paramedial autologous bone graft are placed posteriorly between the atlas and the laminae of the axis; internal fixation with clamps and hooks may enhance the construct.

A reliable method for atlantoaxial arthrodesis consists of a transarticular screw fixation (42). The fixation is achieved by two posteriorly inserted screws, crossing the atlantoaxial joints bilaterally and augmented by a bone graft, placed between the atlas and the spinous process of the axis (Fig. 65.4). In cases of a bifid, broken, or osteoporotic ring of the atlas, the bone graft may be packed directly into the atlantoaxial joint.

Biomechanical stability tests and clinical follow-up studies, combined with extensive clinical experience (26,60), showed that this transarticular screw technique is suitable for C1-C2 arthrodesis in RA provided that there is good bone in the lateral masses. It is not suitable, however, when one of the lateral masses has been resorbed as part of the rheumatoid process. With this technique, immediate postoperative multidirectional stability is achieved (35), and for postoperative management, the patient may require only use of a soft collar for 6 weeks.

Occipitocervical Arthrodesis

Cumbersome postoperative external fixation is to be avoided in patients with RA, who usually are hindered by multiple deformities of the extremities. Solid internal fixation is therefore preferred for occipitocervical fusion.

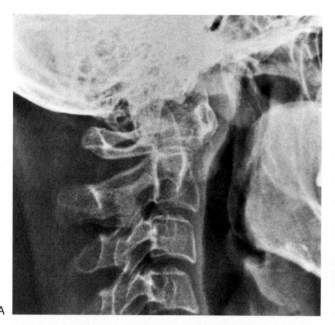
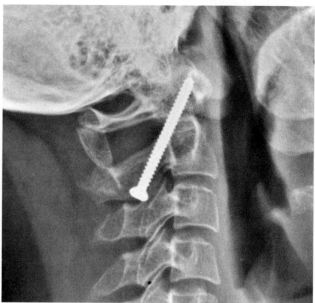

FIG. 65.4. **A:** Isolated atlantoaxial instability in a patient with rheumatoid arthritis. **B:** Posterior fixation with transarticular screws and bone graft allows reduction and firm fixation in an anatomic position.

Several devices are described in the literature: wires (45,61) or screws (62) to fix the bone graft, wires reinforced by bone cement (46,63), metal mesh with or without cement (22), contoured rods (27,50), and plates (56,64).

A Y-plate (54) (Fig. 65.5) combined with transarticular atlantoaxial fixation with a screw has proved a useful tool for occipitocervical arthrodesis (65). The firm fixation of the screw in the midline of the occiput combined with fixation of the atlantoaxial joints provides reliable stability.

Additional bone grafting underneath the plate provides arthrodesis stability against flexion and extension, with rotation being blocked by the transarticular screws. For arthrodesis that must be extended into the lower cervical spine, a long version of the plate may be cut to the appropriate length and fixed by lateral mass screws. Thus, a "custom-made" implant for each case can be provided individually. Because the plate is made of titanium, postoperative imaging with MRI is possible.

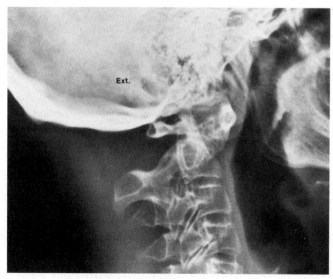
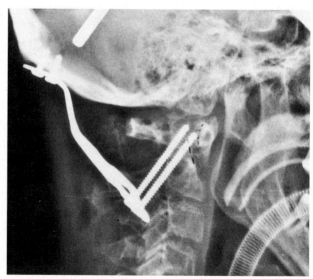

FIG. 65.5. Same patient as in Figure 65.3. **A:** Preoperative. **B:** After transoral decompression with removal of the dens, posterior occipitocervical fixation with a Y-plate and transarticular screws was performed at one time.

CONCLUSION

The goal of operative management of the cervical spine in RA is to relieve pain, reduce deformity, and prevent disease progression. This goal may be achieved by posterior arthrodesis combined with decompressive procedures, if necessary. Internal fixation should provide sufficient immediate postoperative stability to avoid placing the generally impaired patient into a cumbersome halo or halo vest postoperatively. The operation should be performed at an early stage in the disease process; less deformity requires less operative correction. In patients with early neurologic deficit, recovery is likely; advanced damage to the neurologic structures decreases the possibility of good recovery.

Comparison of recently published results of operative intervention in the cervical spine of patients with RA with previous data shows that satisfactory outcomes are more common, mortality rates are decreasing, and fewer complications are reported, due to improved techniques. This should encourage surgeons dealing with the complexity of the cervical spine in RA and widen the indications for stabilization in the early stage of the disease.

REFERENCES

1. Boyle AC. Ernest Fletcher Memorial Lecture: the rheumatoid neck [Abridged]. *Proc R Soc Med* 1971;64:1161.
2. Nakano KK. Neurologic complications of rheumatoid arthritis. *Orthop Clin North Am* 1975;6:861.
3. Weissman BN, Aliabadi P, Weinfield MS, et al. Prognostic features of atlanto-axial subluxation in rheumatoid arthritis patients. *Radiology* 1992;144:745.
4. Henderson FC, Geddes JF, Crockard HA. Neuropathology of the brainstem and spinal cord in end stage rheumatoid arthritis: implications for treatment. *Ann Rheum Dis* 1993;52:639.
5. Stevens JM, Kling Chong W, Barber C, et al. A new appraisal of abnormalities of the odontoid process associated with atlanto-axial subluxation and neurological disability. *Brain* 1994;117:133.
6. Rogers MA, Crockard HA, Moskovich R, et al. Nystagmus and joint position sensation: their importance in posterior occipitocervical fusion in rheumatoid arthritis. *Spine* 1994;19:16.
7. Howard RS, Henderson F, Hirsch NP, et al. Respiratory abnormalities due to craniovertebral junction compression in rheumatoid disease. *Ann Rheum Dis* 1994;53:134.
8. Jankovic J, Padro R. Segmental myoclonus. *Arch Neurol* 1986;43:1025.
9. Shivapour E, Teasdall RD. Spinal myoclonus with vacuolar degeneration of anterior horn cells. *Arch Neurol* 1980;37:451.
10. Ranawat CS, O'Leary P, Pellicci P, et al. Cervical spine fusion in rheumatoid arthritis. *J Bone Joint Surg Am* 1979;61:1003.
11. Casey AT, Bland JM, Crockard HA. Development of a functional scoring system for rheumatoid arthritis patients with cervical myelopathy. *Ann Rheum Dis* 1996;55:901–960.
12. Fries JF, Spitz P, Kraines RG, et al. Measurement of patient outcome in arthritis. *Arthritis Rheum* 1980;23:137.
13. McGregor M. The significance of certain measurements of the skull in the diagnosis of basilar impression. *Radiology* 1948;21:171.
14. Redlund-Johnell I. Posterior atlanto-axial dislocation in rheumatoid arthritis. *Scand J Rheumatol* 1984;13:337.
15. Redlund-Johnell I, Pettersson H. Radiographic measurements of the craniovertebral regions. Designed for evaluation of abnormalities in rheumatoid arthritis. *Acta Radiol Diag* 1984;25:23.
16. Boden SD, Dodge LD, Bohlman HH, et al. Rheumatoid arthritis of the cervical spine. A long term analysis with predictors of paralysis and recovery. *J Bone Joint Surg Am* 1993;75:1282.
17. Dvorak J, Grob D, Baumgartner H, et al. Functional evaluation of the spinal cord by magnetic resonance imaging in patients with rheumatoid arthritis and instability of upper cervical spine. *Spine* 1989;14:1057.
18. Crockard HA, Calder I, Ransford AO. One stage transoral decompression and posterior fixation in rheumatoid atlanto-axial subluxation. *J Bone Joint Surg Br* 1990;72:682.
19. Casey ATH, Crockard HA, Bland JM, et al. Surgery on the rheumatoid cervical spine for the bed-bound, no ambulant myelopathy—too much, too late? *Lancet* 1996;347:1004–1007.
20. Santavirta S, Konttinen YT, Laasonen E, et al. Ten year results for rheumatoid cervical spine disorders. *J Bone Joint Surg Br* 1991;73:116.
21. Isdale I, Conlon P. Atlantoaxial subluxation. A six year follow-up report. *Ann Rheum Dis* 1971;30:387.
22. Lipson S. Rheumatoid disease of the cervical spine: surgical treatment. In: Camins M, O'Leary P, eds. *Disorders of the cervical spine*. Baltimore: Williams & Wilkins, 1992:565.
23. Pellici P, Ranawat C, Tsairis P, et al. A prospective study of the progression of rheumatoid arthritis of the cervical spine. *J Bone Joint Surg Am* 1981;63:343.
24. Breig A. *Adverse mechanical tension in the central nervous system.* New York: Wiley, 1978:61.
25. Clark CR, Goetz DD, Menezes AH. Arthrodesis of the cervical spine in rheumatoid arthritis. *J Bone Joint Surg Am* 1989;71:381.
26. Grob D. Operative dorsale Stabilisierungen der oberen Halswirbelsäule und des craniocervicalen Ueberganges. Thesis. University of Zurich, Medical Faculty, Zurich, Switzerland, 1992.
27. Malcolm GP, Ransford AO, Crockard HA. Treatment of non-rheumatoid occipitocervical instability. Internal fixation with the Hartshill-Ransford loop. *J Bone Joint Surg Br* 1994;76:357.
28. Sherk HH, ed. *The cervical spine: an atlas of surgical procedures.* Philadelphia: JB Lippincott, 1994.
29. Garrod AE. *A treatise on rheumatism and rheumatoid arthritis.* London: Griffin, 1890.
30. Mixter SJ, Osgood RB. Traumatic lesions of the atlas and axis. *Ann Surg* 1910;51:193.
31. Lane WF. Fracture (dislocation) of the spine. Reduction, temporary recovery. *Lancet* 1892;2:661.
32. Hadra BE. Wiring of the spinous processes in Pott's disease. *Trans Am Orthop Assoc* 1891;4:206.
33. Gallie WE. Fractures and dislocations of the cervical spine. *J Bone Joint Surg Am* 1939;46:495.
34. Brooks AL. Atlanto-axial arthrodesis by the wedge compression method. *J Bone Joint Surg Am* 1978;60:279.
35. Grob D, Crisco J, Panjabi MM, et al. Biomechanical evaluation of four different posterior atlanto-axial fixation techniques. *Spine* 1991;17:480.
36. White AA, Panjabi MM. *Clinical biomechanics of the spine.* Philadelphia: JB Lippincott, 1990.
37. Guyotat J, Perrin G, Pelissou I, et al. Utilization due matériel de Cotrel-Dubousset dans les instabilés C1/C2 (French). *Neurochirurgie* 1987;33:236.
38. Holness RO, Huestis WS, Howes WS, et al. Posterior stabilization with an interlaminar clamp in cervical injuries: technical note and review of the long term experience with the method. *Neurosurgery* 1984;14:318.
39. Barbour JR. Screw fixation in fracture of the odontoid process. *South Aust Clin* 1971;5:20.
40. Grob D, Magerl D. Operative Stabilisier ung bei Frakuren can C1 und C2. *Orthopade* 1987;16:46.
41. Grob D, Magerl D, Seemann P. *Operative atlantoaxiale Stabilisierung.* Berlin: Springer Verlag, 1988.
42. Magerl F, Seemann P. Stable posterior fusion of the atlas and axis by transarticular screw fixation. In: Kehr P, Weidner A, eds. *Cervical spine.* New York: Springer-Verlag, 1986:322.
43. Foerster O. *Die Leitungsbahnen des Schmerzgefü und die chirurgishe Behandlung der Schmerzzustände* (German). Berlin: Urban und Schwarzenberg, 1927.
44. Brattström H, Granholm L. Atlantoaxial fusion in rheumatoid arthritis. *Acta Orthop Scand* 1973;47:619.
45. Wertheim SB, Bohlman HH. Occipito-cervical fusion. *J Bone Joint Surg Am* 1987;69:833.
46. Gschwend N. Die operative Behandlung der cervico-occipitalen Instabilitäten bei Polyarthritis. *Akt Rheumatol* 1987;12:120.

47. Steiger U, Gschwend N. Surgical treatment for instability in cranio-cervical bones and their joints in rheumatoid arthritis. In: Voth D, Glees P, eds. *Diseases in the cranio-cervical junction.* New York: De Gruyter, 1987:241.
48. Flint GA, Hockley AD, McMillan JJ, et al. A new method of occipitocervical fusion using internal fixation. *Neurosurgery* 1987;21:947.
49. Itoh T, Tsuji H, Katoh Y, et al. Occipito-cervical fusion reinforced by Luque's segmental spinal instrumentation for rheumatoid diseases. *Spine* 1988;11:1234.
50. Ransford A, Crockard H, Pozo J, et al. Craniocervical instability treated by a contoured loop fixation. *J Bone Joint Surg Br* 1986;68:173.
51. Brattström H, Granholm L. Chirurgie der Halswirbelsäule bei Patienten mit rheumatoider Arthritis. *Orthopade* 1973;2:118.
52. Cantore GP, Ciapetta P, Delfini R, et al. Experiences in the use of methacylaten in the stabilization of the cervical spine and the craniocervical junction. *Acta Neurochir* 1982;66:140.
53. Grob D, Dvorak J, Gschwend N. *Die Chirurgie der subaxialen Halswirbelsäule bei chronischer Polyarthritis.* Interlaken: ARO Klausurtagung, 1990.
54. Grob D, Dvorak J, Gschwend N. Posterior occipitocervical fusion. *Spine* 1991;26:S17.
55. Grob D, Dvorak J, Panjabi MM, et al. Die dorsale atlanto-axial Verschraubung. Ein Stabilitätstest *in vitro* und *in vivo. Orthopade* 1991; 20:154.
56. Privat JM. Instabilités rhumatismales du rachis sous-occipital. Indications, et résultants de la plaque occipito-rachidienne monobloc (French). In: Privat J, ed. *Ostheosynthèse Rachidienne.* Monpellier: Sauramps Médical, 1988:159.
57. Ferlic D, Clayton M, Leidholt J. Surgical treatment of the symptomatic unstable cervical spine in rheumatoid arthritis. *J Bone Joint Surg Am* 1975;57:349.
58. Fielding JW, Hawkins RJ, Ratzan SA. Spine fusion for atlanto-axial instability. *J Bone Joint Surg Am* 1976;58:400.
59. Larsson S, Toolanen G. Posterior fusion for atlantoaxial subluxations in rheumatoid arthritis. *Spine* 1986;1:525.
60. Grob D, Jeanneret B, Aebi M, et al. Atlanto-axial fusion with transarticular screw fixation. *J Bone Joint Surg Br* 1991;73:972.
61. Meijers KA, Cats A, Kremer HPE, et al. Cervical myelopathy in rheumatoid arthritis. *Clin Exp Rheumatol* 1984;2:239.
62. Castaing J, Gouaze A, Plisson JL. Technique de l'arthrodese cervico-occipitale par greffon visse dans l'occipital (French). *Rev Chir Orthop* 1963;49:123.
63. Brattström H, Brandt L, Ljungren B. Atlanto-axial dislocation in rheumatoid arthritis—signs and symptoms, radiographic pathology, operative techniques and results. In: Voth D, Glees P, eds. *Diseases in the cranio-cervical junction.* Berlin: De Gruyter, 1987:262.
64. Roy-Camille R, Camus JB, Sailant GD, et al. Luxation atloidoaxodienne avec impression basilaire et signes medullaires du cours d'un rheumatisme inflammatoire chronique (French). *Rev Chir Orthop* 1983; 69:81.
65. Grob D, Dvorak J, Manohar M, et al. The role of plate and screw fixation in occipitocervical fusion in rheumatoid arthritis. *Spine* 1994;19:2545.

CHAPTER 66

Subaxial Cervical Involvement in Rheumatoid Arthritis

Adam C. Lipson and Stephen J. Lipson

PATHOPHYSIOLOGY

Rheumatoid arthritis (RA) in the cervical spine results in an erosive arthropathy due to the synovitic destruction of the joints, ligaments, and bone. In the cervical subaxial spine, the diarthrodial cartilaginous facet joints are directly destroyed by rheumatoid pannus, which can extend to adjacent structures. The interspinous ligaments are affected, with attenuation resulting in laxity. The intervertebral cervical discs exhibit destruction through spondylodiscitis. In bone, abnormal anatomy may result from osteoporosis and direct erosion by the pannus, resulting in a loss of skeletal integrity. There is evidence of destructive change through each of the mechanisms. One hypothesized mechanism is the initial destruction through synovitis in the neurocentral joints, with erosion of the disc and adjacent bone causing subluxation (1). Another suggested mechanism is that primary facet arthritis and ligamentous instability causes chronic discovertebral trauma, resulting in destructive changes (2). There is also involvement of interspinous bursae, with spinous process destruction and hypermobile segments associated with disc destruction (3).

Autopsy series indicate that cervical myelopathy results from repeated traction injury due to compression, stretch, and movement, and not due to inflammation (4). Other factors contributing to myelopathy include inward bulging of the ligamentum flavum (5), infolding of the dura (6,7), an intraspinal mass of granulations (8,9), and constrictive band formation (8,10,11). Spinal cord responses to subluxations include pachymeningitis, arachnoiditis, and medullary compression.

Instability of the rheumatoid cervical spine commonly manifests as atlantoaxial subluxation, vertical atlantoaxial subluxation resulting in basilar invagination or cranial settling, and subaxial subluxation (SAS). SAS is evident in 10% to 22% of patients with RA cervical subluxations (12). SAS predominates at the C2-C3 and C3-C4 segments, typically exhibiting a lack of osteophyte production and often appearing at multiple levels in a "staircase" fashion (13,14). End-plate erosions are evident in 12% to 15% of patients with RA (13–15). Discovertebral destruction may not always accompany SAS.

Other patterns of subaxial disease that result in neurologic disturbance are subluxations below higher fusions (as many as 36% of patients with occipitocervical fusions develop SAS postoperatively after an average of 2.6 years, as opposed to only 5.5% of patients with atlantoaxial fusions after an average of 9 years), anterior spondylodiscitis causing spinal cord compression, intracanal rheumatoid granulations, and a hyperlordotic cervical spine (16,17).

CLINICAL AND LABORATORY EVALUATION

Clinical manifestations of cervical RA include pain, neurologic disturbance, and death. Involvement of the subaxial spine causes neck pain and referral into the paracervical, suprascapular, and interscapular areas. Local tenderness and crepitation may be noted in affected subaxial levels. Occipitocervical pain usually implicates involvement of the craniocervical structures. SAS can cause varying states of myeloradiculopathy depending on the prevalence of more central spinal cord compression versus foraminal radicular compression and inflammation. Patients with myelopathy will exhibit predominant signs of upper motor neuron disturbance in a radicular distribution.

The history and physical examination will lead to the diagnosis of the state of myeloradiculopathy predominating and to the level of suspicion for subaxial involvement. The neurologic symptoms may be vague and can be multiple.

Subjective symptoms of diffuse paresthesias in the hands may implicate myelopathy, whereas a radicular distribution of sensory and motor disturbance may predominate in SAS in its earlier stage. An electric shock sensation, usually on flexion, radiating into the body (Lhermitte's phenomenon), as well as a feeling of weakness or loss of endurance, may occur with SAS causing spinal cord compression. Posterior column signs may be evident, with loss of vibratory and proprioceptive sensation. Physical examination may be confounded by peripheral rheumatoid disease causing weakness from articular involvement, tenosynovitis, tendon rupture, rheumatoid myopathy, and rheumatoid peripheral neuropathy.

Neurologic assessment of rheumatoid myelopathy is graded on the Ranawat scale (Table 66.1) to enable evaluation in the setting of musculoskeletal dysfunction due to rheumatoid polyarthropathy, although the system must be viewed with the caveat that it is only a very rough indicator of the severity of a patient's neurologic deficit (18). Functional assessments may be useful for grading of myelopathy, such as the Nurick scale, Japanese Orthopedic Association scale, the Myelopathy Disability Index scale, and the European Disability Index scale. Somatosensory evoked potential (SSEP) testing is particularly helpful in distinguishing myelopathic symptoms from radicular or neuropathic or articular etiologies, given the limitations of assessment by physical examination in patients with extensive disease. Motor evoked potentials may also be beneficial. However, electrophysiologic evaluation is not as reliable as serial examination and imaging in our experience.

Occasionally, symptoms of posterior circulation arterial insufficiency have been reported secondary to vertebral artery compression, meriting evaluation of vision and brainstem function, as well as transcranial Doppler evaluation if indicated by patient history.

Cervical SAS is associated with a more severe degree of systemic RA and has been correlated with a higher serum level of C-reactive protein (>3.7 mg/dL), a greater number of joints with radiographic erosive changes, a greater degree of hand involvement (mean carpal height ratio 0.36), and disease subset based on serum C1q levels (12% more erosive disease, and 39% mutilating disease subsets) (19, 20). Younger patient age (<55 years), longer duration of disease (>10 years), and higher doses or longer duration of

corticosteroid administration are also thought to be important risk factors for myelopathy.

RADIOLOGIC EVALUATION

In the patient with SAS, plain radiographs are the starting point for evaluation of lesions contributing to the patient's symptoms. They should ideally be part of the routine screening and follow-up of patients with RA to identify patients with cervical involvement before the onset of symptoms. End-plate erosions are present in 12% to 15% and subluxations are present in 10% to 20% of patients with RA (14,21,22). A neutral lateral radiograph alone is not adequate to determine whether subluxations are present at any level. Flexion and extension lateral views are essential to determine the presence and degree of instability.

A measurement of cervical height, the cervical height index (CHI), is made by the ratio of the height of the subaxial spine from the center point of the C2 pedicle to the base of C7 normalized to the distance of the posterior wall of C2 to the tip of the spinous process of C2. The CHI is strongly predictive for myelopathy from SAS, where subluxation and lordosis contribute to spinal cord dysfunction from subaxial spine disease. When the CHI is less than 2.00, the specificity and sensitivity of CHI and subluxation approach 100% (23).

A progression of anterior slip more than 20%, axial shortening, spinous process erosion, apophysial joint erosion, and intervertebral disc collapse has been correlated with a neurologic deterioration (24). Vertebral displacement of greater than 3 mm is considered abnormal, and indicative of SAS on flexion-extension views. A subaxial canal diameter less than 14 mm is a strong correlate of cord compression, and is a threshold for worsening neurologic function (25,26).

Because plain radiographs cannot estimate the soft tissue contributions of granulations and ligamentum flavum, neuroradiologic evaluation must be used if the compression is to be definitively examined. That evaluation can be accomplished with myelography and enhanced with computed tomography (CT). Magnetic resonance imaging (MRI) is currently the most valuable technique for evaluation of the canal for cord compression, and sagittal flexion-extension (also referred to as functional) MRI within a conventional neck coil defines the role of subluxations and cord compression further on sagittal views. The subarachnoid space available for the cord at the atlantoaxial and subaxial level below C2 has been correlated with cord compression on active flexion views (27). CT evaluation permits evaluation of erosive changes and articular involvement. MRI evaluation with the addition of gadolinium enhancement helps to elaborate the soft tissue components, such as inflammatory soft tissue proliferations, joint effusion, and hypervascular synovial changes, and is most sensitive at detecting early changes. Pannus formation in the subaxial spine is rare, although it has been reported (28). There is, however, a poor correlation between neurologic findings and MRI findings (29).

TABLE 66.1. *The Ranawat Scoring of Myelopathy for Spinal Cord Compression*

Ranawat class	Neurologic status
I	No deficit; includes paresthesias
II	Subjective weakness with hyperreflexia
IIIA	Objective weakness and long tract signs, ambulatory
IIIB	Objective weakness and long tract signs, nonambulatory

NONSURGICAL MANAGEMENT

RA of the cervical spine begins early in the course of a patient's disease, particularly in the atlantoaxial joint. Early, aggressive, and persistent medical management is therefore of major importance. Nonoperative measures are directed at the suppression of active synovitis. These techniques are supportive and primarily oriented to provide comfort for patients with cervical subluxation without objective neurologic signs. Cervical collars are commonly used, but no study we are aware of supports their effectiveness against subluxations at any level or against neurologic progression. One study demonstrated failure to meet these goals (30). Collars can be used for psychological support, pain relief, warmth, and a feeling of stability. Rigid orthoses have not been shown to have specific advantages. Intermittent halter traction may permit comfort, but will not maintain reduction of subluxations or correct neurologic deficits.

Pain relief can be sought (anecdotal) through use of transcutaneous nerve stimulation. Cervical epidural steroid injections may play a role in SAS-induced pain, but should be used with caution. Nontraditional medical techniques, such as acupuncture, may be used, but spinal manipulative techniques are contraindicated in all cervical RA subluxations.

Although cervical myelopathy is generally considered an indication for surgical intervention, an improvement in functional deficit from SAS has been reported using prolonged cervical traction and immobilization with a halo vest, and may be considered an independent nonoperative measure for patients at high operative risk (31).

SURGICAL MANAGEMENT

Indications

The primary indication for surgical intervention is neurologic deficit and intractable pain. As surgical and anesthetic techniques have improved, surgeons no longer delay surgery because of the fear of perioperative death and paralysis. The presence of subluxation per se is not an indication for surgery, because there is a poor correlation between atlantoaxial or subaxial subluxation and neurologic signs (18). The diagnosis of "impending neurologic deficit" has been introduced to designate patients who, although asymptomatic, have markedly abnormal neuroradiographic findings and will have a better outcome if operated on before neurologic deficits manifest (32). In the patient with SAS, more than 4 mm subluxation or thecal sac compression defines impending neurologic deficit.

Complications are minimized and outcomes are improved in patients who undergo surgery at lower Ranawat grades, with one study reporting as many as 58% of grade IIIA patients improving to grade I or II, versus only 20% of nonambulatory grade IIIB patients (33). Neurologic improvement, generally referring to a reduction of myelopathy by one Ranawat grade, in 45% to 94% of patients and a reduction in pain in 90% to 97% of patients have been reported (16,34). For arthrodeses of all types, nonunion rates of 20% to 33% have been reported in varying series. Long-term failure may result from adjacent level instability and subluxation, pseudoarthrosis, lateral joint collapse, and angulation deformity.

Perioperative Management

The difficulties confronting the surgeon anticipating cervical spine surgery focus on the overall status of the RA patient. Such patients tend to be severely afflicted with RA. They are debilitated and crippled; have fragile skin; poor wound healing; and osteopenic bone, making fixation to the spine difficult and bone grafting mechanically inadequate; with problematic rates of nonunion following arthrodeses and increased susceptibility to infection. Perioperative mortality remains high at 5% to 10%, varying according to the degree of preoperative disability (35,36). To avoid complication, careful preoperative assessment and planning is imperative. Nutritional issues and smoking cessation should be addressed prior to any surgical procedure.

Perioperative airway management in cervical RA patients is problematic. A study of 128 RA patients undergoing posterior cervical spine surgery demonstrated a 14% prevalence of upper airway obstruction if patients were not intubated with fiberoptic assistance, as compared with 1% in patients who had been intubated fiberoptically (37). Awake intubation and SSEP monitoring enhance safety to the spinal cord during manipulation for induction and positioning. Intraoperative fluoroscopy should be utilized during patient positioning to monitor skeletal alignment.

Preoperative skeletal traction is recommended to relieve pain, reduce subluxations, arrest or reverse neurologic deterioration, and restore sagittal alignment for deformity correction (12,19,38–42). It is of special value in grade IIIB patients with acute-onset quadriparesis (36). Nonambulatory patients have a far worse outcome of surgery than ambulatory patients (33); thus, arresting and possibly reversing this neurologic status may be particularly beneficial before surgery is attempted. The senior author (SJL) has found the halo wheelchair to be an excellent device to accomplish these goals (43). In a study of 44 procedures in 40 RA patients, subaxial instability was treated in 22 cases using preoperative halo wheelchair traction (44). Halo-dependent traction and the halo-Ilizarov distraction casting are also useful in achieving gradual correction of preoperative deformity (45). Traction is generally applied parallel with the deformity to distract and "unlock" the involved joint, with gradual adjustments directed at correction of vertical deformity first, followed by rotational deformity, with an emphasis placed on time in traction rather than an increase in weight, up to 4 weeks preoperatively.

Most patients experience a reduction in pain and in their myelopathy, and many have reduction of their subluxation, even if it is not fully reduced. The advantages are that the patient is upright, with better skin integrity, has improved swallowing, more easily urinates and defecates, has improved pulmonary toilet, and has a better psychological status. The improved neurologic status and comfort make the timing of surgery more elective. The correction of deformity makes surgical exposure and instrumentation easier. Patients are then placed in a halo vest for stabilization prior to fusion. Botulinum toxin injections or sternocleidomastoid release maneuvers may be necessary adjuncts to accomplish reduction.

Operative Management

The primary goal of surgery is stabilization and relief of cord compression, either via reduction of subluxation or by surgical decompression. Posterior arthrodesis at affected levels is the most common procedure performed. Internal fixation allows earlier mobilization, fewer cervical orthoses, improved pain relief, and increased rates of fusion (38,46,47). Vascular insufficiency in the setting of intermittent compression due to the unstable segment is implicated in rheumatoid myelopathy, offering a pathophysiologic explanation of why arthrodesis or stabilization alone may result in neurologic improvement (48). Stabilization may also enable regression of the inflammatory pannus, reinforcing the idea that the pannus is a reactive fibrous tissue resulting from instability (49).

The role of laminectomy is debated (50), although arthrodesis is necessary when it is performed (51). The senior author (SJL) performed laminectomies when reduction could not be achieved, when persistent spinal cord compression was present, or if no neurologic improvement occurred during preoperative traction. A series of 55 subaxial cervical spine arthrodeses yielded 82% neurologic improvement, and 92% had notable pain reduction (23). A lack of postoperative reduction was associated with a lack of neurologic improvement. Duration of neurologic symptoms was the most significant factor in neurologic outcome.

Lateral mass screw-plate instrumentation via the Magerl technique is effective for stabilization, although joint destruction of the lateral masses may add to the technical complexity, and the poor bone quality may limit adequate purchase. If screw fixation is unattainable, then posterior cervical wiring with sublaminar or spinous process wiring may be used for stabilization. Sublaminar wiring may be dangerous if the subluxation is not reduced. Lateral mass screws likely provide better results in comparison with sublaminar wiring with regard to stabilization and pain control (52), although redundant fixation with both screw and posterior wiring procedures may be beneficial. In circumstances in which the posterior elements are largely deficient or absent, facet wiring may be performed to achieve arthrodesis.

Bone grafting, preferably with cortical and cancellous iliac crest bone, is necessary to achieve fusion, even with methylmethacrylate enhancement of internal stabilization (26,32,46). Metal-mesh backing of the bone graft has been used to make the often-osteoporotic bone graft more substantive (53). The patient is then kept in a halo vest for 3 to 4 months postoperatively to maintain stability. The need to fuse has been challenged in the literature for occipitocervical stabilization (but not for isolated rheumatoid subaxial instability) by the argument that there is very little subaxial instability following occipitocervical stabilization without bone grafting, and that osseous incorporation does not alter outcome in terms of neurologic deficit and postoperative stability of pain for patients with advanced RA (54).

The role of anterior surgery is also controversial. Anterior surgery may risk graft resorption and progressive collapse (51,55) and failure to achieve improvement (56), but is advocated by some surgeons to achieve a better decompression (26), with potentially better fusion results via anterior-posterior stabilization given the poor bone quality (54). In addressing ventral pathology, posterior decompression and stabilization should be considered the primary treatment for compression arising from rheumatoid pannus or degenerative disc osteophytes in the setting of SAS. Anterior versus combined (or staged) anterior/posterior decompression and arthrodesis should be considered if there is severe kyphotic angulation contributing to the cord compression that cannot be corrected using preoperative halo traction. Postinflammatory ankylosis may necessitate anterior release maneuvers.

CONCLUSION

Clinical outcomes in patients with cervical RA have improved because of earlier recognition of disease, more aggressive and innovative medical treatment, and earlier referral to surgery for evaluation of cervical disease. Comparison of patient cohorts between 1974–1982 and 1991–1996 demonstrate fewer patients with severe grade IIIB myelopathy (34% vs. 7%), and marked improvements in early postoperative mortality (9% vs. 0%) and surgical complication rates (50% vs. 22%) (57). A proposed algorithm for the workup and management of SAS is outlined in Figure 66.1. Controversy still exists regarding the necessity of fusion, the timing of surgical intervention, and the choice of approach and instrumentation. The major advances in medical treatments for RA have made substantial contributions to what appears to be a declining incidence of cervical subaxial disease. Combined with earlier recognition, better diagnostic tools, and improved surgical and perioperative management, these factors will continue to make a significant impact on the development of severe myelopathy in rheumatoid patients.

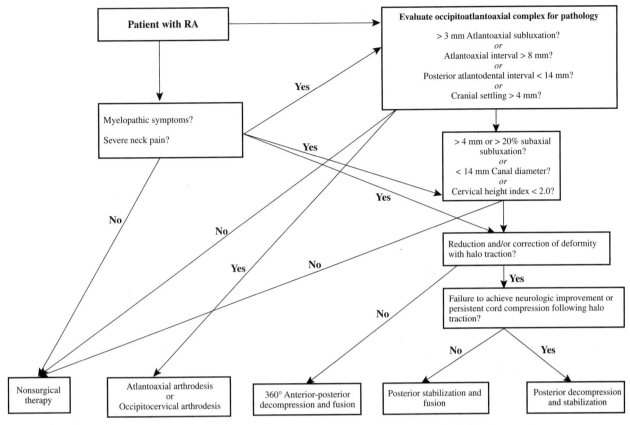

FIG. 66.1. Proposed treatment algorithm for rheumatoid cervical disease.

REFERENCES

1. Martel W. Pathogenesis of cervical discovertebral destruction in rheumatoid arthritis. *Arthritis Rheum* 1977;20:1217–1225.
2. Ball J, Sharp J. Rheumatoid arthritis of the cervical spine. In: Hill AGS, ed. *Modern trends in rheumatology,* vol. 2. London: Butterworth, 1971: 117–138.
3. Bywaters EGL. Rheumatoid arthritis and other disease of the cervical interspinous bursae, and changes in the spinous processes. *Ann Rheum Dis* 1982;41:361–70.
4. Klein JD, Hey LA, Wattenmaker I, et al. Arthrodesis of the subaxial cervical spine in rheumatoid arthritis. *Orthop Trans* 1994;18: 705.
5. Hopkins JS. Lower cervical rheumatoid subluxation with tetraplegia. *J Bone Joint Surg Br* 1967;49:46–51.
6. Euderlink F, Maijers KAE. Pathology of the cervical spine in rheumatoid arthritis: a controlled study of 44 spines. *J Pathol* 1976;120:91–108.
7. Jeffereys E. The cervical spine in rheumatoid disease. In: *Disorders of the cervical spine.* London: Butterworth, 1980:106–118.
8. Kudo H, Iwano K, Yoshizaki H. Cervical cord compression due to extradural granulation tissue in rheumatoid arthritis. A review of five cases. *J Bone Joint Surg Br* 1984;66:426–430.
9. Polyzoides AJ, Pearson JR. Tetraplegia in rheumatoid arthritis with complete recovery after surgery. *Br J Surg* 1973;60:327–329.
10. Kataoka O, Hirohata K, Kurihara A. The surgical treatment of myelopathy secondary to rheumatoid arthritis of the lower cervical spine. *Int Orthop* 1979;3:103–110.
11. Yonezawa T, Itoh T. Radiologic observation of rheumatoid lesions of the posterior elements in the lower cervical spine. *J Jpn Joint Surg* 1991;10:53–60.
12. Thompson RC, Meyer TJ. Posterior surgical stabilization for atlantoaxial subluxation in rheumatoid arthritis. *Spine* 1985;10:597–601.

13. Park WM, O'Neill MO, McCall CI. The radiology of rheumatoid involvement of the cervical spine. *Skeletal Radiol* 1979;4:1–7.
14. Sharp J, Purser JW, Lawrence S. Rheumatoid arthritis of the cervical spine in the adult. *Ann Rheum Dis* 1958;17:303.
15. Conlon PW, Isdale IC, Rose BS. Rheumatoid arthritis of the cervical spine. *Ann Rheum Dis* 1972;31:431.
16. Kraus DR, Peppelman WC, Agarwal AK, et al. Incidence of subaxial subluxation in patients with generalized rheumatoid arthritis who have had previous occipital cervical fusions. *Spine* 1991;16(Suppl):S486–S489.
17. Lipson SJ. Patterns of rheumatoid subaxial disease causing myelopathy and strategies of management. *Orthop Trans* 1994;12:55.
18. Pellicci PM, Ranawat CS, Tsairis P, et al. A prospective study of the progression of rheumatoid arthritis of the cervical spine. *J Bone Joint Surg Am* 1981;63:342–350.
19. Fujiwara K, Fujimoto M, Owaki H, et al. Cervical lesions related to the systemic progression in rheumatoid arthritis. *Spine* 1998;23:2052–2056.
20. van der Heijde DM. Joint erosions and patients with early rheumatoid arthritis. *Br J Rheumatol* 1995;34(Suppl 2):74–78.
21. Blan JH. Rheumatoid arthritis of the cervical spine. *Bull Rheum Dis* 1967;18:471–476.
22. Meikle JA, Wilkinson M. Rheumatoid involvement of the cervical spine. *Ann Rheum Dis* 1971;30:154.
23. Klein JD, Hey LA, Lipson SJ. Predictors of preoperative neurologic deficit and postoperative outcome in patients with rheumatoid arthritis of the subaxial cervical spine. *Orthop Trans* 1994;18:716.
24. Yonezawa T, Tsuji H, Matsui H, et al. Subaxial lesions in rheumatoid arthritis: radiographic factors suggestive of lower cervical myelopathy. *Spine* 1995;20:208–215.
25. Boden SD. Rheumatoid arthritis of the cervical spine. Surgical decision making based on predictors of paralysis and recovery. *Spine* 1994;19:2275–2280.

26. Boden SD, Dodge LD, Bohlman HH, et al. Rheumatoid arthritis of the cervical spine. A long term analysis and predictors of paralysis and recovery. *J Bone Joint Surg Am* 1993;75:1282–1297.

27. Reijnierse M, Breedveld FC, Kroon HM, et al. Are magnetic resonance flexion views useful in evaluating the cervical spine of patients with rheumatoid arthritis? *Skeletal Radiol* 2000;29:85–89.

28. Shiratori K, Mennel HD, Bien S. Intraspinal pannus formation at C6 in a patient with rheumatoid arthritis causing severe cervical cord compression. A case report. *Rheumatol Int* 2003;23:192–194.

29. Stiskal MA, Neuhold A, Szolar DH, et al. Rheumatoid arthritis of the craniocervical region by MR imaging: detection and characterization. *AJR Am J Roentgenol* 1995;165:585–592.

30. Smith PH, Benn RT, Sharp J. Natural history of rheumatoid cervical luxations. *Ann Rheum Dis* 1972;31:431–439.

31. Oostveen JC, Van de Laar MA, Geelen JA, et al. Successful conservative treatment of rheumatoid subaxial subluxation resulting in improvement of myelopathy, reduction of subluxation, and stabilization of the cervical spine. A report of two cases. *Ann Rheum Dis* 1999;58:126–129.

32. Clark CR, Goetz DD, Menezes AH. Arthrodesis of the cervical spine in rheumatoid arthritis. *J Bone Joint Surg Am* 1989;71:381–392.

33. Casey ATH, Crockard HA, Steven J, et al. Surgery on the rheumatoid cervical spine for the non-ambulant myelopathic patient—too much too late? *Lancet* 1996;347:1004–1007.

34. Matsunaga S, Ijiri K, Koga H. Results of a longer than 10-year follow-up of patients with rheumatoid arthritis treated by occipitocervical fusion. *Spine* 2000;25:1749–1753.

35. Moscovich R, Crockard HA, Shott S, et al. Occipital stabilization for myelopathy in patients with rheumatoid arthritis: implications of not bone grafting. *J Bone Joint Surg Am* 2000;82:349–365.

36. Peppelman WC, Kraus DR, Donaldson III WF, et al. Cervical spine surgery in rheumatoid arthritis: improvement of neurologic deficit after cervical spine fusion. *Spine* 1993;18:2375–2379.

37. Wattenmaker I, Concepcion M, Hibberd P, et al. Upper-airway obstruction and perioperative management of the airway in patients with posterior operations on the cervical spine for rheumatoid arthritis. *J Bone Joint Surg Am* 1994;76:360–365.

38. Ferlic DC, Clayton ML, Leidholt JD, et al. Surgical treatment of the symptomatic unstable cervical spine in rheumatoid arthritis. *J Bone Joint Surg Am* 1975;57:349–354.

39. Fielding JW, Hawkins RJ, Ratzan SA. Spine fusion for atlanto-axial instability. *J Bone Joint Surg Am* 1976;58:400–407.

40. McAfee PC, Cassidy JR, Davis RF, et al. Fusion of the occiput to the upper cervical spine. A review of 37 cases. *Spine* 1991;16:S491–S494.

41. Meijers KAE, VanBeusekom GT, Luyendijk W, et al. Dislocation of the cervical spine with cord compression in rheumatoid arthritis. *J Bone Joint Surg Br* 1974;56:668–680.

42. Zoma A, Sturrock RD, Fisher WD, et al. Surgical stabilization of the rheumatoid cervical spine. *J Bone Joint Surg Br* 1987;69:8–12.

43. Stagnara P. Traction cranienne par le halo de Rancho Los Amigos. *Rev Chir Orthop Repar Appar Mot* 1971;57:287–300.

44. Cove J, Lipson SJ. The role of preoperative management by halo-wheelchair traction in patients with rheumatoid arthritic subluxations of the cervical spine. *Orthop Trans* 1996–1997;20:436.

45. Graziano GP, Hensinger R, Patel CK. The use of traction methods to correct severe cervical deformity in rheumatoid arthritis patients: a report of five cases. *Spine* 2001;26:1076–1081.

46. Bryan WJ, Inglis AE, Sculco TP, et al. Methylmethacrylate stabilization for enhancement of posterior cervical arthrodesis in rheumatoid arthritis. *J Bone Joint Surg Am* 1982;64:1045–1050.

47. Thomas WH. Surgical management of the rheumatoid cervical spine. *Orthop Clin North Am* 1975;6:793.

48. Stanley D, Laing RJ, Forster DMC, et al. Posterior decompression and fusion in rheumatoid disease of the cervical spine: redressing the balance. *J Spinal Dis* 1994;7:439–443.

49. Grob D, Wursch R, Grauer W, et al. Atlantoaxial fusion and retrodental pannus in rheumatoid arthritis. *Spine* 1997;22:1580–1583.

50. Christensson D, Saveland H, Zygmunt S, et al. Cervical laminectomy without fusion in patients with rheumatoid arthritis. *J Neurosurg* 1999;90:186–190.

51. Lipson SJ. Rheumatoid arthritis in the cervical spine. *Clin Orthop* 1989;239:121–127.

52. Shad A, Shariff SS, Teddy PJ, et al. Craniocervical fusion for rheumatoid arthritis: comparison of sublaminar wires and the lateral mass screw craniocervical fusion. *Br J Neurosurg* 2002;16:483–486.

53. Tsahakis PJ, Lipson SJ. Occipito-cervical fusion with metal mesh backing in rheumatoid cervical spine disease. *Orthop Trans* 1993;16:789.

54. Olerud C, Larsson BE, Rodriguez M. Subaxial cervical spine subluxation in rheumatoid arthritis. A retrospective analysis of 16 operated patients after 1–5 years. *Acta Orthop Scand* 1997;68:109–115.

55. Yone K, Sakou T, Yoshikuni N, et al. Surgical management of lower cervical spine lesions in rheumatoid arthritis. *Orthop Trans* 1994;18:704–705.

56. Ranawat CS, O'Leary P, Pellicci P, et al. Cervical fusion in rheumatoid arthritis. *J Bone Joint Surg Am* 1979;61:1003–1010.

57. Hamilton JD, Gordon MM, McInnes IB, et al. Improved medical and surgical management of cervical spine disease in patients with rheumatoid arthritis over 10 years. *Ann Rheum Dis* 2000;59:434–438.

CHAPTER 67

Ankylosing Spondylitis

John A. Glaser and Craig D. Brigham

INTRODUCTION

Ankylosing spondylitis (AS) is an inflammatory rheumatologic disease that can severely affect the spine. The lack of a serum marker groups AS with other arthritides such as psoriatic arthritis, Crohn's disease, ulcerative colitis, and Reiter's syndrome, known collectively as seronegative spondyloarthropathies.

Epidemiology: Ankylosing Spondylitis and HLA-B27

The B27 allele on the HLA loci is found in 8% of American white people, but is present in about 90% of those with AS. Only 10% to 20% of individuals with B27 will develop some type of spondyloarthropathy. Epidemiologic studies have shown that the prevalence of AS within an ethnic group is proportional to the prevalence of the B27 antigen in that population. The presence of the B27 antigen (found on chromosome 6 and part of the major histocompatibility antigen complex) does not confirm the diagnosis of ankylosing spondylitis. The diagnosis of AS is based on clinical and radiographic criteria and can be extremely difficult to confirm in a patient with early manifestations.

Clinical Manifestations

Ankylosing spondylitis causes an inflammation and later ossification of the entheses (tendinous insertions into bone). It is not known why the entheses of the spine and the sacroiliac joints are preferentially affected. Ankylosis and osteopenia of the spine creates a pathological condition that predisposes patients to kyphosis and fracture.

Nonsurgical Treatment

Recent studies have suggested that a monoclonal antibody (infliximab) to tumor necrosis factor (TNF) has potential as a treatment for AS and rheumatoid arthritis. Synovial biopsies taken from AS patients treated with infliximab showed less inflammation and proliferation than controls (1). TNF-α promoter alleles have been found to correlate with disease activity in people who are HLA-B27 positive. High amounts of TNF-α mRNA have been found in sacroiliac joint biopsies of patients with AS (2). Other studies have shown short-term clinical improvements in AS patients treated with infliximab (3). Researchers continue to explore the genetic basis for AS and other autoimmune diseases in order to understand their pathogenesis and thus allow for more precise therapeutic intervention.

The mainstay of treatment for AS remains the judicious use of nonsteroidal antiinflammatory drugs. A 6-week randomized, double-blinded, placebo-controlled trial of celecoxib (100 mg twice a day) in 246 patients found that this cyclooxygenase-2 inhibitor was significantly better than placebo in improving AS patients' pain and function (4). The use of sulfasalazine remains controversial. A randomized, prospective, double-blind, multicenter study found that 2,000 mg per day of SSZ was no more effective than placebo (5).

Patients initially diagnosed with AS should be advised to abstain from smoking, avoid sleeping with large pillows that place their neck in kyphosis, and exercise regularly. Uhrin and associates (6) conducted a prospective longitudinal study of 220 AS patients. They found that patients who did regular exercise (especially if they had suffered with their disease for less than 15 years) scored better on functional and pain questionnaires than did those patients who did not exercise. The severity of symptoms and disability associated with spondylitis is extremely variable, making long-term prognosis difficult at the time of diagnosis. Spinal and sacroiliac ankylosis usually manifests by the third decade in patients with AS. Patients with spinal disease secondary to one of the other seronegative spondyloarthropathies may not demonstrate spine ankylosis until the sixth decade (7). Most patients benefit from nonsteroidal antiinflammatory medications, indomethacin being the first drug of choice. Calcium (1,200 mg daily) and vitamin D supplementation is important for women with AS, who are more likely to develop osteoporosis with advanced age. Bone density studies may indicate consideration of the use of alendronate.

FRACTURES

Literature Review

The literature supports the following statements regarding AS patients with cervical spine fractures:

- The prevalence of fracture is greater in patients with AS than in the general population. Fractures often occur in the sixth to eighth decades of life and can be sustained from minimal trauma (8–10).
- Fractures are often unstable. The ankylosed spine fractures in atypical ways: Fractures are more like those that occur in tubular long bone (11–13). Even a nondisplaced fracture can displace suddenly if cervical extension is performed for cardiopulmonary resuscitation or for purposes of immobilization. Acute quadriparesis has been reported in patients with AS as a result of cervical spine fractures that occurred while the patients were undergoing intubation, undergoing emergency immobilization for transport from a trauma setting, being treated in traction, or being placed in a halo vest (9,12,14–20). A nondisplaced or minimally displaced fracture, if not adequately immobilized, may allow gradual accumulation of epidural hematoma and spinal cord compression that can occur hours, days, or even weeks later (21). Persistent micromotion of a nondisplaced fracture through the relatively avascular calcified disc space may lead to nonunion or deformity (8,22).
- Neurologic compromise is common and often severe. Angulation, displacement, or distraction of the spine at the fracture site can cause severe spinal cord injury. Progressive neurologic deficit can occur if an expanding epidural hematoma occurs (23). Spinal cord injury, especially complete quadriplegia, in AS patients portends a grave prognosis (9,10,24).
- Delay in diagnosis is common. Patients with AS are often used to living with chronic neck pain, and an increase in their pain after trivial trauma will not prompt them to seek treatment until symptoms of myelopathy occur. Interpretation of plain radiographs is complicated by osteopenia. Kyphosis makes visualization of the lower cervical spine difficult due to superimposition of the shoulders.
- Management of such patients is difficult, and high rates of morbidity and mortality are reported regardless of treatment methods. Good results have been reported with nonoperative treatment, but in many series cases of worsening neurologic deficit during treatment are reported. Special techniques and close observation are needed when these patients are placed in traction or in a halo orthosis.

- Surgery has been most often recommended for patients with worsening neurologic deficit, which makes it difficult to assess the role of internal fixation as a necessary adjunct to treatment in patients who present with "unstable" fractures. Emergency laminectomy for evacuation of hematoma will not always reverse neurologic deficit, and worsening of a deficit after surgery has been reported. Surgical immobilization both with and without the use of a halo orthosis after surgery has been reported (24,25).
- Patients who have incomplete ossification of the posterior ligaments may sustain low-energy compression fractures that are "stable" but allow progressive kyphosis to occur, in the absence of neurologic deficit.
- Type II odontoid and hangman-type fractures have been reported in patients with AS in whom spontaneous fusion of the occiput to C1 had previously occurred. There is no consensus regarding treatment for this problem (8,26–28).

Evaluation and Treatment of Cervical Spine Fractures

No Neurologic Deficit

A high index of suspicion and aggressive use of imaging studies are required for patients with AS who report increased neck pain, even if there is no history of significant trauma. If a patient presents without signs or symptoms of neurologic injury and without a history of significant trauma, relative stability of the fracture is assumed. The patient is placed in a cervical collar, and plain radiographs are obtained. If a fracture is not clearly evident, computed tomography (CT) with two-dimensional reconstructions or planar tomography is indicated (Fig. 67.1). Due to kyphosis, patients often require large bolsters under their body and legs to allow proper cervical spine imaging in a CT scanner. Imaging studies should clearly define the bony anatomy of the cervical and upper thoracic spine to exclude additional nondisplaced fractures around the cervicothoracic junction. If no fracture is detected but the clinical picture is suspicious, the patient is kept in a hard collar until a bone scan with single photon emission CT (SPECT) is obtained. If the bone scan shows increased uptake, a fracture is presumed to be present and the patient wears a hard collar until symptoms subside. Repeat CT or tomography may disclose the fracture after initial healing has occurred (29).

Neurologic Deficit

If a patient with AS presents with signs or symptoms of myelopathy or a history of significant trauma (especially head trauma), immediate immobilization is essential. Severe instability of the cervical spine must be assumed, and great care must be used in placing the patient in traction or an orthosis. Immobilization of the neck should be initiated by a clinical assessment of the patient's prefracture sagittal alignment. Family members can often help determine the amount of cervical kyphosis that the patient had before in-

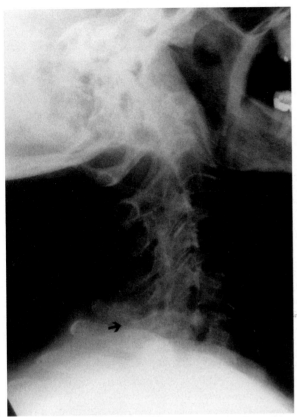

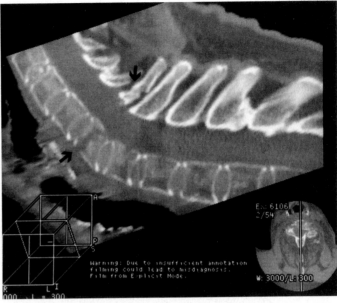

FIG. 67.1. A: Lateral radiograph obtained in the emergency department. A neurologically normal 78-year-old woman with ankylosing spondylitis reported neck pain after sustaining an acetabular fracture in a motor vehicle accident. A fracture of the C6 spinous process was evident, but further definition of the fracture was obscured by the shoulders. **B:** Midsagittal computed tomographic two-dimensional reconstruction clearly showed a three-column fracture that extended anteriorly through the upper body of C6. The overall spinal canal alignment was acceptable. The woman was treated nonoperatively for both her acetabular fracture and cervical fracture. She wore a hard collar for 3 months, achieved a solid union, and remained neurologically normal.

jury. Recent preinjury photographs of the patient can provide useful information in assessing the interval of space between the patient's chin and chest.

Traction, using tongs or a halo, is used to counterbalance the weight of the head and to realign the spine (which is most often in kyphosis relative to the long axis of the trunk), not to utilize the reduction effect of ligamentotaxis. Weights of less than 10 pounds are recommended. Special beds such as the circle-electric or Roto-bed are especially helpful to allow the patient to change position without altering the line of traction on the neck (Fig. 67.2). The line of traction is rarely parallel to the ground with the patient supine, because many patients are unable to lie supine due to kyphosis of the cervical, thoracic, or lumbar spine. Hip flexion contractures are also common in patients with AS. Great care must be taken to prevent overdistraction, which can create irreversible spinal cord ischemia and neurologic deficit (17).

A lateral cervical spine radiograph may not adequately visualize the fracture in the acute setting, due to osteopenia and shoulder interference. If an incomplete neurologic in-

jury is present, magnetic resonance imaging (MRI) is the preferable initial study to define spinal cord compression due to alteration in the bony canal or epidural hematoma. An epidural hematoma will not enhance, whereas an area of long-standing spondylodiscitis is usually characterized by hypointensity on the T1-weighted sequences unless subacute hemorrhage exists (30). Imaging studies should satisfactorily delineate the cause of a neurologic deficit.

Management of Cervical Fractures

After adequate imaging studies have been obtained, the surgeon must consider three factors when outlining a treatment plan. In order of importance, these are as follows:

1. Cause of progression of a neurologic deficit
2. Fracture pattern and its stability
3. The patient's condition

Patients with marked angulation or displacement of the spine should be reduced either by traction or by immediate application of a halo vest. For those with a complete

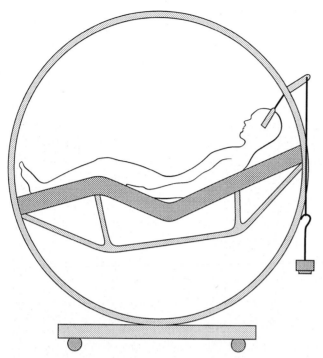

FIG. 67.2. A patient in traction while in a circle-electric bed. This accommodates the patient's thoracic kyphosis and allows cervical traction to be maintained in prefracture alignment. Altering body position for skin pressure relief will not change the angle of traction. To prevent the potentially disastrous consequences of overdistraction, only weight sufficient to counterbalance the head is recommended.

neurologic deficit, the prognosis is poor, with mortality rates as high as 100% reported (10). Treatment in a halo vest should result in union in 3 to 4 months (9).

Motion at the fracture site is most likely responsible for worsening neurologic deficit in patients with AS. This motion can cause spinal cord compression in two ways. An expanding epidural hematoma can occur with motion, even if the spine has acceptable alignment for union (31). Greater amounts of motion can allow bony impingement of the cord by angulation or translation at the fracture site. The patient who presents with an increasing neurologic deficit requires adequate immobilization with spinal alignment as close to its preinjury position as possible. If the patient is already in appropriate immobilization, low-weight traction, or a halo vest, then surgical intervention is indicated. Laminectomy will render the fracture less stable; therefore, some type of internal fixation is desirable after laminectomy. Fixation should span well above and below the fracture (or laminectomy) site. Most patients should be protected in a halo vest or rigid orthosis postoperatively.

Treatment of patients with incomplete quadriparesis and stable neurologic deficit is the most controversial; however, adequate immobilization of the fracture is the primary goal. If the fracture pattern suggests a high degree of instability, with translation, angulation (not reducible in traction), or comminution, performing open reduction and internal fixa-

tion is probably the best way to protect the spinal cord (25). Multiple injuries necessitating surgery (e.g., a laparotomy) represent a relative indication for internal fixation of a cervical spine fracture. A limited laminectomy may be indicated at the time of internal fixation if an epidural hematoma or cord swelling is present. If traction or a halo vest appears to immobilize the spine adequately in an anatomic alignment, nonoperative management is likely to result in union, and significant neurologic improvement has been reported (9,10,13).

In patients with no neurologic deficit, prompt recognition of the fracture and treatment in a halo vest or other rigid orthosis will usually result in a good outcome. Patients may tolerate a halo vest better than a rigid collar orthosis that puts pressure on the chin and occiput. A lack of neurologic deficit implies that severe displacement or angulation of the fracture has not occurred and that the condition is therefore relatively more stable. It is in this group of patients that a high index of suspicion of fracture is needed so that immobilization can be initiated before micromotion and an enlarging epidural hematoma or sudden angulation can cause spinal cord compression. Surgical fixation of the fracture can be performed for patients in whom a halo orthosis is not indicated or for the indications mentioned previously.

In patients with incomplete ossification and kyphotic deformity due to a compression fracture, traction that gently regains their sagittal alignment may be applied before their immobilization in a halo vest. For patients with preexistent severe kyphosis or a healed compression fracture, elective osteotomy may be offered. Patients with circumferential ossification of the spine who sustain a nondisplaced hyperextension-type fracture are probably best treated by immediate placement in a halo orthosis (12). Frequent lateral cervical spine radiographs are required to assess whether reduction of the fracture is maintained during movement of the patient while in the halo. Patients often must be examined every week for minor adjustments of their halo orthosis until 4 to 6 weeks after injury. They should be informed regarding the symptoms of radiculopathy or myelopathy and encouraged to return emergently if any such symptoms occur. Most patients will be comfortable by 6 weeks and at that time may be monitored every 2 to 3 weeks for pin-site checks. Twelve weeks of halo immobilization is usually recommended.

CERVICAL FLEXION DEFORMITY IN ANKYLOSING SPONDYLITIS

Although the incidence is not well documented, a small percentage of patients with AS will develop a severe flexion deformity of the cervical spine at or near the cervicothoracic junction. A retrospective study found that 7 (0.2%) of 3,464 patients being followed for AS underwent cervical osteotomy, but it did not document what percentage had severe flexion deformity (32).

Many of these patients will have had long-standing disease but will develop the severe deformity over a relatively short period. Some will also report that the deformity developed after minor trauma to the cervical spine (22). It may be that this chin-on-chest deformity is actually a result of trauma in a patient with AS rather than part of the natural history of the disease. This has treatment implications, because it may be possible to treat this more acute situation without surgery or with less surgery. The patient will typically present with a chief complaint of worsening deformity, pain, and inability to see straight ahead. Neurologic deficit is uncommon. The ability to perform activities of daily living decreases. Weight loss due to interference with eating has been reported (33,34).

Patient Evaluation

After an assessment of the patient's general physical and psychological health, factors specific to the deformity must be addressed. Defining the primary site of deformity is critical. Hip flexion contracture is not uncommon in AS, and deformity of the lumbar and thoracic spine is also well described (8,34,35). These should certainly be addressed if they are the primary source of deformity.

The chin-brow to vertical angle has been described as a method of quantifying flexion deformity (Fig. 67.3). This is evaluated with the patient standing with the hips and knees fully extended if possible. It may be of benefit in planning correction once the primary site of deformity is defined, but it is not specific to the cervical spine, nor does it provide reliable guidelines as to operative candidates. The decision to intervene should be based on the type and extent of the deformity, the functional limitations of the patient, the surgeon's assessment of the risks and benefits, and the patient's willingness to take those risks.

High-quality radiographic studies are necessary and often difficult to obtain. Dynamic lateral radiographs can help evaluate for instability. If standard imaging studies do not visualize the lower cervical and upper thoracic spine adequately, tomography or CT scanning should supplement them. If there is any question of recent fracture, MRI can also be helpful in defining this. If the anterior column is incompletely ossified, nonoperative correction of the deformity with traction has been reported (36).

Nonoperative Intervention

Although it has been mentioned in the literature, closed manipulation (osteoclasis) of a fixed deformity is not recommended (37).

Mehdian (36) and Graziano (38) and associates have reported success with gradual reduction of deformity. Halo traction was used in one report and a halo-Ilizarov apparatus in the other. Arthrodesis was then performed without the need for osteotomy. Although this technique has not been widely used, it seems to hold some promise for the unusual case of a deformity that is not fixed, such as a subacute fracture.

Operative Intervention

When surgical intervention is indicated, posterior osteotomy is the procedure of choice. Although not the first to perform a spinal osteotomy, Smith-Petersen is generally given credit for devising corrective osteotomy of the spine for flexion deformity (39,40). Along with Larson and Aufranc, he reported on the theory and results of a posteriorly based wedge osteotomy of the spine in 1945. The philosophy they presented, which has continued to this day, was that "[a]ny surgical procedure for correction of flexion deformity must . . . be aimed at the facets, articular processes, and adjacent laminae; osteotomy of these structures, with excision of sufficient bone, should allow corrective leverage to be transmitted to the intervertebral discs and longitudinal ligaments, overcoming whatever resistance these may present." Urist, in 1958, reported using the technique for cervical flexion deformity under local anesthesia in the sitting position. This was performed at the C7-T1 level. He noted at the time of correction that the patient gave a "muffled cry inside of the anesthesia mask" (37). The actual osteotomy portion of the procedure has changed little since then (8,33,41).

If operative intervention is planned and instrumentation is not going to be used, halo immobilization should be applied preoperatively. Simmons has written that a halo vest is inadequate; a halo cast applied preoperatively is necessary (8).

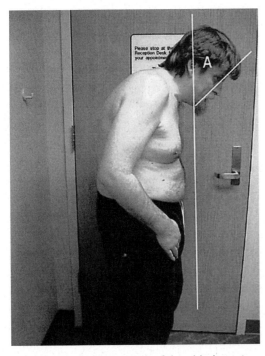

FIG. 67.3. Illustrated photograph of the chin-brow to vertical angle.

Anesthetic and Positioning

The procedure has been performed under local anesthetic with supplemental sedation as well as under general anesthesia. Proponents of local anesthesia note a high complication rate in early series that used general anesthesia, the ability of an awake patient to report any neurologic problems immediately, the technical difficulties involved with endotracheal intubation in these patients, and the ability to "fine tune" the position of the head after surgery (8,37). The sitting position is used with this technique, and halo cast or vest immobilization is applied preoperatively (Fig. 67.4).

Those favoring general anesthesia note the advances in fiberoptic intubation and spinal cord monitoring as well as the advantage of the prone position and document, in a small series of patients, a complication rate equivalent to that of local anesthesia (33,42). All series except that of Simmons, however, are relatively small, so the actual relative safety of either form of anesthetic is not truly known. Table 67.1 reviews the English-language series of patients undergoing cervical osteotomy and documents the type of anesthetic used.

Spinal cord monitoring, either by contact with an awake patient or by evoked potentials, should be used routinely.

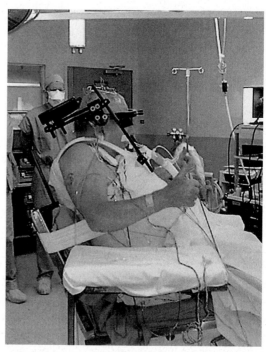

FIG. 67.4. Awake patient in the upright position prior to osteotomy. (Photograph courtesy of Dr. Todd Albert, with permission.)

TABLE 67.1. *Review of Published Series of Cervical Osteotomy*

Author	Year	No. of cases	Anesthetic	Hardware	Position	Complications	Other
Mason et al.	1953	1	General	None	Prone	None	Included vertebral body
Urist	1958	1	Local	None	Sitting	None	
Herbert	1959	3	Not specified	Not specified	Not specified	None	
Law	1969	20	Not specified	Not specified	Not specified	1 death	Discussing Smith-Petersen series
Simmons	1989	101	Local	None	Sitting	4 nonunion; 1 central cord; 13 C8 Sx; 1 CN IX and X lesion; 1 PE; 1 MI	One patient required intraoperative dural splitting
Hyman et al.	1990	1	General	None	Sitting	Pseudarthrosis	Failed local
Shimizu et al.	1996	1	General	Sublaminar/ Hartshill, C4 to T3	Prone	None	
McMaster	1997	15	General	3 pts Luque rectangle/ spinous process wires	Prone	2 C8 palsy; 1 delayed quadriparesis; 1 nonunion; 4 anterolisthesis	
Albert et al.	1998	1	Not specified	Screw/plate, C5 to T3	Not specified	None	
Mehdian et al.	1999	1	General	Screw/ malleable rod, C3 to T3	Prone	None	No postoperative halo

Sx, subluxation; CN, cranial nerve; PE, pulmonary embolism; MI, myocardial infarction.

Surgical Technique

The actual osteotomy technique has changed little since it was first described. It should be performed at the cervicothoracic junction. At this level, the primary nerve root at risk is C8. Injury to this root will cause less disability than it would to more cephalad roots. The vertebral artery is also not yet tethered in the transverse foramen, passing anterior to the transverse process of C7. After wide posterior exposure is performed, the entire lamina of C7, the superior half of T1, and the inferior half of C6 are removed. The decompression should then be expanded laterally through the lateral mass of C7 and the transverse process of T1 so that the roots of C8 are free from any potential bony compression at the time of correction (Fig. 67.5). Enough of the pedicle of C7 should also be removed to prevent compression. McMaster recommended removal of the pedicle of T1 as well (33). The height of the osteotomy in the lateral region over the C8 nerve root should be approximately 1.5 centimeters. The dorsal edges of this area should come into contact with each other when the osteotomy is closed.

If instrumentation is not used, the next step is osteoclasis. For patients under local anesthesia, a short-acting sedative can be given at this point. The halo ring is held by an assistant or the surgeon through sterile drapes, disconnected from the uprights of the halo apparatus, and the head is extended while the osteotomy is visualized. The dura will be seen to wrinkle, and a snap can often be heard or felt as the anterior column fails (Fig. 67.6). The connections of the halo apparatus are then tightened securely. Neurologic sta-

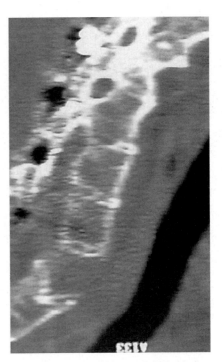

FIG. 67.6. Postoperative sagittal computed tomographic scan showing correction opening of the anterior column. (Photograph courtesy of Dr. Todd Albert, with permission.)

tus is assessed and radiographs obtained. If there is a new deficit, options include readjusting the position of the head and administering systemic steroids. Simmons has also described splitting the dura in this situation if it appears to be tethered (8).

If instrumentation is to be used, it can be applied before or after the decompression. Both manual correction and correction using the implanted hardware have been described (33,42). Utilizing the hardware for controlled correction is theoretically appealing and may decrease the risk of sagittal plane translation during correction (Fig. 67.7).

Spinous process wires, sublaminar wires, and screw fixation have all been described (Table 67.1). Screw fixation, especially lateral mass fixation superior to the osteotomy site, has the advantage of biomechanical strength and should not enter the spinal canal (43). Pedicle screw fixation of the cervical spine can be employed. Although this has mechanical advantages, placement of the screws is difficult and not without risk. A cadaveric study (44) tested three different methods of placement of cervical pedicle screws and found the rate of "critical breaches" to be between 10.6% and 65.5%; others have shown significant variability in the anatomy and morphology of the pedicles of the cervical spine (45). Fixation inferior to the osteotomy site can also vary. Spinous process wires can be placed with relative ease but do not resist sagittal plane rotation well (46). Screws across the base of the transverse processes of T1 and T2 can be employed as well as pedicle screws (47,48). A hybrid plate–rod system can also be used that

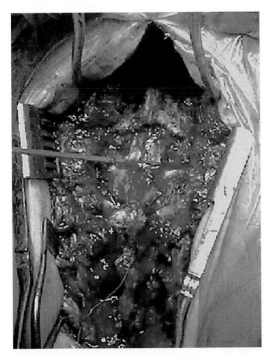

FIG. 67.5. Intraoperative photograph of osteotomy technique. (Photograph courtesy of Dr. Todd Albert, with permission.)

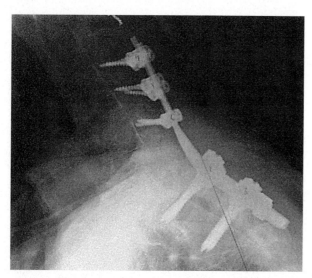

FIG. 67.7. Postoperative lateral radiograph after osteotomy with instrumentation. (Photograph courtesy of Dr. Christopher Shaffrey, with permission.)

allows for screw fixation above the osteotomy site with hooks and/or wires below (49).

The optimal length of instrumentation is also not well defined, although the argument is stronger for longer rather than shorter fixation. Longer fixation will not immobilize previously mobile motion segments because all motion segments are already ankylosed prior to the surgery. Longer fixation will also better resist deforming flexion moments (46).

The purpose of spinal instrumentation must be kept in mind. In this situation, arthrodesis is likely with or without hardware, so the purpose of additional instrumentation should be to allow for rapid mobilization with less external bracing and to prevent displacement at the osteotomy site. Because a large controlled series does not exist to help in deciding whether to use fixation and, if so, what kind to use, the surgeon's experience and capabilities must guide him or her rather than a standard "cookbook" approach.

Management after surgery should include careful observation of the neurologic status and the airway. Early removal of the endotracheal tube is not recommended because of the difficulty of reinsertion. Protection of the uninstrumented osteotomy site is done with halo immobilization until healing is evident, usually at 3 to 6 months. Most patients can be mobilized soon after surgery. If pseudarthrosis does occur, this can be treated with anterior arthrodesis.

REFERENCES

1. Baeten D, et al. Immunomodulatory effects of anti-tumor necrosis factor alpha therapy on synovium in spondyloarthropathy: histologic findings in eight patients from an open-label pilot study. *Arthritis Rheum* 2001;44:186–195.
2. Braun J, et al. Use of immunohistologic and *in situ* hybridization techniques in the examination of sacroiliac joint biopsy specimens from patients with ankylosing spondylitis. *Arthritis Rheum* 1995;38:499–505.
3. Brandt J, et al. Successful treatment of active ankylosing spondylitis with the anti-tumor necrosis factor alpha monoclonal antibody infliximab. *Arthritis Rheum* 2000;43:1346–1352.
4. Dougados M, et al. Efficacy of celecoxib, a cyclooxygenase 2-specific inhibitor, in the treatment of ankylosing spondylitis: a six-week controlled study with comparison against placebo and against a conventional nonsteroidal antiinflammatory drug. *Arthritis Rheum* 2001;44:180–185.
5. Clegg DO, et al. Comparison of sulfasalazine and placebo in the treatment of ankylosing spondylitis. A Department of Veterans Affairs Cooperative Study. *Arthritis Rheum* 1996;39:2004–2012.
6. Uhrin Z, Kuzis S, Ward MM. Exercise and changes in health status in patients with ankylosing spondylitis. *Arch Intern Med* 2000;160:2969–2975.
7. Calin A. Ankylosing spondylitis. *Clin Rheum Dis* 1985;11:41.
8. Simmons EH. The surgical correction of flexion deformity of the cervical spine in ankylosing spondylitis. In: Sherk HH, Dunn EJ, Eismont FJ, eds. *The cervical spine.* Philadelphia: JB Lippincott, 1989:573.
9. Graham B, Van Peteghem PK. Fractures of the spine in ankylosing spondylitis. Diagnosis, treatment, and complications. *Spine* 1989;14:803–807.
10. Hunter T, Dubo HI. Spinal fractures complicating ankylosing spondylitis. A long-term followup study. *Arthritis Rheum* 1983;26:751–759.
11. Woodruff FP, Dewing SB. Fracture of the cervical spine in patients with ankylosing spondylitis. *Radiology* 1963;80:17.
12. Surin VV. Fractures of the cervical spine in patients with ankylosing spondylitis. *Acta Orthop Scand* 1980;51:79–84.
13. Rowed DW. Management of cervical spinal cord injury in ankylosing spondylitis: the intervertebral disc as a cause of cord compression. *J Neurosurg* 1992;77:241–246.
14. Broom MJ, Raycroft JF. Complications of fractures of the cervical spine in ankylosing spondylitis. *Spine* 1988;13:763–766.
15. Detwiler KN, et al. Management of cervical spine injuries in patients with ankylosing spondylitis. *J Neurosurg* 1990;72:210–215.
16. Gravallese EM, Kantrowitz FG. Arthritic manifestations of inflammatory bowel disease. *Am J Gastroenterol* 1988;83:703–709.
17. Murray GC, Persellin RH. Cervical fracture complicating ankylosing spondylitis: a report of eight cases and review of the literature. *Am J Med* 1981;70:1033–1041.
18. Podolsky SM, Hoffman JR, Pietrafesa CA. Neurologic complications following immobilization of cervical spine fracture in a patient with ankylosing spondylitis. *Ann Emerg Med* 1983;12:578–580.
19. Salathe M, Johr M. Unsuspected cervical fractures: a common problem in ankylosing spondylitis. *Anesthesiology* 1989;70:869–870.
20. Weinstein PR, et al. Spinal cord injury, spinal fracture, and spinal stenosis in ankylosing spondylitis. *J Neurosurg* 1982;57:609–616.
21. Bohlman HH. Acute fractures and dislocations of the cervical spine. An analysis of three hundred hospitalized patients and review of the literature. *J Bone Joint Surg Am* 1979;61:1119–1142.
22. Bailey R. Dislocations of the cervical spine. In: Cervical Spine Research Society, eds., *The cervical spine.* Philadelphia: JB Lippincott, 1983:362–387.
23. Grisolia A, Bell RL, Peltier LF. Fractures and dislocations of the spine complicating ankylosing spondylitis. A report of six cases. *J Bone Joint Surg Am* 1967;49:339–344.
24. Fox MW, Onofrio BM, Kilgore JE. Neurological complications of ankylosing spondylitis. *J Neurosurg* 1993;78:871–878.
25. Taggard DA, Traynelis VC. Management of cervical spinal fractures in ankylosing spondylitis with posterior fixation. *Spine* 2000;25:2035–2039.
26. Baron M, Tator CH, Little H. Hangman's fracture in ankylosing spondylitis preceded by vertical subluxation of the axis. *Arthritis Rheum* 1980;23:850–855.
27. Gartman JJ Jr, Bullitt E, Baker ML. Axis fracture in ankylosing spondylitis: case report. *Neurosurgery* 1991;29:590–594.
28. Miller FH, Rogers LF. Fractures of the dens complicating ankylosing spondylitis with atlantooccipital fusion. *J Rheumatol* 1991;18:771–774.
29. Fishman EK, Magid D. Cervical fracture in ankylosing spondylitis: value of multidimensional imaging. *Clin Imaging* 1992;16:31–33.
30. Goldberg AL, et al. Ankylosing spondylitis complicated by trauma: MR findings correlated with plain radiographs and CT. *Skeletal Radiol* 1993;22:333–336.

31. Fitt G, Hennessy O, Thomas D. Transverse fracture with epidural and small paravertebral hematomata, in a patient with ankylosing spondylitis. *Skeletal Radiol* 1992;21:61–63.

32. Koh WH, Garrett SL, Calin A. Cervical spine surgery in ankylosing spondylitis: is the outcome good? *Clin Rheumatol* 1997;16:466–470.

33. McMaster MJ. Osteotomy of the cervical spine in ankylosing spondylitis. *J Bone Joint Surg Br* 1997;79:197–203.

34. Simmons EH. Kyphotic deformity of the spine in ankylosing spondylitis. *Clin Orthop* 1977;128:65–77.

35. Simmons EH. The surgical correction of flexion deformity of the cervical spine in ankylosing spondylitis. *Clin Orthop* 1972;86:132–143.

36. Mehdian H, Jaffray D, Eisenstein S. Correction of severe cervical kyphosis in ankylosing spondylitis by traction. *Spine* 1992;17:237–240.

37. Urist M. Osteotomy of the cervical spine: report of a case of ankylosing rheumatoid spondylitis. *J Bone Joint Surg Am* 1958;40:833–843.

38. Graziano GP, Herzenberg JE, Hensinger RN. The halo-Ilizarov distraction cast for correction of cervical deformity. Report of six cases. *J Bone Joint Surg Am* 1993;75:996–1003.

39. Mayer L. The significance of the iliocostal fascial graft on the treatment of paralytic deformities of the trunk. *J Bone Joint Surg Am* 1944;26:257–271.

40. Smith-Petersen MN, Larson CB, Aufranc OE. Osteotomy of the spine for correction of flexion deformity in rheumatoid arthritis. *J Bone Joint Surgery* 1945;27:1–11.

41. Law WA. Ankylosing spondylitis and spinal osteotomy. *Proc R Soc Med* 1976;69:715–720.

42. Shimizu K, et al. Correction of kyphotic deformity of the cervical spine in ankylosing spondylitis using general anesthesia and internal fixation. *J Spinal Disord* 1996;9:540–543.

43. An HS. Internal fixation of the cervical spine: current indications and techniques. *J Am Acad Orthop Surg* 1995;3:194–206.

44. Ludwig SC, et al. Placement of pedicle screws in the human cadaveric cervical spine: comparative accuracy of three techniques. *Spine* 2000;25:1655–1667.

45. Shin EK, et al. The anatomic variability of human cervical pedicles: considerations for transpedicular screw fixation in the middle and lower cervical spine. *Eur Spine J* 2000;9:61–66.

46. Krag MH. Biomechanics of thoracolumbar spinal fixation. A review. *Spine* 1991;16(Suppl 3):S84–S99.

47. Chapman JR, et al. Posterior instrumentation of the unstable cervicothoracic spine. *J Neurosurg* 1996;84:552–558.

48. Heller JG, Shuster JK, Hutton WC. Pedicle and transverse process screws of the upper thoracic spine. Biomechanical comparison of loads to failure. *Spine* 1999;24:654–658.

49. Vaccaro R, et al. A plate-rod device for treatment of cervicothoracic disorders: comparison of mechanical testing with established cervical spine *in vitro* load testing data. *J Spinal Disord* 2000;13:350–355.

SECTION IX

Degenerative Diseases

CHAPTER 68

Cervical Degenerative Disease: Overview and Epidemiology

Eeric Truumees

Over time, degenerative changes become more common in the cervical spine and may represent normal aging. Often, patients exhibiting radiographic evidence of degeneration do not have symptoms (Fig. 68.1). However, symptomatic degeneration is common. The term *cervical degenerative disease* encompasses a spectrum of clinical syndromes associated with neck pain and neurologic dysfunction. The standard continuum of cervical degenerative disorders includes (a) spondylotic degeneration with neck pain, (b) disc displacement ("soft" disc) with radiculopathy; (c) spondylotic ("hard" disc) radiculopathy; and (d) cervical spondylotic myelopathy (CSM).

Many patients exhibit clinical features of several of these syndromes at once. Given the prevalence of degeneration in the population, a detailed history and physical examination are critical. Imaging findings are then correlated with the history and examination. If a clinical syndrome of cervical spondylosis has been identified, a clear understanding of the natural history of the disease process allows rational treatment decisions to be made.

This chapter provides an overview of these clinical syndromes, with a special emphasis on epidemiology, and an overview of the basic pathophysiology, natural history, symptoms, and treatment of symptomatic cervical spondylosis. Subsequent chapters expand on these topics.

In that lumbar degeneration is more common and more familiar to many practitioners than its cervical counterpart, anatomic and clinical comparisons between these entities are a useful starting point (Tables 68.1 and 68.2).

HISTORICAL BACKGROUND

Our understanding of the biochemical and mechanical pathogenesis of cervical degenerative disease is evolving rapidly. This evolution has been well summarized by Lestini and Wiesel (1) and by Montgomery and Brower (2). Key provided the first description of spondylotic myelopathy in 1838. He reported myelopathic symptoms in a patient with a spondylotic bar projecting into and reducing the area of the spinal canal by one third. In 1911, Bailey and Caramajor described five cases of spinal cord compression in patients with cervical spondylosis. They postulated that disc degeneration led to abnormal motion, with subsequent osteophyte formation occluding the neuroforamina and spinal canal. In 1926, Elliott described radicular symptoms arising from foraminal narrowing. Stookey provided the first clear description of spinal nerve and cord compression from "extradural chondromas" in 1928. After Schmorl's classic description of disc protrusion in 1929, these "chondromas" were seen to be both soft and hard disc herniations. In 1934, Peet and Echols, along with Mixter and Ayer, recognized that disc protrusions can cause radicular, or less commonly, myelopathic symptoms. By 1940, Stookey had outlined three clinical syndromes arising from disc protrusions (3).

The clinical evaluation of cervical neurocompressive pathology was refined with the introduction of Pantopaque in 1944 (2). In 1947, Brain differentiated the presentation of acute disc protrusion from chronic, osteophytic compression (4). Subsequent authors more clearly established sources of compression. For example, Bull described the importance of osteophytes from the neurocentral joints of Luschka in the evolution of spondylotic radicular compression in 1948.

In 1952, Brain and others described the syndrome of CSM in 45 patients (5). The role of anterior spinal artery compression as a cause of cord injury was reported by Mair and Druckman in 1953 (6). Also that year, Taylor described

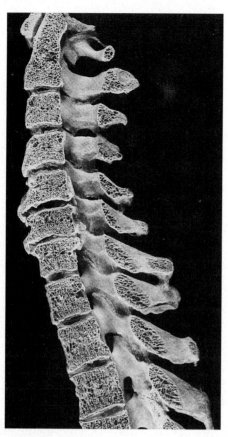

FIG. 68.1. Macerated sagittal section of the cervical spine from a 67-year-old man specimen demonstrating typical degenerative changes such as osteophyte formation and loss of disc height and lordosis. (From Bulloch PG, Boachie-Adjei O. *Atlas of spinal diseases.* Philadelphia: JB Lippincott, 1993, with permission.)

TABLE 68.1. *Similarities Between Cervical and Lumbar Disease*

Three Joint Complex
Disc and posterolaterally oriented diarthrodial joints positioned to maximize mobility while protecting neurologic structures
Laterally placed neuroforamina
Posterior ramus innervation of posterolateral musculoskeletal structures
Anterior ramus innervation of a single extremity
Size and orientation of structures related to biomechanical loads commonly encountered
Good resistance to compression but low resistance to bending/twisting moments
Degenerative disease and disc injury frequently associated with nerve compression
Genetic predisposition to degeneration
Axial pain typically improves spontaneously

CERVICAL DISC DEGENERATION

With age, the nucleus pulposus begins to desiccate and loses its mechanical competence (10). Effective load transmission is no longer possible. Increased strain on the annulus leads to tearing and protrusion. This disc collapse translates into excess motion in the zygapophyseal joints posteriorly and increased strain in the supporting ligaments (1). Degenerative changes affect all cervical levels, but are less common above C3-C4 (2,11).

Radiographically, the C5-6 disc space is most commonly involved, followed by C6-7.

Most authors conclude that the primary pain generator in cervical spondylosis is the intervertebral disc. This cervical degenerative disc "disease" typically presents with axial neck pain and loss of range of motion. Interscapular and upper brachial sclerotomal pain radiation are also common (12). This pain is mechanical in nature and worsens with flexion and extension.

In some patients, facet joint degeneration may lead to spondylotic pain, which worsens with extension (13). Occasionally, cervical spondylosis leads to cervicogenic headache or dysphagia. Night or rest pain should alert the examiner to the possibility of tumor or infection (Fig. 68.2).

a pincer effect of the ligamentum flavum posteriorly and disc protrusions and osteophytes anteriorly as a cause of spinal cord dysfunction (7). In 1957, Payne and Spillane described the increased risk for spinal cord dysfunction in patients with both cervical spondylosis and a congenitally narrow spinal canal (8). Clark and Robinson further distinguished CSM from the syndrome of myelopathy after acute disc herniation (9).

TABLE 68.2. *Differences Between Cervical and Lumbar Disease*

Condition	Cervical	Lumbar
Motion	three planes (sagittal, coronal, axial)	two planes (sagittal/coronal)
UMN injury	common (spinal cord vulnerable)	unlikely (cord ends at L_{1-2})
Muscular support	paravertebral muscles dominant	paravertebral and abdominals
Biomechanical role	linked to shoulder	linked to hip/pelvis
Associated PNE	common (carpal, cubital tunnel, etc)	unusual
Long term disability	less common	more common
Troublesome Tasks	sitting, computer work	manual labor

PNE, peripheral nerve entrapment; UMN, Upper motor neuron

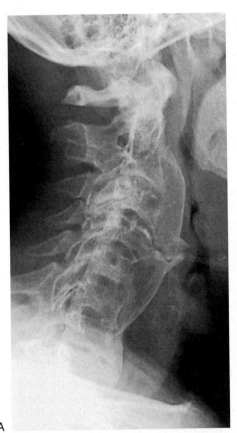
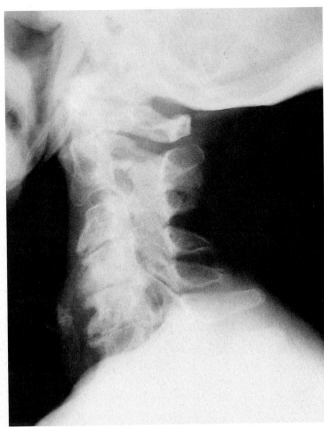

A

B

FIG. 68.2. Two radiographic examples of cervical spondylosis. **A:** Severe disc height loss is accompanied by large osteophyte formation, end-plate sclerosis, and loss of lordosis in a patient complaining of axial neck pain and limited motion. **B:** Flowing osteophytes in a patient with relatively preserved disc height is most typical of diffuse idiopathic skeletal hyperostosis (DISH). This patient complained of mild neck pain and difficulty swallowing.

Clear clinical identification of the pain generator in cervical disc disease remains problematic. The distinction of pathologic change from normal aging is impossible, but an emerging concept of cervical disc disease as early, extensive, painful degeneration is useful.

CERVICAL DISC PROLAPSE

In younger patients, disc material can prolapse through tears in the annulus, causing root, or less commonly, cord impingement. This soft disc herniation causes nerve dysfunction both directly and through vascular compromise of radicular feeders. Patients present with sensory (radicular pain or numbness) or motor (weakness) dysfunction, or both.

Although there is considerable individual variation, each nerve root supplies a unique dermatome. Therefore, a characteristic combination of sensory, motor, and reflex changes can often be identified. The diagnosis is secured with imaging studies.

In the cervical spine, the exiting root is most commonly affected by disc protrusion. Because the C1 root exits between the occiput and C1, the exiting root is named from the inferior vertebral body. Just as the C5-6 interspace exhibits the earliest and greatest degree of degeneration on plain radiography, the C6 root is the most commonly affected by disc protrusion (2). C7 and C5 radiculopathies are also common. A typical patient with a C5-6 soft disc protrusion may complain of radiating lacerating pain down the biceps and into the radial forearm. Muscular complaints often include weakness of the wrist extensors, biceps, and triceps. Diminution of the brachioradialis reflex may be noted. Radicular pain from soft disc protrusion may be intensified with a Valsalva maneuver, rotation and flexion of the head toward the side of symptoms, and axial compression of the skull. Abduction of the shoulder often eases radicular pain (Fig. 68.3).

CERVICAL SPONDYLOTIC RADICULOPATHY

About 10 years after the disc itself begins to degenerate, the mechanical incompetence of the motion segment becomes evident, with spondylotic degeneration of the facets and uncovertebral joints (14). As the disc loses height, the uncovertebral joints come into contact, and osteophytes form.

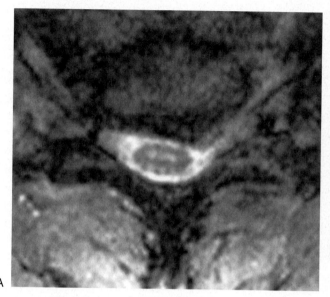

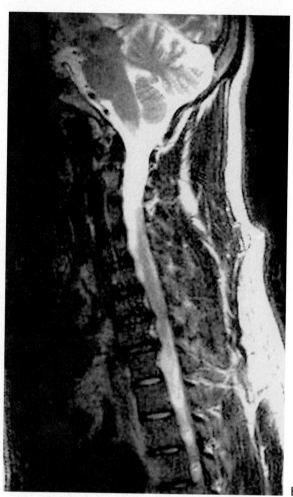

A

B

FIG. 68.3. Axial (**A**) and parasagittal (**B**) T2-weighted magnetic resonance imaging studies of a patient with soft disc herniation who complained of the acute onset of severe left arm pain, predominantly down the radial aspect of the forearm.

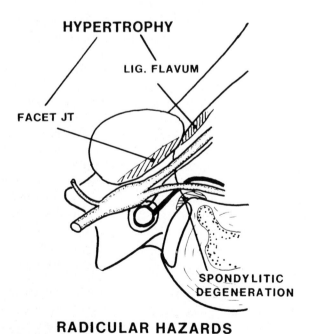

FIG. 68.4. Various causes of spondylotic radiculopathy. (From Parke WW. Correlative anatomy of cervical spondylotic myelopathy. *Spine* 198813(7):831–837, with permission.)

Posteriorly, the zygapophyseal (facet) joints override and also form osteophytes. In the absence of a true disc protrusion, these osteophytes, or hard disc protrusions, can compress the nerve root, leading to a syndrome of radiculopathy similar to that seen with soft disc protrusions (Fig. 68.4).

A patient with C6-7 neuroforaminal stenosis may present complaining of C7 radiculitis, with pain radiating along the posterior shoulder and arm to the posterolateral forearm and into the middle finger. Motor disturbance, including triceps and wrist extensor weakness, may be present, as may a depressed triceps reflex.

Symptoms may develop more gradually in spondylotic radiculopathy patients; however, patients often recall a particular overuse episode as the precipitating factor for pain intensification. Spondylotic radiculopathy patients are more likely to complain of multilevel or bilateral radicular symptoms (1,2) (Fig. 68.5).

CERVICAL SPONDYLOTIC MYELOPATHY

As degeneration of the cervical spine continues, osteophytes may combine with other pathoanatomic changes to

944

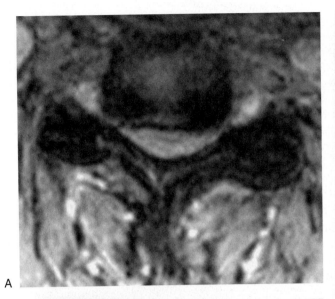

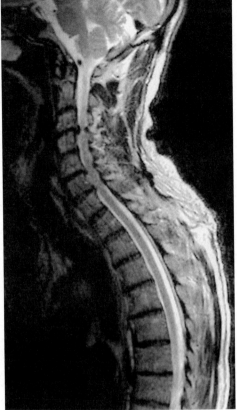

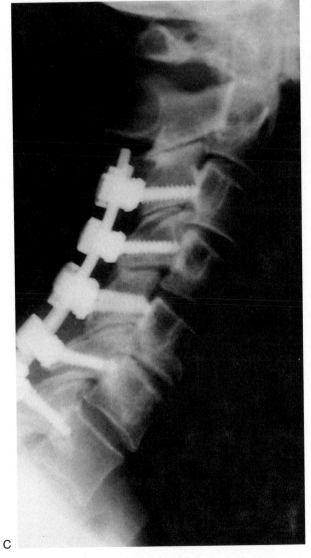

FIG. 68.5. Axial (**A**) and parasagittal (**B**) T2-weighted magnetic resonance imaging studies of a patient with myeloradiculopathy who complained of the gradual onset of diffuse upper extremity pain, paresthesias, and weakness with progressive gait ataxia. This patient had excellent functional recovery and pain relief after a multilevel posterior laminectomy with foraminotomies (**C**).

compress the central spinal canal (Fig. 68.6). The resultant stenosis of the central canal affects cord function through both vascular insufficiency and direct mechanical pressure on the neural elements. The effects of spondylotic canal narrowing may be magnified by spondylolisthesis or dynamic factors.

Cervical spondylosis accounts for more than half of all cases of cervical myelopathy (3) and is the most common cause of spinal cord dysfunction in patients older than 55 years of age (5). Cervical myelopathy usually presents insidiously in the sixth decade, and complete symptomatic reversal is rare after myelopathy occurs.

Although C3-4 and C4-5 have greatest mobility in the elderly spine and thus the greatest tendency to spondylolisthesis, like radiculopathy, myelopathy is most common at C5-6, then at the C4-5, C6-7, and C3-4 levels (15,16) (Fig. 68.7). Five categories of cervical spondylotic myelopathy have been described, based on the predominant neurologic findings (16):

1. The involvement of corticospinal and spinothalamic tracts seen in *transverse lesion syndrome* is the most common. This compression leads to upper motor neuron weakness with gait difficulties and lower extremity spasticity.
2. Primary involvement of the corticospinal or anterior horn cell yields *motor syndrome*. For these patients, sensory complaints are rare, but motor weakness and gait difficulties can be profound.
3. *Central cord syndrome* predominantly affects the central gray matter of the cord and leads to greater upper extremity motor and sensory involvement. The lower extremities are spared. Posterior column deficits may lead to painful dysesthesias of the hands.
4. *Brown-Séquard syndrome* describes a unilateral cord lesion with ipsilateral hemiparesis from corticospinal tract involvement. Contralateral pain and temperature analgesia are reported below the level of the lesion. This syndrome has the best prognosis for recovery.
5. *Brachialgia cord syndrome* typically presents with predominant upper limb pain with some associated long tract involvement. This syndrome is, in essence, a myeloradiculopathy or a combination of radicular and myelopathic findings. Lower motor neuron flaccid weakness in the upper extremities may be combined with spastic upper motor neuron lower extremity involvement.

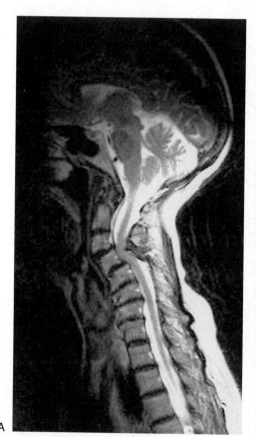

A

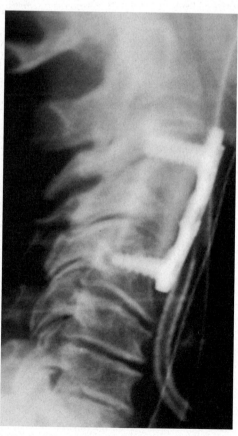

B

FIG. 68.6. A: Parasagittal T2-weighted magnetic resonance imaging study of a patient with cervical spondylolisthesis and stenosis who complained of axial neck pain and electric shock sensations into all four extremities with neck flexion (Lhermitte sign). **B:** This patient had excellent symptom relief and improved gait and grasp after undergoing a cervical corpectomy with plate fixation.

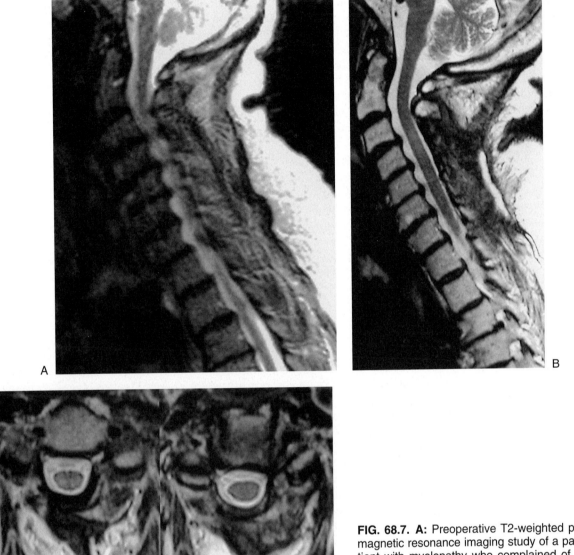

FIG. 68.7. A: Preoperative T2-weighted parasagittal magnetic resonance imaging study of a pain-free patient with myelopathy who complained of increasing difficulty with hand numbness and clumsiness. Post-laminoplasty axial (**B**) and sagittal (**C**) images demonstrating cord decompression.

Less common manifestations of cervical myelopathy include primary sensory loss in a glovelike distribution or symptoms of vertebrobasilar insufficiency with dizziness and nausea. Tandem spinal stenosis (i.e., simultaneous involvement of both cervical and lumbar spines) presents as a triad of neurogenic claudication, complex gait abnormality, and a mixed pattern of upper and lower motor neuron signs (2).

Delayed diagnosis is common owing to the lack of pain and the wide array of often bizarre symptoms seen with cervical myelopathy. One common clinical scenario involves a 70-year-old patient reporting episodic progression of gait disturbance, shuffling, frequent falls, and clumsiness. The patient may complain that hand numbness and decreased grip strength have led to the inability to button a shirt. The patient may describe a Lhermitte phenomenon of electric shocks coursing through the extremities with neck motion. Physical examination is often nonspecific but may reveal hyperreflexia, including the Hoffman or Babinski sign. Wasting of the hand with ulnar deviation of the little finger on finger extension may be noted.

EPIDEMIOLOGY

When describing the epidemiology of cervical disc degeneration, it is useful to remember that *incidence* refers to the number of new cases of a disease or disorder over a period of time (17). Incidence data are therefore useful as a rate of change, describing the number of new cases over the number of persons at risk in a given period of time.

Incidence is often expressed as cases per 1,000 or 100,000 of the population at risk.

Prevalence, on the other hand, refers to the number of existing cases of disease in a given population in a given period of time (17). Point prevalence enumerates cases of a given disease in a given geographic area at one point in time. Period prevalence describes the number of people with a given disease in a given geographic area over a set period of time (e.g., lifetime risk). Thus, prevalence = incidence × duration.

Unfortunately, true incidence data for most syndromes of cervical spondylosis are not available. This is because of difficulties differentiating and objectively "confirming" individual syndromes. For example, many patients have radiographic changes of cervical degeneration without significant symptoms referable to the neck. On the other hand, a younger patient with an acute disc herniation may have only subtle loss of disc height on plain radiographs, or no finding at all (1).

Radiographic Degeneration

A number of plain radiograph studies have been undertaken to understand the evolution of radiographic cervical senescence in various patient populations. By the sixth decade, more than three fourths of individuals have degenerative changes, but many are asymptomatic. Lawrence, for example, found radiographic changes in more than 90% of his patients older than 65 years of age, but peak prevalence of pain was only 9% (18). In another group of 50 men older than the age of 56 years, 76% had degenerative changes on plain radiography (19). In a third study, radiographs demonstrated spondylotic changes in 87% of those older than age 52 years (20). Finally, one paper reported that 25% of asymptomatic patients in their fifth decade, as opposed to 75% of those in their seventh decade, demonstrated cervical degeneration (21) (Fig. 68.8).

The clinical implications of these radiographic changes are not clear. Brain found no consistent association between radiographs and symptoms (4). Gore and co-workers selected 205 patients who had been seen at least 10 years previously for a neck complaint (22). Their follow-up radiographic examination and interview failed to identify a significant relationship between the degree of spinal degeneration and patient symptoms at either initial evaluation or follow-up.

Tapiovaara and Heinivaara found that changes in the posterolateral margins of the vertebral body, neurocentral joints, and narrowing of the foramina were the only radiographic parameters associated with neck symptoms (23). In a similar study by Friedenberg and Miller, these radiographic findings failed to distinguish the symptomatic group from the asymptomatic group, only narrowing of the disc space in the central spine was more common in the symptomatic group (21).

In that plain radiographs do not consistently identify symptomatic disease, a number of studies employing advanced neuroimaging techniques have been undertaken. In one asymptomatic group undergoing myelography for evaluation of acoustic neuroma, 37% had abnormal cervical myelograms, usually from a disc abnormality (24). A study by Boden and co-workers revealed magnetic resonance imaging (MRI) evidence of cervical degeneration in 90% of males older than 50 years of age and in 90% of females older than age 60 years (25). In those younger than 40 years of age, 25% had degenerative disc disease (DDD), and 4% had foraminal stenosis. In those older than 40 years, almost 60% had DDD, and 20% had foraminal stenosis, by MRI. True disc herniations were seen in 10% of asymptomatic

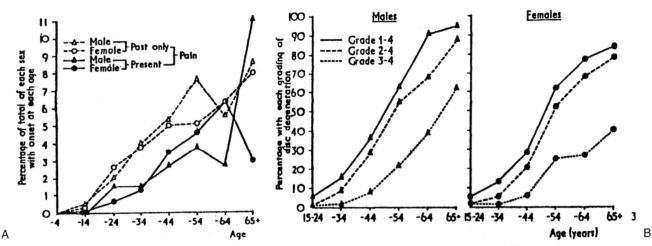

FIG. 68.8. Graphic representation of the increasing incidence of (**A**) symptomatic and (**B**) radiographic cervical degeneration in both men and women. Note that radiographic changes are much more common than symptoms.

individuals aged younger than 40 years, but in only 5% of those older than 40 years.

Spines selected randomly from routine necropsy cases have also been analyzed for degenerative changes. In one study of 120 cervical spines removed from elderly cadavers, degenerative changes increased with age (14). Degeneration was found at an earlier age in men. Mild disease was seen at mean age of 60.5 years, and severe lesions were recorded at a mean age of 72 years. The authors concluded that the earliest cervical degeneration typically precedes more severe changes by a decade. The authors noted that on some occasions only slight histologic change was seen in specimens with severe change on radiographs. They concluded that this discrepancy might explain the absence of symptoms in some patients with radiographically evident degeneration.

Symptomatic Degeneration

Chronic neck pain and neurologic dysfunction are far less common than radiographic change. Overall, neck, shoulder, and related brachial pain have a prevalence of 9% with a yearly incidence of 3% (18). A Finnish study of 8,000 adults reported that 9.5% of men and 12.5% of women complained of chronic neck pain (26). A 1994 study of 10,000 Norwegians found that the overall frequency of neck pain was 24.4% (27). Chronic neck pain was defined as symptoms lasting longer than 6 months. The prevalence of chronic neck pain was 13.8% and increased with age.

Others report neck pain prevalence of 9% to 12% of the general population (28). One third of those questioned were able to recall at least one painful episode. A group of 700 patients were evaluated with cervical spine radiographs, visual analog pain scale (VAS), neck disability index, and questionnaires (29). In this group, there was a significant relationship between number of levels of disc degeneration and chronicity of cervical spine pain. VAS correlated with prior neck trauma and chronicity of symptoms, but radiographic changes were not related to prior trauma or gender. Overall, most episodes were short lived.

Cervical radiculopathy is less common than axial neck pain or lumbar radiculopathy. In the United States, cervical radiculopathy occurs at an annual incidence rate of 85 per 100,000 (30). A door-to-door survey of 7,653 Sicilians identified 27 subjects affected by cervical radiculopathy for an overall prevalence of 3.5% (31). Complaints increased with age to a peak between 50 and 59 years, decreasing thereafter. Another population-based survey in Rochester, Minnesota from 1976 to 1990 identified 561 patients (332 men and 229 women) with radiculopathy, for an annual incidence of 85 per 100,000 (30).

The true incidence of myelopathy is not known, but CSM may be the most underdiagnosed spinal disease (2). CSM is the most common cause of nontraumatic tetraplegia, representing nearly one fourth of cases (32).

Age of Onset

Kelsey and others found that acute disc prolapse was most common in the third decade (33). In some series, cervical radiculopathy occurs in a slightly older age group than lumbar radiculopathy (34). Others report identical age ranges (33). In Lawrence and co-workers' study of disc degeneration, the prevalence of neck, shoulder, and brachial pain progressed in a near linear fashion, beginning in the second decade of life (18). Radiographic change was much more common but also exhibited a linear increase with age. In the mid-20s, disc degeneration had a prevalence of 10%, increasing through the age of 65 years, when it approached 95% prevalence.

Spondylotic changes are increasingly common in those older than 40 years, more than 70% (35). The Rochester study included patients from 13 to 91 years of age (30). The mean age for onset of radicular complaints was similar for men (48.2 years) and women (47.7 years). The age-specific annular incidence rate per 100,000 population reached a peak of 202.9 for the age group between 50 and 54 years.

Therefore, radiographic evidence of cervical degeneration becomes increasingly common with age. Soft disc protrusion causing radiculopathy reaches a peak incidence in the third decade. After this point, disc desiccation becomes increasingly important, and in patients older than 40 years, soft disc protrusions are less likely. On the other hand, the incidence of spondylotic radiculopathy increases.

RISK FACTORS

A number of factors increasing the risk for clinically relevant spondylosis have been identified (Table 68.3). These risk factors, such as driving and lifting, often are found in tandem. Clear isolation of primary etiologic factors is therefore difficult. Based on available evidence, risk factors

TABLE 68.3. *Risk Factors for Cervical Degeneration*

Strongly Implicated
1. Cigarette smoking
2. Axial load bearing
3. High risk occupation: Meat carriers, dentists, professional drivers
4. Prior lumbar radiculopathy
5. Metabolic disturbance possible
6. Prior cervical trauma
7. Vibrational exposure
8. Diet/Nutritional Factors
9. Genetic Factors
10. Racial Factors
11. Gender
12. Atherosclerosis
13. Autoimmune Factors
No Role Identified
1. Repeated turning of the neck
2. Sports
3. Sedentary occupations

are grouped according to strong, possible, or no association with cervical degeneration.

Strong Associations

Several studies have implicated nicotine in the acceleration of disc degeneration. In epidemiologic studies, smoking cigarettes, but not cigars or pipes, is associated with higher rates of spondylosis (4). Cranial load bearing very likely increases the rate and extent of cervical degeneration. In a study of 225 Ghanaians who typically carried loads on their head, 143 (63.6%) were noted to have cervical spondylosis. Only 29 of the 80 people (36%) who did not carry loads on their head had cervical spondylosis (36). Similarly, frequent diving from a board is thought to increase cervical spondylosis (33).

A number of occupations have been identified as having increased risk for cervical spondylosis. As many as 75% of dentists have significant spondylotic change (35,37). Meat carriers, miners, and "heavy workers" also had significantly higher rates of cervical spondylosis compared with a reference group (37). Meat carriers had the highest overall risk for cervical spondylosis at 88% (37). In this study, 40% of the general manual laborers had spondylosis. Like meat carriers, professional drivers have been identified as a risk group because of their exposure to heavy lifting, long sedentary positioning, vibrational exposure, continuous acceleration and deceleration, and whiplash (38).

Prior lumbar radiculopathy also predicts for cervical disease. In a retrospective analysis of 200 patients requiring cervical disc surgery, more than 31% had undergone lumbar disc surgery (39). In patients who had not undergone lumbar surgery, a high number demonstrated abnormal lumbar radiographs or myelograms. Bulging discs were noted in 78, 100 had major root defects, 78 had minor root defects, 8 had spinal stenosis, and 7 had spondylolisthesis. Only 22 of 200 lumbar myelograms were normal in patients with cervical radiculopathy. In the Rochester study, a past history of lumbar radiculopathy was present in 41% of patients with cervical radiculopathy (30).

Metabolic factors accelerate cervical degeneration as well. Destructive spondylotic arthropathy is seen in dialysis patients and represents an accelerated course of cervical articular destruction (40).

Congenital stenosis of the central spinal canal or the neuroforamina significantly increases the risk for symptomatic cervical degenerative disease. The normal anteroposterior diameter of the cervical canal from C3 to C 7 is 17 to 18 mm (41,42). Given that the spinal cord averages 10 mm in size through the midportion of the cervical spine, there is substantial room for spondylotic change in the normal population. Payne and Spillane measured canal size in those with spondylotic myelopathy and found a mean diameter of 14 mm (8). In these patients, smaller degrees of spondylosis cause compression of the neural elements and their vascular supply, predisposing to the development of cervical myelopathy and radiculopathy (43).

Possible Role

The role of vibrational exposure is controversial. Some studies have documented that long-term exposure of vibration accelerates disc degeneration and herniation; others have not (33,44). Similarly, the role of prior cervical spine trauma in development of spondylosis is disputed (9). Repetitive subclinical trauma probably influences the onset and rate of progression of spondylosis. In one epidemiologic study, however, only 14.8% of cases of radiculopathy were preceded by a traumatic event (30).

Diet and nutritional status also affect the rate and degree of cervical degeneration. In both Japanese and Korean studies, consuming vegetable protein in favor of meat and increased salt intake were risk factors for ossification of the posterior longitudinal ligament (OPLL) (45,46). Similarly, atherosclerosis and autoimmune factors have been identified as possible pathogenic agents in cervical degenerative disease. The relationship between spondylosis and decreased range of cervical motion is clear. However, it is not known whether the pain and osteophyte formation of spondylosis limit the range of motion (ROM) or whether limited ROM accelerates spondylotic degeneration (44).

The impact of gender on cervical spine disease varies based on the clinical syndrome. Although there are no anatomic differences in the cervical spine between men and women, women demonstrate more variability in spinal canal dimensions, and perhaps have smaller spinal canals overall (34). Gender predominance for various degenerative conditions of the cervical spine vary by series. Unfortunately, the underlying conditions being sought are not always well delineated. Both male (29,30) and female (47) predominance have been reported for neck pain. In one study, women had more episodes lasting longer than 1 month (27). Another study found that radiographic degeneration was more severe in men than in women (35). Kelley postulated that neck pain might be more common in females because of hormonally derived ligamentous laxity (34).

The incidence of cervical radiculopathy is probably similar between the genders (34,48). However, men are more likely to be treated operatively (34). Although data are limited, myelopathy appears to be more common in men (9).

The presence of a familial predisposition to cervical spondylosis is of increasing interest to researchers in search of gene therapies to halt or reverse the process. In one study of patients older than 50 years of age, those with normal cervical spine radiographs were statistically significantly more likely to have a sibling with a normal or mildly abnormal study (49). Further, a statistically significant concordance of radiologic features in monozygous and, to a lesser extent, dizygotic twin pairs has been identified. Another study selected 85 pairs of male monozygotic twins based on exposure to suspected risk factors for disc degeneration (50). In this group, two intragenic polymorphisms of the vitamin D receptor gene revealed an association with disc degeneration, as demonstrated on T2-weighted sagittal MRI studies. Also, patients with anterior longitudinal ligament ossification (disseminated idiopathic skeletal hyperostosis, or DISH) or OPLL have higher rates of ossification of other ligaments and spondylosis, perhaps signaling an increased tendency to form osteophytes (51,52).

Given the likely influence of genetics on cervical spondylosis, it is reasonable to assume that racial factors affect cervical degeneration. Taitz examined 214 cervical spines from both black and white skeletons (53). In his study, blacks were significantly less affected by degenerative changes than whites. In the black specimens, osteophytes affected *either* the vertebral body or zygapophyseal joints. By contrast, in the whites, both sites are often affected on the same vertebra. Taitz concluded that this pattern of spondylosis in whites made them more likely to have radicular dysfunction.

No Clear Role

A number of previously identified factors have since been found not to increase significantly the risk for spondylosis. For example, Kelsey found that sedentary jobs or jobs requiring twisting of the neck did not increase the incidence of spondylosis (33). Further, Mundt and others reviewed risk factors for cervical disc herniation in athletes. No increased risk for herniation was seen in any sport, including weightlifting (48). They concluded that sports may actually be protective of the cervical spine.

NATURAL HISTORY

Most episodes of neck and arm pain resolve spontaneously. In fact, most cases of neck pain are related to soft tissue sprains and strains, not cervical spondylosis *per se*. Underlying cervical degeneration probably increases the time course of healing for minor neck strains (54). Ultimately, unlike other orthopedic trauma, the disability related to neck pain depends more on the chronicity of symptoms than the inciting event.

Although neck and back pain together account for up to 65% of cases of disability (55), cervical and lumbar pain disorders differ clinically. Neck pain less frequently leads to disability claims. Whereas patients with chronic low back pain have difficulties with heavy labor and transmission of load from the hands through the trunk, chronic neck pain patients have more difficulty with sedentary jobs. In particular, patients with neck pain have difficulty with persistent static positioning (sitting, writing, computer, driving) and with upper extremity activities (reaching, pushing over shoulder).

Overall, most authors report a favorable natural history for cervical radiculopathy as well. The spinal nerve root is composed of secondary motor neurons, which have the capacity for recovery (56). For about half of patients with cervical radiculopathy, symptoms resolve after 6 to 12 weeks. Only 10% to 15% have continuing substantial impairment (57). Gore and others followed 205 patients presenting with neck pain for a minimum of 10 years. In this nonoperatively treated group, 79% were improved or asymptomatic at follow-up; 13% were unchanged, and 8% were worse. Nearly one third still rated their pain as moderate to severe (22).

Lees and Turner followed 57 patients with radiculopathy for up to 19 years (58). Almost half of this group (45%) had only one painful episode and no further recurrence. Thirty percent reported mild continuing symptoms. Only 25% complained of persistent or worsening symptoms. In their series, no patient developed myelopathy if not present initially. In the Rochester study, on the other hand, cervical radiculopathy patients were followed for 4.9 years (30). Symptoms recurred in 31.7%. At last follow-up, 90% were asymptomatic or only mildly incapacitated owing to cervical radiculopathy.

Myelopathy has a less favorable natural history. Lees and Turner published their findings on a series of 44 patients with cervical myelopathy (58). Symptoms and disability were rapidly progressive in only 5% of cases. On the other hand, of 15 patients with severe disability, 14 remained severely disabled at long-term follow-up. Three fourths reported episodic increase in symptoms. In 20%, the symptoms were slowly progressive. In this series, age greater than 60 years was a poor prognostic feature. Nurick reported on 56 patients with myelopathy treated nonoperatively over 20 years (59). Of 27 patients with mild symptoms, 18 cases remained mild. Of 9 with moderate or severe symptoms, 6 remained stable. Nurick concluded that myelopathy with mild disability had the best prognosis. Overall, cervical spondylotic myelopathy was associated with a prolonged course with long periods of nonprogressive disability.

TREATMENT AND HEALTH CARE UTILIZATION

Despite the favorable natural history of most syndromes of cervical degeneration, vast economic resources are directed toward the evaluation and treatment of chronic neck problems. Aside from the direct costs of imaging and treatment, indirect costs such as lost productivity and early retirement are multiples of the direct expenditures.

An outpatient course of nonoperative treatment is attempted initially in all patients with neck pain, radiculopathy, or mild myelopathy (60). In 1985, there were 6,293,000 office visits for neck problems. Females presented 3,669,000 times, males 2,624,000 times. Of these clinical encounters, 3,153,000 were related to injuries, the remainder of cases were mainly degenerative problems.

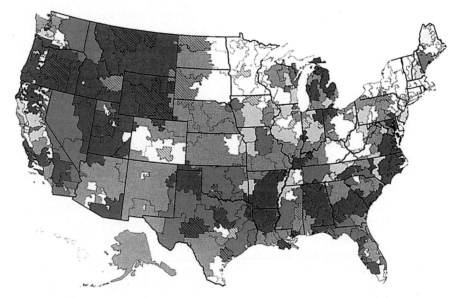

Map 2.2. Cervical Spine Surgery (1996-97)

In 74 hospital referral regions, rates of cervical spine surgery were at least 30% higher than the national average. In 75 hospital referral regions, rates were more than 25% below the average.

Ratio of Rates of Cervical Spine Surgery to the U.S. Average
by Hospital Referral Region (1996-97)

- ◼ 1.30 to 3.52 (74)
- ◼ 1.10 to < 1.30 (40)
- ◼ 0.90 to < 1.10 (74)
- ◻ 0.75 to < 0.90 (40)
- ◻ 0.32 to < 0.75 (75)
- Not Populated
- ◤ Statistically Imprecise
- Suppressed for Confidentiality

    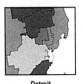

A   San Francisco   Chicago   New York   Washington-Baltimore   Detroit

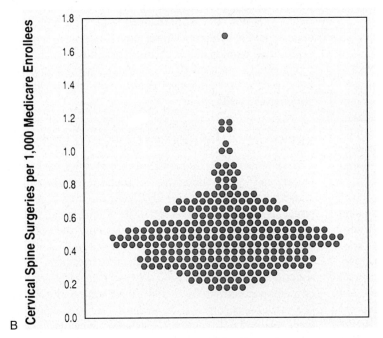

B

FIG. 68.9. There is wide geographic variability in the rates of cervical spine surgery. **A:** Rate of cervical spine surgery by hospital referral region as compared with the U.S. national average. **B:** Rates of cervical spine surgery per 1,000 Medicare enrollees. (From Weinstein JN, Birkmeyer JD. *Dartmouth atlas of musculoskeletal health care.* Chicago: AHA Press, 2000:28–40, with permission.)

Disease education is the first goal of treatment in this patient group. For patients with substantial discomfort, nonsteroidal antiinflammatory medications and other analgesics are added. In cases of more intractable pain, nerve root injections, cervical collar, cervical traction, or pain clinic may be recommended. For patients with multiple recurrences or more severe debility, physical therapy is instituted. For those with acute pain, start with passive modalities. When the acute symptoms subside, institute dynamic and isometric neck stretching and strengthening exercises. Aerobic exercise is encouraged throughout management.

For patients with intractable symptoms, hospitalization is occasionally required. Between 1993 and 1995, cervical spine conditions consumed 696,000 bed-days during 161,000 hospitalizations, with an average 4.3-day stay (60). About 13,000 men were admitted, more commonly with trauma diagnoses; 17,000 women were admitted, more commonly with degenerative conditions. Overall, hospital utilization for cervical spine problems has changed between the catalog periods of 1985 to 1988 and 1993 to 1995. During this interval, total hospital days have decreased 51.3%, and length of stay has decreased 31.7%. On the other hand, office visits have increased 20.5%.

Although most symptomatic cervical degenerative disease responds to nonoperative management, surgery is indicated for patients with intractable pain or severe or progressive neurologic deficits. Arm pain responds better to surgical intervention than neck pain. In the Rochester series, 26% of patients with cervical radiculopathy underwent surgery. A combination of radicular pain, sensory deficits, and objective muscle weakness were predictors for decision to operate (30).

Goals of cervical spine surgery in patients with degenerative disease include decompression and stabilization. A number of techniques provide decompression of the cervical spine, including discectomy, corpectomy, laminoforaminotomy, laminectomy, and laminoplasty.

Unlike the lumbar spine, the presence of the spinal cord and greater likelihood of postdecompression spinal deformity (such as kyphosis) have increased the utilization of anterior approaches. These anterior approaches typically include decompression with fusion. A posterior arthrodesis is occasionally performed with laminectomy to prevent iatrogenic instability.

Degenerative disorders account for most cervical spine surgeries done each year (61); however, there is substantial regional variation (62) (Fig. 68.9). Between 1996 and 1997, 88,000 spine surgeries were performed in the United States. Of these, of these, 27,000 were performed on the cervical spine (Fig. 68.10). Disc and stenosis surgeries represented 83% of this group. The other 17% of surgeries included all diagnostic groups: tumor, infection, and trauma.

In 1996, 3,011 orthopedic surgeons and 2,934 neurosurgeons performed spine surgery (62) (Fig. 68.11). However,

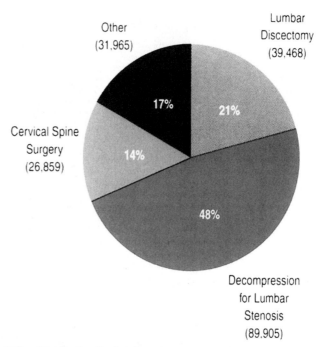

FIG. 68.10. Cervical spine surgery as a percentage of spine surgery overall. (From Weinstein JN, Birkmeyer JD. *Dartmouth atlas of musculoskeletal health care.* Chicago: AHA Press, 2000:28–40, with permission.)

64% of the total procedures were performed by neurosurgeons. Geography significantly affects this balance. In Akron, Ohio, neurosurgeons performed 19% of the spine operations. In Rapid City, South Dakota, neurosurgeons performed 99%. Overall, neurosurgeons performed 85% of the cervical spine procedures but only 59% of the lumbar procedures.

Rates of spine surgery in general have increased 57% during the 10 years from 1988 to 1997 (62). This represents an increase from 2.1 to 3.4 cases per 100,000 in the Medicare population. Cervical spine surgery alone increased from 0.16 to 1.72 per 100,000 Medicare recipients. Rates of spine surgery vary geographically by a factor of 6 from 1.4 per 100,000 in the Bronx to 8.6 per 100,000 in Bend, Oregon (Fig. 68.12).

Over time, there has been an increasing use of arthrodesis techniques (62). Arthrodeses were included in 23% of cervical spine procedures in 1993 and 29% in 1997. Similarly, there has been an increase in the use of internal fixation from 50% to 60% over the same interval. Neurosurgeons are less likely to fuse and instrument the spine. Forty-two percent of neurosurgical spine cases were decompression only; 32% included an arthrodesis without implants; 27% were listed as arthrodeses with instrumentation. For orthopedic spine surgeons, on the other hand, 25% were decompression alone, 32% were arthrodesed without implants, and 42% were listed as arthrodeses with instrumentation.

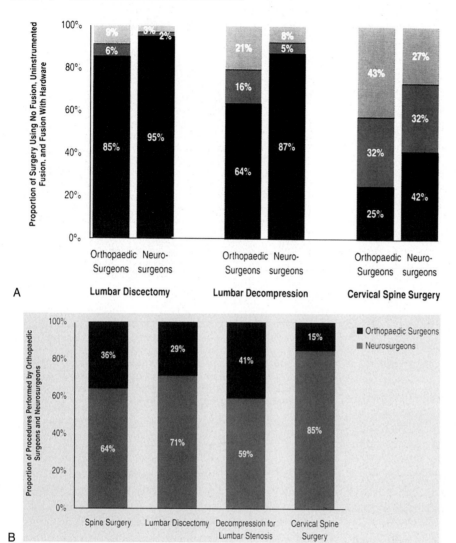

A

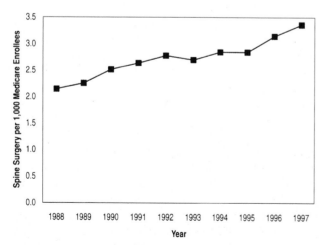

B

FIG. 68.11. Bar graphs depicting the differences in practice between orthopaedic and neurosurgical spine surgeons in terms of the use of fusion (**A**) and overall proportion of surgery (**B**). (From: Weinstein JN, Birkmeyer JD. *Dartmouth atlas of musculoskeletal health care*, Chicago: AHA Press, 2000:28–40, with permission.)

FIG. 68.12. The increasing rate of cervical spine surgery in the United States (per 1,000 enrollees). (From Weinstein JN, Birkmeyer JD. *Dartmouth atlas of musculoskeletal health care.* Chicago: AHA Press, 2000:28–40, with permission.)

CONCLUSION

Cervical spine degeneration is a common feature of aging. In some cases, degenerative changes lead to symptoms. Depending on the predominant complaint, these symptoms are classified into the clinical syndromes of degenerative disc disease, cervical radiculopathy, and cervical myelopathy. Neck pain alone in the face of cervical disc degeneration is termed cervical degenerative disc disease. Occasionally, a syndrome of painful facet joint spondylosis is identified. Patients with significant arm pain or radicular dysfunction from nerve root impingement from disc protrusions or osteophytes are said to have cervical radiculopathy. Myelopathy from spinal cord compression leads to a wide array of neurologic manifestations, often including hand numbness, gait difficulty, and spastic weakness. There is considerable overlap between these clinical syndromes.

Cervical degenerative problems lead to at least 3 million new patient encounters per year. Although the natural history for most of these problems is favorable, there are vast direct and indirect expenditures required both to evaluate and manage these patients and to compensate for lost productivity. Most patients are initially treated nonoperatively with disease education, physical therapy, medications, and steroid injections. In some patients, neurologic deficits prove progressive, or pain is intractable. Surgery is indicated in these patients and may consist of either anterior or posterior decompression and, possibly, surgical stabilization.

REFERENCES

1. Lestini WF, Wiesel SW. The pathogenesis of cervical spondylosis. *Cervical Orthop Relat Res* 1989;239:69–93
2. Montgomery DMM, Brower RS. Cervical spondylotic myelopathy. *Orthop Clin North Am* 1992;23:487–493.
3. Stookey B. Compression of the spinal cord and nerve roots by herniation of nucleus pulposus in cervical region. *Arch Surg* 1940;40:417.
4. Brain WR. Rupture of the intervertebral disk in the cervical region. *Proc R Soc Med* 1948;49:509.
5. Brain WR, Northfield D, Wilkinson M. The neurological manifestations of cervical spondylosis. *Brain* 1952;75:187–225.
6. Mair WG, Druckman R. The pathology of spinal cord lesions and their relations to the clinical features in the protrusion of cervical intervertebral discs. *Brain* 1953;76:70.
7. Taylor AR. Mechanism and treatment of spinal cord disorders associated with cervical spondylosis. *Lancet* 1953;1:717.
8. Payne EE, Spillane JD. The cervical spine. An anatomico-pathologic study of 70 specimens with particular reference to the problem of cervical spondylosis. *Brain* 1957;80:571.
9. Clark E, Robinson PK. Cervical myelopathy: a complication of cervical spondylosis. *Brain* 1956;79:483–570.
10. Hendry NG. The hydration of the nucleus pulposus and its relation to the intervertebral disc derangement. *J Bone Joint Surg Br* 1958;40:132.
11. Friedenberg ZB, Edeiken J, Spencer N, et al. Degenerative changes in the cervical spine. *J Bone Joint Surg Am* 1959;45:1171.
12. Aprill C, Dwyer A, Bogduk N. Cervical zygapophyseal joint pain patterns. II. A clinical evaluation. *Spine* 1990;15(6):458–461.
13. Aprill C, Bogduk N. The prevalence of cervical zygapophyseal joint pain. A first approximation. *Spine* 1992;17(7):744–747.
14. Holt S, Yates PO. Cervical spondylosis and nerve root lesions. Incidence at routine necropsy. *J Bone Joint Surg Br* 1966;48(3):407–423.
15. Hayashi H, Okada K, Hashimoto J, et al. Cervical spondylotic myelopathy in the aged patient. A radiographic evaluation of the aging changes in the cervical spine and etiologic factors in myelopathy. *Spine* 1988;13:618–625.
16. Crandall PH, Batzdorf U. Cervical spondylotic myelopathy. *J Neurosurg* 1966;25:57–66.
17. Skovron NL. Clinical epidemiology. In: Kasser JR, ed. *Orthopaedic knowledge update*, 5th ed. Chicago: American Academy of Orthopaedic Surgeons, 1996:71–73.
18. Lawrence JS. Disc degeneration: its frequency in relationship to symptoms. *Ann Rheum Dis* 1969;28:121–137.
19. Horwitz T. Degenerative lesions in the cervical portion of the spine. *Arch Intern Med* 1940;55:1178.
20. Kellgren JH, Lawrence JS. Rheumatism in miners. II. X-ray study. *Br J Indust Med* 1952;9:197
21. Friedenberg ZB, Miller WT. Degenerative disc disease of the cervical spine. *J Bone Joint Surg Am* 1959;41:61.
22. Gore DR, Sepic SB, Gardner GM, et al. Neck pain: a long-term follow-up of 205 patients. *Spine* 1987;12(1):1–5.
23. Tapiovarra J, Heinovaara O. Correlation of cervico-brachalgias and roentgenographic findings. *Ann Chir Gynaecol* 1954;43-S:436.
24. Hitselberger WE, Witten R. Abnormal myelograms in asymptomatic patients. *J Neurosurg* 1968;28:204.
25. Boden SD, McCowin PR, Davis DO, et al. Abnormal magnetic-resonance scans of the cervical spine in asymptomatic subjects. A prospective investigation. *J Bone Joint Surg Am* 1990;72(8):1178–1184.
26. Makela M, et al. Prevalence, determinants and consequences of chronic neck pain in Finland. *J Epidemiol* 1991;134:1356–1367.
27. Bovim G, Schrader H, Sand T. Neck pain in the general population. *Spine* 1994;19:1307–1309.
28. Wilson PR. Chronic neck pain and cervicogenic headache. *Clin J Pain* 1991;7:5–11.
29. Marchiori DM, Henderson CN. A cross-sectional study correlating cervical radiographic degenerative findings to pain and disability. *Spine* 1996;21(23):2747–2751.
30. Radhakrishnan K, Litchy WJ, O'Fallon WM. Epidemiology of cervical radiculopathy. A population-based study from Rochester, Minnesota, 1976 through 1990. *Brain* 1994;117(Pt 2):325–335.
31. Salemi G, Savettieri G, Meneghini F, et al. Prevalence of cervical spondylotic radiculopathy: a door-to-door survey in a Sicilian municipality. *Acta Neurol Scand* 1996;93(2–3):184–188.
32. Moore AP, Blumhardt LD. A prospective survey of the causes of non-traumatic spastic paraparesis and tetraparesis in 585 patients. *Spinal Cord* 1997;35(6):361–367.
33. Kelsey JL, Githens PB, Walter SD, et al. An epidemiological study of acute prolapsed cervical intervertebral disc. *J Bone Joint Surg Am* 1984;66:907–914.
34. Kelley LA. In neck to neck competition are women more fragile? *Clin Orthop* 2000;(372):123–130.
35. Rahim KA, Stambough JL. Radiographic evaluation of the degenerative cervical spine. *Orthop Clin North Am* 1992;23(3):395–403.
36. Jumah KB, Nyame PK. Relationship between load carrying on the head and cervical spondylosis in Ghanaians. *West Afr J Med* 1994;13(3):181–182.
37. Hagberg M, Wegman DH. Prevalence rates and odds ratios of shoulder-neck disease in different occupational groups. *Br J Indust Med* 1987;44:602–610.
38. Jensen MV, Tüchsen F, Ørhede E. Prolapsed Cervical Intervertebral Disc in Male Professional Drivers in Denmark, 1981–1990. A longitudinal study of hospitalizations. *Spine* 1996;21(20):2352–2355.
39. Jacobs B, Ghelman B, Marchisello P. Coexistence of cervical and lumbar disc disease. *Spine* 1990;15(12):1261–1264.
40. Abumi K, Ito M, Kaneda K. Surgical treatment of cervical destructive spondyloarthropathy (DSA). *Spine* 2000;25(22):2899–2905.
41. Burrows EH. The sagittal diameter of the spinal canal in cervical spondylosis. *Clin Radiol* 1963;14:77–86.
42. Hayashi H, Okada K, Hamada M, et al. Etiologic factors of myelopathy. A radiographic evaluation of the aging changes in the cervical spine. *Clin Orthop* 1997;214:200–209.
43. Humphreys SC, Hodges SD, Patwardhan A, et al. The natural history of the cervical foramen in symptomatic and asymptomatic individuals aged 20–60 years as measured by magnetic resonance imaging: a descriptive approach. *Spine* 1998;23(20):2180–2184.
44. Hagen KB, Harms-Ringdahl K, Enger NO, et al. Relationship between subjective neck disorders and cervical spine mobility and motion-related pain in male machine operators. *Spine* 1997;22(13):1501–1507.
45. Morisu M. Influence of food on the posterior longitudinal ligament of the cervical spin and serum sex hormones. *J Jpn Orthop Assoc* 1994;68:1056–1058.
46. Wang P-N, Chen S-S, Liu H-C, et al. Ossification of the posterior longitudinal ligament of the spine: a case-control risk factor study. *Spine* 1999;24(2):142–144.
47. Schellhas KP, Smith MD, Gundry CR, et al. Cervical discogenic pain. Prospective correlation of magnetic resonance imaging and discography in asymptomatic subjects and pain sufferers. *Spine* 1996;21(3):300–311; discussion, 311–312.
48. Mundt DJ, Kelsey JL, Golden AL, et al. An epidemiologic study of sports and weight lifting as possible risk factors for herniated lumbar and cervical discs. *Am J Sports Med* 1993;21:854–860.
49. Ball J, El Gammal T, Popham M. A possible genetic factor in cervical spondylosis. *Br J Radiol* 1969;42:9–16.
50. Videman T, Leppävuori J, Kaprio J, et al. 1998 Volvo Award winner in basic science studies: intragenic polymorphisms of the vitamin D receptor gene associated with intervertebral disc degeneration. *Spine* 1998;23(23):2477–2485.
51. Ono K, Ota H, Tada A, et al. Ossification of the posterior longitudinal ligament. A clinicopathologic study. *Spine* 1977;2:126–138.
52. Resnich D, Guerra J, Robinson CA, et al. Association of diffuse skeletal hyperostosis (DISH) and ossification of the posterior longitudinal ligament. *AJR Am J Roentgenol* 1978;313:1049–1053.

53. Taitz C. Osteophytosis of the cervical spine in South African blacks and whites. *Clin Anat* 1999;12(2):103–109.

54. Mayer TG. Functional restoration of patients with chronic spinal pain. In: Fardon DE, Garfin SR, eds. *Orthopaedic knowledge update*: spine 2. Rosemont, IL: American Academy of Orthopaedic Surgeons, 2002:230–231.

55. Weinstein JN. Neck and back pain. In: *Physical medicine and rehabilitation state of art review*. Philadelphia: Hanley & Belfus, 1990:201–214.

56. Rydevik B, Hasue M, Wehling P. Etiology of sciatic pain and mechanisms of nerve root compression. In Wiesel SW, et al, eds. *The lumbar spine*, 2nd ed. Philadelphia: WB Saunders, 1996:123–141.

57. Ellenberg MR, Honet JC, Treanor WJ. Cervical radiculopathy. *Arch Phys Med Rehabil* 1994;75(3):342–352.

58. Lees F, Turner JWA. Natural history and prognosis of cervical spondylosis. *BMJ* 1963;2:1607–1610.

59. Nurick S. The pathogenesis of the spinal cord disorder associated with cervical spondylosis. *Brain* 1972;95(1):87–100.

60. Praemer A, Furner S, Rice DP. *Musculoskeletal conditions in the United States*. Rosemont, IL: American Academy of Orthopaedic Surgeons, 1999:27–70.

61. Zeidman SM, Ducker TB, Raycroft J. Trends and complications in cervical spine surgery: 1989–1993. *J Spinal Disord* 1997;10(6):523–526.

62. Weinstein JN, Birkmeyer JD. *The Dartmouth atlas of musculoskeletal health care*. Chicago: AHA Press, 2000:28–40.

CHAPTER 69

Pain and Neurologic Dysfunction

Eeric Truumees

Cervical degenerative disease, or spondylosis, represents a spectrum of clinical entities directly affecting the cervical spine. The intervertebral disc undergoes degeneration with height loss and, possibly, protrusion. The vertebrae themselves exhibit osteophyte formation and facet joint degeneration. The longitudinal ligaments and ligamentum flavum calcify, overgrow, or fold into the canal. These changes to the spinal column may directly compress the neural elements or disrupt the blood supply to the spinal cord and nerve roots.

Cervical spine degeneration tends to progress with age and often develops at multiple interspaces. Many of the morphologic changes thought of as degenerative disease are indistinguishable from the universal effects of aging (1). Unlike the development of wrinkles, debilitating symptoms may arise, at which time a disease process is identified. The distinction between aging and disease is more easily made in patients with neurologic dysfunction than in those with axial pain alone.

Cervical spondylosis is a common condition, estimated to represent 2% of all hospital admissions in the United States (2). Mechanical neck pain arising from spinal arthritis is much more common than neurologic dysfunction. Such cervical degenerative disc disease often presents with a decreased range of motion or referred somatic pain. Radicular symptoms may result from chemical mediators from the disrupted disc, vascular embarrassment, or nerve root compression from disc protrusions or osteophytes. These radicular symptoms include pain (radiculitis) or nerve root dysfunction (radiculopathy). In younger patients, symptoms tend to arise acutely from disc protrusion. In older patients, more gradual symptom onset stems from spondylotic narrowing of the foramina or central canal. Compression of the spinal cord, or its vascular supply, may cause cord dysfunction and myelopathy, often leading to upper motor neuron findings such as spastic weakness and ataxia. Developmental size of the spinal canal and host metabolic factors affect the likelihood of symptom progression (3).

When considering clinical syndromes associated with cervical spine degeneration, it is useful to remember the four cardinal attributes that define a disease (4):

- Cause (etiology)
- Mechanism of development (pathogenesis)
- Structural alterations induced in cells and tissues (morphology)
- Functional consequences observed clinically (signs and symptoms)

In this chapter, the available cervical degenerative disease pathophysiology literature is reviewed in light of these four properties. Much of what is known about radicular dysfunction stems from animal sciatic nerve models, and relevant research is discussed. Mechanisms of spinal cord dysfunction derived from spinal cord injury research will also be included.

PATHOGENESIS OF DISC DEGENERATION

Buckwalter described cervical spine degeneration as a cascading process beginning in the intervertebral disc (5). Susceptibility is likely genetically coded and accelerated by repeated, subclinical traumas to the joints of the spine. Biochemical degeneration leads to mechanical destabilization, and additional, abnormal stresses are borne by the spinal articulations. Lost disc height and changes in mobility lead to a vicious cycle of progressive degeneration.

These biochemical changes begin in the nucleus pulposus. The nucleus is a three-dimensional lattice of collagen fibrils and a protein–polysaccharide complex (1). The polysaccharides impart hydrophilia, causing the disc to imbibe water. The normal nucleus pulposus acts as a contained fluid (6). Axial loads to the spine are converted to tensile strain on annular fibers and are then transmitted to the vertebral end plates. With continuous loading, the nucleus exhibits creep.

With age, this gel structure degenerates. Starting in the second decade of life, the collagen content of the disc increases while glycoprotein content decreases (7). The loss of glycoproteins decreases imbibation pressure. When relaxed, the degenerated disc can imbibe fluid, but when pressure is reapplied, this fluid is not retained. Over time, disc hydration decreases from 88% weight by volume to 69% (8) (Fig. 69.1).

The normal function of the annulus is to contain the nucleus and convert compressive stress to tangential stress. When the nucleus fails to maintain its hydration, strain changes occur at the nucleus–annulus interface. The overall mechanical effectiveness of the disc decreases with its decreasing state of hydration (9). The disc is no longer able to generate increased intradiscal pressures and is therefore unable to distribute force effectively (8). The central annular lamellae buckle under constant compressive loading. The disc subsequently collapses, causing the external concentric bands of the annulus fibrosis to bulge outward (Fig. 69.2).

Increased annular stress leads to fibrillation and tearing of the annular fibers. In younger patients, nuclear material can protrude through these defects. Thus, disc herniation is part of a continuum of degeneration leading to more advanced spondylosis (9). If herniation does not occur early, it becomes less likely as the nucleus progressively dehydrates. Although acute disc herniation may also complicate chronic spondylotic changes, annular degeneration and protrusion predominate in older patients. With loss of disc height, the facets override. With decreasing facet competence, segmental motion increases, further hastening the disc degeneration (9).

The intervertebral discs are the largest avascular tissues in the human body (10). Disc nutrition derives from diffusion across the cartilaginous end plates. Normally, oxygen tension drops at the center of the disc. With spinal degeneration, the end plates become sclerotic, thereby decreasing nutrient exchange. This sclerosis further accelerates disc degeneration as part of a vicious cycle.

A number of factors influence the rate and degree of disc degeneration, including loading, genetics, and local autocrine factors. High rates of disc degeneration occur only in lordotic portions of the spine, implicating axial loading (11). When static compressive stress exceeds the disc's swelling pressure, water is forced out of the disc, altering intradiscal stress distribution, resulting in a number of harmful, dose-dependent responses (6). Nuclear cells exhibit apoptosis and an associated loss of cellularity. Collagen II and aggrecan gene expression is down-regulated, and the annulus fibrosis becomes increasingly disorganized.

The cells of the intervertebral disc are metabolically active and are capable of responding to biochemical stimuli. These autocrine factors function as local cellular signals to either increase or decrease disc degeneration. For example, matrix metalloproteinases decompose aggregating proteoglycans, contributing to destruction of both the articular cartilage and intervertebral disc. Cells of the intervertebral discs increase their production of matrix metalloproteinases

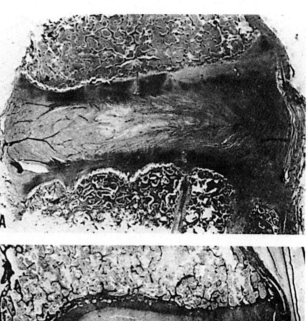

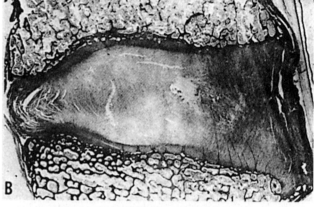

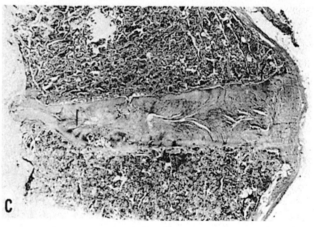

FIG. 69.1. The intervertebral disc sections at various ages, demonstrating progressive degeneration. **A:** A 6-year-old boy (original magnification × 4). **B:** A 54-year-old man (original magnification × 2.5). **C:** A 70-year-old man. (From Coventry MB, Ghormley RK, Kernohan JW. The intervertebral disc. Its microscopic anatomy and pathology. I. Anatomy, development and physiology. *J Bone Joint Surg* 1945; 27:105, with permission.)

when stimulated by interleukin-1 (12). Endogenously produced nitric oxide strongly inhibits the production of interleukin-6, suggesting that autocrine mechanisms play an important role in the regulation of disc cell metabolism. Using immunohistologic staining, one study found that the

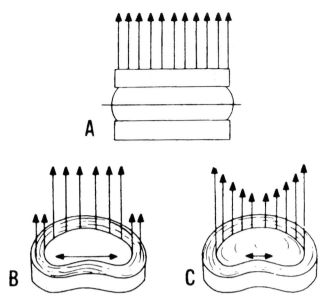

FIG. 69.2. Representations of normal and abnormal force transfer through the intervertebral disc. **A:** Schematic of even pressure distributed over the disc. **B:** Force transfer through the normal nucleus and annulus. The *horizontal arrows* depict the conversion of axial loads into transverse shear. **C:** Force transfer through the degenerated nucleus. The nucleus is now less effective in transmitted load, and more axial load is borne with less conversion into tensile force. (From Eyring EJ. The biochemistry and physiology of the intervertebral disk. *Clin Orthop* 1969;67:16, with permission.)

matrix metalloproteinase-3-positive cell ratio correlated with the degree of degeneration on magnetic resonance imaging (MRI) (13). Further, degenerated discs exhibited matrix metalloproteinase-3 but no metalloproteinase tissue inhibitor. For cervical intervertebral discs, the matrix metalloproteinase-3-positive cell ratio correlated with osteophyte size. These authors concluded that intervertebral disc degeneration is caused by a disturbance in the equilibrium of matrix metalloproteinase-3 and tissue inhibitor of metalloproteinase-1. Cathepsins and other proteolytic enzymes are also involved in disc degeneration, forming clefts that separate the discs from their vertebral bodies (14).

DEGENERATIVE CHANGES OUTSIDE THE DISC

The disc is part of a three-point articulated support system, including two zygapophyseal, or facet, joints posteriorly (15). The zygapophyseal joint is a classic synovial joint serving as part of a tripod that can resist most physiologic moments, allowing a large arc of motion without a significant decrease in the space for the neural elements.

Forces applied to the intervertebral disc produce coupled motions in the facets. Kirkaldy-Willis and colleagues found that, in the lumbar spine, the development of degenerative changes in the disc are mirrored by similar processes in the facets (15). However, load bearing in the cervical spine

differs from that in the lumbar spine. Unlike the lumbar spine, where 80% of axial load passes through the disc (16), in the cervical spine, axial load is distributed almost equally between the disc anteriorly and each articular pillar posteriorly (16).

Cervical spondylosis is a slowly progressive phenomenon. Early degeneration in the disc typically precedes major bony change by 10 years (17). Ultimately, with decreasing disc height, facet mechanics are altered, increasing mechanical stress at the cartilaginous end plates (18–21). Much like synovial joint degeneration elsewhere, findings include cartilage space narrowing, sclerosis of the bony margins, and osteophyte formation (1). Facet osteophytes tend to occlude the neuroforamen rather than the central canal.

In some cases, mechanical incompetence of a disc and facets leads to spondylolisthesis (22). The superior joint surfaces slip backward, eroding into the lamina below. Alternatively, osteophytes can form to stabilize the vertebral motion segment (18–21). Biochemically, receptors for bone morphogenetic proteins (BMPs) have been found to move from cartilage cells to fibrous cells during the course of disc degeneration. This new receptivity to BMPs may promote osteophyte formation (23).

Osteophytes increase the weight-bearing surface of the vertebral end plates in proportion to the square of the new vertebral radius (24,25). Mechanically, this increased surface area decreases effective force per unit area. Osteophytes also lead to decreased motion, acting as a "limiting mechanism" against further deterioration. In some cases, osteophytes effectively "autofuse" the degenerated segment (1).

In one series of 260 patients with suspected cervical spine disorders, instability was identified on the flexion-extension radiographs of 14.5% (150) of motion segments (26). This cervical segmental instability correlated with early or moderate degeneration as seen on MRI. Others have also reported increased mobility in mildly degenerated discs rather than in normal or severely degenerated discs (15). These findings support Kirkaldy-Willis' hypothesis of three phases of degeneration:

- Dysfunction
- Unstable phase
- Stabilization

Disc degeneration also leads to changes in cervical alignment. Normal vertebral bodies are bigger posteriorly and smaller anteriorly. Therefore, the normal cervical lordosis is maintained by the relatively larger disc height anteriorly (1). As discs lose height, the cervical spine loses lordosis. Uncovertebral joints begin to touch posteriorly, preventing further posterior height loss and continued, preferential anterior loss (27). Uncovertebral joint apposition also leads to osteophyte formation (Fig. 69.3).

Changes in spinal alignment and motion also affect cervical ligaments. These ligaments lose elasticity and thicken with age (28). Disc collapse increases tension on the surrounding ligaments, and the ligamentum flavum buckles

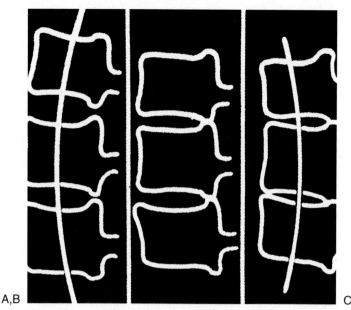

A,B

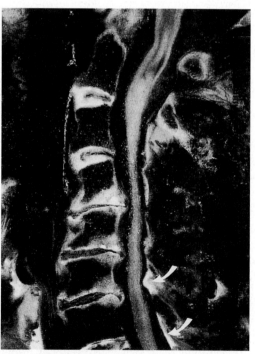

C

FIG. 69.3. Depiction of the gradual loss of cervical lordosis seen with disc degeneration. **A:** Initially, lordosis is created by greater anterior than posterior disc height. **B:** With disc degeneration, height is initially lost symmetrically, but eventually the uncovertebral joints meet posteriorly. **C:** Further degeneration will take place only anteriorly, leading to relative cervical kyphosis. (From MacNab I. Cervical spondylosis. *Clin Orthop* 1975;109:69, with permission.)

inward (Fig. 69.4). The increased tension of the attachments of the anterior longitudinal ligament (ALL) and posterior longitudinal ligament (PLL) to bone leads to a periosteal reaction with bone growth in the form of osteophytes (1,29,30). In a rabbit model, induced disc degeneration led to osteophyte formation by metaplasia of the deep annular fibers and subsequent enchondral ossification (30).

PATHOPHYSIOLOGY OF NECK PAIN

Most patients present to a spine physician because of pain. Ultimately, the relationship between this pain and the underlying degenerative change is affected by the subjective aspects of the pain experience. For example, suffering is the emotional response to nociceptive input and may be affected by many factors outside the cervical spine itself (e.g., sleep disorders and depression). In general, the purpose of pain is to signal actual or impending tissue damage. Common pain patterns in patients with cervical spine disorders include nociceptive pain, neuropathic pain, and chronic pain (31–33).

Nociceptive pain arises from the musculoskeletal system through nociceptors widely distributed in cutaneous tissue, bone, muscle, connective tissue, vessels, and viscera. Nociceptive pain is typically described as sharp, dull, aching,

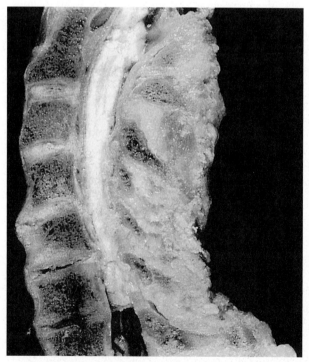

A

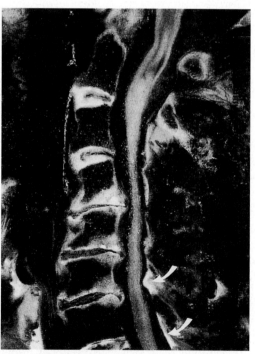

B

FIG. 69.4. Gross pathology photographs of sagittally sectioned, spondylotic cervical spines. **A:** Specimen from a 67-year-old man with central stenosis, particularly at the C5 to C6 level. Note the combination of posterior compression from osteophytes and anterior compression from disc-level osteophytes. **B:** A cryomicrotome section demonstrating both disc space narrowing and buckling of the ligamentum flavum *(arrows)*. (**A** from Bulloch PG, Boachie-Adjei O. *Atlas of spinal diseases.* Philadelphia: JB Lippincott, 1993, with permission; **B** from An HS, Simpson JM. *Surgery of the cervical spine.* London: Martin Dunitz, 1994, with permission.)

or throbbing in character and often responds to nonsteroidal antiinflammatory drugs (NSAIDs) and opioids. Neuropathic pain, on the other hand, refers to pain that arises from injury or disease of the nervous system. Neuropathic pain is associated with burning and hyperalgesia and does not typically respond to NSAIDs (31,34).

Chronic pain differs from acute pain in that is has extended beyond the period of normal tissue healing. Over time, pain behaviors become globalized and less closely associated with the inciting nociceptive input. Frequently, a discrete pain generator cannot be identified despite sophisticated imaging techniques. Treatment of the pain generator is no longer adequate to resolve this chronic pain pattern. In these patients, multidisciplinary rehabilitation and pain management are preferred to surgery (34,35).

Pain Pathways

Cervical spine degenerative disease leads to pain through one of several pathways. First, the receptor relays an impulse to the primary afferent nerve. The primary afferent feeds into the spinal nerve (nerve root), which conveys signals to the spinal cord and ultimately the brain (Fig. 69.5). Most nociceptive pain is mediated through mechanical, thermal, or chemical receptors and unmyelinated or lightly myelinated afferents, such as A-delta and C fibers. These small primary afferents exhibit little or no spontaneous activity. Discharge frequency increases with increased stimulus intensity and correlates with the pain response (36). Local tissue injury leads to persistent, spontaneous bursting activity from the primary afferents at the site (36).

Nociceptive neurotransmitters include glutamate, substance P, vasoactive intestinal polypeptide (VIP), and somatostatin. Most small primary afferents have multiple transmitters. Typically, amino acid neurotransmitters, such

as glutamate, result in rapid, short-lasting depolarization, whereas peptide neurotransmitters, such as substance P, cause delayed, long-lasting depolarization (37).

These primary afferent sensory nerves converge at the spinal nerve root, which then supplies the dorsal horn neurons of the spinal cord. Like the primary afferents, the spinal nerve does not normally produce spontaneous discharges (38–40). The dorsal horn neurons are second-order nociresponsive elements classified by their firing threshold (41, 42). Nociceptive-specific neurons fire in an all-or-nothing pattern to detect the presence of a nociceptive signal. Wide dynamic range (WDR) neurons, on the other hand, have the ability to encode stimulus intensity. These WDR neurons may be activated by stimulation from a variety of organ systems. For example, the same WDR neuron is excited by both cutaneous and deep input within a dermatome. Therefore, the T5 dermatomal receptors excite the same WDR as the coronary arteries, causing the brain to perceive coronary occlusion as left arm pain (41,42).

In the spinal cord, sensory signals pass and coalesce into several fiber tracts, including the tract of Lissauer, a small C-fiber tract. Large afferents are typically conveyed into the dorsal columns. These fibers typically pass rostrally on the ipsilateral side for several segments before crossing to the contralateral side (36,42). Cervical spine afferents may collateralize less and be more level specific on entering the cord than lumbar afferents (43).

Nociceptive signals are processed in the midbrain and cortex. Brainstem processing includes the medullary reticular formation, which acts as a relay station. This medullary relay also incorporates nociceptive input into the autonomic system. In the cortex, there are two important somatosensory areas, SI and SII. SII is more important in pain perception. The limbic system controls the affective-motivational component of pain response. Lesions here cause the subject

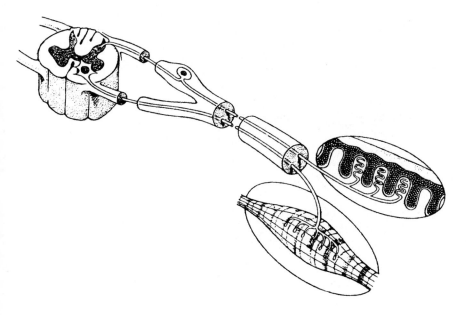

FIG. 69.5. A single spinal cord segment with end organs. The motor root is ventral with terminals on skeletal muscle. The sensory root is dorsal, passing from the receptors in the skin to the dorsal root ganglion and into the cord. (From Lundborg G. Nerve regeneration and repair. *Acta Orthop Scand* 1987;58:145–169, with permission.)

to dissociate reported stimulus intensity with its affective component (34,42).

Nociceptive Response Modulators

Subacute pain stems from exaggerated neuronal discharge in response to subthreshold stimuli. Factors released into the periterminal milieu after local tissue injury mediate this effect. Important factors include amines, kinins, lipidic acids, cytokines, and peptides. A number of modulators on the terminal of the primary afferent also function to inhibit the release of afferent neurotransmitters. For example, agonists of the opiate or α_2-adrenoreceptors lead to blockade of C-fiber transmission and thus local analgesia (44,45). Li and Zhou found that multiple receptor agonists and antagonists, including glutamate and serotonin, affect conduction rates in sensory nerves (46).

Modulators at the nerve root level have been closely studied in order to develop pharmacologic interventions for chronic radicular pain. The tachykinins are neuropeptides such as substance P, neurokinin A, and neurokinin B, which bind to dorsal horn receptors (47). Substance P increases synaptic transmission in nociceptive pathways by affecting calcium release from intracellular stores (48,49). Peripheral nerve transection or chronic compression leads to decreased levels of substance P in the cord (41,48).

N-methyl-D-aspartate (NMDA) receptors bind the neurotransmitter glutamate and are found throughout the central nervous system (CNS), including the dorsal horn. These receptors may mediate synaptic plasticity and some forms of memory (50). Blocking these receptors reduces spinal nociception (51). Nitric oxide (NO) functions as a secondary mediator of many of these effects, increasing the responsivity of dorsal horn neurons to nociceptive afferents (52,53). NO has been found in the cerebrospinal fluid (CSF) of chronic pain patients (41). Intracutaneous NO injection evokes pain in a dose-dependent manner (41). NSAIDs may decrease pain by blocking the mediators. These agents inhibit cyclooxygenase and therefore the production of prostaglandins from arachidonic acid in cell membranes (54). Whereas an intrathecal substance P injection leads to hyperalgesia, an intrathecal NSAID injection antagonizes this effect (37).

Modulation of nociceptive input occurs at the dorsal horn level as well. Repetitive stimulation leads to windup and somatotopic remodeling wherein the receptive field of the dorsal horn enlarges and responds more vigorously to modestly aversive stimuli (55). These changes are affected through descending inhibitory and excitatory pathways modulated by interneurons at the spinal level. Over time, altered sensory input changes the processing patterns of afferent information in the dorsal horn of the cord (48).

Severing the afferent nerve has this effect, but long-term blockade with tetrodotoxin does not (55). This difference implies that chemical or metabolic factors, not the electrical impulses themselves, are responsible for cord reorganization. A redistribution of central terminals of thick, myeli-nated afferents from low-threshold mechanoreceptors is observed. This shift could lead to inappropriate responses to innocuous peripheral stimuli and may explain the intractability of neuropathic pain (56).

Over time, modulation of afferent impulses is also mediated through differential gene expression in dorsal horn neurons. For example, the C-fos protein acts as a third messenger in stimulus–transcription coupling in neurons (41). That is, *c-fos* encodes transcription factors that regulate target gene expression. Genes for neuropeptides such as the tachykinins and enkephalins are affected (32). This gene-level modulation can be blocked by morphine.

PAIN GENERATORS

There are many potential pain generators in the cervical spine. The intervertebral disc is believed by many authors to be a primary generator of axial cervical spine pain. Parke concluded that distinguishing between the confluence of nerve fibers supplying the disc, the PLL, and the periosteum was difficult, but that the outer portions of disc were likely innervated by sinuvertebral nerve complex (7,57). The occurrence of nerve endings below the outer lamellae of the annulus is still controversial (58).

The sinuvertebral nerve emerges just distal to the dorsal root ganglion whereupon it reenters the foramen. The sinuvertebral nerve then arborizes over two levels on the PLL. This overlapping, dual innervation usually provides a less precise anatomic basis for the pain-referral patterns seen during discography. The sinuvertebral nerve conveys information from a combination of receptors on mechanical

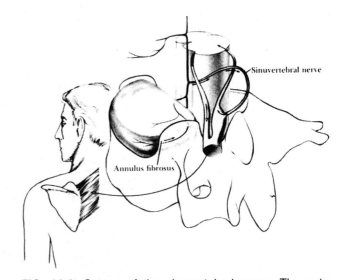

FIG. 69.6. Course of the sinuvertebral nerve. The outer annulus is innervated. With disc degeneration, pain can be referred along the same sclerotome to the interscapular musculature. (From Lestini WF, Wiesel SW. The pathogenesis of cervical spondylosis. *Cervical Orthop Relat Res* 1989; 239:69–93, with permission.)

deformation and position. Overstimulation of the sinuvertebral nerve complex causes the surrounding muscles to go into spasm (59,60) (Fig. 69.6).

Zygapophyseal joint degeneration may indirectly cause pain through subchondral bone fracture, ligament attenuation, and excessive muscle strains and injury (61). The facets are richly innervated by the posterior primary rami, including substance P–containing fibers (61,62). Encapsulated mechanoreceptors respond to capsular distention, ligamentous instability, and direct trauma (Fig. 69.7). Periarticular receptors respond to chemical stimuli. The facet meniscoid represents a highly vascularized and innervated infolding of the capsule (63). The meniscoid atrophies and disappears with age.

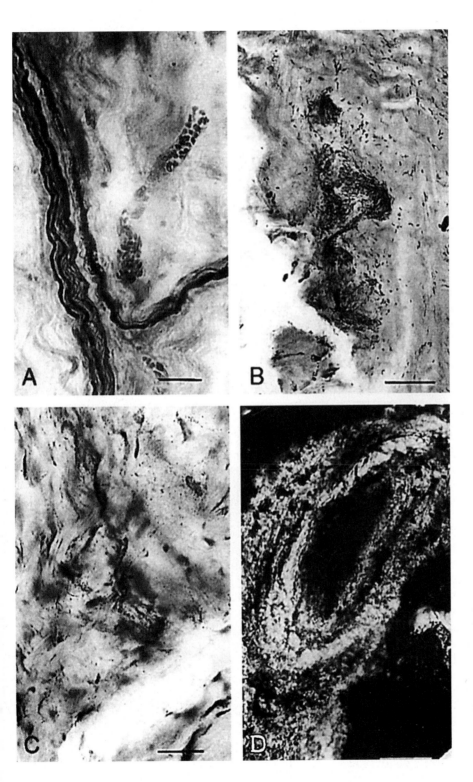

FIG. 69.7. A silver impregnation technique is used to demonstrate nerve endings within the human facet joint capsule. **A:** Three-micron nerve fibers. **B:** Ruffini-type nerve ending. **C:** Free nerve endings with parent nerve fiber. **D:** The distinctive onionskin appearance of a pacinian corpuscle. (From Rydevik B, Hasue M, Wehling P. Etiology of sciatic pain and mechanisms of nerve root compression. In: Wiesel SW, et al, eds. *The lumbar spine,* 2nd ed. Philadelphia: WB Saunders, 1996: 123–141, with permission.)

Stimulation of zygapophyseal joint afferents produces a discrete referral pattern that can mimic cervical radiculopathy (64). Marked reduction in nerve activity can be achieved with lidocaine facet injections (61).

The bone of the cervical spine is a metabolically active composite tissue affected by a variety of physiologic processes. Subchondral sclerosis is an example of a dynamic response to injury. Fine nerve endings are found in the marrow, periosteum, and cortex. Pain-related neuropeptides have been localized to these fine nerve fibers and may play a direct role in bone pain, triggering intraosseous hypertension or ischemia (24,62).

The cervical spine ligaments, such as the PLL, are also richly innervated. Although there is a significant interdigitation of annular fibers and the PLL fibers, the nerve endings in the PLL are more numerous and varied (57). Mechanical distortion or disruption of fibers in the posterolateral aspect of the intervertebral disc is a likely source of pain in disc protrusion or rupture as well as in cases of segmental instability in which disc mechanics are significantly altered.

Muscular pain and spasm are a common component of neck pain and may result directly from injury or indirectly from overuse, inflammation, or ischemia. Pain receptors in the muscle may be either chemonociceptive or mechanonociceptive. Damaged tissues release vascular permeability factors and attract inflammatory cells. Edema, inflammation, and irritation of the injured muscle triggers muscle spasms and involuntary contractions. Gross muscular contractions further affect load-damaged or spondylotic discs and facets (65).

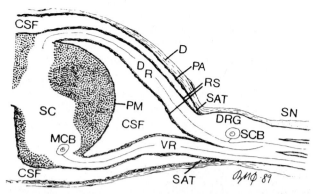

FIG. 69.8. Schematic of the spinal nerve root anatomy. The spinal nerve (SN) is made up of afferent and efferent contributions. Ventral root axons enter the cord through the ventral ramus (VR) and terminate at the cell bodies of the motor axons (MCB). Dorsal root axon cell bodies are housed in the dorsal root ganglion (DRG). Postganglionic fibers pass from the dorsal ramus (DR) and terminate in the posterior horns of the cord. Coverings of the neural elements include pia mater (PM), which covers the cord and continues over the spinal nerve as the root sheath (RS) reflecting into the single pia arachnoid (PA) at the subarachnoid triangle (SAT). Before the reflection, the dura (D) is continuous with one portion of the PA, the space between the two halves contains the cerebrospinal fluid (CSF). SC, spinal cord. (From Rydevik B, Hasue M, Wehling P. Etiology of sciatic pain and mechanisms of nerve root compression. In: Wiesel SW, et al, eds. *The lumbar spine*, 2nd ed. Philadelphia: WB Saunders, 1996:123–141, with permission.)

PATHOPHYSIOLOGY OF RADICULOPATHY

Each nerve has two functions: electrical impulse propagation and axonal transport of proteins and organelles. Both of these functions require energy and can be blocked by local ischemia or root compression (38,66–68). Disruption of these functions is based on different cellular mechanisms. That is, axonal transport can be maintained over a nerve segment that does not conduct impulses.

The nerve root (spinal nerve) has two parts. Its ventral efferent roots convey motor information. The dorsal, afferent roots convey sensory information. These elements are contained together in the root sleeves, which are extensions of the dura. Within the root sleeve, these elements are soaked in CSF (41). The spinal nerve lacks the perineurium and epineurium of peripheral nerves (68) (Fig. 69.8).

The dorsal root fibers' cell bodies are contained in the dorsal root ganglion (DRG). This structure is important in the synthesis of neuropeptides such as substance P and calcitonin-related peptide (CRP) (41). The DRG typically lies in the neuroforamen, but its position is not constant. Occasionally, the DRG is found in the spinal canal or outside the foramen (69). DRG size varies with the vertebral level, and the structure is covered with a tight capsule (41).

The blood supply of spinal nerves is sparser than that of peripheral nerves (41,42). On the other hand, the extension of CSF around the proximal portion of the nerve confers partial nutrition from diffusion (70). The blood–nerve barrier limits the flow of albumin and makes the spinal nerve more susceptible to edema than peripheral nerves (71).

Radicular blood supply is carried through segmental arteries. Outside the spine, these arteries divide into three branches when approaching the foramen (41). The anterior branch supplies visceral structures anterior to the spinal column. The posterior branch supplies the paraspinal muscles and facets. The intermediate branch supplies the spinal canal contents. The intermediate branch arborizes to supply the DRG, ventral root, dorsal root, and vasocorona of the cord itself (72). These vessels run parallel to the nerve roots, but there is no apparent connection with them (73,74).

The nerve root receives vascular supply from two directions: the intermediate branch distally and the vasocorona of the cord proximally. These vessels run in the epipials, the outer layer of root sheath, and anastomose at a point two thirds of the nerve root length from the cord (75,76). This watershed anastomosis region is vulnerable to insufficiency (75) (Fig. 69.9).

The absence of an epineurium and a perineurium renders spinal nerves susceptible to mechanical injury (77). With an elastic limit 15% of their resting length, ultimate load and stiffness are 10% and 20% of that of peripheral nerves, re-

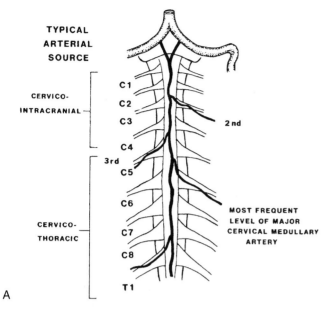

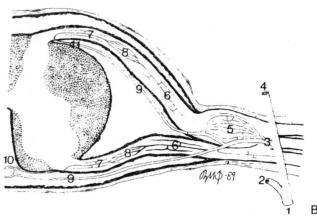

B

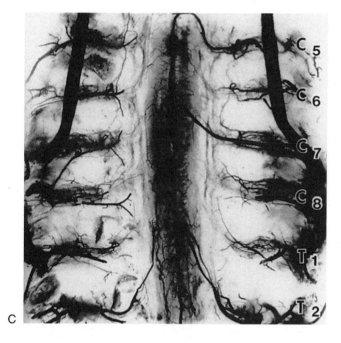

C

FIG. 69.9. Depictions of the radicular vascular supply. **A:** Main sources of arterial blood for the nerve roots and the cord. In the upper cervical spine (C1 to C4), the cord is supplied by the anterior spinal artery from intracranial sources. From C5 to T1, the anterior spinal artery is supplied by a unilateral medullary feeder, usually near C6. Alternatively, this feeder may arise from C3 or C4. **B:** Local blood supply at the root level. The intermediate branch of the segmental artery (1) enters the canal dividing into an anterior spinal canal branch (2), a nervous system branch (3), and a posterior spinal canal branch (4). A ganglionic plexus (5) is created where the lateral-ward nervous system branch joins the nerve root and meets the medial-ward supply from the caudal nerve root arteries (7) in the cranial half of the root (8). Other segments of the nervous system branch pass medially to become medullary feeder arteries (9). One branch passes anteriorly to contribute to the anterior spinal artery (10). The other branch contributes to one of the two dorsal spinal arteries (11). **C:** Photograph of an injected neonatal spinal cord. Note that the anterior spinal artery receives thoracic and cervical level medullary feeders. Lesser degrees of supply pass through the segmentals at each foramen. (**A** from Parke WW. Correlative anatomy of cervical spondylotic myelopathy. *Spine* 1988;13(7):831–837, with permission; **B** from Rydevik B, Hasue M, Wehling P. Etiology of sciatic pain and mechanisms of nerve root compression. In: Wiesel SW, et al., eds. *The lumbar spine*, 2nd ed. Philadelphia: WB Saunders, 1996:123–141, with permission; **C** from Parke WW. Correlative anatomy of cervical spondylotic myelopathy. *Spine* 1988;13(7):831–837, with permission.)

spectively (78). Human thoracic nerves have an ultimate load of 5N to 33N (77). The mechanical properties of spinal nerves are also variable relative to their position. These nerves are stronger in foramen than in thecal sac. A lower collagen content also increases susceptibility to compression (79,80). Further, spinal nerves have a parallel fiber pattern, unlike the sturdier plexiform pattern seen in peripheral nerves (81).

Nerve Root Compression

Each root is partially fixed at its origin from the surface of the cord, in the dural sheath, and by an adventitial leash

as it passes through the foramen (41). Mechanical forces distort the fixed nerve root by stretching the nerve between these points or by compressing the nerve directly between two firm surfaces. Typical sites of compression include the region of passage over the intervertebral disc, the intervertebral foramen, and the paravertebral areas directly adjacent to the external neural foramen.

There are four common biomechanical settings for nerve root compression: acute disc herniation in the absence of spondylosis, acute disc herniation in the context of spondylosis, subacute compression from spondylotic osteophytes, and chronic radiculopathy. Acute herniation in patients without significant prior spondylosis typically occurs

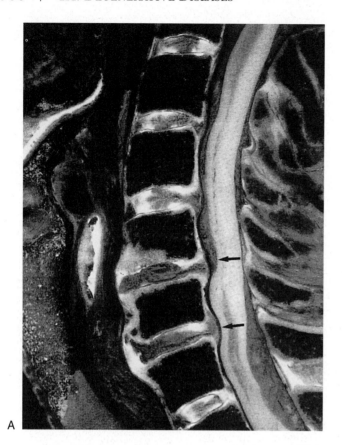

A

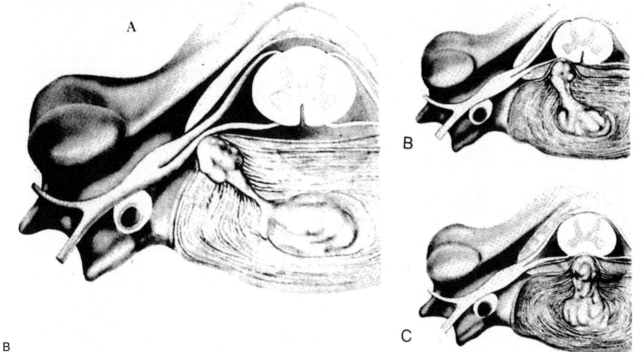

FIG. 69.10. Examples of soft disc herniation. **A:** Photograph of a midsagittal cryomicrotome section of a mildly degenerative cervical spine with herniation of the nucleus pulposus at the C5-C6 and C6-C7 levels *(arrows)*. In this case, spinal cord impingement results. **B:** Stookey's types of soft disc protrusion: intraforaminal (A), ventrolateral (B), and midline (C). (**A** from An HS, Simpson JM. *Surgery of the cervical spine.* London: Martin Dunitz, 1994, with permission; **B** from Lestini WF, Wiesel SW. The pathogenesis of cervical spondylosis. *Cervical Orthop Relat Res* 1989; 239:69–93, with permission.)

in younger patients. In high-energy injuries, these disc displacements may be associated with vertebral end-plate fracture and typically include both nuclear and annular material (1).

Acute herniation in patients with prior spondylosis represents an exacerbation of prior annular incompetence with new protrusion of disc material and can occur with minor trauma. Subacute radiculopathy develops in patients with long-standing spondylosis. A gradual progression of radicular symptoms of one or more roots occurs with no single traumatic event. Symptoms are often precipitated by overuse or an inflammatory mediator. In patients with chronic radiculopathy, symptoms develop insidiously after periods of increased or unusual activity.

Anatomic Basis

Nerve root compression can occur with static compression by soft disc herniation. *Soft disc herniation* refers to extradural compression by annular and nuclear material and is the cause of most acute radiculopathies (Fig. 69.10). Stookey described three morphologic patterns of herniation: intraforaminal, ventrolateral, and midline (82). Intraforaminal herniations are the most common and cause greater sensory than motor disturbance. Typically, paresthesias, hyperesthesias, and hyperalgesias in the neck, shoulder, and affected dermatome are reported. With ventrolateral protrusions, motor symptoms predominate, leading to weakness, decreased tone, and atrophy. Large midline herniations produce myelopathic symptoms and are rarely associated with root compression.

The nucleus pulposus represents 15% of the total disc volume (1). Therefore, if the entire volume of the nucleus extrudes, a 0.7 cm diameter sphere is generated. This volume is insufficient to create significant cord compression in midline herniations. In a more contained space, such as with foraminal herniation, this volume is sufficient to cause radiculopathy.

In spondylotic radiculopathy, nerve root compression is mediated by a hard disc formation. A *hard disc* refers to an osteophyte protrusion into the foramina from the facets and uncovertebral joints and is the cause of most chronic radiculopathies. As disc degeneration occurs, the uncinate process overrides and hypertrophies, compromising the ventrolateral portion of the foramen. Facet hypertrophy decreases dorsolateral foraminal volume. At the disc level, marginal osteophytes and disc protrusions develop. Together, the concentric foraminal narrowing engendered by these osteophytes compresses the spinal nerve, leading to radiculopathy (1). Additional stresses such as trauma or chronic, heavy use exacerbate this process (Fig. 69.11).

Exogenous compression affects all of the tissue components of the nerve, including the nerve fibers themselves, the connective tissue, and the blood vessels. Each of these tissues has different mechanical properties. Below the threshold force of the nerve, no change in function is noted. Above this threshold, functional, and later structural, changes occur. Distortion of the radicular vascular

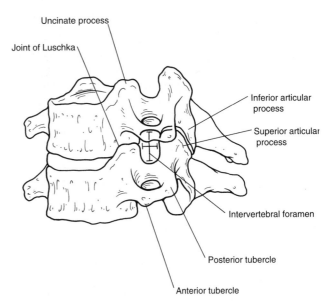

FIG. 69.11. The boundaries of the cervical intervertebral foramen. (Modified from Lestini WF, Wiesel SW. The pathogenesis of cervical spondylosis. *Cervical Orthop Relat Res* 1989;239:69–93, with permission.)

supply may compound any primary mechanical effect on the nerve function. The amount of nerve compression can be indirectly affected by mechanical factors, such as head position, increased intraabdominal pressure (cough, sneeze, Valsalva), or shoulder abduction (83).

The severity of neurologic symptoms accompanying cervical soft disc herniation is inversely related to the sagittal diameter and the area of the bony cervical spinal canal. Although nerves can be compressed without pain and patients with foraminal narrowing may be asymptomatic, 97% of patients with radiculopathy have roentgenographic evidence of foraminal narrowing (25).

Patients with developmentally smaller foramina or spinal canals are more likely to experience symptomatic radiculopathy or myelopathy because there is less reserve volume for the osteophytes or disc protrusions to occupy. When patients undergoing soft cervical discectomy surgery were compared with healthy age-matched individuals, the symptomatic patients had significantly smaller sagittal canal diameters, intervertebral foramen diameters, and cross-sectional canal areas (84). Similarly, patients with spondylotic radiculopathy had smaller foraminal heights, widths, and areas than asymptomatic volunteers (85).

Compression causes pain through both direct and indirect mechanisms. Direct pain generation occurs through deformation of the rich nervous plexus around the spinal nerve and ventral dura (43). These fibers travel with the root's vascular elements and convey both somatic and sympathetic information through the sinuvertebral nerve as well as directly to the DRG (73). The dorsal root and dura, on the other hand, have very few nerve fibers (86).

The dorsal root ganglion is even more sensitive to direct pressure. The normal DRG does not produce spontaneous discharges. Unlike the root, which produces long discharges only when inflamed, the DRG generates prolonged neural discharges after only brief compression (39).

Parke and Whalen's study of the vascular architecture of the DRGs revealed a consistent pattern of internal arterialization and superficial venous drainage (81). This vascular architecture renders the DRG vulnerable to ischemia and, with compression, compartment syndrome. With chronic compression, the DRG changes shape from oval to triangular or crescentic (17).

Radicular symptoms may also be generated through anterior horn cell dysfunction in the ventral spinal cord. This compression is mediated by mechanical compression from spondylotic lipping, disc protrusion, or an associated vascular effect (88).

Chronic compression structurally changes the nerve root. A postmortem study of patients with chronic nerve root compression found demyelination, degeneration, regeneration of nerve fibers, atrophy of DRG cells, prominent venous changes, and fibrosis (89). This nerve and DRG swelling can be seen on computed tomography (CT) myelography and gadolinium-enhanced MRI in patients with disc herniation (90,91). These structural changes in the root may be the source of chronic radiculopathy (33,92).

Role of Inflammation

Only irritated or inflamed roots elicit pain by compression or traction (93). Therefore, secondary mechanisms must play a role in pain production. Cytokines may biochemically induce pain. The presence of cytokines increases spontaneous nerve root activity after compression (94). Epineurally applied cytokines also impair peripheral nerve function (94,95).

The nucleus pulposus has a similar inflammatory effect (96). Autologous porcine nucleus pulposus induces inflammatory reactions as well as structural and functional changes in nerve roots (96–99). Phospholipase A_2 and synovial cytokines may leak from the degenerative facet or disc to the nerve root and cause a chemical radiculitis (44,100). Yabuki and colleagues found that application of nucleus pulposus to the DRG induced vascular changes similar to a compartment syndrome (101). Brisby and co-workers studied the modulators of this inflammatory neuromodulation and reported that a significant portion of this increased activity could be reduced by inhibition of NO synthase (102).

This inflammatory effect is not completely understood, but may explain why some patients have a classic radicular pain pattern in the absence of clear neurocompressive pathology and why other patients with long-standing spinal stenosis suddenly develop leg pain. In one hypothesis, facet synoviocytes or disc chondrocytes become activated and synthesize neutral proteases, prostaglandins, and cytokines

(78). These mediators diffuse to nerve roots, nerve endings, and receptors around spinal joints. These mediators produce pain directly or indirectly by making nerve responsive to minimal compressive forces.

Radicular symptoms may resolve or become chronic. On one hand, a vicious cycle of chronic pain develops in which abnormal inputs up-regulate neural responses, amplifying the incoming signal (41). On the other hand, radicular symptoms resolve after removal or resorption of compressive forces, nerve atrophy leading to decreased space demands, or plastic deformation of the nerve allowing conformation to the space available.

Nonoperative treatment of radiculopathy, based on the elimination of excess motion, cervical distraction, and local and systemic antiinflammatory agents, may arrest this self-perpetuating cycle of irritation by allowing spontaneous resolution of anatomic compression. Lees and Turner followed patients with radiculopathy treated without surgery (103). Half of these patients were stable or improved, one fourth had limited symptoms, and one fourth developed progressive disability.

PATHOPHYSIOLOGY OF MYELOPATHY

Cervical spondylosis accounts for more than half of the cases of cervical myelopathy. However, the cellular pathophysiology is not yet well understood (1,104). Myelopathy results from the interacting effects of developmental and acquired stenosis with vascular and neurologic compression from spondylotic transverse bars, hypertrophic facets, and ligamentum flavum (105). This stenosis affects, in variable degrees, the gray and white matter at various levels of the cord, producing a clinical picture of an incomplete cord lesion involving particular cord elements in a patchy distribution (1,104) (Table 69.1).

Five clinical syndromes of spondylotic myelopathy have been characterized by Crandall and Batzdorf, each of which may have a different underlying pathoanatomy and prognosis (106):

1. *Transverse lesion syndrome* is the most common and involves the posterior column, spinal thalamic, and cortical spinal tracts. Anterior horn cells are also often involved in this syndrome.
2. *Motor system syndrome* preferentially affects the cortical spinal tract, producing upper and lower extremity weakness, gait disturbance, and spasticity, but minimal sensory complaints.
3. *Central cord syndrome* results in greater upper extremity weakness. Painful dysesthesias of the hands may be present.
4. *Brown-Séquard syndrome* causes the development of cross-motor and sensory dysfunction related to unilateral compression of the spinal cord. Pain and temperature analgesia is seen one to two levels below the highest

TABLE 69.1. *Pathophysiology of Cervical Spondylotic Myelopathy (129,134)*

- Mechanical factors
  - Static
    - Developmental Canal stenosis
    - Osteophytes
    - Disk herniations
    - Ossification of the posterior longitudinal ligament
    - Uncovertebral joint spurs
    - Apophyseal joint deformation
    - Ligamentum flavum infolding
  - Dynamic
    - Normal and Abnormal Motion
      - Changes in flexion: spinal cord lengthens causing increased tension on dorsal fiber tracts
      - Changes in extension
    - Loads
    - Hypotonic ligamentum flavum
- Role of Ischemia
  - Pathological evidence
    - Changes in cord predominantly in the distribution of the anterior spinal artery
    - Hyalinization and thickening of walls of anterior spinal artery and perforating vessels
    - Possible role of periradicular fibrosis
  - Experimental evidence
    - Compression of cord with fogerty balloon catheter causes ischemia due to compression/stretching of transversely placed intramedullary vessels
    - Microangographic, autoradiographic and hydrogen clearance evidence of ischemia due to compression
    - Pathophysiological effects of ischemia are additive with compression

level of motor involvement. This syndrome has the best prognosis.

5. *Brachialgia cord syndrome* combines upper extremity root compression with myelopathic long tract findings. Clinically, a mixed cervical myeloradiculopathy is encountered. The classic example of this mixture of upper and motor neuron findings is the inverted radial reflex. Radicular compression on the lower motor neuron decreases the brachioradialis reflex, but cord compression of the upper motor neuron leads to a pathologic spread to the finger flexors, and often to an increased triceps reflex.

Anatomic Basis

The anatomic basis of cervical myelopathy stems from static and dynamic circumferential compromise of the cord from spondylosis and osteophyte production.

Although asymptomatic cord compression has been noted in the literature (107–109), in most cases of cervical myelopathy, greater degrees of cord compression are closely related to worsening neurologic symptoms (110, 111). Penning and others found that long tract signs were only present when the transverse area of the canal was reduced by more than 30%, or a transverse area less than 60 mm² (112). De-

creasing canal dimensions are significantly related to impaired electrophysiologic responses (113).

Static compression arises chiefly from large osteophytic bars along the anterior canal, disc bulging, and infolding of the hypertrophied ligamentum flavum. Decreased intervertebral disc height increases disc diameter at the expense of canal diameter. Disc herniations magnify this effect (Fig. 69.12).

Osteophytic and disc compression is magnified by compression from ligamentous hypertrophy. In early life, the ligamentum flavum is only a few millimeters thick. With age and degeneration, abnormal motion and loss of disc height lead to buckling and thickening (114). In a study of 45 patients undergoing canal expansive procedures for cervical spondylotic myelopathy (CSM), preoperative space available for the cord correlated well with modified Japanese Orthopaedic Association (JOA) scores. Bony canal measurements alone were not as predictive because of the significant role of ligamentous hypertrophy in the degree of canal stenosis (115).

These elements are often coupled with a kyphotic deformity and affect both the spinal cord and its vascular supply (104). The triangular geometry of the canal explains the predominance of motor over sensory symptoms despite the larger degree of canal encroachment from anterior osteophytes (25). Yu and others reported that a triangular canal was associated with severe cord signs, marked pyramidal weakness, and sphincter disturbance (116). In an electrophysiology study, the lateral quarter compression ratio more sensitively predicted spinal cord evoked potentials (SCEPs) than central canal compression (113).

Effects of Developmental Stenosis on Myelopathy

Cervical spondylosis alone does not usually result in myelopathy. The cervical cord is fairly uniform in size from C1 to C7 at 10 mm in diameter (range, 8.5 to 11.5 mm) (117). The normal cervical canal diameter from C3 to C7 is 17 to 18 mm (118,119). From C4 to C7, one fourth of the canal is unoccupied and can accommodate spondylotic spurs without cord compression (Fig. 69.13).

Individuals with developmentally smaller spinal canals have less reserve volume. Thus, congenital stenosis predisposes these patients to myelopathy (118,120). Although a congenitally narrow canal does not necessarily doom a person to myelopathy, symptomatic disease rarely develops in individuals with canals that are larger than 13 mm. In patients with cervical spondylosis, a sagittal diameter of 12 mm or less predicted the development of myelopathy (121,122).

In 1952, Boijsen defined the measurement of canal diameter as the distance from the midpoint of the back of the vertebra to the nearest point of the same vertebral lamina as projected on lateral radiographs (123). Pallis and others noted that spondylotic myelopathy occurred in patients with canal diameter averaging 14 mm (124). Payne

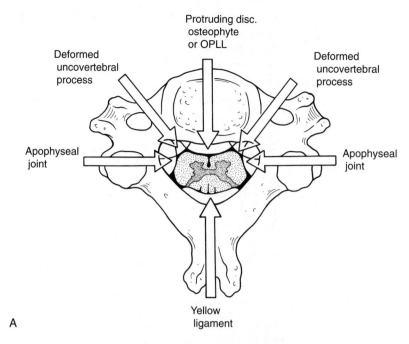

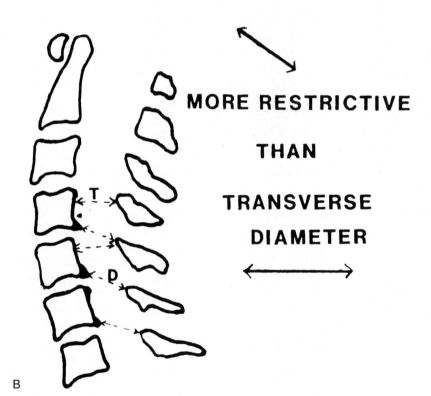

DIAGONAL DIAMETER

MORE RESTRICTIVE

THAN

TRANSVERSE

DIAMETER

FIG. 69.12. Spinal canal narrowing. **A:** Axial schematic depicting sources of stenosis. **B:** Sagittal schematic illustrating the tight constriction in a diagonal direction. (**A** Used with permission; **B** from Parke WW. Correlative anatomy of cervical spondylotic myelopathy. *Spine* 1988;13(7):831–837, with permission.)

and Spillane measured cervical spinal canal diameters from C4 to C7. In patients with myelopathy, the canal was, on average, 3 mm smaller than in nonmyelopathic patients (117).

Several authors have noted the limitations of direct canal diameter measurement from lateral plain radiographs, cit-ing differences in patient size and target-to-film distance (125–127). These studies have established ratios of canal to vertebral width between 0.80 and 0.85 as predictive of the development of myelopathy (127). A recent study found that a low Torg-Pavlov ratio was the most sensitive predictor in differentiating spondylotic and myelopathic patients

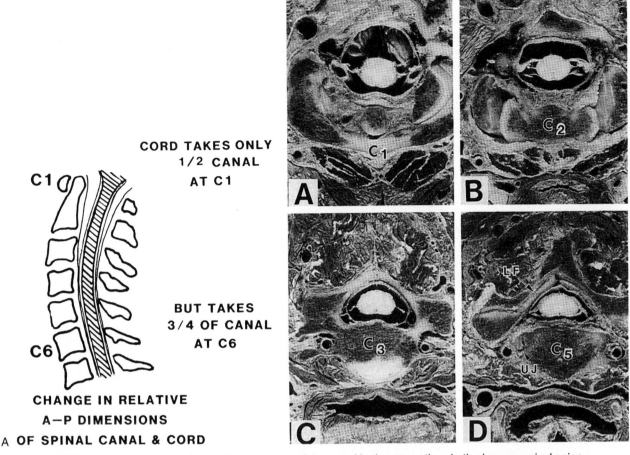

FIG. 69.13. The cord occupies relatively less of the canal in the upper than in the lower cervical spine. **A:** Sagittal schematic. **B:** Axial cryomicrotome photographs from a 68-year-old man. At the C1 level, the dens and the cord each occupy one third of the canal, leaving one third unoccupied (A). Proceeding caudally, there is progressively less room from C2 (B), to C3 (C), to C5 (D). Note the additional decrease in canal diameter at C5 from the infolded ligamentum flavum (LF). (From Parke WW. Correlative anatomy of cervical spondylotic myelopathy. *Spine* 1988;13(7):831–837, with permission.)

from nonspondylotic, nonmyelopathic patients (128) (Fig. 69.14).

Effects of Spine Motion on Myelopathy

Degeneration of the motion segment also leads to instability. At rest, spondylolisthesis decreases canal dimensions. In patients with a mobile spondylolisthesis, this effect is magnified, leading to a so-called guillotine effect on the cord (129). Even in the absence of segmental instability, flexion and extension accentuate the degree of spinal cord compression. White and Panjabi reviewed the role of the dentate ligament in holding the cord against the spurs anteriorly (129). More recently, dentate ligaments have not been considered a major contributor in CSM.

The cervical spinal cord itself changes in diameter through neck motion. During flexion, the spinal cord lengthens and thins but is stretched over ventral osteophytic bars. An autopsy study confirmed focal points of compression over anterior bars (130). In extension, the cord's cross-sectional are increases while its length decreases. Vertebral

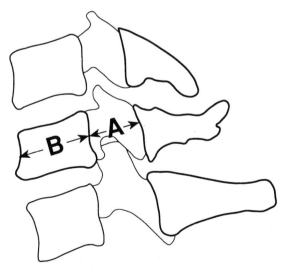

FIG. 69.14. Ratio between the sagittal diameter of the spinal canal (**A**) and the vertebral body (**B**). (From Law M, Bernhardt M, White A. Evaluation and management of cervical spondylotic myelopathy. *J Bone Joint Surg Am* 1994;76: 1420–1433, with permission.)

971

body retrolisthesis may occur along the plane of facet inclination, leading to 2 to 3 mm of additional spinal canal narrowing (22). This motion further approximates the two closest points of the cervical canal: the posteroinferior vertebral edge of the superior vertebra and the superior central laminar edge of the inferior vertebra. Moreover, ligamentum flavum infolding increases with extension (117) (Fig. 69.15).

Motion also affects cord vascularity. Whereas the *pincher movement* between the flavum and the anterior osteophytes compresses the cord directly, it also affects the anterior spinal and vertebral arteries (131,132). Moreover, the flattening of the cord with motion results in transverse widening, affecting the internal arteriole system. This decreased canal size, coupled with increased cord size, further endangers the blood supply. The relative decrease in canal size with motion increases with age and spondylosis (133).

Effects of Vascular Compromise on Myelopathy

The role of spinal cord ischemia in the pathophysiology of CSM was first proposed by Brain in 1948 (134). The histopathologic changes that are observed in CSM frequently involve gray matter, with minimal white matter involvement. This pattern is more consistent with ischemic

insult than with direct, mechanical compression (130). Further, symptoms often extend to cord levels cranial to the source of compression (135). Vascular embarrassment can arise as a result of direct compression of the anterior spinal artery, distortion of the sulcal arteries, or compression of the segmental feeders in the foramen (Fig. 69.16).

Mair and Druckman observed hyalinization and thickening of the walls of the anterior spinal artery and in the parenchymal arterioles (136). Thrombus formation in the artery itself is rare (1). In many patients with cervical spondylosis, major symptoms are those of vertebrobasilar insufficiency. The vertebral arteries become tortuous, and flow is restricted by head position, particularly rotation (137).

The gray matter and medial white matter are typically affected early in the course of CSM. Their blood supply arises from transverse perforating vessels that arborize from the sulcal arteries and pass transversely through the substance of the cord. With flattening of the cord, these vessels are stretched, thereby decreasing luminal volume. Areas of the cord that are typically affected only late in CSM have differing vascular trees. The subpial portion of dorsal columns, for example, is resistant to ventral compression because posterior spinal arteries zigzag and are not put under tension when the cord elongates in cervical flexion (138). Similarly, the anterior columns are supplied by

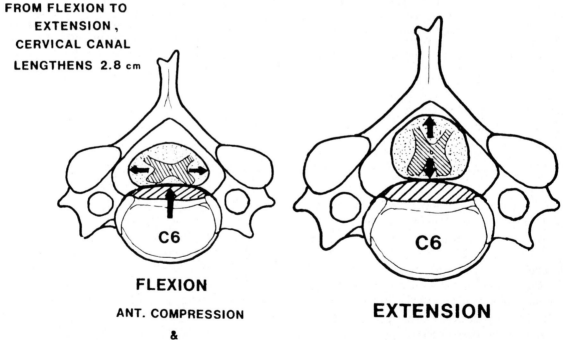

FIG. 69.15. Changes in the degree of stenosis with cervical flexion and extension. **A:** In flexion, the spinal cord lengthens 2.8 cm. In the process, it is flattened against the spondylotic bars anteriorly. **B:** In extension, the cord decreases in length and increases in diameter, increasing the degree of posterior compression. (From Parke WW. Correlative anatomy of cervical spondylotic myelopathy. *Spine* 1988; 13(7):831–837, with permission.)

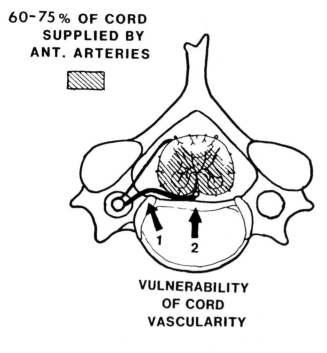

60-75% OF CORD SUPPLIED BY ANT. ARTERIES

VULNERABILITY OF CORD VASCULARITY

1. LAT. HYPERTROPHIES

2. CENTRAL "BARS"

FIG. 69.16. Spondylotic threats to spinal cord vascularity include uncovertebral joint hypertrophy (1) and disc-level spondylotic bars (2). (From Parke WW. Correlative anatomy of cervical spondylotic myelopathy. *Spine* 1988;13(7):831–837, with permission.)

arteries running in an anteroposterior direction and are thus not affected by stresses flattening the cord itself.

Experimental evidence of ischemia in animal models of CSM is based on microangiography, autoradiography, and hydrogen clearance experiments (139–141). Doppman and others used a Fogerty balloon catheter to compress the anterior, posterior, and lateral cord (142). Anterior compression compromised cord perfusion through the transverse arterioles arising from the anterior sulcal arteries. When the cord was compressed posteriorly, perfusion was reduced to the intramedullary branches in the central gray matter. Accordingly, stretching the cord laterally or flattening the cord elongates and interrupts the transverse intramedullary arteries, decreasing perfusion to the gray matter in adjacent lateral columns. Shimomura and associates studied the effect of ischemia in conjunction with compression of the cervical cord in dogs and demonstrated that obstruction of the peripial arterial plexus could cause intramedullary cavitation (143). The oligodendroglia are particularly vulnerable to ischemic injury. Ischemia therefore accounts for the demyelination that occurs in chronic CSM (111).

The role of foraminal occlusion in the pathogenesis of myelopathy is more debatable. Taylor suggested that radicular arteries to the cervical spinal cord were interrupted by fibrosis in the intervertebral foramina (144). The radicular arteries within the dural sleeves tolerate compression and repetitive minor trauma poorly. The dominant vessels enter in the lower cervical spine at the same levels prone to spondylotic foraminal narrowing. Wilkinson and colleagues demonstrated a relationship between foraminal narrowing and myelopathy (25). On the other hand, in Crandall and Batzdorf's study, no evidence of foraminal narrowing was noted in 58% of their patients with myelopathy (106). None of Lee and Turner's patients with radiculopathy went on to develop myelopathy despite the fact that at least some of these patients would be expected to have foraminal stenosis (103). Even the Wilkinson study found that canal diameter was a greater predictor of myelopathy than foraminal volume (25).

It is likely that ischemia and compression have additive effects on spinal cord dysfunction. Gooding and associates examined the combined effects of anterior spinal cord compression and segmental artery ligation in dogs (145). Ischemia exacerbated the pathologic effects of compression on the spinal cord, particularly in the vulnerable corticospinal tracts. Kobrine and colleagues studied vascular effects on the spinal evoked potentials in monkeys and concluded that although both mechanical compression and vascular compromise of the cord were factors in neurologic dysfunction, compression of neurologic elements was more important (146).

Pathoanatomy of Myelopathy

The natural history of cervical myelopathy is not as favorable as that of radiculopathy. Typically, patients follow a slow and insidious course with gradual, stepwise increases in dysfunction. Accelerated progression is occasionally noted, particularly in patients with abnormal motion, such as those with degenerative spondylolisthesis (1).

In the series by Clark and Robinson, no patient ever returned to a normal state (147). Three fourths of patients demonstrated episodic worsening. In 20%, slow, steady progression was seen. Five percent had a rapid onset followed by lengthy disability. Lees and Turner characterized stepwise progression with periods of quiescent stability between exacerbations (103). Nurick noted that the degree of disability was often established early in the disease (148). Roberts studied 24 patients with cervical myelopathy for up to 6½ years (149). In his series, about one third improved, one third remained the same, and one third deteriorated. Roberts found that motor symptoms tended to be much more progressive and less likely to improve than sensory abnormalities.

Indicators for poor prognosis include duration of symptoms longer than 6 months at time of presentation, vertebral canal-to-body ratio of less than 0.8, and cord compression ratio after surgery of less than 0.4 (150). These natural history and prognosis data are supported by a histologic analysis of cadaver specimens with chronic cord compression. In

TABLE 69.2. *Pathology of Cervical Spondylotic Myelopathy (134) Central Gray and Medial White Matter Most Severely Affected*

- Wallerian degeneration of posterior columns cephalad to site of compression
- Wallerian degeneration of corticospinal tracts caudal to site of compression
- Relative sparing of anterior column
- Progression of pathologic changes varies with severity of compression
  - Lateral corticospinal tracts most vulnerable
  - Anterior horn cell loss or localized infarction of gray matter associated with severe compression
  - Extensive infarction of gray and white matter associated with anterior-posterior compression ratio of < 20%

these specimens, the central gray and medial portions of the myelinated long tracts are affected most severely with cystic cavitation, gliosis, and demyelination (139). Wallerian degeneration of the posterior columns and posterolateral tracts occurred cephalad to the site of compression. Anterior horn cell dropout occurred at the site of compression, and the corticospinal tracts underwent degeneration, with loss of myelin staining caudal to the site of compression (Table 69.2).

In one autopsy examination of spinal cord tissue from seven patients with cervical spondylotic myelopathy, atrophy of the anterior horn and intermediate zone of the gray matter was seen in the compressed segments in all cases (151). Atrophy and myelin pallor in the lateral and posterior funiculi were observed in six patients. The lateral funiculi of two were severely affected. Many thin myelinated fibers and denuded axons were demonstrated ultrastructurally in the damaged white matter, suggesting that demyelinating and remyelinating processes occur in cervical spondylotic myelopathy. A common pattern of lesion progression in cervical spondylotic myelopathy was inferred:

- Atrophy and neuronal loss in the anterior horn and intermediate zone develops first.
- This is followed by degeneration of the lateral and posterior funiculi.
- Eventually, marked atrophy develops throughout the entire gray matter, and severe degeneration occurs in the lateral funiculus.

Ono and associates (152) and Ogino and co-workers (111) reported similar necropsy findings in patients with

myelopathy documented premortally. Again, extensive destruction of both gray and white matter was noted, with demyelinization above and below the lesions. Posterolateral white matter fibers, including the lateral corticospinal tracts, were most susceptible to minor degrees of compression. Anterior horn cell loss and localized infarction of the gray matter were associated with more severe degrees of compression. The anterior and medial dorsal columns were remarkably resistant to degeneration. A good correlation was noted between compression ratio and areas of most severe cord infarction, with extensive infarct in areas with anteroposterior compression ratios of less than 20%. Ono and associates (152) concluded that the spastic paralysis seen clinically was from descending pyramidal tract involvement and that sensory changes precipitated from ascending posterior funiculus lesions (Fig. 69.17).

Implications of Spinal Cord Injury Research to the Pathophysiology of Cervical Spondylotic Myelopathy

In that there is only limited information about the pathophysiology of CSM at the cellular level, Fehlings and Skaf correlated research findings from the pathophysiology of acute spinal cord injury (134). Myelopathy and traumatic cord injury may hold several factors at the cellular level in common, including glutamate-mediated cell death, free radical injury, cationic injury, and cellular apoptosis (Table 69.3).

In both acute and chronic neurologic diseases, increased extracellular glutamate has been proposed as a mechanism of neuronal cell death. There are two varieties of glutamate receptors: inotropic and metabotropic. Ionotropic receptors gate entry of Na^+ and Ca^{2+} ions and include subgroups gated by compounds such as 2-Amino-3 (3-Hydroxy-5-Methylisoxasol-4yl)-Proprionic Acid (AMPA), kainate, and NMDA. Metabotropic receptors are coupled to guanosine triphosphate–binding proteins. Agonists impair intracellular energy metabolism and increases neuronal vulnerability to glutamate. Therefore, blocking these receptors may have therapeutic value.

Free radical and lipid peroxidation reactions have a role in the pathophysiology of traumatic and ischemic injury to the CNS. The modest effects of high-dose steroids in spinal cord injury may be mediated by blocking this peroxidation (153,154). Similarly, the delayed anterior horn cell loss in CSM may partially involve free radical–mediated injury. If

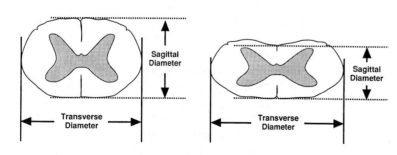

FIG. 69.17. The measurement of cord compression ratio by dividing the sagittal diameter over the transverse diameter. (From Law M, Bernhardt M, White A. Evaluation and management of cervical spondylotic myelopathy. *J Bone Joint Surg Am* 1994;76:1420–1433, with permission.)

TABLE 69.3. *Mechanisms of Traumatic Spinal Cord Injury of Potential Relevance to Cervical Spondylotic Myelopathy (134)*

- mechanical factors (static/dynamic)
- ischemia
- free-radical mediated cell injury
- cation-mediated injury (NA^+/Ca^{++})
  - linked to protease activation (calpain)
- glutamatergic cell injury
  - ionotropic glutamate receptors
    - NMDA (anterior horn cell injury)
    - AMPA/kainite (white matter injury)
  - Metabotropic receptors (coupled to G proteins)
    - Group 1 mGluRs (linked to rises in Ca^{++} through PLC)
    - Group 2,3 mGluRs (negatively coupled to cAMP)
- Apoptosis (programmed cell death)
  - Proaptotic genes: Bax, Bcl-xS, c-fos, c-jun, p75NGFR, and ICE-like proteases
  - Genes that block apoptosis: Bcl-2 and Bcl-xl

so, antioxidants and free radical scavengers may be useful in the treatment of myelopathic patients.

Cationic-mediated injury occurs in states of energy depletion. Failure of the Na^+-K^+-ATP pump results in accumulation of axonal Na^+. This accumulated cation, in turn, reverses normal Na^+/Ca^{2+} exchange, leading to Ca^{2+} overload. Additional calcium activates several calcium-dependent enzymes, including calpain, phospholipase, and protein kinase C, resulting in cytoskeletal injury. Given that CSM involves both compressive and ischemic injury, cationic-mediated cell injury may play a role, particularly with regard to destruction of the myelinated tracts.

Apoptosis refers to programmed cell death as a distinct form of controlled cellular degeneration. Apoptosis is distinguished from necrosis by the absence of inflammation, by internucleosomal DNA cleavage, and by its regulation through specific genes. Apoptosis serves physiologic functions, such as cellular population control, during development and deletion of abnormal cells. A number of genes have been identified that promote apoptosis (*Bax, Bcl-xS, c-fos, c-jun, p75NGFR*, and Interleukin Converting Enzyme [ICE]-like proteases) and block apoptosis (*Bcl-2* and *Bcl-xl*) (134). In acute spinal injury, both secondary degeneration at the site of injury and chronic demyelination of tracts distant to the site of injury are mediated by apoptosis. The delayed degeneration of anterior horn cells seen in CSM may also reflect apoptosis. Apoptotic-signaling pathway blockers may someday be useful in the treatment of CSM.

A recent study of the histologic changes of chronic compression included a mouse myelopathy model as well as a histochemical analysis of human cadaveric material (155). Apoptotic cells were observed in the chronically compressed spinal cord in both the autopsy of a human patient and in model mice. Descending degeneration in the anterior and lateral columns and ascending degeneration in the posterior column were observed, with a resulting irreversible neurologic deficit. These histologic factors may explain the variable clinical recovery seen after decompressive surgery (156).

CONCLUSION

Degenerative changes are nearly ubiquitous in the aging cervical spine. In some patients, these changes lead to pain or neurologic dysfunction, resulting in the clinical syndrome of degenerative disc disease, radiculopathy, and myelopathy. Often, these syndromes overlap.

Susceptibility to degenerative change is genetically encoded. Biochemical changes in the nucleus result in desiccation and alteration of the mechanical properties of the motion segment. The annulus may tear, leading to protrusion of disc material and radiculopathy. In others, abnormal motion and osteophyte formation are encountered. In patients with congenitally narrowed foramina and central spinal canals, compression on the cord, nerve root, or their vascular supply leads to pain and dysfunction. Over time, compression permanently changes the structure of the roots and cord.

REFERENCES

1. Lestini WF, Wiesel SW. The pathogenesis of cervical spondylosis. *Cervical Orthop Relat Res* 1989;239:69–93.
2. Praemer A, Furner S, Rice DP. *Musculoskeletal conditions in the United States.* Rosemont, IL: American Academy of Orthopaedic Surgeons, 1999:27–70.
3. Abumi K, Ito M, Kaneda K. Surgical treatment of cervical destructive spondyloarthropathy (DSA). *Spine* 2000;25(22):2899–2905.
4. Cotran RS, Kumar V, Robbins SL. *Pathologic basis of disease,* 5th ed. Philadelphia: WB Saunders, 1994:1–2.
5. Buckwalter JA. Aging and degeneration of the human intervertebral disk. *Spine* 1995;20:1307–1314.
6. Lotz, JC, Colliou OK, Chin JR, et al. 1998 Volvo Award Winner in Biomechanical Studies. Compression-induced degeneration of the intervertebral disc: an in vivo mouse model and finite-element study. *Spine* 1998;23(23):2493–2506.
7. Hendry NG. The hydration of the nucleus pulposus and its relation to the intervertebral disc derangement. *J Bone Joint Surg Br* 1958;40:132.
8. Nachemson A. Lumbar intradiscal pressure. Experimental studies on postmortem material. *Acta Orthop Scand* 1960;43-S:]9.
9. Hunt WE. Cervical spondylosis. Natural History and rare indications for surgical decompression. *Clin Neurosurg* 1980;27:466.
10. Urban JPG, Holm S, Maroudas A, et al. Nutrition of the intervertebral disc. *Clin Orthop* 1977;129:101–114.
11. Lindblom K. Intervertebral disc degeneration considered as pressure atrophy. *J Bone Joint Surg Am* 1957;39:933–945.
12. Kang JD, Stefanovic-Racic M, McIntyre LA, et al. Toward a biochemical understanding of human intervertebral disc degeneration and herniation contributions of nitric oxide, interleukins, prostaglandin E₂, and matrix metalloproteinases. *Spine* 1997;22(10):1065–1073.
13. Kanemoto M, Hukuda S, Komiya Y, et al. Immunohistochemical study of matrix metalloproteinase-3 and tissue inhibitor of metalloproteinase-1 in human intervertebral discs. *Spine* 1996;21(1):1–8.
14. Ariga K, Yonenobu K, Nakase T, et al. Localization of cathepsins D, K, and L in degenerated human intervertebral discs. *Spine* 2001;26(24):2666–2672.
15. Kirkaldy-Willis WH, Wedge JH, Young-Hing K, et al. Pathology and pathogenesis of lumbar spondylosis and stenosis. *Spine* 1978;3:319.
16. Pal GP, Sherk HH. The vertical stability of the cervical spine. *Spine* 1988;13:447–449.
17. Holt S, Yates PO. Cervical spondylosis and nerve root lesions. Incidence at routine necropsy. *J Bone Joint Surg Br* 1966;48(3):407–423.
18. Coventry MB. Anatomy of the intervertebral disc. *Clin Orthop* 1969;67:9.
19. Coventry MB, Ghormley RK, Kernohan JW. The intervertebral disc. Its microscopic anatomy and pathology. I. Anatomy, development and physiology. *J Bone Joint Surg* 1945;27:105.

20. Coventry MB, Ghormley RK, Kernohan JW. The intervertebral disc. Its microscopic anatomy and pathology. II. Changes in the intervertebral disc concomitant with age. *J Bone Joint Surg* 1945;27:233.

21. Coventry MB, Ghormley RK, Kernohan JW. The intervertebral disc. Its microscopic anatomy and pathology. III. Pathological changes in the intervertebral disc. *J Bone Joint Surg* 1945;27:460.

22. Penning L. Some aspects of plain radiography of the cervical spine in chronic myelopathy. *Neurology* 1962;12:513.

23. Takae R, Matsunaga S, Origuchi N, et al. Immunolocalization of bone morphogenetic protein and its receptors in degeneration of intervertebral disc. *Spine* 1999;24(14):1397.

24. Ten Have HA, Eulderink F. Degenerative changes in the cervical spine and their relationship to its mobility. *J Pathol* 1980;132:133.

25. Wilkinson HA, LeMay ML, Ferris EJ. Clinical-radiographic correlation in cervical spondylosis. *J Neurosurg* 1969;30:313.

26. Dai L. Disc degeneration and cervical instability: correlation of magnetic resonance imaging with radiography. *Spine* 1998;23(16):1734–1738.

27. MacNab I. Cervical spondylosis. *Clin Orthop* 1975;109:69.

28. Parke WW. Correlative anatomy of cervical spondylotic myelopathy. *Spine* 1988;13(7):831–837.

29. Lind B, Sihlbom H, Nordwall A, et al. Normal range of motion of the cervical spine. *Arch Phys Med Rehabil* 1989;70(9):692–695.

30. Lipson SJ, Mujir H. Vertebral osteophyte formation in experimental disc degeneration. Morphologic and proteoglycan changes over time. *Arthritis Rheum* 1980;23:319.

31. Bannister G, Gargan M. Prognosis of whiplash injuries. A review of the spine. In: *State of the art reviews*. Philadelphia: Hanley & Belfus;, 1993:557–570.

32. Coderre TJ, Katz J, Vaccarrino AL, et al. Contribution of central neuroplasticity to pathological pain. Review of clinical and experimental evidence. *Pain* 1993;52:259–285.

33. Jayson MIV, Keegan A, Million R, et al. A fibrinolytic defect in chronic back pain syndromes. *Lancet* 1984;2:1186–1187.

34. Wilson PR. Chronic neck pain and cervicogenic headache. *Clin J Pain* 1991;7:5–11.

35. Ellenberg MR, Honet JC, Treanor WJ. Cervical radiculopathy. *Arch Phys Med Rehabil* 1994;75(3):342–352.

36. Olmarker K, Myers RR. Pathogenesis of sciatic pain. Role of herniated nucleus pulposus and deformation of spinal nerve root and dorsal root ganglion. *Pain* 1998;78:99–105.

37. Malmberg AB, Yaksh TL. Hyperalgesia mediated by spinal glutamate or substance P receptor blocked by spinal cyclooxygenase inhibition. *Science* 1992;257:1276–1279.

38. Rydevik B, McLean WG, Sjostrand J, et al. Blockage of axonal transport induced by acute, graded compression of the rabbit vagus nerve. *J Neurol Neursurg Pscychiatry* 1980;43:690–698.

39. Howe JF, Loeser JD, Calvin WH. Mechanosensitivity of dorsal root ganglia and chronically injured axons. A physiologic basis for the radicular pain of nerve root compression. *Pain* 1977;3:25–41.

40. Wall PD, Devor M. Sensory afferent impulses originate from dorsal root ganglia as well as from the periphery in normal and nerve impaired rats. *Pain* 1983;17:321–329.

41. Rydevik B, Hasue M, Wehling P. Etiology of sciatic pain and mechanisms of nerve root compression. In: Wiesel SW, et al., eds. *The lumbar Spine*, 2nd ed. Philadelphia: WB Saunders, 1996:123–141.

42. Rydevik B, Brown MD, Lundborg G. Pathoanatomy and pathophysiology of nerve root compression. *Spine* 1984;9:7–15.

43. Yamada H, Honda T, Kikuchi S, et al. Direct innervation of sensory fibers from the dorsal root ganglion of the cervical dura mater of rats. *Spine* 1998;23(14):1524–1529.

44. Marshall LL, Trethewie ER, Curtain CC. Chemical radiculitis. A clinical, physiological, and immunological study. *Clin Orthop* 1977;129:61–67.

45. Mendell LM. Modifiability of spinal synapses. *Physiol Rev* 1984;64:260–324.

46. Li P, Zhou M. Cholinergic, noradrenergic, and serotonergic inhibition of fast synaptic transmission in spinal lumbar dorsal horn of rat. *Brain Res Bull* 2001;54(6):639–647.

47. Nakanishi S. Mammalian tachykinin receptors. *Ann Rev Neurosci* 1991;14:123–136.

48. Hokfelt T. Neuropeptides in perspective. The last ten years. *Neuron* 1991;7:867–879.

49. Womack MD, MacDermott AB, Jessell TM. Sensory transmitters regulate intracellular calcium in dorsal horn neurons. *Nature* 1988;334:351–353.

50. Collingridge GL, Singer W. Excitatory amino acid receptors and synaptic plasticity. *Trends Pharmacol Sci* 1990;11:290–296.

51. Dickenson AH, Ayday E. Antagonism at the glycine site on the NMDA receptor reduces spinal nociception in the rat. *Neurosci Lett* 1991;121:263–266.

52. Meller ST, Gebhart GF. Nitric oxide and nociceptive processing in the spinal cord. *Pain* 1993;52:127–136.

53. Snyder SH, Bredt DS. Biological roles of nitric oxide. *Sci Am* 1992; May:28–35.

54. Clark CR. Degenerative conditions of the spine: Differential diagnosis and non-surgical treatment. In: Frymoyer JW, ed. *The adult spine: principles and practice*. New York: Raven Press, 1991:1154–1164.

55. Devor M, Wall PD. Plasticity in the spinal cord sensory map following peripheral nerve injury. *J Neurosci* 1981;1:671–684.

56. Woolf CJ, Shortland P, Coggeshell RE. Peripheral nerve injury triggers central sprouting of myelinated afferents. *Nature* 1992;355:75–77.

57. Parke WW. Applied anatomy of the spine. In: Rothman R, Simeone F, eds. *The spine*. Philadelphia: WB Saunders, 1975:36.

58. Heller JG. The syndromes of degenerative cervical disease. *Orthop Clin North Am* 1992;23(3):381–394.

59. Barnsley L, Lord S, Wallis B, et al. False-positive rates of cervical zygapophysial joint blocks. *Clin J Pain* 1993;9(2):124–130.

60. Bogduk N, Windsor M, Inglis A. The innervation of the cervical intervertebral discs. *Spine* 1988;13(1):2–8.

61. Cavanaugh JM, Ozaktay AC, Yamashita HT, et al. Lumbar facet pain: biomechanics, neuroanatomy and neurophysiology. *J Biomech* 1996; 29(9):1117–1129.

62. Giles LG, Harvey AR. Immunohistochemical demonstration of nociceptors in the capsule and synovial folds of human zygapophyseal joints. *Br J Rheumatol* 1987;26(5):362–364.

63. Dvorék J. Epidemiology, physical examination, and neurodiagnostics. *Spine* 1998;23(24):2663–2672.

64. Dwyer A, April C, Bogduk N. Cervical zygapophyseal joint pain patterns. I. A study in normal volunteers. *Spine* 1990;15(6):453–457.

65. April C, Dwyer A, Bogduk N. Cervical zygapophyseal joint pain patterns. II. A clinical evaluation. *Spine* 1990;15(6):458–461.

66. Dahlin LB, Rydevik B, McLean WG, et al. Changes in fast axonal transport during experimental nerve compression at low pressures. *Exp Neurol* 1984;84:29–36.

67. Leone J, Ochs S. Anoxic block and recovery of axoplasmic transport and electrical excitability of nerve. *J Neurobiol* 1978;9:229–245.

68. Kikuchi S, Sato K, Konno S, et al. Anatomic and radiographic study of dorsal root ganglia. *Spine* 1994;19:6–11.

69. Haller ER, Low FN. The fine structure of the peripheral nerve root sheath in the subarachnoid space in the rat and other laboratory animals. *Am J Anat* 1971;131:1–20.

70. Jacobs JM, Macfarlande RM, Cavanaugh JB. Vascular leakage in the dorsal root ganglia of the rat studied with horseradish peroxidase. *J Neurol Sci* 1976;29:95–107.

71. Olsson Y. Topographical differences in the vascular permeability of the peripheral nervous system. *Acta Neuropathol* 1968;10:26–33.

72. Lazorthes G, Gouaze A, Zadeh JO, et al. Arterial vascularization of the spinal cord. Recent studies of the anatomic substitution pathways. *J Neurosurg* 1971;35:253–262.

73. Parke WW, Watanabe R. The intrinsic vasculature of the lumbosacral spinal nerve roots. *Spine* 1985;10:508–515.

74. Pettersson CAV, Olsson Y. Blood supply of spinal nerve roots. An experimental study in the root. *Acta Neuropathol* 1989;78:455–461.

75. Parke WW, Gammell K, Rothman RH. Arterial vascularization of the cauda equine. *J Bone Joint Surg Am* 1981;63:52–62.

76. Waggoner JD, Beggs J. The membranous coverings of neural tissues. An electron microscopic study. *J Neuropathol* 1967;26:412–426.

77. Sunderland S, Bradley KC. Stress-strain phenomena in human spinal nerve roots. *Brain* 1961;84:120–125.

78. Baratz ME, Georgescu HI, Evans CH. Studies on the autocrine activation of a synovial cell line. *J Orthop Res* 1991;9:651–657.

79. Stodieck LS, Beel JA, Luttges MW. Structural properties of spinal nerve roots. Protein composition. *Exp Neurol* 1986;91:41–51.

80. Gamble HJ. Comparative electron-microscopic observations on the connective tissues of a peripheral nerve and a spinal nerve root in the rat. *J Anat* 1964;98:17–25.

81. Murphy RW. Nerve roots and spinal nerves in degenerative disc disease. *Clin Orthop* 1977;129:46–60.

82. Stookey B. Compression of the spinal cord and nerve roots by herniation of nucleus pulposus in cervical region. *Arch Surg* 1940;40:417.

83. Davidson RI, Dunn EJ, Metzmaker JN. The shoulder abduction relief test in the diagnosis of radicular pain in cervical extradural compressive monoradiculopathies. *Spine* 1981;6:441.

84. Debois V, Herz R, Berghmans D, et al. Soft cervical disc herniation: influence of cervical spinal canal measurements on development of neurologic symptoms. *Spine* 1999;24(19):1996.

85. Humphreys SC, Hodges SD, Patwardhan A, et al. The natural history of the cervical foramen in symptomatic and asymptomatic individuals aged 20–60 years as measured by magnetic resonance imaging: a descriptive approach. *Spine* 1998;23(20):2180–2184.

86. Groen GJ, Baljet B, Drukker J. The innervation of the spinal dura mater. Anatomic and clinical implications. *Acta Neurochir* 1988;92: 39–46.

87. Parke WW, Whalen JL. The vascular pattern of the human dorsal root ganglion and its probable bearing on a compartment syndrome. *Spine* 2002;27:247–352.

88. Alexander JT. Natural history and nonoperative management of cervical spondylosis. In: Menezes AH, Sonntag VKH, et al, eds. *Principles of spinal surgery*, Vol 1. New York: McGraw-Hill, 1996: 547–557.

89. Watanabe R, Parke WW. The vascular and neural pathology of lumbosacral spinal stenosis. *J Neurosurg* 1986;64:64–70.

90. Takata K, Inoue S, Takahishi K, et al. Swelling of the cauda equine in patients who have herniation of a lumbar disc. *J Bone Joint Surg Am* 1988;70:361–368.

91. Toyone T, Takahishi K, Kitahara H, et al. Visualization of symptomatic nerve roots. *J Bone Joint Surg Br* 1993;75:529–533.

92. Cooper RG, Mitchell WS, Illingworth KJ, et al. The role of epidural fibrosis and defective fibrinolysis in the persistence of postlaminectomy back pain. *Spine* 1991;16:1044–1048.

93. Smyth MJ, Wright V. Sciatica and the intervertebral disc. An experimental study. *J Bone Joint Surg Am* 1958;40:1401–1418.

94. Wehling P, Bandara G, Evans CH. Synovial cytokines impair the function of sciatic nerve in rats. *Neuro Orthop* 1989;7:55–59.

95. Wehling P, Pak MA, Cleveland SJ, et al. The influence on spinal cord evoked potentials of chymopapain applied to the rat lumbar spinal canal. *Spine* 1989;14:65–67.

96. Olmarker K, Rydevik B, Nordberg D. Autologous nucleus pulposus induces neurophysiologic and histologic changes in porcine cauda equine nerve roots. *Spine* 1993;18:1425–1432.

97. Anzai H, Hamba M, Onda A, et al. Epidural application of nucleus pulposus enhances nociresponses of rat dorsal horn neurons. *Spine* 2002;27:E50–55.

98. Iwabuchi M, Rydevik B, Kikuchi S, et al. Effects of anulus fibrosus and experimentally degenerated nucleus pulposus on nerve root conduction velocity: relevance of previous experimental investigations using normal nucleus pulposus. *Spine* 2001;26(15):1651–1655.

99. Takebayashi T, Cavanaugh JM, Cuneyt Ozaktay A, et al. Effect of nucleus pulposus on the neural activity of dorsal root ganglion. *Spine* 200115;26(8):940–945.

100. Saal JS, Franson RC, Dobrow R, et al. High levels of inflammatory phospholipase A activity in lumbar disc herniations. *Spine* 1990;15: 674–678.

101. Yabuki S, Igarashi T, Kikuchi S. Application of nucleus pulposus to the nerve root simultaneously reduces blood flow in dorsal root ganglion and corresponding hindpaw in the rat. *Spine*. 2000;25(12):1471–6.

102. Brisby H, Byrod G, Olmarker K, et al. Nitric oxide as a mediator of nucleus pulposus-induced effects on spinal nerve roots. *J Orthop Res* 2000;18(5):815–820.

103. Lees F, Turner JWA. Natural history and prognosis of cervical spondylosis. *BMJ* 1963;2:1607–1610.

104. Law M, Bernhardt M, White A. Evaluation and management of cervical spondylotic myelopathy. *J Bone Joint Surg Am* 1994;76:1420–1433.

105. Bohlman HH, Emery SE. The pathophysiology of cervical spondylosis and myelopathy. *Spine* 1988;13:843–846.

106. Crandall PH, Batzdorf U. Cervical spondylotic myelopathy. *J Neurosurg* 1966;25:57–66.

107. Boden SD, McCowin PR, Davis DO, et al. Abnormal magnetic-resonance scans of the cervical spine in asymptomatic subjects. A prospective investigation. *J Bone Joint Surg Am* 1990;72(8):1178–1184.

108. Matsumoto M, Fujimura Y, Suzuki N, et al. MRI and cervical intervertebral discs in asymptomatic subjects. *J Bone Joint Surg Br* 1998; 80;19–24.

109. Teresi LM, Lufkin RB, Reicher MA, et al. Asymptomatic degenerative disk disease and spondylosis of the cervical spine: MR imaging. *Radiology* 1987;164(1):83–88.

110. Okada Y, Ikata T, Yamada H, et al. Magnetic resonance imaging study on the results of surgery for cervical compression myelopathy of the cervical spine. *Spine* 1993;18:2024–2029.

111. Ogino H, Tada K, Okada K, et al. Canal diameter, anteroposterior compression ratio, and spondylotic myelopathy of the cervical spine. *Spine* 1983;8:1–15.

112. Penning L, Wilmink JT, van Woerden HH, et al. CT myelographic findings in degenerative disorders of the cervical spine: clinical significance. *AJR Am J Roentgenol* 1986;146(4):793–801.

113. Kanchiku T, Taguchi T, Kaneko K, et al. A correlation between magnetic resonance imaging and electrophysiological findings in cervical spondylotic myelopathy. *Spine* 2001;26(13):e294–e299.

114. Yoshia M, Shima K, Taniguchi Y, et al. Hypertrophied ligamentum flavum in lumbar spinal stenosis. *Spine* 1992;17:1353.

115. Hagen KB, Harms-Ringdahl K, Enger NO, et al. Relationship between subjective neck disorders and cervical spine mobility and motion-related pain in male machine operators. *Spine* 1997;22(13): 1501–1507.

116. Yu YL, Boulay JM, Stevens JM, et al. Computer-assisted myelography in cervical spondylotic myelopathy and radiculopathy. *Brain* 1986;109:259–278.

117. Payne EE, Spillane JD. The cervical spine. An anatomico-pathologic study of 70 specimens with particular reference to the problem of cervical spondylosis. *Brain* 1957;80:571.

118. Hayashi H, Okada K, Hamada M, et al. Etiologic factors of myelopathy. A radiographic evaluation of the aging changes in the cervical spine. *Clin Orthop* 1997;214:200–209.

119. Burrows EH. The sagittal diameter of the spinal canal in cervical spondylosis. *Clin Radiol* 1963;14:77–86.

120. Edwards WC, LaRocca H. The developmental segmental sagittal diameter of the cervical spinal cord in patients with cervical spondylosis. *Spine* 1983;8:20–27.

121. Adams CB, Logue V. Studies in cervical spondylotic myelopathy. II. The movement and contour of the spine in relation to the neural complications of cervical spondylosis. *Brain* 1971;94:568–586.

122. Arnold JGJ. The clinical manifestations of spondylochondrosis (spondylosis) of the cervical spine. *Ann Surg* 1955;141:872–889.

123. Boijsen E. Cervical spinal canal in interspinal expansive processes. *Acta Radiol* 1954;42:101–115.

124. Pallis C, Jones AM, Spillane JD. Cervical spondylosis: incidence and implications. *Brain* 1954;77:274–289.

125. Chrispin AR, Lees F. The spinal canal in cervical spondylosis. *J Neurol Neurosurg Psychiatry* 1963;26:166–170.

126. Ehni G. Developmental variations, including shallowness of the cervical spinal canal. In: Post MJ, ed. *Radiographic evaluation of the cervical spine*. New York: Mason, 1980:469–474.

127. Pavlov H, Torg JS, Robie B, et al. Cervical spinal stenosis: determination with vertebral body ratio method. *Radiology* 1987;164:771–775.

128. Yue W-M, Tan S-B, Tan M-H, et al. The Torg-Pavlov ratio in cervical spondylotic myelopathy: a comparative study between patients with cervical spondylotic myelopathy and a nonspondylotic, nonmyelopathic population. *Spine* 2001;26(16):1760–1764.

129. White AA, Panjabi MM. Biomechanical considerations in the surgical management of cervical spondylotic myelopathy. *Spine* 1988;13: 856–860.

130. Breig A, Turnbull I, Hassler O. Effects of mechanical stresses on the spinal cord in cervical spondylosis. *J Neurosurg* 1966;24:45.

131. Penning L, Zwaag PVD. Biomechanical aspects of spondylotic myelopathy. *Acta Radiol* 1966;5:1090–103.

132. Wilkinson M. The morbid anatomy of cervical spondylosis and myelopathy. *Brain* 1960;83:589–616.

133. Hayashi K, Yabuki T. Origin of the uncus and of Luschka's joint in the cervical spine. *J Bone Joint Surg Am* 1985;67:788.

134. Fehlings MG, Skaf G. A review of the pathophysiology of cervical spondylotic myelopathy with insights for potential novel mechanisms drawn from traumatic spinal cord injury. *Spine* 1998;23(24): 2730–2736.

135. Hayashi H, Okada K, Hashimoto J, et al. Cervical spondylotic myelopathy in the aged patient. A radiographic evaluation of the aging changes in the cervical spine and etiologic factors in myelopathy. *Spine* 1988;13:618–625.

136. Mair WG, Druckman R. The pathology of spinal cord lesions and their relations to the clinical features in the protrusion of cervical intervertebral discs. *Brain* 1953;76:70.

137. Hutchinson EC, Yates PO. The cervical portion of the vertebral artery. A clinico-pathological study. *Brain* 1956;79:319.

138. Murone I. The importance of the sagittal diameters of the cervical spinal canal in relation to spondylosis and myelopathy. *J Bone Joint Surg Br* 1974;56:30–36.

139. Hoff J, Nishimura M, Pitts L, et al. The role of ischemia in the pathogenesis of cervical spondylotic myelopathy: a review and new microangiographic evidence. *Spine* 1972;2:100–108.

140. Gooding MR, Wilson CB, Hoff JT. Experimental cervical myelopathy: autoradiographic studies of spinal cord blood flow patterns. *Surg Neurol* 1976;5:233–239.

141. al-Mefty O, Harkey HL, Marawi I, et al. Experimental chronic compressive cervical myelopathy. *J Neurosurg* 1993;79(4):550–561.

142. Doppman JL. The mechanism of ischemia in anteroposterior compression of the spinal cord. *Invest Radiol* 1975;10:543–551.

143. Shimomura Y, Hukuda S, Mizuno S. Experimental study of ischemic damage to the cervical spinal cord. *J Neurosurg* 1968;28:565–581.

144. Taylor AR. Mechanism and treatment of spinal cord disorders associated with cervical spondylosis. *Lancet* 1953;1:717.

145. Gooding MR, Wilson CB, Hoff JT. Experimental cervical myelopathy. Effects of ischemia and compression of the canine cervical spinal cord. *J Neurosurg* 1975;43:9–17.

146. Kobrine AI, Evans DE, Rizzoli H. Correlation of spinal cord blood flow and function in experimental compression. *Surg Neurol* 1978;10:54–59.

147. Clark E, Robinson PK. Cervical myelopathy: a complication of cervical spondylosis. *Brain* 1956;79:483–570.

148. Nurick S. The natural history and the results of surgical treatment of the spinal cord disorder associated with cervical spondylosis. *Brain* 1972;95:101–108.

149. Roberts AH. Myelopathy due to cervical spondylosis treated by collar immobilization. *Neurology* 1966;16:951–959.

150. Fujiwara K, Yonenobu K, Ebara S, et al. The prognosis of surgery for cervical compressive myelopathy. An analysis of factors involved. *J Bone Joint Surg Br* 1989;71:393–398.

151. Ito T, Oyanagi K, Takahashi H, et al. Cervical spondylotic myelopathy: clinicopathologic study on the progression pattern and thin myelinated fibers of the lesions of seven patients examined during complete autopsy. *Spine* 1996;21(7):827–833.

152. Ono K, Ota H, Tada K, et al. Cervical myelopathy secondary to multiple spondylotic protrusions. A clinico-pathologic study. *Spine* 1977;2:109–125.

153. Bracken MB, Shepard MJ, Collins WF, et al. Methylprednisolone or naloxone treatment after acute spinal cord injury: 1-year follow-up data. Results of the second National Acute Spinal Cord Injury Study. *J Neurosurg* 1992;76(1):23–31.

154. Bracken MB, Shepard MJ, Holford TR, et al. Administration of methylprednisolone for 24 or 48 hours or tirilazad mesylate for 48 hours in the treatment of acute spinal cord injury. Results of the Third National Acute Spinal Cord Injury Randomized Controlled Trial. National Acute Spinal Cord Injury Study. *JAMA* 1997;277:1597–604.

155. Yamaura I, Yone K, Nakahara S, et al. Mechanism of destructive pathologic changes in the spinal cord under chronic mechanical compression. *Spine* 2002;27(1):21–26.

156. Fujiwara K, Yonenobu K, Ebara S, et al. The prognosis of surgery for cervical compressive myelopathy. An analysis of factors involved. *J Bone Joint Surg Br* 1989;71:393–398.

CHAPTER 70

Molecular Biology: Applications to the Cervical Spine

Christian Lattermann, Lars G. Gilbertson, and James D. Kang

The etiology and pathophysiology of degenerative disc disease (DDD) are still unknown. However, it is believed that DDD is the result of a complex interaction between biologic and mechanical factors.

New biologic techniques allow for addressing intervertebral disc degeneration in the cervical spine on a molecular level. Recent advances in recombinant DNA technology have led to the decoding of many human genes that appear to be attractive for the scientific and clinical use in musculoskeletal disorders (1,2). Growth factors and embryogenic differentiation factors have been isolated and studied for many musculoskeletal conditions. Bone morphogenetic proteins (BMPs), for example, are being used successfully to enhance bone healing and fusion in humans (3). Other growth factors, such as transforming growth factor-β (TGF-β) and insulin-derived growth factor-1 (IGF-1), have been shown to influence the proliferation and extracellular matrix production of various different musculoskeletal tissues (4–6).

After this brief overview, we will introduce several novel approaches involving molecular genetic techniques and how their use can be advantageous in the treatment of degenerative disc disease in the cervical spine.

IDENTIFICATION OF GENES FOR TARGETED GENE MANIPULATION

Intervertebral disc disease occurs as a result of a complex interaction of cells, cell products, inflammatory cytokines, and degradative processes occurring in the intervertebral disc. All the mechanisms identified to date are naturally occurring processes designed to maintain the intervertebral disc homeostasis. One or multiple unknown triggers mark the beginning of disc degeneration by causing a shift of the anabolic–catabolic equilibrium. The goal of any bio-

logic therapy for degenerative disc disease, therefore, must be to reinstate the equilibrium or slow down the shift of the anabolic–catabolic equilibrium. Based on present knowledge, there are three critical mechanisms that could be amenable to a targeted protein or gene therapy approach aimed at restoration or containment of the status quo within the intervertebral disc.

To identify the different pathways in which a gene therapy protocol would be able to intervene toward a slowing of the degenerative process, one has to understand the process of disc degeneration. Although there are still many secrets to be solved in the complex process of disc degeneration, it appears that a fundamental concept of homeostasis is gradually disrupted during the degeneration of the intervertebral disc. To facilitate the understanding of the complex process of intervertebral disc degeneration and the possible avenues of therapeutic intervention, one can group the different mechanisms responsible for maintenance of disc homeostasis into two major categories: nutritional and catabolic.

Nutritional Mechanisms

One of the first steps in disc degeneration may be the increase in fibrochondrocytes along the annulus fibrosus. This increased fibrosis has been observed parallel to a decrease in diffusion of substances throughout the intervertebral disc. This, in turn, may be responsible for the declining oxygen tension within the intervertebral disc. A decrease in oxygen tension most likely will result in impairment of cellular function within the nucleus and thus may lead to a decrease in matrix synthesis. Decreased matrix synthesis leads to a favored production of the smaller, less complex keratan sulfate, shifting the equilibrium toward a higher concentration of nonaggregated proteoglycans that bind fewer water molecules (7–9). As a result, the overall capacity of the nucleus pulposus to imbibe water decreases. In addition, abundant smaller proteoglycan fragments appear in early disc degeneration as a result of the collapse of adequate matrix proteoglycan production. These smaller, nonaggregate proteoglycans and breakdown products decrease the fluid flow throughout the disc and thus further inhibit the diffusion capacity of nutrients throughout the disc. This again limits the oxygen tension and nutrient supply to and from the intervertebral disc cells.

A further cascade involved in disruption of normal disc homeostasis is the constant maintenance of different collagen types within the intervertebral discs. The intervertebral disc is predominantly composed of type I and II collagen. The annulus is predominantly composed of type I collagen fibers. Type II collagen is mainly found in the nucleus pulposus. The distribution shows a small gradient toward the periphery, with the concentration of collagen type II decreasing and type I collagen fibers increasing toward the annulus. Despite the fact that this collagen scaffold does not appear to change substantially during the aging process, degenerative disc disease shows substantial alteration of the collagen composition early on. In early degeneration, more type II and type I collagen is expressed, together with an increase in minor collagen types (III, V, and VI). During the course of further degeneration, collagen type II disappears in the nucleus and is replaced by collagen type 1. The minor collagen types of fibrosis (III, IV, and X) become more abundant within the nucleus pulposus, gradually leading to loss of elasticity.

Catabolic Mechanisms

An inflammatory component has been discussed as a major entity in degeneration of the intervertebral disc. Nitric oxide (NO), interleukin-1 (IL-1), IL-6, and prostaglandin E_2 (PGE_2) are powerful inflammatory mediators that have been shown to be elevated in degenerated human intervertebral discs. Although the mechanisms are not fully understood, NO, IL-6, and PGE_2 appear to be up-regulated in response to the main inflammatory cytokine IL-1. It is likely that these inflammatory mediators have multiple functions; however, one of their functions is to support the breakdown of proteoglycans mediated by degradative enzymes called *metalloproteinases* (MMPs). These MMPs are a family of enzymes responsible for the breakdown of collagens and extracellular matrix. The MMPs include well-known enzymes, such as collagenase I, II, and III; gelatinase; stromelysin; and aggrecanase. These powerful catabolic enzymes are able to break down different sizes of matrix proteoglycans and collagens and show a significantly higher activity in degenerated intervertebral disc cells than in normal discs. It is surprising, however, that the actual amount of MMPs is not increased in the degenerated intervertebral disc. In fact, the increase in proteo-

glycan breakdown may be more likely a result of the lack of inhibition of the MMPs.

In a normal intervertebral disc, MMPs are inhibited by molecules called *tissue inhibitors of metalloproteinases* (TIMPs). The concentration of the TIMPs is greatly decreased in degenerated intervertebral discs. This mechanism, therefore, suggests a breakdown of the anticatabolic system within the intervertebral disc during degeneration.

Strategies that result in a net increase in proteoglycans may have therapeutic potential in altering the natural history of disc degeneration. These strategies could involve increasing the production of proteoglycans, blocking their catabolic degradation, or a combination of both.

POSSIBLE TARGETS FOR GENE OR PROTEIN TRANSFER

One common way to increase the productivity of cells in the presence of impaired function uses small proteins called growths factors. These growth factors have the ability to override and steer cellular protein synthesis in a less than optimal surrounding. Naturally occurring, these growth factors offer a way in which intervertebral disc cells can be influenced and guided to produce extracellular matrix and collagen in the face of disc degeneration and thus counteract the degradation of the intervertebral disc.

Several promising growth factors have been isolated that have the ability to increase extracellular matrix and collagen production in intervertebral disc cells. TGF-β1 and BMPs are two examples of growth factors (out of many) with strong potential for altering intervertebral disc biology. Thompson and colleagues studied the *in vitro* response of canine intervertebral disc tissue to the following growth factors: human recombinant IGF-1, epidermal growth factor (EGF), fibroblast growth factor (FGF), and TGF-β1 (10). Incorporation rates by the tissue regions of up to five times the control rate were reported, with the nucleus and transition zone responding more than the annulus. TGF-β1 and EGF elicited greater response than FGF, whereas IGF-1 produced only a marginally significant response in the nucleus and no response in the annulus and transition. Our group showed that the use of TGF-β1 and BMP-2 led to higher levels of proteoglycan production in degenerative human and rabbit nucleus pulposus cells (6). Takegami and associates studied the effect of human recombinant osteogenic protein (hrOP-1) on cell proliferation as well as on proteoglycan production and collagen synthesis (11). They showed a dose-dependent increase in proliferation rate as well as in collagen and proteoglycan production of rabbit intervertebral disc cells treated with hrOP-1. They also demonstrated the restoration of proteoglycan in previously proteoglycan-depleted cultures of intervertebral disc cells treated with hrOP-1. Our laboratory recently showed that the treatment of degenerative intervertebral disc cells with TIMP-1 increases proteoglycan production and the rate of proteoglycan synthesis by a factor of 5.

The critically important issue for the delivery of growth factors is the length of therapeutic effect of these exogenous growth factors to targeted cells in the intervertebral disc. The normal half-life for most of these growth factors *in vivo* is about 20 minutes. Therefore, the therapeutic effect of injecting growth factors directly into the intervertebral disc may be too transient to have a major long-lasting effect on a chronic disorder such as DDD, and repeated injections may not be practical or well tolerated by patients.

THE CONCEPT OF GENE TRANSFER

An elegant way to deliver sustained levels of growth factors to musculoskeletal tissues has been shown to be gene transfer technology. Particularly, the use of viral vectors appears to be highly efficient in the delivery of the desired transgene to most mesenchymal tissues.

Gene transfer is a novel technique in which genes of interest are inserted into target cells, causing them to synthesize the protein encoded by the inserted gene. This technique can be used as an approach for treating genetic diseases by compensating for mutant genes or, more recently, as a means of delivering a therapeutic substance to the area of interest.

Protein synthesis within a mammalian cell involves several steps. At first a gene consisting of specific DNA sequence is transcribed into a complementary chain heterogeneous nuclear RNA. This is then processed into messenger RNA (mRNA) by a series of modifications that include capping, splicing, and the addition of a polyadenosine tail. The mature mRNA leaves the nucleus of the cell and is translated by ribosomes into a sequence of amino acids that form the protein. When an exogenous gene is introduced into the nucleus of a cell, it is also transcribed into mRNA and thus produces the protein encoded by the gene. The cell may normally not make this protein of interest, or it may be made in insufficient amounts. There are different techniques available that aid the insertion of a foreign gene into the genome of a mammalian cell. Gene transfer to cells normally requires the assistance of a vehicle or vector, which may be viral or nonviral in nature. The nonviral techniques typically use small particles like liposomes or spheroblasts carrying the gene of interest. These particles have the ability to fuse with the target cell or to enter the cell by endocytosis. Other techniques, such as electroporation and microparticle bombardment, use physical strain or electrical shock to break small temporary defects into the cell wall without severely damaging the cell, allowing the DNA strand to travel into the cell. Another approach uses a direct microinjection of the gene into the cell. These methods tend to be inefficient (5).

Viral-based vectors generally use the inherent capacity of a virus to attach to the surface of a cell through specific receptors and to insert its genome into the cell (Fig. 70.1). For safety reasons, the viral vector must be altered to render the virus incapable of replicating. Hence, viral vectors are engi-

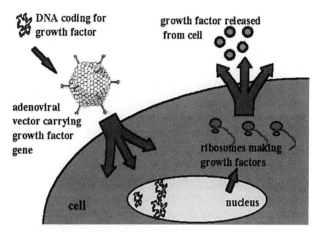

FIG. 70.1. The DNA coding for a growth factor is engineered into a vector (i.e., adenoviral vector capsid). The vector is applied to the tissue or cell culture and attaches to the cell membrane. The DNA is inserted into the cell and travels to the nucleus, where it integrates episomally or integrates into the chromosome. The inserted DNA then uses the regular transcription and translation process of the host cell and is translated into the protein of interest. The treated cell goes on to produce the protein of interest in high amounts.

neered such that endogenous gene sequences required for replication and pathology are removed. The ideal viral vector, therefore, carries the genes of interest into cells with high efficiency, but does not replicate or cause pathology.

By far the most commonly used vectors are retroviral, and most are based on the Molony murine leukemia virus. Retroviral vectors specifically infect dividing cells with a very high efficiency. They insert their genes into the chromosomes of the target cell. This leads to reproduction of the inserted gene each time the infected cell divides. Clinical trials have already been successfully initiated using retroviral vectors. Although retroviral vectors are the most commonly used vectors in human clinical trials at present, there are certain disadvantages to their use. For example, retroviruses do not infect nondividing cells. Furthermore, there is a theoretical risk for mutagenesis due to the random integration of the viral DNA into the chromosome of the target cell. If chromosomal integration occurs near a site of an oncogene, activation may occur, causing the cell to transform. Because of this potential risk, most investigators have used the retroviral vectors in an *ex vivo* approach (see later). To date, however, there are no reports of malignancy caused by gene therapy using retroviral vectors.

The second most commonly used viral vector is derived from the adenovirus. This is a DNA virus that is highly infectious to a number of different cell types. The adenoviral vector infects dividing as well as nondividing cells and can be prepared in high titers. In contrast to the retroviral vectors, the genome of the adenoviral vector is not integrated into the chromosome of the target cell. The adenoviral vector inserts its genome as an episome within the nucleus of the target cell. Thus, the inserted genes will not be automatically passed on during cell division. As a result, the percentage of infected daughter cells rapidly decreases as a result of dilution with every cell generation. Because of the random nature of retroviral integration into the host genome, gene therapy using retroviral vectors possesses the potential for disruption of normal gene expression. Therefore, most retrovirus-based gene therapy studies have been initiated using *ex vivo* delivery of transduced cells to target tissues.

Alternatively, adenoviral vectors can infect nondividing as well as dividing cells. There is no integration of the viral genome or the passenger therapeutic gene into the host chromosomes; however, after repeated cell division, copies of the transgene can be lost. In addition, adenoviral vectors are highly antigenic and initiate strong immune responses. Likewise, herpes viral vectors, which can include multiple transgenes, are also antigenic and often cytotoxic to the host cell or tissues. Currently, new generations of viral-based vectors are underdevelopment that increase the efficiency of transduction of both dividing and nondividing cells. The most promising of these are based on adeno-associated virus (AAV), herpes simplex virus (HSV), and the retrovirus Lentivirus. These vectors show a high infectivity and may provide a long-term expression. The goal is to generate new viral vectors that can escape the surveillance of the host immune system and express the desired gene product in a tissue-specific manner.

Gene transfer can be accomplished by two main approaches, *ex vivo* and *in vivo*, to transduce target cells. The *ex vivo* approach transduces target cells after harvest and culture *in vitro* under sterile conditions. The cells are transduced and selected in culture and then prepared for injection into the recipient tissue. Because no viral particles enter the human body, *ex vivo* gene therapy provides a measure of safety that is not found with *in vivo* gene delivery.

In vivo transduction is a more straightforward procedure. The vector is directly applied into the tissue of interest by catheter or needle injection. This approach does not allow control over the rate of target cell transduction. Because of the direct introduction of viral particles into the body, safety concerns are higher. The choice of the approach to achieve target cell transduction is dependent on the desired longevity of gene expression, the viral vector chosen, the anatomy and physiology of the target organ, safety considerations, and the underlying cause of the disease to be treated. Generally, the *ex vivo* approach is employed when using retroviral vectors because of the necessity for high rates of cell division and safety concerns surrounding the injection of retrovirus into the body. Because of their high infectivity and ability to infect nondividing cells, adenoviral vectors are often used experimentally in the *in vivo* approach (5).

GENE TRANSFER TO THE INTERVERTEBRAL DISC

Several authors have previously shown successful transfer of exogenous genes to musculoskeletal tissues. In our laboratory, we have pioneered the viral gene transfer to the intervertebral disc using adenoviral and retroviral gene transfer protocols.

Wehling and co-workers reported the successful gene transfer of the *LacZ* marker gene as well as the interleukin receptor antagonist gene *(IRAP)* to bovine intervertebral disc cells (12). Subsequently, Nishida and associates showed that the adenoviral transfer of the *LacZ* marker gene to the rabbit intervertebral disc is feasible and will lead to long-term expression of the marker gene (13). This has since been shown to be the case with different viral vectors, including the AAV vector (Figs. 70.2 and 70.3). Surprisingly, the intervertebral disc allowed for long-term gene

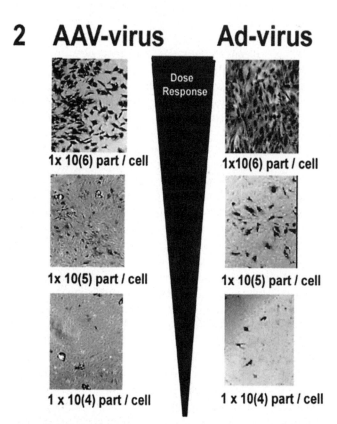

FIG. 70.2. *In vitro* transduction of human intervertebral disc cells with two different viral vectors. The adeno-associated virus (AAV) vector and the adenoviral (ad) vector both transfer the *LacZ* marker gene to human intervertebral disc cells. Both viruses show a clearly dose-dependent transduction efficacy. The adenoviral vector is overall more efficient. Adenoviral vectors have the advantage of efficient transduction of nondividing cells. The AAV shares this advantage but in addition is much less immunogenic and is not associated with any known disease in humans. Thus, the AAV vectors may be potentially safer than adenoviral or retroviral vectors.

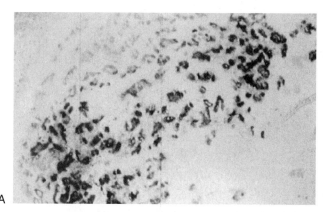
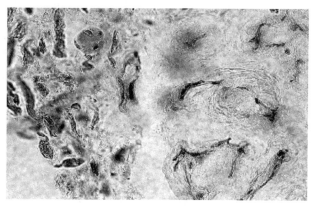

A

B

FIG. 70.3. *In vivo* transduction of intervertebral disc cells in rabbits can be achieved using a simple injection technique. Adenoviral gene transfer of the *LacZ* marker gene (3A) at 6 weeks can be traced for as long as 1 year after injection. The in vivo delivery of the *LacZ* marker gene using the novel AAV vector (3B) can be detected for at least 6 weeks after injection.

expression after utilization of an adenoviral vector, suggesting that the intervertebral disc may be an immune-privileged site within the human body. This observation has since been underlined by Park and co-workers, who found an unusually high expression of Fas ligand, a suppressor of cellular immunity, within the intervertebral disc (14). In a follow-up study, Nishida transferred the gene for TGF-β to rabbit intervertebral discs *in vivo* and showed that the overall proteoglycan production of the intervertebral disc cells increased (15). Moon and colleagues investigated the effect of different growth factors transferred to human intervertebral disc cells using an adenoviral vector. They demonstrated synergism between the expression of TGF-β, BMP-2, and IGF-1 with respect to the overall proteoglycan production in culture (6). In a recently published study, Yung and associates applied a pellet culture technique to grow intervertebral disc cells in a three-dimensional matrix. Transduction of these pellet cultures with Ad-BMP-2 led to an increase in proteoglycan synthesis and total proteoglycan content (16).

FUTURE PERSPECTIVES

Clearly, there are still many obstacles to overcome before a viral or nonviral gene transfer protocol can be used as a viable treatment option in degenerative disc disease. Molecular biologists and surgeons, however, are feverishly working to develop safer methods of gene transfer in order to influence the biologic environment within soft tissues such as the intervertebral disc. We know from animal experimental data that the approach is feasible *in vivo*. Safety studies are underway to determine whether these technologies may be applicable to humans.

In addition to the development of novel and safe vectors, researchers are developing new models to mimic intervertebral discs *in vitro* and *in vivo*.

Finally, it is important to understand the goal of any therapeutic approach to disc degeneration. The major issue to overcome at this time is still the early detection of disc degeneration. Remaining questions address the time course of degeneration: When is it too degenerated for therapy? How much regeneration potential does a degenerated disc have? How well does the MRI signal change correlate with the biologic activity of the intervertebral disc? All these questions have to be addressed before a broad-based attempt can be made to treat this disease using gene therapy. To date, we still do not know the exact cause of disc degeneration. It is certainly not feasible to treat everyone's discs prophylactically at all levels with a gene therapy approach. It is therefore important to focus treatment using this new technology to very limited and clearly defined problems. One of these problems, for example, is disc degeneration occurring above and below fusions in the cervical spine. At the time of arthrodesis, an injection into the adjacent discs could be performed without any problems.

In conclusion, gene transfer technology offers an elegant way to influence the biochemical environment inside the degenerated intervertebral disc and may be a useful tool to treat this highly prevalent disease in the future. The transfer of growth factors to the intervertebral disc may be able to limit disc degeneration or prevent disc degeneration if the gene transfer is done prophylactically in a junctional level at the time of posterior spinal fusion. Viral or nonviral gene transfer is an emerging technology that offers exciting new perspectives in research and treatment of intervertebral disc disease.

REFERENCES

1. Evans CH, Scully SP. Orthopaedic gene therapy. *Clin Orthop* 2000; 379[Suppl]:S2.
2. Jaffurs D, Evans CH. The Human Genome Project: implications for the treatment of musculoskeletal disease. *J Am Acad Orthop Surg* 1998; 6(1):1–14.

3. Boden SD, Zdeblick TA, Sandhu HS, et al. The use of rhBMP-2 in inter-body fusion cages. Definitive evidence of osteoinduction in humans: a preliminary report. *Spine* 2000;25(3):376–381.
4. Puolakkainen PA, Twardzik DR, Ranchalis JE, et al. The enhancement in wound healing by transforming growth factor-beta 1 (TGF-beta 1) depends on the topical delivery system. *J Surg Res* 1995;58(3):321–329.
5. Gruber HE, Hanley EN Jr. Human disc cells in monolayer vs 3D culture: cell shape, division and matrix formation. *BMC Musculoskelet Disord* 2000;1(1):1.
6. Moon SH, Gilbertson LG, Nishida K, et al. Human intervertebral disc cells are genetically modifiable by adenovirus-mediated gene transfer: implications for the clinical management of intervertebral disc disorders. *Spine* 2000;25(20):2573–2579.
7. Lipson SJ, Muir H. 1980 Volvo Award in basic science. Proteoglycans in experimental intervertebral disc degeneration. *Spine* 1981;6(3):194–210.
8. Pearce RH, Grimmer BJ, Adams ME. Degeneration and the chemical composition of the human lumbar intervertebral disc. *J Orthop Res* 1987;5(2):198–205.
9. Stevens RL, Ryvar R, Robertson WR, et al. Biological changes in the annulus fibrosus in patients with low-back pain. *Spine* 1982;7(3):223–233.
10. Thompson JP, Oegema TR Jr, Bradford DS. Stimulation of mature canine intervertebral disc by growth factors. *Spine* 1991;16(3):253–260.
11. Takegami K, Thonar EJ, An HS, et al. Osteogenic protein-1 enhances matrix replenishment by intervertebral disc cells previously exposed to interleukin-1. Spine 2002;27(12):1318–1325.
12. Wehling P, Schulitz KP, Robbins PD, et al. Transfer of genes to chondrocytic cells of the lumbar spine. Proposal for a treatment strategy of spinal disorders by local gene therapy. Spine 1997;22(10):1092–1097.
13. Nishida K, Kang JD, Suh JK, et al. Adenovirus-mediated gene transfer to nucleus pulposus cells. Implications for the treatment of intervertebral disc degeneration. *Spine* 1998;23(22):2437–2442.
14. Park JB, Chang H, Kim KW. Expression of Fas ligand and apoptosis of disc cells in herniated lumbar disc tissue. *Spine* 2001;26(6):618–621.
15. Nishida K, Kang JD, Gilbertson LG, et al. Modulation of the biologic activity of the rabbit intervertebral disc by gene therapy: an in vivo study of adenovirus-mediated transfer of the human transforming growth factor beta 1 encoding gene. *Spine* 1999;24(23):2419–2425.
16. Yung Lee J, Hall R, Pelinkovic D, et al. New use of a three-dimensional pellet culture system for human intervertebral disc cells: initial characterization and potential use for tissue engineering. *Spine* 2001;26(21):2316–2322.

CHAPTER 71

Cervical Spondylotic Myelopathy and Radiculopathy: Natural History and Clinical Presentation

John K. Houten and Thomas J. Errico

Although new technologies allow for exquisitely detailed imaging of degenerative disease of the cervical spine, there is, perhaps, no area in medicine where the clinician's history taking and physical examination are more crucial. Degenerative disease is ubiquitous; few asymptomatic individuals older than 50 years are without abnormalities on magnetic resonance imaging (MRI), and some even have evidence of severe neural compression. How, then, is the clinician to decide which patient needs treatment and what therapeutic measures are appropriate? It is within the details of the clinical presentation and findings of the physical examination that answers may be found.

Degenerative disease of the cervical spine may lead to compression of the spinal cord, causing the upper motor neuron signs and symptoms associated with myelopathy, and to compression of cervical nerve roots, producing signs and symptoms of lower motor neuron dysfunction, including radicular pain. Occasionally, a large disc herniation or spondylotic ridge may compress both the spinal cord and nerve root, resulting in both radicular and myelopathic findings. Although the term *myeloradiculopathy* is used in connection with such clinical presentations, it does not represent a distinct clinical entity but, rather, the signs and symptoms of coinciding upper and lower motor neuron compression.

MYELOPATHY

Symptoms

Cervical spondylotic myelopathy (CSM) results from spinal cord compression that may be caused by spondy-losis, ossification of the posterior longitudinal ligament (OPLL), or soft disc herniation. Spondylosis, however, is by far the most frequently seen cause. Early symptoms are abnormal sensation in the hands, gait deterioration, and impairment in the use of the hands for tasks requiring fine motor skills (1).

At surgical presentation, the average age of patients with CSM was reported to be in the middle to late 50s (1–3). Symptoms typically evolve slowly and insidiously, although many patients describe periods of stability with interspersed episodes of deterioration. The duration of symptoms until surgical treatment may range widely from several months to several years (1,3). Hand sensory complaints usually are described by patients as numbness or tingling in the hands that start in the fingertips and generally remain confined to the hands. Patients occasionally relate feeling as if their hands are gloved (4). It is noteworthy that these complaints occur in all fingers and do not follow a dermatomal pattern, underscoring that they arise from the spinal cord and are not radicular symptoms attributable to a specific nerve root.

Deterioration in gait usually follows closely the overall severity of CSM and is usually more the consequence of spasticity than muscle weakness. Patients may complain of a sensation of heaviness in their legs or an inability to make their legs do what they want. Those with very early symptoms of CSM may complain of gait dysfunction that, although it may be noticeable to the patient, is too subtle to be appreciated on physical examination. Patients with more pronounced myelopathy may develop severe gait instability and present to the physician already unable to ambulate without a walker or wheelchair.

A history of deterioration in hand use is often subtle and may be elicited with directed questioning. Difficulty is usually noticed in tasks requiring fine movements such as buttoning shirt buttons and sorting change from a change purse. As the disease progresses, patients may notice a change in the appearance of their handwriting. Worsening hand weakness may ultimately cause severe impairment in the ability to write, drive, or attend to personal care.

Other less frequent symptoms include upper and, rarely, lower extremity pain. Patients with CSM may experience pain in a radicular pattern when spondylotic ridges produce compression of an exiting nerve root in addition to the spinal cord (Fig. 71.1A and B). Sphincter and sexual dysfunction are relatively infrequent and are generally associated with advanced myelopathy (1). Bladder dysfunction may manifest with irritative symptoms of urgency and intermittent incontinence, obstructive symptoms, or a combination of both (4).

Some patients relate a history of experiencing Lhermitte sign, a sudden, generalized electrical shock–like sensation in the arms and back caused by spinal cord compression and occurring with jarring motion or during neck flexion. For example, one recent patient described a ride in a off-road vehicle over rough terrain during which he felt "shocks" in his hands every time the vehicle passed over a bump.

Suboccipital headache has been reported in association with cervical spondylosis (5). Mechanisms for this phenomenon have been postulated to relate to either nuchal muscle contraction (6) or pain referred from pain generators emanating from the disc or posterior longitudinal ligament. No features definitively distinguish these headaches from those of common tension headaches and, given the frequency of headaches in the general population, symptoms of headache are unhelpful in the diagnosis of cervical myelopathy.

The clinical presentation of OPLL is generally similar to that of CSM (7). The posterior longitudinal ligament generally occurs in the midline and produces central compression on the spinal cord and, thus, uncommonly produces radicular symptoms. The mean age at presentation is older than that in soft disc herniation but slightly younger than in CSM, and OPLL is significantly more common in men. Although once thought to be exceptional in the non-Asian population, it has been well established to occur in general population as well (8,9).

Soft disc herniation produces predominantly radicular symptoms, with pure myelopathy seen in fewer than 10% of patients (10). The clinical presentation in these patients differs from that in patients with spondylosis and OPLL in that it has a shorter duration and more rapid development of symptoms. Uncommonly, soft disc herniation may present with symptoms of acute myelopathy.

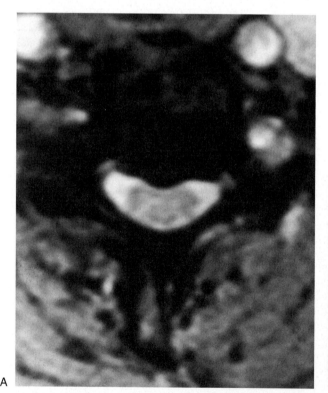

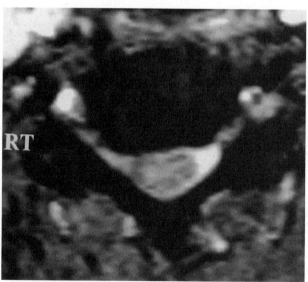

A
B

FIG. 71.1. A: Axial T2-weighted magnetic resonance imaging (MRI) study of a patient with signs and symptoms of cervical myelopathy demonstrating spinal cord compression. **B:** Axial T2-weighted MRI study of a different patient who complained of right arm pain in addition to symptoms characteristic of myelopathy. Note that the spondylotic ridge not only is compressing the spinal cord but is also impinging on the lateral portion of the spinal canal and is producing compression of the nerve root.

Signs

Muscle weakness occurs in CSM in a characteristic pattern. The hand intrinsic and triceps muscles are typically the earliest and most severely impaired. Lower extremity weakness manifests in the proximal musculature, primarily affecting the iliopsoas.

The pattern of muscle weakness is a consequence of spinal cord compression rather than compression of discrete nerve roots. This becomes evident on review of the upper extremity innervation. Given the high frequency of spondylosis at C5-6, one would expect to find many patients with weakness in the biceps, innervated primarily by the C6 nerve root. Yet, this muscle group is seldom affected in CSM. Moreover, the pattern of demonstrated muscle weakness and symptoms tends to remain consistent without regard to which cervical level is most severely affected (1) (Fig. 71.2).

Signs of spasticity are characteristic features of cervical myelopathy. Spasticity rather than weakness is usually the underlying cause of the patient's complaints of gait dysfunction. As a consequence, gait problems may persist postoperatively in patients in whom substantial improvement is seen in lower extremity strength (1). Hyperreflexia is an early sign of spinal cord compression, although it is occasionally found in normal individuals. A positive Hoffman reflex consists of a reflex contraction of the thumb and index finger in response to flicking the tip of the middle finger and is an extremely useful sign in detecting cervical spinal cord compression (11,12). In our experience, this sign is present in about half of patients undergoing surgical decompression for CSM and OPLL and may even be present in patients with minimal deficits. Other signs of spasticity usually seen in more advanced myelopathy include the Babinski reflex and ankle clonus.

Muscle wasting is a relatively uncommon finding in cervical myelopathy and is the end result of long-standing spinal cord compression with loss of anterior horn motor neurons. Muscle fasciculation, a sign of denervation of the lower motor neuron, is not a feature of CSM.

Natural History

Although the natural history of cervical spondylotic myelopathy has been the subject of debate in the literature (13), recent studies of both surgically treated and nonoperatively managed patients indicate that it is a disorder that is slowly progressive; however, many individuals may experience lengthy periods of relative stability or intermittent episodes of acute deterioration. Lees and Turner published in 1963 a series of 44 patients in whom they observed that CSM was a disease with a lengthy course of static symptomatology and that deterioration was seen only in the exceptional patient (14). These findings were supported by Nurick's 1972 report of 91 patients with CSM, of whom 37 were treated conservatively. Despite the fact that Nurick appreciated better outcomes in patients undergoing laminectomy, he concluded that CSM is "generally a benign disorder caused by compression of the cord in which disability develops in an initial phase of variable duration" and that "the disability remains static except in older patients, in whom it may progress" (15).

This view of CSM as a benign condition, however, was challenged by authors noting the severity of disability and lack of improvement so often seen (16,17). In addition, patient series studied after the advent of computed tomography (CT) myelography and MRI that allowed for the exclusion of disorders that may produce various signs and symptoms similar to those seen in cervical myelopathy, including multiple sclerosis, normal pressure hydrocephalus, syringomyelia, and spinal cord tumors tended to document a course of more progressive symptoms leading to substantial disability (1,18–21). As a possible explanation for this progressive deterioration, Barnes and Saunders observed that functional decline was noted in the subset of patients with a total range of motion of the head and neck of more

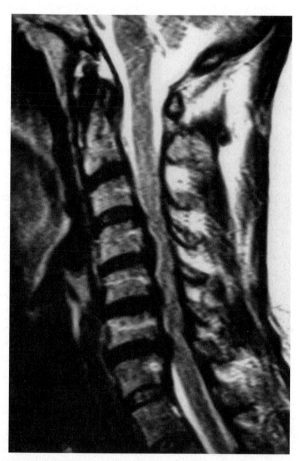

FIG. 71.2. Sagittal T2-weighted magnetic resonance imaging study of the cervical spine of a patient with complaints of hand numbness, clumsiness, and gait deterioration. Severe spinal cord compression is seen at C4-5, C5-6, and C6-7, with mild compression at C3-4. The only notable findings on neurologic examination were hand intrinsic weakness, increased bilateral deep tendon reflexes, and bilateral Hoffman reflexes.

than 62 degrees, but not in patients with more limited neck movement, indicating that the deterioration in CSM may be related to repetitive trauma to the spinal cord (21).

In conclusion, cervical myelopathy from degenerative spine disease is a consequence of chronic spinal cord compression, although radicular symptoms from coexisting nerve root compression are sometimes also seen. The most frequent symptoms are hand numbness or paresthesia, gait difficulty, and impairment of fine hand movements. Muscle weakness occurs in a characteristic pattern, with the hand intrinsics, triceps, and iliopsoas muscles most frequently and severely affected. Most patients have evidence of spasticity, and this is the underlying cause of most gait complaints. Although it has been the subject of controversy, many recent authors describe the natural history of CSM as one of progressive deterioration interspersed with periods of relative stability or accelerated functional decline.

RADICULOPATHY

Signs and Symptoms

Cervical radiculopathy results from impingement on a nerve root by either spondylotic narrowing of the neural foramen or a lateral intervertebral disc herniation. Frequent complaints include painful neck movements, radicular pain, paraspinal muscle spasm, muscle weakness, and diminished deep tendon reflexes (22). The nerve roots most commonly affected are C6 and C7, reflecting the predilection for the development of degenerative disease at the C5-6 and C6-7 levels (1,10,23–25). A male predominance is found in a large number of clinical series (26–29). The location of pain and paresthesias may be difficult to attribute clearly to a single root, owing to overlap of innervation of adjacent roots, intradural connections between dorsal nerve rootlets, and anatomic variability from individual to individual (30–32). Muscle innervation, however, is fairly constant and has greater specificity than either cutaneous sensation or reflex examinations.

Radiculopathy tends to produce substantial limitation of movement of the head and neck. Patients with cervical radiculopathy may have reproduction of radicular pain with axial compression of the head with neck extension and rotation toward the side of pain. This maneuver, also known as the Spurling maneuver or axial compression test, serves to

diminish the size of the neural foramen and accentuate disc bulging and, when present, was found to be highly specific for nerve root compression (33,34). The shoulder relief sign produces temporary relief of lower cervical radiculopathy upon arm abduction, presumably caused by impingement on the lower cervical nerve roots (35,36).

Symptoms of a disc rupture frequently arise abruptly, although rarely is a specific traumatic event identified (29). Some patients first notice symptoms upon waking up in the morning. Often, paresthesias are the initial symptom with nerve root compression, and sharp pain ensues with subsequent nerve inflammation. The sharp pain may be described as "stabbing," is worse on coughing, and may be associated with a more constant deep ache radiating over the shoulder and down the arm. Patients often complain of headache and after several weeks may notice wasting of the muscles innervated by the compressed root. The symptoms of foraminal stenosis generally differ from soft disc herniation in that they tend to develop gradually, although for reasons often poorly understood, they may acutely become troublesome.

Impingement on individual cervical nerve roots generally produces complaints and findings on physical examination that are characteristic of the affected nerve's root pattern of innervation, and, thus, signs and symptoms are easiest to describe together (Table 71.1).

Compression of C3 and C4 does not produce perceptible muscle weakness and can be difficult to diagnose. C3 may cause suboccipital and neck pain, whereas C4 produces pain on one side of the neck and superior shoulder pain aggravated by movement, complaints that can easily be confused with the more common neck and shoulder muscular strain (37–39). Compression of C5 causes weakness of the deltoid and rotator cuff muscles, resulting in weakness and fatigue in shoulder abduction. This deficit is particularly disabling because it impairs the ability to perform multiple common tasks such as combing and brushing hair, dressing, and hailing a taxi. Although C5 makes a contribution to the biceps, this is rarely perceptible when C6, its major innervation, is unimpaired.

C6 compression results in complaints of pain radiating across the top of the shoulder and along the anterolateral aspect of the arm and forearm to the middle and index finger. Weakness affects the biceps, infraspinatus, serratus anterior, supinator, extensor pollicis, and extensor carpi radialis muscles. The physical examination typically elicits weak-

TABLE 71.1. *Patterns of Signs and Symptoms in Cervical Radiculopathy*

Level	Nerve root involved	Distribution of pain	Motor deficits	Reflex change
C3/4	C4	Back of the neck sometimes radiating to the upper chest	None	None
C4/5	C5	Base of the neck to the shoulder and area above the deltoid	Deltoid	None
C5/6	C6	Lateral arm and forearm to the index finger and thumb	Biceps and brachioradialis	Biceps
C6/7	C7	Middle of the forearm to the middle finger	Triceps	Triceps
C7/T1	C8	Medial forearm to ulnar aspect of the hand	Hand intrinsics	None

ness in elbow flexion, forearm supination, and wrist extension. C6 impingement also results in a diminished biceps and supinator jerk.

Compression of the C7 root causes pain radiating across the back of the shoulder, across the triceps, and down the posterior arm to the middle finger. C7 contributes to the innervation of the triceps, pectoralis major, latissimus dorsi, and extensors of the wrist, thumb, and fingers. On examination, the most striking motor deficit is weakness of elbow extension. In contrast to deltoid weakness that is readily apparent to patients, triceps weakness may not be noticed until the deficit is profound. An absent triceps jerk is another useful and early clinical sign of C7 compression.

The C8 nerve root is compressed by degeneration of the C7-T1 level. Cutaneous innervation is provided to the medial hand, including the fifth and a portion of the fourth digits. Pain, however, is an infrequent complaint in relation to the hand weakness produced by a C8 radiculopathy. C8 innervates the interosseous muscles of the hand as well as the opponens pollicis, abductor digiti minimi, and flexor digitorum profundus. Examination often demonstrates weakness in finger abduction and extension, hand grip, wrist flexion, and thumb opposition. Patients may thus complain of experiencing difficulty in operating tools and in holding a pen to write.

Although patients with pure radiculopathy should not exhibit signs of myelopathy such as spastic gait, increased deep tendon reflexes, or sphincter dysfunction, they may occur in those in whom a large paracentral disc herniation or spondylotic ridge compresses both the spinal cord and the exiting nerve root.

Natural History

Remarkably little literature exists describing the natural history of cervical radiculopathy. The prognosis is generally more favorable in patients with pure soft disc herniation compared with that secondary to foraminal stenosis from spondylosis or hard disc because spontaneous symptomatic improvement is frequently seen that can be correlated with desiccation and regression of the herniation (40). The distinction between hard and soft disc, however, may be difficult to make definitively except at surgery.

Various studies have shown that nonoperative management of cervical radiculopathy leaves a substantial minority of patients with persistently troublesome symptoms (14,41, 42). Lees and Turner found that in two thirds of patients, symptoms tend to persist in the absence of surgical treatment (14). DePalma and Subin found that of 255 patients treated nonoperatively, only 29% experienced complete symptom relief (22,41). Better outcomes with nonoperative management, however, have been observed in studies that were based in physiotherapy centers than those from surgical series (22).

In conclusion, cervical radiculopathy is usually caused by later herniation of the intervertebral disc, spondylotic narrowing of the intervertebral foramen, or a combination of both. Signs and symptoms are those of unilateral lower motor neuron dysfunction related to compression of a discrete nerve root that usually can be identified on the physical examination. The Spurling test and the shoulder abduction test either exacerbate or relieve pressure on a nerve root in the neural foramen and provide supportive evidence for foraminal compression. Most patients with acute radiculopathy from soft disc herniation experience some remission of symptoms. The natural history of radiculopathy from spondylotic foraminal stenosis and chronic lateral disc herniation is unknown, although there appear to be a substantial minority of patients who endure persistent symptoms.

REFERENCES

1. Chiles BW 3rd, Leonard MA, Choudhri HF, et al. Cervical spondylotic myelopathy: patterns of neurological deficit and recovery after anterior cervical decompression. *Neurosurgery* 1999;44(4):762–769; discussion, 9–70.
2. George B, Gauthier N, Lot G. Multisegmental cervical spondylotic myelopathy and radiculopathy treated by multilevel oblique corpectomies without fusion. *Neurosurgery* 1999;44(1):81–90.
3. Kumar VG, Rea GL, Mervis LJ, et al. Cervical spondylotic myelopathy: functional and radiographic long-term outcome after laminectomy and posterior fusion. *Neurosurgery* 1999;44(4):771–777; discussion, 7–8.
4. Voskuhl RR, Hinton RC. Sensory impairment in the hands secondary to spondylotic compression of the cervical spinal cord. *Arch Neurol* 1990;47(3):309–311.
5. Heller JG. The syndromes of degenerative cervical disease. *Orthop Clin North Am* 1992;23(3):381–394.
6. Iansek R, Heywood J, Karnaghan J, et al. Cervical spondylosis and headaches. *Clin Exp Neurol* 1987;23:175–178.
7. Nakanishi T, Mannen T, Toyokura Y, et al. Symptomatic ossification of the posterior longitudinal ligament of the cervical spine. Clinical findings. *Neurology* 1974;24(12):1139–1143.
8. Ramos-Remus C, Russell AS, Gomez-Vargas A, et al. Ossification of the posterior longitudinal ligament in three geographically and genetically different populations of ankylosing spondylitis and other spondyloarthropathies. *Ann Rheum Dis* 1998;57(7):429–433.
9. Klara PM, McDonnell DE. Ossification of the posterior longitudinal ligament in Caucasians: diagnosis and surgical intervention. *Neurosurgery* 1986;19(2):212–217.
10. Bucciero A, Vizioli L, Cerillo A. Soft cervical disc herniation. An analysis of 187 cases. *J Neurosurg Sci* 1998;42(3):125–130.
11. Denno JJ, Meadows GR. Early diagnosis of cervical spondylotic myelopathy. A useful clinical sign. *Spine* 1991;16(12):1353–1355.
12. Sung RD, Wang JC. Correlation between a positive Hoffmann's reflex and cervical pathology in asymptomatic individuals. *Spine* 2001;26 (1):67–70.
13. Rowland LP. Surgical treatment of cervical spondylotic myelopathy: time for a controlled trial. *Neurology* 1992;42(1):5–13.
14. Lees F, Turner J. Natural history and prognosis of cervical spondylosis. *BMJ* 1963;2:1607–1610.
15. Nurick S. The natural history and the results of surgical treatment of the spinal cord disorder associated with cervical spondylosis. *Brain* 1972;95(1):101–108.
16. Phillips DG. Surgical treatment of myelopathy with cervical spondylosis. *J Neurol Neurosurg Psychiatry* 1973;36(5):879–884.
17. Symon L, Lavender P. The surgical treatment of cervical spondylotic myelopathy. *Neurology* 1967;17(2):117–127.
18. Sadasivan KK, Reddy RP, Albright JA. The natural history of cervical spondylotic myelopathy. *Yale J Biol Med* 1993;66(3):235–242.
19. Montgomery DM, Brower RS. Cervical spondylotic myelopathy. Clinical syndrome and natural history. *Orthop Clin North Am* 1992; 23(3):487–493.

20. Wang YL, Tsau JC, Huang MH. The prognosis of patients with cervical spondylotic myelopathy. *Kaohsiung J Med Sci* 1997;13(7):425–431.
21. Barnes MP, Saunders M. The effect of cervical mobility on the natural history of cervical spondylotic myelopathy. *J Neurol Neurosurg Psychiatry* 1984;47(1):17–20.
22. Radhakrishnan K, Litchy W, O'Fallon W, et al. Epidemiology of cervical radiculopathy. *Brain* 1994;117:325–335.
23. Odom G, Foinney W, Woodhall B. Cervical disk lesions. *JAMA* 1958; 166:23–28.
24. Lunsford LD, Bissonette DJ, Zorub DS. Anterior surgery for cervical disc disease. 2. Treatment of cervical spondylotic myelopathy in 32 cases. *J Neurosurg* 1980;53(1):12–19.
25. Dubuisson A, Lenelle J, Stevenaert A. Soft cervical disc herniation: a retrospective study of 100 cases. *Acta Neurochir* 1993;125(1–4):115–119.
26. Cloward R. The anterior approach for removal of ruptured cervical discs. *J Neurosurg* 1958;15:602–617.
27. Espersen JO, Buhl M, Eriksen EF, et al. Treatment of cervical disc disease using Cloward's technique. I. General results, effect of different operative methods and complications in 1,106 patients. *Acta Neurochir* 1984;70(1–2):97–114.
28. Grisoli F, Graziani N, Fabrizi AP, et al. Anterior discectomy without fusion for treatment of cervical lateral soft disc extrusion: a follow-up of 120 cases. *Neurosurgery* 1989;24(6):853–859.
29. Scoville WB, Dohrmann GJ, Corkill G. Late results of cervical disc surgery. *J Neurosurg* 1976;45(2):203–210.
30. Slipman CW, Plastaras CT, Palmitier RA, et al. Symptom provocation of fluoroscopically guided cervical nerve root stimulation. Are dynatomal maps identical to dermatomal maps? *Spine* 1998;23(20): 2235–2242.
31. Tanaka N, Fujimoto Y, An HS, et al. The anatomic relation among the nerve roots, intervertebral foramina, and intervertebral discs of the cervical spine. *Spine* 2000;25(3):286–291.
32. Yoss R. Significance of symptoms and signs in localization of involved root in cervical disc protrusion. *Neurology* 1957;7:373–383.
33. Spurling R, Scoville W. Lateral rupture of the cervical intervertebral discs. *Surg Gynecol Obstet* 1944;78:350–358.
34. Viikari-Juntura E, Porras M, Laasonen EM. Validity of clinical tests in the diagnosis of root compression in cervical disc disease. *Spine* 1989;14(3):253–257.
35. Fast A, Parikh S, Marin EL. The shoulder abduction relief sign in cervical radiculopathy. *Arch Phys Med Rehabil* 1989;70(5):402–403.
36. Farmer JC, Wisneski RJ. Cervical spine nerve root compression. An analysis of neuroforaminal pressures with varying head and arm positions. *Spine* 1994;19(16):1850–1855.
37. Chen TY. The clinical presentation of uppermost cervical disc protrusion. *Spine* 2000;25(4):439–442.
38. Jenis LG, An HS. Neck pain secondary to radiculopathy of the fourth cervical root: an analysis of 12 surgically treated patients. *J Spinal Disord* 2000;13(4):345–349.
39. An HS. Cervical root entrapment. *Hand Clin* 1996;12(4):719–730.
40. Bush K, Chaudhuri R, Hillier S, et al. The pathomorphologic changes that accompany the resolution of cervical radiculopathy. *Spine* 1997; 22:183–186.
41. DePalma A, Subin D. Study of the cervical syndrome. *Clin Orthop* 1965;38:135–134.
42. Rothman R, Rashbaum R. Pathogenesis of signs and symptoms of cervical disc degeneration. *AAOS Instructional Course Lectures* 1978; 27:203–215.

CHAPTER 72

Nonoperative Treatment of Radiculopathy and Myelopathy

Steven E. Weber and Glenn Rechtine II

The treatment of cervical spine disorders should be based on accurate knowledge of the condition as well as the natural history of the disease process. The natural histories of radiculopathy and myelopathy are not the same. Although these processes may occur simultaneously, they are considered separately in this chapter. Outcomes of operative and nonoperative management should be compared to the natural history of the disease before definitive treatment is recommended.

CERVICAL RADICULOPATHY

Natural History

The natural history of cervical radiculopathy has been reviewed by multiple authors (1,2). Radiculopathy generally presents with pain, numbness, or weakness in a dermatomal distribution. Causative factors include an acute nucleus pulposus herniation, spondylitic changes around the foramen causing nerve compression, or a combination of these. Cadaver studies document the natural progression of disc disease with aging (3). The pathomechanial cause of radicular symptoms may be secondary to direct compression or stretching of the nerve root. Spontaneous regression of a herniated nucleus pulposus has been demonstrated in the cervical spine (4). Disc degeneration is related to many factors. The patient's generalized health, occupation, genetics, and adverse health habits are all contributory factors (*). The natural history may also be affected by a lack of patient motivation due to secondary gain issues, depression, substance abuse, financial problems, or aberrant social dynamics. Nonoperative treatment frequently leads to resolution of symptoms while avoiding the risks of surgery.

Treatment

The goals of any treatment plan should be well defined. Specifically, it should be the goal of the treating physician to relieve pain, improve function, and prevent recurrence.

Although some symptomatic patients meet surgical criteria, most patients are clearly candidates for nonoperative treatment. The surgeon should educate the patient regarding the condition as well as the role of various treatments. Chronic cervical disease may entail psychological modifiers that may adversely affect outcomes. Likewise, secondary gain issues may complicate outcomes. Treatment modalities for radiculopathy include rest, medications, physical therapy, manipulation, injections, and patient education.

Rest

Patients with acute exacerbations of lumbar radicular symptoms may benefit from a short period of rest. A randomized clinical trial revealed that outcomes for patients who had 48 hours of bed rest were at least equivalent to those who had 7 days of bed rest (5). Longer periods of inactivity contribute to diminished muscle strength (6), further deconditioning, decreased bone mineral density (6,7), and a negative nitrogen balance. This should be similar with cervical radiculopathy. The patient should be mobilized after no more than 2 days of bed rest to maximize the rehabilitation potential.

Medications

Pharmacologic agents treat the underlying condition and provide symptomatic relief. The various classes of medications used to treat radiculopathy include steroids, nonsteroidal antiinflammatory drugs (NSAIDs), muscle relaxants, narcotics, and antidepressants (8). It is crucial to differentiate between acute and chronic pain. Some therapies that may be beneficial for acute pain management may be detrimental or addictive for patients suffering from chronic pain.

Steroids have a potent antiinflammatory effect and may be indicated for short-term initial management of radiculopathy. A multitude of undesirable side effects can occur with these medications and are amplified with prolonged use. Contraindications include congestive heart failure, heart disease, peptic ulcer disease, hypertension, infections, diabetes, glaucoma, osteoporosis, and psychosis.

NSAIDs have become common for use in the initial treatment of cervical radiculopathy. These medications interfere with prostaglandin synthesis, inhibiting the inflammatory cascade that accompanies the condition. There are substantial side effects with regard to the renal, hepatic, gastrointestinal, cardiovascular, and hematologic systems. Recently, cyclooxygenase-2 (COX-2) inhibitors have been released, with reported benefits of fewer gastrointestinal side effects and decreased antiplatelet effects. Cost may preclude these medications from being first-line therapy if traditional NSAIDs may be used effectively.

Muscle relaxants have been shown to provide relief for associated muscle spasm that may occur with cervical disc disease (9). In general, the use of a centrally acting agent that does not produce sedation is optimal. Use of medications that cause relaxation of all skeletal muscles should be avoided because they produce fatigue and may have abuse potential.

Narcotic medications are indicated for short-term use in patients with acute radicular symptoms. Adverse effects include constipation, sedation, and addiction. Long-term use of narcotics for the treatment of chronic neck or radicular symptoms should be avoided.

Antidepressant agents may be helpful in the treatment of radiculopathy. They may be useful for treating depression as a result of prolonged pain (10).

Physical Therapy

Physical therapy is an important element in the treatment algorithm for cervical radiculopathy. It includes both passive and active modalities. Physical therapy addresses all three treatment goals. Some recommend initiation in the first 3 to 5 days of treatment (11). During the initial evaluation by the physical therapist, patients are educated regarding their condition.

Passive Modalities

Passive modalities include heat, cryotherapy, mechanical traction, ultrasound, massage, and the use of a soft cervical collar (11). However, well-designed studies that show an advantage for any of these treatments over placebo are lacking. Heat is divided into superficial and deep compo-

nents. Superficial heat is thought to reduce pain at trigger points (12) and to reduce muscle spasms (13). Deep heat is produced by ultrasound, which is thought to provide relief of radicular pain through mechanical stimulation of neural pathways (14). Cryotherapy is used as an adjunct to increase the pain threshold, decrease muscle guarding, and reduce acute inflammation. Cervical traction has been postulated to distract joints, relieve pressure off nerve roots and discs, improve epidural blood flow, and reduce inflammation, pain, and muscle spasm. Unfortunately, well-designed studies proving long-term benefits for this modality do not exist. Likewise, massage provides mechanical stimulation to increase circulation and promote muscle relaxation, but no clinical study shows its efficacy in the treatment of cervical disc disease. Soft cervical collars may provide a feeling of increased support during the initial phase of treatment but have never revealed any statistical improvement over placebo (11).

Active Modalities

Active modalities include isometrics, aerobic conditioning, range-of-motion exercises, and dynamic muscle training. Isometric exercises entail a static training regimen that permits the strengthening of the paravertebral muscles without invoking spinal motion. This prevents loss of muscle tone and is indicated in the acute phase of pain, when neck motion is not well tolerated. Aerobic conditioning is necessary to regain endurance, increase oxygen consumption, and increase strength for the deconditioned patient. It may be the most important factor in the prevention of future recurrences once the patient has reached a pain-free state. High-impact aerobics are to be avoided in the acute phase of pain. Patients should be limited to walking or riding a stationary bike 20 to 30 minutes three times a week. The patient then progresses into range-of-motion exercises as pain permits. These should be performed in conjunction with an aerobic program, and segue into resistance exercises. These dynamic maneuvers allow for strength training and should focus on the paravertebral, shoulder, and upper truck musculature. These are important in the prevention of symptom recurrence, the last goal of treatment (15).

Manipulation

Manipulation may be undertaken in many forms, from soft tissue mobilization to high-velocity thrusting techniques. Although reliable studies do exist for the treatment of the lumbar spine, quality data in controlled studies are lacking for cervical radiculopathy. Neurologic complications have occurred but are extremely rare (16) and almost exclusively related to high-velocity thrusting techniques. Spinal root compromise is also a contraindication for high-velocity techniques (17). Soft tissue mobilization may be beneficial in the acute phase of pain but should only be performed by the appropriate trained specialist (18).

Injection Therapy

Nerve root injections may be useful for diagnostic and sometimes palliative treatments, but this is based on anecdotal evidence at best. Well-controlled studies for epidural steroid injections are lacking for cervical radiculopathy. Serious complications from these treatments have occurred (19,20). Trigger point treatments probably work by direct mechanical stimulus, and although they may have minimal associated side effects, their efficacy in long-term management of radicular symptoms has not been proved.

Other Treatments

Electrical stimulation has been shown to help eliminate the symptoms of neck pain, but scant literature is available regarding cervical radiculopathy (21). Electrical stimulation fails to address long-term relief or the prevention of recurrent episodes. Muscle stimulation has not been studied in well-controlled settings for cervical radiculopathy.

CERVICAL MYELOPATHY

Cervical myelopathy is defined as symptomatic spinal cord compression typically due to a decrease in the diameter of the spinal canal. It may be a result of a large central disc herniation or, more commonly, may be due to degenerative changes in the cervical spine. Myelopathy may have an acute or insidious onset, with the latter being more common (22). The mere radiographic appearance of spinal cord compression does not in itself indicate the presence of myelopathy. Indeed, striking degrees of cord compression may occur without neurologic compromise. A change in the spinal cord itself must occur for symptomatic myelopathy to occur. Sudden alterations in the cord compression, as often seen in acute disc herniation or trauma, allow less time for adaptation and are more likely to be associated with serious neurologic sequelae. On the contrary, in longstanding cervical spondylosis, the spinal cord has time to adapt to the compression. Thus, neurologic changes may be insidious in onset. However, even a trivial injury in the patient with acquired cervical stenosis may have a devastating effect on an already compromised spinal cord.

Natural History

Although there is some debate with regard to the natural history, it is well accepted by most clinicians that the general course of cervical myelopathy is that of a nonlinear decline in function (23). Some patients experience a plateau in their symptoms, but spontaneous improvement is rare. Other patients may show a fairly rapid decline. Several attempts have been made to correlate the clinical course with radiographic or clinical indicators, but no reproducible predictor has been discovered. High signal intensity regions on T2 MRI films were hypothesized to be predictive of perma-

nent neurologic damage, but this has not been consistent (24,25).

Unlike focal nerve root compression in radiculopathy, the physical findings of myelopathy vary considerably. Gait disturbance and spasticity are common, as is the so-called myelopathic hand. Various spinal cord syndromes may occur. Physical exam may reveal multiple pathologic reflexes. It is important to remember, however, that the differential diagnosis for myelopathy extends well beyond cervical spinal cord compression.

Treatment

For the patient who is blatantly myelopathic, any therapeutic modalities should be adjunctive to surgical intervention. Physical therapy with modalities may be used in the perioperative period to assist with rehabilitation and endurance as well as pain control. Likewise, medications may be used to help control pain. The use of a neck brace for patients with a biomechanical component to their clinical process may be of benefit. Epidural steroids in this condition are not likely to be helpful and may present increased risk in an already compromised spinal canal.

A somewhat more difficult predicament occurs in the patient with asymptomatic spinal cord compression. Again, the previously mentioned treatments may assist with pain modulation. Patient education in this scenario is paramount. Potential outcomes of various treatments, both operative and nonsurgical, must be reviewed in detail along with associated risks in order to formulate a treatment plan.

CONCLUSION

Cervical radiculopathy is often treated successfully by nonoperative means (26). The occurrences of radiculopathy and myelopathy are not mutually exclusive. The presence of myelopathy may persuade the surgeon to consider operative intervention. Nonoperative modalities in frank cervical myelopathy should be adjunctive to surgical intervention. Chronic pain, workers' compensation, and litigation cases may evoke modulating circumstances (27). Patient education is important in the treatment of both entities.

REFERENCES

1. Lees F, Aldren Turner JW. Natural history and prognosis of cervical spondylosis. *BMJ* 1963;2:1607.
2. Nurick S. The natural history and the results of surgical treatment of the spinal disorder associated with cervical spondylosis. *Brain* 1972; 95:101–108.
3. Coventry M, Ghormley R, Kernohan J. The intervertebral disc: its microscopic anatomy and pathology. Part 1. *J Bone Joint Surg Am* 1945; 27:105.
4. Maigne JY, Deligne L. Computed tomography follow-up study of 21 cases of non-operatively treated cervical intervertebral soft disc herniation. *Spine* 1994;19:189–191.
5. Deyo R, Diehl A, Rosenthal M. How many days of bed rest for acute low back pain? A randomized clinical trial. *N Engl J Med* 1986;315: 1064.

6. Krolner B, Toft B. Vertebral bone loss: unheeded side effect of thera- peutic bed rest. *Clin Sci* 1983:64:537.
7. Hansson T, Roos B, Nachemson A. Development of osteopenia in the fourth lumbar vertebrae during prolonged bed rest after operation for scoliosis. *Acta Orthop Scand* 1975;46:621.
8. Dillin W, Uppal G. Analysis of medications used in the treatment of cervical disc degeneration. *Orthop Clin North Am* 1992;23:421.
9. Cullen A. Carisoprodol (Soma) in acute back conditions: a double- blind randomized placebo controlled study. *Curr Ther Res Clin Exp* 1976;20:557.
10. Malloy P. Tricyclic antidepressants for resistant rheumatic pain. *Intern Med* 1991;12:35.
11. Tan J, Nordin M. Role of physical therapy in the treatment of cervical disk disease. *Orth Clin North Am* 1992;23:435.
12. McGray RE, Patton NJ. Pain relief at trigger point injections: a com- parison of moist heat and short wave diathermy. *J Orthop Sports Phys Ther* 1984;5:175.
13. Fountain FP, Gerstein JW, Sengu O. Decrease in muscle spasm pro- duced by ultrasound, hot packs, and infrared radiation. *Arch Phys Med Rehabil* 1960;41:293.
14. Ziskin MC, McDiarmid T, Michlovitz SL. Therapeutic ultrasound. In: Michlovitz S, ed. Thermal agents in rehabilitation. Philadelphia: FA Davis, 1990;2:134.
15. Astrand P. Exercise physiology and its role in disease prevention and rehabilitation. *Arch Phys Med Rehabil* 1987;68:305.
16. Livingston M. Spinal manipulation causing injury (a three year study). *Clin Orthop* 1971;81:82.
17. Kleynhans AM. Complications and contraindications to spinal manip- ulative therapy. *In* Haldeman S, ed. Modern developments in the prin- cipals and practice of chiropractic. Norwalk, CT: 1980:359.
18. Brodin H. Cervical pain and mobilization. *Int J Rehabil Res* 1984; 7:190.
19. Hodges SD, Castleberg RL, Miller T, et al. Cervical epidural steroid injection with intrinsic spinal cord damage. *Spine* 1999;11:1170.
20. McLain RF, Fry M, Hecht JT. Transient paralysis associated with epidural steroid injection. *J Spinal Disord* 1997;5:441–444.
21. Deyo R, Walsh N, Martin D, et al. A controlled trial of transcutaneous electrical nerve stimulation and exercise for chronic low back pain. *N Engl J Med* 1990;322:1627.
22. Bernhardt M, Hynes RA, Blume HW, et al. Cervical spondylotic myelopathy: current concepts review. *J Bone Joint Surg Am* 1993;75: 119.
23. Orr RD, Zdeblick TA. Cervical spondylotic myelopathy. *CORR* 1999; 359:58.
24. Ota K, Ikata T, Katoh S. Implication of signal intensity on T1 weighted MR image on the prognosis of cervical spondylotic myelopathy. *Orthop Trans* 1996;20:443.
26. Wiesel S, Cuckler J, DeLuca F, et al. Acute low back pain: an objec- tive analysis of conservative therapy. *Spine* 1980;5:324.
27. Anderson G. Epidemiologic aspects of low back pain in industry. *Spine* 1981;6:53.
25. Wada E, Ohmura M, Yonenobu K. Intramedullary changes of the spinal cord in cervical spondylotic myelopathy. *Spine* 1995;20: 2226.

CHAPTER 73

Differential Diagnosis of Cervical Radiculopathy and Myelopathy

Richard S. Brower

Neck and back pain are very common reasons for patients to seek medical care. There are many diagnostic entities that may cause pain of the neck, shoulder girdle, and arm. It is not unusual for such patients to have more than one diagnosis. For example, many patients with neck pain develop shoulder pain as well, and often the patient with rotator cuff disease or a "frozen" shoulder develops concomitant neck pain. It is essential to perform a thorough history and physical examination to come to a definitive diagnosis. In cases in which there are several diagnoses identified, it is necessary to identify the main cause of the symptoms and to direct any medical interventions toward the main offenders.

The personal situation of the patient may have a profound effect on the presentation of neck and arm pain. Headache is a very common complaint in this group of patients. Establishing the differential diagnosis for these individuals can be a very confusing process. Workers' compensation issues, motor vehicle crashes, and emotional instability all too often further cloud the clinical picture. This chapter is intended to help sort out some of the clinical situations that present as neck and arm pain.

PHYSICAL EXAMINATION OF THE PATIENT WITH NECK AND ARM PAIN

As with any other musculoskeletal disorder, evaluation of a patient presenting with neck and arm pain starts with a detailed history and physical examination. There are some special maneuvers that should be included in the physical examination of these individuals, along with a thorough neurologic examination.

Cervical Radiculopathy

The term *radiculopathy* refers to the signs and symptoms of nerve root dysfunction. Root dysfunction may result from mechanical deformation of the nerve root, such as is caused by a herniated disc or a bone spur, or it may be idiopathic. Classically, root dysfunction manifests as changes in sensory, motor, and reflex function in the course of the nerve root involved. In the lumbar spine, it is often easy to identify the nerve root involved. Because of the subtle variability of the branching of the brachial plexus, it may be difficult to identify the affected nerve root in a patient with neck and arm pain. Young patients with a single-level soft disc herniation may exhibit a classic single-level radicular pattern with acute onset of symptoms. Older patients with extensive degenerative changes often exhibit signs and symptoms of more than one level of root involvement, especially if there is an element of spinal cord compression. In this setting, the radiculopathy is usually chronic in nature, with a gradual onset of symptoms.

C3 Radiculopathy

The third cervical nerve root is rarely involved in degenerative disease of the cervical spine, owing to the normally limited amount of motion at the C2-3 disc. The dermatomal pattern of this root radiates over the posterior upper neck onto the occiput and the ear. There is no distinct motor function for this root, and numbness is unusual. Headache pain may be confused with a C3 radiculopathy.

C4 Radiculopathy

The C3-4 disc has more motion than C2-3 and is therefore more commonly involved in radicular pain. The pattern of

C4 root pain is at the base of the neck, out over the medial shoulder, and inferior to the level of the scapula. The fourth root lacks a definitive motor function, but pain may be provoked by neck extension. Although the fourth root controls diaphragm function and is of concern in a patient with a spinal cord injury, radicular problems of the fourth root rarely affect diaphragmatic function.

C5 Radiculopathy

Herniation of the C4-5 disc (Fig. 73.1) is uncommon but is more common than at the levels above. Degenerative changes of this level occur third most commonly, after C5-6 and C6-7. Radiculopathy of the fifth root may be difficult to differentiate from shoulder pathology. The sensory distribution is from the base of the neck out over the top of the shoulder and down onto the lateral upper arm (so-called epaulet pattern). A thorough evaluation of shoulder motion is necessary along with the neurologic examination to differentiate cervical disease from shoulder pathology. Most importantly, internal and external rotation of the shoulder, along with strength testing of the rotator cuff muscles, must be documented. Some patients with fifth root pathology may develop a frozen shoulder as a consequence of their radicular pain. The exact etiology of this phenomenon is uncertain.

The deltoid is innervated primarily by the fifth root, so that motor involvement results in weakness of shoulder abduction. This may appear similar to an acute rotator cuff tear, but without tenderness over the shoulder. Complete paralysis of the deltoid may be quite disabling because the patient has difficulty using the affected arm for daily activities, especially those that require overhead motion. Careful examination may demonstrate weakness of external shoulder rotation (supraspinatus and infraspinatus), but this is less reliable. There may also be an element of biceps weakness with C5 root lesions and possible suppression of the biceps reflex. A patient with profound weakness of the deltoid and disability related to daily activities as a result of cervical disc disease may require a more aggressive surgical approach.

C6 Radiculopathy

The C5-6 disc (Fig. 73.2) is most commonly affected by degenerative disc disease and, along with the C6-7 disc, represents one of the two most common levels for disc herniation. The pain of a sixth root lesion radiates from the base of the neck, along the biceps muscle and lateral forearm, and onto the dorsum of the hand and fingers on the radial side, involving the tips of the first two digits. Patients may note tenderness of the biceps muscle during examination. Biceps weakness is often subtle and unnoticed by the patient until demonstrated by examination and may be accompanied by weakness of wrist extension. More subtle muscular changes involve the infraspinatus, serratus anterior, supinator, and extensor pollicis. The biceps reflex is mediated primarily by the sixth root and provides additional objective evidence of an anatomic lesion. The clinical picture often includes pain in the proximal arm, with numbness into the hand.

C7 Radiculopathy

C7 radiculopathy is a common occurrence because of the frequency of both disc herniations and degenerative changes at the C6-7 level (Fig. 73.3). Although sensory distribution is variable among individuals, pain or numbness involving the middle finger is a hallmark of seventh root lesions, with some possible overlap onto the bordering digits. Patients trace the pain distribution across the poste-

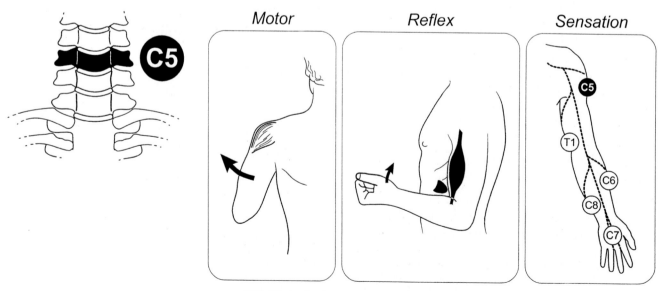

FIG. 73.1. C5 neurological level.

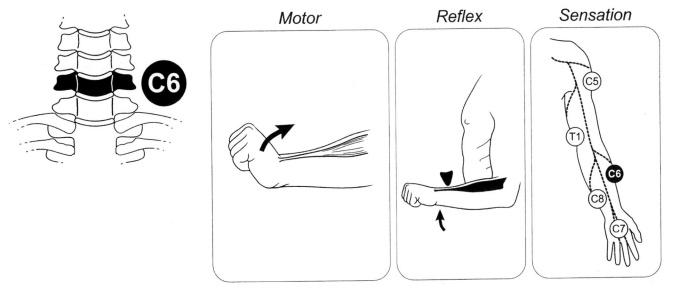

FIG. 73.2. C6 neurological level.

rior shoulder, along the triceps and posterolateral forearm, to the middle digit. Loss of the triceps reflex is a reliable indicator of seventh root dysfunction.

Triceps weakness is often quite profound but may not be noticed by the patient. For a spinal cord injured patient, the triceps is vital for push-off function in order to live independently, but gravity can provide elbow extension in persons with normal leg function. An athletically involved patient whose sport involves forceful elbow extension or a manual laborer who performs overhead activities may notice triceps weakness. The examiner must be careful not to be fooled by a patient who tries to substitute internal rotation of the humerus to compensate for triceps weakness.

The C7 root also provides some motor function to the pectoralis major muscle that may be evaluated by testing humeral adduction. Additional muscles that may be included in the C7 neurologic level are the pronator, extensor digitorum, and latissimus dorsi, along with wrist flexion, primarily from the flexor carpi radialis.

C8 Radiculopathy

Herniation of the disc at the C7-T1 level is unusual, but it does occur. The C8 nerve root provides sensation to the ulnar side of the hand, primarily the fourth and fifth digits, and to the ulnar side of the forearm. Pain and numbness are

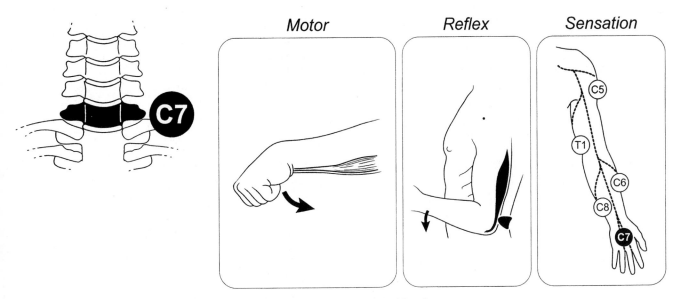

FIG. 73.3. C7 neurological level

distributed the same as with an ulnar nerve lesion at the elbow.

Strength testing of the C8 root involves primarily the small muscles of the hand. Finger flexion, as powered by the flexor digitorum profundus and superficialis muscles, is under control of the eighth root. In addition, the intrinsic muscles, especially the interossei, which control finger abduction, are innervated by C8 and T1. Loss of motor function can be very disabling, with weakness of the power grip, normally from the ulnar side of the hand. There may also be difficulties with turning keys or holding small objects owing to weakness, especially of the first dorsal interosseous muscle.

Upper Motor Neuron Examination

Any time there is a clinical situation of neck and arm pain, it is important to evaluate the function of the upper motor neurons as well. The differential diagnosis may change substantially depending on the results of the complete physical examination. Some patients also have more than one diagnosis.

When evaluating the neurologic function of the upper extremity, the examiner can assess the coordination of the limb just by observation. It may be a subtle finding, but some patients tend to have difficulty cooperating with strength testing, not for lack of effort, but because of loss of coordination. During the reflex examination, observation of an inverted radial reflex should alert the examiner to the possibility of cervical cord compression. Examination should always include looking for the Lhermitte sign, which suggests a dynamic compression of the cervical cord related to head position. The Hoffman sign may be nonspecific but can be an indicator of upper motor neuron disease or cervical cord compression.

Even if the clinical problem involves only the upper extremity, the lower extremities should be examined for hyperreflexia and spasticity. I usually do a quick reflex examination of the lower extremities and check the ankle for clonus. Should there be any suggestion of upper motor neuron disease detected, a more detailed examination may be conducted. One of the best ways to assess the function of the patient's central nervous system is to observe him or her walking. Spasticity may be seen as a wide-based, unsteady gait. The patient's gait tends to deteriorate with faster walking and with walking greater distances. Family members of the patient with an early myelopathic gait often complain of the patient bumping into them frequently while walking together.

CLINICAL SYNDROMES

Disc Herniation

Clinical presentations of cervical disc herniation are quite variable, depending on the level involved. Generally, patients note the onset of neck pain followed by radiation of the pain into the characteristic dermatomal pattern of the nerve root involved. Weakness is often not noted immediately because pain inhibition markedly limits activities. Just as in individuals with shoulder pain, these patients are more comfortable sleeping in a reclining chair than in a bed. Some present with a torticollis rotating away from the painful side in an unconscious effort to open the neuroforamen and lessen the arm pain. Extension of the cervical spine exacerbates pain for almost any patient with cervical spine disease, whether soft disc herniation or degenerative disc disease. Patients with acute disc herniation may present in a very characteristic posture with the shoulder abducted and the forearm resting on top of the head. This promotes lateral flexion toward the opposite side to open the affected neuroforamen, and the abduction relieves tension on the nerve root. During examination, rotating the head and laterally bending toward the symptomatic side (Spurling test) exacerbates the arm pain. Routine neurologic examination reveals the changes characteristic of the involved nerve root, as discussed earlier.

Immobilization of the cervical spine often provides substantial relief of pain. Again, extension is quite painful; therefore, if a soft collar is used, wearing it backward (with the Velcro in front) is more comfortable because the neck is held in a flexed position. This is very useful for sleeping.

Mechanical Neck Pain

Patients with degenerative disc disease of the cervical spine complain of activity-related axial pain. The pain may be referred along sclerotomal lines into the shoulder and upper arm, but the overwhelming complaint is of neck pain. Activities that involve cervical extension, such as painting the ceiling, exacerbate symptoms. Many patients complain of grinding or crepitation with cervical motion. Driving may be difficult for a number of reasons. It requires a substantial amount of motion to watch for traffic and to park. In addition, the vibration of the vehicle may induce substantial discomfort, especially over rough roads. Rest and immobilization should relieve symptoms of mechanical neck pain.

Differential Diagnosis

Tumors

Tumors of a number of structures may produce pain in the neck or arm. The pain distribution produced depends on the nature and location of the lesion. Benign tumors may exert their effects by causing structural problems such as vertebral collapse and deformity or by compressing the neurologic structures. Osteoid osteoma may cause local pain that is relieved with nonsteroidal antiinflammatory drugs (NSAIDs). Osteoblastoma has a predilection for the posterior elements of children and rarely causes neurologic symptoms. Eosinophilic granuloma can produce vertebra plana and cause neurologic symptoms, but it more frequently causes axial pain. Giant cell tumors and aneurysmal bone cysts are associated with large soft tissue masses and therefore cause neurologic symptoms such as spinal cord compression.

Unilateral radicular pain may result from several benign tumors. Schwannomas are usually intradural, developing from the sensory root, and most characteristically cause unilateral radicular pain. The pain may be multidermatomal if the lesions are multiple, as in neurofibromatosis, and they may grow so large as to cause myelopathic symptoms. Oblique films show the foraminal enlargement characteristic of these lesions. Meningiomas of the cervical spine, which generally occur in middle-aged women, have a similar origin and clinical presentation.

In the adolescent age group, rapid growth of osteochondromas in the posterior elements may cause a monoradicular pattern of pain. The larger soft tissue mass of aneurysmal bone cysts may cause radicular or myelopathic symptoms.

Malignant lesions cause nonmechanical pain that is of a deep burning or boring character. These patients complain of pain keeping them awake at night and that they cannot find a comfortable position. They may be restless in the examination room, unable to sit still for any length of time. The pain is constant in nature but is more tolerable during the day when patients have more sensory input to mask their discomfort. As the lesion grows, these symptoms of bone destruction may evolve into radicular or myelopathic-type symptoms. This change is very sudden and can be catastrophic if bone collapse and deformity cause acute neurologic compromise (Fig. 73.4). Any patient with a history of malignancy and complaints of spine pain should

have a nuclear bone scan to rule out metastases. The character of the lesion may make detection difficult because very lytic tumors to which the body has no chance to mount an osteoblastic response may produce a false-negative bone scan. The classic example of this is multiple myeloma, but it may be imitated by a variety of malignancies, such as renal cell carcinoma and lung tumors.

Extraspinal malignancies may mimic cervical disc disease by the development of shoulder and arm pain. Lesions in any part of the shoulder girdle skeleton may cause weakness through pain inhibition or biomechanical abnormality. Soft tissue lesions also can present with characteristics of neck or arm pain or weakness. The classic example is a Pancoast tumor of the apex of the lung. Direct extension of the tumor mass can invade the brachial plexus and be missed on routine chest films. Apical lordotic films may demonstrate the lesion, but a computed tomography (CT) scan of the chest is more reliable. These patients present with shoulder girdle pain and weakness, along with Horner syndrome (ipsilateral miosis, pseudoptosis, and enophthalmos), which is due to the disruption of the sympathetic chain (Fig. 73.5). Other lesions of the pharynx or upper mediastinum may result in invasion of the spine, chest wall, or brachial plexus.

Intracerebral lesions may also mimic radicular symptoms from cervical disc disease. Tumors or vascular phenomena may result in paralytic symptoms or dysesthesia. The presence of upper motor neuron abnormalities such as a hyper-reflexic jaw jerk should lead the examiner to consider the brain as the source of the problem.

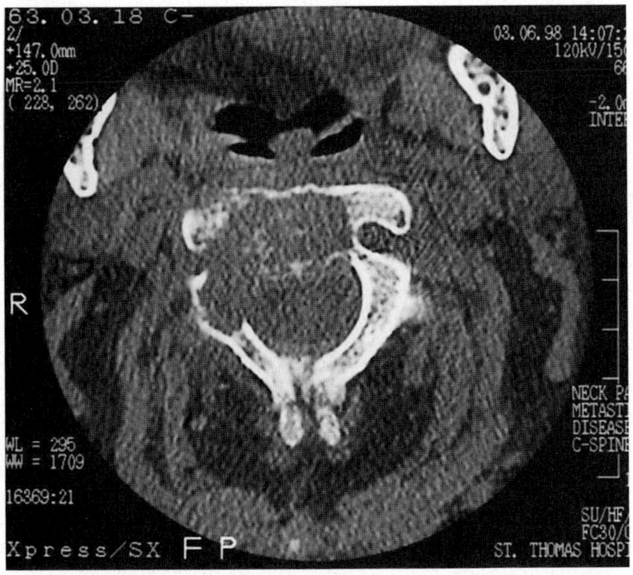

FIG. 73.4. Computed tomography scan of C4 in a patient with neck pain due to metastatic breast cancer. The vertebral body, right pedicle, and facet have been destroyed.

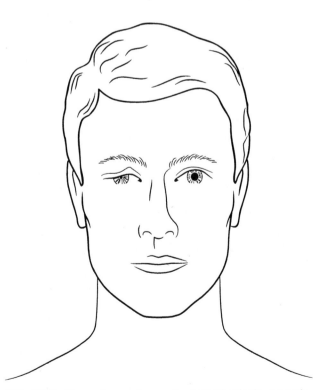

FIG. 73.5. Horner's syndrome (ipsilateral miosis, pseudoptosis, and enophthalmos).

Neurologic Disease

A number of central nervous system conditions may result in pain and weakness similar to those seen in cervical radiculopathy. A cerebrovascular accident can cause paralytic symptoms of the shoulder girdle. Although weakness is the predominant presenting complaint, pain may be substantial.

Multiple sclerosis (MS) and amyotrophic lateral sclerosis (ALS) are neurologic conditions that are described later in this chapter (see Motor Neuron Disease).

Guillain-Barré syndrome is an ascending paralysis and paresthetic condition of the peripheral nerves that first affects the lower and then the upper extremities. It is also known as *acute idiopathic polyneuritis*. The degree of motor paralysis is more advanced than the sensory changes.

Idiopathic Brachial Neuritis

This very painful condition is thought to be caused by a viral infection of the motor nerves and is quite sudden in onset. The syndrome starts with severe pain into the arm that is worse with movement. Within 2 weeks, the pain abates and is followed by profound upper extremity weakness that may result in a flail arm without any sensory changes. There is usually spontaneous recovery of function, but recovery may not be full. It is easily differentiated from radiculopathy by the lack of sensory changes and the involvement of multiple nerve roots. Electromyogram (EMG) examination shows signs of neurogenic atrophy.

Brachial Plexopathy

Stretch injury to the brachial plexus (Fig. 73.6) can occur in high-velocity motor vehicle crashes with sudden depression of the shoulder and lateral bending of the neck to the opposite side. This represents a spectrum of syndromes from the minor stretch of a single nerve root to the complete avulsion of multiple roots from the cervical spinal cord. Brachial plexopathy may also result from surgical misadventure, particularly from procedures for thoracic outlet syndrome (TOS) or from sternal splitting procedures such as coronary artery bypass. As with any nerve injury, reflex sympathetic dystrophy may be seen in the aftermath of the acute injury. Missile injuries such as gunshot or knife wounds and radiation to the area of the brachial plexus such as for breast carcinoma are other etiologies of plexopathy. Chances for recover and clinical outcome are determined by the severity of the initial injury.

Upper Extremity Nerve Entrapment Syndromes

Thoracic Outlet Syndrome

TOS involves either vascular or neurologic symptoms or a combination of both as a result of compression of the vascular tree or the brachial plexus as it passes from the base of the neck through the axilla. Vascular symptoms are related to compression of the subclavian or axillary artery or the accompanying veins and affect the radial side of the hand. Neurologic symptoms are caused by compression of C8 and T1, the lower two roots of the brachial plexus, and commonly affect the ulnar side of the hand. These symptoms

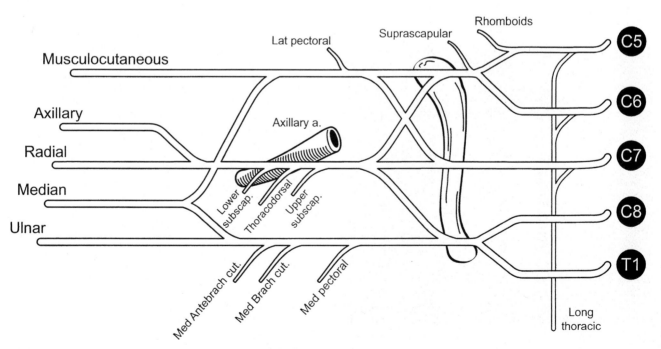

FIG. 73.6. Brachial plexus.

may be related to compression by bony elements such as cervical ribs, the first thoracic rib, and the clavicle, or by muscles such as the scalenus anticus and the pectoralis minor.

There is substantial individual variation in the points of insertion of the scalenes onto the first rib after their origin from the transverse processes of the third through sixth cervical vertebrae. First-rib elevation can further narrow the available space for the neurovascular bundle. To perform Adson's test, the arm is abducted, externally rotated, and extended while palpating the radial pulse. If the pulse diminishes as the patient turns his or her head toward the affected side, it indicates compression of the subclavian artery.

Once past the scalene muscles, the vessel may be compressed between the clavicle and the first rib—the costoclavicular syndrome. This may be tested for by pulling the shoulders downward and backward to see if symptoms are reproduced. The potential space between the clavicle and the first rib may be narrowed by malunion of the clavicle, exostoses of the first rib, or congenital anomalies. The final area of possible compression is between the pectoralis minor muscle anteriorly and the first rib posteriorly. The result is hyperabduction syndrome—the neurovascular bundle is compressed with the shoulders in the fully abducted and extended position. Asking the patient to place his or her hands behind the head and push the elbows backward may reproduce symptoms.

Vascular TOS can be differentiated from cervical radiculopathy because there is no muscular weakness at rest. Signs and symptoms of vascular disease should be overwhelming in the clinical presentation without any clear sensory or reflex changes. Major arterial TOS may be the result of an aneurysm formation in the subclavian artery, most commonly caused by the presence of a cervical rib. Examination shows asymmetric pulses in the upper extremities with a supraclavicular bruit. Patients may exhibit Raynaud phenomenon and complain of muscle fatigue. Sudden progression of symptoms, along with ischemic pain or ulceration in the fingers, may be the harbinger of arterial emboli that could cause loss of the limb. This is better managed on an elective basis before reaching this stage. Surgical treatment consists of excision of the aneurysm and primary anastomosis or vascular grafting.

Minor arterial TOS is not an immediate danger to the viability of the upper extremity because it is not associated with aneurysm formation or with embolic events. It is much more common than major arterial TOS. Patients complain of numbness, weakness, and paresthesias as the artery is compressed between the clavicle and the first rib. Symptoms are provoked by working overhead and are relieved by lowering the arms.

Venous TOS results from compression of the subclavian vein between the scalenus anticus muscle, the clavicle, and the first rib. Symptoms are similar to those of a subclavian vein thrombosis, with cyanosis and swelling of the upper extremity. Venous TOS should be positional in nature and relieved by rest.

Neurogenic TOS is a rare entity characterized by weakness and atrophy of the intrinsic musculature of the hand, with the most severe involvement in the lateral thenar muscles. The lower trunk of the brachial plexus is the structure involved, and symptoms consist of pain, paresthesias, and numbness over the medial upper arm, forearm, and hand. There are several different anatomic anomalies associated with neurogenic TOS, including a cervical rib or elongated transverse process of C7. Some patients have a tough fibrous band from the tip of the anomalous bone to the first rib. Symptoms are less positional in nature and much more common in women than in men. Because the neurologic symptoms stem from more proximal compression, the symptoms are less distinct than those of ulnar neuropathy. Sensory changes in ulnar neuropathy divide the ring finger in half, but this does not occur in TOS. There are also median nerve symptoms, with weakness of the lateral thenar muscles. As opposed to C8 and T1 radiculopathies, the interossei are less affected in TOS. Neurogenic TOS should demonstrate abnormalities on the EMG.

Treatment of TOS usually consists of postural exercises, and it may take time for improvement to occur. Resection of the bony anomaly such as a cervical rib may be considered if therapy fails to improve the symptoms. Surgical resection of the first rib is rarely indicated and may result in injury to the brachial plexus.

Dorsal Scapular Nerve Entrapment

The dorsal scapular nerve originates from the upper trunk of the brachial plexus and is composed of nerves from the C8 root. It passes through the scalenus medius muscle and at this point may be kinked. This nerve supplies the rhomboid muscles with motor function. Traction on the nerve may present as unilateral rhomboid pain, and over time, the patient may note weakness of the shoulder girdle and complain of pain into the arm. Turning the head toward the affected extremity and flexing laterally in the opposite direction may reproduce the symptoms. Surgical decompression is rarely indicated, and the first line of treatment is a strengthening program for the shoulder girdle musculature. A traction strain of this nerve may result from a whiplash-type injury.

Long Thoracic Nerve Entrapment

The long thoracic nerve forms from the uniting of the fifth and sixth cervical roots after they enter the scalenus medius muscle. As this branch exits the muscle, a branch from the C7 root joins it. The nerve supplies motor function to the serratus anterior muscle, and loss of function appears as a winging of the scapula. Treatment consists of an exercise program to stabilize the scapula and waiting for the nerve to recover.

Suprascapular Nerve Entrapment

The suprascapular nerve is a pure motor nerve that originates from the upper trunk of the brachial plexus, specifically the C5 and C6 roots, and supplies motor function to the supraspinatus and infraspinatus muscles. The nerve passes through the suprascapular notch of the scapula, where it is found deep to the transverse ligament. The clinical picture can be very cloudy and may involve repetitive trauma such as throwing or may be associated with frozen shoulder syndrome. Patients complain of activity-related shoulder pain, and examination shows weakness to shoulder abduction and external rotation, along with atrophy of the supraspinatus and infraspinatus muscles. The diagnosis may be made with EMG evaluation or more simply by blocking the nerve with local anesthetic in the suprascapular notch. Occasionally, surgical decompression is a consideration.

Median Nerve Entrapment

Pronator Syndrome

As the median nerve passes from the upper to the lower arm, there are four main places of potential nerve entrapment. The first is the ligament of Struthers, which originates from a supracondylar process of the humerus. Next is the lacertus fibrosus, which crosses the nerve at the level of the elbow joint. The third is the pronator teres muscle, which may be substantially hypertrophied. The final area of possible nerve entrapment is at the origin of the flexor digitorum superficialis muscle. The area of compression may be identified by physical examination. If the symptoms are aggravated by flexion of the elbow against resistance between 120 and 135 degrees of flexion, the ligament of Struthers is the most likely source. Pain with active flexion of the elbow while holding the forearm in pronation is likely caused by the lacertus fibrosus. With the wrist held in flexion to relax the flexor digitorum superficialis, pain with resisted pronation of the forearm indicates that the pronator muscle is the culprit. The flexor digitorum superficialis is the source of symptoms if there is pain with resisted flexion of the superficialis to the middle finger.

The clinical picture of pronator syndrome consists of pain in the proximal volar forearm and sensory signs and symptoms in the radial three and one half digits. There may be weakness of all the median nerve–innervated muscles because the compression is proximal to the branching of the anterior interosseous nerve. The sensory symptoms most closely imitate a C6 or C7 radiculopathy but do not involve the radial nerve–innervated muscles from these roots such as the triceps, wrist extensors, and wrist flexors.

Initial treatment usually consists of modification of activities. Before surgical exploration, the diagnosis ideally should be verified by EMG. Surgical release for pronator syndrome normally includes a release of all the areas of potential compression.

Anterior Interosseous Syndrome

The anterior interosseous nerve is a pure motor branch of the median nerve. Compression of this nerve results in vague pain in the distal forearm that is exacerbated by activity and relieved by rest. Examination should show weakness of the flexor pollicis longus, the flexor digitorum profundus of the index finger, and the pronator quadratus. Attempts by the patient to exert a strong pinch with the thumb and index finger result in hyperextension of the distal interphalangeal joint of the index finger and the interphalangeal joint of the thumb. There is often not a distinct structure causing this compression; thus, surgical exploration, if indicated, should start in the proximal forearm and follow the anterior interosseous nerve into the deep volar compartment. The origin of the flexor digitorum muscle appears to be the most common source of this syndrome.

Carpal Tunnel Syndrome

Carpal tunnel syndrome results from compression of the median nerve within the carpal canal. The etiology of the nerve compression may be thickening of the transverse carpal ligament or any space-occupying lesion within the carpal canal, including a ganglion cyst, malunion of distal radius fractures, carpal dislocation, or rheumatoid arthritis. Carpal tunnel syndrome is very common in pregnancy but usually subsides after delivery. Common symptoms are weakness or clumsiness of the hand, especially with vigorous activity, hypesthesia, paresthesia, or awakening with hand numbness. Sensory complaints should involve the radial three and one half digits, although patients often complain of whole hand numbness in the initial stages. There can be proximal radiation of the pain all the way up to the shoulder level. Carpal tunnel syndrome is more common in women and in individuals involved with repetitive use of the hand and wrist. Symptoms may be reproduced with the Phalen test (Fig. 73.7) or Tinel sign. The sensory symptoms may mimic a C6 or C7 radiculopathy, but without any associated proximal muscle weakness. In the advanced state, thenar weakness may mimic a T1 radiculopathy, but the first dorsal interosseous and hypothenar muscles are intact because they are innervated by the ulnar nerve.

Treatment begins with splinting the wrist in a neutral position, especially at night or during activities that exacerbate the symptoms. Injection of steroid and local anesthetic into the carpal canal can help make the diagnosis and may provide pain relief, at least temporarily.

Palmar Cutaneous Nerve

This sensory nerve originates from the radial side of the median nerve proximal to the wrist and innervates the skin of the thenar eminence. Injury to the palmar cutaneous nerve may have some of the sensory characteristics of a C6 radiculopathy, but without any associated muscle weakness. The

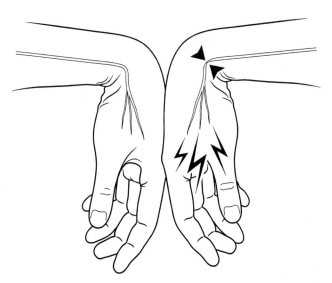

FIG. 73.7. Phalen's test reproduces pain and numbness in the patient with carpal tunnel syndrome.

nerve often lies between the palmaris longus and the flexor carpi radialis tendons and may be injured during injection of the carpal tunnel or during carpal tunnel release.

Ulnar Nerve Entrapment

Cubital Tunnel Syndrome

The most common location of entrapment of the ulnar nerve is the elbow. The clinical presentation of cubital tunnel syndrome starts with pain on the medial side of the elbow, with radiation of the pain and paresthesias down the ulnar forearm to the small finger and the ulnar side of the ring finger. Symptoms are reproducible with sustained hyperflexion of the elbow, and the Tinel sign should be positive at the elbow. Muscle atrophy is present early in the clinical course. Weakness is seen in the muscles innervated by the ulnar nerve distal to the elbow, including the flexor carpi ulnaris, flexor digitorum profundus to the long and ring fingers, and interossei and hypothenar muscles. The clinical syndrome may be difficult to differentiate from C8 and T1 radiculopathies. The difference can be seen on examination by normal strength in the C8 and T1 muscles that are not innervated by the ulnar nerve, such as the flexor pollicis longus, the thenar muscles, and the flexors of the index and long fingers.

The ulnar nerve arises as a continuation of the medial cord of the brachial plexus. The cubital tunnel forms behind the medial epicondyle of the humerus. The nerve lies beneath a fascial arcade, and at its distal end, the nerve passes between the two heads of the flexor carpi ulnaris to lie on the volar surface of the flexor digitorum profundus. Nerve conduction tests should show velocities with a reduction greater than 33%. Surgical treatment may be considered if nighttime bracing of the elbow in extension fails to improve

the pain. Surgical treatment generally consists of submuscular or subcutaneous transposition of the ulnar nerve at the elbow.

Guyon Canal Syndrome

Compression of the ulnar nerve within the Guyon canal can be from a number of anatomic causes. Ganglion cysts, thrombosis of the ulnar artery, or repetitive trauma causing hypothenar hammer syndrome are all common causes. The dorsal cutaneous branch of the ulnar nerve forms in the forearm, so that dorsal sensation over the ulnar side of the hand should be intact in this entity. Within the canal, the nerve splits into deep motor and dorsal sensory branches. The motor branch supplies the hypothenar muscles, the interossei, and the adductor pollicis. It should not be confused with C8 or T1 radiculopathies because the thenar muscles should be intact, and there should be normal sensation over the dorsal surface of the ulnar digits.

Radial Nerve Entrapment

The radial nerve passes through the lateral intermuscular septum at the junction of the middle and distal thirds of the humerus. In the anterior compartment, it lies between the brachialis and the brachioradialis muscles. At the radial head, the nerve branches into the superficial sensory branch that runs beneath the tendon of the brachioradialis to the distal forearm, where it supplies sensation to the dorsum of the hand. The deep motor branch enters the radial tunnel at the arcade of Frohse, passing between the superficial and deep heads of the supinator, and branches to supply the extensor digitorum communis, extensor carpi ulnaris, abductor pollicis longus, and extensor pollicis longus muscles. There are four main regions for compression within the radial tunnel. The first are fibrous bands anterior to the radial head at the entrance to the radial tunnel. Next is the leash of Henry, a fan-shaped leash of arteries crossing the nerve on their way to the brachioradialis and the extensor carpi radialis longus muscles. The third site is the tendinous margin of the extensor carpi radialis brevis. The fourth and most common site of radial nerve compression is the arcade of Frohse, a ligamentous band over the deep radial nerve as it enters the supinator.

Patients complain of aching in the extensor muscle mass that radiates to the distal forearm. Pain may be elicited by full flexion of the elbow with the forearm in supination and the wrist in a neutral position. The alternative maneuver is to flex the wrist with the forearm in full pronation. This can be differentiated from a C7 radiculopathy because the triceps should be spared because it is innervated in the upper arm.

Cervical radiculopathy may be imitated by many different disease entities. Careful history and physical examination are key to preventing one from falling into a diagnostic trap. Without listening to and examining the patient, it is all too easy to start proposing surgical procedures for anatomic abnormalities seen on sensitive tests such as magnetic resonance imaging (MRI) that are in fact asymptomatic.

As mentioned earlier, the complete examination should include evaluation for possible upper motor neuron disease. Upper motor neuron disease may be a secondary diagnosis picked up only by subtle findings on the physical examination. In the next section of this chapter, there may be considerable crossover with the radiculopathy section. It often requires good detective work to sort out these patients.

CERVICAL MYELOPATHY

Many different diagnostic entities may result in the clinical syndrome of cervical myelopathy. The term *myelopathy* refers to a very diverse symptom complex that may include spasticity or weakness of the upper and or lower extremities, loss of sensation, incoordination, and sphincter disturbance. There may be considerable crossover of symptoms with cervical radiculopathy, depending on the etiology of the myelopathy. Because of the wide variety of clinical presentations, the diagnosis is very often missed for considerable periods of time. It is not unusual for the myelopathic patient to have been seen by several different physicians and to have a number of differing diagnoses before the proper diagnosis is made.

Myeloradiculopathy

Myeloradiculopathy is characterized by the clinical presentation of both upper motor neuron signs and symptoms along with lower motor neuron symptoms as discussed earlier in the section on radiculopathy. This syndrome is seen most often in patients with cervical spinal canal stenosis in which there is compression of both the cord and the nerve roots. The result is a very confusing picture of weakness, pain, and spasticity. The lower motor neuron symptoms, like weakness, are seen more commonly in the upper extremities and are caused by stenosis in the upper cervical levels. Upper motor neuron symptoms such as spasticity and incoordination are more prevalent in the lower cervical levels and lower extremities.

Patients with myeloradiculopathy are most commonly older and have cervical spinal stenosis from degenerative disc disease. The combination of central canal narrowing and foraminal narrowing results in deformity of the cord and individual nerve roots. It is not unusual for these patients to have had at least a workup, if not surgery, for carpal tunnel syndrome before seeing a spine surgeon. Because of their age, many of these patients have some evidence of median nerve slowing by nerve conduction velocity, but the main problem may well be in the neck. I have found myelopathy to be a common cause of failed carpal tunnel releases.

Cervical Spondylotic Myelopathy

Degeneration of the intervertebral disc is inevitable in humans as we age. The loss of water content in the nucleus of the disc results in loss of height of the disc. As the disc flattens, the annulus may bulge outward from its usual profile, resulting in narrowing of the spinal canal. At the same time, there is usually degeneration of the facet joint located posterior to the cord. As the facets degenerate and enlarge, the spinal canal is narrowed further. For the patient with a narrow canal, on a genetic basis, there is a limited ability to accommodate these intrusions, and the result is deformity of the spinal cord. Once the cord deformity reaches a critical level, myelopathic symptoms may ensue. It is not unusual for traumatic incidents to trigger the onset of symptoms, or they may appear without an inciting event.

For the patient with advanced degenerative changes and a narrow spinal canal, a fall with hyperextension of the cervical spine is the classic cause of central cord syndrome. As the neck is forced into hyperextension during the traumatic episode, the cord is trapped between the osteophytes located at the posterior aspect of the vertebral end plates and the infolding ligamentum flavum located posteriorly.

The injury to the cord involves the medial aspect of the lateral corticospinal tract, thus causing motor paralysis of the upper extremity distal to the lesion. The sparing of the lateral aspect of the lateral corticospinal tract allows for better strength in the lower extremities. Depending on the severity of the injury, these patients often experience some recovery. Immediate surgery does not appear to be of much value for these patients, and steroids are recommended if they can be started within 8 hours of the incident.

Patients with degenerative changes leading to cervical stenosis are the most common group of patients presenting with myelopathy. A thorough history and physical examination are needed to raise the suspicion of myelopathy as a possible diagnosis. Regular x-rays should always be done first to look for structural problems. The next step is often an MRI. Many surgeons still consider the myelogram with a postmyelogram CT scan to be the gold standard for diagnosis of cervical spinal canal stenosis (1).

Herniated Disc

Very large herniated cervical discs may cause myelopathic symptoms (Fig. 73.8). The patient population that seems most prone to this situation are young patients who still have a large amount of material in their discs and a congenitally narrow canal. In this situation, there is a large amount of disc material available to herniate into the canal and a very limited canal area to contain both the cord and the herniation. If the herniation is in the midline, the clinical presentation may demonstrate little if any arm pain but pure weakness and spasticity distal to the level of the blockage. Should the fragment be more to one side of the canal,

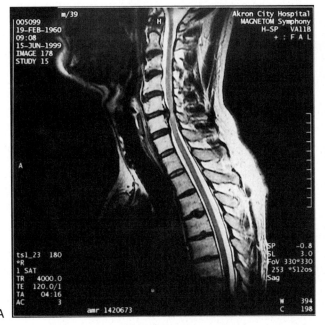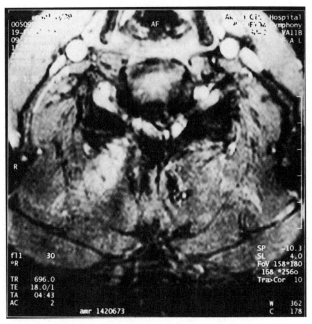

FIG. 73.8. A: Sagittal T2-weighted magnetic resonance imaging (MRI) study of a 39-year-old man who presented with weakness and incoordination in all four extremities. **B:** Axial MRI study of the same patient showing nearly complete blockage of the spinal canal.

arm pain and lower motor neuron symptoms may be seen at the level of the herniation. Fortunately, herniated discs large enough to cause myelopathy are rare.

Ossification of the Posterior Longitudinal Ligament

OPLL is seen most commonly in Asia, particularly in Japan; however, it is not unusual to see it in the United States. As the ligament is ossified with cortical bone, it continues to grow and occupy more space in the spinal canal. Over time, the cord may become quite compressed, and myelopathic symptoms may ensue. These patients have a fairly stiff spine, providing some protection of cord function because there is limited mechanical stimulation of the cord. Myelopathic symptoms may appear gradually, or they may appear with a traumatic incident. Men and women are affected equally. Because the compression of the cord is from cortical bone, it may be seen better by CT than by MRI, which does not visualize lamellar bone well.

Instability

Many different disease processes can lead to instability of the cervical spine. The spine has two essential tasks: to maintain posture and to protect the neurologic elements. Anytime the spine is unable to fulfill its normal function, it may be considered unstable. As the cervical spine subluxes out of normal alignment, the cord and nerve roots

may be compressed or irritated. The mechanical stimulation can result in myelopathic symptoms.

Trauma

Trauma can trigger myelopathy by a number of mechanisms. These are linked by the common thread of narrowing of the spinal canal and mechanical deformation of the neurologic elements. We have already discussed central cord syndrome in which the cord is compressed by the anterior osteophytes and posterior ligamentum flavum. This is seen most commonly without fracture or dislocation.

In cases of trauma, patients may suffer an injury to the posterior ligaments or a fracture that is unrecognized. These patients may present a considerable time after the injury with complaints of myelopathic symptoms due to the continued cord compression and irritation from posttraumatic instability. It is essential to review plain film before ordering neuroradiographic imaging to rule out the possibility of instability. Dynamic films can be helpful if there is a high index of suspicion and static films fail to reveal the diagnosis. The occipitocervical junction must be examined carefully for abnormalities, such as pseudoarthrosis of the dens, that are easy to miss without careful inspection. Posttraumatic transverse atlantal ligament instability is an unusual injury that is recognized on dynamic films. It may also cause myelopathy.

A traumatic incident may be the trigger to recognizing chronic patterns of instability like those changes common to rheumatoid arthritis or other inflammatory diseases. It is typical for patients to ignore what they consider to be common pain. Films taken after a minor accident may reveal long-standing but previously unrecognized instability patterns. Patients with ankylosing spondylitis are at increased risk for late instability of deformity caused by unrecognized fractures, occasionally from seemingly minor trauma.

Os Odontoideum

Os odontoideum is a rounded ossicle of bone in the normal location of the odontoid process of the axis. The etiology of os odontoideum remains uncertain, but a traumatic cause seems most likely. Although this disorder may be asymptomatic, it may become symptomatic at virtually any time of life. It can be differentiated from an acute fracture of the dens in that the sharp fracture lines seen with acute fracture are absent. The os has smooth, rounded borders and a considerable gap between the ossicle and the body of the axis. There may be considerable instability seen on flexion and extension films. With flexion, the cord may be caught between the body of the axis anteriorly and the posterior aspect of the ring of C1. Patients may present with mechanical neck pain or with the onset of myelopathy. If it becomes symptomatic, surgical stabilization is necessary.

Congenital Anomalies of the Atlantoaxial Joint

Dwarfing conditions may be associated with congenital abnormalities of the atlantoaxial joint that can lead to instability. Down syndrome is the most common of these genetic abnormalities with the instability pattern of atlantoaxial subluxation. The question of screening these children for participation in sports is a controversial topic. It is clear that for the patient with a symptomatic C1-C2 instability, stabilization is the appropriate treatment. Children with Morquio syndrome (mucopolysaccharidosis type IV) have a high prevalence of atlantoaxial instability due to odontoid hypoplasia.

Klippel-Feil Syndrome

Patients with Klippel-Feil syndrome have congenital fusions in the cervical spine. The classic triad used to identify Klippel-Feil syndrome includes a short neck, a low posterior hairline, and a limited range of motion of the neck. The radiographic changes may be difficult to identify in the young child until there is sufficient ossification of the cervical spine. Cineradiography may be used to study the biomechanics of cervical motion in order to identify which levels have abnormal mechanics. There are many other abnormalities associated with the syndrome, including scoliosis, cleft lip and palate, facial asymmetry, cardiovascular anomalies, and urogenital anomalies, most commonly unilateral absence of the kidney. Myelopathy develops from the associated basilar invagination or more commonly from hy-

permobility at the levels adjacent to the congenitally fused segments.

Chiari Malformation

Chiari malformations are the extension of the cerebellum through the foramen magnum into the spinal canal. Asymptomatic Chiari malformations may be seen as an incidental finding on MRI. Type I malformations become symptomatic in young adults and adolescents who do not have myelomeningocele. They often present with lower cranial nerve palsies, vertigo, ataxia, headache, and syncope during Valsalva maneuver. If there is an associated syringomyelia, the patient often has sensory loss and atrophy, especially in the hands. Type II lesions are associated with myelomeningocele and often become symptomatic in infancy with respiratory difficulties. Either type may become symptomatic with a clinical picture of myelopathy, and both types are best diagnosed by MRI.

Rheumatoid Arthritis

Rheumatoid arthritis has a predisposition to affect the cervical spine. The topic is covered exhaustively elsewhere in this text. The main cervical manifestations of rheumatoid arthritis are cranial invagination (basilar invagination), atlantoaxial subluxation, and subaxial subluxation. They may be present individually or in combination with each other. In general, these are patients with long-standing disease with substantial manifestations of their disease involving other joints. When myelopathic signs and symptoms develop in a patient with rheumatoid arthritis, a careful series of radiographic study must be undertaken. MRI and CT scans may be needed to evaluate the bony landmarks, the space available for the cord, and for the presence of significant pannus formation.

Infection

Infection of the cervical spine may occur for a number of reasons. The infection may form from hematogenous seeding from another infection in the body. Recent surgery, trauma, or the presence of malignancy creates an area that is more easily susceptible to secondary infection. Infection may also be the result of direct inoculation during medical procedures, such as discography or surgery. Patients with compromised immune systems are at greater risk. These include elderly patients and patients with diabetes mellitus, human immunodeficiency virus (HIV) infection, rheumatoid arthritis, alcoholism, and intravenous drug use. It may require a high index of suspicion in immunocompromised patients to diagnose infection because they may demonstrate only weakness and pain with little in the way of constitutional symptoms. The usual hallmarks of infection such as fever, chills, elevated white cell count, and elevated sedimentation rate may be absent. A careful history of antecedent infection may be important in identifying the virulent organism. Workup of these patients should include pan culturing to look for other sites of infection.

Myelopathy may be seen as a consequence of disc space infection or osteomyelitis of the spine. Infection that progresses to the formation of an epidural abscess may create a surgical emergency because the myelopathic syndrome develops over a very short period of time and may progress rapidly to full quadriparesis and death. For the patient with an acute infection, myelopathy develops from the mass effect caused by the abscess. In the case of a more long-standing infection, deformity and instability from destruction of the bony elements may well be part of the problem. Infection in the cervical spine may also result from direct extension of infection from the pharynx or mediastinum.

HIV infection may cause myelopathy because of opportunistic infection of the brain or spinal cord. The HIV virus has been associated with the development of a vacuolar degeneration and demyelinization of the cord itself. The etiology of this process is uncertain.

Tumors

Tumors of the brain or spinal cord may be the cause of myelopathy. Benign skeletal lesions may induce symptoms because they are space-occupying lesions and may compress the brain or cervical cord. Metastatic disease is the most common cause of myelopathy from tumor. These may be identified on plain radiograph or bone scan, but neuroradiographic imaging is needed to assess the degree of cord compression. MRI is very sensitive for identifying the marrow changes of tumor in the bone, but CT is the better modality to grade the amount of bone destruction present. Evaluation of bony destruction is essential in determining whether surgical stabilization is needed. For the patient with myelopathy but minimal changes seen in the cervical spine, imaging of the brain is appropriate.

Neurofibroma

Neurofibromas, also known as *schwannomas*, originate from the Schwann cell of the sensory nerve root and form a fusiform dilation of the root. When they straddle the neuroforamen, the appearance is that of the classic dumbbell lesion. When the lesions are large enough, they may compress the cervical cord, resulting in myelopathy. Because the root is involved first, it is common for radiculopathy to develop, followed by myelopathy.

MRI is the procedure of choice to identify these lesions. On plain film, neurofibromas frequently cause widening of the foramen of the involved root, and the cord may be shifted toward the opposite side. They are isointense on T1-weighted images and are likely to have increased signal on T2-weighted images.

Meningiomas

Another intradural but extramedullary tumor, a meningioma often originates in the area of the dentate ligament. It is thought to arise from arachnoid villi cells near the nerve root sleeve. Meningiomas are more likely solitary but may be multiple, and a small minority may be extradural. A high percentage of meningiomas have progesterone receptors that make them sensitive to changes in levels of female sex hormones. Clinical presentation is similar to neurofibromas, with radiculopathy in the early stages and myelopathy seen later.

Intramedullary Tumors

A number of intramedullary tumors can cause myelopathy. Detailed discussion of them can be found elsewhere in this text.

Syringomyelia

The term *syringomyelia* is used to describe all abnormal fluid-filled cavities in the spinal cord except small nonenlarging cavities secondary to trauma or necrosis. There is a strong association with both types of Chiari malformations, and they may form after a significant spinal cord injury. The etiology of these cysts is still uncertain. They may become symptomatic at any point of life, and the clinical presentation depends on the location of the cyst within the cord substance. In children, scoliosis is often the first manifestation of syringomyelia, whereas adults have pain and numbness. Patients may also present with Charcot joints in the upper extremity as their first symptom. The natural history is uncertain, as is the timing of surgical intervention, if appropriate. Syringomyelia is best diagnosed by MRI but may also be seen on postmyelogram CT views if there is a delay after the myelogram.

Radiation Myelopathy

Patients who have had radiation to the cervical spine may develop myelopathic symptoms a year or more after the radiation exposure. The patients are often quite ill to start with because the radiation is used to treat a cord tumor or metastatic disease. The symptoms are often progressive after their initial insidious appearance. There is no satisfactory treatment for this entity.

Motor Neuron Disease

Amyotrophic Lateral Sclerosis

ALS is a progressive disease of both the upper and lower motor neurons. ALS appears in the fourth to the sixth decades. It usually presents in adults with symmetric muscular weakness of the shoulder with atrophy and fasciculations, all without any loss of sensation. The first manifestations are often in the hands, with progression up to the shoulder girdle. Fasciculations of the tongue are a hallmark of the physical examination. EMG demonstrates denervation atrophy, whereas nerve conduction velocities are relatively unaffected. Neuroradiographic images fail to identify any cervical lesions, and cerebrospinal fluid chemistry is normal. The disease progresses relentlessly to death in 2 to 5 years with few exceptions. There is no effective treatment for this disease.

Multiple Sclerosis

MS traditionally presents with visual changes and upper motor neuron lesions, but it can appear just like a disc herniation in the cervical spine, with pain and weakness. The typical age of onset is between 20 and 40 years, and MS is slightly more common in women. MS is more common in temperate climates; thus, there may be environmental factors involved in this disease. The plaques of MS can be found in the cervical spinal cord as well as in the brain. Usually, multiple nerve roots are involved. The diagnosis is aided by the presence of visual changes, paresthesias, and spasticity. The clinical picture includes waxing and waning of the symptoms without much predictability. As mentioned earlier in the chapter, MS can have virtually any clinical presentation, from upper to lower motor neuron symptoms. It should be considered especially in young patients with onset of spasticity, weakness, and myelopathy. MRI is the imaging modality of choice to visualize the spinal cord and brain.

CONCLUSION

History and physical examination are both key to making the correct diagnosis. Although many of these clinical syndromes are rare, they do exist. In the myelopathic patient in whom no structural lesion can be found on cervical imaging, medical causes must be considered. It requires perseverance to make the correct diagnosis for many of these patients. Especially in cases of cervical myelopathy, the patients may be very frustrated because of the number of physicians they have seen without a real diagnosis. Many feel better just to know what they have.

REFERENCE

1. Shafaie FF, Wippold FJ II, Gado M, et al. Comparison of computed tomography myelography and magnetic resonance imaging in the evaluation of cervical spondylotic myelopathy and radiculopathy. *Spine* 1999; 24(17):1781–1785.

CHAPTER 74

Discogenic Neck Pain

Timothy A. Garvey

Smith and Robinson described anterior cervical discectomy and fusion (ACDF) as a treatment option for cervical disc degeneration in patients suffering from a cervical disc syndrome. This syndrome featured chronic pain in the posterior part of the neck, shoulder, occiput, and arm; paresthesias in the arm; limitation of movement of the neck; and roentgenographic evidence of cervical disc degeneration (1–3). This description appears to encompass the continuum of pain symptoms that can be generated from a cervical motion segment. This includes axial mechanical localized neck pain, referred symptoms ranging from the occiput to the interscapular region, and radicular pain into the upper extremity along the course of the ventral rami. In patients with radicular pain and objective neurologic compression or loss of neurologic function, whether radicular or myelopathic, there is little controversy about the reasonableness of ACDF as a treatment option (2–24). The focus of this chapter is on patients who have localized neck pain, with or without referred symptoms, as their chief complaint, who present for evaluation of potential surgical options. The goal is provide an understanding of the surgical literature that affects rational decision making regarding the surgical option for such patients.

EPIDEMIOLOGY

Although another chapter in this textbook details the epidemiology of the degenerative process, a brief review of neck pain is useful. Bovim and colleagues reported on a prevalence study in which 35% of the general Norwegian population reported neck pain complaints within the previous year (25). Fourteen percent of the respondents reported that their neck pain lasted more than 6 months. A similar population-based study in Finland noted that about 9.5% of men and 13.5% of women reported a chronic neck pain syndrome (26). A more recent report by Cote on the Saskatchewan Health and Back Pain Survey revealed that

54% of respondents experienced neck pain in the previous 6 months; almost 5% of these respondents perceived their neck pain as highly disabling (27). It appears, therefore, that neck pain of some magnitude, with a minority of about 5% to 10% of cases being severe or chronic in nature, may affect the general human population.

NATURAL HISTORY

Although most of those with neck pain complaints noted in questionnaire studies likely do not present for medical evaluation, many patients do so. We have an appreciation for the natural history of these cases. Gore reported on the long-term follow-up of 205 patients with neck pain (28). In this study with, an average 15.5-year follow-up, nonoperative management led to 79% of patients noting improvement, with 43% being pain free and 32% having moderate to severe persistent pain (28). Specific injury and severity of initial symptoms were reported to be more indicative of an unsatisfactory outcome.

Rothman, despite now being a nonadvocate of surgical intervention in those with axial cervical spine pain, stated, "It does not appear that cervical disc degeneration is a brief self-limiting disorder, but rather a chronic disease, productive of significant pain and incapacity over an extended period of time" (29). DePalma and Subin reported on a series of patients with neck or neck and radicular pain, of which only 45% of those treated nonoperatively had a satisfactory long-term outcome (30). DePalma, Rothman, and colleagues reported on another series of patients with significant cervical disc degeneration, dominant neck pain, and no gross radiculopathy; in these patients, nonoperative care led to complete relief in 21%, partial relief in 49%, and no relief in 22% at 3 months of follow-up (9). Rothman noted at a 5-year follow-up study that 23% of patients who had significant cervical symptoms from disc degeneration remained partially or totally disabled (20). However, in the surgical group treated for dominant neck pain, little functional difference was noted at the 5-year point, which led to his adopting a "most conservative posture in the treatment of the nonneurogenic syndromes" (20).

Lees in the 1960s (31) and Dillin in the 1980s (32) reported on the natural history and prognosis of cervical radiculopathy. Their work demonstrated that radiculopathy typically does not progress to myelopathy, but that in almost two thirds of those treated nonoperatively, there is persistent symptomatology (although not severe in all).

It thus seems that as a ballpark estimate for the education of a patient seeking consultation regarding treatment options, natural history studies would predict a minority of about 20% to 30% of individuals who present with complaints referable to cervical degenerative conditions to have persistent symptomatology of moderate to severe enough magnitude to interfere with the activities of daily living. It is in this smaller group that the surgeon needs to evaluate whether surgical management is a viable option.

TRAUMATIC ETIOLOGY

A substantial number of patients who present for surgical evaluation have a specific traumatic event as the initiating factor of their symptoms, whereas for others, a gradual onset would go along with a slowly progressive degenerative disorder. Many patients present with a classic rear-end mechanism of injury, that is, a whiplash injury. The Quebec Task Force preferred the terminology whiplash-associated disorder (WAD) in its monograph (33). It concluded that WAD is almost always self-limited and rarely results in permanent harm (33). In their review and methodologic critique of the literature, however, Freeman and colleagues determined, "There is no epidemiologic or scientific basis in the literature for the following statements; whiplash injuries do not lead to chronic pain, rear impact collisions that do not result in vehicle damage are unlikely to cause injury, and whiplash trauma is biomechanically comparable with common movements of daily living" (34).

Ian MacNab, one of the founding members of the Cervical Spine Research Society, summated his experience with whiplash injuries: "about 10–20% are left with discomfort of sufficient severity to interfere with their ability to do work or to enjoy themselves in leisure hours" (35). Although this was more of his gestalt, he specifically commented on a total of 266 patients, of an original 575 group series, 2 years after the settlement of court actions (36,37). Of these 266 patients, 145 were available for review, and 121 had persistence of symptoms. Therefore, a minimum of 45% (121 of 266) of patients 2 years after court settlement had persistence of symptoms.

In Hohl's 5-year follow-up of 146 patients with soft tissue injuries to the neck, 43% of patients, who had no *pre-existing degenerative changes*, had persistent symptomatology, although no comment as to the magnitude of that symptomatology is given (38).

A continuing series from Bristol has assessed prognostic factors in soft tissue injuries of the cervical spine (39–41). At 2-years' follow-up, 66% of subjects had complaints of neck pain, and 43% had headaches (40). At 10.8-years' follow-up, Gargan and Bannister noted that residual symptoms were intrusive in 28% and severe in 12% (39).

Hildingsson and Toolanen reported on a prospective series of 93 patients regarding the outcome of soft tissue neck injuries suffered in car crashes (42); 42% of patients reported complete recovery, and 58% reported continued symptoms. Of the total 93 patients, 41 (44%) had substantial complaints, whereas 13 (14%) complained of only mild discomfort. Jonsson and associates reported on a prospective 5-year evaluation of 50 patients with whiplash-type neck distortions (43). Fourteen of 50 (28%) had persistent symptoms, with an average visual analog score (VAS) of 3.1. Another 6 of 26 (23%) who originally had improved at 6 weeks redeveloped neck symptoms.

Finally, Freeman and co-workers reported on an interesting study of major spinal injury resulting from low-level acceleration—a case series of roller coaster injuries (44). Major spinal injuries occurred at a rate of 13 per 100,000 exposures despite the calculated generated forces of the roller coaster being similar in level and duration to those generated by a 3- to 4-mile per hour rear-impact collision.

From this review of the literature, it appears that McNab's observations are accurate (33,35,45,46). I counsel patients that about 60% of patients have complete or nearly complete resolution of symptoms, most within the first few months, and that roughly 40% have persistent symptoms. Of an original injury group, about 10% to 20% have symptoms of sufficient nature to limit markedly their occupational or recreational activities. Instead of using the Quebec Task Force wording that patients "almost always" get better, and "rarely have permanent harm," I prefer counseling patients that "usually" or "most often" their symptoms will resolve, and that in only "a smaller percentage" of cases will long-term significant symptoms or permanent damage become evident.

OFFICE EVALUATION

The key to any care is the initial establishment of a solid patient–physician relationship. This is accomplished with a careful attainment of the patient's history, a review of the patient's self-intake documentation (e.g., pain diagram, self-reported functional scales, SF36), and performance of a thorough physical examination. A patient with discogenic neck pain often has a history of trauma, usually complains of pain with forward flexion, usually has increasing symptoms with driving (whole-body vibration), and usually experiences some relief with postural changes. The social history is often of particular importance, so that specific documentation of compensation and litigation issues is undertaken. Indicators of depression on intake evaluation forms or noted on examination are documented. The neurologic examination, which may appear less important in this group with dominant axial neck pain, should nonetheless be detailed because it is still imperative to correlate lesser radicular symptoms and signs clinically, with the available anatomic imaging studies.

Although the classic incongruency signs were validated for low back pain, I use a similar approach in evaluating patients with a chief complaint of neck pain (47). If light touching of the skin causes violent complaints of pain, if whole-arm numbness or multiroot breakaway weakness is noted, or if the patient exhibits pain behavior consistent with overreaction, I then formalize the psychosocial evaluation. This is done with an MMPI study or referral for a formal psychological assessment. For example, a patient with overreacting chronic pain behavior of grimacing and "owching," with breakaway weakness and complaints of pain with light palpation, and with documented disillusionment with the medical profession or depressive tendencies on our intake forms would not be initially considered a candidate for surgical workup and would be encouraged to participate in a multidisciplinary pain program.

In patients who have failed an active nonoperative program, who generally have symptoms of at least 12 to 18 months' duration, and who have no apparent psychosocial contraindication, I then evaluate the imaging studies for potential objectification of a surgical level. This includes plain radiographs with flexion-extension views and typically magnetic resonance imaging (MRI). Specific neurologic compression or lack thereof, morphologic status of the intervertebral disc spaces, and presence or absence of mechanical instability are recorded. If the leading differential diagnosis is established as discogenic neck pain, I then recommend cervical discography. This is done after a careful explanation to the patients that this is a quality-of-life issue. Patients must assess whether their symptoms affect their daily activity to such a degree that an approximate 70% to 80% chance of substantial improvement of pain (which is what we estimate based on our experience and the literature) justifies the risk of surgery. In general, younger patients are considered for one- or two-level procedures, whereas multilevel procedures are considered if the patient's physiologic status appears to predict a decreased physical demand on the cervical spine.

NONOPERATIVE MANAGEMENT

Although nonoperative management is also detailed in another chapter of this text, a brief comment regarding the philosophy of our center is in order. Our focus is on active patient participation in aerobic conditioning, active range-of-motion exercises, cervical strengthening, and upper and lower extremity strengthening. We recommend education regarding body posture and mechanics. For the patient with chronic pain, I find little or no role for passive physical therapy or chiropractic treatments alone (48–50). I do recommend medications if they improve the patient's symp-

toms. These generally includes a nonsteroidal antiinflammatory drug as well as acetaminophen and may include a mild narcotic agent. If work site issues are a concern, a therapist or other professional may be suggested to visit the work site and make specific ergonomic recommendations in order to maximize the patient's function. I generally do not recommend placing the patient off duty, but rather on restricted duty, allowing the patient and the employer to work out the details. This type of approach, even in the chronic phase, can help certain patients avoid a surgical workup.

DISCOGRAPHY

It appears that use of the diagnostic tool of discography still emotes controversy. What it really comes down to is how discography is used in the decision-making process to recommend or not recommend surgery, thus affecting the clinical outcome that is perceived by the patient. If one is to undertake the surgical care of a patient with discogenic neck pain, then it is imperative to include discography to maximize the surgical success rate (51–53). Zeidman and Thompson eloquently reviewed the subject in the third edition of *The Cervical Spine*, but an update is pertinent (54).

Most of what we call "degeneration" of the cervical spine comes from our interpretation of anatomic imaging studies. When there are discrete signs and symptoms of cervical radiculopathy, anatomic imaging that confirms our clinical diagnosis of a specific nerve root compressive lesion may suffice as the surgical roadmap for operative intervention. However, using anatomic imaging alone as a blueprint for a cervical reconstructive procedure in an individual with axial mechanical pain will likely lead to a large number of clinical failures owing to the number of asymptomatic individuals with abnormalities documented on other imaging studies (55–61).

Friedenberg documented with routine radiographs that 25% of asymptomatic patients have degenerative changes by the fifth decade, and that by the seventh decade, 75% have such changes (57).

In the quest to better document anatomic findings, myelography, computed tomography (CT), and MRI have been developed. However, it is the presence of positive studies, in asymptomatic individuals, that precludes their isolated use (55–61). Hitselberger noted a 21% incidence of filling defects in 300 individuals who were asymptomatic at the time of study (these patients had myelograms to assess for acoustic tumors) (59). Boden noted a 19% incidence of herniated nucleus pulposus in a younger asymptomatic population and, as suspected, a greater percentage of morphologic disc abnormalities in successive age groups (56).

Schellhas and colleagues published a study on the prospective correlation of MRI and discography in asymptomatic subjects and pain sufferers (62). They concluded that annular tears often escape MRI detection and that MRI cannot reliably identify the source of discogenic pain (62). Although

TABLE 74.1.

	Clinical subjects	Asymptomatic volunteers	
Positive discogram	19	3	22
Negative discogram	21	37	58
	40	40	80

TABLE 74.3. *Clinical Outcome by Discography Results*

Discography type	Good/Excellent	Fair/Poor	Total
Classic	32	3	35
Non Classic	21	10	31
Not Done	18	3	21

many asymptomatic individuals had degenerative change, only 3 of the 40 discs studied in the group elicited a pain response, suggesting a high specificity and positive predictive value (63) (Table 74.1). The use of cervical discography at our center usually is ordered at multiple levels and mirrors the experience recently reported by Grubb and Palit (51–53). The key is to have a substantial (greater than 6 of 10) concordant reproduction of pain at the affected levels, with little or no pain at the adjacent level. This concordant pain means the type of pain that the patient feels on a daily basis and that which the patient wishes to be addressed with surgical intervention.

A note should be made about analgesic discography (64). Roth reported on selecting the surgical level by injecting 1 mL of 2% local anesthesia into the suspected disc. If excellent relief occurred, this was considered positive. He reported 93% good to excellent results in 71 patients over a 2-year period.

Regarding complications, the published rates of discitis are very low, less than 1% (52,54,62). However, this likely depends on the technical expertise of the individual doing the discography, the size of the needle used, and the use of antibiotics.

SURGICAL OUTCOMES FOR DISCOGENIC NECK PAIN

What it really comes down to for most patients is, did the surgical procedure, based on whatever selection criteria were used, make a discernible, worthwhile impact at the 2- to 5-year follow-up that would lead the patient to make the same decision again? Although prospective randomized trials are laudable, useful information does come from review of the current surgical literature (65–67). Our results, similar

to those reported by other authors, support the surgical approach here advocated (Table 74.2). These studies, although not prospective, randomized, nor double blind, do have merit and would be considered grade II to III (scale, I to III) evidence by the U.S. Preventative Service Task Force (68). I will comment first on our surgical series for axial mechanical neck pain, then on other similar series, as well as on the classic historical perspective (1–3,11,13,21,51–53,64,69,70–77).

We have reported on a consecutive series of 112 patients who had an anterior cervical discectomy and arthrodesis for dominant neck pain (51). Eighty-seven of those patients had long-term follow-up averaging 4.8 years. Sixty-seven had one- or two-level procedures; 20 had three- or four-level arthrodesis. We reported by arthrodesis level as well as etiology of symptoms, but noted no statistical difference among the groups. The overall average VAS decreased from 8.4 preoperatively to 3.8 postoperatively. The patients reported about 50% improvement in self-perceived function, as measured by a modified Oswestry disability index and a modified Roland and Morris disability index. Seventy-six of the 87 (87%) would definitely or probably have the same treatment again. Seventy-one of 87 (82%) self-rated their outcome to be good, very good, or excellent. We found no negative correlation with the presence or absence of compensation or litigation. These 112 patients represent about 4% of the total surgical practice of the involved attending surgeons over the time frame of acquisition.

We assessed outcome based on discography. It appeared that a clean pattern of provocative discography was predictive of a better surgical outcome (Table 74.3). We define "clean" as substantial concordant reproduction of pain at the affected levels, all of which were removed, with little or no pain at a validating level at the adjacent segment. Thirty-two of 35 patients with clean discography reported good to

TABLE 74.2.

Study	No. of patients	Reported outcome
Garvey et al., 2002 (26)	87	82% good or excellent, 16% fair, 2% poor
Palit et al., 1999 (55)	38	79% satisfactory, 21% not satisfactory
Whitecloud & Seago, 1977 (76)	34	70% good or excellent, 12% fair, 18% poor
Roth, 1976 (62)	71	93% good or excellent, 1% fair, 6% poor
White et al., 1973 (74)	28	62% good or excellent, 23% fair, 23% poor
Riley et al., 1969 (59)	93	72% good or excellent, 18% fair, 10% poor
Simmons et al., 1969 (66)	30—neck pain 51—neck and arm pain	78% good or excellent, 15% fair, 7% poor
William et al., 1968 (77)	15	1 excellent, 3 good, 5 fair, 6 poor
Dohn, 1966 (19)	34	62% good or excellent, 24% fair, 15% poor
Robinson et al., 1962 (61)	56	73% good or excellent, 22% fair, 5% poor

excellent outcome, whereas only 21 of 31 with a nonclean pattern reported good outcome. This was statistically different ($p = 0.016$) using chi-squared analysis.

Palit and associates recently reported on ACDF in the management of neck pain (53). They reported on 38 patients (a small percentage of their overall surgical series) using discography in the selection process. There mean VAS went from 8.3 to 4.1, with functional scales improving about 30% and overall satisfaction being 79%. They also noted no statistical association with compensation-related surgical patients.

We can learn much from the pioneers of this technique, Robinson and Smith (1–3). In 1958, they reported on 14 patients, all of whom had preoperative discography, which was "useful in those patients in whom there were multiple disc narrowing and in whom it was not clear which of the multiple levels was the source of the major complaint" (3). Some of these patients had neck and referred pain alone. The patient outcomes were rated 9 excellent, 2 good, 2 fair, and 1 poor. In dealing with patients with cervical disc syndrome, they reported, "If conservative treatment fails to relieve the pain, or if the pain becomes excessively burdensome to the patient, then surgery is indicated" (3).

When reporting their continued experience in 1962, Robinson reported on 56 patients, 38 of whom had a traumatic etiology, with 25 being indirect, such as a rear-end automobile crash (2). Neck pain was present in 45 of the 56 patients, occipital pain in 25 of the 56 patients, and interscapular pain in 26 of the 56 patients. Discography was done in 47 of 56 patients, with 24 being preoperative and 23 being intraoperative, with a switch to the latter, secondary to the patient complaints of pain with the actual discographic procedure! Of the 56 patients, 73% consider themselves to have good or excellent results, with 5.5% rating the outcome poor and 22% rating the outcome fair. Nine of 56 patients had a pseudarthrosis noted on flexion-extension views, with only 4 of those being symptomatic. The authors concluded, "When other treatment seems impractical, anterior interbody fusion appears to be a good surgical treatment for degenerative joint and disc disease of the cervical spine" (3).

Cloward, also reporting in 1958, described his dowel technique of anterior discectomy and fusion in a series of 47 patients with 6 to 18 months' follow-up (8,69). All 47 patients were studied with discography. Cloward reported that the pain was completely relieved in 42 of 47 patients and improved in 5 patients. He reported 8 patients whose pain was not relieved or was made worse by the initial procedure and required reoperation, with 3 of 47 patients having graft resorption.

Dohn reported on 210 anterior cervical arthrodesis done at the Cleveland clinic in a 1966 paper (11). Thirty-four were done for discogenic pain, that is, axial mechanical cervical spine pain, with 137 for radicular symptoms and 39 for myelopathy. Discography was done in 49% of the cases, litigation was in progress in 63 cases, and emotional problems were often a seemingly aggravating factor. In the cervical discogenic group (neck pain), 85% of outcomes were considered satisfactory and 15% poor.

Williams is generally quoted as showing that patients with nonradicular symptoms do not do as well and thus should be considered less for operative intervention (24). In a group of only 15 patients with nonradicular symptoms, 1 had excellent results, 3 good, 5 fair, and 6 poor. This equates to a 63% satisfactory rate. The radicular group of Williams represented 45 patients, who showed 8 excellent, 25 good, 4 fair, and 8 poor results. Thus, 82% had satisfactory and 18% had poor outcomes. Thirty-six patients had "technically adequate" discograms. The authors stated that no correlation could be made between an abnormal discogram and final outcome, but in 30 patients whose disc was excised at the level of pain reproduction on discography, 23 of 30 (77%) had satisfactory outcomes, and 7 of 30 (23%) had poor outcomes. Eight of 48 patients (16%) with available roentgenograms had a pseudarthrosis, with 5 requiring a second procedure.

Riley and colleagues in 1969 reported on 93 consecutive patients who were "without objective clinical evidence of nerve root or spinal cord compression" (75). Discography was done in 87 of the 93 patients, most intraoperatively. Results showed 39 of 93 (42%) excellent, 28 of 93 (30%) good, 7 of 93 (8%) fair, and 9 of 93 (10%) poor outcomes. When only one or two levels were fused, 75% of patients reported good or excellent outcomes, but only 58% did so when three or more levels were fused. Twenty-two of 93 (23%) patients had a pseudarthrosis, with 14 of 22 requiring no additional procedure. He noted that if three or more levels were involved, the results, although acceptable, were less satisfactory. He also noted that emotional and environmental factors should be evaluated.

Riley in a review paper of 1969 noted that surgical treatment should not be denied "the rare individual who has not responded to conservative treatment, for prolonged pain is associated with a definite emotional response which may be more disabling than the pain itself" (74). He reviewed a personal series of patients with chronic neck pain, who as a group were depressed and irritable, who were not prone to generate warm physician–patient relationships, but who did respond to surgical intervention, with the disappearance of their emotional characteristics following successful relief of their pain (74).

Simmons reported on a series of 84 patients with specific reference to the keystone-type graft technique (21). He noted that despite criticisms, when discography is properly performed, "It is the most valuable single guide to the level of the causative lesion." Thirty of the 84 patients had chronic neck pain alone, whereas 51 had neck pain and objective neurologic findings. Overall, he reported 78% good or excellent, 15% fair, and 7% poor results, with a higher percentage of good or excellent results occurring in a one-level procedure, as well as better results in the keystone group versus the dowel technique group.

White and co-workers reported on their experience for the relief of pain by anterior cervical spine arthrodesis in spondylosis (22). Eighty-eight percent of patients rated themselves as better, much better, or cured, with 12% being the same or worse. In patients with radicular symptoms, 75% of outcomes were rated good or excellent, whereas in the neck pain alone group, 57% of patients rated their outcomes good or excellent. White stated that favorable factors included radicular symptoms, positive roentgenographic findings at only one level, concordant myelographic defects, and the achievement of a solid arthrodesis without collapse. "None of these factors, however, were indispensable to a good result."

In his paper describing cervical analgesic discography, Roth reported that of 71 consecutive discogenic patients who had an anterior cervical arthrodesis, 93% reported good or excellent results (64). Roth noted, "The sudden cessation of chronic, debilitating pain brought about dramatic reversals of personality traits to normal in patients who because of their emotional response to chronic pain, had been depressed, irritable, anxious and agitated" (64).

Whitecloud reported on a group of 34 patients who had cervical discogenic syndrome and underwent anterior cervical discectomy and arthrodesis based on the results of provocative discography (23,77). Eighty-two percent had improvement, whereas 18% did not. The results showed 11 of 34 (32%) excellent, 13 of 34 (38%) good, 4 of 34 (12%) fair, and 6 of 34 (18%) poor. Whitecloud noted that 8 of 38 (21%) had a pseudarthrosis, with only 2 of the 8 requiring a second procedure. Whitecloud noted, "Better surgical results can be anticipated if a single level is found to be abnormal on discography and an arthrodesis is obtained."

Light undertook a contemporary review of the Simmons keystone technique in a series of 35 patients (72). The results showed 74% good or excellent, 14% fair, and 11% poor outcomes. Eight of the patients underwent the procedure for "painful joint complex" alone, just more than half of the patients had two- or three-level procedures, and 3 of 35 (9%) developed pseudarthrosis.

The surgical series of DePalma and Rothman reported in 1972 included 229 patients, of whom 63% had good or excellent results, 29% fair, and 8% poor. The series included both those with radicular symptoms and those with neck pain alone (9).

ADJACENT SEGMENT

One of the big concerns regarding doing a cervical arthrodesis for discogenic neck pain is whether this alters the mechanics sufficiently to increase the rate of adjacent segment degeneration so rapidly that it creates a pathway for a patient that leads to multiple future procedures. This is an important concern because many of the potential surgical patients for discogenic neck pain have multiple-level degenerative change. Grubb noted three or more abnormal disc levels in more than half of the patients he studied with discography for potential surgical intervention in those with discogenic neck pain (52). He recommended surgically approaching those with one or two levels of involvement. Philosophically, this agrees with the approach at our center. In physiologically young patients, our primary indication is to approach those with one or two levels of involvement, and consideration can be made for those with multilevel involvement. If one does not address all of the levels of involvement on discography, then there likely is a higher chance of early return of symptoms; therefore, my approach in this population has been to approach all of the levels of involvement or none. That is, taking out one or two obviously degenerative levels while leaving other abnormalities that are positive on discography does not predictably relieve the patients' symptoms in my experience (51).

Clements and colleagues reported on 94 patients who had treatment directed at their radicular complaints and in whom they did not address the adjacent segment, which had visible anatomic spondylosis (7). Overall, the investigators noted 88% good or excellent results, but with only 60% (p = 0.01) in those with the adjacent segment degenerative changes. They did not recommend addressing those adjacent segments primarily; however, if symptoms did develop, then an additional surgical procedure could be considered, and that in their series, this salvage attempt was usually successful. In my practice, we would discuss including the obviously spondylotic level with the patient.

Hilibrand and associates recently reported on the adjacent segment progression of spondylosis in the Case Western experience over a 20-year period (78). "Symptomatic adjacent segment pathology occurred at a relatively constant incidence of 2.9% per year during the 10 year period after the operation. Survivorship analysis predicted that 25.6% of the patients who had an ACDF would have new disease at an adjacent level within 10 years after the operation." They noted that contrary to their hypothesis, the risk for developing adjacent-level pathology was significantly lower after a multilevel procedure than after a one-level procedure.

SUMMARY

It appears that the available surgical literature does support a potential surgical option of an ACDF for those with discogenic neck pain. Although all neck pain is not discogenic and all patients with discogenic neck pain do not require surgical management, for the small minority with chronic neck pain substantially interfering with their activities of daily living, who have not benefited from active rehabilitative programs, there is a rational surgical approach. It does not appear reasonable to counsel this group that "nothing can be done." If these patients have had a careful evaluation, have failed an active nonoperative program, and have no apparent psychosocial contraindication, a diagnostic workup including discography may yield a surgical option with an approximate 70% to 80% chance of satisfactory "good to excellent" outcome for many of these patients.

REFERENCES

1. Robinson R, Smith G. Anterolateral cervical disc removal and interbody fusion for cervical disc syndrome. *Bull Johns Hopkins Hosp* 1955;96:223–224(abst).
2. Robinson R, Walker E, Ferlic D, et al. The results of anterior interbody fusion of the cervical spine. *J Bone Joint Surg Am* 1962;44(8):1569–1587.
3. Smith G, Robinson R. The treatment of certain cervical-spine disorders by anterior removal of the intervertebral disc and interbody fusion. *J Bone Joint Surg Am* 1958;40(3):607–624.
4. Aronson N. The management of soft disc protrusions using the Smith-Robinson approach. *Clin Neurosurg* 1973;20:253–258.
5. Aronson N, Filtzer D, Bagan M. Anterior cervical fusion by the Smith-Robinson approach. *J Neurosurg* 1968;29:396–404.
6. Bailey R, Badgely C. Stabilization of the cervical spine by anterior fusion. *J Bone Joint Surg Am* 1960;42(4):565–594.
7. Clements D, O'Leary P. Anterior cervical discectomy and fusion. *Spine* 1990;15:1023–1025.
8. Cloward R. Cervical diskography technique, indications and use in diagnosis of ruptured cervical disks. *AJR Am J Roentgenol* 1958;79(4):563–574.
9. DePalma A, Rothman R, Lewinnek G, et al. Anterior interbody fusion for severe cervical degeneration. *Surg Gynecol Obstet* 1972;134:755–758.
10. Dillin W, Watkins R. Cervical myelopathy and cervical radiculopathy. *Semin Spine Surg* 1989;4:200–208.
11. Dohn D. Anterior interbody fusion for treatment of cervical disk condition. *JAMA* 1966:897–900.
12. Emery S, Bolesta M, Banks M, et al. Robinson anterior cervical fusion: comparison of the standard and modified techniques. *Spine* 1994;19(6):660–663.
13. Gore D, Sepic S. Anterior cervical fusion for degenerated or protruded discs: a review of 146 patients. *Spine* 1984;9:667–671.
14. Herkowitz H. A comparison of anterior cervical fusion, cervical laminectomy and cervical laminoplasty for surgical management of multiple level spondylitic radiculopathy. *Spine* 1988;13:774–780.
15. Hirsch C, Wickbum I, Lidstrom A, et al. Cervical disc resection. A follow-up of myelographic and surgical procedure. *J Bone Joint Surg Am* 1964;46:1811–1821.
16. Jacobs B, Krueger E, Leivy D. Cervical spondylosis with radiculopathy. Results of anterior diskectomy and interbody fusion. *JAMA* 1970;211:2135–2139.
17. Lunsford L, Bissonette D, Janetta P, et al. Anterior cervical surgery for cervical disc disease. I. Treatment of lateral cervical disc herniation in 253 cases. *J Neurosurg* 1980;53:1–11.
18. Matwijecky C, Guyer R. Degenerative disorders of the cervical spine. Anterior microdiscectomy and multilevel anterior fusion. *Spine: State of the Art Reviews* 1991;5(2):259–272.
19. Odom G, Finney W, Woodhall B. Cervical disk lesions. *JAMA* 1958;166(1):23–28.
20. Rothman R, Rashbaum R. Pathogenesis of signs and symptoms of cervical disc degeneration. In: *American Academy of Orthopaedic Surgeons*. St. Louis: CV Mosby 1978;203–215.
21. Simmons E, Bhalla S, Butt W. Anterior cervical discectomy and fusion. A clinical and biomechanical study with eight-year follow-up. With a note on discography: technique and interpretation of results. *J Bone Joint Surg Br* 1969;51:225–237.
22. White A, Southwick W, Deponte R, et al. Relief of pain by anterior cervical spine fusion for spondylosis. *J Bone Joint Surg Am* 1973;55:525–534.
23. Whitecloud T. Management of radiculopathy and myelopathy by the anterior approach. In: The Cervical Spine Research Society, ed. *The cervical spine*. Philadelphia: JB Lippincott, 1989;644–658.
24. William J, Allen M, Harkess J. Late results of cervical discectomy and interbody fusion. Some factors influencing the results. *J Bone Joint Surg Am* 1968;50:277–286.
25. Bovim G, Schrader H, Sand T. Neck pain in the general population. *Spine* 1994;19(12):1307–1309.
26. Makela M, Heliovaara M, Sievers K, et al. Prevalence, determinants and consequences of chronic neck pain in Finland. *Am J Epidemiol* 1991;134:1356–1367.
27. Cote P, Cassidy J, Carroll L. The factors associated with neck pain and its related disability in the Saskatchewan population. *Spine* 2000;25(9):1109–1117.
28. Gore D, Sepic S, Gardner G, et al. Neck pain: a long term follow-up of 205 patients. *Spine* 1987;12:1–5.
29. Rothman R, ed. *The spine*. Philadelphia: WB Saunders, 1982:477.
30. DePalma A, Subin D. Study of the cervical syndrome. *Clin Orthop* 1965;38:135–141.
31. Lees F, Turner J. Natural history and prognosis of cervical spondylosis. *BMJ* 1963;2:1607–1610.
32. Dillin W, Booth R, Cuckler J, et al. Cervical radiculopathy: a review. *Spine* 1986;11:988–991.
33. Quebec Task Force on Whiplash-Associated Disorders. Scientific monograph of the Quebec Task Force on Whiplash-Associated Disorders. *Spine* 1995;20(8S):3s–73s.
34. Freeman M, Croft A, Rossignol A, et al. A review and methodologic critique of the literature refuting whiplash syndrome. *Spine* 1999;24:86–98.
35. MacNab I, McCulloch J. Neck ache and shoulder pain. In: *Whiplash injuries of the cervical spine*. Baltimore: Williams & Wilkins, 1994.
36. MacNab I. Acceleration injuries of the cervical spine. *J Bone Joint Surg Am* 1964;46:1797–1799.
37. MacNab I. The "whiplash syndrome". *Orthop Clin North Am* 1971;2:389–403.
38. Hohl M. Soft-tissue injuries of the neck in automobile accidents. Factors influencing prognosis. *J Bone Joint Surg Am* 1974;56(8):1675–1682.
39. Gargan M, Bannister G. Long-term prognosis of soft-tissue injuries of the neck. *J Bone Joint Surg Br* 1990;72(5):901–903.
40. Norris S, Watt I. The prognosis of neck injuries resulting from rear-end vehicle collisions. *J Bone Joint Surg Br* 1983;65(5):608–611.
41. Watkinson A, Gargan M. Prognostic factors in soft tissue injuries of the cervical spine. *Injury* 1991;23:307–309.
42. Hildingsson C, Toolanen G. Outcome after soft-tissue injury of the cervical spine. A prospective study of 93 car accident victims. *Acta Orthop Scand* 1990;61:357–359.
43. Jonsson H, Cesarini K, Sahlstedt B, et al. Findings and outcome in whiplash-type neck distortions. *Spine* 1994;19(24):2733–2743.
44. Freeman M, Nicodemus N, Croft A, et al. Significant spinal injury resulting from low-level accelerations: a case series of roller coaster injuries. Presented at Cervical Spine Research Society, Charleston, South Carolina, 2000.
45. Bannister G, Gargan M. Prognosis of whiplash injuries: a review of the literature. *Spine: State of the Art Reviews* 1993;7(3):557–569.
46. Barnsley L, Lord S, Bogduk N. The pathophysiology of whiplash. *Spine: State of the Art Reviews* 1993;7(3):329–353.
47. Waddell G, McCulloch J, Jummel E, et al. Non-organic physician signs in low back pain. *Spine* 1980;5:117–130.
48. Bronfort G, Evans R, Nelson B, et al. A randomized clinical trial of exercise and spinal manipulation for patients with chronic neck pain. *Spine* 2001;26(7):788–999.
49. Hoving J, Gross A, Gasner D, et al. A critical appraisal of review articles on the effectiveness of conservative treatment for neck pain. *Spine* 2001;26(2):196–205.
50. Koes B, Bouter L, VanMamegen H, et al. The effectiveness of manual therapy, physiotherapy, and treatment by the general practitioner for nonspecific back and neck complaints. A randomized clinical trial. *Spine* 1992;17(1):28–35.
51. Garvey T, Transfeldt E, Malcolm J, et al. Outcome of anterior cervical discectomy and fusion as perceived by patients treated for dominant axial-mechanical cervical spine pain. *Spine* 2002;27(17).
52. Grubb S, Kelly C. Cervical discography: clinical implications from 12 years of experience. *Spine* 2000;25(11):1382–1389.
53. Palit M, Schofferman J, Goldthwaite N, et al. Anterior discectomy and fusion for the management of neck pain. *Spine* 1999;24(21):2224–2228.
54. Zeidman S, Thompson K. Cervical discography. In: The Cervical Spine Research Society, ed. *The cervical spine*. Philadelphia: Lippincott-Raven Publishers, 1998:205–216.
55. Bell G, Ross J. Diagnosis of nerve root compression: myelography, computed tomography and MRI. *Orthop Clin North America* 1992;23(3):405–419.

56. Boden S, McCowin P, Davis D, et al. Abnormal magnetic resonance scans of the cervical spine in asymptomatic subjects. *J Bone Joint Surg Am* 1990;72:1178–1184.

57. Friedenberg Z, Miller W. Degenerative disc disease of the cervical spine. *J Bone Joint Surg Am* 1963;45:1171–1178.

58. Gore D, Sepic S, Gardner, G. Roentgenographic findings of the cervical spine in asymptomatic people. *Spine* 1986;11:521–524.

59. Hitselberger W, Witten R. Abnormal myelograms in asymptomatic patients. *J Neurosurg* 1968;28:204–206.

60. Peter C, Christenson M. The radiologic study of the normal spine. *Radiol Clin North Am* 1977;15:133–154.

61. Spitzer W, Bayne J, Charnon K, et al. Canadian Task Force on Periodic Health Examination. The periodic health examination. *Can Med Assoc J* 1979;21:1193–1254.

62. Schellhas K, Smith M, Gundry C, et al. Cervical discogenic pain: prospective correlation of magnetic resonance imaging and discography in asymptomatic subjects and pain sufferers. *Spine* 1996;21(3): 300–311.

63. Smith M, Schellhas K, Johnson L. Cervical discography in symptomatic and asymptomatic individuals: a prospective study. *Bull Minn Spine Center* 1994;4(1):10–11(abst).

64. Roth D. A new test for the definitive diagnosis of the painful-disk syndrome. *JAMA* 1976;235(16):1713–1714.

65. Garvey T, Marks M, Wiesel S. A prospective randomized double blind evaluation of trigger-point injection therapy for low back pain. *Spine* 1989;14:962–964.

66. Jhanjee R, Wood K, Butterman G, et al. Operative vs nonoperative treatment of thoracolumbar burst fractures without neurological deficit: a randomized, prospective study. *J Bone Joint Surg Am* 2002.

67. Montella B, Garvey T, Wood K, et al. Patient perceived outcome following instrumented posterolateral spinal fusion with and without cancellous posterior lumbar interbody fusion for dominant mechanical low back pain. Presented at North American Spine Society, New York, New York, 1997.

68. U.S. Preventive Services Task Force. *Guide to clinical preventive services.* Prepublication Copy 1989. Practice Parameter Advisory Committee and Minnesota Department of Health, 1994.

69. Cloward R. The anterior approach for ruptured cervical discs. *J Neurosurg* 1958;15:602–617.

70. Connelly E, Seymore R, Adams J. Clinical evaluation of anterior cervical fusion for degenerative cervical disc. *J Neurosurg* 1965;23:431–437.

71. Green P. Anterior cervical fusion: a review of 33 patients with cervical disc degeneration. *J Bone Joint Surg Br* 1977;59:236–240.

72. Light K, Simmons E. Simmons keystone anterior cervical discectomy and fusion. *Surg Rounds Orthop* 1989;Oct:13–21.

73. Metzger C, Schlitt M, Quindlen E. Small central cervical disc syndrome: evaluation and treatment of chronic disabling neck pain. *J Spinal Disord* 1989;2:234–237.

74. Riley L. Various pain syndromes which may result from osteoarthritis of the cervical spine. *Maryland State Med J* 1969;18:103–105.

75. Riley L, Robinson R, Johnson K. The results of anterior interbody fusion of the cervical spine. *J Neurosurg* 1969;30:127–133.

76. Southwick W, Robinson R. Surgical approaches to the vertebral bodies in cervical and lumbar regions. *J Bone Joint Surg Am* 1957;39: 631.

77. Whitecloud T, Seago R. Cervical discogenic syndrome. Results of operative intervention in patients with positive discography. *Spine* 1987;12(4):313–316.

78. Hilibrand A, Carlson G, Palumbo M, et al. Radiculopathy and myelopathy at segments adjacent to the site of a previous anterior cervical arthrodesis. *J Bone Joint Surg Am* 1999;81(4):519–528.

CHAPTER 75

Surgical Management of Cervical Radiculopathy: Anterior Procedures

Part A
Anterior Cervical Discectomy and Fusion

Jeffrey S. Fischgrund

Cervical disc degeneration is a normal function of aging, occurs in most of the population, and is usually asymptomatic. Symptoms, when they do occur, can present as neck pain, radiculopathy, or myelopathy. Although both axial neck pain and cervical radiculopathy are usually treated successfully nonoperatively, surgical treatment may be necessary for the patient with symptomatic cervical radiculopathy, which is nonresponsive to conservative measures. Surgical options for the treatment of cervical radiculopathy include both anterior and posterior procedures.

The first part of this chapter focuses on anterior cervical discectomy and fusion (ACDF). Radiographic evaluation, surgical indications, and surgical procedures and outcome are highlighted.

RADIOGRAPHIC EVALUATION

Routine cervical spine radiographs taken for the evaluation of degenerative disc disease and cervical radiculopathy include lateral, anteroposterior, and oblique views. Degenerative changes observed include intervertebral disc space narrowing, osteoarthritis of the apophyseal joints, and uncovertebral arthrosis (Fig. 75.1). If degenerative subluxation is noted on standard lateral radiographs, flexion-extension views can be helpful in determining the degree of instability by noting translation as well as angular motion.

Routine radiographs will obviously not directly visualize the neural elements; however, spinal cord compression can be indirectly visualized on the lateral radiograph by determining the space available for the spinal cord. Generally, the space available for the spinal cord ranges from 14 to 23 mm, averaging 17 to 18 mm (1). Congenital spinal stenosis can be seen frequently in asymptomatic individuals and can be measured using the Pavlov or Torg ratio (2) (Fig. 75.2). The spinal canal diameter is the distance from the midpoint of the posterior aspect of the vertebral body to the nearest point on the corresponding spinal laminar line. This number is then divided by the anteroposterior width of the vertebral body. Using this method of measurement, a spinal canal–to–vertebral body ratio of less than 0.8 is indicative of cervical spinal stenosis. Additional hints of neural compression can be noted on the oblique x-rays by evaluating the amount of neural foraminal narrowing. Finally, arthrosis of the uncovertebral joints can lead the practitioner to suspect cervical nerve root compression.

Because radiographs only indirectly visualize the neural elements, further imaging studies are necessary to assess the degree of neural compression. The use of water-soluble, nonionic, myelographic agents provides excellent visualization of the entire spinal canal, although this test is relatively invasive and somewhat nonspecific. It is often difficult to distinguish the cause of neural compression on a myelogram, with difficulty differentiating between a hard disc herniation (osteophyte formation) and a soft disc herniation. Accuracy rates for myelography are greatly improved

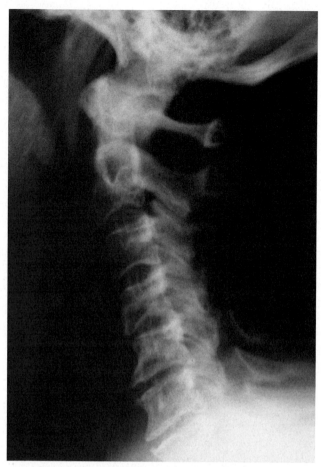

FIG. 75.1. Lateral radiograph demonstrating narrowing of the C4-5 and C5-6 interspaces. Additionally, there is anterior and posterior osteophyte formation at these levels.

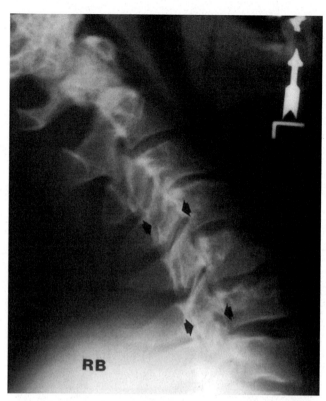

FIG. 75.2. Lateral radiograph denoting congenital spinal stenosis. The *arrows* indicate the space available for the spinal cord. Pavlov's ratio is determined by measuring this distance and dividing by the anteroposterior width of the corresponding vertebral body. A ratio of less than 0.8 indicates spinal stenosis.

with the addition of computed tomography (CT) scans and range anywhere from 70% to 90% (3).

Magnetic resonance imaging (MRI) of the cervical spine is noninvasive, does not involve radiation exposure, and provides excellent resolution of the cervical disc and neural elements. However, this test and cervical CT myelograms must be interpreted with caution because there is a high rate of false-positive readings. It is very important to correlate the patient's symptoms with findings on these tests and then make the appropriate treatment recommendations. Boden and colleagues (4) found that 19% of 63 asymptomatic patients had major abnormalities on cervical spine MRI studies.

Cervical radiculopathy is often caused by a disc herniation, which is easily seen on MRI. However, MRI is also useful for distinguishing infectious processes from metastatic disease. Additionally, major compression on the spinal cord can cause physiologic changes within the cord, leading to myelomalacia, which can be visualized by MRI (Fig. 75.3).

SURGICAL INDICATIONS

Initial indications for anterior cervical discectomy and arthrodesis were popularized by Smith and Robinson for the surgical treatment of cervical disc disease in 1958 (5). Their initial indication for surgical treatment was the failure of conservative treatment in a patient with persistent upper extremity radicular symptoms. Current indications for surgery in cervical radiculopathy include (a) persistent or recurrent arm pain, nonresponsive to a trial of conservative treatment (6 to 12 weeks); (b) progressive neurologic deficit; (c) static neurologic deficit associated with major radicular pain; and (d) confirmatory imaging studies consistent with clinical findings.

SURGICAL TECHNIQUE

ACDF is usually performed under general anesthesia. Proper positioning of the endotracheal tube will assist the surgeon, especially with upper cervical disc herniations. If the surgeon chooses to perform the procedure on the left side of the patient's neck, the tube should generally be taped on the right side of the patient's face. A small rolled towel is then placed between the scapulae to allow

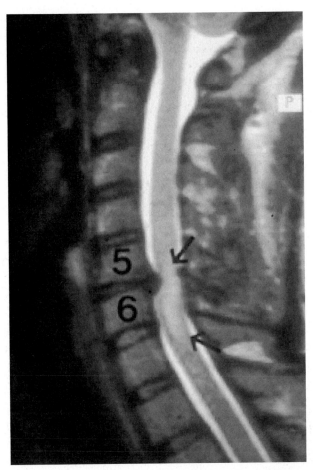

FIG. 75.3. Sagittal magnetic resonance imaging (MRI) study demonstrating disc protrusion at C5-6. Note the increased signal intensity of the spinal cord outlined by the *arrows*. This indicates myelomalacia within the cord, due to longstanding compression from this cervical disc rupture.

for *slight* hyperextension of the neck (Fig. 75.4A and B). Care should be taken, however, when performing this maneuver in a patient with myelopathy. Cervical myelopathy is often worse with neck hyperextension, and this position should be avoided during positioning if the patient developed marked symptoms while hyperextending the neck during examination before the surgical procedure. Finally, traction should be placed in a downward position on the shoulders, with surgical tape. Although this helps in patient positioning, it is most helpful for visualizing the lower cervical spine intraoperatively with radiographs because the shoulders often obscure the lower cervical spine when they are in the neutral position.

Many spine surgeons recommend the procedure be performed on the left side of the neck to decrease the risk for injury to the recurrent laryngeal nerve. The nerve leaves the carotid sheath on a variable level on the right side of the neck and then courses anteriorly behind the thyroid, thereby leaving itself susceptible to injury. On the left side of the neck, the nerve predictably enters the thorax within the carotid sheath, then loops under the aortic arch and ascends into the neck beside the trachea and esophagus. Numerous studies (6) have shown that the risk for injury to the recurrent laryngeal nerve can be decreased by a left-sided approach. Newer investigations have disputed the anatomic basis for injury to the recurrent laryngeal nerve and have proposed the idea that retractor displacement of the larynx against the shaft of the endotracheal tube impinges on the intralaryngeal segment of the recurrent laryngeal nerve. It has been suggested that deflation of the endotracheal cuff can decrease the rate of injury to the recurrent laryngeal nerve (6), thereby decreasing the rate of postoperative voice changes.

A transverse incision is generally used for one- or two-level discectomy and may even be used for more extensive

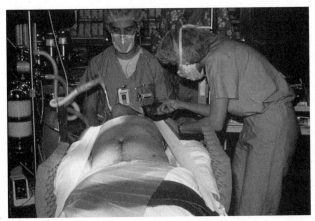

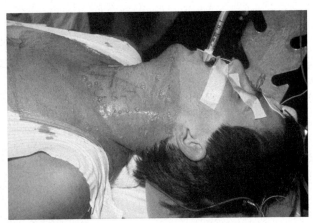

FIG. 75.4. A, B: Proper positioning for an anterior cervical discectomy and fusion note that for a left-sided approach, the endotracheal tube is taped on the patient's right side of the mouth. Traction on the shoulders is provided by 3-inch wide tape to assist in securing the patient and to allow intraoperative visualization of the lower cervical spine with radiographs.

procedures. A longitudinal incision can be used for a more extensive procedure such as multilevel corpectomies. An attempt should be made by the surgeon to place the incision at the appropriate level of neural compression. Superficial landmarks such as hyoid bone can be palpated at about the level of C3. The thyroid cartilage is located at C4-C5, whereas the cricoid cartilage lies at the level of C6 (Fig. 75.5). Incisions on the lower cervical spine (C7-T1) can be better accessed through a longitudinal incision because the inferior thyroid vessels are frequently visible at this level and can be managed more readily through this approach.

After the skin incision, hemostasis should be obtained along the skin edges with electrocautery. The two edges of the skin can then be elevated with hand-held retractors, and

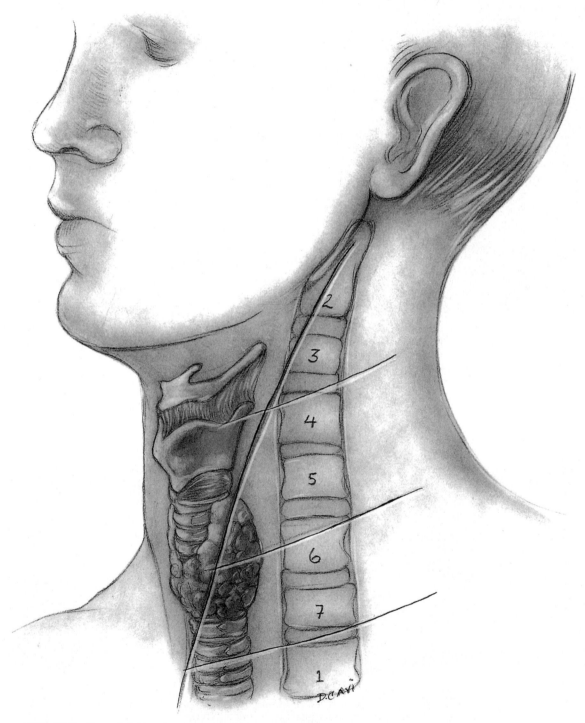

FIG. 75.5. Superficial landmarks are helpful in placing the skin incision. The hyoid bone is at the level of C3. The thyroid cartilage is at C4-5, and a cricoid cartilage is opposite C6.

dissection continues until the fascia above the platysma muscle is identified. After incision of this fascial layer, the platysma muscle is generally incised in line with the original incision by placing a blunt curved hemostat underneath the platysma muscle, again using electrocautery (Fig. 75.6). Once the incision through the platysma muscle is complete, the sternocleidomastoid muscle is visualized, and the ap-

proach should proceed in a medial direction between the carotid sheath laterally and the trachea and esophagus medially. This interval can usually be defined by manual palpation, and the anterior vertebral bodies are usually easily palpated in the midline. Retraction at this level should be obtained with blunt hand-held retractors because sharp edges can injure either the carotid vessels or the esophagus (Fig. 75.7). The superior and

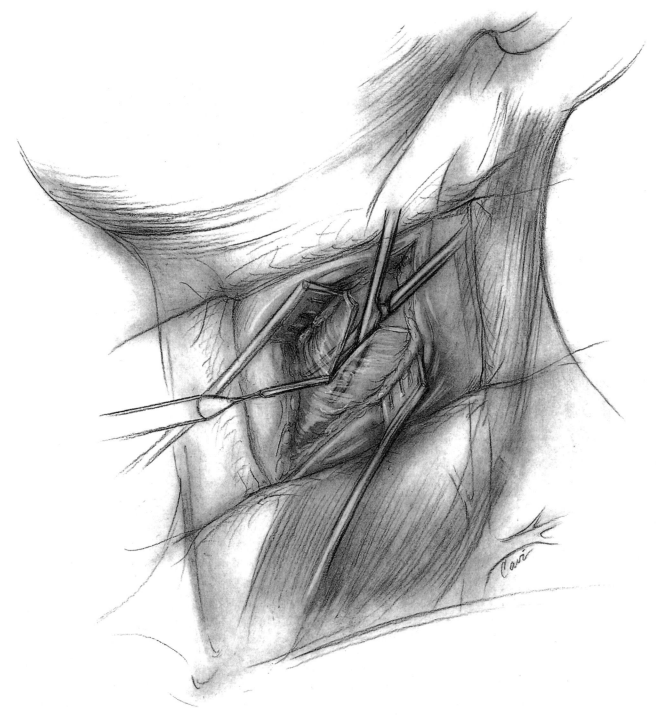

FIG. 75.6. Transverse skin incision exposing the platysma muscle, which is incised in line with the original incision with electrocautery.

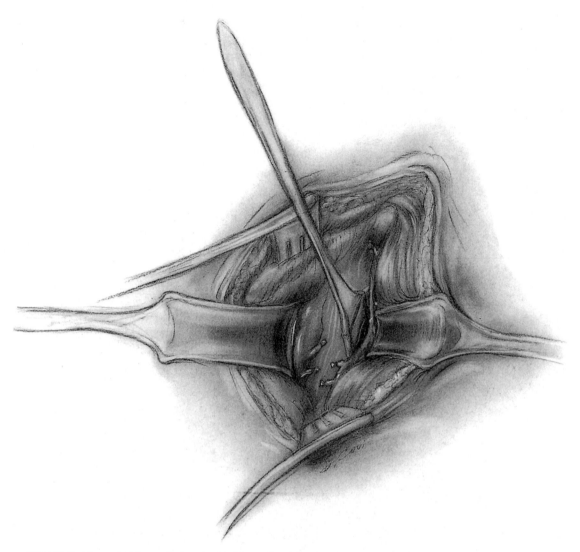

FIG. 75.7. The carotid sheath is retracted laterally while the esophagus and trachea are retracted medially. A subperiosteal dissection of the longus colli muscle is completed with elevators and electrocautery.

inferior thyroid vessels arise from the carotid artery and can be observed crossing this interval; they occasionally may need to be ligated or divided. Additionally, the omohyoid muscle is usually visualized with extensive longitudinal incisions and may need to either be retracted or divided.

After palpating the vertebral body in the midline, prominent disc spaces can be identified. The prevertebral fascia over the anterior vertebral body is divided, and the longus colli muscles are easily visualized. Elevation of the longus colli muscles, bilaterally, is accomplished with a combination of electrocautery and mild blunt dissection. Correct level identification should be done before disc removal through the use of intraoperative lateral radiographs.

After correct level identification, the anterior longitudinal ligament, which overlies the disc space, should be incised with a No. 15 scalpel blade in a rectangular fashion (Fig. 75.8). Through this opening, pituitary rongeurs can be used to remove the superficial anterior portion of the interverte-

bral disc. After disc material can no longer be easily removed with a pituitary rongeur, small curettes are used to remove the cartilaginous end plates and attached intervertebral disc. After enough disc has been removed, a small intervertebral spreader can be placed between the two bodies, thereby affording distraction and easy removal of the remaining disc material and cartilaginous end plates (Fig. 75.9). Alternatively, pins can be placed in the adjacent vertebral bodies and then specialized distracters placed to distract the disc space. To improve visualization, large overhanging anterior osteophytes may need to be removed with either a rongeur or burr to allow access to the disc space. The surgeon should note the angle of the disc space on the intraoperative localization film, and care should be taken to perform the disc removal along the angle of the end plates to avoid inadvertent penetration of the vertebral bodies.

The discectomy then continues from an anterior to a posterior direction, and the uncinate processes, as well as the

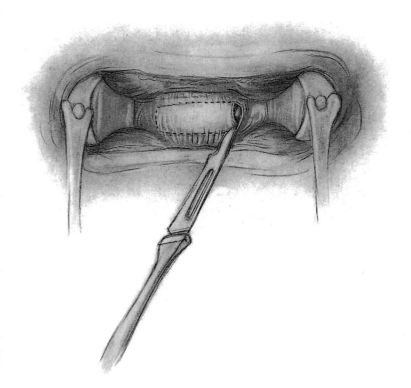

FIG. 75.8. Exposure of the disc space is complete, and a scalpel is used to initiate disc removal.

posterior longitudinal ligament (PLL), are visualized. Although MRI can be helpful for determining whether or not a sequestered disc fragment is present, visualization of the PLL is necessary. If there is no preoperative suspicion of a sequestered fragment and the PLL appears intact, it is generally not necessary to remove the PLL or the posterior osteophytes. However, if preoperative studies do indicate a sequestered fragment or there is a tear in the posterior longitudinal ligament, the tear should be probed with a nerve hook and then opened up with a micro-Kerrison rongeur to allow visualization and search for a free disc fragment. Posterior osteophytes generally do not need to be removed unless they are causing substantial spinal cord or nerve root compression.

After the decompression is complete, the disc space is ready for insertion of the graft. Before graft insertion, the disc space should be measured from an anteroposterior direction, using either a calibrated nerve hook or a small wire. Generally, the disc can accept a block of bone up to 10 mm high (usually 5 to 8 mm), 10 to 15 mm wide, and 12 to 17 mm deep. It is recommended that the depth of the graft be several millimeters less than the actual depth of the disc space, to avoid spinal cord compression.

Before graft insertion, bleeding bone should be obtained on the end plates to increase the chances of a successful bony union. This can be accomplished by either of two means. A small angled curette can be used to make several holes in both the end plates of the previous prepared disc space; alternatively, the end plates can be partially removed with a burr. The disc space is then distracted again, either manually by the anesthesiologist or mechanically with a

disc space distractor. The bone graft can then be placed into position and tamped with a mallet. If an anterior cervical plate is not part of the procedure, the bone graft should be countersunk 1 to 2 mm in relation to the anterior margin of the adjacent vertebral bodies to decrease the chance of graft extrusion. If the surgeon's preference is to add an anterior cervical plate, then countersinking of the graft is frequently not necessary (Fig. 75.10). A lateral intraoperative radiograph is then obtained to confirm correct graft placement as well as hardware placement, if used.

Frequently, a soft drain is placed in the wound, with the fascia over the platysma closed with simple absorbable sutures, and the skin is closed with a running absorbable subcuticular suture.

Postoperative management considerations are in a state of transition. Before the widespread use of anterior cervical instrumentation, it was generally recommended that patients be placed in a rigid collar for 6 weeks after the surgical procedure. However, newer rigid anterior instrumentation systems have led several surgeons to discontinue the routine use of postoperative immobilization. If adequate internal fixation is obtained, generally, a soft collar can be used for a short period of time in the initial postoperative period. All patients are usually ambulatory on the day of surgery, and most are discharged on postoperative day one. Typical follow-up of these patients includes an office visit at 1 week, with routine anteroposterior and lateral radiographs. By 6 weeks, lateral flexion-extension views usually show that the fusion construct is stable, such that the patient is allowed to begin range of motion and strengthening exercises. Most patients can

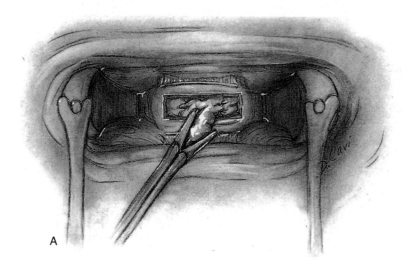

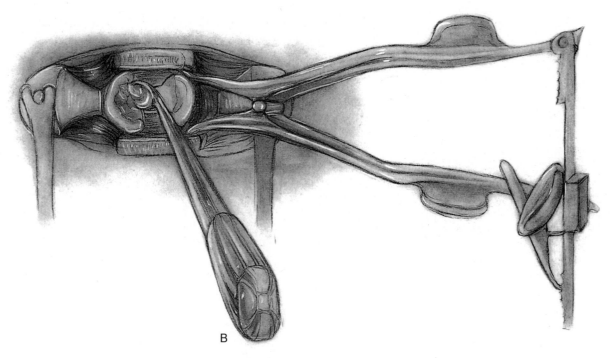

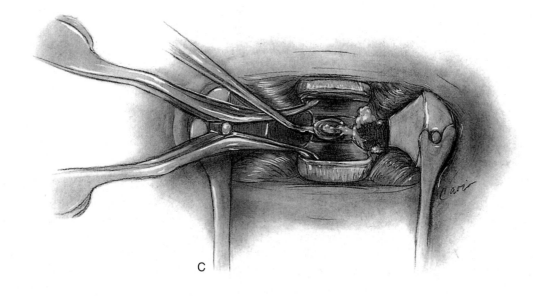

FIG. 75.9. The disc cartilage end plates were removed with a combination of pituitary rongeurs and curettes. A small lamina spreader improves the exposure by distracting the disc space, thereby affording better visualization of the uncinate processes at the posterior margin of the vertebral bodies.

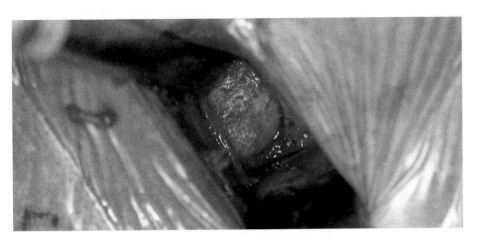

FIG. 75.10. Intraoperative photograph of a tricortical graft inserted into the disc space. Note the intact iliac crest cortex anteriorly in the disc space.

expect return to full activity within 3 to 4 months after the surgical procedure.

ANTERIOR CERVICAL PLATING

To increase the fusion rate after anterior cervical discectomy and arthrodesis, several investigators have advocated the routine use of anterior cervical instrumentation. Although the anterior cervical plate provides increased stability after decompression, as well as an increased fusion rate, the risks of this procedure, as well as the additional cost, must be weighed against the benefits before its use can be widely recommended.

The earliest description of an anterior cervical place was by Bohler in the mid-1960s (7). This initial plating system was a modification of available hardware that was primarily used in the extremities. The indication for anterior cervical plating was restoration of cervical stability following a traumatic injury. Currently, the use of an anterior cervical plate has been advocated to increase postoperative stability, decrease the prevalence of graft extrusion, improve the fusion rate, and obviate the need for postoperative halo-brace placement after extensive multilevel corpectomies. Early systems used bicortical screw fixation, which required the use of intraoperative fluoroscopy to avoid overpenetration of the screws into the epidural space. Contemporary systems use unicortical screws with various locking systems that secure the screw to the plate, thereby decreasing the postoperative complication of screw loosening.

Biomechanical testing of bicortical anterior cervical instrumentation after one-level discectomy has shown a marked reduction in motion compared with the intact specimen (8). Additional testing by Grubb and coworkers (9) has shown that the unicortical Cervical Spine Locking Plate System (Synthes, Paoli, PA) is biomechanically equivalent and in some cases more stable than the Caspar System (bicortical) for fixation of a severe compression flexion injury. Finally, Spivak et al.'s (10) study has shown that locking screws significantly increase rigidity of the hardware systems initially and after cyclic loading. Based on a combination of biomechanical and clinical studies, most surgeons recommend the use of unicortical plating systems.

The clinical effectiveness of anterior cervical plate fixation must be judged not only by the successful fusion rate but also by the clinical outcome. Connolly and colleagues (11) reported on 43 patients treated for cervical spondylosis with anterior cervical discectomy and arthrodesis using autogenous iliac crest bone graft. Group I consisted of 25 consecutive patients treated with anterior cervical discectomy and arthrodesis as well as an anterior cervical plate. In this group, the overall success rate was 72%, with all patients obtaining a solid fusion an average of 12 weeks after surgery. Group II consisted of 18 consecutive patients treated without plate fixation; the overall success rate was 83%, with 88% achieving a successful fusion. The authors noted no difference in the overall clinical results between these two groups. Additionally, the fusion rate of a one-level cervical fusion was not statistically improved with anterior cervical plate fixation. The authors did note, however, that the overall graft complication rate in multilevel arthrodesis was decreased with anterior cervical plate fixation.

McLaughlin and associates (12) reported a cost analysis of 64 patients who underwent a two-level anterior cervical discectomy and arthrodesis for radiculopathy. They compared the costs of rigid internal fixation for a two-level arthrodesis with a similar population of patients who had an identical procedure, without instrumentation. Again, they noted no difference in the clinical outcome between the two groups, with both groups obtaining a 92% excellent or good result using the Odom criteria. However, the authors did note that patients who underwent rigid plating returned to light activities, driving, and unrestricted work sooner than noninstrumented patients. Although the overall cost was higher for those patients in the instrumentation group, the investigators felt that the increased cost was justified because of the substantial advantage for patients and insurance disability providers of early mobilization and return to work.

Caspar and colleagues (13) and Geisler and coworkers (14) described 365 patients who underwent a one- or two-level cervical arthrodesis performed both with and without anterior cervical plate stabilization. The goal of this study was to determine whether the use of an anterior cervical plate decreased the need for a second surgical procedure. Although the patients were not randomized and there was a mix of autograft and allograft procedures, as well as multiple level arthrodeses, the investigators reported that 22 patients required a second surgical intervention, with 20 of these in the noninstrumented group.

With proper surgical technique, the use of an anterior cervical plate rarely leads to additional intraoperative complications. Frequently, no additional exposure is necessary for placement of the plate because the width of the corpectomy or discectomy defect is usually similar to the width of the anterior cervical plate. Additionally, with the use of unicortical screws, the risk to the spinal cord is minimized. Vertebral artery injury is extremely rare and occurs only with extreme screw misplacement (Fig. 75.11). Finally, placement of the cervical plate usually adds only 15 to 30 minutes to the surgical procedure.

Although the successful fusion rate may be higher with the use of instrumentation, clinical outcomes have not yet significantly improved with the addition of hardware. As the complexity of cervical reconstructive procedures increases, the use of cervical plates appears to be justified because of the higher fusion rate with multilevel disease.

RESULTS

The first large series of patients treated with anterior interbody arthrodesis for cervical degenerative disc disease was reported by Robinson and colleagues (15) in 1962. They performed discectomy and anterior interbody arthrodesis on 107 interspaces, in 55 patients. The length of follow-up ranged from 2 to 73 months, with 46% of the patient outcomes recorded as excellent, 27% good, 22% fair, and 6% poor. Patients who underwent surgery at more than one level had worse results than those who had one-level surgery. Seventeen of 18 patients who had surgery at a single level had an excellent or good result, whereas only 8 of 16 patients with three or more levels fused had an excellent or good result.

Robinson noted that there was no clear correlation after operation between the presence of a pseudarthrosis and clinical outcome. Of the 9 patients who developed a nonunion, only 4 continued to have complaints of pain that was thought to result from a lack of union. Additionally, only 1 of 46 patients who had solid fusion needed additional surgery (Fig. 75.12). Robinson's technique preserved the

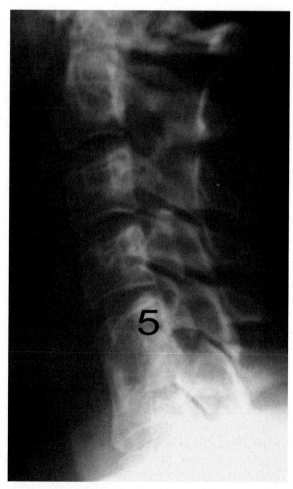

FIG. 75.12. An anterior cervical fusion at C5-6 using tricortical iliac crest graft.

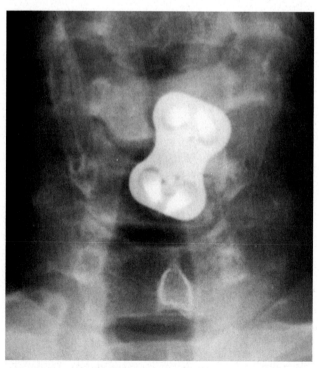

FIG. 75.11. Malalignment of an anterior cervical plate. Although the plate was not oriented properly in the vertical plane, this patient experienced no adverse clinical sequelae.

subchondral bone plate above and below the graft, which led him to conclude that preservation of the subchondral bone left a bearing surface for the graft to help maintain the height of the intervertebral space during healing. This technique contrasts with that by Emery and associates (16), who reported a low pseudarthrosis rate of only 4.4% in 29 patients treated with a modified Robinson technique, in which end-plate burring was used to expose the subchondral bone.

The clinical effect of the pseudarthrosis on patient outcome remains controversial. Patients who have a successful fusion will theoretically have improved cervical alignment, continued foraminal distraction, and prevention of collapse into kyphosis. The pseudarthrosis rate after one-level surgery ranges from 0% to 20% (17,18), with the rates approaching 50% for those patients undergoing multiple-level surgery (19,20).

Phillips and coworkers (21) attempted to determine the natural history, risk factors, and treatment outcomes in a large population with documented pseudarthrosis after anterior cervical discectomy and arthrodesis. They reported on 48 patients with radiographically proven pseudarthrosis, at an average of 5 years from the initial surgical procedure. Sixty-seven percent of the patients were symptomatic at latest follow-up or at the time of a second surgical intervention. Several patients had a symptom-free period of up to 2-years after the anterior cervical discectomy and arthrodesis before redeveloping cervical symptoms after a minor traumatic episode. Analysis of the results reveals that patients who have surgery at a younger age had an increased likelihood of the pseudarthrosis becoming symptomatic. Fourteen of 16 patients had a successful repair of the pseudarthrosis through an anterior approach, whereas 6 patients underwent posterior cervical arthrodesis, with all going on to successful fusion. In patients in whom fusion was achieved with a second operation, the results were excellent in 19 and good in 1. The authors concluded that the surgical repair of the pseudarthrosis with either an anterior or posterior approach does result in a higher likelihood of a successful clinical outcome.

The etiology of pseudarthrosis following anterior cervical surgery is multifactorial. Various authors have cited multilevel procedures, cigarette smoking, and revision surgery as relative risk factors for the development of pseudarthrosis. Multiple studies of lumbar spine arthrodeses have shown that cigarette smoking adversely effects fusion. Hilibrand and colleagues (22) compared the long-term radiographic and clinical results of smokers and nonsmokers who had undergone arthrodesis with autogenous bone graft following multilevel anterior cervical decompression for the treatment of cervical radiculopathy, myelopathy, or both. One hundred ninety patients were followed clinically and radiographically for at least 2 years after either corpectomy or multiple discectomies and interbody grafting. A subset of 40 of these patients were smokers who had undergone a cervical arthrodesis, and only 20 had a solid fusion at all levels, whereas 69 of the 91 nonsmokers had a solid fusion at all levels ($p < 0.02$). This difference was more significant among patients who had a two-level interbody grafting procedure. They concluded that smoking had a significant negative impact on healing and clinical recovery after multilevel anterior cervical decompression and arthrodesis with autogenous interbody graft for radiculopathy or myelopathy.

Long-term follow-up studies of patients treated with anterior cervical discectomy and arthrodesis have shown that about 10% of patients underwent reoperation at an adjacent level because of progressive spondylolysis or a new disc herniation (23–26). This adjacent segment disease has been theorized to be secondary to the increased biomechanical stresses on an unfused level adjacent to a solid fusion. Whether the biomechanical forces alone are sufficient to cause new disease or this is just a progression of the natural history of cervical spondylosis in a patient with substantial degenerative changes remains to be determined. However, treatment of this adjacent level disease is theoretically more difficult because achievement of a solid fusion in these patients is hindered by the long lever arm of the prior fusion acting across the adjacent level.

A retrospective review of all patients surgically treated for adjacent segment disease of the cervical spine over a 20-year period was performed to evaluate the effect of adjacent segment disease of the cervical spine (26). Thirty-eight patients were identified who underwent surgical treatment for multilevel adjacent segment disease by either discectomy with interbody grafting or corpectomy with strut grafting. The authors found that the rate of arthrodesis in 24 patients treated with discectomy was only 63%, which is much lower than that reported in the literature for patients undergoing a primary cervical procedure, whereas those patients treated with corpectomy and strut grafting had a fusion rate of 100%. The authors concluded that the use of subtotal corpectomy (in patients who have had previous cervical surgery) has a higher fusion rate with strut grafting techniques. They believed that the strut of bone passing through a trough in the intermediate vertebrae across multiple motion segments may provide greater stability than multiple smaller pieces of tricortical iliac crest at each disc space. Secondarily, strut grafting requires bony union across only two surfaces, compared with four or six surfaces for either two- or three-level discectomy and arthrodesis procedures, respectively.

A review of the literature has demonstrated that the results of anterior cervical surgery are usually reported in terms of successful fusion rate. Although there are indications that a successful fusion correlates with a successful clinical outcome, radiographic results alone are an insufficient parameter for determining the success of the surgical procedure. Recent orthopaedic literature has shown the value of measuring quality-of-life parameters after surgical intervention. Both clinicians and patients alike can benefit from this information. Additionally, this information can be used to convince insurance carriers of the benefit of surgical intervention.

Recently, Klein and associates (27) reviewed the outcomes of 28 patients with cervical radiculopathy treated with one- or two-level anterior cervical discectomy and arthrodesis using a health status questionnaire. The survey was self-administered and evaluated at an average follow-up interval of 21.8 months. The authors noted statistically significant improvement in postoperative scores for bodily pain, physical function, role function, and social function and concluded that this is a highly reliable surgical procedure for the management of cervical radiculopathy.

COMPLICATIONS

The complication rate of anterior surgery for cervical disc disease is quite low. When complications do occur, they can be divided into those occurring in the neck and those occurring at the graft site. Robinson et al.'s (15) initial report described no complications in 48 of 56 patients; 4 patients had a temporary unilateral paralysis of the vocal cords, 2 patients had marked temporary dysphasia, and 2 patients had a transient Horner syndrome. DePalma and coworkers (28) reported that the most common complications occurred at the graft donor site. They noted that hematomas developed in 9% of the patients and that 36% of the patients continued to have persistent donor site pain, 1 year after surgery. Persistent pain at the donor sites can be minimized by limiting surgical exposure with careful dissection of both the inner and outer table of the iliac crest. The incision should be a minimum of 2 fingerbreadths lateral to the anterosuperior iliac spine to avoid the lateral femoral cutaneous nerve (29). Obviously, the prevalence of iliac crest donor site pain can be eliminated through the use of allograft.

Flynn (30) compiled the results of 704 neurosurgeons describing 36,657 anterior cervical interbody arthrodeses. He noted that the most common neurologic complication was recurrent laryngeal nerve palsy, which occurred in 52 cases, constituting nearly 20% of all neurologic complications. As described previously, the risk to the recurrent laryngeal nerve can be decreased by using a left-sided approach and possibly by deflation of the endotracheal cuff.

The single most feared neurologic complication following any type of spine surgery is spinal cord injury. Flynn (30) re-

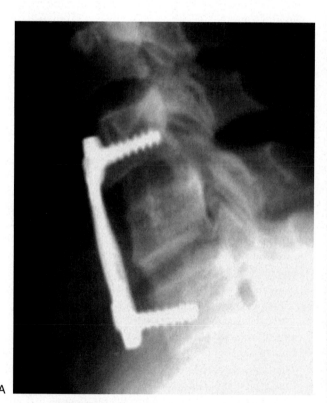

A

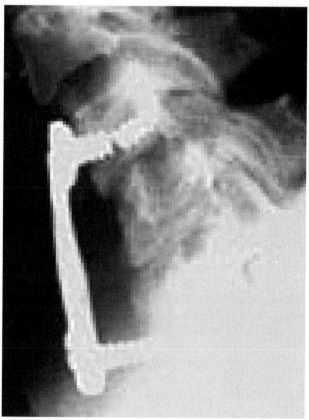

B

FIG. 75.13. A: Anterior cervical plating following a two-level anterior cervical discectomy and fusion. Initial postoperative radiographs demonstrate that the inferior portion of the plate is anterior to the vertebral body. **B:** After 1 month, pull-out of the inferior portion of the cervical plate is seen, with breakage of the superior screws.

ported that there were 100 cases of permanent myelopathy or myeloradiculopathy in his large series. Of these, 75% of the patients had immediate deficit postoperatively, whereas 25% developed a neurologic deficit in the immediate postoperative recovery period. Analysis of these data led Flynn to conclude that regardless of the etiology of the myelopathy, reoperation had little effect on the ultimate status of the neurologic deficit. In addition, most surgeons were unable to determine the etiology of the neurologic deterioration.

Perhaps the most common problem to occur postoperatively is a transient sore throat or difficulty in swallowing (31,32). Although most practitioners believe this complication is relatively insubstantial, many patients do complain of difficulty swallowing for several weeks, with a frequent need to chew their food completely in order to swallow. The risk for injury may be decreased by the use of blunt retractors. Perforation injuries to the esophagus are extremely rare but can be life threatening. Newhouse and colleagues (33) reported that the prevalence of esophageal perforation was 0.25% in more than 10,000 cases of anterior cervical surgery. One third of the perforations were noted at the time of surgery and related to sharp or motorized instruments. Late perforation is usually related to the loosening or pullout of an anterior plate or screws (Fig. 75.13). If the perforation is noted at the time of surgery, all attempts should be made for an acute repair. Late perforations are usually more difficult to repair and often require the prolonged use of nasogastric suction as well as parenteral hyperalimentation.

AUTOGRAFT VERSUS ALLOGRAFT

In an attempt to eliminate donor site problems while maintaining acceptable fusion rates, many surgeons have advocated the use of allograft instead of autogenous bone for anterior cervical arthrodesis. Allograft obviously eliminates the necessity for a second procedure to obtain the graft, thereby decreasing operative time, morbidity, and pain at the donor site.

One of the earliest studies comparing allograft to autograft bone for anterior cervical fusion was reported by Brown and associates in 1976 (34). They noted no difference in fusion rates between the two types of graft. However, there was noted a substantial difference in graft collapse rate, with 28% of the patients receiving allograft demonstrating radiographic collapse, compared with 16% of patients receiving autograft. This trend was found to be true only for multiple level fusions.

Fernyhough and associates (35) retrospectively reviewed 126 patients who either had autogenous or allograft fibular strut graft used for arthrodesis after decompression for multilevel cervical spondylosis. The combined nonunion rate for both groups ranged from 21% for a two-level arthrodesis up to 50% for a four-level arthrodesis. Overall, the allo-

graft group had a statistically significant higher rate of nonunion (41%) than the autograft group (27%). However, there was noted to be no association between the clinical results and the rate of union in this study.

Zdeblick and Ducker (36) reviewed 88 consecutive patients who underwent a Smith-Robinson anterior cervical arthrodesis. Sixty of these patients had an autogenous iliac crest graft placed, and freeze-dried iliac crest grafts were inserted in 27 patients. The delayed union rate and nonunion rate were noted to be significantly higher in the allograft group compared with the autograft group. However, when examining one-level arthrodeses, the nonunion rates at 1 year were similar. In two-level arthrodeses, the union rate was dramatically lower with allograft (38% versus 83%). Additionally, the freeze-dried allograft was more frequently collapsed. The clinical results between the two groups were noted to be similar. These authors concluded that the use of freeze-dried iliac crest allograft in Smith-Robinson cervical arthrodeses is not recommended in multilevel arthrodeses. When freeze-dried iliac crest graft is used for one-level arthrodeses, radiographic collapse or lucency may persist despite clinical success.

Recently, Bishop and colleagues (37) evaluated the results of 132 patients after nonplated anterior cervical fusions who had at least 1 year of follow-up. Of the 83 patients who received autograft, 94% achieved a solid one-level fusion, whereas 87% achieved fusion after multilevel anterior cervical discectomy and arthrodesis. Patients who received allografts had a lower fusion rate of 73% for one-level and 53% for multilevel procedures.

Until recently, the most common type of allograft used was tricortical iliac crest harvested from cadaver iliac crest, similar in fashion to the autograft harvest. Several surgeons have recently advocated the use of grafts with superior structural properties such as fibula and patella. Theoretically, the superior structural properties of such grafts make them less likely to collapse than iliac crest autograft (38). MacDonald and coworkers (39) reported on 36 patients who had anterior cervical arthrodesis using fibular strut allograft. Although 15 of these patients did undergo internal fixation, at 2-year follow-up, 96% had a solid fusion. An even larger study by Martin and colleagues (40) evaluated the use of freeze-dried fibular allograft in 269 patients, of whom 242 patients eventually achieved a solid radiographic fusion for a union rate of 90% at 2 years of follow-up. A subset of these patients, those who underwent a two-level arthrodesis, achieved a fusion rate of only 72%.

During the past decade, there has been a substantial change in the testing of donor patients as well as the sterilization techniques of allograft bone. Because of the increased availability and improved safety profile, the use of allograft bone and anterior cervical surgery continues to improve. With the addition of an anterior cervical plate, union rates will most likely approach those of autograft even in multilevel arthrodeses. Although allograft has not yet replaced autograft as the gold standard for anterior cervical surgery, its use should be discussed with patients before surgical procedures.

ANTERIOR DISCECTOMY WITHOUT ARTHRODESIS

Anterior cervical discectomy without arthrodesis developed as an alternative technique to cervical arthrodesis, based on the premise that if successful results of anterior fusions occur with pseudarthrosis, then discectomy can be performed without arthrodesis. Several papers have advocated anterior cervical discectomy without arthrodesis, reporting success rates similar to those with fusion (41–43). Murphy and Gadd (42) reported 26 patients who underwent one- or two-level anterior cervical discectomy for "radiculitis" secondary to a herniated cervical disc. Good results (neurologic deficit improved, pain alleviated, and patient able to return to normal activities) were reported in 24 of 26 patients. The 2 patients with poor results required reoperation within 2 weeks of the initial procedure. The authors noted that 72% of the patients developed a spontaneous fusion at the discectomy level and that all 20 patients developed some degree of postoperative kyphosis.

The studies by Murphy and Gadd (42) and others (41) neglected to mention the postoperative prevalence of neck pain. Transient postoperative severe neck pain after cervical discectomy without arthrodesis has been noted by several authors (44–46). This procedure defeats the principle of successful anterior cervical surgery that is based on the premise of neuroforaminal distraction and reduction of buckling of the ligamentum flavum. In addition, by its very nature, this surgery is designed to create a pseudarthrosis that may lead to a less satisfactory result. Theoretically, the results of this surgery may be more successful for soft disc herniation than for patients with spondylolysis, but there is an unacceptably high rate of persistent postoperative neck pain. Most series to date have a limited clinical follow-up and poor radiographic correlation to determine the development and importance of instability or kyphotic angulation.

Recent studies of anterior cervical discectomy with and without arthrodesis (47,48) have demonstrated that the procedure without arthrodesis does decrease hospital cost and hospital stay as well as surgical morbidity. However, these early economic benefits must be weighed against long-term outcomes.

Review of these studies leads to the conclusion that patients who undergo arthrodesis at the same time of anterior cervical discectomy have better long-term outcomes. The risks and pain associated with autograft harvest can obviously be reduced with bone graft substitutes. Although allograft is used most commonly, future ceramics and composites materials, either with or without bone morphogenic proteins, can provide the benefit of a solid fusion without morbidity of bone graft harvesting. The more widespread introduction of anterior cervical instrumentation has decreased the need for brace use and increased fusion rates; although in the short-term it has increased operative costs, its long-term economic benefits can be realized by earlier patient mobilization and return to normal activity levels.

REFERENCES

1. Brain L, Wilkinson M, eds. *Cervical spondylolisthesis and other disorders of the cervical spine,* 1st ed. Philadelphia: WB Saunders, 1967.
2. Torg JS, Pavlov H, Genuario SE, et al. Neuropraxia of the cervical spinal cord with transient quadriplegia. *J Bone Joint Surg Am* 1986; 68:1354–1370.
3. Bell GR, Ross JS. Diagnosis of nerve root compression. *Orthop Clin North Am* 1992;22:405–419.
4. Boden SC, McCowin PR, Davis DO, et al. Abnormal magnetic-resonance scans of the cervical spine in asymptomatic subjects. *J Bone Joint Surg Am* 1990;72:1178–1184.
5. Smith G, Robinson R. The treatment of certain cervical spine disorders by anterior removal of the intervertebral disc and interbody fusion. *J Bone Joint Surg Am* 1958;40:607–624.
6. Apfelbaum RI, Kriskovich MD, Haller JR. On the incidence, cause, and prevention of recurrent laryngeal nerve palsies during anterior cervical spine surgery. *Spine* 2000;25(22):2906–2912.
7. Bohler J. Sofort-und Fruhbehandlong traumatischer querschnitt lahmungen. *Zeitschr Orthopad Grenzgebiete* 1967;103:512–528.
8. Schulte K, Clark C, Goel V. Kinematics of the cervical spine following discectomy and stabilization. *Spine* 1989;14:1116–1121.
9. Grubb M, Currier B, Shih J, et al. Biomechanical evaluation of anterior cervical spine stabilization. *Spine* 1998;23:886–892.
10. Spivak J, Chen D, Kummer F. The effect of locking fixation screws on the stability of anterior cervical plating. *Spine* 1999;24:334–338.
11. Connolly PJ, Esses SI, Kostuik JP. Anterior cervical fusion: outcome analysis of patients fused with and without anterior cervical places. *J Spinal Disord* 1996;9:202–206.
12. McLaughlin MR, Purighalla V, Pizzi FJ. Cost advantages of two-level anterior cervical fusion with rigid internal fixation for radiculopathy and degenerative disease. *Surg Neurol* 1997;48:560–565.
13. Caspar W, Geisler FH, Pitzen T, et al. Anterior cervical plate stabilization in one- and two-level degenerative disease: over-treatment or benefit? *J Spinal Disord* 1998;11:1–11.
14. Geisler FH, Caspar W, Pitzen T, et al. Re-operation in patients after anterior cervical plate stabilization in degenerative disease. *Spine* 1998; 23:911–920.
15. Robinson R, Walker A, Ferlic D. The results of anterior interbody fusion of the cervical spine. *J Bone Joint Surg Am* 1962;44:1569–1587.
16. Emery SE, Bolesta MJ, Banks MA, et al. Robinson anterior cervical fusion. Comparison of standard and modified techniques. *Spine* 1994; 19:660–663.
17. Aronson N, Filtzer DL, Bagan M. Anterior cervical fusion by the Smith-Robinson approach. *J Neurosurg* 1968;29:397–404.
18. Riley LH, Robinson RA, Johnson KA, et al. The results of anterior interbody fusion of the cervical spine. *J Neurosurg* 1969;30:127–133.
19. Connolly ES, Seymour RJ, Adams JE. Clinical evaluation of anterior cervical fusion for degenerative cervical disc disease. *J Neurosurg* 1965;23:431–437.
20. White AA, Southwick WO, DuPonte R, et al. Relief of pain by anterior cervical spine fusion for spondylosis. *J Bone Joint Surg Am* 1968; 55:525–534.
21. Phillips FM, Carlson G, Emery SE, et al. Anterior cervical pseudarthrosis: natural history and treatment. *Spine* 1997;22:1585–1589.
22. Hilibrand AS, Fye MA, Emery SE, et al. Impact of smoking on the outcome of anterior cervical arthrodesis with interbody or strut-grafting. *J Bone Joint Surg Am* 20001;83:668–673.
23. Bohlman HH, Emery SE, Goodfellow DB, et al. Robinson anterior cervical discectomy and arthrodesis for cervical radiculopathy: Long-term follow-up of one-hundred-and-twenty-two patients. *J Bone Joint Surg Am* 1993;75:1298–1301.

24. Gore DR, Sepic SB. Anterior cervical fusion for degenerated or protruded discs. *Spine* 1984;9:667–671.
25. Clements DH, O'Leary PF. Anterior cervical discectomy and fusion. *Spine* 1990;15:1023–1025.
26. Hilibrand AS, Yoo, JU, Carlson GD, et al. The success of anterior cervical arthrodesis adjacent to a previous fusion. *Spine* 1997;22:1574–1579.
27. Klein GR, Vaccaro AR, Albert TJ. Health outcome assessment before and after anterior cervical discectomy and fusion for radiculopathy: a prospective analysis. *Spine* 2000;25:801–803.
28. DePalma A, Rothman R, Lewinnek G, et al. Anterior interbody fusion for severe cervical disc degeneration. *Surg Gynecol Obstet* 1972;134:755–758.
29. Kurz LT, Garfin SR, Booth RE. Harvesting autogenous iliac bone grafts. *Spine* 1989;12:1324–1331.
30. Flynn T. Neurologic complications of anterior cervical interbody fusion. *Spine* 1982;7:536–539.
31. Herkowitz H. The surgical management of cervical spondylotic radiculopathy and myelopathy. *Clin Orthop* 1989;239:94–108.
32. Whitecloud T. Complications of anterior cervical fusion. In: *Instructional course lectures*, Vol XXVII. St. Louis: CV Mosby, 1978.
33. Newhouse K, et al. Esophageal perforation following anterior cervical spine surgery. *Spine* 1989;14:1051–1056.
34. Brown M, Malinin T, Davis P. A roentgenographic evaluation of frozen allografts versus autografts in anterior cervical spine fusions. *Clin Orthop* 1976;119:231–326.
35. Fernyhough J, White J, LaRocca H. Fusion rates in multilevel cervical spondylosis comparing allograft fibula with autograft fibula in 126 patients. *Spine* 1991;16:5561–5564.
36. Zdeblick T, Ducker T. The use of freeze-dried allograft bone for anterior cervical fusions. *Spine* 1991;16:726–729.
37. Bishop RC, Moore KA, Hadley MN. Anterior cervical interbody fusion using autogenic and allogenic bone graft substrate: a prospective comparative analysis. *J Neurosurg* 1996;85:206–210.
38. Malloy KM, Hilibrand AS. Autograft versus allograft in degenerative cervical disease. *Clin Orthop Relat Res* 2002;394:27–38.
39. MacDonald RL, Fehlings MG, Tator CH, et al. Multilevel anterior cervical corpectomy and fibular allograft fusion for cervical myelopathy. *J Neurosurg* 1997;86:990–997.
40. Martin GJ, Haid RW, MacMillian M, et al. Anterior cervical discectomy with freeze-dried fibula allograft. *Spine* 1999;24:852–859.
41. O'Laire S, Thomas D. Spinal cord compression due to prolapse of cervical intervertebral (herniation of nucleus pulposus). *J Neurosurg* 1983;59:846–853.
42. Murphy M, Gadd M. Anterior cervical discectomy without interbody bone graft. *J Neurosurg* 1972;37:71–74.
43. Rosenorn J, Hansen E, Rosenorn M. Anterior cervical discectomy with and without fusion. *J Neurosurg* 1983;59:252–255.
44. Benini A, Krayenbuhl H, Bruder R. Anterior cervical discectomy without fusion: microsurgical technique. *Acta Neurochir* 1982;61:105–110.
45. Kadoya S, Nakamura T, Kwak R. A microsurgical anterior osteophytectomy for cervical spondylotic myelopathy. *Spine* 1984;9:437–441.
46. Wilson D, Campbell D. Anterior cervical discectomy without bone graft. *J Neurosurg* 1977;47:551–555.
47. Watters WC III, Levinthal R. Anterior cervical discectomy with and without fusion: Results, complications and long-term follow-up. *Spine* 1994;19:2343–2347.
48. Wirth FP, Dowd GC, Sanders HF, et al. Cervical discectomy: a prospective analysis of three operative techniques. *Surg Neurol* 2000;53:340–348.

Part B
Posterior Laminoforaminotomy

Paul Klimo, Jr. and Ronald I. Apfelbaum

Degenerative cervical disc disease is common in adults. Interestingly, it was originally thought to be caused by a tumor, termed an "enchondroma" by Oppenheim and Krause in 1907 (1). This notion remained unchallenged until 1934 when Mixter and Barr correctly identified the herniated nucleus pulposus as the more likely cause (2). Disc degeneration and herniation can present with a variety of symptoms: neck pain, shoulder or arm pain, paresthesias or dysesthesias in a radicular distribution, hypesthesia, and upper extremity weakness. In severe cases, myelopathy with long tract signs may also occur. Patients who present with radicular symptoms in a dermatomal distribution that is resistant to nonoperative measures and in whom imaging studies show a herniated disc at the appropriate level are the typical surgical candidates.

Approaches to the herniated cervical disc are classified as either anterior or posterior. In this section of the chapter,

we explore the history of the posterior laminoforaminotomy technique, its indications, complications, and operative nuances, and we review the relevant literature on the effectiveness of this technique.

HISTORY AND INDICATIONS

In 1934, Nachlas (3) described in detail the typical symptoms of cervical radiculopathy caused by a laterally herniated disc, followed by Stookey in 1940 (4) and Semmes and Murphey in 1943 (5). Pain and stiffness of the neck are usually the first symptoms. A patient may also present with headaches, often emanating from the occipital region; interscapular or rhomboid pain; chest pain (so called "cervical angina"); and even retroocular pain. Many patients give a history of first developing pain in the neck or rhomboid region upon awakening one particular day followed by arm pain (6,7). Murphey and colleagues concluded that the pain in the neck, rhomboid region, and anterior chest was referred pain from the disc and therefore that a ruptured disc at any level could cause these symptoms (6,7). The neck and arm pain is aggravated by movements such as coughing, sneezing, and Valsalva maneuver. The term *radiculopathy* refers to the signs and symptoms of nerve root dysfunction, which are manifested as changes in sensory, motor, and reflex function in a dermatomal distribution. The C3 and C4 roots are rarely involved. Radiculopathy of the third cervical root manifests as pain in the upper cervical and occipital region. The fourth cervical root presents with pain over the medial shoulder and inferior to the level of the scapula. There are no identifiable reflexes or motor functions attributed to the C3 and C4 roots. (The symptoms and signs referable to the individual roots from C5 to T1 are outlined in Table 75.1.)

In 1966, Scoville classified cervical disc lesions into five categories: (a) lateral soft disc, (b) lateral hard or osteophyte disc, (c) central bar or ridge, (d) central soft disc, and (e) fracture-dislocations with disc protrusions (8). Of the 741 cases Scoville reviewed, 82% were lateral soft discs, and 13% were lateral hard discs (8). Thus, 95% of all operable disc lesions in his series were laterally placed. Today, disc herniations are classified as either hard or soft by their radiographic features and intraoperative appearance. Many herniations have features of both.

In 1934, Mixter and Barr described the use of a posterior laminectomy to treat 19 cases of intervertebral disc herniation, including four ruptured cervical discs (2). In 1946,

Scoville presented the so-called keyhole foraminotomy technique at the annual Harvey Cushing meeting. This was followed in 1951 by his report on 115 patients treated using this technique (9). The anterior approach was first described in the 1950s by Cloward (10) and by Robinson and Smith (11). Both the anterior and posterior approaches were increasingly employed as improved neurodiagnostic modalities were developed. Despite being developed after the posterior approach, the anterior approach has been widely adopted for many cervical conditions and often is used for cervical radiculopathy. Although it is clear that excellent results can be obtained by a competent surgeon using either approach, there are clear indications for the posterior technique.

The ideal operative candidate for a posterior laminoforaminotomy is a patient with a painful single-level radicular syndrome, corresponding neurologic findings, and concordant preoperative imaging demonstrating disc disease in a lateral or foraminal location (Fig. 75.14A and B) (8,9,12–25). Fager did not believe that symptomatic radiculopathy could occur simultaneously at more than one level and thus argued that multilevel foraminotomies should be avoided (12,13). However, it may be difficult to distinguish C6 and C7 radiculopathy clinically. This, according to Fager, would be the only reason to operate on more than one level at the same time. Many surgeons agree that the operation should not be performed for isolated nonsegmental pain of the shoulder and neck (8,14–17,). Both hard and soft lateral discs can be treated with the posterior approach, although the results in patients with hard discs may not be as good (14,15).

TABLE 75.1. *Root Lesions in the Arm*

Roots	C5	C6	C7	C8	T1
Sensory supply	Lateral border upper arm to elbow	Lateral forearm including thumb and index finger	Over triceps, mid-forearm and middle finger	Medial forearm to include little finger	Axilla down to the olecranon
Sensory loss	As above, over deltoid	As above over thumb and radial border of hand	Middle finger, front and back of hand	Little finger Heal of hand to above wrist	In axilla (usually minimal)
Area of pain	As above and medial scapula border, neck, occasionally anterior chest, shoulder	As above, especially thumb and index finger, neck, shoulder, medial border of scapula, occasionally anterior chest, lateral aspect of arm and dorsum of forearm	As above and areas involved in C6 radiculopathy	Neck, medial border of scapula, sometimes anterior chest, down medial aspect of upper arm and forearm	Deep aching in shoulder and axilla to olecranon
Reflexes affected	Biceps and brachioradialis jerk	Supinator, brachioradialis and biceps	Triceps jerk	Finger and triceps jerk	None
Motor deficit	Deltoid, supraspinatus, infraspinatus, rhomboid	Pronators and supinators of the forearm, biceps, brachioradialis, brachialis	Triceps, wrist extensors, wrist flexors, latissimus dorsi, pectoralis major	Triceps, wrist flexors and extensors, finger flexors and extensors, intrinsic muscles of hand	All small hand muscles (Note: May have Horner's Syndrome)

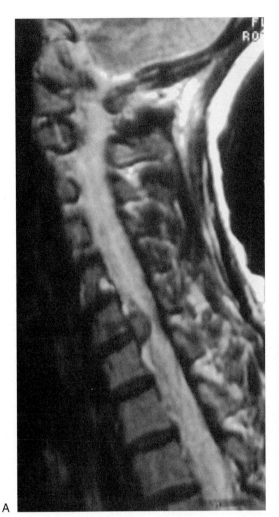

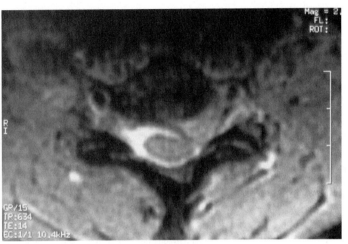

FIG. 75.14. A: Sagittal T2-weighted magnetic resonance imaging study showing left lateral disc herniation at the C6-7 interspace. **B:** Axial T2-weighted image showing large left lateral soft disc herniation with severe nerve root compression.

The posterior approach has several advantages over the anterior. Raynor compared the anterior and posterior approaches in cadaveric specimens (26). He found that resecting up to one half of the facet joint easily allowed 3 to 5 mm of the sensory root to be exposed. Although the same amount of root could be exposed with the anterior approach, it could only be achieved with aggressive dissection laterally beyond the line of direct vision using up-angled curettes. However, in his study, Raynor did not employ the operating microscope or apparently remove a portion of the uncinate process. Other advantages of the posterior approach are avoidance of major neck structures such as the trachea, esophagus, carotid and vertebral arteries, and the recurrent laryngeal nerve; preservation of the remaining disc and motion segment; and elimination of potential morbidities associated with arthrodesis such as pseudoarthrosis, accelerated spondylotic disease at adjacent levels, graft harvest complications, and subsidence and hardware failures. Despite the advantages of the posterior approach, the ante-

rior approach can be used effectively any time the posterior approach is contemplated, but the reverse is not true. The anterior approach continues to dominate the posterior approach because of its broader application. The anterior approach can be used not only in the ideal posterior patient but also in one who has less favorable features, such as midline pathology (hard or soft disc), kyphotic deformity, disc herniation associated with an unstable or traumatic cervical spine, and multilevel disease, and in those with primarily axial neck pain. The classic posterior approach also involves more muscle dissection and retraction and may be associated with more postoperative pain.

SURGICAL TECHNIQUE

Most laminoforaminotomies today are still performed in the same manner that Scoville described in 1951. Many surgeons still prefer to position the patient in a sitting position

(13–16,22,27,28). This provides a relatively dry field with precise identification of the nerve roots. A combination of a precordial Doppler and an end-tidal CO_2 monitor may be used for early detection of air emboli. Raising venous pressure by Valsalva maneuver prevents further entrainment of air and reveals its source by back bleeding, thus allowing the entry site of the air to be sealed. The patient's head is fixated with a Mayfield head holder and kept in a straight, neutral, erect position. When using the sitting position, adequate assessment and maintenance of intravascular volume is necessary. The patient's legs should be kept elevated rather than flexed and dependent. Amazingly, Scoville performed all of his procedures on patients who were sitting upright under local anesthetic block (8,9,26). More recently, the prone position has been favored by some surgeons (20,21,23, 24). Again, the head can be placed in the Mayfield head holder system with the neck in a neutral position. Regardless of which position is used, intraoperative radiology is used to confirm the adequacy of positioning and the abnormal level.

The most common approach used in the past has been through a midline incision. A 4- to 5-cm incision is usually adequate for a one-level decompression. Williams stated that he found a 1-inch incision to be adequate for a two-level foraminotomy using a microsurgical approach (27). The incision is carried precisely through the avascular midline raphe to the spinous processes. The cervical musculature is then dissected away from the bone on the diseased side only, in a careful subperiosteal manner using monopolar electrocautery to avoid excessive bleeding and to expose the facet complex fully (Fig. 75.15).

Once the facet joint complex of the affected level is exposed, bone removal begins. This is usually done with a high-speed drill but can also be done with a hand-held perforator, an instrument used to make holes in bone. Fager used a cranial perforator and burr to place burr holes at the lateral margins of the lamina (13). The bone is often thinned first with the drill and definitively removed with other instruments such as curettes and Kerrison rongeurs to avoid mechanical or thermal injury to the nerve root (Figs. 75.16 and 75.17). Under the microscope or loupe magnification, one third of the upper and lower laminae is drilled away. Laterally, one third, but never more than one half, of the medial facet joint is removed. The bone where the superior articular facet of the inferior vertebra meets the pedicle is also removed to gain access to the nerve root axilla. Fager favored a full hemilaminectomy from the inferior border of lamina below to the superior border of lamina above, leaving a portion of lamina medially (12,13). Because, in his experience, the nerve root and overlying dura and epidural veins are always tightly compressed against bone, the hemilaminectomy provided a superior decompression. After bone removal, the ligamentum flavum is first separated from underlying structures using a Woodson dental tool and then removed by incising with a knife followed by small Kerrison rongeurs (Fig. 75.18). After coagulation of the epidural veins, the nerve root is identified. Such an exposure is termed a "keyhole" foraminotomy.

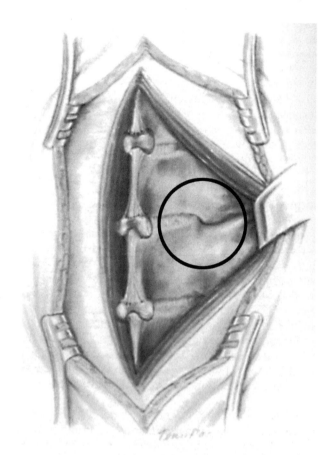

FIG. 75.15. The initial exposure with the classic approach. The paracervical muscles have been dissected free, revealing the laminae and facet complex. The *black circle* represents the exposure obtained with the newer technique utilizing sequential dilators. (From Collias JC, Roberts MP. Posterior surgical approaches for cervical disk herniation and spondylotic myelopathy. In: Schmidek HH, Sweet WH, eds. *Operative neurosurgical techniques: indications, methods and results,* 4th ed. Philadelphia: WB Saunders, 2000: 2016–2027, with permission.)

The sensory and motor nerve roots can now be seen within their separate dural sleeves as they enter the neural foramen. The motor nerve root, which may be smaller than the sensory root, is located anterior and caudal to the larger sensory root. It should be carefully identified to avoid mistaking it for a disc fragment. By elevating the nerve roots superiorly, a small microsurgical blunt nerve hook can be passed beneath the nerve root and the dura, in the region of the axilla of the nerve, and with a 360-degree sweeping motion, herniated disc fragments that breached the PLL can be safely removed (Figs. 75.19 and 75.20). If the fragments are located behind the PLL, it is incised in an inferolateral direction, away from the spinal cord and nerve root sleeve. Instruments can then be introduced through the defect, and the fragments may be "milked out like toothpaste" according to Scoville and associates (9). Although most fragments are located in the axilla of the nerve root, a thorough exploration must be conducted above, below, and medial to the nerve. Many disc herniations have both soft and hard features. Osteophytes can be removed with a drill,

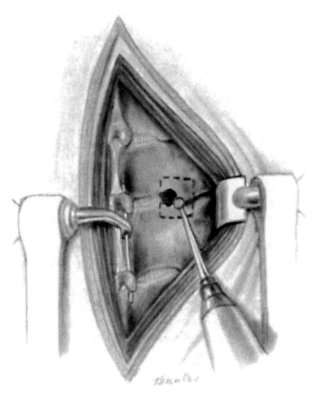

FIG. 75.16. A drill is used to begin removal of the medial facet complex and the lateral portions of the superior and inferior laminae. (From Collias JC, Roberts MP. Posterior surgical approaches for cervical disk herniation and spondylotic myelopathy. In: Schmidek HH, Sweet WH, eds. *Operative neurosurgical techniques: indications, methods and results,* 4th ed. Philadelphia: WB Saunders, 2000:2016–2027, with permission.)

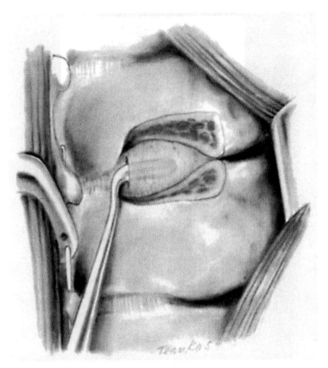

FIG. 75.18. A Woodson dental tool is used to dissect the ligamentum flavum free of any underlying structures. (From Collias JC, Roberts MP. Posterior surgical approaches for cervical disk herniation and spondylotic myelopathy. In: Schmidek HH, Sweet WH, eds. *Operative neurosurgical techniques: indications, methods and results,* 4th ed. Philadelphia: WB Saunders, 2000:2016–2027, with permission.)

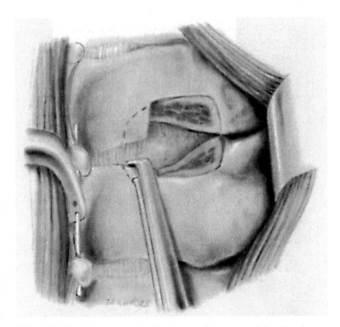

FIG. 75.17. A rongeur is then used to complete the bone removal. (From Collias JC, Roberts MP. Posterior surgical approaches for cervical disk herniation and spondylotic myelopathy. In: Schmidek HH, Sweet WH, eds. *Operative neurosurgical techniques: indications, methods and results,* 4th ed. Philadelphia: WB Saunders, 2000:2016–2027, with permission.)

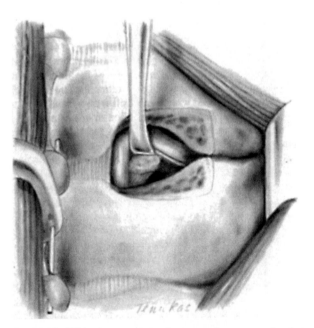

FIG. 75.19. With the nerve root exposed, a nerve hook is placed in the axilla, and the root (both sensory and motor components) is elevated, revealing the herniated disc. (From Collias JC, Roberts MP. Posterior surgical approaches for cervical disk herniation and spondylotic myelopathy. In: Schmidek HH, Sweet WH, eds. *Operative neurosurgical techniques: indications, methods and results,* 4th ed. Philadelphia: WB Saunders, 2000:2016–2027, with permission.)

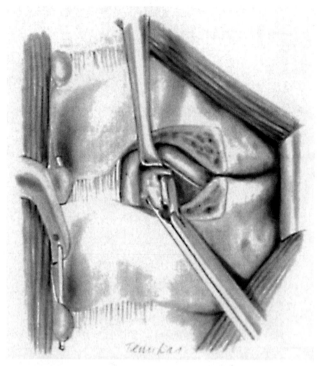

FIG. 75.20. A disk rongeur is used to remove the herniated disc fragment.

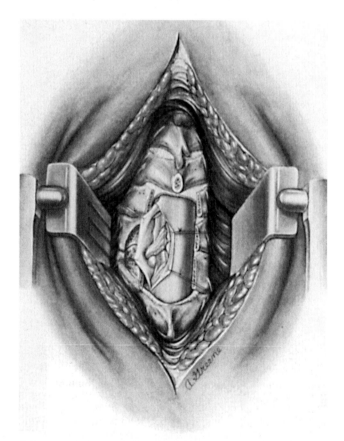

FIG. 75.21. The exposure for a transdural resection of a medially herniated disc. Note the more extensive bone removal and curved lateral dural incision. (From Fager CA. Posterolateral approach to ruptured median and paramedian cervical disk. *Surg Neurol* 1983;20:443–452, with permission.)

rongeurs, or curettes. Some surgeons prefer to decompress the nerve root without removing the osteophytes (14,16,22,29,). A formal discectomy is never performed. In this procedure, only extruded disc fragments, if present, are removed, but the disc space is not entered to avoid enlarging the opening in the annulus. The decompression is complete when a probe can be placed through the foramen without difficulty and gentle manipulation reveals the nerve root to be loosened.

Hemostasis and thorough irrigation of the wound is then performed. The wound is closed with absorbable material in multiple layers including the paraspinal musculature, overlying fascia, subcutaneous layer, and skin. We do not use antibiotics or steroids perioperatively or a collar postoperatively. We have found that a combination of scheduled ketorolac and diazepam for no more than 48 hours provides substantial relief of postoperative incisional pain and muscle spasm. The patient is encouraged to perform cervical range-of-motion exercises as soon as possible. When we perform this classic approach, the patient is usually discharged on the first postoperative day.

Some surgeons have modified the posterior approach to remove a central disc herniation. Both Scoville and Fager described a combined intraextradural technique for central soft disc lesions (8,16,28). Once the nerve root is exposed, the dura is opened by an incision extending superior and inferior to the nerve root (Fig. 75.21). The extruded fragment should then come into view, distending and thinning the anterior dura. A second dural incision is then made anteriorly to remove these fragments (Fig. 75.22). Although elevation

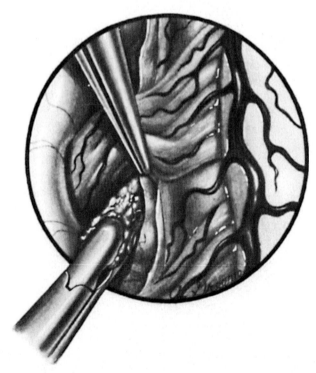

FIG. 75.22. Removal of disc fragments through an incision in the ventral dura. (From Fager CA. Posterolateral approach to ruptured median and paramedian cervical disk. *Surg Neurol* 1983;20:443–452, with permission.)

or retraction of the spinal cord is not prohibited, it is rarely necessary, according to Fager. No attempt is made to close the defect in the anterior dura, and the posterior durotomy is easily sealed. More recently, Fujimto and coworkers described a very similar technique, although it was done on 31 patients who, in addition to the disc herniation, had developmental canal stenosis or multilevel posterior compression from ligamentous hypertrophy and were myelopathic (30). Patients with monoradiculopathy from lateral disc herniations underwent keyhole foraminotomies. The intradural approach was combined with a multilevel laminoplasty. The ventral and dorsal dura were closed with 6–0 nylon sutures.

Hunt and Miller appear to have been the first to advocate a paramedian, muscle-splitting approach (31). They believed that this approach produced less postoperative pain and placed the wound under little tension. With this technique, patients are placed in a lateral forward oblique position, the involved side up, and the head resting on a pad. A 5-cm diagonal incision is then made parallel to the trapezius fibers. The incision passes over the articulation of the desired interspace. The multiple layers of muscles are sequentially split until the two laminae and facet complex are exposed. A keyhole laminotomy and nerve root decompres-

sion are then performed as described earlier. The trapezius fascia, subcutaneous tissue, and skin edges are then closed.

In 1998, Adamson (17) developed a technique modeled on the microendoscopic discectomy (MED) approach to lumbar disc herniations by Smith and Foley (32). This technique has gained in popularity and is the approach we, and others, currently use (33,34). The patient is placed in the sitting position with the head fixed in a Mayfield frame. Localization of the operative site is first confirmed by passing a spinal needle under fluoroscopic guidance to the facet complex. A C-arm fluoroscope can be placed arching in front of the patient to image the spine. In the sitting position, the shoulders descend, allowing easy localization down to the cervicothoracic junction. A 15- to 20-mm vertical incision 2 cm off midline is then carried down to the subcutaneous tissue. A K wire is then passed through the incision to the facet complex. Adamson and others prefer using either a sequence of circular dilators to atraumatically split the paracervical musculature around the K wire; or alternatively, narrow, flat-bladed, speculum-type tractors may also be used (17,33) (Fig. 75.23). Again, the lateral portions of the superior and inferior laminae and the medial portion of the corresponding facet joint is exposed, but with less dissection and trauma to the cervical musculature, as with the more classic approach

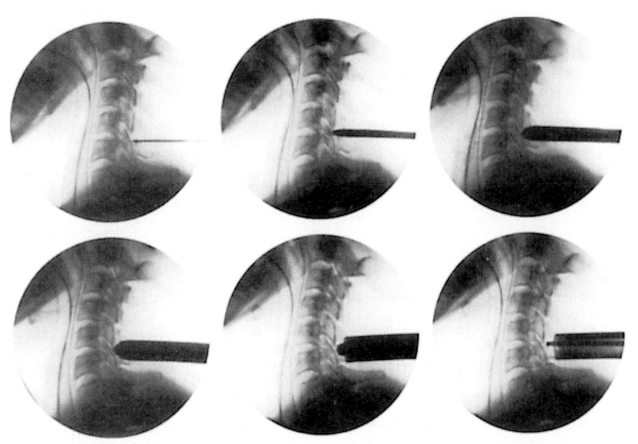

FIG. 75.23. Sequence of intraoperative fluoroscopy images showing the progression of larger dilators directed at the C5-6 interspace. The final picture shows an instrument being passed through the dilator. (From Adamson TE. Microendoscopic posterior cervical laminoforaminotomy for unilateral radiculopathy: results of a new technique in 100 cases. *J Neurosurg (Spine 1)* 2001;95:51–57, with permission.)

described earlier (see *circle* drawn on Fig. 75.15). At this point, we prefer to use the operative microscope to provide the necessary magnification and illumination. Others have found success using an endoscope (17,33,34). After thinning and resecting the bone with air drills, rongeurs, and curettes, the nerve root is exposed, and any disc fragments found are removed in same manner as described above. The wound is closed in two layers (subcutaneous layer and skin).

BIOMECHANICAL CONSIDERATIONS

White and Panjabi have provided a useful and widely used definition of spinal instability (35): "Clinical instability is the loss of the ability of the spine under physiologic loads to maintain its pattern of displacement so that there is no initial or additional neurological deficit, no major deformity, and no incapacitating pain." The effects of resecting the lamina and varying degrees of the zygapophyseal joints have been investigated (17,36). Raynor and colleagues tested 14 single cervical segments with their ligaments intact (36). Five were fresh-frozen cadavers specimens with intact facets, and 9 were formalin-fixed specimens that had undergone bilateral facetectomies (removing 50% of the facets or less in 5 of these specimens and 70% in 4). Their purpose was to study bone strength under shear stress as a function of the amount of bone removed from the facets. The vertebral body end plates were fixated to aluminum plates with methylmethacrylate, and a shear force was applied. There were two types of failures: fixation and fracture. A fixation failure occurred when the cement was unable to hold the vertebral body on the mounting plate. When the remaining facet joint fractured and the vertebral bodies dislocated in relation to each other, this was termed a *fracture failure*. In three of the four 70%-facetectomized specimens, failures occurred because of fractures occurring in the remaining facet joint. Only one of the five 50%-facetectomized specimens failed because of facet fracture, and none in the intact specimens. The rest of the failures occurred when the vertebral body tore loose from the acrylic cement attaching it to the mounting plate. The authors did not test specimens with unilateral facetectomies. Based on their results, the authors concluded that no more than 50% of the joint should be resected because it may fracture "under loads in the physiologic range."

Zdeblick and coworkers, however, questioned this study, stating that the model used by Raynor and colleagues did not accurately reflect physiological conditions (37). Instability after a partial facetectomy, according to Zdeblick, is not due to a fracture of the remaining facet but to progressive subluxation, and therefore testing osseus failure is inappropriate. Zdeblick and coworkers analyzed 12 fresh-frozen human cervical spines that were rigidly fixated at the third and seventh bodies and that had undergone non-destructive testing. The spines were tested intact, after a full bilateral laminectomy of the fifth vertebra, and with progressive bilateral facetectomies of the C5-C6 joint (25%,

50%, 75%, and 100% of the facet joint and capsule). The tests consisted of an axial load of 200 Newton, a torsional moment of 5 Newtons-meter with 100 Newtons of applied axial preload, and a flexion-extension moment. They calculated mean axial stiffness, torsional stiffness, and flexural displacement. Axial stiffness did not change with progressive facetectomies. Torsional hypermobility occurred after resection of more than 50% of the facet joint. Flexural displacement, as measured by the change in length between the posterior elements of the fourth and sixth cervical vertebrae, increased with removal of 50% or more of the facets. Again, the conclusion was that segmental hypermobility might occur if more than 50% of the facet is resected.

Cusick and colleagues performed increasing compression-flexion loads on 12 cadaveric specimens that were first tested intact, then after a complete unilateral facetectomy, and then after a bilateral facetectomy (38). They found that unilateral facetectomy diminished the strength of the spine by 31% and that bilateral facetectomy diminished the strength by 53%. In another study, Voo and associates analyzed the effect of progressive unilateral and bilateral facetectomies using a C4 to C6 finite element model subjected to a pure-moment load in flexion, extension, lateral bending, and axial torsion (39). In general, the amount of rotation between C4 and C6 compared with an intact model increased as the degree of resection increased. The maximum increases were 11.5% for bilateral facetectomy and 5% for unilateral facetectomy with lateral bending and 100% facet resection. The increase in motion after a complete unilateral facetectomy was still less than that created after a 75% bilateral facetectomy.

Recently, Chen and coworkers used a computer-generated, three-dimensional, nonlinear finite element model to evaluate the change in flexibility of C5-C6 after a posterior foraminotomy, anterior foraminotomy with discectomy, and anterior discectomy with fusion (40). The keyhole procedure was modeled by removing 50% of the facet and inferior layer of the C5 lamina along with the superior layer of the C6 lamina on the right side. The primary motions of their intact model closely matched those of a cadaveric specimen. Each model was tested in flexion, extension, torsion, and lateral bending. As expected, the anterior foraminotomy and discectomy without fusion model produced the greatest amount of additional motion. The anterior discectomy with fusion model decreased motion by 50% to 100%. The keyhole foraminotomy caused little added movement, the most being 18% with right lateral bending compared with the intact model.

Based on these studies, the current recommendations are to avoid removing more than 50% of the facet complex. This is based on cadaver models in which bilateral facetectomies and a complete laminectomy were performed. To our knowledge, no cadaver study has been performed to evaluate the biomechanical effects of a standard unilateral posterior laminoforaminotomy. However, as discussed later, postoperative instability has never been reported. Therefore, it is safe to assume that a one-level laminoforaminotomy limiting the resection of the facet complex to 50% or less will have little affect on stability.

RESULTS AND COMPLICATIONS

There are many reports in the literature on the effectiveness of the posterior laminoforaminotomy technique. However, some of these reports lack a substantial follow-up period or provide little detail on the patients' functional outcome, and the methods of measuring success vary. Recently, there has been a movement to create a standardized system for evaluating patient outcome. Odom and colleagues provided definitions for the terms *excellent, good, satisfactory,* and *poor* that incorporate not only symptomatic relief but also how the surgery affected the patients' daily activities (41) (Table 75.2). Prolo and associates devised a system to evaluate the success of posterior lumbar interbody fusion cases that incorporated anatomic, economic, and functional features (42). The economic scale measured the patient's capacity for gainful employment or other comparable pursuits, whereas the functional scale ranked pain responses and the effect of pain on the activities of living (Table 75.3). The sum of the responses between the two scales ranged from 2 to 10. Table 75.4 summarizes the data from the literature that is reported herein.

In 1951, Scoville first published a report of 115 cases (9). All but three patients had lateral herniations, with the C6-C7 disc being the most common level. Myelograms were done on all patients and were positive in 99% of the patients, usually revealing a minimal defect in the root sleeve. All patients returned to work, and only two patients had recurrences. Scoville cited no follow-up and simply concluded that the procedure was "proven economically more satisfactory than the previously used conservative treatment" and that it should be used in all patients with arm pain who are unable to sleep or work. Scoville then published a somewhat more detailed report in 1976 (28). Of 246 patients who had lateral disc herniations, 72% had soft discs, and 28% had hard discs. Of the 246 patients, follow-up was available in 171 and ranged from 5 to 33 years, with a mean of

TABLE 75.2. *Criteria for the Evaluation of Surgery from Odom et al. (32)*

Results of surgery	Criteria
Excellent	No complaints referable to cervical disc disease. Daily occupations are carried out without impairment.
Good	Intermittent discomfort related to cervical disc disease. Daily occupations are carried out without significant impairment.
Satisfactory	Subjective improvement but physical activities are significantly limited.
Poor	Unchanged or worse compared to condition before operation.

21 years. Ninety-five percent of patients reported their quality of recovery as being excellent or good. One third of patients returned to work within 2 weeks, and 96% of men and 100% of women eventually returned to their previous jobs. No complications were reported.

In 1973, Murphey and colleagues published one of the largest series (6): 648 cases seen over more than 30 years. Of those, 380 had follow-up, ranging from 1 to 28 years. Ninety percent of the patients preoperatively awoke in the morning with pain in the neck or rhomboid region, which was followed by arm pain, and 20% of the patients had anterior chest pain. All patients were operated in the prone position, usually with local anesthesia. Of the 648 cases, 393 were at the C6-C7 level and 171 at the C5-C6 level. The patients who were available for follow-up were asked to estimate their postoperative improvement and its effect on their occupation. Three hundred sixteen, or 84%, reported that they had more than 90% relief of their preoperative symptoms. Nine patients rated the relief between 50% and 59%, but Murphey noted that all of these patients had other reasons to have shoulder, arm, or neck pain, and the most common site of pathology was in the shoulder (e.g., bursitis). Only 4% of patients had to seek new jobs after their operations because of pain. Six patients developed early or late recurrences that required reoperation. Contrary to the belief of many other surgeons, Murphey believed that osteophytes alone rarely, if

TABLE 75.3. *Economic-Functional Rating System by Prolo et al. and Modified by Davis (33,37)*

Economic status	Functional status
E1: Complete invalid	F1: Total incapacity (or worse than before operation)
E2: No gainful occupation (including ability to do housework or continue retirement activities)	F2: Persistent neck and arm pain, persistent paresthesias, motor weakness same as prior to operation (able to perform tasks of daily living)
E3: Ability to work, but not at previous occupation; able to perform housework, school and retirement activities	F3: Moderate neck and arm pain, persistent paresthesias, minimal motor weakness
E4: Working at previous occupation part-time or with limited status	F4: No neck or arm pain, persistent paresthesias in fingers, no motor weakness
E5: Able to work at previous occupation with no restrictions	F5: No neck or arm pain, no paresthesias, no motor weakness, complete recovery, able to perform previous sports activities

TABLE 75.4. *Review of the Posterior Laminoforaminotomy Literature*

Authors	Number of PTS	Number of procedures	Follow up (available patients)	Position	Outcome	Complications
Aldrich (41)	36	36	Avg. = 26 mo	Prone	All had resolution of pain and weakness	None
Collias and Roberts (40)	2035	N/A	N/A	Sitting	96% excellent or good	0.2%
Grieve et al. (42)	77	86	Avg. = 40 mo (60)	Prone	70% had complete or >75% resolution of pain. Mean pt satisfaction score = 7.5/10	1.3%: 1-C6 paresis
Henderson et al. (34)	736	846	Avg. = 2.8 yrs	Sitting	91% excellent or good	1.5%: 13-wound infections
Krupp et al. (14)	230	254	Avg. = 3.5 yrs (161)	Sitting	94% excellent or good	5%: 1-tetraparesis, 1-worsened weakness, 2 durotomies, 4 DVTs, 2 PEs
Murphey et al. (6)	648	648+ 4 pts had "multiple" levels	Range = 1–28 yrs (380)	Prone	84% of pts had over 90% relief of their preop sxs	2.6%: 1-increased deficit, 6-"causalgia", 6-recurrences
Rodrigues et al. (39)	51	51	Avg. = 46 mo	Prone	All had resolution of pain	None
Scoville (9)	115	115	N/A	Sitting	All pts returned to work	1.7%: 2-recurrences
Scoville (17)	246	246	Avg. = 21 yrs (171)	Sitting	95% excellent or good	None
Silveri et al. (35)	84	102	Avg. = 6.1 yrs (60)	Prone	93% excellent	1.67%: 1-wound infection
Tomaras et al. (43)	183	185	Avg. = 19 mo	Sitting	Non workers' comp. group: 93% excellent or good Workers' comp. group: 78% excellent or good	None
Williams (18)	235	585	Followed over 10 years (Mean and range not given)	Sitting	All patients had complete resolution of radicular pain by six weeks	11%: 19-transient sxs, 5-prolonged paresis, 1-wound infection, 5-recurrences
Witzmann et al. (36)	67	79	Avg. = 3.1 yrs	Sitting	93% excellent or good	1.5%: 1-wound infection
Zeidman and Ducker (15)	172	243	Two or more years in 77% of pts, one year in 23%	Sitting	97% of pts had relief of radicular pain	3%: 4-air emboli, 1-central cord syndrome

ever, produce radiculopathy and that if they are present, there is always a concomitant acute disc fragment.

Henderson and coworkers published their experience with 736 patients between 1963 and 1980 (43). A total of 846 procedures were performed, all in the sitting position. Of the patients reported, 626 had only one procedure, 103 had two, and 7 had three. Surprisingly, in 45% of the cases, the pain and paresthesias were in a nondermatomal pattern. Sixty-eight percent had demonstrable motor weakness, and 828 procedures were preceded by cervical myelography. Among these, there was a 73% correlation between the myelographically diagnosed space and the space actually thought to be most importantly involved. Interestingly, the authors decompressed the nerve roots, but never removed any disc material or osteophytes. The mean follow-up was

2.8 years. Patients were asked to rate their symptoms using a modification of the criteria developed by Odom and colleagues (41). Postoperative resolution of the radicular symptom complex, which included arm, neck, scapular, and anterior chest pain as well as weakness and headache, was "good or excellent" in 91% of cases. Twenty-four patients (3.3%) developed a recurrence and required a reoperation. Thirty-two patients with one or more posterior procedures required an anterior interbody fusion for ongoing symptoms. No instability was mentioned. The average time to return to work or "normal activities" was 9.4 weeks. A morbidity rate of 1.5% (13 cases) was reported, and all due to wound infections or breakdowns.

Several other authors have used the Odom criteria in evaluating the success of the procedure. Krupp and colleagues described 203 patients, 208 of whom underwent a one-level foraminotomy; 21 patients underwent a two-level foraminotomy, and 1 patient had four nerve roots exposed (14). All were performed in the sitting position. Sixty-five percent of patients had soft discs, 14% had hard discs, and 21% had features of both. Of the 203 patients, 161 were available for follow-up, which averaged 3.5 years. Ninety-four percent of patients had a good or excellent result from their surgery. When the patients were divided based on their disc morphology, 98% of those with a soft disc had good to excellent result, compared with 84% with hard discs and 91% with combined features. Ninety-two percent of patients resumed normal working capability. A perioperative morbidity rate of 5% was reported, and 80% of patients went on to a full recovery. More recently, Silveri and associates described their study, which used the Odom criteria (18). They reported 84 patients who underwent a total of 102 decompressions. Sixty patients with a total of 69 foraminotomies were available for follow-up, with an average follow-up of 6.1 years. Using the Odom criteria, 56 of 60 patients reported excellent results, and three reported good results. All patients were able to return to daily activities within 2–3 weeks, and the average time to return to work was 4.7 weeks. Twenty-five patients underwent flexion/extension films, which showed no instability.

Three studies have been reported that used the scale developed by Prolo and colleagues. Witzmann and associates reported 67 patients who underwent a total of 79 decompressions (19). Average follow-up was 3.1 years (range, 1.5 to 7 years). Eighty-five percent of patients judged the result of their operation as excellent, 7% were good, and 7% were fair or poor. Based on the Prolo scale, 90% of patients showed excellent economic outcome. Seventy-nine percent of the patients returned to their previous occupation. Davis reported 170 patients seen over a 30-year period (29). Ninety-one percent presented with neck and arm pain, and 94% had weakness. All patients had concordant imaging studies, which was a criterion for surgery. Of the 170 patients, 164 were available for follow-up (range, 1 to 32 years; average, 15 years). The mean scores for the economic and functional scales and the overall mean total score were 4.7, 4.2, and 8.9, respectively. Total Prolo scores of 8, 9, and 10 were classified as a good result, and the percentage of patients in these groups were 5%, 38%, and 43%, respectively. The perioperative morbidity rate was 1.2%. One patient developed an axillary nerve injury due to positioning, and another had a transient paresis due to manipulation of the C5 nerve root. Woertgen and associates operated on 54 patients, 50 of whom were available for an average follow-up of 1 year (20). In addition to the Prolo scale, the investigators used a pain-grading scale and asked patients about their overall health and quality of life. Using the Prolo scale, 78% of the patients were classified as a good outcome (total sum, 8 to 10), and 80% reported an improvement in their quality of life. However, they found that patients who had symptoms and neurologic deficits for longer than 2 to 3 months

had an increased risk for a poor outcome. Therefore, the authors recommended early surgery.

Zeidman and Ducker reviewed their results with 172 patients who underwent a total of 243 procedures, all operated on in the sitting position (15). Forty-three patients (25%) underwent a one-level decompression without discectomy, and 60 patients (35%) had disc fragments removed. The remaining 68 patients (40%) were operated on at multiple levels. Follow-up was 2 years or more in 77% of the patients and 1 year for the rest. Ninety-seven percent of patients had relief of their radicular pain, and 93% had improvement in their motor weakness. The patients who underwent multiple decompressions had significant pain relief, but only 5.8% had any improvement in their weakness, and the degree to which their sensation improved was not to the level of those with the one-level decompressions. Four patients developed air emboli without any major consequences, and one patient developed a central cord syndrome postoperatively that improved, but not completely.

Recently, Rodrigues and coworkers reported 51 patients with one-level unilateral radiculopathy (21). Follow-up ranged from 18 to 108 months, with an average of 46 months. All patients had resolution of their radicular pain, and 93% had regained their strength. No complications were reported, and follow-up films were obtained, which showed no instability. The largest series to date that we are aware of is by Collias and Roberts (22). In their review of 2,035 cases, 85% of the cases were soft discs, 11% were hard discs, and 4% were soft central discs. Many of these patients were Scoville's. Ninety-six percent of the patients had good to excellent result, although these terms are not defined, and the same percentage returned to work. The authors reported one recurrence and a 0.2% morbidity rate, but failed to elaborate. Two cases of air emboli occurred causing severe brain damage, and two major postoperative neurologic deficits related to the surgery occurred, one of which was related to cord retraction when a transdural approach was being used for a more medial disc herniation. The authors subsequently abandoned this approach for central discs.

Finally, most recently, Adamson (17) reported on 100 patients with unilateral cervical radicular syndromes, 57% at the C6-C7 level and 30% at C5-C6. All patients were operated on in the sitting position. Ninety patients were discharged the day of their operation, and the rest stayed a single night. Sixty patients were able to return to work or resume normal activity within 1 week or less, 24 within 6 to 8 weeks. The follow-up period ranged from 6 to 31 months, with an average of 14.8 months. Ninety-one patients had excellent outcomes, six were good, two fair, and one poor. Two of these patients were professional football players. Both were able to return to aerobic exercise and strength training within 1 week. One returned to full contact after 3 weeks and played in a game after 4 weeks. There was one case of a superficial wound infection and two asymptomatic durotomies.

CONCLUSION

Posterior laminoforaminotomy is an excellent and effective procedure for the patient with a monoradiculopathy and a laterally located soft disc. If disc degeneration is otherwise modest (at this level), this may be the procedure of choice because it decompresses the root and spares the motion segment. Minimal incision approaches improve patient comfort, may offer a quicker return to normal activities, and shorten hospitalization and recovery without sacrificing effectiveness. The procedure is probably not indicated in multilevel (greater than two) pathology or in patients who would benefit from a fusion and correction of a kyphotic angulation. Roots compressed by hard discs can be decompressed dorsally. Using the posterior approach to remove an anteriorly located hard disc may be more risky than just decompressing the root. Therefore, roots compressed by large hard discs may be better decompressed by an anterior approach, which will allow fuller resection of the hard disc (osteophyte) and performance of an anterior foraminotomy to enlarge the neural foramina as needed. The anterior approach may also be safer for hard and soft discs that are not purely lateral in location.

REFERENCES

1. Oppenheim H, Krause F. Uber zwer operativ geheilte Faelle von Geschwuelsten am Halsmark. *Muenchen med Wchnschr* 1909;56:1134–1136.
2. Mixter WJ, Barr JS. Rupture of the intervertebral disc with involvement of the spinal canal. *N Engl J Med* 1934;211:210–215.
3. Nachlas IW. Pseudo-angina pectoris originating in the cervical spine. *JAMA* 1934;103:323–325.
4. Stookey B. Compression of spinal cord and nerve roots by herniation of the nucleus pulposus in the cervical region. *Arch Surg* 1940;40:417–432.
5. Semmes RE, Murphey F. Syndrome of unilateral rupture of sixth cervical intervertebral disk, with compression of seventh cervical nerve root; report of 4 cases with symptoms simulating coronary disease. *JAMA* 1943;121:1209–1214.
6. Murphey F, Simmons JCH, Brunson B. Surgical treatment of laterally ruptured cervical disc: review of 648 cases, 1939 to 1972. *J Neurosurg* 1973;38:679–683.
7. Murphey F, Simmons JCH, Brunson B. Ruptured cervical discs: 1939 to 1972. *Clin Neurosurg* 1973;20:9–17.
8. Scoville WB. Types of cervical disk lesions and their surgical approaches. *JAMA* 1966;196:105–107.
9. Scoville WB, Whitcomb BB, McLaurin RL. The cervical ruptured disc: report of 115 operative cases. *Trans Am Neurol Assoc*, 1951;76:222–224.
10. Cloward RB. The anterior approach for removal of ruptured cervical discs. *J Neurosurg* 1958;15:602–614.
11. Robinson RA, Smith GW. Anterolateral disc removal and interbody fusion for cervical disc syndrome. *Bull Johns Hopkins Hosp* 1955;96:223–224(abst).
12. Fager CA. Posterior surgical tactics for the neurological syndromes of cervical disc and spondylotic lesions. *Clin Neurosurg* 1978;25:218–244.
13. Fager CA. Management of cervical disc lesions and spondylosis by posterior approaches. *Clin Neurosurg*, 1977;24:488–507.
14. Krupp W, Schattke H, Müke R. Clinical results of the foraminotomy as described by Frykholm for the treatment of lateral cervical disc herniation. *Acta Neurochir* 1990;107:22–29.
15. Zeidman SM, Ducker TB. Posterior cervical laminoforaminotomy for radiculopathy: review of 172 cases. *Neurosurgery* 1993;33:356–362.
16. Scoville WB, Dohrmann GJ, Corkill G. Late results of cervical disc surgery. *J Neurosurg* 1976;45:203–210.
17. Adamson TE. Microendoscopic posterior cervical laminoforaminotomy for unilateral radiculopathy: results of a new technique in 100 cases. *J Neurosurg (Spine 1)* 2001;95:51–57.
18. Silveri CP, Simpson JM, Simeone FA, et al. Cervical disk disease and the keyhole foraminotomy: Proven efficacy at extended long-term follow-up. *Orthopedics* 1997;20:687–692.
19. Witzmann A, Hejazi N, Krasznai L. Posterior cervical foraminotomy. A follow-up study of 67 surgically treated patients with compressive radiculopathy. *Neurosurg Rev* 2000;23:213–217.
20. Woertgen C, Holzschuh M, Tothoerl RD, et al. Prognostic factors of posterior cervical disc surgery: a prospective, consecutive study of 54 patients. *Neurosurgery* 1997;40:724–729.
21. Rodrigues MA, Hanel RA, Prevedello DMS, et al. Posterior approach for soft cervical disc herniation: a neglected technique? *Surg Neurol* 2001;55:17–22.
22. Collias JC, Roberts MP. Posterior surgical approaches for cervical disk herniation and spondylotic myelopathy. In: Schmidek HH, Sweet WH, eds. *Operative neurosurgical techniques: indications, methods and results,* 4th ed. Philadelphia: WB Saunders, 2000:2016–2027.
23. Aldrich F. Posterolateral microdiscectomy for cervical monoradiculopathy caused by posterolateral soft cervical disc sequestration. *J Neurosurg* 1990;72:370–377.
24. Grieve JP, Kitchen ND, Moore AJ, et al. Results of posterior cervical foraminotomy for treatment of cervical spondylotic radiculopathy. *Br J Neurosurg* 2000;14:40–43.
25. Tomaras CR, Blacklock JB, Parker WD, et al. Outpatient surgical treatment of cervical radiculopathy. *J Neurosurg* 1997;87:41–43.
26. Raynor RB. Anterior or posterior approach to the cervical spine: an anatomical and radiographic evaluation and comparison. *Neurosurgery* 1983;12:7–13.
27. Williams RW. Microcervical foraminotomy: a surgical alternative for intractable radicular pain. *Spine* 1983;8:708–716.
28. Fager CA. Posterolateral approach to ruptured median and paramedian cervical disk. *Surg Neurol* 1983;20:443–452.
29. Davis RA. A long-term outcome study of 170 surgically treated patients with compressive cervical radiculopathy. *Surg Neurol* 1996;46:523–533.
30. Fujimto Y, Baba I, Sumida T, et al. Microsurgical transdural discectomy with laminoplasty. *Spine* 2002;27:715–721.
31. Hunt WE, Miller CA. Management of cervical radiculopathy. *Clin Neurosurg* 1986;33:485–502.
32. Smith M, Foley K. Microendoscopic discectomy. *Tech Neurosurg* 1997;2:301–307.
33. Burke RH, Caputy A. Microendoscopic posterior cervical foraminotomy: a cadaveric model and clinical application for cervical radiculopathy. *J Neurosurg (Spine 1)* 2000;93:129–129.
34. Roh SW, Kim DH, Cardoso AC, et al. Endoscopic foraminotomy using a microendoscopic discectomy system in cadaveric specimens. *Neurosurg Focus* 1998;4(2):Article 2.
35. White AA, Panjabi MM. *Clinical biomechanics of the spine,* 2nd ed. Philadelphia: JB Lippincott, 1990.
36. Raynor RB, Pugh J, Shapiro I. Cervical facetectomy and its effect on spine strength. *J Neurosurg* 1985;63:278–282.
37. Zdeblick TA, Zou D, Warden KE, et al. Cervical stability after foraminotomy. *J Bone Joint Surg Am* 1992;74:22–27.
38. Cusick JF, Yoganandan N, Pintar F, et al. Biomechanics of cervical spine facetectomy and fixation techniques. *Spine* 1988;13:808–812.
39. Voo LM, Kumaresan S, Yoganandan N, et al. Finite element analysis of cervical facetectomy. *Spine* 1997;22:964–969.
40. Chen BH, Natarajan RN, An HS, et al. Comparison of biomechanical response to surgical procedures used for cervical radiculopathy: posterior keyhole foraminotomy versus anterior foraminotomy and discectomy versus anterior discectomy with fusion. *J Spinal Disord* 2001;14:17–20.
41. Odom GL, Finney W, Woodhall B. Cervical disc lesion. *JAMA* 1958;161:23–28.
42. Prolo DF, Oklund SA, Butcher M. Toward uniformity in evaluating results of lumbar spine operations. A paradigm applied to posterior interbody fusions. *Spine* 1986;11:601–606.
43. Henderson DM, Hennessy RG, Shuey HM, et al. Posterior-lateral foraminotomy as an exclusive operative technique for cervical radiculopathy: a review of 846 consecutively operated cases. *Neurosurgery* 1983;13:504–512.

CHAPTER 76

Treatment of Cervical Myelopathy

Part A
Laminectomy

Nancy E. Epstein and Joseph A. Epstein

Cervical laminectomy is valuable for the management of congenital or acquired multilevel cervical spinal stenosis associated with spondylosis, ossification of the posterior longitudinal ligament (OPLL), and ossification of the yellow ligament (OYL). The cervical lordotic curvature must be preserved in these patients. In addition, when instability is present or threatened, a posterior facet wiring and arthrodesis or lateral mass arthrodesis should be performed.

ANATOMY

The spinal cord and nerve roots may become compressed in a canal narrowed in its anteroposterior (AP) dimension by absolute or relative stenosis, other forms of stenosis being associated with congenitally shortened pedicles (achondroplasia) and lowered laminar arches (1). The normal AP diameter of the spinal canal between the C3 and C7 levels is 17 mm. In absolute (congenital) stenosis, this is often narrowed to 10 mm or less, whereas in relative (acquired) stenosis, it typically measures about 13 mm (2). When taking into consideration the AP dimensions of the spinal cord (0.8 to 1.3 cm) and the 2 to 3 mm occupied by the soft tissues (posterior longitudinal ligament, yellow ligament, epidural fat, venous plexus), there remains little to no residual "available space" for the neural tissues (1). Disc disease, spondyloarthrosis, and hypertrophy or ossification of the posterior longitudinal or yellow ligaments further contribute to radicular or myelopathic syndromes. Although chronic, microtrauma contributes to slowly progressive changes; acute hyperextension injury may result in the rapid evolution of irreversible cord damage.

PATHOLOGY

In spinal stenosis, two major mechanisms of neural injury have been invoked: direct mechanical compression and indirect vascular insufficiency. These two processes contribute to the varied extent and location of cord changes often located several levels proximal or distal to the sites of maximal compression (3). Specifically, in the study by Ono and colleagues of five cadavers, atrophy, demyelination, and vascular infarction involving gray and white matter, including ascending and descending long tracts, frequently occurred far removed from major sites of disc, spondylotic, or OPLL intrusions (3).

CLINICAL PRESENTATION

Patients with absolute stenosis typically present in their 40s or 50s, whereas those with relative stenosis with secondarily acquired spondyloarthrosis become symptomatic in their 60s or 70s (4–10). Males tend to outnumber females by a 2:1 ratio. Although a subset of patients may also exhibit radiculopathy alone, most present with myelopathy with or without radiculopathy once the AP diameter of the canal has been narrowed by more than 50%.

Myelopathy may be rated using different grading systems. In the United States, the Nurick Myelopathy Grading System is commonly used: grade 0—intact, grade I—mild myelopathy, grade II—mild to moderate myelopathy, grade III—moderate myelopathy, grade IV—moderate to severe myelopathy, and grade V—severe myelopathy (6–10). Alternatively, the Japanese

Orthopaedic Association (JOA) score, most typically used in Japan, assigns 17 points to both upper and lower extremity function (11,12). Most patients indicated for laminectomy with or without posterior arthrodesis present with moderate to severe myelopathy (Nurick grades III and IV). Neurologic deficits in the upper extremities often present with the so-called useless hand syndrome. This is characterized by diffuse atrophy, weakness of the hands, and loss of dexterity with often-superimposed higher or more cephalad radicular deficits (C4, C5). Proximal lower extremity weakness is most often associated with severe myelopathy; the cord changes are further confirmed by the presence of ataxia, spasticity and hyperreflexia, and bilateral Babinski responses. Accompanying sensory deficits may include numbness and loss of proprioception, impaired vibratory appreciation, and varying sensory levels. Changes in the lower extremities reflect underlying dorsal column dysfunction, characterized by a positive Romberg sign and the inability to walk in a tandem fashion. Sphincter function is compromised only late in the clinical course.

DIFFERENTIAL DIAGNOSES

Differential diagnoses for cervical myelopathy include multiple sclerosis (MS), amyotrophic lateral sclerosis (ALS), paraneoplastic syndromes, toxic-metabolic disorders (diabetes, alcoholism, vitamin B_{12} deficiency), and others (5). Studies that help differentiate between cervical myelopathy and these other entities include magnetic resonance imaging (MRI), which demonstrates demyelinating plaques in the brain in up to 85% of MS patients. Cerebrospinal fluid evaluation may demonstrate monoclonal bands with myelin-based protein and gamma globulin levels compatible with MS, whereas positive cytology may confirm the presence of a tumor. Although an electromyogram (EMG) may indicate a diagnosis of ALS or peripheral neuropathy, blood tests may identify other metabolic disorders. An additional 10% of patients presenting with lumbar stenosis have tandem cervical cord compression with myelopathy (13).

BIODYNAMICS

Flexion and Extension X-rays

Brieg and colleagues (1), along with Reed (14), evaluated how flexion and extension maneuvers alter the conformation of the cervical spinal cord and canal. In flexion, although the canal actually enlarges, increased axial tension narrows the AP diameter of the cord, deforms the lateral columns and anterior horns, and contributes to ischemia. Conversely, hyperextension narrows the spinal canal and thickens the cord with infolding of the yellow ligament, thereby reducing available space but improving cord perfusion by releasing axial tension.

Laminectomy and Varying Degrees of Facetectomy

Instability may follow laminectomy if accompanied by varying degrees of facetectomy. Raynor and associates determined how critical it was to preserve most of the facet joint (i.e., removing only the medial 25% of the facet) to maintain stability (15). They successively resected 25%, 50%, 75%, and 100% of the facet joint and capsule in a cadaveric model and showed significantly increased mobility with removal of more than 50% of the facet joint and capsule (16). The biomechanical advantages of different cervical spinal stabilization methods were also assessed in cadaveric models (17,18) and in clinical settings (19–21). Denervation of the erector spinae muscles by overdissection and traction contributes to instability as well.

NEURODIAGNOSTIC STUDIES

Plain X-rays

Plain x-rays are useful in the evaluation of the patient with cervical spinal stenosis. On a 6-foot lateral film, one may directly measure the AP diameter of the spinal canal, which normally should be about 17 mm. Other "quick" ways to assess for stenosis include observing where the posterior margin of the facet joints intersect the dorsal interlaminar line: (a) if these two lines are directly superimposed, significant canal stenosis exists; and (b) where a wide margin exists between the two lines, stenosis is usually absent. If the width of AP dimension of the canal is less than the AP dimension of the vertebra itself, stenosis may be present; if, however, the AP dimension of the canal is larger than that of the vertebral body, stenosis is likely absent. Various published ratios based on x-ray studies help confirm the presence of stenosis. Stenosis can also be confirmed not only on static but also on dynamic MRI examinations.

Lordosis, Kyphosis, Instability

Cervical alignment, the extent of lordosis, kyphosis, or presence of instability may also be visualized on static and dynamic lateral radiographs. At a minimum, a lordotic curvature of at least 10 degrees is needed to allow the cord to migrate away from ventrally situated osteophytes or OPLL (11). Instability may be defined in three parts: (a) greater than 3.5 mm of subluxation on dynamic radiographs, (b) greater than 20 degrees of angulation, and (c) greater than 4 mm of motion between the tips of the spinous processes.

Magnetic Resonance Imaging

MRI is uniquely valuable for evaluating intrinsic cord and attendant soft tissue pathology in patients with cervical spondylotic myelopathy (CSM) or myelopathy associated with OPLL, or OYL (2,22–25). The sagittal, coronal, or transaxial images readily demonstrate areas of maximal spinal cord or nerve root compression, while also revealing abnormal signals in the cord indicating the presence of demyelination, edema, or myelomalacia. On T1-weighted images, the cerebrospinal fluid (CSF) remains hypointense, whereas the vertebral bodies themselves are isointense to hyperintense, and the cord is isointense. On the T2-weighted images, CSF becomes hyperintense, therefore providing a "myelographic" effect. Another advantage of the T2-weighted images is the ability to visualize intrinsic changes within the cord, increased cord signals indicating the presence of edema, myelomalacia, demyelination, or other conditions. Additionally, increased cord signals on T2-weighted images seen in patients with CSM are poorer prognostic indicators than in patients with OPLL. Further MRI evidence of intramedullary cystic necrosis or degenerative syrinx formation, indicating irreversible cord injury, is a relative contraindication for surgery (22).

Shortcomings of MRI interpretation include the frequent underestimation of the bony abnormalities associated with spondylostenosis or OPLL. This is largely due to the hypointense appearance of the bone and the hyperintense or "positive" image, reflecting the location of fat in the bone marrow. Bony abnormalities are better identified on computer tomography (CT).

Computed Tomography

CT scans have the advantage in CSM and OPLL of directly visualizing bony structures. Sagittal, coronal, and transaxial images, along with two- and three-dimensional reconstructions, best demonstrate the extent of bony pathology. The addition of intrathecal contrast (the CT myelogram) may further facilitate detailed analysis of cord or root compression. Myelography should not be performed in patients with maximal cord compression or edema because this may lead to acute neurologic deterioration.

NONOPERATIVE MANAGEMENT OF CERVICAL STENOSIS

Nonoperative management of cervical stenosis includes the use of antiinflammatory medication (steroidal, nonsteroidal), biofeedback, orthoses (limited), epidural steroid injections (risk associated with intrathecal or intramedullary injection), and supportive care by a physiatrist. In addition, a referral to a neurology consultant or to a multimodality pain center may be indicated.

Performing surgery in asymptomatic patients with severe radiographic evidence of spondylostenosis or OPLL is controversial. For younger patients with severe cord compromise, the advantages of prophylactic surgical decompression include the avoidance of an acute cord injury and chronic neurologic deterioration; the major disadvantage is the risk for postoperative quadriplegia. Alternatively, nonoperative management may be appropriate for older patients, particularly those presenting with "fixed"

moderate to severe spastic cervical myeloradicular syndromes. Those with long-standing deficits (>6 months) and intrinsic cord changes on T2-weighted MRI studies reflecting irreversible cord damage often do not benefit from surgery.

Poor Prognostic Factors

Poor prognostic factors in patients being considered for surgery include the presence of significant medical comorbidities, which typically include age over 70 years, cardiac disease, peripheral vascular disease, obstructive pulmonary disease in heavy smokers, diabetes, stroke, hypertension, and alcoholism (9,10,26). Patients with significant prior cardiovascular abnormalities, or older individuals (>70 years) should undergo preoperative thallium stress testing to determine whether cardiac stenting or bypass is required before surgery. Other risk factors include a history of atrial fibrillation, transient ischemic attack, or stroke; mechanical valvular disease; deep venous thrombosis; and pulmonary embolism. For these conditions, patients require either antiplatelet therapy or full anticoagulation. Unfortunately, these contribute to postoperative wound hematomas or breakdown, with increased neurologic deficits if therapy is begun too soon after surgery. Individuals with a mechanical heart valve may require a "heparin window" before surgery if they are taking warfarin sodium (Coumadin). Patients with a history of deep venous thrombosis or pulmonary embolism may need a prophylactic inferior vena cava filter placed preoperatively.

PATIENT SELECTION FOR LAMINECTOMY OR LAMINOPLASTY

Cervical Lordosis and Kyphosis

To be optimal candidates for laminectomy or laminoplasty with or without arthrodesis, a patient needs to have adequate lordosis without kyphosis. Yamazaki and coworkers measured the acceptable range of lordosis and kyphosis and the AP dimension of OPLL in 38 patients undergoing laminoplasty and correlated these findings with the adequacy of cord decompression (27). Postoperatively, ventral compression was relieved in 15 patients with at least 10 degrees of lordosis and less than 7 mm of AP OPLL. For the 23 patients with residual ventral cord compression, less than 10 degrees of lordosis and greater than 7 mm of ventral OPLL was present. Similarly, when selecting patients for laminoplasty, Ishida and colleagues found that for 63 patients with CSM and 31 with OPLL, laminoplasty had to produce more than a 14-mm AP canal diameter for those with CSM; however, for those with OPLL, a 17-mm AP canal diameter was needed, and the transverse decompression had to extend across 70% of the mediolateral canal (28).

LAMINECTOMY

Anesthesia: Awake Intubation and Positioning

Patients undergoing laminectomy with or without arthrodesis usually require an awake nasoendotracheal fiberoptic intubation performed by an experienced anesthesiologist. The patient is then turned prone with a hard cervical collar in place, while still awake, and while still undergoing somatosensory evoked potential (SSEP) monitoring.

Other Adjuncts

At the time of surgery, arterial line monitoring is routinely employed along with the use of alternating compression antiembolism devices and Foley catheterization. Patients are administered 1 g of methylprednisolone at the time of induction along with prophylactic antibiotics (1 g of ceftazidime in the penicillin-nonallergic patient).

In the sitting or Concorde position, a Doppler device and a central venous catheter are used to monitor for the presence of air embolism, along with monitoring of end-tidal CO_2 levels. If an air embolism is detected, the wound is irrigated and packed, whereas the site of venous bleeding is coagulated or covered with microfibrillar collagen or Gelfoam. Valsalva maneuvers may assist in identifying bleeding sites. Only rarely is it necessary to bring the patient's head down and turn the table with the left side down to lock air in the right atrium.

Operative Positioning

Sitting Position

Cervical laminectomy may be performed in the sitting position, with the head immobilized in a Mayfield three-pin head holder. Advantages of this position include decreased bleeding and a drier operative field. Although this may not be critical when dealing with simple stenosis, foraminal disc or spur excision is greatly facilitated by use of this position. After awake intubation, patients are positioned awake, with local anesthesia injected at the three-pin sites of the Mayfield head holder. After the patient is seated for 10 minutes, having remained neurologically intact while demonstrating no SSEP changes, induction follows. Disadvantages of this position include the risk for air embolism, the requirement for a central venous catheter, and the combined risks for hypotension, stroke, and cord ischemia, particularly in older patients (29–31). Proper perfusion of the cord must be maintained.

Prone Position

Cervical laminectomy alone or laminectomy with fusion may be readily performed in the prone position. The patient is intubated and positioned awake with SSEP monitoring. The patient is then turned prone onto either bilateral chest rolls or a Wilson frame. Once prone, the three-pin head holder is applied after injecting local anesthesia (1% lidocaine with 1:200,000 epinephrine solution, 5 mL) at each pin site. The head holder is then attached to the operating room table, and the patient's SSEPs and neurologic examination are monitored until stable (5 to 10 minutes). Induction then follows.

Surgery

The laminectomy is initiated by injecting the skin and paracervical musculature with 0.5% bupivacaine with 1:200,000 epinephrine (30 mL). A midline cervical incision is made from C2 to T1 using a No. 10 blade knife, and the cautery is then used to deepen the incision. Subperiosteal dissection of the ligamentum nuchae and the paracervical muscles from the spinous processes of C3 through C7 is then completed, exposing the inferior spinous process of C2 and superior spinous process of T1. All efforts should be made to leave a bulk of the muscular attachments to these structures intact. Laterally, the dissection should be carried to the medial aspect of the facet joints, and the facet joint capsules should be preserved when laminectomy alone is being performed. Alternatively, when exposing for facet wiring or lateral mass arthrodesis techniques, the facet joints are exposed bilaterally, and the capsules are removed and later decorticated. One should avoid denervating the erector spinae muscles by intermittently releasing the retractors, especially for long procedures.

Cervical laminectomy should typically extend two levels above and two levels below the site of maximal cord compression. This degree of dissection allows for maximal dorsal cord migration away from ventrally situated osteophytes or OPLL. However, dorsal cord migration takes place only if the patient has an adequate cervical lordosis, typically a minimum of 10 degrees, or when the ventral osteophyte or OPLL mass is less than 7 mm in AP dimension.

After the initial exposure is complete, the lamina medial to the facet joints is gently scored with a 4-mm diamond bit using a lower-speed drill with a diamond burr to perforate the outer laminar cortex lightly (Figs. 76.1 and 76.2). Higher-speed drills risk rapid penetration of both the anterior and posterior cortices of the laminae, with resultant inadvertent dural or root penetration. This may be particularly true in extremely spondyloarthrotic deformed laminae in individuals in whom the yellow ligament is atretic or absent, the dura is densely adherent to the undersurface of the lamina, or the dura has become ossified in conjunction with ossification of the yellow ligament.

With the surgeon using magnified vision or microscope visualization, bilateral troughs are fashioned extending the full length of the laminectomy. To facilitate drilling, one half of the spinous processes should be removed. If bone is to be harvested for a fusion, this should be done with a small rongeur after all soft tissues have been stripped. After perforating the dorsal cortex, the inferior cortex in the lateral

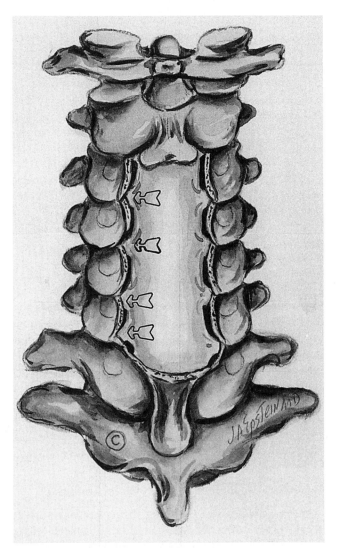

FIG. 76.1. This illustration of a cervical laminectomy includes the C3 to C7 levels, with undercutting of C2. Bilaterally, a diamond bit is used initially to create "channels" in the posterior laminar cortex, just medial to the facet joints. The remaining ventral cortex is then removed using either a diamond drill or a 2-mm Kerrison rongeur. The laminae are sequentially elevated away from the thecal sac as the ligamentum flavum is freed from either side. After laminectomy, medial facetectomy and foraminotomy may be accomplished at respective levels *(arrows)*.

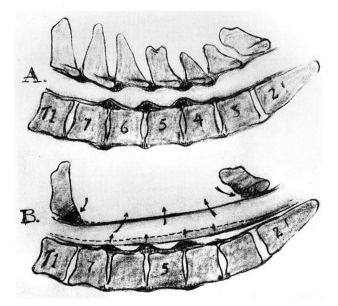

FIG. 76.2. At least 10% of the cervical lordotic curvature should be present when choosing to perform a cervical laminectomy. **A:** Additionally, ventral intrusions, particularly those associated with ossification of the posterior longitudinal ligament (OPLL), must be smaller than 7 mm in anteroposterior dimension. **B:** Laminectomy *(two large curved arrows)* should then be successful because now the thecal sac *(three large curved arrows)* migrates away from ventrally situated osteophytes *(four small arrows)*.

After the laminae have been removed, medial facetectomy and foraminotomy are accomplished bilaterally using again the rotating 2-mm Kerrison rongeur. Dissection is carried out from inferiorly (C6-C7), to superiorly (C2-C3). Great care is exercised to preserve the lateral 75% of the facet joint to avoid postoperative instability.

Nerve Roots

Nerve roots in the seated patient are typically displaced horizontally or upward, whereas in the prone position, they are directed downward. In about 30% of patients, the two roots are separate structures, the dorsal sensory nerve root being invested by a thicker white dura, the ventral root by a thinner, more grayish dura.

When significant foraminal stenosis is present, unroofing of the foramen is accomplished using an undercutting technique with a 2-mm rotating Kerrison rongeur. Adequate foraminal dissection allows for greater dorsal migration of the thecal sac away from the ventrally situated osteophytes and perineural adhesions. A sharp, undercutting curette may also be helpful in this regard. However, in most circumstances, simple foraminal decompression alone may be adequate (15,32).

After sufficient foraminal decompression, a small nerve hook may be carefully inserted parallel to the thecal sac,

gutters may now be carefully perforated using a small 4-mm diamond drill, or rotating (360-degree) 2-mm Kerrison rongeur. When the bone–yellow ligament dural margin is indistinct, the lamina is thinned, and the rongeur rather than the drill is used. After the dissection is completed bilaterally, allowing the laminae to "float," the yellow ligament is directly incised in either gutter using the rotating 2-mm Kerrison rongeur. Lifting the lamina at each segment away from the cord from caudad to cranial levels is facilitated by placing a sweetheart clamp on the residual spinous process. No instrument is placed under the lamina overlying the spinal cord.

under the superiorly exiting nerve root. In this fashion, adhesions are freed, allowing the nerve hook to be replaced by a small down-biting curette for disc or osteophyte excision. Here, the addition of EMG to SSEP monitoring may avoid injuring the exiting motor root.

If bleeding occurs during dissection, hemostatic agents, such as microfibrillar collagen (Avitene) or Gelfoam may be placed epidurally for tamponade. After adequate decompression, the dura bulges back into the decompressed site and often helps restrict bleeding from the epidural venous plexus, so long as no CSF leak is present. Next, large strips of microfibrillar collagen are placed in the lateral gutters, and a larger pledget of Gelfoam is placed centrally overlying the thecal sac. Direct hemostasis of the paraspinal muscles is followed by the placement of an epidural closed-drainage system. Once a dry sterile dressing is in place, a hard collar or cervicothoracic orthosis (CTO) is applied. The patient is transferred to a stretcher in the supine position, is immediately assessed neurologically, and is extubated if fully awake and neurologically intact. For those individuals with severe preoperative deficits, intraoperative complications, or other comorbidities precluding extubation (e.g., pulmonary disease), intubation is maintained. Postoperatively, following a laminectomy alone, a hard collar is employed for 4 to 6 weeks, whereas the patient undergoing an arthrodesis is placed in a CTO until fusion is documented, typically 3 to 5 months after surgery.

MONITORING OF CERVICAL SURGERY

Continuous Intraoperative Somatosensory Evoked Potential Monitoring

Intraoperative SSEP monitoring involves the continuous evaluation of median or ulnar and posterior tibia potentials throughout the duration of surgery (33). This entire technique is noninvasive and presents minimal to no risk to the patient. For patients undergoing laminectomy with or without attendant arthrodesis, monitoring a potential from both the upper and lower extremities is necessary because evaluation of the median or ulnar potentials alone will miss significant cord changes and may result in a higher rate of irreversible neurologic injury. Potentials are monitored using skin electrodes applied along the median or ulnar aspect of the wrist and over the posterior tibial nerve at the level of the medial malleolus of the ankle. Recordings are then made over the somatosensory cortex. Significant changes are defined by a more than 50% loss of amplitude or greater than 10% prolongation of latency. If significant changes occur, both medical (increased oxygenation, decreased inhalation or intravenous anesthetic, warming of irrigating solutions, induction of hypertension, addition of peroxide) and surgical (decrease or release of distraction, cessation of manipulation) resuscitative measures may be invoked. It is important to use microfibrillar collagen for hemostasis in the lateral gutter and to avoid placing Oxycel

or Gelfoam into confined spaces where they may expand and contribute to neurologic compromise. Additionally, when performing a cervical laminectomy in the seated position, the patient's amplitude and latency may decline significantly, although the systemic blood pressure (with the monitor at the level of the neck) appears to be normal. In these cases, a "relative hypotension is inferred," calling for the artificial induction of hypertension to 20% to 30% above baseline. In most of these cases, significant SSEP changes will resolve, and the patient will not be left with a neurologic deficit. Of interest, such relative hypotension with resultant SSEP changes may also be observed in the prone or Concorde position; similarly, responding by elevating the blood pressure in these cases serves to avoid the evolution of a permanent deficit.

Intraoperative Electromyographic Monitoring

When working in and around compromised neural foramina, whether due to attendant disc disease or spondyloarthrosis, additional monitoring with an intraoperative EMG may be useful. In instances in which a foraminal disc is being excised in conjunction with a decompressive laminectomy for stenosis, this may help indicate whether the dissection is too aggressive. Alternatively, if during the performance of a facet wiring or posterior wiring and arthrodesis there is too much tension on the wire, EMG changes may alert the surgeon to modify the procedure accordingly.

Intraoperative Motor Evoked Potential Monitoring

MEPs may also be employed intraoperatively to supplement or supplant SSEPs. Here, direct evaluation of the motor pathways facilitates ventral cord manipulation (34).

Laminoforaminotomy for Radiculopathy

Laminoforaminotomy addresses radicular complaints related to either spondylotic osteophyte formation or disc disease (9,10). The "keyhole" laminoforaminotomy may be performed alone or in conjunction with a multilevel laminectomy; its aim is focal nerve root decompression. Zeidman and Ducker evaluated 172 patients undergoing laminoforaminotomies over a 7-year period and found this to be an effective means of managing monoradicular syndromes without arthrodesis (35).

Dentate Section with Laminectomy

The dentate ligaments transmit cephalocaudal axial stresses between the spinal cord and dura but do not "tether" the cord in a specific ventral or dorsal position in the spinal canal (14). Therefore, the concept that the dentate ligaments should be resected is based on a misconception that this maneuver will allow the cord to migrate further away from ventrally situated osteophytes. Furthermore, opening up the dura to section these ligaments leads to significant intraoperative and postoperative complications (pneumocephalus, postoperative hematoma, postoperative CSF fistula, and others), while increasing the potential for postoperative adhesive arachnoiditis and meningitis.

POSTERIOR ARTHRODESIS TECHNIQUES AFTER LAMINECTOMY

Patients undergoing laminectomy and arthrodesis for instability may be successfully managed using different facet arthrodesis techniques (13,36–38). Braided titanium cables employed for facet wiring lead to successful facet fusion 96% of the time, with limited morbidity (21,39–41) (Fig. 76.3). Ninety percent of patients studied by Maurer and col-

leagues underwent successful fusion by use of a posterior Luque rectangle facet arthrodesis technique (37). Fusion rates for lateral mass plates employing bicortical screw fixation approached 100% in some series, with limited morbidity (6.1% screw malposition or pullout, 1.8% frequency of nerve root injury) and lateral mass fractures (18,36,41–43). Alternatively, using lateral mass plates with pedicle screw fixation, 83% of Abumi and Kaneda's 26 patients undergoing laminectomy had fusion without kyphosis (36). Miyazaki and colleagues documented fusion in 79% of 46 patients undergoing noninstrumented facet arthrodesis after laminectomy (38).

Facet Wiring and Fusion Technique

For patients who demonstrate significant spinal instability at single or multiple levels, bilateral facet wiring and arthrodesis may be appropriate (Fig. 76.3). Hamanishi and Tanaka evaluated 69 patients with CSM, 34 of whom also had posterolateral arthrodesis for focal instability and found that clinical outcomes (an average of 3.5 years later) were comparable for both groups, including those undergoing additional arthrodesis (11). Wiring of the facet joints requires removing the articular cartilage of each facet joint, resecting about one fourth to one third of the superior articular facet, and carefully preserving the inferior articular facet and its cortical rim. A 2- to 3-mm dental right-angle burr is then employed to make a hole in the exposed inferior articular process. Next, the smooth end of a braided titanium cable is passed through the hole in the inferior articular facet into the superior facet defect, then pulled outward with an empty needle holder. It is necessary to push and pull the wire slowly through the hole, rather than pulling upward, because the latter maneuver allows the wire to escape through the inferior articular facet. With this technique, wires are passed cephalad to caudad on each side of the laminectomy defect. A continuous wire technique or second technique employing separate wire fixation of each inferior articular facet to a fibula strut structural allograft may be employed for multilevel fixation. In both circumstances, the wires are hand-tightened and individually crimped.

Arthrodesis with Facet Wiring and Allograft Fibula

Facet wiring using allograft fibula requires that a separate wire be passed through each inferior articular facet. It is then passed through a fibula allograft strut, which has been split and perforated with the dental drill (10). On each side, the braided cable through each facet is then hand-tightened and crimped after decorticating the underlying facet joints. Autogenous bone from the removed laminae is then covered with inductive-conductive matrix (non-water-soluble and impregnated with 70% cancellous and 30% cortical bone).

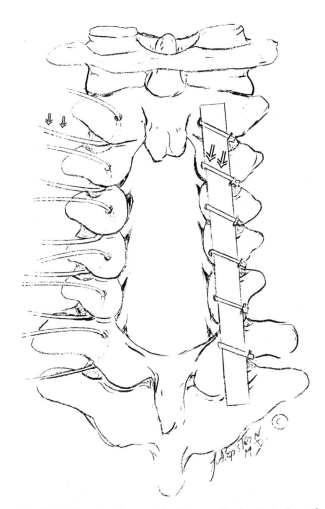

FIG. 76.3. Facet wiring and fusion to a fibula strut allograft. After laminectomy, a dental drill is used to perforate each inferior articular facet *(small arrows)*. A braided titanium cable is passed through each hole *(small arrows)* and again through holes placed in a split fibula strut allograft; wires are then sequentially tightened *(large arrows)*. In this type of facet wiring and fusion, the facet joint capsule is removed along with a portion of the superior articular facet adjacent to the joint to facilitate wire passage.

Arthrodesis with Lateral Mass Plates

Bicortical lateral mass plating systems has long been available, and now, some systems are introducing unicortical rod-screw design. Evaluating the long-term efficacy of cervical laminectomy supplemented with posterior lateral mass plates for the management of CSM, Kumar and associates studied 25 patients over a 2-year period (44). Using the SF-36 patient-based outcome questionnaire, they determined that 80% of patients experienced good outcomes and 76% demonstrated improvement in myelopathy scores. Eight percent had complications directly related to the surgery.

Although the bilateral fixation afforded by these plates limits flexion, extension, and rotation when compared with the use of wire, complications can occur. Heller and associates reported complications after the application of lateral mass screws and plates in 78 patients followed for more than 2 years (43). Of 654 screws placed (average, 8.4 screws per patient), complications included nerve root injury in 0.6%, facet violation in 0.2%, broken screws in 0.3%, screw avulsion in 0.2%, and screw loosening in 1.1%. Other complications included cord injury (2.6%), iatrogenic foraminal stenosis (2.6%), broken plates (1.3%), loss of reduction (2.6%), adjacent segment degeneration (3.8%), infection (1.3%), and pseudarthrosis (1.4%). Recently, Wellman and co-workers observed no complications after placement of 281 screws in 43 patients followed an average of 25 months (45).

Pedicle Screw Fixation Technique Using Lateral Mass Plates or Rods

Lateral mass pedicle screw fixation techniques offer another alternative for arthrodesis after laminectomy (36,46). Abumi and associates employed a one-stage posterior decompression and reconstructive technique in 46 patients (46). In 190 screw insertions, 5.3% perforated the cortex of the pedicles, indicating the risk posed by this technique to neurovascular structures.

Complications of Laminectomy with or without Arthrodesis

The prevalence of cord injury resulting from laminectomy varies from 0% to 3%, whereas the frequency of root injury can be as high as 15% (26,47). Cord damage is most frequently due to the inadvertent introduction of an instrument under the central lamina, which is why lateral entry into the spinal canal is recommended. Most cord injuries, however, are more likely vascular and ischemic in etiology, owing to intraoperative hypotension or overdistraction.

Radiculopathy after Cervical Laminectomy

Postoperative motor root deficits, particularly involving the C5 distribution, have more frequently been reported after dorsal than anterior decompression of the cervical spinal canal. Root injuries are variously attributed not only to direct manipulation and lateral dissection but also to root traction associated with spontaneous migration after cord decompression (26). Dai and associates followed 287 consecutive patients after multilevel laminectomy and observed a 12.9% rate (37 patients) of postoperative new radicular deficits (48). Radiculopathy, typically involving the C5 or C6 motor distributions, developed within 4 hours to 6 days after surgery. Note that these are the most mobile segments of the cervical spine. The average time for recovery of function was 5.4 months, varying from 2 weeks to 3 years, with enhanced recovery in spondylotic patients compared with those with OPLL.

OUTCOMES

Outcomes after Laminectomy

Adequate postoperative outcomes have been observed after laminectomy for multilevel cervical spondylosis or OPLL in older patients (>65 years of age) with an adequately preserved lordotic or hyperlordotic curvature (Figs. 76.4 to 76.8). After laminectomy with foraminotomy in 90 patients, Snow and Weiner observed that 77% of patients improved, 13% remained unchanged, and 10% deteriorated (none in the immediate postoperative period) (49). Kato and colleagues observed a 23% prevalence of delayed deterioration after laminectomy performed in 44 patients with OPLL, who had been followed for an average of 14 years (50). The original neurologic recovery rate of 44%, observed 1 year after surgery, was 43% 5 years after surgery. Significant worsening occurred between postoperative years 5 and 10 when the recovery rate deteriorated to 33%. Multivariate analysis of risk factors indicated that poor preoperative prognostic factors included advanced age at the initial surgery (>70 years of age), dense initial myelopathy, and a history of new trauma. Although deterioration was initially attributed to OPLL progression observed in 70% of patients, it was actually responsible for increased neurologic dysfunction in only one individual. Evidence of progressive kyphosis serves as a relative contraindication to performing these procedures (Fig. 76.9).

Outcomes after Laminectomy for Central Cord Syndromes

The efficacy of delayed laminectomy for the management of patients presenting with central cord syndromes remains controversial. Levi and associates evaluated 20 patients, averaging 54 years of age, undergoing laminectomy delayed by an average of 17 days (until plateauing occurred) for central cord injury (51). Patients had C2 to C7 laminectomies and were followed an average of 28 months. Three months after injury, 12 patients

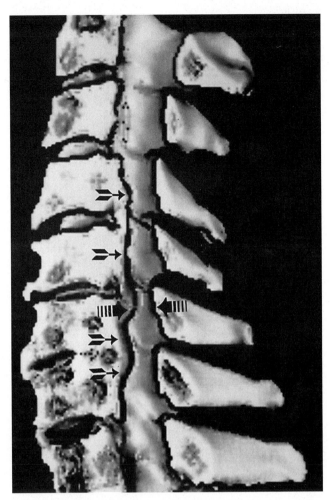

FIG. 76.4. On this slightly paramedian sagittal three-dimensional computed tomography study, the patient exhibited 10 degrees of residual lordosis, congenital stenosis (anteroposterior diameter < 10 mm), maximal at the C5-C6 level *(large double arrows),* and continuous C4 to C7 ossification of the posterior longitudinal ligament (OPLL; *multiple arrows*).

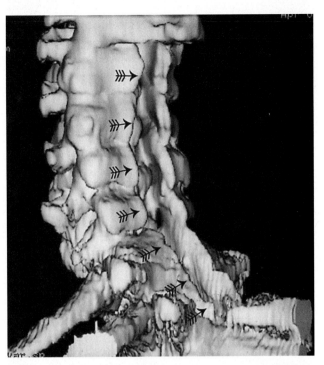

FIG. 76.5. Cervical laminectomy *(arrows)* with medial facetectomy and foraminotomy on this dorsal-oblique three-dimensional computed tomography scan, obtained 3 months postoperatively, provided adequate decompression.

had improved, 7 remained unchanged, and one worsened. MR studies were repeated postoperatively, attempting to correlate the degree of cord decompression with the extent of neurologic recovery. The two did not correlate, however, because despite adequate cord decompression in 12 patients, only 8 exhibited significant recovery of function.

Outcomes after Laminoplasty

Laminoplasty is an alternative to laminectomy. Its theoretical advantages include a reduction of postlaminectomy complications, including instability (12). Kohno and associates performed a 5-year follow-up study on 22 patients undergoing LOP for CSM, OPLL, or both (52). Postoperative improvement was observed in 18 of the 22 patients.

Poor prognostic factors included high intrinsic cord signals on T2-weighted MRI with underlying cord atrophy, long symptom duration, age over 70 years, worsening secondary to trauma, severe cord compression, radiculopathy, and kyphosis. Poor candidates for laminoplasty included those with MRI evidence of irreversible cord damage. Lee, Manzano, and Green concluded that poor prognostic factors in 25 patients undergoing expansive cervical laminoplasty included a recent history of trauma, age over 60 years, long duration of symptoms (18 months), preoperative sphincteric dysfunction, and lower extremity dysfunction (53).

Outcomes after Laminectomy or Laminoplasty for Ossification of the Posterior Longitudinal Ligament

More rapid progression of OPLL after dorsal spinal decompression has been variously reported. Specifically, Takatsu and associates observed the accelerated progression of OPLL after laminoplasty (25 patients) and laminectomy (16 patients) compared with those managed conservatively (56 patients) (54).

Lesser degrees of neurologic recovery were reported after laminectomy or laminoplasty than after anterior surgery for OPLL. In two series in which up to 25% of North Americans had myelopathy attributed to OPLL, those undergoing

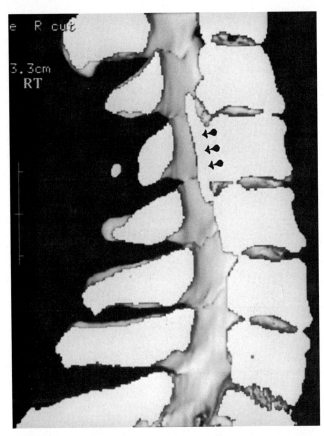

FIG. 76.6. Parasagittal three-dimensional computed tomography scan of cervical stenosis in a patient demonstrating adequate preservation of the cervical lordosis with less than 7 mm of ossification of the posterior longitudinal ligament (OPLL) extending into the canal from the C3-C4 through C4-C5 levels *(multiple arrows)*, managed with cervical laminectomy.

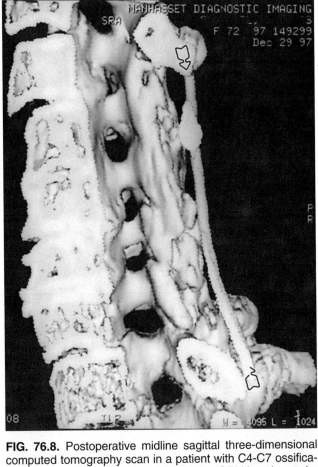

FIG. 76.8. Postoperative midline sagittal three-dimensional computed tomography scan in a patient with C4-C7 ossification of the posterior longitudinal ligament (OPLL) and spondylostenosis, where posterior facet wiring *(arrows)* and fusion helped maintain the lordotic curvature.

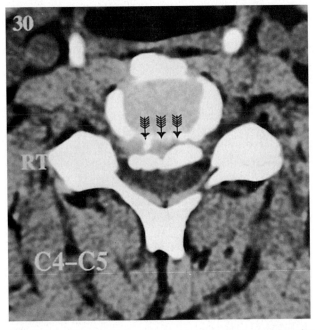

FIG. 76.7. Transaxial noncontrast computed tomography scan obtained in the same patient as in Fig. 76.6 with less than 7 mm of anterior intrusion resulting from ossification of the posterior longitudinal ligament (OPLL) at the C4-C5 level *(arrows)*. Laminectomy with facet fusion provided adequate decompression while inhibiting anticipated accelerated postlaminectomy OPLL regrowth.

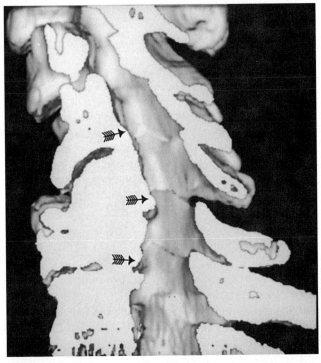

FIG. 76.9. Severely kyphotic *(arrows)* patients were not candidates for laminectomy.

anterior discectomy or corpectomy with arthrodesis demonstrated better neurologic recovery than those having laminectomy. Better outcomes after anterior procedures were obtained in 41 patients, as compared with 10 undergoing laminectomy (6–8). Kawano and colleagues similarly observed better outcomes in 75 patients presenting with OPLL managed with anterior corpectomy and arthrodesis (14 patients) with 78% improvement, compared with laminoplasty or laminectomy (61 patients) with 46% improvement (55). Long-term recoveries were better for those who had anterior operations, whereas those undergoing dorsal decompressions exhibited further more rapid deterioration. Banerji and co-workers also reported the benefits of multilevel anterior rather than posterior surgery in patients with OPLL (4).

Outcomes after Laminectomy or Laminoplasty for Cervical Spondylotic Myelopathy

Ebersold, Pare, and Quast studied long-term outcomes after anterior decompression and arthrodesis (49 patients) and laminectomy (51 patients) surgery for CSM (56). Of those managed anteriorly, 72% improved, whereas 68% treated posteriorly improved. In the anterior group, 12% required secondary posterior procedures, whereas 14% of those having initial posterior surgery required additional anterior surgery. One (2%) patient showed early deterioration in the anterior group, compared with 5 (10%) in the posterior group. Late deterioration (average follow-up, 7.35 years) occurred in 6 patients in the anterior group, whereas 18 of 33 remained improved, and 9 were unchanged. For the 51 laminectomy patients, 19 improved, 13 were unchanged, and 19 deteriorated. The data from this series indicate that the risk for acute postoperative deterioration, as well as long-term worsening, is greatest for those undergoing laminectomy compared with anterior surgery. Nevertheless, for those patients identified with adequate lordotic curvatures attended by preoperative evidence of frank instability on flexion-extension x-rays, adequate results may be achieved by performing laminectomy with simultaneous facet wiring and arthrodesis (Figs. 76.10 to 76.18).

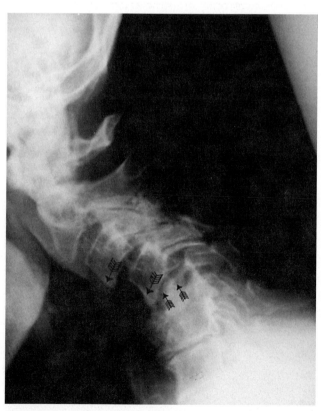

FIG. 76.10. Acquired spinal stenosis and instability were demonstrated at the C3-C4 (active grade II olisthy) and C4-C5 levels (active grade I olisthy) *(arrows)* on this lateral flexion radiograph.

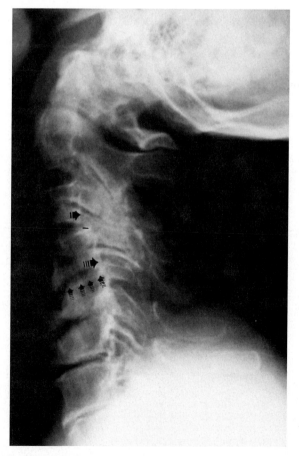

FIG. 76.11. Both C3-C4 and C4-C5 subluxation (shown in Fig. 76.10) adequately reduced *(arrows)* on this lateral extension radiograph.

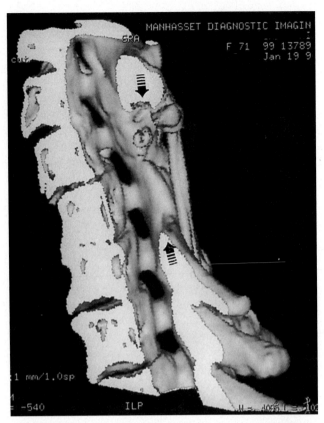

FIG. 76.12. The midline three-dimensional computed tomography scan shows that the cervical alignment was adequately corrected after a C3-C5 cervical laminectomy with facet wiring and fusion *(arrows)* performed to maintain the patient (shown in Figs. 76.10 and 76.11) in extension.

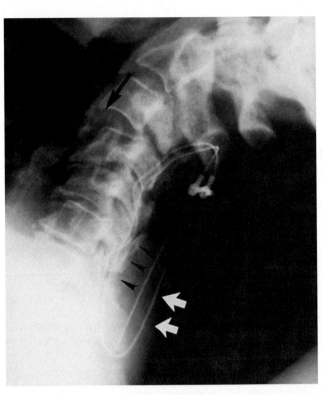

FIG. 76.14. Lateral extension radiograph confirming stabilization of olisthy at C3-C4, where spontaneous bony bridging occurred *(large black arrow)* after braided titanium cable *(multiple white arrows)* spinous process (C2, C7) and facet wiring and fusion (C3 to C6) *(multiple black arrows)* demonstrating stabilization.

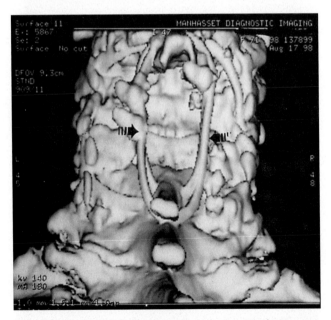

FIG. 76.13. Dorsal three-dimensional computed tomography view demonstrating the C3-C5 laminectomy defect with fusion of bilateral facet joints *(arrows)* following posterior wiring and facet fusion (see Figs. 76.10 to 76.12).

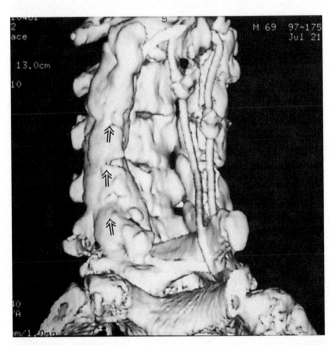

FIG. 76.15. Postoperative three-dimensional computed tomography scan 6 months later confirms adequate bilateral facet fusion *(arrows)* after a C3-C6 laminectomy with facet wiring and fusion.

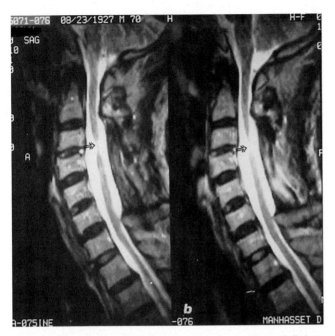

FIG. 76.16. Magnetic resonance imaging with gadolinium DTPA study obtained 6 months after C3 to C6 laminectomy with facet wiring and fusion demonstrates complete cord decompression as well as atrophy within the laminectomy site *(arrow)*.

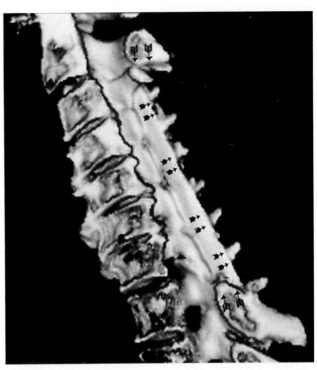

FIG. 76.18. Stabilization of kyphosis (Fig. 76.17) demonstrated on parasagittal three-dimensional computed tomography scan obtained 4 months after a C3 to C7 laminectomy *(two sets of arrows)* with facet wiring and fusion using a fibula strut allograft and braided titanium cables *(multiple arrows)*.

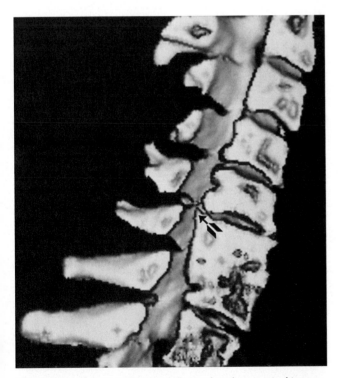

FIG. 76.17. Parasagittal three-dimensional computed tomography study demonstrating cervical spondylostenosis associated with mild kyphosis *(arrow)*.

REFERENCES

1. Brieg A, Turnbull I, Hassler O. Effects of mechanical stresses on the spinal cord in cervical spondylosis: a study of fresh cadaver material. *J Neurosurg* 1966;25:45–48.
2. Epstein JA, Epstein NE. The surgical management of cervical spinal stenosis, spondylosis, and myeloradiculopathy by means of the posterior approach. In: The Cervical Spine Research Society Editorial Committee, ed. *The cervical spine*, 2nd ed. Philadelphia: JB Lippincott, 1989:625–643.
3. Ono K, Ikata T, Yamada H, et al. Cervical myelopathy secondary to multiple spondylotic protrusions. *Spine* 1977;2:218–221.
4. Banerji D, Acharya R, Behari S, et al. Corpectomy for multi-level cervical spondylosis and ossification of the posterior longitudinal ligament. *Neurosurg Rev (Germany)* 1997;20(1):25–31.
5. Epstein NE. Ossification of the posterior longitudinal ligament: Diagnosis and surgical management. *Neurosurg Q* 1992;2:223–241.
6. Epstein N. The surgical management of ossification of the posterior longitudinal ligament in 51 patients. *J Spinal Disord* 1993;6(5):432–454.
7. Epstein NE. The surgical management of ossification of the posterior longitudinal ligament in 43 North Americans. *Spine* 1994;19(6):664–672.
8. Epstein NE. Advanced cervical spondylosis with ossification into the posterior longitudinal ligament and resultant neurological sequelae. *J Spinal Disord* 1996;9(6):477–484.
9. Epstein NE. Circumferential surgery for the management of cervical ossification of the posterior longitudinal ligament. *J Spinal Disord* 1998;11(3):200–207.
10. Epstein NE. The value of anterior cervical plating in preventing vertebral fracture and graft extrusion following multilevel anterior cervical corpectomy with posterior wiring/fusion: indications, results, and complications. *J Spinal Disord* 2000;13:9–15.

11. Hamanishi C, Tanaka S. Bilateral multilevel laminectomy with or without posterolateral fusion for cervical spondylotic myelopathy: relationship to type of onset and time until operation. *J Neurosurg* 1996;85(3):447–451.

12. Hirabayashi K, Bohlman H. Multilevel cervical spondylosis. Laminoplasty versus anterior decompression. *Spine* 1995;10(15): 1732–1734.

13. Epstein NE, Epstein JA, Carras R, et al. Coexisting cervical and lumbar stenosis: diagnosis and management. *Neurosurgery* 1984;15:489–496.

14. Reed JD. Effects of flexion-extension movements of the head and spine upon the spinal cord and nerve roots. *J Neurol Neurosurg Psychiatry* 1960;23:214–216.

15. Raynor RB, Pugh J, Shapiro I. Cervical facetectomy and its effect on spine strength. *J Neurosurg* 1985;63:278–282.

16. Zdeblick TA, Zou D, Warden KE, et al. Cervical stability after foraminotomy. A biomechanical in vitro analysis. *J Bone Joint Surg* 1992;74(1):22–27.

17. Coe JD, Warden KE, Sutterlin CE 3rd, et al. Biomechanical evaluation of cervical spinal stabilization methods in human cadaveric model. *Spine* 1989;14(10):1122–1131.

18. Grubb MR, Currier BL, Stone J, et al. Biomechanical evaluation of posterior cervical stabilization after a wide laminectomy. *Spine* 1997;22(17):1948–1954.

19. Cooper PR. Posterior stabilization of the cervical spine. *Clin Neurosurg* 1993;40:286–320.

20. Graham AW, Swank ML, Kinard RE, et al. Posterior cervical arthrodesis and stabilization with a lateral mass plate. Clinical and computed tomographic evaluation of lateral mass screw placement and associated complications. *Spine* 1996;12(3):323–328.

21. Lovely TJ, Carl A. Posterior cervical spine fusion with tension-band wiring. *J Neurosurg* 1995;83(4):631–635.

22. Al-Mefty O, Harkey LH, Middleton TH, et al. Myelopathic cervical spondylotic lesions demonstrated by magnetic resonance imaging. *J Neurosurg* 1988;68:217–222.

23. Burgerman R, Rigamonti D, Randle JM, et al. The association of cervical spondylosis and multiple sclerosis. *Surg Neurol* 1992;38:265–270.

24. Matsuda Y, Miyazaki K, Tada K, et al. Increased MR signal intensity due to cervical myelopathy. Analysis of 29 surgical cases. *J Neurosurg* 1991;74:887–892.

25. Okada Y, Ikata T, Yamada H, et al. Magnetic resonance imaging study on the results of surgery for cervical compressive myelopathy. *Spine* 1993;18:2024–2029.

26. Saunders RL, Pikus HJ, Ball P. Four-level cervical corpectomy. *Spine* 1998;23(33):2455–2461.

27. Yamazaki A, Homma T, Uchiyama S, et al. Morphologic limitation of posterior decompression by midsagittal splitting method for myelopathy caused by ossification of the posterior longitudinal ligament in the cervical spine. *Spine* 1999;24(1):32–34.

28. Ishida Y, Ohmori K, Suzuki K, et al. Analysis of dural configuration for evaluation of posterior decompression in cervical myelopathy. *Neurosurgery* 1999;44(1):91–95.

29. Albin MS, Carroll RG, Maroon JC. Clinical considerations concerning detection of venous air embolism. *Neurosurgery* 1978;3:380–384.

30. Matjasko J, Petrozza P, Cohen M, et al. Anesthesia and surgery in the seated position: analysis of 554 cases. *Neurosurgery* 1985;17:695–702.

31. Standefer M, Bay JW, Trusso R. The sitting position in neurosurgery: a retrospective analysis of 488 cases. *Neurosurgery* 1984;14:649–658.

32. Henderson CM, Henessey RG, Shuey HM, et al. Posterior lateral foraminotomy as an exclusive operative technique for cervical radiculopathy. A review of 846 consecutively operated cases. *Neurosurgery* 1983;13:504–512.

33. Epstein NE, Danto J, Nardi D. Somatosensory evoked potential monitoring during 100 cervical operations. *Spine* 1993;18:737–747.

34. Maertens de Noodhout A, Remacle JM, Pepin JL, et al. Magnetic stimulation of the ventral motor cortex in cervical spondylosis. *Neurology* 1991;41:75–80.

35. Zeidman SM, Ducker TB. Posterior cervical laminoforaminotomy for radiculopathy: review of 172 cases. *Neurosurgery* 1993;33(3):356–362.

36. Abumi K, Kaneda K. Pedicle screw fixation for non-traumatic lesions of the cervical spine. *Spine* 1997;22(16):1853–1863.

37. Maurer PK, Ellenbogen RG, Ecklund J, et al. Cervical spondylotic myelopathy: treatment with posterior decompression and Luque rectangle bone fusion. *Neurosurgery (US)* 1991;28(5):680–683.

38. Miyazaki K, Tada K, Matsuda Y, et al. Posterior extensive simultaneous multisegment decompression with posterolateral fusion for cervical myelopathy with cervical instability and kyphotic and/or S-shaped deformities. *Spine* 1989;14(11):1160–1170.

39. Brodsky AE, Khalil MA, Sassard WR, et al. Repair of symptomatic pseudarthrosis of anterior cervical fusion. Posterior versus anterior repair. *Spine* 1992;17(10):137–143.

40. Weiland DJ, McAfee PC. Posterior cervical fusion with triple-write strut graft techniques; one hundred consecutive patients. *J Spinal Disord* 1991;4(10):15–21.

41. Weiss JC, Cunningham BW, Kanayama M, et al. In vitro biomechanical comparison of multistrand cables with conventional cervical stabilization. *Spine* 1996;21(18):2108–2114.

42. Ebraheim NA, Rupp RE, Salvolaine ER, et al. Posterior plating of the cervical spine. *J Spinal Disord* 1995;8(2):111–115.

43. Heller JG, Silcox DH 3rd, Sutterline CE 3rd. Complications of posterior cervical plating. *Spine* 1995;20(22):2442–2248.

44. Kumar VG, Rea GL, Mervis LJ, et al. Cervical spondylotic myelopathy: functional and radiographic long-term outcome after laminectomy and posterior fusion. *Neurosurgery* 1999;44(4):771–777.

45. Wellman BJ, Follett KA, Traynelis VC. Complications of posterior articular mass plate fixation of the subaxial cervical spine in 43 consecutive patients. *Spine* 1998;23(2):193–200.

46. Abumi K, Kaneda K, Shono Y, et al. One-stage posterior decompression and reconstruction of the cervical spine by using pedicle screw fixation systems. *J Neurosurg* 1999;90[1 Suppl]:19–26.

47. Yonenobu K, Hosono N, Iwasaki M, et al. Neurologic complications of surgery for cervical compression myelopathy. *Spine* 1991;16(11): 1277–1282.

48. Dai L, Ni B, Yuan W, et al. Radiculopathy after laminectomy for cervical compression myelopathy. *J Bone Joint Surg Br* 1998;80(5):846–849.

49. Snow RB, Weiner H. Cervical laminectomy and foraminotomy as surgical treatment of cervical spondylosis: a follow-up study with analysis of failures. *J Spinal Disord* 1993;6(3):245–250.

50. Kato Y, Iwasaki M, Fuji T, et al. Long-term follow-up results of laminectomy for cervical myelopathy caused by ossification of the posterior longitudinal ligament. *J Neurosurg* 1998;89(2):217–223.

51. Levi L, Wolf A, Mirvis S, et al. The significance of dorsal migration of the cord after extensive cervical laminectomy for patients with traumatic central cord syndrome. *J Spinal Disord* 1995;8(4):289–295.

52. Kohno K, Kumon Y, Oka Y, et al. Evaluation of prognostic factors following expansive laminoplasty for cervical spinal stenotic myelopathy. *Surg Neurol* 1997;48(3):237–245.

53. Lee TT, Manzano GR, Green BA. Modified open-door cervical expansive laminoplasty for spondylotic myelopathy: operative technique, outcome, and predictors for gait improvement. *J Neurosurg* 1997;86 (1):64–68.

54. Takatsu T, Ishida Y, Suzuki K, et al. Radiological study of cervical ossification of the posterior longitudinal ligament. *J Spinal Disord* 1999;12(3):271–273.

55. Kawano H, Hand Y, Ishii H, et al. Surgical treatment for ossification of the posterior longitudinal ligament of the cervical spine. *J Spinal Disord* 1995;8(2):145–150.

56. Ebersold MJ, Pare MC, Quast LM. Surgical treatment for cervical spondylotic myelopathy. *J Neurosurg* 1995;82(5):745–751.

Part B
Laminoplasty

Kazuo Yonenobu, Eiji Wada, and Keiro Ono

The posterior approach to the cervical spine was the primary method of access to the spinal canal until the anterior approach was developed by Robinson and Smith (1) and Cloward (2). Posterior decompression was performed by removing the spinous processes, laminae, and articular processes. With the accumulation of experience in posterior decompression for CSM, successful laminectomy was possible only when a lordotic alignment of the cervical spine, wide and extensive decompression for adequate posterior shift of the spinal cord (3), and stability of the spine (4,5) were achieved. Thick fibrous tissue formation secondary to a hematoma after laminectomy occasionally led to an unfavorable outcome.

The insertion of surgical instruments such as a Kerrison rongeur or a curette into the spinal canal without awareness of the degree of canal stenosis, or uneven decompression of the spinal cord during resection of the laminae, can impinge or distort the spinal cord and result in deterioration of neurologic function. Several investigators have indicated that there is a hazard of postoperative loss of neural function after surgical intervention (6–8).

Because of the poor results of conventional laminectomy for cervical compressive myelopathy, Kirita and Miyazaki developed an extensive simultaneous multisegment decompression laminectomy to avoid distortion of the spinal cord by the edges of the resected laminae (9,10).

Oyama and colleagues (11) devised an expansive Z-shaped laminoplasty in which a posterior wall of the spinal canal was preserved by Z plasty of the thinned laminae. They thus attempted to prevent the invasion of scar tissue, that is, the so-called laminectomy membrane, which was believed to be a cause of late neurologic regression. They also anticipated that the laminae reconstructed by Z plasty would provide support for the spine. The introduction of a high-speed air drill allowed the successful development of this procedure.

In 1977, Hirabayashi and colleagues (12) introduced an epoch-making laminoplasty, the expansive open-door laminoplasty. They described the advantages of this procedure: multiple levels of the spinal cord can be decompressed simultaneously, better postoperative stability of the neck allows earlier mobilization of the patients, postoperative kyphotic deformity of the cervical spine can be prevented, and mobility of the cervical spine is reduced

postoperatively, which helps to prevent late neurologic deterioration as well as the progression of OPLL.

After the introduction of the laminoplasty of Hirabayashi, various modifications and supplementary procedures have been devised for further improvement of safety and efficacy of decompression and for stability of the spine.

AIMS, ADVANTAGES, AND DISADVANTAGES OF LAMINOPLASTY

The aims of the laminoplasty are to expand the spinal canal, to secure spinal stability, and to preserve the protective function of the spine. Preservation of mobility of the spine is also a goal of this procedure for multiple-level involvement.

The maximum expansion of the canal is obtained at its central part in the bilateral hinge type of laminoplasty and at its opening side in the unilateral hinge type. Posterior migration of the spinal cord after both types of laminoplasty has been confirmed using CT myelography (13,14). Sodeyama and associates reported the spinal cord moved a mean of 3 mm (0 to 6.6 mm) posteriorly at the C5 or C6 level. In the unilateral hinge type, decompression can be extended along the nerve root on the opening side by partial facetectomy.

Preservation of the posterior spinal structures permits reinsertion of the nuchal muscles and the spinal ligaments after they have been completely or partially detached. This prevents kyphosis or listhesis of the cervical spine, which often develops after laminectomy, particularly in subjects younger than 50 years of age. Reattaching muscles or ligaments to the spinous processes after the laminoplasty may improve the dynamic stability of the spine.

The development of kyphosis and a thick peridural scar subsequent to laminectomy is a notorious cause of late neurologic worsening. The spared laminae preserve the protective function of the spine, shielding the spinal cord from the pressure of hematoma during the early postoperative period and preventing the invasion of scar tissue in the late convalescent period.

Advantages of laminoplasty include that the spinal cord can be decompressed without the removal of spondylotic protrusions impinging on the neural tissue. Removal of osteocartilaginous protrusions encroaching on the already compromised neural tissue is the most hazardous portion of the procedure when surgeons use the anterior approach to CSM. A second advantage is that laminoplasty facilitates obtaining hemostasis around the affected spinal cord. Anterior surgery for CSM and OPLL often demands more careful and meticulous procedures for hemostasis. These procedures may threaten the spinal cord or the nerve root, which is already distressed. A third advantage is that laminoplasty allows additional procedures for nerve root decompression or reinforcement of spinal stability. Partial facetectomy for nerve root decompression is optional except for the facets on the hinge side of the laminae. Bone graft for stabilization in either single or multiple segments is easily applicable.

There are two disadvantages of laminoplasty. First, the range of motion (ROM) of the cervical spine is reduced, particularly in extension, lateral bending, and rotation. This becomes more marked when laminotomy or hinges are located at the facet in either expansive open-door laminoplasty or spinous process–splitting laminoplasty. Second, discomfort of the neck may result after laminoplasty. This is one of the most discouraging problems. Not placing a gutter for the hinge directly at the facet, avoiding too much muscle detachment during surgery, and encouraging mobilization of the neck as early as possible are all believed to lessen the postoperative discomfort (15).

INDICATIONS AND CONTRAINDICATIONS FOR LAMINOPLASTY

Generally, laminoplasty can be indicated for myelopathy secondary to developmental spinal canal stenosis (AP canal diameter < 13 mm), continuous or mixed type of OPLL, multisegmental spondylosis associated with a narrow spinal canal, and the distal type of cervical spondylotic amyotrophy (16) with canal stenosis.

Laminoplasty should be considered first for patients who have multisegmental spondylotic myelopathy with a relatively narrow spinal canal (AP canal diameter of 13 to 14 mm) (17). When this condition is associated with spinal instability, laminoplasty should be supplemented by spinal arthrodesis.

For one- or two-level spondylosis without developmental spinal canal stenosis, anterior discectomy and arthrodesis is the treatment of choice. Anterior removal of the segmental type of OPLL is more radical than posterior decompression, as well as very technically demanding.

In cervical disc herniation, the consensus has been that anterior discectomy and spinal fusion (ASF) is preferred for one or two vertebral segments. However, for patients with narrowed spinal canals (<13 mm), laminoplasty has had favorable results because it avoids adjacent segment degeneration and bone graft complications. Resorption of herniated disc fragments has been confirmed in follow-up MRI studies (18,19).

Spinal cord tumors can also be extirpated by laminoplasty in combination with ultrasonic suction. For younger patients, laminoplasty should be borne in mind. Laminoplasty is preferable to laminectomy because of the lower

risk for postoperative kyphosis and instability. Laminoplasty with stabilization (arthrodesis) has been widely indicated for myelopathy secondary to multilevel subaxial subluxation in patients with rheumatoid arthritis (RA).

At present, no type of laminoplasty can correct a fixed kyphotic deformity to a lordotic curve. Accordingly, a kyphotic cervical spine is a contraindication for laminoplasty. However, laminoplasty, combined with a formal arthrodesis procedure, can be indicated for myelo(radiculo)-pathy secondary to multisegmental spondylosis associated with athetoid cerebral palsy provided that the athetoid movements of the neck can be adequately controlled with a halo vest in the postoperative period.

The age of the patient does not place a limit on laminoplasty because the invasiveness of the procedure is similar to that of laminectomy. Laminoplasty is beneficial, even in patients older than 75 years of age, in improving neurologic function and ability to engage in activities of daily living (20). The average operating time in our series was 2.1 hours, and the average blood loss was 225 mg. Hirabayashi reported an average operating time of 2 hours and an average blood loss of 362 mL, respectively (21).

TECHNIQUES OF LAMINOPLASTY AND SUPPLEMENTARY PROCEDURES

The basic concept of each surgical procedure is similar to that of the expansive open-door laminoplasty already described. Therefore, this procedure is described in more detail. Further details of other procedures should be obtained from the original articles (21–26). No procedure has been proved statistically superior to any others with regard to the neurologic and radiographic results.

The patient is placed in the prone position on a laminectomy frame to decrease the abdominal pressure. A three-point pin fixation device such as Mayfield tongs is strongly recommended to secure the head and maintain cervical alignment in the neutral position or in slight extension. When spinal arthrodesis is required, the cervical spine is adjusted to its proper alignment after laminoplasty.

Through a posterior midline incision, the nuchal ligament is divided at the midline. Typically, in CSM, the extent of decompression is from C3 to C7 for complete posterior migration of the spinal cord. Decompression should also be wide enough for the spinal cord to migrate posteriorly. However, surgeons differ regarding placement of the laminotomy for the opening and the gutter for the hinge. Both of these factors are believed to be related closely to the nature and prevalence of the complications of this procedure.

Unilateral Hinge Laminoplasty

Expansive Open-Door Laminoplasty of Hirabayashi

The spinous processes are exposed from C2 to T1, with care taken not to damage the supraspinous and interspinous ligaments (21) (Fig. 76.19). A gutter is then created at the

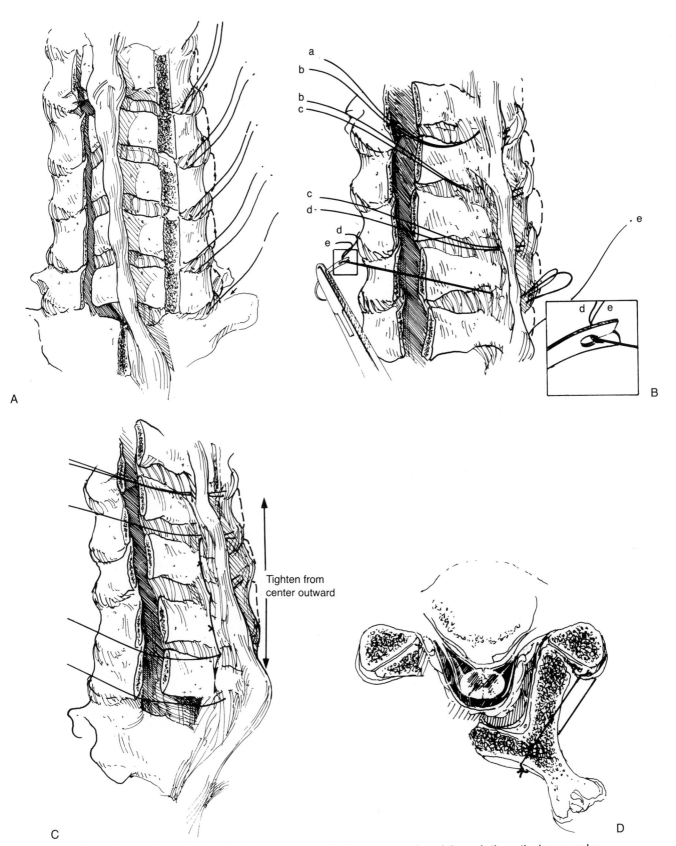

FIG. 76.19. Expansive open-door laminoplasty. **A:** Sutures are placed through the articular capsules and surrounding soft tissues on the hinge side. **B:** Both ends of the suture placed through the capsules are pulled out through the superior and inferior interspinous ligaments to the open side. **C:** The threads are ligated to prevent the lifted laminae from closing. **D:** Transverse section. (From Hirabayashi K. Expansive open door laminoplasty. In: Shark HH, et al., eds. *The cervical spine. An atlas of surgical procedures.* Philadelphia: JB Lippincott, 1994:233–250, with permission.)

junction of the articular processes and the laminae with a steel burr followed by a diamond burr. The laminae are then cut along the gutter with a thin-bladed Kerrison rongeur. Next, another gutter is created on the hinge side with a steel burr, being set more laterally than the gutter on the opening side. Opening of the laminae is secured by sutures placed on the facet joint capsules on the hinge side and the corresponding laminae.

If the lifted laminae are not fixed firmly, the enlargement of the spinal canal may be reduced. A bone graft used to support the lifted lamina was devised by Itoh and Tsuji (23) to avoid loss of enlargement in the so-called en-bloc laminoplasty. Use of a Kerrison rongeur can present another pitfall because insertion of even a thin-bladed rongeur into the spinal canal may cause spinal cord or vascular (epidural venous plexus) injury and lead to neurologic deficit or heavy bleeding. We use a steel burr to cut the outer cortex and cancellous bone of the laminae and then thin the inner cortex progressively with a diamond burr. With adequate irrigation and suction, the color of the cortex can be seen to change from ivory to dark red as the epidural venous plexus becomes evident. Because the cranial part of each lamina is thicker than the caudal part and is covered by the caudal portion of the lamina above, it requires more grinding than the caudal part to equalize the thickness of the inner cortex. Then a scalp clip holder is inserted into the gutter and opened to separate both edges of the gutter by fracturing the thinned inner cortex (Fig. 76.20). With this technique, no instruments need to be inserted into the canal.

En Bloc Laminoplasty of Itoh and Tsuji

Through a conventional posterior midline approach, the spinous processes are cut at their bases and kept for bone grafting (23). Two gutters are made in the laminae just medial to each articular process. Tunnels for wiring are made within the laminae and the inferior articular processes at C4 and C6 using a specially designed awl and pusher. After en bloc lifting of the laminae, usually from C3 to C7, prop grafts made of the resected spinous processes are placed between the articular processes and the edges of laminae at C4 and C6 to support the lifted laminae. The laminae and bone grafts are then secured in position with steel wires (Fig. 76.21).

Foraminotomy on the opening side can be combined with this technique. If spinal arthrodesis is required, a block bone graft from the ileum is placed to bridge the segments to be fused and is secured with wire (Fig. 76.22). However, wiring for fixation of the laminae and grafts makes this procedure complicated and also makes it difficult to obtain postoperative MRI scans. We use a nonabsorbable synthetic suture material for fixation and place sutures only on the opening side unless the hinges are stable.

Bilateral Hinge Laminoplasty

Spinal arthrodesis can also be performed with this bilateral hinge laminoplasty, but foraminotomy is usually impossible to perform.

French-Door Laminoplasty

After resection of the spinous processes, gutters for the hinges are made at the transitional area between the articular processes and laminae on both sides (27) (Fig. 76.23). The laminae are then cut at the midline, opened bilaterally, and sutured to the capsule. When spinal arthrodesis is indicated, bone chips from the resected spinous processes are placed in the gutter as well as between the laminae and the articular processes. However, the protective function of the

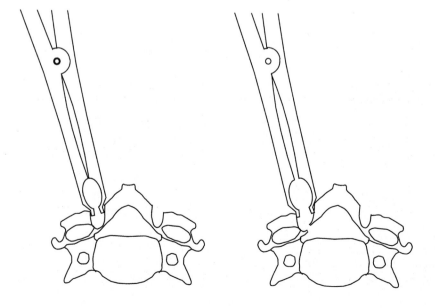

FIG. 76.20. Laminotomy. After making the inner cortex equally thin with a diamond burr, a scalp clip holder is inserted into the gutter and opened to separate both edges of the gutter by fracturing the thinned inner cortex.

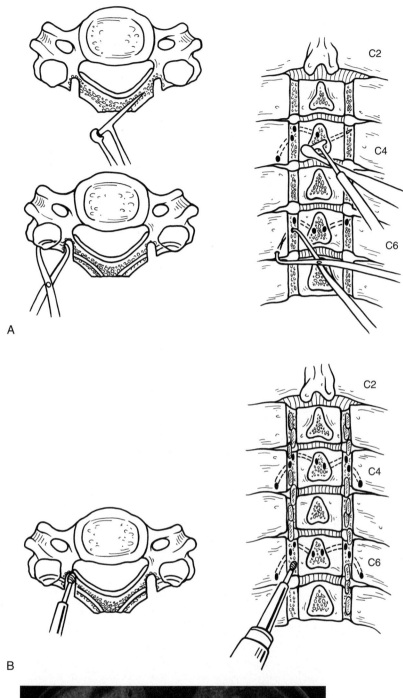

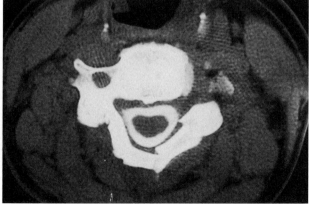

FIG. 76.21. En bloc laminoplasty. **A:** Tunnels for wiring are made within the laminae and the inferior articular processes at C4 and C6 using a specially designed awl and pusher. **B:** Stabilization of the lifted laminae with bone graft. **C:** Postoperative computed tomography scan. (From Itoh T, Tsuji H. technical improvements and results of laminoplasty for compressive myelopathy in the cervical spine. *Spine* 1985; 10:729–736, with permission.)

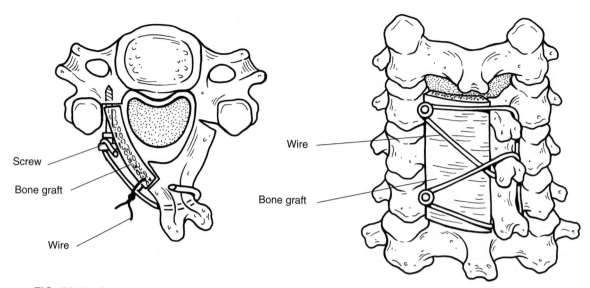

FIG. 76.22. Cervical expansive laminoplasty with posterolateral hemifusion for cervical spine. (From Matsuzaki H, Hoshino M, Kiuchi T, et al. Dome-like expansive laminoplasty for the second cervical vertebra. *Spine* 1989;14:1198–1203, with permission.)

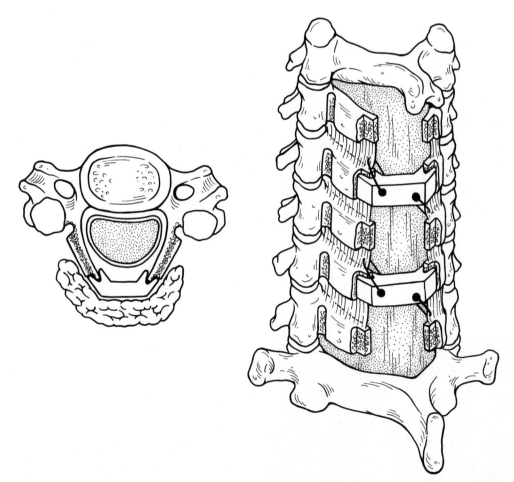

FIG. 76.23. French door laminoplasty with ceramic laminas. (From Hase H, Watanabe T, Hirasawa Y, et al. bilateral open laminoplasty using ceramic laminas for cervical myelopathy. *Spine* 1991;16:1269–1276, with permission.)

neural arch is not completely restored by this procedure. To prevent the loss of decompression and to fill the defect between the separated laminae, an artificial lamina made of ceramic has been developed (22).

Spinous Process–Splitting Laminoplasty of Kurokawa

The dorsal part of each spinous process is removed (25) (Fig. 76.24), and the fragments are used as bone grafts in the space made by spinous process splitting. Gutters for the hinge are created as in the French-door laminoplasty. The laminae are then cut at the midline with a diamond burr, and bone grafts from the spinous processes or ileum are shaped to fit the spaces. When spinal arthrodesis is required, a long bone block is positioned to connect the desired spinous processes. A ceramic spacer can also be substituted for an autogenous bone graft (28).

Tomita modified the process of spinous process splitting by using a threadwire-saw (T-saw laminoplasty) (29). The author reported that this technique shortened the mean time of surgery by 63 minutes and lessened the mean blood loss by 70 mL compared with original procedure.

Supplemental Procedures to Laminoplasty

The nuchal muscles and ligaments are believed to be an indispensable structure helping to stabilize the cervical spine in lordosis. In fact, the nuchal muscles are displaced laterally and ventrally in patients who develop kyphotic deformity after laminectomy, indicating that these muscles and ligaments play an important role in stabilization of the cervical spine. A recent morphologic study with coronal view of MRI also revealed that repair of semispinalis cervicis is important for maintenance

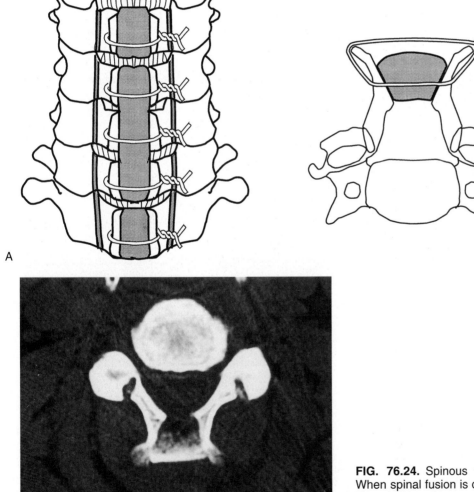

FIG. 76.24. Spinous process–splitting laminoplasty. **A:** When spinal fusion is desired, a block bone graft from the ileum is placed between the segments to be fused and is secured with wire. **B:** Postoperative computed tomography scan.

of cervical lordosis after laminoplasty (30). Therefore, the following procedures have been performed to attempt to reconstruct soft tissue for restoration of stability in lordosis.

Reattachment of the Nuchal Muscles to the Spinous Process of the Axis

The rectus major, inferior oblique, and semispinalis cervicis muscles originally attached to the spinous process of the axis are detached from their origins along with small fragments of the spinous process tip, and the lamina and articular processes of C3 are exposed by retracting the semispinalis cervicis muscles laterally (Fig. 76.25). After laminoplasty, the muscles are reattached to their origins by suturing the bony fragments to the tip of the spinous process. The other nuchal muscles are also repositioned and sutured to each other to form a suspensory nuchal ligament.

Preservation of the Spinous Process–Ligament–Muscle Complex

In this procedure, the laminae on one side are exposed, and the nuchal, supraspinous, and interspinous ligaments are preserved intact (Fig. 76.26). The spinous processes are then cut at their bases, and the laminae on the opposite side are exposed by retracting the nuchal muscles laterally with the resected spinous processes.

POSTOPERATIVE MANAGEMENT

A couple of days after surgery, patients are allowed to leave the bed wearing a Philadelphia collar. We used to recommend 4 weeks of neck immobilization with a collar after surgery. Recently, we are trying to minimize the immobilization period to improve the cervical motion and to lessen the postoperative discomfort of the neck. Patients are encouraged to do active mobilization of the neck followed by isometric neck muscle exercises. When spinal arthrodesis is required, the neck should be immobilized with a collar for 2 months.

RESULTS AND OUTCOMES

Neurologic Results

We operated on 854 patients with cervical compressive myelopathy from 1970 to 1993 (Table 76.1). The characteristics of patients with at least 2-year postoperative follow-up are reviewed in Table 76.2.

Since the JOA proposed a scoring system for cervical myelopathy in 1975, Japanese orthopedic surgeons have used this system (the JOA system). Recently, new scoring systems have been proposed to improve the assessment of shoulder and elbow function and to subdivide the assessment scale for sensory function (31,32). Neurologic results were assessed by the JOA system and evaluated from the postoperative score and the recovery rate determined by the method of Hirabayashi and colleagues (12).

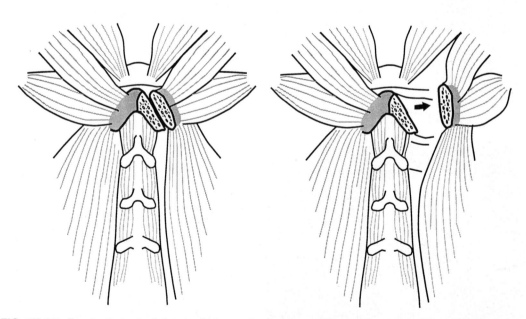

FIG. 76.25. Reattachment of the nuchal muscles to the spinous process of the axis. The rectus major, inferior oblique, and semispinalis cervicis muscles attached to the spinous process of the axis are detached from their origins along with small fragments of the tip of the spinous process. After laminoplasty, the muscles are reattached to their origins by suturing the bony fragments to the tip of the spinous process.

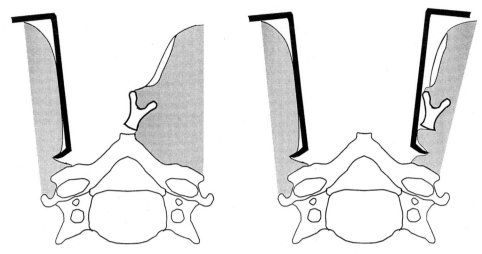

FIG. 76.26. Preservation of the spinous process–ligament–muscle complex. The laminae on one side are exposed while preserving the nuchal, supraspinous, and interspinous ligaments intact. Then the spinous processes are cut at their bases, and retracting the nuchal muscles laterally with the resected spinous processes exposes the laminae on the opposite side.

TABLE 76.1. *Number of Patients by Procedure and Disease*

| | Pathology | | | |
Procedure	CSDH	CSM	OPLL	Total
Laminoplasty				
En-bloc		72	43	115
Spinous process splitting		59	29	88
Laminectomy		41	74	115
Subtotal corpectomy and arthrodesis	13	116	80	209
Discectomy and arthrodesis	155	156	16	327
Total	168	444	242	854

CSDH, myelopathy due to cervical soft disc herniation; CSM, cervical spondylotic myelopathy; OPLL, myelopathy due to ossification of the posterior longitudinal ligament.

TABLE 76.2. *Results of Surgery: Average Postoperative Japanese Orthopedic Association (JOA) Score and Recovery Rate*

| | CSDH | | CSM | | OPLL | |
Procedure	Postop. JOA score	Recovery rate(%)	Postop. JOA score	Recovery rate(%)	Postop. JOA score	Recovery rate(%)
Laminoplasty						
En bloc			12.8	51.2	12.4	44.4
Splitting			12.9	49.0	NA	NA
Laminectomy			11.7	38.7	12.1	41.2
Subtotal corpectomy and arthrodesis	NA	NA	13.4	55.2	14.0	57.7
Discectomy and arthrodesis	15.0	72.5	12.8	45.3	NA	NA

CSDH, myelopathy due to cervical soft disc herniation; CSM, cervical spondylotic myelopathy; OPLL, myelopathy due to ossification of the posterior longitudinal ligament; NA, data not available.

Little study has been done with respect to issue of differences in surgical outcome based on the particular procedure used. Tsuzuki and associates (33,34) employed six different procedures for CSM and reported no difference in the degree of improvement of the long tract signs of CSM. We compared the results of two procedures, en bloc laminoplasty with reconstruction of the nuchal muscle attachments and spinous process–splitting laminoplasty in patients with multisegmental spondylotic myelopathy (Table 76.2). The average recovery rate of the en bloc laminoplasty group was 51.2%, and that of the spinous process–splitting laminoplasty group was 49.0%. There was no significant difference between the two groups. It is very difficult to compare the results of various procedures, even if the outcome is evaluated using the same scale. However, the recovery rate after various laminoplasties is reported to range from 50% to 70%. So far, no procedure to our knowledge has been proved statistically superior to the others, suggesting that the outcomes are likely to be the same provided that the procedure is done properly.

An issue is whether there is any difference in surgical outcomes between procedures done for spondylosis and OPLL. Miyazaki and colleagues (35) reported that 87% of OPLL patients treated with extensive simultaneous laminectomy showed useful improvement, as compared with 76% of patients with CSM after the same procedure. They also reported that increased instability of the spine after laminectomy influenced the surgical results and therefore added posterolateral arthrodesis to laminectomy. When this was combined with posterolateral arthrodesis, the results improved and were better than those for OPLL (35). Kawai and associates (24) analyzed the results of expansive Z laminoplasty and reported superior results in patients with spondylotic myelopathy over those in patients with OPLL. Therefore, better surgical results have been demonstrated in spondylotic myelopathy when laminoplasty was properly performed. The severity of the myelopathy will certainly influence the surgical results.

Decompression of the nerve roots is usually impossible when the bilateral open type of laminoplasty is selected. With unilateral open laminoplasty, however, foraminotomy or facetectomy can be performed on the side. Herkowitz (36) compared the results of anterior cervical arthrodesis, laminectomy, and laminoplasty for multilevel spondylotic radiculopathy and concluded that although anterior cervical arthrodesis provided the best results, laminoplasty provided an effective alternative to anterior arthrodesis. However, the results of laminoplasty for radiculopathy associated with myelopathy have not been reported to our knowledge. In our series, eight patients reported pain on the radial side of the arm and forearm that was believed to be of radicular origin before surgery. Six of the eight patients showed reduction of radicular symptoms after en bloc laminoplasty without facetectomy. Four patients with weakness of the deltoid and biceps brachii as well as myelopathic symptoms underwent en bloc laminoplasty and facetectomy of C4-C5 and C5-C6; two of four had some reduction in weakness. Thus, radiculopathy (mainly radicular pain) can be relieved

with laminoplasty as part of spinal cord decompression, probably because the spine is stabilized by laminoplasty. However, the results of laminoplasty with facetectomy for advanced radiculopathy causing muscle atrophy have not been consistent.

Roentgenographic Outcomes

Laminoplasty aiming to maintain or restore spinal stability should be evaluated by both the radiographic outcome and the clinical outcome.

Kyphotic deformity after laminectomy is a notorious problem, especially when the procedure is carried out in young patients (37). The prevalence of kyphotic deformity after laminectomy for CSM, developmental cervical canal stenosis, and OPLL is probably lower than is believed. Mikawa and coworkers (38) reported that no deformity developed after multilevel laminectomy for spondylosis and that deformity developed more often in OPLL. In our series, 21% of laminectomy patients showed deterioration of neurologic symptoms due to cervical spine instability. About half of them had a straight spine before surgery, and their symptoms worsened in association with the development of kyphosis triggered by minor trauma.

Assessment of cervical spinal alignment is not easy because it cannot be described by simple numeric values. We measured the distance between the center of the cervical curve and the line connecting the posterior edge of the odontoid process and the posteroinferior edge of the seventh vertebral body. Lordotic alignment was defined as a distance of 2 mm or more, and other cases were defined as kyphotic alignment. All the patients with kyphotic alignment before surgery showed worsening of their alignment after laminectomy, whereas no patient with lordotic alignment before surgery showed deterioration after en bloc laminoplasty with reconstruction of the nuchal muscle attachment. The degree of lordosis in the patients with lordotic alignment before surgery decreased slightly, but no patient developed kyphotic deformity of the cervical spine. After spinous process–splitting laminoplasty in our series, 27% of the patients showed deterioration of spinal alignment. Hirabayashi and associates (39) did not note any postoperative malalignment of the cervical spinal lateral curvature after expansive open-door laminoplasty. The reason for the difference between the procedures is not clear. There has been controversy about whether postoperative malalignment leads to poor surgical results. Kawakami and associates (40) evaluated sagittal alignment of the spinal cord and the cervical spine with MRI. They reported that, although sagittal alignment of the cervical spine did not influence the surgical results, patients with a kyphotic spinal cord tended to have a low recovery rate.

A patient with OPLL of the cervical spine tends to be kyphotic, although the reason for this is not clear. Fortunately, few patients deteriorated as a result of kyphotic deformity after laminoplasty. Formed laminae prevent infiltration of scar tissue into the spinal canal and maintain room for the spinal cord. Hirabayashi and associates (39) reported the progression of OPLL after laminectomy and suggested the usefulness of laminoplasty in this respect. Although progression of OPLL (defined as growth in thickness or length of 2 mm or more) was also observed in about 60% of patients who underwent laminoplasty, none reported worsening of their neurologic symptoms secondary to this progression.

Little is known with regard to listhesis because laminoplasty originally was not indicated for patients with marked spinal instability. In our series, all patients with instability as defined by White and Panjabi (41) had improved stability, and their results were not different from those of the patients without instability.

To our knowledge, no procedure has been proved to prevent further progression of kyphotic deformity of the cervical spine completely (Fig. 76.27) or to create cervical lordosis in patients with a preexisting kyphotic deformity. Except when supplemented with spinal arthrodesis, no type of laminoplasty can guarantee lifelong spinal stability. To obtain a more consistent outcome after laminoplasty, procedures to reconstruct the supporting soft tissues must be further developed, as must rehabilitation programs.

Postoperatively, ROM of the neck usually decreases, with the extent of the decrease ranging from 30% to 70%. The type of laminoplasty, the extent of exposure, the position of laminotomy, the use of bone grafting, and the postoperative rehabilitation program, including the period of neck immobilization, may all influence the degree of ROM loss. Many surgeons believe that the loss of ROM has a favorable effect on the neurologic outcome by partially stabilizing the spine. Few patients complain of the inconvenience of decreased ROM of the neck that generally occurs after multisegmental anterior spinal fusion. Therefore, patient complaints of decreased ROM reduction after laminoplasty may derive from a combination of stiffness and neck discomfort.

Long-Term Results

Laminoplasty was developed in the late 1970s, and various modifications were reported in the early 1980s (Fig. 76.28). Recently, several long-term (>10 years) follow-up studies have been published. Miyazaki and associates (35) performed a study with a mean of 12 years 11 months of follow-up and reported that improvement after surgery was maintained. Kawai and colleagues (24) monitored patients having a Z laminoplasty for 10 years on the average and reported that patients with spondylotic myelopathy were stable, in contrast to the results of patients with OPLL. Seichi and associates (42) also reported that 91% of patients with CSM were stable over 10 years after spinous process–splitting laminoplasty, in contrast to 81% of patients with OPLL. The reasons for this difference were not

described in detail. However, patients with OPLL frequently have diabetes mellitus and ossification of spinal ligaments in the thoracic and lumbar spine, which also causes myelopathy. These factors may influence the long-term results of surgical treatment to varying degrees. Wada and associates (43) compared the long-term outcomes of open-door laminoplasty and subtotal corpectomy for multilevel CSM and found no difference between the two procedures. Neurologic recoveries in both groups generally last more than 10 years.

COMPLICATIONS

Generally, the complications of laminoplasty are similar to those of laminectomy. However, nonneurologic complications are relatively rare compared with other procedures, including laminectomy. Delayed healing or dehiscence of the surgical wound may occur slightly more frequently after laminoplasty than with laminectomy, and this may be related to the bulk of the elevated laminae. The prevalence of neurologic complications attributed to laminectomy is less in laminoplasty because of simultaneous decompression and the use of air-driven instruments. There are, however, complications characteristic to this procedure: nerve root palsy and axial (neck and shoulder) pain.

Neurologic deterioration due to hematoma has decreased because reconstructed or preserved laminae still have a protective function, diminishing blood pooling and soft tissue swelling after surgery. We have experienced this complication in only 0.3% of patients undergoing laminoplasty, as compared with 2.4% of patients undergoing laminectomy.

Fracture of a hinge or loss of spinal canal enlargement due to insufficient fixation of the lifted laminae is reported to cause nerve root or spinal cord palsy when a lamina migrates into the spinal canal. CT is useful for delineating the pathology in this case, and complete or partial removal of the lifted lamina is necessary. The prognosis is usually good if salvage is performed promptly. For prevention, the inner cortex of the lamina destined to be the hinge should be thinned gradually while its mobility is assessed.

Nerve root palsy due to thermal damage or mechanical injury to the nerve root occasionally develops after posterior decompression, and a different type of nerve root palsy is reported to occur after laminoplasty (33,34,44). The initial symptom is severe pain in the shoulder and upper arm, followed by paresis or paralysis of the deltoid and biceps brachii muscles. There is a motor-dominant type of nerve root paralysis. The former symptom is the more frequent form of this complication. It occurs on postoperative day 1, 2, or 3, and not immediately after surgery. The fifth cervical nerve root is most frequently involved, followed by the sixth and seventh in order. The eighth nerve root is rarely affected. Of 203 laminoplasty patients in our series, 12 patients developed fifth

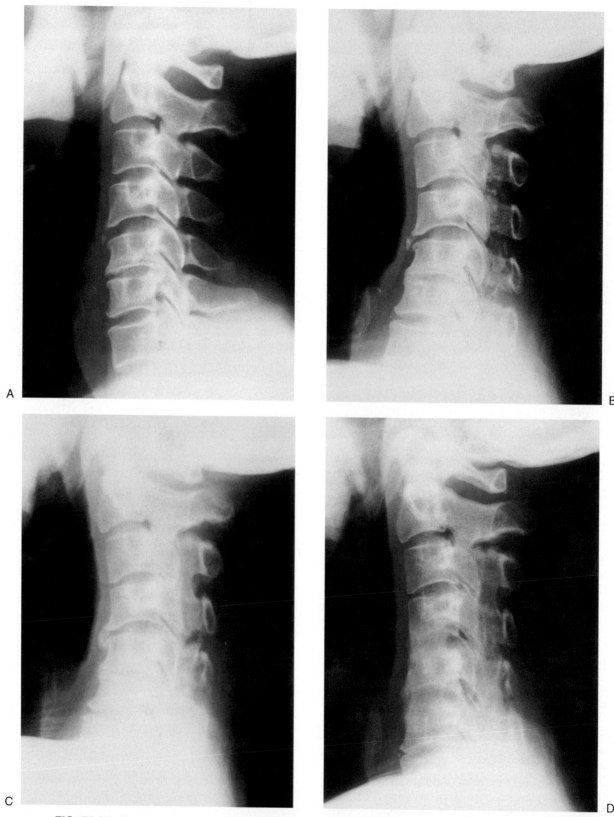

FIG. 76.27. Kyphotic deformity after en bloc laminoplasty. The patient is a 58-year-old man who had en bloc laminoplasty for myelopathy due to narrow spinal canal. **A:** Lateral x-ray before surgery showed a narrow spinal canal. The spine is in straight alignment. **B:** Because of regression of neurologic symptoms 3 months after surgery, the x-ray revealed kyphotic deformity of the cervical spine. Deterioration of the patient's symptoms was triggered by a minor trauma. **C:** The patient was referred to us for fusion. **D:** Multiple-level discectomy and fusion.

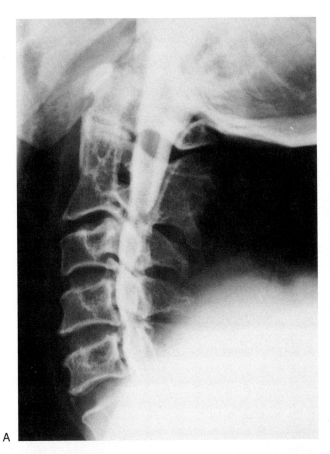

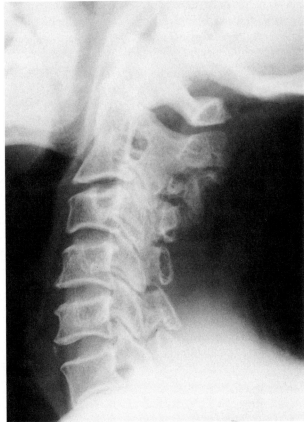

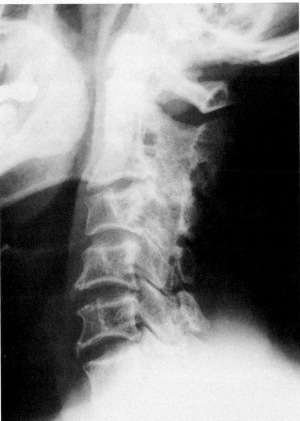

FIG. 76.28. Case presentation. **A:** The patient is a 54-year-old man who presented with complaints of difficulty walking and loss of dexterity. The Japanese Orthopedics Association (JOA) score at the first visit was 8 points. Myelogram showed indentation against the cord at multiple levels and spinal canal stenosis. **B:** The spinal canal was enlarged, and lordosis of the cervical spine was kept 6 months after surgery. **C:** Neurologic recovery has been preserved 9 years after surgery. Roentgenographic study showed slight progression of spondylosis, but the enlargement of the canal and the cervical lordosis were still maintained.

or sixth nerve root palsy, three patients had seventh nerve root involvement, and one patient had an eighth root complication. The long tract signs and symptoms are usually improved, and no regression of the long tract signs and symptoms can be detected. The prevalence of nerve root palsy varies. Tsuzuki and co-workers (34) studied its prevalence in relation to the surgical procedure in their own series. They used the following six different procedures: laminectomy, French-door laminoplasty, spinous process–splitting laminoplasty without facetectomy, laterally enlarged closed laminoplasty without facetectomy, medially enlarged closed laminoplasty with multiple foraminotomy (C4-C5, C5-C6), and laterally enlarged closed laminoplasty with multiple foraminotomy (C4-C5, C5-C6). The total frequency of this complication was 11%. The motor-dominant type of paralysis occurred in 9%, and the sensory-dominant type occurred in 2%. A higher prevalence of nerve root palsy was evident in both closed types of laminoplasty with foraminotomy (C4-C5, C5-C6), whereas the closed laminoplasties without foraminotomy or facetectomy were associated with a lower prevalence.

This complication has been reported to occur rarely after laminectomy, and its mechanism has not yet been fully clarified. Nerve root tethering due to posterior migration of the spinal cord has been suggested to be the major cause (33,34,44).

This entity may be differentiated from nerve root or spinal cord palsy due to mechanical compression by CT scanning with or without contrast medium. Pain can be controlled with nonsteroidal antiinflammatory drugs (NSAIDs), analgesics, or both. Neck traction in the neutral position may also reduce pain. The motor paralysis usually recovers to normal or good grade in 12 months or less. Severe spondylotic changes, especially at the root tunnel, and spinal cord atrophy are believed to be predisposing factors for nerve root palsy (Fig. 76.29). Although the alignment of the cervical spine, the relative position of the facets to the vertebral body, and the distance from the cord to the dura—nerve root junction were all analyzed, no factor was proved a sole predictor of this complication.

Foraminotomy or facetectomy has not been proved a preventive measure. However, controlled opening of the lamina may prevent this problem, although a definitive method for control of opening has not been devised.

Postoperatively, patients with laminoplasty report various axial symptoms such as nuchal pain and stiffness of the neck and shoulder muscles. Neck stiffness usually appeared on the hinge side in our series of en bloc laminoplasties. In our series, 60% of patients who underwent laminoplasty reported some axial symptoms within 1 year of surgery, as compared with 27% of patients who underwent laminectomy and 19% of those who underwent subtotal corpectomy and arthrodesis. After spinous process–splitting laminoplasty, a few patients reported neck or shoulder pain or both. The symptoms were usually distributed on both sides and their cause was not clear. However, changes in and around the facet joints caused by surgical intervention may have been the cause. These symptoms resolved by about 1 year after surgery in

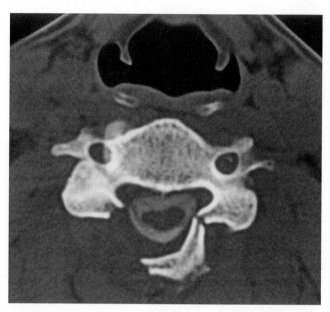

FIG. 76.29. Computed tomography scan of the patient with C5 nerve root palsy. Note the marked dorsal shift of the spinal cord after laminoplasty.

most patients. Axial symptoms are the chief complaint in some patients, and their cause should also be clarified. Thermal therapy and active mobilization of the neck and shoulder are recommended for treatment. NSAIDs and muscle relaxant drugs have little effect. Recently, several surgeons have started to assess the usefulness of various postoperative muscle exercise and neck motion programs to prevent these complaints and to maintain or create a cervical lordosis after laminoplasty, but none of these programs has been proved useful.

REFERENCES

1. Robinson RA, Smith GW. Anterolateral cervical disc removal and interbody fusion of the cervical spine. *Johns Hopkins Med J* 1955;96: 223–224.
2. Cloward RB. The anterior approach for removal of ruptured cervical discs. *J Neurosurg* 1958;15:602–617.
3. Rogers L. The surgical treatment of cervical spondylotic myelopathy. Mobilization of the complete cervical cord into an enlarged canal. *J Bone Joint Surg Br* 1961;43:3–6.
4. Yonenobu K, Fuji T, Ono K, et al. Choice of surgical treatment for multisegmental cervical spondylotic myelopathy. *Spine* 1985;10:710–716.
5. Yonenobu K, Okada K, Fuji T, et al. Causes of neurological deterioration following surgical treatment of cervical myelopathy. *Spine* 1986;11:818–823.
6. Bohlman HH. Cervical spondylosis with moderate to severe myelopathy. *Spine* 1977;2:151–162
7. Graham JJ. Complications of cervical spine surgery. In: Shark HH, et al., eds. *The cervical spine*, 2nd ed. Philadelphia: JB Lippincott, 1989:831–837.
8. Mayfield FH. Complications of laminectomy. *Clin Neurosurg* 1976; 23:435–439.
9. Kirita Y. Posterior decompression for cervical spondylosis and ossification of the posterior longitudinal ligament [in Japanese]. *Shujutu* 1976;30:287.
10. Miyazaki K, Kirita Y. Extensive simultaneous multisegment laminectomy for myelopathy due to the ossification of the posterior longitudinal ligament in the cervical lesion. *Spine* 1986;11:531–542.

11. Oyama M, Hattori S, Moriwaki N. A new method of posterior decompression [in Japanese]. *Chubuseisaisi* 1973;16:792.
12. Hirabayashi K, Miyagawa J, Satomi K, et al. Operative results and postoperative progression of ossification among patients with ossification of cervical posterior longitudinal ligament. *Spine* 1981;6:354–364.
13. Aita I, Hayashi K, Wadano Y, et al. Posterior movement and enlargement of the spinal cord after cervical laminoplasty. *J Bone Joint Surg Br* 1998;80:33–37.
14. Sodeyama T, Goto S, Mochizuki M, et al. Effect of decompression enlargement laminoplasty for posterior shifting of the spinal cord. *Spine* 1999;24:1527–1532.
15. Hosono N, Yonenobu K, Ono K. Neck and shoulder pain after laminoplasty: a noticeable complication. *Spine* 1996;21:1969–1973.
16. Ebara S, Yonenobu K, Fujiwara K, et al. Myelopathy hand characterized by muscle wasting. A different type of myelopathy hand in patients with cervical spondylosis. *Spine* 1988;13:785–791.
17. Yonenobu K, Hosono N, Iwasaki M, et al. Laminoplasty versus subtotal corpectomy. A comparative study of results in multisegmental cervical spondylotic myelopathy. *Spine* 1992;17:1281–1284.
18. Iwasaki M, Ebara S, Miyamoto S, et al. Expansive laminoplasty for cervical radiculomyelopathy due to soft disc hernia. A comparative study between laminoplasty and anterior arthrodesis. *Spine* 1996;21:32–38.
19. Yoshida M, Tamaki T, Kawakami N, et al. Indication and clinical results of laminoplasty for cervical myelopathy caused by disc herniation with developmental canal stenosis. *Spine* 1998;23:2391–2397.
20. Matsuda Y, Shibata T, Oki S, et al. Outcomes of surgical treatment for cervical myelopathy in patients more than 75 years of age. *Spine* 1999;24:529–534.
21. Hirabayashi K. Expansive open door laminoplasty. In: Shark HH, et al., eds. *The cervical spine. An atlas of surgical procedures.* Philadelphia: JB Lippincott, 1994:233–250.
22. Hase H, Watanabe T, Hirasawa Y, et al. Bilateral open laminoplasty using ceramic laminas for cervical myelopathy. *Spine* 1991;16:1269–1276.
23. Itoh T, Tsuji H. Technical improvements and results of laminoplasty for compressive myelopathy in the cervical spine. *Spine* 1985;10:729–736.
24. Kawai S, Sunago K, Doi K, et al. Cervical laminoplasty (Hattori's method). Procedure and follow-up results. *Spine* 1988;13:1245–1250.
25. Kurokawa T, Tsuyama N, Tanaka H, et al. Enlargement of spinal canal by the sagittal splitting of the spinous process [in Japanese]. *Bessatsu Seikeigeka* 1982;2:234–240.
26. Matsuzaki H, Hoshino M, Kiuchi T, et al. Dome-like expansive laminoplasty for the second cervical vertebra. *Spine* 1989;14:1198–1203.
27. Hukuda S, Mochizuki T, Ogata M, et al. Operations for cervical spondylotic myelopathy. A comparison of the results of anterior and posterior procedures. *J Bone Joint Surg* 1985;67:609–615.
28. Nakano K, Harata S, Suetsuna F, et al. Spinous process-splitting laminoplasty using hydroxyapatite spinous process spacer. *Spine* 1992;17:S41–43.
29. Tomita K, Kawahara N, Torihata Y, et al. Expansive midline T-saw laminoplasty (modified spinous process-splitting) for the management of cervical myelopathy. *Spine* 1998;23:32–37.
30. Iizuka H, Shimizu T, Tateno K, et al. Extensor musculature of the cervical spine after laminoplasty. *Spine* 2001;26:2220–2226.
31. Yamauchi Y, Hirabayashi K. The criteria for evaluation of treatment of cervical myelopathy by the Japanese Orthopaedic Association. *J Jpn Orthop Assoc* 1994;68:490–503.
32. Yonenobu K, Abumi K, Nagata K, et al K. Inter- and intra-observer reliability of the Japanese Orthopaedic Association Scoring System for evaluation of cervical compression myelopathy. *Spine* 2001;26:1890–1894.
33. Tsuzuki N, Zhogshi L, Abe R, et al. Paralysis of the arm after posterior decompression of the cervical spinal cord. 1. Anatomical investigation of the mechanism of paralysis. *Eur Spine J* 1993;2:191–196.
34. Tsuzuki N, Abe R, Saiki K, et al. Paralysis of the arm after posterior decompression of the cervical spinal cord. 2. Analyses of clinical findings. *Eur Spine J* 1993;2:197–202.
35. Miyazaki K, Hirohuji E, Ono S, et al. Extensive simultaneous multisegmental laminectomy and posterior decompression with posterolateral fusion [in Japanese]. *J Jpn Spine Res Soc* 1994;5:167.
36. Herkowitz HN. A comparison of anterior cervical fusion, cervical laminectomy, and cervical laminoplasty for the surgical management of multiple level spondylotic radiculopathy. *Spine* 1988;3:774–779.
37. Yasuoka S, Peterson HA, Maccarty CS. Incidence of spinal column deformity after multilevel laminectomy in children and adults. *J Neurosurg* 1982;57:441–445.
38. Mikawa Y, Shikata J, Yamamuro T. Spinal deformity and instability after multilevel cervical laminectomy. *Spine* 1987;12:6–11.
39. Hirabayashi K, Watanabe K, Wakano K, et al. Expansive open-door laminoplasty for cervical spinal stenotic myelopathy. *Spine* 1983;8:693–699.
40. Kawakami N, Tamaki T, Iwasaki H, et al. A comparative study of surgical approaches for cervical compressive myelopathy. *Clin Orthop* 2000;381:129–136.
41. White AA, Panjabi MM. The problem of clinical instability in the human spine. *Clinical biomechanics of the spine*, 2nd ed. Philadelphia: JB Lippincott, 1990.
42. Seichi A, Takeshita K, Ohishi I, et al. Long-term results of double-door laminoplasty for cervical stenotic myelopathy. *Spine* 2001;26:479–487.
43. Wada E, Suzuki S, Kanazawa, et al. Subtotal corpectomy versus laminoplasty for multilevel cervical spondylotic myelopathy. A long-term follow-up over 10 years. *Spine* 2001;26:1443–1448.
44. Yonenobu K, Hosono N, Iwasaki M, et al. Neurological complications of surgery for cervical compression myelopathy. *Spine* 1991;16:1277–1282.

Part C
Anterior Approach

Chetan K. Patel, Eeric Truumees, and Harry N. Herkowitz

Chronic disc degeneration with protrusion, posterior vertebrae body osteophytes, disc herniation, OPLL, hypertrophied uncovertebral or apophyseal joints, and hypertrophied ligamentum flavum may cause myelopathy (spinal cord compression), radiculopathy (nerve root compression), or myeloradiculopathy (both cord and root compression). CSM is the most common type of spinal cord dysfunction in patients older than 55 years of age. For these patients, the most likely etiology of stenosis is bony compression, whereas soft disc herniation is the most likely etiology in those younger than 55 years of age (1). The most common level of involvement is C5-C6, followed by C6-C7; C5-C6 exhibits the greatest motion of any cervical level below C2 (2,3). Most cases of spondylotic myelopathy have an insidious onset, leading to static disability followed by episodic worsening (4–6).

SURGICAL INDICATIONS

The severity of symptoms upon presentation and the correlation of radiographic findings with history and physical examination are of utmost importance. Spinal cord abnormality correlates with the severity of clinical disease (7). The AP compression ratio represents the AP diameter of the cord divided by its lateral diameter. This ratio correlates with the degree of pathologic findings. Pathologic findings in severe cases of compression include extensive destruction of both white and gray matter with demyelination of ascending and descending tracts above and below the lesion. A low ratio suggests significant cord narrowing and pathologic change. Fujiwora and coworkers found that results of decompressive surgery are poor if the preoperative cord area is less than 30 mm² (8). Okada and associates reported that atrophy of the spinal cord predicts unsatisfactory clinical results (9). Good prognostic factors for surgery include young age, symptom duration of less than 1 year, fewer levels involved, unilateral motor deficit, and the presence of Lhermitte sign. Surgery is indicated in patients with moderate to severe myelopathy and in those who have an unsatisfactory lifestyle and substantial restriction in activities of daily living.

SURGICAL OPTIONS

An anterior approach is usually preferred for disease involving up to three motion segments and predominant anterior abnormalities. For one- or two-level abnormalities confined to the level of the discs, anterior cervical discectomy and arthrodesis is recommended. Given that the pseudoarthrosis rate increases with the number of levels that are arthrodesed, a corpectomy is often considered for three- and four-level procedures (10–14). A corpectomy and arthrodesis requires that only two surfaces, as opposed to six in a three-level anterior cervical discectomy and fusion (ACDF), heal. When osteophytes are present posterior to the vertebral body, adequate and safe decompression often requires total or partial corpectomy instead of an ACDF.

Multilevel anterior corpectomy and discectomy procedures are associated with higher rates of graft and soft tissue complications than one-level procedures. For longer stenotic segments, a posterior exposure is technically easier and does not require retraction of the vulnerable anterior viscera. Therefore, patients with neutral or lordotic sagittal alignment and compression at more than three motion segments should be considered for a posterior approach (15). In those with a kyphotic sagittal alignment, adequate decompression is not possible with a posterior-only approach (15,16). In this group, either anterior alone or a combined anterior and posterior approach should be considered.

Another option for the anterior approach is anterior cervical discectomy without arthrodesis. Advocates of this approach cite the advantage of avoiding graft harvest morbidity. This procedure in essence is a planned pseudoarthrosis. The disadvantages of a discectomy without arthrodesis are postoperative neck pain, kyphosis, lack of foraminal distraction, and continued growth of osteophytes and restenosis (17–19). For these reasons, we do not consider this procedure a viable option.

ANTERIOR CERVICAL DISCECTOMY AND FUSION

In 1955, Smith and Robinson described ACDF as a means of decompressing the cervical canal as well as providing stability to the diseased segment (20). This procedure allows direct and indirect decompression of the spinal cord and nerve roots. Direct decompression is performed by removing the offending disc and osteophytes. Spinal stabilization may lead to osteophyte resorption and prevention of recompression. Interspace grafting indirectly decompresses the neuroforamina by distraction and decompresses the spinal canal by decreasing ligamentum flavum infolding. The degree to which foraminal distraction and resorption contribute to clinical outcomes continues to be debated (21–23). The disadvantages of ACDF include immobilization, graft dislodgment, pseudoarthrosis, accelerated adjacent segment degeneration, donor site morbidity, and the potential morbidity of an anterior approach to the cervical spine.

Surgical Technique

There are two surgical goals: adequate decompression and solid fusion. Decompression is addressed by complete removal of the disc and the offending osteophytes (Fig. 76.30). Some authors advocate leaving the posterior osteophytes in place, assuming that they will resorb with fusion. In the face of significant myelopathy or a preoperative motor deficit, complete osteophyte resection is recommended (4,24,25). An ACDF is performed using the standard Smith-Robinson anterior approach to the cervical spine. A left-sided approach is typically used to decrease the potential of injury to the shorter, more oblique, and less predictable course of the right recurrent laryngeal nerve (26,27). However, we are aware of no conclusive randomized prospective study that demonstrates the suspected superiority of the left-sided over the right-sided approach (28–30).

During the decompression, osteophytes on the end plates are identified and resected directly. Undercutting or reaching around bony margins of the vertebrae may further compress the cord and is contraindicated. A partial corpectomy

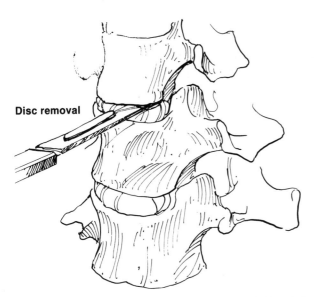

FIG. 76.30. The anterior longitudinal ligament (ALL) and the annulus are incised with a knife to begin the discectomy. (From Sherk HH, Larson SJ, eds. *The cervical spine: an atlas of surgical techniques.* Philadelphia: JB Lippincott, 1999:191, with permission.)

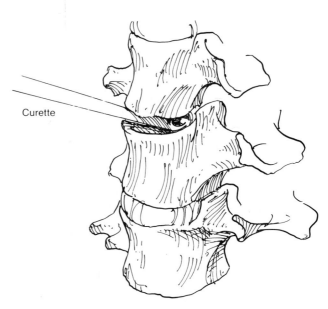

FIG. 76.31. The end plates are curetted to remove all cartilage. (From Sherk HH, Larson SJ, eds. *The cervical spine: an atlas of surgical techniques.* Philadelphia: JB Lippincott, 1999:191, with permission.)

is necessary if adequate decompression requires substantial resection cranial or caudal to the disc level. Before beginning the decompression, the uncinate processes are identified, and midline is marked to help maintain orientation throughout the decompression. In the severely degenerative cervical spine, these landmarks may be difficult to visualize, but safe lateral decompression requires clear definition of the anatomy. Decompression of the uncinate process and the associated osteophytes can be safely carried out by burring the posterior 5 mm of the uncinate, followed by the use of a 1-mm Kerrison to complete the foraminal decompression anterior to the nerve root. A fine nerve hook or ball-tipped probe can be used to verify the decompression. The instrument should pass unobstructed into the neural foramen.

Once decompression has been achieved and verified, the spine is prepared for arthrodesis. The end-plate cartilage is completely removed and breached to enhance vascular ingrowth by perforating the end plate with a small angled curette or by decortication with a burr (Fig. 76.31). Aggressive burring may diminish the end plate's ability to support the graft structurally, leading to postoperative collapse (4). With the end plate prepared, distraction is applied, and graft height, width, and depth, are measured. The graft should be 2 to 4 mm greater than the preoperative disc height and must be at least 5 mm thick to prevent resorption while restoring the disc and foraminal height (31,32). If too large of a graft is used, overdistraction can occur. Overdistraction leads to decreased posterior column load transmission and increased load on the graft and the vertebral body, leading to graft failure (33). Many choices are available in terms of fashioning the graft, which are described in the following section. Either an autograft or an allograft can be used.

Once the graft is cut to the appropriate dimensions, lordosis may be built into the graft by creating a graft that tapers to a lower height posteriorly. This can help recreate the natural lordotic alignment of the cervical spine. After the graft is ready, distraction of the disc space may be achieved by a Caspar retractor, a vertebral spreader introduced laterally in the disc space, by a head halter, or manually. The graft should be countersunk 1 or 2 mm to help prevent extrusion (34) (Figs. 76.32 and 76.33). At this point, a cervical plate may be added to provide a more rigid construct in addition to providing a physical block to graft extrusion.

The surgical technique for a multilevel ACDF is identical to that for a one-level ACDF. An oblique instead of the usual transverse incision may have to be considered when more than a two-level surgery is performed to allow adequate exposure.

Postoperatively, a firm cervical collar is used for 6 weeks if no instrumentation is added and for 1 to 2 weeks if instrumentation is used. Radiographs are recommended at regular intervals after surgery until union in achieved.

Grafting Techniques

The graft technique described earlier is the most commonly performed with a Smith-Robinson horseshoe graft. However, many other variations exist (Fig. 76.34). Cloward described direct visualization and decompression of the neural elements followed by cutting of the end plates with a trephine drill to a preset depth (35). A precut dowel-shaped graft is then tapped into place. This technique does not allow for the distraction provided by the Smith-Robinson horseshoe graft. The Bailey and Badgely technique consists of a shallow trough cut into

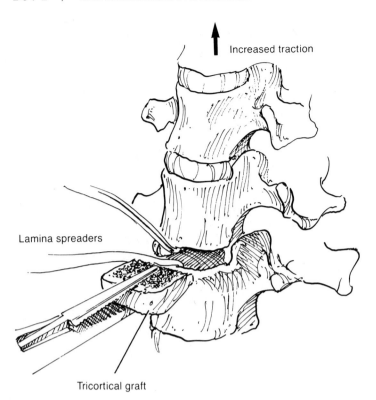

FIG. 76.32. Placement of a Smith-Robinson type of tricortical graft. (From Sherk HH, Larson SJ, eds. *The cervical spine: an atlas of surgical techniques.* Philadelphia: JB Lippincott, 1999:193, with permission.)

the anterior aspect of the vertebral bodies (36). This technique does not describe any visualization of the posterior longitudinal ligament (PLL) or direct decompression. Simmons and Bhalla described a keystone graft, which has a longer height posteriorly than anteriorly (37). This variation was designed to be more stable than other graft designs. The horseshoe graft has been shown to have more compressive strength than both the Bailey-Badgely and the Simmons-Bhalla grafts (38,39).

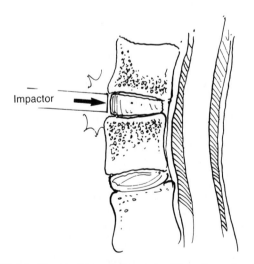

FIG. 76.33. The graft is countersunk with an impactor. (From Sherk HH, Larson SJ, eds. *The cervical spine: an atlas of surgical techniques.* Philadelphia: JB Lippincott, 1999:193, with permission.)

Results

High rates of symptomatic relief and neurologic and functional recovery are expected after ACDF. Important technical variables affecting outcomes include grafting technique, decompression effort, disc space distraction, graft type (including allograft versus autograft), and the use of instrumentation. Several classification systems have been used in the literature to grade the degree of neurological impairment. The Nurick and JOA scoring system are two examples that allow repeated measures of the global effects of myelopathy. Nurick created a myelopathy grading system from 0 to 5 that focused on progressively worsening gait abnormalities (6,40). The JOA scoring system, on the other hand, is based on upper and lower extremity motor function, sensory function, and sphincter function (18,41).

The first large series of ACDF that we are aware of was reported by Robinson et al. in 1962. They reported good to excellent results in 73% of his 52 patients. The worst outcome was noted in multilevel procedures (13). In 1972, DePalma and coworkers reported 63% satisfactory results in 229 patients (42). Their series included a 12% pseudarthrosis rate, which did not always correlate with poor outcome. They postulated that a stable, fibrous union might account for the lack of neck pain in many pseudarthrosis patients (42). In 1977, Bohlman reported improvement in the functional status in 16 of his 17 patients (24). No effort was made to remove the osteophytes or the PLL in this study.

In 1983, Zhang and colleagues reported an improvement in 91% of 121 patients (43). Most patients underwent three

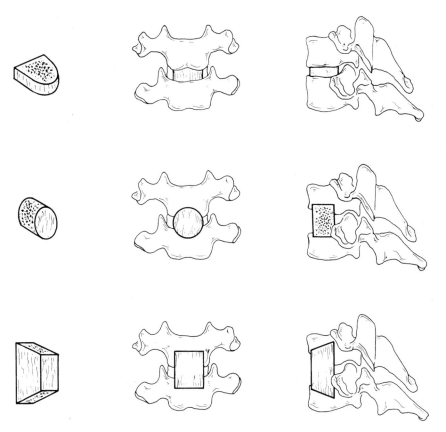

FIG. 76.34. The Smith-Robinson (**top**), Cloward (**middle**), and Simmons-Bhalla grafts (**bottom**). (From Bridwell KH, Dewald RL, eds. *The textbook of spinal surgery*, 2nd ed. Philadelphia: Lippincott—Raven, 1997:1386, with permission.)

or more levels of decompression and arthrodesis with either allograft or autograft. The fusion rate was 82% for iliac crest autograft as opposed to 50% for iliac crest allograft. They noted poor results in patients with pseudoarthroses (43). In 1984, Kadoya and colleagues reported an improvement of at least one Nurick grade in 91% of their 43 patients (44). They removed the PLL and the offending osteophytes in all cases and did not note any neurologic worsening.

In 1987, Yang and coworkers reported an improvement in functional status in 90% of 214 cases (45). No attempt was made to remove the osteophytes, with an average of 3.1 levels arthrodesed. The pseudoarthrosis rate was 37%, with no correlation between pseudoarthrosis and clinical outcome. Patients with prolonged duration of symptoms preoperatively had a poorer outcome.

Although ACDF with an autograft remains the gold standard, its associated donor site morbidity and increased operative time have led to increasing use of allograft. Up to 15% of patients have donor site pain lasting more than 3 months and up to 10% of patients sustain an injury to the lateral femoral cutaneous nerve (46). Allografts, on the other hand, are associated with prolonged healing times and higher pseudoarthrosis rates. Without instrumentation, nonunion rates and collapse are higher for allograft than autograft in multilevel discectomies and arthrodeses. Fusion rates appear to be similar for a one-level fusion between allograft and autograft (14). In 1991, Zdeblick and Ducker reported on 87 patients who underwent 60 autograft and 27 allograft

ACDFs, with resolution of pain in 95% of the autograft group and 93% of the allograft group. In patients who underwent a one-level ACDF, there was no difference in the fusion rates. In two-level procedures, the allograft group had a significantly lower fusion rate (38% versus 83%). In both cases, more collapse was noted with allograft.

The rate of nonunion increases as the number of levels arthrodesed increases (10–14,42). This has led to the increased use of instrumentation over time. With the addition of a cervical plate in a multilevel construct, fusion rates appear to increase for allograft and autograft, although we are aware of no data from prospective randomized trials (47–50). With internal fixation, the period of postoperative external immobilization may also be truncated. Conversely, instrumentation increases operative time and costs and subjects the patient to hardware complications such as loosening and failure. Placement of anterior cervical plates requires greater soft tissue retraction, which may increase the risk for dysphagia and dysphonia. Plates may lead to stress shielding of the involved vertebrae and possibly increase the stress on adjacent segments.

ANTERIOR CERVICAL CORPECTOMY AND FUSION

ACDF provides decompression that is limited to the intervertebral disc space. It also has the drawback of decreasing fusion rates in multilevel cases. Thus, in patients with multilevel spondylotic disease in which compression occurs beyond the disc space and dorsal to the vertebral body, removal of the vertebral body may be necessary to gain adequate decompression.

Surgical Technique

Preoperative assessment of voluntary neck range of motion is important in determining the amount of neck extension that can be safely used during intubation and the surgical procedure. In highly stenotic patients or in those for whom symptoms are magnified by moderate extension, fiberoptic intubation is recommended. Gardner-Wells tongs may be useful in providing intraoperative traction and is recommended when kyphosis is present. Next, a standard left-sided anterior cervical approach is carried out. Although a transverse incision may be acceptable for a one- or two-level corpectomy, a longitudinal incision should be considered for a more extensive decompression. After the exposure, the midline can be marked superior and inferior to the intended levels of decompression to help maintain orientation as the decompression progresses. Typically, the longus colli muscles are elevated 2 to 3 mm laterally to allow placement of self-retaining retractors. The uncovertebral joints provide a good landmark to define the lateral borders. Dissection and decompression should not extend beyond the elevation of the longus colli to avoid injury to the vertebral artery.

First, discectomies are carried out at all of the involved levels (Fig. 76.35). Next, a Leksell rongeur is used to create a trough in the central part of the body. The trough is widened and deepened with a 5-mm high speed bur (Figs. 76.36 and 76.37). Judicious use of bone wax can help control the bleeding and improve visualization. In severely spondylotic patients, destruction of typical landmarks and increased vertebral artery tortuosity increase the risk for vertebral artery injury during lateral decompression (51). Vaccaro and colleagues demonstrated that a 19-mm wide central decompression can be carried out at C6 with a 5-mm safety margin to the foramen transversarium (52). To maintain this safety margin, only a 15-mm central decompression could be carried out at C3. A preoperative CT myelogram or MRI is useful for surgical planning and to assess the course of the vertebral arteries.

After the posterior cortex is thinned, a small curette is used to breach the cortex along the lateral portion of the trough. This opening is then enlarged with small curettes and 1- to 2-mm Kerrison rongeurs to remove all of the remaining bone. It is important always to elevate the bone away from the dura and the compressed spinal cord. The corpectomy trough should be at least 16 mm wide to provide adequate decompression (53). Routine removal of the PLL is not necessary unless ossification of the ligament is noted to be compressing the cord. Because of the risk for an absent dura in severe OPLL, leaving small isolated islands of OPLL has been described to avoid a large defect in the dura (54).

After the decompression has been completed and verified, the defect is stabilized with a structural graft. The use

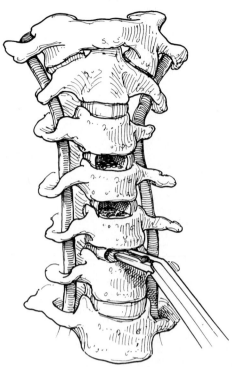

Disc removal, anteroposterior view

FIG. 76.35. Discectomy is performed at all involved levels. (From Sherk HH, Larson SJ, eds. *The cervical spine: an atlas of surgical techniques.* Philadelphia: JB Lippincott, 1999:201, with permission.)

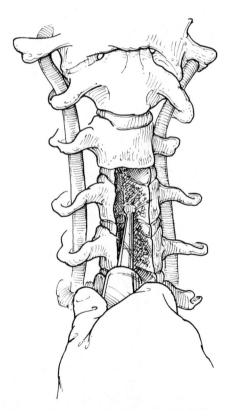

FIG. 76.36. Anteroposterior view of the high-speed burr creating the corpectomy trough. (From Sherk HH, Larson SJ, eds. *The cervical spine: an atlas of surgical techniques.* Philadelphia: JB Lippincott, 1999:204, with permission.)

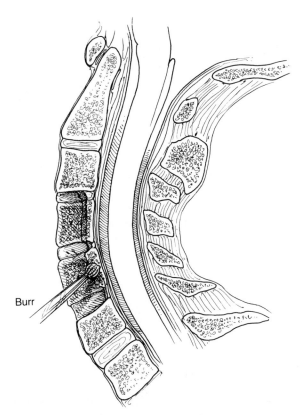

FIG. 76.37. Lateral view of the high-speed burr creating the corpectomy trough. (From Sherk HH, Larson SJ, eds. *The cervical spine: an atlas of surgical techniques.* Philadelphia: JB Lippincott, 1999:191, with permission.)

of a structural autograft, such as an autogenous fibula or a large iliac crest strut, is decreasing because of donor site morbidity. Other options include cages packed with autogenous cancellous bone graft (55,56).

At this point, a cervical plate may be added to provide a more rigid construct in addition to providing a physical block to graft extrusion. Biomechanical studies have confirmed the increased stiffness after addition of an anterior plate to a multilevel corpectomy model (57–59). Although a rigid plate decreases the graft force in flexion, it increases the force in extension compared with the graft construct without a plate. According to the *in vitro* study by Isomi and associates, the stability afforded by the plate may decrease with fatigue loading, and this may explain the increased rate of hardware failure in multilevel constructs (60,61). For multilevel constructs, failure is noted both clinically and biomechanically, most often at the caudal end of the construct (62,63). Consequently, some authors have advocated the use of a small inferior antikick plate. Early reports have noted graft extrusions with this method, and the use of this plate is not recommended (64,65). The most recent proposed solution is the use of a dynamic plate. The idea is that a dynamic plate provides stability while allowing the graft-plate construct to settle and thus maintains contact between the graft and the end plates. In an *in vitro* study performed

by Brodke and colleagues, dynamic cervical plates load share more effectively than locked plates in the setting of 10% graft subsidence (66). This may lead to improved graft healing rates. Clinical data on these dynamic plates are still lacking.

During a corpectomy, the time of soft tissue retraction should be minimized to decrease the prevalence of dysphagia and dysphonia, which are the two most frequent complaints after the procedure. It may be useful to release retraction of soft tissues for a short period of time if a long retraction time is anticipated. Meticulous hemostasis should be obtained to decrease the risk for a postoperative hematoma and respiratory difficulty.

With the addition of instrumentation, a firm cervical collar is used postoperatively for 6 to 12 weeks. Without instrumentation, a halo should be considered for increased external immobilization to protect the graft during healing. Long-term follow-up, including periodic flexion-extension radiographs, is recommended to assess graft incorporation, particularly when allograft is used.

Grafting Techniques

Many options exist for grafting the corpectomy defect. Both fibular shaft and the iliac crest are viable options for one- and two-level corpectomy. The anatomy of the fibular shaft is better suited for the larger corpectomy defects. Whitecloud and LaRocca described the H graft to prevent graft dislodgment in the larger corpectomy defects (67). The superior and inferior end plates of the vertebral bodies to be arthrodesed, as well as both ends of the fibular strut, are notched (Fig. 76.38). By extension of the neck, the notched fibular strut can be delivered into the notched end plates and locked into place by flexing the neck (Fig. 76.39). One cortex of the fibular strut remains anterior to the arthrodesed vertebral bodies with this technique. Postoperatively, extension is avoided to prevent extrusion of the graft.

One variation of this technique is to notch the end plates only, leaving the fibular graft intact without notching. The fibula is delivered into the notched end plates with the neck in extension and is locked into place by flexing the neck (68). Thus, the graft comes to lie recessed entirely within the end plates, unlike the H graft. A 5-mm depth should be achieved in seating the graft, especially at the inferior end plate. The disadvantage of notching the end plates is the loss of structural support from the end plate, leading to graft collapse. If the end plates are maintained to prevent collapse with the graft only relying on the interference fit with the end plates, a higher graft migration rate may be expected. When a cervical plate is added to a one- or two-level corpectomy defect, a lordotic graft may be fashioned and tamped into place flush against the decorticated end plates without notching.

In all cases, traction can be used to assist placement of the graft. Traction is especially useful in reconstruction of a kyphotic cervical spine. Both preoperative and intraoperative traction may be useful to correct the deformity.

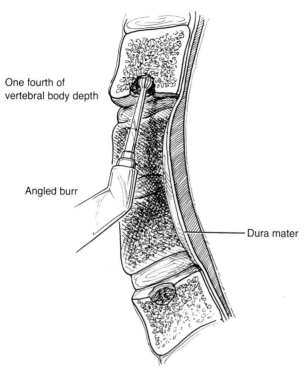

FIG. 76.38. Lateral view demonstrating the notching of vertebral endplates for graft placement. (From Sherk HH, Larson SJ, eds. *The cervical spine: an atlas of surgical techniques.* Philadelphia: JB Lippincott, 1999:206, with permission.)

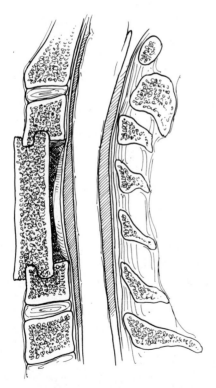

FIG. 76.39. Final position of the H graft. (From Sherk HH, Larson SJ, eds. *The cervical spine: an atlas of surgical techniques.* Philadelphia: JB Lippincott, 1999:209, with permission.)

Results

After an ACCF, satisfactory results can be expected in 75% to 90% of patients (16,69–73). In 1984, Boni and associates reported 53% good results and 39% moderate results in 29 patients undergoing ACCF (73). Three or more levels were decompressed in all cases, and iliac crest autograft was used in this study. In 1986, Hanai and co-workers reported 100% satisfaction in 30 patients with an improvement in the mean JOA score from 8.9 to 13.9 after an ACCF (74). In 1987, Bernard and Whitecloud reported at least one Nurick functional grade improvement in 76% of 21 patients (70). They had performed three or more levels of decompression and stabilization with a fibular autograft in all cases. Outcome was inferior in those patients with symptoms for more than 1 year and a high-grade preoperative disability.

In 1998, Emory and associates reported a 2- to 17-year follow-up of patients who underwent either discectomy or corpectomy along with fusion for myelopathy (12). Of the 87 patients with a preoperative motor deficit, 62% noted complete recovery. Thirty percent had a partial recovery. Thirteen of the 16 pseudoarthroses were in patients undergoing multilevel discectomies. Only 1 patient with an autologous fibular strut had a nonunion. Only 1 patient (1%) worsened after surgery, and 6 (6%) remained unchanged.

In 2002, Hilibrand and colleagues reported a retrospective study of 190 patients undergoing two or more disc levels with either ACDF or ACCF using autogenous bone grafting without instrumentation (74). The fusion rate was 93% in the ACCF group versus 66% in the ACDF group. However, the higher fusion rate was at the cost of 10% graft dislodgment or extrusion rate. Eight percent of patients in the ACCF group required a revision for graft complications, compared with none in the ACDF group. Good and excellent results were reported in 88% of patients with ACCF and 84% of patients with ACDF. Pseudoarthrosis did correlate with a poorer clinical outcome in this study.

With arthrodesis procedures, just as in fracture healing, nonunion and clinical failure rates increase in smokers (75). Elderly patients undergoing anterior cervical procedures for myelopathy likely have some level of degeneration at the adjacent disc levels. Degeneration at adjacent levels may be accelerated by a solid fusion, resulting in the deterioration of the long-term results of decompression and arthrodesis. Within 10 years, as many as 25% of patients may develop significant degenerative changes adjacent to a cervical fusion (76). These patients often respond to nonoperative treatment. Those that fail nonoperative treatment can be successfully treated with extension of the arthrodesis anteriorly to the degenerated level (77).

SUMMARY

Once the decision is made to pursue surgical intervention for myelopathy, the patient's clinical presentation and radiographic findings must be matched to the risks and benefits of each surgical option. Isolated disc pathology at one, two, or three levels is often best treated with an ACDF. ACCF should be considered for patients with abnormalities that extend beyond the disc level and in those with three contiguous levels of abnormality. Posterior approaches should be considered in patients with three or more levels of stenosis, particularly in those with global conditions, such as continuous OPLL or congenital stenosis. Posterior approaches should not be performed in those with a kyphotic neck. Overall, anterior decompression and arthrodesis is a safe procedure with a high rate of pain relief, neurologic recovery, and functional improvement.

REFERENCES

1. Simeone FA, Dillin W. Treatment of cervical disc disease. Selection of operative approach. *Contemporary Neurosurgery* 1986;8:1–6.
2. Brown MD. The pathophysiology of disc disease. *Orthop Clin North Am* 1971;2:359–370.
3. DePalma AF, Rothman RH. *The intervertebral disc.* Philadelphia: WB Saunders, 1970:37–38.
4. Epstein JA, Epstein NE. The surgical management of cervical spinal stenosis, spondylosis and myeloradiculopathy by means of the posterior approach. In: Sherk HH, eds. *The cervical spine,* 2nd ed. Philadelphia: JB Lippincott, 1989:625–643.
5. Lees F, Turner JWA. Natural history and prognosis of cervical spondylosis. *BMJ* 1963;2:1607–1610.
6. Nurick S. The natural history and the results of surgical treatment of the spinal cord disorder associated with cervical spondylosis. *Brain* 1972;95:101–105.
7. Ono K, Ota H, Tada K, et al. Cervical myelopathy secondary to multiple spondylotic protrusions. *Spine* 1977;2:218.
8. Fujiwara K, Yonenobu K, Ebara S, et al. The prognosis of surgery for cervical compression myelopathy. *J Bone Joint Surg Br* 1985;71:393–398.
9. Okada K, Shiraski N, Hayashi H, et al. Treatment of cervical spondylotic myelopathy by enlargement of the spinal canal anteriorly, followed by arthrodesis. *J Bone Joint Surg Am* 1991;73:352–364.
10. Bohlman HH, Emery SE, Goodfellow DB, et al. Robinson anterior cervical discectomy and arthrodesis for cervical radiculopathy: long term followup of one hundred and twenty two patients. *J Bone Joint Surg* 1992;75:1298–1307.
11. Emery SE, Fisher JR, Bohlman HH. Three-level anterior cervical discectomy and fusion: radiographic and clinical results. *Spine* 1999;22:2622–2624.
12. Emery SE, Bohlman HH, Bolesta MJ, et al. Anterior cervical decompression and arthrodesis for the treatment of cervical spondylotic myelopathy. Two to seventeen year follow-up. *J Bone Joint Surg* 1998;80:941–951.
13. Robinson RA, Walker AE, Ferlic DC, et al. The results of anterior interbody fusion of the cervical spine. *J Bone Joint Surg* 1962;44:1569–1587.
14. Zdeblick TA, Ducker TB. The use of freeze-dried allograft bone for anterior cervical fusions. *Spine* 1991;16:726–729.
15. Herkowitz H. A comparison of anterior cervical fusion, cervical laminectomy, and cervical laminoplasty for the surgical management of multiple level spondylotic radiculopathy. *Spine* 1988;13:774.
16. Herkowitz H. The surgical management of cervical spondylotic radiculopathy and myelopathy. *Clin Orthop* 1989;239:94.
17. Wilson DH, Campbell DD. Anterior cervical discectomy without bone graft. *J Neurosurg* 1977;47:551–555.
18. Benini A, Krayenbuhl H, Bruder R. Anterior cervical discectomy without fusion. Microsurgical technique. *Acta Neurochir* 1982;61:105–110.
19. Hukuda S, Mochizuki T, Ogata M, et al. Operations for cervical spondylotic myelopathy. *J Bone Joint Surg Br* 1985;67:609–615.
20. Smith GW, Robinson RA. The treatment of certain cervical spine disorders by anterior removal of the intervertebral disc and interbody fusion. *J Bone Joint Surg Am* 1958;40:607–624.
21. Albert TJ, Smith MD, Bressler E, et al. An in vivo analysis of the dimensional changes of the neuroforamen after anterior cervical diskectomy and fusion. A radiologic investigation. *J Spinal Disord* 1997;10(3):229–233.
22. Bayley JC, Yoo JU, Kruger DM, et al. The role of distraction in improving the space available for the cord in cervical spondylosis. *Spine* 1995;20(7):771–775.
23. Murphy MA, Trimble MB, Piedmonte MR, et al. Changes in the cervical foraminal area after anterior discectomy with and without a graft. *Neurosurgery* 1994;24(1):93–96.
24. Bohlman H. Cervical spondylosis with moderate to severe myelopathy. *Spine* 1977;2:151–162.
25. Connelly ES, Seymour RJ, Adams JE. Clinical evaluation of anterior cervical fusions for degenerative cervical disc disease. *J Neurosurg* 1965;23:431–437.
26. Netterville JL, Koriwchak MJ, Winkle M, et al. Vocal fold paralysis following the anterior approach to the cervical spine. *Ann Otol Rhinol Laryngol* 1996;105:85–91.
27. Weisberg NK, Spengler DM, Netterville JL. Stretch-induced nerve injury as a cause of paralysis secondary to the anterior cervical approach. *Otolaryngol Head Neck Surg* 1997;116:317–326.
28. Beutler WJ, Colleen A, Sweeney MA, et al. Recurrent laryngeal nerve injury with anterior cervical spine surgery. *Spine* 2001;26(12):1337–1342.
29. Heeneman H. Vocal cord paralysis following approaches to the anterior cervical spine. *Laryngoscope* 1973;83:17–21.
30. Moepeth JF, Williams MF. Vocal fold paralysis after anterior cervical diskectomy and fusion. *Laryngoscope* 2000;110(1):43–46.
31. An HS, Evanich CJ, Nowicki BH, et al. Ideal thickness of Smith-Robinson graft for anterior cervical fusion. A cadaveric study with computed tomographic correlation. *Spine* 1993;18:2043–2047.
32. Bohlman H. Degenerative arthrosis of the lower cervical spine. In: Evarts CM, ed. *Surgery of the muskuloskeletal system,* 2nd ed. New York: Churchill Livingstone, 1983:25–55.
33. Olsewski JM, Garvey TA, Schendel MJ. Biomechanical analysis of facet and graft loading in Smith-Robinson type cervical spine model. *Spine* 1994;19:2540–2544.
34. Kurz LT, Herkowitz HN. Surgical management of myelopathy. *Orthop Clin North Am* 1992;23:495–504.
35. Cloward RB. The anterior approach for removal of ruptured cervical discs. *J Neurosurg* 1958;15:602–614.
36. Bailey RW, Badgley CE. Stabilization of the cervical spine by anterior fusion. *J Bone Joint Surg Am* 1960;42:565–594.
37. Simmons EH, Bhalla SK. Anterior cervical discectomy and fusion (Keystone Technique). *J Bone Joint Surg Br* 1969;51:225–237.
38. White A, Hirsch C. An experimental study of the immediate load bearing capacity of some commonly used iliac bone grafts. *Acta Orthop Scand* 1971;42:482–490.
39. Wittenberg RH, Moeller J, Shea M, et al. Compressive strength of autologous and allogenous bone grafts for thoracolumbar and cervical spine fusion. *Spine* 1990;15:1073–1078.
40. Nurick S. The pathogenesis of the spinal cord disorder associated with cervical spondylosis. *Brain* 1972;95:87–100.
41. Hirabayashi K, Miyakawa J, Satomi K, et al. Operative results and postoperative progression of ossification among patients with ossification of cervical posterior longitudinal ligament. *Spine* 1981;6:354–364.
42. DePalma AF, Rothman RH, Lewinnek G, et al. Anterior interbody fusion for severe cervical disc degeneration. *Surg Gynecol Obstet* 1972;134:755–758.
43. Zhang Z, Yin H, Yang K, et al. Anterior intervertebral disc excision and bone grafting in cervical spondylotic myelopathy. *Spine* 1983;8:16–19.
44. Kadoya S, Nakamura T, Kwak R. A microsurgical anterior osteophytectomy for cervical spondylotic myelopathy. *Spine* 1984;9:437–441.
45. Yang KC, Lu XS, Cai QL, et al. Cervical spondylotic myelopathy treated by anterior multilevel decompression and fusion. *Clin Orthop* 1987;221:161–164.
46. Kurz LT, Garfin SR, Booth R. Harvesting autogenous iliac bone graft. A review of complications and techniques. *Spine* 1993;14:1324–1331.
47. Geer CP, Papadopoulos SM. The argument for single-level anterior cervical discectomy and fusion with anterior plate fixation. *Clin Neurosurg* 1999;45:25–29.
48. Bose B. Anterior cervical instrumentation enhances fusion rates in multilevel reconstruction in smokers. *J Spinal Disord* 2001;14:3–9.

49. Wang JC, McDonough PW, Kanim LE, et al. Increased fusion rates with cervical plating for two-level anterior cervical discectomy and fusion. *Spine* 2000;25:41–45.

50. Wang JC, McDonough PW, Kanim LE, et al. Increased fusion rates with cervical plating for three-level anterior cervical discectomy and fusion. *Spine* 2001;26:643–646.

51. Oga M, Yuge I, Terada K, et al. Tortuosity of the vertebral artery in patients with cervical spondylotic myelopathy. Risk factor for the vertebral artery injury during anterior cervical decompression. *Spine* 1996;21(9):1085–1089.

52. Vaccaro A, Ring D, Seuderi G, et al. Vertebral artery location in relation to the vertebral artery as determined by two-dimensional computed tomography evaluation. *Spine* 1994;19;2637.

53. Goto S, Mochizuki M, Watanabe T, et al. Long term follow up study of anterior surgery for cervical spondylotic myelopathy with special reference to the magnetic resonance imaging findings in 52 cases. *Clin Orthop* 1993;291:142–153.

54. Epstein N. The surgical management of ossification of the posterior longitudinal ligament in 51 patients. *J Spinal Disord* 1993;6:432–455.

55. Majd ME, Vadhva M, Holt RT. Anterior cervical reconstruction using titanium cages with anterior plating. *Spine* 1999;24:1604–1610.

56. Iew KD, Rhee JM. The use of titanium mesh cages in the cervical spine. *Clin Orthop Relat Res* 2002;394:47–54.

57. DiAngelo DJ, Foley KT, Vossel KA, et al. Anterior cervical plating reverses load transfer through multilevel strut-grafts. *Spine* 2000;7:783–795.

58. Foley KT, DiAngelo DJ, Rampersaud R, et al. The in vitro effects of instrumentation on multilevel cervical strut-graft mechanisms. *Spine* 1999;24:2366–2376.

59. Wang J, Panjabi MM, Isomi T. The role of bone graft force in stabilizing the multilevel anterior cervical spine plate system. *Spine* 2000;13:1649–1654.

60. Isomi T, Panjabi M, Wang J, et al. Stabilizing potential of anterior cervical plates in multilevel corpectomies. *Spine* 1999;24:2219–2223.

61. Vaccaro AR, Falatyn SP, Scuderi GJ, et. al. Early failure of long segment anterior cervical plate fixation. *J Spinal Disord* 1998;11:410–415.

62. Lowery GL, McDonough RF. The significance of hardware failure in anterior cervical plate fixation: patients with 2- to 7-year follow up. *Spine* 1998;23:181–187.

63. Panjabi MM, Isomi T, Wang J. Loosening at the screw-vertebrae junction in multilevel anterior cervical plate constructs. Spine 1999;22:2383–2388.

64. MacDonald RL, Fehlings MG, Tator CH, et al. Multilevel anterior cervical corpectomy and fibular allograft fusion for cervical myelopathy. *J Neurosurg* 1997;86:990–997.

65. Riew KD, Sethi NS, Devney J, et al. Complications of buttress plate stabilization of cervical corpectomy. *Spine* 1999;24:2404–2410.

66. Brodke DS, Gollogly S, Alexander M, et al. Dynamic cervical plates: biomechanical evaluation of load sharing and stiffness. *Spine* 2001;26:1324–1329.

67. Whitecloud T, LaRocca H. Fibular strut graft in reconstructive surgery of the cervical spine. *Spine* 1976;1:33.

68. Zdeblick T, Bohlman H. Myelopathy, cervical kyphosis and treatment by anterior corpectomy and strut grafting. *J Bone Joint Surg Am* 1989;71:170.

69. Bernard TN, Whitecloud TS. Cervical spondylotic myelopathy and myeloradiculopathy. Anterior decompression and stabilization with autogenous fibula strut graft. *Clin Orthop* 1987;221:149–160.

70. Flynn T. Neurologic complications of anterior cervical interbody fusion. *Spine* 1982;7:536.

71. Saunders R, Bernini P, Shireffs T, et al. Central corpectomy for cervical spondylotic myelopathy. A consecutive series with long-term follow-up evaluation. *J Neurosurg* 1991;74:163.

72. Boni M, Cherubino P, Benazzo F. Multiple subtotal somatectomy. Technique and evaluation of a series of thirty-nine cases. *Spine* 1984;9:358–362.

73. Hanai K, Fujiyoshi F, Kamei K. Subtotal vertebrectomy and spinal fusion for cervical spondylotic myelopathy. *Spine* 1986;11:310–315.

74. Hilibrand AS, Fye MA, Emery SE, et al. Increased rate of arthrodesis with strut grafting after multilevel anterior cervical decompression. *Spine* 2002;27:146–151.

75. Hilibrand AS, Fye MA, Emery SE, et al. Impact of smoking on the outcome of anterior cervical arthrodesis with interbody or strut grafting. *J Bone Joint Surg* 2001;83(5):668–673.

76. Hilibrand AS, Carlson GD, Palumbo MA, et al. Radiculopathy and myelopathy at segments adjacent to the site of a previous anterior cervical arthrodesis. *J Bone Joint Surg* 1999;81(4):519–528.

77. Hilibrand AS, Yoo JU, Carlson GD, et al. The success of anterior cervical arthrodesis adjacent to a previous fusion. *Spine* 1997;22(14):1574–1579.

CHAPTER 77

Approach to the Cervical Spine: Anterior versus Posterior Indications

Sanford E. Emery

Operative procedures for degenerative disorders of the cervical spine generally include one or more of the following surgical goals: (a) decompress impinged neural structures, either nerve root or spinal cord; (b) maintain or provide stability; and (c) maintain or correct alignment. These surgical efforts are designed to achieve the clinical goals of decreasing pain, correcting neurologic deficits, and improving patient function. These surgical and clinical goals can often be met by an anterior, posterior, or circumferential (360-degree) approach to the spine.

Some patients are candidates for either type of procedure, and some are best treated by one approach and not the other. The surgeon's choice will primarily depend on (a) the pathoanatomy of the individual patient; (b) the relative success of the chosen approach for achieving the goals of surgery, given the specific pathoanatomy; (c) the relative risk for complications (short and long term) accompanying each approach; (d) the patient's symptoms; and (e) the surgeon's experience. These factors relate to guidelines used to assist the surgeon in choosing the best surgical treatment option for his or her patient.

CERVICAL RADICULOPATHY

The pathoanatomy of cervical radiculopathy is root compression, usually from a soft disc herniation or cervical spondylosis. The latter can cause root impingement due to a hard disc, uncovertebral hypertrophy, or hypertrophic posterior facet joints. Surgical options for cervical radiculopathy typically comprise anterior cervical discectomy and fusion (ACDF) or laminoforaminotomy with discectomy.

The best candidates for ACDF techniques include patients in whom cord impingement requires an anterior approach for safe and adequate decompression (Fig. 77.1A). Posterior approaches cannot directly remove anterior abnormalities because the spinal cord cannot be retracted without incurring iatrogenic deficits. Given the same reasoning, patients with lateral soft disc herniations may be excellent candidates for laminotomy and discectomy (Fig. 77.1B) because no cord retraction is needed to retrieve a lateral disc fragment. This avoids the short-term risks for nonunion and the longer-term risks for adjacent segment degeneration that exist with arthrodesis procedures.

Aldrich in 1990 (1) published a series of 36 patients treated with microsurgical laminoforaminotomy techniques for lateral disc herniations. These patients had severe radicular pain and usually weakness, mild neck pain, and a herniated disc fragment lateral to the dural sac. Sequestered fragments were removed after a laminotomy, and the dura was not retracted, nor was the disc entered. Clinical results were excellent, with a follow-up range of 4 to 42 months and mean of 26 months. The author stressed the success of this approach for lateral disc herniations, as opposed to central or paracentral compressive lesions that might best be approached anteriorly. Similar conclusions and recommendations were published by Zeidman and Ducker in their larger series of 172 patients (2). Excellent results have been reported by other authors using a posterior foraminotomy-discectomy approach (1–4) or even laminoplasty (5). Patients with significant cervical spondylosis have also been successfully treated with posterior foraminotomies (2,6,7). These spondylotic patients, however, typically have preoperative axial pain symptoms, and I believe they may be better served with anterior discectomy and fusion. This option restores disc space height, opens the foramen, and relieves pain from the spondylotic motion segment (8–11).

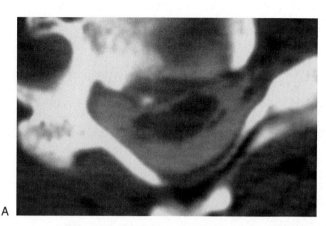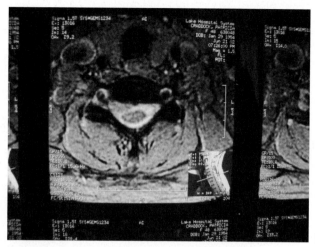

FIG. 77.1. A: This computed tomography myelogram demonstrates typical spondylotic changes of disc material and osteophytic ridging producing posterolateral compression on the spinal cord. This pathology is too medial to be removed through a posterior approach and would best be treated with anterior decompression and arthrodesis. **B:** This transverse magnetic resonance imaging slice shows a lateral soft disc herniation that caused severe C7 root compression in this patient. Note that there is no cord deformation because of the far lateral position of the herniation. This patient is an excellent candidate for laminoforaminotomy and excision of the disc fragment.

CERVICAL MYELOPATHY AND STENOSIS

Patients with multilevel degenerative changes or ossification of the posterior longitudinal ligament (OPLL) can develop cervical stenosis. This may be severe enough to produce the clinical syndrome of myelopathy. Typically, this manifests as gait disturbance, weakness, numbness, long tract signs, or any combination of the above. Radicular symptoms with pain may be present as well. The underlying pathoanatomy is usually hard disc herniations with osteophytes or OPLL, either of which may be complicated by kyphosis or subluxation at one or more levels. These patients are the focus of most discussions for anterior versus posterior surgical approaches to treat disorders of the cervical spine. Options include corpectomies with strut grafting, laminoplasty, laminectomy, laminectomy with arthrodesis fusion, or a combination of anterior and posterior approaches for a circumferential decompression and stabilization. Simple, right?

The decision-making factors involved in reaching a surgical treatment plan for this patient population involve several aspects of the pathoanatomy present in the cervical spine. Planning also involves to some degree the patient's preoperative symptoms, such as the presence of significant axial neck pain. The pathoanatomy is perhaps more compelling in that a relative contraindication to one approach may exist and become the determining factor in choice of approach. Here are some of the most important considerations:

1. What is the overall sagittal alignment of the cervical spine? Is there normal lordosis? Is the spine straight or kyphotic? If kyphotic, how much? Is it mild (10 degrees or less), moderate, or severe kyphosis? Patients with nor-

mal lordosis or at least a straight cervical spine are potential candidates for laminoplasty; however, as kyphosis increases, the anterior approach becomes a better option. If kyphosis is severe, circumferential approaches may be preferable. If the kyphosis is very flexible, a posterior approach alone with arthrodesis may suffice, given more rigid instrumentation systems available today.

2. How many levels are involved? Will two disc levels need to be addressed (i.e., a one-level corpectomy), or would a three- or four-level corpectomy need to be performed if an anterior approach is chosen? As an anterior strut graft gets longer, the risk for graft dislodgment increases; thus, patients needing long decompressions may do better with a posterior approach if the other pieces of the puzzle fit. Patients considered for three- or four-level corpectomy procedures with strut grafting may be better candidates for circumferential arthrodesis.

3. Is there static subluxation evident on plain films? Is there dynamic subluxation evident on flexion-extension views? Any demonstrable instability would exclude laminectomy alone as an option and arguably tip the scales in favor of arthrodesis as part of the procedure.

4. What is the pathoanatomic picture of the spinal cord compression? Does the patient have congenital narrowing of the spinal canal with diffuse stenosis from C3 to C7? This pattern typically produces flattening of the cord anteriorly and circumferential narrowing, which responds well to laminoplasty. Or is there more focal anterior compression of the cord from a disc herniation or osteophyte producing a kidney bean–shaped deformation of the cord, which would best be decompressed through an anterior approach? This question requires

high-quality neuroradiologic imaging with magnetic resonance imaging (MRI) or often computed tomography (CT) myelography for finer detail.

5. What is the patient's bone quality? Anterior grafts are at higher risk in extremely osteoporotic patients. This may weigh in favor of a posterior approach or a circumferential procedure to achieve the goals for that patient.

ADVANTAGES AND DISADVANTAGES OF SURGICAL APPROACHES

Anterior Corpectomies and Strut Grafting

Anterior cervical corpectomy procedures evolved through the 1980s and have become a significant advance in the treatment of cord compression and myelopathy in the cervical spine. As neuroradiologic imaging became more advanced with CT and then MRI, the pathology causing spinal cord compression became clearer. Typically, cord compression in this patient population is caused by anterior structures such as disc herniations, central and uncovertebral osteophytes, and OPLL (12). Anterior corpectomies provide a very direct approach to this anterior cord compression and allow removal of the offending pathology (Fig. 77.2). Neurologic recovery or improvement typically occurs in the 80% to 90% of patients with myelopathy following anterior decompression and arthrodesis (13–18). Not only does an anterior approach allow for direct decompression of the canal centrally, but also removal of uncovertebral spurs can successfully treat radicular symptoms (13).

The other main advantage of anterior corpectomies with strut grafting is arthrodesis of the spine. This treats any instability and prevents late kyphosis. It also allows for correction of preoperative kyphosis. Small amounts of residual cervical kyphosis (≤10 degrees) in my experience have not been a clinical problem. However, more severe sagittal deformity typically produces neck pain and could logically contribute to adjacent segment instability.

Another potential advantage of corpectomies with arthrodesis relates to postoperative pain relief. Arthrodesis does not give a patient a new cervical spine, but studies have shown good pain relief after decompression and arthrodesis, particularly in the patient with cervical spondylotic myelopathy (15,16,19). Patients with long segmental or continuous OPLL are stiff and nearly autofused and do not appear to have the preoperative pain levels of many patients with degenerative spondylosis.

The relative disadvantages of anterior corpectomies and strut grafting include the technical demands of the procedure. This is particularly true with multilevel corpectomies and patients with OPLL. Although the abnormal bone and disc material that is compressing the cord is lifted up and away from the dura in a no-touch technique, great care is still needed to avoid inadvertent manipulation or pressure on the already compromised cord. This is certainly true in severe cases of myelopathy in which a ribbon-like cord is present. Severe OPLL can ossify the dura and lead to spinal fluid leakage (20). This can be problematic, requiring fascial patching and lumbar cerebrospinal fluid drainage. With appropriate training and experience, these intraoperative problems are uncommon but certainly enter into the decision-making process regarding choice of approach.

The most common problem with anterior corpectomy and strut grafting concerns graft complications (15,20–23). The use of strut graft requires meticulous technique to sculpt the docking sites and the graft itself. This minimizes complications; however, dislodgment or nonunion is still a potential problem. Displaced grafts typically fracture the inferior vertebrae and displace anteriorly. This usually requires revision surgery. The quality of the vertebra body bone is very important in minimizing these complications and is a significant factor in decision making, as mentioned earlier. Patients with prior multisegment laminectomies have a high rate of graft dislodgment (24); although the use of anterior plating alone has been reported (25), these patients may best be treated by circumferential arthrodesis.

Other disadvantages of the anterior approach with arthrodesis include the need for postoperative airway monitoring (26,27), postoperative bracing, and loss of motion. As instrumentation has improved, bracing requirements have lessened, but some restrictive orthosis is needed for long strut graft procedures. Fusions provide stability, but there is some risk for adjacent segment degeneration (28). Whether this risk is greater than the natural history of disc degeneration in and of itself is not totally clear, but it seems logical to assume there is some increased stress at adjacent levels above or below stiffened segments. This probably is of more concern in the younger patient with a congenitally narrow canal as opposed to the octogenarian with a stiff spine who would be at lower risk for long-term adjacent segment problems.

Posterior Approach

One major advantage of posterior solutions for cervical stenosis and myelopathy include the relative degree of technical difficulty for the surgeon. It is often easier and faster to perform a laminoplasty, laminectomy, or even a laminectomy plus arthrodesis compared with a multilevel anterior corpectomy and strut grafting. This is especially true in large, heavy patients with thick necks. There should also be less of a risk for any spinal fluid leakage in OPLL patients using a posterior approach. This is not to say that these procedures are easy or should be taken lightly; a great deal of skill and training are certainly a requirement, and neurological complications (such as C5 root palsies) are possible. Relatively speaking, however, posterior procedures are less demanding for multilevel pathology. Perhaps the greatest advantage is that these approaches avoid the potential graft complications present in strut grafting procedures (Fig. 77.3).

A significant disadvantage of multilevel laminectomy procedures is the risk for postlaminectomy kyphosis. A

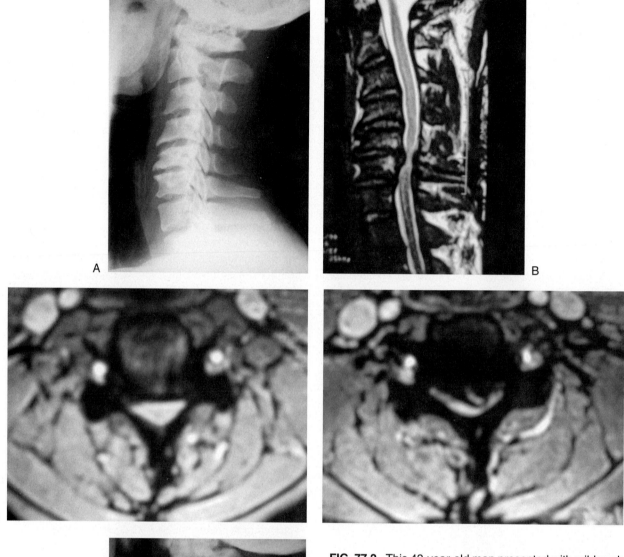

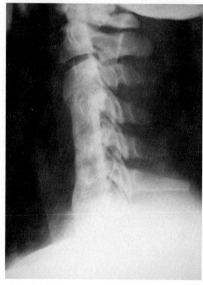

FIG. 77.2. This 43-year-old man presented with mild neck pain and evidence of severe myelopathy with marked gait disturbance, bilateral upper extremity weakness, unilateral leg weakness, and spasticity evident on exam. **A:** This lateral plain film demonstrates mild cervical kyphosis with severe spondylotic changes. The patient has severe disc narrowing and posterior osteophytes at multiple levels along with a narrow spinal canal. **B:** The patient's sagittal magnetic resonance imaging study shows the cord draped over the posterior osteophytes and disc material with the kyphotic deformity. **C, D:** Two cross sections at C4-C5 and C5-C6 show severe anterior deformation of the spinal cord. **E:** The patient underwent a three-level anterior cervical corpectomy and autogenous fibular strut grafting from C3 to C7. An anterior approach alone was used, and the patient was treated postoperatively in a two-poster-type brace. This postoperative lateral plain film shows correction of the kyphosis to neutral and a healed graft. The patient's pain is relieved and his myelopathy has improved to the point of normal function.

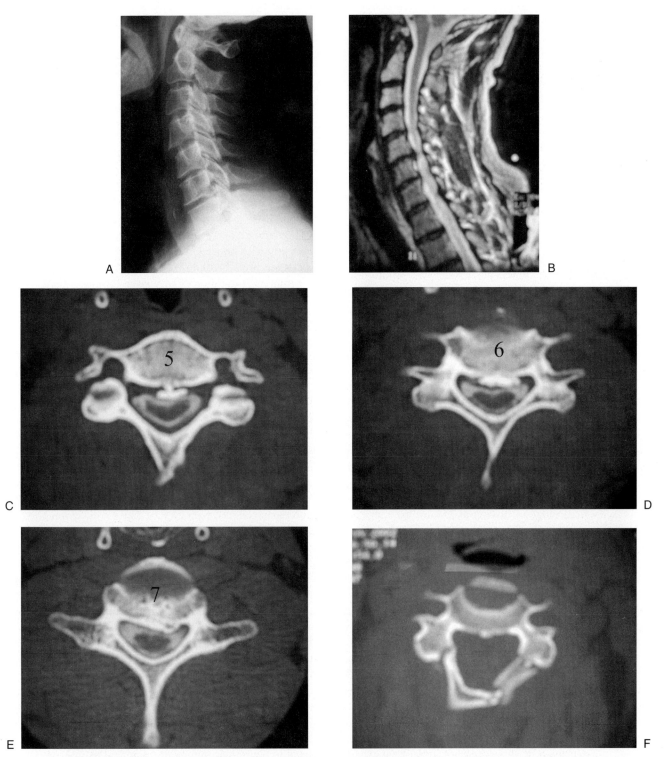

FIG. 77.3. This 50-year-old man had symptoms of gait disturbance, numbness, and weakness. He had evidence of cervical myelopathy on physical examination. He had no neck pain and no radiculopathy. **A:** This lateral plain film shows some mild to moderate cervical spondylotic changes with normal lordosis. **B:** The patient's sagittal magnetic resonance imaging study shows diffuse canal stenosis over multiple levels with a moderate disc protrusion at C5-C6. He has some evidence of myelomalacia. **C–E:** These three transverse cuts of the patient's computed tomography (CT) myelogram taken sequentially at C5, C6, and C7 show cord compression from segmental ossification of the posterior longitudinal ligament (OPLL). **F:** The patient's postoperative CT scan, taken after the patient underwent a C3 to C7 laminoplasty procedure, demonstrates the canal expansion with the bone graft in place to maintain the open-hinged trap door. The patient has recovered from his myelopathy and has not developed neck pain in the postoperative period.

consistent percentage of patients who are expected to have this complication is difficult to document in the literature, probably because of slightly different patient populations (e.g., OPLL versus spondylosis), different degrees of facet resection, and the long-term nature of the problem. Several authors have discussed the problem of postlaminectomy kyphosis (29,30) as well as the related complication of late neurologic deterioration (31). Laminoplasty techniques were developed in part to avoid postlaminectomy kyphosis (32). Although an improvement, laminoplasty does not appear to eliminate the risk for postoperative kyphosis. Inone and colleagues noted that about 10% of their patients with cervical spondylotic myelopathy developed increasing kyphosis after laminoplasty at an average postoperative follow-up of 8 years, although many of these individuals had some preoperative kyphosis (33). A similar percentage was reported by Yonenobu and associates after laminoplasty (23). Baba and coworkers noted that a higher prevalence (35%) of their patients developed kyphosis postoperatively, although without neurologic sequelae (34).

Decreased range of motion has been noted in nearly all series of patients after laminoplasty, although controversy exists about whether this is a problem or benefit. Kimura and colleagues (35), Morio and associates (36), and others (37) believe that less motion will be beneficial to existing myelopathy symptoms and perhaps prevent late deterioration. Other authors stress the importance of preserving motion in patients (38,39). A longer-term follow-up study by Satomi and associates documented a steady decrease in cervical range of motion over several years, with final range of motion at 35% of preoperative values (40). Although motion decreased, clinical deterioration did not occur.

The limitations of laminoplasty or laminectomy are largely related to the pathoanatomic factors to be considered in the decision-making process. Because the compressive abnormality is usually anterior, posterior approaches are an indirect method of decompressing the spinal canal. It is necessary for the spinal cord to be able to translate posteriorly to relieve pressure and allow for functional recovery. Spinal cord compression will persist in a patient with preoperative cervical kyphosis even after a laminoplasty or laminectomy because the cord will be draped over discs, osteophytes, and vertebral bodies and remain compressed. If the deformity is flexible, then a posterior laminectomy and arthrodesis of the patient in extension will allow the cord to drift backward, allowing a better chance of success. Preoperative instability or subluxation may worsen after a posterior decompression procedure alone such as laminectomy or laminoplasty, and laminectomy plus posterior fusion may be the treatment of choice. Although the rate of spinal cord injury in posterior approaches for treating stenosis should be extremely low, the problem of C5 nerve root palsies is higher after laminoplasty (41) than after anterior decompression procedures.

Combined Anterior and Posterior Approaches

The use of combined approaches to the cervical spine can minimize some of the disadvantages of either an anterior or posterior approach alone, while maintaining the potential advantages of each method. A multilevel anterior corpectomy and strut grafting procedure followed by a posterior arthrodesis will allow for direct decompression of the canal, correction of deformity, treatment of axial pain symptoms, and limitation of potential graft complications by the rigidity of an instrumented posterior arthrodesis fusion. This decreases postoperative bracing requirements as well and should essentially eliminate the risk for pseudarthrosis. It is, however, a bigger procedure for the patient to tolerate in this often elderly population. Time between the anterior and posterior procedures ("flip time") must be added to the setup time, breakdown time, and operative duration to quantitate the duration of anesthesia for that patient.

SUMMARY

Although no randomized surgical trial comparing anterior versus posterior operative treatment of cervical myelopathy or myeloradiculopathy exists that I am aware of, several studies have looked at their experience using these two approaches. Herkowitz in 1988 (7) compared anterior interbody fusion, laminectomy, and laminoplasty in patients with multilevel radiculopathy from cervical spondylosis. The results showed anterior decompression and fusion similar to laminoplasty in good to excellent outcomes (92% versus 86%). Laminectomy procedures were less successful (66% good to excellent), with 25% of patients developing kyphosis within 2 years after surgery. Hukuda and associates (42) reported on 191 cases of spondylotic myelopathy. Anterior arthrodesis procedures were a mix of Cloward-type and Smith-Robinson-type interbody arthrodeses, with a small number of subtotal spondylectomies. Twelve patients had laminectomies, and 13 underwent laminoplasties. Their anterior arthrodesis was better for symptoms involving arm pain with pathology over one or two levels, and posterior procedures were best for trunk and leg symptoms plus three-level or more pathology. Edwards and associates (43) recently looked at matched cohorts of patients with cervical myelopathy who underwent multilevel corpectomy or laminoplasty procedures. Although the groups were small (13 patients in each), similar improvement was noted with respect to neurologic symptoms, gait, and pain. Analgesic requirements were statistically greater for arthrodesis patients at follow-up. More perioperative complications were noted in the anterior arthrodesis group as well. Sagittal motion decreased 57% after arthrodesis and 38% after laminoplasty. The authors favored laminoplasty as their procedure of choice for multilevel cervical myelopathy in the absence of kyphosis. Tani and coworkers (44) retrospectively compared anterior subtotal corpectomy procedures with laminoplasty in the treatment of myelopathy from massive OPLL. Four of 12 patients undergoing laminoplasty had postoperative cord deficits that improved but did not resolve. They recommended the anterior approach for this subset of OPLL patients.

Yonenobu and others at his institution compared anterior and posterior approaches in several articles. In 1985, they reported on 91 patients treated by either laminectomy, anterior interbody fusion, or subtotal corpectomy procedures (30). Subtotal spondylectomy fared better and was recommended for three disc levels or less, whereas extensive laminectomy was preferred for four disc levels or more. In 1992, Yonenobu and colleagues reviewed subtotal corpectomy patients treated from 1976 to 1983 and laminoplasty patients treated after 1984 (23). Neurologic recovery was similar for both groups. Some patients developed radiographic instability after laminoplasty, but were not symptomatic. C5 root palsies did occur after laminoplasty in 7% of patients, but all recovered. Twelve patients (29%) in the corpectomy population had perioperative complications, 10 of which were graft related. Laminoplasty was thought to provide satisfactory neural recovery with less perioperative morbidity. Iwasaki and coworkers (45) from the same institution published a series comparing laminoplasty to anterior discectomy and fusion for soft disc herniations causing myeloradiculopathy. Both approaches were equally effective, but the anterior fusion patients again had more complications. Hosono and associates (46) compared 72 patients having laminoplasty with 26 patients having subtotal corpectomy and strut grafting, focusing more on pain outcomes than in their earlier work. Postoperative axial (neck or shoulder) pain symptoms were significantly higher after laminoplasty (60%) than after anterior fusion (19%). Wada and coworkers (47), again from Osaka University, reexamined their subtotal corpectomy and laminoplasty groups for spondylotic myelopathy with 10- to 14-year follow-up. Again, neurologic recovery remained equivalent for both approaches. Anterior arthrodesis patients had some graft-related complications, including symptomatic pseudarthroses. Axial neck pain was more prevalent in the laminoplasty group (40%) than the arthrodesis group (15%). Range of motion was reduced 49% for the arthrodesis patients and more for the laminoplasty patients (69%). In-

creased degenerative changes were noted at adjacent levels in the anterior arthrodesis patients, but only one patient needed surgery for recurrent myelopathy.

These studies suggest that for appropriately selected patients, either anterior corpectomies with strut grafting or posterior laminoplasty can successfully treat myelopathy. Although many of the benefits are similar, each approach has its own set of potential short- and long-term risks. The major advantages and disadvantages of anterior or posterior approaches to treat cervical stenosis and myelopathy are summarized in Table 77.1. As described earlier, however, there are many factors to consider in this decision, including the surgeon's confidence and expertise with a given approach or technique. Clinical and surgical judgment are always needed in patient selection for the treatment approach, and in many cases, either approach will achieve good clinical outcomes. For me, the ideal candidate for anterior corpectomies and strut grafting is a patient with focal anterior cord compression as opposed to generalized congenital stenosis; one or two corpectomy levels; a neutral or kyphotic sagittal alignment; preoperative subluxation; and significant preoperative axial neck pain. The ideal candidate for a laminoplasty would be someone with normal lordosis, no instability, generalized canal stenosis over multiple levels, ossification of the posterior longitudinal ligament, and mild preoperative neck pain. An arthrodesis can be added if the patient has a flexible deformity that can be held in extension by posterior instrumentation and bone grafting, or if multiple anterior procedures preclude safe access from another anterior approach (Fig. 77.4). The ideal candidates for a combined anterior and posterior procedure include patients with osteoporosis who require a multilevel anterior approach (Fig. 77.5); postlaminectomy patients; some patients with three-level corpectomies and any four-level corpectomy procedures; those with moderate to severe preoperative kyphotic deformity; and patients who are difficult to brace secondary to obesity or immobility. These "ideal" candidates represent guidelines to think about the options for any given patient. The fact that we have options in treating this patient population should be considered a positive feature rather than a frustration for our subspecialty. These guidelines certainly will (and should) evolve over time as clinical experience and research accumulate.

TABLE 77.1. *Advantages and Disadvantages of Anterior and Posterior Approaches*

	Advantages	Disadvantages
Anterior Approach	1. Direct decompression 2. Stabilization with arthrodesis 3. Correction of deformity 4. Axial lengthening of spinal column 5. Good axial pain relief	1. Technically demanding 2. Graft complications 3. Need for postoperative bracing 4. Loss of motion 5. Adjacent segment degeneration
Posterior Approach	1. Less loss of motion 2. Not as technically demanding 3. Less bracing needed 4. Avoids graft complications	1. Indirect decompression 2. Preoperative kyphosis and/or instability limitations 3. Inconsistent axial pain results 4. Late instability

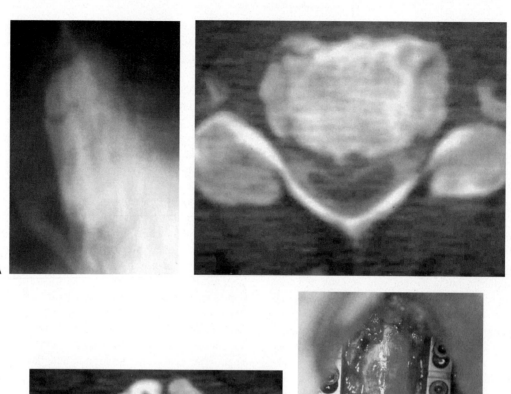

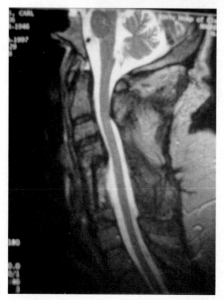

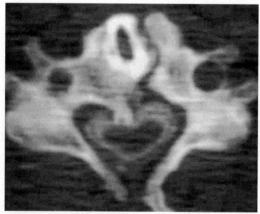

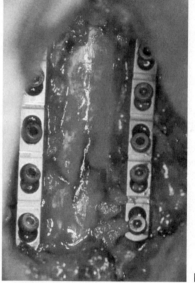

FIG. 77.4. This 48-year-old man presented with persistent neck pain and cervical myelopathy. He had undergone multiple anterior procedures elsewhere and still had a nonunion of an anterior strut graft, a contracted longitudinal right-sided scar, a thick bull-neck, and a postoperative unilateral vocal cord paralysis. **A:** This lateral tomogram shows the nonunion of the superior pole of the fibula strut graft. **B:** This transverse cut of the computed tomography (CT) myelogram just above the attempted decompression shows persistent spinal cord deformation. **C:** This transverse CT myelogram cut shows an area of inadequate decompression from the prior anterior approaches. Given the multiple anterior attempts, vocal cord paralysis, nonunion, and the patient's body habitus, the decision was made to salvage this patient posteriorly with a multilevel laminectomy and fusion with lateral mass plating. **D:** This intraoperative photograph demonstrates the exposed dura after the laminectomy with the lateral mass plates visible bilaterally. **E:** A postoperative magnetic resonance imaging study demonstrates satisfactory decompression of the cord. The patient's myelopathy improved, but his hand numbness and some pain symptoms persisted.

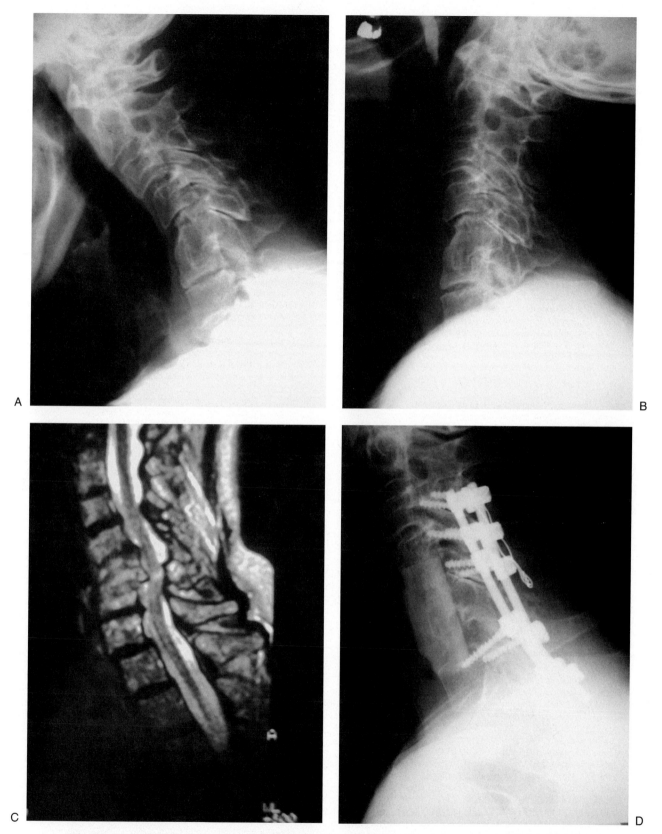

FIG. 77.5. An 82-year-old woman, otherwise healthy, presented with neck pain and frank myelopathy. Ambulation required use of a walker. **A, B:** The lateral plain film flexion and extension views demonstrate cervical kyphosis and compensatory subluxation. The patient has relative osteoporosis. **C:** The sagittal magnetic resonance imaging study shows severe compression, particularly behind the vertebral body just below the subluxation. Myelomalacia changes are evident. Because of the osteoporosis, moderately severe kyphosis and instability, we opted for a circumferential approach. The patient underwent a two-level anterior cervical corpectomy, allograft fibular strut grafting, and same-day posterior instrumentation and fusion from C3 to T1. She has done well postoperatively with resolution of her pain and myelopathy.

REFERENCES

1. Aldrich F. Posterolateral microdiscectomy for cervical monoradiculopathy caused by posterolateral soft cervical disc sequestration. *J Neurosurg* 1990;72:370–377.
2. Zeidman SM, Ducker TB. Posterior cervical laminoforaminotomy for radiculopathy: review of 172 cases. *Neurosurgery* 1993;33:356–362.
3. Henderson CM, Hennessy RG, Shuey HM Jr, et al. Posterior-lateral foraminotomy as an exclusive operative technique for cervical radiculopathy: a review of 846 consecutively operated cases. *Neurosurgery* 1983;13:504–512.
4. Herkowitz HN, Kurz LT, Overholt DP. Surgical management of cervical soft disc herniation: a comparison between the anterior and posterior approach. *Spine* 1990;15:1026–1030.
5. Herkowitz HN. Cervical laminaplasty: its role in the treatment of cervical radiculopathy. *J Spinal Disord* 1988;1:179–188.
6. Grieve JP, Kitchen ND, Moore AJ, et al. Results of posterior cervical foraminotomy for treatment of cervical spondylotic radiculopathy. *Br J Neurosurg* 2000;14:40–43.
7. Herkowitz HN. A comparison of anterior cervical fusion, cervical laminectomy, and cervical laminoplasty for the surgical management of multiple level spondylotic radiculopathy. *Spine* 1988;13:774–780.
8. Bohlman HH, Emery SE, Goodfellow DB, et al. Robinson anterior cervical discectomy and arthrodesis for cervical radiculopathy: long-term follow-up of one hundred and twenty-two patients. *J Bone Joint Surg Am* 1993;75:1298–1307.
9. Gore DR, Sepic SB. Anterior cervical fusion for degenerated or protruded discs: a review of one hundred forty-six patients. *Spine* 1984;9:667–671.
10. Shapiro S, Connolly P, Donnaldson J, et al. Cadaveric fibula, locking plate, and allogeneic bone matrix for anterior cervical fusions after cervical discectomy for radiculopathy or myelopathy. *J Neurosurg* 2001;95:43–50.
11. Wang JC, McDonough PW, Endow KK, et al. Increased fusion rates with cervical plating for two-level anterior cervical discectomy and fusion. *Spine* 2000;25:41–45.
12. Bohlman HH, Emery SE. The pathophysiology of cervical spondylosis and myelopathy. *Spine* 1988;13:843–846.
13. Bernard TN Jr, Whitecloud TS. Cervical spondylotic myelopathy and myeloradiculopathy: anterior decompression and stabilization with autogenous fibula strut graft. *Clin Orthop* 1987;221:149–160.
14. Chiles BW, Leonard MA, Choudhri HF, et al. Cervical spondylotic myelopathy: patterns of neurological deficit and recovery after anterior cervical decompression. *Neurosurgery* 1999;44:762–770.
15. Emery SE, Bohlman HH, Bolesta MJ, et al. Anterior cervical decompression and arthrodesis for the treatment of cervical spondylotic myelopathy: two to seventeen-year follow-up. *J Bone Joint Surg Am* 1998;80A:941–951.
16. Hanai K, Fujiyoshi F, Kamei K. Subtotal vertebrectomy and spinal fusion for cervical spondylotic myelopathy. *Spine* 1986;11:310–315.
17. Okada K, Shirasaki N, Hayashi H, et al. Treatment of cervical spondylotic myelopathy by enlargement of the spinal canal anteriorly, followed by arthrodesis. *J Bone Joint Surg Am* 1991;73:352–364.
18. Saunders RL, Bernini PM, Shirreffs TG, et al. Central corpectomy for cervical spondylotic myelopathy: a consecutive series with long-term follow-up evaluation. *J Neurosurg* 1991;74:163–170.
19. Mayr MT, Subach BR, Comey CH, et al. Cervical spinal stenosis: outcome after anterior corpectomy, allograft reconstruction, and instrumentation. *J Neurosurg* (Spine 1) 2002;96:10–16.
20. Smith MD, Bolesta MJ, Leventhal M, et al. Postoperative cerebrospinal-fluid fistula associated with erosion of the dura: findings after anterior resection of ossification of the posterior longitudinal ligament in the cervical spine. *J Bone Joint Surg Am* 1992;74:270–277.
21. MacDonald RL, Fehlings MG, Tator CH, et al. Multilevel anterior cervical corpectomy and fibular allograft fusion for cervical myelopathy. *J Neurosurg* 1997;86:990–997.
22. Vaccaro AR, Falatyn SP, Scuderi GJ, et al. Early failure of long segment anterior cervical plate fixation. *J Spinal Disord* 1998;11:410–415.
23. Yonenobu K, Hosono N, Iwasaki M, et al. Laminoplasty versus subtotal corpectomy: a comparative study of results in multisegmental cervical spondylotic myelopathy. *Spine* 1992;17:1281–1284.
24. Riew KD, Hilibrand AS, Palumbo MA, et al. Anterior cervical corpectomy in patients previously managed with a laminectomy: short-term complications. *J Bone Joint Surg Am* 1999;81:950–957.
25. Herman JM, Sonntag VK. Cervical corpectomy and plate fixation for postlaminectomy kyphosis. *J Neurosurg* 1994;80:963–970.
26. Emery SE, Smith MD, Bohlman HH. Upper-airway obstruction after multilevel cervical corpectomy for myelopathy. *J Bone Joint Surg Am* 1991;73:544–551.
27. Epstein NE, Hollingsworth R, Nardi D, et al. Can airway complications following multilevel anterior cervical surgery be avoided? *J Neurosurg* 2001;94:185–188.
28. Hilibrand AS, Carlson GD, Palumbo MA, et al. Radiculopathy and myelopathy at segments adjacent to the site of a previous anterior cervical arthrodesis. *J Bone Joint Surg Am* 1999;81:519–528.
29. Albert TJ, Vacarro A. Postlaminectomy kyphosis. *Spine* 1998;24:2738–2745.
30. Yonenobu K, Fuji T, Ono K, et al. Choice of surgical treatment for multisegmental cervical spondylotic myelopathy. *Spine* 1985;10:710–716.
31. Yonenobu K, Okada K, Fuji T, et al. Causes of neurologic deterioration following surgical treatment of cervical myelopathy. *Spine* 1986;11:818–823.
32. Hirabayashi K, Satomi K. Operative procedure and results of expansive open-door laminoplasty. *Spine* 1988;13:870–876.
33. Inoue H, Ohmori K, Ishida Y, et al. Long-term follow-up review of suspension laminotomy for cervical compression myelopathy. *J Neurosurg* 1996;85:817–823.
34. Baba H, Maezawa Y, Furusawa N, et al. Flexibility and alignment of the cervical spine after laminoplasty for spondylotic myelopathy: a radiographic study. *Int Orthop* 1995;19:116–121.
35. Kimura I, Shingu H, Nasu Y. Long-term follow-up of cervical spondylotic myelopathy treated by canal-expansive laminoplasty. *J Bone Joint Surg Br* 1995;77:956–961.
36. Morio Y, Yamamoto K, Teshima R, et al. Clinicoradiologic study of cervical laminoplasty with posterolateral fusion or bone graft. *Spine* 2000;25:190–196.
37. Yoshida M, Otani K, Shibasaki K, et al. Expansive laminoplasty with reattachment of spinous process and extensor musculature for cervical myelopathy. *Spine* 1992;17:491–497.
38. Morimoto T, Matsuyama T, Hirabayashi H, et al. Expansive laminoplasty for multilevel cervical OPLL. *J Spinal Disord* 1997;10:296–298.
39. Shaffrey CI, Wiggins GC, Piccirilli CB, et al. Modified open-door laminoplasty for treatment of neurological deficits in younger patients with congenital spinal stenosis: analysis of clinical and radiographic data. *J Neurosurg* 1999;90:170–177.
40. Satomi K, Nishu Y, Kohno T, et al. Long-term follow-up studies of open-door expansive laminoplasty for cervical stenotic myelopathy. *Spine* 1994;19:507–510.
41. Chiba K, Toyama Y, Matsumoto M, et al. Segmental motor paralysis after expansive open-door laminoplasty. *Spine* 2002;27:2108–2115.
42. Hukuda S, Mochizuki T, Ogata M, et al. Operations for cervical spondylotic myelopathy: a comparison of the results of anterior and posterior procedures. *J Bone Joint Surg Br* 1985;67:609–615.
43. Edwards CC, Heller JG, Murakami H. Corpectomy versus laminoplasty for multilevel cervical myelopathy: an independent matched-cohort analysis. *Spine* 2002;27:1168–1175.
44. Tani T, Ushida T, Ishida K, et al. Relative safety of anterior microsurgical decompression versus laminoplasty for cervical myelopathy with a massive ossified posterior longitudinal ligament. *Spine* 2002;27:2491–2498.
45. Iwasaki M, Ebara S, Miyamoto S, et al. Expansive laminoplasty for cervical radiculomyelopathy due to soft disc herniation: a comparative study of laminoplasty and anterior arthrodesis. *Spine* 1996;21:32–38.
46. Hosono N, Yonenobu K, Ono K. Neck and shoulder pain after laminoplasty: a noticeable complication. *Spine* 1996;21:1969–1973.
47. Wada E, Suzuki S, Kanazawa A, et al. Subtotal corpectomy versus laminoplasty for multilevel cervical spondylotic myelopathy: a long-term follow-up study over 10 years. *Spine* 2001;26:1443–1447.

CHAPTER 78

Ossification of the Posterior Longitudinal Ligaments: Prevalence, Presentation, and Natural History

Shunji Matsunaga and Takashi Sakou

Ossification of the posterior longitudinal ligament (OPLL) is a hyperostotic condition of the spine associated with severe neurologic deficit (1–5). This disease was first reported about 160 years ago (6). OPLL was previously considered specific to Asian peoples (7) and did not attract attention in Europe or the United States. However, because of reports that this disease occurs in white peoples (8–16) and that about half of patients with diffuse idiopathic skeletal hyperostosis (DISH), which is well known in Europe and the United States, had OPLL, this disease has come to be recognized as a subtype of DISH (17,18).

This chapter summarizes the prevalence of OPLL and clinical findings regarding this unique entity.

PREVALENCE

OPLL was found to occur in 1.5% to 2.4% (19–26) of adult outpatients with cervical disorders at several university hospitals in Japan (Table 78.1). In the same survey of foreign countries, the prevalence of OPLL was 0.4% to 3.0% in Asian countries (27–31). In a review of plain cervical spine films by Yamauchi (27,32) and Izawa (26), the prevalence of OPLL was 2.1% among Japanese patients (143 per 6,994), 1.0% in Koreans, 0.1% in North Americans, and 0.1% in Germans. A survey in Italy in 1984 by Terayama (33), however, revealed a high prevalence of OPLL (Table 78.2). Our survey in a Utah university hospital (34) revealed OPLL in the cervical spine in 8 of 599 subjects (1.3%).

To determine the actual incidence of OPLL in various countries around the world, an epidemiologic study of the general population has been encouraged. The incidence of OPLL in the general Japanese population was reported to be 1.9% to 4.3% (35–40) among people older than 30 years (Table 78.3). However, a few overseas studies have analyzed the general population. We performed an overseas study in Taiwan on 1,004 Chinese and 529 Takasago tribe people older than 30 years (41,42). The incidence of OPLL was 0.2% in Chinese and 0.4% in the Takasago tribe, evidently lower than that of Japanese people. Recently, Tomita and associates (43) carried out an epidemiologic study of OPLL in China involving 2,029 Chinese and 500 Mongolian people. According to this study, the prevalence of OPLL was 1.6% in Chinese and 1.8% in Mongolians.

Resnick et al. (17) reported DISH as a common disorder characterized by bone proliferation in axial and extraaxial sites. The most characteristic abnormalities in this condition are ligamentous calcification and ossification along the vertebral body (18). Changes in extraspinal locations are also frequent, including ligament and tendon calcification and ossification, paraarticular osteophytes, and bony excrescence at sites of ligament and tendon attachment to bone. In his study of a group of 74 patients with DISH, 37 (50%) patients had concomitant OPLL on cervical radiographs (44). A similar figure of OPLL in 43% of 40 patients with DISH was reported from France (45). Whereas DISH is a fairly common disease of the general population in whites older than 50 years, its frequent association with OPLL suggests that OPLL itself cannot be a rare disease in whites.

In 1992, Epstein proposed a new concept about OPLL (12). Epstein examined computed tomography scans of the cervical spine in whites and noted hypertrophy of the posterior longitudinal ligament with punctuate calcification. This finding was described as *ossification of the posterior longitudinal ligament in evolution* (OEV). Epstein noted that the

TABLE 78.1. *OPLL in Outpatient Clinic for Cervical Disorders in Japan*

Reporter		Location of survey	Subjects(n)	Age of subject	OPLL(n)	Incidence of OPLL (%)
Okamoto	(1967)[19]	Okayama	1,000	ND	21	2.1
Yanagi	(1967)[20]	Nagoya	1,300	>20	31	2.4
Onji et al.	(1967)[21]	Osaka	1,800	ND	31	1.7
Shinoda et al.	(1971)[22]	Sapporo	3,747	>10	55	1.5
Harata	(1976)[23]	Hirosaki	2,275	ND	33	1.5
Sakou et al.	(1978)[24]	Okinawa	1,969	>30	30	1.5
Kurihara et al.	(1978)[25]	Kobe	9,349	>15	183	2.0
Izawa	(1980)[26]	Tokyo	6,944	>20	143	2.1

Superscript figures indicate the reference number. n; number, ND; not detailed
(Reprinted with permission of Yonenobu K, Sakou T, Ono K: OPLL, First ed., Tokyo, Springer-Verlag, 1997, p13)

prevalence of OPLL among whites with cervical myelopathy has recently increased from 2% to 25% (46). Epidemiologic surveys of OPLL by Japanese researchers were done using plain radiographs of the cervical spine to detect the OPLL. Most Japanese researchers did not include OEV on their OPLL surveys. Furthermore, there is controversy about the definition of OPLL between Japanese researchers and North American researchers.

PRESENTATION

Several papers on the clinical characteristics of OPLL have been published (4,5,47–49). The clinical characteristics of patients with OPLL in papers of Japanese and foreign researchers have been similar. Terayama, member of the Investigation Committee on Ossification of the Spinal Ligaments of Japanese Ministry of Public Health and Welfare, et al. performed the first national survey of OPLL in 1975 (48). Investigators abstracted 880 hospitals, including university hospitals, for this survey, and 2,142 OPLL patients were registered. Based on the results of this survey, OPLL typically developed in patients older than 40

years and carried a male predominance of 2:1 to 3:1. The average age of onset was 51.2 years in men and 48.9 years in women. Sixty-seven percent of patients were 45 to 65 years old. Ninety-five percent of patients had some clinical symptoms, but 5% of patients were free of symptoms. Initial complaints typically consisted of cervical discomfort in conjunction with numbness of the upper extremity. The typically recognized symptoms of OPLL were as follows: sensory and motor dysfunction of upper and lower extremities, hyperreflexia of tendon reflexes, pathologic reflexes, and bladder dysfunction. As many as 16.8% of patients needed assistance in activities of daily living; 5.4% of patients showed a rapid aggravation of symptoms; and 11.4% of patients showed a chronic aggravation. Symptoms spontaneously appeared and continually progressed. Initial complaints typically consisted of cervical discomfort in conjunction with numbness or myeloradiculopathy, typically characterized by symmetric upper and lower extremity findings. In cases in which quadriparesis had rapidly evolved, sphincteric dysfunction was often also noted (49). As many as 9.7% of patients also had diabetes mellitus. As for the glucose tolerance test, 29% of patient showed

TABLE 78.2. *OPLL in Outpatient Clinic in the World*

	Reporter		Country	Subjects(n)	Age of subject	OPLL(n)	Incidence of OPLL (%)
Asia	Yamauchi	(1978)[27]	Korea	529	>20	5	1.0
	Kurokawa	(1978)[28]	Taiwan	395	>40	12	3.0
			Hong Kong	498	>40	2	0.4
	Yamaura et al.	(1978)[29]	Philippine	332	ND	5	1.5
	Tezuka	(1980)[30]	Taiwan	661	>20	14	2.1
	Lee et al.	(1991)[31]	Singapore	5,167	>30	43	0.8
Europe & USA	Yamauchi et al.	(1979)[32]	West Germany	1,060	>27	1	0.1
	Terayama and Ohtsuka	(1984)[33]	Italy	1,258	>35	22	1.7
	Izawa	(1980)[26]	U.S.A. (Minnesota)	840	>30	1	0.1
			U.S.A. (Hawaii)	490	>20	3	0.6
	Firoozmia et al.	(1982)[14]	U.S.A. (New York)	1,000	>20	7	0.7
	Ijiri et al.	(1996)[34]	U.S.A. (Utah)	599	>30	8	1.3

USA; United States of America, Superscript figures indicate the reference number. n; number, ND; not detailed

(Reprinted with permission of Yonenobu K, Sakou T, Ono K: OPLL, First ed., Tokyo, Springer-Verlag, 1997, p13)

TABLE 78.3. *Incidence of OPLL of General Population in Japan*

Reporter	Location of survey	Subjects (M, F)	Age of subjects	OPLL(n)	Incidence of OPLL (%)
Ikata and Sakou (1979)[35]	Tokushima	705 (330, 366)	>20	21	3.0
Ohtani et al. (1980)[36]	Yaeyama	1,046 (578,468)	>20	21	2.0
Yamauchi et al. (1982)[37]	Kamogawa	788 (408, 379)	>40	20	2.5
	Kofu	383 (169, 214)	>40	13	3.4
Sakou and Morimoto (1982)[38]	Kagoshima	585 (195, 390)	>30	11	1.9
Ohtsuka et al. (1984)[39]	Yachiho	1,058 (440, 618)	>50	34	3.2
Ikata et al. (1985)[40]	Tokushima	415 (122, 293)	>30	18	4.3

Superscript figures indicate the reference number. F, Female; M, Male; n, number
(Reprinted with permission of Yonenobu K, Sakou T, Ono K: OPLL, First ed., Tokyo, Springer-Verlag, 1997, p14)

diabetes mellitus pattern, and this prevalence was very high compared with that (5%) of an age-equivalent group without OPLL. Also, 23% of patients had a history of trauma to the cervical region. Trauma in the cervical spine may have precipitated the onset of symptoms, which, in some cases, included quadriparesis (50–52). However, the prevalence of trauma that caused symptoms was only 15% (48).

A genetic survey of OPLL patients has revealed a higher rate of occurrence among families (53,54). A nationwide survey in Japan of 347 families of OPLL, evaluated by Terayama (53,54), revealed that OPLL was radiographically detected in 24% of the second-degree or closer blood relatives and in 30% of OPLL patients' siblings. The authors looked at another 220 of the second-degree or closer blood relatives of 72 patients with OPLL and determined that 32 families (44%) were indeed predisposed to this condition (55). A nationwide study in Japan by the Committee, including 10 sets of twins (8 monozygotic twin pairs and 2 dizygotic twin pairs) who exhibited OPLL, was performed (56). Six of the 8 monozygotic twin pairs had OPLL. This suggested or implicated a genetic factor, contributing to the frequency of this disease amongst the twins. HLA (a human leukocyte antigen) haplotype analysis provides a useful means for studying genetic backgrounds of diseases and was performed in patients with OPLL (57). Specific HLA haplotype of OPLL could not be found in this study, but a very interesting finding was that if a sibling had both the

same haplotypes as the proband, the prevalence of OPLL was much higher than if the sibling had only one of the haplotypes the same as the proband (58). If neither of the haplotypes was seen in the proband, the occurrence was almost nil (Table 78.4). The HLA gene is located on the short arm of chromosome 6. DNA analysis was therefore performed in the region of HLA genes on chromosome 6. Genetic linkage evidence of the genetic susceptibility of OPLL mapped to the HLA complex of chromosome 6 by a nonparametric genetic linkage study with 91 affected sib-pairs with OPLL revealed that collagen α2(XI) is a candidate gene for OPLL (59,60).

OPLL was mostly found at the C4, C5, and C6 levels (Fig. 78.1). The level with the maximal thickness of OPLL was often C5. OPLL in the cervical spine may be radiographically classified into four types (49,58), based on the findings on a lateral radiograph: continuous, mixed, segmental, and other (Fig. 78.2). When ossification is interrupted at the intervertebral disc levels but continuous behind the vertebral bodies, this is characterized as segmental type.

TABLE 78.4. *Relationship Between the Share of Identical HLA Haplotypes and Existence of OPLL in 61 Siblings*

	Two strands identical (n = 19)	One strand identical (n = 21)	Not identical (n = 21)
OPLL	10 (53%)	5 (24%)	1 (5%)

*The percentage represents the rate of existence of OPLL on X-ray and CT in each group. The rate of existence of OPLL in two strands identical group is significantly higher than other two groups. (P<0.05)
OPLL, ossification of the posterior longitudinal ligament; HLA, human leukocyte antigen
Reprinted with permission from Shunji Matsunaga: *Spine,* 24:937–938, 1999, Lippincott Williams & Wilkins

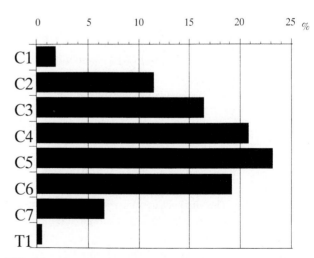

FIG. 78.1. Level of ossification of the posterior longitudinal ligament (OPLL); C1 to C7 represents the level of vertebral body of cervical spine, and T1 represents the level of the first thoracic spine. The percentages indicate the rates of OPLL in the vertebral levels, respectively.

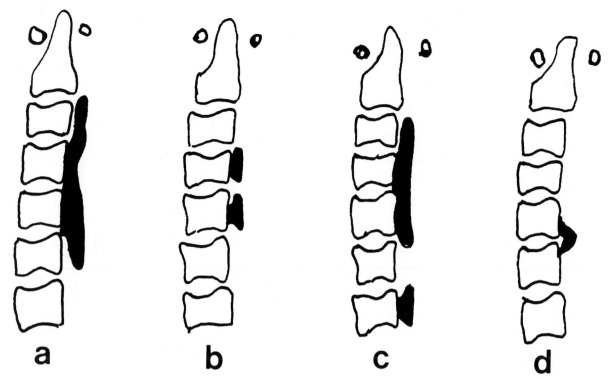

FIG. 78.2. Classification of ossification of the posterior longitudinal ligament (OPLL) by the Investigation Committee on the Ossification of the Spinal Ligaments, Japanese Ministry of Health and Welfare; *black areas* represent OPLL. **A:** Continuous type—ossification over several vertebral bodies continuously. **B:** Segmental type—interrupted ossification of one or more vertebral bodies. **C:** Mixed type—continuous-type ossification associated with segmental-type ossification. **D:** Other type—restricted ossification within the intervertebral disc level.

If ossification is not interrupted, this constitutes the continuous type. The mixed type is characterized by skip areas intervening between continuous and segmental types. A small ossification seen crossing the intervertebral disc space alone may alternatively be termed the "other" type. In the nationwide survey in Japan, the segmental type was recognized in 39%, continuous in 27%, mixed in 26%, and other in 7%. The sagittal diameter of the spinal canal is measured as the distance from the posterior aspect of the vertebral body to the anterior edge of the base of the spinous process on the lateral view. This distance is regarded as the anteroposterior diameter of the cervical canal. The percentage of the thickness of the ossification to the anteroposterior diameter of the spinal canal is then regarded as the spinal canal stenosis rate (Fig. 78.3). The maximum spinal canal stenosis rate, as determined at the thickest point of the ossified area, was 38% on average in cases with myelopathy and 27% in cases without myelopathy. The thickness of ossification was not always associated with the degree of neurologic dysfunction, that is, paralysis. Even if ossification is severe within the canal, neurologic symptoms are sometimes mild.

OPLL in the cervical spine is often accompanied by ossification in the thoracic or lumbar spine and may be complicated by ossification of the ligamentum flavum in the thoracic spine or ankylosing vertebral hyperostosis (61). In our series of 166 cases of OPLL in the cervical spine, 28 (17%) were complicated by thoracic OPLL and 85 (51%) by ossification of the ligamentum flavum in the thoracic or lumbar spine. Sixty-eight cases (41%) had radiographic features of ankylosing vertebral hyperostosis (stage II changes by Forestier classification, affecting more than

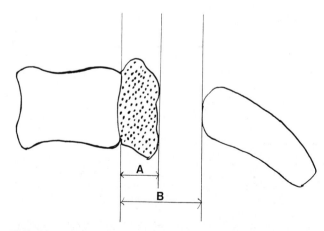

FIG. 78.3. The measurement of spinal canal stenosis rate; *dotted area* shows the ossification of the posterior longitudinal ligament. Spinal canal stenosis rate (%) equals A/B × 100.

three vertebral bodies). Furthermore, ligamentous ossification of hip and ankle joints may also be found in these individuals, suggesting that they are indeed systemically predisposed to diffuse ossification of ligaments.

OPLL is usually visible as a signal-free or low-signal area on MRI studies. However, hypointense, isointense, and hyperintense areas may also be noted in portions of ossified tissue (62), representing small medullary cavities actively involved in bone marrow production. Hypertrophy of the posterior longitudinal ligament has been evaluated using magnetic resonance imaging (MRI). A dilated signal-free area in the posterior aspect of the vertebral bodies is visible in some without OPLL. Some investigators considered this as an early sign of ligamentous hypertrophy preceding OPLL. Sakamoto et al. (63) compared MRI studies with histopathologic findings and noted that the dilated low-signal areas around the ossified lesion on T1-weighted images corresponded to ligamentous hypertrophy in conjunction with proliferating chondrocytes. A high-intensity area in the spinal cord on the T2-weighted images, observed in 25% to 45% patients with OPLL (64–66), likely corresponds to irreversible intrinsic changes within the cord, that is, myelomalacia (65). Abe et al. reported that myelopathy is most likely to be severe in instances in which such high signals are visualized within the cord (67).

Computed tomography (CT) provides an excellent axial view of the spinal canal, yielding valuable information concerning the ossified area and its median or paramedian location (Fig. 78.4). Three-dimensional CT studies

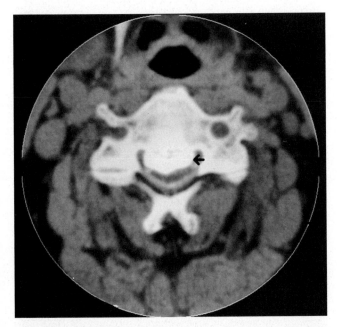

FIG. 78.4. Computed tomography (CT) associated with myelogram of patients with ossification of the posterior longitudinal ligament (OPLL). Remarkable OPLL *(arrow)* is recognized in the posterior site of the C4 vertebral body, and the spinal cord is compressed by this OPLL.

provide excellent documentation of the three-dimensional morphology of OPLL involving the cervical spinal canal. One may use these evaluations for operative planning for OPLL decompression (68).

NATURAL HISTORY

Few studies have prospectively evaluated the progression of OPLL. One hundred twelve patients with OPLL, who had been treated conservatively, were studied (75 men and 37 women) (69). They ranged in age from 27 to 78 years (mean, 54.5 years), and they were followed for 1 to 16.9 years. Progression of ossification in length was demonstrated in 24% of patients and in thickness, in 13% of patients in the group followed over 5 years. However, the amount of progression was small. The maximum progression in length was 43 mm over 10 years in one case of continuous OPLL (equivalent to the height of two vertebral bodies), and 3.4 mm in thickness. The type of ossification changed in some instances. The continuous type changed to the mixed type in three cases. The segmental type changed to the mixed type in three cases and to the continuous type in three cases, whereas the mixed type was altered to continuous type in one instance. In our biomechanical study, progression of OPLL was recognized at the site of increased strain in intervertebral disc (70). Progression of ossification did not always lead to exacerbation of symptoms, although there were some instances of worsening.

The course of ossification in 94 patients who had surgery was carefully followed. There were 75 men and 19 women included in this cohort, whose ages ranged from 23 to 79 years (mean, 54.8 years). Follow-up periods varied from 8.9 years for anterior decompressions and arthrodesis, 2.5 years for laminoplasties, and 6.6 years after laminectomy. Ossification progressed markedly and at a higher rate in laminectomy- (40%) and in laminoplasty-treated (35%) patients and appeared in relatively shorter intervals after these surgical procedures, that is, earliest within 2 months after surgery and most often within 6 months. The frequency of the ossification progression was shown to be higher in laminectomy- or laminoplasty-treated patients when compared with conservatively treated individuals (71,72). Possible explanations include (a) mechanical stress becoming increased in the cervical spine due to destruction of the posterior supportive elements, and (b) biologic stimulation produced by the laminoplasty or laminectomy.

The prognosis of patients with OPLL has generally been thought to be disappointing. The authors examined the natural course of this disease (73). In our recent personal study, a total of 450 patients, averaging 74.6 years of age at last evaluation, were prospectively followed for an average of 17.6 years (10 to 30 years) to discern the natural history of disease progression. Myelopathy was originally recognized in 127 patients, 91 of whom were managed surgically. The remaining 36 myelopathic patients were treated nonoperatively, and an increase in

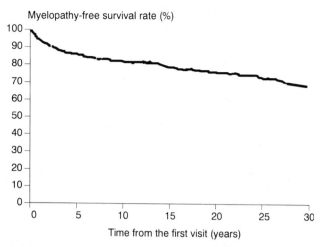

Myelopathy-free survival rate (%)

Time from the first visit (years)

FIG. 78.5. Kaplan-Meier estimate of myelopathy-free survival among patients who had no myelopathy at the first examination.

myelopathy was observed in 23 (65%) of these individuals. For the 323 patients without original myelopathy, 64 (20%) became myelopathic during the follow-up interval. The Kaplan-Meier estimates (74) of myelopathy-free survival among patients without myelopathy at the first visit was 71% at 30 years follow-up (Fig. 78.5). Forty-five patients with more than 60% of the spinal canal compromised by OPLL were all myelopathic. The range of motion of the cervical spine was calculated by dynamic x-rays. The range of motion was significantly larger in patients with myelopathy and with less than 60% of the canal compromised with OPLL (Table 78.5). Although myelopathy was recognized in all patients with more than 60% of the spinal canal compromised by OPLL, small OPLL at first examination rarely developed to large OPLL with more than 60% stenosis during the follow-up. Therefore, one cannot simply say that myelopathy develops with OPLL. Rather, dynamic factors (range of motion) appear to be very important for the evolution of myelopathy in patients with less than 60% of the canal compromised with OPLL (75). Data from this long-term prospective analysis indicate that prophylactic surgery for nonmyelopathic patients with OPLL may not be neces-

sary, particularly because the course of symptomatic progression appears milder than anticipated.

ACKNOWLEDGMENT

The presented studies were supported in part by a grant-in-aid for the Investigation Committee on the Ossification of the Spinal Ligaments of the Japanese Ministry of Public Health and Welfare.

REFERENCES

1. Bakay L, Cares HL, Smith RJ. Ossification in the region of the posterior longitudinal ligament as a cause of cervical myelopathy. *J Neurol Neurosurg Psychiatr* 1970;33:263–268.
2. Minagi H, Gronner AT. Calcification of the posterior longitudinal ligament: a cause of cervical myelopathy. *Am J Roentgenol* 1969;105:365–369.
3. Nagashima C. Cervical myelopathy due to ossification of the posterior longitudinal ligament. *J Neurosurg* 1972;37:653–660.
4. Ono K, Ota H, Tada K, et al. Ossified posterior longitudinal ligament. A clinicopathologic study. *Spine* 1977;2:126–38.
5. Tsuyama N. Ossification of the posterior longitudinal ligament of the spine. *Clin Orthop* 1984;184:71–84.
6. Key GA. On paraplegia depending on the ligament of the spine. *Guy Hosp Rep* 1838;3:17–34.
7. Matsunaga S, Sakou T. *Epidemiology of ossification of the posterior longitudinal ligament.* In: Yonenobu K, Sakou T, Ono K, eds. *OPLL.* Tokyo: Springer–Verlag, 1997:3–17
8. Hanna M, Watt I. Posterior longitudinal ligament calcification of the cervical spine. *Br J Radiol* 1979;52:901–905.
9. Wennekes MJ, Anten HWM, Korten JJ. Ossification of the posterior longitudinal ligament. *Clin Neurol Neurosurg* 1984;87:297–302.
10. Lecky BFR, Britton JA. Cervical myelopathy due to ossification of the posterior longitudinal ligament. *J Neurol Neurosurg Psychiatry* 1984;47:1355–1361.
11. Trojan DA, Pokrupa R, Ford RM, et al. Diagnosis and treatment of ossification of the posterior longitudinal ligament of the spine: report of eight cases and literature review. *Am J Med* 1992;92:296–306.
12. Epstein NE. Ossification of the posterior longitudinal ligament: diagnosis and surgical management. *Neurosurg Q* 1992;2:223–241.
13. Epstein NE. Ossification of the posterior longitudinal ligament in evolution in 12 patients. *Spine* 1994;19:673–681.
14. Firooznia H, Benjamin VM, Pinto RS, et al. Calcification and ossification of posterior longitudinal ligament of spine. Its role in secondary narrowing of spinal canal and cord compression. *NY State J Med* 1982;82:1193–1198.
15. Klara PM, McDonnel DE. Ossification of the posterior longitudinal ligament in Caucasians: diagnosis and surgical intervention. *Neurosurgery* 1986;19:212–217.
16. McAfee PC, Regan JJ, Bohlman HH. Cervical cord compression from ossification of the posterior longitudinal ligament in non-Orientals. *J Bone Joint Surg Br* 1987;69:569–573.
17. Resnick D, Shaul SR, Robinsons JM. Diffuse idiopathic skeletal hyperostosis (DISH): Forestier's disease with extraspinal manifestations. *Radiology* 1975;115:513–524.
18. Resnick D, Guerra J Jr, Robinson CA, et al. Association of diffuse idiopathic skeletal hyperostosis (DISH) and calcification and ossification of the posterior longitudinal ligament. *Am J Roentgenol* 1978;131:1049–1053.
19. Okamoto Y. Ossification of the posterior longitudinal ligament of cervical spine with or without myelopathy. J Jpn Orthop Assoc 1967;40:1349–1360.
20. Onji Y, Akiyama H, Shimomura Y, et al. Posterior paravertebral ossification causing cervical myelopathy: a report of eighteen cases. *J Bone Joint Surg Am* 1967;49:1314–1328.
21. Yanagi T, Yamamura Y, Andou K, et al. Ossification of the posterior longitudinal ligament in the cervical spine: a clinical and radiological analysis of thirty-seven cases [in Japanese]. *Rinsho Shinkei* 1977;7:727–735.

TABLE 78.5. *Range of Motion of Cervical Spine in Patients with Less Than 60% of the Spinal Canal by OPLL*

	With myelopathy (n = 111)	Without myelopathy (n = 93)	P value
Range of motion of cervical spine (degree)	51 ± 17.5	39 ± 9.5	<0.01

Results are expressed as mean ±SD. OPLL, ossification od the posterior longitudinal ligament

22. Shinoda Y, Hanzawa S, Nonaka K, et al. Ossification of the posterior longitudinal ligament [in Japanese]. *Seikeigeka* 1971;22:383–391.
23. Harata S. Research report on ossification of the posterior longitudinal ligament [in Japanese]. *Investigation Committee 1975 report on the ossification of the spinal ligaments of the Japanese Ministry of Public Health and Welfare,* 1976:43–48.
24. Sakou T, Tomimura K, Maehara T, et al. Epidemiological study of ossification of the posterior longitudinal ligament in the cervical spine in Okinawa prefecture [in Japanese]. *Investigation Committee 1977 report on the ossification of the spinal ligaments of the Japanese Ministry of Public Health and Welfare,* 1978:172–173.
25. Kurihara A, Kataoka O, Maeda A, et al. Clinical picture and course of the ossification of posterior longitudinal ligament of the cervical spines [in Japanese]. *Seikeigeka* 1978;29:745–751.
26. Izawa K. Comparative radiographic study on the incidence of ossification of the cervical spine among Japanese, Koreans, Americans, and Germans [in Japanese]. *J Jpn Orthop Assoc* 1980;54:461–474.
27. Yamauchi H. Epidemiological and pathological study of ossification of the posterior longitudinal ligament of the cervical spine [in Japanese]. *Investigation Committee 1977 report on the ossification of the spinal ligaments of the Japanese Ministry of Public Health and Welfare,* 1978: 21–25.
28. Kurokawa T . Prevalence of ossification of the posterior longitudinal ligament of the cervical spine in Taiwan, Hong Kong, and Singapore [in Japanese]. *Investigation Committee 1977 report on the ossification of the spinal ligaments of the Japanese Ministry of Public Health and Welfare,* 1978:8–9.
29. Yamaura I, Kamikozuru M, Shinomiya K. Therapeutic modalities and epidemiological study of ossification of the posterior longitudinal ligament of the cervical spine [in Japanese]. *Investigation Committee report on the ossification of the spinal ligaments of the Japanese Ministry of Public Health and Welfare,* 1978:18–20.
30. Tezuka S. Epidemiological study of ossification of the posterior longitudinal ligament of the cervical spine in Taiwan [in Japanese]. *Investigation Committee 1977 report on the ossification of the spinal ligaments of the Japanese Ministry of Public Health and Welfare,* 1980:19–23.
31. Lee T, Chacha PB, Orth MCh, et al. Ossification of posterior longitudinal ligament of the cervical spine in non-Japanese Asians. *Surg Neurol* 1991;35:40–44.
32. Yamauchi H Izawa K, Sasaki K, et al. Radiological examination by plain film of the cervical spine in West Germany [in Japanese]. *Investigation Committee 1978 report on the ossification of the spinal ligaments of the Japanese Ministry of Public Health and Welfare,* 1979:22–23.
33. Terayama K, Ohtsuka Y. Epidemiological study of ossification of the posterior longitudinal ligament on Bologna in Italy [in Japanese]. *Investigation Committee 1983 report on the ossification of the spinal ligaments of the Japanese Ministry of Public Health and Welfare* 1984 ;55–62.
34. Ijiri K, Sakou T, Taketomi E, et al. Epidemiological study of ossification of posterior longitudinal ligament in Utah [in Japanese]. *Investigation Committee 1995 report on the ossification of the spinal ligaments of the Japanese Ministry of Public Health and Welfare,* 1996:24–25.
35. Ikata T, Tezuka S . Epidemiological study on the prevalence of ossification of the posterior longitudinal ligament [in Japanese]. *Investigation Committee 1978 report on the ossification of the spinal ligaments of the Japanese Ministry of Public Health and Welfare,* 1979;24–27.
36. Ohtani K, Higuchi M, Watanabe T, et al. Epidemiological study of ossification of the posterior longitudinal ligament of the cervical spine in Yaeyama islands of Okinawa [in Japanese]. *Investigation Committee 1979 report on the ossification of the spinal ligaments of the Japanese Ministry of Public Health and Welfare,* 1980:17–18.
37. Yamauchi H, Issei K, Endou A, et al. Comparative study on the prevalence of OPLL by plain X-ray film and heavy metal content of hair between Chiba and Yamanashi [in Japanese]. *Investigation Committee 1981 report on the ossification of the spinal ligaments of the Japanese Ministry of Public Health and Welfare,* 1982:15–19.
38. Sakou T, Morimoto N. Epidemiological study of the cervical OPLL on islands of Kagoshima [in Japanese]. *Investigation Committee 1981 report on the ossification of the spinal ligaments of the Japanese Ministry of Public Health and Welfare,* 1982:20–23.
39. Ohtsuka Y, Terayama K, Wada K, et al. Epidemiological study of ossification of the spinal ligament on Yachiho in Nagano prefecture [in Japanese]. *Investigation Committee 1983 report on the ossification of the spinal ligaments of the Japanese Ministry of Public Health and Welfare,* 1984:63–67.
40. Ikata T, Takada K, Murase M, et al. Epidemiological study of ossification of the posterior longitudinal ligament of the cervical spine [in Japanese]. *Investigation Committee 1984 report on the ossification of the spinal ligaments of the Japanese Ministry of Public Health and Welfare,* 1985:61–65.
41. Sakou T, Morimoto N, Oh S, et al. Epidemiological study of ossification of the posterior longitudinal ligament of the cervical spine in general population in Taiwan [in Japanese]. *Investigation Committee 1984 report on the ossification of the spinal ligaments of the Japanese Ministry of Public Health and Welfare,* 1985:66–70.
42. Sakou T, Taketomi E, Sameshima T. Epidemiological study of ossification of the posterior longitudinal ligament of the cervical spine on Takasago-tribe in Taiwan [in Japanese]. *Investigation Committee 1987 report on the ossification of the spinal ligaments of the Japanese Ministry of Public Health and Welfare,* 1988:8–9.
43. Tomita T, Harata S, Ueyama K, et al. Epidemiological study of ossification of the posterior longitudinal ligament (OPLL) of cervical spine and cervical spondylotic changes in China [in Japanese]. *Investigation Committee 1993 report on the ossification of the spinal ligaments of the Japanese Ministry of Public Health and Welfare,* 1994:101–105.
44. Resnick D, Niwayama G. Radiographic and pathologic features of spinal involvement in diffuse idiopathic skeletal hyperostosis (DISH) *Radiology* 1976;119:559–568.
45. Arlet J, Pujol M, Buc A, et al. Role del hyperostose vértebrale dans les myélopathies cervicales. *Rev Rheum* 1976;43:167–175.
46. Epstein NE. The surgical management of ossification of the posterior longitudinal ligament in 43 North Americans. *Spine* 1994;19:664–672.
47. Yanagi T. Ossification of the posterior longitudinal ligament. A clinical and radiological analysis of forty-six cases [in Japanese]. *Brain Nerve* 1970;22:909–921.
48. Terayama K, Kurokawa T, Seki H. National survey of ossification of the posterior longitudinal ligament [in Japanese]. *Investigation Committee 1975 report on the ossification of the spinal ligaments of the Japanese Ministry of Public Health and Welfare* 1976:8–33.
49. Tsuyama N. Ossification of the posterior longitudinal ligament of the spine. *Clin Orthop* 1984;184:71–84.
50. Takeda T, Arima T. A case report of ossification of posterior longitudinal ligament with tetrapalsy by mild trauma [in Japanese]. *Rinsho Seikei-geka* 1972;7:949–953.
51. Katoh S, Ikata T, Hirai N, et al. Influence of minor trauma to the neck on the neurological outcome in patients with ossification of the posterior longitudinal ligament (OPLL) of the cervical spine. *Paraplegia* 1995;33:330–333.
52. Fujimura Y, Nakamura M, Toyama Y. Influence of minor trauma on surgical results in patients with cervical OPLL. *J Spinal Disord* 1998; 11:16–20.
53. Terayama K. Family study of ossification of the posterior longitudinal ligament [in Japanese]. *Investigation Committee 1986 report on the ossification of the spinal ligaments of the Japanese Ministry of Public Health and Welfare,* 1987:10–11.
54. Terayama K. Genetic studies on ossification of then posterior longitudinal ligament of the spine. *Spine* 1989;14:1184–1191.
55. Uehara H, Sakou T, Morimoto N, et al. Familial study of ossification of the posterior longitudinal ligament in the cervical spine [in Japanese]. *Seikeigeka to Saigaigeka* 1988;36:800–802.
56. Miura Y, Furusho T, Ibaraki K, et al. Genetic studies for OPLL: analysis of twin [in Japanese]. *Investigation Committee 1991 report on the ossification of the spinal ligaments of the Japanese Ministry of Public Health and Welfare* 1992:5–7.
57. Sakou T, Taketomi E, Matsunaga S, et al. Genetic study of ossification of the posterior longitudinal ligament in the cervical spine with human leukocyte antigen haplotype. *Spine* 1991;6:1249–1252.
58. Matsunaga S, Yamaguchi M, Hayashi K, et al. Genetic analysis of ossification of the posterior longitudinal ligament. *Spine* 1999;24:937–938.
59. Koga H, Sakou T, Taketomi E, et al. Genetic mapping os ossification of the posterior longitudinal ligament of the spine. *Am J Genet* 1998; 62:1460–1467.
60. Maeda S, Koga H, Matsunaga S, et al. Gender-specific haplotype association of collagenα 2(X1) gene in ossification of the posterior longitudinal ligament of the spine. *J Hum Genet* 2001;46:1–4.
61. Forestier J, Lagier R. Ankylosing hyperostosis of the spine. *Clin Orthop* 1971;74:65–83.
62. Saitou Y. Magnetic resonance imaging and ossification of the posterior longitudinal ligament [in Japanese]. *Gazou-shindan* 1989;9:1446–1452.

63. Sakamoto R, Ikata T, Murase M, et al. Magnetic resonance imaging and histologic study of ossification of the spinal ligaments [in Japanese]. *Seikeigeka* 1993;44:1091–1099.

64. Iwahashi T, Tamaki T, Kawakami M, et al. Changes of signal intensity on MRI and spinal cord symptom in cervical OPLL [in Japanese]. *Investigation Committee 1990 report on the ossification of the spinal ligaments of the Japanese Ministry of Public Health and Welfare*, 1991:57–59.

65. Kameyama T, Yanagi T, Yasuda T, et al. MRI evaluation of spinal cord lesions for cervical spondylosis and OPLL. *Investigation Committee 1990 report on the ossification of the spinal ligaments of the Japanese Ministry of Public Health and Welfare*, 1991:42–48.

66. Yone K, Sakou T, Yanase M, et al. Preoperative and postoperative magnetic resonance image evaluations of the spinal cord in cervical myelopathy. *Spine* 1992;17:S388–S392.

67. Abe H, Koyanagi I, Iwasaki Y, et al. Relationship between the neurological deficits and MRI findings in the case of cervical OPLL [in Japanese]. *Investigation Committee 1994 report on the ossification of the spinal ligaments of the Japanese Ministry of Public Health and Welfare,* 1995:175–180.

68. Terada A, Taketomi E, Matsunaga S, et al. 3-Dimensional computed tomography analysis of ossification of spinal ligament. *Clin Orthop* 1997;336:137–142.

69. Taketomi E. Progression of ossification of the posterior longitudinal ligament in the cervical spine. *J Jpn Spine Res Soc* 1997;8:359–366.

70. Matsunaga S, Sakou T, Taketomi E, et al. Effects of strain distribution in the intervertebral discs on the progression of ossification of the posterior longitudinal ligaments. *Spine* 1996;21:184–189.

71. Ichimoto H, Kawai S, Oda H, et al. Postoperative progression pattern of ossification of the posterior longitudinal ligament in cervical spine [in Japanese]. *Investigation Committee 1980 report on the ossification of the spinal ligaments of the Japanese Ministry of Public Health and Welfare*, 1981:199–200.

72. Miyazaki K, Hirofuji E, Onozaki A, et al. Follow-up studies on the development of ossification of the posterior longitudinal ligament in the cervical region after simultaneous multisegmental laminectomy [in Japanese]. *Spine Spinal Cord* 1993;6:905–910.

73. Matsunaga S, Sakou T, Taketomi E, et al. The natural course of myelopathy caused by ossification of the posterior longitudinal ligament in the cervical spine. *Clin Orthop* 1994;305:168–177.

74. Kaplan EL, Meier P. Nonparametric estimation from incomplete observations. *J Am Stat Assoc* 1958;53:457–481.

75. Matsunaga S, Kukita M, Hayashi K, et al. Pathogenesis of myelopathy on the patients with ossification of the posterior longitudinal ligament. *J Neurosurg* (in press).

CHAPTER 79

Surgery for Ossification of the Posterior Longitudinal Ligament

Part A
Thinning and Anterior Floating

Isakichi Yamaura and Keiro Ono

The technique of cervical vertebrectomy was originally developed to treat trauma and tumors. When the anterior cervical approach was introduced in the 1950s, it became apparent that direct removal of compressive structures anteriorly was technically easy and safe for the patient (1–4). The vertebrectomy through the anterior approach has since been widely indicated not only for localized lesions but also for multisegmental lesions, especially as surgical techniques have become more refined and have been supported by the development of surgical devices and improved image technology (5).

Direct access to compressive structures impinging on the spinal cord—along with decompression consisting of excision or minimizing of the compressive structure—have become feasible over time. An ingenious technique has been developed in Japan for the surgical treatment of ossification of the posterior longitudinal ligament (OPLL) (6,7). For greater safety, hard compressive structures (OPLL) are cut very thin and allowed to float away from the dural sack without removing it.

This technique of decompression of the spinal cord and nerve roots underneath the multisegmental OPLL has become widely accepted for patients presenting with cervical myelopathy (8,9).

PREOPERATIVE SURGICAL PLANNING

In the surgical technique, the vertebral bodies are extensively excised, leading to a quadrilateral trough aligned with the midline of the cervical spine (Fig. 79.1). The size (length and width) of the trough should encompass the main portion of the OPLL compressing the spinal cord. To determine the size of the main portion or structure of the OPLL, plain radiography, tomography (frontal, lateral, and computed transverse), and computed tomography (CT) myelography are used. As imaging technology advances, magnetic resonance imaging is replacing CT myelography for this purpose.

1. The upper and lower margins of the trough are situated at the end of the uncompromised area of the subarachnoid space, as identified by the MRI or CT myelogram. For various practical reasons, the vertebrectomy is limited to C2 cranially to T3 caudally. OPLL at C2 and above is rarely harmful to the spinal cord.

2. The width of the trough should be determined with great caution so that the vertebral artery will not be damaged. To locate the vertebral foramen, a CT scan is indispensable. During the trough-shaped excision of the vertebral body, the junction between the body and the pedicle can provide an indication of the width limit at the vertebral level. At the intervertebral disc level, on the other hand, the joint of Luschka is used as the width limit.

3. Within the deep trough longitudinally situated in the vertebrae, a typical lesion of the OPLL is cut paper thin and transversely divided 5 mm above the base of C2 cranially and at the upper third of C7 caudally. For lateral decompression, the width of excision of the vertebral body is preferably expanded to 23 mm, or nearly the transverse diameter of the spinal canal.

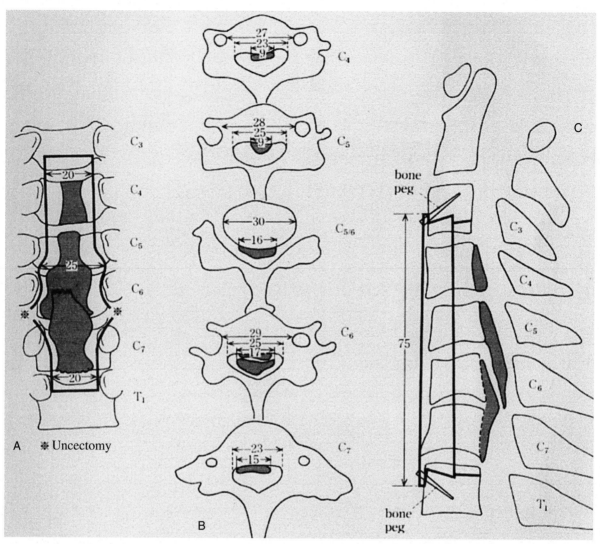

FIG. 79.1. Surgical planning. **A:** Extent of vertebrectomy. A trough-shaped excision map is drawn on an anteroposterior tomogram. **B:** Transverse diameter of the trough at each vertebral level: distance between the foramen vertebrale, right and left, on computed tomography; width of the trough to be excised at each vertebral level; width of the ossification of the posterior longitudinal ligament at each vertebral level. **C:** Height and design of the strut graft to be inserted in the trough.

POSITIONING AND TRACTION

The patient is properly positioned, and traction in slight extension is applied for a multisegmental vertebrectomy in the cervical spine.

During division of the uppermost lesion of the OPLL at C2, a head-down position and a microscope are required for obtaining an adequate view of the lesion, which is located behind the C2 body. On the contrary, a head-up position is preferable for dividing the lower portion of the OPLL at the C7 body. During this positional change, the patient should be fixed firmly to the surgical frame, and traction should not be loosened.

The appropriateness of the alignment of the cervical spine and location, as well as the depth of the surgical in-

struments, must be checked at each step by intraoperative roentgenography or fluoroscopic examination.

POSTOPERATIVE MANAGEMENT

Postoperatively, the patient should be evaluated for respiratory distress and difficulty in expectoration of sputum; difficulty in swallowing (or any sign suggesting injury to the esophagus); dislodging of the strut graft; leakage of cerebrospinal fluid; and any sign of spinal cord injury or postoperative infection.

For prevention of graft dislodgment and early return to active life, the use of a halo vest apparatus is recommended.

SURGICAL TECHNIQUE

For a typical OPLL extending from C2 to T7, an oblique skin incision made along the border of the sternocleidomastoid on the left side of the neck is recommended. If it is a short or segmental OPLL expanding over three vertebral bodies, a horizontal skin incision is sufficient (as in the case with disc herniation). The interval between the carotid sheath and the esophagus and trachea is developed after skin incision. When the anterior aspects of the cervical vertebrae are exposed using blunt dissection, the correct cervical disc level must be identified using a spinal needle with a stopper along with lateral roentgenography. To secure enough space to access the expansive lesion and provide a relatively bloodless field, the upper and lower thyroid vessels and the omohyoid muscle are ligated and divided. Cardinal tissues, such as the recurrent nerve, the laryngeal nerve, the phrenic nerve, the subclavian vein, and the apex of the lung, should be carefully retracted.

Retractor Application

After the precervical fascia is excised, the anterior portion of the vertebral column exposed, and the indexed disc confirmed, the medial edge of the longus colli muscles are elevated away from the midline of the vertebrae using both a periosteal elevator and electric cautery. Cloward retractors are set up carefully on these edges so as not to injure the esophagus, the trachea, and the carotid sheath. Because the total surgical intervention often lasts more than 3 hours, the previously mentioned structures should be protected from prolonged compression. Retractors should be released once an hour, and any discoloration of these structures should be allowed to return to normal before reapplication of the instrument.

Disc Removal

Keeping the proper level for disc removal in mind, the disc material is removed from C2-C3 to C6-C7 thoroughly with a rongeur, a pituitary forceps, or a curette until the posterior longitudinal ligament is visible (Fig. 79.2). The bilateral joints of Luschka are exposed and curetted cautiously. This ensures correct midline access to the spinal canal during the subsequent vertebrectomy and excision of spondylotic bony spurs originating from the joints. To prevent severe disruption of the total spine after removal of multiple disc materials, each empty disc space should be packed with a block of gauze.

Vertebrectomy

The vertebrectomy is begun with drilling bilateral holes in the joints of Luschka and nibbling the vertebral body. As shown in Figures 79.3 and 79.4, bilateral drill holes in each disc space are useful for intraoperative marking of

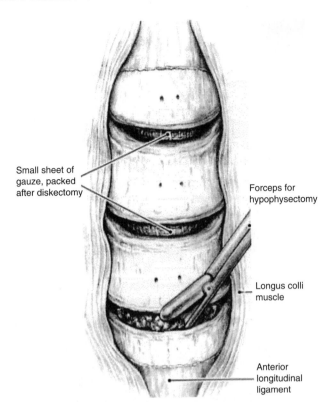

Small sheet of gauze, packed after diskectomy

Forceps for hypophysectomy

Longus colli muscle

Anterior longitudinal ligament

FIG. 79.2. Discectomy.

the quadrilateral trough, which was planned preoperatively on roentgenograms of the cervical spine. The width of the trough should extend 20 mm or attain nearly the width of the spinal canal.

Employing a power drill and a rongeur, a major portion of the vertebrectomy can be performed through expansion and deepening of the vertebral body resection to include the end plate and spondylotic protrusion (Fig. 79.5). The vertebrectomy allows access and ensures a wide view of the OPLL; therefore, the bony resection should not extend beyond the posterior annulus and the posterior longitudinal ligament at this stage (Fig. 79.6).

Thinning and Division of the Ossification of the Posterior Longitudinal Ligament

After wide resection of the vertebral bodies from C3 to C6 and partial resection of C2 caudally and C7 cranially, thick masses of the OPLL are cut thinly in a canoe shape, with a maximum depth on the midline (Fig. 79.7). The accurate location of the drill head should be confirmed on lateral roentgenography during the cutting procedure. During this procedure, a surgical microscope is employed to allow identification of the boundary of each structure, such as bone, cartilage, and ligament, and for discrimination between the thin cortex of the vertebra and the ligamentous tissue inserted between the OPLL and the posterior aspect of the vertebral body. The ossified posterior ligament often

T-shaped measure for measuring width
of bone resection during surgery

Specially designed ronger

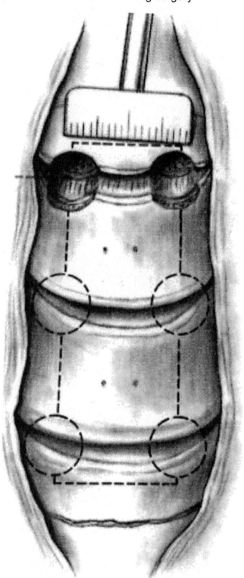

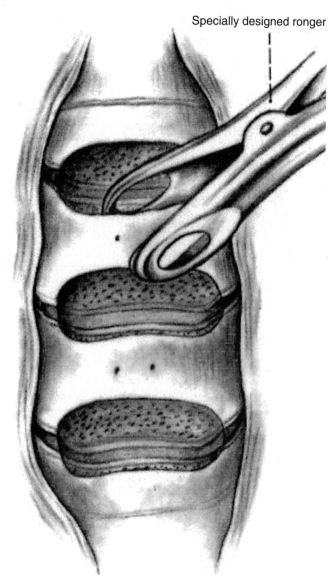

FIG. 79.4. Nibbling of vertebral body with a specially designed rongeur, reserving small chips of cancerous bone for grafting.

FIG. 79.3. Vertebrectomy begins with bilateral drilling centered on the joints of Luschka.

contains unossified ligamentous tissue within the mass. Such unossified tissue must be identified precisely to allow for safe completion of this procedure.

Thinning of the ossified mass is always carried out evenly from the center to the periphery (Fig. 79.8); otherwise, perforation may occur, causing heavy bleeding and spinal cord injury.

Until the ossified mass is adequately evenly thinned and divided craniocaudally at the C2 and C7 levels, respectively, it should not be divided at its lateral margin joining with the posterior cortex of the cervical vertebra (Fig. 79.7; see asterisks).

In summary, the anterior floating of the OPLL is carried out according to a certain order: (a) bilateral drilling cen-

tered on the Luschka joint (at the lateral margin of the mass, the spinal cord is not present in the bottom); (b) trough-shaped excision of the vertebral body and the bony and cartilaginous end plate and disc materials, according to the preoperative plan; (c) even thinning of both the posterior cortex of the vertebra and the OPLL, from the center to the periphery (the ossified mass with maximum thickness in the midline should be cut thin in the shape of a canoe); (d) dividing of the thinned mass transversely at C2 and C7 levels (Fig. 79.9), where the spinal cord is confirmed to be separated with only a short distance of subarachnoid fluid space; and (e) finally, dividing of the ossified mass at its lateral margin safely. If the OPLL were divided from its margin before extensive thinning was accomplished, the ossified mass would float partially and unevenly so that further decompression would be unattainable.

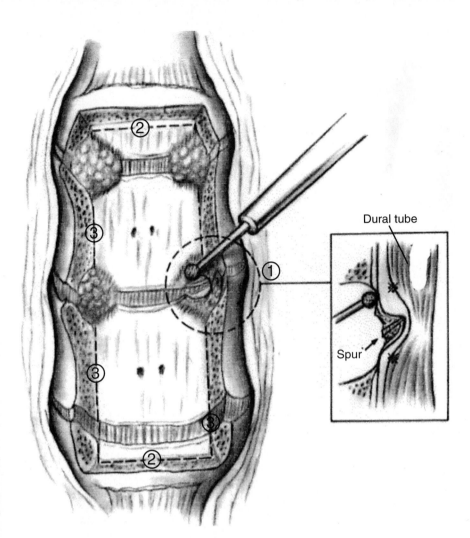

FIG. 79.5. After the trough-shaped vertebrectomy, thin cortices of the vertebral bodies are visualized at the bottom. Spondylotic bony protrusions, the bony ridge of the uncinate processes, and the corresponding portions of the posterolateral corner of the vertebra are carefully excised using power drill and curette. The *dotted line* indicates demarcation of the thin cortex where it will be divided, craniocaudally and laterally.

Width of trough should be adjusted when vertebral foramens are situated closer to midline of vertebra.

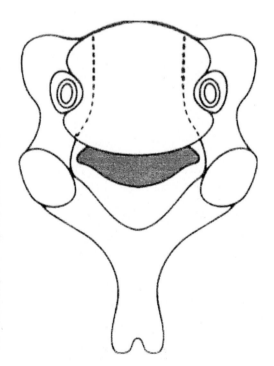

FIG. 79.6. Cross-sectional view of the vertebra associated with ossification of the posterior longitudinal ligament where vertebrae foramens are situated more centrally so that vertebrectomy should start with a narrower trough and expand as excision advances below the foramens, terminating not less than the width of spinal canal.

1103

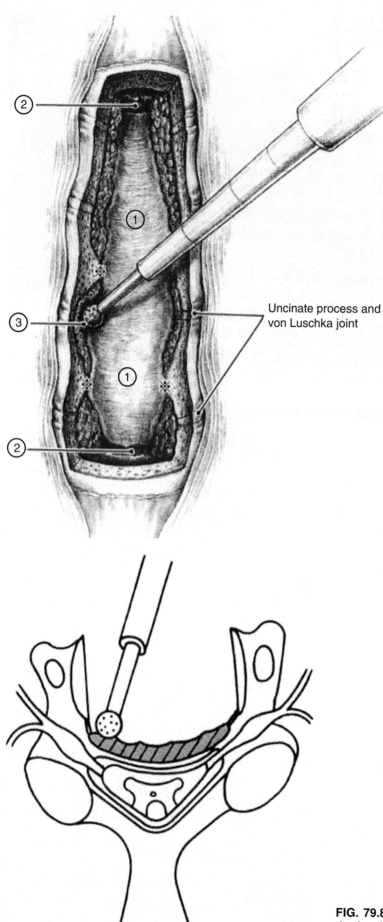

Uncinate process and
von Luschka joint

FIG. 79.7. Behind thin cortices, the ossification of the posterior longitudinal ligament (OPLL) is further cut papery thin with the deepest apex at midline. The OPLL finally assumes a canoe shape. Spondylotic protrusion or any lateral extension of ossified mass should be divided at the joints of Luschka. The longitudinal OPLL mass should be divided craniocaudally at C2 and C7, respectively. Until final division at the posterolateral vertebral wall *(asterisk),* however, the entire OPLL mass is unfloatable.

FIG. 79.8. Cross-sectional view of ossification of the posterior longitudinal ligament thinning and dividing at the lateral margin where vertebra, pedicle, and costotransverse process conjoin.

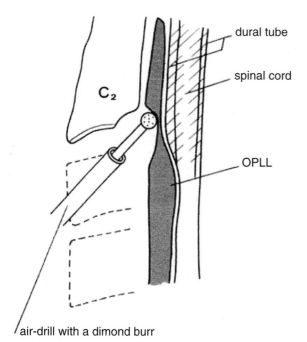

FIG. 79.9. Behind C2, the ossification of the posterior longitudinal ligament is divided transversely after vertebrectomy.

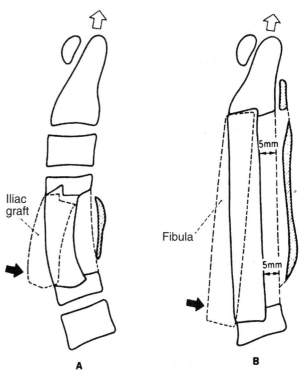

FIG. 79.10. Strut bone grafting employing iliac crest (**A**) or fibula (**B**). Fibular bone graft is recommended when more than two vertebral bodies are to be removed. The length and width of fibula necessary for grafting can be estimated by measuring the size of trough. The allograft is then cut with a power saw to a length slightly longer than trough, and is prepared using a power burr. A spike structure or wedge design is preferable so that the graft does not dislodge from the trough. The bottom of C2 and top of C7 are undercut for graft seating, as illustrated in **B**. For enabling anterior floating of ossified mass, there should be a space of 5 mm behind the allograft after its final insertion. Once the floor of the trough and the allograft are completely prepared for insertion, the cervical spine is extended moderately by using a head halter or skull tong for smooth insertion of graft.

Bleeding from the cancerous bone can be controlled with bone wax. Bleeding from the epidural venous plexus should be controlled with cauterization, meticulous application of a hemostatic agent, or both.

If anterior floating of the ossified mass is unsatisfactory or limited, incomplete division at the margin—craniocaudal or bilateral—should be checked. Additional division is carried out using a spatula for microsurgery. If division at the margin is found to be unsatisfactory, then a small hook can be used for picking the OPLL out for floating. Further floating can be expected during the recovery period if thinning and dividing has been carried out satisfactorily.

Application of Strut Bone Graft from C2 to C7

A fibular bone graft is recommended when more than two vertebral bodies are to be removed (10–13). The length and width of the fibula necessary for grafting can be estimated by measuring the size of the trough. The allograft is then cut with a power saw to a length slightly longer than the trough and is prepared using a power burr. A spike structure or wedge design is preferable for the graft not to dislodge from the trough. The bottom of C2 and top of C7 are undercut for graft seating, as illustrated in Fig. 79.10. To enable anterior floating of the ossified mass, there should be a space of 5 mm behind the allograft after the final insertion of it. Once the floor of the trough and the allograft are prepared for insertion, the cervical spine is extended moderately by using a head halter or a skull tong for smooth insertion of the graft.

Immobilization of the Cervical Spine

A halo vest apparatus is preferable for immobilization of the cervical spine. For postoperative care of the wound and to ensure adequate respiration and swallowing, this apparatus is recommended. The apparatus should be applied before surgery; during surgery, the apparatus is disconnected at the junction between the halo and the vest. The halo ring remains attached to the skull and is used for fixation to the surgical table and for traction, if necessary.

OTHER POSTOPERATIVE CONSIDERATIONS

Postoperatively, the ossified mass migrates anteriorly, as long as thinning and disconnection from the longitudinal ligament (craniocaudally) and the vertebra (laterally) was accomplished (Fig. 79.11). Ballooning of the dural sack is found to cause such an anterior floating of the

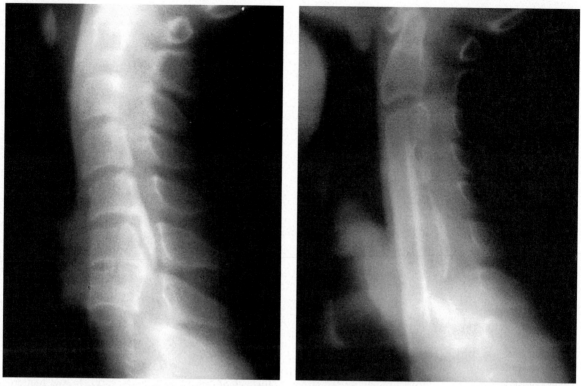

FIG. 79.11. A: A preoperative lateral tomography shows the apex of ossification of the posterior longitudinal ligament (OPLL) at C6, extraordinarily protruded into the spinal canal (>80% of the anteroposterior diameter of canal). **B:** A postoperative lateral tomogram taken 1 year after surgery. The anterior migration of OPLL *(asterisks)* is noticeable, and no regrowth of residual ossification can be observed. Fibular strut graft was well incorporated in the vertebral trough so that the cervical spine was fused from C3 to T1. External immobilization with a halo vest apparatus was required for about 2 months after surgery.

OPLL because the cervical spinal cord that was decompressed and the subarachnoid space recovers after surgery. In our experience, the spinal canal expands after 4 to 8 weeks, and anterior floating can be confirmed by lateral roentgenography (preferably CT).

Through a follow-up study (14,15), we learned that the ossified mass shifted anteriorly, uniting with the C2 and C7 bodies at both ends. In addition, it did not regrow, but rather became thinner 1 year later, as long as the strut graft was well situated in the vertebrectomy trough.

REFERENCES

1. Bailey RW, Badgley CE. Stabilization of the cervical spine by anterior fusion. *J Bone Joint Surg* 1960;42:565.
2. Cloward RB. The anterior approach for removal of ruptured cervical disks. *J Neurosurg* 1958;15:602.
3. Crandall PH, Batzdorf U. Cervical spondylotic myelopathy. *J Neurosurg* 1966;25:57.
4. Smith GW, Robinson JT. The treatment of cervical spine disorders by anterior removal of the intervertebral disc and interbody fusion. *J Bone Joint Surg Am* 1958;40:607.
5. Sakou T, Matsunaga S, Epstein N. Ossification of the posterior longitudinal ligament (OPLL): epidemiology, pathology, etiology, diagnosis and treatment. In: Ono K, Dvorak J, Dunn E, eds. *Cervical spondylosis and similar disorders.* Singapore: World Scientific, 1998:701–753.
6. Yamaura I, Isobe Y, Kamikozuru M, et al. Evaluation of surgical treatment of ossification of the posterior longitudinal ligament in the cervical spine: anterior decompression [in Japanese]. *Seikeigeka* 1976;27:87–95.
7. Yamaura I. Anterior approach (anterior floating method) and its surgical results for cervical myelopathy caused by ossification of the posterior longitudinal ligament (OPLL). *J West Pac Orthop Assoc* 1990;17:47–55.
8. Yamaura I, Kurosa Y, Matsuoka T. Anterior approach (anterior floating method) and its surgical results for cervical myelopathy caused by ossification of the posterior longitudinal ligament. In Yonenobu K, Sakou T, Ono K, eds. *OPLL: ossification of the posterior longitudinal ligament.* Tokyo: Springer-Verlag, 1997:165–172.
9. Yonenobu K, Sakou T, Ono K. *OPLL: ossification of the posterior longitudinal ligament.* Tokyo: Springer-Verlag, 1997.
10. Bernard TN Jr, Whitecloud TS. Cervical spondylotic myelopathy and myeloradiculopathy: anterior decompression and stabilization with autogenous fibula strut graft. *Clin Orthop* 1987;221:149.
11. Bohlman HH. Cervical spondylosis with moderate to severe myelopathy: a report of 17 cases treated by Robinson anterior cervical discectomy. *Spine* 1977;2:151.
12. Whitecloud TS. Multilevel cervical vertebrectomy and stabilization using cortical bone. In: Sherk HH, ed. *The cervical spine: an atlas of surgical procedures.* Philadelphia: JB Lippincott, 1997:197–212.
13. Zdeblick TA, Bohlman HH. Cervical kyphosis and myelopathy. Treatment by anterior corpectomy and strut grafting. *J Bone Joint Surg* 1989; 71:170.
14. Matsuoka T, Yamaura I, Kurosa Y, et al. Long-term results of the anterior floating method for cervical myelopathy caused by ossification of the posterior longitudinal ligament. *Spine* 2001;26:241–248.
15. Yamaura I, Kurosa Y, Matsuoka T, et al. Anterior floating method for cervical myelopathy caused by ossification of the posterior longitudinal ligament. *Clin Orthop* 1999;359:27–34.

Part B
Posterior Approach

Kazuhiko Satomi

Spinal cord compression by OPLL can be decompressed by either an anterior or a posterior surgery. Although anterior extirpation or floatation of the ossified mass followed by vertebral body arthrodesis is a method of treatment (1, 2), technical difficulties are associated with the treatment, including intraoperative nervous tissue damage, the need for long-term bed rest or external support, and prolongation of graft bone healing. Yamaura and associates reported that floating surgery was indicated even in cases with continuous-type or mixed-type OPLL, and they reported good operative results without neurologic deterioration after surgery (2).

In my view, anterior surgery is indicated only in cases in which OPLL involves fewer than three discs, whereas posterior decompressive surgery is indicated in cases in which OPLL involvement extends to three or more disc levels. This means that almost all OPLL cases will be treated by posterior surgery. The choice of surgery was anterior in 20% of the patients and posterior in 80% in my clinic. Furthermore, a two-stage combined operation was indicated in cases with mixed OPLL having locally prominent ossified masses. In this operation, posterior decompression is performed first, followed by anterior decompression and arthrodesis within 3 to 6 weeks of the first surgery, or both operations can be performed on the same day (3,4).

CONCEPT OF SURGICAL POSTERIOR DECOMPRESSION

Posterior decompression is achieved by shifting the spinal cord posteriorly after either laminectomy or laminoplasty (5,6) (Fig. 79.12). Preoperative or postoperative lordotic positioning of the cervical spine is necessary to realize effective posterior decompression. It is thought that better decompression can be achieved in the lordotic cervical spine than in the normal or kyphotic cervical spine. In that sense, laminoplasty is preferable to laminectomy because kyphotic changes can occur in the cervical spine postoperatively after laminectomy (7).

Oyama and colleagues were the first to devise an expansive Z laminoplasty in 1973 (8). However, the procedure has not come into widespread use because it requires a very high level of surgical technique. Hirabayashi initiated unilateral open-door laminoplasty in 1977, and this procedure is reported to be simpler and safer than that used in the Z laminoplasty (9,10). The technique was further modified in 1982 into midsagittal splitting (bilateral open-door) laminoplasty with or without bone grafting (11,12). The two methods, unilateral and bilateral open-door laminoplasty, have been widely used for posterior decompression of the cervical cord (13,14). Further modifications have been made using artificial lamina for spacers in the opened spaces instead of bone spacers (15–18) (Fig. 79.13) and using a T-saw instead of pneumatic drills for making bone gutters in both methods (19).

I performed conventional unilateral open-door laminoplasty until 1993 (20). Since then, I carried out unilateral open-door laminoplasty using hydroxyapatite lamina spacers to prevent closure of the opened lamina and to facilitate early ambulation, thus resulting in good alignment of the cervical spine postoperatively (17).

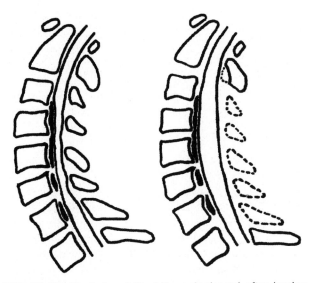

FIG. 79.12. Posterior shift of the spinal cord after laminoplasty.

A. BILATERAL OPEN LAMINOPLASTY

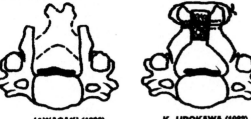

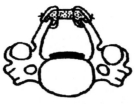

IAWASAKI (1982)   **K UROKAWA (1982)**   **HASE (1991)**

B. UNILATERAL OPEN LAMINOPLASTY

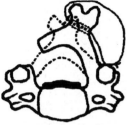

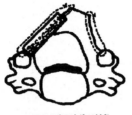

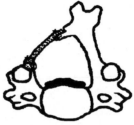

HIRABAYASHI (1978)   **ITO & TSUJI (1982)**   **SATOMI (1993)**

FIG. 79.13. Schematic representation of various laminoplasties. Bone blocks are used for spacers in the methods shown in the middle column, and hydroxyapatite blocks are used in the methods shown in the right column.

SURGICAL TECHNIQUE OF UNILATERAL OPEN-DOOR LAMINOPLASTY WITH LAMINA SPACERS FROM C3 TO C7

The patient, with the head fixed by the Mayfield three-pin system, is placed in the prone position, tilted cranially upward at an angle of 30 degrees to minimize blood loss from congestion of the epidural vessels during surgery. The neck is flexed to a straight position of the cervical spine, and the nuchal level is maintained horizontally. The prominent spinous processes of C6 and C7 are the landmarks of the midline and can be easily identified by palpation.

A midline approach between the paraspinal muscles must be performed correctly to minimize local bleeding. Muscles attached to the spinous process of C2 are reflected bilaterally together with a small bone mass from the process for later reattachment of the muscles in the final stage of the operation (Fig. 79.14). Then, the paraspinal muscles are separated from the spinous processes to the bilateral facets between C2 and T1. Both supraspinous and interspinous ligaments must be preserved without damage, including the ligaments between C2-C3 and C7-T1.

First, a partial laminectomy is made in the lower half of the C2 lamina bilaterally, which is referred to as a domelike laminectomy (21). Using a steel burr on a pneumatic drill, a bony gutter is created in the open side (usually on the left) from C2 and C7. In the final stage of fashioning the gutter, a diamond burr should be used to avoid damaging the dural tube or cervical root sheath. The interlaminar ligamentum flavum and fibrous tissue are cut using a microscissors or a thin-blade Kerrison rongeur on the open side. The exposed ligamenta flava between the laminae at both the upper and lower ends of the laminoplasty are then removed bilaterally.

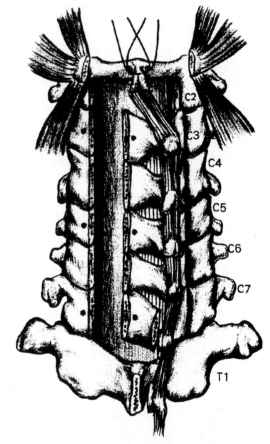

FIG. 79.14. Schematic representation of unilateral open-door laminoplasty. Muscles attached to the C2 spinous process are reflected bilaterally. The caudal half of the C2 lamina is laminectomied, referred to as *dome laminectomy*. Interlaminal ligaments between C2 and C3, and between C7 and T1, are resected; however, interspinous ligaments between these are preserved. The base of the spinous processes is cut transversely in C7 and T1.

The bony gutter on the hinge side is then drilled slightly more laterally than on the hinge side to prevent the laminar hinge from becoming unstable or from dislodging. After a preliminary bony gutter has been made, the spinous processes are pushed tentatively to check the stability of the hinge (Fig. 79.15). If the medial wall is too thick for the laminae to be opened, this cortex should be redrilled thinner with the diamond burr (22). When the laminar doors are ready to be opened, stay sutures are stitched around the spinous processes of C4 and C6 and into the capsules around the facets used for keeping the laminae open. It is very difficult to do this once the laminar door has been opened.

Holes are made in the facets and laminae on the open side of C3, C5, and C7 using a small steel burr to attach the hydroxyapatite lamina spacers. The base of the spinous process of T1 is cut transversely to make the laminae open more easily, and that of C7 is sometimes also cut when the spinous process is long (Fig. 79.14). The laminar door is then opened. The resected border of the lamina is elevated, just like opening a door, using a large Kerrison rongeur as if the corner of the rongeur were the fulcrum of a lever. When each lamina has been elevated, the remaining ligamentum flavum and any adhesive fibrous bands between the dura mater and the inner surface of the laminae are divided with scissors from the open side.

After the dural pulsation is clearly visualized, lamina spacers are tied with two threads on the facet side and one thread in the opened lamina at the C3, C5, and C7 levels. Additionally, the stay sutures are tied around the bases of the spinous processes through the ligamentum flavum to hold the lamina door open at the C4 and C6 levels (Fig. 79.16). Five spacers, one for each opened lamina, would provide

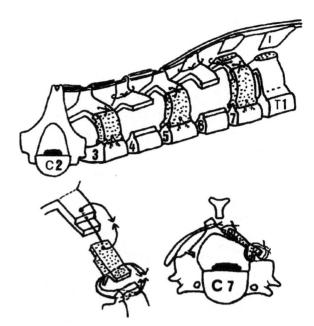

FIG. 79.16. Schematic representation of cervical spine fixed by lamina spacers at C3, C5, and C7.

better stability in the opened laminae; however, this would require significantly more surgical time. Generally, three spacers are sufficient to provide stability in the opened laminae, already supporting the C4 and C5 laminae by threads (Fig. 79.17).

Before closing the paraspinal muscles and skin, muscles attached to the C2 spinous process are reattached firmly to the spinous process.

Postoperatively, the patients should remain in bed for 2 to 5 days and then should ambulate with a cervical brace for 2 months.

OPERATIVE RESULTS

One hundred and six patients (88 men and 18 women, average age of 57 years) with myelopathy were treated by unilateral open-door laminoplasty between 1977 and 1997. Of these, 38 recent patients were operated on by laminoplasty using lamina spacers, as mentioned in the previous section. In these patients, postoperative complications were examined, including motor paresis of the upper extremities.

Postoperative improvement of clinical symptoms was assessed with respect to recovery rate calculated based on scores according to the Japanese Orthopaedic Association (JOA) scoring system (23) in 55 patients with an average age of 56 years, who were followed for 5 years or longer (average, 9 years; range, 5 to 17 years). The average presurgery duration of symptoms was 36.6 months. The average sagittal diameter of the cervical spinal canal was 13.7 mm, which was measured from the interlaminar line to the back of the vertebral body.

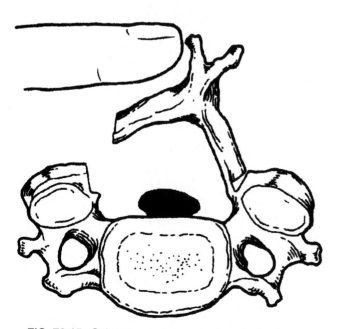

FIG. 79.15. Spinous process pushed gently by finger.

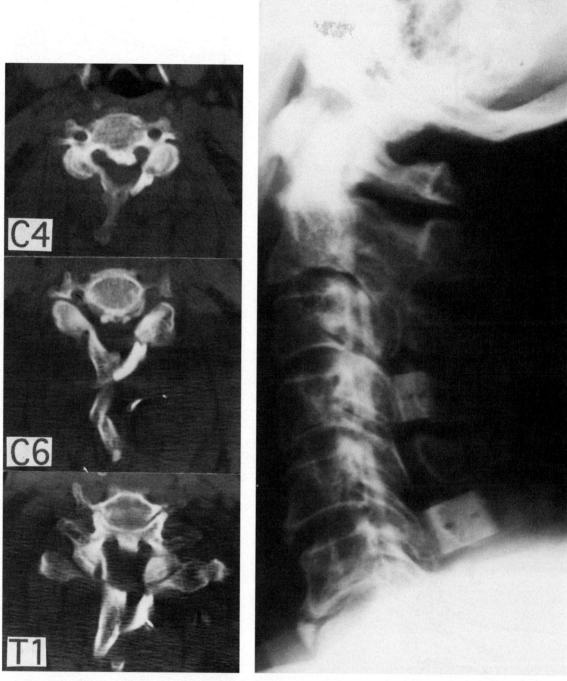

FIG. 79.17. A: Lateral radiograph showing mixed type of ossification of the posterior longitudinal ligament in 60-year-old man. **B:** The ossified mass and flattening of spinal cord are well documented on computed tomography myelogram. **C:** Postoperative radiograph shows widening of spinal canal after laminoplasty from C3 to T1 with lamina spacers. **D:** Hydroxyapatite lamina spacers are seen at C4, C6, and T1 with widening of the spinal canal.

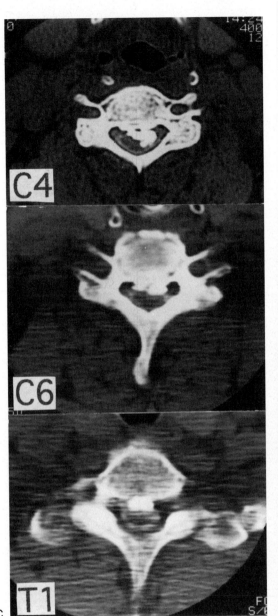

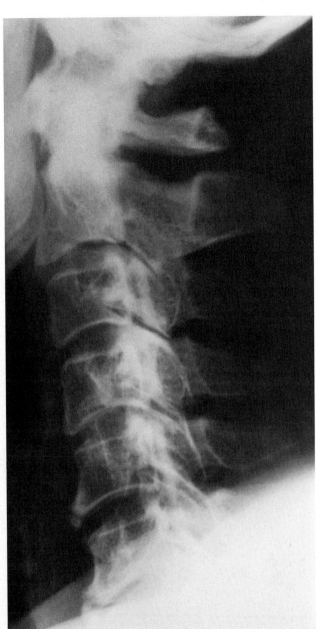

FIG. 79.17. *Continued*

The recovery rate with respect to clinical symptoms was 50.3% immediately after surgery, 68.2% at 3-year follow-up, and 61.3% at the final follow-up. Widening of the sagittal canal by 3 to 5 mm was achieved (Fig. 79.18), which remained stable throughout the postoperative period.

COMPLICATIONS

Postoperative complications included muscle weakness of the upper extremities in 10 patients (9.6%), closure of the opened laminae in 3 patients (2.8%), and pseudomeningocele in 1 patient (0.9%); however, these rates have decreased in recent years. The 3 patients with postoperative closure of opened laminae and neurologic deterioration later experi-

enced a slight improvement in symptoms after an additional laminectomy immediately performed on the same level that underwent laminoplasty in the initial surgery. The patient with a postoperative cervical pseudomeningocele was successfully treated by subcutaneous lumbar drainage of the cerebrospinal fluid.

Postoperative weakness occurred in the shoulder girdle muscles in 9 patients and in the intrinsic muscles in 1 patient. The side of weakness was located on the open side in 5 patients, on the hinge side in 4, and on both sides in 1 patient. Eight patients were aware of weakness the day after the operation, and 2 patients noted weakness more than 2 days after operation. The weakness resolved to a level of 4 or 5 out of 5 for manual muscle testing in 7 patients within

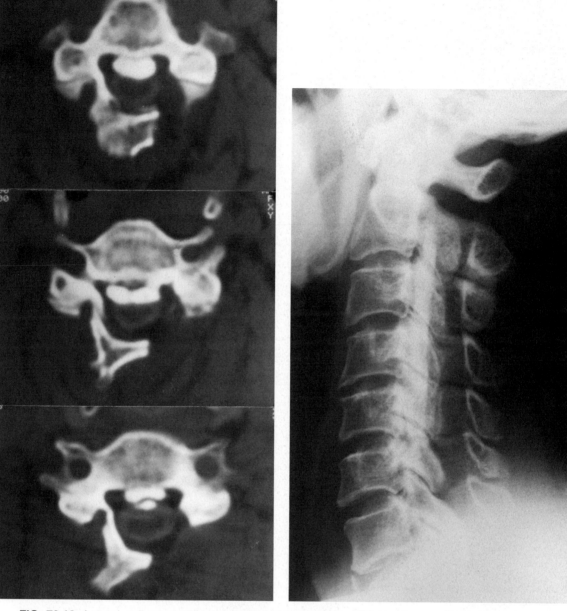

FIG. 79.18. Lateral radiograph (**A**) and computed tomography (CT) myelogram (**B**) showing mixed-type ossification of the posterior longitudinal ligament in 57-year-old man. Postoperative radiograph (**C**) and CT myelogram (**D**) showing widening of spinal canal and enlargement of spinal cord after conventional unilateral open-door laminoplasty between C2 and C7.

4 years without the need for any additional surgery. The weakness did not resolve in 3 patients, who were not followed beyond 3 years after surgery.

The causes of motor paresis are not known with certainty. However, these may be secondary to operative trauma (10, 24), a tethering effect of the roots following the posterior shift of the spinal cord (24), intramedullary lesions due to rapid blood perfusion following decompression of the spinal cord (25), and displacement of the lamina on the hinge side (26).

FACTORS INFLUENCING OPERATIVE RESULTS

Preoperative Factors

A number of preoperative factors have been reported to influence the final operative results. These include age at operation, duration of myelopathic symptoms before surgery, onset with or without trauma, a stenotic condition of the spinal canal, and cervical curvature of the spine (10). Patient age less than 60 years at the time of operation and more than 1 year's duration of symptoms before surgery

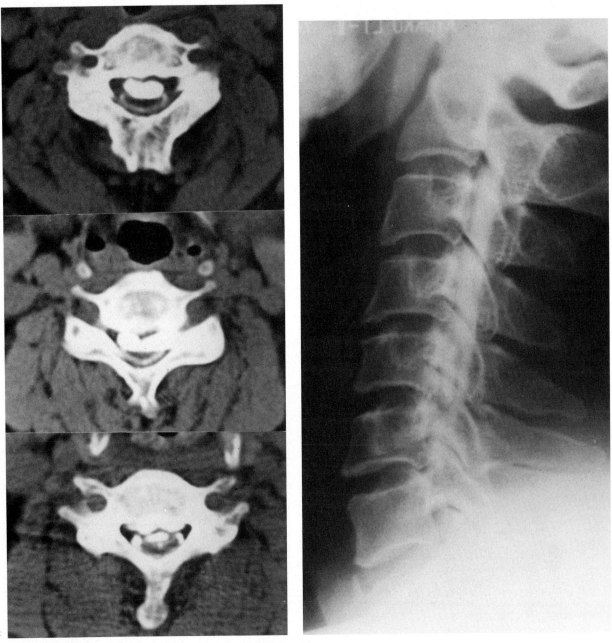

FIG. 79.18. *Continued*

were significantly correlated with the recovery rate of clinical symptoms in this series. The recovery rate was not correlated with either preoperative function judged by the JOA score or spinal sagittal diameter (26).

Intraoperative Factors

Intraoperative damage to nerve roots or to the spinal cord could result in postoperative muscle weakness of the upper extremities or spinal cord injury. Closure of the opened laminae could result in neurologic deterioration, and displacement of lamina into the spinal canal on the hinge side

could result in damage to the nerve roots. However, these complications have decreased substantially since I began using lamina spacers in laminoplasty.

Postoperative Factors

A wide range of postoperative factors can be seen to influence the final results, including aging, ossification in either longitudinal or transverse direction, developments in OPLL in the thoracic spine, cervical curvature, changes in the range of motion in the cervical spine, and trauma. The recover rate tends to decrease beyond 3 years after surgery, possibly because of an increased ossified mass, new OPLL developments in the thoracic spine, and an increase in the patient's age.

CONCLUSION

Most patients with myelopathy due to OPLL can be treated successfully by unilateral open-door laminoplasty, although the ossified mass can persist in the canal after surgery. Full recovery of clinical symptoms is occasionally observed in many patients after posterior decompression. Posterior decompressive surgery using laminectomy and various methods of laminoplasty have been reported, and good operative results have been described. However, laminectomy should be avoided whenever possible as a treatment for OPLL because the cervical spine can develop a kyphotic deformity postoperatively (7).

Although good operative results are not always achieved in some patients because of inevitable preoperative factors or technical intraoperative problems, careful operative techniques and early operative intervention may improve operative outcomes.

REFERENCES

1. Sakou T, Miyazaki A, Tomimura K, et al. Ossification of the posterior longitudinal ligament of the cervical spine: subtotal vertebrectomy as a treatment. *Clin Orthop* 1979;140:58–65.
2. Yamaura I, Kurosa Y, Matuoka T, et al. Anterior approach (anterior floating methods) and its surgical results for cervical myelopathy caused by ossification of the posterior longitudinal ligament. In: Yonenobu K, Sakou T, Ono K, eds. *Ossification of the posterior longitudinal ligament*. Tokyo: Springer-Verlag, 1997:165–172.
3. Hirabayashi K, Satomi K, Toyama Y. Surgical management of OPLL: anterior versus posterior approach. Part II. In: Clark CR, ed. *The cervical spine,* 3rd ed. Philadelphia: Lippincott-Raven, 1998:876–887.
4. Satomi K, Hirabayshi K, Itoh Y, et al. Staged posterior and anterior decompressive surgery for cervical spondylotic myelopathy with narrow spinal canal [in Japanese]. *Seikeigeka* 1977;28:1618–1626.
5. Aita I, Hayashi K, Wadano T, et al. Posterior movement and enlargement of the spinal cord after cervical laminoplasty. *J Bone Joint Surg Br* 1998;80:33–37.
6. Satomi K, Hirabayashi K. Ossification of the posterior longitudinal ligament. In: Herkowitz HN, et al., eds. *The spine,* 4th ed. Philadelphia: WB Saunders, 1999:565–580.
7. Sim FH, Svien HJ. Swan-neck deformity following extensive cervical laminectomy. *J Bone Joint Surg Am* 1994;56:564–580.
8. Oyama M, Hattori S, Moriwaki N, et al. A new method of cervical laminectomy [in Japanese]. *Chubu Seisei-shi* 1973;16:792–794.
9. Hirabayashi K. Expansive open-door laminoplasty for cervical spondylotic myelopathy [in Japanese]. *Shujutu* 1978;32:1159–1163.
10. Hirabayashi K, Toyama Y, Chiba K. Expansive laminoplasty for myelopathy in ossification of the longitudinal ligament. *Clin Orthop* 1999;359:35–48.
11. Iwasaki Y. Cervical expansive laminoplasty [in Japanese]. *Bessatsu Seikeigeksa* 1982;2:228–33.
12. Kurokawa T. Enlargement of spinal canal by the sagittal spitting of the spinal process laminoplasty (in Japanese). *Bessatsu Seikeigeksa* 1982;2:234–240.
13. Itoh T, Tsuji H. Technical improvements and results of laminoplasty for compressive myelopathy in the cervical spine. *Spine* 1985;10:729–736.
14. Yoshida M, Otani K, Shibasaki K, et al. Expansive laminoplasty with reattachment of spinous process and extensor musculature for cervical myelopathy. *Spine* 1992;17:491–497.
15. Hase H, Watanabe T, Hirasawa Y, et al. Bilateral open laminoplasty using ceramic laminae for cervical myelopathy. *Spine* 1991;16:1269–1276.
16. Lee TT, Manzono GR, Green BA. Modified open-door cervical expansive laminoplasty for spondylotic myelopathy: operative technique, outcome, and predictors for gait improvement. *J Neurosurg* 1997;86:64–68.
17. Satomi K, Miyasaka Y, Hoshi T, et al. Cervical expansive open-door laminoplasty with hydroxyapatite lamina spacers [in Japanese]. *Bessatu Seikeigeka* 1996;29:69–73.
18. Tsuzuki N, Abe R, Saiki K, et al. Tension-band laminoplasty for cervical spine. *Int Orthop* 1996;20:275–284.
19. Tomita K, Kawahara N, Toribatake Y, et al. Expansive midline-T saw laminoplasty (modified spinous process-splitting) for the management of cervical myelopathy. *Spine* 1998;23:32–37.
20. Satomi K, Nishi Y, Kohno T, et al. Long-term follow-up studies of open-door expansive laminoplasty for cervical stenotic myelopathy. *Spine* 1994;19:507–510.
21. Matsuzaki H, Hoshino M, Kiuchi T, et al. Dome-like expansive laminoplasty for the second cervical vertebra. *Spine* 1987;12:6–11.
22. Hirabayashi K, Satomi K. Operative procedure and results of expansive open-door laminoplasty. *Spine* 1988;13:870–876.
23. Japanese Orthopaedic Association. Scoring system for cervical myelopathy. *Nippon Seikeigeka Gakkai Zasshi* 1991;65:431–440.
24. Tsuzuki N, Abe R, Saiki K, et al. Extradural tethering effects as one mechanism of radiculopathy complicating posterior decompression of the cervical spinal cord. *Spine* 1996;21:203–211.
25. Shimizu T, Shimada H, Edakuni H. Post-laminoplasty palsy of upper extremities, with special reference to the spinal cord factor [in Japanese]. *Seikeigeka* 1996;29:188–193.
26. Satomi K, Ogawa J, Ishii Y, et al. Short-term complications and long-term results of expansive open-door laminoplasty. *Spine J* 2001;1.

CHAPTER 80

Spinal Instrumentation in Degenerative Disorders of the Cervical Spine

Lukasz Curylo and Howard S. An

HISTORICAL PERSPECTIVE

Spinal arthrodeses were originally performed primarily for stabilization of spinal tuberculosis. Studies in 1911 by Albee (1) and Hibbs (2) reported a high complication and death rate (40%). Such arthrodeses were performed as stand-alone structural grafts and required prolonged bedrest or cast immobilization. Early reports of cervical arthrodesis were published by Cloward (3), Smith and Robinson (4,5), and others (6) and involved noninstrumented cervical spine arthrodeses with a high nonunion rate.

The use of anterior cervical plate and screw fixation was first reported by Bohler in 1967 (7). Anterior cervical instrumentation was initially used in cervical trauma. However, because of the obvious benefits of this instrumentation, the indications for its use have been expanded to degenerative cases, including patients with multilevel decompressions, those with allograft use, and those who smoke. The mechanical design of anterior cervical plating initially involved nonconstrained designs. Subsequently, owing to the increased failure rate of nonconstrained implants, a "locking" screw design has been incorporated into contemporary anterior plates (8). Multiple designs of anterior plates exist, including both static and dynamic designs. Most recently, load-bearing devices have been investigated in cervical spine arthrodeses. Multiple anterior cervical arthrodesis cage designs are undergoing clinical trials as stand-alone devices (9,10).

Posterior spine arthrodesis attempts were initially published in nondegenerative cases. Initially, wiring was reported for treatment of Potts' disease by Hadra in 1891 (11). Rogers and colleagues published the first report of posterior interspinous wiring in 1942, describing fixation of cervical fractures and dislocations (12,13). Since then, numerous reports of various posterior interspinous and facet wiring techniques have been published. Even today, this simple technique remains a viable option for enhancing posterior arthrodesis, either as a stand-alone construct or in combination with posterolateral mass plating.

Posterior cervical plate fixation is a relatively more recent technique. It was initially used by Roy-Camille in 1970 (14) and popularized by Cooper and associates in 1988 (15). Initially reported in the trauma literature, its uses have since been expanded to primary and revision degenerative disorders. Since then, several variants of lateral mass plating technique haves been published by An and associates, Magerl and coworkers, and Anderson and associates (16,17). Initial reports involved the use of nonconstrained systems. Recently, fixed-angle or locking rod-screw polyaxial designs, such as the Synthes StarLock or Stryker-Howmedica Summit systems, are gaining popularity because of increased stability and ease of application.

ANTERIOR CERVICAL FIXATION

Indications

With the recent advances in surgical technique and material engineering, anterior cervical instrumentation is gaining popularity. It offers several benefits over noninstrumented arthrodeses by increasing the likelihood of a solid union, decreasing graft-related complications, and allowing for minimum postoperative immobilization.

Anterior plating can neutralize suboptimal biomechanical conditions in multilevel anterior decompressions and arthrodeses. Multilevel discectomies have decreased fusion rates because of the decreased stability and increased micromotion. Graft dislodgment in noninstrumented single-level anterior cervical discectomy and fusion (ACDF) is reported in 2% to 4.6% of cases. It is even higher in noninstrumented multilevel arthrodeses (10% to 29% of cases)

(18). Nonunion occurs in 10% to 12% of one-level ACDF, in 20% to 27% of two-level ACDF, and in an unacceptably high rate of 30% to 63% of three-level ACDF (19,20).

Plating is especially important in suboptimal biologic environments such as in smokers and when using allograft bone. Smoking is a well-known cause of increased pseudoarthrosis rate. The adverse effect of nicotine on graft incorporation and vascular ingrowth into autologous graft has been well demonstrated in animal models (21). Hillibrand and co-workers have shown an overall doubling of the nonunion rate from 19% to 38% in smokers with noninstrumented anterior cervical procedures (22). In this series, the nonunion effect was most pronounced in patients undergoing multilevel anterior cervical discectomy and interbody grafting, where the pseudoarthrosis increased from 24% to 50% in smokers. The effect of nicotine increases the nonunion rate by 27% to 47% (23).

Instrumentation also increases the rate of fusion, often allowing the use of less optimal grafting material such as allograft bone. Thus, donor site morbidity related to bone graft harvesting can be avoided. Fernyhough and colleagues (23a) have demonstrated in a series of 126 patients the increase of nonunion rate in patients with allograft (41%) as compared with autograft (27%). Certainly, a combination of smoking and allograft has an even greater effect on union. Bishop and associates in a prospective study of 132 patients have shown a significantly decreased fusion rate in smokers receiving allograft for cervical interbody arthrodeses (24).

Anterior plating prevents late deterioration of the alignment obtained at surgery and thus prevents delayed neurologic deterioration. This is essential in multilevel arthrodeses. Emery and associates showed a 4.3-degree to 6.5-degree increase in cervical kyphosis in noninstrumented three-level ACDF (25).

Anterior instrumentation can also be used in revision cases involving a psuedoarthrosis. Tribus and co-workers demonstrated an 81% fusion rate in anterior nonunions revised with anterior plating (26). It is indicated especially when allograft bone is used for such nonunion repair (27).

The postoperative course is favorably altered by allowing the use of less constrained cervical orthoses for postoperative immobilization. Rehabilitation time is often shortened, and resultant cost savings are obvious.

One-level ACDF in a nonsmoker with use of iliac crest autograft is usually performed without fixation (Fig. 80.1A). We prefer to use plating in one-level ACDF when using allograft bone or in smokers (Fig. 80.1B). Plating is also used for all multilevel ACDF and for one- and two-level corpectomies (Fig. 80.1C and D). Segmental fixation in such cases is recommended. However, because of potential complications of anterior plating of three- and four-level corpectomies, we prefer in such cases to combine an instrumented anterior strut arthrodesis with a posterior cervical fusion using lateral mass plating or to use rigid postoperative immobilization (two-poster brace,

four-poster brace, or halo vest). Often, corpectomies can be performed at the most severely involved levels and can be combined with ACDF at less involved areas. Thus, more stable segmental fixation constructs can be achieved (Fig. 80.1E).

Rationale

Anterior plates increase the stiffness of arthrodesis constructs and increase fusion rates. They also decrease graft-related complications.

Anterior plating systems have been refined through multiple modifications. Currently used systems allow for more rigid fixation with less risk. Smith and colleagues have demonstrated in biomechanical studies that locking of cervical screws to the plate provides additional stability under large angular displacement when comparing the nonlocking plates with the locking plates (28,29). Bicortical screw placement into the vertebral bodies additionally offers improved pullout strength in flexion-extension as compared with unicortical screws, as shown by Ryken and associates in a cadaveric study (30). Bicortical screw fixation provides additional stability in cyclic loading as compared with unicortical screws (31). However, the Synthes AO-Caspar plate with unlocked bicortical screw purchase offers no additional stability as compared with a locked unicortical screw-plate system, such as the Synthes CSLP plate (32) (Fig. 80.2A). However, multiple studies have demonstrated the high efficacy of locked unicortical screw-plate systems [such as the Sofamor-Danek Orion plate (Fig. 80.2B) or the DePuy-Acromed Peak plate (Fig. 80.2C)] in stabilizing degenerative cervical disorders. More recently, systems allowing dynamic axial compression across a fusion site have been introduced (e.g., Depuy-Acromed DOC Sliding plate, the Aesculap ABC plate, and the Sofamor Danek Premier Anterior plate). Such systems theoretically increase the healing rate by allowing for dynamic graft and end-plate axial compression while maintaining the rotatory and flexion-extension stability comparable to static locking plates (32). Initial clinical results are encouraging and show a 90% to 95.7% fusion rate with 4.3% graft and hardware complications, using dynamic plates in a mixed patient population (33,34). However, these systems may not provide rigid enough fixation for unstable fractures, and more long-term results are needed for three- and four-level fixation after multilevel corpectomy. There is no advantage of these systems in one- and two-level cases (35).

Vanichkahorn and colleagues have reported that the anterior buttress plate technique theoretically may prevent or decrease the prevalence of graft or internal fixation dislodgment in long segmental cervical arthrodeses (36). It must be stressed that three- or four-level corpectomy cases are challenging to restore biomechanical stability with anterior fixation alone, and posterior supplemental fixation should be considered. If posterior segmental fixation is used, anterior

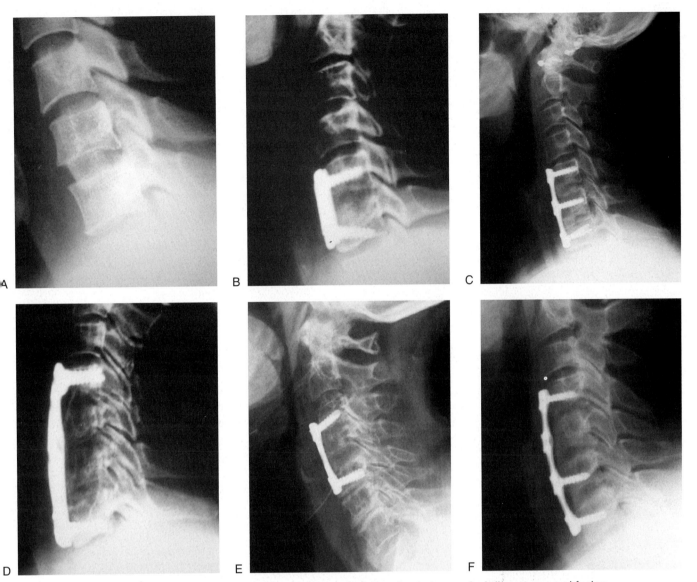

FIG. 80.1. A: Example of a successful nonplated single-level anterior cervical discectomy and fusion (ACDF) using autograft bone. **B:** Example of successful anterior Sofamor Danek Orion plate of a single-level ACDF using allograft bone. **C:** Example of successful anterior DePuy Acromed Peak plate with segmental screws following two-level discectomy and fusion with allograft **D:** Example of anterior Sofamor Danek Orion plate of a three-level ACDF using nonsegmental terminal screws. Use of rigid postoperative immobilization is strongly advised in this case. **E:** Variant of anterior DePuy-Acromed Peak plate with terminal screws of single-level corpectomy and fusion with iliac crest allograft and corpectomy autograft bone chips. **F:** Example of anterior DePuy-Acromed Peak plate with terminal screws and intermediate screws following corpectomy at one level and discectomy at another level with fusion with iliac crest allograft and corpectomy autograft bone chips. This semisegmental fixation gives superior stability over long strut graft with terminal screws alone.

buttress plate or any internal fixation other than bone graft probably is not needed.

Technique

For access to the lower cervical spine, the classic anteromedial Smith-Robinson approach is used (37). Incisions in line with Langer's skin lines are most commonly used and extend from midline to the lateral boarder of the sternocleidomastoid muscle. Occasionally, oblique or longitudinal incisions can be used for access to more than three cervical levels; however, cosmesis is inferior to transverse incisions because of scarring and contractions. The subcutaneous tissue, platysma, and deep cervical fascia are cut in line with the skin incision. The platysma muscle can be undermined cranially and caudally to gain access to more cervi-

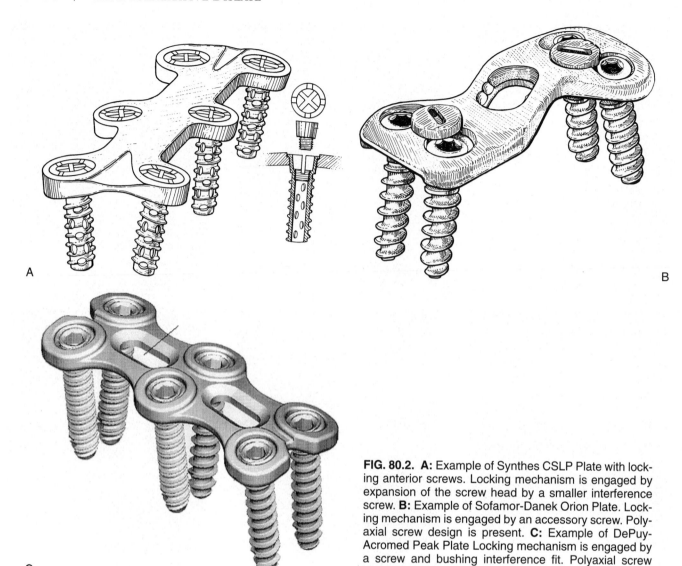

A

B

C

FIG. 80.2. A: Example of Synthes CSLP Plate with locking anterior screws. Locking mechanism is engaged by expansion of the screw head by a smaller interference screw. **B:** Example of Sofamor-Danek Orion Plate. Locking mechanism is engaged by an accessory screw. Polyaxial screw design is present. **C:** Example of DePuy-Acromed Peak Plate Locking mechanism is engaged by a screw and bushing interference fit. Polyaxial screw placement is possible.

cal levels. Care must be taken to avoid bleeding from large branches of the anterior jugular vein by their ligation or careful retraction. Next, gentle finger blunt dissection is done through the interval between the medial sternocleidomastoid muscle and the strap muscles. Once a plane is developed, it can be expanded proximally and distally to increase exposure. Care must be taken to retract the carotid sheath and its contents laterally by palpating the carotid pulse. Also commonly encountered, inferior thyroid artery must be protected or suture-ligated. A smooth retractor is then used to retract the tracheoesophageal structures medially and the sternocleidomastoid muscle laterally. Tension on the retractors allows for visualization of the pretracheal and the prevertebral fascia directly overlying the anterior cervical spine. Both these layers are then bluntly spread in the longitudinal direction to allow for direct surgical access to the discs and vertebral bodies. The longus colli muscle is then subperiostealy undermined. Self-retaining smooth blade retractors are positioned underneath this

muscle to prevent injury to the medially lying tracheoesophageal structures and the lateral carotid sheath. Depending on the level of the skin incision, the levels from C2 to T1 can be visualized with this approach. Next, depending on the degenerative pathoanatomy, decompression is performed by a discectomy or corpectomy, as described elsewhere in the textbook. This is followed by preparation of end plates and graft-docking sites. Next, distraction is applied, and the appropriate length of allograft or autograft is inserted.

The instrumentation phase begins with selection of plate length. Using calipers, the distance from midpoints of terminal vertebrae is measured, and an appropriate length of anterior plate is chosen. An appropriate length of plate should not impinge on disc spaces adjacent to the planned arthrodesis, which are not being arthrodesed. The plate is next contoured to match the radius of cervical lordosis. Anterior osteophytes are removed with a rongeur or burr to enlarge the plate contact surface. Before placement of the plate, the midline of the vertebral bodies is marked, so that it can be aligned with the long axis of the plate. Several landmarks can be used to identify the midline of each vertebral body: the peak of the convex contour of the body (in the mediolateral direction) or the middle of the distance from the right to left longus colli. The plate is then fixed with temporary pins, and the plate alignment is assessed. If necessary, portable radiographs can confirm the plate position. Compression is then applied at the terminal vertebrae either indirectly by removing traction, or through direct compression using a Cloward distractor. Depending on the surgeon's preference, unicortical or bicortical screw holes are then drilled using standard technique. For unicortical screws, a drill stop at 14 to 16 mm is recommended to prevent unwanted posterior cortex penetration (38). Bicortical screws are drilled at 2-mm increments until the posterior cortex is perforated. Tapping is recommended in sclerotic bone. Screws must be parallel to end-plate surfaces and should converge toward midline for optimal stability. Before final tightening, an intraoperative lateral radiograph confirms proper intraosseous screw placement and graft position. Most system manufacturers provide larger-diameter "salvage" or "emergency" screws, if previously misplaced screws need to be redirected and redrilled. During final tightening, the screw-locking mechanism must be engaged and verified.

For anterior access to C1-C2, modified approaches must be used. Either a lateral approach of Whitesides, anterior retropharyngeal approach of McAfee (39), or transoral-transpharyngeal decompressive approach as described by Fang and colleagues (40) can be used. With either approach, anterior C1-C2 fixation can be performed with the Harms plate (41) or by placement of transarticular anterior-to-posterior screws, as described by Vaccaro and colleagues (42).

POSTERIOR CERVICAL FIXATION

Indications

Posterior cervical arthrodeses are often performed in patients with degenerative diseases of the upper and lower cervical spine.

Uncommonly degenerative changes occur at the atlanto-occipital and atlantoaxial facet joints, with a documented 4.8% incidence (43). In such advanced cases, patients often fail conservative treatment. Occipitocervical and C1-C2 fusions can be used in such instances, especially when degeneration is a result of trauma or instability.

More commonly, posterior cervical arthrodeses are done for primary degeneration of the lower cervical spine. Instrumentation is often used to increase rigidity of such arthrodesis constructs and maintain alignment until fusion occurs. Often, posterior arthrodeses are used as salvage techniques in cases of pseudoarthrosis after attempted anterior arthrodeses. Interspinous wiring techniques are indicated for one-

level and multilevel arthrodeses of the lower cervical spine in cases with intact posterior elements. This technique is commonly employed in conjunction with rigid postoperative bracing. Posterior plating using lateral mass or pedicle screw fixation technique provides even stronger stabilization than stand-alone posterior wiring. Lateral mass plating lowers the prevalence of loss of reduction in cases of missing or insufficient posterior elements, which preclude interspinous wire fixation. It is routinely used to stabilize and prevent postoperative kyphosis in multilevel posterior fusions and in cases of posterior decompression by laminectomies and foraminotomies. If posterior elements are intact, plating is often combined with wiring for increased rigidity. Posterior plating is also indicated in circumferential cervical arthrodeses and in cases in which the arthrodesis crosses the cervicothoracic or occipitocervical junction. The need to eliminate or limit external postoperative immobilization and the need for early mobilization are other relative indications (15,17).

We routinely use posterior instrumentation in a lateral mass arthrodesis construct with multilevel laminectomies (Fig. 80.3A and B). This is often performed in patients with multilevel bilateral myeloradiculopathy who present with neck pain, instability, and loss of cervical lordosis. We prefer, however, a noninstrumented laminoplasty technique if symptoms are unilateral or if patients have minimal neck pain and a lordotic cervical spine.

Rationale

Multiple *in vitro* biomechanical studies have investigated the rigidity provided by various posterior fixation methods in the lower cervical spine (44,45).

Coe and colleagues evaluated *in vitro* posterior cervical wiring techniques in the lower cervical spine (46). Their results showed equal stability of interspinous (Bohlman triple wire and Rogers) techniques compared with sublaminar wiring, therefore obviating the need for this more dangerous technique.

Gill and associates evaluated posterior plating techniques with lateral mass fixation (47). They have shown the superior stability of lateral mass plates with bicortical screws as compared with Rogers' interspinous wiring technique and lateral mass plating with unicortical screws. Bicortical lateral mass screws are superior to unicortical screws, as shown by Heller and co-workers (48). Sutterlin and colleagues (44) have demonstrated the increased stiffness of posterior plating when compared with anterior plating techniques.

Posterior plating with pedicle screw fixation provides even higher stability. It is superior to both posterior lateral mass plating and anterior plating (49). Unfortunately, use of this technique is limited by cervical anatomy with narrow pedicles and the possibility of serious neurovascular complications. The only recommended sites for screw placement are the pedicles of C2, C7, and T1.

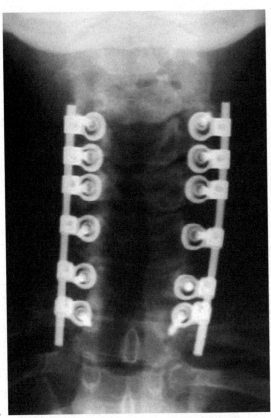

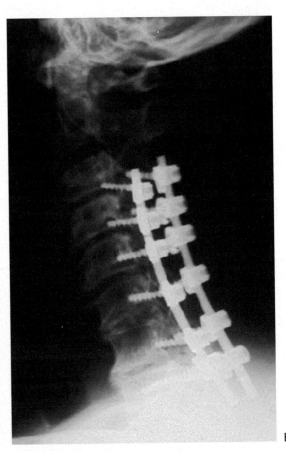

A

B

FIG. 80.3. Example of posterior multilevel fusion using lateral mass screws and rods (Synthesis Cervifix posterior cervical system) following a multilevel laminectomy. Immediate postoperative anteroposterior (**A**) and lateral (**B**) radiographs are shown.

In addition, upper cervical spine fixation methods have been extensively studied *in vitro* (50).

Technique

Posterior fixation is performed under general or local anesthesia with adjunctive intravenous sedation (51). The patient is positioned prone in cranial tong traction or a Mayfield head holder. In cases of myelopathy, severe stenosis or instability fiberoptic intubation is used, and the patient is turned on a Stryker table or rotating Jackson table. Prepositioning and postpositioning neurologic checks are routinely performed. A lateral radiograph ensures optimum positioning because lateral mass plating has minimal ability to correct malalignment. A midline approach through the posterior cervical raphé allows access to the occipital protuberance, spinous processes, and lamina and minimizes intraoperative bleeding. Paraspinal muscles are subperiosteally elevated at the desired levels. During the exposure, care must be taken at the superior margin of the C1 arch. If the dissection is more than 1.5 cm lateral to the midline, a substantial risk for vertebral artery injury exists. Also, the venous plexus between C1 and C2 should carefully be exposed to avoid bleeding.

Multiple sites are available for posterior fixation placement: the occipital bone; the laminae and transverse processes at all cervical levels; the pedicle at C2, C7, and T1; and the lateral masses at C3 to C7.

For occipitocervical arthrodesis, several techniques have been described: the Bohlman triple-wire technique (52), posterior plating, and the Ransford-Crockard loop (53). For purposes of fixation, Heywood and colleagues mapped the occipital bone thickness (54). The thickness ranges from 3 to 17 mm depending on the relations to midline and to the external occipital protuberance. Either unicortical or bicortical 3.5-mm screws can be placed, except for areas at the level of or superior to the external occipital protuberance. The proximity of the superior sagittal sinus and the transverse sinus precludes bicortical screw placement. Typical screw length is 6 to 12 mm. Similarly, wires can be passed through bicortical burr holes and used for fixation to bone graft or contoured rods.

Wire techniques, such as the Brooks or Gallie graft technique or their variations, are popular in the upper cervical spine arthrodeses in cases of C1-C2 arthrosis. They are usually used in conjunction with postoperative halo immobilization. They offer secure fixation without the risks of the Magerl intraarticular screw technique. These wiring techniques can even be employed in cases of severe osteoporosis that otherwise precludes screw fixation.

In the subaxial cervical spine, dissection is continued to the far lateral margin of the facet joints. To prevent postoperative instability and degeneration, care must be taken to preserve facet capsules of joints above and below the planned arthrodesis. Surgical landmarks of the rectangular lateral masses, including the margins and center, must be identified to facilitate screw placement. The medial boundary is the valley at the junction of the lamina and lateral mass. The lateral margin is the far edge of the facet. Adjacent facet joints define inferior and superior boundaries. At the C2 lateral mass, the vertebral artery passes through the superolateral quadrant. At C3 to C7, the relation of lateral masses to nerve roots and vertebral arteries is consistent: the exiting roots are located at level of the superior facet joint anterolaterally, and the vertebral artery lies anterior to the lamina–facet joint junction.

At C2, the pedicle presents with the optimal fixation site without risk for vertebral artery injury. The C2 pedicle medial and superior border should be palpated with a Penfield 4 elevator. The pedicle screw starting point is typically in the midline of the facet joint 3 to 5 mm cranial to the C2-C3 articulation. A 2.5-mm drill bit is used under direct fluoroscopic guidance. The screws typically converge 25 degrees and are aimed 25 degrees cranially. Typical screw length is 20 mm.

Four lateral mass screw techniques have been described in the lower cervical spine by An and associates (16), Anderson and colleagues (17), Jeannert and Magerl and co-workers (55), and Roy-Camille and co-workers (14). Roy-Camille and co-workers use center of the lateral mass as the screw starting point. The bicortical screw is directed straight anteriorly and 10 degrees laterally to avoid vertebral artery injury. The typical Roy-Camille screw length is 16 to 18 mm. Jeannert, Magerl, and co-workers use a starting point 1 to 2 mm medial and 1 to 2 mm cranial to the lateral mass center. They aim the bicortical screw 30 degrees cranially and 15 to 25 degrees laterally. A typical Magerl screw is 18-mm long. An and associates recommend using a starting point 1 mm medial to the lateral mass center and aim the bicortical screw 15 degrees cranially and 30 degrees laterally. Screws are usually 12 to 14 mm long with this technique. This is based on an anatomic study in which screws placed more cranially and medially had an increase risk for neurologic injury. Finally, Anderson and colleagues use a modified Magerl technique. The screw starts similarly 1 mm medial to the lateral mass center. It is aimed 20 to 30 degrees cranially and 10 to 20 degrees laterally. A typical Anderson screw has a depth of 16 to 18 mm. Montesano and associates (55a) showed the Magerl technique to have 40% higher pullout strength than the Roy-Camille screws. Heller and colleagues showed no significantly different morbidities when using different lateral mass screw techniques (56).

Because of the decreased anteroposterior thickness of the C7-T1 lateral mass, as compared with the other cervical levels, the C7-T1 pedicle screw offers often a safer site of fixation. The unique cervicothoracic junction anatomy has been thoroughly investigated by An and associates (57), Xu and colleagues (58), and Jonsson and co-workers (59). The average inner pedicle diameter at C7-T1 is 5 to 6.5 mm, thus easily accommodating a 3.5-mm diameter screw (60,61).

Supplemental posterior interspinous wires or cables can also augment anterior or posterior cervical plating.

CLINICAL RESULTS

Anterior Instrumentation

Abundant literature documents the benefits of internal fixation of the upper and lower cervical spine in degenerative disorders (62).

Anterior plating allows for increased fusion rates and decreased postoperative bracing in patients with multilevel ACDF. Wang and colleagues reported a significant increase of the union rate from 63% to 82% when plating was used in three-level ACDF, and from 75% to 100% when plating was used in two-level ACDF (63,64). However, anterior plating of one-level ACDF offers no significant increase in bony union over noninstrumented arthrodeses, especially in nonsmokers (65,66). However, it eliminates postoperative bracing, allows for allograft use, and increases the fusion rate in smokers. Analysis of stabilizations with anterior plating in smokers shows increased fusion rates and improved outcomes. A series of 106 patients undergoing two-, three-, and four-level ACDF with a 97% fusion rate was reported by Bose (67).

Anterior plating also increases union rates in one- and two-level corpectomy and arthrodesis. Used in conjunction with posterior wiring, anterior plates in patients with a corpectomy gave a 100% fusion rate with no graft-related complications, as compared with 14% graft complications in the nonplated group (68). Eleraky and colleagues demonstrated a 98.8% fusion rate in a mixed population of 185 patients undergoing anterior corpectomy and plating (69).

Use of anterior instrumentation also lowers the reoperation rate. Geisler and co-workers compared a large series of instrumented and noninstrumented one- and two-level fusions and demonstrated a decreased reoperation rate (70).

Anterior plating also maintains postoperatively the desired alignment in cervical lordosis. Katsuura and colleagues compared 30 nonplated to 44 plated multilevel anterior arthrodeses (71). Graft collapse with resultant kyphosis occurred in nine cases in the nonplated group and was not observed in the plated group.

Relatively few reports of anterior interbody cervical arthrodesis cages results have yet been published (9,72–74). Reported success rates for one- and two-level ACDF using the cage device were as high as 97% (75). Recent reports have shown that during 1- to 2-year follow-up, outcomes are similar in one-level arthrodeses with standard anterior cervical graft and plating as compared with patients with interbody cervical cages (76). Despite these favorable results, these implants still remain investigational.

Posterior and Combined Anterior and Posterior Instrumentation

Most reports of clinical results of posterior cervical arthrodeses with instrumentation have been published in the trauma literature. Anderson reported 100% fusion rates in traumatic injuries of the cervical spine arthrodesed with lateral mass plating (17). Also, Fehlings and Cooper reviewed 38 patients with posterior plating and reported a high 93% fusion rate with nonunion and resultant loss of kyphosis in only three patients (77).

Posterior plating is commonly used in multilevel laminectomy. It functions to improve alignment and stabilize the posterior spine, especially in cases of cervical hypolordosis or frank kyphosis. Kumar and colleagues reported long-term follow-up results of multilevel laminectomy and arthrodesis with lateral mass plating for cervical myelopathy (78). They showed improvement of neurologic status and maintenance of alignment.

Combined anterior and posterior cervical arthrodeses also benefit from cervical anterior and posterior fixation. Rogers and associates have shown that fusion rates of posterior plating as an adjunct to noninstrumented multilevel anterior cervical fusion using fibular allograft (socalled 360-degree arthrodeses) can be as high as 100% (79). Also, McAfee and co-workers reported excellent outcomes in circumferential arthrodeses in a series of 100 patients (80).

Finally, several authors have performed general outcome analysis of instrumentation in the cervical spine (81). These reviews have demonstrated the cost advantages and improved patient outcomes of instrumentation. McLaughlin and colleauges showed that the convalescence period was shortened from 136 to 66 days and resultant short-term disability was significantly reduced (82).

COMPLICATIONS

Complications after instrumentation of degenerative cervical disorders can occur at various time points during and after surgery. Such risks exist during the perioperative period, during the early postoperative healing phase, and finally in the late phase (after an established union or nonunion).

Perioperative Complications

Complications during the perioperative period related to exposure and decompressive technique are discussed elsewhere in the text. However, intraoperatively, substantial risks exist related to hardware placement.

Anterior cervical plating can potentially be complicated by neurologic or vascular injuries secondary to inappro-priate screw placement. Potential for nerve root or spinal cord injury related to bicortical screw placement is minimal, as documented by Lesoin and colleagues in 630 patients (83) and by Caspar and associates in 195 cases (84), where the incidence of this complication was 0%. Risk for vascular injury to the vertebral artery is also minimal (1 of 630 cases), as shown by Lesoin. More contemporary plate-screw systems and techniques with unicortical screw purchase offer an even safer alternative. Screws at the terminal end of a fusion construct often are also misplaced into the adjacent inferior or superior disc space. If such penetration occurs, it can be easily identified on intraoperative radiographs. Risks for such misplacement are related to a weaker construct with potential for early pullout failure. Long-term outcome may be affected by such misplaced screws related to premature degeneration of the affected adjacent disc.

Potential for perioperative neurovascular injuries also exists during application of posterior instrumentation. Screws placed during lateral mass plating can injure or impinge on the nerve root if bicortical purchase is obtained, especially when excessively long screws protrude into the neural foramen. The reported prevalence of resultant nerve root injury is low (0.6%) (85). This is more prevalent at the cervicothoracic junction (especially at C7 and T1 vertebrae) where the lateral masses are thinner than at more cephalad vertebrae (86). The complication rate of lateral mass screws is also technique dependent. *In vitro* studies have demonstrated lower risk for penetration with the An technique than with the Magerl and Anderson techniques (87). Most authors have shown that placement of later mass screws is safe and effective (88). Also, cervical pedicle screw placement poses risks for nerve root or vertebral artery injury. A clinical study by Abumi and associates documented a 6.7% prevalence of pedicle penetration; however, only 2 of the 45 misplaced screws were a source of radiculopathy, secondary to iatrogenic foraminal stenosis (89). The high risk for potential complications has also been shown by *in vitro* studies in which the incidence of pedicle penetration was as high as 18% (90). Vertebrae with larger pedicles, such as C2, C7, and T1, can safely accommodate a 3.5-mm pedicle screw (91,92). However, preoperative evaluation of C7 with computed tomography is mandatory because the foramen transversarium of C7 can contain the vertebral artery in 5% of patients (93). Screw placement in the C2 pedicle is also relatively safe provided adequate dissection is present allowing intraoperative verification of anatomic landmarks (usually the medial and superior aspect of the axis pedicle) (94).

Potential for such injuries also exists during transarticular C1-C2 screw placement using the Magerl technique (95). The prevalence of transarticular screw misplacement has been reported in up to 15%; however, resultant neurologic injuries occurred only in 1.2% of misplaced screws (96,97). The twelfth (hypoglossal) cranial nerve can be injured in up to 2.7% of patients if screws placed are too long (98). Neurologic risks for this technique can be minimized by meticulous preoperative evaluation and planning, as emphasized by several clinical and *in vitro* anatomic studies (99–101). Injuries to the vertebral artery (VA) by the Magerl screw technique occur in 8.6%, as reported by Madawi and co-workers (102). Fortunately, serious complications, such as exsanguination, brainstem or cerebellar infraction, and Wallenberg syndrome, are far less common. This is largely dependent on local anatomic factors: the presence of vertebral artery asymmetry (up to 52% prevalence), large VA groove (up to 20% prevalence) (103), VA anomalies (up to 2.3% prevalence) (104), and inadequate thickness of the C2 isthmus (up to 10% prevalence) (105).

Early Postoperative Complications

Complications during the early postoperative period are often graft related. Such complications as graft extrusion, graft settling, and nonunion occur less commonly as a result of additional stability provided by cervical instrumentation. In this phase, however, several hardware-related complications exist. They are mostly related to hardware failure or failure of the bone–screw interface.

Fatigue failure of anterior plates can occur through an established nonunion and has been reported in up to 14% of patients. Such failures are more common if thinner plates are used (Synthes Orozco, Synthes CSLP plate), as opposed to thicker implants, such as the Orion plate (8). Failure of the anterior cervical plate can also occur through fatigue fracture secondary to overcontouring of titanium plates (106).

Screw breakage can occur with several specific screw designs. Fenestrated Morscher and Hallowel screws, despite their theoretical advantage of bone ingrowth (107), have a reported high rate of fatigue failure and have been withdrawn from the market (108). Failure of solid screw designs is far less common and has been reported in up to 4% of cases (8).

Far more common than screw or plate breakage is the failure of the bone–screw interface. This is especially prevalent in patients with decreased bone strength in conditions like osteoporosis or degenerative disease superimposed on metabolic bone disease. Early designs of anterior cervical plates without a screw locking mechanism, such as the AO-Orozco Plate, demonstrated a predictably higher screw-loosening rate in up to 44% of patients (Fig. 80.4B and C). Contemporary locking screw designs are much more constrained (such as AO-CSLP plate or the Orion plate) and expectantly have a significantly decreased incidence of this complication of 18% (8).

Certainly, the rate of loosening is higher for multilevel discectomy constructs. Constructs involving multilevel cervical corpectomy and strut grafting that are instrumented with nonsegmental anterior plate fixation are particularly prone to early failure (109). The existence of a large lever arm, combined with graft pistoning, often results in failure of inferior screw fixation in such a long plate construct (Fig. 80.4A). Cadaveric models have demonstrated that anterior or posterior plating alone excessively loads the long graft with small degrees of motion and increases terminal screw-vertebra loosening, thus promoting failure (110–112). Also, the use of technique of instrumentation described as "antikick" or buttress anterior cervical plating has been reported to fail in an unacceptably high number of patients. Riew and associates (113) reported plate pullout in 2 of 14 of their buttress plates, and MacDonald and colleagues (114) observed a failure in two of two buttress plates. In most cases of backout, no injuries to neurovascular or tracheoesophageal structures occur. Screw backout, however, can result in erosion into the surrounding structures with resultant esophageal perforation (115). Such esophageal perforation can progress to a serious infection. Resultant fistulas of the esophagus can be treated by direct closure or by conservative treatment consisting of intravenous antibiotics, elimination of oral intake, and parenteral nutrition (116). Therefore, careful observation is necessary for such screw backout, with early removal of metallic implant (117). Rarely do such erosions occur without serious complications, but case reports of uneventful passage of hardware into the alimentary tract exist (118, 119). Tracheal injury with resultant catastrophic airway compromise and death can also occur secondary to failed anterior spine fixation. Riew and co-workers (115) reported this complication in 1 of 14 patients undergoing buttress anterior cervical plating for long segment fusions.

Early postoperative infections also occur with instrumentation in the cervical spine. The reported prevalence is up to 5% and is similar to that of instrumented procedures in other anatomic regions.

Late Postoperative Complications

Complications related to hardware after a successful fusion are rare. Certainly, a potential for bacterial seeding of implant with a resultant infection can occur; however, this has not been clinically documented. Rarely, scarring around anterior plates can promote the formation of a pharyngeal pouch (120). Local effects of posterior plating techniques are mostly related to impingement on facet joints of segments adjacent to a successful fusion. Such mechanical impingement may result in early degeneration and instability of adjacent motion segments. However, Hilibrand and colleagues reviewed patients who underwent arthrodesis without instrumentation. They demonstrated that the prevalence of adjacent segment degeneration at 5 years was 14% and at 10 years increased to 26% (121). The prevalence of adjacent segment disease after plating has not been well documented.

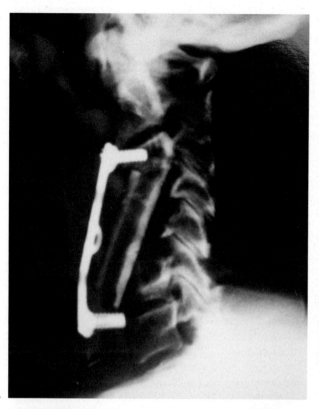

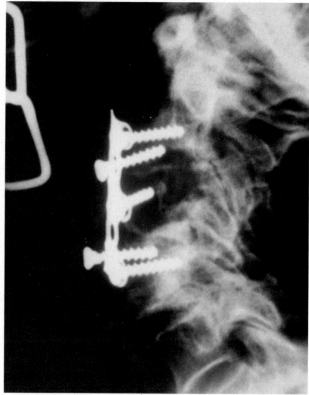

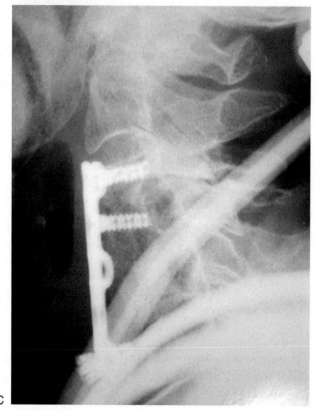

FIG. 80.4. A: Example of an early failure of plating in a case of multilevel corpectomy and fibula strut grafting. Note failure of the distal fixation and inferior graft extrusion, resulting in compression of anterior tracheoesophageal structures. **B:** Example of failure of segmental plate fixation in a multilevel anterior cervical discectomy and fusion (ACDF) case. Note the plate design with nonlocking screws. **C:** Example of failure of nonsegmental plate fixation in a multilevel ACDF case. Note the failure of fenestrated Morscher screws.

CONCLUSION

Instrumentation in degenerative disorders of the cervical spine is a safe and effective means of increasing the fusion rate. It is especially valuable in patients with less than optimal healing conditions, such as smoking or use of allograft. It can also be used for revision surgery in an attempt to repair an established pseudoarthrosis. Instrumentation offers cost savings to the patients and society, improves outcomes, and allows quicker return to work.

REFERENCES

1. Albee F. Transplantation of a portion of the tibia into the spine for Pott's disease: a preliminary report. *JAMA* 1911;57:885.
2. Hibbs PA. An operation for progressive deformities. *NY State J Med* 1911;93:1013.
3. Cloward R. Treatment of acute fractures and fracture dislocations of the cervical spine by vertebral body fusion. A report of 11 cases. *J Neurosurg* 1961;18:205–209.
4. Robinson R, Smith G. Anterolateral cervical disk removing and interbody fusion for cervical disk syndrome. *Bull Johns Hopkins Hosp* 1955;96:223–224.
5. Robinson R, Southwick W. Indications and techniques for early stabilization of the neck in some dislocations of the cervical spine. *South Med J* 1960;53:565.
6. Bailey R, Badgley C. Stabilization of the cervical spine by anterior fusion. *J Bone Joint Surg Am* 1960;42:565–624.
7. Bohler J. Sofort und Frühbehandlung traumatischer Querschnitt Lahmungen. *Z Orthop Ihre Grenzgeb* 1967;103(4):512–529.
8. Lowery G, McDonough R. The significance of hardware failure in anterior cervical plate fixation. Patients with 2 to 7 year follow-up. *Spine* 1998;23(2):181–186.
9. Hacker R, Cauthen J, et al. A prospective randomized multicenter clinical evaluation of an anterior cervical fusion cage. *Spine* 2000;25(20):2646–2654.
10. Kitchel S. Cervical interbody fusion with threaded titanium fusion cages: long term results. Poster presentation #14, Annual CSRS meeting, Seattle, WA, 1999.
11. Hadra B. Wiring of the vertebrae as a means of immobilization in fracture and Potts' disease. *Med Times Reg* 1891;22 [reprinted in *Clin Orthop Relat Res* 1975;112:4–8].
12. Hadra B. Wiring the vertebrae as a means of immobilization in fractures and Pott's disease. *Clin Orthop Relat Res* 1975;112:4–8.
13. Rogers W. Treatment of fracture and dislocations of the cervical spine. *J Bone Joint Surg Am* 1942;24:245–248.
14. Roy-Camille R, Saillant G. Fractures du rachis cervical. In: Judet R, ed. *Actualites de chirurgie orthopedique del'Hospital Raymond-Poincarre*, Vol 8. Paris: Masson & Cie, 1970:175–195.
15. Cooper P, Cohen A. Posterior stabilization of cervical spine fractures and subluxations using plates and screws. *Neurosurgery* 1988;23:300–306.
16. An H, Gordin R, et al. Anatomic considerations for plate screw fixation to the cervical spine. *Spine* 1988;13:813–816.
17. Anderson P, Henley M. Posterior cervical arthrodesis with AO reconstruction plates and bone graft. *Spine* 1991;16S:S72–S79.
18. Zdeblick T, Cooke M, Wilson D, et al. Anterior cervical discectomy, fusion and plating. A comparative animal study. *Spine* 1993;18:1974–1983.
19. Parsons IM, Kang JD. Mechanisms of failure after anterior cervical disk surgery. *Curr Opin Orthop* 1998;9:2–11.
20. Emery S, Fisher J, Bohlman H. Three-level anterior cervical discectomy and fusion: radiographic and clinical results. *Spine* 1997;22(22):2622–2624.
21. Riebel G, Boden S, et al. The effect of nicotine on incorporation of cancellous bone graft in an animal model. *Spine* 1995;20(20):2198–2202.
22. Hillibrand A, Fye M, et al. Impact of smoking on the outcome of anterior cervical arthrodesis with interbody or strut grafting. *J Bone Joint Surg Am* 2001;83(5):668–673.
23. Silcox D, Daftari T, et al. The effect of nicotine on spinal fusion. *Spine* 1995;20(14):1549–1553.
23a. Fernyhough JC, White JI, LaRocca H. Fusion rates in multilevel spondylosis comparing allograft fibula with autograft fibula in 126 patients. *Spine* 1991;16:S561–S564.
24. Bishop R, Moore K, et al. Anterior cervical interbody fusion using autogenic and allogenic bone graft substitute: a prospective comparative analysis. *J Neurosurg* 1996;85:206–210.
25. Emery S, Fisher J, Bohlman H. Three level anterior cervical discectomy and fusion: radiographic and clinical results. *Spine* 1997;22:2622–2625.
26. Tribus C, Corteen D, Zdeblick T. The efficacy of anterior cervical plating in the management of symptomatic pseudoarthrosis of the cervical spine. *Spine* 1999;24(9):860–864.
27. Coric D, Branch C, et al. Revision of anterior cervical pseudoarthrosis with anterior allograft fusion and plating. *J Neurosurg* 1997;86(6):969–974.
28. Grubb M, Currier B, et al. Biomechanical evaluation of anterior cervical spine stabilization. *Spine* 1998;23:886–892.
29. Smith S, Lindsey R, Doherty B, et al. An *in vitro* biomechanical comparison of the Orosco and AO locking plates for anterior cervical spine fixation. *J Spinal Disord* 1995;8(3):220–223.
30. Ryken TC, Goel V, et al. Assessment of unicortical and bicortical fixation in a quasistatic cadaveric model. Role of bone mineral density and screw torque. *Spine* 1995;20(17):1861–1867.
31. Chen I. Biomechanical evaluation of subcortical versus bicortical screw purchase in anterior cervical plating. *Acta Neurochir* (Wien) 1996;138:167–173.
32. Clausen J, Ryken T, et al. Biomechanical evaluation of Caspar and Cervical Spine Locking plate systems in a cadaveric model. *J Neurosurg* 1996;84(6):1039–1045.
33. Brodke D, et al. Dynamic cervical plates: do they load-share at the expense of stability? Poster presentation #65, Annual CSRS meeting, Seattle, WA, 1999.
34. Apfelbaum R, Dailey A, Barbera J. Clinical experience with a new load-sharing anterior cervical plate. Poster presentation #64, Annual CSRS meeting, Seattle, WA, 1999.
35. Fehlin M, Boker D, et al. Clinical and radiological evaluation of the Codman anterior cervical plate: results of a prospective, multicenter study with 2-year follow-up. Poster presentation #63, Annual CSRS meeting, Seattle, WA, 1999.
36. Vanichkachorn J, Vaccaro A, et al. Anterior junctional plate in the cervical spine. *Spine* 1998;23(22):2462–2467.
37. Smith G, Robinson R. The treatment of certain cervical disorders by anterior removal of the intervertebral disc and interbody fusion. *J Bone Joint Surg* 1958;40:607.
38. Ebraheim NA, Fow J, et al. The vertebral body depths of the cervical spine and its relation to anterior plate-screw fixation. *Spine* 1998:2299–2302.
39. McAfee P, Bohlman H. The anterior retropharyngeal approach to the upper part of the cervical spine. *J Bone Joint Surg Am* 1987;69:1371–1383.
40. Fang H, Ong B. Direct anterior approach to the upper cervical spine. *J Bone Joint Surg Am* 1962;44;1588–1604.
41. Harms J, Schmelzle R. Osteosynthesen im occipito-cervicalen Übergang vom transoralen Zugang aus. In: *17th SICOT World Congress Abstracts.* Munich: Demeter Verlag, 1987.
42. Vaccaro A, Ring D, et al. Salvage anterior C1-C2 screw fixation and arthrodesis through the lateral approach in a patient with a symptomatic pseudoarthrosis. *Am J Orthop* 1997;26:349–353.
43. Zapleat J, Valois J. Radiologic prevalence of advanced lateral C1–2 osteoarthritis. *Spine* 1997;21:2511–2513.
44. Sutterlin C, McAfee P. A biomechanical evaluation of cervical spinal stabilization methods in a bovine model. Static and cyclical loading. *Spine* 1988;13(7):795–802.
45. Smith ME, Cibischino M. A biomechanical study of a cervical spine stabilization device: Roy-Camille plates. *Spine* 1997;22(1):38–43.
46. Coe JD, Warden K. Biomechanical evaluation of cervical spinal stabilization methods in a human cadaveric model. *Spine* 1989;14(10):1122–1131.
47. Gill K, Paschal S, et al. Posterior plating of the cervical spine. A biomechanical comparison of different posterior fusion techniques. *Spine* 1988;13(7):813–816.

48. Heller J, Estes B, et al. Biomechanical study of screws in the lateral masses: variables affecting pullout resistance. *J Bone Joint Surg* 1996; 78:1315–1321.

49. Kotani Y, Cunningham B, Abumi K, et al. Biomechanical analysis of cervical stabilization systems. An assessment of transpedicular screw fixation in the cervical spine. *Spine* 1994;19(22):2529–2539.

50. Naderi S, Crawford N. Biomechanical comparison of C1-C2 posterior fixations. Cable, graft, and screw combinations. *Spine* 1998;23(18): 1946–1955.

51. Bohlman, B, Dabb B. Anterior and posterior cervical osteotomy. In: Bradford D, ed. *Master techniques in orthopedic surgery. The spine.* Philadelphia: Lippincott-Raven, 1997:75–88.

52. Wertheim S, Bohlman H. Occipitocervical fusions. *J Bone Joint Surg Am* 1987;69:833–836.

53. Ransford A, Crockard A, et al. Craniocervical instability treated by contoured loop fixation. *J Bone Joint Surg Br* 1986;68:173–177.

54. Heywood A, Learmonth, et al. Internal fixation for occipitocervical fusion. *J Bone Joint Surg Br* 1988;70:708–711.

55. Jeannert B, Magerl F, et al. Posterior stabilization of the cervical spine with hook plates. *Spine* 1991;16S:S56–63.

55a. Montesano PX, Jauch E, Jonsson H Jr. Anatomic and biomechanical study of posterior cervical spine plate arthrodesis: an evaluation of two different techniques of screw placement. *J Spinal Dis* 1992;5:301–305.

56. Heller J, Carlson G, et al. Anatomic comparison of the Roy-Camille and Magerl techniques for screw placement in the lower cervical spine. *Spine* 1991;16S:S552–557.

57. An H, Gordon R, et al. Anatomic consideration for plate screw fixation in the cervical spine. *Spine* 1991;16S:S548–551.

58. Xu R, Ebraheim N. Anatomy of C7 lateral mass and projection of pedicle axis on its posterior aspect. *J Spinal Disord* 1995;8:116–120.

59. Jonsson, Rausching. Anatomical and morphometric studies in posterior cervical spinal screw-plate systems. *J Spinal Disord* 1994;7:429–438.

60. Zindrick M, Wiltse, et al. Analysis of the morphometric characteristics of the thoracic and lumbar pedicles. *Spine* 1987;12:160–166.

61. Misenhimer G, Peck R, et al. Anatomic analysis of pedicle angle and cancellous diameter as related to screw size. *Spine* 1989;14:367–372.

62. Zaveri G, Ford M. Cervical spondylosis: the role of anterior instrumentation after decompression and fusion. *J Spinal Disord* 2001;14(1):10–16.

63. Wang J, McDonough P, et al. Increased fusion rates with cervical plating for three-level anterior cervical discectomy and fusion. *Spine* 2001;26(6):643–646.

64. Wang J, McDonough P, et al. Increased fusion rates with cervical plating for two-level anterior cervical discectomy and fusion. *Spine* 2000;25(1):41–45.

65. Zoega B, Karrholm J, Lind B. One-level cervical spine fusion. A randomized study, with or without plate fixation, using radiostereometry in 27 patients. *Acta Orthop Scand* 1998;69:363–368.

66. Wang J, McDonough P, et al. The effect of cervical plating on single-level anterior cervical discectomy and fusion. *J Spinal Disord* 1999; 12(6):467–471.

67. Bose B. Anterior cervical instrumentation enhances fusion rate in multilevel reconstruction in smokers. Poster presentation #37, Annual CSRS meeting, Seattle, WA, 1999.

68. Epstein N. The value of anterior cervical plating in preventing vertebral fracture and graft extrusion after multilevel anterior cervical corpectomy with posterior wiring and fusion: indications, results, and complications. *J Spinal Disord* 2000;13(1):9–15.

69. Eleraky MA, Llanos C, Sonntag VK. Cervical corpectomy: report of 185 cases and review of the literature. *J Neurosurg* 1999;90S:35–41.

70. Geisler FH, Caspar W, Pitzen T, et al. Reoperation in patients after anterior cervical plate stabilization in degenerative disease. *Spine* 1998; 23:911–920.

71. Katsuura A, Hukuda S, et al. Anterior cervical plate used in degenerative disease can maintain cervical lordosis. *J Spinal Disord* 1996;9(6): 470–476.

72. Profeta G, de Falco R, et al. Preliminary experience with anterior cervical microdiscectomy and interbody titanium cage fusion (Novus CT-Ti) in patients with cervical disc disease. *Surg Neurol* 2000;53(5):417–426.

73. Brooke N, Rorke A, et al. Preliminary experience of carbon fiber cage prostheses for treatment of cervical spine disorders. *Br J Neurosurg* 1997;11(3):221–227.

74. Ashkenazi E, Millgram M. Anterior cervical spine fusion with the aid of threaded C-BAK Cages. Experience in 38 myelopathic patients with a minimum 1 year follow-up. Poster presentation #30, Annual CSRS meeting, Seattle, WA, 1999.

75. Hacker R. A randomized prospective study of an anterior cervical interbody fusion device with a minimum of 2 years of follow-up results. *J Neurosurg* 2000;93S:222–226.

76. David S, David S, Orr R, et al. Prospective comparison of cervical lordotic interbody fusion cages versus plated ACDF for single level fusion. Poster presentation #32, Annual CSRS meeting, Seattle, WA, 1999.

77. Fehlings MG, Cooper P. Posterior plates in the management of cervical instability: long-term results in 44 patients. *J Neurosurg* 1994;81: 341–349.

78. Kumar V, Rea G, et al. Cervical spondylotic myelopathy: functional and radiographic long-term outcome after laminectomy and posterior fusion. *Neurosurgery* 1999;44:771–777.

79. Rogers D, McDonough P, Cortes Z, et al. Combined anterior and posterior fusions in patients requiring 3 or more vertebrectomies. Poster presentation #27, Annual CSRS meeting, Seattle, WA, 1999.

80. McAfee PC, Bohlman H, et al. One-stage anterior cervical decompression and posterior stabilization. A study of one hundred patients with a minimum of two years of follow-up. *J Bone Joint Surg Am* 1995;77:1791–1800.

81. Connoly P, Esses S, et al. Anterior cervical fusion: outcome analysis of patients fused with and without anterior cervical plates. *J Spinal Disord* 1996;9(3):202–206.

82. McLaughlin M, Purighalla V. Cost advantages of two-level anterior cervical fusion with rigid internal fixation for radiculopathy and degenerative disease. *Surg Neurol* 1997;48(6):560–565.

83. Lesoin F, Cama A, et al. The anterior approach and plates in lower cervical posttraumtic lesions. *Surg Neurol* 1984;21:581–587.

84. Caspar W, Barbier D, et al. Anterior cervical fusion and Caspar plate stabilization for cervical trauma. *Neurosurgery* 1989;25:491–502.

85. Heller J, Silcox D. Complications of posterior cervical plating. *Spine* 1995;20(22):2442–2448.

86. Stanescu S, Ebraheim N, et al. Morphometric evaluation of the cervicothoracic junction. *Spine* 1994;19:2082–2088.

87. Xu R, Haman S, et al. The anatomic relation of lateral mass screws to the spinal nerves. A comparison of the Magerl, Anderson, and An techniques. *Spine* 1999;24(19):2057–2061.

88. Wellman B, Follett K, et al. Complications of posterior articular mass plate fixation of the subaxial cervical spine in 43 consecutive patients. *Spine* 1998;23(2):193–200.

89. Abumi K, Shono Y, et al. Complications of pedicle screw fixation in reconstructive surgery of the cervical spine. *Spine* 2000;25(8):962–969.

90. Ludwig S, Kowalski J, et al. Cervical pedicle screws: comparative accuracy of two insertion techniques. *Spine* 2000;25(20):2675–2681.

91. Albert T, Klein G, et al. Use of cervicothoracic junction pedicle screws for reconstruction of complex cervical spine pathology. *Spine* 1998;23(14):1596–1599.

92. Panjabi M, Duranceau J, et al. Cervical human vertebrae: quantitative three-dimensional anatomy of the middle and lower regions. *Spine* 1991;16:861–869.

93. Jovanovic MS. A comparative study of the foramen transversarium of the sixth and seventh cervical vertebrae. *Surg Radiol Anat* 1990; 12:167–172.

94. Ebraheim N, Rollins J, et al. Anatomic consideration of C2 pedicle screw placement. *Spine* 1996;21(6):691–695.

95. Jeannert B, Magerl F. Primary posterior fusion C1/2 in odontoid fractures: indications, technique and results of transarticular screw fixation. *J Spinal Disord* 1992;5(4):464–475.

96. Gebhard I, Jeannert B. Anatomic assessment of atlanto-axial transarticular screw fixation. Presented at 21st Annual CSRS Meeting, New York, Dec 1–2, 1993.

97. Grob D, Jeannert B, Aebi M. Atlanto-axial fusion with transarticular screw fixation: transarticular screw fixation. *J Bone Joint Surg Br* 1991;73:972–976.

98. Ebraheim N, Misson J, et al. The optimal transarticular C1–2 screw length and the location of the hypoglossal nerve. *Surg Neurol* 2000; 53(3):208–210.

99. Nadim Y, Sabry F, et al. Computed tomography in the determination of transarticular C1-C2 screw length. *Orthopedics* 2000;23(4):373–375.

100. Jun B. Anatomic study for ideal and safe posterior C1-C2 transarticular screw fixation. *Spine* 1998;23(15):1703–1707.

101. Dull S, Toselli R. Preoperative oblique axial computed tomographic imaging for C1-C2 transarticular screw fixation: technical note. *Neurosurgery* 1995;37(1):150–152.

102. Madawi A, Casey A, et al. Radiological and anatomical evaluation of the atlantoaxial transarticular screw fixation technique. *J Neurosurg* 1997;86:961–968.

103. Madawi A, Solanki G, et al. Variation of the groove in the axis for the vertebral artery: implications for instrumentation. *J Bone Joint Surg Br* 1997;79:820–823.

104. Tokuda K, Miyasaka K, et al. Anomalous atlantoaxial portions of vertebral and inferior cerebellar arteries. *Neuroradiology* 1985;27:410–413.

105. Mandell I, Kambach B, et al. Morphologic considerations of C2 isthmus dimensions for the placement of transarticular screws. *Spine* 2000;25(12):1542–1547.

106. Baldwin N, Hartman G, et al. Failure of a titanium anterior cervical plate implant: microstructural analysis of failure. Case report. *J Neurosurg* 1995;83(4):741–743.

107. Morscher E, Sutter F, et al. Anterior plating of the cervical spine with the hollow screw-plate system of titanium. *Chirurgie* 1986;57(11):702–707.

108. Hollowell J, Reinartz J, et al. Failure of Synthes anterior cervical fixation device by fracture of Morscher screws: a biomechanical study. *J Spinal Disord* 1994;7(2):120–125.

109. Vaccaro A, Falatyn, et al. Early failure of long segment anterior cervical plate fixation. *J Spinal Disord* 1998;11(5):410–415.

110. Panjabi M, Isomi T, et al. Loosening at the screw-vertebra junction in multilevel anterior cervical plate constructs. *Spine* 1999;24:2383–2388.

111. Foley K, DiAngelo D, et al. The *in vitro* effects of instrumentation on multilevel cervical strut graft mechanics. *Spine* 1999;24:2366–2376.

112. DiAngelo D, Foley K, et al. Anterior cervical plating reverses load transfer through multilevel strut-grafts. *Spine* 2000;25:783–795.

113. Riew D, Sethi N, et al. Complications of buttress plate stabilization of cervical corpectomy. *Spine* 1999;24:2404.

114. MacDonald RL, Fehlings M, et al. Multilevel anterior cervical corpectomy and fibular allograft fusion for cervical myelopathy. *J Neurosurg* 1997;86:990–997.

115. Smith M, Bolesta M. Esophageal perforation after anterior cervical plate fixation. *J Spinal Disord* 1992;5(3):357–362.

116. Newhouse K, Lindsey R, et al. Esophageal perforation following anterior cervical spine surgery. *Spine* 1989;14(10):1051–1053.

117. Hanci M, Toprak M, et al. Oesophageal perforation subsequent anterior cervical spine screw/plate fixation. *Paraplegia* 1995;33(10):606–609.

118. Fujibayashi S, Shikata J, et al. Missing anterior cervical plate and screws: a case report. *Spine* 2000;25:2258–2261.

119. Yee G, Terry AF. Esophageal penetration by anterior cervical fixation device: a case report. *Spine* 1993;18:522–527.

120. Sood S, Henein R, et al. Pharyngeal pouch following anterior cervical fusion. *J Laryngol Otol* 1998;112(11):1085–1086.

121. Hilibrand AS, Carlson GD, Palumbo MA, et al. Radiculopathy and myelopathy at segments adjacent to the site of a previous anterior cervical arthrodesis. *J Bone Joint Surg Am* 1999;81:519–528.

CHAPTER 81

Management of Adjacent Segment Disease following a Prior Cervical Fusion

Robert A. McGuire, Jr.

Degeneration of segments adjacent to a prior fusion of the cervical spine can lead to neural compromise necessitating further surgery. The management of this adjacent segment degeneration can sometimes prove to be difficult. This chapter discusses situations that lead to increased degeneration and methods that can be used to minimize the possibility of adjacent segment problems as well as methods of treatment when these problems become symptomatic.

PATHOPHYSIOLOGY OF ADJACENT SEGMENT DEGENERATION

Yoon and colleagues (1) recently presented data from a study using a three-dimensional nonlinear finite element model of C4 to C7. They were able to vary flexion and extension moments, simulate normal cervical loads, and vary the angles at which these forces were applied. This model allowed the investigators to simulate fusion of the cervical spine in a fixed kyphotic position. The results of this study found significant increases in the adjacent disc motion in both flexion and extension. With the spine fused in kyphosis, it was found that adjacent segments moved less than those fused in the neutral position under the same application of force. To maintain normal cervical movement, the forces required for adjacent segment movement are increased, which places an increased biomechanical demand on the cervical spine. This study suggests a deleterious effect of a kyphotic graft or fusion on adjacent segments during flexion and extension (Fig. 81.1).

This report by Yoon and colleagues is supported clinically by a retrospective review of 60 patients with a mean follow-up period of 4.5 years by Kawakami and associates (2). They found that 18% of this group developed adjacent segment degeneration, with 50% of these having clinically important symptoms. In analyzing the data, the investiga-tors found a local kyphosis and narrowing of the neural foramina at the fused segment more often in patients with symptoms than in those without symptoms.

There is discussion in the literature about whether the adjacent segment degeneration is a result of the continued progression of normal cervical spondylosis, or whether it is triggered by the increased forces across the adjacent segment as a result of internal fixation or fusion. Goffin and co-workers (3) reviewed 120 patients who had been treated with a cervical arthrodesis for either degenerative conditions or trauma situations with no preexisting degenerative spondylosis noted at least 5 years after their initial surgery. They found that 92% of these patients developed degenerative changes at either the superior or inferior segment at follow-up. There was no differential in the percentage of degeneration in those treated with internal fixation compared with those treated with a graft only. These investigators surmised from these data that the fusion itself was the triggering factor rather than the normal progression of preexisting degenerative changes. They also noted that those patients who had been treated with plate fixation had an increased prevalence of ossification of the anterior longitudinal ligament (66% ossification in those treated with a plate as compared with 29% in those treated without plate). This data differed from previous studies, which suggested that degeneration occurs at the adjacent level at a more rapid rate if degenerative changes are present at the time of the initial arthrodesis (4).

Hamburger and colleagues (5) reviewed 249 patients who had a cervical discectomy and interbody fusion with polymethylmethacrylate and were followed for a mean of 12.2 years. Twenty of these patients (8%) had adjacent segment abnormalities requiring further surgery. Eleven of these patients had been symptom free for more than a year, whereas seven had no symptom resolution with the first surgical pro-

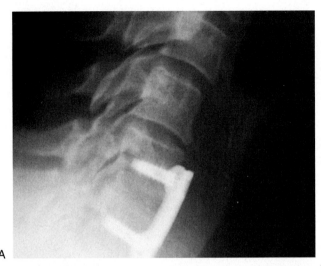
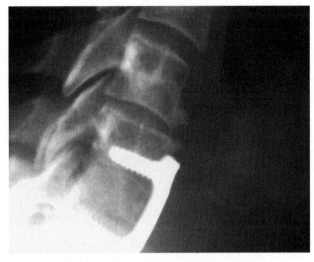

A

B

FIG. 81.1. A: This lateral cervical radiograph reveals degeneration of the segment above the fusion 2 years after the initial fusion. **B:** Continued degeneration is noted by progressive disc space narrowing and osteophyte formation 2 years after Fig. 81.1A was taken. The patient continues to be asymptomatic at this time.

cedure. This suggests that 3% (7 of 249) of this group had two-level disease that should have been addressed initially.

Hilibrand and colleagues (4) found fusion at the C5-C6 level with evidence of preexisting adjacent segment degeneration before initial surgery to increase significantly the risk for new disease onset. In this series of 374 patients followed over a long period, symptomatic adjacent segment disease occurred at a rate of 2.9% per year over a 10-year period. These investigators found the risk for adjacent segment disease to be less in multilevel fusions than in one-level segments. In this population, more than two thirds of patients failed conservative treatment and required surgical intervention.

MANAGEMENT OF SYMPTOMATIC ADJACENT DISEASE

Review of clinical data in patients treated for adjacent segment disease suggests conservative treatment to be effective in 30% to 50% of the cases (2,4). The risk for developing symptomatic adjacent segment disease appears to be related to cervical levels involved initially. The lowest risks per level appear to be at the cervicothoracic and the second and third levels. The risk at the C3-C4 and C4-C5 levels is 3.2 times the lowest level, and the risk is 4.9 times the lowest level at the C5-C6 and C6-C7 levels (4). This information is very important in patients who have a symptomatic C5-C6 disc herniation with radiculopathy and adjacent segment degenerative disease at either C4-C5 or C6-C7 without nerve compression. There is a significant risk for repeat surgery at the adjacent segment within a short period of time after surgery when these levels are not addressed with the initial surgery. Therefore, based on the risks for progression, the adjacent segment may need to be included

with the initial surgery. When discussing possible surgical options with the patients, inclusion of the adjacent segment in the high-risk group should be considered.

In individuals who develop symptomatic adjacent segment disease, nonoperative methods should be tried initially unless there is a progressive neurologic condition. Nonoperative measures consist of physical therapy for stabilization, optimal posturing, and strengthening of the cervical musculature. The use of a soft cervical collar and nonsteroidal antiinflammatory drugs as adjuvants to the physical therapy can be helpful (6–9).

In patients who fail nonoperative treatment, surgical options should be considered. In patients with radiculopathy as a result of a lateral disc herniation, foraminal decompression with removal of the free fragment has been shown to be quite successful (10) (Fig. 81.2). This foraminotomy technique should not be considered in patients with substantial axial pain or instability arising adjacent to a fused segment, as removal of the first is likely to increase instability and potentially worsen pain comparent.

In patients with symptomatic radiculopathy or myelopathy, anterior surgery should be considered. This allows direct decompression of the neural elements and bone grafting with maintenance of anterior column support to reestablish normal cervical lordosis. Hilibrand and associates (11) found in their study of 38 patients treated for adjacent segment disease had a fusion rate of 63% when using tricortical grafting alone. The rate of fusion did not significantly differ in those individuals treated with either one-level or multilevel fusion with grafts at each individual level rather than strut grafting (62% vs. 64%). On the other hand, they found 100% fusion when the patients with multilevel fusion were treated with strut grafting across all segments, as com-

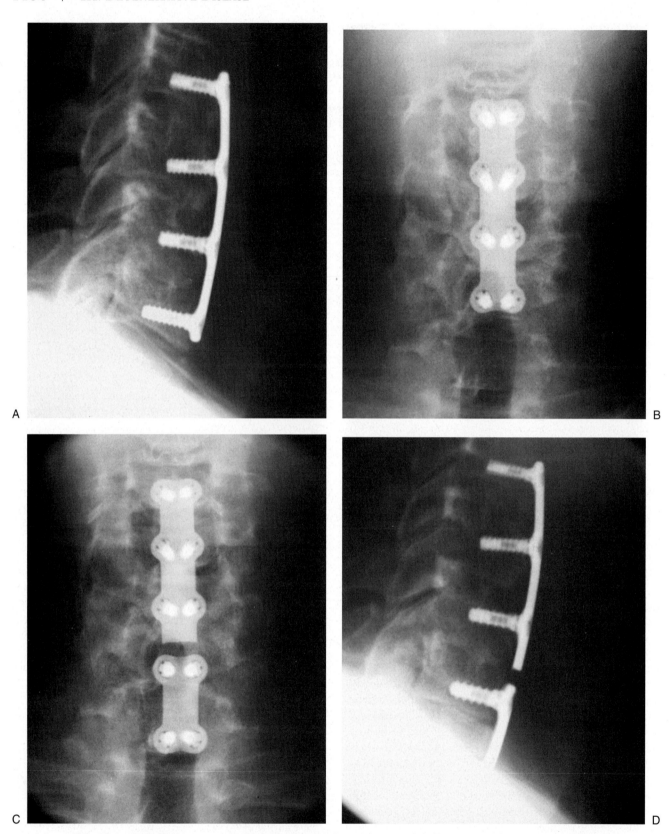

FIG. 81.2. A, B: This anteroposterior and lateral radiograph was taken 9 months after a multilevel anterior cervical discectomy and fusion (ACDF) with anterior plate fixation. The patient subsequently developed a disc herniation at the adjacent C6-C7 segment and needed to have this addressed surgically. **C, D:** To minimize potential problems from exposure required to remove the previous plate, the caudal screws were removed, and the plate was cut off. After decompression and grafting were done, a plate was placed and stabilized with oversized screws in the previous holes cephalad, and regular fixation was achieved in the caudal body. The radiculopathy and axial pain resolved with a good clinical recovery.

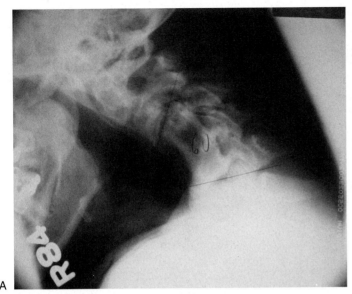
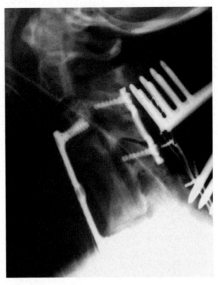

FIG 81.3. A: This patient had previous multiple cervical procedures but was left in significant kyphosis. Instability developed above the fused segment, resulting in myelopathy. Studies have shown significant forces to be developed at the adjacent segment disc space in these situations. **B:** After decompression, reconstruction was accomplished with strut grafts to maintain the angular correction. Because to its length, posterior fixation was also placed to protect the anterior construct.

pared with 63% fusion in those treated with individual tricortical grafts at each segment. These investigators suggested that the difference noted may be that the strut, in passing through a trough in the previous fused segment, provides more bony contact, enhanced stability, and therefore a better arthrodesis. Another possibility suggested by the authors for the increased rate of union in those patients treated with a strut is the fact that bony union is only required over two end-plate surfaces rather than the four or six surfaces required in two- or three-level fusion procedures, therefore increasing the probability of obtaining a solid arthrodesis.

The use of anterior plating has been shown to enhance the fusion rate over grafting alone (12). It does so by increasing the stability across the graft site. When more than three segments are involved, posterior stabilization should also be considered because there has been shown to be a substantial risk for failure with the anterior procedure alone (13) (Fig. 81.3).

CONCLUSION

Adjacent segment disease occurs at a rate of 2.9% per year, and over a 10-year period, 25% of patients develop new adjacent segmental disease. About half require surgical treatment. When a free fragment of disc is present and the patient has radiculopathy only, posterior foraminotomy and disc excision have a good clinical success rate. When the patient has substantial axial pain with instability or myelopathy, anterior decompression and strut grafting or tricortical grafting and plate fixation should be considered. It is im-

portant to reestablish normal cervical lordosis to minimize stress on remaining adjacent segments.

REFERENCES

1. Yoon T, Natarajan R, An H, et al. Adjacent disc biomechanics after anterior cervical diskectomy and fusion in kyphosis. Presented at Cervical Spine Research Society, Charleston, SC, Nov. 30–Dec. 2, 2000.
2. Kawakami M, Tetsuya T, Yoshida M, et al. Axial symptoms and cervical alignments after cervical anterior spinal fusion for patients with cervical myelopathy. *J Spinal Disord* 1999;12:50–56.
3. Goffin J, Geusens E, Vantomme N, et al. Long-term follow-up after interbody fusion of the cervical spine. Present at Cervical Spine Research Society, Charleston, SC, Nov. 30, Dec. 2, 2000.
4. Hilibrand A, Carlson G, Palumbo M, et al. Radiculopathy and myelopathy at segments adjacent to the site of a previous anterior cervical arthrodesis. *J Bone Joint Surg* 1999;4:519–528.
5. Hamburger C, Festenberg F, Uhl E. Ventral discectomy with PMMA interbody fusion for cervical disc disease. Long-term results in 249 patients. *Spine* 2001;26:249–255.
6. Fanciullo GJ, Hanscom B, Seville J, et al. An observational study of the frequency and pattern of use of epidural steroid injection in 25,479 patients with spinal and radicular pain. *Reg Anesth Pain Med* Jan.–Feb., 2001;26:5–11.
7. Ellenger MR, Honet JC, Treanor WJ. Cervical radiculopathy. *Arch Phys Med Rehabil* 1994;75:342–352.
8. Ferrante FM, Wilson SP, Iacobo C, et al. Clinical classification as a predictor of therapeutic outcome after cervical epidural steroid injection. *Spine* 1993;18:730–736.
9. Weinstein SM, Herring SA, Derby R. Contemporary concepts in spine care. Epidural steroid injections. *Spine* 1995;20:1842–1846.
10. Herkowita HN, Kurz LT, Overholt DP. Surgical management of cervical soft disc herniation. A comparison between the anterior and posterior approach. *Spine* 1990;15:1026–1030.
11. Hilibrand AS, Yoo JU, Carlson GD, et al. The success of anterior cervical arthrodesis adjacent to a previous fusion. *Spine* 1997;22:1574–1579.
12. Zdiblick TA, Cooke JE, Wilson D, et al. Anterior cervical discectomy, fusion and plating; a comparative animal study. *Spine* 1993;18:1974–1983.
13. Vaccaro AR, Falatyn SP, Scuderi GJ, et al. Early failure of long segment anterior cervical plate fixation. *J Spinal Disord* 1998;11:410–415.

SECTION X

Complications

CHAPTER 82

Management of Cervical Kyphosis Caused by Surgery, Degenerative Disease, or Trauma

D. Greg Anderson, Jeff S. Silber, and Todd J. Albert

Cervical lordosis is critical to normal sagittal plane balance of the spine. It compensates for thoracic kyphosis and allows the head to be positioned over the trunk. This produces a neutral sagittal vertical axis and minimizes the muscular effort necessary to maintain an upright posture (1). Cervical kyphosis is defined as a forward decompensation of the head in the sagittal plane (2). Segmental kyphosis is present when there is an angular relationship between two vertebrae with a posterior-directed apex. Cervical kyphosis results in a major alteration of biomechanical forces acting on the neck. There are many causes of cervical kyphosis, including trauma, tumor, surgery, congenital deformities, musculoskeletal dysplasias, inflammatory conditions, and degenerative diseases. This chapter focuses on cervical kyphosis due to surgery, degenerative disease, and trauma.

ANATOMY AND BIOMECHANICS

The normal weight-bearing axis of the head (sagittal vertical axis) passes through the middle of the C1 and T1 vertebral bodies and falls behind the vertebral bodies of C2 through C7 (Fig. 82.1) (3). The normal mean sagittal contour of the adult cervical spine is 14.4 degrees of lordosis (4). Biomechanically, the cervical spine is composed of an anterior column made up of the vertebral bodies, discs, and associated ligaments and a posterior column made up of the facet joints, laminae, and posterior ligamentous structures (2,5,6). Compressive loads are supported by a normal lordotic cervical spine by distributing 36% of the load through the anterior column, while each side of the posterior column supports 32% of the load. Thus, the posterior column supports a total of 64% of an applied axial load (7). Ligament sectioning studies have documented the importance of both the anterior and posterior osteoligamentous structures

in maintaining spinal stability. With regard to the development of kyphosis, at least one of the posterior structures in addition to an intact anterior column is required to prevent failure of the spinal segment (5,6).

The competence of posterior column structures, in particular the facet joints, is critical to the maintenance of a lordotic cervical posture. Using finite element analysis, Saito and associates (8) found that loss of one or more posterior elements (such as the spinous process, ligamentum flavum, or intraspinous ligaments) subjected the facet joints to tensile forces rather than the normal compressive loads. Several investigators have documented decreased stiffness and increased motion of the cervical spine following laminectomy (9,10).

Cusick and colleagues (11) found that unilateral facetectomy decreased the strength of the vertebral motion segment by 31%, whereas bilateral facetectomy resulted in a 53% decrease in strength during flexion compression loading. In addition, facetectomy caused anterior displacement of the instantaneous axis of rotation in the sagittal plane, leading to increased compressive loads on anterior column structures (11). Using a finite-element cervical spine model, Kumaresan and associates (12) demonstrated that removal of more than 50% of the facet joints bilaterally transferred high stresses to the annulus fibrosis during flexion and rotation. Raynor and Carter (13) studied the effects of both 50% and 70% facetectomies on the ultimate strength of the cervical motion segment. Fifty percent facetectomy allowed exposure of only 3 to 5 mm of nerve root but did not result in failure at the facet joint. A 70% facetectomy allowed exposure of 8 to 10 mm of nerve root but resulted in failure via a fracture at the facet joint during shear loading. Zdeblick and associates (14,15) studied the effect of progressive losses of either the facet joint or the facet capsule on a single-level laminectomy model and found that both

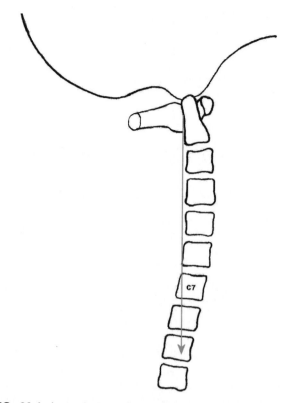

FIG. 82.1. Lateral view of the occiput, cervical, and upper thoracic spine. Notice that due to the normal lordosis of the cervical region, the weight-bearing axis (sagittal vertical axis) begins at the occipital condyles, falls behind the behind the vertebral bodies of C2 to C7, and passes through the vertebral body of T1.

flexional and torsional stability were significantly compromised by loss of more than 50% of either structure. Nowinski and colleagues (16) demonstrated significantly increased motion with resection of as little as 25% of the facet joint in a multilevel laminectomy model.

Loss of anterior column height also can contribute to cervical kyphosis. The discs make up about 15% of cervical height and are normally slightly trapezoidal, with a greater height anteriorly than posteriorly. Loss of disc height due to degenerative arthritis or collapse of a vertebral body secondary to a fracture can shorten the anterior column, leading to a kyphotic deformity. This in turn can alter the weight-bearing axis and transfer tensile and shear forces to the posterior column structures.

The contribution of normal muscle function to the development of cervical kyphosis has been debated. Perry and Nickel (17) felt that posterior cervical muscle paralysis did not necessarily lead to notable instability as long as the bony and ligamentous restraints remained intact. However, Saito and associates (8) demonstrated in an *in vitro* study that any forward shift in the gravitational center of the head promoted cervical kyphosis. Nolan and Sherk (1) studied the extensor musculature and found that the semispinalis cervicis and capitis were primarily responsible for exten-

sion of the spine and head. They emphasized the importance of preserving the attachment of the muscles to the C2 arch whenever possible and demonstrated that about 14 kg of force was required to support the head in a horizontal position. Other authors have emphasized the role of muscle denervation or fibrosis secondary to aggressive retraction that can predispose to the development of a kyphotic deformity (18,19).

Regardless of the initial pathomechanics, cervical kyphosis initiates a vicious cycle of pathological forces that can result in the development of a progressive deformity (3). As the head shifts forward, the weight-bearing axis is translated anteriorly, causing the anterior column to be loaded with increased compression while the posterior column is placed under increased tensile loads. Posterior extensor muscles are placed at a mechanical disadvantage and may become less effective at holding the head upright (1). Chronic tensile forces may result in attenuation of the posterior ligamentous structures and facet capsules. As the deformity progresses, the neural elements are translated forward against the apex of the kyphos, resulting in spinal cord dysfunction (Fig. 82.2). In summary, this can lead to a triad of progressive deformity, neurologic compromise, and further stretching of the posterior soft tissue restraints.

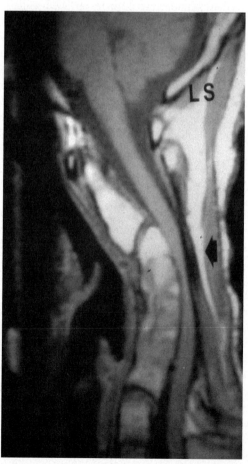

FIG. 82.2. Spinal cord draping over kyphos in postlaminectomy kyphosis.

Spinal cord stresses are generated as the cord is pulled against the apex of the kyphotic deformity, resulting in irritation or dysfunction of the cord or nerve roots or both. A finite amount of spinal cord lengthening can occur without a substantial rise in internal tensile stresses, such as occurs with normal cervical flexion. However, in pathological kyphosis, the posterior cord may be lengthened beyond its elastic limits, resulting in the generation of tensile stresses within the cord. In addition, the anterior spinal cord becomes compressed as the cord is pulled against the apex of the kyphos, bringing it into contact with an osteophyte or protuberant intervertebral disc. The spinal cord may also be subjected to a bending load across the apex of the kyphosis. The additive effect of these internal stresses results in complex changes within the spinal cord. In the anterior cord, compressive stresses predominate, whereas in the posterior cord tensile stresses are predominant. Cord flattening and internal stresses may lead to compromise of cord microvasculature and neuronal ischemia. Variations in cord stresses and ischemia are partly responsible for the wide spectrum of neurologic manifestations observed in patients with a cervical kyphotic deformity (20,21).

CLINICAL PRESENTATION

The symptoms of cervical kyphosis can vary depending on the nature and severity of the underlying condition. The most commonly experienced symptoms include radiculopathy, myelopathy, neck pain, muscle fatigue, and loss of forward gaze.

Patients with postlaminectomy kyphosis often give a history of a honeymoon period with improved symptoms following a posterior laminectomy. However, with the development of forward decompensation of the head, they begin to experience worsening neck pain, muscle fatigue and spasm, neurologic deterioration, and occasionally loss of forward gaze (due to fixed downward head position). In addition to complaints of radicular arm pain, the physician must search for symptoms of spinal cord dysfunction. Myelopathy can present as subtle clumsiness in the hands, gait unsteadiness, or sphincter dysfunction. Signs of hyperreflexia, pathological reflexes such as Hoffmann's and Babinski's signs, and difficulty with tandem gait should be documented.

Myelopathy in the setting of cervical kyphosis tends to be progressive and should be treated to halt spinal cord irritation and dysfunction. Ebersold and associates (22) reported that, of several factors evaluated, only a long duration of myelopathic symptoms predicted a poor neurologic outcome for patients following decompression of cervical spondylotic myelopathy.

Neck pain and gaze difficulty can cause substantial disability for patients. The forward position of the head necessitates constant contraction of the neck extensor muscles to balance the weight of the head against gravity. This leads to muscle fatigue and neck pain that often worsens as the day progresses. Gaze difficulty may be encountered in patients with a severe, fixed cervical kyphotic deformity, especially in patients with ankylosing spondylitis. To look forward, a patient with a kyphotic deformity must compensate by hyperextension at another level, often the occipitocervical junction. If hyperextension is not possible, forward gaze may be limited.

POSTLAMINECTOMY CERVICAL KYPHOSIS

The true prevalence of postlaminectomy kyphosis is difficult to ascertain from the literature due to the heterogeneous nature of the patients undergoing laminectomy, but it is probably the most common cause of cervical kyphosis. Factors such as age, preoperative sagittal alignment, underlying diagnosis, aggressiveness of the posterior procedure, and the location and number of laminae removed all help to define the risk of developing cervical instability.

Iatrogenic instability following a cervical laminectomy often follows a characteristic clinical sequence. In the early postoperative course, there is often good resolution of radicular or myelopathic symptoms due to decompression of the neural elements. As kyphosis begins to develop, the patient will often complain of axial neck pain associated with easy fatigability of neck musculature. As the kyphotic deformity worsens, there is often a recurrence of the old neurologic symptoms or the development of new neurologic complaints. This may cause the patient to return to the use of a cervical collar or lead to manual support of the chin.

Postlaminectomy kyphosis is seen much more frequently in growing children than in adults, with a reported prevalence of 37% to 95% (23–29). After multilevel laminectomy, Bell and colleagues (25) found a 37% prevalence of kyphosis and a 15% prevalence of hyperlordosis. When combining cervical laminectomy with a suboccipital decompression to treat an Arnold-Chiari malformation, Aronson and associates (24) reported a 95% prevalence of cervical kyphosis. Yasouka and co-workers (29) reported the development of kyphosis without preexisting deformity or violation of the facet joints and speculated that the development of kyphosis in children occurred secondary to the effects of growth in the setting of disrupted stabilizing structures. In contrast, McLaughlin and associates (30) found that only 9% of 32 patients developed kyphosis following upper cervical laminectomy and suboccipital craniectomy for treatment of an Arnold-Chiari malformation and emphasized the importance of careful preservation of the facet and soft tissue restraints.

Adults with normal cervical alignment have a much lower prevalence of frank kyphosis following cervical laminectomy. Kato and associates (31) studied patients following multilevel cervical laminectomy for ossification of the posterior longitudinal ligament. Although a postoperative change in cervical alignment (with the cervical spine becoming straight, S-shaped, or kyphotic) was seen in 47% of the patients, none of the patients had neurologic worsening attributed to the presence of the deformity. Mikawa and colleagues

(32) reviewed 64 patients following multilevel cervical laminectomy for a variety of pathologies. Thirty-three patients (52%) demonstrated a change in cervical alignment, and a kyphotic deformity was observed in 9 patients (14%), 2 of whom were children. The adults with postlaminectomy kyphosis failed to exhibit neurologic worsening and thus did not require treatment. Morimoto and associates (33,34) found that some patients with neurologic worsening after a laminectomy have a more subtle form of dynamic instability that can be confirmed by a flexion-extension magnetic resonance imaging study demonstrating cord compression by the laminectomy membrane during neck extension.

Risk factors for the development of instability have been established in several studies. Katsumi and colleagues (35) analyzed 34 patients following cervical laminectomy for the removal of spinal cord tumors. Seven patients (20%) developed instability, defined as segmental motion greater than 12 degrees or subluxation of more than 3.5 mm. Risk factors for instability included younger age, lack of preoperative lordosis, four or more laminae removed, C2 laminectomy, and disruption of facet joints. Patients with instability averaged 2.5 factors, compared with 1.2 factors in patients without instability. Patients ultimately requiring surgery averaged 3 risk factors.

Guigui and associates (36) reviewed 58 patients following cervical laminectomy for spondylotic myelopathy. Eighteen patients (31%) demonstrated a change from their preoperative cervical alignment, and 15 patients (25%) were noted to have increased postoperative sagittal plane translation. Three patients required surgery for neck pain or neurologic worsening or both. Neurologic improvement was unaffected by postoperative alignment but was less satisfactory in patients with sagittal plane translation. Risk factors for instability included younger age, C2 laminectomy, and increased preoperative range of motion. Preoperative kyphotic alignment was not a risk factor for destabilization.

Postlaminectomy kyphosis, when responsible for neurologic deterioration or intractable neck pain, presents a treatment challenge. The goals of correcting postlaminectomy kyphosis include decompression of the neural elements and reestablishing the normal sagittal vertical axis of the spine. Deformity correction can be accomplished by anterior column lengthening, posterior column shortening, or both when neural compression is due solely to the deformity. Bridwell (4) emphasized the importance of balancing the anterior and posterior corrective forces by combining anterior column load sharing with reconstruction of the posterior tension band. Ideally, kyphosis correction is achieved by rotation of the spine through the axis of the middle column using the posterior longitudinal ligament as a hinge (4). To assess flexibility and to assist in gaining partial correction, preoperative traction may be used in severe deformities.

Anterior, posterior, and combined approaches have been reported for treating postlaminectomy kyphosis. Zdeblick and associates (37) included eight patients with postlaminectomy kyphosis in a series of patients treated for myelopathy with anterior corpectomy and strut grafting. Although these patients were treated in a halo device, two experienced graft dislodgment (Fig. 82.3). Riew and colleagues (38) reviewed the complications of 18 patients with postlaminectomy kyphosis treated with anterior cervical corpectomy and strut grafting. Three patients also had anterior cervical plating, while an additional three patients underwent posterior facet wiring. All patients with three- or four-level vertebral resections were immobilized in a halo vest. Complications included four graft extrusions, and three patients experienced progressive kyphosis of more than 10 degrees. Because the halo vest failed to prevent graft extrusion, the authors recommended supplemental internal fixation when performing multilevel corpectomies in a patient with a prior laminectomy kyphosis (38).

Herman and Sonntag (39) reported 20 patients with kyphosis averaging 38 degrees who where treated by corpectomy at an average of 3.8 levels followed by strut grafting and anterior plate fixation. Half the patients also received supplemental halo fixation. At follow-up, the average kyphosis was 16 degrees and most patients experienced neurologic improvement. Although no graft dislodgements were reported in this series, many of the patients had short-segment corpectomies.

Other authors have advocated circumferential surgery for patients with postlaminectomy kyphosis. Advocates of this approach emphasize the biomechanical superiority of rigid posterior instrumentation in reconstructing the deficient tension band (40). DiAngelo and Foley and their co-workers (41,42) have shown that although anterior plating of a long strut construct leads to high stresses at the graft–bone interface, the addition of anterior and posterior instrumentation can serve to normalize the forces on the strut graft and substantially stiffen the overall construct. Sasso and associates (43) found that the addition of posterior instrumentation decreased the rate of construct failure in patients with long corpectomy constructs (Fig. 82.4). Vanichkachorn and colleagues (44) reported no failures among 11 patients with long corpectomy constructs reconstructed with a junctional plate and posterior instrumentation.

Abumi and associates (45) used a posterior approach with pedicle screw fixation in 30 patients to treat cervical kyphosis with myelopathy. Anterior surgery was also used in patients with fixed deformities. The average preoperative kyphosis of 29.4 degrees was corrected to an average of 2.8 degrees at final follow-up, and all patients achieved a solid fusion. Two patients sustained nerve root injuries that required reoperation.

Kyphosis prevention is much easier than treatment of an established deformity. Two alterations of the standard posterior decompression have been used to decrease the prevalence of postlaminectomy kyphosis. First, facet fusion and lateral mass fixation can be performed in conjunction with laminectomy to provide stability and prevent the development of a progressive deformity. Kumar and associates (46) found excellent long-term neurologic improvement in 25

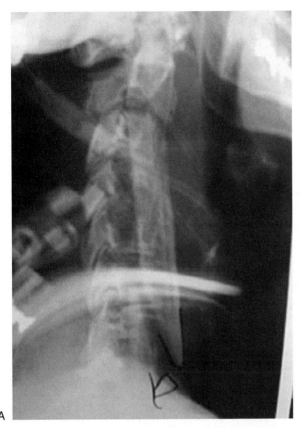

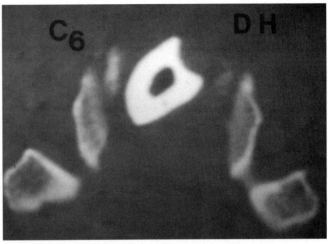

A   B

FIG. 82.3. A: Graft fracture and dislodgement after anterior corpectomy and strut grafting. This is due to 360-degree instability **(B)** after corpectomy in the face of previous laminectomy.

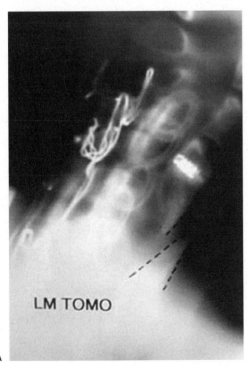

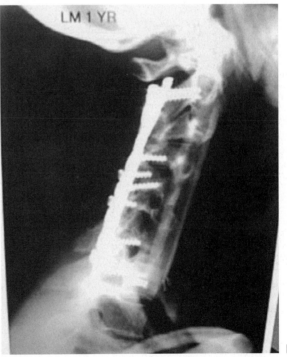

A   B

FIG. 82.4. A: Preoperative lateral tomogram displaying fractured strut graft and retained broken instrumentation in a 50-year-old woman with postlaminectomy kyphosis after 12 prior surgeries. **B:** Postoperative lateral radiograph after anterior multilevel corpectomy and strut grafting followed by posterior segmental fixation. Anterior and posterior surgery is generally necessary in these patients after performing anterior corpectomies.

patients undergoing laminectomy, fusion, and lateral mass fixation.

The other alteration of surgical technique designed to prevent instability is cervical laminoplasty. Although several forms of laminoplasty have been described, the common goal of these procedures is to expand the cervical spinal canal size while maintaining the integrity of the neural arch. These procedures originally gained popularity in Japan, where they have been widely used to treat multilevel cervical spinal cord compression. Nowinski and colleagues (16) compared laminoplasty to multilevel laminectomy in a cadaver model and found that laminoplasty maintained motion characteristics similar to the intact spine. Matsunaga and associates (47) reported a significantly lower prevalence of cervical kyphotic deformity following laminoplasty compared with laminectomy. Herkowitz (48) compared laminoplasty, laminectomy, and anterior decompression and arthrodesis and found a higher rate of good and excellent outcomes in the laminoplasty group (86%) versus the laminectomy-alone group (66%). Heller and co-workers (49) compared similar cohorts of patients undergoing either a laminoplasty or laminectomy with arthrodesis for multilevel cervical myelopathy. Objective and subjective improvement was better in the laminoplasty group, whereas the prevalence of

complications was greater in the fusion group. Critics of the laminoplasty approach argue that laminoplasty patients may experience substantial neck stiffness and axial neck pain. However, a randomized prospective comparison of laminoplasty versus laminectomy and fusion is needed to truly determine the relative merits and incidence of complications of these procedures.

Our preferred surgical approach to postlaminectomy kyphosis in a patient without a fused spine begins with an anterior decompression of the kyphotic segment, often via a multilevel corpectomy. A structural strut graft is used to reconstruct the compressive strength of the anterior column and regain height while allowing kyphosis correction about the axis of the posterior longitudinal ligament. Depending on the length of the anterior construct, a cervical plate or a buttress plate is often applied to prevent graft extrusion during positioning for the posterior procedure. Under the same anesthesia, a posterior facet arthrodesis is performed using rigid segmental lateral mass instrumentation. In certain situations in which decompression of the entire body is not required for decompression, segmental correction can be obtained by interbody grafting in conjunction with anterior plating (Fig. 82.5). In situations in which a major deformity is corrected, we believe that posterior instrumentation and

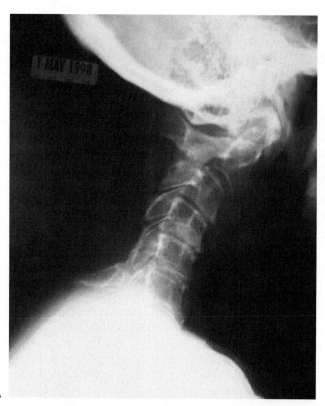
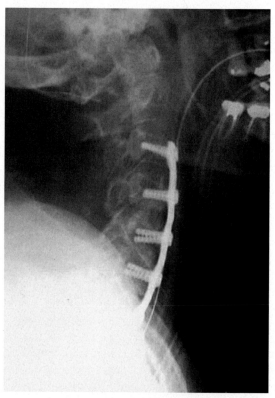

A

B

FIG. 82.5. A: Preoperative lateral radiograph of a 68-year-old woman with postlaminectomy kyphosis, neck pain, and residual myelopathy. **B:** Postoperative lateral radiograph after multilevel segmental correction with autograft and anterior segmental fixation. Note improvement in sagittal alignment with this technique.

facet fusion substantially decreases the rate of construct failure.

In myelopathic patients with a major kyphotic deformity, correction of the spine may place the precarious spinal cord at substantial risk. Therefore, we believe that introspective spinal cord monitoring is necessary. Some patients will not tolerate complete correction of the deformity; in these cases, decompression of the neural elements should take precedence over deformity correction. It is reasonable to consider supplemental halo fixation postoperatively for patients with circumferential instability or with poor bone quality.

DEGENERATIVE CERVICAL KYPHOSIS

Kyphosis due to degenerative disease is the most common cervical deformity in older patients. The pathophysiology usually begins with disc space narrowing or collapse followed by hypertrophic degenerative changes of the uncovertebral and facet joints. Loss of anterior column height leads to tensile forces in the posterior column and ultimately laxity of the posterior soft tissue structures. Minimal degrees of spondylolisthesis or excess mobility in the sagittal plane may accompany this process and further contribute to neural compression and irritation. Ultimately, the combination of degenerative narrowing of the spinal canal, kyphotic deformity, and sagittal plane instability can lead to spinal cord dysfunction and long tract findings (37). The magnitude of kyphosis seen in degenerative conditions is generally less severe than that seen in postlaminectomy kyphosis. In addition to myelopathic complaints, patients often have arm pain related to nerve root compression or irritation. Anterior, posterior, and circumferential decompression and stabilization have been advocated to surgically treat cervical myeloradiculopathy associated with kyphotic degenerative cervical disease.

In patients with straight or lordotic spines, both anterior and posterior surgery can be used successfully to provide decompression of the spinal cord. Ebersold and colleagues (22) reported on 84 patients following decompression for spondylotic myelopathy. Thirty-three patients were treated by anterior decompression and arthrodesis, and 51 patients underwent posterior decompression only. Although no differences in outcomes were found between the two approaches, patients with a longer duration of symptomatic myelopathy had a statistically worse outcome following surgery.

In patients with a fixed kyphotic deformity, posterior decompression is often contraindicated. Therefore, anterior decompression alone or anterior surgery combined with a posterior decompression is required to provide a satisfactory outcome. In treating patients with cervical kyphosis due to degenerative disease, it is important for the surgeon to have a mastery of a variety of surgical techniques to address the specific pathology that is encountered. Therefore, knowledge of both anterior and posterior decompression procedures as well as anterior and posterior instrumentation techniques is necessary.

Anterior decompression and arthrodesis, using either discectomies or corpectomies, is the mainstay of treatment for localized cervical spondylotic myelopathy with a kyphotic deformity (50–56). However, multilevel disease continues to be a challenge. Discectomies at one and two levels are generally successful, but the pseudarthrosis rate is high when discectomies are performed at three or more levels (57,58).

Multilevel cervical corpectomies, although providing an improved rate of fusion, are prone to more instability compared with multilevel discectomies. Sasso and associates (43) reported a 5.5% failure rate following two-level corpectomy with anterior plating but an 83% failure rate following three-level corpectomy with anterior plate fixation. However, when posterior instrumentation was used in conjunction with three-level corpectomies, no failures were observed. Vaccaro and co-workers (59) reported similar results in 45 patients following anterior corpectomies with anterior plating. In this study, a 50% failure rate was observed in three-level corpectomies with anterior plating in spite of halo usage (Fig. 82.6). These studies have led to the recommendation to use posterior supplemental instrumentation when three or more vertebral bodies are resected.

Vanichkachorn and associates (60) used anterior strut grafting, an anterior junctional buttress plate, and posterior lateral mass fixation in 11 patients following a corpectomy at an average of 3.36 levels and experienced no graft or hardware failures. McAfee and colleagues (61) used circumferential cervical arthrodesis in 100 patients, with few complications and a high rate of fusion. Likewise, Schultz and co-workers (62) found a 100% rate of fusion and no graft dislodgement in 72 patients treated with anterior decompression, strut grafting, and anterior plating followed by posterior lateral mass plating.

Older techniques of posterior facet wiring in conjunction with a rib strut graft (63) or Luque rectangle fixation (64) have been supplanted by more rigid lateral mass screw-plate or screw-rod fixation systems. These systems are able to provide construct stiffness well in excess of the intact spinal segment. Lateral mass plating techniques have been shown to provide improved rates of fusion without the need to extend the fusion below the level of decompression (65,66).

Cervical pedicle screws provide a high degree of construct stability, but when used in the C3 through C6 segments present the risk of an iatrogenic injury to the vertebral artery. Abumi and associates (45) reported a 5.3% rate of pedicle perforation in 46 patients undergoing posterior decompression and deformity correction, although none of these patients suffered a neurovascular complication. Ludwig and colleagues (67) reported substantial variability of the pedicle anatomy in a cadaveric spine study and reported an unacceptable rate of C3 through C6 pedicle

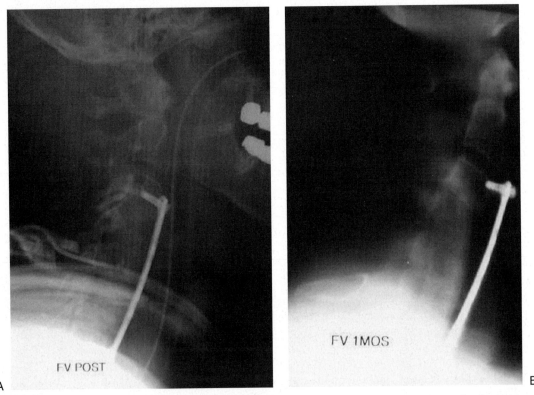

A

B

FIG. 82.6. A 75-year-old man with postlaminectomy kyphosis. **A:** Immediate postoperative lateral radiograph after corpectomy and anterior plate fixation. **B:** One-month postoperative lateral radiograph showing plate dislodgement and settling of construct. Anterior plates should not be used in isolation in this situation without posterior segmental fixation.

breeches even with the use of computer-assisted surgery. However, pedicle fixation was performed safely at the C2 and C7 levels.

Our preferred treatment of cervical spondylotic myelopathy with kyphosis is dependent on the number of levels requiring decompression, as well as the degree and flexibility of the kyphotic deformity. Because the spinal cord is nearly always compressed anteriorly, we utilize an approach to achieve decompression of the neural elements. Discectomies can be used to decompress pathology limited to the disc space at one or two levels. More extensive pathology requires removal of the vertebral bodies. Structural grafting is utilized to lengthen the anterior column and correct the kyphotic deformity, hinging the correction on the posterior longitudinal ligament. Anterior plating or junctional plating is used to provide construct stability. When three or more vertebral bodies are removed or when a large deformity is corrected, supplemental posterior instrumentation and arthrodesis are performed under the same anesthetic. Lateral mass screw-plate or screw-rod fixation is our preferred construct posteriorly to provide maximal construct rigidity and minimize the risk of anterior graft dislodgement. Postoperatively, bracing is dependent on the bone quality, patient reliability, and degree of deformity

that is corrected. A halo jacket orthosis is considered when the balance of these factors amounts to major instability.

POSTTRAUMATIC CERVICAL KYPHOSIS

Traumatic injuries of the cervical spine can lead to the development of a kyphotic deformity due to tension failure of posterior column structures or compression failure of the anterior column structures. The mechanism of injury is critical to understand when analyzing the direction and degree of instability of a given injury. In this regard, we find the classification of Allen and Ferguson (68) to be most useful because it suggests the anatomic structures likely to be disrupted in a given injury (Table 82.1).

The injury mechanisms most prone to the development of kyphosis include distractive flexion (flexion distraction) and compressive flexion (flexion compression) due to the disruption of the posterior stabilizing structures. Other injury patterns with destruction of the posterior stabilizing structures are also prone to the development of kyphosis. White and Panjabi (69), using serial ligament sectioning studies, have shown that destruction of the posterior structures plus one anterior structure allows the spine to assume a sharp angular kyphosis.

TABLE 82.1. *Allen/Ferguson Classification of Cervical Injuries*

Compressive Flexion
Stage 1   Rounded shape to upper end plate due to compression failure
Stage 2   "Beaked" appearance of anterior body due to compression failure of anterior body
Stage 3   Oblique fracture line traversing from anterior body to inferior end plate
Stage 4   Stage 3 plus up to 3 mm of retropulsion of the body
Stage 5   Greater than 3 mm of retropulsion of the body, usually with widening of the posterior elements

Distractive Flexion
Stage 1   Widening of the posterior elements due to soft tissue stretch
Stage 2   Unilateral facet dislocation
Stage 3   Bilateral facet dislocation
Stage 4   Gross displacement (usually greater than 50% translation) of the upper segment of the spine

Vertical Compression
Stage 1   "Cupping" of either superior or inferior end plate due to compression failure
Stage 2   Failure of both end plates, with or without vertical fracture line between end plates
Stage 3   Comminution of body with radial displacement of the fracture fragments

Compressive Extension
Stage 1   Unilateral vertebral arch fracture (pedicle, facet, or lamina); may have rotational displacement
Stage 2   Bilateral lamina fracture, often at multiple contiguous levels
Stage 3   Stage 2 with partial forward displacement of the superior vertebral body
Stage 4   Stage 2 with gross forward displacement of the superior vertebral body

Distractive Extension
Stage 1   Widening of the anterior disc space
Stage 2   Widening of the anterior disc space with posterior subluxation of upper vertebral body

Lateral Flexion
Stage 1   Unilateral compression failure of vertebral body and posterior elements
Stage 2   Stage 1 combined with contralateral widening between adjacent vertebrae

Traumatic instability has the potential for a more rapidly progressive kyphotic deformity compared with kyphosis secondary to surgery or degenerative disease, leading to either worsening of the patient's neurologic status or chronic neck pain. Jenkins and associates (70) found that kyphosis of 20 degrees or more was strongly associated with cervical pain in 96 patients following cervical fusion for trauma.

The length of time since the injury is important to consider when contemplating correction of a posttraumatic cervical deformity. Recent injuries often remain mobile, allowing significant correction with the use of cervical traction. Injuries older than 4 to 6 weeks are difficult to correct by closed techniques and may require surgical release to obtain correction. Often, these complex cases may require a "back, front, back" approach (Fig. 82.7). This begins with a posterior approach to release or osteotomize the healed posterior elements, followed by an anterior decompression and deformity correction with strut grafting procedure. The posterior aspect of the spine is then reexposed to allow segmental rigid internal fixation and facet fusion to be performed.

Even in seemingly innocuous injuries, it is important to be vigilant regarding the possibility of a developing deformity due to an occult ligamentous injury. This subacute instability has been described by Herkowitz and Rothman (71) in patients who initially appear to have a stable cervical spine but are subsequently noted to develop instability and a cervical deformity. To avoid missing these injuries, the authors recommended maintaining immobilization until muscle spasm has subsided, allowing good-quality flexion-extension lateral radiographs to be taken to rule out instability (71). In addition, patients with continued neck symptoms should be followed at regular intervals for up to a year to avoid missing late instability.

High-grade distractive and compressive flexion injury patterns tend to be highly unstable and may displace even in a halo vest orthosis (72,73). Due to the loss of the posterior stabilizing structures, it is logical to reconstruct the posterior tension band. Coe and associates (74) tested multiple forms of fixation in a human cervical facet dislocation injury model and verified that posterior fixation is indeed superior to anterior plating for this injury pattern. Clinically, success has been reported with both posterior and anterior approaches. Laporte and colleagues (75) reported good results with lateral mass fixation in 44 patients with instability following a severe posterior ligament sprain. Shapiro and co-workers (76) found similar clinical results in patients following facet dislocations treated with either posterior wiring or lateral mass fixation, but noted less segmental kyphosis in the group treated with lateral mass fixation. Razack and associates (77) were successful in 21 of 22 patients with a bilateral facet dislocation treated with anterior

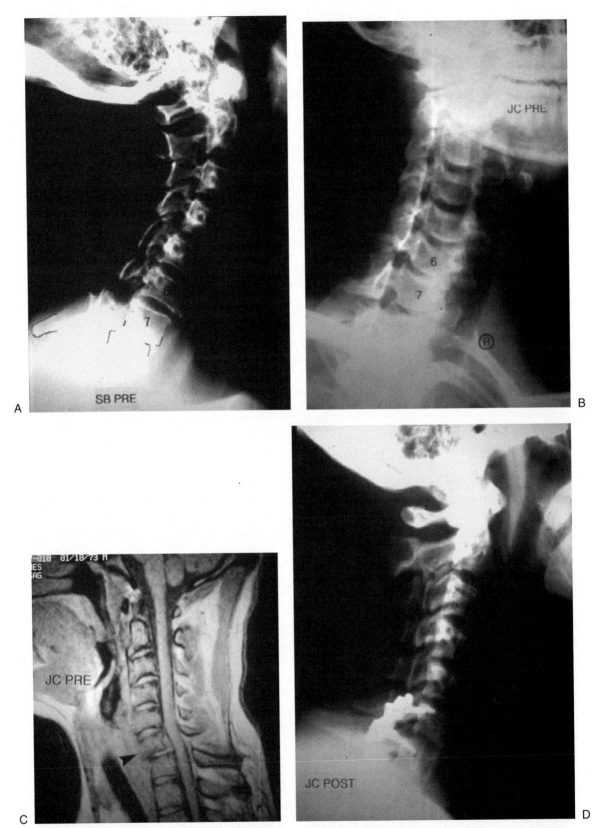

FIG. 82.7. A 22-year-old man was injured in a motor vehicle accident. He was transferred 3 months after the accident with ongoing pain and a neglected fracture dislocation at C6-C7. **A:** Lateral radiograph of the cervical spine. **B:** Oblique radiograph showing perched versus dislocated unilateral (left) facet joint. **C:** Magnetic resonance imaging clearly shows malalignment. **D:** An anterior/posterior/anterior sequence was utilized to relocate the neglected fracture. A facet fracture fragment was retained, causing nerve root compression.

grafting and unicortical plate fixation. Signoret and colleagues (78) successfully used a posterior reduction and plate-screw fixation technique to treat eight patients with high-grade flexion compression (flexion teardrop) injuries. High-grade distraction extension injuries also tend to demonstrate a high prevalence of progressive instability when treated nonoperatively. Lifeso and associates (79) reported uniform failure with a posterior approach but success with anterior discectomy and plating in a clinical series with this injury pattern.

The vertical compression injury pattern often demonstrates segmental kyphosis due to loss of the structural integrity of the vertebral body in association with retropulsion of bone into the spinal canal. Posterior soft tissue restraints may or may not be disrupted, depending on the severity of the energy dissipation and the magnitude and direction of secondary injury vectors. Overall canal occlusion tends to be significantly worsened by fast loading rates, as shown by Carter and associates (80). Although an anterior approach with strut grafting is required for decompression of the neural elements, Do Koh and colleagues (81) found that posterior plating provided a substantially more stable construct, especially in flexion, than anterior plating alone.

Late injuries with major kyphosis are considerably more challenging to treat and require an individualized approach. The location of neural compression, the magnitude of deformity, and the neurologic status of the patient must all be considered when designing a treatment plan. Old traumatic deformities are generally fixed and therefore require a release of the ankylosed segments prior to attempting any deformity correction. It is also crucial to adequately decompress the spinal cord prior to attempting a deformity correction. Therefore, the case may begin with a release of the deformity on one side of the spine, followed by a decompression and release of the deformity on the opposite side of the spine. This allows the deformity to be corrected, followed by appropriate grafting, arthrodesis, and circumferential instrumentation. Good spinal cord monitoring is advisable in neurologically intact patients undergoing significant deformity corrections. Postoperative immobilization is generally required to supplement the overall construct and minimize the chance of construct failure.

In summary, vigilance should be applied to cervical injuries so that progressive deformity can be detected early. Acute management of a cervical injury should be based on a good understanding of the disrupted anatomy. To facilitate this, we find a mechanistic injury classification useful. Late injuries with major kyphosis are a major challenge and require an individualized approach with a good working knowledge of both anterior and posterior decompression, instrumentation, and arthrodesis techniques.

SUMMARY

Cervical kyphosis regardless of the cause results in a pathologic shift in the normal sagittal vertical axis of the head. The clinical result is often severe axial neck pain and progressive neurologic compromise. Treatment strategies are based on decompressing the neural elements and restoring normal cervical biomechanics by correction of the deformity. To achieve success, a good understanding of anterior and posterior cervical decompression, instrumentation, and arthrodesis techniques is required.

REFERENCES

1. Nolan JP, Sherk HH. Biomechanical evaluation of the extensor musculature of the cervical spine. *Spine* 1988;13:9.
2. White AA, Panjabi MM, Thomas CL. The clinical biomechanics of kyphotic deformity. *Clin Orthop* 1977;128:8.
3. Spivak JM, Giordano CP. Cervical kyphosis. In: Bridwell KH, DeWald RL, eds. *The textbook of spinal surgery*, 2nd ed., vol. 1. Philadelphia: Lippincott–Raven, 1997:1027.
4. Bridwell KH. Sagittal spinal balance. Presented at a meeting of the Scoliosis Research Society, AAOS section IV, New Orleans, LA, 1994.
5. White A, Johnson RM, Panjabi MM, et al. Biomechanical analysis of clinical stability in the cervical spine. *Clin Orthop* 1975;109:85.
6. Panjabi MM, White A, Keller D, et al. Stability of the cervical spine under tension. *J Biomechanics* 1978;11.
7. Gaya PP, Sherk HH. The vertical stability of the cervical spine. *Spine* 1988;13:447.
8. Saito T, Yamamuro T, Shikata J, et al. Analysis and prevention of spinal column deformity following cervical laminectomy. I. Pathogenetic analysis of postlaminectomy deformities. *Spine* 1991;16:494.
9. Goel VK, Clark CR, Harris KG, et al. Kinematics of the cervical spine: effects of multiple total laminectomy and facet wiring. *J Orthop Res* 1998;6:611.
10. Cusick JF, Pintar FA, Yoganandan N. Biomechanical alterations induced by multilevel cervical laminectomy. *Spine* 1995;20:2392.
11. Cusick JF, Yoganandan N, Pintar F, et al. Biomechanics of cervical spine facetectomy and fixation techniques. *Spine* 1988;13:808.
12. Kumaresan S, Yoganandan N, Pintar FA, et al. Finite element modeling of cervical laminectomy with graded facetectomy. *J Spinal Disord* 1997;10:40.
13. Raynor RB, Carter FW. Cervical spine strength after facet injury and spine plate application. *Spine* 1991;16:558.
14. Zdeblick TA, Zou D, Warden KE, et al. Cervical stability after foraminotomy. *J Bone Joint Surg Am* 1992;74:22.
15. Zdeblick TA, Jean-Jacques A, Kunz DN, et al. Cervical stability after sequential capsule resection. *Spine* 1993;18:2005.
16. Nowinski GP, Visarius H, Nolte LP, et al. A biomechanical comparison of cervical laminoplasty and cervical laminectomy with progressive facetectomy. *Spine* 1993;18:1995.
17. Perry J, Nickel VL. Total cervical spine fusion for neck paralysis. *J Bone Joint Surg* 1959;41:37.
18. Epstein JA. The surgical management of cervical spinal stenosis, spondylosis, and myeloradiculopathy by means of the posterior approach. *Spine* 1988;13:864.
19. Heller JG, Silcox DH. Postlaminectomy instability of the cervical spine: etiology and stabilization technique. In: Frymoyer JW, ed. *The adult spine: principles and practice*, 2nd ed. Philadelphia: Lippincott–Raven, 1997.
20. Breig A. *Adverse mechanical tension in the central nervous system*. New York: John Wiley & Sons, 1978.
21. Panjabi M, White A. Biomechanics of nonacute cervical spinal cord trauma. *Spine* 1988;13:838.
22. Ebersold MJ, Pare MC, Quast LM. Surgical treatment for cervical spondylitic myelopathy. *J Neurosurg* 1995;82:745.
23. Yasouka S, Peterson HA, Laws ES, et al. Pathogenesis and prophylaxis of postlaminectomy deformity of the spine after multiple level laminectomy: difference between children and adults. *Neurosurgery* 1995;9:145.
24. Aronson DD, Kahn RJ, Canady A. Cervical spine instability following suboccipital decompression and cervical laminectomy for Arnold-Chiari syndrome. Presented at the 56th annual meeting of the American Academy of Orthopaedic Surgeons, Las Vegas, NV, 1989.

25. Bell DF, Walker JL, O'Conner G, et al. Spinal deformity after multiple-level cervical laminectomy in children. *Spine* 1994;4:406.

26. Cattell HS, Clark GL. Cervical kyphosis and instability following multiple laminectomies in children. *J Bone Joint Surg* 1977;59:991.

27. Lonstein JE. Post-laminectomy kyphosis. *Clin Orthop* 1977;128:93.

28. Taddonio RF, King AG. Atlantoaxial rotatory fixation after decompressive laminectomy: a case report. *Spine* 1982;7.

29. Yasouka S, Peterson HA, MacCarty CS. Incidence of spinal deformity after multilevel laminectomy in children and adults. *J Neurosurg* 1982;57:441.

30. McLaughlin MR, Wahlig JB, Pollack IF. Incidence of postlaminectomy kyphosis after Chiari decompression. *Spine* 1997;22:613.

31. Kato Y, Iwasaki M, Fuji T, et al. Long-term follow-up results of laminectomy for cervical myelopathy caused by ossification of the posterior longitudinal ligament. *J Neurosurg* 1998;89:217.

32. Mikawa Y, Shikata J, Yamamuro T. Spinal deformity and instability after multilevel cervical laminectomy. *Spine* 1987;12:6.

33. Morimoto T, Okuno S, Nakase H, et al. Cervical myelopathy due to dynamic compression by the laminectomy membrane: dynamic MR imaging study. *J Spinal Disord* 1999;12:172.

34. Morimoto T, Ohtsuka H, Sakaki T, et al. Postlaminectomy cervical spinal cord compression demonstrated by dynamic magnetic resonance imaging. Case report. *J Neurosurg* 1998;88:155.

35. Katsumi Y, Honma T, et al. Analysis of cervical instability resulting from laminectomies for removal of spinal cord tumor. *Spine* 1998;14:1171.

36. Guigui P, Benoist M, Deburge A. Spinal deformity and instability after multilevel cervical laminectomy for spondylotic myelopathy. *Spine* 1998;23:440.

37. Zdeblick TA, Bohlman HH. Cervical kyphosis and myelopathy: treatment by anterior corpectomy and strut-grafting. *J Bone Joint Surg Am* 1989;71:170.

38. Riew KD, Hilibrand AS, Palumbo MA, et al. Anterior cervical corpectomy in patients previously managed with a laminectomy: short-term complications. *J Bone Joint Surg Am* 1999;81:950.

39. Herman J, Sonntag V. Cervical corpectomy and plate fixation for postlaminectomy kyphosis. *J Neurosurg* 1994;80:963.

40. Albert TJ, Vacarro A. Postlaminectomy kyphosis. *Spine* 1998;23:2738.

41. DiAngelo DJ, Foley KT, Vossel KA, et al. Anterior cervical plating reverses load transfer through multilevel strut-grafts. *Spine* 2000;25:783.

42. Foley KT, DiAngelo DJ, Rampersaud YR, et al. The *in vitro* effects of instrumentation on multilevel cervical strut-graft mechanics. *Spine* 1999;24:2366.

43. Sasso RC, Ruggiero RA, Reilly TA. Reconstruction failures after multilevel cervical corpectomy. Cervical Spine Research Society, 2000.

44. Vanichkachorn JS, Vaccaro AR, Silveri CP, et al. Anterior junctional plate in the cervical spine. *Spine* 1998;23:2462.

45. Abumi K, Shono Y, Taneichi H, et al. Correction of cervical kyphosis using pedicle screw fixation systems. *Spine* 1999;24:2389.

46. Kumar VG, Rea GL, Mervis LJ, et al. Cervical spondylotic myelopathy: functional and radiographic long-term outcome after laminectomy and posterior fusion. *Neurosurgery* 1999;44:771.

47. Matsunaga S, Sakou T, Nakanisi K. Analysis of the cervical spine alignment following laminoplasty and laminectomy. *Spinal Cord* 1999;37:20.

48. Herkowitz HN. A comparison of anterior cervical fusion, cervical laminectomy and cervical laminaplasty for the surgical management of multiple level spondylotic radiculopathy. *Spine* 1988;13:870.

49. Heller JG, Edwards CC II, Murakami H, et al. Laminoplasty versus laminectomy and fusion for multilevel cervical myelopathy: an independent matched cohort analysis. *Spine* 2001;26:1330.

50. Macdonald RL, Fehlings MG, Tator CH, et al. Multilevel anterior cervical corpectomy and fibular allograft fusion for cervical myelopathy. *J Neurosurg* 1997;86:990.

51. Hanai K, Fujiyoshi F, Kamei K. Subtotal vertebrectomy and spinal fusion for cervical spondylotic myelopathy. *Spine* 1986;11:310.

52. Saunders RL, Bernini PM, Shirreffs TG Jr, et al. Central corpectomy for cervical spondylotic myelopathy: a consecutive series with long-term follow-up evaluation. *J Neurosurg* 1991;74:163.

53. Saunders RL. Anterior reconstructive procedures in cervical spondylotic myelopathy. *Clin Neurosurg* 1991;37:682.

54. Bernard TN Jr, Whitecloud TS 3rd. Cervical spondylotic myelopathy and myeloradiculopathy. Anterior decompression and stabilization with autogenous fibula strut graft. *Clin Orthop* 1987;221:149.

55. Yang KC, Lu XS, Cai QL, et al. Cervical spondylotic myelopathy treated by anterior multilevel decompression and fusion. Follow-up report of 214 cases. *Clin Orthop* 1987;221:161.

56. Zhang ZH, Yin H, Yang K, et al. Anterior intervertebral disc excision and bone grafting in cervical spondylotic myelopathy. *Spine* 1983;8:16.

57. Emery SE, Fisher JR, Bohlman HH. Three-level anterior cervical discectomy and fusion: radiographic and clinical results. *Spine* 1997;22:2622.

58. Bolesta MJ, Rechtine GR II, Chrin AM. Three- and four-level anterior cervical discectomy and fusion with plate fixation: a prospective study. *Spine* 2000;25:2040.

59. Vaccaro AR, Falatyn SP, Scuderi GJ, et al. Early failure of long segment anterior cervical plate fixation. *J Spinal Disord* 1998;11:410.

60. Vanichkachorn JS, Vaccaro AR, Silveri CP, et al. Anterior junctional plate in the cervical spine. *Spine* 1998;23:2462.

61. McAfee PC, Bohlman HH, Ducker TB, et al. One-stage anterior cervical decompression and posterior stabilization. A study of one hundred patients with a minimum of two years of follow-up. *J Bone Joint Surg Am* 1995;77:1791.

62. Schultz KD, McLaughlin MR, Haid RW, et al. Single-staged anterior-posterior decompression and stabilization for complex cervical spine disorders. *J Neurosurg* 2000;93:214.

63. Callahan RA, Johnson RM, Margolis RN, et al. Cervical facet fusion for control of instability following laminectomy. *J Bone Joint Surg Am* 1977;59:991.

64. Cusick JF, Pintar FA, Yoganandan N, et al. Wire fixation techniques of the cervical facets. *Spine* 1997;22:970.

65. Heller JG, Silcox DH 3rd, Sutterlin CE 3rd. Complications of posterior cervical plating. *Spine* 1995;20:2442.

66. Fehlings MG, Cooper PR, Errico TJ. Posterior plates in the management of cervical instability: long-term results in 44 patients. *J Neurosurg* 1994;81:341.

67. Ludwig SC, Kramer DL, Balderson RA, et al. Placement of pedicle screw in the human cadaveric cervical spine. *Spine* 2000;25:1655.

68. Allen BL, Ferguson RL, Lehmann TR, et al. A mechanistic classification of closed, indirect fractures and dislocations of the lower cervical spine. *Spine* 1982;7:1.

69. White AA, Panjabi MM. *Clinical biomechanics of the spine*. Philadelphia: JB Lippincott, 1978.

70. Jenkins LA, Capen DA, Zigler JE, et al. Cervical spine fusions for trauma. A long-term radiographic and clinical evaluation. *Orthop Rev* 1994(Suppl):13.

71. Herkowitz HN, Rothman RH. Subacute instability of the cervical spine. *Spine* 1984;9:348.

72. Sears W, Fazl M. Prediction of stability of cervical spine fracture managed in the halo vest and indications for surgical intervention. *J Neurosurg* 1990;73:478.

73. Glaser JA, Whitehill R, Stamp WG, et al. Complications associated with the halo-vest. A review of 245 cases. *J Neurosurg* 1986;65:762.

74. Coe JD, Warden KE, Sutterlin CE 3rd, et al. Biomechanical evaluation of cervical spinal stabilization methods in a human cadaveric model. *Spine* 1989;14:1122.

75. Laporte C, Laville C, Lazennec JY, et al. Severe hyperflexion sprains of the lower cervical spine in adults. *Clin Orthop* 1999;363:126.

76. Shapiro S, Snyder W, Kaufman K, et al. Outcome of 51 cases of unilateral locked cervical facets: interspinous braided cable for lateral mass plate fusion compared with interspinous wire and facet wiring with iliac crest. *J Neurosurg* 1999;91:19.

77. Razack N, Green BA, Levi AD. The management of traumatic cervical bilateral facet fracture-dislocations with unicortical anterior plates. *J Spinal Disord* 2000;13:374.

78. Signoret F, Jacquot FP, Feron JM. Reducing the cervical flexion teardrop fracture with a posterior approach and plating technique: an original method. *Eur Spine J* 1999;8:110.

79. Lifeso RM, Colucci MA. Anterior fusion for rotationally unstable cervical spine fractures. *Spine* 2000;25:2028.

80. Carter JW, Mirza SK, Tencer AF, et al. Canal geometry changes associated with axial compressive cervical spine fracture. *Spine* 2000;25:46.

81. Do Koh Y, Lim TH, Won You J, et al. A biomechanical comparison of modern anterior and posterior plate fixation of the cervical spine. *Spine* 2001;26:15.

CHAPTER 83

Complications of Anterior Cervical Plating

Jeffrey D. Coe and Alexander R. Vaccaro

OVERVIEW

Since the introduction of anterior cervical surgery in the 1950s and the anterior cervical plate in the 1960s and 1970s, there has been a progressive increase in the number of cervical arthrodesis and, in particular, anterior cervical arthrodesis with plating (1,2). Abraham and Herkowitz (1) noted a 289% increase in the incidence of cervical fusion surgery between 1985 and 1996 (from 38,000 cases in 1985 to 110,000 cases in 1996) based on data from the Health Care Financing Administration. In the early 1990s, the Cervical Spine Research Society (CSRS) initiated a study to compare prospectively the clinical and radiographic outcomes as well as complications associated with anterior cervical surgery with the specific goal of obtaining comparative data between plated and nonplated anterior arthrodesis cases. In the three years of patient entry in this multicenter study, 349 (82.5%) of the 423 patients who underwent anterior arthrodesis surgery were plated, whereas 74 (17.5%) were not (2).

The goal of anterior cervical plate fixation is to increase the stability of the surgical construct, thereby increasing the union rate, decreasing the need for external immobilization, and decreasing the need for supplemental posterior surgery. Wang and co-workers (3) have demonstrated a statistically significant increase in fusion rates for patients undergoing two-level anterior cervical discectomy and fusion (ACDF) procedures with and without anterior cervical plates. Seven of the 28 nonplated patients developed nonunions, whereas none of the 32 plated patients developed nonunions. In a separate report, however, these same authors were unable to demonstrate any significant difference between plated and nonplated single-level ACDF patients (4).

Many authors have attested to the decreased need for immobilization, both in terms of type and duration, in plated ACDF and corpectomy patients (5–23). Many of these same authors have also asserted that anterior plating may obviate the need for posterior arthrodesis and instrumenta-

tion in certain spinal disorders (5,6,12–18,20,23–25). Some authors have suggested that plating of an anterior cervical arthrodesis may permit the use of allograft in lieu of autograft, obviating iliac crest donor site pain and associated complications (20–22,26). Collectively, these benefits ostensibly result in a decrease in overall surgical morbidity, decreased hospitalization, and increased return to function, all of which may partially or completely offset the cost of these implants (12,18–20). Several authors, however, have called into question the routine use of anterior cervical plate fixation and believe that these devices are not cost effective and are potentially fraught with complications (27,28).

The use of anterior cervical plate fixation in any given case must be tempered with a thorough understanding of the complications that are unique to anterior cervical instrumentation in the specific pathoanatomy under treatment. These complications include implant loosening, prominence, and migration resulting in dysphagia or esophageal erosion or injury; graft/plate failure with dislodgement; implant (screw, rod, or plate) breakage; and implant malposition resulting in vascular or neurologic injury.

History

Bohler (29,30) reported what was likely the first use of anterior cervical plate fixation when he described in 1967 the use of a long-bone plate in a patient who had sustained cervical spinal trauma. In 1975, Herrmann (31) reported three cases of traumatic cervical instability that were successfully treated with AO (Arbeitsgemeinschaft für Osteosynthesefragen) long-bone plates. Also in the 1970s, Orozco and Houet (32) described the use of a one-third tubular plate in the anterior cervical spine and subsequently designed custom "H" and "HH" plates that were adopted by the AO for use throughout Europe in anterior cervical surgery, primarily for traumatic injuries. In 1980, Caspar developed a "trapezoidal" plate for use in the cervical spine (33). He described the use of this plate for multiple indications, including trauma, tumors, inflammatory diseases, myelopathy, multilevel radiculopathy, and revision surgery (9,11,24,33,34).

The first reports of the use of anterior cervical plates in the United States that we are aware of appeared in 1983 (35,36). Bremer and Nguyen (35) reported the 3-month results of six patients with traumatic instability treated with anterior cervical decompression, arthrodesis, and stabilization using Osteo plates (Richards Manufacturing, Memphis, TN). Gassman and Seligson (36) reported on 13 cases (seven degenerative, five traumatic, and one infection) using their design of an anterior cervical plate. In 1987, de Oliviera (25) reported on the use of his anterior cervical plate in 40 cases of cervical spine trauma. With the exception of the Osteo plate in the Bremer and Nguyen series, all of these early devices required penetration of the posterior cortex of the vertebral body for adequate bicortical screw fixation. (Fig. 83.1). The fear of dural penetration and subsequent neurologic catastrophe delayed acceptance of the use of these devices worldwide, particularly in the United States, despite reassurances from the developers that this complication did not occur in their series (25,32,33,36).

It was not until the introduction of the titanium Cervical Spinal Locking Plate (CSLP) by Morscher in 1986 that anterior cervical plating began to gain widespread acceptance (37). This device was a modification of the Orozco plate and used a screw originally developed by Raveh for use in mandibular reconstruction that introduced two unique features: (a) the use of a conical expansion bolt placed in an expandable screw head in order to lock the screw to the plate and prevent

screw loosening and migration, and (b) the use of a plasma-sprayed hollow screw to allow bone ingrowth, thereby increasing screw purchase over time (17,37). This device obviated the need for posterior vertebral cortical screw purchase, increasing the perception of its safety. Biomechanical studies supported the stability of this device as compared with the nonlocking plates, although some studies suggested that the Morscher plate was somewhat susceptible to loosening with fatigue testing as compared with the Caspar device (38–40). The AO subsequently adopted this plate, and its use soon became widespread, with many series reporting excellent clinical results (17,19,21,22,41). Reports of screw breakage, together with a biomechanical study by Hollowell and associates (42) in 1994 indicating the relative weakness of the hollow plasma-sprayed screw and lack of demonstrated benefit of bone ingrowth, led to the abandonment of the original Morscher screw in favor of a solid locking screw for use with the CSLP device (17,22,43). Other cervical locking plates were developed in the late 1980s and the early 1990s as plating became more popular throughout North America (44–48).

Reports of graft plate failure, particularly in long multilevel corpectomy cases using plates with rigid screw-plate locking mechanisms, began to appear in the mid-1990s, raising concerns about the limitations of these devices (49). Biomechanical studies also called into question the use of these devices in long corpectomy cases (16,50). New plates and devices described as "hybrid" or "translational" have since been developed that allow for rotational and/or cephalocaudal translational motion of some or all of the screws with respect to the plate or device while still remaining "locked" to the longitudinal component of the anterior fixation device (47,51,52). Early reports indicate that these devices may overcome some of the deficiencies of the more rigid plates in long multilevel corpectomy cases (52).

Many different anterior cervical implant systems are currently available on the market. Most of these systems use some type of mechanism to lock the screw to the device. Examples include the original CSLP system with solid locking screw (Synthes Spine, Paoli, PA), the Orion plate (Medtronic Sofamor Danek, Memphis, TN), the Reflex plate (Stryker, Howmedica, Osteonics, Allendale, NJ), and the fixed DOC plate (DePuy AcroMed, Cleveland, OH). "Hybrid" devices, which allow rotation of the screws with respect to the plate or device while preventing screw backout with various locking mechanisms, include the PEAK plate (DePuy AcroMed, Cleveland, OH), as well as the Atlantis plate (Medtronic Sofamor Danek, Minneapolis MN). Translational devices available on the market include the dynamic DOC device (DePuy AcroMed, Cleveland, OH), the ABC plate (Aesculap, San Francisco, CA), and the Premier plate (Medtronic Sofamor Danek, Minneapolis MN).

Biomechanics

In order to understand well the nature and types of complications associated with anterior cervical instrumentation,

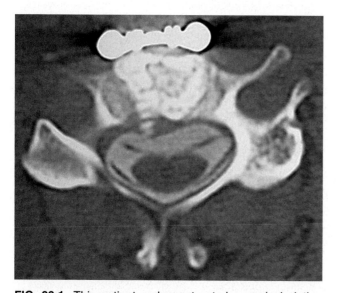

FIG. 83.1. This patient underwent anterior cervical plating with a bicortical screw of excessive length. Note that the screw intrudes 3 to 4 mm into the spinal canal and indents (but does not penetrate) the dura. Fortunately, this patient did not have significant central stenosis and did not develop a neurologic deficit.

a basic understanding of cervical biomechanics is necessary. In clinical situations of major posterior instability, anterior cervical arthrodesis alone often is inadequate to restore necessary spinal stability. Van Peteghem and Schweigel (53) reported a 50% cervical graft dislodgement rate in their series of 12 patients with posterior instability due to trauma. None of their patients underwent anterior cervical plating. Biomechanical studies by Sutterlin (54), Coe (11), Ulrich (55), and Montesano (56) and their associates have demonstrated that posterior fixation provides greater stiffness and strength in cadaveric and animal spines than does anterior fixation. All of these studies have demonstrated that the use of anterior cervical fixation does enhance the stability of posteriorly unstable spines when compared with the destabilized spines. Furthermore, with regard to torsional and extensile forces, cervical construct stiffnesses with anterior fixation applied are superior to the intact spine. From a clinical standpoint, multiple clinical studies have supported the efficacy of anterior cervical plating in traumatic cases (13–15,25,29,30,32, 33,57,58).

Schulte and colleagues (59) reported a biomechanical study using human cadaveric spines stabilized with anterior cervical plates and bone grafts. They demonstrated a significant reduction in motion with anterior plate fixation as compared with bone grafting alone. In contrast to the previously discussed biomechanical studies, which examined primarily posterior instability (traumatic) models, the model used by Schulte and co-workers utilized an anterior discectomy instability model.

Several studies have also compared different types of plating systems, in particular the CSLP system and the Caspar plate. Clausen and associates (38) reported the results of a study in which 15 human cadaveric spines were tested using an anterior spinal column instability model before and after fatigue loading. The CSLP device stabilized the specimens significantly in flexion before, but not after, fatigue failure and remained unstable in extension both before and after fatigue failure. The Caspar system stabilized the specimens significantly in flexion and extension both before and after fatigue. They attributed the difference in test results between these two systems to differences in bone screw fixation. Spivak and colleagues (60) evaluated two locked anterior cervical plates (the Orion and the CSLP plates) and one nonlocking plate (Acroplate). The locking plates were tested locked and unlocked, and the Acroplate was tested with both unicortical and bicortical screw purchase. These investigators concluded that locking screws significantly increased the rigidity of the unicortical (locking plate) screw systems before and after cyclical loading. They noted, however, that the highest rigidity was in specimens utilizing bicortical screw fixation.

Grubb and co-workers (39) performed a biomechanical study in porcine and human cadaveric cervical spines comparing the Caspar plate and the CSLP system. In contrast to Clausen's study, they noted higher rigidity with the CSLP system than the Caspar plate; however, they did not perform

fatigue testing in their study. Richman and associates (40) performed a study in porcine cervical spines using a corpectomy model and methylmethacrylate grafts stabilized anteriorly with either a CSLP or a Caspar plate and posteriorly with two lateral mass plates. Maximum stability was noted with lateral mass plating and anterior grafting, but all instrumented specimens demonstrated stiffness greater than that of the intact spine. There was no significant difference between the stability achieved by the CSLP (unicortical, locked) system and the Caspar (bicortical, unlocked) plate.

Chen (61) performed a study in nine porcine cervical spines that had been anteriorly stabilized with Orozco "H" plates and screws with either bicortical or unicortical (subcortical) screw purchase. He noted comparable stability in the constructs plated with screws either unicortically or bicortically before cyclical loading. However, he noted deterioration in the unicortical constructs as compared with the bicortical constructs after cyclical loading of 100 cycles.

Zdeblick and colleagues (62) performed an animal study in which 35 alpine goats divided into five groups of seven underwent three-level anterior cervical discectomies with the following treatment variables: no graft, autograft alone, autograft and plate, allograft alone, and allograft and plate. They noted a significant difference in the stiffnesses of the harvested specimens (harvested at 12 weeks) between the plated and nonplated groups, but did not note a significant difference in the fusion rates between the plated and nonplated groups. There was a significant difference in the fusion rates between the allograft and autograft groups, however.

Plate and screw materials and design characteristics have also been studied. Hollowell and associates (42) performed cyclic studies of the plasma-sprayed fenestrated Morscher screws designed for use with the CSLP system as compared with a nonfenestrated solid screw design. These investigators noted that the mean cycles to failure for the fenestrated screws was 1,115, whereas the solid screws survived over 10,000 cycles, at which time testing was discontinued. The hollow screw failures always occurred by fracture through the plane of the fenestrations. Baldwin and co-workers (63) performed electron microscopic analysis of a failed titanium plate to evaluate the mode of failure. No metallurgic flaw was noted. The failure point was at the intermediate screw hole, which was presumed to be the weakest part of the plate. They attributed this plate's failure to preimplantation contouring resulting in microfracture that theoretically continued to propagate following implant placement. The authors recommended that the site of implantation be shaved with an air drill to minimize the need for contouring. They also suggested that if plate contouring becomes necessary, a cam-bending device be utilized in order to bend the plate at a site other than through a screw hole.

The biomechanics of anterior cervical plates in long strut corpectomies have been studied in some detail by several authors (16,64–67). Kirkpatrick and associates (66) performed flexibility testing in 11 human cadaveric cervical spine specimens in the following conditions: the intact spine; following a three-level corpectomy and strut grafting; following subsequent anterior (Orion) plating; and following removal of the anterior plate and placement of lateral mass (posterior) plating with the Axis (Medtronic Sofamor Danek, Memphis, TN) plating system. The most rigid construct was determined to be the posteriorly plated construct, followed by the anteriorly plated construct, the intact spine, and then the nonplated strut graft corpectomy specimens. The authors concluded that either anterior or posterior plating increases the stability of multilevel corpectomy constructs.

Isomi and co-authors (16) performed a comparative biomechanical study evaluating one-level and three-level corpectomies in seven human cadaveric cervical spines stabilized with CSLP anterior plates. Flexibility testing in flexion, extension, bilateral torsion, and lateral bending in varying moments before and after 100-cycle fatigue loading was performed. These investigators noted no significant difference in construct stability between the one-level and three-level constructs before fatigue; however, they noted a significant decrease in the stability of the three-level constructs compared with the one-level construct after fatigue loading.

Foley and colleagues (65) evaluated the biomechanical stability of six human cadaveric cervical spines following various corpectomy and reconstruction strategies. These included a three-level corpectomy and strut graft composite stabilized with either an anterior plate, a posterior plate, or both. Forces were measured with a force-sensing strut graft. It was noted that the anteriorly plated construct was unloaded in flexion and loaded in extension, in contrast to the unplated spine, in which the anterior graft was loaded in flexion and unloaded in extension. Posteriorly plated constructs markedly loaded the anterior strut graft in flexion as compared with the unplated spines, while extension in the posterior plated specimens resulted in unloading of the strut graft. The combined anterior-posterior plated specimens demonstrated less strut graft loading as compared with the anterior or posterior plated specimens alone.

In a related study from the same laboratory, DiAngelo and associates (64) supported the results of their previous study by noting that anterior cervical plating, while increasing global stiffness and decreasing local motion of a strut-grafted three-level human cadaveric corpectomy, reversed load transfer to the strut graft as compared with the unplated specimen. The magnitudes of the increased loads in extension approached that of the compressive strength of the vertebral end plates. The authors suggested that clinical failures of anteriorly plated strut-grafted multilevel corpectomies occur when excessive loads are transferred to the graft in extension, resulting in strut graft pistoning, plate loosening, and vertebral end plate failure. These same authors (68) reported the results of a similar study in which a translational (dynamic) anterior cervical plate (Premier; Medtronic Sofamor Danek, Memphis, TN) was compared with a constrained (static) anterior cervical plate (Orion; Medtronic Sofamor Danek, Memphis, TN) in five human cadaveric spines using the same corpectomy model as in their previous studies. Both constructs were noted to have

increased graft loads in extension and decreased graft loads in flexion. The dynamically plated constructs, however, were noted to have decreased graft loads in extension as compared with the statically plated constructs, and these loads were not significantly different than the graft-alone constructs. The authors concluded that the dynamic plates were biomechanically advantageous as compared with static plates in multilevel corpectomy constructs.

Wang and associates (67) performed a biomechanical study on eight human cadaveric specimens in which corpectomies were performed followed by anterior plating. The authors measured the "stability potential index," a determinate of spinal construct stability defined as the decrease in motion in the test specimens compared with the intact spine. They confirmed the results of Foley and colleagues (65) and DiAngelo and co-workers (64) and indicated that their plated corpectomy specimens experienced a graft force decrease in flexion and a graft force increase in extension. They also noted that fatigue loading decreased graft force and thus the stability of both plated one-level and three-level corpectomy constructs, attributed to screw and plate loosening with fatigue. This loss of stability was greater and statistically significantly in the three-level constructs.

IMPLANT COMPLICATIONS

The evolution of anterior cervical plating has led to implants that are low profile and designed to minimize the risk of implant dislodgement in order to avoid dysphagia or esophageal erosion/perforation. Most of the plates available on the market today lock the screws to the plate in order to minimize implant loosening. The effect of these design changes was addressed in detail in a 1998 review by Lowery and McDonough (46), who evaluated implant failure in 109 patients who were treated with three different types of anterior cervical plates (Orozco, CSLP, and Orion). There was a 44% failure rate with the Orozco plate, a 23% failure rate with the CSLP system, and a 12% failure rate with the Orion plate, for an overall failure rate of 35%. When the Orion and CSLP data are combined, the overall failure rate for the locked systems was 18%. Although no tracheoesophageal erosion or neurovascular compromise as a result of implant failure was noted, 4 patients (2%) in this series had marked prominence of failed hardware that eventually required implant removal. The other 27% of patients with loose implants were judged to have minimal loosening (less than 2 mm); these patients were observed without further complications developing. Lowery and McDonough (46), as well as others (69), have interpreted the data from this study as indicating that cervical implant migration of less than 5 mm can usually be safely observed.

In a series published in 1997 from the same institution [and perhaps including some of the same patients as the series of Lowery and McDonough (46)], Swank and associates (43) reported on 64 consecutive patients who underwent anterior cervical fusion for degenerative disease at one or more levels with anterior cervical plating of various plating types. There were 27 patients (42%) with implant complications.

This included 8 patients (13%) with screw or plate loosening, 11 patients (17%) with screw fracture, and 8 patients (13%) with plate fracture.

Anterior cervical plating has been used to stabilize long corpectomy constructs in the hope of obviating the need for posterior arthrodesis with mixed results (Figs. 83.2 and 83.3). In 1998, Vaccaro and associates (49) reported a retrospective multicenter study of 45 patients who underwent two-level (33 patients, 73%) or three-level (12 patients, 27%) corpectomies for a variety of indications, primarily degenerative. The Synthes CSLP system was used in all but one patient in this series. Thirty-one patients (69%) were immobilized in a halo vest for 12 weeks. The remaining patients were immobilized in a hard collar for 12 weeks postoperatively. They reported 9 patients in the total series (20%) with

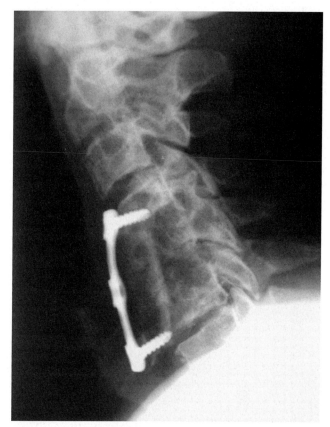

FIG. 83.3. This patient, who underwent anterior cervical corpectomy fusion and plating at two vertebral levels, is noted to have graft and plate failure at the caudal end of his construct. He subsequently underwent revision by extending his fusion to the C7 level and supplementing his reconstruction with a posterior fusion. (Photograph courtesy of Dr. Ian Farey, with permission.)

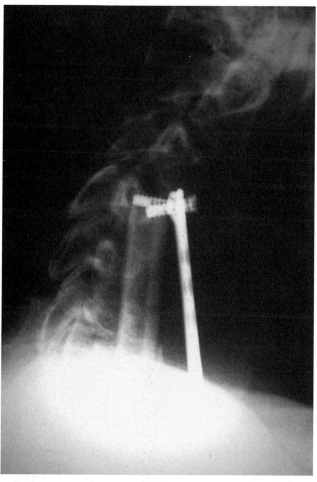

FIG. 83.2. This lateral cervical radiograph demonstrates complete failure of an anterior cervical construct, with the graft telescoping completely through the C3 vertebral body into the C2-3 intervertebral disc, having pushed one screw into the disc with the other screw backing out, despite use of a locking plate (Synthes CSLP). The plate has lifted away from the anterior spine as well, and most likely has failed at the caudal end of the construct (image obscured by shoulders). Note that his patient has had a prior laminectomy and therefore has little in the way of posterior ligamentous tension band that would aid in stability and prevent kyphotic malalignment.

graft/plate dislodgement: 6 of the 12 patients in the three-level corpectomy group and 3 patients (9.1%) in the two-level corpectomy group. This difference was statistically significant ($p < 0.05$). Complications related to graft/plate failure included screw penetration in the disc space in 1 of the 3 patients in the two-level corpectomy group and 3 of the 12 patients in the three-level corpectomy group. Two of the 12 patients in the three-level corpectomy group also had screws incompletely tightened to the plate as demonstrated on an initial postoperative film. Four patients in the three-level corpectomy group developed plate loosening. One patient in the three-level corpectomy group developed anterior graft and plate dislodgement 1 week after posterior instrumentation and fusion. The authors suggested that further clinical and laboratory investigation was needed in order to determine the degree of spinal stabilization necessary to ensure an acceptably low rate of plate loosening after multilevel anterior cervical reconstruction.

With the exception of the "outlier" series of Lowery and McDonough (46) and Swank and colleagues (43), and the multilevel corpectomy series of Vaccaro and associates (49), the prevalence of most implant and graft complications appears to be reasonably low (Tables 83.1 and 83.2).

TABLE 83.1. *Implant Complications in Published Consecutive Series of Anterior Fusion with Plating (N ≥ 30)*

First author (reference no.)	Publication year	N	Major diagnostic category	Plate type	Posterior fusion?	Fixation complications (percentage of patients)							Comments
						Screw or plate loosening	Screw fracture	Plate fracture	Plate/graft displacement or Fx	Implant malposition	Revision for implant complications	Total fixation complications	
Lesoin (90)	1984	145	Trauma	Multiple	N	1.4%	0.0%	0.0%	0.0%	0.0%	0.0%	1.4%	
Aebi (5)	1986	50	Trauma	Orozco	N	4.0%	2.0%	0.0%	0.0%	0.0%	0.0%	6.0%	
Caspar (33)	1989	60	Trauma	Caspar	N	5.0%	0.0%	0.0%	1.7%	0.0%	1.7%	6.7%	
Goffin (14)	1989	41	Trauma	Caspar	N	4.9%	0.0%	0.0%	0.0%	0.0%	4.9%	4.9%	
Aebi (6)	1990	86	Trauma	Orozco	N	1.2%	1.2%	0.0%	0.0%	0.0%	0.0%	2.3%	
Randle (138)	1990	54	Trauma	Caspar	N	3.7%	0.0%	0.0%	0.0%	0.0%	1.9%	3.7%	Plate removed to treat esophageal fistula
Jonsson (76)	1991	40	Trauma	CSLP	Y (29)	0.0%	0.0%	0.0%	0.0%	2.5%	0.0%	2.5%	Screw removed in one patient
Ripa (57)	1991	92	Trauma	Orozco	N	4.3%	1.1%	1.1%	0.0%	6.5%	1.1%	13.0%	
Schweighofer (118)	1992	171	Trauma	Multiple	Rare	1.2%	0.0%	0.6%	0.0%	0.0%	1.2%	1.8%	Patients with screws in disc had plate loosening
Kostuik (17)	1993	42	Degenerative	CSLP	N	4.8%	4.8%	0.0%	0.0%	4.8%	2.4%	9.5%	
Papadopoulos (20)	1993	160	Degen, OPLL	CSLP	N	5.6%	1.3%	0.0%	1.3%	0.0%	3.1%	8.1%	2 Plates removed for infection (distantly seeded)
Johnston (139)	1995	50	Degenerative	CSLP	N	0.0%	4.0%	0.0%	4.0%	0.0%	4.0%	8.0%	
Katsuura (92)	1996	44	Degenerative	CSLP, Caspar	N	9.1%	9.1%	0.0%	0.0%	0.0%	0.0%	18.2%	
Paramore (80)	1996	49	Degenerative	Caspar	N	10.2%	6.1%	1.1%	4.1%	0.0%	8.2%	20.4%	
Shapiro (21)	1996	88	Degenerative	CSLP	N	2.6%	0.0%	0.0%	0.0%	0.0%	0.0%	3.4%	
McLaughlin (92)	1997	39	Degenerative	CSLP	N	2.6%	5.1%	2.6%	0.0%	0.0%	2.6%	10.3%	
Shapiro (122)	1997	195	Degenerative	CSLP	N	1.0%	0.5%	0.5%	0.5%	0.0%	0.0%	2.6%	
Swank (43)	1997	64	Degenerative	Mixed	N	12.5%	17.2%	12.5%	0.0%	0.0%	7.2%	42.2%	
Bose (8)	1998	97	Degenerative	Caspar	N	10.3%	7.2%	0.0%	0.0%	0.0%	0.0%	17.5%	
Caspar (9)	1998	146	Degenerative	Multiple	N	0.7%	0.7%	0.0%	0.0%	0.0%	0.0%	1.4%	
Geisler (94)	1998	182	Degenerative	Caspar	N	0.5%	0.0%	0.0%	0.0%	0.0%	0.0%	0.5%	
Heidecke (44)	1998	96	Degenerative	Orion	Y (6)	1.0%	0.0%	0.0%	0.0%	0.0%	0.0%	2.1%	
Lowery (46)	1998	109	Degenerative	Multiple	N	*	*	*	*	*	*	34.9%	
—	—	70		Orozco	N	10.0%	4.0%	14.0%	0.0%	0.0%	8.3%	44.3%	
—	—	22		CSLP	N	4.0%	0.0%	9.0%	0.0%	0.0%	0.0%	22.7%	
—	—	17		Orion	N	0.0%	3.0%	0.0%	0.0%	0.0%	0.0%	11.8%	
Vaccaro (69)	1998	45	Degenerative	CSLP	Y (3)	8.9%	0.0%	0.0%	20.0%	8.9%	20.0%	20.0%	All Patients
—	—	33		CSLP	N	0.0%	0.0%	0.0%	9.1%	3.0%	9.1%	9.1%	2-Level Corpectomy Sub-group
—	—	12		CSLP	Y (3)	33.3%	0.0%	0.0%	50.0%	41.7%	50.0%	50.0%	3-Level Corpectomy Sub-group
Eleraky (74)	1999	185	Degenerative	Multiple	N	3.9%	0.0%	0.0%	3.9%	0.0%	*	7.8%	
Caspar (24)	1999	37	Failed Surgery	Caspar	N	8.1%	0.0%	0.0%	0.0%	0.0%	0.0%	8.1%	
Caspar (34)	1999	30	Tumor	Caspar	Y	0.0%	0.0%	0.0%	0.0%	0.0%	0.0%	0.0%	
Majid (47)	1999	34	Degenerative	Orion	N	0.0%	0.0%	0.0%	0.0%	0.0%	0.0%	0.0%	Cages used in all 34 patients; 4 patients not plated
Schneeberger (140)	1999	35	Degenerative	Orozco	N	0.0%	0.0%	0.0%	0.0%	0.0%	0.0%	0.0%	
Wang (4)	1999	44	Degenerative	CSLP?	N	0.0%	0.0%	0.0%	0.0%	0.0%	0.0%	0.0%	
Schultz (99)	2000	72	Degenerative	Multiple	Y	0.0%	0.0%	0.0%	1.4%	0.0%	0.0%	1.4%	
Wang (3)	2000	32	Degenerative	CSLP?	N	0.0%	0.0%	0.0%	0.0%	0.0%	0.0%	0.0%	
Shapiro (85)	2001	246	Degenerative	CSLP	N	0.0%	0.0%	0.8%	0.0%	0.4%	0.0%	1.2%	
Bose (95)	2001	106	Degenerative	Multiple	N	8.5%	5.7%	0.0%	0.9%	0.0%	5.7%	15.1%	
Zaveri (134)	2001	47	Degenerative	CSLP	Y (9)	4.3%	2.1%	2.1%	0.0%	4.3%	0.0%	12.8%	Unicortical fixation

*Data not retrievable from paper

TABLE 83.2. *Implant Complications in Published Consecutive Series of Anterior Fusion with Plating (N < 30)*

First author (reference no.)	Publication year	N	Major diagnostic category	Plate type	Posterior fusion?	Fixation complications (percentage of patients)							Comments
						Screw or plate loosening	Screw fracture	Plate fracture	Plate/graft displacement or Fx	Implant malposition	Revision for implant complications	Total fixation complications	
Brown (72)	1989	13	Degenerative	Orozco	N	15.4%	0.0%	0.0%	7.7%	7.7%	15.4%	23.1%	
Mann (78)	1990	16	Trauma	Various	N	0.0%	6.3%	6.3%	6.3%	12.5%	18.8%	18.8%	
Suh (41)	1990	13	Degen, Trauma	CSLP	N	0.0%	0.0%	0.0%	0.0%	0.0%	0.0%	23.1%	
Seifert (128)	1991	22	Degenerative	Orozco (?)	N	9.1%	0.0%	0.0%	0.0%	0.0%	0.0%	9.1%	
Garvey (13)	1992	14	Trauma	Caspar	Y (2)	7.1%	7.1%	0.0%	0.0%	0.0%	0.0%	14.3%	
Brockmeyer (91)	1995	11	Trauma	Caspar, CSLP	N	0.0%	0.0%	0.0%	9.1%	0.0%	0.0%	9.1%	
Ebraheim (71)	1995	25	Degenerative	Orozco	N	12.0%	0.0%	0.0%	4.0%	8.0%	20.0%	20.0%	
Herman (75)	1995	20	Kyphosis	CSLP, Caspar	N	5.0%	0.0%	0.0%	0.0%	0.0%	0.0%	5.0%	
McAfee (98)	1995	17	Tumor	Caspar, CSLP	Y	0.0%	0.0%	0.0%	0.0%	0.0%	0.0%	0.0%	
Connolly (12)	1996	25	Degenerative	CSLP	N	4.0%	4.0%	0.0%	0.0%	8.0%	0.0%	16.0%	
Coric (93)	1997	19	Nonunion	CSLP, Caspar	N	0.0%	0.0%	0.0%	0.0%	0.0%	0.0%	0.0%	
Vanichkachorn (23)*	1998	11	Degenerative	CSLP, Orion	Y (6)	0.0%	0.0%	0.0%	9.1%	0.0%	0.0%	9.1%	Graft fracture due to intragraft screw placement
Riew (97)*	1999	14	Degen, OPLL	CSLP, Orion	Y (3)	0.0%	0.0%	0.0%	14.3%	0.0%	0.0%	14.3%	Death due to graft/plate extrusion & resp. arrest
Tribus (88)	1999	16	Nonunion	Caspar	N	0.0%	0.0%	0.0%	0.0%	6.3%	0.0%	6.3%	
Bolesta (70)	2000	15	Degenerative	CSLP	N	6.7%	13.3%	6.7%	0.0%	0.0%	13.3%	26.7%	
Epstein (100)	2000	22	OPLL	Orion	Y	0.0%	0.0%	0.0%	4.5%	0.0%	0.0%	4.5%	
Razack (81)	2000	22	Trauma	CSLP	N	0.0%	0.0%	4.5%	0.0%	0.0%	0.0%	4.5%	
Boockvar (86)	2001	14	Degenerative	CSLP	N	0.0%	0.0%	0.0%	21.4%	0.0%	0.0%	21.4%	

*Buttress or junctional plates used in these series

Note: References 51, 58, 73, 87, 89, 123, 141, and 142 not included as implant complications were not reported in these series.

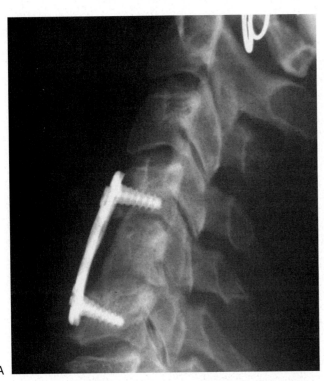
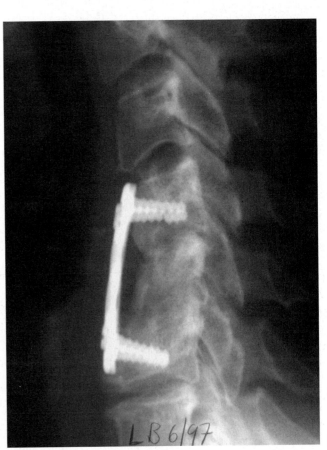

A   B

FIG. 83.4. This 42-year-old woman underwent a subtotal corpectomy of C5 for two-level disc disease. She developed a nonunion and a fracture of one of her cephalad screws and was subsequently noted to have a solid arthrodesis 1 year after posterior wiring and fusion.

The prevalence in the literature of screw and plate loosening was between 0% and 15.4%, the prevalence of screw fracture (Fig. 83.4) was between 0% and 13.3%, the prevalence of plate fracture was between 0% and 6.7%, the prevalence of plate and graft displacement (with or without graft fracture) was between 0% and 21.4%, and the prevalence of implant malposition (screws in discs, plating of unfused segments, etc.) was between 0% and 12.5%. The prevalence of all implant complications in some series was as high as 26.7% (70), and the overall revision rate for implant complications was as high as 20% (71). These data should be interpreted with caution for many reasons: (a) most of the large complication percentages are in series with relatively small numbers of patients, and may be somewhat high due to the learning curve of the involved surgeons (Table 83.2); (b) several of the published reports are from the same investigators or institutions, and therefore some of the same subsets of patients may be reported in different publications; and (c) there is a great deal of variability in these many reports with regard to diagnostic categories, numbers of discectomies performed, numbers of corpectomies performed, plating techniques, bone graft types, postoperative immobilization (length and type), and follow-up length, all of which make most of the series very

difficult to compare directly (5,6,8,21,24,33,34,36,46,52, 54–56,58,59,71–89).

Implant Fixation Complications

In 1984 Lesoin and co-authors (90) reported on a 290-patient series of traumatic injuries to the lower cervical spine, of which 145 were treated anteriorly with decompression, fusion, and instrumentation with iliac crest autograft. Loose screws were noted in 2 patients; otherwise, there were no implant-related complications. The plates used in this case were variable, but the predominant type was the Orozco ("H") plate, with some of the patients in this series treated with a new type of expansion screw. One hundred patients (34.5%) in the entire series of 290 patients were quadriplegic. Two (1.4%) of the plated patients developed screw loosening.

In 1989 Goffin and associates (14) reported a prospective series of 41 patients with fractures and/or dislocations of the cervical spine treated with an anterior cervical arthrodesis and stabilization with a Caspar plate. Four patients (10%) died within the first 3 months, all from cardiac arrest as a result of neurologic injury or a preexisting serious neuromuscular disorder. There were only 2 cases (5%) of plate and screw loosening requiring revision. The authors attributed these failures to overdistraction of notably unstable motion segments. In a separate report, these same authors reported their 5- to 9-year follow-up in 1995 of 25 patients who were a subset of their original series (15). They noted fracture of one plate occurring at 53 months postoperatively. They also noted 15 patients (60%) with radiographic degeneration of disc levels adjacent to the fused segments. No patient experienced neurologic deterioration.

In 1995, Brockmeyer and colleagues (91) reported a series of 24 pediatric cervical spine procedures that involved anterior cervical plate stabilization. Eleven cases were traumatic and were treated with either Caspar plates (10 patients) or the CSLP system (1 patient). One of the anteriorly plated patients in this series (9%) was noted to have graft and plate dislodgement requiring revision. Herman and Sonntag (75) reported a series of 20 patients who underwent cervical corpectomy and plate fixation for postlaminectomy kyphosis. Seventeen patients (85%) underwent fixation with the Caspar system, and 3 patients (15%) underwent anterior plating with the CSLP system. One patient (5%) was noted to have screw loosening, and 3 patients (15%) were noted to have transient recurrent laryngeal nerve palsy. There was no neurologic deterioration in this series. The authors determined that all patients were solidly fused at final follow-up.

In 1996, Connolly and colleagues (12) reported a series of 43 patients surgically treated for cervical spondylosis with anterior cervical discectomy and arthrodesis with autograft. Twenty-five of these patients underwent anterior cervical plating with the CSLP system using the Morscher hollow titanium plasma-sprayed screws. The authors reported a 100% fusion rate in the plated group, which was not statistically significantly different, however, from the fusion rate in the 18 patients (83.3%) who were not plated. Implant-related complications included two patients (8%) with malpositioned screws in the disc space, one (4%) loose screw, and one (4%) broken screw. Four patients (16%) had implant-related complications. There were also two patients (8%) with transient dysphagia.

Also in 1996, Katsuura and co-workers (92) reported a series of 44 patients who underwent multilevel anterior cervical arthrodesis with cervical plating. Thirty-three patients (75%) had degenerative disease, whereas 11 patients (25%) had ossification of the posterior longitudinal ligament (OPLL) as their presenting diagnosis. These patients were plated with either the CSLP (11 patients; 25%) or the Caspar plate (33 patients; 25%). The mean follow-up was 38 months. Forty-two (95.5%) of the 44 patients went on to solid fusion. A total of 8 (18%) patients had minor implant-related complications: 4 patients (9%) had loose screws and 4 patients (9%) had broken screws. As compared with a series of 30 historical controls, there was less kyphosis and a lower incidence of persistent neck pain in this series of plated patients. The types of screws used were not reported. Paramore and co-authors (80) reported a series of 49 patients treated for mixed diag-

noses with one-level or more fusions using Caspar anterior plate and either autograft or allograft depending on length of fusion and number of corpectomy levels. They reported only one case of nonunion at follow-up. The authors noted a total of 10 patients (20%) with implant-related complications, including 5 patients (10%) with screw loosening, 3 patients (6%) with screw fracture, and 2 patients (4%) with screw back-out. All of these patients were treated with the Caspar plating system. They correlated the prevalence of implant failure and pseudoarthrosis with increasing patient age and plate length. Shapiro (21) reported on 88 patients who were treated with anterior cervical decompression and arthrodesis with fibular allograft with a CSLP device for degenerative discs at one or more levels. With the exception of minor screw loosening in 2 patients (2%), they reported no significant complications at a mean follow-up of 22 months. One patient did develop a plate fracture 6 months after a multilevel fusion as a consequence of a motor vehicle accident. The overall implant complication rate in this series was 3%. The authors compared this series of patients with a historical series of 100 similar patients fused with autologous iliac crest and noted significantly fewer graft-related complications and less graft collapse in the plated/allograft fibular group.

In 1997, Coric and co-workers (93) reported their series of revision anterior cervical surgical procedures for pseudoarthrosis using allograft and anterior plating in 19 patients. Ten patients were arthrodesed with the CSLP system and 10 were arthrodesed with the Caspar plate. All patients went on to union. There were no implant-related complications.

In 1998, Caspar and associates (9) reported their comparison study of 356 patients who underwent one- or two-level anterior cervical discectomy and arthrodesis procedures for degenerative disease. Of this group, 210 patients did not undergo plating, and 146 patients underwent plating with either the Caspar plate, the CSLP, or the Orion plate. All 11 (3%) of the revisions in this series were for nonunion. Of the 146 plated patients, only 1 (0.7%) required revision, whereas 10 (5%) of the 210 patients without plating required revision. Two patients (1%) experienced minor implant complications in this series, one (8%) each with screw loosening and screw fracture. Geisler and associates (94) reported on a series of 402 patients from two institutions who underwent anterior cervical discectomy and arthrodesis at one or more levels for degenerative disease. One hundred and eighty-two of these (45%) were anteriorly plated with the Caspar plate. A mixture of allograft and autograft was used in this series. One patient (0.5%) underwent revision surgery for implant complications (screw loosening and back-out causing dysphagia). Another patient (0.5%) in the plating group underwent revision surgery for pseudoarthrosis. The authors noted a statistically significant decrease in the rate of revision surgery in the plated group (2 of 182, or 1.1%) as compared with the nonplated group (20 of 220, or 9.1%).

Bolesta and co-authors (70) reported in 2000 their prospective series of 15 patients who underwent a modified

Smith-Robinson anterior cervical discectomy and fusion and plating with the CSLP system at three or four levels for cervical radiculopathy or myelopathy. Solid arthrodesis was achieved at all levels in only 7 of their 15 patients. They noted four hardware complications in their series, two of which required revision. One of the two revision cases included one loose plate, in which the plate was removed and the patient went on to uneventful fusion. The other patient developed a nonunion and a fractured plate; the plate was removed, and a posterior arthrodesis was performed under the same anesthetic. One patient with a solid fusion was noted to have a fractured screw at 30 months follow-up. Another patient with a fractured screw went on to develop a nonunion at one level that was successfully revised with posterior grafting and fusion 18 months after the initial operation. Although not specifically stated by the authors, it appeared from illustrations and radiographs in the manuscript that the nonfenestrated screws were utilized in the patients in this series. Two additional patients required revision surgery for nonunion.

In 2000, Wang and colleagues (3) reported a series of 32 patients who underwent anterior cervical discectomy and fusion and plating for two-level cervical disc herniations. All 32 patients (100%) went on to solid fusion, and no implant complications were reported. They reported good to excellent results in 88% of these patients. They compared these 32 patients with a concurrent, but nonrandomized, series of 28 patients who were arthrodesed without plates. It was noted that 7 (25%) of these 28 patients had pseudoarthrosis that ultimately required revision. The mean follow-up of the combined series (60 patients) was 32.4 months. A year earlier in a series from the same institution, Wang and associates (4) reported on the results on 44 patients who underwent single-level anterior cervical discectomy and arthrodesis with plating with a mean follow-up of 42 months. In contrast to their multilevel series, the fusion rate was 92%. There were no implant-related complications in this series as well. Concurrent, but nonrandomized, controls in this series consisted of 30 non-plated patients, 33 (92%) of whom went on to a solid fusion. The authors concluded that there was no significant difference in the fusion rates between single-level nonplated versus plated fusions. Good to excellent results were 91% in the plated group and 89% in the nonplated group.

Bose (95) reported in 2001 a comparison study of smokers and nonsmokers who underwent anterior cervical discectomy and arthrodesis with plating at one or more levels. Of the 106 patients evaluated, 20 patients had a one- or two-level corpectomy. Ninety patients were arthrodesed with iliac crest autograft, and 16 patients were arthrodesed with fibular allograft. Caspar, Synthes (CSLP), and Codman plates were used in this series. The fusion rate was 97% at final follow-up (mean not stated). Nine patients (9%) developed screw loosening, and 6 patients (6%) had screw frac-

ture, for an overall implant complication rate of 14% (15 patients). Only 6 patients (6%), however, required revision surgery for implant complications. Other surgical complications included 3 patients (3%) with dysphagia; 4 patients (4%) with transient C5 motor weakness, all resolving by 6 months postoperative; 2 patients (2%) with airway obstruction, one with sleep apnea syndrome who required tracheostomy for 1 month; and 3 patients (3%) with recurrent laryngeal nerve palsies, all of whom recovered. There was no difference in the fusion rate between the smokers and nonsmokers in this study.

The problems and challenges of anterior instrumentation at the cervicothoracic junction were documented by Boockvar and associates (96) in their 2001 series of 14 patients who underwent anterior cervical stabilization at the cervicothoracic junction. Most of these patients were treated for degenerative disease; however, two of these patients only had nonunion that required posterior revision. Two patients had graft fractures and were treated with posterior fusion and lateral mass plating, while another patient had graft migration that was treated with a halo vest. One patient developed a hematoma and had respiratory arrest from which he recovered. The mean follow-up in this series was 21.8 months.

Buttress or Junctional Plating

Vanichkachorn and co-authors (23) reported in 1998 a novel technique using a single-level anterior cervical locking plate (CSLP or Orion) as a junctional or buttress plate at one end (usually caudal) of a multilevel corpectomy and arthrodesis construct. They reported the results of this technique in 16 patients with a mean follow-up of 30.8 months. All but one patient (90%) fused. The one patient who did not fuse had early failure of a fibula strut graft. All patients underwent posterior lateral mass plating during the same anesthetic. Postoperatively, the patients were immobilized in a rigid cervical collar. The only instrumentation-related failure was a graft fracture due to intragraft screw placement, requiring a second surgery for revision. No patient experienced neurologic deterioration postoperatively. The authors suggested that it was unclear if this technique would obviate the need for simultaneous posterior fixation procedure because it was performed in all patients in the current study.

In 1999, Riew and colleagues (97) reported a series of 14 patients who underwent two- or three-level corpectomies with fibula strut grafting (autograft in 4 and allograft in 10) for myelopathy (spondylosis or OPLL) followed by buttress plate stabilization with either the Orion plate or the CSLP system. In contrast to the series of Vanichkachorn and associates (23), only 3 patients underwent subsequent posterior stabilization. Although all 13 of the surviving patients in this series experienced neurologic improvement, only 10 went on to solid union (mean follow-up of 27.8 months). Only two of the three nonunions, however, were revised. The authors indicated that they have subsequently abandoned the use of buttress plate stabilization in multilevel corpectomies.

Posterior Stabilization

Several studies appear to document a decreased prevalence of anterior fixation complications in patients who also undergo posterior stabilization. Jonsson and co-authors (76) reported in 1991 a series of 40 patients with 19 fractures and 21 fracture dislocations who underwent anterior cervical arthrodesis and plating at one or more levels. The plates used in this series were the CSLP with titanium hollow plasma-sprayed screws. Twenty-nine of these patients (73%) underwent supplemental posterior arthrodesis. There were two deaths in this series (5%) for reasons not specified. One patient had a malpositioned implant that was not revised. Another patient developed an esophageal fistula that was treated by primary repair and removal of the anterior plate. There was no implant loosening in this series. All 36 patients at mean follow-up of 24 months had a solid fusion rate. McAfee and associates (98) in 1995 reported their series of 100 patients who underwent single-stage anterior cervical decompression and posterior stabilization. Fifty-five (55%) of these patients had a neoplasm with pathological fracture and/or a neurologic deficit. Seventeen patients (17%) underwent adjunctive anterior cervical plate fixation for stabilization, of which 9 had a diagnosis of neoplastic disease. None of the anteriorly plated patients developed any implant-related complications.

In 2000, Schultz and co-workers (99) reported a series of 72 patients who underwent anterior decompression with anterior plate stabilization (CSLP, Orion, or Codman) combined with posterior lateral mass plating. The predominant diagnosis was spondylosis and spinal stenosis in 32 patients. Allograft fibula was used anteriorly, and autograft morcellized iliac crest bone was used posteriorly. Fusion was determined to be successful in all 72 patients with a minimum of 2-year follow-up. With the exception of 2 patients (2.8%) with OPLL who experienced transient neurologic worsening, there were no new neurologic deficits. Six patients (8.3%) experienced difficulty swallowing, with 2 patients (2.7%) with dysphagia not improving to baseline. Hoarseness was noted in 7 patients (9.7%), resolving in all but 1 patient (1.4%). There was only one anterior plate-related complication—an anterior cervical plate in 1 patient (1.4%) that pulled out due to screw loosening. Interestingly, 16 (3.1%) of 516 lateral mass screws partially backed out. However, none of the posterior or anterior constructs required revision in this series.

In another series published that same year, Epstein (100) reported on 22 cases of OPLL treated with anterior decompression and strut grafting with anterior plating with the Orion plate followed by posterior fusion and wiring. There was one late graft extrusion occurring 4 months after a four-level procedure. The authors noted a marked reduction in the revision rate for acute graft extrusions as compared with a series of 22 patients treated similarly with the exception that no anterior plating was performed. This historical series had graft extrusions in 3 patients (14%) within 24 hours of surgery. There was one (4.5%) cerebrospinal fluid (CSF) leak that required reexploration, dural grafting, and a postoperative lumbar drain.

Dynamic Plates

In 1999, Apfelbaum and associates (101) reported preliminary results of anterior cervical discectomy and fusion in 149 patients who were fused for degenerative disease (43%), trauma (38%), and several other indications and who underwent stabilization with the dynamic ABC system (Aesculap, San Francisco, CA). These authors noted that 70% of the levels had fused by 3 months follow-up. Those patients who were followed at least 6 months were noted to have 86% of all levels fused. There was vertebral settling noted in nearly all patients in this series before 3 months, but none after 3 months. Allograft was used in 56% and autograft in 44% of the patients in this series. There were no implant-related complications.

In 2001, Epstein (102) reported the results of 80 patients with spinal stenosis due to OPLL who were treated with two- to four-level corpectomies and strut graft fusion with (58 patients) or without (22 patients) anterior cervical plating. The plated patients all received fresh frozen fibula strut grafts, and the unplated patients received autologous iliac crest grafts. All patients underwent posterior wiring and arthrodesis during the same anesthetic. Of the 58 plated patients, the Orion plate was used in 22, the Atlantis (hybrid) plate was used in 16, and the ABC (dynamic) plate was used in 20. The graft extrusion rate was 14% (3 patients) in the unplated group, 9% (2 patients) in the Orion plated group, 19% (3 patients) in the Atlantis plated group, and 0% (no patients) in the ABC plated group.

That same year, Zdeblick and Herkowitz (52) reported their series of 108 patients at 12- to 24-month (18-month average) follow-up who had undergone anterior cervical decompression fusion and plating with a translational anterior cervical plate (Premier; Medtronic Sofamor Danek, Memphis, TN) without supplemental posterior arthrodesis (Fig. 83.5). Most of these patients (85%) had degenerative disease and were operated on at one to four levels. These authors noted no implant complications and an initial fusion rate of 95%. Subsidence occurred only between surgery and 6 weeks after surgery, often within the first few days, with maintenance of lordosis.

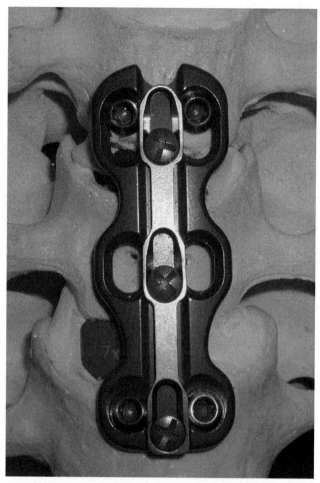

FIG. 83.5. A dynamic (translational) cervical plate. Note that the screws can translate vertically in the slotted holes but are restrained from backing out by the sliding lock.

OTHER COMPLICATIONS OF ANTERIOR CERVICAL PLATING

The nonimplant-related surgical complications from major published series of anterior cervical fusion and plating are summarized in Table 83.3. Although some of these complications can have a direct relationship to anterior cervical implants (for example, dysphagia and esophageal perforation), the relationship between most of these complications and the presence of anterior cervical plates is unclear.

Dysphagia

The early literature regarding complications of anterior cervical surgery contains little or nothing on dysphagia as a complication of these procedures (103–105). Zeidman and associates (106), in their 1997 report on CSRS complications, noted that esophageal dysfunction was more of a problem than previously recognized, but were unable to relate this complication to anterior internal fixation of the cervical spine. The incidence of dysphagia in anterior plate fixation cases has been reported to be as high as 28% (71). Dysphagia is one of the primary symptoms of plate and/or screw loosening; thus, complaints of persistent or worsening swallowing dysfunction should stimulate radiographic evaluation. If anterior implant loosening is greater than 2 to 5 mm (Fig. 83.6), revision surgery may need to be considered (46,69).

The effect of satisfactorily placed anterior implants on swallowing function and dysphagia is unclear because there is little in the literature on this subject. Speech and swallowing specialists, however, have noted an increased prevalence of dysphagia associated with the increased use of anterior cervical instrumentation (79). Winslow and colleagues (107), in a single-institution study in which questionnaires were mailed to 497 patients who had undergone anterior cervical arthrodesis and/or discectomy, reported complaints of dysphagia in 60%, as compared with 23% of 150 unoperated controls sent the same questionnaires ($p < 0.01$). This qualitative questionnaire revealed that difficulty eating solid foods or odynophagia (painful swallowing) was notably more common following the anterior approach to the cervical spine. Admitted limitations of the study include lack of objective data regarding swallowing function. Furthermore, these authors did not relate their findings to the presence or absence of anterior cervical plates.

Bazaz and Yoo (108) reported the results of their study of 190 patients who underwent anterior cervical surgery and were followed with questionnaires at 1, 2, and 6 months postoperatively. They noted that 51% of the patients complained of dysphagia at 1 month, 31% at 2 months, and 15% at 6 months. Only two patients complained of moderate to severe dysphagia symptoms at 6 months. Higher rates of dysphagia were seen with revision surgery and with an increased number of levels arthrodesed. Like the Winslow study (107), this study is limited by lack of objective data.

Donnelly and associates (109) reported a prospective study of 16 patients who underwent multilevel anterior cervical arthrodesis using the Smith-Robinson technique followed by anterior cervical plating. All patients underwent otolaryngologic evaluation pre- and postoperatively. Four of their patients had swallowing problems postoperatively. Two patients had postoperative studies documenting abnormalities, including one with an obstruction at the distal esophageal sphincter and another with a "shelf" and retropharynx felt to be consistent with scar formation or a mechanical obstruction at the proximal end of the plate. Both of these patients had normal swallowing studies preoperatively. The other two patients with swallowing problems resolved their symptoms spontaneously.

TABLE 83.3. *Other Surgical Complications in Published Consecutive Series of Anterior Fusion with Plating*

First author (reference no.)	Publication year	N	Type	#	%	Comments
Aebi (5)	1986	50	RLN Palsy	2	4.0%	
Brown (72)	1989	13	Dysphagia	2	15.4%	One revision for prominent implants and dysphagia
Caspar (33)	1989	60	Dysphagia	1	1.7%	Dysphagia resolved
Mann (78)	1990	16	Dysphagia	1	6.3%	
Randle (138)	1990	54	Infection	1	1.9%	
Suh (41)	1990	13	Dysphagia	0	0.0%	
Jonsson (76)	1991	40	Esophageal Inj.	1	5.9%	Plate removed to treat esophageal fistula
Ripa (57)	1991	92	Dysphagia	1	1.1%	Dysphagia resolved after screw removal
Seifert (128)	1991	22	Sup. Infection	1	4.5%	
Garvey (13)	1992	14	Dysphagia	2	14.3%	
Schweighofer (118)	1992	171	Infection	4	2.3%	
—	—	—	Vertebral Artery Inj.	1	0.6%	
—	—	—	Nerve Root Injury	1	0.6%	
—	—	—	Dysphagia	1	0.6%	
Kostuik (17)	1993	42	Dysphagia	3	7.1%	
—	—	—	RLN Palsy	1	2.4%	
Papadopoulos (20)	1993	160	Infection	2	1.3%	2 Plates removed for infection (distantly seeded)
—	—	—	Dysphagia	4	2.5%	1 Plate removed for dysphagia
Ebraheim (71)	1995	25	Dysphagia	7	28.0%	6 of 7 dysphagia cases resolved
Herman (75)	1995	20	RLN Palsy	3	15.0%	
Johnston (139)	1995	50	Dysphagia	6	12.0%	2 of 6 dysphagia cases required gastrostomy for 1 month
Connolly (12)	1996	25	Dysphagia	2	8.0%	
Paramore (80)	1996	49	Dysphagia	4	8.2%	
Coric (93)	1997	19	Hoarseness	2	10.5%	Hoarseness resolved, attributed to hematoma in one patient
McLaughlin (19)	1997	39	Infection	1	2.6%	Re-exploration in one patient for epidural hematoma
Swank (43)	1997	64	New Neuro Deficit	1	1.6%	Deltoid weakness, "gradually improved"
—	—	—	Dysphagia	2	3.1%	Dysphagia resolved
—	—	—	RLN Palsy	1	1.6%	RLN palsy resolved
Bose (8)	1998	97	Dysphagia	5	5.2%	Dysphagia resolved
—	—	—	RLN Palsy	3	3.1%	RLN palsy resolved
—	—	—	C5 Motor Weakness	2	2.1%	Weakness resolved
Caspar (9)	1998	146	Dysphagia	1	0.7%	
Geisler (94)	1998	182	Dysphagia	1	0.5%	
Heidecke (44)	1998	96	Dysphagia	7	7.3%	
Eleraky (74)	1999	185	Infection	8	4.3%	
—	—	—	Vertebral Artery Inj.	4	2.2%	None were due to implants
—	—	—	New Neuro Deficit	6	3.2%	Neurologic deteriorations were all transient
—	—	—	Dysphagia	14	7.6%	Dysphagia resolved
—	—	—	CSF Leak	12	6.5%	All CSF leaks successfully treated with lumbar drain
—	—	—	Esophageal Inj.	3	1.6%	Esophageal tear repaired primarily, NPO for 4 days postop
—	—	—	RLN Palsy	4	2.2%	RLN palsy resolved
Caspar (34)	1999	37	RLN Palsy	1	2.7%	RLN palsy resolved?
Caspar (24)	1999	30	RLN Palsy	2	6.7%	RLN palsies resolved
Majid (47)	1999	34	Cage Extrusion	1	2.9%	Cages used in all 34 patients; 4 patients not plated
—	—	—	Radiculopathy	1	2.9%	
Riew (97)	1999	14	CSF Leak	1	7.1%	CSF leak treated with repair & lumbar drain
—	—	—	Resp. Arrest	1	7.1%	Death due to graft/plate extrusion & resp. arrest
Schneeberger (140)	1999	35	Dysphagia	1	2.9%	
Bolesta (70)	2000	15	Dysphagia	1	6.7%	
Epstein (100)	2000	22	CSF Leak	1	4.5%	CSF leak treated with repair (patch graft) and lumbar drain
Schultz (99)	2000	72	Dysphagia	6	8.3%	Permanent in 2 patients (2.7%)
—	—	—	New Neuro Deficit	2	2.8%	Neurologic deteriorations were all transient
—	—	—	Hoarseness	7	9.7%	Hoarseness was transient in 7 patients
—	—	—	RLN Palsy	1	1.4%	Permanent RLN palsy in one patient
Boockvar (96)	2001	14	Resp. Arrest	1	7.1%	Respiratory arrest due to hematoma (patient recovered)
Shapiro (26)	2001	246	Hoarseness	2	0.8%	Hoarseness was transient in both patients
Bose (95)	2001	106	Dysphagia	3	2.8%	Outcome of dysphagia not specified
			C5 Motor Weakness	4	3.8%	Weakness resolved by 6 months
			Airway Obstruction	2	1.9%	One patient required tracheostomy for 1 month
			RLN Palsy	3	2.8%	RLN palsies resolved
Zaveri (134)	2001	47	Dysphagia	2	4.3%	Dysphagia improved after 6 months

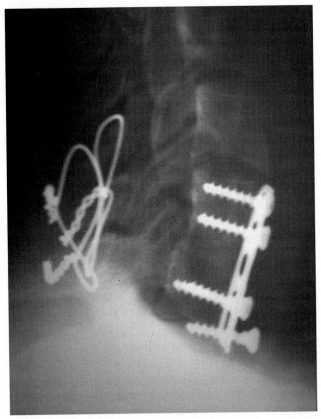

FIG. 83.6. A Caspar plate after a single-level fusion is noted to have loosening of one of the caudal screws that had been placed into the caudal (unfused) disc. It backed out 4 mm but did not cause dysphagia. The patient, however, developed a nonunion and was revised with posterior wiring and fusion.

Esophageal Injuries

Esophageal ruptures or tears are dreaded but rare complications of anterior cervical surgery. Smith and Bolesta (86) reported two cases of esophageal complication due to migration of screws after plate fixation of the cervical spine. Hanci and associates (110) also reported three cases of esophageal perforation due to pressure necrosis following anterior instrumentation of the cervical spine. The onset of symptoms was delayed between 4 and 360 days in these five cases. All of these complications were attributable to pressure necrosis from the spinal implants. Gaudinez and co-workers (111) reported a series of 44 patients with cervical spinal injuries and subsequent esophageal perforations. Thirty-four (77%) of these patients had esophageal injuries directly related to operations performed for their cervical fractures. Twenty-eight (82%) of these 34 patients had anterior cervical plates implanted at the time of their surgery. Although some of these injuries were associated with prominent implants, the authors did not state how many of these perforations were directly attributable to the implants. In 22 (79%) of these patients, treatment included implant removal.

Not all reports of esophageal injuries, however, are directly related to anterior cervical implants. Kelly and colleagues (112) reported four cases of esophageal perforation attributable to pressure necrosis from graft displacement. All four of these patients reported odynophagia (painful swallowing) as their first symptom. No instrumentation was used in these cases. Van Berge Henegouwen and associates (113) reported three cases of intraoperative esophageal perforation, of which one case was recognized at the time of surgery and the other two cases diagnosed 4 and 6 days postoperatively. Whitehill and co-authors (114) reported a case of esophageal perforation occurring 2.5 months postoperatively because of laceration by the sharp edge of an autologous bone graft that had minimally extruded. In their report of esophageal perforations compiled from a survey of CSRS members in 1987, Newhouse and co-authors (115) noted that 4 of the 16 reported cases that occurred postoperatively were related to the presence of anterior cervical implants. Six (27%) of the 22 reported cases, however, were the direct result of intraoperative injury. Occasionally an esophageal perforation results in no apparent morbidity. Fujibayashi and associates (116) reported a case of a "missing" anterior cervical plate and screws occurring between 1 and 3 months after implantation, with the implants presumably passing, without notice and without apparent morbidity, through the gastrointestinal tract. Whole-body fluoroscopy demonstrated no evidence of the plate and screws. A barium swallow failed to demonstrate an esophageal fistula. Geyer and Foy (117) reported a case of "oral extrusion" of a locking screw from a CSLP that had been placed 5 years earlier to support an anterior cervical arthrodesis for myelopathy.

In order to avoid the high morbidity associated with most unrecognized esophageal perforations, Smith and Bolesta (86) have suggested the routine application of 20 to 30 mL of dilute indigo carmine solution into the hypopharynx and proximal esophagus using a small soft catheter before closure and after removal of self-retaining retractors. If bright blue fluid is then detected in the wound, a diligent search for and repair of an esophageal perforation is performed. Seven days of nasogastric suction along with broad-spectrum parenteral antibiotics (including anaerobic coverage) is then employed. Delayed perforation can be avoided by careful clinical and radiographic monitoring of patients after anterior cervical surgery, particularly those cases at high risk for graft and/or implant extrusion.

Clinical signs and symptoms of missed esophageal perforation or delayed esophageal rupture include increasing neck and throat pain, odynophagia, erythema, swelling, tenderness, induration, crepitus, subcutaneous emphysema, unexplained tachycardia, and sepsis (86,109,111,113,115). The diagnosis can be confirmed by barium swallow esophagogram (Fig. 83.7); however, the false-negative rate of imaging studies may be as high as 27% (111), requiring esophagoscopy for diagnosis (Fig. 83.8). Treatment consists of surgical exploration with primary repair, or localized sternocleido-

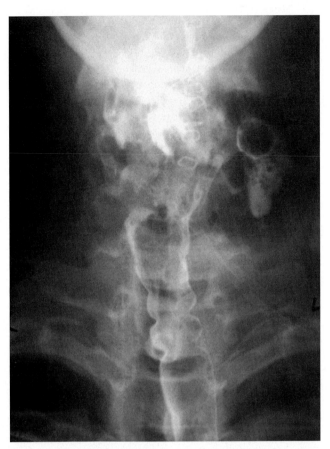

FIG. 83.7. This barium swallow esophagogram in a 43-year-old woman who was noted to have anterior neck swelling, subcutaneous emphysema, fever, and odynophagia 11 days after anterior-posterior fusion for C3-C4 vertebral osteomyelitis demonstrates an esophageal perforation, with contrast noted in the left anterior neck at the level and side of her anterior fusion. The esophagus was successfully repaired, but the patient required feeding gastrostomy for several weeks.

mastoid muscle flap coverage for large unrepairable defects (86,111). Seven or more days of gastric diversion (nasogastric tube or gastrostomy tube) postoperatively are usually necessary. Total parenteral nutrition and broad-spectrum antibiotics are also initiated postoperatively.

Vertebral Artery Injury

The exact prevalence of vertebral artery injury in anterior cervical surgery is unknown; however, most series report a prevalence of 0.6% or less (43,78,118). The highest incidence was 2.2% in the 185-patient series reported by Eleraky and associates (74). Although vertebral artery injury is a well-documented complication of posterior cervical instrumentation, particularly C1-C2 transarticular screw fixation (18), there are few reports of vertebral artery injury due directly to the implantation of an anterior cervical plate. Smith and colleagues (119) reported 10 cases of vertebral artery injury during anterior decompression of the cervical spine. The use of motorized drills was responsible for 6 of the injuries in this series. Three of the injuries were due to "instrumentation"; however, the authors did not elaborate on whether a drill, tap, or screw caused the injury. Control of the bleeding was achieved with tamponade, direct exposure and electrocoagulation, transosseous suture, open suture, or open placement of a vascular clip. Half of their patients were noted to have new postoperative neurologic deficits, with most resolving. These authors felt that pathological, weakened bone resulted in increased risk of vertebral artery injury. They recommended that these injuries be treated by direct exposure and control of the vertebral artery, followed by repair of the vertebral injury (Fig. 83.9).

Curylo and associates (120) performed a 222-specimen cadaveric study in which a 2.7% prevalence of a tortuous

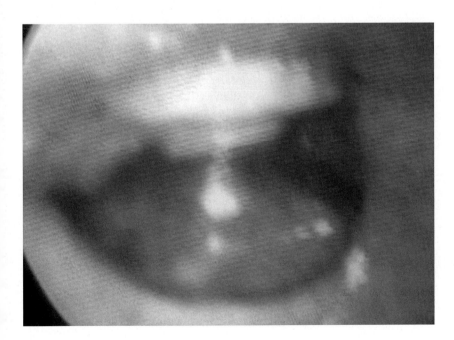

FIG. 83.8. This endoscopic view demonstrates a loose screw that has eroded through the posterior esophageal wall. This patient had the screw retrieved endoscopically, but he required open repair of the esophagus and 7 days of nasogastric suction.

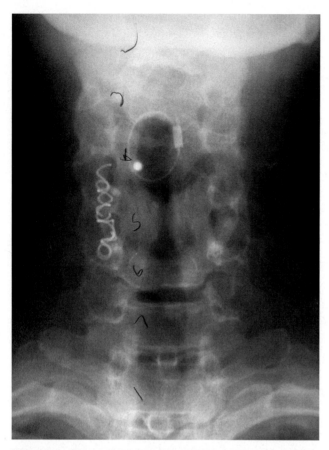

FIG. 83.9. This patient developed acute hemorrhage in the anterior neck 17 days after anterior-posterior cervical fusion for vertebral osteomyelitis complicated by a right vertebral artery laceration treated by packing at the time of surgery. She underwent successful coil embolization and did not develop a neurologic deficit.

vertebral artery coursing was noted (Fig. 83.10). This type of anomaly was noted also in three anteriorly operated patients, one of whom had a vertebral artery laceration and subsequent repair. In the other two cases, these anomalies were recognized preoperatively and the surgical procedures were modified to minimize the risk of this complication. These authors indicated that preoperative axial imaging studies are helpful in identifying vertebral artery tortuosity.

Recurrent Laryngeal Nerve Palsy

The prevalence of recurrent laryngeal nerve injury associated with anterior cervical discectomy has been reported to be between 0.07% and 11% (29). Winslow and colleagues (107) have suggested that the prevalence of temporary vocal cord paralysis may be much higher. Vocal cord paralysis is due to injury to one or both of the recurrent (inferior) laryngeal nerves that branch from the vagus nerve. Anatomically, there is asymmetry in the course of the recurrent laryngeal nerve. On the right side, the recurrent laryngeal nerve exits the main trunk of the vagus nerve and passes underneath the subclavian artery from anterior to posterior. It then ascends in the tracheoesophageal groove. It may bifurcate before entering the larynx. On the left side, the recurrent laryngeal nerve descends parallel to the carotid artery but then passes underneath and posterior to the aorta at the ligamentum arteriosum. The nerve then ascends in the tracheoesophageal groove somewhat more medially than on the right side. Nonrecurrence of the inferior laryngeal nerve on the left side is rare, but on the right side it occurs with an prevalence of 1%, with the inferior laryngeal nerve arising from the main trunk of the vagus. This anomaly is associated with an aberrant subclavian artery.

Surgeons have used both the more medial ascending course of the recurrent laryngeal nerve on the left side and

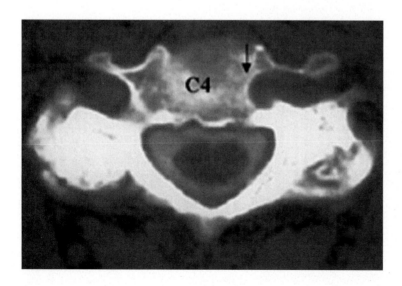

FIG. 83.10. This postmyelogram computed axial tomogram demonstrates a very medialized foramen transversarium (*arrow*), indicating a tortuous vertebral artery course. The risk of vertebral artery injury is especially high, particularly if this radiographic finding is overlooked. (From, Curylo LJ, Mason HC, Bohlman HH, et al. Tortuous course of the vertebral artery and anterior cervical decompression: a cadaveric and clinical case study. *Spine* 2000;25: 2860–2864, with permission.)

the possibility of a nonrecurring inferior laryngeal nerve on the right side as justification for routinely approaching the anterior cervical spine from the left side. This rationale may not be warranted. Beutler and associates (121) reviewed a series of 328 anterior cervical fusion procedures and noted an overall prevalence of recurrent laryngeal nerve symptoms of 2.7%: 2.1% in anterior cervical discectomy and arthrodesis and 3.5% in corpectomy procedures. They also reported a 3% prevalence of recurrent laryngeal nerve dysfunction symptoms with instrumentation and a 9.5% prevalence with reoperative anterior surgical procedures. They reported no association, however, between the laterality of the approach and the prevalence of recurrent laryngeal nerve symptoms in their series. Although the highest reported incidence of recurrent laryngeal nerve palsy we are aware of is 15% in plated anterior cervical arthrodesis (75), there is little or no evidence that this complication is directly related to the implantation or presence of anterior cervical plates.

Apfelbaum and associates (122) reported a decreased prevalence of vocal cord paralysis in a consecutive series of 900 patients who underwent anterior cervical fusion and plating and those patients who had repositioning of their endotracheal tube after placement of self-retaining retractors (deflation and reinflation of the endotracheal tube cuff). The prevalence of temporary paralysis decreased from 6.4% to 1.69% after institution of this maneuver. They hypothesized that recurrent laryngeal nerve injury is due to displacement of the larynx into the unyielding shaft of the endotracheal tube fixed distally by the balloon cuff and proximally by tape at the mouth (Fig. 83.11). These authors supported their hypothesis by demonstrating recentering of the endotracheal tube within the endolarynx with cuff deflation and reinflation in a cadaveric study (122). This study may suggest an indirect relationship to anterior cervical plating, since these procedures typically require longer operating time than equivalent unplated procedures, and

therefore a longer endotracheal tube cuff inflation time (if not repositioned).

Respiratory and Airway Complications

Although the relationship to anterior cervical plating remains unclear, there have been several studies documenting an increased risk of respiratory and airway complications associated with multilevel anterior cervical surgery (123–125). Edema and/or hematoma can result in serious airway compromise in these patients. The studies all suggested that maintenance of the endotracheal tube overnight in high-risk patients may prevent the need for reintubation or subsequent airway complications (123–125). Riew and colleagues (125) reported a study of 256 patients in which the authors used prospective criteria to determine whether it was safe to extubate patients after anterior cervical procedures. They suggested that it may be safe to extubate patients who undergo an anterior cervical procedure that lasts less than 3 hours with a retraction time of less than 2.5 hours. If the patient is difficult to intubate or is morbidly obese, or both, he or she should be kept intubated overnight unless the procedure is less than 90 minutes in length. These authors also reported four patients in this series who developed symptomatic airway obstruction 30 to 48 hours postoperatively secondary to hematoma formation, suggesting that vigilance in observing for airway complications needs to last up to 3 days postoperatively.

Apart from the obvious direct relationship of airway complications associated with anterior plate dislodgement (97), there may be an indirect relationship of this complication to anterior cervical plating resulting from longer operating times in these procedures as compared with equivalent unplated procedures. Fujibayashi and associates (126) described a bilateral phrenic nerve palsy as a very rare complication of anterior cervical surgery in a 57-year-old man with OPLL, requiring ventilatory support for 3 months postoper-

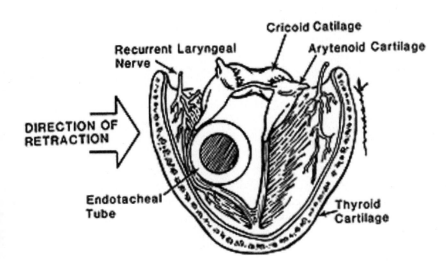

FIG. 83.11. A cross-sectional view of the larynx that demonstrates the endotracheal tube compressing the vulnerable endolaryngeal portion of the recurrent laryngeal nerve. (From, Apfelbaum RI, Kriskovich MD, Haller JR. On the incidence, cause, and prevention of recurrent laryngeal nerve palsies during anterior cervical spine surgery. *Spine* 2000; 25:2906–2912, with permission.)

atively. Plate fixation was not used. This complication was attributed to either bilateral C4 nerve root stretch injury or spinal cord injury (either due to direct trauma, secondary to edema or a vascular insult, or secondary to spinal cord shift and reimpingement).

Cerebral Spinal Fluid Leak

A CSF leak is a rare complication of anterior cervical surgery [0.4% prevalence per the CSRS data as reported by Zeidman and colleagues (106)]. This complication in plated series ranges from 7.1% in the small (14-patient) series of Riew and associates (97) to 6.5% in the larger, 165-patient series of Eleraky and co-workers (74). Most authors state that CSF leaks are best managed, if detected intraoperatively, with primary repair if possible or fibrin glue sealing if not. In large defects (such as those encountered during surgery for OPLL), dural patching may be necessary.

If the CSF leak cannot be controlled at the time of surgery, or if the CSF leak is detected postoperatively, a diverting drain (127) is very successful in preventing CSF wound drainage after anterior cervical surgery. This technique is performed by placing an epidural-type catheter in the subarachnoid space via a lumbar puncture. Two hundred to 300 mL of CSF is drained into a blood collection bag for each 24-hour period. A new bag is used each day and changed under sterile conditions. The patient is kept in a supine position and allowed to log roll from side to side. Daily CSF samples are obtained for culture cell count differential and determination of glucose and protein levels to monitor for the development of meningitis. The catheter is left in for approximately 4 days and then removed, with the patient being kept supine for an additional 24 hours to allow the puncture site to seal. In the series reported by Kitchel and associates (126), successful healing occurred in all 3 patients (of the total of 19 patients in their series) who underwent closed subarachnoid drainage. All of the reported cases of CSF leakage following anterior cervical arthrodesis with plate fixation resolved with closed lumbar subarachnoid drainage (74,97,100). There is no evidence that the prevalence of this complication is directly related to the implantation of anterior spinal plates.

Infection

Infections after anterior cervical spine surgery are uncommon. They are usually prevented by meticulous surgical technique, wound drainage, and the administration of prophylactic antibiotics. The prevalence of acute postoperative infection is reported to be between 0% and 5% (106,112). The highest reported prevalence we are aware of in a plated series is 4.5% (128). Clinical signs and symptoms of infection are those typical of any wound infection (erythema, edema, purulent wound drainage, tenderness, fever, elevated erythrocyte sedimentation rate,

elevated white blood cell count, and increasing pain). Treatment is with wound irrigation and debridement (after obtaining appropriate cultures), leaving the implant and bone grafts in place. Parenteral antibiotics are administered for 10 to 14 days for superficial infections and for 6 weeks or more for deep infections (112). In some cases, the treatment of established infection will require implant removal (20).

Anterior cervical plating appears to be safe, even in the face of a tracheostomy. Northrup and co-authors (129) reported a series of 11 patients who had undergone an anterior cervical fusion in the presence of an existing tracheostomy. Anterior cervical plates were implanted in 5 (45%) of these patients. Meticulous care was taken to isolate the tracheostomy from the surgical field. No patient developed a wound infection, although 3 developed culture-positive "excessive secretions" treated successfully with antibiotics. Apart from the aforementioned risk of esophageal perforation and infection from prominent anterior spinal implants, there has been no evidence that the presence of anterior cervical plates increases the prevalence of infection in anterior cervical surgery (Table 83.2) (112).

Neurologic Injury

The prevalence of spinal cord injury in anterior cervical surgery is quite low [0.4% according to the CSRS data as reported by Zeidman and associates (106)]. These injuries often are due to iatrogenic compression or vascular injury, but deformity and instability also can result in quadriparesis (77). Most often the source of iatrogenic compression is a posteriorly displaced bone graft. When compression is recognized, intravenous steroids should be administered according to the National Acute Spinal Cord Injury Study II protocol (130). Imaging studies can be considered; however, the time taken to obtain these studies may result in an excessive delay in returning the patient to the operating room for surgical exploration and removal of the graft. Neurophysiologic monitoring with somatosensory evoked potentials and/or motor evoked potentials may play a role in the prevention and timely diagnosis of serious neurologic injuries.

Nerve root injuries also occur at a very low incidence [0.6% according to the CSRS data as reported by Zeidman and associates (106)]. The most affected nerve root is C5. Saunders (131) attributed the relatively high prevalence of C5 nerve root injury in cervical corpectomy cases to traction on the root caused by shifting of the spinal cord as a consequence of a wide anterior decompression. In the vast majority the deficit resolved within 6 weeks. He noted a marked decreased incidence of this complication with diminished width of decompression in the later cases in his series. The largest prevalence in plated series was 3.2% (74). No reported evidence of a neurologic injury directly due to placement of bicortical anterior cervical screws has been reported. Overall, there appears to be little or no direct relationship between neurologic complications and anterior cervical plating.

Transitional Degeneration

Long-term complications of anterior cervical procedures include transitional degeneration of adjacent spinal segments. This is a common problem, particularly in multilevel fusions (13,76,132–134). Katsuura and co-authors (133) have correlated the prevalence of transitional degeneration with postoperative kyphosis, ostensibly a factor that can be prevented or reduced with anterior cervical plating. In the series of Garvey and associates (13), however, 5 of 14 patients (all anteriorly fused and plated for cervical trauma) were noted to have spondylotic changes above and/or below the instrumented levels at follow-up (mean of 30 months) despite minimal residual deformity. Three of these patients developed new-onset hypermobility that met radiographic criteria for instability. All 5 of the patients, however, remained relatively asymptomatic.

Goffin and colleagues (132) reported a series of 120 patients who had undergone an anterior cervical fusion primarily for traumatic and degenerative indications. At a mean follow-up time of 98.7 months, 92% of their patients demonstrated adjacent segment deterioration (many of these with clinical deterioration as well). These findings were equal between those patients who had been fused for trauma and those who had been fused for degenerative conditions. The authors reported an increased prevalence of ossification of the anterior longitudinal ligament at adjacent segments in those patients treated with anterior cervical plates (66%) as compared with those without (29%) ($p < 0.001$).

In the series of Jonsson and co-authors (76), of 40 patients with fractures and/or fracture dislocations who underwent anterior cervical fusion and plating at one or more levels, 8 patients (20%) developed degenerative changes in adjacent discs. Unintended partial fusion caused by anterior bone overgrowth occurred in 4 patients (10%) in this series. Twenty-nine (73%) of the patients in this series, however, underwent supplemental posterior fusion that may have contributed to these adjacent segment problems. Ten (35%) of these patients developed extension of their fusions to adjacent segments due to exuberant bony overgrowth. The patients who had anterior-posterior plating had a higher prevalence of neck pain and a decrease in the average range of cervical motion at final follow-up as compared with those patients who had undergone anterior plating alone.

In the series of Zaveri and Ford (134), 7 of 47 patients demonstrated evidence of adjacent segment degeneration at a follow-up (mean 40.8 months). Three of these patients were symptomatic in spite of spinal cord and/or cervical root compression at the transitional level confirmed by gadolinium-enhanced magnetic resonance imaging. One patient responded to nonoperative treatment, but the other two patients required one or more operations.

SUMMARY

Complications of anterior cervical instrumentation can range from minor screw loosening to graft and plate dislodgement that results in respiratory arrest and death. At the present time, the "perfect plate" does not exist, as evidenced by the vast array of designs available on the market today. These available plating systems have evolved substantially over time, and most can be safely implanted without any significant risk to the patient. Avoidance of complications requires careful preoperative planning, meticulous attention to surgical technique, appropriate postoperative immobilization, and close clinical and radiographic monitoring postoperatively (Fig. 83.12). An adequate understanding of the biomechanics of cervical instrumentation is required in order to avoid pushing the envelope too far and asking too much from one plate and four screws, particularly in corpectomies of three or more levels. Thus, until the

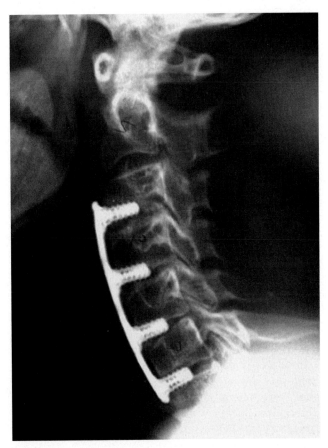

FIG. 83.12. Plate and screw malposition as seen in this lateral cervical radiograph should be completely avoidable with meticulous surgical technique and intraoperative radiographic monitoring. (Photograph courtesy of Dr. Robert Hacker, with permission.)

published clinical results of series using dynamic (hybrid and/or translational) implants indicate that these devices adequately stabilize corpectomies of three or more levels, prudence suggests that these patients should also be stabilized posteriorly at the same time they are decompressed and stabilized anteriorly. Buttress or junctional plates should be used cautiously and virtually always supplemented with posterior stabilization.

Patients who complain of persistent or worsening dysphagia should undergo radiographic evaluation. If implant migration is more than 5 mm, revision should be strongly considered in order to obviate the devastating complication of esophageal perforation. Despite the suggestions of some investigators that a plate can fracture in a solidly fused patient (21), evidence of implant fatigue should alert one to the potential of a nonunion until proved otherwise (Fig. 83.13). Close monitoring of these patients, at the very least, is indicated. Radiographic monitoring of all plated patients should be carried out on a regular basis until solid healing is confirmed since late screw loosening can occur at any time (117). When considering surgical options for patients re-

quiring anterior cervical decompression and arthrodesis, one must counsel the patient as to the unique risks associated with anterior cervical plating (implant loosening, fracture, and/or dislodgement) and those other risks that are potentially increased as a result of anterior plating (dysphagia, esophageal perforation, and respiratory problems) so that he or she can make an intelligent decision as to his or her treatment options.

FUTURE TRENDS

Without a doubt, there are new and improved techniques on the horizon for treating patients with degenerative, traumatic, neoplastic, inflammatory, congenital, and/or developmental disorders of the cervical spine. The development of dynamic anterior cervical plates and devices appears to show great promise in improving clinical results and reducing implant complications (25,51,52). These results so far are preliminary, and further study with longer-term follow-up is needed with these new types of devices. There are encouraging reports that anterior cervical cages with local bone autograft (104,135,136) may be just as effective as structural iliac autograft in achieving solid fusion and clinical results; but again, further study is required. An integrated plate-cage device has been developed and used for anterior cervical reconstruction in a series of 29 patients (83). The use of cages introduces a new variable into the risk equation for anterior cervical surgery, however (136).

Bone morphogenetic protein (BMP) has been recommended for approval by the Food and Drug Administration Advisory Panel for use in anterior lumbar fusion. Although so far there has been little published on the use of BMP in the cervical spine, almost certainly there is a future for this technology in cervical spine surgery.

An emerging technology, cervical disc replacement, may obviate fusion in the future and (it is hoped) transitional degeneration in some patients now treated with anterior cervical discectomy and fusion (137). The use of these new and potentially improved technologies in the anterior cervical spine, however, must be approached with caution, because all of them will carry with them a learning curve as well as unique complications.

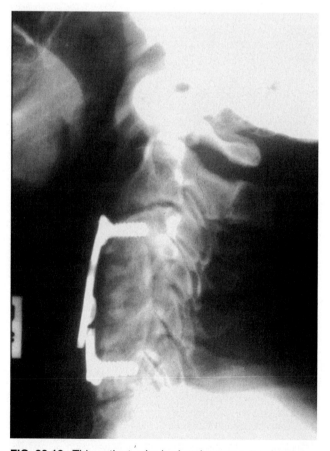

FIG. 83.13. This patient, who had undergone a two-level corpectomy 15 months previously, was noted to have recurrent neck and arm pain but no dysphagia. He underwent posterior revision for his nonunion. The anterior plate was left in place. (Photograph courtesy of Dr. Ian Farey, with permission.)

REFERENCES

1. Abraham D, Herkowitz H. Indications and trends in use in cervical spine fusions. *Orthop Clin North Am* 1998;29:731–744.
2. Ben-Debba M. Personal communication.
3. Wang JC, McDonough PW, Endow KK, et al. Increased fusion rates with cervical plating for two-level anterior cervical discectomy and fusion. *Spine* 2000;25:41–54.
4. Wang JC, McDonough PW, Endow KK, et al. The effect of cervical plating on single-level anterior cervical discectomy and fusion. *J Spinal Disord* 1999;12:467–471.
5. Aebi M, Mohler J, Zach GA, et al. Indications, surgical technique and results of 100 surgically-treated fractures and fracture-dislocations of the cervical spine. *Clin Orthop* 1986;203:244–257.

6. Aebi M, Zuber K, Marchesi D. Treatment of cervical spine injuries with anterior plating: indications, techniques, and results. *Spine* 1991 (Suppl);6:S30–S45.

7. Barros Filho TE, Oliviera RP, Grave JM, et al. corpectomy and anterior plating in cervical spine fractures with tetraplegia. *Rev Paul Med* 1993;111:375–377.

8. Bose B. Anterior cervical fusion using Caspar plating: analysis of results and review of the literature. *Surg Neurol* 1998;49:25–31.

9. Caspar W, Geisler FH, Pitzen T, et al. Anterior cervical plate stabilization in one- or two-level degenerative disease: overtreatment or benefit? *J Spinal Disord* 1998;11:1–11.

10. Castro FP Jr, Holt RT, Majd M, et al. A cost analysis of two anterior cervical fusion procedures. *J Spinal Disord* 2000;13:511–514.

11. Coe JD, Warden KE, Sutterlin CE, et al. Biomechanical evaluation of cervical spinal stabilization methods in a human cadaveric model. *Spine* 1989;14:1122–1131.

12. Connolly PF, Esses SI, Kostuik JP. Anterior cervical fusion: outcome analysis of patients fused with and without anterior cervical plates. *J Spinal Disord* 1996;9:202–206.

13. Garvey TA, Eismont FJ, Roberto LJ. Anterior decompression, structural bone grafting, and Caspar plate stabilization for unstable spine fractures and/or dislocations. *Spine* 1992;17(Suppl):431–435.

14. Goffin J, Plets C, van den Bergh R. Anterior cervical fusion and osteosynthetic stabilization according to Casper: a prospective study of 41 patients with fracture and/or dislocations of the cervical spine. *Neurosurg* 1989;25:865–871.

15. Goffin J, van Loon J, Van Calenbergh F, et al. Long-term results after anterior cervical fusion and osteosynthetic stabilization for fractures and/or dislocations of the cervical spine. *J Spinal Disord* 1995;8: 499–508.

16. Isomi T, Panjabi MM, Wang JL, et al. Stabilizing potential of anterior cervical plates in multilevel corpectomies. *Spine* 1999;24:2219–2223.

17. Kostuik JP, Connolly PJ, Esses SI, et al. Anterior cervical plate fixation with the titanium hollow screw plate system. *Spine* 1993;18: 1273–1278.

18. McCullen GM, Garfin SR. Spine update: cervical spine internal fixation using screw and screw-plate constructs. *Spine* 2000;25:643–652.

19. McLaughlin MR, Purighalla V, Pizzi FJ. Cost advantages of two-level anterior cervical fusion with rigid internal fixation for radiculopathy and degenerative disease. *Surg Neurol* 1997;48:560–565.

20. Papadopoulos SM. Anterior cervical instrumentation. *Clin Neurosurg* 1993;40:273–282.

21. Shapiro S. Banked fibula and the locking anterior cervical plate in anterior cervical fusions following cervical discectomy. *J Neurosurg* 1996;84:161–165.

22. Shapiro SA, Snyder W. Spinal instrumentation with a low complication rate. *Surg Neurol* 1997;48:566–574.

23. Vanichkachorn JS, Vaccaro AR, Silveri CP, et al. Anterior junctional plate in the cervical spine. *Spine* 1998;23:2462–2467.

24. Caspar W, Pitzen T, Papavero L, et al. Anterior cervical plating for the treatment of neoplasms in the cervical vertebrae. *J Neurosurg* 1999; 90(Suppl 1):27–34.

25. de Oliviera JC. Anterior plate fixation of traumatic lesions of the lower cervical spine. *Spine* 1987;12:324–329.

26. Shapiro S, Bindal R. Femoral ring allograft for anterior cervical interbody fusion: technical note. *Neurosurgery* 2000;47:1457–1459.

27. Boni M. Stabilization of cervical spine: problems and techniques. *J Neurosurg Sci* 1984;28:167–171.

28. Branch CL Jr. Anterior cervical fusion: the case for fusion without plating. *Clin Neurosurg* 1999;45:22–24 .

29. Bohler J, Gaudernak T. Anterior plate stabilization for fracture dislocation of the lower cervical spine. *J Trauma* 1980;20:203–205.

30. Bohler J. Sofort-und Fruhbehandlong traumatischer querschnitt lahmungen (German). *Zeitschr Orthopad Grenzgebiete* 1967;103:512–528.

31. Herrmann HD. Metal plate fixation after anterior cervical fusion for unstable fracture dislocations of the cervical spine. *Acta Neurochir (Wien)* 1975;32:101–111.

32. Orozco DR, Houet J. Osteosintesis en los traumaticos y degenerativos de la columna vertebral. *Traumotol Cirvjia Rehabil* 1971;1:45–52.

33. Caspar W, Barbier DD, Klara PM. Anterior cervical fusion and Caspar plate stabilization for cervical trauma. *Neurosurgery* 1989;25:491–502.

34. Caspar W, Pitzen T. Anterior cervical fusion and trapezoidal plate stabilization for re-do surgery. *Surg Neurol* 1999;52:345–351.

35. Bremer AM, Nguyen TQ. Internal metal plate fixation combined with anterior interbody fusion in cases of cervical spine injury. *Neurosurgery* 1983;12:649–653.

36. Gassman J, Seligson D. The anterior cervical plate. *Spine* 1983;8: 700–707.

37. Morscher E, Sutter F, Jennis M, et al. Die vordere verplattung der Halwirbel-saule meit dem Holschrauben-platten-system (German). *Der Chirurg* 1986;57:702–707.

38. Clausen JD, Ryken TC, Traynelis VC, et al. Biomechanical evaluation of Caspar and cervical spine locking plate systems in a cadaveric model. *J Neurosurg* 1997;84:1039–1045.

39. Grubb MR, Currier BL, Shih JS, et al. Biomechanical evaluation of anterior cervical spine stabilization. *Spine* 1998;15:886–892.

40. Richman JD, Daniel TE, Anderson DD, et al. Biomechanical evaluation of cervical spine stabilization methods using a porcine model. *Spine* 1995;20:2192–2197.

41. Suh PB, Kostuik JP, Esses SI. Anterior cervical plate fixation with the titanium hollow screw plate system. A preliminary report. *Spine* 1990; 15:1079–1081.

42. Hollowell JP, Reinarts J, Pintar FA, et al. Failure of Synthes anterior cervical fixation device by fracture of the Morscher screws. A biomechanical study. *J Spinal Disord* 1994;7:120–125.

43. Swank ML, Lowery GL, Bhat AL, et al. Anterior cervical allograft arthrodesis and instrumentation: multilevel interbody grafting or strut graft reconstruction. *Eur Spine J* 1997;6:138–143.

44. Heidecke V, Rainov NG, Burkert W. Anterior cervical fusion with the Orion locking plate system. *Spine* 1998;23:1796–1803.

45. Lettice JJ, Coe JD, Seago RL, et al. Subtotal corpectomy with autologous iliac strut graft fusion and anterior cervical plating for multilevel cervical disc disease. Paper presented at the Cervical Spine Research Society 25th annual meeting, December 1997, Rancho Mirage, CA.

46. Lowery GL, McDonough RF. The significance of hardware failure in anterior cervical plate fixation. Patients with 2- to 7-year follow-up. *Spine* 1998;23:181–186.

47. Majid ME, Vadhva M, Holt RT. Anterior cervical reconstruction using titanium cages with anterior plating. *Spine* 1999;24:1604–1610.

48. Vaccaro AR, Balderston RA. Anterior plate instrumentation for disorders of the subaxial cervical spine. *Clin Orthop* 1997;335:112–121.

49. Vaccaro AR, Falatyn ST, Scuderi GJ, et al. Early failure of long segment anterior cervical plate fixation. *J Spinal Disord* 1998;11:410–415.

50. Panjabi MM, Isomi T, Wang JL. Loosening at the screw-vertebra junction in multilevel anterior cervical plate constructs. *Spine* 1999;24: 2383–2388.

51. Epstein NE. The management of one level anterior cervical corpectomy with fusion using Atlantis hybrid plate: preliminary experience. *J Spinal Disord* 2000;13:324–328.

52. Zdeblick A, Herkowitz HN. Translational cervical plating: early clinical results. Paper presented at the Cervical Spine Research Society 29th annual meeting, November–December 2001, Monterey, CA.

53. Van Peteghem PK, Schweigel JF. The fractured cervical spine rendered unstable by anterior cervical fusion. *J Trauma* 1979;19:110–114.

54. Sutterlin CE 3rd, McAfee Pc, Warden KE, et al. A biomechanical evaluation of cervical spinal stabilization methods in a bovine model. Static and cyclical loading. *Spine* 1988;13:795–802.

55. Ulrich C, Arand M, Nothwang J. Internal fixation on the lower cervical spine—biomechanics and clinical practice of procedures and implants. *Eur Spine J* 2001;10:88–100.

56. Montesano PX, Juach EC, Anderson PA, et al. Biomechanics of cervical spine internal fixation. *Spine* 1991;16:S10–S16.

57. Ripa DR, Kowall MG, Meyer PR Jr, et al. Series of ninety-two traumatic cervical spine injuries stabilized with anterior ASIF plate fusion technique. *Spine* 1991;16:S46–S55.

58. Tippets RH, Apfelbaum RI. Anterior cervical fusion with the Caspar instrumentation system. *Neurosurg* 1988;22:1008–1013.

59. Schulte K, Clark C, Goel V. Kinematics of the cervical spine following discectomy and stabilization. *Spine* 1989;14:1116–1121.

60. Spivak JM, Chen D, Kummer FJ. The effect of locking fixation screws on the stability of anterior cervical plating. *Spine* 1999;15:334–338.

61. Chen IH. Biomechanical evaluation of subcortical versus bicortical screw purchase in anterior cervical plating. *Acta Neurochir (Wien)* 1996;138:167–173.

62. Zdeblick TA, Cooke ME, Wilson D, et al. Anterior cervical discectomy, fusion, and plating. A comparative animal study. *Spine* 1993;18: 1974–1983.

63. Baldwin NG, Hartman GP, Weiser MW, et al. Failure of titanium anterior cervical plate implant: microstructural analysis of failure. Case report. *J Neurosurg* 1995;83:741–743.

64. DiAngelo DJ, Foley KT, Vossel KA, et al. Anterior cervical plating reverses load transfer through multilevel strut-grafts. *Spine* 2000;25: 783–795.

65. Foley KT, DiAngelo DJ, Rampersaud YR, et al. The *in vitro* effects of instrumentation on multilevel cervical strut-grafts mechanics. *Spine* 1999;24:2366–2376.

66. Kirkpatrick JS, Levy JA, Carillo J, et al. Reconstruction after multilevel corpectomy in the cervical spine. A sagittal plane biomechanical study. *Spine* 1999;24:1186–1191.

67. Wang JL, Panjabi MM, Isomi T. The role of bone graft force in stabilizing the multilevel anterior cervical spine plate system. *Spine* 2000; 25:1649–1654.

68. DiAngelo DJ, Foley KT, Liu W, et al. Biomechanical testing of a translational anterior cervical plate with a constrained anterior cervical plate. Paper presented at the Cervical Spine Research Society 29th annual meeting, November–December 2001, Monterey, CA.

69. Vaccaro AR. Point of view. *Spine* 1998,23:186–187.

70. Bolesta MJ, Rechtine DR 2nd, Chrin AM. Three- and four-level anterior cervical discectomy and fusion with plate fixation: a prospective study. *Spine* 2000;25:2040–2056.

71. Ebraheim NA, DeTroye RJ, Rupp RE, et al. Osteosynthesis of the cervical spine with an anterior plate. *Orthop* 1995;18:141–147.

72. Brown JA, Havel P, Ebraheim N, et al. Cervical stabilization by plate and bone fusion. *Spine* 1988;13:236–240.

73. Cabanela CA, Ebersold MJ. Anterior plate stabilization for bursting teardrop fractures of the cervical spine. *Spine* 1988;13:888–891.

74. Eleraky MA, Llanos C, Sonntag VK. Cervical corpectomy: report of 185 cases and review of the literature. *J Neurosurg* 1999;90:35–41.

75. Herman JM, Sonntag VK. Cervical corpectomy and plate fixation for postlaminectomy kyphosis. *J Neurosurg* 1994;80:963–970.

76. Jonsson H Jr, Cesarini K, Petren-Mallmin M, et al. Locking screw-plate fixation of cervical spine fractures with and without ancillary posterior plating. *Arch Orthop Trauma Surg* 1991;111:1–12.

77. Kraus DR, Stauffer ES. Spinal cord injury as a complication of elective anterior cervical fusion. *Clin Orthop* 1975;112:130–141.

78. Mann DC, Bruner BW, Keene JS, et al. Anterior plating of unstable cervical spine fractures. *Paraplegia* 1990;28:564–572.

79. Martin-Harris B. Personal communication.

80. Paramore CG, Dickman CA, Sonntag VK. Radiologic and clinical follow-up review of Caspar plates in 49 patients. *J Neurosurg* 1996; 84:957–961.

81. Razack N, Green BA, Levi AD. The management of traumatic cervical bilateral facet fracture-dislocations with unicortical anterior plates. *J Spinal Disord* 2000;13:374–381.

82. Rezai AR, Woo HH, Errico TJ, et al. Contemporary management of spinal osteomyelitis. *Neurosurgery* 1999;44:1018–1026.

83. Samandouras G, Shafafy M, Hamlyn PJ. A new anterior cervical instrumentation system combining an intradiskal cage with an integrated plate: an early technical report. *Spine* 2001;26:1188–1192.

84. Segal H. Anterior plate failure. *J Neurosurg* 1996;84:537–538.

85. Shapiro S, Connolly P, Donnaldson J, et al. Cadaveric fibula, locking plate, and allogeneic bone matrix for anterior cervical fusions after cervical discectomy for radiculopathy or myelopathy. *J Neurosurg* 2001; 95(Suppl 1):43–50.

86. Smith MD, Bolesta MI. Esophageal perforation after anterior cervical plate fixation. A report of two cases. *J Spinal Disord* 1992;5:357.

87. Tominaga T, Koshuy K, Mizoi D, et al. Anterior cervical fixation with the titanium locking screw-plate: a preliminary report. *Surg Neurol* 1994;42:408–413.

88. Tribus CB, Corteen DP, Zdeblick TA. The efficacy of anterior cervical plating in the management of symptomatic pseudoarthrosis of the cervical spine. *Spine* 1999;24:860–864.

89. Tuite GF, Papadopoulos SM, Sonntag VK. Caspar plate fixation for the treatment of complex hangman's fractures. *Neurosurgery* 1992;30: 761–764.

90. Lesoin F, Cama A, Lozes G, et al. The anterior approach and plates in lower cervical post traumatic lesions. *Surg Neurol* 1984;21: 581–587.

91. Brockmeyer D, Apfelbaum R, Tippets R, et al. Pediatric cervical spine instrumentation using screw fixation. *Ped Neurosurg* 1995;22:147–157.

92. Katsuura A, Hukuda S, Imanada T, et al. Anterior cervical plate used in degenerative disease can maintain cervical lordosis. *J Spinal Disord* 1996;9:470–476.

93. Coric D, Branch CL Jr, Jenkins D. Revision of anterior cervical pseudoarthrosis with anterior allograft fusion and plating. *J Neurosurg* 1997;86:969–974.

94. Geisler FH, Caspar W, Pitzen T, et al. Reoperation in patients after anterior cervical plate stabilization in degenerative disease. *Spine* 1998;23:911–920.

95. Bose B. Anterior cervical instrumentation enhances fusion rates in multilevel reconstruction in smokers. *J Spinal Disord* 2001;14:1–9.

96. Boockvar JA, Philips MF, Telfeian AE, et al. Results and risk factors for anterior cervicothoracic junction surgery. *J Neurosurg* 2001;94 (Suppl 1):12–17.

97. Riew KD, Sethi NS, Devney J, et al. Complications of buttress plate stabilization of cervical corpectomy. *Spine* 1999;24:2404–2410.

98. McAfee PC, Bohlman HH, Ducker TB, et al. One-stage anterior cervical decompression and posterior stabilization. A study of one hundred patients with a minimum of two years of follow-up. *J Bone Joint Surg Am* 1995;77:1791–1800.

99. Schultz KD Jr, McLaughlin MR, Haid RW Jr, et al. Single-stage anterior-posterior decompression and stabilization for complex cervical spine disorders. *J Neurosurg* 2000;93:214–221.

100. Epstein NE. The value of anterior cervical plating in preventing vertebral fracture and graft extrusion after multilevel anterior cervical corpectomy with posterior wiring and fusion: indications, results, and complications. *J Spinal Disord* 2000;13:9–15.

101. Apfelbaum RI, Dailey AT, Barbera J. Clinical experience with a new load-sharing anterior cervical plate. Paper presented at the Cervical Spine Research Society 27th annual meeting, November–December 1999, Seattle, WA.

102. Epstein NE. Graft and plate failures following circumferential cervical surgery in 80 patients. Paper presented at the Cervical Spine Research Society 29th annual meeting, November–December 2001, Monterey, CA.

103. Cloward RB. Complications of anterior cervical disc operation and their treatment. *Surgery* 1971;69:175–182.

104. Graham JA. Complications of cervical spine surgery. *Spine* 1989;14: 1046–1050.

105. Tew JM Jr, Mayfield FH. Complications of surgery of the anterior cervical spine. *Clin Neurosurg* 1976;23:424–434.

106. Zeidman SM, Ducker TB, Raycroft J. Trends and complications in cervical spine surgery: 1989–1993. *J Spinal Disord* 1997;10:523–526.

107. Winslow CP, Winslow TJ, Wax MK. Dysphonia and dysphagia following the anterior approach to the cervical spine. *Arch Otolaryngol Head Neck Surg* 2001;127:51–55.

108. Bazaz R, Yoo JU. Incidence of dysphagia following anterior cervical spine surgery. Paper presented at the Cervical Spine Research Society 29th annual meeting, November–December 2001, Monterey, CA.

109. Donnelly RE, O'Brien MF, Dart D, et al. Dysphagia after multilevel cervical arthrodesis: a clinical and cineradiographic evaluation. Paper presented at the Cervical Spine Research Society 29th annual meeting, November–December, 2001, Monterey, CA.

110. Hanci M, Toprok M, Sarioglu AC, et al. Oesophageal perforation subsequent to anterior cervical spine screw/plate fixation. *Paraplegia* 1995;33:606–609.

111. Gaudinez RF, English GM, Gebhard JS, et al. Esophageal perforations after anterior cervical surgery. *J Spinal Disord* 2000;13: 77–84.

112. Kelly MF, Spiegel J, Rizzo KA, et al. Delayed pharyngoesophageal perforation: a complication of anterior spine surgery. *Ann Otol Rhinol Laryngol* 1991;100:201–205.

113. Van Berge Henegouwen DP, Roukema JA, et al. Esophageal perforation during surgery on the cervical spine. *Neurosurgery* 1991;29: 766.

114. Whitehill R, Sirna EC, Young DC, et al. Late esophageal perforation from an autogenous bone graft. *J Bone Joint Surg Am* 1985;67: 644.

115. Newhouse KE, Lindsey RW, Clark CT, et al. Esophageal perforation following anterior cervical spine surgery. *Spine* 1989;14:1051–1053.

116. Fujibayashi S, Shikata J, Kamiya N, et al. Missing anterior cervical plate and screws. *Spine* 2000;25:2258–2261.

117. Geyer TE, Foy MA. Oral extrusion of a screw after anterior cervical spine plating. *Spine* 2001;26:1814–1816.
118. Schweighofer F, Passler JM, Wildburger R, et al. Interbody fusion of the lower cervical spine: a dangerous surgical method? *Langenbecks Arch Chir* 1992;377:295–299.
119. Smith, MD, Emery SE, Dudley A, et al. Vertebral artery injury during anterior decompression of the cervical spine. A retrospective review of ten patients. *J Bone Joint Surg Br* 1993;75:410–415.
120. Curylo LJ, Mason HC, Bohlman HH, et al. Tortuous course of the vertebral artery and anterior cervical decompression: a cadaveric and clinical case study. *Spine* 2000;25:2860–2864.
121. Beutler WJ, Sweeney CA, Connolly PJ. Recurrent laryngeal nerve injury with anterior cervical spine surgery risk with laterality of surgical approach. *Spine* 2001;26:1337–1342
122. Apfelbaum RI, Kriskovich MD, Haller JR. On the incidence, cause, and prevention of recurrent laryngeal nerve palsies during anterior cervical spine surgery. *Spine* 2000;25:2906–2912.
123. Epstein NE, Hollingworth R, Nardi D, et al. Can airway complications following multilevel anterior cervical surgery be avoided? *J Neurosurg* 2001;94(Suppl 2):185–188.
124. Harris OA, Runnels JB, Matz PG. Clinical factors associated with unexpected critical care management and prolonged hospitalization after elective cervical spine surgery. *Crit Care Med* 2001;29:1989–1902.
125. Riew KD, Won DS, DellaRocca GJ, et al. Parameters for maintaining intubation postoperative following anterior cervical procedures. Paper presented at the Cervical Spine Research Society 29th annual meeting, November–December 2001, Monterey, CA.
126. Fujibayashi S, Shikata J, Yoshitomi H, et al. Bilateral phrenic nerve palsy as a complication of anterior decompression and fusion for cervical ossification of the posterior longitudinal ligament. *Spine* 2001;26:E281–E286.
127. Kitchel SH, Eismont FJ, Green BA. Closed subarachnoid drainage for management of cerebrospinal fluid leakage after an operation on the spine. *J Bone Joint Surg Am* 1989;71:984–987.
128. Seifert V, Stolke D. Multisegmental cervical spondylosis: treatment by spondylectomy, microsurgical decompression, and osteosynthesis. *J Neurosurg* 1991;29:498–503.
129. Northrup BE, Vaccaro AR, Rosen JE, et al. Occurrence of infection in anterior cervical fusion for spinal cord injury after tracheostomy. *Spine* 1995;20:2449–2453.
130. Bracken MB, Shepard MJ, Collins WF, et al. A randomized, controlled trial of methylprednisolone or naloxone in the treatment of spinal-cord injury. Results of the second National Acute Spinal Cord Injury Study. *N Engl J Med* 1990;322:1405–1411.
131. Saunders RL. On the pathogenesis of the radiculopathy complicating multilevel corpectomy. *Neurosurgery* 1995;37:408–412.
132. Goffin J, Geusens E, Vantomme N, et al. Long-term follow-up after interbody fusion of the cervical spine. Paper presented at the Cervical Spine Research Society 28th annual meeting, November 2000, Charleston, SC.
133. Katsuura A, Hukuda S, Saruhashi Y, et al. Kyphotic malalignment after anterior cervical fusion is one of the factors promoting the degenerative process in adjacent intervertebral levels. *Eur Spine J* 2001;10:320–324.
134. Zaveri GR, Ford M. Cervical spondylosis: the role of anterior instrumentation after decompression and fusion. *J Spinal Disord* 2001;14:10–16.
135. Hacker RJ. A randomized prospective study of an anterior cervical interbody fusion device with a minimum of 2 years of follow-up results. *J Neurosurg* 2000;93(Suppl 2):222–226.
136. Whitecloud TS III, Ricciardi JE, Werner JG Jr. Bone graft, hardware, and halo fixator-related complications. In: Clark CR, et al., eds. *The cervical spine*, 3rd ed. Philadelphia: Lippincott–Raven, 1998:903–921.
137. Goffin J, Kehr P, Lind B, et al. Early clinical experience with the Bryan cervical disk prosthesis in single-level patients. Paper presented at the Cervical Spine Research Society 29th annual meeting, November–December 2001, Monterey, CA.
138. Randle MJ, Wolf A, Levi L, et al. The use of anterior Caspar plate fixation in acute cervical spine injury. *Surg Neurol* 1991;36:181–189.
139. Johnston FG, Crockard HA. One-stage internal fixation and anterior fusion in complex cervical spinal disorders. *J Neurosurg* 1995;82:234–238.
140. Schneeberger AG, Boos N, Schwarzenbach O, et al. Anterior cervical interbody fusion with plate fixation for chronic spondylitic radiculopathy: a 2- to 8-year follow-up. *J Spinal Disord* 1999;12:215–220.
141. Lifeso RM, Colucci MA. Anterior fusion for rotationally unstable cervical spine fractures. *Spine* 2000;25:2028–2034.
142. Thalgott JS, Fritts K, Guiffre JM, et al. Anterior interbody fusion of the cervical spine with coralline hydroxyapatite. *Spine* 1999;24:1295–1299.

CHAPTER 84

Postoperative Infection

Christopher M. Bono, Christopher P. Kauffman, and Steven R. Garfin

Despite the use of perioperative antibiotics and improved surgical technique, infection remains one of the most disconcerting complications of cervical spine surgery. Generally less frequent than after lumbar surgery, postoperative neck infections continue to occur with a definite, albeit low, prevalence (1,2). Various factors influence the development of infection, including choice of surgical approach (3), nutritional and immune status of the patient (4–6), use of surgical implants such as instrumentation or methylmethacrylate (7–9), and the meticulousness of surgical technique with early recognition of intraoperative iatrogenic injuries such as esophageal tears (10,11). Although prevention is optimal, attentive clinical examination with judicious use of laboratory and imaging modalities is crucial to early diagnosis. Although nonoperative measures may have a role in the management of some infections, surgical débridement along with culture-specific antibiotics remains the accepted treatment for more serious cases.

PREVALENCE

The rate of infection after cervical spine surgery has varied between 0% and 18% (10,12–20). Overall infection rates for anterior and posterior surgery are probably comparable, although most spine surgeons perceive the posterior approach to be more prone to infection (3). Some reported rates for posterior surgery are as high as 15% to 18%. Many of these series represent patients who are immunocompromised, such as those with rheumatoid arthritis or Down syndrome, in whom posterior surgery is more commonly performed (4,13).

The standard anterior approach to the cervical spine has resulted in infection in between 1% and 3% of cases (12, 15,16,21). Most surgeons attribute this to a relatively atraumatic dissection and clear tissue planes compared with posterior surgery. The transoral approach to the upper cervical spine, by necessity, crosses a grossly contaminated region of

the nasopharynx. Early reports indicated infection rates as high as 66% (22). With more meticulous surgical technique, watertight closures, and specific antibiotic prophylaxis, more recent series have documented more encouraging results (21, 23). A more in-depth discussion of the influence of surgical approaches is presented later in this chapter.

RISK FACTORS FOR INFECTION

As with any surgical procedure, there are numerous influences on the development of postoperative infection. Some of these are intrinsic to the patient, whereas others are more dependent on the surgeon, technique, and choice of implants.

Intrinsic Factors

Systemic Disorders

Wimmer and associates (24) detected substantially higher infection rates in patients with diabetes, obesity, a history of smoking, or a history of alcohol abuse. Diabetics are a high-risk group (24,25). Attention to preoperative glucose levels is crucial, because uncontrolled disease may increase the infection risk; this warrants a delay for elective procedures (24).

Cervical spine surgery is commonly performed in patients with rheumatoid arthritis (6,13,26). These patients may be at increased risk due to prolonged chemotherapeutic treatment as well as general systemic illness. Many are on long-term steroid regimens, which in itself is a known risk factor (24). Clark and associates (26) reviewed the results of posterior cervical arthrodesis in 41 patients with rheumatoid arthritis. Three (7.3%) developed a superficial wound infection, with no reports of deep infection or osteomyelitis. Interestingly, the authors successfully managed

1170

these complications with antibiotics alone without surgical debridement.

Genetic and congenital disorders are believed to increase the infection risk (4,19). Infections in this population can be devastating. Segal and colleagues (19) studied a series of 10 patients with Down syndrome who underwent posterior arthrodesis for atlantoaxial instability. The overall complication rate was high, with infection at either the wound or halo pin sites in 3 patients (30%). Multiple wound debridements were necessary for eradication of the infected wounds. In a series of 15 Down's syndrome patients, Doyle and associates (4) observed one case each of wound infection and dehiscence. The wound infection resolved after surgical debridement.

After Organ Transplantation

The advancement of solid organ transplant technology has led to an increase in the number of these life-saving procedures being performed. Patients are living longer and with a greater quality of life, so their demands for elective surgery, such as total joint arthroplasty, are expected to increase. A major concern is the increased risk for infection (27,28). Chronic immunosuppression is no longer a contraindication to elective surgery (27). Few reports of spine surgery in renal transplant recipients exist. Dunn and Aiona (27) documented successful operative treatment of scoliosis in a renal allograft recipient. The patient healed her wounds with no signs of infection. When operating on a posttransplantation individual, the surgeon must keep in mind that skin, integument, and soft tissues may be thin and attenuated from chronic corticosteroid therapy. Modifications of prophylactic antibiotic regimens to include more broad-spectrum coverage should also be considered, especially for those on renal dialysis. These individuals may be especially prone to infection due to *Pseudomonas aeruginosa*.

Human Immunodeficiency Virus and Acquired Immunodeficiency Syndrome

The population of patients infected with human immunodeficiency virus (HIV) continues to rise worldwide. As a result, an increasing number of these individuals will undergo both elective and emergent surgery (29). Although not specifically addressed in the spine literature, surgery in this population may result in higher infection rates than the general population (29). It behooves surgeons to be familiar with the pertinent values used to gauge the degree of immunocompromise. One such value is the helper T-cell count, more popularly referred to as the CD4 count. It is currently believed that patients with values greater than 600 to 700 are at no greater risk for infectious complications than HIV-negative subjects, while those with 200 or less have a significantly higher risk (29). Although some operations in those with a CD4 count of less than 200 are emergent, elective

cases in such patients might benefit from delay until the immune system is more fortified. As the population of HIV-positive individuals remains healthier for longer periods of time as a result of improvements in treatment and prophylaxis, these issues become more relevant to spinal surgeons who perform elective cervical operations.

Extrinsic Factors

There are various "controllable" risk factors for infection after cervical spine surgery. These are related to surgical approach, technique, implants, antibiosis, nutrition, and postoperative care.

Surgical Approach

The relative rates of infection after anterior versus posterior surgery are probably comparable, despite differences in some reported series. Each approach has unique features that must be recognized in order to avoid infection.

The anterior cervical approach is used for a variety of diagnoses, including traumatic, degenerative, and congenital disorders. Perhaps the most common indication is degenerative disc disease with or without associated neurologic deficit. In these cases, the infection rate is typically low. In a series of 253 patients who underwent anterior disc surgery, Lunsford and colleagues (16) reported an overall rate of 1%. The highest rate was after arthrodesis for a "hard" disc herniation (8%). Bohlman and associates (12) reported no postoperative infections in 122 patients after anterior cervical discectomy and fusion, whereas Bertalanffy and Eggert (1) documented 8 infections (1.6%) in 450 cases of discectomy without arthrodesis.

Cervical surgery is often necessary in a patient with a tracheostomy. Because of the proximity of the surgical wound to the tracheostomy site, it is thought that there is an increased risk for wound infection. Northrup and associates (30) examined this question in a retrospective series of 11 patients undergoing an anterior cervical approach following a tracheostomy that had been made an average of 27 days before the anterior cervical surgery. With follow-up ranging from 6 to 51 months, no case of wound infection was documented. Of note, the authors had studied a select group of patients with cervical cord damage resulting from blunt injury.

In the standard anterior approach to the cervical spine, surgical dissection proceeds through a clear plane between the esophagus and carotid sheath. Although vascular penetration is alarmingly detected at the time of surgery, esophageal injury offers a less dramatic sentinel (31). In addition to making an effort to avoid perforating this structure, it should be carefully inspected in all cases before closure of the wound. Early detection and repair of a tear can dramatically reduce the risk of infection (11). Van Berge Hengouwen and associates (11) described three cases of esophageal perforation during anterior cervical surgery for elective discectomy and fusion. In two cases, infection was avoided by repair within 6 hours of the initial surgery. In a third case, the esophageal tear was diagnosed 4 days after the initial surgery, resulting in a deep abscess, local tissue necrosis, and a 55-day hospital stay. In a survey of the Cervical Spine Research Society, Newhouse and associates (32) studied a series of 22 cases of esophageal tears. Six were recognized intraoperatively and repaired without further complication, and 6 were detected and treated within the first postoperative week. The remaining cases were delayed weeks to years and required repeat surgery and prolonged hospital stays. Predisposing factors for esophageal perforation included the use of surgical instrumentation, polymethylmethacrylate, sharp bone edges, graft extrusion, scar tissue, and radiation treatment. Fuji and colleagues (31) diagnosed an esophagocutaneous fistula 3 months after anterior corpectomy and strut grafting and attributed this complication to a missed esophageal tear at the time of the index procedure. Upon exploration of the wound, a hole in the posterior esophagus directly communicated with the bone graft. Effective management included debridement, irrigation, repair of the tear, and interposition of the sternocleidomastoid muscle as a flap between the esophagus and the anterior cervical spine. Nonoperative treatment, including placement of a feeding tube and prolonged intravenous antibiotic therapy, has also been used (32). In the authors' opinion, this is an option only in those patients who remain too unstable to return to the operating room. Injection of indigo carmine through a nasogastric tube may help detect an occult tear prior to closure. If infection occurs, esophagoscopy should be considered preoperatively to help localize the site.

The transoral approach to the upper cervical spine is not commonly performed because the technique crosses a grossly contaminated region of the oropharyngeal pathway. Documented infection rates after this approach have varied. Early in its development, Fang and Ong (22) reported a wound infection in four of six patients in whom they utilized this approach. More recent, larger series have documented rates between 0% and 3% (21,23), similar to other cervical approaches. Specific antibiotic prophylaxis, multilayer closure, and avoidance of surgical implants may be responsible for these improved results.

In comparison to the clean surgical planes of the anterior approach, the posterior approach to the cervical spine, as in the thoracolumbar spine, is a muscle stripping procedure that can devascularize large areas of musculotendinous tissue. Judicious debridement of obviously devitalized areas might decrease the likelihood of secondary contamination within necrotic regions; however, this is rarely actually performed because of concern of inadequate bony coverage and increased bleeding. As discussed, many series of posterior surgery include patients who are systemically compromised. This may account for the relatively higher infection rates documented for posterior versus anterior cervical surgery. In series of uncompromised patients, however, the prevalence is comparable. In one report of 20 cases of cer-

vical fractures treated by posterior stabilization with plates and screws, 1 (5%) case of infection was documented (14). Wellman and co-workers (2) documented a 5% prevalence of wound infection after lateral mass plating for a variety of diagnoses. Treatment with surgical debridement and intravenous antibiotics was successful in these cases without removal of the implants. The rate of infection in children may be lower. McGrory and associates (33) reported no infections (0%) after posterior arthrodesis for cervical trauma in children aged 1 to 15 years.

Surgical Technique

Although surgical contamination is theoretically preventable, it remains a common source of infection during elective surgery. Strict adherence to sound principles of scrubbing, gowning, draping, and surgical field preparation is important. Traffic in and out of the room should be kept to a minimum. Self-retaining retractors should be periodically removed or released, and the wound irrigated with copious amounts of saline. Meticulous hemostasis with either electrocautery or pharmacologic agents (thrombin-soaked Gel-Foam, Surgicel, Avitene) minimizes the chance of hematoma formation and secondary bacterial seeding. If this cannot be ensured, a temporary closed suction drain system should be considered. This may be removed between 24 to 48 hours after surgery. Drains indwelling for longer periods may act as a route of secondary bacterial contamination.

Implants

In an extensive review of the literature, the authors could find no prospective study comparing infection rates in instrumented versus noninstrumented cases. However, reported rates appear to be slightly higher with the use of metallic implants (2,14). As a foreign body, indwelling instrumentation can cause a persistent subacute inflammatory reaction (34). In addition, use of instrumentation systems can increase operative time, especially if the surgeon is unfamiliar with its application. Undue length of procedure should be avoided, as this may increase the risk of infection (24).

Some authors believe that the use of polymethylmethacrylate (PMMA) might be a risk factor (3). This may be partially attributed to its more common use in systemically compromised patients with cancer, rheumatoid arthritis, and osteoporotic bone. In an early series, Bryan and associates (13) reported two wound infections in 11 patients treated with a PMMA-augmented posterior arthrodesis for instability secondary to rheumatoid arthritis. In one case the wound could not be closed until a layer of bone cement had been removed. It appears that this may have been an issue of an amount of cement that placed the skin closure under tension. Regardless, the infection rate was relatively high, although it is unclear if the predisposing factor was the cement or the immunocompromised state of the patient population. In contrast, a number of series have documented a 2% to 3% rate of infection with the use of PMMA when used to stabilize acute cervical trauma in otherwise healthy individuals (7,8). Branch and colleagues (7) diagnosed three infections in 99 cases of lower cervical fractures instrumented with wires and PMMA. Likewise, Duff and associates (8) reported only one infection in 52 cases of treated fractures. These fractures were fixed through a posterior approach, making definite conclusions regarding the influence of PMMA itself on the prevalence of infection difficult to draw.

Nutrition

The role of nutrition on the postoperative infection rate after spine surgery has been well established. Stambough and Beringer (35) noted that 16 of 19 patients with deep wound infections after spine surgery were malnourished. Clinical indicators of malnutrition were a total lymphocyte count of less than 2,000 cells/mm³ or a serum albumin level of less than 3.5 g/dL. Similar findings were documented by Jevesar and Karlin (36) in patients with cerebral palsy. Staged anterior and posterior procedures are frequently performed in the cervical spine. There are data indicating that a sufficient period of time between procedures should be allowed in order for the nutritional status of the patient to rebound (37,38).

Prophylactic Antibiotics

As recently as the mid-1980s, routine antimicrobial prophylaxis was not universally supported. In 1984, Mader and Cierny (39) believed it was "indicated only under specific surgical settings." Administration of preincision prophylactic antibiotics is currently accepted as routine (40,41). Maximal effectiveness is obtained if administered before incision and continued for 24 to 48 hours postoperatively (42). In a retrospective study of 531 cases of lumbar disc surgery, Horowitz and Curtin (42) found an infection rate of 1% in those receiving antibiotics versus 9.3% in those who did not receive prophylaxis. Furthermore, patients who received both preincision and postoperative therapy had an infection rate of 0.6%, whereas those who were given only postoperative antibiotics had a 2.7% rate of infection. Similarly, Keller and Pappas (43) documented a decrease from 2.7% to 0% with the use of perioperative prophylactic antibiotics. Although these were not randomized, prospective investigations, they offer compelling evidence of the value of routine preincisional antibiotic prophylaxis. In both series, however, various antibiotics were used. Despite a lack of similar studies in cervical spine surgery, the authors strongly encourage this practice.

The most commonly used agents in cervical spine surgery are cephalosporins because of their excellent coverage of typical gram-positive skin contaminants (*Staphylococcus aureus, Staphylococcus epidermidis*). With a reported 10%

concordance with penicillin allergy, cephalosporins may be relatively contraindicated in some allergic patients. Alternative coverage should be considered, such as clindamycin or vancomycin. Clindamycin has excellent bone penetration, but is only bacteriostatic. Vancomycin offers excellent coverage of skin flora contaminants, but is more expensive and must be carefully followed with serial laboratory evaluation of blood levels to ensure therapeutic levels. However, this is less a factor for perioperative use than when used for long-term treatment.

Perioperative antibiotics should not be used in treating an existing spinal infection for which definitive culture and sensitivity information is not yet available. In these circumstances, infusion of the agent should be delayed until an adequate open biopsy of the lesion has been obtained in the operating room. Other situations in which prophylactic antibiotics might be delayed, or excluded, are for patients in whom the potential toxicity of available agents would outweigh the risks of its use (for example, vancomycin with renal insufficiency). Fortunately, these situations are rare.

The routine use of cephalosporins alone must be contemplated in each surgical case. In some scenarios, concomitant infectious risks may warrant additional agents. For example, intraoperative esophageal perforation could introduce gram-negative organisms into the wound. Thus, coverage must be tailored for each situation. However, routine use of broad-spectrum medications is contraindicated, because this practice fosters the emergence of resistant bacterial strains. Patients undergoing a transoral exposure should receive prophylaxis with agents such as nafcillin for gram-negative oral flora (23).

Postoperative Care

In addition to careful wound management and sterile dressing changes, distant sites of contamination should be eliminated. Indwelling Foley catheters should be removed 1 to 2 days postoperatively. In the spinal cord–injured or bed-bound patient, decubitus precautions can minimize breakdown and hematogenous seeding through the ulcer. Oral alimentation should be initiated when safe. Until then, tube feeding through a nasogastric or percutaneous endogastric site should be used, because enteral feedings decrease bacterial translocation into the blood through the gut. If this is not possible, nutritional support through parenteral alimentation should be considered (44). Wound healing is improved if the absolute lymphocyte count is maintained above 1,500 cells/mm³ and albumin concentration is at least 3.5 g/dL (5).

CLASSIFICATION

Classification of cervical spinal wound infections is not frequently discussed (45). The authors present this discussion to help the reader organize various "descriptors" of the infection. In doing so, a sense of outcome and management may help better guide the practitioner.

Superficial

There is no clear definition of superficial wound infection. It is reasonable, however, to state that it involves the more superficial layers of fascia, including the epidermis, dermis, and overlying muscle fascia. Such infections can present with increasing erythema, pain, and discharge. It is difficult to discern a superficial from deep wound infection without exploration. Typically, a superficial infection presents 3 to 4 days postoperatively.

Deep

A deep wound infection extends past the layer of the dermis and involves the muscle and its underlying compartments. A deep infection directly communicates with the instrumentation, bone, and exposed neural elements. Pus can be loculated in compartments. Thorough surgical inspection is necessary. Although it may be associated with osteomyelitis, bone infection is not a necessary component of a deep wound infection, particularly if treated early. Presentation is usually between 7 to 14 days postoperatively, but may be longer.

Osteomyelitis (Deeper)

The bony components of the vertebrae can eventually be contaminated by a deep wound infection. This, however, rarely occurs. Alternatively, contamination of the bone hematogenously, lymphatically, or at the time of surgery can occur. Postoperative osteomyelitis requires ablative treatment including removal of all devitalized bone back to a bleeding surface.

Abscess

A collection of pus can develop within any part of a surgical wound. An abscess does not communicate with the outer incision and is not self-decompressing. Most concerning is an abscess that forms within the epidural space. Direct spinal compression can occur, resulting in neurologic compromise. A high index of suspicion for a deep spinal abscess must be maintained, because this form of postoperative infection yields the least external wound manifestations.

Necrotizing

Particular organisms such as group A streptococci can lead to necrotizing fascial infections. This entity causes quick and expansive regions of tissue death. Involvement of the muscle is more likely with *Clostridia* species. Sometimes, aerobic and anaerobic organism act in con-

cert to form a synergistic necrotizing infection. Although an exceedingly rare complication, such a case has been documented after spinal surgery (46). Necrotizing wound infections are surgical emergencies because they are life-threatening conditions.

Discitis

Discitis is a low-grade infection of the disc space that typically occurs following cervical discectomy, corpectomy, or discograms. This is perhaps the most benign of postoperative spinal infections, with highly effective conservative treatment and a generally good prognosis. The usual offending organisms are *S. aureus* and *S. epidermidis*.

DIAGNOSIS

History and Physical Examination

In the immediate postsurgical period, it is sometimes difficult to discern complaints related to an infection from those usual in the postoperative period. Varying degrees of pain occur at the surgical site after cervical surgery. Pain that is progressively increasing, especially in the area of the wound, is an important alerting feature. Night sweats, in addition to general malaise, can also indicate a brewing infection.

As stated previously, drains should usually be removed 1 to 2 days after surgery. After the initial dressing change, the wound should be covered daily until all drainage has stopped. Suspicious wound drainage is cloudy, puslike, or foul smelling. Wound edges are normally erythematous after surgery. With suspicion of a wound infection, the rim of erythema should be marked daily. If this edge is advancing away from the incision line, a wound infection may be developing. Fluctuance can indicate hematoma or an infectious collection. Typically, a sterile hematoma is not associated with increased pain or rubor. However, a persistent hematoma can become secondarily seeded with bacteria. Gross pus that is expressible from the wound edge is incontrovertible evidence of infection. Fluid cultures should be obtained carefully so as to avoid contamination from normal skin flora. Unfortunately, they often merge.

Fevers may be low grade. Temperature spikes, either at home or in the hospital, after surgery are a red flag. In the first 2 to 3 days after surgery, fevers are most likely related to poor pulmonary clearance and atelectasis. However, fevers after this point should be regarded more seriously.

Laboratory Tests

Blood cultures should be drawn at the peak of temperature spikes. Additional workup includes a complete blood count with differential, erythrocyte sedimentation rate (ESR), and C-reactive protein (CRP) levels. Leukocyte elevation with a definite shift toward polymorphonuclear cells is an indication of postoperative infection. Although the ESR is elevated immediately after surgery, it peaks by 4 days and usually returns to normal levels by 14 days (47). At 2 weeks, values should be less than 30, and at 6 weeks the ESR should be less than 20. A rising ESR after the fourth postoperative day is highly suggestive of an infectious process. CRP levels usually peak on postoperative day 2 and quickly return to preoperative levels. Infection can cause a persistently elevated CRP, or a second peak after surgery.

ESR and CRP levels may be persistently elevated in the presence of metallic hardware. In a prospective investigation, Takahashi and associates (34) demonstrated that CRP levels peaked on postoperative day 2 in both instrumented and noninstrumented cases. Although these levels returned to preoperative levels by 4 weeks in noninstrumented patients, those in instrumented patients remained elevated for more than 6 weeks. ESR levels peaked on day 4 in the non-instrumented group and day 11 in the instrumented group. Similarly, the ESR remained elevated substantially longer with the presence of hardware. In their cases of infection, CRP was the most sensitive and earliest parameter, with a second peak between 7 to 11 days.

If a fluctuance is present, multiple aspirations after sterile preparation of the skin can be considered. The fluid should be analyzed by Gram staining, aerobic and anaerobic cultures, and antibiotic sensitivities. Early isolation and identification of the infectious organism is beneficial, especially if formal debridement and biopsy is delayed.

Imaging

Plain film radiography is unlikely to be helpful in the diagnosis of an acute postoperative infection. Bone loss must be substantial before it is detectable on a radiograph. Enlarging soft tissue shadows might represent fluid or edema response. In more delayed infections, lucency around grafts, hardware, or within the vertebrae is suggestive. Air in the soft tissues can suggest an esophageal tear or a gas-forming fascial infection. In the absence of these findings, the cervical spine series is useful to ensure maintenance of spinal alignment and hardware or graft position.

Modalities such as computed tomography (CT) and magnetic resonance imaging (MRI) normally show dramatic changes after surgery. Edema, seroma, and hematoma are difficult, if not impossible, to differentiate from infection. If these modalities are obtained, the surgeon must consider that the radiologist's interpretation will include infection in the differential diagnosis (48). Thus, the diagnosis more heavily relies on appearance of the wound, laboratory studies, and clinical judgment. CT-guided biopsy may be of utility in the presence of a suspicious lesion or fluid collection.

Postoperative discitis begins to be evident on plain films weeks to months after onset. The changes are characteristic, including bony reaction at the borders of the disc space and loss of detail at the end plates. Chronic discitis demonstrates bony erosion or sclerotic lesions indicative of progression to frank osteomyelitis. MRI can detect changes much earlier (48). Characteristic features include blunting of the transition between disc and end plate, increased signal on T2 images, and decreased intensity on T1 images.

TREATMENT

Management of postoperative infection of the cervical spine is particular to the type. Some, such as discitis or a mild superficial wound infection (such as suture abscess), may be effectively treated with nonsurgical modalities. Most infections, however, require surgical débridement, irrigation, and confirmation of spinal stabilization. Depending on the severity, surgery may be required on an urgent to emergent basis, as with epidural abscesses or necrotizing fascial or myonecrotic processes.

Wound Infections

Initial management of superficial and deep wound infections consists of culture-sensitivite and Gram stain–specific antibiotics. If aspiration is not possible, the patient should be placed on a broad-spectrum antibiotic to cover likely organisms, unless urgent surgery is planned. If antibiotics are started before a return to the operating room, they should be held 24 hours prior to surgery, if possible, in order to increase the yield of a positive specimen at the time of surgery. The regimen can be restarted in the operating room as soon as tissue is obtained.

After medical optimization of the patient's overall status, surgical debridement and irrigation should be planned as soon as possible for all wound infections. The incision should be reopened along its original planes and inspected at every level for fluid loculation. Necrotic and fibrinous material should be sharply debrided from all fascial planes. Muscles should be inspected for viability by contraction with stimulation by electrocautery. Devitalized tissue is debrided as needed.

Posterior wounds can be associated with devitalized paraspinal muscle. Anterior wound infections are more likely to be so-called dead space infections; however, the longus colli and sternocleidomastoid muscles should be carefully scrutinized. Particular attention should also be paid to the esophagus. Tears can be an occult source of contamination. At the time of irrigation and debridement, a tear should be identified and oversewn. This site should not lie directly over the exposed surface of the vertebral body, which may predispose to fistula formation. If this occurs, the sternocleidomastoid muscle should be mobilized as a flap and interposed between the esophagus and the spine (31). Injection of indigo carmine through the esophagus may show the location of the tear by dye leakage in the field.

Along with debridement, an equally important principle is maintaining spinal stability when treating spinal infections. Spinal implants should be thoroughly inspected after exposure. Loose instrumentation should be removed and replaced if necessary for stability. If not grossly contaminated, autogenous and allogenous bone grafts should remain in place. If the graft is removed, it should be replaced to adequately stabilize the spine. In the anterior spine, prominent hardware that may erode into the esophagus should be revised (32).

Wound management can be effected by primary closure or healing by secondary intention. It is the authors' preference to primarily close the surgical wound when possible. A nonbraided absorbable suture is optimal. Closed suction drains are placed at each fascial level and maintained until drainage decreases below 40 mL every 8 hours. It is the authors' protocol to routinely culture the effluent from the drain bulb 2 days after surgery, as well as the drain tip upon removal. If cultures of the effluent (or the tip) are positive, the infection is probably not adequately treated and a return to the operating room for repeat irrigation and debridement should be considered. If no gross purulence is noted at the time of surgery, closure over a drainage tube can again be considered.

Wounds that cannot be closed primarily are left open. Wet to dry dressings are applied daily until granulation tissue has filled the void. Alternatively, a vacuum-assisted wound closure device can be employed (49). This consists of continuous suction delivered through a sponge material. An advantage of this over standard wet to dry dressings is the need for less frequent dressing changes (approximately three times per week). A disadvantage is the negative pressure cavity created, making it more practical for posterior, rather than anterior, cervical wounds. Culture-specific antibiotics should be continued for approximately 6 weeks. They are discontinued pending clinical resolution of infection and normalization of laboratory values.

Vertebral Osteomyelitis

The treatment of postoperative osteomyelitis follows standard principles of primary bone infection. After safe exposure of the involved area, necrotic bone is removed by curette, Kerrison rongeur, or burr until a healthy bleeding surface is exposed. The neural elements are protected at all times. The wound is copiously irrigated to remove all loose pieces. Stability should then be ascertained. Anterior defects from corpectomy or discectomy must be reconstructed. Both allograft and autograft appear suitable for this purpose, even in the presence of active infection. Posterior instrumentation and arthrodesis should be performed to stabilize the motion segments after the acute infection has been controlled with antibiotics; usually a 2-week delay is appropriate.

Bone infection generally requires a more prolonged course of postoperative antibiotics. The authors recommend a 6- to 12-week course of intravenous therapy. Oral antibiotics may be recommended for longer periods. Installation of peripheral intravenous indwelling catheters (PIC lines) can facilitate drug administration. Repeat debridements may be planned depending on the extent of involvement and the surgeon's confidence in removal of all necrotic material.

Necrotizing Fascial Infections

We are aware of only one case report of necrotizing infection after spinal surgery (46). Although it is a rare complication, urgent and massive surgical debridement is the necessary treatment. Dead fascia and muscle must be sharply removed in serial operations. Repeat surgery is the rule and should continue until intraoperative examination reveals no further tissue necrosis. Hyperbaric oxygenation may be of benefit. Culture-specific antibiotics, with repeat cultures at each debridement, are necessary to maintain control of the infection.

Epidural Abscess

In contrast to other types of surgical infections, preoperative imaging with MRI is beneficial in planning decompression of a postoperative epidural abscess. The abscess is typically approached according to its location: posterior or lateral abscesses via laminectomy, anterior abscesses via the anterior approach. High anterior cervical lesions may be better accessed through a transoral exposure. Epidural abscesses must be drained, completely debrided, and the wound irrigated in a standard manner. Instability after laminectomy or anterior column resection must be reconstructed. With no associated osteomyelitis or deep wound infection, culture-sensitive antibiotics should be administered for 7 to 10 days, pending clinical response. Serial ESR levels are useful in documenting resolution of infections.

Discitis

More accurately termed a *disc space infection,* postoperative discitis can occur after discectomy, corpectomy, or minimally invasive procedures such as a discogram (50, 51). Involvement of the remaining avascular disc material, particularly the lateral annulus, can allow contaminant bacteria to flourish. Typical infecting organisms are skin flora such as *S. aureus* and *S. epidermidis*, although other organisms such as *Escherichia coli* have also been implicated (52). The reported rate of disc space infection after a discogram is 3.2% (53).

Standard initial treatment of postoperative cervical disc space infection is bedrest, hard collar, and intravenous antibiotics. Antibiotics are usually administered empirically, although some surgeons may opt to obtain tissue culture from a percutaneous biopsy (54). Typically, antibiotics are continued for approximately 6 weeks. Oddly, it is often noted that the normal disc is avascular, with little antibiotic penetrance to its substance (55). Despite this, antibiotic therapy is frequently successful. Surgical treatment is indicated in some situations: failure of nonoperative treatment, severe intractable pain positively associated with the infection, or septicemia secondary to the disc space infection. Plain radiography may demonstrate end plate changes with postoperative discitis, suggesting bony involvement. This not does not always lead to consideration for open surgical debridement, because these changes are often responses to the infection rather than frank osteomyelitis. However, it is worrisome.

SUMMARY

Postoperative infections after cervical spine surgery are best treated by prevention. In these rare but unfortunate cases, the surgeon should always consider the possibility in the differential diagnosis of postsurgical pain and wound tenderness. With virtually no pathognomonic radiographic, laboratory, or physical signs, sound and prudent clinical judgment is the best tool in early detection. Prompt treatments including culture, antibiotics, and surgical debridement when indicated affords the best possible outcome. If a decision has to be made, early surgical intervention may be better than watching and waiting.

REFERENCES

1. Bertalanffy H, Eggert HR. Complications of anterior cervical discectomy without fusion in 450 consecutive patients. *Acta Neurochir (Wien)* 1989;99:41–50.
2. Wellman BJ, Follett KA, Traynelis VC. Complications of posterior articular mass plate fixation of the subaxial cervical spine in 43 consecutive patients. *Spine* 1998;23:193–200.
3. Ghanayem AJ, Zdeblick TA. Cervical spine infections. *Orthop Clin North Am* 1996;27:53–67.
4. Doyle JS, Lauerman WC, Wood KB, et al. Complications and long-term outcome of upper cervical spine arthrodesis in patients with Down syndrome. *Spine* 1996;21:1223–1231.
5. Jensen JE, Jensen TG, Smith TK, et al. Nutrition in orthopaedic surgery. *J Bone Joint Surg Am* 1982;64:1263–1272.
6. Saway PA, Blackburn WD, Halla JT, et al. Clinical characteristics affecting survival in patients with rheumatoid arthritis undergoing cervical spine surgery: a controlled study. *J Rheumatol* 1989;16:890–896.
7. Branch CL, Kelly DL, Davis CH, et al. Fixation of fractures of the lower cervical spine using methylmethacrylate and wire: technique and results in 99 patients. *Neurosurgery* 1989;25:503–512.
8. Duff TA, Khan A, Corbett JE. Surgical stabilization of cervical spinal fractures using methylmethacrylate. Technical considerations and long-term results in 52 patients. *J Neurosurg* 1992;76:440–443.
9. Talmi YP, Knoller N, Doley M, et al. Postsurgical prevertebral abscess of the cervical spine. *Laryngoscope* 2000;110:1137–1141.
10. Kuriloff DB, Blaugrund S, Ryan J, et al. Delayed neck infection following anterior spine surgery. *Laryngoscope* 1987;97:1094–1098.
11. van Berge Hengouwen DP, Roukema JA, de Nie JC, et al. Esophageal perforation during surgery on the cervical spine. *Neurosurgery* 1991; 29:766–768.
12. Bohlman HH, Emery SE, Goodfellow DB, et al. Robinson anterior cervical discectomy and arthrodesis for cervical radiculopathy. *J Bone Joint Surg Am* 1993;75:1298–1307.
13. Bryan WJ, Inglis AE, Sculco TP, et al. Methylmethacrylate stabilization for enhancement of posterior cervical arthrodesis in rheumatoid arthritis. *J Bone Joint Surg Am* 1982;64:1045–1049.
14. Cooper PR, Cohen A, Rosiello A, et al. Posterior stabilization of cervical spine fractures and subluxations using plates and screws. *Neurosurgery* 1988;23:300–306.
15. Cuatico W. Anterior cervical discectomy without interbody fusion: an analysis of 81 cases. *Acta Neurochir* 1981;57:269.
16. Lunsford LD, Bissonette DJ, Jannetta JP, et al. Anterior surgery for cervical disc disease. I: Treatment of lateral cervical disc herniation in 253 cases. *J Neurosurg* 1980;53:1–11.
17. Martins AN. Anterior cervical discectomy with and without interbody bone graft. *J Neurosurg* 1976;44:290.
18. Schaerer JP. Anterior cervical disk removal and fusion. *Arch Suisses Neurol Neurochir Psych* 1968;102:331.
19. Segal LS, Drummond DS, Zanotti RM, et al. Complications of posterior arthrodesis of the cervical spine in patients who have Down's syndrome. *J Bone Joint Surg Am* 1991;73:1547–1554.
20. Weiland DJ, McAfee PC. Posterior cervical fusion with triple-wire strut graft technique: 100 consecutive patients. *J Spinal Disord* 1991;4:15.
21. Louis R. Anterior surgery of the upper cervical spine. *Chir Organi Mov* 1992;77:75–80.
22. Fang HSY, Ong GB. Direct anterior approach to the upper cervical spine. *J Bone Joint Surg Am* 1962;44:1588.
23. Merwin GE, Post JC, Sypert GW. Transoral approach to the upper cervical spine. *Laryngoscope* 1991;101:780–784.
24. Wimmer C, Gluch H, Franzreb M, et al. Predisposing factors for infection in spine surgery: a survey of 850 spinal procedures. *J Spinal Disord* 1998;11:124–128.
25. Bendo JA, Spivak J, Moskovich R, et al. Instrumented posterior arthrodesis of the lumbar spine in patients with diabetes mellitus. *Am J Orthop* 2000;29:617–620.
26. Clark CR, Goetz DD, Menezes AH. Arthrodesis of the cervical spine in rheumatoid arthritis. *J Bone Joint Surg Am* 1989;71:381–392.
27. Dunn HK, Aiona MD. Spinal instrumentation and fusion for idiopathic scoliosis in a renal-transplant patient: a case report. *Spine* 1982; 7:177–179.
28. Hirsche BL, Woods JE. Experience with elective surgery in renal allograft recipients. *Am J Surg* 1974;127:730–732.
29. Luck JV, Logan LR, Benson DR, et al. Human immunodeficiency virus infection: complications and outcome of orthopaedic surgery. *J Am Acad Orthop Surg* 1996;4:294–304.
30. Northrup BE, Vaccaro AR, Rosen JE, et al. Occurrence of infection in anterior cervical fusion for spinal cord injury after tracheostomy. *Spine* 1995;20:2449–2453.
31. Fuji T, Kuratsu S, Shirasaki N, et al. Esophagocutaneous fistula after anterior cervical spine surgery and successful treatment using a sternocleidomastoid muscle flap. *Clin Orthop* 1991;267:8–13.
32. Newhouse K, Lindsey RW, Clark CR, et al. Esophageal perforation following anterior cervical spine surgery. *Spine* 1989;14:1051–1053.
33. McGrory BJ, Klassen RA. Arthrodesis of the cervical spine for fractures and dislocations in children and adolescents. A long-term follow-up study. *J Bone Joint Surg Am* 1994;76:1606–1616.
34. Takahashi J, Ebara S, Kamimura M, et al. Early-phase enhanced inflammatory reaction after spinal instrumentation surgery. *Spine* 2001; 26:1698–1704.
35. Stambough JL, Beringer D. Postoperative wound infections complicating adult spine surgery. *J Spinal Disord* 1992;5:277.
36. Jevasar DS, Karlin LI. Perioperative nutritional status and postoperative complications after operation for scoliosis in patients who have cerebral palsy. *J Bone Joint Surg Br* 1993;75:880.
37. Dick J, Boachie-Adjei O, Wilson M. One-stage versus two-stage anterior and posterior spinal reconstruction in adults. *Spine* 1992;17:S310.
38. Mandelbaum BR, Tolo VT, McAfee PC, et al. Nutritional deficiencies after staged anterior and posterior spinal reconstructive surgery. *Clin Orthop* 1988;234:5.
39. Mader JT, Cierny G. The principles of the use of preventative antibiotics. *Clin Orthop* 1984;190:75–82.
40. Riley LH. Prophylactic antibiotics for spine surgery: description of a regimen and its rationale. *J South Orthop Assoc* 1998;7:212–217.
41. Rimoldi RL, Haye W. The use of antibiotics for wound prophylaxis in spinal surgery. *Orthop Clin North Am* 1996;27:47–52.
42. Horowitz NH, Curtin JA. Prophylactic antibiotics and wound infections following laminectomy for lumbar disc herniation. *J Neurosurg* 1975;43:727–731.
43. Keller RB, Pappas AM. Infections after spinal fusion using internal fixation instrumentation. *Orthop Clin North Am* 1972;3:99–11.
44. Klein JD, Garfin SR. Nutritional status in the patient with spinal infection. *Orthop Clin North Am* 1996;27:33–36.
45. Thalgott JS, Cotler HB, Sasso RC, et al. Postoperative infection in spinal implants. Classification and analysis—a multicenter study. *Spine* 1991;16:981–984.
46. Kauffman CP, Bono CM, Vessa P, et al. Postoperative synergistic gangrene after spinal fusion. *Spine* 2000.;25:1729–1732.
47. Jonsson B, Soderholm R, Stromqvist B. Erythrocyte sedimentation rate after lumbar spine surgery. *Spine* 1991;16:1049–1050.
48. Ross JS. Magnetic resonance imaging of the postoperative spine. *Semin Musculoskeletal Radiol* 2000;4:281–291.

49. Yuan-Innes MJ, Temple CL, Lacey MS. Vacuum-assisted wound closure: a new approach to spinal wounds with exposed hardware. *Spine* 2001;26:E30–33.

50. Darden BV, Connor PM. Cervical discography complications and clinical efficacy. *Spine* 1993;18:2035.

51. Schweighofer F, Passler JM, Wildburger R, et al. Interbody fusion of the lower cervical spine: a dangerous surgical method? *Langenbecks Arch Chir* 1992;377:295–299.

52. Iversen E, Nielsen VAH, Hansen LG. Prognosis in postoperative discitis, a prospective study of 111 cases. *Acta Orthop Scand* 1992;63:305–309.

53. Connor PM, Darden BV. Cervical discography complications and clinical efficacy. *Spine* 1993;18:2035–2038.

54. Fouquet B, Goupille P, Jattiot F, et al. Discitis after lumbar surgery, features of aseptic and septic forms. *Spine* 1992;17:356–368.

55. Eismont FJ, Wisel SW, Brighton CT, et al. Antibiotic penetration into rabbit nucleus pulposus. *Spine* 1987;12:254–256.

CHAPTER 85

Complications and Treatment of Occipitocervical Internal Fixation Devices

Christopher D. Kager and Iain H. Kalfas

Occipitocervical internal fixation and arthrodesis have been used for the management of instability of the occipitocervical junction for more than 70 years. Although a solid, osseous bone fusion between the occiput and the cervical spine remains the primary objective of this procedure, a variety of fixation devices have evolved to facilitate this process. These devices provide immediate, internal immobilization to the occipitocervical junction to minimize the potential for pseudoarthrosis. Although it is generally considered to have a relatively low morbidity, a variety of complications can arise from the use of these fixation devices in this region.

MANAGEMENT OF OCCIPITOCERVICAL INSTABILITY

The primary indication for arthrodesis and fixation of the occipitocervical region is biomechanical instability. A variety of pathologic processes can result in destruction or injury to the critical bony or ligamentous structures that serve to stabilize this region. The disorders that can lead to occipitocervical instability include rheumatoid arthritis, trauma, neoplasm, infection, congenital deformity, and iatrogenic causes (such as occipital condyle resection) (1–3). The development of instability in this region can subsequently result in intractable pain with or without neurologic deficit.

Early management options of occipitocervical instability consisted primarily of extended bed rest and external bracing. These options frequently proved to be ineffective because of the presence of substantial ligamentous injury or destruction as the primary reason for instability in this region. Although these conservative measures may be effective in managing spinal instability that is due primarily to bone injury, they are less effective when used to manage significant ligamentous pathology. This conservative approach is also compromised by the sophisticated anatomy and motion capabilities as well as the biomechanical demands of the occipitocervical region. External bracing of the occipitocervical junction is generally ineffective in substantially limiting the complex motion in this region to the degree necessary to allow for sufficient healing of bone or ligamentous pathology (3).

The surgical management of occipitocervical instability has evolved during the past several decades. Initial surgical approaches focused primarily on the placement of bone grafts across the occipitocervical junction (4). These grafts were typically rib or iliac crest autografts that were secured to the occiput and upper cervical vertebrae with wire (5,6). The use of polymethylmethacrylate has also been described for this condition (7,8). Postoperatively, these patients were managed with long periods of external bracing with varying degrees of clinical and radiographic success.

The inconsistent results associated with these earlier surgical approaches eventually led to the development and evolution of a variety of internal fixation devices for this region (2,3,9–12). The fixation devices now available to help manage occipitocervical instability include braided cables, precontoured metal loops, and a collection of sophisticated fixation devices that offer a combination of screws, rods, and plates to secure the occiput to the upper cervical spine and facilitate the development of a solid bone fusion. Each of these devices offers a more rigid degree of occipitocervical immobilization than can be provided by external bracing alone or by some of the earlier surgical options. Although these advanced devices and techniques help improve the long-term outcome of occipitocervical surgery, a variety of complications can still occur during the management of instability in this region. Although some complications are common to all spinal arthrodesis and fixation procedures, other complications can occur as a direct result of using internal fixation in the occipitocervical region. The ability of the spinal surgeon to recognize and understand these complications is important to the successful outcome of occipitocervical arthrodesis and fixation.

COMPLICATIONS OF OCCIPITOCERVICAL FIXATION

As with surgery in other regions of the spinal column, complications in the occipitocervical region can result from a failure to recognize the proper extent of the pathology, errors in preoperative planning, technical mistakes made intraoperatively, and suboptimal management of the patient postoperatively. Each complication that develops contributes to the potential failure of surgery in this complex anatomic region.

Pseudoarthrosis

Achieving a successful fusion of the occipitocervical junction has always been more challenging than obtaining a fusion in other levels of the spinal column. The complex anatomy, motion, and biomechanical forces transferred across this region create numerous obstacles to the fusion process. Failure to achieve fusion in the occipitocervical region is typically more common than in other regions of the spinal column, with pseudoarthrosis rates ranging from 4% to 50% (10,13–16). Although the development and use of advanced fixation devices have helped improve on the high pseudoarthrosis rates associated with the earlier fusion techniques, they do not serve as a substitute for a meticulous approach to the bone grafting process in this region. Careful preparation of the graft bed, the preferential use of autograft, and the achievement of sufficient occipitocervical immobilization are all important factors in avoiding pseudoarthrosis in this region.

Pseudoarthrosis rates are generally higher in patients with rheumatoid arthritis because of the associated use of steroids and nonsteroidal antiinflammatory medications. Fusion can also be compromised in patients with neoplastic disorders who have received radiation therapy to the occipitocervical region. These patients require an even more meticulous approach for both the bone grafting technique and as the internal fixation method selected. Although many of the current fixation devices allow for the elimination of halo fixation following occipitocervical surgery, patients with severe rheumatoid arthritis or neoplastic disorders may require the additional support of external immobilization to minimize the complication of a failed fusion.

Wound Infection

The reported prevalence of postoperative wound infection following occipitocervical fusion and fixation ranges from 5% to 10% (4,9,17). This rate of wound infection is slightly higher than for surgeries performed in other regions of the spinal column. This may relate to the duration of occipitocervical procedures as well as to the nutritional and immunocompromised status of many of the patients undergoing these procedures. The use of fixation devices introduces the element of a foreign body, which can also contribute to this higher infection rate.

As with other spinal procedures, the incidence of wound infection can be minimized by the perioperative use of antibiotics and the careful handling of tissues during surgery. The use of excessive electrocautery should be avoided to minimize the presence of necrotic tissue within the wound. The nutritional status in compromised patients should ideally be optimized preoperatively and maintained in the immediate postoperative recovery period. The use of steroids should be stopped or, if this is not feasible, substantially reduced before and immediately after surgery.

As with other surgical wound infections, superficial infections in this region can typically be managed with local care, whereas deeper, subfascial infections require open débridement with or without the removal of all fixation devices and loose, nonfused bone graft.

Occipitocervical Malalignment

Malalignment of the occipitocervical junction is a rare but important complication of arthrodesis and fixation in this region. It may result from improper positioning of the patient on the operative table immediately before beginning the surgery. A patient can be inadvertently fixated and arthrodesed in an abnormally flexed, extended, or rotated position. If abnormally flexed, problems with respiration and swallowing can occur (Fig. 85.1). If abnormally extended or rotated, difficulties with vision and balance can develop. An abnormal alignment of this region may also contribute to the development of postoperative kyphosis and subaxial subluxation (18,19). Abnormal alignment or "buckling" of cervical vertebrae spanned by the fixation device may occur if they are not included in the construct (Fig. 85.2). Finally, with either extreme flexion or extension or with malalignment of the occipitocervical junction, narrowing of the spinal canal may result in major neurologic sequelae (20).

Problems with occipitocervical malalignment can be avoided by careful positioning of the patient on the operative table. I prefer securing a patient's head in a three-point headholder. This allows for a precise positioning of the patient's head and neck preoperatively. It also helps maintain the proper position during surgery when subtle forces applied to the occipitocervical anatomy during instrumentation may result in an inadvertent movement and malalignment of these structures. When satisfactory preoperative positioning has been achieved, a lateral radiograph of the head and neck should be obtained to verify the intended positioning of the head and neck before proceeding with fixation and arthrodesis (21).

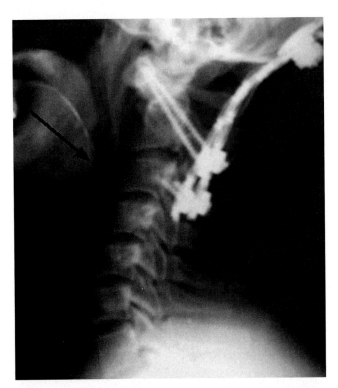

FIG. 85.1. Lateral radiograph demonstrating occipitocervical malalignment after posterior fixation and fusion. The head and neck are in mild flexion producing a slight kinking of the trachea and esophagus *(arrow)*. This patient had difficulty swallowing postoperatively and required a revision of the internal fixation.

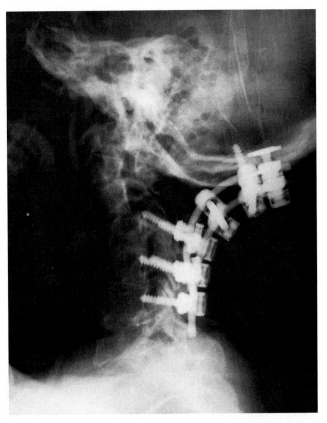

FIG. 85.2. Lateral radiograph demonstrating subluxation of C1 and C2 after occipitocervical fixation. Failure to include C1 and C2 in the construct contributed to this problem.

Fixation Failure

Internal fixation of the occipitocervical junction provides rigid immobilization of the unstable spinal segments to decrease the potential for pseudoarthrosis. However, the application of these devices can be associated with a variety of complications related to either their insertion or failure. The earliest attempts at fixation in this region consisted of stainless-steel wires used to secure bone grafts in place. Several studies demonstrated that the rate of wire breakage was as high as 13% (8,9,17,22,23). More recently, braided titanium cables have replaced the use of wire because of their potentially greater tensile strength and resistance to breakage. In addition to securing bone grafts in place, cables are used to attach contoured rods to both the occiput and the cervical spine. Although they are stronger then conventional wire, cables can also potentially loosen or break. This may subsequently lead to fixation failure and pseudoarthrosis (Fig. 85.3).

In addition to cables, fixation screws are commonly used to secure plates or rods to both the occipital bone and the lateral masses of the cervical spine. Complications related to these screws can occur as a result of either improper positioning, screw pullout, or screw fracture (Fig. 85.4). Although screws properly positioned in the occiput generally have suf-

ficient pullout strength, variations in occipital bone anatomy make the precise placement of these screws critical.

The thickest portion of the occipital bone is in the midline at the level of the external occipital protuberance. Longer screws in the range of 10 to 12 mm can be safely placed into this occipital keel without violating the underlying dura. However, moving laterally from the midline, the thickness of the occipital bone decreases substantially. The lateral margins of the occipital bone can frequently be as thin as 4 to 6 mm, necessitating the use of shorter screws. The use of these shorter screws, which reduces the potential for injury to the underlying cerebellum, also reduces the pullout strength of the construct and increases the potential of screw breakage and construct failure.

Haher (24) evaluated the biomechanical factors of various screw purchases in the occipital bone. This study demonstrated that the greatest pullout strength was at the occipital protuberance for all fixation types. Although bicortical screw placement had a 50% greater pullout strength than wire or unicortical screw placement, screws placed through only the outer cortex at the occipital protuberance offered acceptable pullout strength without the potential complications of bicortical screw or wire passage. Other studies have supported this conclusion (25,26).

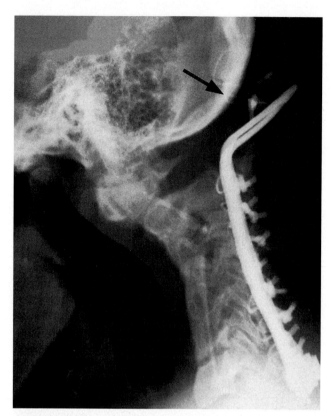

FIG. 85.3. Lateral radiograph demonstrating broken cables in the occiput. A pseudoarthrosis and failure to correct the deformity in the upper cervical spine during the initial procedure contributed to this problem.

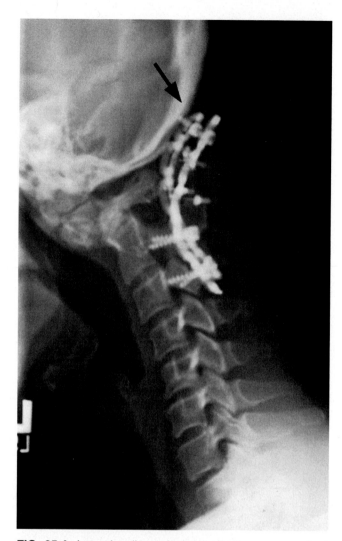

FIG. 85.4. Lateral radiograph demonstrating screw pullout from the lateral margins of the occipital bone. Lateral occipital screw placement necessitated the use of short screws, increasing the risk for screw pullout in this patient.

To take advantage of these biomechanical and anatomic data, several current fixation systems use a customized occipital plate that can be attached to the occiput with several longer screws placed into the central occipital keel. The nonattached limbs of the plate extend bilaterally, providing a platform and site of attachment for two rods or plates that are secured to the cervical spine.

In the cervical spine, options for placing fixation screws include the lateral masses of the subaxial vertebrae, the pedicle of C2, and across the facet joints at the C1-C2 level. Each of these screw placements can be associated with screw fracture or pullout. In general, screws placed into the lateral mass are shorter and, therefore, more prone to failure by pullout. However, by properly positioning the screws and increasing the number of cervical levels included in the construct, the failure of lateral mass screws can be minimized. Screws placed through the pedicle of C2 or across the facet at C1-C2 are generally longer than lateral mass screws and less likely to fail. If they do fracture or pullout, it is typically related to the presence of a notable pseudoarthrosis.

Fracture of the rod or plate component of an occipitocervical construct is rare. The forces that are required to achieve this generally cause the attached screws or cables to fracture first. The failure of the weakest link of the construct prevents the fracture of the stronger rod or plate. An exception to this point is when an extreme bend in the rod or plate has been made to fit it appropriately to the sagittal occipitocervical contour. These extreme bends in the titanium rods or plates create a stress riser or point of weakness in the metal that subjects it to a potential fracture. This occurs because titanium is notch sensitive. An acute bend creates a crease in the metal. If a bend is needed in the rod or plate, it should be applied evenly in smaller increments over a longer section to minimize the development of a stress riser.

Construct Design

The preoperative planning and design of an occipitocervical construct is a critical factor in preventing complications in this region. Many instances of "hardware failure" can be traced back to the surgeon's lack of recognizing the degree of occipitocervical instability and understanding the capabilities and limitations of the hardware selected to manage this instability. In general, there is a tendency to provide too little instrumentation as opposed to providing too much. Construct design complications can also be associated with the failure to correct a major occipitocervical deformity before instrumentation as well as the surgeon's unrealistic reliance on the hardware instead of the incorporation of a solid osseous fusion.

Neural and Vascular Injury

Although injury to the underlying neural and vascular structures in the occipitocervical region can occur during the dissection and decompression stages of the surgery, such injuries occur more commonly as a result of applying internal fixation. These injuries, although rare, typically occur during the insertion of either cables or screws.

When cables are used to secure contoured rods, they are typically placed through burr holes in the occipital bone and passed beneath the lamina in the cervical spine. Passage of these cables brings them into direct contact with the underlying dura and makes the inadvertent passage of these cables through the dura, with subsequent injury to the cerebellum or spinal cord, a remote possibility. Violation of the dura by incorrect cable placement may also result in the development of a cerebrospinal fluid fistula.

Injury to the dura and neural elements during cable placement can be avoided by first creating a generous burr hole or laminotomy at the site of the cable insertion. The underlying dura should be inspected to ensure a clear plane between it and the occipital bone or cervical lamina. As an added safety measure, a suture can be passed through the burr hole or laminotomy first, attached to the cable, and used to draw the cable into position. When performing this maneuver, even tension should be applied to both the suture and the cable during the passage to prevent the cable from "bowing" toward the dura.

Injury to the neural and vascular structures in the occipitocervical region can also occur as a result of improper fixation screw trajectory. Placement of occipital screws, lateral mass screws, C2 pedicle screws, or C1-C2 transarticular screws places the cerebellum, spinal cord, exiting cervical nerve roots, and vertebral arteries at risk. These injuries can be avoided by the surgeon having a thorough knowledge of the appropriate anatomy and techniques for occipitocervical screw insertion, preoperatively assessing each individual patient's occipitocervical anatomy through the use of reformatted computed tomography (CT) images (Fig. 85.5) and, for upper cervical screw placement, using intraoperative fluoroscopy with or without the addition of image-guided spinal navigation technology (Fig. 85.6).

Injury to the vertebral artery is a potentially catastrophic event. It can occur while drilling or tapping a

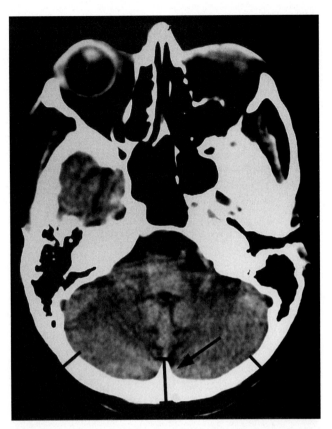

FIG. 85.5. Reformatted sagittal computed tomography image of the upper cervical spine demonstrating the width of the C2 par interarticularis (arrows). The vertebral artery lies immediately anterior to the pars interarticularis. This information is used preoperatively to determine the anatomic feasibility and safety of placing transarticular screws at C1-C2.

hole for screw placement. Although rare, it is more commonly encountered during the placement of transarticular screws at C1-C2. If injury to one vertebral artery occurs, it can be initially managed by either a direct repair approach or a more practical method of tamponading the bleeding by insertion of the screw along the selected trajectory. Although this latter approach does not correct the problem of vessel damage, it does minimize the additional blood loss that can occur with a direct repair approach.

It is also important to recognize that if a vertebral artery injury occurs during the placement of the first of two screws, placement of the second screw should be aborted. Although the loss of one vertebral artery is generally well tolerated because of the continued blood flow in the contralateral vertebral artery, the loss of both arteries can be fatal. If a vertebral artery injury does occur, a postoperative vertebral angiogram should be obtained to rule out the presence of a false aneurysm or vessel dissection at the site of injury. If present, such an injury may necessitate anticoagulant therapy postoperatively to minimize the potential of a cerebrovascular embolic event.

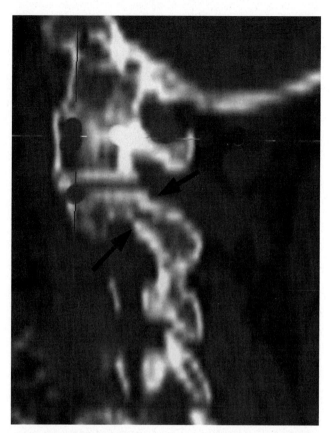

FIG. 85.6. Image-guided spinal navigation screen demonstrating the trajectory for a C1-C2 transarticular screw. Orientation to the pertinent cervical and vascular anatomy is obtained in multiple planes during the procedure. The selected trajectory (*black lines* in the two lower quadrants) and screw tip position at selected insertion depths (*black cursor* in upper left quadrant) are displayed in real time and can be adjusted as needed.

When using lateral mass screws, injury to the vertebral artery can often be avoided by aiming the screw trajectory laterally. The vertebral artery on the side of screw insertion lies directly anterior to the junction of the lamina at that level with its corresponding articular pillar. A lateral trajectory that has an entry point in the center of this articular mass will avoid the vertebral artery. It is also important to avoid using lateral mass screws that go beyond the measured depth of the hole drilled because this may risk injury to the exiting nerve root at that level (27).

The use of fixation screws in the occipital bone can also cause injury to the underlying neural or vascular structures. The cerebellum can be injured if longer screws are placed laterally. The underlying transverse venous sinus can be injured with bicortical screws placed at or above the level of the nuchal ridge. A preoperative CT scan of the occipitocervical region can demonstrate the thickness of the occipital bone and provide information regarding the optimal length and position of these screws. If used, occipital screws should be placed as close to the midline as possible and preferably below the nuchal ridge.

CONCLUSION

Fixation and fusion of the occipitocervical junction can be a demanding procedure. Although the development and evolution of a variety of fixation devices has greatly improved the management of instability in this region, complications can still occur. It is imperative that spinal surgeons performing these procedures have an understanding of all potential pitfalls and are able to recognize and manage them appropriately.

REFERENCES

1. Bejjani GK, Sekhar LN, Riedel CJ. Occipitocervical fusion following the extreme lateral transcondylar approach. *Surg Neurol* 2000;54(2): 109–116.
2. Pait TG, Al-Mefty O, Boop FA, et al. Inside-outside technique for posterior occipitocervical spine instrumentation and stabilization: preliminary results. *J Neurosurg* 1999;90[1 Suppl]:1–7.
3. Vale FL, Oliver M, Cahill DW. Rigid occipitocervical fusion. *Neurosurg Focus* 1999;6(6):1–12.
4. Elia M, Mazzara JT, Fielding JW. Onlay technique for occipitocervical fusion. *Clin Orthop* 1992;280:170–174.
5. McAfee PC, Cassidy JR, Davis RF, et al. Fusion of the occiput to the upper cervical spine. A review of 37 cases. *Spine* 1991;16[10 Suppl]: 490–494.
6. Wertheim SB, Bohlman HH. Occipitocervical fusion. Indications, technique, and long-term results in thirteen patients. *J Bone Joint Surg Am* 1987;69(6):833–836.
7. Brattstrom H, Granholm L. Atlanto-axial fusion in rheumatoid arthritis. A new method of fixation with wire and bone cement. *Acta Orthop Scand* 1976;47(6):619–628.
8. Zygmunt SC, Christensson D, Saveland H, et al. Occipito-cervical fixation in rheumatoid arthritis: an analysis of surgical risk factors in 163 patients. *Acta Neurochir* 1995;135(1–2):25–31.
9. Clark CR, Goetz DD, Menezes AH. Arthrodesis of the cervical spine in rheumatoid arthritis. *J Bone Joint Surg Am* 1989;71(3):381–392.
10. Smith M, Anderson P, Grady S. Occipitocervical arthrodesis using contoured plate fixation. An early report on a versatile fixation technique. *Spine* 1993;18:1984–1990.
11. Sasso RC, Jeanneret B, Fischer K, et al. Occipitocervical fusion with posterior plate and screw instrumentation. A long-term follow-up study. *Spine* 1994;19(20):2364–2368.
12. Schultz KD Jr, Petronio J, Haid RW, et al. Pediatric occipitocervical arthrodesis. A review of current options and early evaluation of rigid internal fixation techniques. *Pediatric Neurosurg* 2000;33(4): 169–181.
13. Crockard A. Evaluation of spinal laminar fixation be a new, flexible stainless steel cable: early results. *Neurosurgery* 1994;35:892–898.
14. Dickman CA, Sonntag VK. Surgical management of atlantoaxial nonunions. *J Neurosurg* 1995;83(2):248–253.
15. Dormans J, Drummond D, Sutton L, et al. Occipitocervical Arthrodesis in children. *J Bone Joint Surg Am* 1995;77:1234–1240.
16. Jain V, Takayasu M, Singh S, et al. Occipito-axis posterior wiring and fusion for atlantoaxial dislocation associated with occipitalization of the axis. *J Neurosurg* 1993;79:142–144.
17. Rodgers WB, Coran DL, Emans JB, et al. Occipitocervical fusions in children. Retrospective analysis and technical considerations. *Clin Orthop* 1999;364:125–133.
18. Matsunaga S, Onishi T, Sakou T. Significance of occipitoaxial angle in subaxial lesion after occipitocervical fusion. *Spine* 2001;26(2):161–165.
19. Matsunaga S, Sakou T, Sunahara N, et al. Biomechanical analysis of buckling alignment of the cervical spine. Predictive value for subaxial subluxation after occipitocervical fusion. *Spine* 1997;22(7):765–771.

20. Nakashima C. Long-term follow-up of acrylic fixation for atlantoaxial dislocation-with technical note on the normalization procedure of the clivo-axial angle. *Neurosurgeons* 1985;4:237–249.

21. Phillips FM, Phillips CS, Wetzel FT, et al. Occipitocervical neutral position. Possible surgical implications. *Spine* 1999;24(8):775–778.

22. Fehlings MG, Errico T, Cooper P, et al. Occipitocervical fusion with a five-millimeter malleable rod and segmental fixation. *Neurosurgery* 1993;32(2):198–208.

23. Robertson SC, Menezes AH. Occipital calvarial bone graft in posterior occipitocervical fusion. *Spine* 1998;23(2):249–255.

24. Haher TR, Yeung AW, Caruso SA, et al. Occipital screw pullout strength. A biomechanical investigation of occipital morphology. *Spine* 1999;24(1):5–9.

25. Papagelopoulos PJ, Currier BL, Stone J, et al. Biomechanical evaluation of occipital fixation. *J Spinal Disord* 2000;13(4):336–344.

26. Roberts A, Wickstrom J. Prognosis of odontoid fractures. *Acta Orthop Scand* 1973;44(1):21–30.

27. Heller JG, Silcox DH, Sutterlin CE. Complications of posterior cervical plating. *Spine* 1995;20:2442–2448.

CHAPTER 86

Complications of Cervical Spine Pedicle Screw Placement

Steven C. Ludwig

Pedicle screws provide stabilization until biologic fusion occurs. Posterior cervical fixation has become increasingly popular in recent years. Dissatisfaction with lateral mass fixation, especially at the cervicothoracic junction, has led to the use of cervical pedicle screw fixation for reconstruction in a number of different cervical spine disorders. Pedicle screw fixation in the cervical spine has been considered too risky for the neurovascular structures with the exception of the C2 and C7 levels. Many surgeons who feel comfortable placing pedicle screws in the C2 and C7 pedicles hesitate to place them in the C3 to C6 pedicles and recommend the use of lateral mass fixation.

Pedicle screw fixation can be a pragmatic solution to the treatment of unusual cervical reconstructive disorders. In circumstances in which posterior wiring or lateral mass fixation cannot be achieved, pedicle fixation may afford optimal stabilization of an unstable motion segment. Anatomic feasibility studies looking at pedicle screw insertion techniques concluded that advanced techniques are required to select the necessary starting point and trajectory for the safe insertion of a cervical pedicle screw (1–3). Studies investigating the morphology of the cervical pedicles appropriately raised concerns about whether transpedicular fixation can be applied safely (4). Above C7, pedicle screw insertion poses a risk to the spinal cord, nerve roots, and vertebral arteries. This risk is further amplified by the trend toward smaller pedicles as the cervical spine ascends cephalad.

Abumi has perhaps the greatest clinical experience in placing pedicle screws in the cervical spine (5–10). The prevalence of clinically important complications caused by his specific pedicle screw insertion technique are low (8). Based on his operative experience, complications associated with cervical pedicle screws are thought to be minimized by a thorough knowledge of the posterior cervical anatomy, sufficient preoperative imaging studies of the pedicles, and strict control of screw insertion with the use of intraoperative fluoroscopy.

The potential complications of cervical pedicle screw insertion are well understood given the proximity of the pedicle to vital surrounding neurovascular structures. When reconstructive dilemmas arise in which cervical pedicle screw fixation becomes a necessary means of stabilization, it is important for a spine surgeon to investigate various methods of cervical pedicle screw insertion to enhance the margin of safety. Critical structures such as the vertebral artery, nerve root, and spinal cord observed *in vitro* have been shown to have a higher rate of injury than those observed clinically. Thus, it appears that the human cervical pedicle is tolerant to screw violation. Regardless of this tolerance, the potentially catastrophic complications that may be incurred should be respected.

INDICATIONS

The goals of a fixation device used in the spine are to: (a) assist in correcting or preventing additional changes in spinal alignment, (b) enhance fusion rates, and (c) allow early mobilization of the patient without the need for cumbersome external immobilization. Three-column fixation using transpedicular screws has increased stability and strength and thus appears to be a useful stabilizing procedure for the reconstruction of the cervical spine (11).

The indications for pedicle screw fixation of the cervical spine have not been clearly defined. Clinically, pedicle screw fixation may be applied as a posterior stabilization device in both traumatic and atraumatic reconstruction procedures (Fig. 86.1). Pedicle screws can be useful in situations with multilevel instabilities, postlaminectomy kyphosis correction, and disorders that require long fixa-

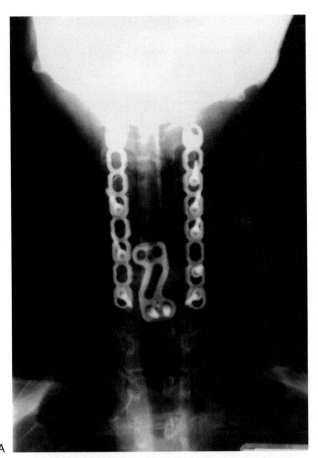
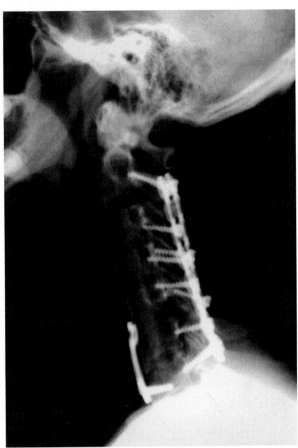

A

B

FIG. 86.1. Anteroposterior and lateral plain radiographs. **A:** Anterior C3 to C7 corpectomies, fibula strut, with anterior junctional buttress plate. **B:** Posterior C2 to C7 fusion with instrumentation and pedicle screws at the C2 and C7 levels.

tion, such as fixation from the occiput to the lower cervical spine. In cases in which the lamina or spinous processes are destroyed, pedicle screws can be a useful alternative for stabilization.

SURGICAL TECHNIQUE

Several different methods of pedicle screw insertion have been reported (1–3,5,10,12). Most comparative surgical data reported are based on human cadaver models. The use of posterior anatomic topography alone has been shown to result in a substantial rate of critical injuries to the spinal cord, nerve roots, or vertebral artery (1,2). Because of the variability in morphology of the human cervical pedicles, in addition to the difficulties inherent in a surgeon's ability to reproduce intended trajectories, anatomic landmarks alone are an insufficient means of placing cervical pedicle screws. Advanced techniques employing computer-assisted image-guided surgery, fluoroscopic guidance, and direct palpation of the cervical pedicle through a laminoforaminotomy technique may improve accuracy.

The C2 pedicle is unique and has the largest pedicle diameter (13). Its superior and medial border can be dissected and directly visualized and palpated without performing a laminoforaminotomy. Thus, a C2 pedicle screw should be safer than insertion of screws into the subaxial pedicles. The drilling angle is directed 10 to 15 degrees medially and 35 degrees superiorly to avoid injury to the vertebral artery (12,13). The safest method for C2 pedicle screw placement employs drilling guided by direct palpation of the medial and superior aspect of the individual C2 pedicle.

A laminoforaminotomy technique allows the surgeon to palpate the pedicle directly (Fig. 86.2). Human cadaver–based studies report 39.6% injuries to the spinal cord, nerve root, or vertebral artery in the subaxial spine with this technique (1). Albert and colleagues reported on 21 patients in whom cervical pedicle screw fixation was used at C7 alone (14). All pedicle screws were placed after direct palpation of the pedicle with a nerve hook following a laminoforaminotomy at the C6-C7 level. The authors reported no neurologic complications related to pedicle screw placement. At 1 year of follow-up, no failures of fixation or complications related to pedicle fixation occurred.

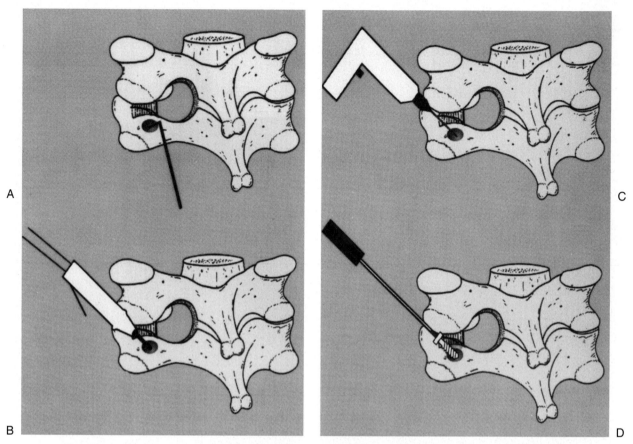

FIG. 86.2. Laminoforaminotomy technique for placing pedicle screws. **A:** A keyhole foraminotomy is performed at the correct level, and a nerve hook palpates the pedicle both superiorly and medially. **B:** A 2-mm burr is used to create a starting hole in the previously palpated pedicle. **C:** A power drill is used with a stop set at 18 mm to drill through the pedicle into the vertebral body. **D:** After the screw hole is tapped, a 20-mm screw is placed into the pedicle.

The authors concluded that pedicle screws in C7 placed with a laminoforaminotomy technique appeared to be safe and efficacious.

The largest clinical series I am aware of reporting the use of cervical pedicle screws have been performed by Abumi and associates (5–10) (Fig. 86.3). The entry point of screw insertion was described as slightly lateral to the center of the lateral mass and close to the posterior proximal margin of the superior articular surface. An insertion hole with a 2-mm burr is made, and the bleeding cancellous bone of the pedicle is directly visualized. The surgeon then cannulates the pedicle using a hand-guided probe. This is performed with the assistance of lateral fluoroscopy. The probe is directed with a medial inclination of about 25 to 45 degrees. According to the clinical results reported by Abumi and associates, the rates of pedicle breach by inserted screws were between 5.3% and 6.7% (5–10). Even with lateral wall perforation, no clinical complications involving the vertebral artery were apparent. Human cadaver studies with the Abumi technique

have shown a 12% injury rate to the vertebral artery, nerve root, or spinal cord (3).

COMPLICATIONS

Transpedicular cervical spine screw insertion is associated with obvious risks to major neurovascular structures, including the spinal cord, nerve root, and vertebral arteries. A laterally placed pedicle screw places the vertebral artery at risk if the screw substantially encroaches into the foramen transversarium (Fig. 86.4). A medially directed screw poses a risk to the spinal cord, and a superiorly or inferiorly directed screw could injure an exiting nerve root. Complications not directly attributable to pedicle screw insertion may also occur, including infection, pseudarthrosis, loss of reduction, and implant breakage.

Previous human cadaver studies comparing the accuracy of different pedicle screw insertion methods (anatomic topography, laminoforaminotomy, computer-assisted image-guided surgical systems, and the Abumi technique) revealed

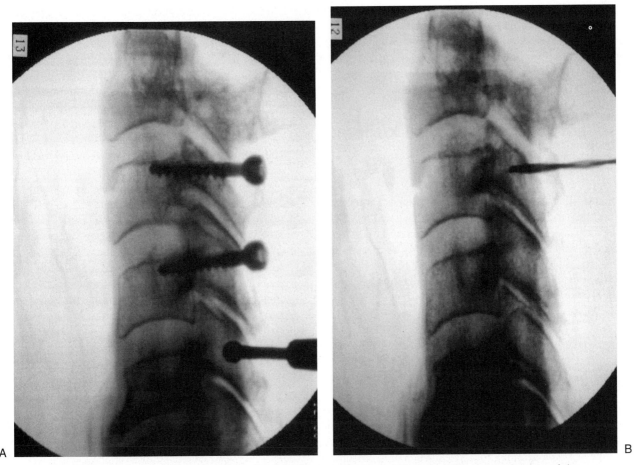

A

B

FIG. 86.3. Abumi technique for cervical pedicle screw placement. **A:** Lateral fluoroscopic view of the cervical spine. A 2-mm burr is decorticating the C5 lateral mass to obtain the appropriate starting position. Note the pedicle screws placed at the C3 and C4 levels. **B:** Lateral fluoroscopic view of the cervical spine. Sounding the cervical pedicle is done using a 1.25-mm handheld probe.

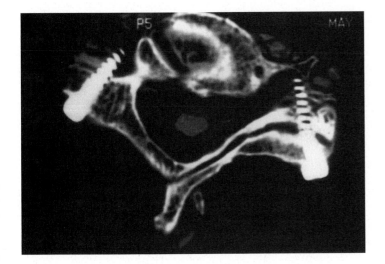

FIG. 86.4. Postoperative computed tomography scan performed in a human cadaver study. Note the bilateral violation of the foramen transversarium. Open dissection revealed complete transection of the vertebral artery on the right side and perforation of the vertebral artery on the left side.

a rate of injury to these critical structures ranging between 11% and 66% (1–3). In these anatomic studies, any violation of the foramen transversarium or medial aspect of the pedicle was regarded as a potential injury to the vertebral artery or spinal cord. Regardless of the method employed, the vertebral artery is the most likely structure to be injured, followed by the exiting nerve root.

Neurologic Complications

Pedicle screw instrumentation in the cervical spine should be performed with intraoperative neurophysiologic monitoring. Somatosensory and motor evoked potentials should be used. Any substantial deviation from baseline potentials following the placement of a pedicle screw should be treated as a presumptive neurologic injury. Spinal cord injury related to a malpositioned cervical spine pedicle screw has never been reported. If faced with substantial changes in the spinal cord monitoring, reversal of the maneuver that caused the change, such as removing the instrumentation or changing the corrective forces placed on the cervical spine, should be performed immediately. In addition, spinal cord injury dosing of methylprednisolone, 30 mg/kg bolus, followed by 5.4 mg/kg per hour for 23 hours, should also be started immediately. Postoperatively, the patient should be placed in an intensive care unit to observe the patient's neurologic status. Advanced imaging studies such as magnetic resonance imaging (MRI) or computed tomography (CT) myelogram should be performed to look for any evidence of neurocompression or cord contusion.

Cervical nerve roots run about 45 degrees anterolaterally in relation to the coronal plane and 10 degrees downward or caudally in relation to the transverse plane (11,15). Within the neuroforamen, the root is located in the inferior half. Thus, there is some room between the neural elements and surface of the medial and inferior pedicle walls. This anatomic configuration allows for slight "safe" perforation of the pedicle wall by screw threads in the medial or inferior direction. Postoperatively, the patient who complains of any radicular symptoms or has objective neurologic changes from the baseline examination requires advanced imaging studies to rule out an injury due to a malpositioned pedicle screw. CT myelogram (with 1-mm cuts) with coronal and sagittal reconstruction may identify a screw invading the neuroforamen. Patients with clinically important postoperative neurologic changes require immediate removal of the instrumentation to maximize the potential for neural recovery. Clinically, Abumi and colleagues reported on only 2 of 45 screws penetrating the pedicle and causing a transient radiculopathy (8). None of these patients required revision or removal of their instrumentation.

Vascular Complications

Classically, the vertebral artery is divided into four segments. The first extends from the subclavian artery, anterior to C7, to the foramen transversarium of C6. The second extends through the foramina transversaria of C6 to C1. The third is from the superior aspect of the arch of the atlas to the foramen magnum. The fourth is from the foramen magnum to the point at which the vertebral artery unites with the corresponding vertebral artery from the contralateral side to form the basilar artery. The paired vertebral arteries compose the posterior circulation of the brain, which includes the occipital lobes, the brainstem, and the labyrinthine branches to the inner ear.

The second segment of the vertebral artery is the region where the artery is most susceptible to injury during placement of cervical spine pedicle screws. In the transverse foramina, the structures transmitted include the vertebral vascular bundle, which is composed of a single artery and multiple veins, and the sympathetic nervous plexus. When a vertebral artery is injured in the subaxial cervical region, the patient with an inadequate blood flow in the contralateral vertebral artery is at risk for the development of a lateral medullary infarction (Wallenberg syndrome). Clinically, this may result in decreased pin sensation in the ipsilateral face and contralateral limbs, nystagmus, ataxia, dysmetria in the ipsilateral limbs, and Horner syndrome on the ipsilateral side.

The vertebral veins are located medial to the arteries. It is difficult to determine their relative risk for injury as compared with the artery with respect to pedicle screw placement. Fortunately, judicious use of thrombostatic agents, cotton patties, and suction usually controls bleeding from these venous structures. Because there is no neurologic deficit associated with operative vertebral vein injuries, I am aware of no published data on the prevalence of injuries to the vertebral veins.

If a vertebral artery injury occurs during the placement of a pedicle screw, various management options are available. The single most important point to understand is that the surgeon should abandon the placement of a pedicle screw on the contralateral side to prevent bilateral injury and subsequent death. Options to obtain hemostasis include the use of a thrombostatic agent, direct ligation and repair, and the placement of the screw in the side of injury to tamponade the bleeding. Because of the limited operative exposure from a posterior approach, direct ligation, repair, or even performing a microvascular bypass is technically challenging. Endovascular techniques of therapeutic embolization have emerged and are helpful for managing these injuries.

After intraoperative vascular control of a vertebral artery injury is achieved, it is important to obtain radiographic imaging confirmation of the adequacy of hemostasis. This may be performed through angiography or magnetic resonance angiography (MRA). Because a pedicle screw may cause an unacceptable artifact, MRA can be difficult to interpret. Thus, angiography remains the study of choice. Admitting the patient to an intensive care unit after surgery for close monitoring of neurologic function is important. Further management based on the etiology of the abnormality detected, such as embolization for persistent bleeding or anticoagulation with partial occlusion, may be indicated.

In most patients, the vertebral artery is absent from the foramen transversarium of C7. Studies have shown that the foramen transversarium of C7 contains the vertebral artery, vein, and associated nerve fibers in about 5% of patients (16). Therefore, advanced imaging studies before pedicle screw placement in the C7 vertebra looking for a dysplastic foramen transversarium is necessary (Fig. 86.5). The largest series of a single surgeon's clinical experience I am aware of (180 patients, 669 pedicle screws) revealed one vertebral artery injury without neurologic sequelae (<1%) (8). Thus, even in those cases with lateral wall perforation, no complication of the vertebral artery was clinically apparent. Because the vertebral artery does not occupy the whole part of the foramen transversarium, a minimal violation of the foramen transversarium may not be as risky as initially thought.

Ludwig and co-workers (3) performed an analysis of the accuracy of cervical pedicle screw placement, looking at cervical pedicle diameter, regardless of cervical level. In this human cadaver series, they found a critical pedicle diameter of 4.5 mm, below which injuring a critical structure (vertebral artery) occurred 33% of the time. However, at those pedicles with a diameter greater than 4.5 mm instrumented with a 3.5-mm screw, a 98% likelihood of safe screw placement was noted (Fig. 86.6). Because the screws inserted had a 3.5-mm diameter, the decreasing diameter of a pedicle eventually imposes an unacceptable margin for error.

Spine surgeons attempting to place pedicle screws in the cervical spine should therefore use specific methods to avoid misinsertion. These include a thorough understanding of the patient's cervical spine anatomy, careful analysis of preoperative advanced imaging studies to define anatomic anomalies, preoperative measurement of the pedicle diameter (>4.5 mm), and the use of either an image-guided

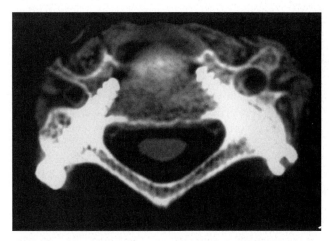

FIG. 86.6. Postoperative computed tomographic scan performed in a human cadaver study. Bilateral pedicle screws are well positioned and extend into the vertebral body.

surgical system or fluoroscopic imaging to assist in the placement of the screws.

CONCLUSION

Successful placement of a pedicle screw in the cervical spine requires a sufficient three-dimensional understanding of pedicle morphology to allow accurate identification of the ideal screw axis. Several advanced techniques have emerged to assist the surgeon in the placement of a cervical spine pedicle screw. Performing a laminoforaminotomy has been shown to be safe for the placement of pedicle screws at the C7 level. The Abumi method offers a safe

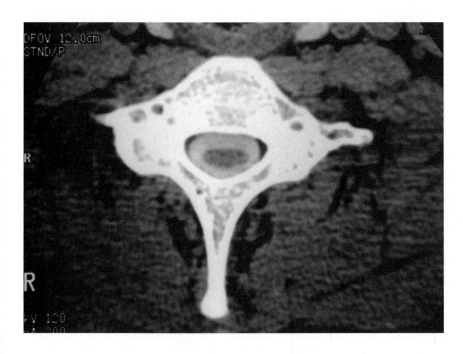

FIG. 86.5. Computed tomography scan through the C7 pedicle showing a dysplastic foramen transversarium.

alternative. Unfortunately, its clinical success has only been reported by the surgeon who developed the technique. Centers with access to a computer-assisted image-guided surgical system may use this technique to assist in placing these screws.

Numerous clinical reports attest to the effectiveness and success of pedicle fixation at the C2 and C7 levels. Elsewhere in the subaxial cervical spine, pedicle screw insertion poses a more substantial challenge. The dimensions of the pedicles are smaller, so that the margins for error are less.

Theoretical injuries to critical structures in human cadaver studies have been reported. However, the clinical success of using pedicle screws in the cervical spine with rare neurovascular complications contradicts these *in vitro* data. Because the pedicles at C3 to C6 are closer to the spinal cord, nerve roots, and vertebral artery, less margin for error exists. At the C2 and C7 levels, lateral masses are not well formed, and the pedicles are large, allowing for better screw accommodation than at other levels.

Conventional methods of posterior cervical instrumentation such as wiring or lateral mass fixation remain the preferred initial techniques to consider. However, when circumstances arise that make these methods unfeasible, the cervical pedicle screw may be an alternative point of fixation. When using this technique, the spine surgeon must be aware of the potential neurovascular complications that may occur. Early recognition and aggressive treatment of these complications may minimize any further morbidity.

REFERENCES

1. Ludwig SC, Kramer DL, Balderston RA, et al. Placement of pedicle screws in the human cadaveric cervical spine: comparative accuracy of three techniques. *Spine* 2000;25(13):1655–1667.
2. Ludwig SC, Kramer DL, Vaccaro AR, et al. Transpedicle screw fixation of the cervical spine. *Clin Orthop Relat Res* 1999;359:77–88.
3. Ludwig SC, Kowalski J, Edwards C, et al. Cervical pedicle screws: comparative accuracy of two insertion techniques. *Spine* 2000;25(20):2675–2681.
4. Panjabi MM, Duranceau J, Goel V, et al. Cervical human vertebrae: quantitative three-dimensional anatomy of the middle and lower regions. *Spine* 1991;16:861–869.
5. Abumi K, Itoh H, Taneichi H, et al. Transpedicular screw fixation for traumatic lesions of the middle and lower cervical spine: description of the techniques and preliminary report. *J Spinal Disord* 1994;7:19–28.
6. Abumi K, Kaneda K. Pedicle screw fixation for nontraumatic lesions of the cervical spine. *Spine* 1997;22:1853–1863.
7. Abumi K, Kaneda K, Shono Y, et al. One stage posterior decompression and reconstruction of the cervical spine by using pedicle screw fixation systems. *J Neurosurg* 1999;90:19–26.
8. Abumi K, Shono Y, Ito M, et al. Complications of pedicle screw fixation in reconstructive surgery of the cervical spine. *Spine* 2000;25(8):962–969.
9. Abumi K, Shono Y, Taneichi H, et al. Correction of cervical kyphosis using pedicle screw fixation systems. *Spine* 1999;24(22):2389–2396.
10. Abumi K, Shono Y, Kotani K, et al. Indirect posterior reduction and fusion of the traumatic herniated disc using a cervical pedicle screw system. *J Neurosurg* 2000;92:30–37.
11. Pech P, Daniels DL, Williams AL, et al. The cervical neural foramina: correlation of microtomy and CT anatomy. *Radiology* 1985;155:143–146.
12. Roy-Camille R. Rationale and techniques of internal fixation in trauma of the cervical spine. In: Errico T, Bauer RD, Waugh T, eds. *Spinal trauma.* Philadelphia: JB Lippincott, 1991:163–191.
13. Kotani Y, Cunningham BW, Abumi K, et al. Biomechanical analysis of cervical stabilization systems. An assessment of transpedicular screw fixation in the cervical spine. *Spine* 1994;19:2529–2539.
14. Albert T, Klein G, Joffe D, et al. Use of cervicothoracic junction pedicle screws for reconstruction of complex cervical spine pathology. *Spine* 1998;23:1596–1599.
15. Daniels DL, Hyde JS, Kneeland JB. The cervical nerves and foramina: local-coil MRI imaging. *AJNR Am J Neuroradiol* 1986;7:129–133.
16. Jovanoic MS. A comparative study of the foramen transversarium of the sixth and seventh cervical vertebrae. *Surg Radiol Anat* 1990;12:167–172.
17. Ebraheim N, Rollins JR, Xu R, et al. Anatomic consideration of C2 pedicle screw placement. *Spine* 1996;21(6):691–695.

CHAPTER 87

Complications Related to the Management of Dens Fractures

Rick C. Sasso

Care of the patient with a dens (odontoid) fracture may be fraught with difficulty. From the initial evaluation, when the fracture may be missed, to the definitive treatment, either operative or nonoperative, complications can occur. As our society ages, the special dilemma and specific complications of the elderly patient with a dens fracture will likely become more common. This chapter outlines the range of complications related to the management of dens fractures and offers guidance to minimize the magnitude and frequency of possible complications.

ANATOMY

Many complications related to the management of dens fractures stem from an underappreciation of the complex anatomy of the occipitocervical junction. The upper cervical spine represents a transition zone between the rigid skull base and the mobile cervical spinal column. It consists of the occiput and paired occipital condyles, the foramen magnum, atlas, axis, and an interconnected array of stabilizing ligaments. As a result, axis (C2) fractures should be viewed not as an isolated bony injury but as an injury of the craniovertebral junction. The odontoid process extends as a vertical post from the body of the axis and serves as the primary bony stabilizer of the atlantoaxial complex. It articulates with the posterior aspect of the anterior arch of the atlas as a synovial joint. The C1-C2 facet joints, in conjunction with the dens, form a unique architecture, which allows about 50% of all cervical rotation and 12% of cervical flexion-extension (1). Embryologic development of the axis is complex. Three different sclerotomes compose C2. The lowest occipital sclerotome (proatlas) forms the tip of the dens, whereas the body of the C1 sclerotome separates during ontogeny to join with the axis, forming the odontoid process. Finally, the C2 sclerotome forms the remaining body of the axis.

The primary ligamentous stabilizers of the occipitocervical complex include the transverse atlantal ligament (which passes immediately posterior to the dens and attaches to tubercles on the inner aspect of each lateral mass of the atlas) and the tectorial membrane (a continuation of the posterior longitudinal ligament, attaching to the anterior aspect of the foramen magnum). Accessory ligaments include the paired alar ligaments (attaching the superior lateral aspect of the dens to the inner aspect of the occipital condyles) and the rudimentary apical ligament (attaching the tip of the dens to the anterior margin of the foramen magnum).

A thorough understanding of the bony anatomy of the dens is particularly important to avoid complications of anterior or posterior instrumentation. Histomorphometric analysis has revealed high-density trabecular bone located in the center tip of the dens as well as in the weight-bearing lateral masses beneath the superior facets. The anterior base of the body of C2, where the anterior longitudinal ligament attaches, is composed of thickened cortical bone. However, the upper portion of the C2 body and the base of the dens consist of relatively weaker, fine trabecular bone (2). Because bone quality is a crucial determinant of screw purchase, these factors affect dens fracture fixation. Optimal anterior dens screw placement obtains strong purchase at the entry site (anteroinferior border of C2 body) and exit site (dens tip), traversing the weak, hypodense bone in the body of C2. If the entry site is too cephalad along the anterior body of C2, the screw may cut out of this weak bone. If the screw does not exit engaging the cortical bone at the tip of the dens, poor purchase of the dens fragment may result.

The projection angle of the dens is the most variable dimension of the axis, ranging from −2 degrees (tilting anterior) to 42 degrees (tilting posterior), with a mean of 13 degrees (3). This variability can make the assessment of fracture reduction difficult. The diameter of the dens may be less than 6 mm, preventing placement of two 3.5-mm anterior odontoid screws (3,4). Patient body size correlates poorly as a predictor of the dens size (5).

The vascular supply of the dens is provided primarily by the paired right and left posterior and anterior ascending arteries of the axis, which are branches of the vertebral arteries between the second and third cervical vertebrae (6). These also anastomose with horizontal arteries from the internal carotid arteries, forming a rich local vascular network, leading some investigators to conclude that a dens fracture nonunion is not primarily due to an inadequate vascular supply (7,8). In the axis, the vertebral artery groove is located near the pars, along the inferior portion of the superior facet. Because

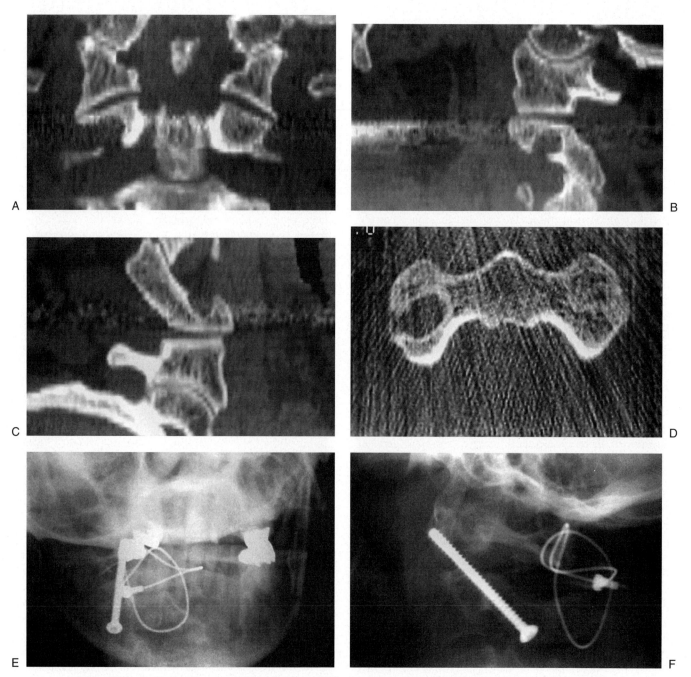

FIG. 87.1. A: Coronal computed tomography (CT) scan with a medial and high-riding vertebral artery groove on the right and with normal vascular anatomy on the left. **B:** Sagittal CT of the right C1-C2 lateral mass region showing a high-riding vertebral artery groove without enough space for a transarticular screw. **C:** Sagittal CT on the left showing adequate room for a transarticular screw. **D:** Axial CT through the lateral mass of C2 showing an anomalous vertebral artery groove on the right side with a normal left side. **E:** Postoperative anteroposterior x-ray with the left C1-C2 transarticular screw in place. **F:** Postoperative lateral X-ray with the transarticular screw and modified Gallie cable construct.

the C2 body is relatively narrow, the vertebral artery is more medial in the axis, ultimately traveling in a lateral direction as it heads cephalad into the transverse foramen of the atlas. Paramore and co-workers (9) showed that up to 18% of patients have unilateral anomalous vertebral artery positions, forming a high-riding transverse foramen that substantially narrows the pedicle and lateral mass of C2. This effectively precludes safe placement of a posterior C1-C2 transarticular screw on the corresponding side (Fig. 87.1).

BIOMECHANICS

The great mobility of the atlantoaxial articulation results in substantial forces being imparted on the odontoid at the extremes of motion. Human cadaveric testing has demonstrated that dens fractures occur as a result of a combination of horizontal shear and vertical compression force (7). When the shear component is applied in a direct sagittal plane (extension), a type III fracture pattern is created (10). Mouradin and associates believed this was due to simultaneous forces exerted by the alar, apical, and tectorial membrane ligaments (11). When the shear force is applied more obliquely (laterally), a type II fracture occurs, possibly owing to the lateral mass of the atlas impinging on the base of the odontoid (10,11). A forward flexion moment, with resultant anterior displacement, is believed to account for 60% to 80% of dens fractures (12–14). Similarly, an extension moment has been shown to lead to posterior displacement, found more commonly among elderly patients (13–16).

A finite element model of the occipitoatlantoaxial complex predicts that force loading that puts the head in extension, coupled with lateral shear or compression, leads to a type I fracture (17). This finite element analysis also showed that axial rotation and lateral shear can produce type II fractures. Moreover, flexion provided a protective mechanism against force application that would otherwise cause a higher risk for odontoid failure (17).

The biomechanics of dens fracture internal fixation deserves special attention. The strength of the anterior dens screw construct is dependent on the interdigitation of the fracture fragments. An anatomically reduced fracture with the fracture fragments maximally lagged together provides stability in excess of the isolated strength of the screw. Isolated screws loaded to failure are much weaker than dens fracture constructs in which one or two screws are used for fixation (18). It is thus very important to ensure that anatomic reduction is present if internal fixation is performed. This maximizes the surface area at the fracture site. Even 1 mm of displacement profoundly diminishes the surface area available for interdigitation. Also, it is important that the fracture fragments are lagged together. This can be done by a lag technique with the body fragment overdrilled to the outer diameter of the screw, or by using a partially threaded screw. If a partially threaded "lag" screw is used, however, it is important that all of the threads be in the odontoid fragment to ensure compression across the fracture.

EPIDEMIOLOGY

Dens fractures represent a common spinal injury, constituting nearly 60% of axis fractures and 7% to 18% of all traumatic cervical spine fractures. Despite their relative frequency, significant controversy exists regarding appropriate surgical and nonsurgical treatment options in the management of these injuries.

Because there is a proportionally greater amount of space available for the spinal cord in the upper cervical spine, the prevalence of neurologic deficit in dens fractures is believed to be relatively low (18% to 26%). These injuries can range from greater occipital nerve injury to a high tetraparesis with respiratory dysfunction (14,15,19,20).

Although dens fractures occur in all age groups, there tends to be a bimodal distribution, with a mean age of 47 years. In younger patients, this injury is usually secondary to high-energy trauma, with motor vehicle crashes being the most common cause (14,19,20). Among this group, concomitant spinal injuries are present in up to 34% of patients. Of the concomitant fractures, 85% occur in the cervical spine, with the atlas most commonly also injured (15,21,22). A frequent source of complications related to the management of dens fractures is either missing a noncontiguous spinal injury or not appreciating the severity of a contiguous injury. Atlas fractures and transverse atlantal ligament injuries in particular are major factors in the prognosis and treatment options for type II dens fractures.

Dens fractures, however, are not uncommon among the elderly, accounting for the second prevalence peak (23). Although the prevalence of subaxial spine fractures decreases with age, that of dens fractures increases with age (24), representing the most common cervical spine fracture in patients older than 70 years (16,25–27). These injuries are usually the result of low-energy trauma, such as falls from a standing height in which the forehead strikes an object. In these instances, associated spinal trauma is much less common (21,28).

CLASSIFICATION

The most widely used classification system for dens fractures is that of Anderson and D'Alonzo (20). First described in 1974, it has withstood the test of time because the classification is useful in predicting outcome and selecting treatment methods (25). This system divides fractures into three types based on the anatomic location of the fracture. Type I is a small, oblique fracture of the tip of the dens, believed to be due to avulsion by the alar ligament. This may be confused with an ossiculum terminale, a congenital anomaly in which the previously discussed proatlas fails to fuse with the dens. This is a rare fracture pattern, accounting for 1% to 5% of dens fractures, with some authors doubting its existence. However, if present, it may be associated with an occipitoatlantal dislocation (29). Type II is the most common (38% to 80%), a horizontal fracture occurring at the junction of the odontoid process with the C2 body. Hadley and colleagues proposed an additional IIA subtype, defined as a type II fracture with marked comminution at the base, due to its inherently increased instability (30). Finally, a type III fracture extends into the body of C2, accounting for 15% to 40% of all dens fractures.

ERRORS IN EVALUATION

Initial evaluation and management of patients with suspected dens process fractures is similar to that of all cervical spine trauma patients. This includes employing early cervical orthosis immobilization (usually with a rigid cervical collar) and maintaining spinal immobilization during airway management and particularly during transfers for radiographic evaluation. A halo traction ring or a Gardner-Wells tong may be placed to apply 10 to 15 pounds of traction (starting with 5 to 10 pounds and radiographically verifying that occipitocervical instability is not present). This is particularly useful if there is any dens displacement, in order to obtain reduction and verify that reduction, in fact, can be accomplished. If it cannot be reduced with adequate traction and surgery is contemplated, this will preclude some instrumentation options (such as an anterior dens screw or posterior C1-C2 transarticular screws). If a halo ring or tongs are applied before complete imaging, magnetic resonance imaging (MRI)-compatible devices should be chosen because MRI may be required to assess for associated upper cervical ligamentous injury or cord compression.

A comprehensive diagnostic approach in the assessment of suspected upper cervical spine injuries remains controversial, particularly in the presence of polytrauma and in obtunded patients. Initial cervical spine imaging consists of the three-view trauma series: anteroposterior, lateral, and open-mouth view radiographs (31). This series reveals 65% to 90% of axis fractures (32–34). Several studies have demonstrated that the anteroposterior view provides little additional information (35,36). As noted previously, careful evaluation of the entire upper cervical and subaxial spine is required because of the substantial prevalence of associated spinal injuries (15,21,22,31). Some studies have reported up to a 16% rate of noncontiguous fractures (37). Thin-slice helical computed tomography (CT) scanning has been shown to be the best study for evaluating C2 bony injuries in patients with inadequate plain films and for differentiating acute dens fracture from chronic nonunion and congenital anomalies (38,39). This imaging study has been found to be more sensitive than plain films in the C1-C2 area, which is the location of most initially undetected cervical fractures (39). However, CT may underestimate soft tissue and associated ligamentous injuries. More recently, passive dynamic flexion-extension real-time fluoroscopic examination has been proposed as a method to identify occult ligamentous injuries in patients who had otherwise normal radiographs but could not be clinically cleared because of an altered sensorium (40).

MRI, like CT, has been shown to be more sensitive than radiographs in revealing some forms of subtle dens trauma and is especially effective in assessing ligamentous structures (39,41,42). In one recent review, 10% of all dens fracture patients had an associated transverse atlantal ligament disruption (42). Evaluating the integrity of the transverse atlantal ligament in dens fractures is important because its incompetence alters treatment options and substantially increases the risk for dens nonunion (42). Anterior dens screw fixation may achieve osseous union in these patients, but it will not restore atlantoaxial stability. Catastrophic neurologic decline may occur if this is not realized.

TREATMENT

A variety of treatment methods are available in the management of dens fractures, both surgical and nonsurgical. These include rigid cervical orthoses, SOMI (skull, occiput, mandibular immobilization) and Minerva jackets, halo vest orthoses, anterior dens screw fixation, and posterior atlantoaxial arthrodesis. Specific treatment choice should be guided by a number of factors, including fracture type, presence of associated injuries, patient age, and patient comorbidity.

Type I

The rare type I fracture is a stable injury, with several of the accessory ligaments remaining intact, including the transverse atlantal ligament. These may be managed by simple cervical collar immobilization. Initial assessment, however, should include careful evaluation for possible association with an occipitoatlantal dislocation (19–21,29). Devastating neurologic complications may occur if occipitocervical instability is overlooked.

Type III

Because of their large cancellous fracture surface, type III injuries are generally regarded to heal uneventfully with nonoperative management, provided closed reduction is obtained (15). Immobilization in a halo vest or rigid cervical orthoses for 8 to 14 weeks has been reported to result in successful union in 92% to 100% of cases (20,22,43,44). Clark and White, however, described a nonunion rate of up to 13% for these fractures, with a trend toward nonunion in fractures with more than 5 mm of displacement (14). These authors recommended treatment with halo immobilization.

The high type III fracture subset with a shallow base may act like a type II fracture with a higher complication rate and increased incidence of nonunion without operative treatment (45).

Type II

Despite the relative frequency of type II injuries, their treatment remains highly controversial (24,26). Substantial complications can occur by managing these fractures operatively or nonoperatively.

Nonoperative

Nonoperative management yields reported rates of nonunion ranging from 26% to 85% (8,14,19,23,26). Although some studies suggest this high rate of nonunion is secondary to the disruption of the dens process vascular supply (6), other investigators have demonstrated adequate blood flow from above and below the odontoid process base (7,8). Other factors potentially contributing to nonunion include the difficulty of maintaining an adequate fracture reduction of the dens relative to the body of the axis as well as the predominantly intersynovial location of the dens itself (15, 25,46). The prevalence of type II fracture nonunion has been shown to correlate with initial displacement of 4 to 6 mm (14,19,47,48), with several studies concluding such displacement to be the most important single factor in determining the success of nonsurgical management. Similarly, posterior displacement, age over 60 years, delay in diagnosis greater than 3 weeks, and angulation greater than 10 degrees have all been associated with an increased rate of nonunion (8,14,19,22,23,43,48,49).

Pseudarthrosis

The possible complications associated with a nonunion of a type II dens fracture include pain and functional deficit from limited range of motion and muscle spasm; however, the most dreaded concern is a progressive myelopathy from brainstem compression. Late-onset progressive myelopathy secondary to dens nonunion is probably uncommon, but it is a real and catastrophic complication of odontoid fracture management (50). Lynch and associates also recently presented the occurrence of delayed myelopathy in five nonrheumatoid patients after nonunion of type II dens fractures. They conclude that the initial failure to treat type II dens fractures in asymptomatic patients or deferred treatment in an initially unrecognized fracture may lead to delayed development of cervicomedullary compression (51).

Halo

The standard method of nonoperative treatment for type II dens fractures is halo immobilization. Although it is the most stable form of nonoperative immobilization of the upper cervical spine (52), profound complications can occur with this modality. Application of a halo should not be considered as always the most "conservative" form of treatment, and especially for elderly patients, operative stabilization many times is more conservative than halo immobilization. The use of halo immobilization in type II fractures presents several distinct disadvantages, including pin-site infections, skin breakdown, facet joint stiffness, dysphagia, and loss of reduction (19,53). Additional major

halo-related complications include a documented decrease in pulmonary function, brain abscess, hygiene problems, and difficulty interpreting follow-up radiographs (54–57). Glaser and co-workers evaluated 245 patients who wore a halo and found a complication rate of 26%, with 23 patients losing reduction and 24 patients with an unstable cervical spine despite 3 months in the halo (53). Pin-site infections, cerebrospinal fluid leak from a pin site, and death from pneumonia also occurred. Garfin and colleagues evaluated 179 patients in a halo and found that 36% had pin loosening, 20% had pin-site infections, 11% had pressure sores under the vest, and 18% had severe pin site discomfort (58). They also documented nerve injury, dural penetration, dysphagia, and cosmetically disfiguring scars. Recently, new-onset generalized tonic-clonic seizures were found to be due to an epileptic focus of scar tissue in the brain that developed secondary to halo pin penetration of the skull in a 29-year-old man treated in a halo for a C7 fracture without spinal cord deficit (59).

The management of dens fractures in the elderly patient deserves special mention. Although some investigators have not found age to be a risk factor for nonunion with halo immobilization (14,26,47,60), many others have noted a significant effect of age on outcome (16,19,27,48,49,61). Dunn and Seljeskog reported a 78% nonunion rate with halo immobilization in patients aged 65 years or older with a type II dens fracture (48). Pepin and colleagues found a nonunion rate of 54% in elderly patients treated nonoperatively and reported a high rate of complications with external immobilization (16). Ryan and Taylor reviewed 35 patients older than 60 years with a type II dens fracture treated nonoperatively and found a nonunion in 77% (27). Seybold and Bayley found that patients over 60 years of age with a dens fracture had a higher complication rate and lower cervical range of motion when treated with a halo (26). In a case-control study, Lennarson and co-workers found that patients older than 50 years were 21 times more disposed to failure of halo immobilization than patients younger than 50 years of age (24). Primary surgical treatment of type II fractures has been advocated in this group with increased risk for nonunion to decrease in-hospital mortality and avoid higher complication rates associated with halo use in elderly patients (16,24,27,28,59, 62). Bednar and associates reported an in-hospital mortality rate of 42% in 19 patients aged 50 years and older treated nonoperatively with a halo for a type II dens fracture without neurologic deficit (28). With a prospective protocol of early surgical stabilization and no halo immobilization postoperatively, these investigators were able to decrease the in-hospital mortality rate to 0% in this elderly population. Hanigan and colleagues also documented the dangers of treating older patients (≥80 years) nonoperatively (63). They defined a primary in-hospital mortality rate of 26.3% in 19 patients without spinal cord injury, with substantial respiratory complications in 33% of survivors treated with recumbency. They reported no morbidity or mortality in older patients treated with a primary surgical C1-C2 arthrodesis. Muller and colleagues also reviewed the management of dens fractures in elderly patients (64). They found the in-hospital mortality rate in patients 70 years and older treated nonoperatively to be 38% with a complication rate of 61%, whereas only 33% of the patients younger than 70 years experienced a complication. Their operative procedure of choice was anterior dens screw fixation. They recommend that elderly patients undergo early internal stabilization. Bednar and associates concluded that an aggressive primarily applied surgical management protocol significantly decreases and potentially eliminates in-hospital mortality in elderly and debilitated type II dens process fracture patients (28).

When a dens nonunion develops, either due to failure of conservative treatment or as a late presentation, some authors recommend operative intervention to prevent the development of late myelopathy (50,65). Alternatively, Hart and co-workers recently reported on five asymptomatic elderly patients with a mobile dens nonunion, who were managed conservatively in a Philadelphia collar; none developed a neurologic deficit through their latest follow-up (66). Some authors have recommended using a Philadelphia collar in elderly patients with an acute type II dens fracture because of the major complications reported with halo immobilization in this population. Polin and colleagues retrospectively evaluated the success rates of halo and Philadelphia collar treatment for 36 type II dens fractures (67). Twenty patients had a halo, whereas 16 were immobilized in a collar. The success rate of those in a halo was 74%, but only 53% healed in a cervical collar. The authors reported that no significant difference existed between these two groups based on the numbers available (67). In a classic study, Johnson and associates clearly demonstrated the superiority of the halo vest over all other external immobilization devices in limiting motion at the occipitocervical junction (52). The halo vest was found to limit 75% of flexion-extension motion at C1-C2, whereas the best cervical brace restricted only 45% (52).

Most scientific evidence focused on the appropriate treatment of the elderly patient with a type II dens fracture is class III data from poorly controlled retrospective case reviews. The only series that we are aware of that provides class II evidence (from a case-control study) is from Lennarson and colleagues (24). Because of the very high rate of complications and failure from nonoperative halo immobilization, they recommended surgical intervention in patients 50 years or older if it could be accomplished with acceptable risk for morbidity.

Operative

Because of the relatively high rates of nonunion associated with nonoperative management of these injuries, many investigators have recommended primary internal fixation for these fractures believed to be at high risk for nonunion (14,15,20–22,30,47,48,68). This includes type II and shallow type III fractures with substantial initial displacement (greater than 4 to 6 mm), most subtype IIA fractures (30), posterior fracture displacement, fracture angulation of more than 10 degrees, patient age more than 40 to 50 years, and inability to obtain or maintain a stable reduction. Additionally, surgical intervention may be warranted in a polytrauma patient, a patient with a spinal cord injury, and a patient unable to tolerate a halo and redisplacement despite halo immobilization. Ideally, the use of internal fixation in the treatment of dens fractures should provide immediate stability, allow rapid patient mobilization, improve rates of successful arthrodesis, and minimize the requirement of rigid external immobilization. This may be achieved by posterior atlantoaxial arthrodesis or direct anterior dens internal fixation.

C1-C2 Arthrodesis

Traditional methods of atlantoaxial arthrodesis (AAA) include posterior C1-C2 wiring constructs such as the Gallie (69), Brooks-Jenkins (70), or interspinous method (71). Because of the substantial mobility of the C1-C2 segment, most reported studies have been performed using supplemental halo-vest immobilization with these techniques to improve fusion rates (69,71–75). Documented failure rates for AAA with these methods have subsequently ranged from 3% to 80% (14,19,21,28,71–76). Biomechanical studies have demonstrated that the Brooks-type fixation, with its wedge-compression grafting and sublaminar wire position at C2, is more stable than the modified Gallie methods (75,77,78). Posterior C1-C2 wiring constructs, however, may loosen after cyclical loading and allow substantial increases in C1-C2 rotational and translational motion (75, 79). Intraoperative reduction sometimes is lost during the healing period. Especially prone to failure are posterior displaced odontoid fractures treated with posterior wire technique (Fig. 87.2). Clinical series have demonstrated little difference in fusion rates obtained between these two methods (14,49,70,72,80). Flexible cables have increased the ease of sublaminar wire passage, and their use may thus decrease the rate of iatrogenic neurologic deficit during wire passage, reported to be 5% to 7% (72,74). As noted previously, dens fractures often occur with concomitant atlas fractures; a deficient C1 posterior arch prevents use of these AAA methods.

In 1979, Magerl and Seemann (81) described the posterior C1-C2 transarticular screw fixation technique as an alternative in the surgical management of patients with atlantoaxial instability. This method requires an anatomic reduction intraoperatively to avoid complications of vertebral artery injury, neurologic deficit, and inadequate bony purchase. A precise drill trajectory is needed, entering at the posterior cortex of the C2 inferior articular process about 2 mm above the C2-C3 facet joint and 2 to 3 mm lateral to the medial border of the C2-C3 facet. This is then directed superiorly, down the axis of the C2 pars, aiming toward the

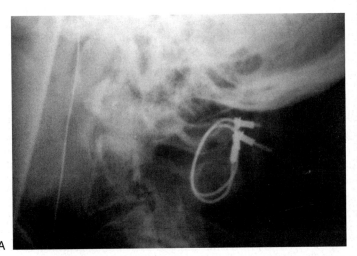
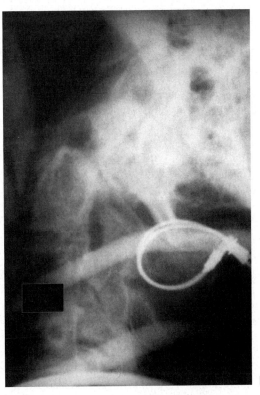

FIG. 87.2. **A:** Postoperative lateral x-ray of Brooks-type C1-C2 arthrodesis with anatomic reduction of the type II dens fracture. **B:** Six-week postoperative x-ray with posterior displacement of the dens fracture.

anterior arch of C1 (as viewed in a lateral image), with a 0- to 10-degree medial angulation. This is performed under biplane fluoroscopic imaging or with the use of a frameless stereotactic image-guidance system. This method of internal fixation does not require an intact posterior arch of C1 but, when used in conjunction with a posterior C1-C2 wiring, creates a very rigid three-point fixation system, providing immediate multidirectional stability (77,82). Biomechanical studies have demonstrated this method of internal fixation to be more rigid than posterior wiring techniques, particularly in rotation, where transarticular screws were noted to be 10-fold stiffer (77,82,83). Clinical results have reported fusion rates of up to 100% with this method of AAA, along with the additional advantage that it avoids the need for any supplemental halo-vest immobilization (76,81,84,85). As previously discussed, C1-C2 transarticular screws may be contraindicated unilaterally in up to 18% because of anomalous vertebral artery anatomy (9). However, Song and co-workers noted a 95% fusion rate among patients who underwent unilateral transarticular screw fixation due to anatomic constraints (86). Grob and associates (85), in one of the largest series studying transarticular C1-C2 screws, reported no instance of vertebral artery or spinal cord injury, a 6% rate of other screw-related complications, and a pseudarthrosis rate of less than 1%. However, despite its clinical and biomechanical advantages, this technique is technically demanding. In one recent survey, the risk for vertebral artery injury with this method was 4%, although the risk for subsequent neurologic deficit after vascular injury was reported to be only 0.2% (87).

An alternative technique for atlantoaxial instrumentation entails placing a screw into the lateral mass of the atlas and connecting it with a rod to a pedicle screw in C2 (88,89). The advantages of this method include the ability to obtain stable internal fixation without first anatomically reducing the atlantoaxial articulation and more easily avoiding a high-riding vertebral artery groove in C2. Because the C2 pedicle screw can be inserted in the mediocranial aspect of C2, it is further away from the vertebral artery groove than a transarticular screw, which must be started more inferolaterally in the posterior aspect of C2. Also, the C1-C2 articulation must be anatomically reduced before implanting the transarticular screw. With this rigid screw-rod construct between C1 and C2, patients can be mobilized without a halo postoperatively just as those treated with transarticular screw fixation.

Regardless of technique, AAA is an indirect method of treating atlantoaxial instability secondary to odontoid fractures (unless accompanied by an associated transverse atlantal ligament injury). Because of the functionally important mobility provided by the C1-C2 articulation, AAA will result in some decreased cervical range of motion postoperatively.

Studies have indicated restricted motion of 30 to 50 degrees, particularly with 50% loss of axial rotation (90–92).

Anterior Dens Screw Fixation

An alternative approach to AAA is that of anterior dens screw fixation, initially described independently by Nakanishi (93) and Bohler (94) in the early 1980s. Direct anterior osteosynthesis of the dens can provide immediate postoperative stability, while preserving C1-C2 motion. Henry and colleagues reported on 61 patients with dens fractures who underwent anterior dens screw fixation (95). Of these, 71% showed a full cervical range of motion postoperatively, whereas only 10% had a decrease of greater than 25%. Jeanneret and co-workers found that 39% of their dens screw patients retained completely normal atlantoaxial mobility in a postoperative CT scan study (91). Similar to AAA with C1-C2 transarticular screws, anterior dens screw fixation has demonstrated a high clinical success rate (85% to 100%) without the need for supplemental halo-vest immobilization (23,45,68,94). Additional advantages of anterior screw fixation over posterior AAA methods are that anterior odontoid instrumentation does not require autologous bone graft harvest [which itself may be associated with complication rates approaching 20% to 30% (90,96,97)], nor does it require an intact posterior C1 arch. Before proceeding with anterior dens screw fixation, an anatomic reduction of the fracture must be obtained (90,98). This may be assessed preoperatively with lateral radiographs or fluoroscopic imaging after reduction techniques with Gardner-Wells tong traction; inability to achieve an anatomic reduction is a contraindication to this procedure (99).

Under biplane fluoroscopy, anatomic reduction is obtained. Depending on the amount of flexion required for reduction, the anteroposterior view might be best shot through the mouth. If appropriate, a radiolucent bite block or a wad of gauze in the mouth can facilitate the visualization of the odontoid. A Steinman pin is placed alongside the neck to ensure proper trajectory under lateral fluoroscopy while clearing the sternum. The cervical spine may need to be protracted (translated anteriorly), while keeping the occipitocervical junction in a reduced position in order to clear the chest.

The surgical approach for this method involves a standard anterior Smith-Robinson approach to the C5-C6 level through a transverse skin incision. Blunt dissection is accomplished cephalad to the C2-C3 disc. The entry point is in the anterior aspect of the inferior end plate of C2. A 2.5-mm drill bit is directed through the center of the dens, exiting the cortical tip of the dens. The body fragment is then overdrilled with a 3.5-mm bit up to, but not across, the fracture. A 3.5-mm tap is placed through the gliding hole to the fracture, and the dens fragment is tapped, including the strong cortex at the tip. One 3.5-mm fully threaded cortical screw is pushed through the gliding hole, engaging the dens

fragment. The proper screw length is important to accomplish a lag effect. As the screw head contacts the strong cortical inferior end plate, pulling the dens fragment down, compression occurs across the fracture. A cannulated technique may be used, but meticulous attention to the possibility of the K wire shearing, binding, and driving into spinal canal is necessary to avoid complications.

Starting the screw in the anterior cortex of C2 leads to an increased risk for failure by screw cutout as a result of the previously discussed odontoid bone anatomy with poor hypodense cancellous bone in the midbody of C2 (2). Also, by starting the screw in the anterior body of C2, a shallow trajectory across the fracture site usually results in very poor purchase in the dens fragment (Fig. 87.3). To obtain the appropriate steep trajectory, this procedure requires manipulation of instruments nearly parallel to the long axis of the cervical spine under biplane fluoroscopic guidance. As such, ideal drill trajectory can be hindered by certain body habitus and are relative contraindications to this technique, including morbid obesity, large "barrel chest," short neck, fixed kyphosis at the cervicothoracic junction, and fracture patterns that require a flexed position to obtain reduction (91,99).

Because of the cervical extension that may be required during this procedure, caution must be exercised when dealing with elderly patients who may have significant cervical spondylosis and stenosis. Relative contraindications also include osteoporosis and an established nonunion. It is imperative that the dens process is perfectly visualized on both the anteroposterior and lateral intraoperative fluoroscopic views. Osteopenia combined with dental implants and the requirement to hyperflex or extend the neck to obtain reduction may cause substantial difficulty in obtaining an appropriate anteroposterior image. The procedure should be abandoned if radiographic visualization is not satisfactory and posterior C1-C2 fusion may be contemplated. Excellent visualization of the dens in both planes is mandatory.

Although some initial studies favored anterior dens screw fixation using two screws (45,94,98), several more recent reports have demonstrated the adequacy and safety of using only one screw (18,68,100). Compared with one-screw fixation, the placement of two screws is technically more difficult and offers no biomechanical advantage, as demonstrated by Sasso and associates (18) and others (68, 90,100). In a biomechanical dens fracture model, stability after internal fixation was 50% that of the unfractured dens, regardless of whether one or two 3.5-mm screws were used (18); accurate reduction of the odontoid fracture bed provides stability in excess of the isolated strength of the screw (10). Therefore, it is important to engage the far cortex of the dens tip, to ensure secure purchase and the ability to create interfragmentary compression across the fracture site. This lag effect may be achieved by overdrilling the proximal fragment (gliding hole) and using a fully threaded

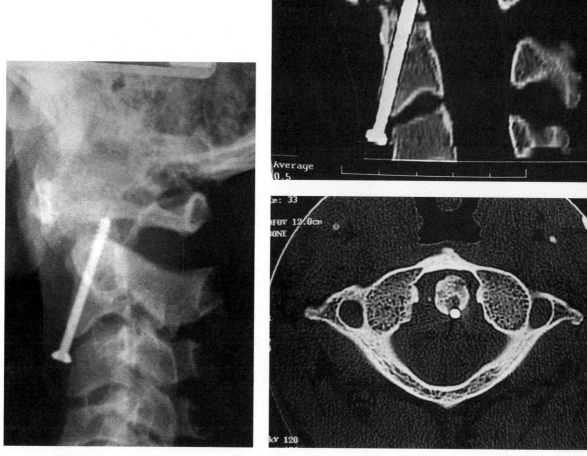

FIG. 87.3. A: Postoperative lateral x-ray after anterior odontoid screw performed with very poor entry site. The screw was started too anterior in the very weak anterior body of C2. When started in this manner, the trajectory across the fracture is too flat. **B:** Sagittal CT reconstruction demonstrating the poor purchase in the odontoid fragment when this anterior entry point is used. **C:** Axial CT scan showing the excessive posterior position of the screw in the odontoid fragment. With the horizontal trajectory across the fracture, the screw cannot obtain purchase into the tip of the odontoid where the strong cortical bone is present. Notice the cutout of the screw posteriorly due to the poor bone quality in the base of the odontoid process.

screw or a partially threaded "lag" screw (in which case great care must be taken to ensure that none of the threads cross the fracture line, thus preventing compression). If a partially threaded lag screw is used, a high fracture may not allow the threads to be completely contained in the dens fragment. These threads across the fracture site will keep the fracture fragments distracted. The tip of a partially threaded screw may be cut to shorten the length of threads if too long.

Type II injuries with an oblique fracture line extending from posterosuperior to anteroinferior in the sagittal plane are also a relative contraindication to this technique. Inter-

fragmentary compression in this instance leads to shear forces across the fracture, which may cause anterior displacement of the odontoid fragment (45). This complication can be avoided by driving the screw through a one-hole plate or washer to buttress the odontoid fragment as the screw is seated.

Several series reporting on anterior dens screw fixation have demonstrated an aggregate fusion rate of 94.5% along with a low complication rate, 2% screw malposition, 1.5% screw breakout, and no incidence of neurologic or vascular injury (45,90,94,99,101). In the presence of associated transverse atlantal ligament injury, anterior odontoid screw

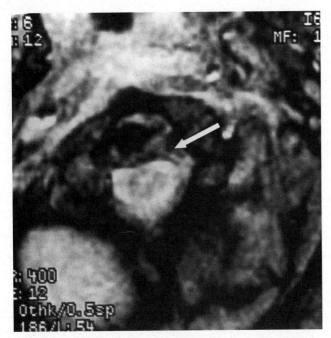

FIG. 87.4. Preoperative axial MRI with a disrupted transverse atlantal ligament. This is a contraindication for isolated anterior odontoid screw internal fixation to prevent the complication of atlantoaxial instability after odontoid instrumentation.

fixation will not restore atlantoaxial stability (42). Therefore, this should be carefully assessed preoperatively with MRI (Fig. 87.4) or under controlled flexion-extension dynamic fluoroscopic imaging intraoperatively after anterior odontoid screw fixation (21,40,42).

CONCLUSION

The management of type II dens fractures is difficult and fraught with complications. Both operative and nonoperative treatment may lead to major complications, and the appropriate treatment is dependent on many factors and characteristics of the patient and the surgeon. Patient age, fracture pattern, amount of displacement, associated injuries, anatomic and fracture characteristics, and surgeon experience are all very important. Acute type II or high (with a shallow base) type III dens fractures with greater than 6 mm of initial radiographic displacement have a very high prevalence of nonunion despite immobilization in a halo for 3 months. Direct anterior screw fixation of a dens fracture results in very high primary healing rates without the complications of halo immobilization and bone graft donor site morbidity. If anatomic closed reduction is possible, it is reasonable to consider direct fixation of the fracture. Because anterior dens screw stabilization is not highly effective for established nonunions, if halo treatment fails, then the only surgical alternative is posterior C1-C2 arthrodesis with subsequent loss of 50% of cervical axial rotation. Although the data for the use of an anterior odontoid screw

for the treatment of acute type II fractures are compelling, there does not exist a prospective study critically assessing the results. A prospective, controlled study is needed to solve this dilemma definitively.

REFERENCES

1. White AA, Panjabe MM. The clinical biomechanics of the occipito-atlantal complex. *Orthop Clin North Am* 1978;9:867–878.
2. Heggeness MH, Doherty BJ. The trabecular anatomy of the axis. *Spine* 1993;18:1945–1949.
3. Doherty BJ, Heggeness MH. Quantitative anatomy of the second cervical vertebra. *Spine* 1995;20:513–517.
4. Heller JG, Alson MD, Schaffler MB, et al. Quantitative internal dens morphology. *Spine* 1992;17:861–866.
5. Schaffler MB, Alson MD, Heller JG, et al. Morphology of the dens: a quantitative study. *Spine* 1992;17:738–743.
6. Schiff DC, Parke WW. Arterial supply of the odontoid process. *J Bone Joint Surg Am* 1973;55:1450–1456.
7. Althoff B. Fracture of the odontoid process: an experimental study. *Acta Orthop Scand* 1979;177S:1–95.
8. Schatzker J, Rorabeck CH, Waddell JP. Nonunion of the odontoid process: an experimental investigation. *Clin Orthop* 1975;108:127–133.
9. Paramore CG, Dickman CA, Sonntag VKH. The anatomic suitability of the C1/C2 complex for transarticular screw fixation. *J Neurosurg* 1996;95:221–224.
10. Doherty BJ, Heggeness, MH, Esses SI. A biomechanical study of odontoid fractures and fracture fixation. *Spine* 1993;18:178–184.
11. Mouradin WH, Fietti VG, Cochran GVB, et al. Fractures of the odontoid: a laboratory and clinical study of mechanisms. *Orthop Clin North Am* 1978;9:985–1001.
12. Przybylski GJ. Management of odontoid fractures. *Contemp Spine Surg* 2000;1:21–25.
13. Sherk HH, et al., and the Cervical Spine Research Society, eds. *The cervical spine*. Philadelphia: JB Lippincott, 1989.
14. Clark CR, White AA. Fractures of the dens: a multicenter study. *J Bone Joint Surg Am* 1985;67:1340–1348.
15. Southwick WO. Current concepts review: the management of fractures of the dens. *J Bone Joint Surg Am* 1980;62:482–486.
16. Pepin JW, Bourne RB, Hawkins RJ. Odontoid fractures, with special reference to the elderly patient. *Clin Orthop* 1985;193:178–183.
17. Puttlitz CM, Goel VK, Clark CR, et al. Pathomechanisms of failures of the odontoid. *Spine* 2000;25:2868–2876.
18. Sasso RC, Doherty BJ, Crawford MJ, et al. Biomechanics of odontoid fracture fixation: comparison of the one- and two-screw technique. *Spine* 1993;18:1950–1953.
19. Appuzo ML, Heiden JS, Weiss MH, et al. Acute fractures of the odontoid process. *J Neurosurg* 1978;48:85–91.
20. Anderson LD, D'Alonzo RT. Fractures of the odontoid process of the axis. *J Bone Joint Surg Am* 1974;56:1663–1674.
21. Chutkan NB, King AG, Harris MB. Odontoid fractures: Evaluation and management. *J Am Acad Orthop Surg* 1997;5:199–204.
22. Greene KA, Dickman CA, Marciano FF, et al. Acute axis fractures: analysis of management and outcomes. *Spine* 1997;22:1843–1852.
23. Marchesi D. Management of odontoid fractures. *Orthopedics* 1997;20:911–916.
24. Lennarson PJ, Mostafavi H, Traynelis VC, et al. Management of type II dens fractures: a case-control study. *Spine* 2000;25:1234–1237.
25. Ryan MD, Taylor TF. Odontoid fractures: a rational approach to treatment. *J Bone Joint Surg Br* 1982;64:416–421.
26. Seybold EA, Bayley JC. Functional outcome of surgically and conservatively managed dens fractures. *Spine* 1998;23:1837–1846.
27. Ryan MD, Taylor TK. Odontoid fractures in the elderly. *J Spinal Disord* 1993;6:397–401.
28. Bednar D, Parikh J, Hummel J. Management of type II odontoid process fractures in geriatric patients. *J Spinal Disord* 1995;8:166–169.
29. Scott EW, Haid RW, Peace D. Type I fractures of the odontoid process: implications for atlantoaxial instability. *J Neurosurg* 1990;72:488–492.
30. Hadley MN, Browner CM, Liu SS, et al. New subtype of acute odontoid fractures (IIA). *Neurosurgery* 1988;22:67–71.

31. Hu RW. Evaluation and assessment of the polytrauma patient for spinal injuries. In: Kellam JF, Fischer TJ, Tornetta P, et al., eds. *Orthopaedic knowledge update: trauma II.* Rosemont, IL: American Academy of Orthopaedic Surgeons, 2000:319–328.

32. Walter J, Doris PE, Shaffer MA. Clinical presentation of patients with acute spinal cord injury. *Ann Emerg Med* 1984;13:512–515.

33. Spain DA, Trooskin S, Flancbaum L, et al. The adequacy and cost effectiveness of routine resuscitation-area cervical spine radiographs. *Ann Emerg Med* 1990;19:276–278.

34. Vandemark RM. Radiology of the cervical spine in trauma patients. *AJR Am J Roentgenol* 1990;155:465–472.

35. Schaffer M, Doris P. Limitation of the cross table lateral view in detecting cervical spine injuries. *Ann Emerg Med* 1981;10:1065–1070.

36. Holliman C, Mayer J, Cook R, et al. Is the AP radiograph of the cervical spine necessary in the evaluation of trauma? *Ann Emerg Med* 1990;19:483–484.

37. Vaccaro AR, An HS, Sun S, et al. Noncontiguous injuries of the spine. *J Spinal Disord* 1992;5:320–329.

38. Blacksin MF, Lee J. Frequency and significance of fractures of the upper cervical spine detected by CT in patients with severe neck trauma. *AJR Am J Roentgenol* 1995;165:1201–1204.

39. Blacksin MF, Avagliano P. Computed tomographic and magnetic resonance imaging of chronic odontoid fractures. *Spine* 1999;24:158–162.

40. Harris MB, Waguespack AM, Kronlage S. Clearing cervical spine injuries in polytrauma patients. *Orthopedics* 1997;20:903–907.

41. Dickman CA, Mamourian A, Sonntag VKH. Magnetic resonance imaging of the transverse atlantal ligament for the evaluation of atlantoaxial instability. *J Neurosurg* 1991;71:642–647.

42. Greene KA, Dickman CA, Marciano FF, et al. Transverse atlantal ligament disruption associated with odontoid fractures. *Spine* 1994;19:2307–2314.

43. Hadley MN, Browner C, Sonntag VKH. Axis fractures: a comprehensive review of management and treatment in 107 cases. *Neurosurgery* 1985;17:281–290.

44. Wang GJ, Mabie KN, Whitehill R, et al. The nonsurgical management of odontoid fracture in adults. *Spine* 1984;9:229–233.

45. Aebi M, Etter C, Coscia M. Fractures of the odontoid process: treatment with anterior screw fixation. *Spine* 1989;14:1065–1070.

46. Bucholz RW, Burkhead WZ. The pathological anatomy of fatal atlanto–occipital dislocations. *J Bone Joint Surg Am* 1979;61:248–250.

47. Hadley MA, Dickman CA, Browner CM, et al. Acute axis fractures. *J Neurosurg* 1989;71:642–647.

48. Dunn ME, Seljeskog EL. Experience in the management of odontoid process injuries. *Neurosurgery* 1986;18:306–310.

49. Schatzker J, Rorabeck CH, Waddell JP. Fracture of the dens: an analysis of 37 cases. *J Bone Joint Surg Br* 1971;53:392–404.

50. Crockard HA, Heilman AE, Stevens JM. Progressive myelopathy secondary to odontoid fractures. Clinical, radiological and surgical features. *J Neurosurg* 1993;78:579–586.

51. Lynch JJ, Duke DA, Krauss WE. Remote development of cervicomedullary dysfunction after untreated odontoid type II fractures [Abstract]. 13th Annual North American Spine Society, October 1998.

52. Johnson R, Hart D, Simmons E. Cervical orthoses: a study comparing their effectiveness in restricting cervical motion in normal subjects. *J Bone Joint Surg Am* 1977;59:332–339.

53. Glaser JA, Whitehill R, Stamp W, et al. Complications associated with the halo vest: a review of 245 cases. *J Neurosurg* 1986;65:762–769.

54. Clark CR. *The cervical spine,* 3rd ed. Philadelphia: Lippincott-Raven, 1998:415–429.

55. Vaccaro AR, Madigan L, Ehrler DM. Contemporary management of adult odontoid fractures. *Orthopedics* 2000;23:1109–1113.

56. Rosenblum D, Ehrlich L. Brain abscess and psychosis as a complication of a halo orthosis. *Arch Phys Med Rehabil* 1995;76:865–867.

57. Lind BL, Bake B, Lundquist C, et al. Influence of halo vest treatment on vital capacity. *Spine* 1987;12:449–452.

58. Garfin SR, Botte MJ, Waters RL, et al. Complications in the use of the halo fixation device. *J Bone Joint Surg Am* 1986;68:320–325.

59. Nottmeier EW, Bondurant CP. Delayed onset of generalized tonic-clonic seizures as a complication of halo orthosis. Case report. *J Neurosurg* 2000;92:233–235.

60. Schweigel JF. Management of the fractured odontoid with halo-thoracic bracing. *Spine* 1987;12:838–839.

61. Ekong C, Schwartz ML, Tator CH, et al. Odontoid fracture: management with early mobilization using the halo device. *Neurosurgery* 1981;9:631–637.

62. Weller SJ, Malek AM, Rossitch E. Cervical spine fractures in the elderly. *Surg Neurol* 1997;47:274–280.

63. Hanigan WC, Powell FC, Elwood PW, et al. Odontoid fractures in elderly patients. *J Neurosurg* 1993;78:32–35.

64. Muller EJ, Wick M, Russe O, et al. Management of odontoid fractures in the elderly. *Eur Spine J* 1999;8:360–365.

65. Paradis G, Jane J. Posttraumatic atlantoaxial instability: the fate of the odontoid process fracture in 46 cases. *J Trauma* 1973;13:359–366.

66. Hart R, Saterbak A, Rapp T, et al. Nonoperative management of dens fracture nonunion in elderly patients without myelopathy. *Spine* 2000;25:1339–1343.

67. Polin RS, Szabo T, Bogaeu CA, et al. Nonoperative management of types II and III odontoid fractures: the Philadelphia collar versus halo vest. *Neurosurgery* 1996;38:450–456.

68. Jenkins JD, Coric D, Branch CL. A clinical comparison of one- and two-screw odontoid fixation. *J Neurosurg* 1998;89:366–370.

69. Gallie WE. Fracture and dislocations of the cervical spine. *Am J Surg* 1939;46:495–499.

70. Brooks AL, Jenkins EB. Atlantoaxial arthrodesis by the wedge compression method. *J Bone Joint Surg Am* 1978;60:279–284.

71. Dickman CA, Papadopoulos SM, Sonntag VK, et al. The interspinous method of posterior atlanto-axial arthrodesis. *J Neurosurg* 1991;74:190–198.

72. Fielding JW, Hawkins RJ, Ratzan SA. Spine fusion for atlanto-axial instability. *J Bone Joint Surg Am* 1976;58:400–407.

73. Fried LC. Atlanto-axial fractures. Failure of posterior C1 to C2 fusion. *J Bone Joint Surg Br* 1973;55:490–496.

74. Griswold DM, Albright JA, Schiffman E. Atlantoaxial fusion for instability. *J Bone Joint Surg Am* 1978;60:258–292.

75. Dickman CA, Crawford NR, Paramore CG. Biomechanical characteristics of C1-C2 cable fixations. *J Neurosurg* 1996;85:316–321.

76. Coyne TJ, Fehlings MG, Wallace CM. C1-C2 posterior cervical fusion: long-term evaluation of results and efficacy. *Neurosurgery* 1995;37:688–692.

77. Grob D, Crisco JJ, Panjabi MM, et al. Biomechanical evaluation of four different posterior atlanto-axial fixation techniques. *Spine* 1992;17:480–490.

78. Hajeck PD, Lipka J, Hartline P, et al. Biomechanical study of C1-C2 posterior arthrodesis techniques. *Spine* 1993;18:173–177.

79. Crawford NR, Hurlbert RJ, Choi WG, et al. Differential biomechanical effects of injury and wiring at C1-C2. *Spine* 1999;24:1894–1902.

80. Waddell JP, Reardon GP. Atlantoaxial arthrodesis to treat odontoid fractures. *Can J Surg* 1983;26:255–258.

81. Magerl F, Seeman PS. Stable posterior fusion at the atlas and axis by transarticular fixation. In: Kehr P, Weidner A, eds. *Cervical spine I.* New York: Springer-Verlag, 1985:322–327.

82. Hanson PB, Montesano PX, Sharkey NA, et al. Anatomic and biomechanical assessment of transarticular screw fixation for atlanto-axial instability. *Spine* 1991;16:1141–1145.

83. Jeanneret B, Magerl F. Primary posterior fusion C1/C2 in odontoid fractures: indications, techniques and results of transarticular screw fixation. *J Spinal Disord* 1992;5:464–475.

84. Marcotte P, Dickman CA, Sonntag VK, et al. Posterior atlantoaxial screw fixation. *J Neurosurg* 1993;79:234–237.

85. Grob D, Jeanneret B, Aebi M, et al. Atlantoaxial fusion with transarticular screw fixation. *J Bone Joint Surg Br* 1991;73:972–976.

86. Song GS, Theodore N, Dickman CA, et al. Unilateral posterior atlantoaxial transarticular screw fixation. *J Neurosurg* 1997;87:851–855.

87. Wright NM, Lauryssen C. Vertebral artery injury in C1/C2 transarticular screw fixation: results of a survey of the AANS/CNS section on disorders of the spine and peripheral nerves. *J Neurosurg* 1998;88:634–640.

88. Melcher RP, Ruf M, Harms J. The direct posterior C1-C2 fusion technique with polyaxial head screws. Twenty-eighth Annual Meeting Cervical Spine Research Society. Charleston, SC, November 30–December 2, 2000.

89. Christensen DM, Lynch J, Currei, R, et al. C1 anatomy and dimensions relative to lateral mass screw placement. Twenty-eighth Annual

Meeting Cervical Spine Research Society. Charleston, SC, November 30–December 2, 2000.

90. Subach BR, Morone MA, Haid RW, et al. Management of acute odontoid fractures with single-screw anterior fixation. *Neurosurgery* 1999; 45:812–819.

91. Jeanneret B, Vernet O, Frei S, et al. Atlantoaxial mobility after screw fixation of the odontoid: a computerized tomographic study. *J Spinal Disord* 1991;4:203–211.

92. Penning L. Normal movements of the cervical spine. *AJR Am J Roentgenol* 1979;130:317–326.

93. Nakanishi T. Internal fixation of odontoid fractures. *Orthop Trauma Surg* 1980;23:399–406.

94. Bohler J. Anterior stabilization for acute fractures and nonunions of the dens. *J Bone Joint Surg Am* 1982;64:18–27.

95. Henry AD, Bohl J, Grosse A. Fixation of odontoid fractures by an anterior screw. *J Bone Joint Surg Br* 1999;81:472–477.

96. Fernyhough J, Schmandle J, Weigel M, et al. Chronic donor site pain complicating bone graft harvesting from the posterior iliac crest for spinal fusion. *Spine* 1992;17:1474–1480.

97. Younger E, Chapman M. Morbidity at bone graft donor sites. *J Orthop Trauma* 1989;3:192–195.

98. Geisler F, Cheng C, Poka A, et al. Anterior screw fixation of posteriorly displaced type II odontoid fractures. *Neurosurgery* 1989;25:30–38.

99. Sasso RC, Reilly TM. Odontoid and hangman's fractures. In: Kellam JF, Fischer TJ, Tornetta P, et al., eds. *Orthopaedic knowledge update: trauma II.* Rosemont, IL: American Academy of Orthopaedic Surgeons, 2000:337–346.

100. Graziano G, Jaggers C, Lee M, et al. A comparative study of fixation techniques for type II fractures of the odontoid process. *Spine* 1993; 18:2283–2387.

101. Montesano PX, Anderson PA, Schehr F, et al. Odontoid fractures treated by anterior odontoid screw fixation. *Spine* 1991;16:533–537.

CHAPTER 88

Management of Symptomatic Cervical Pseudarthrosis

William C. Welch, Peter C. Gerszten, Arthur P. Nestler, and James P. Burke

In the fifth edition of Astley Cooper's *Treatise on Dislocations and Fractures of the Joints* published in 1842, observations were reported that are fully valid even today. On the development of a nonunion and of false joints, he wrote the following: "There is no difficulty, for example, in understanding that the materials effused for the consolidation of a fracture can never be converted into a bony callus, if subjected to frequent motion and disturbance." He recommends the following to the doctor engaged in healing a nonunion: "to ensure all the mechanical conditions which are essential for the consolidation of callus, comprising perfect rest and immobility, and contact and pressure of the broken surfaces against each other." Nine years before the discovery of x-rays, Bruns recommended the following classification of disturbed fracture union: (a) delayed consolidation, and (b) pseudarthrosis. Witt, in 1952, recommended autogenous bone transplantation as that operation for pseudarthroses that promises the greatest success (1). In 1955, Robinson and Smith first described anterior cervical arthrodesis (2). In 1962, Robinson and colleagues reported on four patients with symptomatic pseudarthrosis of an anterior cervical arthrodesis. Revision surgery was performed and was successful in three of the four patients (3).

Pseudarthrosis is a potential complication that can occur after attempted arthrodesis of the cervical spine. The prevalence of pseudarthrosis is variable and depends on type and severity of pathology, surgical technique, use of immobilization, instrumentation, and host factors (4). Although in some cases the pseudarthrosis may not cause substantial symptoms, patients who have abnormal movement at the surgical site may experience severe neck pain along with radicular or myelopathic signs or symptoms. The treatment options in management of symptomatic cervical pseudarthrosis should include a continuum of intervention, from pain manage-

ment to possible surgical repair to rehabilitation. Numerous considerations are important with regard to these treatment options. These include whether the patient smokes, the number of involved vertebral levels, and what surgical approach, technique, and materials were used. Management should focus on circumvention of those variables that may prevent optimal individual care.

DEFINITION

Derived from Greek, *pseudarthrosis* literally means "false joint." Strictly speaking, a pseudarthrosis is not a false joint. The term implies the persistence of a motion segment resulting from failure of bony fusion (5). When looking at a cervical pseudarthrosis as a failure to achieve bony union, a number of integral factors should be considered. The surgical approach (anterior vs. posterior), the type of bone graft (autogenous vs. allograft), the number of vertebral levels involved, and the type of instrumentation can all affect the success of interbody cervical fusion. The patient's postoperative course, compliance with activity restriction as well as with the external immobilization, and proclivity for cigarette smoking may be factors effecting fusion. The importance of these factors has been, and most likely will continue to be, debated. Nonetheless, they deserve consideration when investigating fusion failure, especially when considering surgical repair of a symptomatic cervical pseudarthrosis. A cervical pseudarthrosis is generally considered symptomatic when a patient complains of cervical pain, which may be in conjunction with radicular or myelopathic symptoms. It is therefore important to note that even though the impact of a pseudarthrosis on the clinical outcome is questionable, and that its full clinical implication remains controversial, its role in postoperative morbidity is well documented (6,7).

Fusion can be defined as no abnormal motion, no lucency, and the presence of bony trabeculation at the operative site (8). Pseudarthrosis without motion, or fibrous union, indicates no abnormal motion, lucency, and no trabeculation or bony bridging. Pseudarthrosis with motion, or instability, refers to the presence of abnormal motion, lucency, and no trabeculation (9). Instability involves the spine's loss of ability to maintain normal vertebral relationships under a physiologic load, in such a way that the spine no longer prevents damage to the cord or nerve roots or prevents incapacitating deformity or pain. Successful spinal arthrodesis requires a local environment that has sufficient surface area of decorticated host bone, sufficient graft material, absence of excessive motion, and a rich vascular supply. Failure to provide such an environment increases the risk for pseudarthrosis (10).

DIAGNOSIS

Even with radiographic evidence of a cervical pseudarthrosis, if the spinal cord and nerve roots are not compromised, the patient may be asymptomatic. Radiographic diagnosis alone would not be a sufficient indication for operative intervention. After an anterior cervical discectomy, the bone graft may increase the size of the neural foramen, acting as a spacer, thus relieving nerve root compression. The decision to reoperate for repair of a pseudarthrosis needs to be made on clinical information as well as radiographic confirmation (11).

Investigators have reported pseudarthrosis rates ranging from 3% to 36% after anterior cervical arthrodesis. Traditionally, the diagnosis of pseudarthrosis has been based on the clinical triad of pain, radiographic evidence of instability, and loss of correction or fixation (6). However, not all patients diagnosed with pseudarthrosis experience pain to the level of considering undergoing reoperation. In the series by Newman, 7 of 23 patients elected not to undergo a second procedure (7). All seven had persistent neck pain, but none thought the symptoms were sufficient to warrant another surgery.

Most often, after anterior cervical discectomy and arthrodesis, if fusion has not occurred after 6 months, it is considered delayed and deemed a failure after 12 months. Diagnosis can be based on serial flexion and extension x-rays that display a radiolucent gap between the graft and the vertebral body, typically in extension. A lack of continuous bridging between the vertebrae at the operative site may also prompt the diagnosis (11). Symptomatic patients may require further imaging if the x-rays do not provide clear-cut evidence of pseudarthrosis. Single-photon emission computed tomography (SPECT) has the potential to confirm the diagnosis of pseudarthrosis reliably but may be limited when used as a screening tool because of a paucity of information documenting the natural history of arthrodesis on SPECT images after surgical fusion (6). Albert and associates, in their prospective study examining the accuracy of SPECT scanning in diagnosing a pseudarthrosis, could not recommend the use of SPECT scanning alone (12). They did point out, however, that SPECT scanning may be more accurate in diagnosing pseudarthrosis in the noninstrumented spine (12). When dealing with a lumbar arthrodesis, surgical inspection is considered by some to be the best method of determining its solidity but is impractical because of its morbidity and cost (13). Computed tomography (CT) scans can assist in confirming the diagnosis. Lang and colleagues found two- and three-dimensional tomography studies to be superior to x-rays in demonstrating the presence of fusion in posterior lumbar arthrodesis patients (14). Interestingly, in regard to a postoperative cervical arthrodesis, Epstein showed that three-dimensional CT study provided little additional information when compared with routine flexion and extension x-rays (9) (Fig. 88.1).

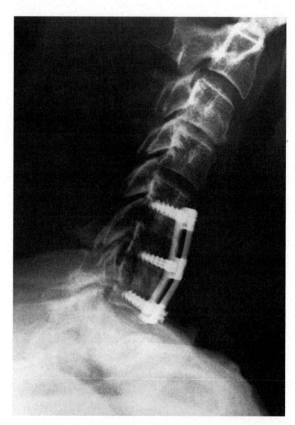

FIG. 88.1. Although surgical inspection may be considered the most effective way to diagnose pseudarthrosis, radiographs still provide a fairly effective and easily attainable method of diagnosing nonunion. This cervical X-ray demonstrates bony fusion despite instrumentation failure in the form of inferior screw backout.

RISK FACTORS

Numerous potential risk factors can affect the progression toward solid fusion and influence the surgeon's choice of subsequent treatment. Factors influencing the development of a solid fusion are patient or surgeon specific. Smoking, renal disease, diabetes, thyroid dysfunction, obesity, and advanced age are patient-specific factors that may influence the development of pseudarthrosis (15,16). The choice of autogenous bone graft, the use of spinal instrumentation, and the preparation of the fusion bed are important measures in decreasing the occurrence of pseudarthrosis after cervical fusion (16).

NONSURGICAL MANAGEMENT

It is reasonable for a patient who does not experience substantial neck or upper extremity pain, but who has a radiographic radiolucency indicative of a pseudarthrosis, to be followed with serial imaging. As previously noted, the clinical importance of a pseudarthrosis is controversial. Bohlman and colleagues believe, based on their long-term follow-up study of 122 patients with anterior cervical discectomy and arthrodesis, that the best clinical results are related to achieving a solid fusion (17). The clinical series by Newman further supports the relationship between obtaining a solid cervical fusion and having a positive clinical result (7). For a patient with a symptomatic pseudarthrosis presenting with substantial neck or upper extremity pain or weakness, nonsurgical management becomes more challenging. Although the rate of successful fusion after a second operation is fairly high, a patient may decide to avoid further surgery, opting for more conservative measures. These may include analgesia control or other pain relief modalities, physical therapy, and psychological counseling. The role of pain in a patient's socioeconomic situation and psychological functioning should not be underestimated.

SURGICAL CONSIDERATIONS

When alternative modalities fail to maintain a patient within his or her desired level of daily functioning, and the possibility of surgical repair has been agreed on, reoperation to correct symptomatic cervical pseudarthrosis is a valid option.

Before deciding on a particular surgical approach to treat a symptomatic pseudarthrosis, the surgeon must attempt to identify those factors that may have led to the nonunion. For example, unrecognized posterior instability and segmental motion or shear stresses may contribute to the development of a pseudarthrosis; therefore, consideration should be given to performing a revision posterior procedure and supplementing it with internal fixation, respectively. The surgeon

should also consider the possibility of an underlying metabolic abnormality (10). Surgical indications for cervical pseudarthrosis include radiographic diagnosis plus the presence of pain or radicular and myelopathic symptoms, generally 12 months after the initial surgery.

Possible causes of pseudarthrosis include inadequate immobilization, patient noncompliance, graft extrusion, graft fracture, methods of bed preparation, type of bone graft, number of levels fused, and smoking (18). These causes are also important to consider when deciding to proceed with another surgery.

SURGICAL OPTIONS

The benefits of particular surgical approaches and the efficacy of an anterior versus posterior approach have been the focus of much discussion and deserve consideration. In 1990, Farey and colleagues reported solid posterior fusion in each of the 19 patients they treated for symptomatic cervical pseudarthrosis (11). In 1991, Brodsky and associates performed a randomized study that compared posterior repair with anterior repair for symptomatic pseudarthrosis after anterior cervical arthrodesis (18). Seventeen patients received anterior repair. Sixteen of 17 patients who received posterior repair showed radiographic fusion, and 1 patient continued to have pseudarthrosis. In the anterior repair group, 13 achieved successful fusion, and 4 had persistent pseudarthrosis. They concluded that a posterior cervical arthrodesis was more effective than an anterior cervical repair of a symptomatic pseudarthrosis. In 1995, Lowery and co-workers concluded that the high probability of fusion, coupled with good clinical results and few complications, supports the use of a posterior cervical arthrodesis and lateral mass plating for failed anterior cervical arthrodesis (19). Phillips and colleagues in 1997 reported on their series of patients that underwent repair for a pseudarthrosis. Sixteen patients had a repeat anterior procedure and fusion, which was successfully achieved in 14 of the patients. Six patients underwent primary posterior repair, and a successful fusion occurred in all patients (5). In 1998, Siambanes and Miz treated 14 patients suffering from nonunion after an anterior cervical discectomy by means of the Roger wiring technique, and radiographic union was achieved in all patients (20). They recommend the use of posterior stabilization but advocate an anterior procedure in the face of continued or residual neural compression, graft dislodgment, or cervical kyphosis (Fig. 88.2).

Using an anterior revision approach has been successful as well. Zdeblick and colleagues in 1997 reported on 35 patients whom they treated for failed anterior cervical discectomy and arthrodesis (21). Operative treatment involved a repeated anterior Robinson arthrodesis. Their results were reported as excellent for 29 patients, good for 1, fair for 4,

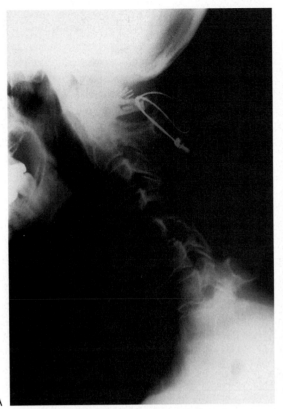
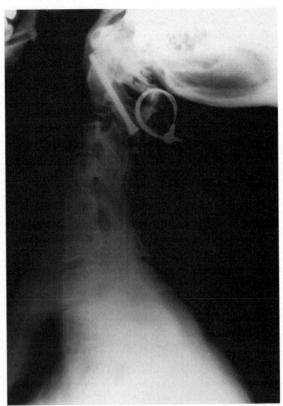

FIG. 88.2. A: This lateral cervical x-ray demonstrates posterior instrumentation failure evidenced as loosened wiring. **B:** A postoperative x-ray after posterior surgical revision shows well-purchased screw placement in addition to secure posterior wiring.

and poor for 1. They concluded that, in patients who have persistent symptoms following an anterior cervical arthrodesis, an excellent result can be achieved with repeat anterior decompression and autogenous bone-grafting. Also in 1997, Coric and co-workers used an anterior revision using an interbody allograft and anterior plating (6). They reported successful fusion in each of the 19 patients they treated. They believe an anterior revision to be a safe and efficacious procedure. In 1999, Tribus and colleagues reported on 16 patients with symptomatic pseudarthrosis treated with an anterior resection of the pseudarthrosis, decompression, autogenous iliac crest bone grafting, and cervical plating with a titanium locking screw-plate system (22). They reported that stability was obtained as demonstrated on flexion-extension views in all 16 patients, and 11 patients rated their pain as improved from pre-revision status. They also believe that anterior revision surgery has several advantages to offer, including direct visualization and removal of the pseudarthrosis, direct decompression of the neural elements, and aversion of posterior stripping of the paraspinal musculature.

Vaccaro and associates presented an illustrative case of a salvage anterior C1-C2 screw fixation and arthrodesis through a lateral approach in a patient with a symptomatic pseudarthrosis (23). Using the Whitesides lateral approach,

they showed the efficacy of an alternative approach that could be valuable when standard anterior or posterior exposures prove to be inadequate.

In view of these reports, it would be difficult to select a superior approach. The technique that is subsequently selected should be chosen following careful consideration of the relative benefits, drawbacks, and indications of each approach, and determining which would provide the most benefit when applied to a particular patient's condition.

Surgical options also include the choice of fusion substrate as well as the decision if it is to be used at all. Fuji and associates, in their series of nine patients who had unsuccessful anterior interbody fusion or subtotal spondylectomy and fusion for cervical spondylosis and were treated by interspinous wiring without bone grafting, concluded that satisfactory bone union could be obtained by this technique if applied to properly selected patients (24). When using a fusion substrate, choosing between autograft and allograft remains a debated issue. Rish and colleagues, in 1976, completed a comparative study of autogenous and homologous bone grafts in Smith-Robinson-type anterior cervical fusions that revealed no significance difference between the two with regard to clinical and radiographic results (25). An allograft is advantageous in that it avoids donor-site complications (26). More recently, in 1996, Bishop and colleagues found that tricortical iliac crest

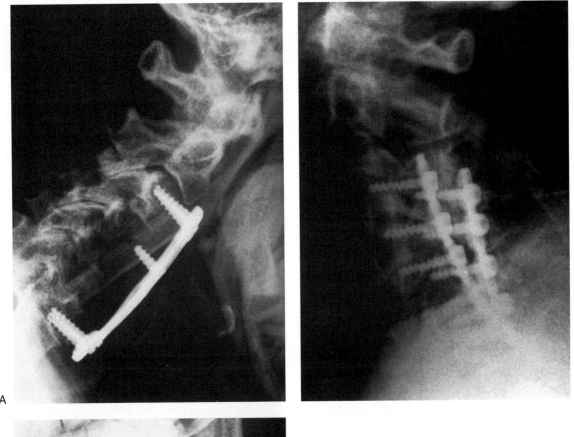

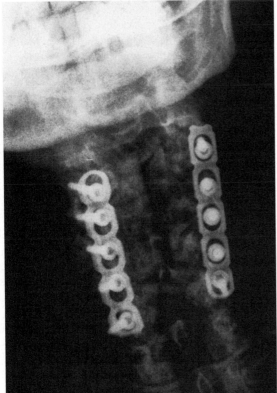

FIG. 88.3. A: Obvious anterior plate failure can be seen in this initial postoperative cervical spine x-ray. Postoperative x-rays after surgical revision to ensure fusion demonstrates a solid posterior fusion construct in a lateral view (B) and in an anteroposterior view (C).

autograft for interbody fusion following one-level and multilevel anterior cervical discectomy was superior to allograft tricortical iliac crest material. They also found a higher failure of fusion rate in smokers, and it was particularly apparent in smokers treated with allograft (15). Bone grafts may be classified according to source of graft (autograft, allograft, xenograft), tissue composition (cortical, corticocancellous, cancellous), anatomic site of origin, blood supply (nonvascularized, revascularized), and preservation method (fresh, frozen, freeze dried, or irradiated). Each of these considerations affects the biomechanical and physiologic properties of the graft and thus affects the clinical usefulness and the choice of bone graft material. No single bone graft preparation is ideal for all spinal applications. Iliac crest graft material, both as a strut graft and as a cancellous inductive material, remains the biologic and biomechanical standard with which other alternatives are compared (27). With these factors in mind, including route of surgical approach, type of fusion substrate, and whether the patient smokes, the surgeon constructs a surgical plan that optimizes the chance of fusion in the face of a pseudarthrosis.

Reports of failure at attempted interbody fusion after an anterior cervical discectomy and arthrodesis have been higher after multilevel surgery than after one-level surgery (5). Brunton and colleagues noted an increased nonunion rate after a two-level arthrodesis (30%) compared with a one-level arthrodesis (16.6%) (28). When considering surgical treatment for revision of a pseudarthrosis, operating on multiple levels may often influence operative fusion technique. Immobilization is another factor. During healing, relative immobilization is required. Under certain circumstances, strut grafts alone may be sufficient; however, additional immobilization may be accomplished by wiring, by plates, screws, and rods, or by bracing. Unsolved issues include how strong and rigid the immobilization should be and how long it is required (27) (Figs. 88.3).

SURGICAL ADJUNCTS

Bone possesses a variety of electrical and mechanical properties (29). As an organ, bone has complex interrelationships between physical and biologic properties, the very architecture of bone being a response to the mechanical demands placed on it. This is one manifestation of Wolff's law that was described numerous decades ago. Also, electromechanical and electrochemical properties of bone are thought to play an important role in its growth and remodeling (30). Becker, and later Friedenberg and Brighton, showed that the site of injury or fracture has a negative charge and that altering the electric potential also alters the progression of healing. The culmination of this work was the clinical use of electric fields to induce healing of nonunions and delayed unions (31). Although external electrical stimulation has been indicated for treatment of a pseudarthrosis, a preferred method includes débridement of the interven-

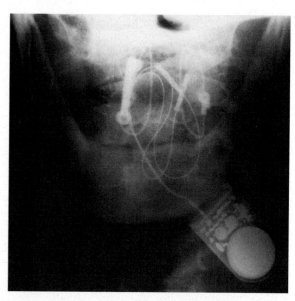

FIG. 88.4. Placement of an internal bone growth stimulator can be viewed in this cervical spine x-ray. This patient was 1 of 14 who participated in a study conducted by several of the authors that looked at the efficacy of electrical bone growth stimulation in the cervical spine.

ing scar tissue, autogenous bone grafting, and rigid internal fixation. This is then supplemented with electrical stimulation; either an implantable device or an external one (16). Kucharzyk, in 1999, reported on a series of patients, 65 who underwent lumbar instrumentation without electrical stimulation, with an 87% fusion rate, and 65 who underwent instrumentation and electrical stimulation, with a 95% fusion rate (32). Although mostly reported with respect to lumbar fusion, it appears reasonable that electrical stimulation may be considered a surgical adjunct when trying to accomplish solid cervical fusion. Recently, the author (Welch) conducted a pilot study with 14 patients that was designed to examine the use of an implantable direct current bone growth stimulator (IDCBGS) as an adjunct to cervical arthrodesis in patients at high risk for nonunion after cervical arthrodesis from the occiput to C3. Each of the 14 were deemed at high risk for non-union because of advancing age, rheumatoid arthritis, infection, failed prior fusion attempt, or immunosuppressive drug use. The follow-up was quite short, with a mean of 18 months and a range of 2 to 44 months. All 14 patients demonstrated radiographic evidence of fusion at follow-up as well as stabilization or improvement in both symptoms and neurologic status (S. Willis, personal communication, March 2003) (Fig. 88.4).

CONCLUSION

Symptomatic cervical pseudarthrosis can be a challenging clinical dilemma. Although some controversy surrounds the impact of pseudarthrosis on clinical outcome, results are generally better if arthrodesis is achieved. Conservative measures may assist some symptomatic patients in continuing their accustomed level of functioning. If not, revision surgery can be considered. Neck pain, extremity pain, weakness, paresthesias, and possibly myelopathic symptoms can be a result of a cervical pseudarthrosis. Consideration of what factors may have contributed to the pseudarthrosis is important before proceeding with reoperation. However, patients with physiologic risk factors for an increased incidence of pseudarthrosis should not be denied surgery solely on that basis (16). Successful fusion can be accomplished through an anterior or posterior approach, with different types of graft, and with various combinations of instrumentation. Once reoperation becomes the course of treatment, and solid fusion is the goal, there are numerous surgical options that can be chosen based on the individual considerations of the patient.

REFERENCES

1. Weber BG, Cech O. *Pseudarthrosis: pathophysiology, biomechanics, therapy, results.* New York: Grune & Stratton, 1976:12.
2. Robinson RA, Smith GW. Anterolateral cervical disc removal and interbody fusion for cervical disc syndrome. *Bull Johns Hopkins Hosp* 1955;96:223–224.
3. Robinson RA, Walker AE, Ferlic DC, et al. The results of anterior interbody fusion of the cervical spine. *J Bone Joint Surg Am* 1962;44:1569–1586.
4. Cotler JM, Simpson JM, An HS. Principles, indications, and complications of spinal instrumentation: a summary chapter. In: An HS, Cotler JM, eds. *Spinal instrumentation* Williams & Wilkins, Baltimore, 1992:435–456.
5. Phillips FM, Carlson G, Emery SE, et al. Anterior cervical pseudarthrosis: natural history and treatment. *Spine* 1997;22:1585–1589.
6. Coric D, Branch CL, Jenkin JD. Revision of anterior cervical pseudarthrosis with anterior allograft fusion and plating. *J Neurosurg* 1997;86:969–974.
7. Newman M. The outcome of pseudarthrosis after cervical anterior fusion. *Spine* 1993;18:2380–2382.
8. White AA, Panjabi MM. The problem of clinical instability in the human spine: a systematic approach. In: *Clinical biomechanics of the spine.* Philadelphia: JB Lippincott, 1990:277–378.
9. Epstein NE. Evaluation and treatment of clinical instability associated with pseudarthrosis after anterior cervical surgery for ossification of the posterior longitudinal ligament. *Surg Neurol* 1998;49:246–252.
10. Steinman JC, Herkowitz HN. Pseudarthrosis of the spine. *Clin Orthop Relat Res* 1992;284:80–90.
11. Farey ID, McAfee PC, Davis RF, et al. Pseudarthrosis of the cervical spine after anterior arthrodesis. *J Bone Joint Surg Am* 1990;72:1171–1177.
12. Albert TJ, Pinto M, Smith MD, et al. Accuracy of SPECT scanning in diagnosing pseudarthrosis: a prospective study. *J Spinal Disord* 1998;11:197–199.
13. Brodsky AE, Kovalsky ES, Khalil MA. Correlation of radiologic assessment of lumbar spine fusions with surgical exploration. *Spine* 1991;16:S262–S265.
14. Lang P, Genant HK, Chafetz N, et al. Three dimensional computed tomography and multiplanar reformations in the assessment of pseudarthrosis in posterior lumbar fusion patients. *Spine* 1988;13:69–75.
15. Bishop RC, Moore KA, Hadley MN. Anterior cervical interbody fusion using autogenic and allogenic bone graft substrate: a prospective comparative analysis. *J Neurosurg* 1996;85:206–209.
16. Knight RQ. Immediate and delayed postoperative complications. In: Welch WC, Jacobs GB, Jackson RP, eds. *Operative spine surgery.* Stamford, CT: Appleton & Lange, 1999:238–248.
17. Bohlman HH, Emery SE, Goodfellow DB, et al. Robinson anterior cervical discectomy and arthrodesis for cervical radiculopathy. Long-term follow-up of one hundred and twenty-two patients. *J Bone Joint Surg Am* 1993;75:1298–1306.
18. Brodsky AE, Khalil MA, Sassard WR, et al. Repair of symptomatic pseudarthrosis of anterior cervical fusion: posterior versus anterior repair. *Spine* 1992;17:1137–1143.
19. Lowery GL, Swank ML, McDonough RF. Surgical revision for failed anterior cervical fusions: articular pillar plating or anterior revision? *Spine* 1995;20:2436–2441.
20. Siambanes D, Miz GS. Treatment of symptomatic anterior cervical nonunion using the Rogers interspinous wiring technique. *J Orthop Am* 1998;12:792–796.
21. Zdeblick TA, Hughes SS, Riew DK, et al. Failed anterior cervical discectomy and arthrodesis. *J Bone Joint Surg Am* 1997;79:523–532.
22. Tribus CB, Corteen DP, Zdeblick TA. The efficacy of anterior cervical plating in the management of symptomatic pseudarthrosis of the cervical spine. *Spine* 1999;24:860–864.
23. Vaccaro AR, Ring D, Lee RS, et al. Salvage anterior C1-C2 screw fixation and arthrodesis through the lateral approach in a patient with a symptomatic pseudarthrosis. *Am J Orthop* 1997;26:349–353.
24. Fuji T, Yonenobu K, Fujiwara K, et al. Interspinous wiring without bone grafting for nonunion or delayed union following anterior spinal fusion of the cervical spine. *Spine* 1986;11:982–987.
25. Rish BL, McFadden JT, Penix JO. Anterior cervical fusion using homologous bone grafts: A comparative study. *Surg Neurol* 1976;5:19–21.
26. Kurz LT, Garfin SR, Booth RE. Harvesting autogenous iliac bone grafts: a review of complications and techniques. *Spine* 1989;14:1324–1331.
27. Kaufman HH, Jones E. The principles of bony spinal fusion. *Neurosurgery* 1989;14:264–270.
28. Brunton FJ, Wilkinson JA, Wise KS, et al. Cine radiography in cervical spondylosis as a means of determining the level for anterior fusion. *J Bone Joint Surg* 1982;64:399.
29. Behari J. Electrostimulation and bone fracture healing. *Biomed Eng* 1991;18:1991.
30. Lavine LS, Grodzinsky AJ. Current concepts review: electrical stimulation of repair of bone 1987;69:626.
31. Perry CR. Bone repair techniques, bone graft and bone graft substitutes. *Clin Orthop Relat Res* 1999;360:71–86.
32. Kucharzyk DW. A controlled prospective outcome study of implantable electrical stimulation with spinal instrumentation in a high-risk spinal fusion population. *Spine* 1999;24:465–469.

CHAPTER 89

Salvage of Long Strut Graft Failure Following Multilevel Cervical Corpectomy and Arthrodesis

Rick C. Sasso

A challenging problem that the spine surgeon faces is the patient who has had a multilevel cervical corpectomy reconstruction that has failed. Potential adverse outcomes of continued nonoperative treatment include progressive collapse and kyphosis with radiculopathy resulting from neural foraminal narrowing and myelopathy worsening from the cervical spinal cord being draped over the apex of the deformity. Loss of horizontal gaze and decreased cervical range of motion may result from the kyphosis and damage to the normal disc spaces above and below the reconstruction with cavitation of the construct. Pseudarthrosis and progressive instability may cause severe pain and retard neural recovery from the index decompression. Tracheal, esophageal, and soft tissue structures of the anterior neck may be damaged by impingement by the anterior cervical plate or strut graft.

Operative treatment of this problem is a salvage procedure with considerable risks and possible complications. The appropriate approach, procedure, and timing are critical for an optimal outcome. Should the plate and strut graft be removed? Should posterior instrumentation be inserted? Which should be done first? The underlying goal is to restore normal sagittal alignment and obtain stable internal fixation with basic biomechanical principles. The ideal goal, however, is to prevent this complication in the first place.

FAILURE OF MULTILEVEL CORPECTOMY RECONSTRUCTION

Surgical management of cervical myelopathy is difficult when compressive lesions span multiple motion segments. The controversy does not lie in the universally recognized goal of adequately decompressing the spinal cord, but in the method that least destabilizes the cervical spine and allows the optimal environment for neural recovery. Posterior laminectomy and laminoplasty have been advocated (1–4); however, accepted relative contraindications include preexisting kyphosis and instability. Anterior decompression and reconstruction are highly successful for short segment pathology (5–7). Anterior surgical management of extensive cervical disease, however, is problematic because high failure rates have been reported for multilevel anterior corpectomy reconstruction. A 33% construct failure rate requiring reoperation for graft extrusion of a fibular allograft after a three-level corpectomy (8) has not been improved on even with anterior cervical internal fixation. Vaccaro and associates (9) reported failure rates of 9% for two-level corpectomy reconstructions and 50% for three-level corpectomy arthrodesis with anterior cervical plates. The failure rate exponentially increases with length. Swank and co-workers (10) reported nonunion rates of 10% for one-level corpectomy reconstructions and 44% for two-level fusions. Saunders and colleagues (11) reported a 10% early death rate and a 26% morbidity prevalence after four-level cervical corpectomies. Our results with autogenous iliac crest autograft and a constrained anterior cervical plate demonstrated a 6% failure rate for two-level corpectomy reconstructions and a 71% early failure rate with three-level corpectomy arthrodesis with an anterior-only construct. We had no failures of three-level corpectomy reconstructions when posterior lateral mass screw stabilization was added to the anterior construct.

1212

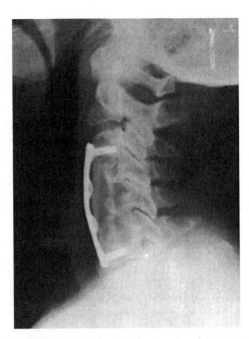

FIG. 89.1. Lateral radiograph of a two-level corpectomy reconstruction with autogenous iliac crest and a constrained plate. This image was taken 3 years after surgery and demonstrates successful fusion and maintenance of physiologic sagittal alignment.

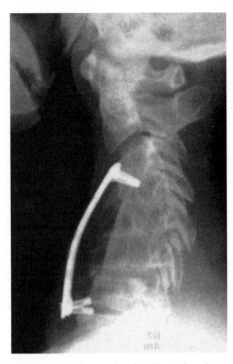

FIG. 89.2. Lateral radiograph of a three-level corpectomy reconstruction with autogenous iliac crest and a constrained plate showing early failure with inferior migration of the graft and displacement of the caudal screws into the disc space as well as anterior displacement of the plate.

The prevalence of failure increases substantially from a two-level corpectomy reconstruction to a three-level construct (Fig. 89.1). The usual method of failure is telescoping of the inferior aspect of the construct (strut graft and plate screws) through the caudal vertebral body and possibly into the subadjacent disc space (Fig. 89.2). Possible complications occurring from this failure are many and range from simple radiographic changes in an asymptomatic patient to death. Riew and co-workers (12) have described profound airway compromise and death from catastrophic multilevel corpectomy reconstruction failure. As the strut graft telescopes inferiorly into the caudal vertebral body, it often also displaces anteriorly. Anterior cervical instrumentation may displace into the retropharyngeal space with the strut graft. Although anterior cervical junctional plates were originally described to be used with posterior cervical instrumentation (13), some surgeons have used the short buttress plate alone without posterior stabilization. This construct may cause tracheal and esophageal compromise if failure occurs.

Spinal cord injury with worsening of the underlying myelopathy may also occur with failure of a multilevel anterior construct. As the strut graft migrates caudally and kicks out anteriorly, the cephalad aspect of the strut graft may displace posteriorly into the spinal canal (Fig. 89.3). Myeloradiculopathy may also result from the acute shortening of the construct with failure, thus narrowing the neural foramen.

Pseudarthrosis of the graft–host junction may or may not cause symptoms, but if a solid fusion does not occur, instrumentation may fail. Long strut grafts may also fracture despite healing at the graft–host junctions (Fig. 89.4). Plate fracture, screw fracture or dislodgment, and uncoupling of the screw–plate interface may also complicate multilevel corpectomy reconstructions.

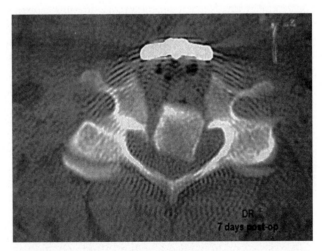

FIG. 89.3. Axial computed tomography scan through the cephalad aspect of multilevel corpectomy reconstruction 7 days after surgery showing displacement of the strut graft posteriorly into the spinal canal with cord compression.

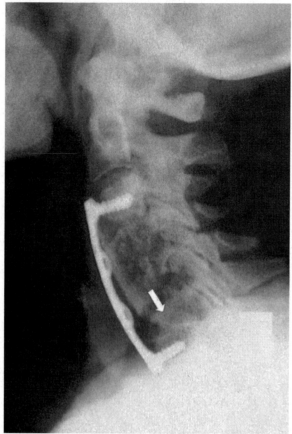

FIG. 89.4. Lateral radiograph of a three-level corpectomy reconstruction with autogenous iliac crest and a constrained plate. Surgical revision revealed fracture of the strut graft *(arrow)* and solid fusion of both graft–host junctions.

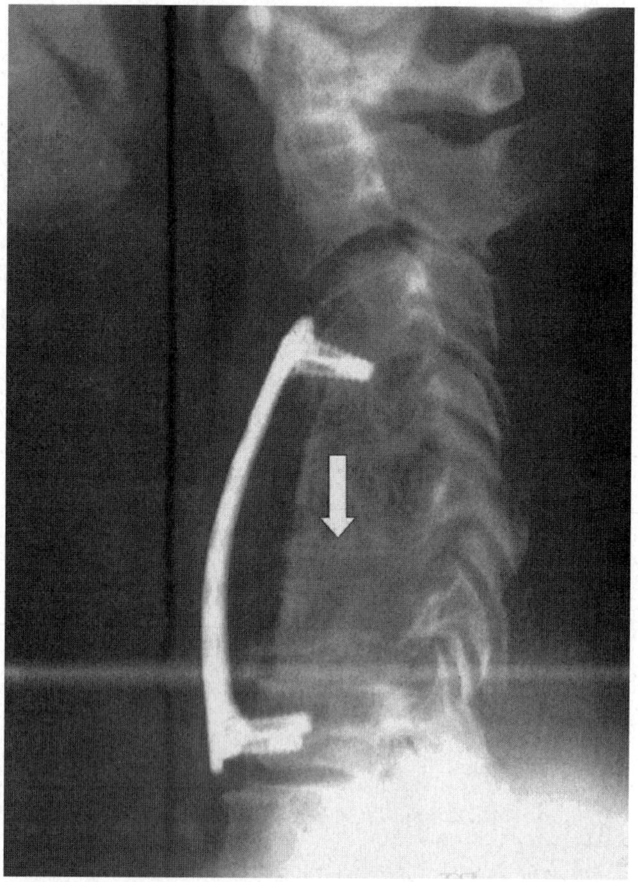

FIG. 89.5. Lateral radiograph of a three-level corpectomy reconstruction with autogenous iliac crest and a constrained plate. Surgical revision revealed fracture of the strut graft *(arrow)* and solid fusion of both graft–host junctions, as in Fig. 89.4.

IMAGING

Plain radiographs usually make the diagnosis of failure after a multilevel corpectomy reconstruction (Fig. 89.5). The lateral x-ray is most useful in catastrophic failures; however, helical computed tomography (CT) scans with sagittal and coronal reconstructions are helpful to detect subtle signs of pseudarthrosis and fracture of the long strut graft. Technically excellent intraoperative and immediate postoperative x-rays are important to compare subsequent films. Only with these studies can initial signs of failure be detected on follow-up x-rays. Comparing the position of the strut graft in relation to the plate and screws may allow early detection of graft migration. Later signs of failure include the inferior screws migrating caudally in the vertebral body.

Long, lateral radiographs of the spine, including the thoracic and lumbar as well as the cervical regions, are useful when planning surgical reconstruction after failure of the construct. Dropping a plumb line from the midbody of C2 and measuring where it falls in relation to the sacral promontory helps in understanding global sagittal align-

ment. If a significant cervicothoracic junction kyphosis is present and the sagittal alignment is markedly displaced anteriorly, then consideration of extending the salvage reconstruction into the upper thoracic spine is important to lessen the biomechanical stresses on the construct by reducing the kyphosis.

BIOMECHANICS

An anterior cervical plate alone is not biomechanically sufficient to stabilize a three-level corpectomy graft adequately in an *in vitro* cervical spine model (14). By including a posterior plate with the anterior reconstruction, a three-level corpectomy of the cervical spine is effectively stabilized (15). The instantaneous axis of rotation (IAR) is shifted anteriorly after application of an anterior plate (Fig. 89.6). The outcome is a reversal of the loading pattern in a long strut graft such that no loading of the graft occurs under flexion moments, and profound, excessive compression of the graft occurs under extension loads (Fig. 89.7). This may result in the

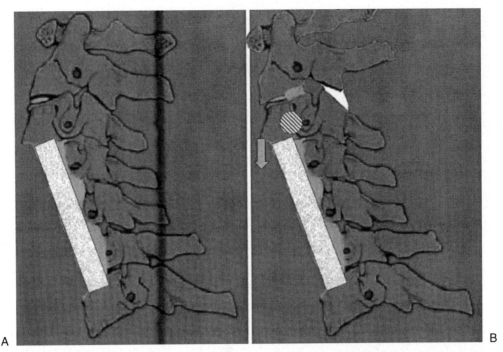

FIG. 89.6. A: Three-level corpectomy reconstruction with a strut graft. **B:** Under flexion loads, the graft is placed under compression because the instantaneous axis of rotation *(ball)* is located in the posterior aspect of the vertebral body axis.

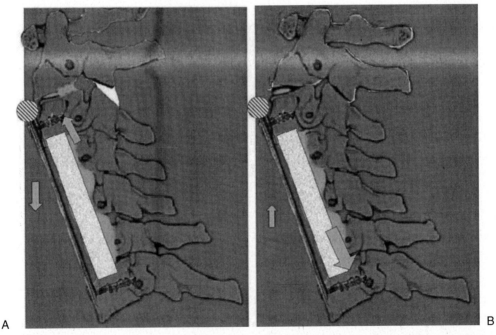

FIG. 89.7. A: Three-level corpectomy reconstruction with a strut graft and anterior plate. The instantaneous axis of rotation is moved anteriorly to the cervical plate so that under flexion loads, the strut graft is unloaded. **B:** Under extension loads, the graft is placed under extreme compression.

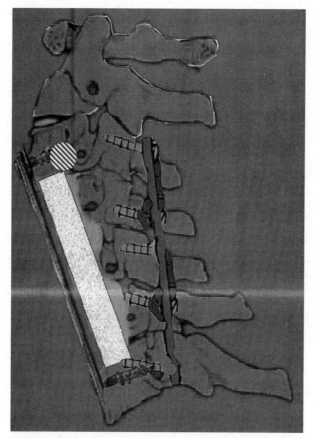

FIG. 89.8. Three-level corpectomy reconstruction with a strut graft, anterior plate, and posterior instrumentation. The instantaneous axis of rotation is moved posteriorly, thus loading the strut graft in a more physiologic manner during flexion and extension.

graft telescoping through the caudal vertebral body and the plate subsequently kicking out of the lower vertebral body. The addition of posterior instrumentation moves the IAR posteriorly, thus approximating its normal location in the posterior aspect of the vertebral body (Fig. 89.8). Biomechanically, this protects the graft from the excessive loads under extension and explains the clinical success of circumferential instrumentation for long segment corpectomy reconstructions.

SALVAGE

The surgical technique of correcting a long strut graft failure following a multilevel corpectomy requires careful consideration. Neurologic and biomechanical issues need to be considered with an approach that is adequate but as minimally invasive as possible to limit morbidity. The approach may be a simple revision anterior procedure with replacement of the strut graft and instrumentation if an anterior cervical plate was not applied during the index operation. Frequently, the vertebral body below and possibly above the construct is damaged as a result of migration of the strut graft or screws pulling out of the vertebral body.

This may require extending the corpectomy an extra level or two.

The surgical approach may consist of a simple posterior stabilization procedure. This is usually most effective if initiation of early failure of the anterior long construct is noticed on postoperative x-rays compared with intraoperative films. These changes may be very subtle, but if a posterior stabilization procedure can be done alone, this is optimal. It is done through usually virgin soft tissue, and the morbidity of a revision anterior approach is avoided. This approach is only possible if there is no significant loss of sagittal alignment and the anterior construct has not displaced into the retropharyngeal space. A posterior-only arthrodesis in the presence of a kyphotic deformity places considerable tension on the instrumentation and bone graft. Large bending moments (stresses) occur when a large kyphotic deformity is present and challenge the corrective forces of the posterior instrumentation.

A posterior followed by an anterior approach may be done if continued anterior collapse is documented after a posterior stabilization. The advantage of this is the assurance that the anterior strut graft is optimally load sharing.

The workhorse approach for failure of a long anterior construct is an anterior revision followed by a posterior stabilization procedure. The anterior strut graft is replaced with or without application of an anterior cervical plate or junctional plate. A biomechanically sound posterior fixation is then done to prevent subsequent failure (Fig. 89.9).

A posterior cervical release followed by an anterior revision of the strut graft followed by posterior fixation may be required if a fixed kyphotic deformity is present. Preoperative traction can be attempted to determine whether the kyphosis is reducible. If the deformity cannot be corrected with traction, this back-front-back technique is required.

If the anterior construct is a hindrance to kyphosis reduction, either because of healing of the strut graft in a kyphotic position or engagement of the screws into solid bone, then an anterior release followed by posterior reduction and fixation followed by anterior strut grafting with or without instrumentation is considered. The advantage of the front-back-front approach is that a laminectomy with excellent visualization of the spinal cord can be done to ensure safety during the reduction maneuver. The initial anterior release allows greater reduction of the kyphotic deformity during the posterior manipulation. It is then important to implant an anterior strut graft after the posterior instrumentation to allow adequate anterior load sharing and thus increase the fusion rate.

Intraoperative and postoperative complications of these salvage procedures can be significant. The infection rate is higher because the approach is through a previously operated surgical field. Neurologic injury is possible due to the cord draping over the apex of a failed, collapsed, kyphotic anterior construct. In addition, the cord is usually attempting to recover from long-standing myelopathy, which was the reason for the index procedure. New spinal cord injury from the catastrophic collapse of the anterior strut graft on

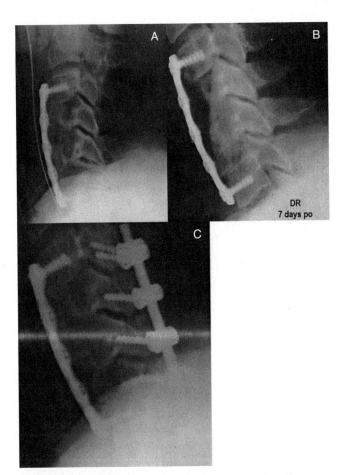

FIG. 89.9. A: Lateral x-ray 1 day after multilevel corpectomy and anterior instrumentation. The autogenous iliac crest strut graft is well placed. **B:** One week after surgery, the strut graft is shown kicking anteriorly at the caudal aspect and posteriorly into the spinal canal at the cephalad end. **C:** Revision with an anterior reconstruction was followed by posterior lateral mass fixation.

an already scarred spinal cord can be disastrous. If reduction of a kyphotic deformity is attempted without direct visualization of the neural elements, spinal cord monitoring is indicated.

CONCLUSION

Salvage of a long anterior cervical strut graft failure is fraught with potential complications. It is best done by a cervical spine surgeon with extensive expertise in circumferential approaches not only of the cervical spine but also of the occipitocervical and cervicothoracic junctions. Appropriate rescue often requires extension to these junctional areas with atraumatic surgical technique and rigid instrumentation. Basic biomechanical principles of restoring normal sagittal alignment and obtaining stable internal fixation

need to be followed. Care must be taken not to overdistract the neural structures.

The most important consideration is to attempt avoidance of complications. Careful planning of the index procedure is paramount. Adequate stabilization is necessary, and if more than a two-level corpectomy defect is reconstructed or if functional posterior instability is present, posterior instrumentation should be added during the index corpectomy. It is interesting to speculate on the issue of a constrained anterior plate–screw interface and whether a semiconstrained (dynamic) plate would result in as high a failure rate in a three-level corpectomy reconstruction. Even further speculation is necessary in considering which type of semiconstrained plate (rotational, translational, or a combination of both) would be most beneficial for these long constructs. Until these clinical and biomechanical issues are resolved, posterior instrumentation should be considered for multilevel corpectomy reconstructions.

REFERENCES

1. Herkowitz H. A comparison of anterior cervical fusion, cervical laminectomy, and cervical laminoplasty for the surgical management of multiple level spondylotic radiculopathy. *Spine* 1988;13:774–780.
2. Hirabayashi K, Bohlman H. Controversy: multilevel cervical spondylosis laminoplasty versus anterior decompression. *Spine* 1995;20: 1732–1734.
3. Hirabayashi K, Miyakawa J, Satomi K, et al. Operative results and postoperative progression of ossification among patients with ossification of cervical posterior longitudinal ligament. *Spine* 1981;6:354–364.
4. Lee T, Manzano G, Green B. Modified open-door cervical expansive laminoplasty for spondylotic myelopathy: operative technique, outcome, and predictors for gait improvement. *J Neurosurg* 1997;86: 64–68.
5. Epstein N. The management of one-level anterior cervical corpectomy with fusion using Atlantis hybrid plates: a preliminary experience. *J Spinal Disord* 2000;13:324–328.
6. Saunders R, Bernini P, Shirreffs T Jr, et al. Central corpectomy for cervical spondylotic myelopathy: a consecutive series with long-term follow up evaluation. *J Neurosurg* 1991;74:163–170.
7. Sukoff M, Harris J, Denenny D, et al. Cervical corpectomy: indications, review of literature, technique, rationale for its use, and presentation of 82 consecutive cases. *Neurosurg Q* 1997;7:209–220.
8. Zdeblick T, Bohlman H. Cervical kyphosis and myelopathy treatment by anterior corpectomy and strut grafting. *J Bone Joint Surg Am* 1989; 71:170–182.
9. Vaccaro A, Falatyn S, Scuderi G, et al. Early failure of long segment anterior cervical plate fixation. *J Spinal Disord* 1998;11:410–415.
10. Swank ML, Lowery GL, Bhat AL, et al. Anterior cervical allograft arthrodesis and instrumentation: multiple interbody grafting or strut graft reconstruction. *Eur J Spine* 1997;6:138–143.
11. Saunders RL, Pikus HJ, Ball P. Four-level cervical corpectomy. *Spine* 1998;23:2455–2461.
12. Riew KD, Sethi NS, Devney J, et al. Complications of buttress plate stabilization of cervical corpectomy. *Spine* 1999;24:2404–2410.
13. Vanichkachorn JS, Vaccaro AR, Silveri CP, et al. Anterior junctional plate in the cervical spine. *Spine* 1998;23:2462–2467.
14. DiAngelo D, Foley K, Vossel K, et al. Anterior cervical plating reverses load transfer through multilevel strut-grafts. *Spine* 2000;25: 783–795.
15. Foley K, DiAngelo D, Rampersaud Y, et al. The *in vitro* effects of instrumentation on multilevel cervical strut-graft mechanics. *Spine* 1999;24:2366–2376.

CHAPTER 90

Cervical Cerebrospinal Fluid Leakage, Durotomy, and Pseudomeningocele

Seth M. Zeidman

Cerebrospinal fluid (CSF) leaks are relatively uncommon after cervical spinal surgery. Cervical laminectomy, discectomy, and corpectomy are all associated with the potential for the development of a postoperative CSF leak. Postoperative leakage may occur at the dural suture line after intradural procedures or can be caused by inadvertent durotomy during discectomy or laminectomy. In the cervical spine, the surgical treatment of ossification of the posterior longitudinal ligament (OPLL) is associated with a notable prevalence of pseudomeningocele and CSF fistula with a reported incidence ranging from 4.5% to 32% (1,2). Midline posterior dural lacerations are readily repaired primarily. However, far-lateral or ventral dural tears are difficult to repair and therefore more problematic.

DUROTOMY, CEREBROSPINAL FLUID LEAK, PSEUDOMENINGOCELE, AND CEREBROSPINAL FLUID FISTULA

CSF leakage poses a risk for substantial morbidity with the potential for development of meningitis as well as late pseudomeningocele formation. Incidental durotomy is defined as an unintended dural laceration or tear. The risk for an incidental durotomy following a laminectomy ranges from 0.3% to 13%. The risk increases to up to 18% with reoperation.

Pseudomeningocele is defined as an extradural CSF collection arising from a dural defect. Teplick and colleagues reported eight cases in 400 symptomatic postlaminectomy patients undergoing computed tomography (CT) (3). In the cervical spine, the surgical treatment of OPLL is associated with a notable rate of pseudomeningocele and CSF fistula. The reported prevalence following this operation ranges from 4.5% to 32% (3).

Pseudomeningocele contents are of CSF density and may or may not have demonstrable communication with the subarachnoid space. Iatrogenic pseudomeningoceles are not necessarily associated with an arachnoid tear, but a dural tear is necessary for one to form. If the arachnoid is not violated, the arachnoid membrane may subsequently herniate through the dural defect, and a CSF-filled arachnoid sac forms. A postsurgical pseudomeningocele forms when CSF extravasates through a dura-arachnoid tear and becomes encysted within the wound, creating a spherical, fluid-filled space with a fibrous capsule lying dorsal to the thecal canal in the laminectomy opening. Because extradural fluid may be contained in either an arachnoid-lined membrane or a fibrous capsule, multiple terms have been used to describe this entity. Most authors prefer the term *pseudomeningocele* because, at least initially, the lesion is not arachnoid lined and therefore does not represent a true meningocele. Pseudomeningoceles have, at various times, been referred to as spurious meningoceles, false cysts, and pseudocysts. Rinaldi and Peach found arachnoidal cells within the capsular membrane of pseudomeningoceles and advocated terming these lesions "true meningoceles" (4). If the proper milieu exists, the extradural fluid collection is reabsorbed, and the communication between the intradural and extradural space is eventually obliterated.

A CSF fistula may result if the extradural fluid communicates with another cavity such as the pleura or if a direct communication exists through the skin. Smith and associates reported that, of 22 patients who had undergone anterior decompression of the spinal canal for OPLL and cervical myelopathy, 7 had absence of the dura adjacent to the ossified part of the ligament. The spinal cord and nerve roots were visible through this defect. Although the arachnoid membrane appeared to be intact and watertight in most

1218

patients, a CSF fistula developed postoperatively in 5, and 3 had a second operation to repair the defect in the dura (2).

Presentation

Incidental durotomy, pseudomeningocele, and CSF fistula can each present with a variety of signs and symptoms. An incidental durotomy is typically asymptomatic but can cause postural headaches, nausea, vomiting, dizziness, photophobia, tinnitus, and vertigo. An exceptional case of cerebellar hemorrhage complicating cervical durotomy has been reported (5). Symptoms resulting from CSF leakage have been classically postulated to result from intracranial hypotension, that is, a decrease in CSF pressure, leading to traction on the supporting structures of the brain. CSF leaking from a dural puncture leads to a loss of CSF pressure in the spine and a loss of buoyancy supporting the brain. When the patient assumes an upright posture, the brain sags, and tension on the meninges and other intracranial structures creates the pain. This explanation is probably overly simplistic. It is likely that as the body assumes a vertical posture, the hydrostatic gradient across the brain increases, forcing more CSF to exit the dural puncture. The body then attempts to compensate for the loss of intracranial volume by vasodilation. Much of the pain is probably related to vascular distention. This process reverses itself when the patient again assumes a supine posture.

Most pseudomeningoceles remain asymptomatic, but they can present with a range of findings, including posture-related headaches, localized neck pain, radiculopathy, and myelopathy. Patients with pseudomeningoceles may also present with symptoms similar to those seen in patients with intracranial hypotension, including photophobia, cranial nerve palsies, and tinnitus. Very frequently, posture-related headaches, relieved in a recumbent position, may be present. Patients may complain of cervical or occipital pain with or without nausea and vomiting while in a standing position. The time interval between the original surgery to the onset of symptoms ranges from days to years. Some pseudomeningoceles may present as a fluctuant mass that can rapidly enlarge with coughing, sneezing, or any Valsalva maneuver. Palpation in the region of the cyst may cause pain, as was seen in all of the patients with pseudomeningoceles studied by Aldrete and Ghaly (6).

Depending on the location of the lesion, patients with a pseudomeningocele can present with a spinal cord syndrome. Horowitz and co-workers reported a patient who presented with Brown-Séquard and Horner syndromes caused by the development of a cervicothoracic pseudomeningocele following an anterior cervical discectomy (7). Pseudomeningoceles can be problematic for a variety of reasons but perhaps most importantly because they can function as a mass lesion. Hanakita and associates reported a case of spinal cord compression due to a postoperative cervical pseudomeningocele (8). Helle and Conley reported a case of delayed myelopathy as a result of a postoperative cervical pseudomeningocele (9).

More rarely, a patient may present with progressive or delayed myelopathy following cervical spine surgery due to spinal cord herniation (10). Goodman and Gregorius reported a patient with progressive myelopathy who was ultimately determined to have spinal cord herniation (11). Intraoperatively, they established that the spinal cord bulged into the cyst with each heartbeat and respiration. The authors concluded that myelopathy related to a cervical pseudomeningocele may result from either spinal cord herniation or focal cord compression. A patient with a CSF fistula can present with this same constellation of symptoms as incidental durotomy or pseudomeningocele (12). He or she can also become symptomatic with wound swelling, headache, and radiculopathy. Finally, a patient with an unrecognized CSF fistula may present with signs and symptoms of acute or chronic meningitis (13,14).

Diagnosis

Magnetic resonance imaging (MRI) is the diagnostic study of choice. Typically, it shows a region of low signal intensity on T1-weighted images and high signal intensity on T2-weighted images consistent with CSF. MRI can delineate the location, extent, and internal characteristics of the lesion and may demonstrate a communication with the thecal sac. It may also elucidate other associated pathologic entities, such as spinal cord compression or nerve root entrapment, as well as differentiate a pseudomeningocele from a syringomyelia, arachnoiditis, or a recurrent tumor (3). Findings noted in spontaneous intracranial hypotension, including intracranial meningeal enhancement, subdural fluid collections, and caudal displacement of the cerebellar tonsils, may also be visualized. CT myelography and radionuclide myelography may provide useful information in difficult cases.

Cutaneous CSF fistulas are often diagnosed by inspection of the wound. If there is a watery discharge that produces a clear halo surrounding a central pink stain, then the fluid is assumed to be CSF until proved otherwise.

Determining the presence or absence of CSF by measuring the glucose level is an unreliable method. Analysis of fluid for β_2-transferrin is highly sensitive in detecting CSF because β_2-transferrin has only been demonstrated in CSF, perilymph, and aqueous humor.

Transferrin is a polypeptide involved in ferrous ion transport. β_1-transferrin is present in serum, nasal secretions, tears, and saliva. β_2-transferrin accounts for 15% of the total transferrin content in CSF. A small sample size of fluid (0.5 mL) is required to detect β_2-transferrin. Proteins in the fluid are separated by polyacrylamide gel electrophoresis and then transferred electrophoretically onto a nitrocellulose sheet. The structural differences between the two forms results in a slower migration of β_2-transferrin toward the cathode. The result is two distinct bands produced during electrophoresis. Serum and other body fluids normally have only one band, represented by β_1-transferrin. The β_2 isoform arises from β_1-transferrin through the loss of sialic acid by the action of neuraminidase. Because neuraminidase is only found in the central nervous system, CSF fluid will have two bands, one representing β_1 and the other representing β_2. Using an antibody reaction (immunoblot), banding patterns are analyzed. Determination of the presence or absence of β_2-transferrin typically takes less than 3 hours.

Management

Preventive

Most pseudomeningoceles and CSF fistulas are the result of iatrogenic durotomy. A watertight dural closure is the key to avoiding these complications. When a pseudomeningocele or CSF fistula is encountered, bed rest, an epidural blood patch procedure, or closed drainage may be attempted (15). If unsuccessful, direct surgical repair may be necessary, and in rare cases, placement of a lumbar peritoneal (LP) drain or shunt may be considered.

If a Valsalva maneuver reveals a persistent leak, a fibrin sealant should be placed over the area of the leak. Analysis of the results obtained in animal studies suggests that fibrin sealant alone can withstand high hydrostatic pressures. However, because it remains *in situ* for only 5 to 7 days, fibrin glue must be supplemented with a dural, muscle, or fat graft placed over the area of the persistent leak. Simply placing Gelfoam or muscle over the dural leak without also applying fibrin glue is ineffective and has been associated with failure to resolve the leak. Paraspinal muscle and overlying fascia should be closed in at least two layers by using No. 0 monofilament with sutures placed 3 to 4 mm apart. Surgically placed drains may lead to the persistence of communication between the intradural and extradural space and may serve as a nidus for infection. Therefore, these drains should not be routinely used in the repair of a dural tear or a pseudomeningocele.

Some authors argue that all cervical spine pseudomeningoceles should be treated surgically, whereas others argue that pseudomeningoceles will resolve with time (16). Horowitz and co-workers reported a case of an anterior cervical pseudomeningocele that resolved after 3 weeks of expectant observation (7). In contrast to lumbar defects, patients with repaired cervical defects may ambulate immediately (15).

Additional recommendations to prevent formation of a CSF fistula when the dura is found to be absent adjacent to an ossified portion of the posterior longitudinal ligament in the cervical spine include use of autogenous muscle or fascial dural patches, immediate lumbar subarachnoid shunting, and modification of the usual postoperative regimen,

such as limitation of mechanical pulmonary ventilation to the shortest time that is safely possible and use of antiemetic and antitussive medications to protect the remaining coverings of the spinal cord.

The role of an LP shunt in the management of pseudomeningocele and CSF fistulas is incompletely defined. There are reports of successful management of CSF fistulas and pseudomeningocele with an LP shunt. However, the placement of permanent hardware should be avoided whenever possible, and other therapies, including surgical repair, should be attempted first. An LP shunt, in general, should be applied only in patients in whom surgical repair failed or in whom surgical repair was not possible because of the location of the defect.

Nonoperative

Most patients with incidental durotomy can be treated effectively with a watertight dural closure and fibrin glue. Patients can be permitted to ambulate immediately after surgery but should be cautioned to lay flat if they develop symptoms. This will reduce the costs related to the hospital stay and missed work. The role of antibiotic therapy in the management of spinal fistulas and pseudomeningocele remains incompletely defined. Traditional management includes bed rest for up to 7 days to eliminate traction and reduce hydrostatic pressure during the healing process. However, use of antibiotics for CSF fistulas and pseudomeningoceles suggests that they do not decrease the short- or long-term incidence of meningitis and are actually associated with development of multidrug resistance.

Epidural blood patches have been applied successfully to treat patients with postlaminectomy CSF fistulas and pseudomeningoceles. Maycock and colleagues have reported on a patient who underwent surgical reexploration for a CSF fistula following a laminectomy; the site of CSF fistula was not found, and the CSF leak continued postoperatively (17). The CSF fistula was subsequently treated successfully using an epidural blood patch. Clot formation and clot strength are known to increase in the presence of CSF. The injection of blood stops CSF leakage by promoting clot formation over the dural tear and raises extradural tissue pressure relative to subarachnoid pressure, thus decreasing the gradient for CSF efflux. Because only a few case reports exist in the literature, the success rate of the epidural blood patch in the treatment of CSF fistulas and pseudomeningoceles is unclear.

The first investigators who treated pseudomeningoceles with closed lumbar subarachnoid catheters used Teflon or polyethylene catheters. These catheters, initially designed for epidural use, were complicated by frequent blockage and kinking and were therefore somewhat difficult to use. In 1992, Shapiro and Scully reported the use of silicone lumbar subarachnoid catheters in 39 patients with spinal CSF fistulas and pseudomeningoceles (18). They reported a 92% success rate after 7 days of drainage alone. Complications included a 24% prevalence of temporary nerve root irritation that resolved after the drain was removed and a 63% prevalence of transient headaches, nausea, and vomiting. There was a 10% prevalence of infection (one wound, two discitis, one meningitis). In an earlier report, Kitchel and colleagues noted a similar success rate of 90% in 17 patients treated with 4 days of drainage (19), but the recurrence rate was higher (18%) when compared with that reported by Shapiro and Scully (8%) (18). The complication rate reported by Kitchel and colleagues (19) was similar to that reported by Shapiro and Scully (18), with a 58% prevalence of headaches, nausea, and vomiting. All patients were successfully treated with adjustment in the rate of CSF drainage, intravenous hydration, and analgesic medication (18). In each study, the authors reported one case of meningitis associated with lumbar subarachnoid drainage, and both cases were successfully treated with antibiotic therapy. McCormack and co-workers reported using an epidural blood patch combined with a brief course of subarachnoid drainage in one patient with spinal implants (20). They speculated that CSF diversion alone in patients with spinal implants may not eliminate the pseudomeningocele because the hardware prevents reapproximation of paraspinal tissues. The blood patch procedure obliterates extradural dead space and provides a substrate for clot formation. Dural healing may thus be optimized because CSF diversion and percutaneous blood patch are complementary in decreasing the CSF pressure differences across the dural breech. Closed subarachnoid drainage, when properly performed and monitored, is a reasonably effective and safe method for treating dural-cutaneous CSF leaks after a spinal operation. It may be considered as a nonoperative alternative to the standard procedure of reoperation and direct repair of the dura. A good result is still possible in patients in whom this technique fails and who eventually need surgical management.

Operative

Management often consists of insertion of a diverting spinal fluid drain and administration of prophylactic or therapeutic antibiotics. In cases of persistent CSF leakage, surgical reexploration is sometimes necessary. It is the usual practice to treat a postoperative CSF leak after an operation on the spine nonoperatively. If conservative treatment fails, surgical intervention usually entails suturing the opening in the dura with or without leaving a fat or muscle graft over the suture line.

The definitive treatment for a CSF fistula and pseudomeningocele is reoperation and dural repair. Surgical indications include failure of nonoperative measures, progressive radiculopathy, and development of a myelopathy. For those with a neurologic deficit, a delay in surgery may put the patient at risk for further neurologic injury. One method of repairing a postsurgical pseudomeningocele includes separation of the dura from the arachnoid, a water-tight dural repair using the operative microscope, and the use of overlapping local muscle flaps to reinforce the dura and obliterate the pseudomeningocele cavity.

The surgery should begin with adequate lighting, and the skin incision should be generous enough to encompass the leak completely. Once the pseudomeningocele is visualized, it must be followed deep into the durotomy site. Often, the pseudomeningocele needs to be resected to identify the region of interest. The durotomy site is protected with a cottonoid, and any necessary bone resection is performed before attempting dural closure to provide adequate room for suturing. Under microscopic magnification, the durotomy site is explored to ensure that nerve root or spinal cord strangulation is not present. In most cases, the dura can be closed primarily, without need of a graft, by using 4–0 to 7–0 nonabsorbable sutures on a taper or reverse cutting, half-circle needle. For a large defect, a local fascial graft or artificial dura may be used to avoid compressing neural elements. For a durotomy that occurs in surgically inaccessible areas, such as a far-lateral durotomy, a small plug of muscle or fat may be introduced through an intentional medial durotomy and pulled into the area of the defect.

Fat is an ideal sealant because it is impermeable to water (21). A thin sheet of autologous subcutaneous fat covers dural repair as well as all exposed dura and can be gently tucked into the lateral recesses. This procedure prevents CSF from seeping around the fat, which may be tacked to the dura with a few sutures. Fibrin glue is spread over the surface of the fat, which is then further covered with Surgicel or Gelfoam. For a ventral dural tear (associated with procedures in which disc material is excised), fat is packed into the disc space to seal off the ventral dural leak. The use of a fat graft is recommended as a rapid, effective means of prevention and repair of a CSF leak after cervical spinal surgery.

In recent years, fibrin glue has gained increasing popularity as a dural sealant (22,23). Fibrin glue is solely suited for dural closure augmentation and is not a substitute for surgical techniques; that is, it should be added to other modalities. The identification of the definite site of CSF leakage is also of great importance and substantially improves the success rate. Muscle graft, in combination with fibrin glue (presumably owing to its adhesive sealing properties), is superior to either muscle packing alone or fibrin glue in isolation.

Shaffrey and associates have reported a 93% effectiveness rate in cases with no preoperative CSF leakage (prophylactic use) and 67% in preestablished CSF fistula (therapeutic use) (24). These investigators treated 15 patients with CSF leakage with fibrin glue and were successful in 10 cases (24). Milde has reported an anaphylactic reaction to fibrin glue (25), and Wilson and colleagues detected one human immunodeficiency virus type 1 (HIV-1) transmission following the use of nonautologous cryoprecipitate (26).

However, a far-lateral tear poses a technically difficult problem for placement of sutures because these sites are inaccessible. In addition, a far-lateral tear that is close to a nerve root is potentially dangerous because the suture may impale neural fascicles or cause traction or scarring of the nerve root.

On the basis of these findings, the use of an autologous fat transplant is recommended as a rapid, effective means for repair of a dural tear or defect that is inaccessible or unsuitable for standard suture technique. Mayfield demonstrated that an autologous fat transplant serves as an excellent water sealant, prevents scar formation, and does not adhere to the neural elements; the fat survives for a long time and becomes revascularized (21).

SUMMARY

Close evaluation of preoperative neuroimaging studies, meticulous surgical technique, and liberal use of microscopic magnification will often avert iatrogenic pseudomeningocele and CSF fistula. All available preoperative neurodiagnostic images should be evaluated for evidence of bone defects caused by possible occult spina bifida or previous surgeries. Each Kerrison rongeur bite should be preceded by the necessary dissection to ensure that the dura mater does not come between the footplate and bone. The movement of the drill is directed laterally so that even with a slip, a dural tear may be avoided. A cottonoid should cover the exposed dura during the drilling. When a dural tear does occur, every attempt should be made to achieve a watertight primary closure. This includes extending the laminectomy, if necessary, to gain better exposure to repair the dura, and using loupe magnification or the operating microscope.

Treatment modalities for CSF fistula and pseudomeningocele includes nonoperative management, placement of an epidural blood patch, lumbar subarachnoid drainage, and surgery.

REFERENCES

1. Epstein NE, Hollingsworth R. Anterior cervical micro-dural repair of cerebrospinal fluid fistula after surgery for ossification of the posterior longitudinal ligament: technical note. *Surg Neurol* 1999;52:511–514.
2. Smith MD, Bolesta MJ, Leventhal M, et al. Postoperative cerebrospinal-fluid fistula associated with erosion of the dura. Findings after anterior resection of ossification of the posterior longitudinal ligament in the cervical spine. *J Bone Joint Surg Am* 1992;74:270–277.
3. Teplick JG, Peyster RG, Teplick SK, et al. CT Identification of post-laminectomy pseudomeningocele. *AJR Am J Roentgenol* 1983;140:1203–1206.
4. Rinaldi I, Peach WF Jr. Postoperative lumbar meningocele. Report of two cases. *J Neurosurg* 1969;30:504–507.
5. Mikawa Y, Watanabe R, Hino Y, et al. Cerebellar hemorrhage complicating cervical durotomy and revision C1-C2 fusion. *Spine* 1994;19:1169–1171.
6. Aldrete JA, Ghaly R. Postlaminectomy pseudomeningocele. An unsuspected cause of low back pain. *Reg Anesth* 1995;20:75–79.
7. Horowitz SW, Azar-Kia B, Fine M. Post-operative cervical pseudomeningocele. *AJNR Am J Neuroradiol* 1990;11:784.
8. Hanakita J, Kinuta Y, Suzuki T. Spinal cord compression due to postoperative cervical pseudomeningocele. *Neurosurgery* 1985;17:317–319.
9. Helle TL, Conley FK. Postoperative cervical pseudomeningocele as a cause of delayed myelopathy. *Neurosurgery* 1981;9:314–316.
10. Hosono N, Yonenobu K, Ono K. Postoperative cervical pseudomeningocele with herniation of the spinal cord. *Spine* 1995;20:2147–2150.
11. Goodman SJ, Gregorius FK. Cervical pseudomeningocele after laminectomy as a cause of progressive myelopathy. *Bull Los Angeles Neurol Soc* 1974;39:121–127.
12. Magliulo G, Sepe C, Varacalli S, et al. Cerebrospinal fluid leak management following cerebellopontine angle surgery. *J Otolaryngol* 1998;27:258–262.
13. Aarabi B, Alibaii E, Taghipur M, et al. Comparative study of functional recovery for surgically explored and conservatively managed spinal cord missile injuries. *Neurosurgery* 1996;39:1133–1140.
14. Romanick PC, Smith TK, Kopaniky DR, et al. Infection about the spine associated with low-velocity missile injury to the abdomen. *J Bone Joint Surg Am* 1985;67:1195–1201.
15. Hodges SD, Humphreys SC, Eck JC, et al. Management of incidental durotomy without mandatory bed rest. A retrospective review of 20 cases. *Spine* 1999;24:2062–2064.
16. Kaar GF, Briggs M, Bashir SH. Thecal repair in post-surgical pseudomeningocoele. *Br J Neurosurg* 1994;8:703–707.
17. Maycock NF, van Essen J, Pfitzner J. Post-laminectomy cerebrospinal fluid fistula treated with epidural blood patch. *Spine* 1994;19:2223–2225.
18. Shapiro SA, Scully T. Closed continuous drainage of cerebrospinal fluid via a lumbar subarachnoid catheter for treatment or prevention of cranial/spinal cerebrospinal fluid fistula. *Neurosurgery* 1992;30:241–245.
19. Kitchel SH, Eismont FJ, Green BA. Closed subarachnoid drainage for management of cerebrospinal fluid leakage after an operation on the spine. *J Bone Joint Surg* 1989;71:984–987.
20. McCormack BM, Taylor SL, Heath S, et al. Pseudomeningocele/CSF fistula in a patient with lumbar spinal implants treated with epidural blood patch and a brief course of closed subarachnoid drainage. A case report. *Spine* 1996;21:2273–2276.
21. Mayfield FH. Autologous fat transplants for the protection and repair of the spinal dura. *Clin Neurosurg* 1980;27:349–361.
22. Nishihira S, McCaffrey TV. The use of fibrin glue for the repair of experimental CSF rhinorrhea. *Laryngoscope* 1988;98:625–627.
23. Pomeranz S, Constantini S, Umansky F. The use of fibrin sealant in cerebrospinal fluid leakage. *Neurochirurgia* 1991;34:166–169.
24. Shaffrey CI, Spotnitz WD, Shaffrey ME, et al. Neurosurgical applications of fibrin glue: augmentation of dural closure in 134 patients. *Neurosurgery* 1990;26:207–210.
25. Milde LN. An anaphylactic reaction to fibrin glue. *Anesth Analg* 1989;69:684–686.
26. Wilson SM, Pell P, Donegan EA. HIV-1 transmission following the use of cryoprecipitated fibrinogen as gel adhesive. *Transfusion* 1991;31:51.

Index